MANAGEMENT OF PEDIATRIC FRACTURES

Associate Editors

Maureen P. Baxter, MD, FRCSC
    Assistant Professor
    Division of Orthopaedics
    Department of Surgery
    University of Ottawa Faculty of Medicine
    Children's Hospital of Eastern Ontario
    Ottawa, Ontario, Canada

Timothy P. Carey, MD, FRCSC
    Assistant Professor
    Division of Orthopaedics
    Department of Surgery
    University of Ottawa Faculty of Medicine
    Children's Hospital of Eastern Ontario
    Ottawa, Ontario, Canada

Jacques D'Astous, MD, FRCSC
    Associate Professor
    Division of Orthopaedics
    Department of Surgery
    University of Ottawa Faculty of Medicine
    Children's Hospital of Eastern Ontario
    Ottawa, Ontario, Canada

James G. Jarvis, MD, FRCSC
    Associate Professor
    Division of Orthopaedics
    Department of Surgery
    University of Ottawa Faculty of Medicine
    Children's Hospital of Eastern Ontario
    Ottawa, Ontario, Canada

Louis J. Lawton, MD, FRCSC
    Assistant Professor
    Division of Orthopaedics
    Department of Surgery
    University of Ottawa Faculty of Medicine
    Children's Hospital of Eastern Ontario
    Ottawa, Ontario, Canada

William McIntyre, MD, FRCSC
    Associate Professor
    Division of Orthopaedics
    Department of Surgery
    University of Ottawa Faculty of Medicine
    Head of Pediatric Orthopaedics
    Children's Hospital of Eastern Ontario
    Ottawa, Ontario, Canada

MANAGEMENT OF PEDIATRIC FRACTURES

EDITED BY

R. MERVYN LETTS, MD, FRCSC

Professor and Head
Division of Orthopaedics
Department of Surgery
University of Ottawa Faculty of Medicine
Surgeon-in-Chief
Children's Hospital of Eastern Ontario
Ottawa, Ontario, Canada

Churchill Livingstone
New York, Edinburgh, London, Madrid, Melbourne, Tokyo

Library of Congress Cataloging-in-Publication Data

Management of pediatric fractures / edited by R. Mervyn Letts.
      p.   cm.
      Includes bibliographical references and index.
      ISBN 0-443-08860-8
      1. Fractures in children. I. Letts, R. Mervyn.
      [DNLM: 1. Fractures—in infancy & childhood. 2. Fractures-
-therapy.   WE 175 M266 1994]
RD732.3.C48M355 1994
617.1'083—dc20
DNLM/DLC
for Library of Congress   93-23427
                                                      CIP

© Churchill Livingstone Inc. 1994

All rights reserved. No part of this publication may be reproduced, stored in a retrieval system, or transmitted in any form or by any means, electronic, mechanical, photocopying, recording, or otherwise, without prior permission of the publisher (Churchill Livingstone Inc., 650 Avenue of the Americas, New York, NY 10011).

Distributed in the United Kingdom by Churchill Livingstone, Robert Stevenson House, 1–3 Baxter's Place, Leith Walk, Edinburgh EH1 3AF, and by associated companies, branches, and representatives throughout the world.

Accurate indications, adverse reactions, and dosage schedules for drugs are provided in this book, but it is possible that they may change. The reader is urged to review the package information data of the manufacturers of the medications mentioned.

The Publishers have made every effort to trace the copyright holders for borrowed material. If they have inadvertently overlooked any, they will be pleased to make the necessary arrangements at the first opportunity.

Copy Editor: *Donna C. Balopole*
Production Supervisor: *Sharon Tuder*
Cover Design: *Paul Moran*
Production services provided by Bermedica Production, Ltd.

Printed in the United States of America

First published in 1994   7 6 5 4 3 2 1

*This book is dedicated to all residents,
emergency medical officers,
and orthopaedic surgeons
who care for traumatized children in hospitals and clinics
in cities, towns, and villages throughout the world.*

Contributors

Peter F. Armstrong, MD, FRCSC
Professor, Division of Orthopaedic Surgery, Department of Surgery, University of Utah School of Medicine; Chief of Staff, Intermountain Unit, Shriners Hospitals for Crippled Children, Salt Lake City, Utah

Anthony Ashworth, MD, FRCSC
Associate Professor, Division of Orthopaedics, Department of Surgery, Queens University Faculty of Medicine; Head, Division of Orthopaedic Surgery, Hotel Dieu Hospital; Attending Staff, Kingston General Hospital, Kingston, Ontario, Canada

John V. Banta, MD
Professor, Department of Orthopaedic Surgery, University of Connecticut School of Medicine, Farmington, Connecticut; Director of Orthopaedic Surgery, Newington Children's Hospital, Newington, Connecticut

Maureen P. Baxter, MD, FRCSC
Assistant Professor, Division of Orthopaedics, Department of Surgery, University of Ottawa Faculty of Medicine, Children's Hospital of Eastern Ontario, Ottawa, Ontario, Canada

Deborah F. Bell, MD, FRCSC
Associate Professor, Department of Orthopedic Surgery, Wayne State University School of Medicine; Assistant Chief of Orthopaedic Surgery, Children's Hospital of Michigan, Detroit, Michigan

John G. Birch, MD
Associate Professor, Department of Orthopaedic Surgery, University of Texas Southwestern Medical Center at Dallas Southwestern Medical School; Staff Orthopedist, Department of Orthopedics, Texas Scottish Rite Hospital for Children, Dallas, Texas

G. Brian Black, MD, FRCSC
Associate Professor, Section of Orthopaedics, Department of Surgery, University of Manitoba Faculty of Medicine; Director of Pediatric Orthopaedics, Section of Orthopaedics, Children's Hospital, Winnipeg, Manitoba, Canada

R. Dale Blasier, MD, FRCSC
Associate Professor, Department of Orthopaedic Surgery, University of Arkansas College of Medicine, Little Rock, Arkansas; Chief of Orthopaedic Traumatology, Arkansas Children's Hospital, Little Rock, Arkansas; Clinical Assistant Professor of Orthopaedic Surgery, Uniformed Services University of the Health Sciences F. Edward Hébert School of Medicine, Bethesda, Maryland

Walter P. Bobechko, MD, FRCSC
Director of Orthopaedic Surgery, Humana Advanced Surgical Institute, Dallas, Texas

Kenneth L.B. Brown, MD, MSc, FRCSC
Associate Clinical Professor, Department of Orthopaedics, University of British Columbia Faculty of Medicine; Pediatric Orthopaedic Surgeon, Department of Orthopaedic Surgery, Bristish Columbia Children's Hospital, Vancouver, British Columbia, Canada

Timothy P. Carey, MD, FRCSC
Assistant Professor, Division of Orthopaedics, Department of Surgery, University of Ottawa Faculty of Medicine, Children's Hospital of Eastern Ontario, Ottawa, Ontario, Canada

Norris Carrol, MD, FRCSC
Professor of Clinical Orthopaedics, Department of Orthopaedic Surgery, Northwestern University Medical School; Martha Washington Professor and Head, Department of Pediatric Orthopaedics, Children's Memorial Hospital, Chicago, Illinois

Stanley M.K. Chung, MD
Associate Professor, Division of Orthopedics, Department of Surgery, University of Hawaii John A. Burns School of Medicine; Chief, Division of Orthopedic Surgery, Department of Pediatric Surgery, Kapiolani Medical Center for Women and Children, Honolulu, Hawaii

Jacques D'Astous, MD, FRCSC
Associate Professor, Division of Orthopaedics, Department of Surgery, University of Ottawa Faculty of Medicine, Children's Hospital of Eastern Ontario, Ottawa, Ontario, Canada

Geoff Dervin, MD, FRCSC
Clinical Fellow, Division of Orthopaedics, Department of Surgery, University of Ottawa Faculty of Medicine, Ottawa General Hospital, Ottawa, Ontario, Canada

Morris Duhaime, MD, FRCSC
Professor, Orthopedic Surgery, Department of Surgery, McGill University Faculty of Medicine; Professor, Division of Orthopedics, Department of Surgery, University of Montreal Faculty of Medicine; Orthopaedic Surgeon, Division of Orthopaedic Surgery, Hôpital Sainte-Justine; Chief of Staff, Shriners Hospital for Crippled Children, Montreal, Quebec, Canada

Francois Fassier, MD, FRCSC
Associate Professor, Division of Orthopedics, Department of Surgery, University of Montreal Faculty of Medicine; Attending Staff, Department of Surgery, Hôpital Sainte-Justine and Shriners Hospital for Crippled Children, Montreal, Quebec, Canada

Allan F. Fehlandt, Jr., DO, MS
Fellow in Sports Medicine, The Children's Hospital, Boston, Massachusetts

Colin Fennell, MD, FRCSC
Assistant Professor, Department of Surgery, University of Calgary Faculty of Medicine; Consultant Division, Orthopaedic Surgery, Foothills Hospital, Calgary, Alberta, Canada

Roger Gallien, MD, FRCSC
Chief of Orthopaedic Surgery, Hôpital Saint-François d'Assise, Quebec City, Quebec, Canada

Robert D. Galpin, MD, FRCSC
Clinical Assistant Professor, Division of Orthopaedics, Department of Surgery, and Department of Paediatrics, University of Western Ontario Faculty of Medicine, London, Ontario, Canada

Robert B. Gledhill, MD, FRCSC
Associate Professor, Orthopedic Surgery, Department of Surgery, McGill University Faculty of Medicine; Head, Department of Orthopedics, Montreal Children's Hospital, Montreal, Quebec, Canada

Walter B. Greene, MD
Professor, Division of Orthopaedic Surgery, Department of Surgery, and Department of Pediatrics, University of North Carolina School of Medicine, Chapel Hill, North Carolina

Curtis R. Gruel, MD
Assistant Professor, Department of Orthopaedic Surgery and Rehabilitation, University of Oklahoma College of Medicine, Oklahoma City, Oklahoma

Kenneth J. Guidera, MD
Assistant Professor, Division of Orthopedic Surgery, Department of Surgery, University of South Florida College of Medicine; Director of Orthopaedic Services, Shriners Hospital for Crippled Children, Tampa, Florida

Alan Gurd, MB, MCh, FRCS
Vice Chairman, Department of Orthopaedics, and Head, Pediatric Orthopaedics, Cleveland Clinic, Cleveland, Ohio

James A. Harder, MD, FRCSC
Clinical Associate Professor, Department of Surgery, University of Calgary Faculty of Medicine; Pediatric Orthopedic Surgeon and Chief of Staff, Surgery, Department of Orthopedics, Alberta Children's Hospital Child Health Centre, Calgary, Alberta, Canada

Douglas Hedden, MD, FRCSC
Associate Professor, Department of Surgery, University of Toronto Faculty of Medicine; Staff Pediatric Orthopaedic Surgeon, Division of Orthopaedics, Department of Surgery, The Hospital for Sick Children, Toronto, Ontario, Canada

John D. Hsu, MD, CM
Clinical Professor, Department of Orthopaedics and Rehabilitation, University of Southern California School of Medicine, Los Angeles, California; Chief of Orthopaedics and Chairman, Department of Surgery, Rancho Los Amigos Medical Center, Downey, California

Walter W. Huurman, MD
Associate Professor Of Orthopaedics and Pediatrics, Department of Orthopaedics, University of Nebraska College of Medicine; Director of Children's Orthopaedics, Department of Pediatric Orthopaedics, University of Nebraska Medical Center, Omaha, Nebraska

Marc Isler, MD, FRCSC
Fellow, Division of Orthopaedic Surgery, Hôpital Sainte-Justine; Fellow, Department of Orthopaedic Surgery, Shriners Hospital for Crippled Children, Montreal, Quebec, Canada

James G. Jarvis, MD, FRCSC
Associate Professor, Division of Orthopaedics, Department of Surgery, University of Ottawa Faculty of Medicine, Children's Hospital of Eastern Ontario, Ottawa, Ontario, Canada

Garth Johnson, MD, FRCSC
Associate Professor, Division of Orthopaedics, Department of Surgery, University of Ottawa Faculty of Medicine; Director of Spine Unit and Head, Department of Orthopaedics, Ottawa Civic Hospital, Ottawa, Ontario, Canada

Gerhard N. Kiefer, MD, FRCSC
Clinical Assistant Professor, Department of Surgery, University of Calgary Faculty of Medicine; Pediatric Orthopedic Surgeon, Department of Orthopedics, Alberta Children's Hospital Child Health Centre, Calgary, Alberta, Canada

Rudolph A. Klassen, MD
Assistant Professor, Department of Orthopedics, Mayo Medical School; Orthopedic Surgeon, Department of Orthopaedics, Mayo Clinic, Rochester, Minnesota

Hubert Labelle, MD, FRCSC
Associate Professor, Division of Orthopedics, Department of Surgery, University of Montreal Faculty of Medicine; Head, Division of Orthopaedic Surgery, Hôpital Sainte-Justine, Montreal, Quebec, Canada

Louis J. Lawton, MD, FRCSC
Assistant Professor, Division of Orthopaedics, Department of Surgery, University of Ottawa Faculty of Medicine, Children's Hospital of Eastern Ontario, Ottawa, Ontario, Canada

R. Mervyn Letts, MD, FRCSC
Professor and Head, Division of Orthopaedics, Department of Surgery, University of Ottawa Faculty of Medicine; Surgeon-in-Chief, Children's Hospital of Eastern Ontario, Ottawa, Ontario, Canada

Randall T. Loder, MD
Assistant Professor, Section of Orthopedics, Department of Surgery, University of Michigan Medical School, Ann Arbor, Michigan

Dennis Lyne, MD
Professor of Orthopaedic Surgery and Pediatrics and Program Director, Department of Orthopaedic Surgery, Michigan State University/Kalamazoo Center for Medical Studies, Kalamazoo, Michigan

William G. MacKenzie, MD, FRCSC
Pediatric Orthopaedic Surgeon, Alfred I. duPont Institute, Wilmington, Delaware; Formerly, Clinical Assistant Professor, Department of Orthopaedic Surgery, University of British Columbia Faculty of Medicine, Vancouver, British Columbia, Canada

Roderick I. Macpherson, MD
Professor, Departments of Radiology and Pediatrics, Medical University of South Carolina College of Medicine, Charleston, South Carolina

Robert F. Martin, MD, FRCSC
Professor, Department of Surgery, and Head, Division of Orthopaedic Surgery, McMaster University School of Medicine, Hamilton, Ontario, Canada

Dominique Marton, MD,
Professor, Department of Radiology, University of Montreal Faculty of Medicine, Hôpital Sainte-Justine, Montreal, Quebec, Canada

Richard E. McCarthy, MD
Arkansas Spine Center, Clinical Associate Professor of Orthopaedic Surgery, University of Arkansas College of Medicine, Little Rock, Arkansas

William McIntyre, MD, FRCSC
Associate Professor, Division of Orthopaedics, Department of Surgery, University of Ottawa Faculty of Medicine; Head of Pediatric Orthopaedics, Children's Hospital of Eastern Ontario, Ottawa, Ontario, Canada

Claude Mercier, MD, FRCSC
Clinical Assistant Professor, Division of Neurosurgery, Department of Surgery, University of Montreal Faculty of Medicine; Chief, Division of Neurosurgery, Hôpital Sainte-Justine, Montreal, Quebec, Canada

Pierre Mercier, MD, FRCSC
Pediatric Orthopedic Surgeon, Hôpital Saint-François d'Assise, Quebec City, Quebec, Canada

Lyle J. Micheli, MD
Associate Clinical Professor, Department of Orthopedic Surgery, Harvard Medical School; Director, Division of Sports Medicine, The Children's Hospital, Boston, Massachusetts

Leslie J. Mintz, MD
Attending Physician, Phoenix Orthopaedic Residency Program, Section of Orthopaedic Surgery, Maricopa Medical Centre, Phoenix, Arizona

Guy Moreau, MD, FRCSC
Chief Resident, Division of Orthopaedics, Department of Surgery, University of Ottawa Faculty of Medicine, Children's Hospital of Eastern Ontario, Ottawa, Ontario, Canada

Benoit Morin, MD, FRCSC
Assistant Clinical Professor, Department of Surgery, University of Montreal Faculty of Medicine; Orthopaedic Surgeon, Division of Orthopaedic Surgeon, Hôpital Sainte-Justine, Montreal, Quebec, Canada

John A. Ogden, MD
Professor of Orthopaedic Surgery and Pediatrics, Division of Orthopedic Surgery, Department of Surgery, University of South Florida College of Medicine; Chief of Staff, Shriners Hospital for Crippled Children, Tampa, Florida

Benoit Poitras, MD, FRCSC
Professor and Chairman, Division of Orthopedics, Department of Surgery, University of Montreal Faculty of Medicine; Attending Staff, Department of Surgery, Hôpital Sainte-Justine and Shriners Hospital for Crippled Children, Montreal, Quebec, Canada

Avrum N. Pollock, MD, FRCPC
Fellow, Department of Radiology, University of Manitoba Faculty of Medicine, Children's Hospital, Winnipeg, Manitoba, Canada

Charles T. Price, MD
Associate Director of Medical Education and Director of Pediatric Orthopedics, Department of Medical Education Orthopedics, Orlando Regional Medical Center, Orlando, Florida

Martin H. Reed, MD, FRCPC
Professor, Departments of Radiology and Pediatrics and Child Health, University of Manitoba Faculty of Medicine; Head, Department of Pediatric Radiology, Children's Hospital, Winnipeg, Manitoba, Canada

Thomas S. Renshaw, MD
Professor, Department of Orthopedics and Rehabilitation, Yale University School of Medicine; Chief of Pediatric Orthopaedic Surgery, Department of Orthopaedic Surgery, Yale-New Haven Hospital, New Haven, Connecticut

Charles H. Rivard, MD, FRCSC
Professor Geographical Full Time, Department of Surgery, University of Montreal Faculty of Medicine; Professor of Orthopaedics and Chief, Department of Surgery, Hôpital Sainte-Justine, Montreal, Quebec, Canada

Eric Robinson, MD, FRCSC
Clinical Fellow, Division of Orthopaedics, Department of Surgery, University of Ottawa Faculty of Medicine, Children's Hospital of Eastern Ontario, Ottawa, Ontario, Canada

Bernard A. Roehr, MD
Assistant Clinical Professor, Department of Surgery, Michigan State University College of Human Medicine, East Lansing, Michigan; Fellow in Adult Reconstructive Surgery of the Hip and Knee, Department of Orthopedic Surgery, Harvard Medical School, Boston, Massachusetts

Kevin Rumball, MD, FRCSC
Clinical Fellow in Orthopaedics, Division of Orthopaedics, Department of Surgery, University of Ottawa Faculty of Medicine, Children's Hospital of Eastern Ontario, Ottawa, Ontario, Canada

Robert B. Salter, OC, MD, MS, FRCSC
University Professor and Professor of Orthopaedic Surgery, Department of Surgery, University of Toronto Faculty of Medicine; Senior Orthopaedic Surgeon, The Hospital for Sick Children, Toronto, Ontario, Canada

John T. Smith, MD
Assistant Professor, Division of Orthopedic Surgery, Department of Surgery, University of Utah School of Medicine; Pediatric Orthopedic Surgeon, Primary Children's Medical Center, Salt Lake City, Utah

William M. Splinter, MD, FRCPC
Clinical Lecturer, Department of Anaesthesia, University of Ottawa Faculty of Medicine; Director of Research, Department of Anaesthesia, Children's Hospital of Eastern Ontario, Ottawa, Ontario, Canada

J. Andy Sullivan, MD
Professor and Don H. O'Donoghue Chair, Department of Orthopedic Surgery and Rehabilitation, University of Oklahoma College of Medicine, Oklahoma City, Oklahoma

Stephen J. Tredwell, MD, FRCSC
Associate Professor, Department of Orthopaedic Surgery, University of British Columbia Faculty of Medicine; Head, Department of Orthopaedic Surgery, British Columbia's Children's Hospital, Vancouver, British Columbia, Canada

Guillermo R. Viviani, MD, FRCSC
Professor of Orthopaedics, Department of Surgery, McMaster University School of Medicine, Hamilton, Ontario, Canada

Dennis S. Weiner, MD
Professor, Department of Orthopaedic Surgery, Northeastern Ohio Universities College of Medicine, Rootstown, Ohio; Chairman, Department of Pediatric Orthopaedic Surgery, Children's Hospital Medical Center of Akron, Akron, Ohio

R. Baxter Willis, MD
Clinical Associate Professor, Division of Orthopaedics, Department of Surgery, University of Western Ontario Faculty of Medicine; Orthopaedic Surgeon, Department of Surgery, Victoria Hospital, London, Ontario, Canada

Foreword

One of my revered teachers in years long gone commented that treating pediatric orthopaedic trauma was the best of all worlds. The fractures were invariably simple and all of them healed—more or less. Treatment modalities were quite unsophisticated. Complications were rare. Remodelling covered all sins. The patients never argued. And no rehabilitation was necessary. The major problems, he said, involved the occasional complication and the frequent confrontation with perplexed parents—requesting further opinions, challenging treatment modalities, doubting your competence, and questioning strange outcomes.

Pediatric orthopaedic trauma does, in fact, manifest these unique characteristics. No one questions that certain childhood fractures may heal faster and with greater equanimity than a comparable fracture in an adult. Consider, for example, a minimally displaced fracture of the distal forearm. There are other common, simple fractures in this category. The diagnosis, management, and results favor the pediatric patient. Regardless, most of these garden variety fractures do perplex the parents!

Children are endowed with a very normal, morphologic phenomenon called "growth." Many factors, trauma included, may inflict venomous wrath upon those growing years of the pediatric patient. Whether focused directly or indirectly on the physis, that innocuous pediatric fracture may develop sinister proportions, not only for the patient but also for those perplexed parents and their lawyer, who has now joined the gallery. Children's fractures are not really the best of every world!

Many pediatric fractures are unique. Compare the different features of adult and pediatric fractures of the distal humerus, elbow, spine, hip, and other joints. Compare the problems with open and closed management, growth plate injuries, and interruption of vascular supply. Finally, the unkindest cut of all—the complications of a fracture in a child more so than in an adult can be very unforgiving. A young person has many places to go, many things to do, and many miles to walk. It is imperative that every responsible physician encountering the pediatric trauma patient be knowledgeable, competent, and skillful in the diagnosis, treatment, and overall care of these young people.

Management of Pediatric Fractures is a compendium of the experiences of many notable, veteran pediatric orthopaedic surgeons and other specialists in the musculoskeletal field. Their words and studies are the composite of what can be verified in personal experience. These authors present the leading edge of current thinking in the management of trauma at the pediatric level.

James Wiley, MD, FRCSC
Associate Dean
University of Ottawa Faculty of Medicine
Ottawa, Ontario, Canada

In no other domain of fracture care has progress been as evident as in that of pediatric traumatology. It is not just a triumph of surgical technique that characterizes these improved results; it is the application of painstakingly documented observations that has allowed the deeper knowledge and understanding of the processes that differentiate the fracture care of children from that of adults.

The end point of treatment in the adult is usually the consolidation of the fracture. However, in pediatric practice much longer follow-up is mandatory to detect and treat possible growth disturbances and other sequelae of injury in the skeletally immature. These long-term observations, in turn, constitute an essential basis for the analysis of treatment regimens and the establishment of improved treatment protocols for fractures in children.

The goal of *Management of Pediatric Fractures* is to disseminate the critically assessed experiences of experts in this field. Dr. Mervyn Letts has succeeded in assembling a group of well-known and respected pediatric orthopaedic surgeons and other specialists in the musculoskeletal field. Many of the contributors are former or present colleagues who have been stimulated by his infectious enthusiasm. The inclusion of residents as co-authors characterizes Dr. Letts's philosophy of encouraging scientific curiosity at an early stage.

This book will permit the practicing orthopaedic surgeon to obtain clear and concrete information when confronted by specific fractures. The clear structure and simple orientation will allow precision in evaluating treatment options and avoiding complications. Residents will find this book of particular value and its didactic presentation will help them acquire the necessary knowledge in an important field of their future practice. The ample reference lists facilitate further in-depth study.

To Dr. Letts and all the associate editors and contributors, I express my deep admiration for a task well done. It is only through this type of high quality academic pursuit by current and future orthopaedic scholars that the specialty of orthopaedic surgery will remain in the forefront of medicine.

Hans K. Uhthoff, MD, FRCSC
Professor and Chairman
Department of Surgery
University of Ottawa Faculty of Medicine
Ottawa, Ontario, Canada

Preface

The objectives in putting together a book on pediatric fractures and dislocations were to produce an authoritative and practical text that (1) would emphasize the management and potential complications of fractures seen in childhood; (2) encompass the full spectrum of childhood fractures including those less commonly encountered, but which frequently pose a dilemma in management; and (3) correlate the characteristic pediatric anatomic characteristics with the type of fracture, displacement, and complications. Thus, it is hoped that *Management of Pediatric Fractures* will function as a front-line reference for pediatric orthopaedic surgeons, pediatric emergentologists, and orthopaedic surgeons who deal with the injured child in a part-time capacity.

To keep pace with the realities of the 1990s chapters have been included on some of the less savory aspects of fracture causation, such as gunshot wounds in children and child abuse. A section has also been included on specific fractures as they relate to certain disease entities in which they are commonly seen, such as osteogenesis imperfecta, severe physical handicap, and myelomeningocele. Emphasis on the avoidance of physeal damage during the reduction and care of all fractures has been provided throughout the text. The inclusion of a chapter on managing physeal bars was felt to be within the purview of those caring for fractures. This should assist in a better understanding of both the mechanism of injury resulting in such bars as well as the treatment available.

Certain fractures have been highlighted that have been a particular problem in management, such as the Chance fracture of the spine, the triplane fracture of the ankle, and intra-articular fractures of the knee. Since fractures about the elbow are fraught with complications and provide major concern to many caregivers dealing with pediatric fractures, these fractures have received special consideration and have been subdivided perhaps more than is usual in fracture texts. This has been done to try and provide the caregiver with an in-depth analysis of elbow trauma in children and to allow full discussion of treatment modalities and the avoidance of potential complications.

Since complications of fractures in growing children are frequently devastating and limb threatening, special consideration has been given to methods of avoidance. In each chapter complications peculiar to that particular fracture are discussed from a prevention and management point of view. Special chapters have been included for the more devastating and vexing complications, such as compartment syndrome, reflex sympathetic dystrophy, and malunions and nonunions.

The text ends with an appendix on a very practical and simple classification system for a pediatric fracture database that was designed by Dr. Jacques D'Astous and is currently being used by the Orthopaedic Service at the Children's Hospital of Eastern Ontario.

It is hoped that *Management of Pediatric Fractures* will become well thumbed and stained with coffee and the pages dog-eared as it sits in a readily accessible place in the emergency departments, libraries, surgeons' offices, and operating rooms in centers dealing with traumatized children.

R. Mervyn Letts, MD, FRCSC

Acknowledgments

The success of bringing together the expertise of numerous individuals into one publication requires the assistance and goodwill of innumerable people. The most onerous task is the documentation of the thoughts and recommendations by each author, and to them I am extremely indebted for their excellence in writing, adherence to the format, and compliance with deadlines! To Drs. Maureen Baxter, Timothy Carey, Jacques D'Astous, James Jarvis, Louis Lawton, and William McIntyre, my colleagues at the Children's Hospital of Eastern Ontario, who acted as associate editors reviewing chapters as well as contributing some of their own, I am particularly grateful. Drs. Jim Wiley and Hans Uhthoff have provided encouragement and suggestions as well as thoughtful generous forewords for which I am grateful. To my secretarial staff, Maureen O'Neil and Sue Ziebell, a special thanks for the immense amount of additional work that was required in getting manuscripts ready for the publisher and maintaining a cheerful demeanor throughout the whole process! A special tribute of appreciation is also very deserved for the Medical Photography Department of the Children's Hospital of Eastern Ontario.

Mary Antoine, Tony Cuillerier, Rick Lane, Ronda Lyle, Natalie Larocque, and John Wladarczyk all worked cheerfully and with considerable expertise in producing artwork, prints, and tables for many of the chapters. Denis Joly, of the Department of Radiology, assisted us in locating superb radiographic examples of many fractures. The Children's Hospital of Eastern Ontario Dominick Conway Library staff, Pat Johnston, Pam LeMoine, and Rose-Marie Mongeon, who obtained numerous reference articles and texts, were invaluable in their assistance and detective work. A most special thanks is due to my wife, Marilyn, for proofreading many of the chapters and restructuring bibliographies when required. To the rest of my family, Ian, Eric, and Daron, my thanks and apology for putting up with manuscripts scattered over the house at various times and odd locations! At Churchill Livingstone, the suggestions and interest of Bob Hurley, former Editor-in-Chief, and the efficient staff, especially Donna Balopole and Jennifer Mitchell, both of whom assisted immensely in bringing the text to a successful completion, were indeed appreciated.

Contents

Section I
General Principles

1. Epidemiology of Children's Fractures / **1**
   Martin H. Reed

2. Epiphyseal Plate Injuries / **11**
   Robert B. Salter

3. Initial Management of the Multiply Injured Child / **27**
   Peter F. Armstrong and John T. Smith

4. Radiologic Diagnosis of Pediatric Skeletal Trauma / **37**
   Roderick I. Macpherson and Martin H. Reed

5. Anesthesia for Children's Fractures / **83**
   William M. Splinter

Section II
Fractures of the Shoulder Girdle

6. Fractures of the Sternum, Scapula, and Ribs / **93**
   Robert B. Gledhill

7. Fractures of the Clavicle / **113**
   John D. Hsu and Colin Fennell

8. Dislocations and Pseudodislocations of the Clavicle / **123**
   Pierre Mercier

9. Fractures of the Proximal Humerus and Humeral Shaft / **137**
   Robert F. Martin

10. Dislocations of the Shoulder / **159**
    R. Baxter Willis and Robert D. Galpin

Section III
Fractures of the Elbow

11. Supracondylar Fractures of the Humerus / **167**
    William McIntyre

12. Transcondylar Fractures of the Distal Humerus / **199**
    Curtis R. Gruel and J. Andy Sullivan

13. Dislocations of the Elbow and Fractures of the Medial Humeral Epicondyle and Condyle / **211**
    Walter W. Huurman

14. Lateral Condylar Fractures of the Humerus / **241**
    William McIntyre

15. Olecranon and Coronoid Fractures / **259**
    R. Dale Blasier

16. Fractures of the Capitellum / **283**
    R. Mervyn Letts and Kevin Rumball

Section IV
Fractures of the Forearm and Wrist

17. Monteggia and Galeazzi Fractures / **295**
    R. Mervyn Letts

18. Fractures of the Midshaft Radius and Ulna / **323**
    Charles T. Price

19. Fractures of the Distal Radius and Ulna / **345**
    Louis J. Lawton

20. Fractures of the Radial Head and Neck / **369**
    Gerhard N. Kiefer

Section V
Fractures of the Hand

21. Fractures of the Carpal Bones / **385**
    R. Mervyn Letts and Geoff Dervin

22. Fractures of the Metacarpals / **407**
    Timothy P. Carey

23. Fractures and Dislocations of the Phalanges / **421**
    Timothy P. Carey

24. Nail Bed and Crush Injuries of the Hand / **441**
    Leslie J. Mintz

Section VI
Fractures of the Pelvis and Hip

25. Fractures of the Pelvis / **453**
    Richard E. McCarthy

26. Fractures of the Hip / **483**
    Stanley M.K. Chung

27. Acute Slipped Capital Femoral Epiphysis / **513**
    Dennis S. Weiner

28. Traumatic Dislocation of the Hip / **523**
    Morris Duhaime, Marc Isler, and Dominique Marton

Section VII
Fractures of the Lower Extremity

29. Fractures of the Femoral Shaft / **539**
    William G. MacKenzie

30. Supracondylar (Nonphyseal) Fractures of the Femur / **563**
    Jacques D'Astous

31. Supracondylar (Physeal) Fractures of the Femur / **569**
    Jacques D'Astous

32. Intra-articular Fractures of the Knee / **593**
    Roger Gallien

33. Fractures and Dislocations of the Proximal Tibia and Fibula / **611**
    James A. Harder

34. Degloving Injuries in Tibial Shaft Fractures / **631**
    R. Mervyn Letts and Eric Robinson

35. The Floating Knee / **661**
    R. Mervyn Letts and Guy Moreau

36. Fractures and Dislocations of the Patella / **671**
    Walter B. Greene

37. Treatment of Posttraumatic Sequelae by the Ilizarov Technique / **695**
    Deborah F. Bell

Section VIII
Fractures of the Ankle and Foot

38. Fractures of the Ankle / **713**
    Anthony Ashworth and Douglas Hedden

39. Tibial Triplane Fractures / **735**
    James G. Jarvis

40. Fractures and Dislocations of the Tarsal Bones / **751**
    Norris Carrol

41. Fractures and Dislocations of the Metatarsals and Phalanges of the Foot / **767**
    Maureen P. Baxter

42. Crush Injuries and Compartment Syndrome of the Foot / **789**
    R. Baxter Willis and Robert D. Galpin

Section IX
Fractures of the Spine

43. Atlanto-Occipital Fractures and Dislocations / **797**
    James G. Jarvis

44. C1-C2 Fractures and Dislocations / **807**
    Francois Fassier

45. C3-C7 Fractures and Dislocations / **833**
    Stephen J. Tredwell

46. Fractures and Dislocations of the Thoracolumbar Spine / **853**
    Rudolph A. Klassen

47. Seat Belt Fractures / **877**
    James G. Jarvis

48. Fractures of the Sacrum and Coccyx / **889**
    Guillermo R. Viviani

49. Acute Spinal Cord Injury / **901**
    Garth Johnson

50. The SCIWORA Syndrome / **919**
    Hubert Labelle and Claude Mercier

Section X
Specific Conditions of Pediatric Fractures

51. Child Abuse Fractures / **931**
    G. Brian Black

52. Extremity Gunshot Fractures / **945**
    Randall T. Loder

53. Stress Fractures / **973**
    Lyle J. Micheli and Allan F. Fehlandt, Jr.

54. Avulsion Fractures / **989**
    Jacques D'Astous

55. Osteochondral Fractures / **1001**
    Benoit Morin

56. Pathologic Fractures / **1027**
    Benoit Poitras and Charles H. Rivard

57. Birth Fractures / **1049**
    Martin H. Reed, R. Mervyn Letts, and Avrum N. Pollock

58. Fractures in the Myelomeningocele Child / **1063**
    John V. Banta

59. Fractures in the Osteogenesis Imperfecta Child / **1079**
    Walter P. Bobechko

60. Fractures in the Severely Handicapped Child / **1105**
    Dennis Lyne and Bernard A. Roehr

Section XI
Complications of Fractures

61. Complications in Children's Fractures / **1111**
    R. Dale Blasier

62. Posttraumatic Physeal Arrest / **1139**
    John G. Birch

63. Reflex Sympathetic Dystrophy / **1155**
    Maureen P. Baxter

64. Compartment Syndrome / **1165**
    Kenneth L.B. Brown

65. Fat Embolism Syndrome / **1177**
    Alan Gurd

66. Operative Fixation of Children's Fractures / **1183**
    Kenneth J. Guidera and John A. Ogden

67. Traumatic Spondylolysis and Spondylolisthesis / **1195**
    Thomas S. Renshaw

Appendix
   Computer Indexing of Fractures / **1213**
   Jacques D'Astous

Index / **1225**

1

Epidemiology of Children's Fractures

Martin H. Reed

The dictionary is the only place where success comes before hard work.

The study of the incidence and distribution of fractures in children—the epidemiology of fractures—is of more than academic interest. It also has some very practical applications[1]; among them the following three are of particular importance:

1. Knowledge of the usual pattern of fractures at a certain age, or in a specific injury situation, can guide the investigation and management of an injured child. For instance, Roshkow and colleagues[2] have shown that the pattern of injuries that children sustain after falls from a height is different from that seen in adults. Therefore, radiographs that might be routine in an adult in such a situation are not necessarily indicated in children. Another example is a study by Weinshel and colleagues,[3] which showed that fractures are very uncommon in wringer washing machine injuries, and that those that occur are usually very minor, suggesting that radiographs are not usually required in the evaluation of limbs injured in this fashion.

2. The study of patterns of injuries, including fractures, in specific types of trauma may also assist in developing preventive measures.[4] A number of studies have shown that head injuries are the major cause of serious morbidity in bicycle accidents in children. This information has stimulated widespread campaigns to encourage the wearing of bicycle helmets by children, and it has been clearly shown that their use does significantly reduce the frequency and severity of head injuries.[5]

3. Epidemiologic studies can be used to help determine the health care costs of injuries.[4,6]

Injuries in general are a very important cause of morbidity in childhood, and they are the leading cause of death in children after 1 year of age. They cause 40 percent of deaths in children ages 1 to 4 years and 70 percent of deaths in older children. Motor vehicle accidents are responsible for almost 50 percent of these trauma-related deaths; homicide is the second most common cause in the United States.[4,7]

Langley and his colleagues[8-13] have undertaken a very valuable longitudinal cohort study of approximately 1,000 children in New Zealand, following them from 1 through 15 years of age. They have shown that children are injured with increasing frequency as they grow older (Table 1-1), and that in any 2-year period, at least 20 percent of children will be injured. Fortunately, most injuries are of mild or moderate severity. Fractures and other orthopaedic injuries comprise a significant number of these mild and moderate injuries[7] (Table 1-1), and the frequency of fractures is second only to contusions, abrasions, and lacerations in children, and to sprains and strains in adolescents.[9-13]

TABLE 1-1. Frequency of Injuries During Childhood

Age (years)	No. of Children	Percentage Injured	No. of Injuries	Fractures (% of Injuries)
6 and 7[9]	1,072	22	273	45 (16)
8 and 9[10]	955	26	283	50 (18)
10 and 11[11]	803	38	413	84 (20)
12 and 13[12]	850	44	550	109 (20)
14 and 15[13]	852	53	657	157 (24)

(Data from Langley[9-13]).

INCIDENCE OF FRACTURES

Fractures occur most frequently in the elderly, and, compared to the last decades of life, the incidence in children is very low.[14] However, as indicated in the previous section, injuries are a very important cause of morbidity in childhood, and fractures comprise a significant and increasing proportion of injuries throughout childhood (Table 1-1). The pattern of fractures seen in children differs significantly from that seen in adults.[14] For instance, fractures of the proximal femur are rare in children, but become increasingly common with age.[14] On the other hand, the peak age for fractures of the clavicle, the supracondylar region of the humerus, and of the tibial shaft is during childhood and adolescence; fractures of the metacarpals and phalanges occur most commonly during adolescence.[14]

A number of studies have evaluated the age and sex distribution, and the sites of fractures, in childhood[15-18]; the most comprehensive of these was an analysis by Landin[19] of 8,682 fractures in Swedish children over a 20-year period. The annual incidence of fractures was 21.2 per 1,000 in Landin's series (children up to the age of 16 years)[19] and 16.0 per 1,000 in the series of Worlock and Stower[15] (children up to the age of 12 years). By determining accumulated risk figures in his series, Landin[19] concluded that 42 percent of boys and 27 percent of girls had had at least one fracture by the age of 16. In all series, boys suffered more fractures than girls[15-18]; the difference was greatest during adolescence when boys had twice as many fractures as girls.[19] Worlock and Stower[15] noted in their study that fractures were rare in infants under 18 months of age.

Upper-extremity fractures are at least three times as common as lower-extremity fractures in children.[15-19] Table 1-2 attempts to compare the frequencies of differ-

TABLE 1-2. Frequency of Fractures at Selected Sites in Children

Anatomic Site	Author				
	Worlock[15] (%)	Wiley[16] (%)	Reed[17] (%)	Iqbal[18] (%)	Landin[19] (%)
Clavicle	6.3	8.4	13.4	15.5	8.1
Humerus (proximal end and shaft)	1.9	3.1	3.4	4.5	
Distal humerus	7.7	6.0		23.4	3.3
Radial neck	2.7	1.7		0.3	1.2
Radius/ulna (shafts)	6.5	4.1	5.6	13.4	3.4
Distal radius/ulna	35.8	28.6	19.8	27.5	22.7
Hand	14.7	18.7	21.5		
Femur	2.0	3.3	6.6	4.5	
Tibia/fibula (shafts)	4.3	9.7	4.6	3.4	5.0
Ankle	4.0	2.3	6.8	4.8	5.5
Foot	7.7	6.5	6.8		
Total fractures	923	2,640	410	291	8,682

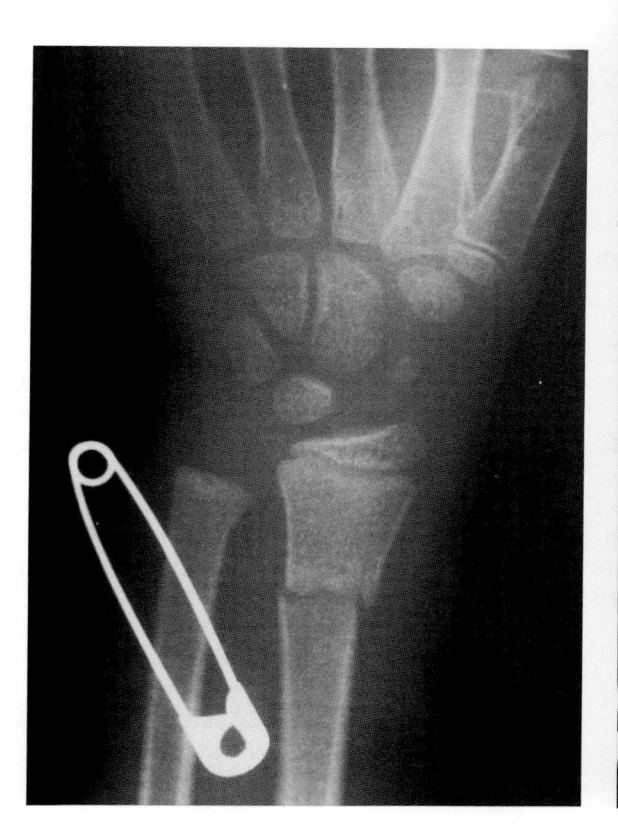

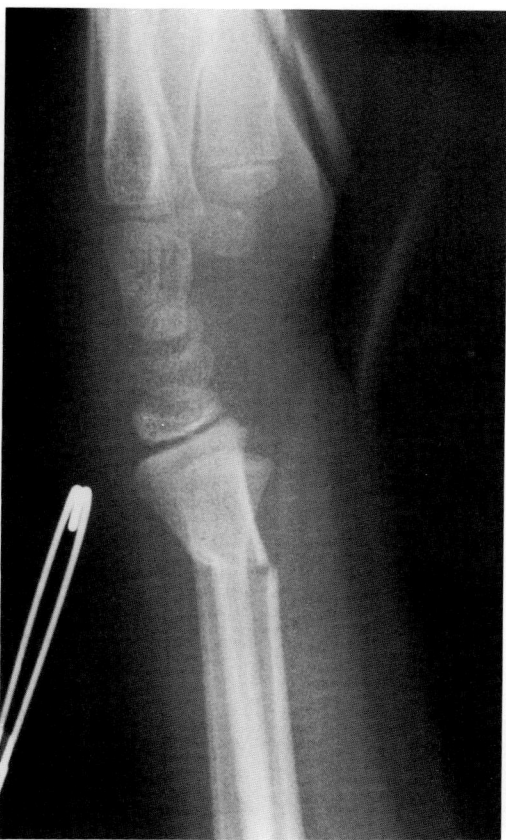

Fig. 1-1. Transverse fracture of the distal radius in a 6-year-old girl.

ent types of fractures in different series. Unfortunately, the figures are not directly comparable because these series reviewed somewhat different age groups; they also included and excluded different types of fractures. These factors explain to some extent the variation in frequency of the different fractures among the series. However, in all series the radius is the bone most frequently fractured in children, and the distal end is the most common site (Fig. 1-1). The hand, followed by the clavicle and the distal humerus are the three other common sites of fractures in the upper extremity. In the lower extremity, fractures appear to occur with approximately equal frequency in the femur, the lower leg, the ankle, and the foot (Table 1-2).

Most of the common fractures, including those of the distal radius and ulna, proximal humerus, ankle, and fingers and toes, follow the general trend and increase in frequency with age, sometimes diminishing in late adolescence.[19] Others, such as those of the tibial and radial and ulnar shafts are less affected by age, whereas fractures of the clavicle and femoral diaphysis occur most commonly in young children.[19] Supracondylar fractures of the humerus peak in incidence between 5 and 10 years of age.[19]

Approximately half the fractures in the series of Worlock and Stower[15] were of the greenstick type, which was the most common type, both in children 5 years of age and younger, and in older children up to 12 years of age. They did not study adolescents. In younger patients, complete fractures—transverse, oblique, and spiral—were the next most common type, but, in older children, epiphyseal fractures were as common as complete fractures.[15]

INCIDENCE OF PHYSEAL INJURIES

Between 18 and 30 percent of pediatric fractures involve the growth plate,[15,20,21] and the frequency of growth plate injuries increases with age.[15] In the series of

TABLE 1-3. Physeal Fractures: Frequency of Salter-Harris Types

Salter-Harris Type	Author		
	Worlock[15] No. (%)	Mann[20] No. (%)	Mizuta[21] No. (%)
I	30 (17.5)	210 (22.3)	30 (8.5)
II	121 (70.8)	483 (51.2)	257 (73.0)
III	5 (2.9)	143 (15.2)	23 (6.1)
IV	15 (8.8)	102 (10.8)	42 (12.0)
V		5 (0.5)	1 (0.1)
Total	171	943	353

Mizuta and coworkers,[21] physeal injuries comprised 10 percent of fractures in infancy (0–5 years), 15 percent of fractures in childhood (6–11 years), and 30 percent of fractures in adolescents (12–17 years). These percentages were similar in males and females.[21] However, the peak age for physeal fractures, overall and at specific sites, generally tends to occur slightly earlier in girls than in boys.[20-22]

Although the large reported series of physeal fractures are not quite comparable in terms of age groups and types of fractures studied, the relative frequencies of the different types of physeal injuries is similar (Table 1-3). The Salter-Harris type II fracture is by far the most common, comprising anywhere from 50 to 75 percent of physeal injuries (Fig. 1-2; Table 1-3). Type I fractures are the next most frequent, in most series. However, it is important to remember that undisplaced type I fractures may be difficult or impossible to diagnose radiologically in the acute situation. Therefore, if radiologic evidence is the sole criterion for diagnosis in a series, the frequency of type I fractures will be underestimated; it is not always clear from the reported series what diagnostic criteria were used. Salter-Harris types III and IV fractures probably occur with similar frequency. Type V fractures are rare. However, because they cannot really be diagnosed acutely, but only when signs of growth arrest appear, their frequency may also be underestimated.

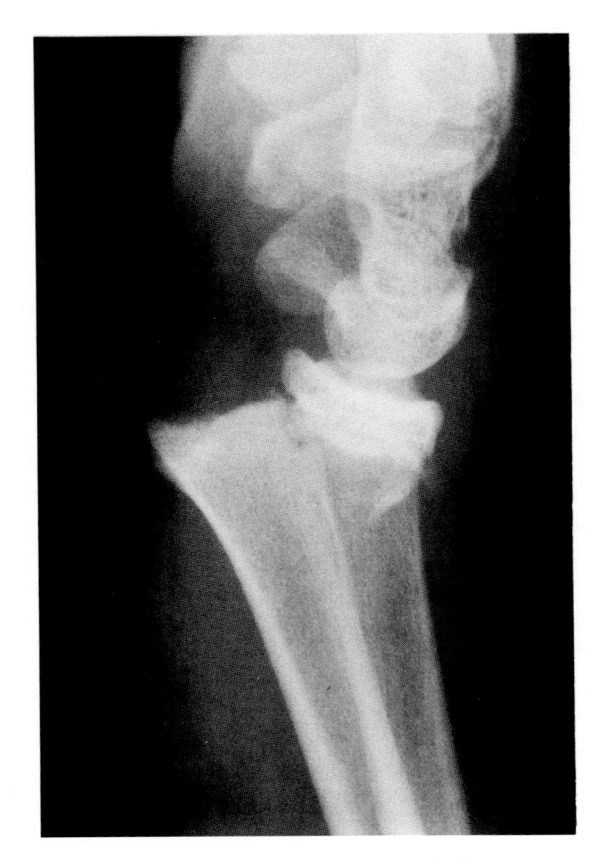

Fig. 1-2. Type II fracture of the distal radius in a 14-year-old girl.

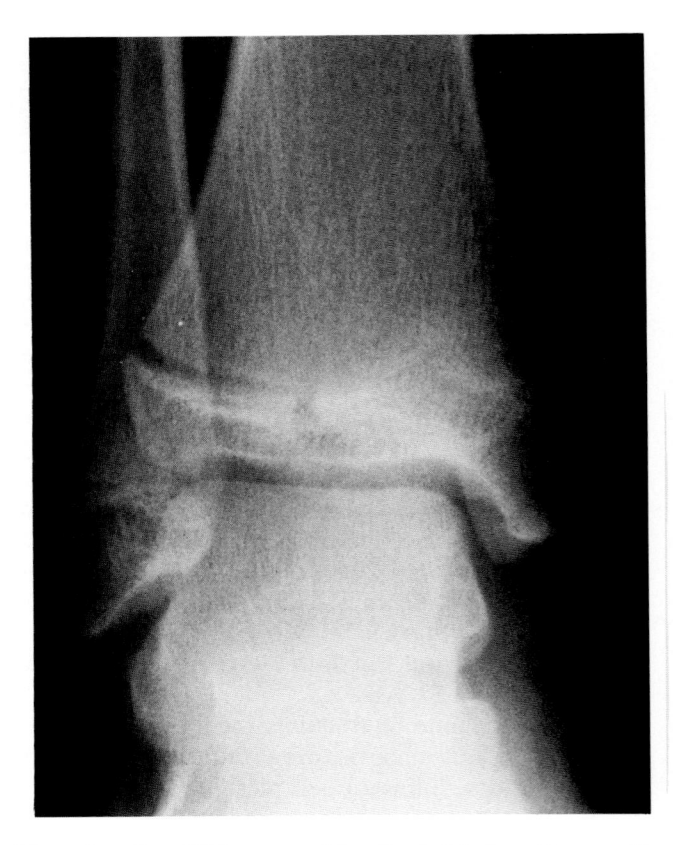

Fig. 1-3. Type III fracture of the distal tibia in a 13-year-old girl.

In the long bones, by far the most common site of a physeal injury, is the distal radius.[20-22] Salter-Harris type I fractures occur most frequently at the distal radius and distal fibula, type II fractures in the distal radius (Fig. 1-2) and distal tibia, type III fractures in the distal tibia (Fig. 1-3), and type IV fractures in the distal humerus and distal tibia.[20,21] Physeal injuries are also very common in the phalanges, both in the fingers and in the toes.[21,22]

FRACTURES ASSOCIATED WITH TYPES OF INJURY

Falls

In most series, falls, both on a level surface and from a height, are the most frequent cause of fractures, and indeed of all types of injuries, in children. Falls from a height have been recognized as a major form of pediatric trauma, particularly in large urban centers, where falls from buildings were found to cause a significant number of severe pediatric injuries.[23] In one series, the fatality rate was 23 percent, the highest of any injury category.[23] The seriousness of this problem has prompted major public education programs and the passage of bylaws mandating guards on windows of apartment buildings.[23] As in most types of pediatric injuries, boys are affected in significantly greater numbers than girls,[23-25] and in most series, approximately 50 percent of affected children are 5 years of age or younger.[2,24,25]

Fractures are the most common type of injury sustained by children in falls from heights. These usually are extremity fractures, and, although figures vary somewhat from series to series, upper and lower extremities are probably affected approximately equally (Table 1-4). In the upper extremity, most fractures involve the radius and ulna, and in the lower extremity, the femur.[2,25] Fractures of the calcaneus, pelvis, and spine are rare (Table 1-4), a pattern very different from adults, in whom fractures at these sites are common.[2] As mentioned earlier, this difference should affect the imaging evaluation of children who have fallen from a height. Radiographic examinations of regions such as the spine and pelvis, which may be standard in adults, are not indicated routinely in children.[2] Head injuries occur very frequently in children as a result of falls from heights, much more so than in adults, probably because of a higher center of gravity in children[2]; they are a major reason for the high morbidity and mortality of this type of accident in children.

Another type of fall that occurs much more frequently in children than in adults, is a fall downstairs. Joffe and Ludwig[26] studied 363 cases of this type of injury. More than 50 percent of the children were 5 years of age and younger. The severity of injury did not appear to relate to the height of stairs the children had fallen down. Although 73 percent of the injuries involved the head and neck, overall there were very few severe injuries. Head injuries were more likely to occur in children under 4 years of age. Extremity injuries were seen in only 28 percent of patients, and only six of these were fractures.[26]

In the investigation of child abuse cases, a frequent explanation proffered for a child's injury is that she or he fell off a bed or similar piece of furniture. Two studies have been reported, surveying the severity of injuries associated with this type of accident, and both of them have shown that serious injuries are very rare, and that extremity fractures are also rare.[27,28] Falls from the top bunk of a bunk bed result in slightly more fractures, but still generally not in significant injuries[29]; a characteristic buckle fracture of the base of the first metatarsal "the bunk bed fracture," has been described as a result of this type of accident.[30]

Road and Off-Road Accidents

Road accidents were the most common cause of injury in one large recently reported series of children admitted to a trauma center; they comprised almost 30

TABLE 1-4. Falls from a Height: Associated Fractures in Children

Fracture Sites	Author			
	Roshkow[2]	Musemeche[22]	Barlow[23]	Smith[24]
Upper extremity	10	20	29	17
Lower extremity	18	5	28	10
Pelvis	2	4	8	1
Spine	1	2	2	
Total patients	45	70	61	66

percent of the cases.[31] In the same series, almost half the deaths occurred in this group of patients.

Motor Vehicle Occupant Accidents

Most traffic-related deaths among children occur in motor vehicle occupant accidents, and the injuries seen in these accidents are among the most severe.[4] In spite of the significance of this type of pediatric trauma, most of the articles dealing with this problem consider only general mortality and morbidity statistics and report only trauma scores[32]; they do not review specific injury patterns. Agran and colleagues[33] studied the injuries in 191 children, who represented a sample of those who were occupants of motor vehicles involved in accidents. These children were all seat-belted; 33 of them were uninjured. There were only five extremity fractures among all the children injured, including three femoral fractures, one fracture of a clavicle, one fracture of a humerus, and one forearm fracture. No spinal fractures occurred.[33] Agran and colleagues,[34] in a separate study, considered the problem of children who were injured while riding in the backs of pickup trucks.[34] Most of these were older children, and, as might be expected, those who were riding in the backs of pickup trucks were more likely to sustain severe injuries than those riding in the cabs. However, only 14 of the 89 who were riding in the back and 10 of the 201 who were riding in the cab, sustained extremity fractures. Most of the injuries involved only the soft tissues, but there were a number of severe head injuries.[34]

Pedestrian Accidents

Pedestrian accidents remain the most frequent cause of death due to trauma in children in the 5- to 9-years age group, which is the peak pediatric age group for this type of accident.[4] In one reported series,[35] extremity injuries occurred approximately as frequently as head injuries in children, whereas they occurred more frequently in adults. In another series,[36] extremity injuries were twice as common as head injuries in children, but the overall frequency of extremity fractures was not provided. In the former series,[35] only 22 of the 60 extremity injuries were fractures; no information was given about the specific fracture sites.

Bell and colleagues[37] discussed a particular type of pediatric motor vehicle accident—children who were run over by slowly moving vehicles. There were 14 children in their series, all but one 6 years of age or under. Most of the injuries in these patients involved the thorax, including fractured ribs in three children, and there were also several severe cranial injuries. There were 12 other skeletal injuries, including 3 femoral fractures, 1 pelvic fracture, and 8 fractures of other bones or joint injuries.[37]

Bicycle Accidents

Another important type of childhood injury is the bicycle accident. Although head and neck injuries comprise only 20 to 30 percent of the injuries in these accidents,[38,39] head injuries are the most important cause of death.[38,40] Bicycle accidents are, in fact, one of the most important causes of significant head injury in childhood.[38] As would be expected, children are most seriously injured in this type of accident when they are hit by a car or some other vehicle.[39,40] Two studies have reviewed general injury patterns that result from bicycle accidents in childhood.[38,39] In one, the upper extremity was more frequently injured than the lower,[38] and in the other, the lower extremity was more frequently injured.[39] Abrasions, lacerations, and contusions comprised more than 50 percent of the injuries. Fractures occurred with almost equal frequency in both series, 14 percent and 13 percent, respectively.[38,39] The authors did not give any more detailed information about the location of the fractures.

Off-Road Vehicle Accidents

Off-road vehicle accidents among children have recently received considerable attention in the literature.[41] The problem was considered serious enough in the United States to justify a ban on the sale of new three-wheel all-terrain vehicles as of January 1988.[41] The most detailed study of the pattern of injuries seen in children involved in accidents while using off-road vehicles was published by Pyper and Black.[42] Their study included children injured in accidents involving minibikes or dirt bikes (40 percent), snowmobiles (31 percent), and all-terrain vehicles (29 percent), most of which were the three-wheeled variety. Among the 233 patients, there were 352 fractures; 60 of these involved the growth plate, almost half Salter-Harris type II, and 34 of the fractures were open. In all three groups, the extremities were by far the most common sites of fractures; they occurred slightly more commonly in the lower extremity than in the upper extremity. In the lower limbs, tibial fractures occurred three times as commonly as femoral fractures in dirt-bike accidents, but with almost equal frequency to femoral fractures in the other two groups. In the upper extremity, the common sites of fractures were the forearm and the humerus, with the former being slightly more frequent than the latter. Fractures of the spine and pelvis were most frequent in all-terrain vehicle accidents, comprising 11 percent of fractures in that group.[42]

Sports and Recreation Injuries

Sports-related injuries become more frequent with increasing age throughout childhood.[10-13,43] A number of studies have reviewed sports-related injuries in children.[1,43-46] Most of these have studied organized sports, but two have compared organized sports to unorganized sports and physical education programs.[43,45] In the series of Kvist and colleagues[43] sports comprised 14 percent of all accidents in the 6- to 10-years age group and 26 percent of all accidents in the 11- to 15-years age group. In all the series sports-related injuries were more common in boys than girls. There was no agreement among the various studies as to which sports were most likely to produce injuries. Fractures comprised between 7 and 26 percent of all injuries in organized sports, depending on the study.[1,43-46] Backx and coworkers[1] found a higher percentage of fractures (18 percent) among the injuries sustained in physical education classes than among those sustained in organized sports (4 percent) or nonorganized sports (8 percent), but Tursz and Monique[45] found no significant difference in the percentage of fractures among these different groups. Upper-extremity fractures are more common than lower-extremity fractures.[1,43,45,46] Only two studies reviewed specific sites of fractures. In the upper limb, the forearm and wrist, and metacarpals and phalanges were the most frequent sites; in the lower limb, the lower leg and the ankle were the most frequent sites.[43,46] Watson's[46] was the only study that specifically discussed the sites of dislocations, all of which occurred in the upper extremity.[46]

Soccer

Very few studies have considered injury patterns among children involved in specific sports. Hoff and Marten[47] compared the frequency and type of injuries occurring in youths playing indoor and outdoor soccer. They found a higher incidence of injuries overall, and a higher frequency of fractures, among players involved in indoor soccer; they provided no information about the specific sites of the fractures.[47]

Downhill Skiing

Upper extremity injuries are more common than lower extremity injuries in adults involved in downhill skiing accidents; this relationship is reversed in children.[48,49] In the upper limb in children, the thumb is particularly susceptible to injury.[48,49] In adults, the knee and ankle are the most common sites of injury in the lower limb, but in children, injuries usually involve the knee and lower leg.[49] Tibial fractures are a particularly frequent lower-extremity injury in children[48,49] (Fig. 1-4); they usually occur because the binding fails to release.[48] The frequency of this type of injury has been decreasing over the years as equipment has improved.[49]

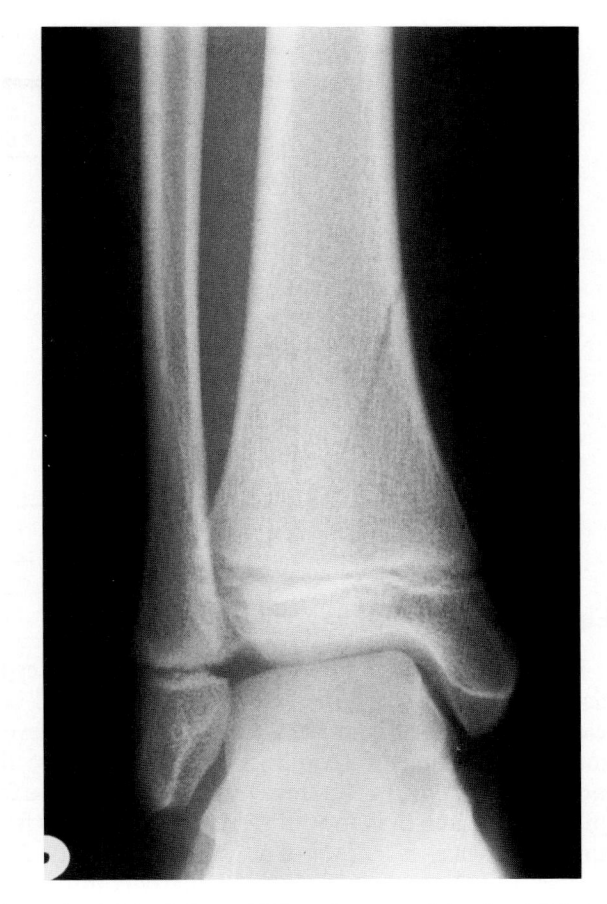

Fig. 1-4. Skiing injury. Oblique fracture of the distal tibia in a 12-year-old girl.

TABLE 1-5. Skateboard Accidents: Associated Fractures in Children

Anatomic Site	Author			
	Illingworth[52]	Cass[53]	Maitra[54]	Allum[55]
Clavicle	5		3	3
Scapula	2			1
Humerus	4	5	2	2
Radius/ulna	42	41	11	12
Scaphoid	14		2	1
Metacarpals/phalanges	10		7	2
Femur	1	7		
Tibia/fibula	7	3	2	2
Metatarsals	5		1	3
Total patients	225	80	59	46

Equestrian Injuries

Equestrian injuries are a particular problem, especially among girls.[43,50] In the series of Kvist and colleagues[43] this sport produced the most moderately severe and severe injuries[43]; head and facial injuries are the most frequent type in children.[50] Fractures are more frequent in children than in adults.[51] Upper-extremity fractures are twice as common as lower-extremity fractures,[50] and the humerus is a particularly common site in this type of accident.[43,51] In the series of Barone and Rogers,[50] there were 10 spinal fractures among 152 injuries in 136 patients; 2 of these involved the cervical spine, 1 resulting in quadriplegia. There were also five pelvic fractures, occurring when the horse fell on the rider.[50]

Skateboarding Injuries

After achieving a peak in popularity in the 1970s, the interest in skateboarding waned, but there has recently been a marked resurgence of skateboarding among the young.[52] A number of studies have documented the injuries that occur as a result of skateboarding accidents. Only one series was restricted to children[53]; the other series included adults, but the vast majority of patients were children.[54-56] Although head injuries occur in these children, they are usually mild.[54] The majority of injuries are fractures (Table 1-5). Upper-limb fractures are by far the most frequent, usually involving the radius and ulna, particularly their distal ends[53-56] (Table 1-5). Fractures of the lower limb commonly involve the tibia and fibula[53-56] (Table 1-5). The peak age incidence for these accidents is between 11 and 15 years.[53,54] Cass and Ross[54] noted that the more serious fractures in their series occurred in children under 10 years of age, but Illingworth and colleagues[53] did not note any significant difference in the severity of injuries comparing children under 10 to those 10 years of age and older. In general, the fractures in these patients were not very serious.

ACKNOWLEDGMENTS

I would like to thank Dr. Dan Wilmot for his critical reading of this chapter and Karen James for her secretarial assistance.

REFERENCES

1. Backx FJG, Beijer HJM, Bol E, Erich WBM: Injuries in high-risk persons and high-risk sports: a longitudinal study of 1818 school children. Am J Sports Med 19:124, 1991
2. Roshkow JE, Haller JO, Hotson GC et al: Imaging evaluation of children after falls from a height: review of 45 cases. Radiology 175:359, 1990
3. Weinshel S, Greydanus W, Glicklich M: Wringer washing machine injuries: criteria for obtaining radiological studies. J Trauma 26:1132, 1986
4. Division of Injury Control, Center for Environmental Health and Injury Control, Centers for Disease Control: Childhood injuries in the United States. Am J Dis Child 144:627, 1990

5. Thompson RS, Rivara FP, Thompson DC: A case-control study of the effectiveness of bicycle safety helmets. N Engl J Med 320:1361, 1989
6. King WD: Pediatric injury surveillance: use of a hospital discharge data base. South Med J 84:342, 1991
7. Chan BSH, Walker PJ, Cass DT: Urban trauma: an analysis of 1,116 paediatric cases. J Trauma 29:1540, 1989
8. Langley J, Dodge J, Silva PA: Accidents in the first five years of life: a report from the Dunedin Multidisciplinary Child Development Study. Aust Paediatr J 15:255, 1979
9. Langley JD, Silva PA, Williams SM: Accidental injuries in the sixth and seventh years of life: a report from the Dunedin Multidisciplinary Child Development Study. N Z Med J 93:344, 1981
10. Langley JD, Silva PA: Injuries in the eighth and ninth years of life. Aust Paediatr J 21:51, 1985
11. Langley JD, Cecchi J, Silva PA: Injuries in the tenth and eleventh years of life. Aust Paediatr J 23:35, 1987
12. Chalmers DJ, Cecchi J, Langley JD, Silva PA: Injuries in the 12th and 13th years of life. Aust Paediatr J 25:14, 1989
13. Lodge JF, Langley JD, Begg DJ: Injuries in the 14th and 15th years of life. J Paediatr Child Health 26:316, 1990
14. Buhr AJ, Cooke AM: Fracture patterns. Lancet 1:531, 1959
15. Worlock P, Stower M: Fracture patterns in Nottingham children. J Pediatr Orthop 6:656, 1986
16. Wiley JJ, McIntyre WM: Fracture patterns in children. p. 159. In: Current Concepts of Bone Fragility. Springer-Verlag, Berlin, 1986
17. Reed MH: Fractures and dislocations of the extremities in children. J Trauma 17:351, 1977
18. Iqbal QM: Long bone fractures among children in Malaysia. Int Surg 59:410, 1974
19. Landin LA: Fracture patterns in children. Acta Orthop Scand, suppl. 54:S202, 1983
20. Mann DC, Rajmaira S: Distribution of physeal and nonphyseal fractures in 2,650 long-bone fractures in children aged 0–16 years. J Pediatr Orthop 10:713, 1990
21. Mizuta T, Benson WM, Foster BK et al: Statistical analysis of the incidence of physeal injuries. J Pediatr Orthop 7:518, 1987
22. Peterson CA, Peterson HA: Analysis of the incidence of injuries to the epiphyseal growth plate. J Trauma 12:275, 1972
23. Musemeche CA, Barthel M, Cosentino C, Reynolds M: Pediatric falls from heights. J Trauma 31:1347, 1991
24. Barlow B, Niemirska M, Gandhi RP, Leblanc W: Ten years experience with falls from a height in children. J Pediatr Surg 18:509, 1983
25. Smith MD, Burrington JD, Woolf AD: Injuries in children sustained in free falls: an analysis of 66 cases. J Trauma 15:987, 1975
26. Joffe M, Ludwig S: Stairway injuries in children. Pediatrics 82:457, 1988
27. Nimityongskul P, Anderson LD: The likelihood of injuries when children fall out of bed. J Pediatr Orthop 7:184, 1987
28. Helfer RE, Slovis TL, Black M: Injuries resulting when small children fall out of bed. Pediatrics 60:533, 1977
29. Selbst SM, Baker MD, Shames M: Bunk bed injuries. Am J Dis Child 144:721, 1990
30. Johnson GF: Pediatric Lisfranc injury: "bunkbed fracture." AJR 137:1041, 1981
31. Peclet MH, Newman KD, Eichelberger MR et al: Patterns of injury in children. J Pediatr Surg 25:85, 1990
32. Agran PA, Dunkle DE: Motor vehicle occupant injuries to children in crash and noncrash events. Pediatrics 70:993, 1982
33. Agran PF, Dunkle DE, Winn DG: Injuries to a sample of seatbelted children evaluated and treated in a hospital emergency room. J Trauma 27:58, 1987
34. Agran PF, Winn DG, Castillo DN: Pediatric injuries in the back of pickup trucks. JAMA 264:712, 1990
35. Derlet RW, Silva J, Holcroft J: Pedestrian accidents: adult and pediatric injuries. J Emerg Med 7:5, 1989
36. Lapidus G, Braddock M, Banco L et al: Child pedestrian injury: a population-based collision and injury severity profile. J Trauma 31:1110, 1991
37. Bell MJ, Ternberg JL, Bower RJ: Low velocity vehicular injuries in children: "run-over" accidents. Pediatrics 66:628, 1980
38. Cushman R, Down J, MacMillan N, Waclawik H: Bicycle-related injuries: a survey in a pediatric emergency department. Can Med Assoc J 143:108, 1990
39. Selbst SM, Alexander D, Ruddy R: Bicycle-related injuries. Am J Dis Child 141:140, 1987
40. Nixon J, Clacher R, Pearn J, Corcoran A: Bicycle accidents in childhood. Br Med J 294:1267, 1987
41. Dolan MA, Knapp JF, Andres J: Three-wheel and four-wheel all-terrain vehicle injuries in children. Pediatrics 84:694, 1989
42. Pyper JA, Black GB: Orthopaedic injuries in children associated with the use of off-road vehicles. J Bone Joint Surg [Am] 70:275, 1988
43. Kvist M, Kujala UM, Heinonen OJ et al: Sports-related injuries in children. Int J Sports Med 10:81, 1989
44. McLain LG, Reynolds S: Sports injuries in a high school. Pediatrics 84:446, 1989
45. Tursz A, Monique C: Sports-related injuries in children: a study of their characteristics, frequency, and severity, with comparison to other types of accidental injuries. Am J Sports Med 14:294, 1986
46. Watson AWS: Sports injuries during one academic year in 6799 Irish school children. Am J Sports Med 12:65, 1984
47. Hoff GL, Martin TA: Outdoor and indoor soccer: injuries among youth players. Am J Sports Med 14:231, 1986
48. Hill SA: Incidence of tibial fracture in child skiers. Br J Sports Med 23:169, 1989
49. Ungerholm S, Engkvist O, Gierup J et al: Skiing injuries in children and adults: a comparative study from an 8-year period. Int J Sports Med 4:236, 1983
50. Barone GW, Rodgers BM: Pediatric equestrian injuries: a 14-year review. J Trauma 29:245, 1989
51. Gierup J, Larsson M, Lennquist S: Incidence and nature of

horse-riding injuries: a one-year prospective study. Acta Chir Scand 142:57, 1976
52. Committee on Accident and Poison Prevention: Skateboard injuries. Pediatrics 83:1070, 1989
53. Illingworth CM, Jay A, Noble D, Collick M: 225 skateboard injuries in children. Clin Pediatr (Phila) 17:781, 1978
54. Cass DT, Ross F: Skateboard injuries. Med J Aust 153:140, 1990
55. Maitra AK: Skateboard injuries. Br J Clin Pract 33:281, 1979
56. Allum RL: Skateboard injuries: a new epidemic. Injury 10:152, 1978

2

Epiphyseal Plate Injuries

Robert B. Salter

Experience is the mother of science.

Injuries involving the epiphyseal plate present special problems in diagnosis and management. The dread complication of serious disturbance of growth is usually predictable and, in certain circumstances, can be prevented. Thus, knowledge of the prognosis for a given injury to the epiphyseal plate in a particular child is of considerable importance to the surgeon, who has the dual responsibility of treating the child and advising the parents.

APPLIED ANATOMY AND HISTOLOGY

Each epiphysis has its own plate through which skeletal growth occurs; it is important that a distinction be made between the epiphysis and the epiphyseal plate (also referred to as the physis).

Histology

A knowledge of the microscopic features of the normal epiphyseal plate is pivotal in understanding the problems associated with the various types of injuries to which it may be subjected. The three main types of injuries are separation of the epiphysis through its epiphyseal plate, fractures that cross the epiphyseal plate, and crushing injuries of the plate itself.

When seen in longitudinal section, four distinct layers can be identified in the normal epiphyseal plate: the layer of resting cells, the layer of proliferating cells, the layer of hypertrophying cells, and the layer of endochrondral ossification (Fig. 2-1). The space between the cells is filled with cartilage matrix or intercellular substance. It is this intercellular substance, and not the cells, that provides the strength of the epiphyseal plate, particularly its resistance to shear. In common with the intercellular substance of other sorts of connective tissues, that of cartilage is made up of collagen fibers embedded in an amorphous cement substance. Because the refractive indexes of these two components are the same, the collagen fibers cannot be identified in ordinary preparations, but they can be seen by special techniques, for instance, phase-contrast microscopy.

These collagen fibers in the matrix of the epiphyseal plate are arranged longitudinally and no doubt play a role similar to that of the steel rods in reinforced concrete. In the first two layers of the plate the matrix is abundant, and here the plate is strong. In the third layer the matrix is scanty, and here the plate is weak. On the metaphyseal side of this layer, however, the matrix is calcified, forming the so-called zone of provisional calcification. The addition of calcification seems to reinforce this part of the third layer, because the plane of cleavage after separation lies in the third layer at approximately the junction of the calcified and uncalcified parts. It seems logical, then, that the constancy of the plane of cleavage is the direct result of the structural details of the normal plate. The significance of the constant location

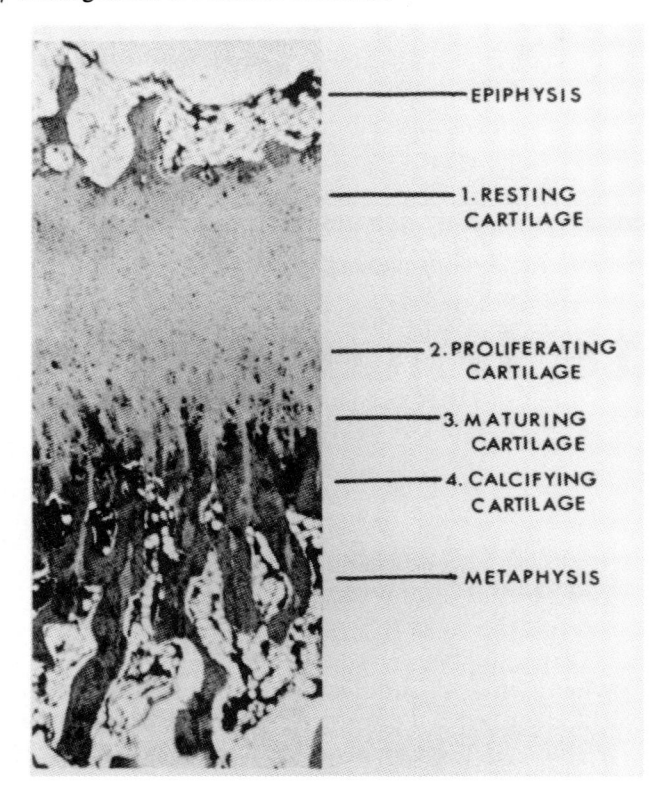

Fig. 2-1. Low-power photomicrograph of an epiphyseal plate from the proximal end of the tibia of a child. (From Salter and Harris,[5] with permission.)

of the plane of cleavage after complete epiphyseal separation is that the growing cells remain attached to the epiphysis. Thus, if the nutrition of these cells is not damaged by the separation, there is no reason why growth should not continue in a normal fashion. The crux of the problem, then, is not the nature of the mechanical damage to the plate, but whether the separation interferes with its blood supply.

Fractures that cross the epiphyseal plate and crushing injuries of the epiphyseal plate present additional problems and are discussed below.

Mechanism of Nutrition

There are two separate systems of blood vessels to the epiphyseal plate. The epiphyseal system arises from vessels in the epiphysis that penetrate the bone plate of the epiphysis and end in capillary tufts or loops in the layer of resting cells of the plate. These vessels are essential to the viability of the chondrocytes of the epiphyseal plate. The metaphyseal system arises in the marrow of the shaft and ends in vascular loops in the layer of endochrondral ossification.

Dale and Harris[1] have demonstrated that the nutrient vessels of the epiphysis (from which the terminal vascular loops to the epiphyseal side of the plate are derived) enter in one of the two ways. The first, and more common, occurs when the sides of the epiphysis are covered with periosteum, as is the case in the distal femoral and proximal tibial epiphyses, in which the nutrient vessels penetrate the side of the epiphysis at a point remote from the epiphyseal plate. The second, and decidedly less common, occurs when the entire epiphysis in intra-articular and hence covered with articular cartilage. In this case, the nutrient vessels enter the epiphysis by traversing the rim of the epiphyseal plate. It is easy to see that the vessels to this type of epiphysis are in danger in the event of epiphyseal separation and might easily be ruptured. The upper femoral epiphysis is the main example of this type; the upper radial epiphysis probably belongs to this group as well.

Relative Strength

The cartilaginous epiphyseal plate is obviously less strong than bone, and yet fractures through bone are much more common in childhood than epiphyseal separations. The probable explanation for this apparent paradox is that only shearing and avulsion forces are capable of separating an epiphysis.

The epiphyseal plate is also less strong than normal tendons and ligaments in adolescents. For this reason, injuries that may result in complete tear of a major ligament in the adult actually produce a separation of the epiphysis in the adolescent. For example, an abduction injury of an adolescent's knee will result in epiphyseal separation rather than a rupture of the medial collateral ligament of the knee. Thus, tears or ruptures of major ligaments are very uncommon in adolescence, and every adolescent suspected of having torn a major ligament should have a radiographic examination to study the epiphyses of the area. By the same token, the epiphyseal plate is not as strong as the fibrous joint capsule, and traumatic dislocations of major joints, such as the knee, during adolescence are thus decidedly less common than epiphyseal separations.

Relative Growth at the Ends of Long Bones

In the lower extremity, more longitudinal growth occurs in the region of the knee than in the regions of the hip or ankle. In the femur, 70 percent of growth occurs in the distal end and 30 percent occurs in the proximal end. In the tibia, 55 percent of growth occurs in the proximal end and 45 percent occurs in the distal end.

DIAGNOSIS

Clinical Diagnosis

Although the accurate diagnosis of epiphyseal plate injuries depends on radiographic examination, suspect such an injury in any child or adolescent who exhibits evidence of a fracture near the end of a long bone, a dislocation, ligamentous rupture, or even a severe sprain of a joint. Remember that an epiphysis may be displaced at the moment of injury and then return to its normal position, in which case clinical examination is likely to be of considerable importance in recognizing the nature of the injury. The history of the mechanism of injury, although often inadequate, may arouse suspicion of a crushing type of epiphyseal plate injury, which is difficult to detect on the radiograph.

Radiographic Diagnosis

Accurate interpretation of the radiographs of adolescent bones and joints necessitates a knowledge of the normal appearance of epiphyses and epiphyseal plates at various ages. Two views at right angles to each other are essential, and often two additional oblique views are required. If in doubt, obtain comparable views of the opposite uninjured extremity.

When the clinical examination suggests an epiphyseal plate injury but the radiographs do not reveal such an injury, stress radiographs taken with the patient under general anesthesia frequently reveal that a separation through the epiphyseal plate has, in fact, occurred and that in the initial radiographs the epiphysis had returned to its normal position.

Late radiographic diagnosis of an undisplaced epiphyseal separation can be made by demonstrating subperiosteal new bone formation in the metaphyseal region 10 days or more after injury.

INJURIES INVOLVING EPIPHYSES

Of all injuries to the long bones during childhood approximately 15 percent involve the epiphyseal plate.[2,3]

Age and Sex Incidence

Although injuries to the epiphyseal plates may occur at any age during childhood, they are somewhat commoner in periods of rapid skeletal growth, in the first year, and during the prepuberty growth spurt. These injuries—and others—are more frequent in boys than in girls, presumably because of the more active physical life of boys.

Site

In general, epiphyseal plates that provide the most growth are most commonly separated by injury. This is not true, however, of two types of epiphyseal injury—fractures that cross or crush the epiphyseal plate.

The lower radial epiphyseal plate is by far the one most frequently separated by injury; indeed, injuries to this

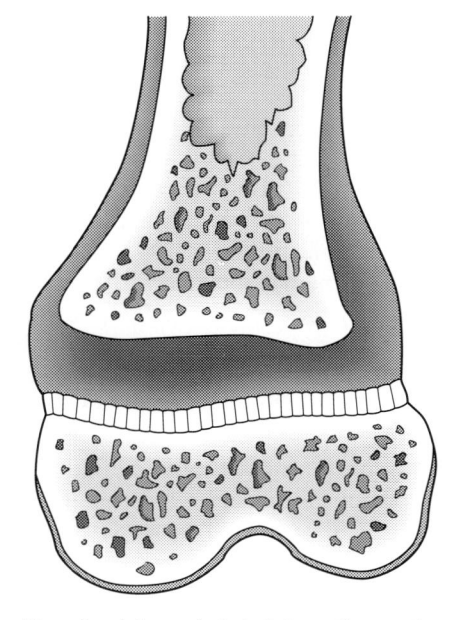

Fig. 2-2. Type I epiphyseal plate injury. Separation of epiphysis. (Adapted from Salter and Harris,[5] with permission.)

Fig. 2-3. Type I separation of the distal fibular epiphysis in a 14-year-old boy. **(A)** This radiograph appears normal because after the injury the fibular epiphysis had returned to its normal position. **(B)** In this stress radiograph (taken while a varus stress is being applied to the ankle joint with the child under anesthetic) there is a tilt of the talus and the separation of the fibular epiphysis is apparent. (From Salter and Harris,[5] with permission.)

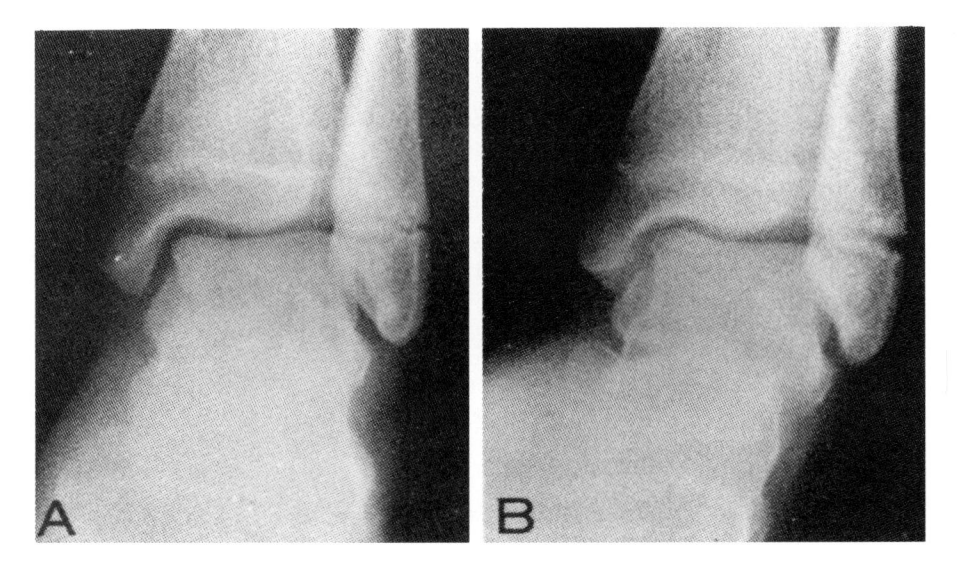

epiphyseal plate are nearly as frequent as all other injuries to the epiphyseal plates combined.[4] In order of decreasing frequency, slipping is found in the lower ulnar, lower humeral (lateral condyle), upper radial (head), lower tibial, lower femoral, upper humeral, upper femoral (head), upper tibial, and phalangeal epiphyseal plates.

POSSIBLE EFFECTS OF EPIPHYSEAL INJURIES

Fortunately, most epiphyseal-plate injuries are not associated with any disturbance of growth. After separation of an epiphysis through its epiphyseal plate there may be a slight and transient acceleration of growth, in which case no significant deformity ensues.

The clinical problem associated with premature cessation of growth depends on several factors, including the bone involved, the extent of involvement of the epiphyseal plate, and the amount of remaining growth normally expected in the involved epiphyseal plate.

If the entire epiphyseal plate ceases to grow, the result is progressive shortening without angulation. However, if the involved bone is one of a parallel pair (such as tibia and fibula or radius and ulna), progressive shortening of the one bone will produce progressive deformity in the neighboring joint. If growth in one part of the epiphyseal plate ceases but continues in the rest of the plate, progressive angulatory deformity occurs.

Cessation of growth does not necessarily occur immediately after injury to the epiphyseal plate, and, indeed, growth arrest may be delayed for 6 months or even longer. Furthermore, there may be a period of retardation before growth ceases completely.

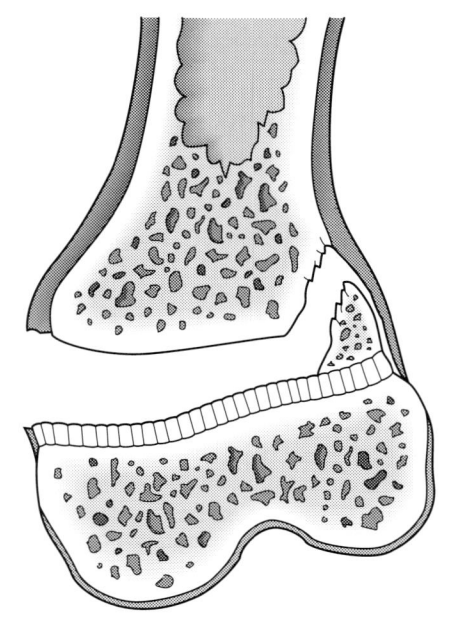

Fig. 2-4. Type II epiphyseal plate injury. Fracture-separation of epiphysis. (Adapted from Salter and Harris,[5] with permission.)

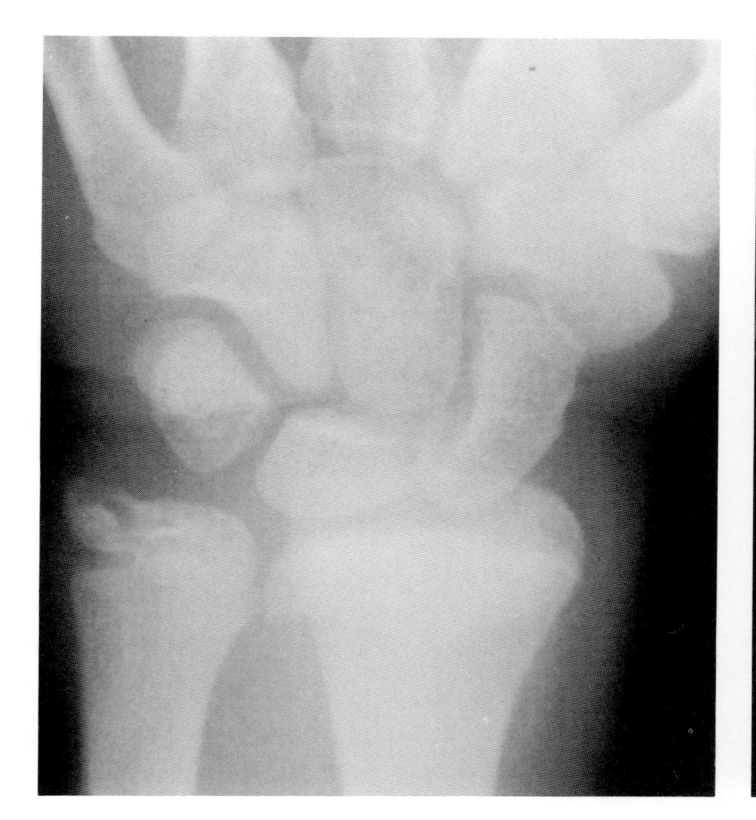

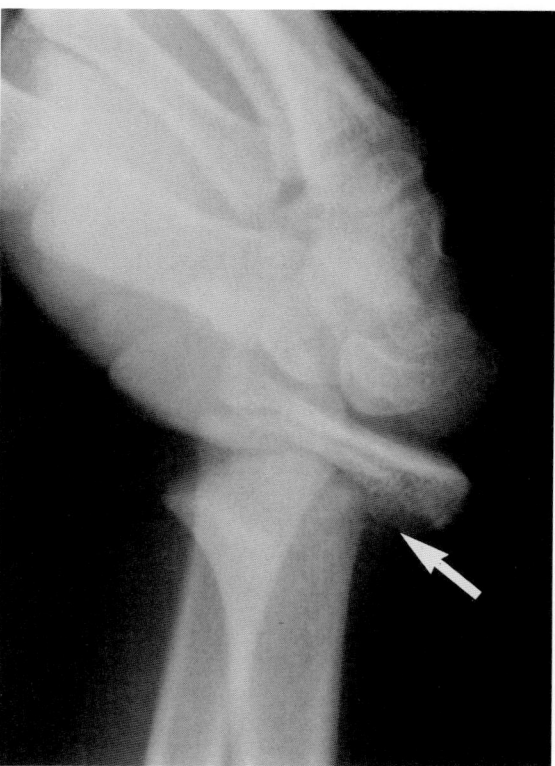

Fig. 2-5. Type II fracture-separation of the distal radial epiphysis. In the anteroposterior projection the epiphyseal plate of the radius is not apparent because the epiphysis is displaced and angulated. In the lateral projection the backward displacement and angulation of the epiphysis are apparent. The *arrow* identifies the small triangular metaphyseal fragment attached to the epiphysis and its epiphyseal plate.

CLASSIFICATION

The following classification, developed by Salter and Harris, is based on the mechanism of injury and the relationship of the fracture line to the growing cells of the epiphyseal plate and is also correlated with the prognosis for growth disturbance.[5-8]

Type I

In a type I epiphyseal plate injury (Figs. 2-2 and 2-3), there is a complete separation of the epiphysis from the metaphysis without any bony fracture. The growing cells of the epiphyseal plate remain with the epiphysis. This type of injury, which is caused by a shearing or avulsion force, is more common in birth injuries and during early childhood, when the epiphyseal plate is relatively thick. It is also seen in pathologic separations of the epiphysis associated with scurvy, rickets, osteomyelitis, and endocrine imbalance. Wide displacement is uncommon because the periosteal attachment is usually intact. Reduction is not difficult, and the prognosis for future growth is excellent unless the epiphysis involved is entirely covered by cartilage (e.g., upper end of the femur), in which case the blood supply is frequently damaged with resultant premature closure of the epiphyseal plate.

Type II

In a type II epiphyseal plate injury (Figs. 2-4 and 2-5), the most common type, the line of separation extends along the epiphyseal plate for a variable distance and then moves out through a portion of the metaphysis, providing the familiar triangular metaphyseal fragment

16 / Management of Pediatric Fractures

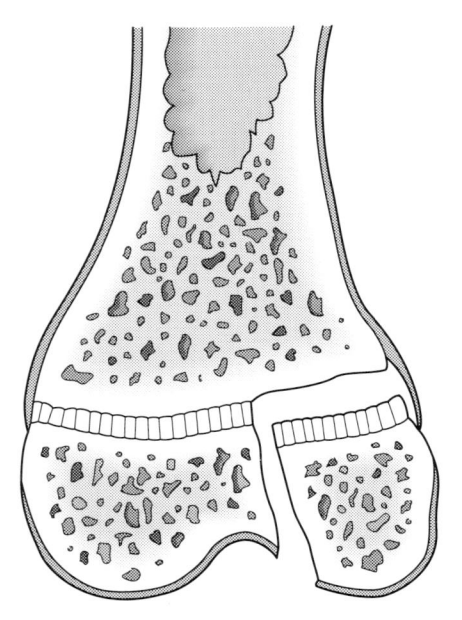

Fig. 2-6. Type III epiphyseal plate injury. Fracture of part of epiphysis. (Adapted from Salter and Harris,[5] with permission.)

sometimes referred to as Thurston Holland's sign. This type of injury usually occurs in children over the age of 10 years and is the result of shearing injury or an avulsion force. The periosteum is torn on the convex side of the angulation but is intact on the concave side, that is, the side on which the metaphyseal fragment is seen. Reduction is relatively easy to obtain and to maintain; because of the intact periosteal hinge and the metaphyseal fragment, overreduction cannot occur. The growing cartilage cells of the epiphyseal plate remain with the epiphysis, and thus the prognosis for growth is excellent, provided the circulation to the epiphysis is intact; it nearly always is.

Type III

In a type III epiphyseal injury (Figs. 2-6 and 2-7), the fracture, which is intra-articular, extends from the joint surface to the weak zone of the epiphyseal plate and then along the plate to its periphery. This type of injury is uncommon, but when it does occur it is usually in the upper or lower tibial epiphyses and is due to an intra-ar-

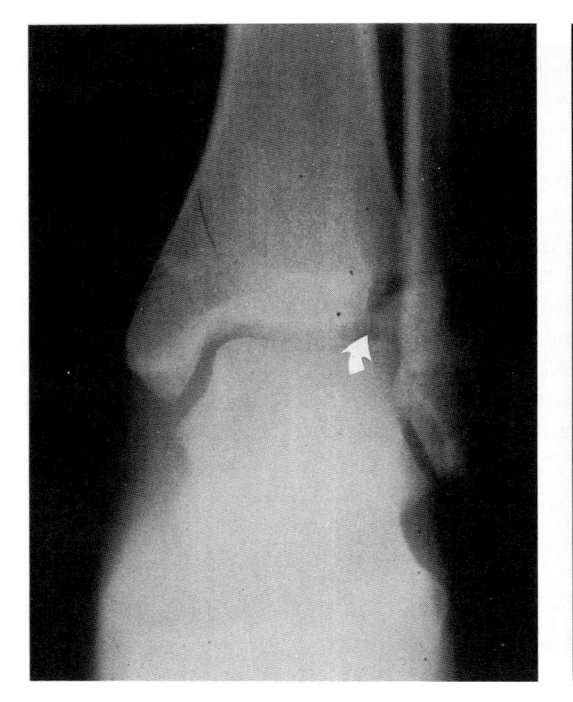

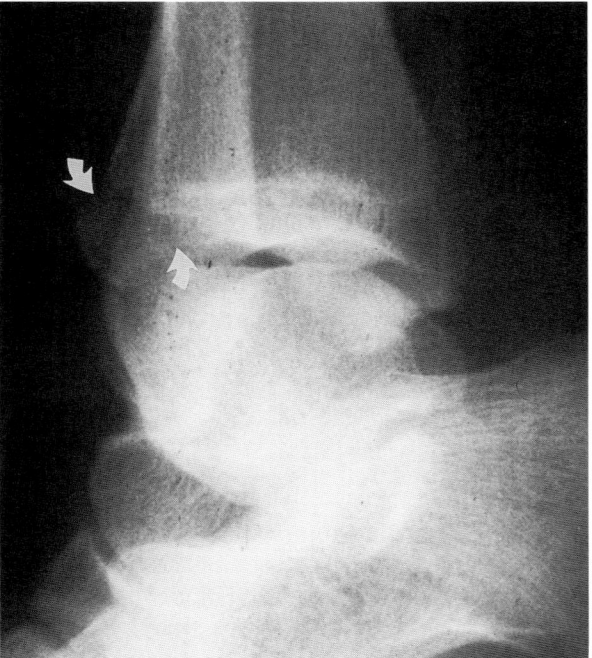

Fig. 2-7. Type III injury of the left distal tibial epiphysis in a 14-year-old boy. Note that the displacement of the anterolateral corner of the epiphysis is more obvious in the lateral projection than in the anteroposterior projection.

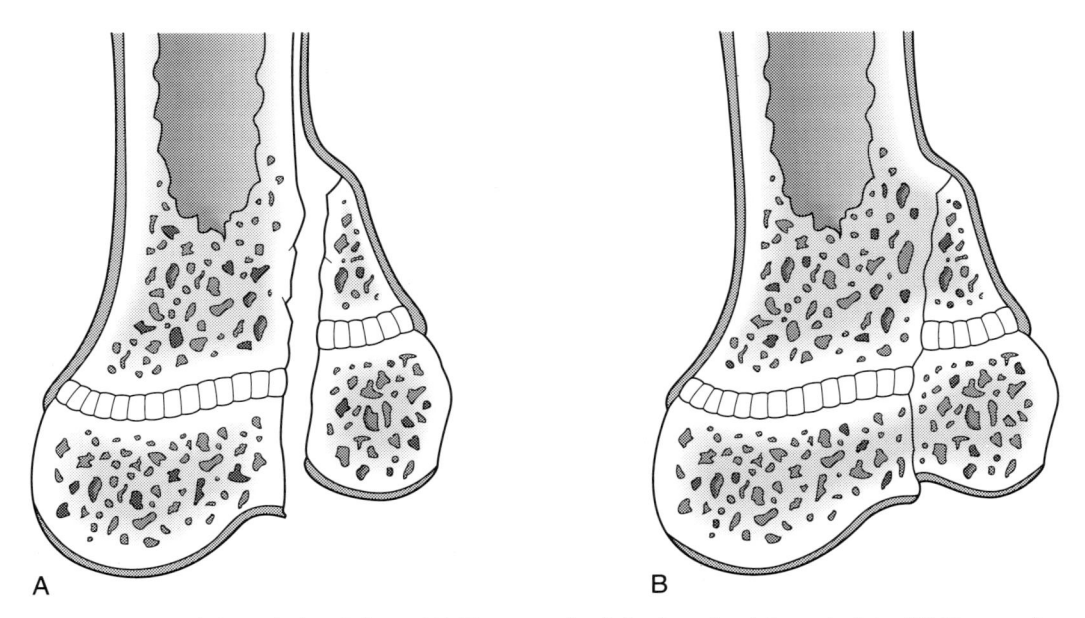

Fig. 2-8. Type IV epiphyseal plate injury. **(A)** Fracture of epiphysis and epiphyseal plate. **(B)** Bony union will cause premature closure of the plate. (Adapted from Salter and Harris,[5] with permission.)

ticular shearing force. Accurate reduction is essential, not so much for the sake of the epiphyseal plate as for the restoration of a smooth joint surface; open operation may be necessary to obtain such reduction. As in types I and II injuries, the prognosis is good, provided the blood supply to the separated portion of the epiphysis is intact.

Type IV

In a type IV epiphyseal injury (Figs. 2-8 to 2-10), the fracture, which is intra-articular, extends from the joint surface through the epiphysis, across the full thickness of the epiphyseal plate, and through a portion of the meta-

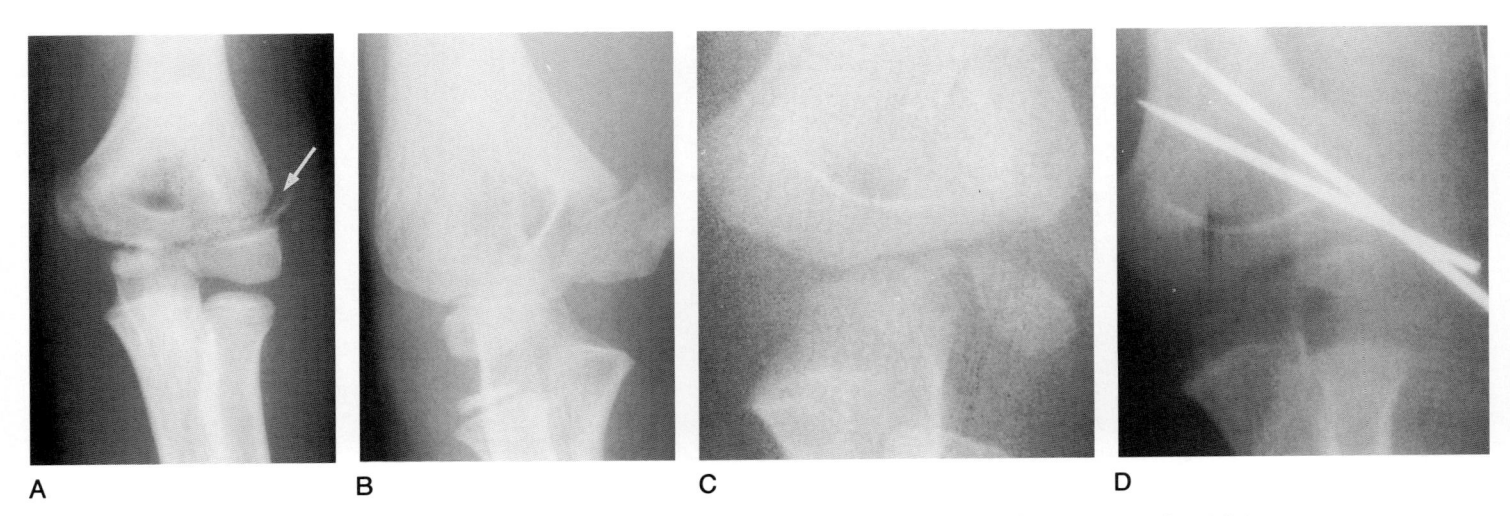

Fig. 2-9. Type IV epiphyseal plate injury. Fracture of the lateral condyle of the humerus in children. **(A)** Relatively undisplaced. **(B)** Moderately angulated. **(C)** Completely distracted and rotated. **(D)** After open reduction and internal fixation of the fracture with Kirschner wires.

Fig. 2-10. Type IV injury of the distal tibial epiphysis. **(A)** Note that the fracture line begins at the joint surface, crosses the epiphyseal plate, and extends into the metaphysis. The entire medial malleolus is shifted medially and proximally. This fracture should have been treated by open reduction and internal fixation. Notice also the type I injury of the distal fibular epiphysis. **(B)** One year after injury a growth disturbance is apparent; the medial part of the distal tibial epiphysis has ceased growing while the lateral part has continued to grow. The varus deformity of the ankle will be progressive. (From Salter and Harris,[5] with permission.)

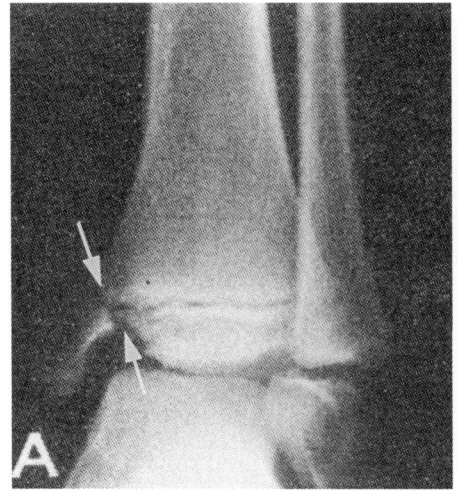

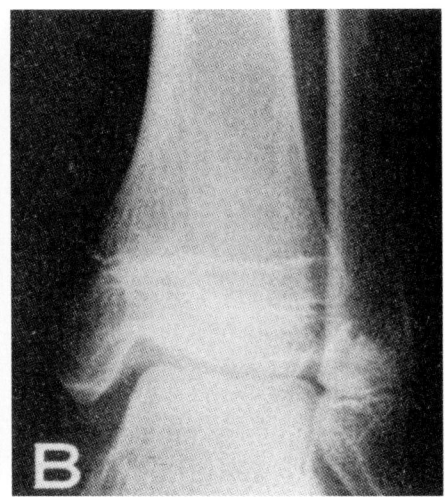

physis, thereby producing a complete split. Perfect reduction of a type IV epiphyseal plate injury is essential, not only for the sake of the epiphyseal plate but also for the restoration of a smooth joint surface. Unless the fracture is undisplaced, open reduction is always necessary. The epiphyseal plate must be accurately realigned in order to prevent bony union across the plate with resultant local premature cessation of growth. If metal fixation is required to obtain stability, preferably place it across the metaphysis, although fine, smooth Kirschner wires that traverse the plate for a few weeks do not interfere with subsequent growth.

Type V

The type V epiphyseal injury (Figs. 2-11 and 2-12), a relatively uncommon type of injury, results from a severe crushing force applied through the epiphysis to one area of the epiphyseal plate. It occurs in joints that move

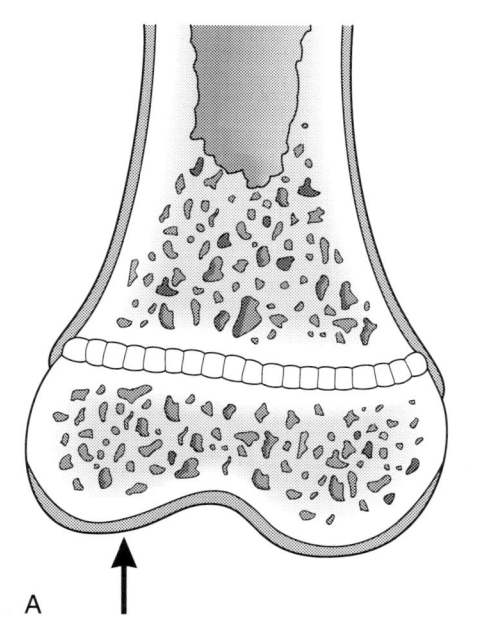

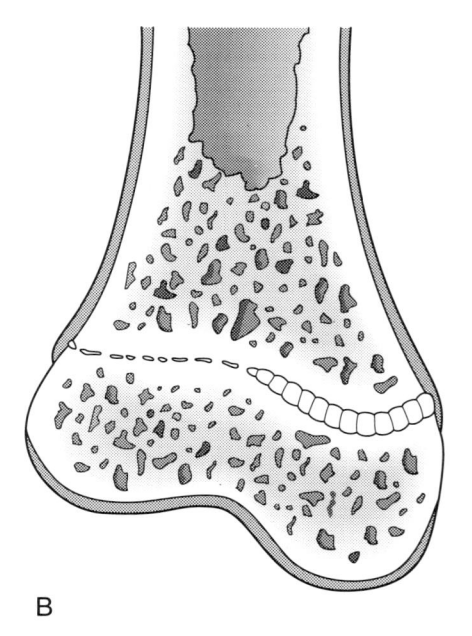

Fig. 2-11. Type V epiphyseal plate injury. **(A)** Crushing of epiphyseal plate. **(B)** Premature closure of the plate on one side with a resultant angulatory deformity. (Adapted from Salter and Harris,[5] with permission.)

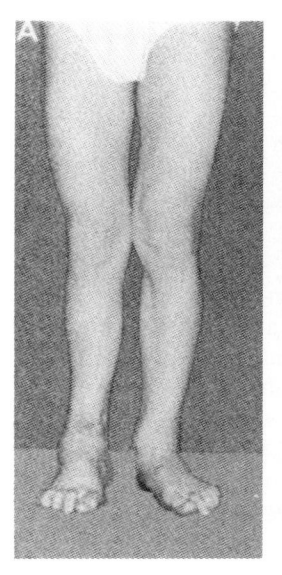

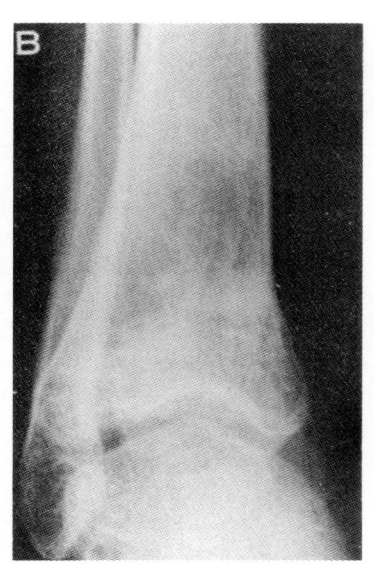

Fig. 2-12. Type V injury of the distal tibial epiphysis. **(A)** Clinical varus deformity of the ankle in a 9-year-old boy 5 years after a fall from a considerable height. He landed on his right foot and was thought to have sustained "only a sprained ankle." One year later he began to develop a progressive deformity of his ankle. Note also the shortening of the right leg. **(B)** A radiograph of the ankle reveals a growth disturbance of the distal tibial epiphysis. Growth had ceased in the medial part of the epiphyseal plate due to a type V crushing injury but had continued in the lateral part and also in the fibular epiphysis with a resultant varus deformity and shortening. (From Salter and Harris,[5] with permission.)

in one plane only, such as the ankle or the knee. A severe abduction or adduction injury to a joint that normally only flexes or extends is likely to produce crushing of the epiphyseal plate, which may then separate. Displacement of the epiphysis under these circumstances is unusual, and the initial radiograph gives little indication of the serious nature of the injury; indeed, the injury may be dismissed as a sprain. Suspect crushing of the epiphyseal plate under such circumstances and prevent weight bearing for 3 weeks in the hope of preventing the almost inevitable premature cessation of growth. The prognosis in type V epiphyseal plate injuries is decidedly poor.

Type VI

To this five-type classification, a sixth type has been added by the author's colleague, Mercer Rang.[9] This type consists of an injury to the perichondrial ring of the epiphyseal plate. If the perichondrial ring is either removed by a sharp object in an open injury or avulsed by an injury to a ligament attached to it, bone will grow across the epiphyseal plate from epiphysis to metaphysis, thereby producing a bony bridge and a resultant progressive angulatory deformity.

Other Classifications

Epiphysical injuries have also been classified by Poland,[10] Aitken and Magill,[11] and more recently by Ogden,[12] but the Salter-Harris classification would seem to be the one most widely used. At the distal end of the tibia near the end of skeletal growth, closure of the epiphyseal plate begins medially and proceeds laterally. While this closure is in progress an injury may produce a "triplane fracture," which combines either a type II and type III injury or even a type IV injury as described by Cooperman and colleagues.[13] The triplane fracture may include either two or three fragments. Radiographic examination may be difficult to interpret and a computed tomography (CT) scan is indicated to determine the nature of the fracture as well as the precise position of the fragments. The type III and type IV components of the triplane fracture require accurate reduction and maintenance of such reduction; this may necessitate open reduction and internal fixation.

FACTORS IN THE PROGNOSIS REGARDING GROWTH DISTURBANCE

Significant growth disturbance follows approximately 10 percent of epiphyseal plate injuries, although minor disturbances are seen in a higher percentage of patients. Although it is not possible in a given patient with a given epiphyseal plate injury to predict the prognosis with absolute accuracy, several factors help considerably in estimating prognosis.

Type of Injury

The anatomic type of injury, described above, is important from the prognostic point of view. In general, types I, II, and III injuries have a good prognosis for growth provided the blood supply of the epiphysis is intact and the injury has not been severe, such as an automobile accident or a fall from a great height. Type IV epiphyseal injuries carry a bad prognosis unless the fracture across the epiphyseal plate is completely reduced. Type V injuries associated with actual crushing of the cartilaginous plate have the worst prognosis.

Age at the Time of Injury

The age of the patient indicates the predicted amount of growth normally expected in the particular epiphyseal plate during the remaining years of growth. Obviously, the younger the patient at the time of injury, the more serious any growth disturbance will be. On the other hand, even a serious injury incurred during the last year of growth will not produce a significant deformity, since so little normal growth potential remains.

Blood Supply to the Epiphysis

The epiphyseal plate is nourished by blood vessels of the epiphysis, and if this blood supply is destroyed, the epiphyseal plate degenerates and growth ceases. Thus, interference with the blood supply to the epiphysis (a common complication of epiphyseal injuries of the femoral and radial heads) is associated with a poor prognosis.

Fortunately, in the region of the knee, the blood vessels enter the distal femoral and proximal tibial epiphyses directly; consequently, separation of these epiphyses does not usually disturb their blood supply.

Severity of the Injury (Velocity and Force)

When a given type of injury occurs in an epiphyseal plate as the result of a violent injury, such as an automobile accident or a fall from a great height, there may be some crushing of the plate even if the injury is a type I, II, or III. The prognosis for subsequent growth may thus be poor, even though with a less severe injury the prognosis might have been good.

Method of Reduction

Unduly forceful manipulation of an epiphysis may injure the epiphyseal plate; this is particularly true if the manipulation is carried out past the tenth day after injury. Likewise, the use of instruments to pry on an epiphyseal plate at the time of open operation crushes the plate; screw nails or threaded wires that traverse the epiphyseal plate also increase the chance of premature cessation of growth. Excessive soft-tissue stripping of an epiphysis at the time of open reduction can lead to avascular necrosis of that epiphysis and the underlying epiphyseal plate with resultant premature cessation of growth.

Closed or Open Injury

Open (formerly called compound) injuries of the epiphyseal plate are uncommon. However, they have a poorer prognosis than do closed injuries because of the added factor of contamination and possible infection. If infection develops at the site of an epiphyseal plate injury, the cartilaginous epiphyseal plate is usually destroyed by the process of chondrolysis, and the prognosis is therefore very poor indeed.

GENERAL PRINCIPLES OF TREATMENT

Gentleness in Reduction

In types I, II, and III epiphyseal plate injuries, in contrast to fractures through bone, one of the fracture surfaces is composed of delicate, vulnerable cartilage of the epiphyseal plate. Consequently, avoid unduly forceful manipulation of such an injury in order to prevent damage to the plate. This principle applies equally to surgical methods of reducing a displaced epiphysis at the time of open operation. No instrument should be used to pry a displaced epiphysis back into place.

Time of Reduction

The best time to reduce an epiphyseal plate injury is the day of the injury, since reduction becomes progressively more difficult with each passing day. Indeed, after about 10 days the fragments, particularly in types I and II injuries, are difficult to shift without using excessive force. Under these circumstances, forceful manipulation may further damage the cartilaginous plate and should be avoided; at this stage it is wiser to accept an imperfect reduction than to risk either forceful manipulation or open operation. Perform a corrective osteotomy later if necessary. In types III and IV injuries, however, delayed reduction, although not desirable, is preferable to leaving the intra-articular fragment displaced.

Method of Reduction

The vast majority of types I and II epiphyseal plate injuries are readily reduced by closed means, and furthermore the reduction is easily maintained. Type III injuries may require open reduction to obtain a smooth joint surface, but displaced type IV injuries nearly always require open reduction. When internal fixation is deemed necessary, it is preferable to place such fixation through the metaphysis rather than through the epiphysis. Never insert screw nails or threaded wires across the epiphyseal plate; fine smooth Kirschner wires that cross the plate at right angles may be used with impunity but should be removed when the injury is healed. Take great care to avoid damage to the blood supply of the epiphysis.

The contour of the epiphyseal plate is such that perfect reduction of type I and II injuries is usually possible. If however, there is residual moderate displacement (anterior, posterior, medial, or lateral) or slight angulation, repeat manipulation is not necessary, since remodeling of the bone from the periosteum is adequate. The criteria for acceptable position are less rigid in the region of a multiplane joint, such as the shoulder, than in the region of a single-plane joint, such as the knee. Types III and IV injuries must be perfectly reduced (see above).

Period of Immobilization

Experience has shown that types I, II, and III injuries unite in approximately half the time required for union of a fracture through the metaphysis of the same bone in the same age group; therefore, the period of immobilization may be correspondingly reduced. Type IV injuries, because of their location, require the same period for union as metaphyseal fractures.

Estimation and Discussion of Prognosis

In a given epiphyseal plate injury, consider the prognosis for growth disturbance at least in the general terms described above. Part of the surgeon's responsibility in the treatment of these injuries is to provide the parents with some indication of the prognosis without causing them undue anxiety. Stress the importance of follow-up examination.

Period of Follow-up Observation

The need for regular follow-up observation of epiphyseal plate injuries is obvious; it is not always obvious just how long a period of observation is required. Since growth disturbance may be delayed, at least in its manifestations, for up to 1 year, this period of observation is the minimum. Six months after injury examine the injured bone and its opposite number in the healthy extremity with radiographs. If little growth has occurred in the uninjured bone during this 6-month period, 6 more months are needed before a definitive prognosis can be made.

COMPLICATIONS OF EPIPHYSEAL INJURIES

Failure of Early Diagnosis

The clinical and radiographic diagnosis of epiphyseal plate injuries has been discussed above and merits emphasis in order to prevent or avoid failure of early diagnosis.

Failure to diagnose a type I injury is difficult to avoid in infants when the involved epiphysis is not yet ossified, for example, in a birth injury that produces a fracture-separation of the unossified proximal femoral epiphysis. Initially, this injury is difficult to differentiate by radiograph from congenital or traumatic dislocation of the hip in the newborn, unless an arthrogram is performed. Within 1 week, however, periosteal new bone formation along the neck of the femur provides a clue. Another example is fracture-separation of the entire unossified distal humeral epiphysis in an infant.

Failure to diagnose an epiphyseal plate injury early means that appropriate treatment is delayed. This can be particularly serious with an unstable type IV injury of the lateral condyle of the humerus, which, if untreated, can go on to a nonunion. Failure to recognize a type IV injury in the knee or ankle can result in a malunion that in turn leads to premature cessation of growth in the involved epiphyseal plate.

Malunion

When a type I or II epiphyseal plate injury has healed in an unsatisfactory position, there may be some spontaneous correction of the deformity, provided the epiphyseal plate continues to grow, the child is young, and the deformity is in the plane of motion of the nearest joint, for example, posterior or anterior angulation in the femur at the site of a distal femoral epiphyseal separation. If the deformity does not, or is unlikely to, correct spontaneously, a corrective osteotomy is required.

Malunion of a type III injury of the distal tibial epiphyseal plate may lead to posttraumatic degenerative

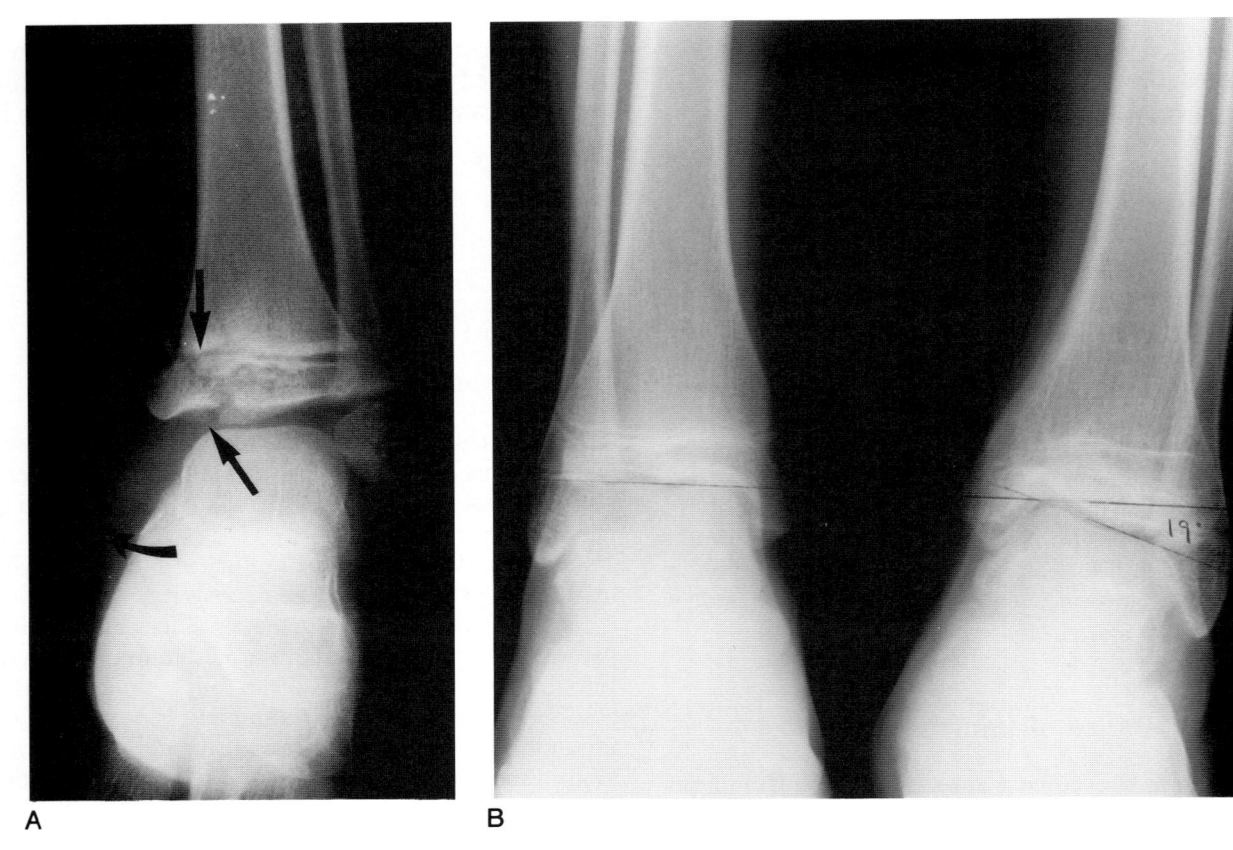

Fig. 2-13. (A) Type IV injury of the medial tibial physis in a 6-year-old child sustained in a fall out of a tree. (B) Malunion of the distal tibia associated with a growth plate arrest possibly augmented by a type V compression injury and varus deformity of ankle 6 years later.

arthritis unless the incongruity of the joint surface is corrected surgically.

Malunion of a type IV injury of, for example, the distal tibial epiphyseal plate, inevitably leads to a premature cessation of growth (Fig. 2-13).

Nonunion

The most common site of nonunion after an epiphyseal plate injury is the type IV fracture-separation of the lateral condyle of the humerus, a complication that in turn leads to additional complications of lateral instability of the elbow joint and, eventually, a tardy ulnar nerve palsy (Fig. 2-14). Displaced type IV injuries of the lateral condyle of the humerus represent an absolute indication for accurate open reduction and internal fixation in order to prevent malunion or nonunion.

Osteomyelitis

An open injury of an epiphyseal plate carries the same risk of osteomyelitis as any open fracture. Osteomyelitis in the region of the epiphyseal plate, however, especially if due to Staphylococcus aureus, may result in chondrolysis of the cartilaginous plate and lead to premature cessation of growth (Fig. 2-15). Therefore, treat such injuries with meticulous debridement and prophylactic antibiotics; leave them open initially with a delayed skin closure.

Neurologic Complications

An unreduced type II injury of the distal radial epiphysis with residual anterior angulation (dorsal tilt of the epiphysis) may cause compression of the median

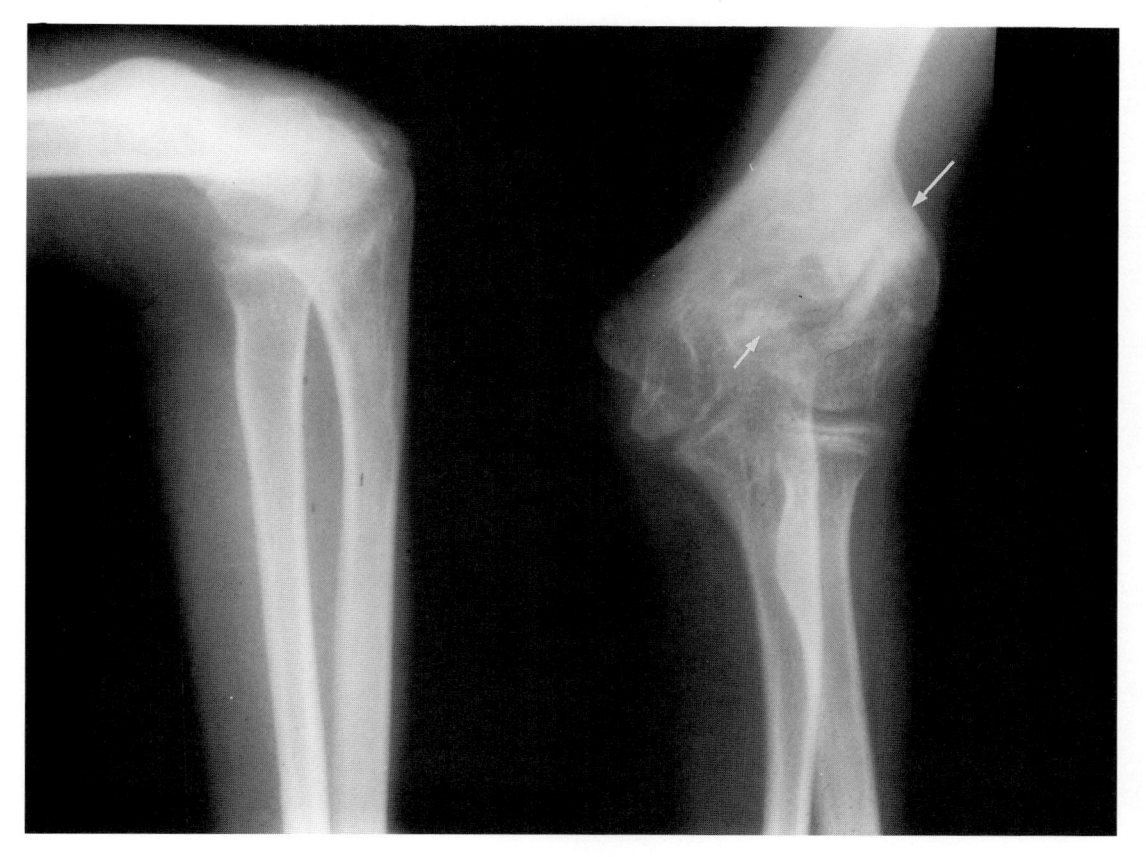

Fig. 2-14. Nonunion of the lateral condyle secondary to an unrecognized fracture of the type IV lateral condyle. Growth plate arrest with subsequent development of a valgus deformity of the elbow and tardy ulnar nerve palsy is a future possibility.

nerve, which is a form of carpal tunnel compression syndrome.

Hyperextension injuries in the region of the knee (type I or II injuries of either the distal femoral or proximal tibial epiphyseal plates) are associated with a risk of serious injury to the medial popliteal nerve, usually of the traction type. Careful neurologic examination and documentation are essential before treatment in order to differentiate between neurologic damage caused by the injury and that caused by the treatment.

Vascular Complications

Vascular injuries are seldom associated with epiphyseal plate injuries except in the region of the knee, where the popliteal artery is at risk along with the medial popliteal nerve for the same types of injuries mentioned above. Indeed, unrecognized intimal tears or disruptions of the popliteal artery secondary to hypertension may even lead to gangrene necessitating amputation.

Avascular Necrosis of Epiphyses

The blood supply to the epiphysis has been discussed above. It is apparent that completely displaced type I injuries of the proximal femoral and proximal radial epiphyses carry a high risk of avascular necrosis of the epiphysis and, even more important, of the related epiphyseal plates. When an epiphyseal plate loses its blood supply, the chondrocytes of the plate die and are replaced by fibrocytes, with resultant cessation of epiphyseal plate growth.

Avascular necrosis of the proximal femoral epiphysis at an early age is therefore associated with failure of the femoral neck to grow in length, continued growth of the greater trochanter, and a functional coxa vara, which

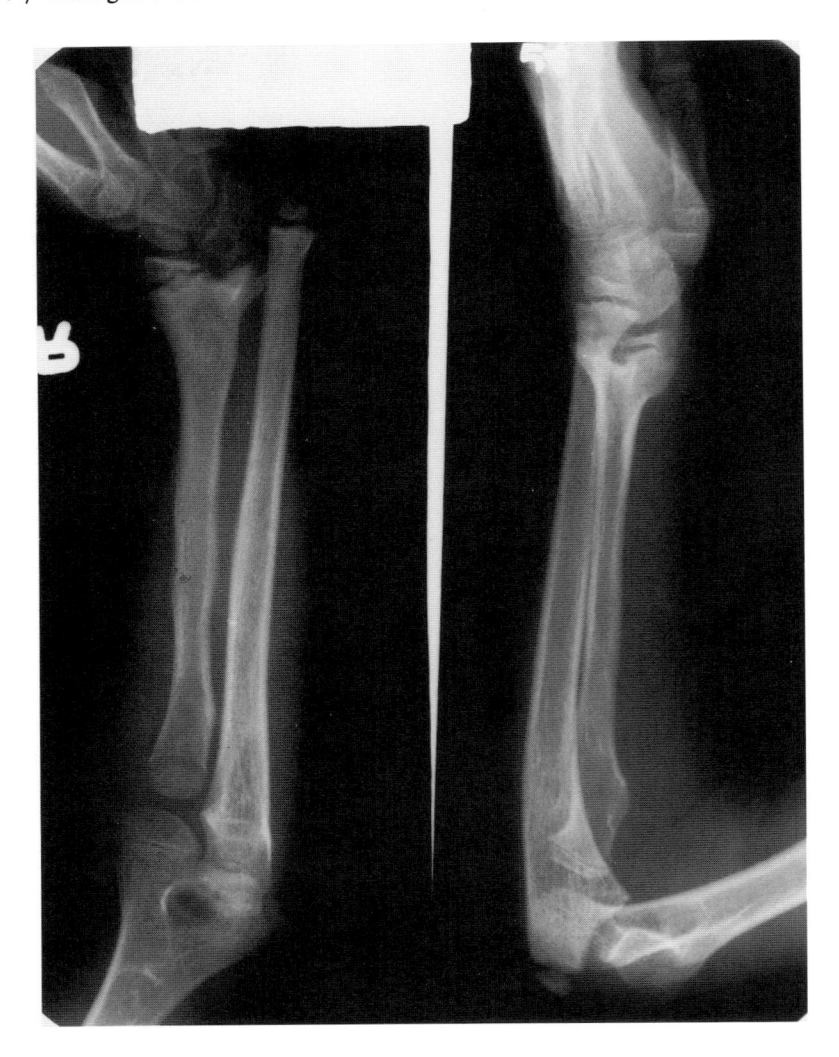

Fig. 2-15. Growth plate arrest of the distal radius in an 8-year-old girl who sustained a septic arthritis of the wrist with osteomyelitis of the distal radius at the age of 3 years secondary to an open fracture of the distal radius.

may necessitate a distal and lateral transfer of the greater trochanter to overcome the associated Trendelenburg limp.

Premature Cessation of Growth and Its Management

The possible effects of epiphyseal injuries on subsequent growth in the injured epiphyseal plate have been described in an earlier section of this chapter.

After an epiphyseal plate injury, local growth may either cease immediately or it may continue at a retarded rate for a variable period before complete cessation; furthermore, the growth disturbance may involve the entire epiphyseal plate or only one part of it (Fig. 2-16). The resultant deformity is progressive until the end of the growing period. Thus, the gravity of the clinical problem depends on several factors; the site of the growth disturbance, the extent of involvement of the epiphyseal plate, and the expected amount of growth remaining in the involved plate. The main types of deformity that may develop are progressive angulation, progressive shortening, or a combination. Considerable judgment is required in planning the most effective management of these progressive deformities.

Retardation or cessation of growth in one area of the epiphyseal plate with continuation of growth in the remainder produces a gradually progressive angulation. Under these circumstances, growth in the remainder of the plate eventually ceases prematurely, and shortening becomes superimposed upon angulation. It is usually preferable to deal with progressive angulation by an open

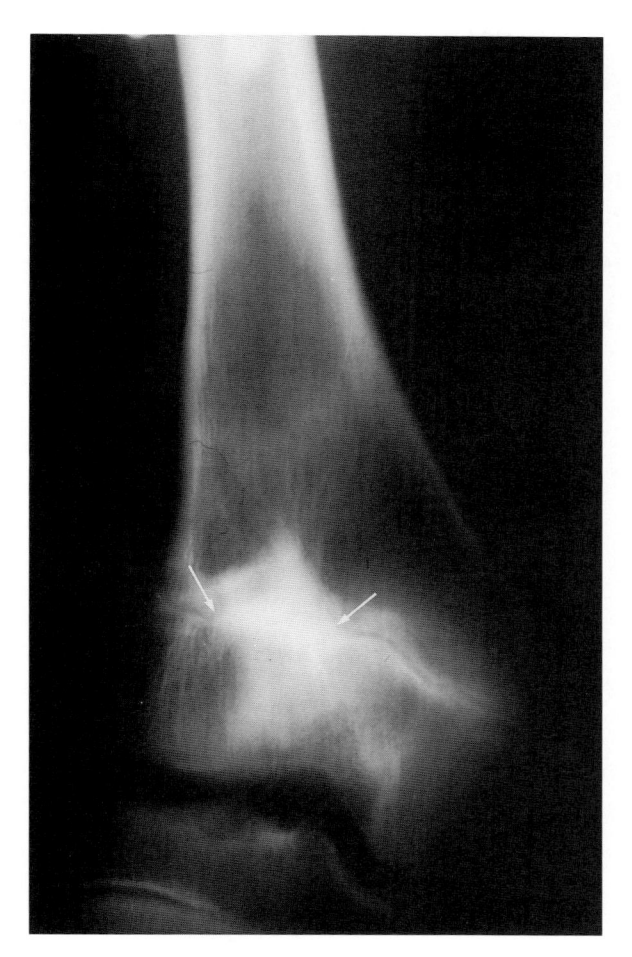

Fig. 2-16. Growth arrest of the distal femur subsequent to a type II fracture of the epiphyseal plate sustained 2 years earlier. This tomogram illustrates a well-developed physeal bar producing a tethering and valgus deformity of the knee.

wedge type of osteotomy in order to preserve the growing potential of the undamaged portion of the epiphyseal plate and to gain some length in the extremity. Unless the entire epiphyseal plate has ceased growing, the osteotomy should overcorrect the deformity to delay its inevitable recurrence. When progressive angulation exists in a child, it may become necessary to repeat the osteotomy more than once. Epiphyseal arrest by stapling may help to correct a progressive angulation, but only if the damaged area of the epiphyseal plate is still growing. This method has the disadvantage, however, of producing further shortening of the involved extremity.

Excision of a posttraumatic bony bridge that crosses the epiphyseal plate and insertion of a free fat graft, as developed by Langenskiold,[14,15] offers hope of preventing a progressive angulatory deformity and even of restoring symmetric longitudinal growth, provided that the bony bridge does not exceed one third of the epiphyseal plate. Using Silastic inserts rather than free-fat grafts, Bright[16] has also had encouraging results (see Ch. 62).

If one of two paired bones (e.g., radius or ulna, tibia or fibula) is the site of premature cessation of growth, the resultant discrepancy in length between the two bones will produce a progressive deformity (varus or valgus) of the nearest joint. For example, premature cessation of growth at the lower radial epiphyseal plate in the presence of continued growth at the lower ulnar epiphysis will produce a progressive valgus or radial deviation of the hand. To overcome this problem it may be necessary to lengthen the shorter bone or shorten the longer bone and at the same time perform an epiphyseal arrest of the growing epiphysis to prevent a recurrence of deformity.

When a single bone (femur or humerus) develops progressive shortening, the resultant problem is one of limb-length discrepancy, which is only significant in the lower extremity. An actual or predicted lower-limb discrepancy of more than 3 cm usually merits surgical lengthening of the involved bone or, alternatively, epiphyseal arrest or surgical shortening of the opposite limb in accordance with the principles of leg-length equalization.

SUMMARY

Epiphyseal injuries add another unique and important dimension to the care of fractures in children. A thorough understanding of the anatomy, histology, and physiology of the growth plate is essential to the provision of optimum treatment for children with fractures.

REFERENCES

1. Dale GG, Harris WR: Prognosis of epiphyseal separation: an experimental study. J Bone Joint Surg [Br] 40:116, 1958
2. Bisgard JD, Martenson Lee: Fractures in children. Surg Gynecol Obstet 65:464, 1937
3. Compere EL: Growth arrest in long bones as a result of fractures that include the epiphysis. JAMA 105:2140, 1935
4. Eliason EL, Ferguson LK: Epiphyseal separation of the long bones. Surg Gynecol Obstet 58:85, 1934
5. Salter RB, Harris WR: Injuries involving the epiphyseal plate. J Bone Joint Surg [Am] 45:587, 1963

6. Salter RB: Injuries of the ankle in children. Orthop Clin North Am 5:147, 1974
7. Salter RB: Epiphyseal injuries in the adolescent knee. p. 77. In Kennedy JC, ed: The Injured Adolescent Knee. Williams & Wilkins, Baltimore, 1979
8. Czitrom A, Salter RB, Willis RB: Fractures involving the distal femoral epiphyseal plate, Int Orthop 4:269, 1981
9. Rang M: Children's Fractures. 2nd Ed. pp. 23 and 315. Williams & Wilkins, Baltimore, 1983
10. Poland J: Traumatic separation of the epiphyses. Smith, Elder, London, 1898
11. Aitken AP, Magill HK: Fractures involving the distal epiphyseal cartilage. J Bone Joint Surg [Am] 34:96, 1952
12. Ogden JA: Skeletal Injury in the Child. Lea & Febiger, Philadelphia, 1982
13. Cooperman DR, Spiegel PG, Taros GS: Tibial fractures involving the ankle joint in children: the so-called triplane spiphyseal fracture. J Bone Joint Surg [Am] 60:1040, 1978
14. Langenskiold A: An operation for partial closure of an epiphyseal plate in children, and its experimental basis. J Bone Joint Surg [Br] 57:325, 1975
15. Langenskiold A: Surgical treatment of partial closure of the growth plate. J Paediatr Orthop 1:3, 1981
16. Bright RW: Operative correction of partial epiphyseal plate closure by osseous bridge resection and silicone rubber implant. J Bone Joint Surg [Am] 56:655, 1974

3

Initial Management of the Multiply Injured Child

Peter F. Armstrong
John T. Smith

> The critical response time for an adult is called the "golden hour," for a child it is the "platinum half hour."

The leading cause of injury and death in children over the age of 1 year is blunt trauma.[1] This is despite significant recent advances in prevention and treatment.[2] Motor vehicle accidents (including pedestrian, passenger, bicycle, etc.) and falls account for most of these deaths.[1,3,4] Many occur because the injuries are so serious that even prompt, thorough resuscitation and treatment are inadequate to sustain life. This is particularly so for serious head injuries. Unfortunately, there are those deaths that could have been prevented with proper medical attention. The real tragedy is when the patient makes it to the hospital with treatable injuries but dies there due to errors in management. Most of these preventable deaths are caused by acute respiratory failure due to airway obstruction or pneumothorax, inadequately treated intra-abdominal bleeding, or secondary brain injury caused by an expanding intracranial hematoma, hypoxia, or shock.[5]

GENERAL CONSIDERATIONS

Care of the injured child requires a systematic, multidisciplinary, *predetermined* approach that will ensure the thorough evaluation of *all* organ systems and the implementation of prompt, appropriate therapy. The processes of evaluation and treatment are carried out *simultaneously*. It also requires a high index of suspicion and frequent repeated examinations to ensure that injuries are not missed. Ignorance of these principles is no excuse. It is our opinion that *any* surgeon involved in the management of acute trauma should be well trained in the principles of initial resuscitation and stabilization. Excellent courses, such as the Advanced Trauma Life Support course provided by the American College of Surgeons, are available to provide this training. Part of this course deals specifically with the pediatric trauma patient.[6]

Patterns of Injury

The patterns of injury in the child differ from those in the adult. Since the child is smaller, the force per unit area may be significantly higher than for the adult. Due to the force being applied to someone with less subcutaneous fat, less elastic connective tissue, and closer proximity of multiple organs, there is a high incidence of multisystem injury.[7]

Head injuries occur in over 80 percent of severely injured children. This is due to the fact that a child's head is large relative to the trunk and, therefore, is often the leading contact point on high-speed impact.

Abdominal injuries are also more frequent because the abdominal viscera are not well protected by the less-developed abdominal muscles. Because of the elasticity of the thoracic cage, fractures of the ribs and sternum are unusual. Nevertheless, severe parenchymal damage to the lungs and heart may occur with little external evidence of injury. Greater mediastinal flexibility allows a more significant lateral shift in instances of tension pneumothorax. This leads to compromised cardiac filling and ventilation of the opposite lung.[8]

Anatomic Considerations

The child's head is large relative to the trunk and, in addition, the cranium is thinner and the brain less myelinated than in adults. As a result, even mild forces may produce severe injuries in the child.[9,10] However, the fact that a younger child has open sutures, a larger subarachnoid space and cisterns, and greater extracellular space in the brain allows children to better tolerate an expanding intracranial mass such as a hematoma or brain swelling.

The glottis in the infant tends to be somewhat more anterior and superior in the pharynx. This, in addition to the fact that children are obligate nose breathers who do not tolerate nasal obstruction well, makes orotracheal intubation better than nasotracheal intubation. The trachea is relatively short, which increases the risk of endobronchial intubation or even inadvertant extubation.

Physiologic Response to Injury

The physiologic response of a child to trauma also differs in some respects from that of an adult. Some of these differences are beneficial to the patient. Usually the child does not have any preexisting disease affecting the major organs. There are usually larger cardiac and pulmonary reserves. The child can withstand longer periods of hypoxia than the adult. The neurologic system shows a phenomenal capacity for recovery following severe injury.

The vascular system is able to maintain the systolic pressure in the normal range despite the existence of significant hypovolemia. This can give a false sense of security, leading to a delay in proper volume replacement. If hypovolemia continues, eventually the pressure can no longer be maintained and it starts to drop, often quite rapidly. Tachycardia does occur early in hypovolemia and should be looked for carefully.

Because of the high ratio of surface area to weight, the child is very prone to develop hypothermia. This causes muscle shivering and peripheral vasoconstriction, leading to lactic acidemia. This can adversely affect the response to the treatment of shock.

MANAGEMENT

The Committee on Trauma of the American College of Surgeons has recommended four distinct phases in the management of the multiply injured patient: primary survey, resuscitation, secondary survey, and definitive care.[6]

Primary Survey and Resuscitation

Attention must obviously be directed first to the immediate threats to the life of the patient—inadequate gas exchange (airway and breathing), and inadequate perfusion of vital organs (circulation). These are well known as the ABCs of trauma management.[6]

History

Obviously, a brief history is necessary. It should include the following:

   Allergies
   Medications
   Past medical history
   Last meal
   Events: details of accident and management received (It is very important to know the neurologic status of the patient at the scene and any changes since then.)

This information can be gathered as the primary survey and resuscitation proceeds.[6]

Every effort should be made to ensure adherence to the principles of universal precautions in the trauma room to minimize the contact with blood or other body fluids.

Airway Management

The incidence of cervical spine injury in children is quite low.[11,12] Nevertheless, it is recommended that all multiply injured children be treated as though they have a cervical spine injury until it is ruled out clinically and radiographically.[6] This is most frequently done using sandbags and taping. Often a rigid collar has already been applied by the ambulance personnel. Since the child has a relatively large occiput, a regular spine board will actually flex the cervical spine. Special pediatric spine boards have been designed with a depression in which the head rests.

CLEARING AND MAINTAINING THE AIRWAY

Airway obstruction is the most frequent source of ventilatory failure. Therefore the establishment and maintenance of a patent airway should receive the highest priority. Obvious foreign material as well as blood, mucus and vomit must be removed from the mouth and oropharynx. Remember that, in infants, it is important to ensure that the nostrils are clear as well. The jaw thrust or lift is helpful in maintaining a clear airway. Insertion of an oral airway in a patient with an intact gag reflex is not recommended, as it may precipitate choking, laryngospasm, or vomiting.

In the unconscious child, the airway is best controlled by the insertion of an uncuffed orotracheal tube.[13] Prior to attempting intubation it is recommended that 100 percent oxygen be administered with a bag-valve mask apparatus. Following intubation there should be a small leak of air around the tube with inflation of the lungs. The diameter of the external nares or the diameter of the little finger are guides to the choice of tube size.

If these methods fail, direct access to the trachea is best achieved by needle cricothyroidectomy. Needle jet insufflation can then be used. This is a temporary, emergency measure only, and a more definitive method to secure an airway should be carried out. This may mean intubation or, in rare circumstances, a tracheostomy. If a tracheostomy is required, it should be performed by someone experienced with the technique and in a controlled environment, such as an operating room.

TRACHEAL INTUBATION

Obviously, tracheal intubation is the most reliable way to gain control of an airway in a child with ventilatory compromise. In those patients that require intubation, the orotracheal route is recommended.[13] As a rough guide, use a tube of similar external diameter to the child's external nares or baby finger. Uncuffed tubes are generally used for all children up to age 8. There should always be a small leak of gas around the tube during inflation. Always check carefully for endobronchial intubation by listening in the axillae for air entry into each lung. The air entry must be reassessed frequently to detect an evolving ventilatory dysfunction. The adequacy of ventilation and oxygenation can be monitored by frequent blood gas determinations, pulse oximetry and/or end-tidal carbon dioxide measurements.

GASTRIC DECOMPRESSION

When stressed, almost all infants and children swallow air, often in large quantities. This gastric dilatation may produce vomiting with the risk of aspiration. It can also cause splinting of the diaphragm and interfere with ventilation. The vena cava may be compressed, resulting in decreased venous return, causing or aggravating hypotension. A nasogastric tube should be used for decompression if there are no contraindications such as facial fractures with damage to the cribriform plate.

Breathing Management

Next to airway obstruction the most common causes of ventilatory failure are pneumothorax and hemothorax.[14] The most immediate life-threatening condition is a tension pneumothorax. This usually produces cyanosis, distended neck veins, mediastinal shift, ipsilateral decreased breath sounds, and hyperresonance. The diagnosis should be made clinically and treated immediately. The patient *should not be sent to x-ray* to confirm the diagnosis prior to treatment!

The tension pneumothorax can be treated quickly by inserting a large-bore intravenous cannula through the second intercostal space in the midclavicular line. This is a temporizing procedure only. Definitive management of the pneumothorax is the insertion of a chest tube through the fifth intercostal space in the anterior to midaxillary line.

Circulation Management

DIAGNOSIS

Significant blood loss in an injured child is a common occurrence. The child, as mentioned previously, has a tremendous physiologic reserve. This is relevant to management because, despite significant hypovolemia, the child is able to maintain reasonably normal vital signs by reflex tachycardia and vasoconstriction. There is a limit to this reserve, and when it is exceeded the vital signs can rapidly deteriorate.[10] By closely monitoring the functions of the heart, kidneys, central nervous system, and skin, the diagnosis is usually not difficult to make. Mon-

30 / Management of Pediatric Fractures

TABLE 3-1. Normal Values for Pediatric Vital Signs in Noncrying Patients

Age (years)	Pulse (rate/min)	Blood Pressure (mmHg)	Respiratory Rate (rate/min)
<1	120–140	70–90	30–40
2–5	100–120	80–90	20–30
6–12	80–100	90–110	15–20

The following formula provides an easy way to estimate a child's systolic blood pressure: (Age in years × 2) + 80.

itoring these functions also allows us to assess the severity of the hypovolemia and follow the response to treatment.

The first sign of hypovolemia is tachycardia. Obviously, it is not the only cause of tachycardia, thus the need to monitor the other systems.

The normal circulating blood volume in a child is 80 ml/kg. The child's weight in kilograms can be roughly estimated by the formula: (Age in years × 2) + 8. A child's vital signs are age-dependent. It is, therefore, very important to know the normal values for the various age groups in order to be able to detect when they are abnormal (Table 3-1). Table 3-2 shows the changes that one sees in the functions of these four organ systems with increasing degrees of blood loss.

Venous Access

Early access to the cardiovascular system should be established. Generally, this is best accomplished by a percutaneous route. Usually, two large-bore intravenous cannulas are inserted in peripheral veins. Central venous lines are good for monitoring response to fluid resuscitation but are not to be the principal route for fluid administration. If attempts to obtain percutaneous venous access fail, a cutdown should be performed. The common sites for a cutdown are:

1. Greater saphenous at the ankle
2. Median cephalic at the elbow
3. Main cephalic higher in the arm
4. External jugular
5. Long bone marrow (intraosseus infusion)

Since the percutaneous route may be difficult to achieve in hypovolemic younger children, intraosseous infusion provides a quick, convenient access to the venous circulation. The technique is effective, easy to learn, can be used in the field, and is most applicable in children up to the age of 6 years.[15] The recommended site is the anterior tibial metaphysis, 2 to 3 cm below the tibial tuberosity. An alternate location is the distal, anterolateral femoral metaphysis, approximately 3 cm above the lateral femoral condyle. The cannula should not be introduced below the site of a fracture as the venous drainage has been partially disrupted by the fracture. A 16- to 18-gauge needle with trochar is introduced at right angles or up to 60 degrees caudad with the bevel up. If marrow is aspirated, the needle is in the correct place. Infusion is at the same rate as the intravenous route.

Fluid Resuscitation

The principles governing fluid resuscitation in the child are virtually the same as those that are applied to the adult. Since the manifestations of clinical shock re-

TABLE 3-2. Systemic Responses to Blood Loss in the Pediatric Patient

Organ System	Early <25% Blood Volume Loss	Prehypotensive 25% Blood Volume Loss	Hypotensive 40% Blood Volume Loss
Cardiac	Weak, thready pulse, increased heart rate	+Tilt test, increased heart rate	Frank hypotension, tachycardia to bradycardia
Central nervous system	Lethargic, irritable, confused, combative	Changes in level of consciousness, dulled response to pain	Comatose
Skin	Cool, clammy	Cyanotic, decreased capillary refill, cold extremities	Pale, cold
Kidneys	Decreased urinary output; increased specific gravity	Increased BUN	No urinary output

quire a blood loss of 25 percent or greater, the initial fluid management is to give a bolus of crystalloid that is approximately one-fourth of the circulating blood volume (20 ml/kg over 10 minutes). The "3-for-1" applies in children as well. Therefore it would take three such boluses to replace a 25 percent loss in circulating blood volume. If there is no response to the first bolus, a second is started, and preparations are made to start administering blood. A surgical opinion is very important at this stage.

Urine output is a valuable way of monitoring response to fluid resuscitation. An infant would be expected to produce 1 to 2 ml/kg/h, a child should produce at least 0.5 to 1 ml/kg/h and an adolescent at least 0.5 ml/kg/h.

BLOOD REPLACEMENT

In the event that the child has not responded to the second crystalloid bolus, blood should be started. If fully crossmatched or type-specific blood is not yet available, O Rh− blood may be given. Packed cells are usually reconstituted with plasma and given as a bolus of 10 mg/kg. If the child does not respond to this bolus, then surgery is very likely indicated, depending on where the site of the ongoing blood loss is felt to be.

Additional Evaluation

The primary survey is completed by performing a brief neurologic evaluation. This is where the Glasgow coma scale is particularly useful. A quick look at pupil size and reaction to light often will identify signs of serious intracranial problems.

It was mentioned earlier that children are prone to develop hypothermia. In addition to warm coverings and heating blankets, warm intravenous fluids and blood warmers are often necessary to prevent hypothermia from developing.

Electrocardiogram (ECG) leads should be applied and oxygen administered. A Foley catheter should be inserted if there are no contraindications. Contraindications include blood at the urethral meatus, high-riding or boggy prostate on rectal examination, or significant perineal or scrotal bruising.

BLOODWORK

Each patient should have blood drawn for a complete blood count (CBC), type and crossmatch, amylase, electrolytes, glucose, blood urea nitrogen (BUN), and creatinine. Arterial blood gases, coagulation screens, and liver enzymes may be ordered if clinically indicated.

DIAGNOSTIC IMAGING

Routine radiographs on all multiple trauma patients should include anteroposterior (AP) and lateral cervical spine films, an AP view of the chest, and an AP view of the pelvis. The computed tomography (CT) scan is often needed to evaluate significant head injury. It is also useful in the investigation of intra-abdominal and pelvic injuries. When used for evaluation of the abdomen, the studies are often done with gastrointestinal and intravenous contrast. Radiographs of the thoracolumbar spine and the limbs are done when indicated.

Secondary Survey and Definitive Management

The secondary survey includes a thorough, systematic physical examination of all the organ systems in addition to appropriate diagnostic imaging. This does not mean that all the life-threatening conditions have been dealt with and can be ignored! The "ABCs" must be regularly monitored and reassessed. The secondary survey usually starts with the head and moves distally. There are special considerations that need to be pointed out for certain organ systems.

Closed Head Injury

The Glasgow coma scale (GCS)[16] (Table 3-3) is very helpful in assessing cortical brain function. Modifications to the verbal response variable of this scale have been developed for the child too young to speak. Decreasing GCS scores should alert you to the urgent need for neurosurgical consultation and care. Anisocoria (unequal pupils) or eye deviation are also important warning signs of significant intracranial pathology.

A CT scan is the most important diagnostic tool in the management of closed head injuries in children.

Hypoxia and hypovolemia will both contribute to the worsening of a closed head injury. They *must* be recognized and treated before any other treatment is initiated.

One of the most effective ways of reducing intracranial pressure is hyperventilation. The arterial Pco_2 should be kept at 3.3 to 4.0 kPa (30 to 40 mmHg) with adequate oxygenation. In the child with a GCS of less than 8 or with signs of brainstem injury or posturing, this is best accomplished by intubation.

Mannitol is reserved for those patients with acute neurologic deterioration or transtentorial herniation and not in shock. It should be used as a lifesaving measure while definitive diagnostic, transport, or surgical options

TABLE 3-3. Glasgow Coma Scale[16]

Variable	Score
Opening of the Eyes	
Spontaneously	4
To speech	3
To pain	2
None	1
Best Verbal Response	
Oriented	5
Confused	4
Inappropriate words	3
Incomprehensible sounds	2
None	1
Children's Best Verbal Response[17]	
Smiles, oriented to sound, follows objects, interacts	*5*
Consolable when crying, interacts inappropriately	*4*
Inconsistently consolable, moans	*3*
inconsolable, irritable, restless	*2*
No response	*1*
Best Motor Response	
Spontaneous (obedience to commands)	6
Localization of pain	5
Withdrawal	4
Abnormal flexion to pain	3
Abnormal extension to pain	2
None	1

are being carried out. Consultation with a neurosurgeon is advised before administering mannitol. The recommended dosage is usually 0.5 to 1 g/kg rapidly intravenously. The use of mannitol is not without risk. It produces changes in electrolytes, dehydration, and increased osmolality. Decadron is not recommended nor are emergency bur holes done by inexperienced personnel.

Spine Trauma

The incidence of cervical spine injury in children 1 to 15 years of age has been estimated at 18.2 per million as compared with an estimated 1,850 pediatric brain injuries per million. The injuries tend to be in the upper cervical spine (C1 to C3) in children under 8 years old and in the C5-C6 or lower regions in the older child. In the younger child, a normal cervical spine radiograph does not preclude a significant spinal cord injury. Of children with traumatic spinal-cord injury, 50 to 60 percent have normal radiographs. A thorough neurologic examination is critical in diagnosing incomplete spinal cord injury. It is recommended that any multiple trauma patient, especially those with an associated head injury, have an AP and lateral view of the cervical spine, including C7 to T1. If a cord injury is suspected in a child with normal radiographs, a magnetic resonance imaging (MRI) or CT myelogram should be performed.

Some measures of neurologic outcome in spinal cord injury patients were found to improve with the administration of methylprednisolone when compared to placebo. The dosage used was 30 mg/kg IV bolus followed by 5.4 mg/kg/h for 23 hours.

Chest Trauma

The flexibility and compliance of the pediatric chest wall has already been mentioned. The significance of this is that a child can sustain major intrathoracic injury with very little external evidence of this injury. The problems of tension pneumothorax and hemopneumothorax are poorly tolerated by the child because of the mobility of the mediastinal structures. When they do occur they must be recognized promptly and managed in exactly the same manner as they would be in the adult. The chest needs to be reevaluated both clinically and radiographically from time to time to prevent overlooking a serious pulmonary contusion that becomes more manifest with time.

Abdominal Trauma

Blunt trauma to the abdomen is very common in the multiply injured child. It can occur in an unrestrained passenger in a car. It can also occur in a child restrained by a lap belt. The abdomen is examined clinically for tenderness, guarding, bowel sounds, and so on. The peritoneal lavage is used infrequently in evaluating the presence of intraperitoneal bleeding. The child is usually assessed by abdominal CT scan and frequent clinical reevaluations. The frequency of gastric distension due to air swallowing has been mentioned. This is best managed by the insertion of a nasogastric tube.

Determination of Injury Severity

The determination of injury severity is important for at least two reasons. It is helpful during the initial period of resuscitation in determining those patients who can be safely managed at the primary treatment facility and those who need to be transported to a designated Level 1 trauma facility. It is also helpful in predicting outcome such as mortality and morbidity.

Several scoring systems are currently used to classify injury severity. The Injury Severity Score (ISS)[18] and the Abbreviated Injury Scale (AIS)[19,20] classify injuries by anatomic site and severity. However, these classification systems are of little clinical value for the triage of trauma victims. The ISS is primarily used for injury classifica-

TABLE 3-4. Pediatric Trauma Score

Variable	+2	+1	−1
Weight (kg)	>20	10–20	<10
Airway patency	Normal	Maintained	Unmaintained
Systolic blood pressure (mmHg)	>90	50–90	<50
Neurologic status	Awake	Obtunded	Comatose
Open wound	None	Minor	Major
Skeletal trauma	None	Closed	Open or multiple

Each variable is given one of the three scores. The scores are totaled (range: −6 to +12). A total ≤8 indicates potentially important trauma.
(From Tepas et al.,[21] with permission.)

tion, research on trauma outcomes, and as a measure for quality assurance. The ISS does have a direct correlation with mortality. Those interested in more information about ISS and AIS are referred to the appropriate articles.[18-20]

Two field scoring systems, the Pediatric Trauma Score (PTS)[21] and the Revised Trauma Score (RTS)[22] are currently used for triage of the severely injured patient.

Pediatric Trauma Score

The Pediatric Trauma Score (Table 3-4) was devised as a means for rapid assessment and triage of the injured child.[21] It was specifically designed to supplement the initial field assessment by providing a schedule of priorities to ensure adequate evaluation of all major body systems. A numerical score is produced that is a reliable predictor of injury severity and subsequent mortality and morbidity. The PTS functions as an effective triage tool ensuring that patients are sent to the appropriate hospital for their specific level of injury.

The PTS assesses six components commonly seen in pediatric trauma and grades them into one of three categories. The sum of the grades from the six components produces the Pediatric Trauma Score. A total score of under 8 is indicative of severe trauma and requires rapid referral to a trauma center.

The six components are as follows.

Weight. Size is the most obvious feature that differentiates the pediatric patient for the adult trauma patient. The PTS is weighted toward identifying the very small child. The smaller child (<10 kg) has an increased body surface to volume ratio and limited physiologic reserve, and therefore presents a greater risk of morbidity and mortality than the larger child. This is due to the increased surface area of skin available for water loss and for thermal stress. In addition, it is more difficult to obtain control of the airway and vascular access in the smaller child.

Airway. The PTS is weighted toward identifying children who need assistance in maintaining a patent airway. Those requiring invasive measures, such as intubation or cricothyroidotomy, receive the greatest emphasis.

Central Nervous System Status. Head injury is often a dominant feature in determining whether a child lives or dies, and also determines the future quality of life. Early response and management in a child with a head injury can minimize central nervous system damage and improve chances for survival. Therefore, the PTS is weighted toward identifying children with significant central nervous system (CNS) injury or the potential for late deterioration.

Circulation. Circulatory and perfusion status in the severely injured child is assessed by physical examination and systolic blood pressure. A child with a systolic blood pressure of less than 50 mmHg or a nonpalpable pulse has obviously sustained severe hemorrhagic injury requiring rapid volume replacement, stabilization, and transfer to the trauma center. Systolic blood pressure is a readily obtainable yardstick of circulatory status in the field and is therefore weighted in the PTS.

Skeletal Injuries. Skeletal injuries play an important role in the early management of the traumatized child in terms of blood loss, pain, and limb dysfunction. Multiple fractures, open fractures, and pelvic and spine injuries correlate with the severity of the overall trauma to the child and are weighted accordingly in the PTS.

TABLE 3-5. Revised Trauma Score

Revised Trauma Score	Glasgow Coma Scale	Systolic Blood Pressure (mmHg)	Respiratory Rate (breaths/min)
4	13–15	>89	10–29
3	9–12	76–89	>29
2	6–8	50–75	6–9
1	4–5	1–49	1–5
0	3	0	0

Each of the three variables is scored (GCS, BP, RR). The scores are totaled (range: 0–12). A total ≤ 11 indicates potentially important trauma.
(From American College of Surgeons, monograph on hospital and prehospital resources for the injured patient.[22])

Cutaneous Injuries. The presence of multiple minor lacerations and abrasions can produce an overall additive effect on survival. The presence of penetrating wounds may indicate more significant injuries that can threaten life and limb. The PTS is weighted to identify these wounds.

The PTS has been shown to accurately predict the degree of injury severity in pediatric trauma victims. Tepas and coworkers[21] showed that there is a statistically significant linear relationship between the Pediatric Trauma Score and the Injury Severity Score. They concluded that the PTS is a useful tool for initial assessment and a reliable predictor of injury severity. Aprahamian and coworkers[23] also found a strong correlation between the PTS and the ISS and recommended that any child with a PTS of 8 or less be transported to a trauma facility.

Revised Trauma Score

The Revised Trauma Score (RTS) is a second commonly used method of rapid assessment of trauma victims in the field.[22] The RTS is based upon a score of 0 to 4 given for each of three variables: Glasgow coma scale, systolic blood pressure, and respiratory rate (Table 3-5). If a patient has a total score of less than 11, referral to a trauma center is recommended.[22] The advantage of the RTS is its simplicity and universal applicability. However, it is *not specific for children.*

The advantage of the PTS in children when compared to other field scoring systems with universal application to children and adults is unclear. Kaufmann and colleagues[24] compared the PTS with the Revised Trauma Score and found that both scores correlated closely with the ISS and survival. However, there was no clear advantage of the PTS over the RTS when applied to children. This was also true for the Trauma Score when compared to the PTS.[25] Eichelberger and colleagues[26] found that a PTS less than 9, RTS less than 12, and TS less than 15 were equally sensitive and specific for pediatric prehospital triage.

It is recommended that copies of the Pediatric Trauma Score and Glasgow coma scale be posted or at least readily available in the Emergency department for use by the physicians who will be managing the pediatric trauma cases.

Orthopedic Management Principles in the Multiply Injured Child

Musculoskeletal injuries are a frequent component of the severely traumatized child. These fractures are rarely life-threatening in themselves. However, proper fracture management from the outset is a key component of optimal care at the time of injury. Obviously, proper fracture management also has a significant impact on the final functional outcome. Neglected fracture care can be a source of significant late morbidity in the severely traumatized child.

A clear treatment plan for the patient's fractures should be established at the initial evaluation and resuscitation. The adage that "all children's fractures heal if they're in the same room" and the assumption that remodeling will correct all inaccuracies of fracture union and alignment in children have no application in the multiply injured patient. These children have special needs and considerations that affect the specific type of fracture treatment selected. Fracture management must improve, not interfere with, the general care of the patient. Therefore, what may be appropriate treatment for an isolated fracture may be contraindicated in this setting.

When establishing a plan for fracture care in the multiply injured child, the following principles should be considered:

1. Make sure that any child with a major long bone fracture is not, in fact, a patient with significant other injuries. Always do a quick "ABC" check on these patients! Remember that a child can maintain a reasonable systolic blood pressure despite significant blood loss, and then, suddenly decompensate. Also remember the high chance of significant lung parenchymal injury despite a paucity of external findings.

2. Early treatment of the fracture should be compatible with the general care of the patient. The child must be accessible to the trauma team. These children often require continuous monitoring, frequent diagnostic tests, and invasive procedures. Arterial and venous access must be available. Injured limbs must be inspected for signs of vascular compromise or compartment syndrome. The type of fracture care chosen should allow the child to be comfortable during these periods of frequent transport to and from diagnostic tests, the operating room, and during routine nursing care. Fracture treatment, that is, multiple limbs in traction, should not obstruct these diagnostic studies.

3. Fracture care should consider the need for early mobilization of the child. The ability to mobilize the multiply injured child has many beneficial aspects. Pulmonary care is facilitated. Joint contractures can be prevented and pressure decubiti avoided. Management of cerebral edema is facilitated if the patient can be positioned with the head elevated. Patients with associated burns and massive soft tissue injuries have specific positioning needs requiring mobility. The ability to mobilize the child allows for early initiation of physical and cognitive rehabilitation. In this setting, the use of a spica cast, or traction, may interfere with the mobility needs of the child. Therefore the judicious use of either internal or external fixation should be considered.

4. Care of the fracture should facilitate management of associated soft tissue injuries. The care of open fractures and soft tissue injuries requires the limbs to be accessible for repeated inspection of the wounds, dressing changes, debridement, and definitive wound closure. Early fracture stabilization is essential for the management of associated soft tissue injuries and is an essential component of soft tissue reconstructive procedures, such as local rotation flaps and free vascularized tissue transfers. Again, either internal or external fixation may be the most appropriate form of treatment.

5. The initial method of treating the fracture should be the definitive method whenever possible. The best opportunity to institute a plan for a given fracture is from the start of treatment. Delaying definitive fracture care or "temporizing" in the multiply injured child often results in missed opportunities and late morbidity. Complications related to other organ systems may prevent or delay further attempts at fracture stabilization.

6. The method of fracture treatment should reflect the specific needs of the patient. In the multiple trauma setting, no single treatment method for a given fracture is applicable to all patients. Fracture care must be carefully individualized. Children's femur fractures are a good example of this. As isolated injuries, femur fractures in children may be managed with traction or an immediate spica cast. Adolescents do well with closed intramedullary nailing and rapid mobilization. However, if the injured child has a head injury or is unconscious, the use of traction has resulted in increased incidence of malunion, shortening, ligamentous instability, and wound problems.[27-31]

Internal fixation, external fixation, and intramedullary nailing may be preferable when the child presents with a closed head injury. If the fracture is open or there are other soft tissue injuries, early stabilization may be beneficial as well.

7. Treat all children as if they are going to survive. Children have a remarkable ability to recover from even the most severe injuries. Children are much more likely to recover from head injury than adults. Bruce and co-workers[31] showed that with aggressive management, 90 percent of children presenting with a closed head injury survived or were moderately disabled, while 8 percent died.[18] All children with a Glasgow coma scale of 5 or greater recovered well. The low incidence of intracranial mass lesions and the high incidence of diffuse intracranial swelling suggested a different pathophysiologic mechanism of response of the child's brain to injury, accounting for improved survival in children following severe closed head injury when compared to adults. These facts should be considered when asked to evaluate a severely injured child with multiple fractures.

CONCLUSION

Children continue to die because serious injuries are missed or managed poorly. The approach to the badly injured child is no different from the ABC approach to the badly injured adult. There are certain anatomic and physiologic differences that should be learned by those who may find themselves managing these children. Use of the systematic, multidisciplinary, predetermined approach should eliminate the tragedy of a preventable death.

REFERENCES

1. Division of Injury Control. Centers for Disease Control: Childhood injuries in the United States. Am J Dis Child 144:627, 1990
2. Greensher J: Recent advances in injury prevention. Pediatr Rev 10:171, 1988
3. Chan B, Walker P, Cass D: Urban trauma: an analysis of 1,116 paediatric cases. J Trauma 29:1540, 1989
4. Tepas JI, DiScala C, Ramenofsky M, Barlow B: Mortality and head injury: the pediatric perspective. J Pediatr Surg 25:92, 1990
5. Dykes E, Spence L, Bohn D, Wesson D: Evaluation of pediatric trauma care in Ontario. J Trauma 29:724, 1989
6. Subcommittee of Advanced Trauma Life Support of the American College of Surgeons Committee on Trauma: Advanced Trauma Life Support Student Manual. 11. Chicago, 1989
7. Lloyd-Thomas AR: ABC of major trauma: paediatric trauma. I. Primary survey and resuscitation. Br Med J 301:334, 1990
8. Leape LL: Progress in pediatric trauma: anatomy and patterns of injury. In Harris BH (ed): The First National Conference on Pediatric Trauma. Nobb Hill Press, Boston, 1985
9. Walker M, Storrs B, Mayer T: Head injuries. In Mayers TA (ed): Emergency Management of Pediatric Trauma. p. 272. WB Saunders, Philadelphia, 1985
10. Kissoon N, Dreyer J, Walia M: Pediatric trauma: differences in pathophysiology, injury patterns and treatment compared with adult trauma. Can Med Assoc J 142:27, 1990
11. Kewalramani L, Kraus J, Sterling H: Acute spinal-cord lesions in a pediatric population: epidemiological and clinical features. Paraplegia 18:206, 1980
12. Hubbard D: Injuries of the spine in children and adolescents. Clin Orthop 100:56, 1974
13. Nakayama D, Gardner M, Rowe M: Emergency endotracheal intubation in pediatric trauma. Ann Surg 211:218, 1990
14. Nakayama D, Ramenofsky M, Rowe M: Chest injuries in childhood. Ann Surg 210:770, 1989
15. Fiser D: Intraosseous infusion. N Engl J Med 322:1579, 1990
16. Teasdale G, Jennet B: Assessment of coma and impaired consciousness. Lancet 2:81, 1974
17. Hahn YS, Chyung C, Barthell MJ, et al: Head injuries in children under 30 months of age: demography and outcome 4:34, 1988
18. Baker S, O'Neill B, Haddon WJ, Long W: The Injury Severity Score: a method for describing patients with multiple injuries and evaluating emergency care. J Trauma 14:187, 1974
19. Civil ID, Schwab CW: The Abbreviated Injury Scale, 1985 revision: a condensed chart for clinical use. J Trauma 28:87, 1988
20. Association for the Advancement of Automotive Medicine: The Abbreviated Injury Scale, 1990 revision. Des Plaines, IL, 1990
21. Tepas JI, Mollitt D, Talbert J, Bryant M: The Pediatric Trauma Score as a predictor of injury severity in the injured child. J Pediatr Surg 22:14, 1987
22. American College of Surgeons: Hospital and Prehospital Resources for Optimal Care of the Injured Patient and Appendices F and J. Chicago, 1986
23. Aprahamian C, Cattey RP, Walker AP et al: Pediatric Trauma Score, predictor of hospital use? Arch Surg 125:1128, 1990
24. Kaufmann CR, Maier RV, Rivara FP, Carrico CJ: Evaluation of the Pediatric Trauma Score. JAMA 263:69, 1990
25. Nayduch DA, Moylan J, Rutledge R: Comparison of the ability of the Adult and Pediatric Trauma Scores to predict pediatric outcome following major trauma. J Trauma 31:452, 1991
26. Eichelberger MR, Gotschall CS, Sacco WJ et al: A comparison of the Trauma Score, the Revised Trauma Score, and the Pediatric Trauma Score. Ann Emerg Med 18:1053, 1989
27. Fry K, Hoffer MM, Brink J: Femoral shaft fractures in brain-injured children. J Trauma 16:371, 1976
28. Porat S, Milgrom C, Meir N et al: Femoral fracture treatment in head-injured children: use of external fixation. J Trauma 26:81, 1986
29. Ziv I, Rang M: Treatment of femoral fracture in the child with head injury. J Bone Joint Surg [Br] 65:276, 1983
30. Gibson JMC: Multiple injuries: the management of the patient with a fractured femur and a head injury. J Bone Joint Surg [Br] 42:425, 1960
31. Bruce DA, Schut L, Bruno LA et al: Outcome following severe head injuries in children. J Neurosurg 48:679, 1989

4

Radiologic Diagnosis of Pediatric Skeletal Trauma

Roderick I. Macpherson
Martin H. Reed

> The moral of x-rays is this—that a right way of looking at things will see through almost anything.
> —Samuel Butler

Despite the highly technologic advances in radiologic imaging of recent years, plain radiography remains the primary method of identifying or excluding significant pediatric skeletal trauma. Unfortunately, however, injuries may easily be overdiagnosed or underdiagnosed on the basis of the radiographic findings. There are several reasons for this. First, there are the technical factors. If the radiologic investigation is performed incorrectly or incompletely, the true nature and extent of the injury may be missed. Second, normal anatomy and its variations in the growing skeleton can mimic fractures and other skeletal injuries. Third, there are nontraumatic diseases that resemble skeletal injuries and, conversely, skeletal injuries that resemble other diseases.

In this chapter, it is our objective to review the major pitfalls in the radiologic diagnosis of pediatric skeletal trauma. After some general comments on the technical factors, normal variants, and nontraumatic pathologic entities involved in the misdiagnosis of pediatric skeletal injuries, the common sources of erroneous diagnosis in each anatomic region of the skeleton will be reviewed.

GENERAL CONSIDERATIONS

Technical Factors in Fracture Diagnosis

Radiographing an injured child can prove to be a difficult and stressful task. Sometimes it is tempting to take radiologic shortcuts in an effort to accelerate the diagnostic process and get on with the treatment. However, while radiographic protocols for trauma victims should be fast and efficient, there are certain principles of pediatric skeletal radiography that should not be forgotten,[1-3] or the clinician will risk encountering some serious pitfalls.

The radiographic examination of the injured part should be composed of at least two views, preferably at 90 degrees one to the other. One will encounter many fractures that are imperceptible on one projection and painfully obvious on the other (Fig. 4-1). There are certain bones, such as the clavicle, where views at right angles to one another are impossible. The compromise in these regions is the use of frontal and tangential views (Fig. 4-2). In certain areas, such as the ankle, the true extent of an injury may not be appreciated in the absence

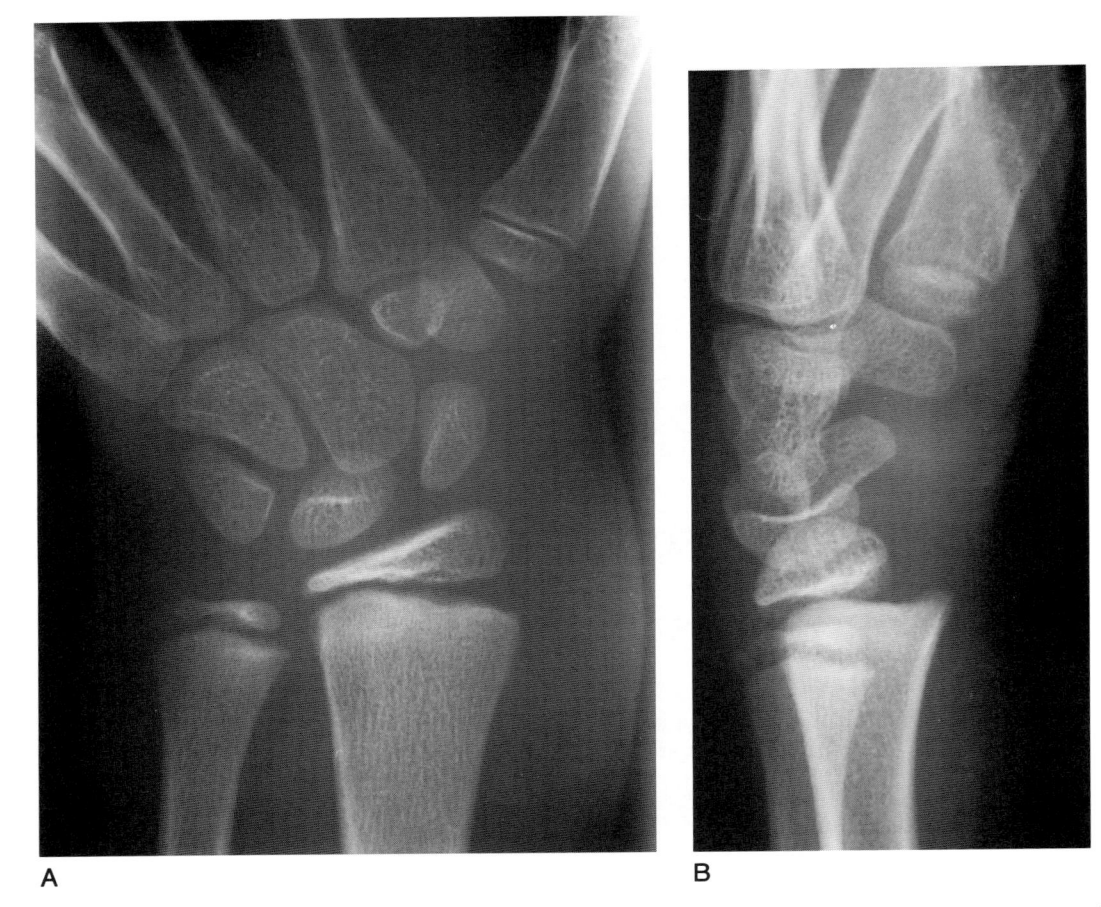

Fig. 4-1. Salter-Harris type I fracture through the distal radial growth plate in a 12-year-old boy. **(A)** AP view. Fracture imperceptible. **(B)** Lateral view. Posterior displacement of distal radial epiphysis.

of oblique projections. The art of skeletal radiography may be found in the creation of axial or tangential views to demonstrate fractures in less accessible locations, such as in tarsal bones or sesamoid bones. We have been impressed with the use of fluoroscopy and spot filming for this purpose. In circumstances where the fracture is in a location difficult to radiograph, and the injured patient cannot be moved, the old technique of stereoscopic imaging can also be resurrected.

The radiographic examination of an injured long bone should include the joints above and below the site of injury. There are many injury patterns where a second lesion will occur remote from the primary injury, for example, fractures of the distal tibia and proximal fibula (see Ch. 34) or Monteggia fractures (see Ch. 17). If the radiographs of these injuries are coned down to the site of the primary fracture, the second injury can be overlooked.

When there is confusion between a fracture and a normal anatomic variant, comparative views of the opposite side can be indispensable. We do not recommend, however, the inclusion of comparative views in routine pediatric skeletal radiography protocols. It has been shown that their utilization by experienced diagnosticians is so infrequent they are a waste of time and money.[4]

There is another form of comparison, however, that is never a wasted effort. If available, any previous radiographs of the affected part should be reviewed in conjunction with the current study. By the same token, the current examination should be saved for future comparison.

A knowledge of symptom patterns in pediatric skeletal trauma will allow a logical progression of the radiologic investigation from one anatomic area to the other. For example, it should be known that hip injuries can

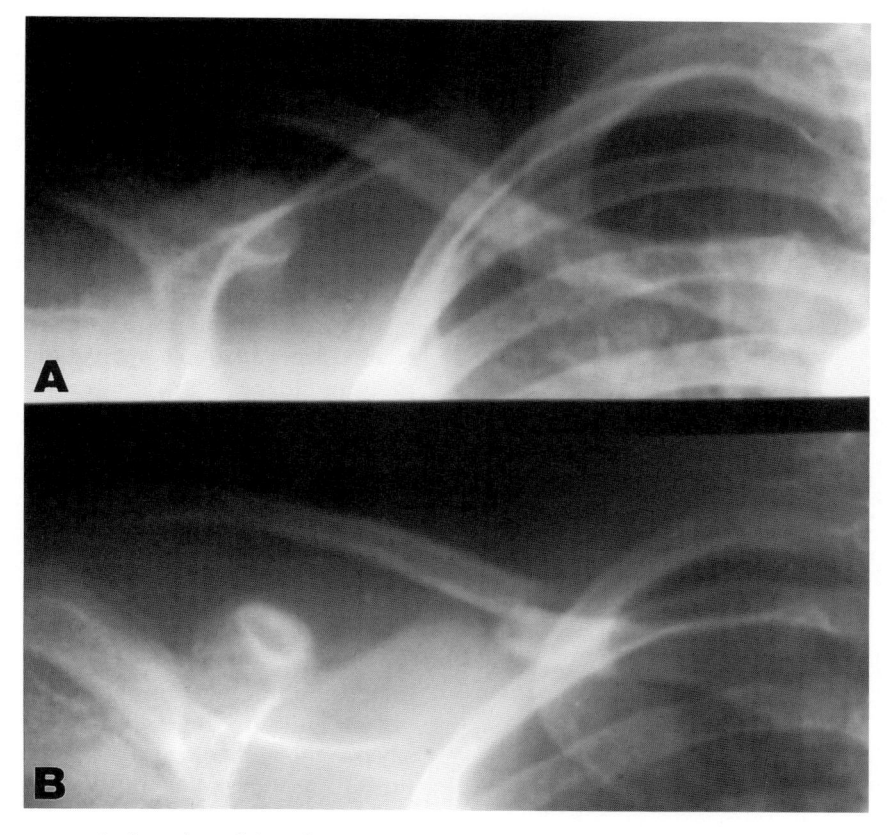

Fig. 4-2. Fracture at the junction of the middle and proximal thirds of the right clavicle in a 13-year-old boy. **(A)** AP view. Fracture imperceptible. **(B)** Tangential view. Fracture clearly visible.

present with knee pain or that fractures through the base of the fifth metatarsal (Fig. 4-3) can mimic ankle injuries. On this basis, if radiographs of the first site are unrewarding, the investigation should proceed to the second.

In addition to symptom patterns, the recognition of certain injury patterns on the initial radiographs should suggest additional investigations. The prime example of this is the discovery of injuries suggestive of child abuse, such as multiple fractures of varying age, metaphyseal fragmentation, or even a simple fracture of a large cylindrical bone without adequate explanation (see Ch. 51). These findings demand further clinical, radiologic, and social investigations, which should be initiated before the patient leaves the health care environment.

There are certain types of acute skeletal injury in children, and certain anatomic locations in the skeleton, where plain radiography cannot be relied upon to provide the definitive diagnostic information. In these instances, one can wait for follow-up radiographs to establish the diagnosis of fracture. In the interim, however, the patient may be at risk for developing serious complications. To avoid this, one must utilize the appropriate alternative imaging modalities to establish an early and confident diagnosis. These include conventional tomography, computed tomography, arthrography, ultrasound, magnetic resonance imaging, and radionuclide studies.

Conventional tomography has been used for many years in the delineation of certain traumatic injuries in children. It is indicated in anatomic locations where a fracture, dislocation, or subluxation can be obscured by adjacent normal structures. For example, the true nature of neural arch and craniocervical lesions (Fig. 4-4) can be clarified by conventional tomography.

In recent years, computed tomography (CT) has been replacing conventional tomography as an alternative imaging modality for a variety of skeletal injuries.[5] It is particularly useful in the evaluation of fractures that involve curved anatomic surfaces, such as the spine (Fig. 4-5A) and the pelvis. It has been used to study the nature and extent of triplane fractures of the distal tibia, sterno-

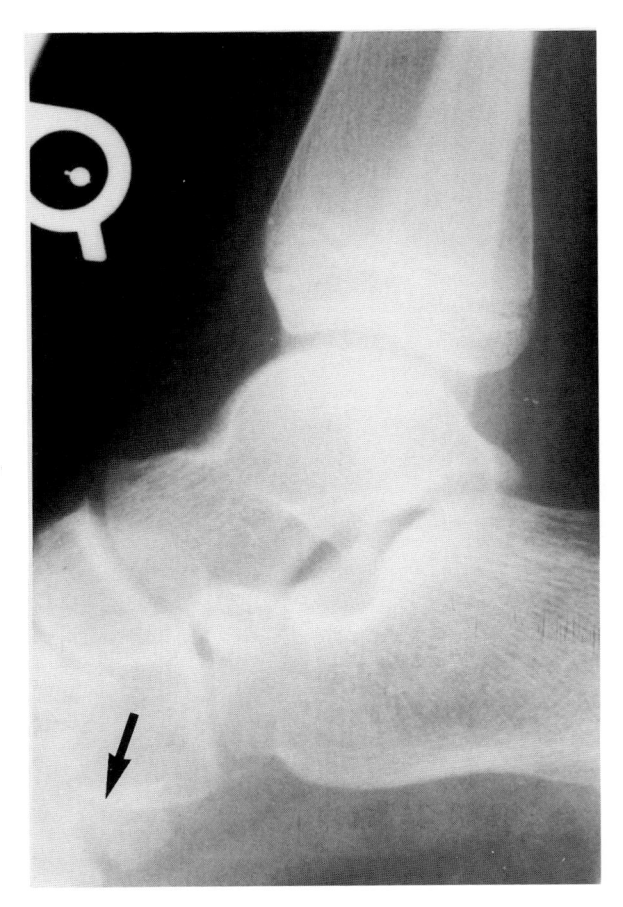

Fig. 4-3. Fracture through the base of the fifth metatarsal in a 14-year-old girl. This "Dancer's fracture" *(arrow)* is discovered as a peripheral finding on the lateral view of an ankle examination.

clavicular separations, and elbow fractures.[6] In addition, it is much better in the assessment of the soft tissue changes of trauma than conventional radiography. From the technical standpoint, CT can be less stressful to the traumatized patient than radiography because the patient does not have to change positions for different views. Also, most casting materials are not a deterrent to a good examination, although metal-containing splints and other hardware can interfere with the quality of the study. Three-dimensional CT offers another perspective in the study of complex injuries in areas with complicated anatomy,[7] such as the craniocervical junction (Fig. 4-5B), pelvis, and ankle.

The diagnosis of Salter-Harris type I growth plate injuries can be difficult to establish, especially prior to the ossification of the epiphysis. Arthrography can be employed to demonstrate fractures of this nature involving the proximal (Fig. 4-6) and distal humerus.[8] Ultrasound[9,10] and magnetic resonance imaging[11,12] can also be used in the diagnosis of occult injuries of this nature.

There are certain sites in the skeleton, such as the ribs, carpal scaphoid, spine, and tibia, where undisplaced fractures remain imperceptible on radiographs, regardless of the projection. ^{99m}Tc-methylene diphosphonate (^{99m}Tc-MDP) bone scans[13] are useful in the delineation of this type of injury (Fig. 4-7). This bone-seeking tracer readily identifies abnormal areas of vascularity or increased bone metabolism. In doing so, it will concentrate in traumatized bone and can demonstrate fractures within hours of the traumatic event. The bone scan is more sensitive than radiography in the detection of occult skeletal injuries, such as subtle fractures of the ribs and long bones.[14] The findings on radiography, however, tend to be more specific for trauma and more useful in assessing the age of the injuries.

There are some pitfalls, however, in the diagnosis of fractures by bone scanning.[14] For example, the child must be carefully positioned for the study, since minor malpositioning can simulate or mask focal abnormalities. In addition, the exposure factors must be precise, since slight overexposure of the images can obscure fractures. The interpreter must be aware of normal scintigraphic anatomy and its variations with age. There is normally preferential uptake of the tracer in the growth plates, the base and sutures of the skull, the temporomandibular joints, the orbits, the costochondral junctions, and the midshafts of the tibiae. In addition to being a site of normal increased uptake of the tracer, growth plates are common sites for pediatric fractures. Because fractures are recognized by increased uptake of the tracer, they may be hard to detect at these sites. If the patient has bilateral fractures, no asymmetry may be detected, and both fractures could be overlooked. As mentioned above, the bone scan provides no information as to the age of the fractures and can miss very early (less than 7 hours old) and completely healed fractures, both of which may be recognized on plain radiographs.

The ^{99m}Tc-MDP bone scan has been used to differentiate between a recent fracture and early osteomyelitis.[13] Gallium scans and radionuclide-labeled white cells may be employed to assist in differentiating between skeletal lesions of traumatic origin and those secondary to neoplasm or infection.

Magnetic resonance imaging (MRI) will never be a substitute for radiography in the diagnosis of fractures.[15] However, it can demonstrate the soft tissue changes of trauma, which might prove useful in the differentiation

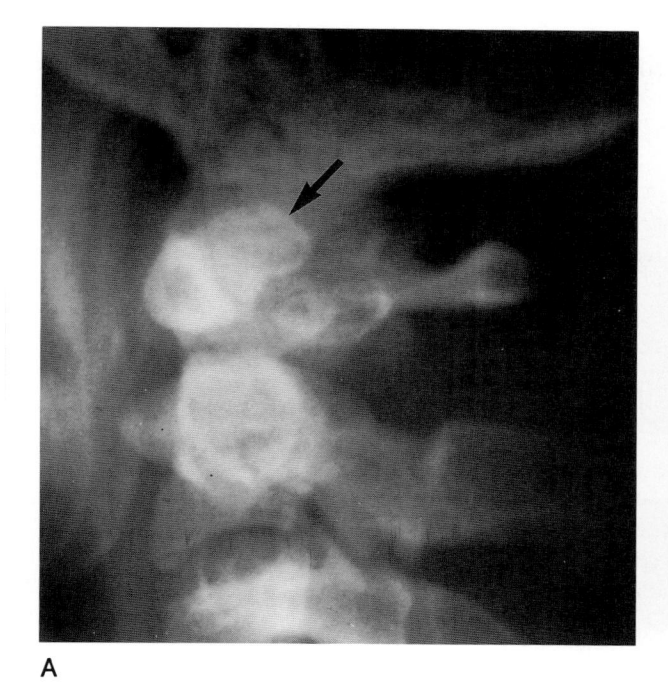

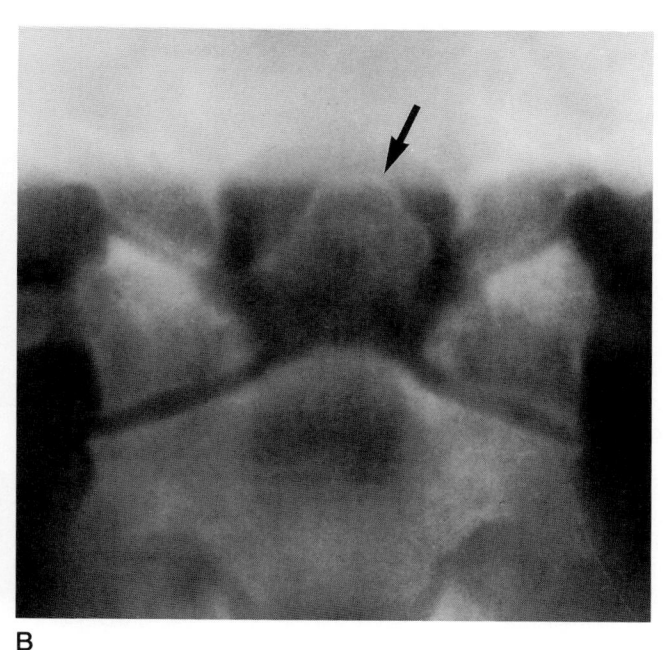

Fig. 4-4. Separate odontoid process in a 16-year-old boy. **(A)** Lateral view and **(B)** AP tomography show the smoothly rounded odontoid process *(arrow)* located behind the anterior arch of the atlas and widely separated from the body of the axis. (From Reed,[23] with permission.)

between physiologic subperiosteal new bone and that secondary to trauma. It has been used in the detection of certain radiographically occult fractures.[11] In addition, MRI has become established as the modality for demonstrating intra-articular and extra-articular ligamentous, tendinous, and cartilaginous injuries.[12] For example, it is a reliable noninvasive method of outlining the meniscus and cruciate ligament tears associated with knee injuries.

Ultrasound plays a minor role in the diagnosis of skeletal trauma in children, but can be used to detect the presence of excess joint fluid in the hip or elbow and to study the nature and extent of soft tissue masses associated with trauma.[16] It has been employed in the demonstration of occult femoral head fractures in the neonate.[9,10]

Normal Anatomy and Its Variants That Mimic Trauma

The radiographic recognition of acute fractures in children is dependent on the identification of breaks, buckles, or bends in the affected bones. Localized soft tissue swelling and adjacent joint effusions are useful secondary signs. Healing fractures are usually recognized by the presence of subperiosteal new bone formation, and the age of a fracture is judged by the maturity of the new bone. The growing skeleton contains a number of normal anatomic structures, as well as many variations in the normal anatomic patterns, that can simulate osseous discontinuity, osseous deformity, or subperiosteal new bone associated with recent or healing fractures.

There are excellent radiologic textbooks[17,18] devoted to the entire issue of normal anatomy and the variants of normal anatomy that can be mistaken for pathology, and we will not try to duplicate these efforts here. In this section, we will categorize and define the common normal structures and normal variants that are involved in the differential diagnosis of pediatric skeletal injuries. Later in this chapter, we will demonstrate some of these as part of our systematic anatomic review of the radiologic pitfalls in the diagnosis of pediatric fractures.

Synchondroses

Synchondroses are junctions between two or more primary centers of ossification in bones of cartilaginous origin. They should not be confused with sutures, the

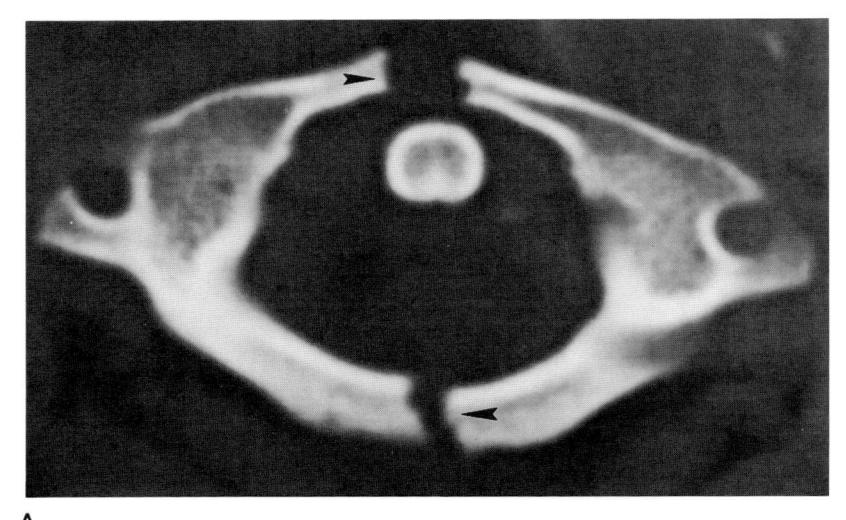

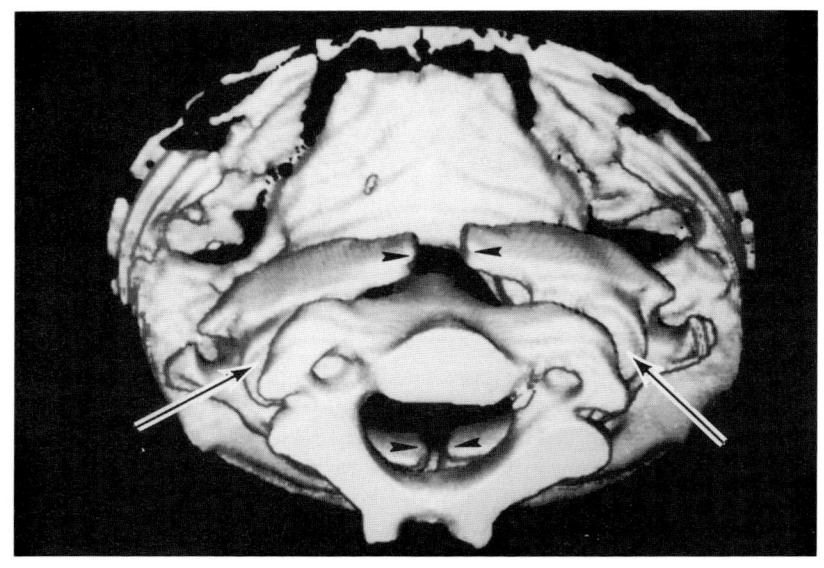

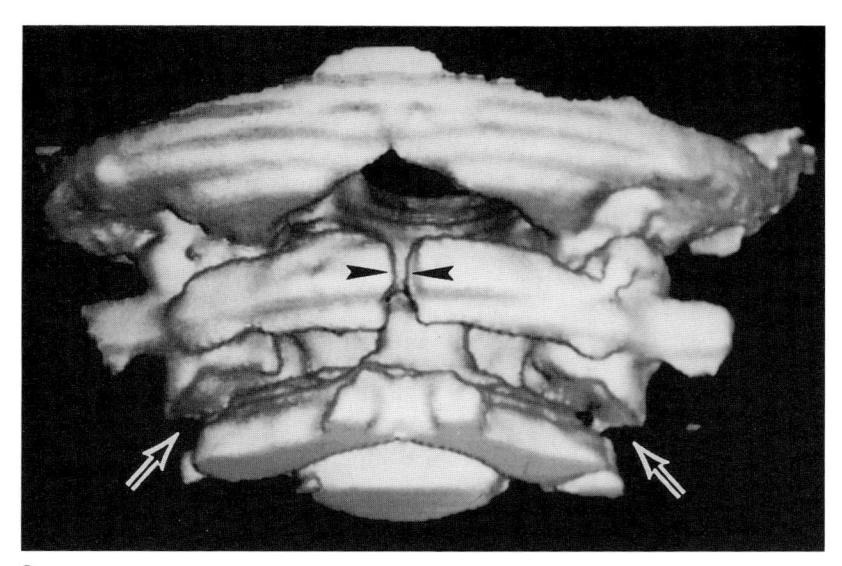

Fig. 4-5. Jefferson fracture in a 7-year-old boy. **(A)** CT of atlas, **(B)** three-dimensional CT of craniocervical junction, viewed from anterior and below, and **(C)** three-dimensional CT viewed from front, showing fractures of the anterior and posterior arches of the atlas *(black arrows)* and offset of atlantoaxial articulation *(black in white arrows)*.

Radiologic Diagnosis of Pediatric Skeletal Trauma / 43

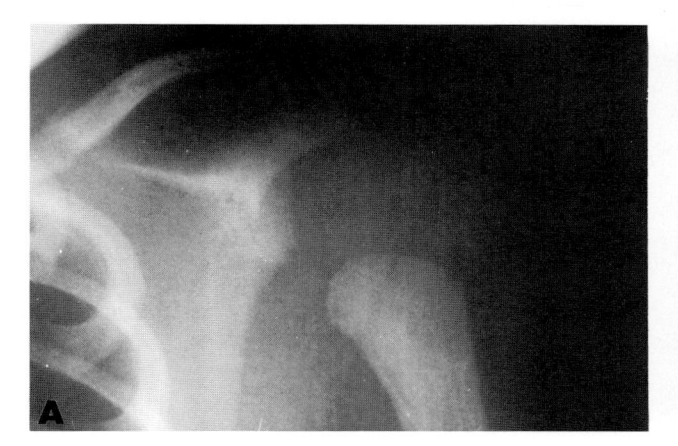

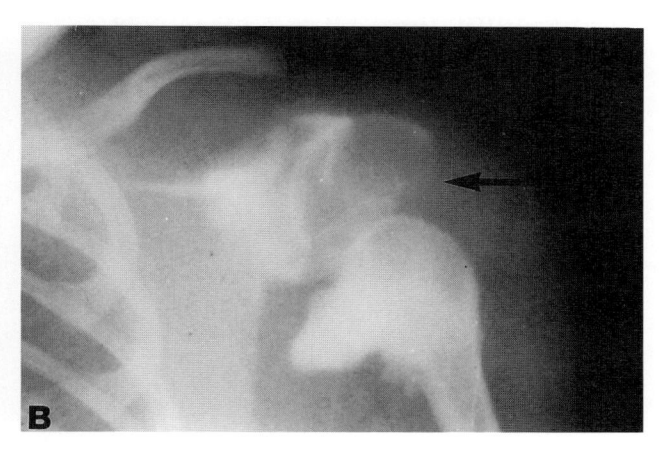

Fig. 4-6. Fracture through proximal left humeral growth plate in newborn male. (A) AP view of shoulder shows clavicular fracture, but humeral fracture imperceptible. (B) Shoulder arthrogram shows separation of cartilaginous humeral head *(arrow)* from shaft. (From Reed,[23] with permission.)

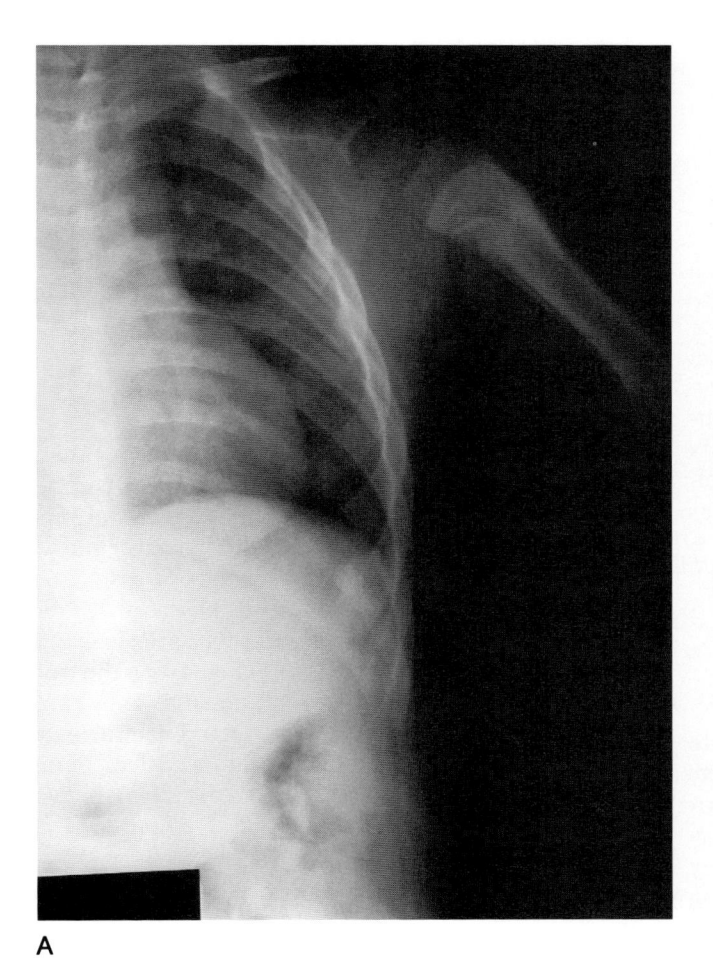

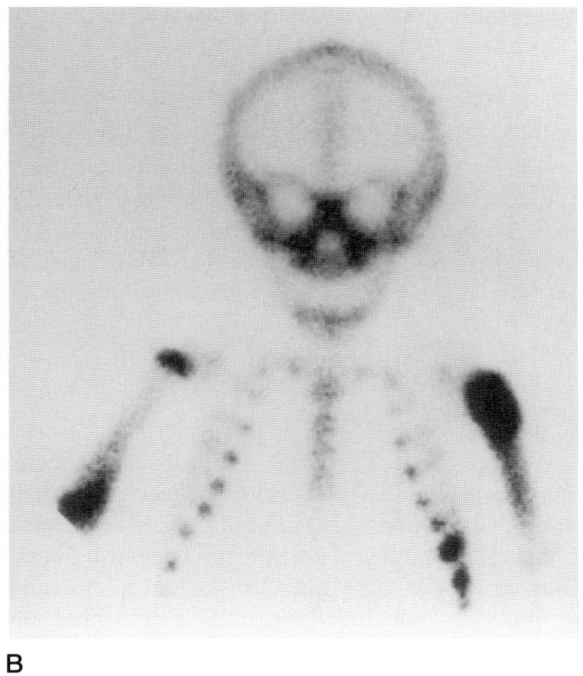

Fig. 4-7. (A) This 13-month-old infant was brought into the emergency department with his mother's complaints that he was favoring his left arm. Radiographs revealed a healing left humeral fracture and a suspicion of rib fractures. (B) ^{99m}Tc scan confirmed rib fractures as well as revealing another healing fracture of the right supracondylar humerus.

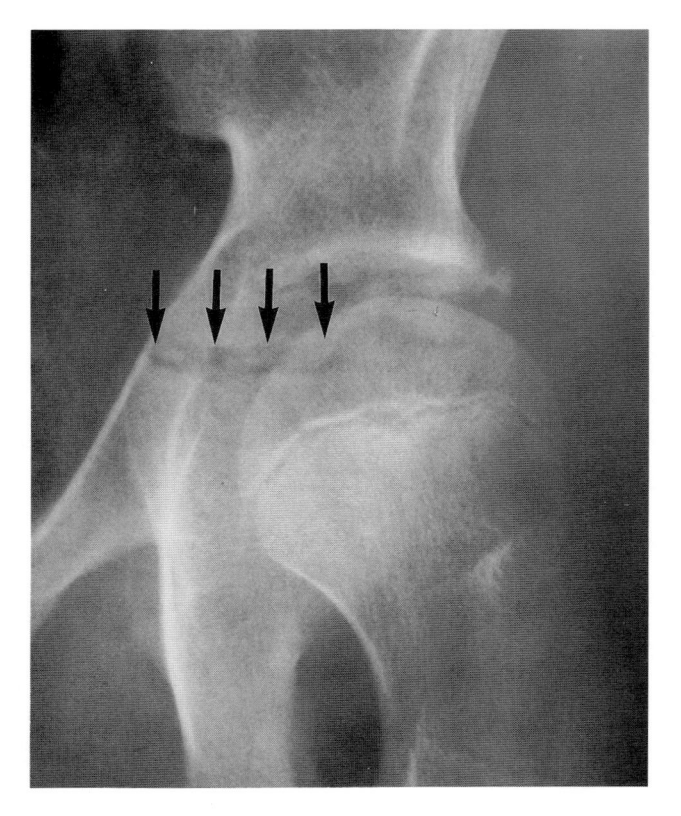

Fig. 4-8. Normal left hip in a 13-year-old girl. The normal triradiate cartilage *(arrows)* could be mistaken for a fracture.

junctions in bones of membranous origin, located exclusively in the skull. Synchondroses are found, primarily in the cranial base, pelvis (Fig. 4-8), and vertebral column. A knowledge of their anatomic locations, as well as the variations in their appearance throughout growth, is important in their radiologic differentiation from fractures.

Growth Plates

Growth plates are the cartilaginous discs that separate primary centers of ossification from secondary centers (epiphyses and apophyses) in bones of cartilaginous origin. They are an integral part of endochondral bone formation and, as a consequence, skeletal growth. They vary in appearance during skeletal development, being relatively wide at birth, gradually narrowing through childhood, and closing when the growth of the bone is complete. Therefore, the appearance of normal growth plates is variable throughout osseous development. As a consequence, certain growth plates, for example, those of the proximal humerus (Fig. 4-9), base of the fifth metatarsal (Fig. 4-10) and about the elbow are frequently mistaken for fractures by unenlightened diagnosticians. This pitfall will be avoided when a thorough knowledge of the radiologic appearances of the growing skeleton is mastered.

Accessory Centers of Ossification

Primary and secondary centers of ossification usually appear as a single ossific nucleus and persist as one center until skeletal growth is completed. Accessory centers of ossification are small extra ossific centers that appear at the periphery of primary or secondary centers of ossification in some children. They are separated from the normal ossification center by a cartilaginous growth plate which can be mistaken for a fracture. The common sites for this normal variant are the medial malleolus (Fig. 4-11), the lateral malleolus, the base of the second metacarpal (Fig. 4-12), and the margins of the acetabulae (Fig. 4-13). Although variable in their appearance from one site to another and from one stage of development to another, they usually occur bilaterally, have a rounded appearance with sclerotic margins, and show a relatively wide gap between them and the rest of the bone. Like other secondary centers of ossification, they usually fuse to the host bone when growth is complete.

Multipartite Centers of Ossification

Centers of ossification that develop from two, three, or more relatively large, simultaneously appearing nuclei are referred to as "bipartite," "tripartite," or "multipartite" centers of ossification. These developmental variants, can be found in primary centers of ossification, such as the patella (Fig. 4-14) and the calcaneus (Fig. 4-15), as well as secondary centers, such as the base of the proximal phalanx of the great toe (Fig. 4-16), the trochlea, and the olecranon process of the ulna. They can be differentiated from fractures by their bilateral occurrence, the smooth, sclerotic appearance of their margins and the relative width of the interval between them.

Irregular Centers of Ossification

In addition to fragmented accessory or partite centers of ossification, one will encounter intact but irregular centers of ossification that can be mistakenly ascribed to trauma or other pathology. This is encountered in pri-

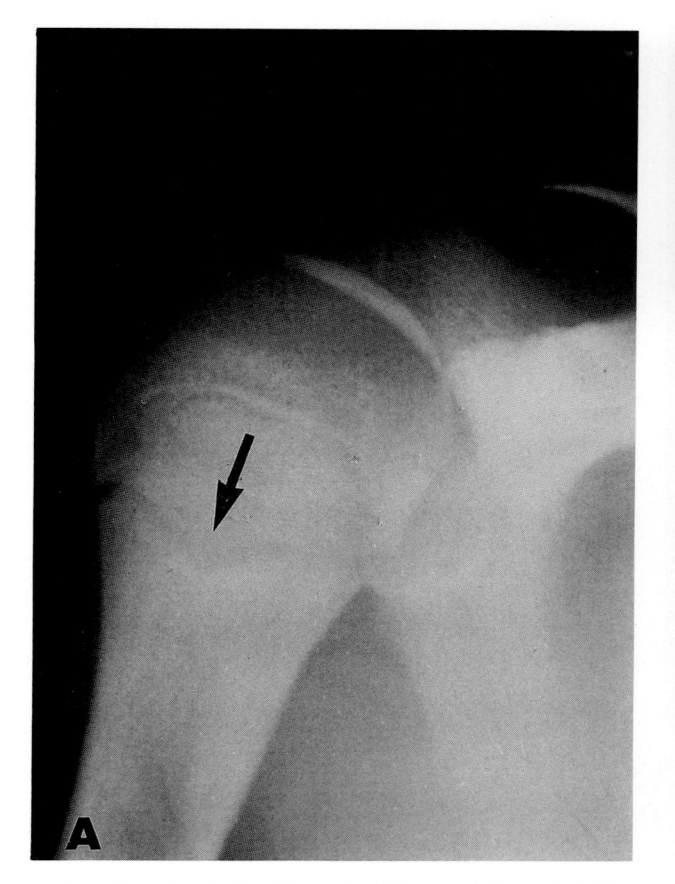

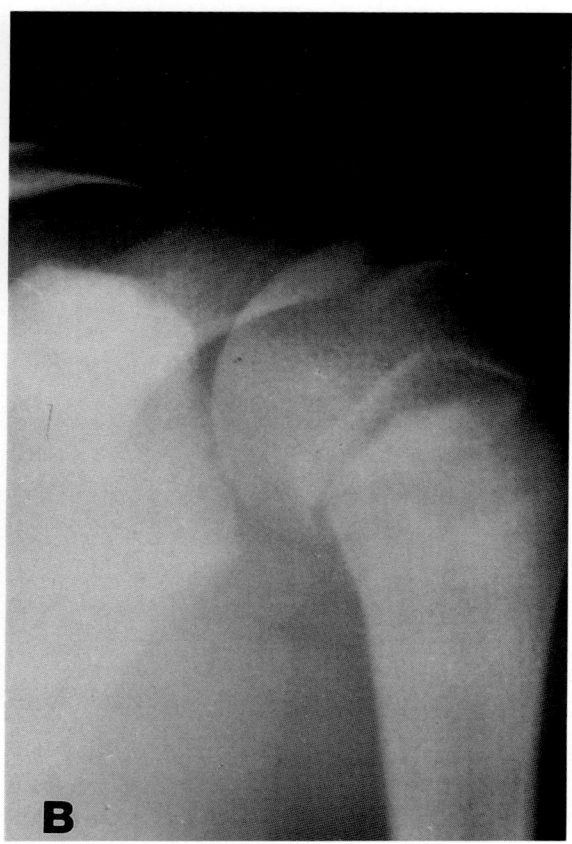

Fig. 4-9. Both shoulders of a 13-year-old boy. **(A)** The normal right proximal humeral growth plate *(arrow)* is often mistaken for fracture. **(B)** The slightly displaced Salter-Harris type I fracture through the proximal left humeral growth plate could be missed.

mary centers of ossification, such as the cuneiforms and the patella (Fig. 4-17), as well as secondary centers, such as the medial aspect of the distal femoral condyle, and the trochlea. These variants tend to have a bilateral occurrence, which will help differentiate them from significant pathology.

Accessory Ossicles

In addition to the well-known normal seven tarsal and eight carpal bones, there a number of other ossicles that can be found on ankle or wrist radiographs in some children. These extra, separate ossifications are called accessory ossicles. Kohler and Zimmer[17] assigned the names to 16 accessory ossicles in the tarsal region (Fig. 4-18) and some 23 in the carpal region. Their predictable locations and rounded appearance will help differentiate accessory ossicles from fractures. Unlike accessory centers of ossification, accessory ossicles persist after growth is complete.

Irregular Growth Plates

Growth plate injuries are common in children, and the radiologic diagnosis of these injuries is often based on the detection of irregularity or fragmentation of the growth plate margins. Spurious growth plate irregularity can be encountered when the wavy cartilaginous plate is viewed obliquely, allowing the back of the epiphysis to be superimposed on the front of the metaphysis, thus simulating a fracture line. Small ossicles are frequently encountered in the periphery of the growth plates of the distal fibula (Fig. 4-19) and distal radius. These can simulate the metaphyseal fragments of a Salter-Harris

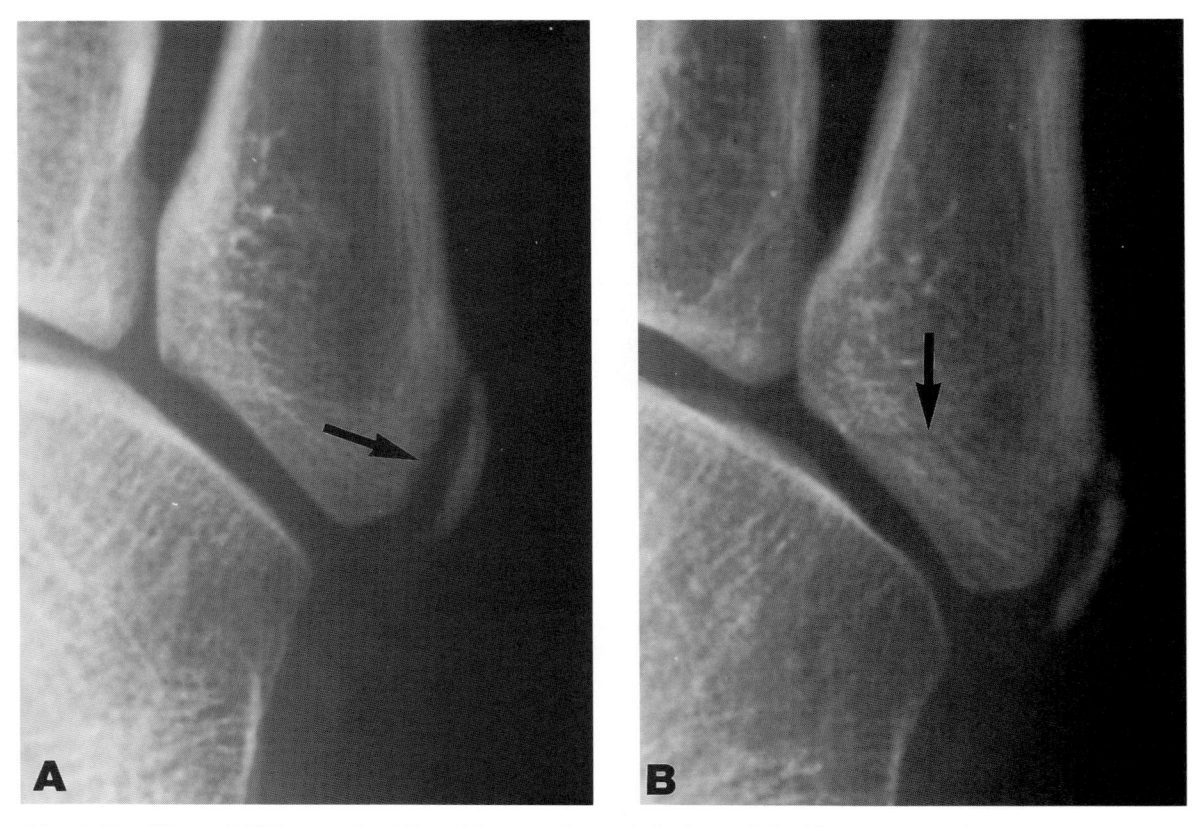

Fig. 4-10. Normal "flake apophysis" and fracture through the base of the fifth metatarsal in a 13-year-old girl. **(A)** The right foot shows a normal flake epiphysis at the base of the fifth metatarsal *(arrow)*. **(B)** The left foot shows the flake epiphysis plus a subtle "Jones's fracture" or "Dancer's fracture" *(arrow)*.

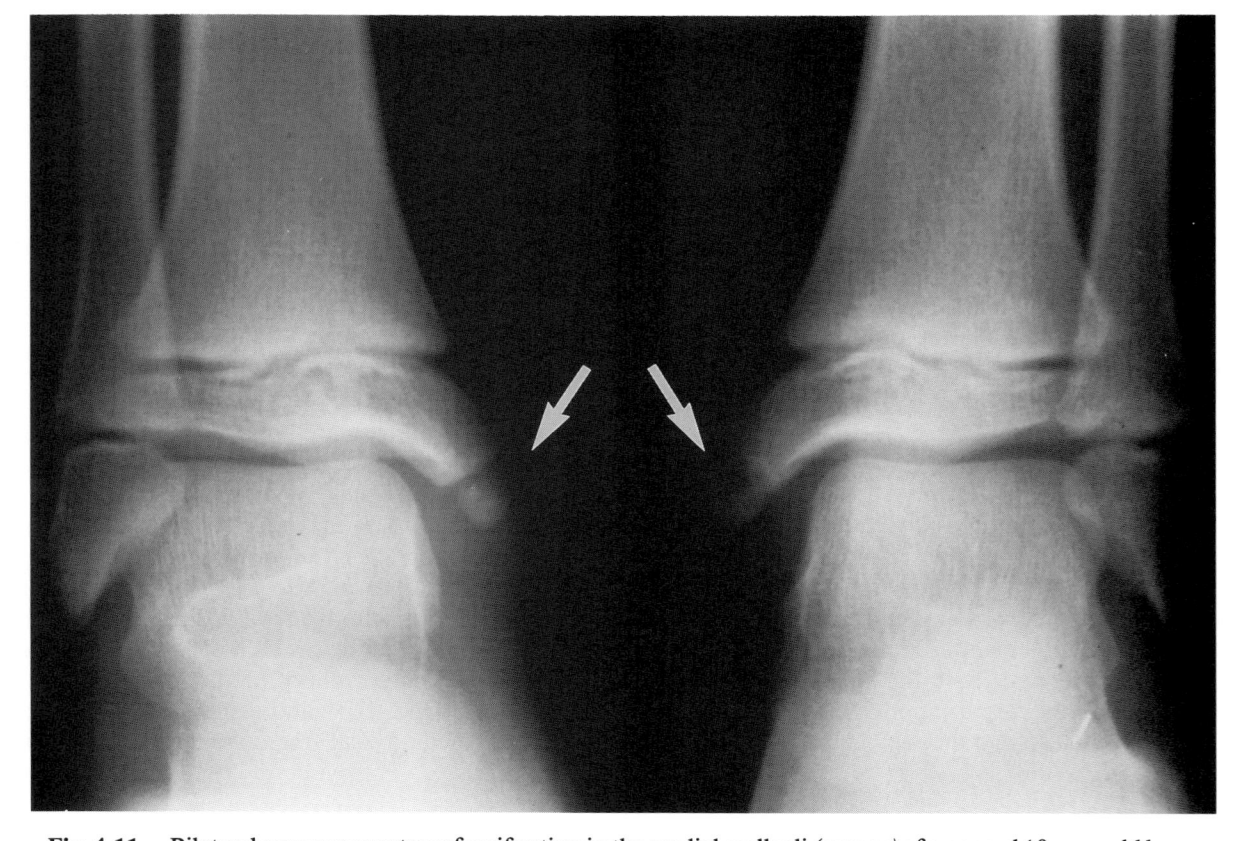

Fig. 4-11. Bilateral accessory centers of ossification in the medial malleoli *(arrows)* of a normal 10-year-old boy.

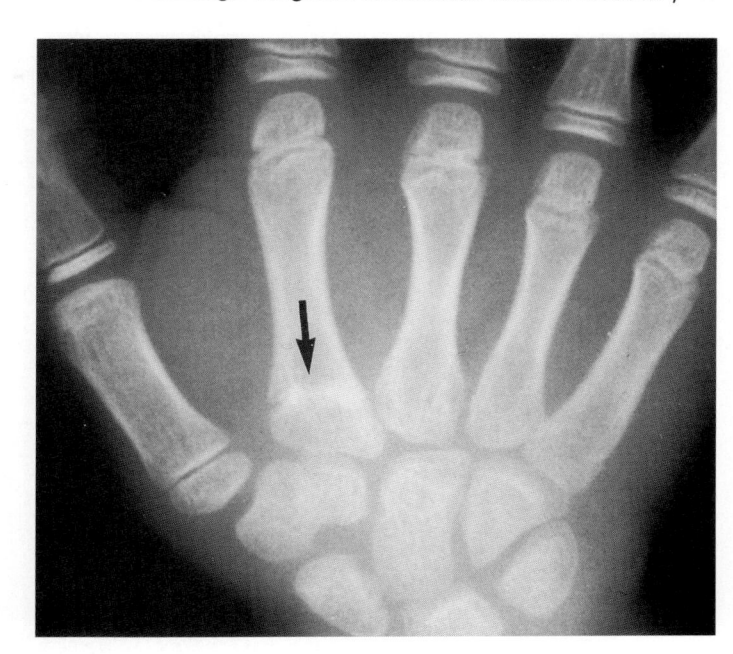

Fig. 4-12. Accessory center of ossification or "pseudoepiphysis" *(arrow)* at the base of the second metacarpal.

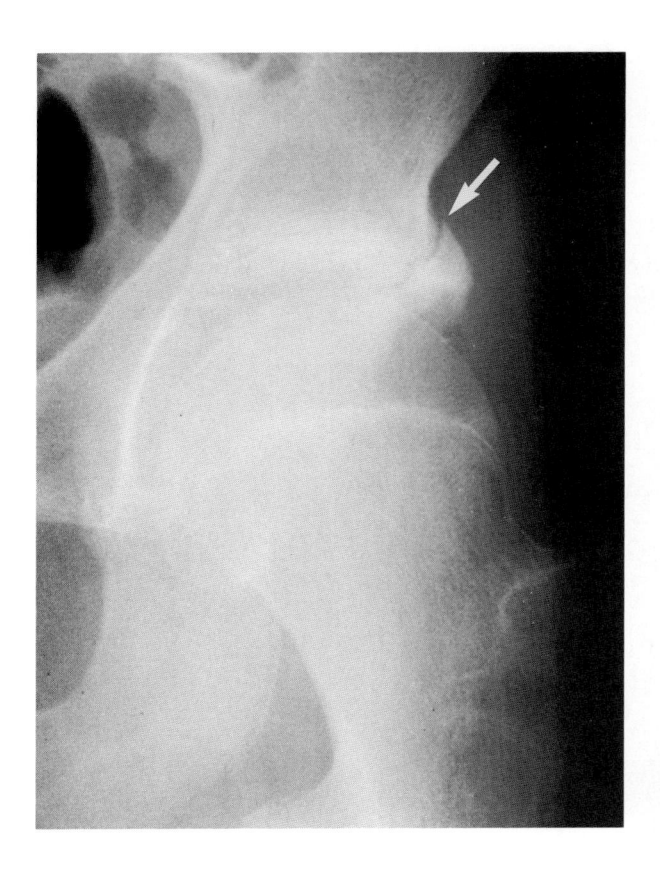

Fig. 4-13. Normal left hip in a 15-year-old boy. The accessory center of ossification or "os acetabuli" *(arrow)* could be mistaken for an acetabular fracture.

48 / Management of Pediatric Fractures

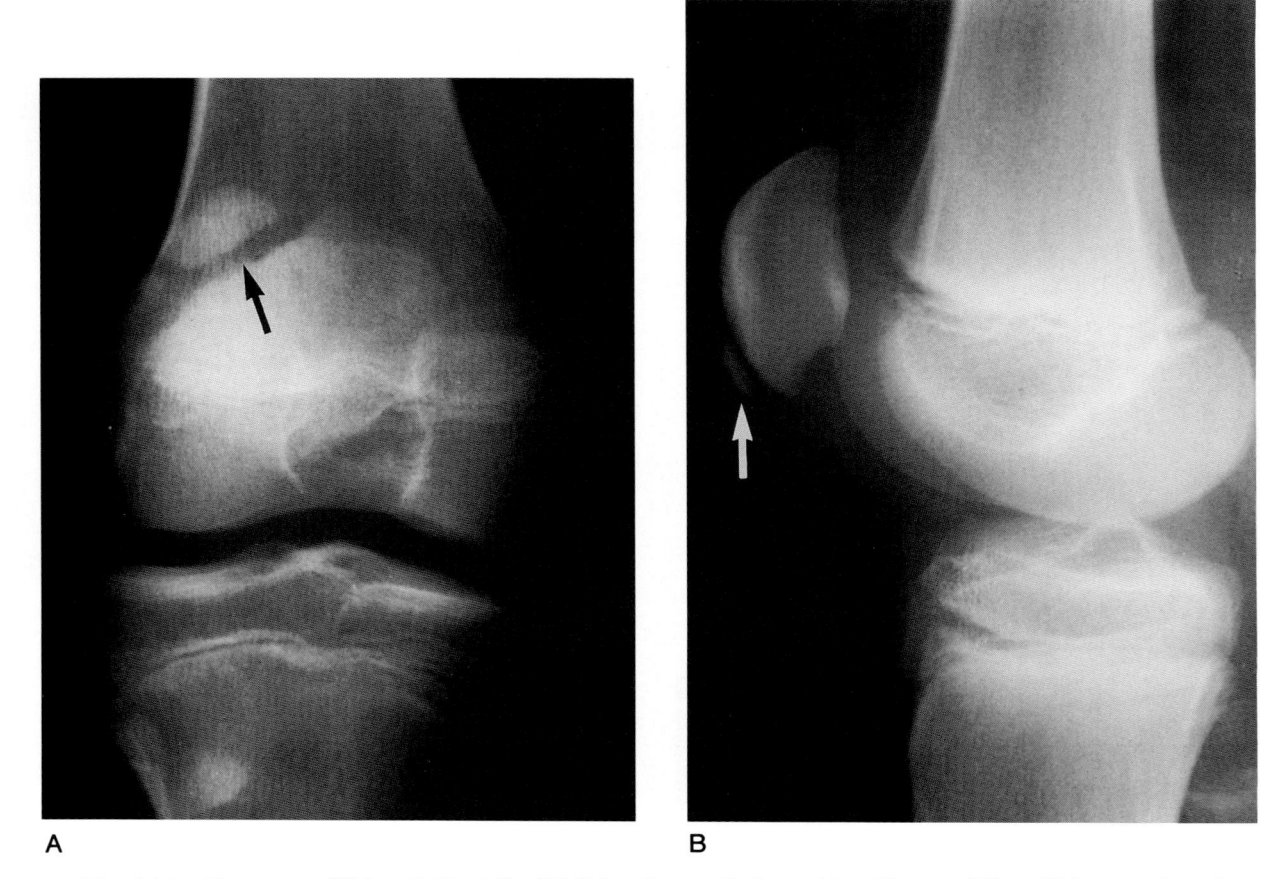

Fig. 4-14. Two types of "bipartite" patella. **(A)** Tripartite patella *(arrow)* in a 12-year-old boy. This superolateral location is the most common site of the accessory centers. **(B)** Bipartite patella *(arrow)* in a 13-year-old boy. This anteroinferior location is uncommon.

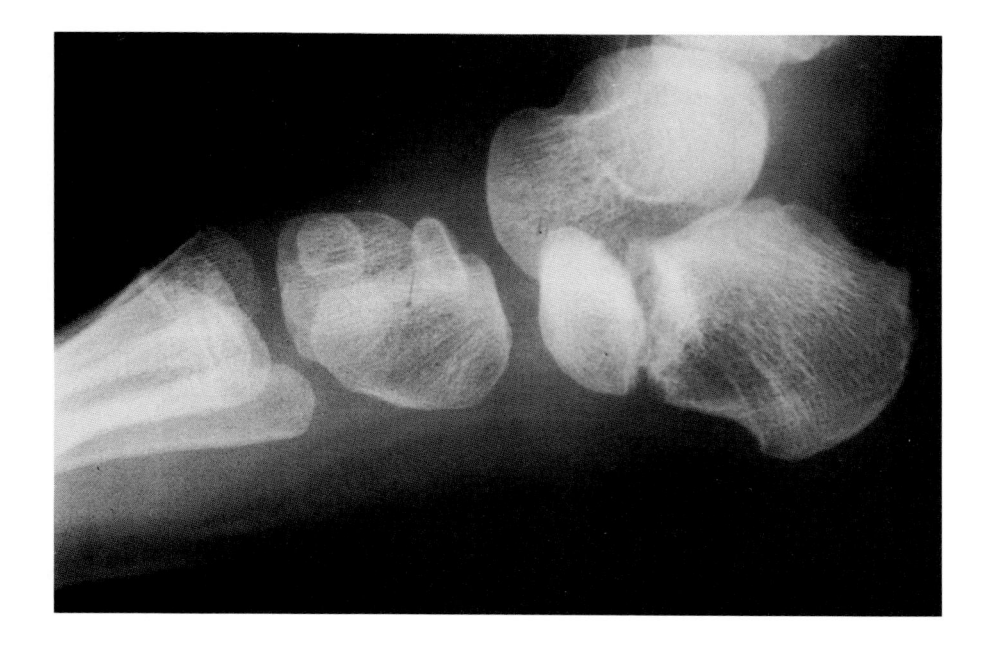

Fig. 4-15. Bipartite primary center of ossification for the calcaneus in a 10-year-old boy.

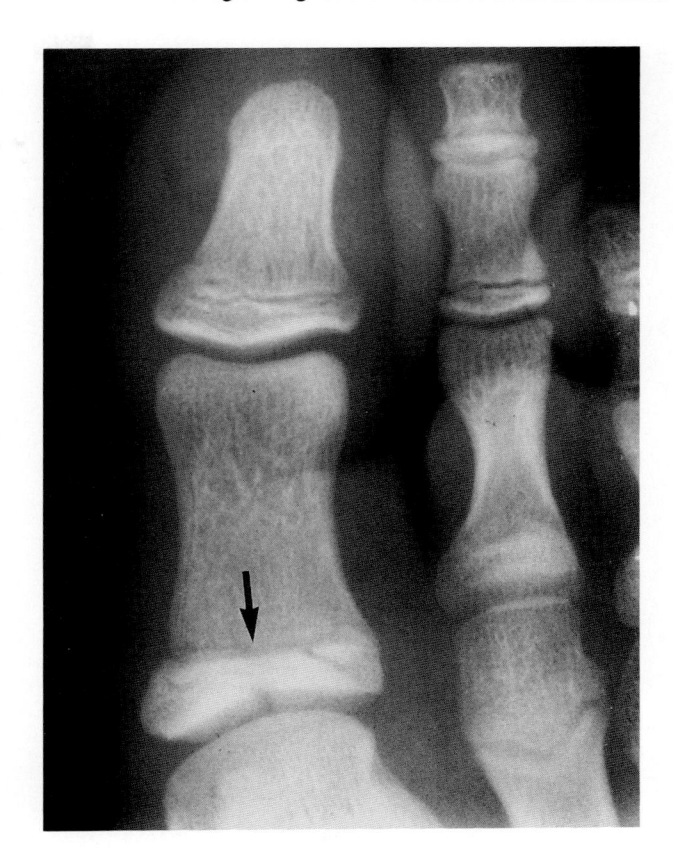

Fig. 4-16. Bipartite secondary center of ossification at the base of the proximal phalanx *(arrow)* of the great toe in a normal 13-year-old boy.

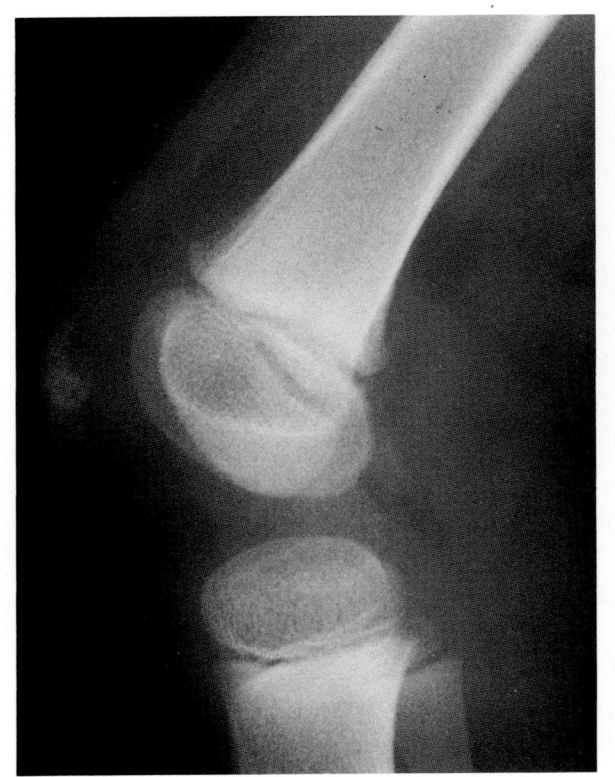

Fig. 4-17. Irregular primary center of ossification in the patella of a normal 6-year-old girl.

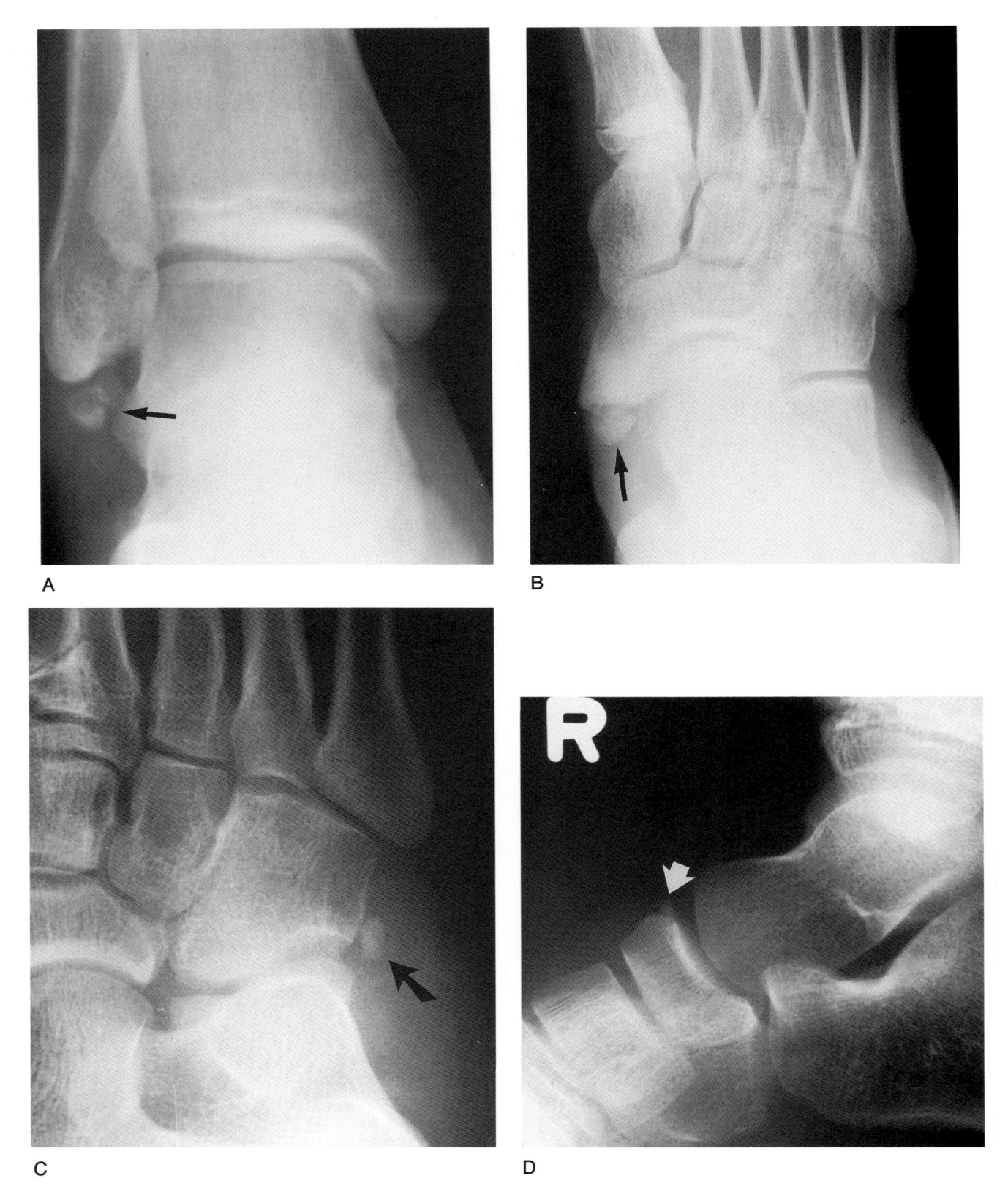

Fig. 4-18. Varieties of accessory ossicles in the ankle. **(A)** Double os subfibulare *(arrow)* in an 18-year-old boy. **(B)** Os tibiale externum *(arrow)* in a 10-year-old girl. **(C)** Os peroneum *(arrow)* in a 14-year-old boy. **(D)** Os supranaviculare *(arrow)* in a 10-year-old boy.

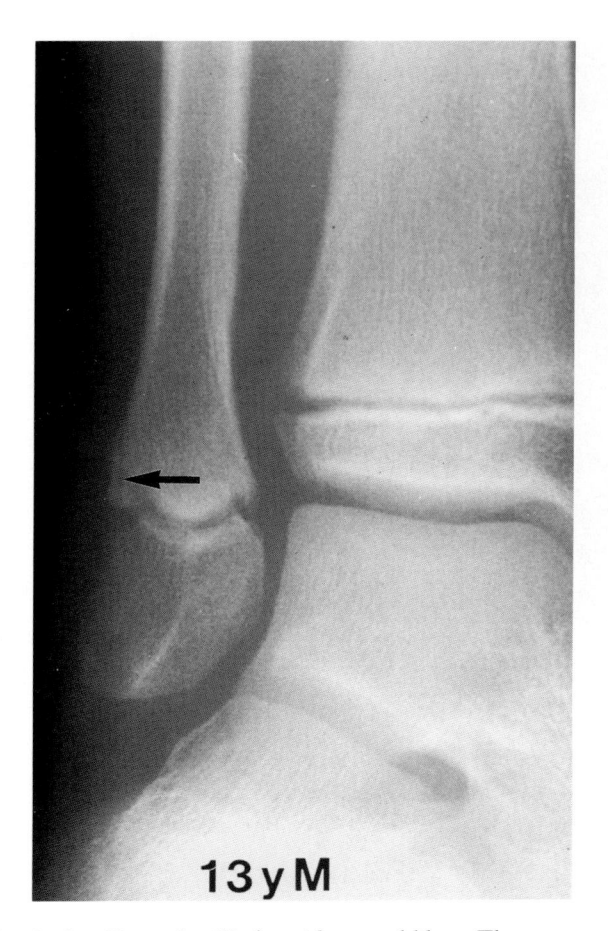

Fig. 4-19. Normal ankle in a 13-year-old boy. The apparent fragment in the lateral aspect of the distal fibular metaphysis *(arrow)* is a normal variant.

type II growth plate injury. In addition, growth plate remnants in the closing distal radial epiphyses are another normal variant that can mimic this type of fracture.[19]

Irregular Metaphyses

Metaphyseal irregularity is seen in adolescents at many sites, including the distal femoral metaphysis (Fig. 4-20), the medial aspect of the proximal humerus, the proximal tibia, and the distal fibula. It can mimic subperiosteal new bone and thus be mistaken for a healing injury. It has been called an "avulsive cortical irregularity," suggesting that it is related to mechanical stress.[20] Keats and Joyce[21] have suggested that these cortical irregularities, in all sites, represent a variation in normal bone growth.

Vascular Grooves

Normal vascular grooves or impressions on bone can cause linear lucencies easily mistaken for fractures. This is most common in the skull, where the meningeal vessels and diploic veins cause grooving of the cortex. In the long cylindrical bones, nutrient arteries can be recognized by their typical oblique course, running "toward the elbow and away from the knee." Nutrient arteries are also seen in the iliac crest as centrally located, stellate linear lucencies.

Neural Grooves

Nerves can cause osseous grooves as well, but only the canal for the supraclavicular nerve (Fig. 4-21), seen on the superior surface of the clavicle, is inclined to be mistaken for a fracture.

Physiologic Metaphyseal Lucent Bands

The term *metaphyseal lucent bands* refers to the widespread, horizontal bands of bone demineralization or destruction found on the diaphyseal side of the zone of provisional calcification in a variety of conditions (Table 4-1), including multiple metaphyseal fractures, such as those associated with child abuse. However, it may be a normal physiologic phenomenon in infancy (Fig. 4-22), occurring when the bands of normal bone formed at the metaphyses during postnatal growth are contrasted with the relatively sclerotic bone that was present at birth.[18]

Physiologic Subperiosteal New Bone Formation

Subperiosteal new bone formation is a reaction to a variety of osseous insults. It can occur as a localized response or as a generalized phenomenon in a variety of disorders. One cause of widespread subperiosteal new bone formation is multiple skeletal trauma, and when this is discovered in an infant, child abuse should be considered. It has been shown, however, that widespread subperiosteal new bone (Fig. 4-23) can be found in 35 percent of normal full-term infants.[22] It is most frequently encountered in the femora and humeri, rarely prior to 1 month of age. It is believed to be a completely benign manifestation of normal periosteal growth, as the new bone is gradually converted into a new cortex. It can be difficult, in infants of this age, to differentiate between this physiologic new bone formation and that which is related to osseous pathology.

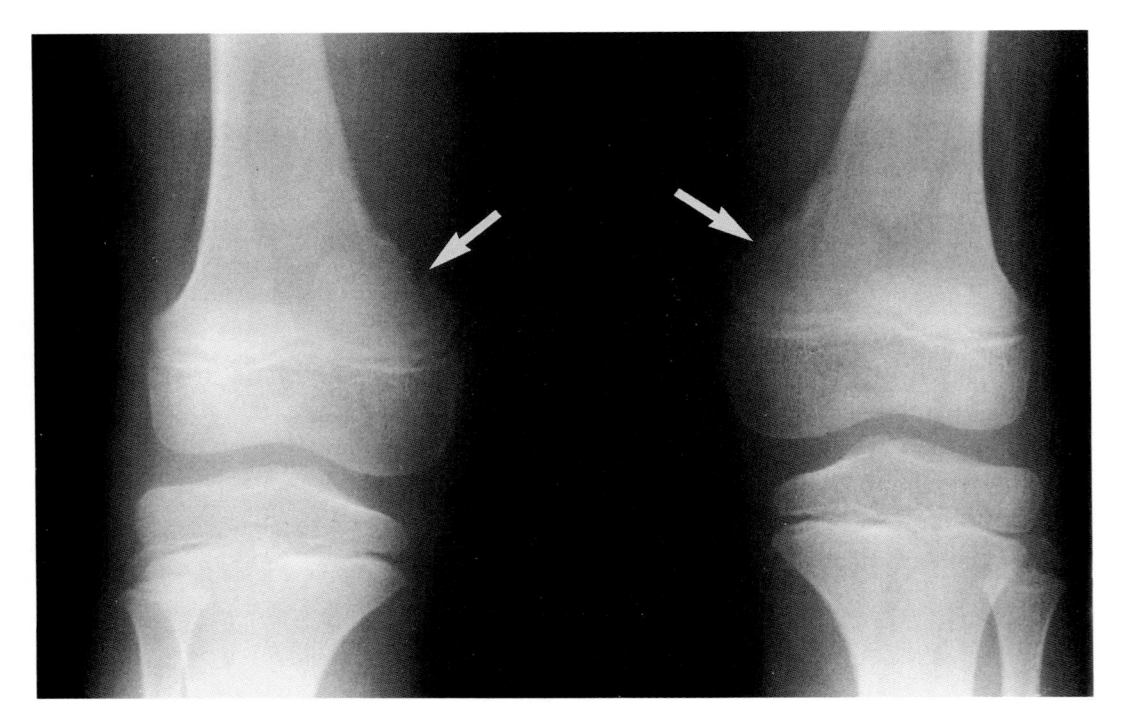

Fig. 4-20. The normal knees in a 6-year-old asymptomatic girl. Note bilateral metaphyseal irregularity *(arrows)* on the medial aspect of both distal femora.

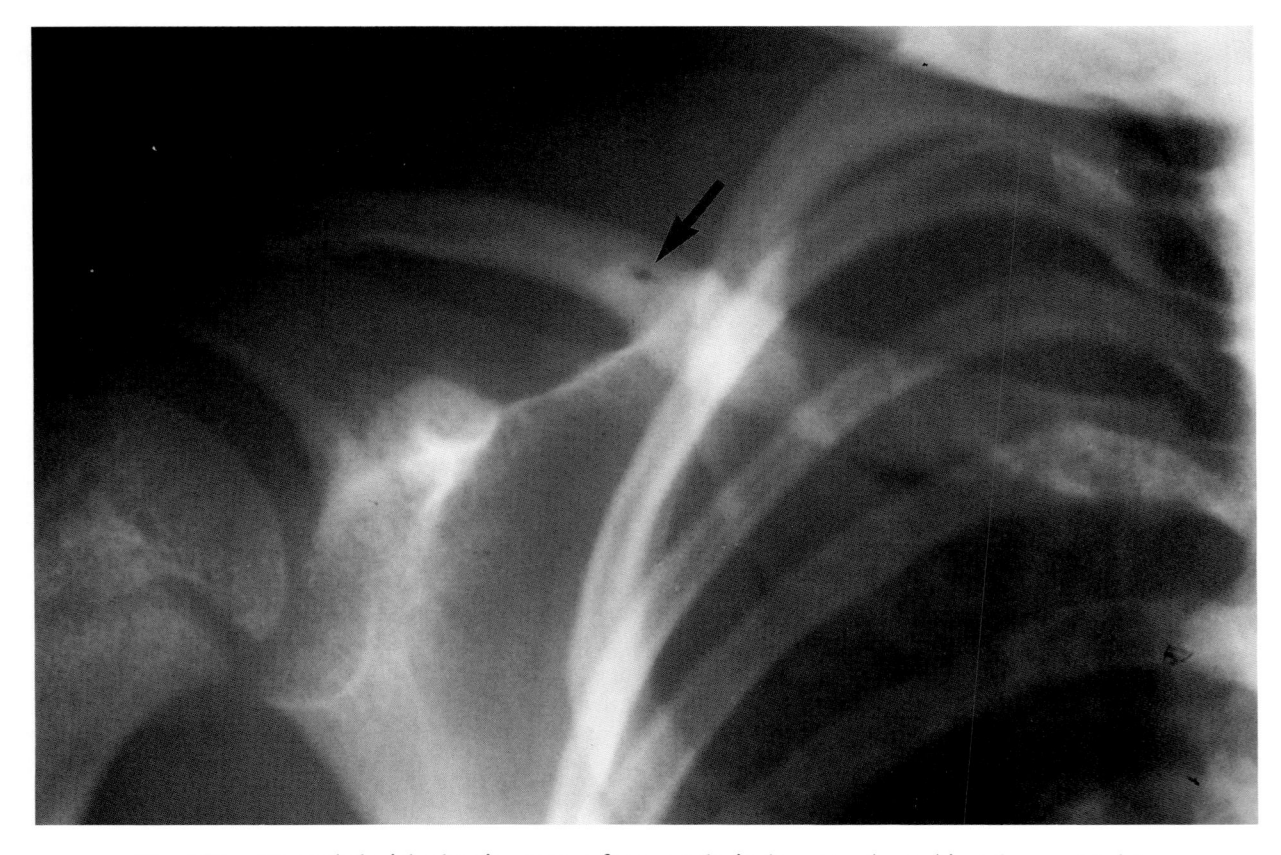

Fig. 4-21. Normal clavicle showing groove for supraclavicular nerve *(arrow)* in a 4-year-old girl.

TABLE 4-1. Causes of Metaphyseal Lucent Bands in Children

Normal
  Physiologic metaphyseal lucent bands
Congenital
  Osteopetrosis
  Osteogenesis imperfecta
Infectious
  Congenital syphilis
  TORCH infections
Trauma
  Multiple metaphyseal fractures
Metabolic
  Scurvy
  Healing rickets
  Hypophosphatasia
  Chronic systemic illnesses
Neoplastic
  Leukemia
  Lymphoma
  Metastases, i.e., neuroblastoma

Nontraumatic Pathology That Can Mimic Trauma

Osseous defects, deformities, and new bone formation are radiologic features of many localized and generalized osseous disorders. As a consequence, trauma enters the differential diagnosis of many skeletal diseases, too numerous to detail here. Nevertheless, we will attempt to catagorize and define some of the common problems.

Congenital Defects

Congenital osseous defects are gaps of variable width that are present from birth and are presumably developmental aberrations. They occur in predictable locations, such as in the neural arches (Figs. 4-24 and 4-25) and the odontoid (see Fig. 4-4). In addition to their characteristic locations, they can be differentiated from recent fractures by their smooth, sclerotic margins, as seen by conventional or computed tomography.

Congenital Pseudarthroses

A congenital pseudarthrosis is a special form of developmental osseous defect in which there is a persistent gap in the affected bone with sclerotic margins simulating an acquired, ununited fracture.[23] Although this abnormality occurs in the femur, clavicle, humerus, first rib, and forearm bones, the most common site is the tibia

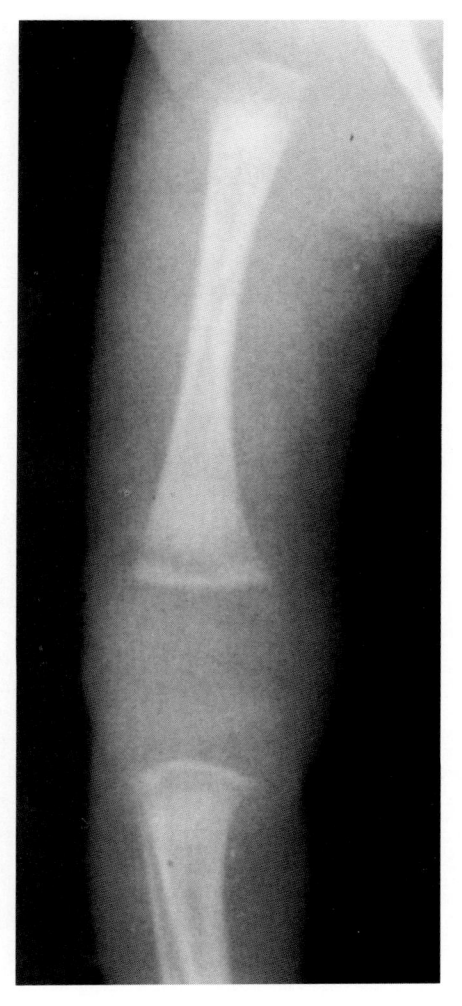

Fig. 4-22. Physiologic metaphyseal lucent bands in the right femur of an 11-day-old premature neonate.

(Fig. 4-26). Pseudarthroses are also found in the subtrochanteric region in proximal focal femoral deficiency and the femoral neck in congenital coxa vara.

Congenital Deformity

Congenital deformities can be defined as skeletal growth disturbances of embryologic or developmental origin that are present from birth. There are a number of congenital osseous deformities that can be mistaken for recent or old fractures, as well as other injuries. For example, the congenital tibial bowing that precedes congenital pseudarthrosis can mimic a "plastic fracture,"

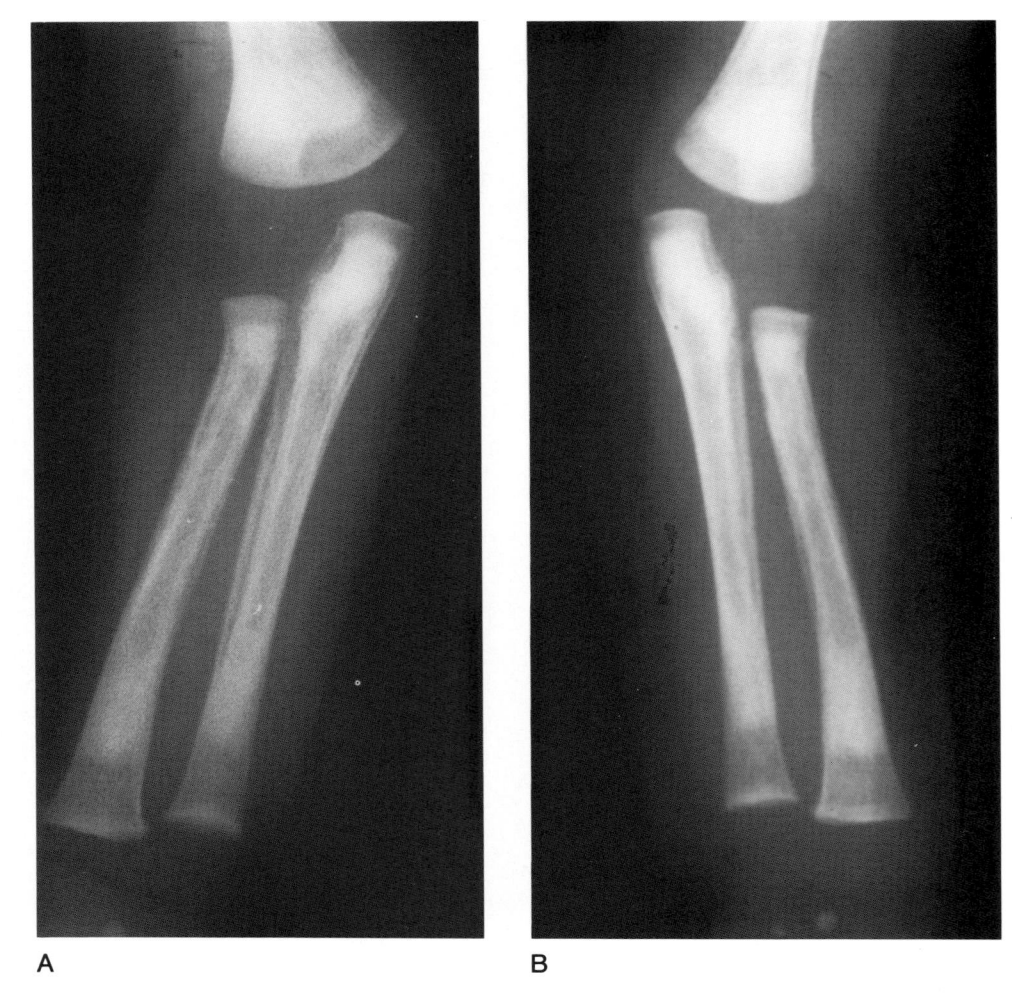

Fig. 4-23. Physiologic subperiosteal new bone along the shafts of the **(A)** right and **(B)** left ulna and radius. Physiologic metaphyseal lucency is also seen. (From Reed,[23] with permission.)

and congenital hypoplastic vertebral bodies can simulate compression fractures.

Pathologic Metaphyseal Lucent Bands

As noted above, metaphyseal lucent bands may be a normal phenomenon, particularly in infancy, but they also occur in a variety of disease processes (Table 4-1). Scurvy and congenital syphilis are two diseases within this group that deserve some discussion because of the close similarity of their radiographic findings to those of child abuse.

Infants with scurvy are usually 6 to 18 months of age and can mimic child abuse clinically by being irritable with swollen, tender extremities and a bleeding tendency.[24] In addition, many of the radiographic features of scurvy, namely, metaphyseal lucent bands, widespread subperiosteal new bone formation, and pathologic fractures (Fig. 4-27), are also seen in child abuse. The symmetry of the metaphyseal changes in scurvy, along with its generalized demineralization, "pencil-line cortices" and "ring epiphyses" will help differentiate this condition from child abuse.

Congenital syphilis[25] has been making a comeback in North America in recent years, and, in our experience, its radiographic findings have been confused with those of child abuse. The destructive metaphyseal lesions of syphilis (Fig. 4-28) can mimic recent metaphyseal fractures, while its diaphyseal periostitis simulates healing fractures. To add to the confusion, pathologic fractures can occur through the metaphyseal lesions. Congenital

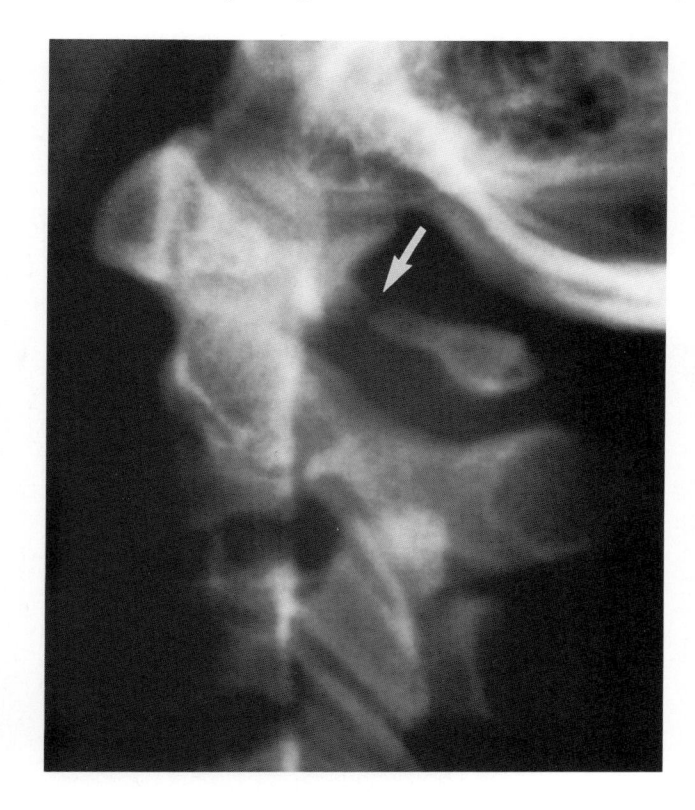

Radiologic Diagnosis of Pediatric Skeletal Trauma / 55

Fig. 4-24. Congenital defects in the atlas in a 14-year-old trauma victim. The lateral view of the cervical spine shows bilateral defects *(arrow)* in the hypoplastic posterior arch of the atlas.

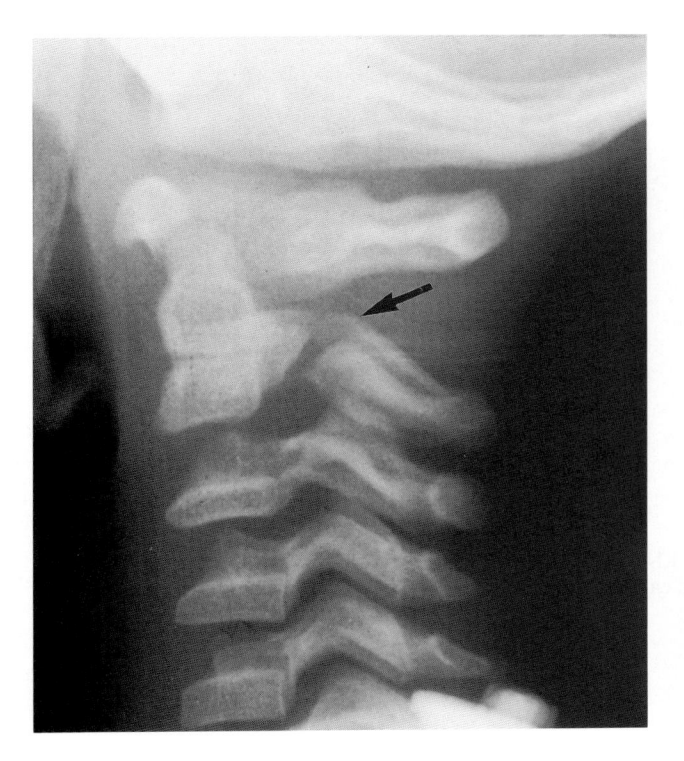

Fig. 4-25. Cervical spondylolisthesis in a 3-year-old trauma victim. The lateral cervical spine film shows bilateral, well-marginated defects *(arrow)* in the neural arch of the axis associated with anterior displacement of C2 on C3. A hangman's fracture was suspected until films made at 3 months of age, showing the same anomaly, were reviewed. (From Reed,[23] with permission.)

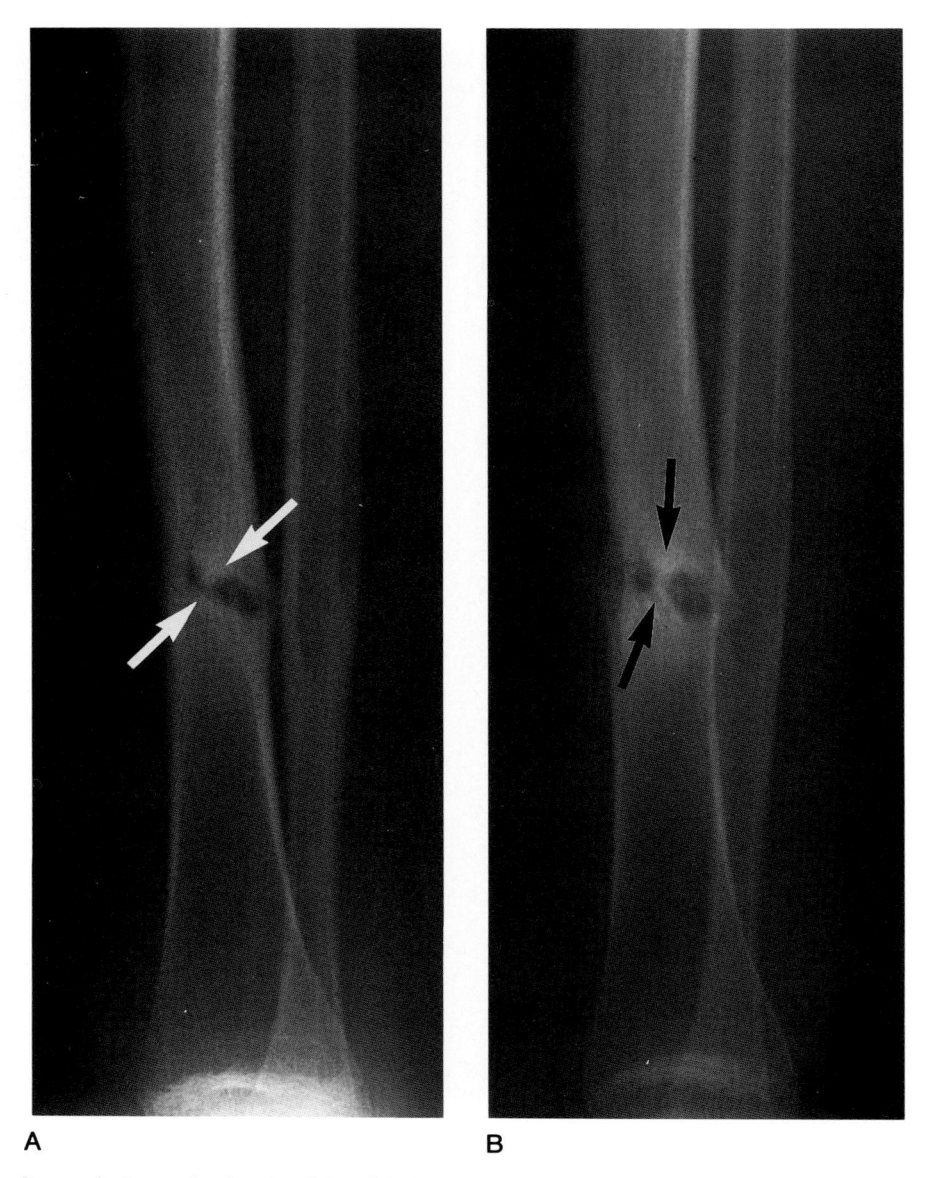

Fig. 4-26. Congenital pseudarthrosis of the tibia in a 12-year-old boy. **(A)** A defect is seen through a sclerotic region in the midtibia. **(B)** Four months later, in spite of casting, the pseudarthrosis is worse. (From Reed,[23] with permission.)

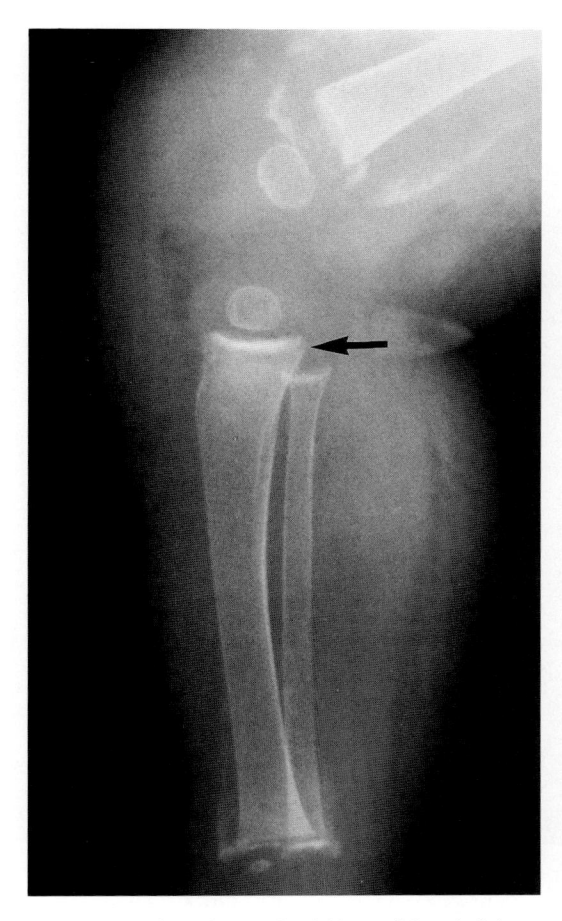

Fig. 4-27. Scurvy in a 6-month-old boy with painful extremities. Lateral radiograph of the left leg shows generalized osseous demineralization with a fine trabecular pattern, metaphyseal lucent bands *(arrow)*, pathologic fractures of distal femur, and distal tibia with adjacent organizing subperiosteal hematomas.

syphilis, however, has a tendency toward symmetric skeletal involvement, which is uncommon in child abuse. Furthermore, the bilateral symmetric, destructive lesions commonly found on the medial aspect of the proximal tibial metaphyses ("Wimberger's sign") is virtually pathognomonic for congenital syphilis.

Metaphyseal Spurs

Metaphyseal spurs are small fragments of bone that project from the margins of the metaphysis into the periphery of the growth plate (Fig. 4-29B&C), mimicking the metaphyseal fragmention that characterizes child abuse. They are found primarily in Menkes syndrome (kinky hair disease), a rare sex-linked recessive disorder of copper metabolism.[26] In this disease, they may actually be fractures, occurring as a result of an altered susceptibility of bone to trauma. In addition, this disease can manifest widespread subperiosteal new bone of the long bones with thickening of the ribs (Fig. 4-29A) and scapulae, further increasing the difficulty in differentiating it from child abuse. The recognition of the other manifestations of the disorder, namely, failure to thrive, psychomotor retardation, seizures, and the kinky hair will help establish the diagnosis, and the detection of a low serum copper level will confirm it.

Pathologic Subperiosteal New Bone Formation

Subperiosteal new bone can be generated by any process that elevates the periosteum, and it is usually a reflection of early reparative efforts on the part of the bone. In addition to trauma, localized subperiosteal new bone can be seen in osteomyelitis, infantile cortical hyperostosis, and bone infarcts, as well as primary and metastatic neoplasms. Although the differentiation between trauma and these other causes can be difficult at times, in the majority of cases the problem is solved when the clinical features are considered in conjunction with the radiographic findings. The alternate imaging modalities can prove useful in difficult cases.

During the first 2 years of life, children with sickle cell disease can present with swollen hands and feet. This "hand-foot syndrome" may be the first indication of sickle cell disease in the child.[27] Radiologically, subperiosteal new bone will be found along the shafts of one or more of the short tubular bones (Fig. 4-30). Although this can resemble fractures, it is usually caused by bone infarction in these patients. The diagnosis of multiple bone infarcts will be established when the presence of sickle cell disease is confirmed.

Widespread subperiosteal new bone formation is a feature of a variety of congenital and acquired osseous diseases, including multiple healing fractures. The majority of the diseases are easily differentiated from traumatic lesions, but infantile cortical hyperostosis or Caffey's disease[28] is an exception. This rare disease of infancy presents with localized or widespread subperiosteal new bone involving any bone, but most commonly the mandible, ribs, scapulae, clavicles, and ulnae (Fig. 4-31). Although its etiology remains uncertain, it is

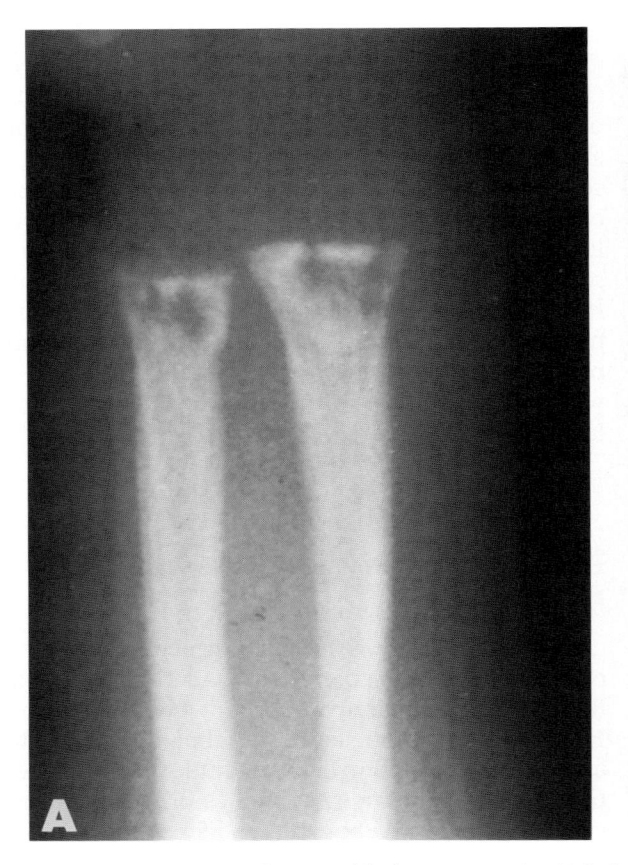

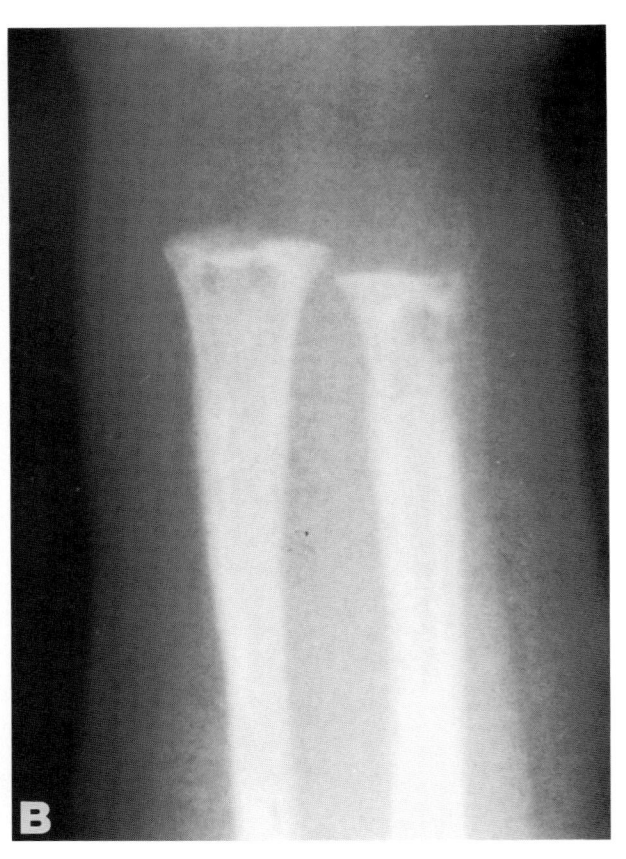

Fig. 4-28. Congenital syphilis in a 1-month-old infant with clinical suspicion of child abuse. Metaphyseal destructive lesions are seen in the distal radius and ulna of the **(A)** right and **(B)** left sides. In addition, subperiosteal new bone was seen along the humeral and femoral shafts. A diagnosis of syphilis was made by serology.

believed to be the result of a viral infection. The affected infants present with swelling and tenderness over the sites of skeletal involvement, associated with low-grade fever and an elevated erythrocyte sedimentation rate. The mandibular involvement is characteristic, and when it occurs in conjunction with the other findings, the diagnosis can be made with ease. Failing this, the diagnosis becomes one of exclusion.

Nontraumatic Dislocations and Subluxations

Traumatic dislocations are relatively uncommon in children, but there are many relatively common nontraumatic causes of joint dislocations and/or subluxations, including congenital hip dysplasia and septic arthritis. The hip is the joint most commonly affected (Fig. 4-32). In addition, there are several syndromes in which neurogenic, neuromuscular, or chronic arthritic processes predispose to joint laxity or contractures and thus to multiple joint dislocations or subluxations.[29]

Traumatic Lesions That Mimic Other Pathology

Just as nontraumatic skeletal pathology can mimic bone and joint injuries, traumatic lesions are frequently mistaken for other disease processes. This applies to the typical acute skeletal injuries that result from accidental trauma, as well as a diverse group of atypical traumatic lesions of childhood, that includes stress-related injuries (Fig. 4-33), neuropathic injuries, osteochondral fractures, and myositis ossificans. The clinical and radiologic features of the majority of these are detailed elsewhere in this text.

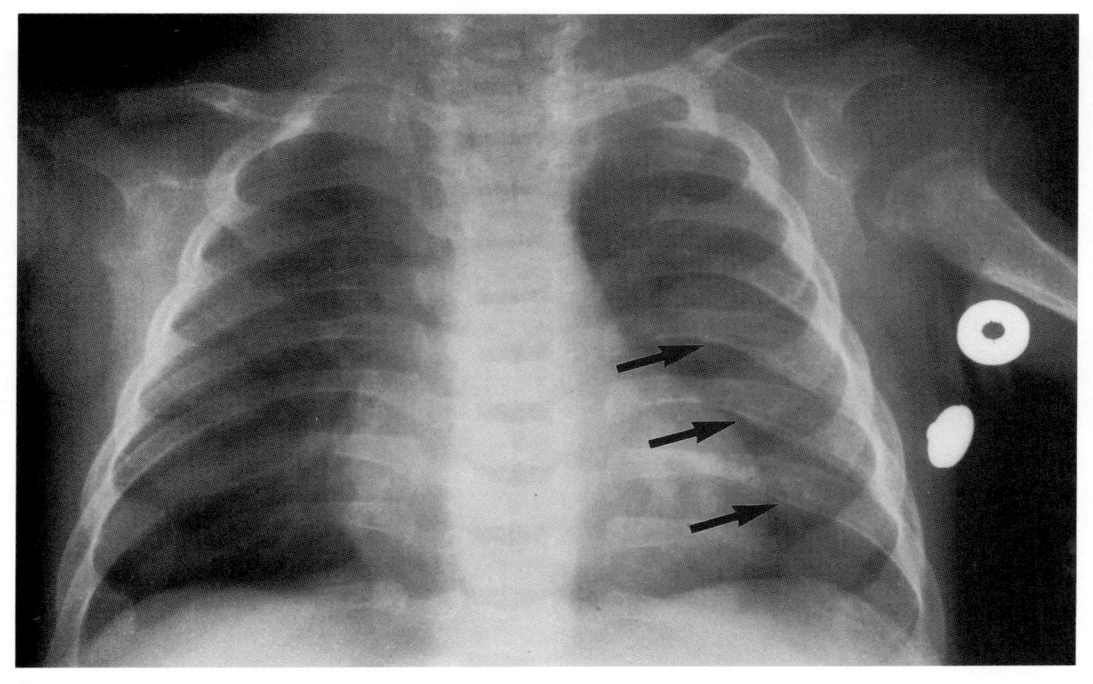

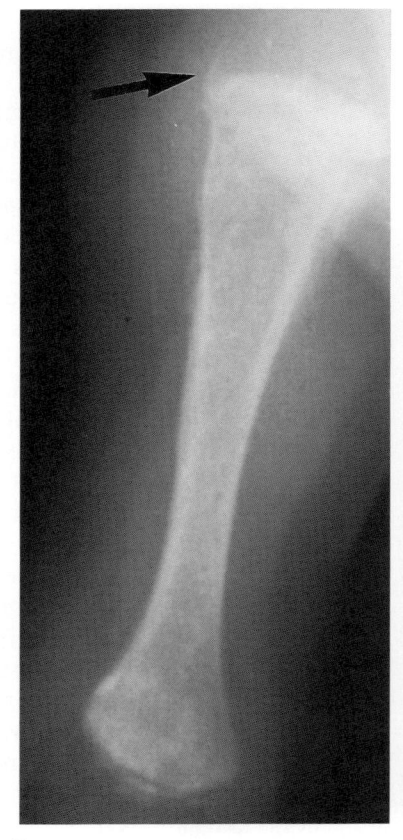

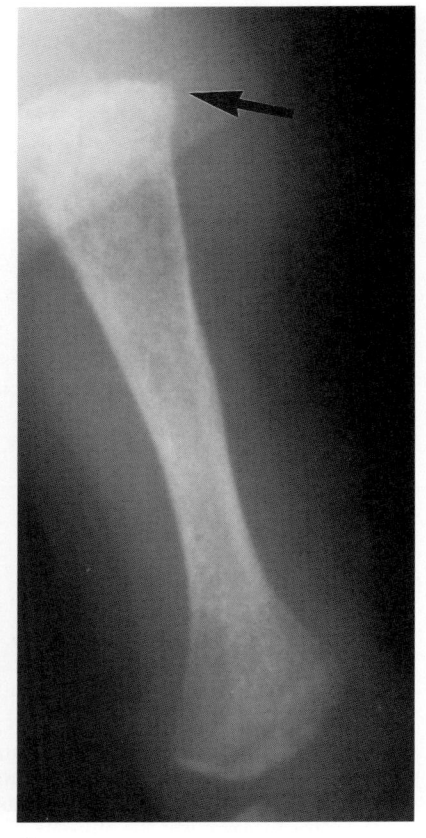

Fig. 4-29. Menkes syndrome in a 4-month-old boy. **(A)** Chest, **(B)** right, and **(C)** left humeral radiographs show subperiosteal new bone formation on the left 6th to 9th ribs *(arrow)* and metaphyseal fragmentation at both ends of the humeri *(arrow)*, mimicking multiple fractures. Child abuse was suspected until the diagnosis of Menkes syndrome was established by low serum copper levels.

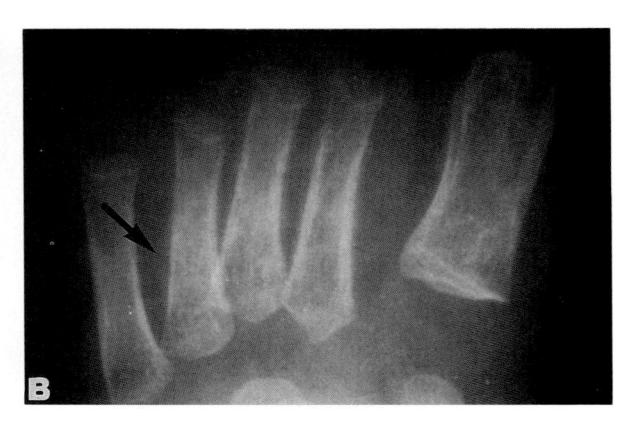

Fig. 4-30. Sickle cell disease with "hand-foot syndrome" in a 2-year-old black boy with swollen hands and feet. **(A)** Right metacarpals and **(B)** metatarsals show mottled rarefaction and fine subperiosteal new bone formation *(arrows)*.

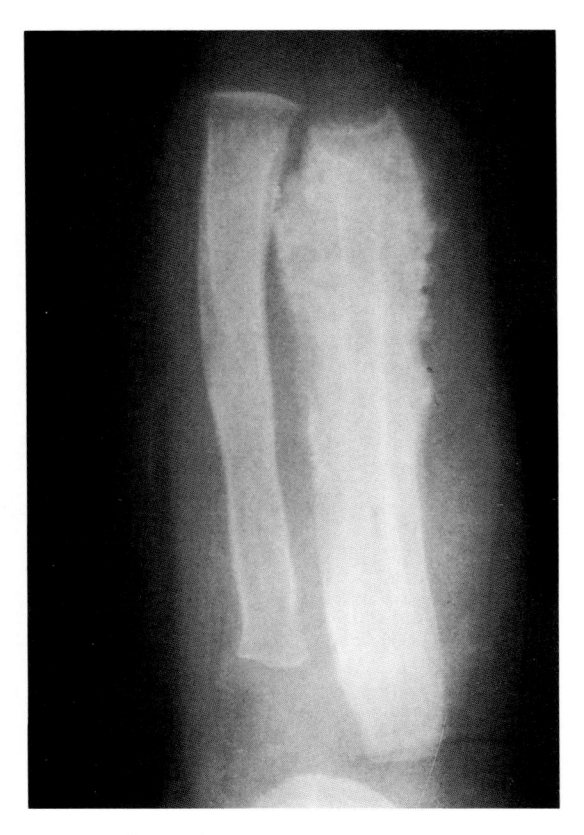

Fig. 4-31. Caffey's disease in a 5-month-old boy with a swollen left forearm. The radiograph shows exuberant periosteal new bone on the ulna and milder changes on the radius. In this child, the forearm was the only site of involvement and healing fractures were difficult to exclude.

THE SHOULDER AND SHOULDER GIRDLE

Technical Pitfalls in Trauma Diagnosis

The shoulder girdle is an anatomic region where it is particularly difficult to get two views at right angles, one to the other. The clavicle is a common site of fracture in children and the two views, anteroposterior and tangential, are essential. When the normal sigmoid-shaped clavicle is viewed obliquely, which can happen with slight shoulder movements in an infant, there may be a spurious appearance of clavicular fracture (Fig. 4-34) or deformity. The second view of the clavicle clarifies the situation. If there is a fracture of a humeral neck or a shoulder dislocation, internal and external rotation of the shoulder may be impossible for the child to perform. One may then have to rely on transthoracic or transaxillary views, which can be difficult to interpret.

The acromioclavicular joint region is often overexposed on clavicular studies in older children, and without increased illumination, fractures through the tip of the clavicle and acromioclavicular separations can hide in the dark. The sternoclavicular joint is difficult to evaluate by conventional radiography at the best of times because of the obliquity of the joint and the overlying adjacent osseous and soft tissue structures. CT is the best imaging modality for assessing injuries at this site.[6]

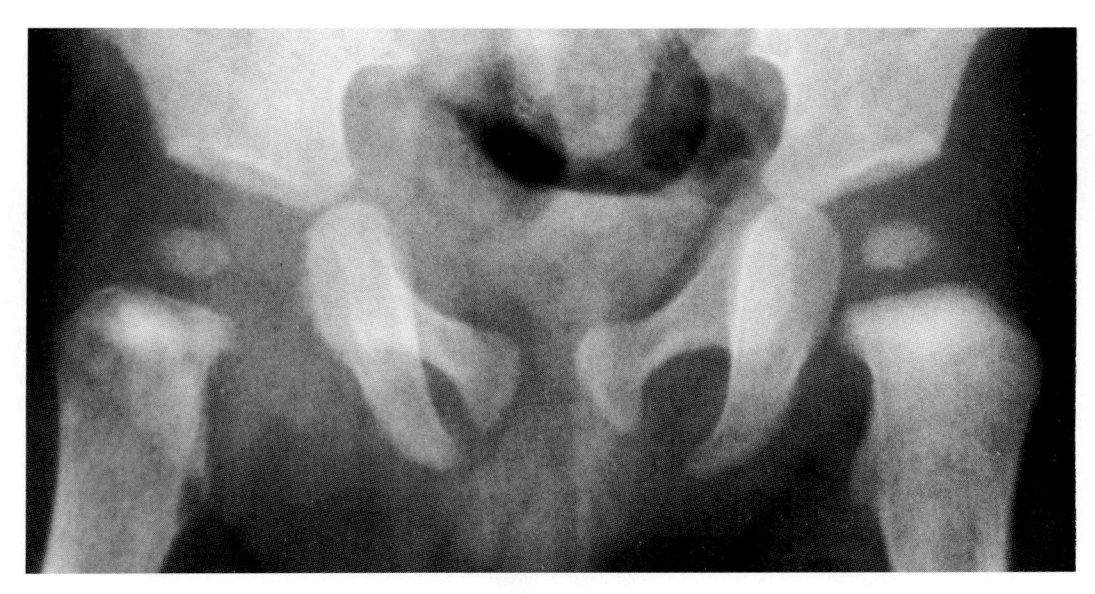

Fig. 4-32. Septic arthritis of the right hip in a 6-month-old infant with a tender immobile right leg. Note the lateral displacement of the right femoral head in the acetabulum. Septic arthritis is the usual etiology of this finding in infants, while trauma is a rare cause.

Normal Anatomy and Its Variants That Can Mimic Trauma

The growth plate for the coracoid process (Fig. 4-35) and the secondary centers of ossification found at both ends of the clavicle, the acromion, the tip of the scapula, and the margins on the glenoid are potential sources of fracture misdiagnosis in adolescents. The canal for the supraclavicular nerve is a groove or pinhole defect on the superior surface of the middle third of the clavicle (Fig. 4-21). It is seen in up to 6 percent of children and should not be misinterpreted as a clavicular fracture. A spurious widening of the acromioclavicular joint can be encountered in normal older children, just before the secondary ossification of the acromion begins. This should not be mistaken for an acromioclavicular separation.

The undulating configuration of the proximal humeral growth plate found in older children (Fig. 4-9A) is frequently mistaken for a humeral neck fracture by the unwary. On the other hand, one must be on guard for Salter-Harris type I growth plate injuries in this location (Fig. 4-9B). The bicipital groove of the proximal humerus, when rotated into profile, may lend an impression of subperiosteal new bone formation. In some normal older children, a notchlike metaphyseal irregularity can be found on the medial aspect of the proximal humeral metaphysis.

Nontraumatic Pathology That Can Mimic Trauma

Congenital pseudarthrosis of the clavicle (Fig. 4-36) is a congenital deformity of uncertain etiology that can mimic a clavicular fracture in children.[30] It usually occurs at the junction of the middle and distal thirds of the clavicle and, unlike a recent fracture, its margins tend to be slightly enlarged, smooth, and rounded. There is no callus or other evidence of healing. It is more common in females, usually affects the right clavicle, and is bilateral in up to 10 percent. Unlike other congenital pseudarthroses, that of the clavicle is not associated with multiple neurofibromatosis.

Cleidocranial dysplasia[31] is a relatively common, autosomal dominant skeletal dysplasia with characteristic cranial, dental, pelvic, and clavicular changes. The clavicular manifestations are that of partial or total aplasia. Clavicular defects, however, similar to that of congenital pseudarthrosis and mimicking ununited fractures can be encountered. The true nature of these defects will be recognized when the other features of the syndrome are uncovered.

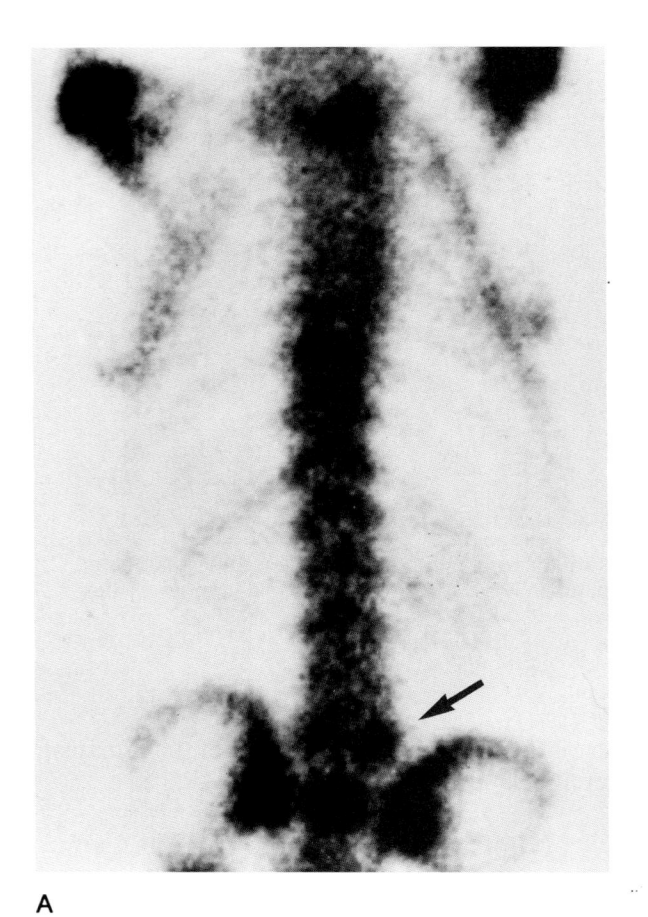

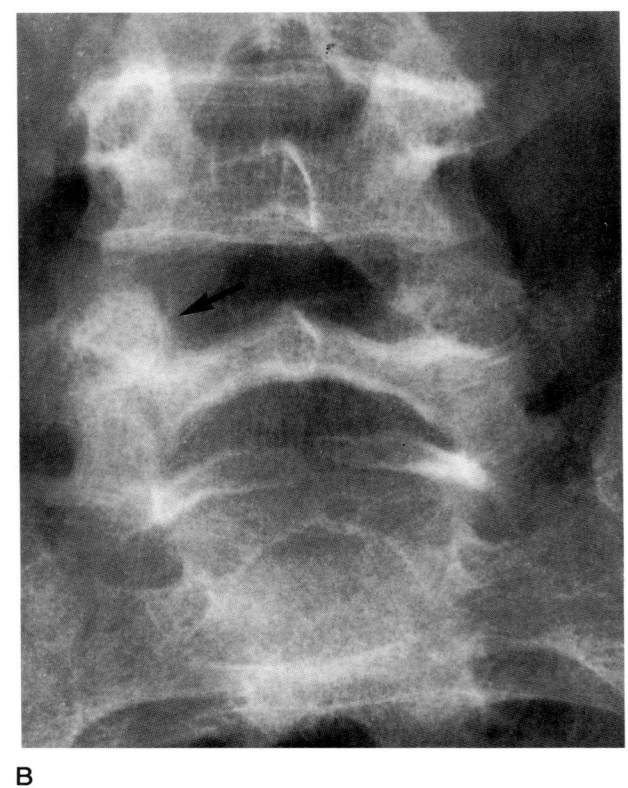

Fig. 4-33. Spondylolysis in an 11-year-old boy with back pain and a history of neuroblastoma. **(A)** ^{99m}Tc-MDP bone scan shows increased activity at the L5 pedicles *(arrow),* right more than left. Metastases were suspected. **(B)** AP view of L5 shows hypertrophied, sclerotic right pedicle *(arrow).* **(C)** Left oblique shows defect in the left pars interarticularis of L5 *(arrow). (Figure continues.)*

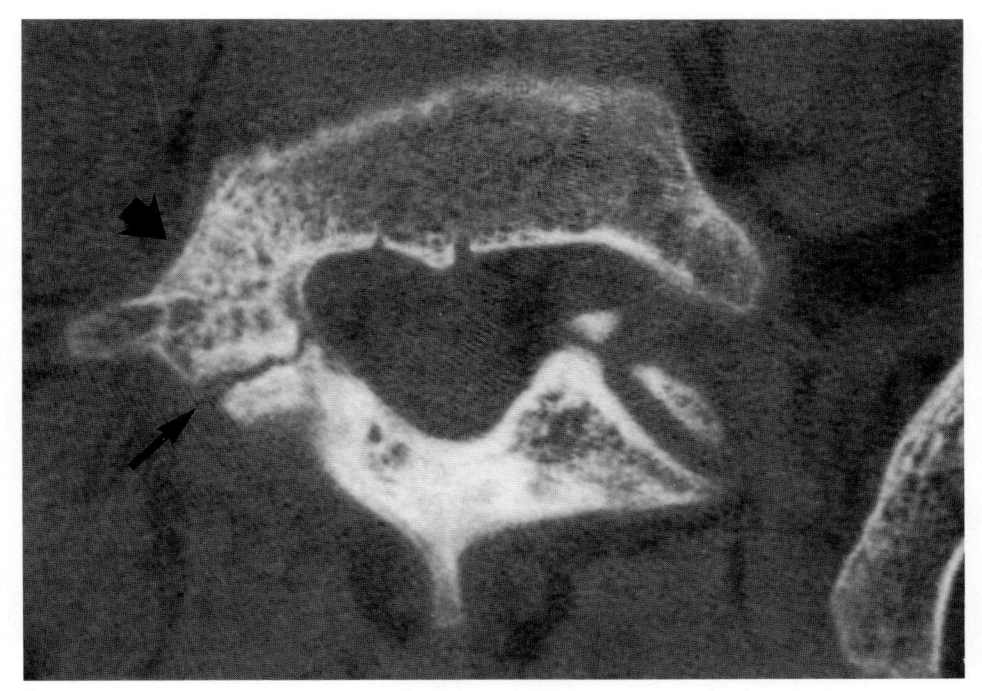

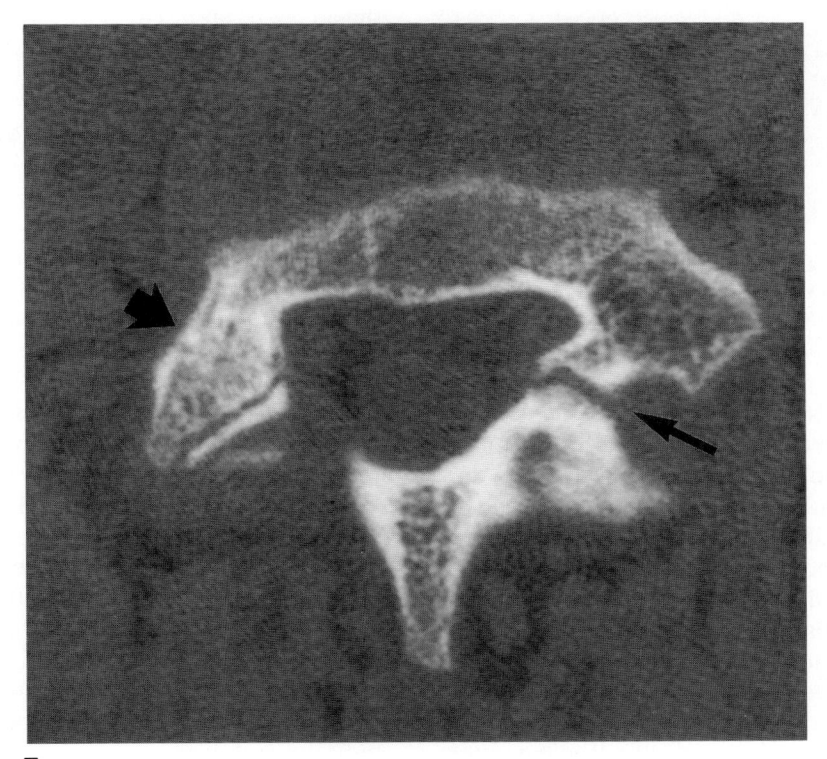

Fig. 4-33 *(Continued).* **(D & E)** Computed tomography of L5 neural arch shows a sclerotic, hypertrophied right pedicle *(wide arrows)* and bilateral defects in the pars interarticularis *(thin arrows)*. These are fractures that mimicked metastases.

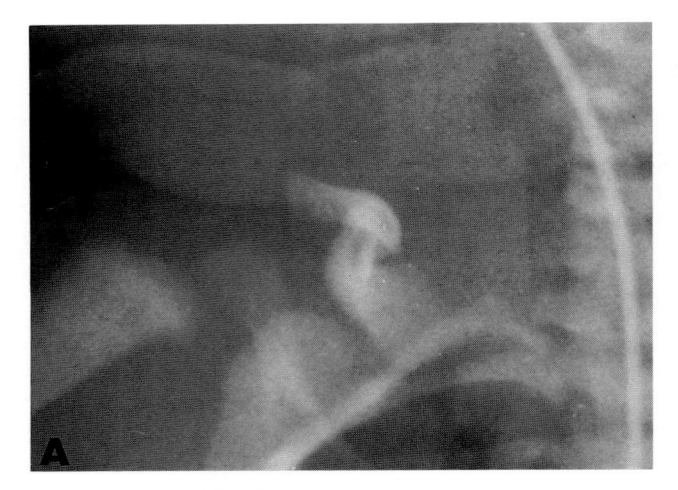

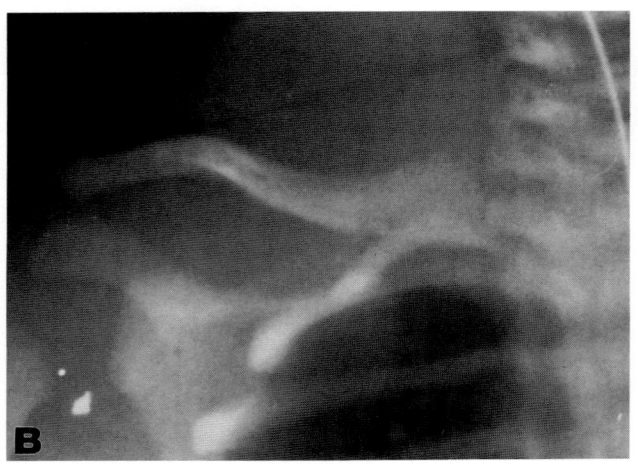

Fig. 4-34. Spurious right clavicular fracture in a newborn infant. **(A)** Oblique view looks like fracture. **(B)** Straight AP view shows normal clavicle.

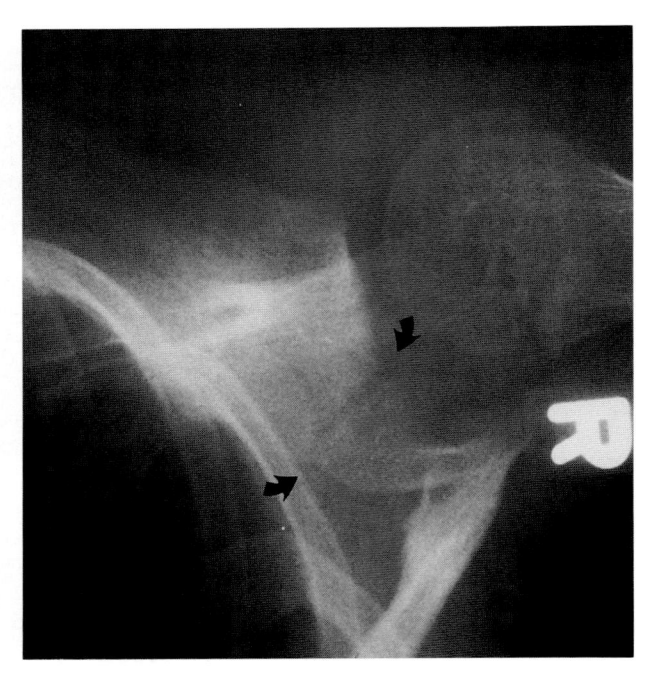

Fig. 4-35. Normal right shoulder in a 9-year-old boy. The growth plate for the coracoid process of the scapula *(arrows)* should not be mistaken for a fracture.

The clavicles and/or scapulae are relatively common sites for the hyperostosis of Caffey's disease[28] and may be the only sites of involvement in some cases. In these cases, it will be difficult to exclude trauma.

The distal and proximal ends of the clavicle are common sites for subchondral resorption of bone in children with hyperparathyroidism, usually secondary to chronic renal failure. These osseous defects should not be mistaken for fractures or joint separations. In addition, children with chronic renal failure can manifest epiphyseal displacements, including that of the proximal humerus.[32] These occur as the result of pathologic metaphyseal fractures secondary to the renal osteodystrophy and, while recognizing the fractures, one must not miss the underlying pathology.

THE ELBOW AND FOREARM

Technical Pitfalls in Trauma Diagnosis

The lateral view of the elbow must be made as a "true lateral" in flexion; if it is not, the anterior and posterior fat-pads cannot be accurately assessed, and it will be difficult to exclude a traumatic elbow joint effusion. The absence of an elbow joint effusion substantially decreases the chances of a significant injury. The presence of a joint effusion, however, should intensify the search for a fracture. If the routine views are unrewarding, additional oblique views may be added in hope of demonstrating a subtle fracture, such as a marginal fracture of the radial head or an undisplaced fracture of the lateral condyle. It has been suggested that a joint effusion is a sign of fracture either visible or occult, and, on this basis, further radiographic investigation is unnecessary. However, it has been shown that only 15 percent of patients with elbow joint effusions, without fracture on the initial films, have clinical or radiographic evidence of an occult fracture on follow-up studies.[33]

Dislocations of the elbow are frequently associated with avulsion fractures of the medial epicondyle, and the

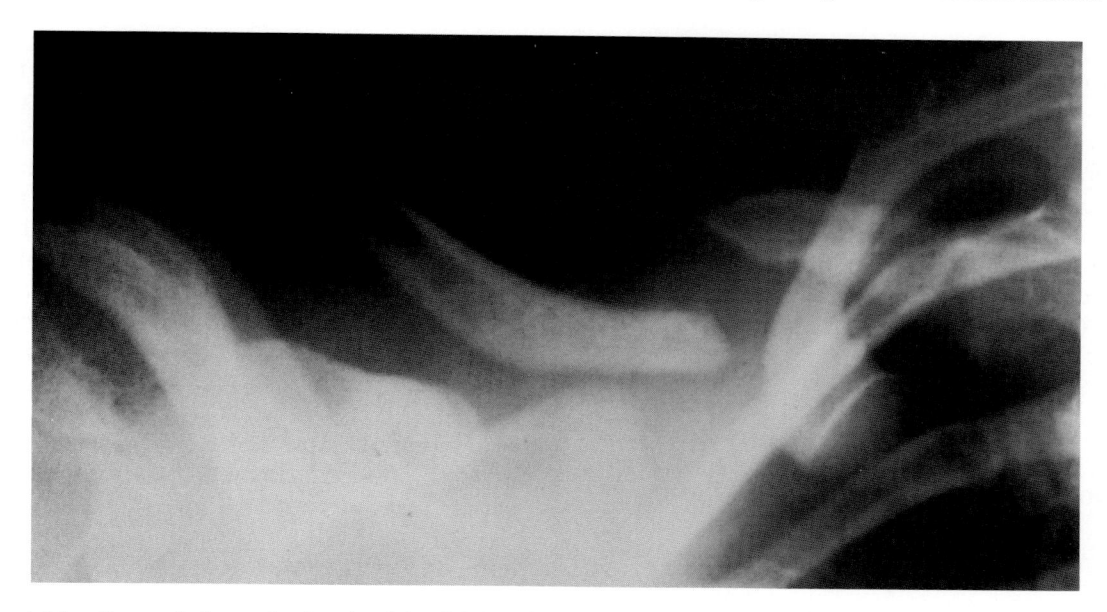

Radiologic Diagnosis of Pediatric Skeletal Trauma / 65

Fig. 4-36. Congenital pseudarthrosis of the right clavicle in a 12-year-old girl. Note the wide gap and smoothly corticated margins.

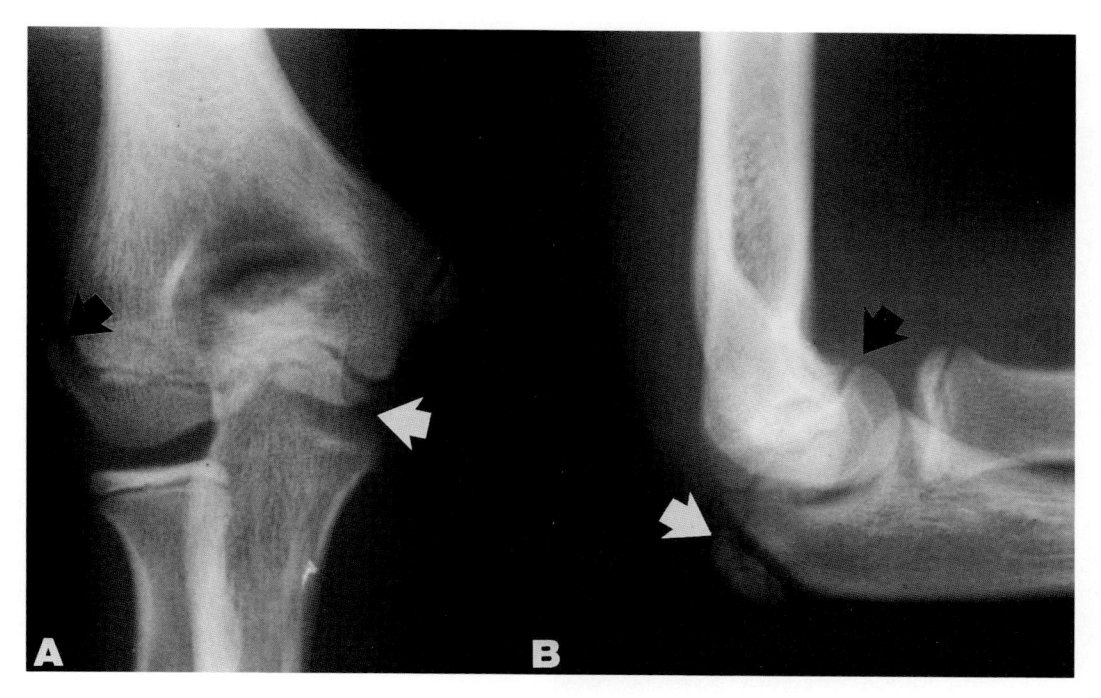

Fig. 4-37. Normal elbow of an 11-year-old boy. **(A)** AP view. The normal lateral epicondyle *(black arrow)* and fragmented trochlea *(white arrow)* can be mistaken for fractures. **(B)** Lateral view. The secondary center for the olecranon *(white arrow)* is often irregular or fragmented. The undisplaced anterior fat-pad *(black arrow)* will help exclude a fracture.

fragment may be trapped in the elbow joint. The radiologic examination of the injured joint, before and after reduction of the dislocation, should be designed to document this possible complication.

If the frontal projection of the forearm is made with the limb pronated, the ulna and radius will be crossed, partially obscuring each other. Also, if the forearm radiographs fail to include the elbow joint, a Monteggia fracture may be missed and if they fail to include the wrist, a Galliazzi fracture can be overlooked (see Ch. 17).

Normal Anatomy and Its Variants That Can Mimic Trauma

The six normal secondary centers of ossification about the elbow can be confused with fracture fragments (Fig. 4-37), particularly if one is unfamiliar with their sequence of appearance and closure. The lateral condyle usually ossifies first, appearing during the first year of life. This is usually followed by the radial head (5 to 6 years), the medial epicondyle (6 to 9 years), the medial condyle (8 to 10 years), the olecranon (10 to 13 years), and, finally, the lateral epicondyle (13 years). The secondary center for the capitellum is usually tilted anteriorly, making the growth plate appear slightly wider posteriorly than anteriorly, simulating a Salter-Harris type I growth plate injury. In addition, the secondary centers, particularly the medial condyle and olecranon (Fig. 4-37), are frequently multipartite or fragmented in appearance, tempting the uninitiated to diagnose a fracture.

A supratrochlear foraminal bone is a separate ossicle that rests posteriorly in the olecranon fossa. It is a normal variant that can simulate a loose fracture fragment in the elbow joint. Also, a tiny sesamoid bone in the triceps tendon (patella cubiti), is occasionally seen adjacent to the olecranon process.

In the forearm bones of the newborn, normal undulations in the contours of the radius and physiologic new bone formation should not be confused with traumatic lesions. In the older child, one must not mistake nutrient vessels for fracture lines or the interosseous ridges of the radius and ulna for subperiosteal new bone.

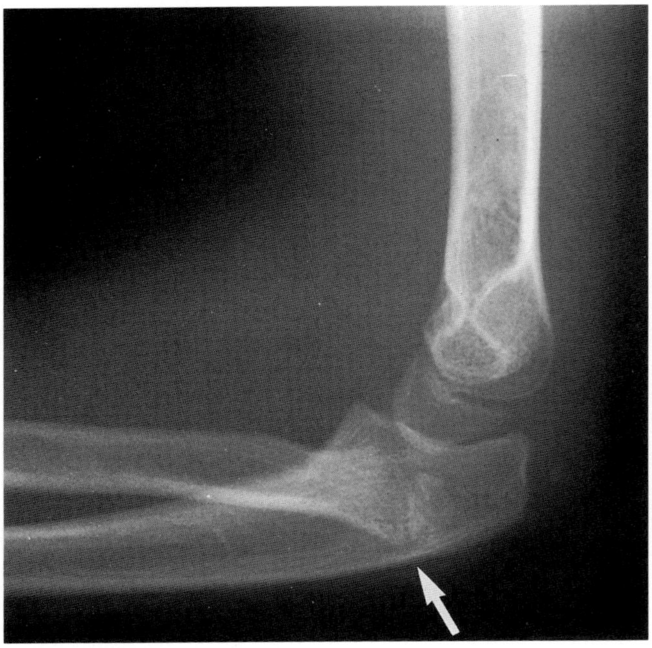

Nontraumatic Pathology That Can Mimic Trauma

Congenital dislocation of radial head[34] is a relatively common congenital anomaly in which the radial head is dislocated anteriorly, posteriorly or, rarely, laterally (Fig. 4-38). It can occur as an isolated anomaly or in association with a number of syndromes. In childhood, it may cause only mild limitation of flexion and extension. Radiologically, the dislocated radial head is dysplastic, while the capitellum is often hypoplastic. These findings are not seen with an acute traumatic dislocation. Often there is an associated proximal radioulnar synostosis and congenital dislocation can be associated with other forearm abnormalities. When present, these will make its differentiation from a long-standing traumatic dislocation less difficult.

Congenital pseudarthrosis of the forearm bones can involve the ulna, the radius or both.[35] Like the more common congenital pseudarthrosis of the tibia, it is often associated with neurofibromatosis and, in reality, an ununited pathologic fracture.

Fig. 4-38. Congenital dislocation of radial head in an 8-year-old girl. The lateral view of the elbow shows posterior displacement of the hypoplastic, deformed radial head *(arrow)*. (From Reed,[23] with permission.)

THE HAND AND WRIST

Technical Pitfalls in Trauma Diagnosis

Anteroposterior, lateral, and oblique views of the hand and wrist are generally reliable in fracture diagnosis. Special views may be necessary to clearly visualize the phalanges and carpal bones in special circumstances. The scaphoid is the most frequently fractured carpal bone, and it is not uncommon for these injuries to be imperceptible on the early radiographs. If one is unwilling to wait for follow-up radiographs to establish the diagnosis, a radionuclide bone scan can be employed (Fig. 4-7B).

Normal Anatomy and Its Variants That Can Mimic Trauma

In the distal radius, there are variations in the normal closure of the growth plate, such as remnants of the growth plate or marginal spurlike projections from the epiphysis, which can mimic fractures.[19] As with the proximal humerus, the undulating growth plate of the distal radius can create overlapping linear shadows that tempt fracture diagnosis. The utilization of the pronator quadratus fat planes helps in excluding injuries in cases such as these.[36] If the fat plane over the pronator quadratus is displaced anteriorly, the suspicion of a fracture should be increased. If the fat plane is undisplaced, a fracture, overt or occult, is virtually excluded.

The carpal bones, particularly the pisiform, can be irregular in shape or bipartite. Accessory ossicles are found less frequently in the wrist than the ankle. Nevertheless, 23 of them have been identified and named.[17] All are normal variants with a potential of being mistaken for fracture fragments. The most common, in our experience, is the accessory ossicle at the tip of the ulnar styloid process ("os ulnostyloideum"), which can be indistinguishable from an ununited fracture.

In addition to the accessory ossicles, one can confuse accessory sesamoid bones with fracture fragments. These normal variants, however, are smooth, rounded ossicles that can occur anterior to the heads of all the metacarpals and most of the terminal interphalangeal joints.

Accessory centers of ossification can be found at the bases of the all the metacarpals, most commonly the second (Fig. 4-12), as well as the head of the first. These "pseudoepiphyses" can be differentiated from fractures by their typical location and appearance.

Nontraumatic Pathology That Can Mimic Trauma

Madelung deformity of the wrist is a congenital deformity characterized by shortening and dorsolateral bowing of the radius, dorsal subluxation of the distal ulna, and a triangular configuration of the carpal bones with the lunate at the apex.[37] It is more common in females, tends to be bilateral and is usually associated with a form of mesomelic dwarfism called "dyschondrosteosis." A similar deformity can develop as an acquired condition if the distal radial growth plate is damaged from trauma or infection.

There are a number of congenital deformities of the fingers that can be misconstrued as results of trauma.[38] These include clinodactyly, camptodactyly, and Kirner's deformity (Fig. 4-39). In the latter, the terminal phalanx of the fifth digit is deformed and incurved, often with a transverse defect across its base that can be mistaken for a fracture.

THE SPINE

Technical Factors in Fracture Diagnosis

The radiographic evaluation of the cervical spine can be difficult in children, particularly for trauma. Frontal and lateral projections of the cervical spine with open-mouth views of the odontoid are the usual routine. However, the lower cervical and upper thoracic segments are frequently imperceptible on routine lateral views, and a "swimmer's view" may have to be added before a fracture can be excluded.

If the lateral view is not a "true lateral," a spurious impression of a facet injury may be obtained. Oblique views are a useful option when a facet injury is suspected. The investigation of this type of injury may not be complete until conventional or computed tomography are utilized.

If instability is suspected at any level of the cervical spine, lateral views made in flexion and extension are helpful. We prefer, however, careful dynamic fluoroscopy of the cervical spine in these cases.

The open-mouth view can be particularly difficult to obtain in struggling children. When suboptimal, this view can promote a spurious diagnosis of odontoid fracture, created by the overlying teeth or occiput. Conventional or computed tomography may be necessary before an odontoid injury can be excluded.

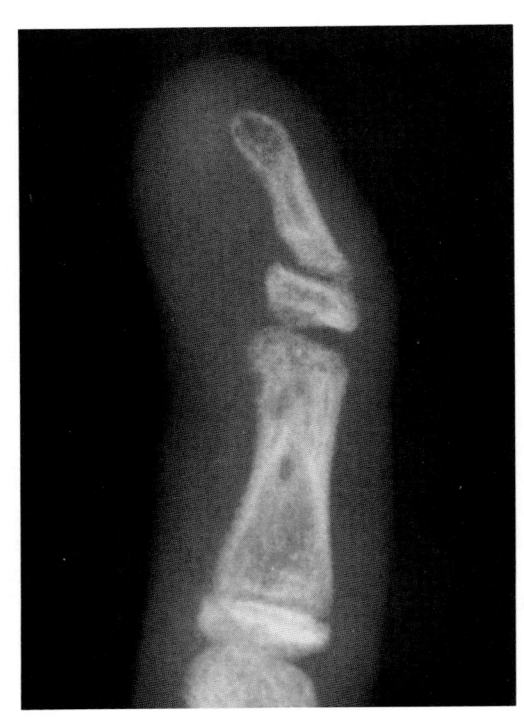

Fig. 4-39. Kirner's deformity of the terminal phalanx of the fifth digit in an 11-year-old boy. The same anomaly was seen in the opposite hand.

The routine radiographic examination of the thoracic and lumbar spines in children is composed of frontal and lateral views. An inability to adequately visualize the upper thoracic vertebrae on the lateral view is a major technical pitfall, and often a "swimmer's view" will be necessary to exclude a fracture. For the same reason, detailed lateral views can be used in the assessment of the lumbosacral junction. Routine oblique views are not necessary in children, but may be used in special circumstances.

Conventional tomography in frontal and lateral planes (Fig. 4-4), thin slice CT with reformatting in the sagittal plane (Fig. 4-40) or three-dimensional CT (Fig. 4-5) can provide definitive diagnostic information at any level of the spine. Magnetic resonance imaging (Fig. 4-41) is best for the assessment of the intervertebral discs, the bone marrow and the spinal contents. In order to obtain the best results, however, sedation may be necessary in small children during all of these procedures.

Normal Anatomy and Its Variants That Can Mimic Trauma

The craniocervical junction is the complex articulation between the vertebral column and the skull. It is made up of the occipital condyles, the atlas, the axis, and the joints between them. Its function is to support the cranium, while permitting flexion, extension, and rotary movements. While there are serious injuries that can occur in this area, there are also a number of pitfalls in trauma diagnosis.

The atlas has no vertebral body or spinous process, being composed of two relatively large lateral masses that join an anterior to a posterior arch. The anterior arch often does not ossify until well into the first year of life, and the central synchondrosis of the posterior arch does not close until the third or fourth year. A normal bipartite superior articular surface of the atlas, as seen on lateral tomography, and the tubercle of the lateral ligament, as seen on open mouth views or tomography,[39] can mimic fractures.

The axis has a unique feature, the odontoid process, which projects superiorly from the body to articulate by a synovial joint with the posterior surface of the anterior arch of the atlas. The odontoid is joined to the body of the axis by a synchondrosis (Fig. 4-42), which does not disappear until around puberty. In addition, there is a secondary center of ossification at the tip of the odontoid (Fig. 4-43) that appears at about 2 years and fuses during adolescence. These normal structures should not be confused with fractures.

The diagnosis of a Jefferson fracture (Fig. 4-5) will be made on open-mouth views of the craniocervical junction, by identifying an offset of the lateral masses of the atlas relative to those of the axis. It should be pointed out, however, that such an offset has been seen in normal children of 3 to 5 years of age.[40]

In the cervical spine, retropharyngeal soft tissue swelling is used as an indicator of significant injury. However, a spurious appearance of retropharyngeal soft tissue swelling can be created if the lateral view of the cervical spine is exposed in expiration. Furthermore, there are many causes of retropharyngeal soft tissue swelling other than trauma.

Deviation from the normal spinal curves cannot be relied upon as an indicator of cervical spine trauma. In infants and children, normal ligamentous laxity can permit anterior displacement of one vertebral body relative to the one below. This so-called "pseudosubluxation" is commonly encountered at the C2-C3 level and can simulate a hangman's fracture[41] (Fig. 4-42).

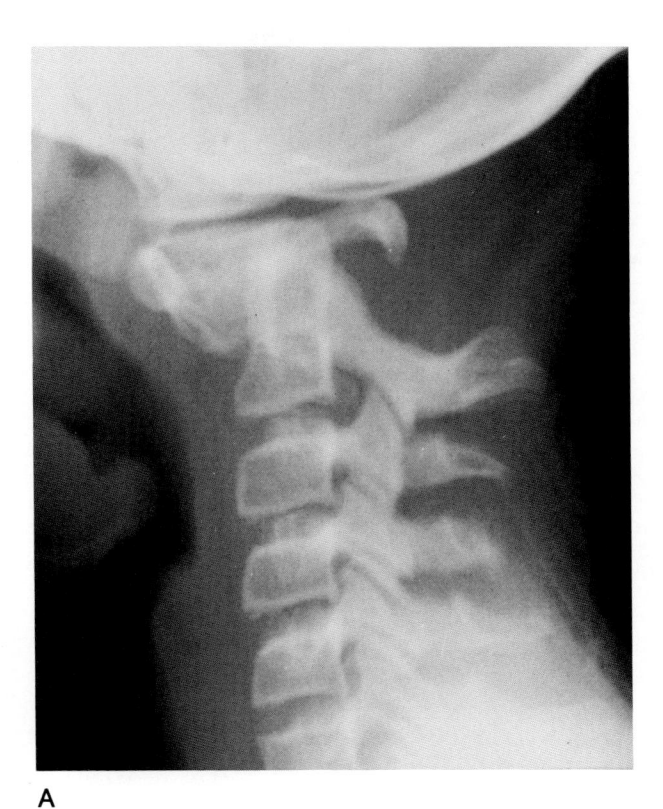

Fig. 4-40. Atlantoaxial instability in a 14-year-old girl with Down syndrome. **(A)** Lateral view and **(B)** CT myelography with sagittal reconstruction shows anterior displacement of the atlas with respect to the axis. The spinal cord *(arrow)* is compressed between the odontoid and the posterior arch of the atlas. (From Reed,[23] with permission.)

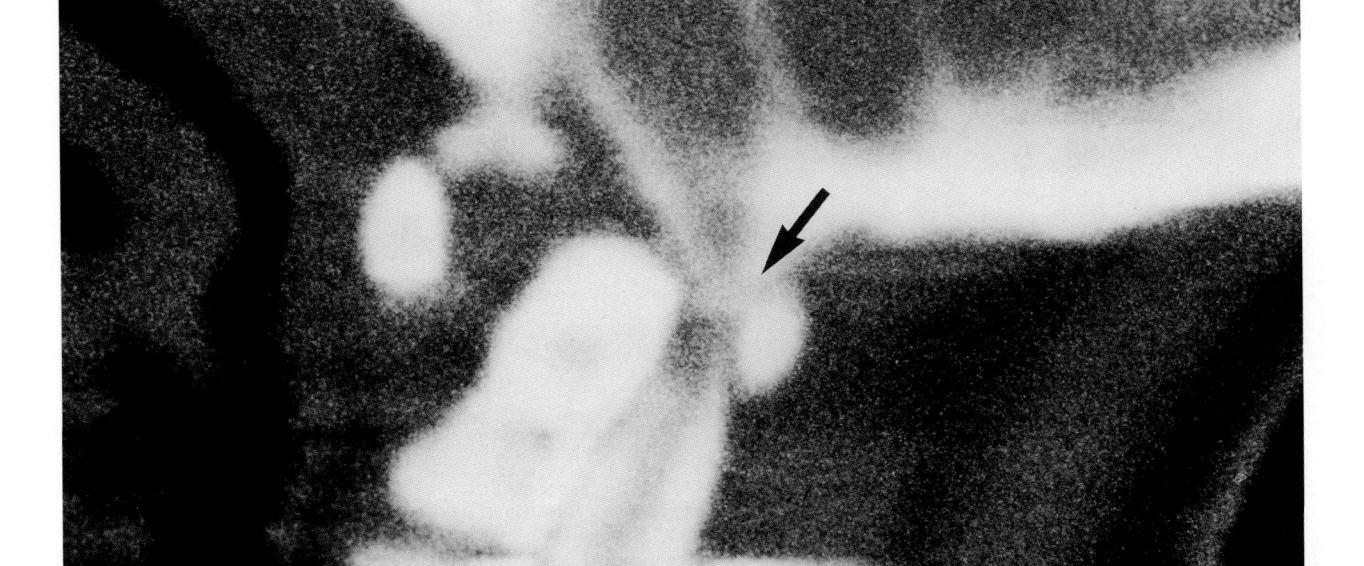

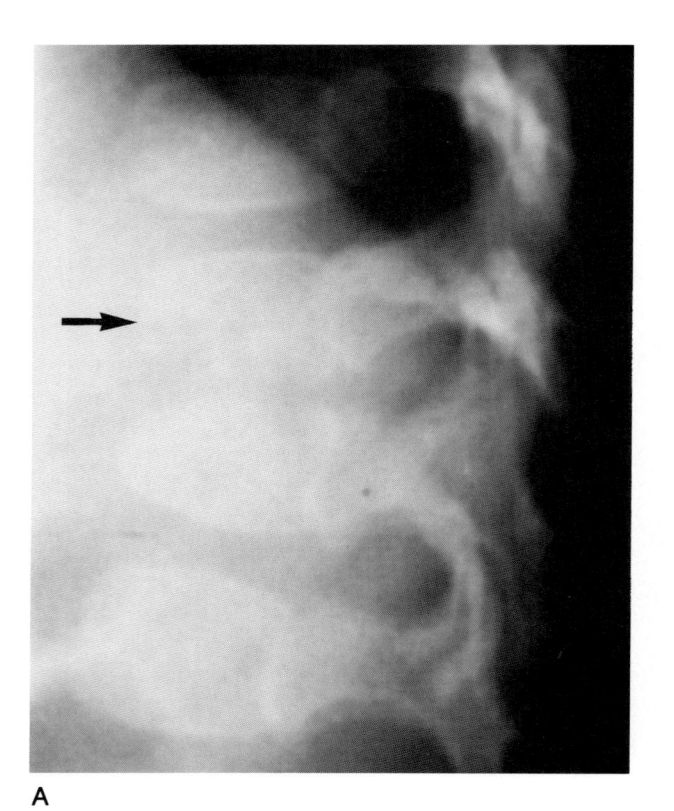

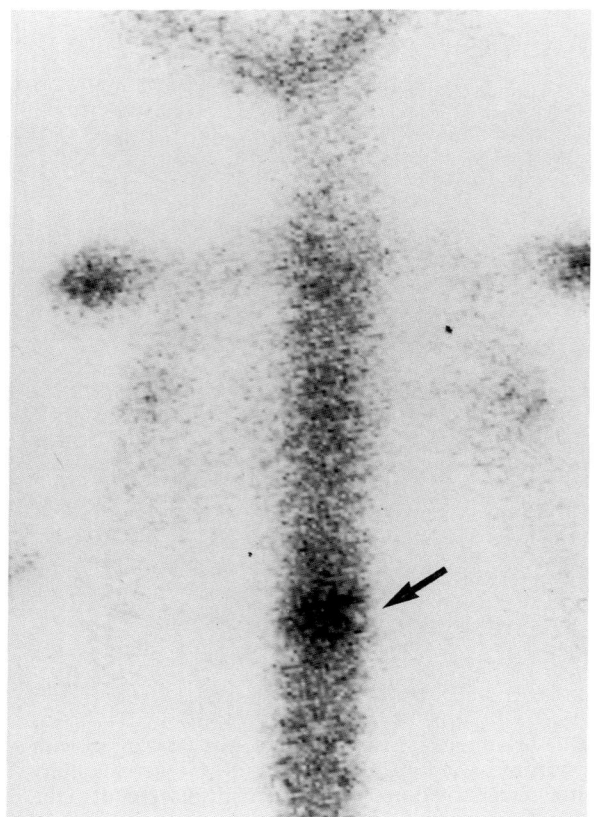

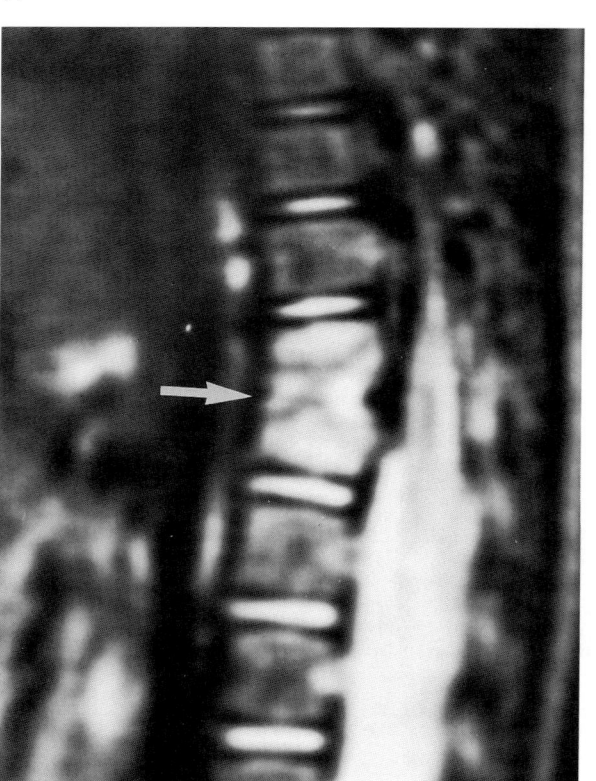

Fig. 4-41. Discitis in a 3-year-old boy. **(A)** Lateral lower thoracic spine film shows narrowing of the T11-T12 disc space *(arrow)* and irregularity of adjacent vertebral endplates. **(B)** ^{99m}Tc-MDP bone scan shows increase uptake of tracer at T11-T12 level *(arrow)*. **(C)** MRI, T2-weighted image. Effacement and loss of height in the T11-T12 disc *(arrow)* with increased signal in adjacent vertebral bodies. (From Reed,[23] with permission.)

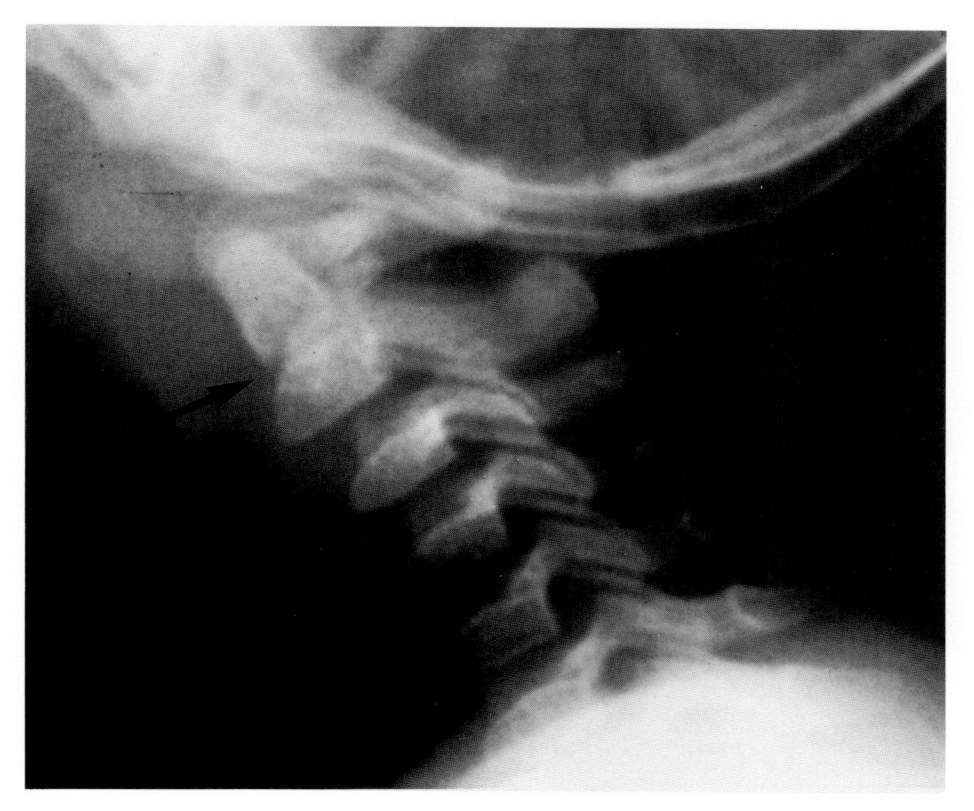

Fig. 4-42. Normal cervical spine in a 1-year-old boy. Note the normal synchondrosis between the odontoid process and the body of the atlas *(arrow)*, the normal anterior tilt of the odontoid and the normal flattened appearance of the cervical vertebral bodies. (From Reed,[23] with permission.)

The diagnosis of vertebral fractures is frequently dependent upon detecting changes in the height and shape of the vertebral bodies. The cervical vertebral bodies in normal children, particularly C3 (Fig. 4-42), can have a flattened or wedged appearance.

The ring apophyses of the cervical spine appear as tiny ossific centers on the anterior aspects of the vertebral bodies in older children. The posterior ring apophyses are less commonly seen.[42] Neither of these normal structures should be confused with fracture fragments.

On the frontal projection of the cervical spine, the spinous processes are expected to line up in an orderly fashion. Deviation from this is regarded as a sign of a cervical fracture or subluxation. Bifid spinous processes, however, can mimic this malalignment.

Nontraumatic Pathology That Can Mimic Trauma

The odontoid process may be separated from the body of the axis, forming a so-called "separate odontoid process" or "os odontoideum."[43] There is debate as to whether this abnormality is a congenital anomaly or an ununited fracture, and there is compelling evidence favoring both concepts. A third theory suggests that it is the result of vascular insufficiency, a pathogenesis that could explain both the congenital and posttraumatic cases.

Since the separated odontoid is attached to the anterior arch of the atlas, there is atlantoaxial instability with a risk of spinal cord compression between the posterior arch of the atlas and the body of the axis. Radiologically, the os odontoideum is a smoothly, rounded ossicle located behind the anterior arch of the atlas and separated from the remainder of the axis by an interval of varying width (Fig. 4-4). There is usually a rounded or pointed mound of hypoplastic odontoid on the body of the axis beneath it. Aplasia and hypoplasia of the odontoid occur less frequently, but have the same clinical implications.

There are other ossicles found in this area that must be differentiated from fractures and an os odontoideum. These include ossiculum terminale and other proatlas

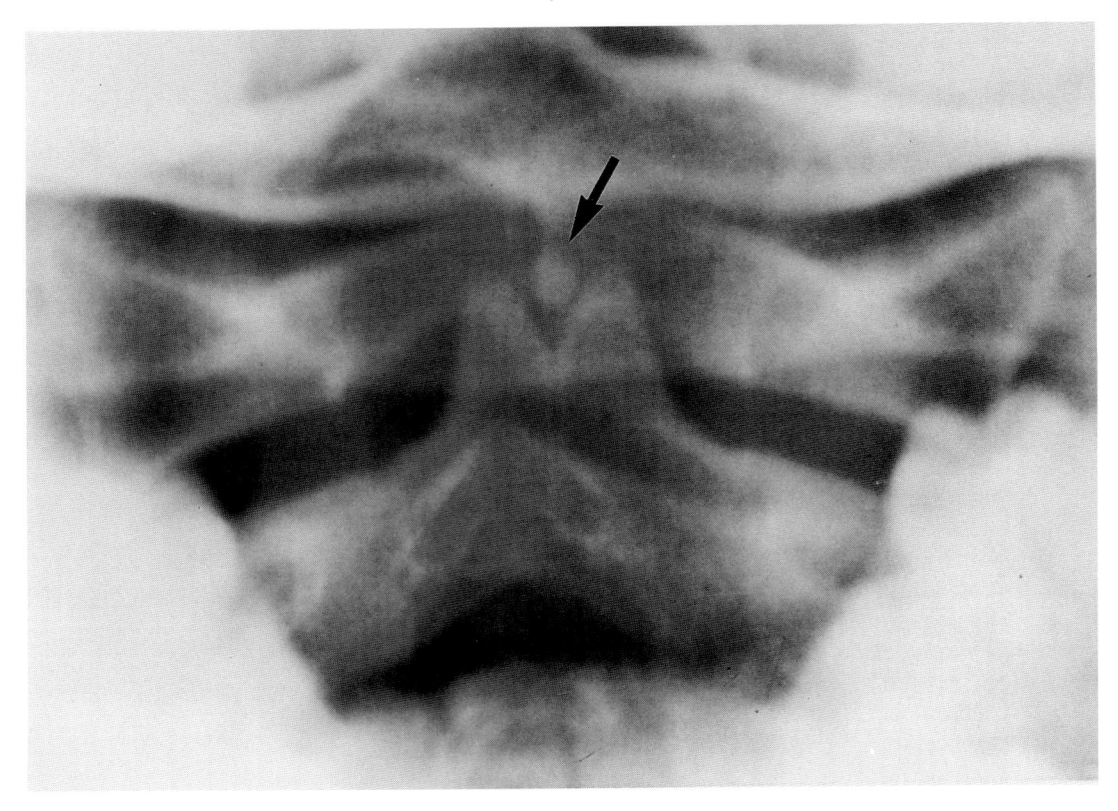

Fig. 4-43. Normal odontoid process in a 6-year-old boy. The diamond-shaped secondary center of ossification (ossiculum terminale) is seen at the tip of the odontoid process *(arrow)*. (From Reed,[23] with permission.)

remnants, as well as accessory ossicles occasionally found in front of the anterior arch of the atlas in older children.[44]

In addition, there are congenital defects and clefts found in the atlas that can simulate serious injuries in the emergency room setting. The posterior arch can be the site of total aplasia, partial aplasia, or clefts (Fig. 4-24). Similar defects in the anterior arch, however, are very rare.

Bilateral, presumably congenital, symmetric clefts can occur in the neural arches of the cervical spine most commonly at C6. The second most common location, however, is the axis, where they can be associated with anterior displacement of the body of the axis or congenital spondylolisthesis[45] (Fig. 4-25). This lesion, which simulates a hangman's fracture, is unstable in itself and has been found in association with certain congenital syndromes, such as pyknodysostosis and Larsen syndrome.

Instability of the atlantoaxial articulation can occur with or without osseous abnormalities. It is gauged by measuring the interval between the odontoid and the anterior arch of the atlas. This interval may measure up to 5 mm. in normal children. Measurements above this are regarded as atlantoaxial instability and the patient is considered at risk of neurologic damage from cord compression. Children with Down syndrome, because of their generalized ligamentous laxity, have a 15 percent chance of atlantoaxial instability[46] (Fig. 4-40). Only 1 to 2 percent, however, are symptomatic and may require spinal fusion to prevent permanent cord damage. The incidence of atlantoaxial instability is lower in adult Down syndrome patients. There are a number of skeletal dysplasias, such as Morquio syndrome and chondrodysplasia punctata, in which there is an increased risk of atlantoaxial instability.[46]

Congenital absence or hypoplasia of vertebral bodies can create deformities resembling trauma. Tsou and colleagues[47] suggested that this group of anomalies result from a vascular insufficiency, occurring after the formation of the membranous analog of the centrum and neural arch, which causes variable degrees of dissolution of the vertebral bodies leaving the neural arches intact. The most extensive vascular compromise causes complete absence of the vertebral body or *asoma*. Lesser vascular deprivation causes "dorsal hemivertebrae" (Fig. 4-44), while the most minor deformity in this group is a *congenital wedge vertebra* (Fig. 4-45), both of which can mimic a vertebral compression fracture. The more common congenital anomalies of the vertebral bodies, such as the classical hemivertebrae, sagittal cleft vertebrae, and coronal cleft vertebrae, are not usually confused with vertebral fractures.

In addition to the cervical defects mentioned above, there are a number of partial deficiencies of the neural arches that can occur at any level of the spine.[48] These include congenital absence of a pedicle or lamina, cleft pedicles (retrosomatic clefts), and cleft lamina (retroisthmic clefts). These defects can be confirmed by CT in the axial plane where they are identified by the smooth margination of the defects.

Cleft spinous processes (spina bifida occulta) are the most common neural arch defect. They are found at the L5, S1, or S2 levels in 23 percent of normal individuals of all ages and in 29 percent of normal people under 40 years of age.[49] Their typical site and appearance results in little likelihood of their being confused with a fracture.

Clefts in the pars interarticularis (spondylolysis) are common neural arch defects most often encountered in the lower lumbar spine.[50] They are usually bilateral and can be associated with spondylolisthesis. While there has been a debate as to whether these defects are congenital or acquired, the current feeling is that the majority are fatigue fractures. An interesting radiologic feature of all the unilateral neural arch defects is the tendency to develop hypertrophy and sclerosis of the opposite pedicle[51] (Fig. 4-33). These enlarged, sclerotic pedicles should not be confused with other forms of spinal pathology.

Compression of vertebral bodies is an expected and common complication of flexion injuries of the spine. There are, however, a number of nontraumatic diseases that can be associated with a loss of vertical height in one or more vertebral bodies. As mentioned above, vertebral bodies can be congenitally wedged (Fig. 4-45). *Vertebra plana*, meaning "flat vertebra," is a term reserved for the solitary flattened vertebral body (Fig. 4-46) that is now recognized as a manifestation of histiocytosis X, usually the eosinophilic granuloma variety.[52] Formerly, this condition was called "Calve's disease" and was believed to be one of the group of osteochondritides. Children with the more widespread *Hand-Schüller-Christian* variety of histiocytosis X can exhibit multiple flattened vertebral bodies.

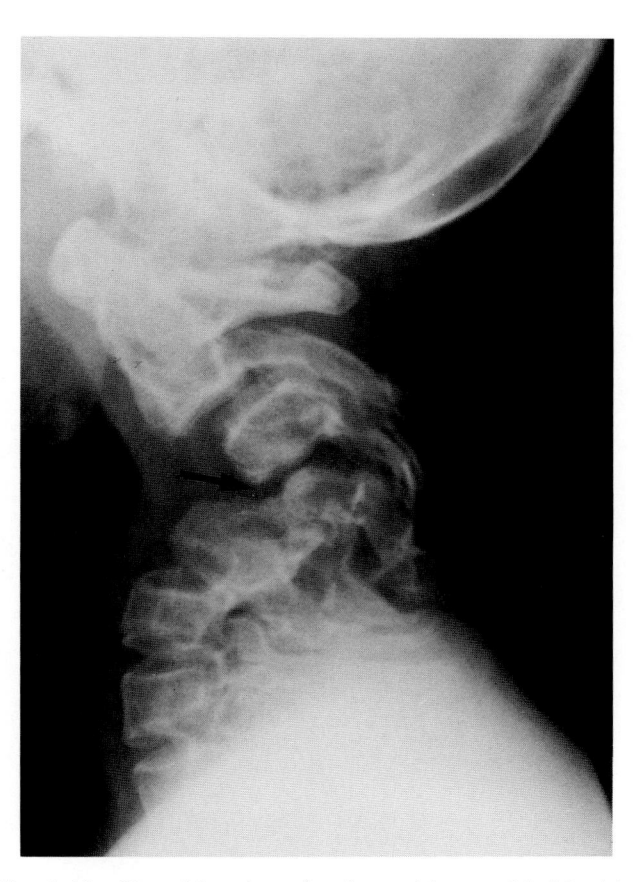

Fig. 4-44. Dorsal hemivertebra in an 11-year-old girl with severe cervical kyphosis. The lateral view of the cervical spine shows a dorsal hemivertebra at C5. This forms the apex of the severe cervical kyphosis. (From Reed,[23] with permission.)

In Scheuermann's disease or juvenile kyphosis,[53] one or several adjacent vertebral bodies may have a wedge shape, simulating compression fractures (Fig. 4-47). The associated disc space narrowing with irregular vertebral endplates will assist in establishing the true nature of the disorder. MRI is ideal for demonstrating the disc changes.

In children with discitis and spinal tuberculosis, some degree of vertebral wedging may be present. Disc space narrowing, vertebral endplate changes and paravertebral soft tissue changes (Fig. 4-41A) are key in the recognition of the true nature of these spinal disorders.[54] A bone scan will show increased activity at the site (Fig. 4-41B). MRI is a superb modality for demonstration of the changes in the disc and adjacent vertebral bodies (Fig. 4-41C).

Platyspondyly is another term used in reference to flattened vertebral bodies, usually in association with

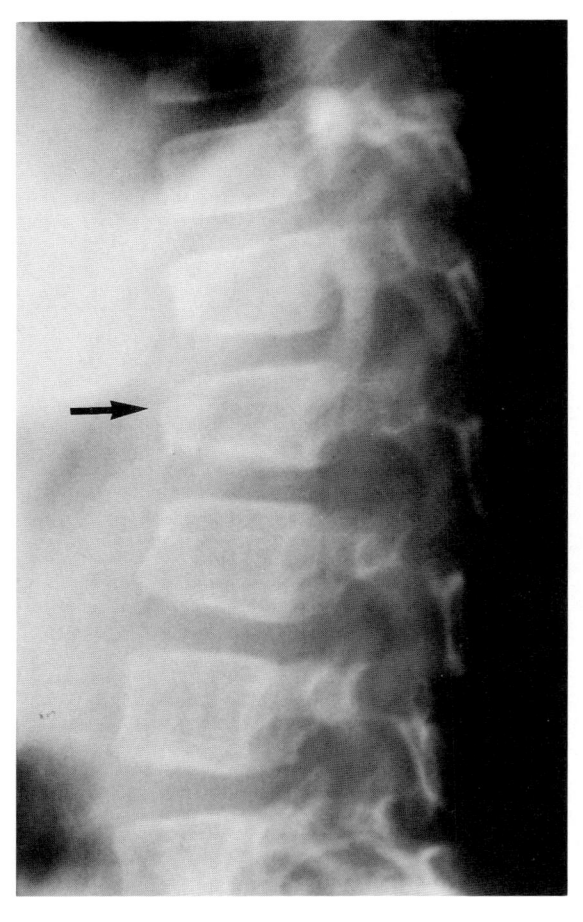

Fig. 4-45. Congenital wedge vertebra in a 17-month-old girl with mild kyphosis. The lateral view of the thoracolumbar spine shows a wedge vertebra at L1 *(arrow)*. (From Reed,[23] with permission.)

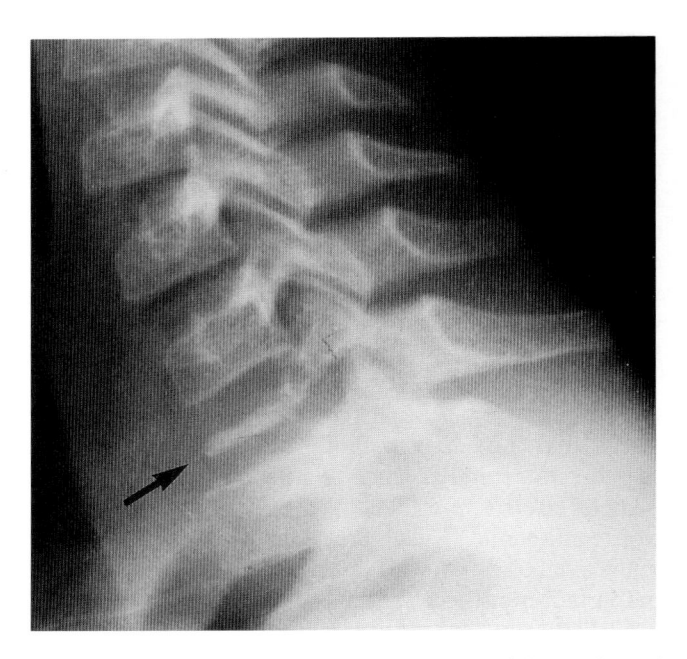

Fig. 4-46. Vertebra plana in an 8-year-old girl. The lateral view of the cervical spine shows a flattened C6 vertebral body. This change, which resembles a compression fracture, is usually indicative of histiocytosis X.

skeletal dysplasias. Universal platyspondyly is a feature of all the congenital spondylodysplasias and, to a certain extent, the mucopolysaccharidoses. The other features of these diseases will be important in their differentiation from multiple fractures.

In generalized skeletal diseases characterized by osteopenia, such as osteogenesis imperfecta and rickets, there can be pathologic compression fractures of one or more vertebral bodies. In this situation, there is the potential pitfall of recognizing the fractures, but missing the underlying pathologic process. If the other clinical and radiographic features do not help in the differentiation between vertebral compression due to trauma and that from other causes, alternate imaging modalities, such as isotope studies may be helpful.

THE THORACIC CAGE

Technical Factors in Fracture Diagnosis

The thoracic cage is composed of the 12 paired ribs and the sternum. The ribs can be evaluated for fractures on frontal and oblique radiographs of the chest, utilizing "rib technique." In young children who are otherwise normal, the presence of rib fractures should raise suspicions of abuse.[23] Undisplaced rib fractures, however, may be imperceptible on rib films until they display ossifying callus as evidence of healing. This can take up to 2 weeks. Because of the obliquity of the ribs, CT is not reliable in the detection of rib fractures. Therefore, in the interim, a radionuclide bone scan may be employed to detect rib injuries.

Normal Anatomy and Its Variants That Can Mimic Trauma

Although the sternum is rarely the site of fractures in pediatric patients, its multiple centers of ossification may be confused with fracture fragments. Normally there are four to six ossification centers perceptible on a

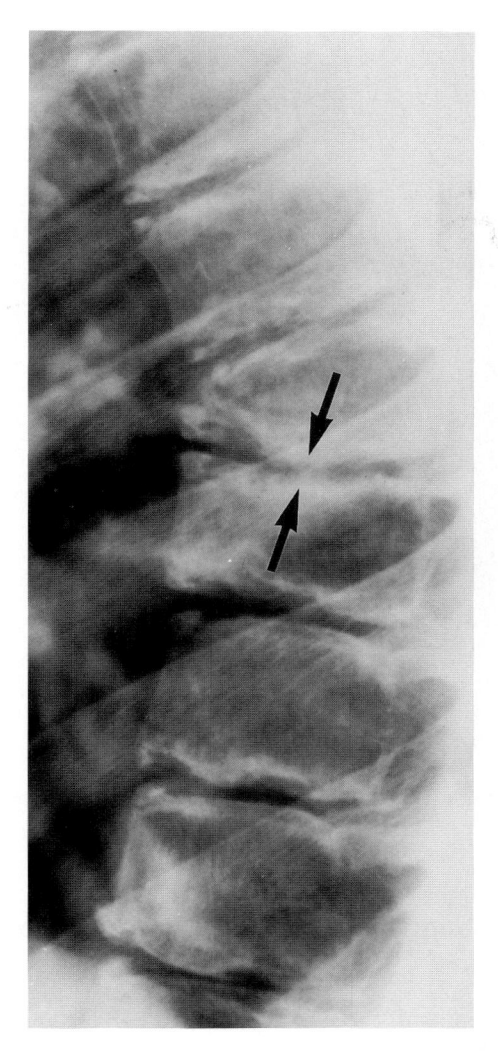

Fig. 4-47. Juvenile kyphosis in a 14-year-old girl. The lateral thoracic spine shows a midthoracic kyphosis with a wedged apical vertebra, disc space narrowing with endplate irregularity *(arrows)*, sclerotic, irregular ring apophyses, and an increase in the depth of the affected vertebrae. (From Reed,[23] with permission.)

lateral or oblique chest radiograph. Occasionally, one or more of these centers are bipartite.

Nontraumatic Pathology That Can Mimic Trauma

The cerebrocostomandibular syndrome is a rare familial syndrome in which mental retardation and micrognathia are associated with multiple rib gaps that can mimic ununited fractures.[55] The ribs are a common site for the hyperostosis of Caffey's disease,[28] prostaglandin administration[56] and Menkes syndrome[26] (Fig. 4-29), all of which could be mistaken for healing fractures. Also, the first rib is a known site for congenital pseudarthrosis.

THE PELVIS AND HIP JOINTS

Technical Factors in Trauma Diagnosis

The radiographic examination of the traumatized pelvis usually begins with a single anteroposterior projection. This is far from all revealing, however. Fractures of the acetabulum, femoral head, obturator ring, ilium, and sacrum may escape detection or be underestimated in their severity. Additional radiographic projections, such as obliques, inlet and outlet views, and conventional tomography may shed more light on the problem. In this day and age, however, CT with imaging in the axial plane,[5] reformatting in other planes imaging modality in the evaluation of pelvic and hip joint injuries. CT is ideal in the evaluation of acetabular fractures, femoral head fractures, and loose fragments in the hip joint. It can be used to determine the nature and extent of hip dislocations and sacroiliac diastasis, as well as fractures involving the curved surfaces of the sacrum, ilium, ischium, and pubic bones.

The potential role of stereoscopic radiography in the identification of hip dislocations should not be forgotten. Also, in the absence of CT, it could be used to better evaluate complex pelvic fractures.

Normal Anatomy and Its Variants That Can Mimic Trauma

The normal synchondroses in the pelvis, namely, the ischiopubic synchondroses (Fig 4-48) and the triradiate cartilages in the acetabuli (Fig. 4-8), vary in appearance during development. As they approach closure, they can mimic fractures. This is particularly true when the closing triradiate cartilage has an inward protrusion. Normal secondary centers of ossification are found along the crest of the iliac bones and at the ischia in older children. In their early stages, they can be confused with avulsion fractures. Accessory centers of ossification at the superolateral margin of the acetabulum (os acetabuli) (Fig. 4-13) are a frequently occurring normal variant. With

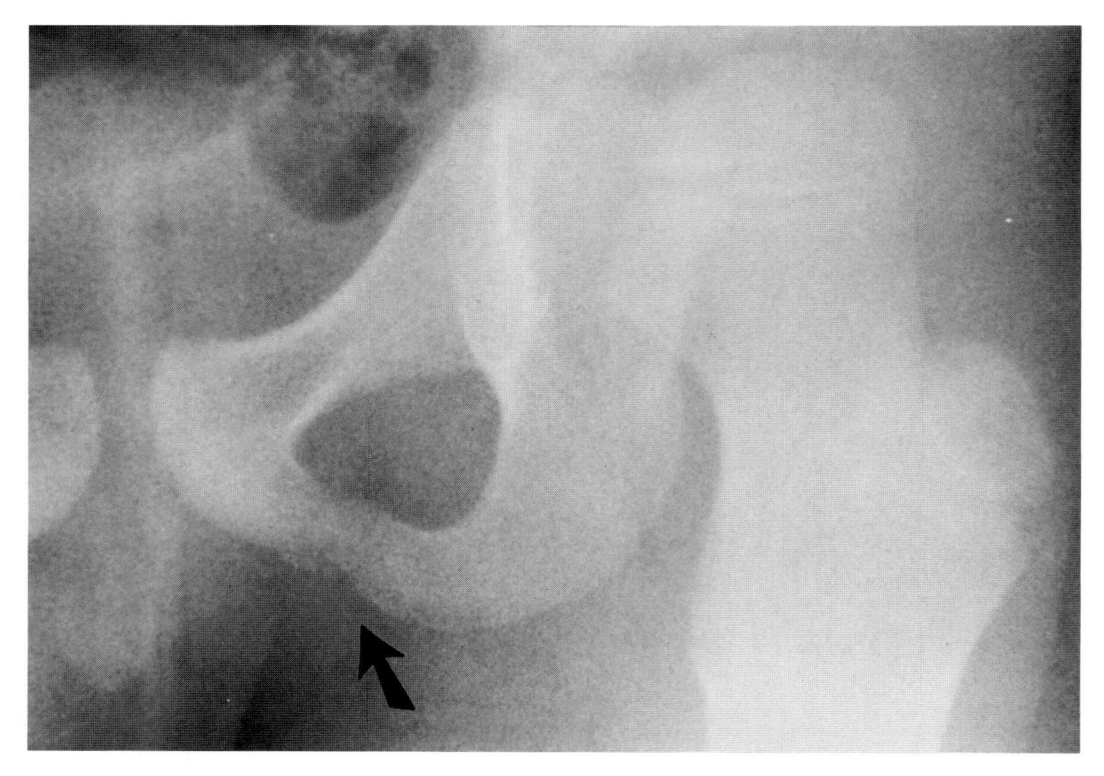

Fig. 4-48. Normal pelvis in a 7-year-old boy. The normal ischiopubic synchondrosis should not be mistaken for a fracture.

further development, they may become incorporated into the rest of the ilium, or they may persist into adulthood as separate ossicles. In addition, accessory centers of ossification are occasionally found on the body of the pubic bones at the inferior margins of the symphysis pubis. Nutrient vessels can create sinuous grooves with sclerotic margins in the body of the iliac bones.

The secondary center of ossification for the femoral head may be bipartite or irregular in shape. In addition, a notch is frequently seen in the femoral head, known as the *fovea capitis*. None of these normal femoral head irregularities should be misinterpreted as traumatic lesions. In addition, the secondary centers of ossification for the greater and lesser trochanters can be quite irregular in appearance, raising the question of avulsion-type injuries.

There are few normal variants in the sacrum and coccyx that can be confused with traumatic lesions. Spina bifida occulta is so common an occurrence as a normal variant at S1, that it is usually recognized as such.[49] The coccyx frequently has an acute anterior angulation that should not be mistaken for a fracture or dislocation.

Nontraumatic Pathology That Can Mimic Trauma

Widening of the symphysis pubis can occur as part of serious pelvic injuries (open-book fractures) in children. It should be remembered, however, that there are many causes of widening of the symphysis pubis (Table 4-2).

Traumatic dislocation or subluxation of the hip is an infrequent occurrence in children. Congenital dislocation, however, is quite common. The dysplastic changes in the acetabulum and femoral head associated with congenital hip dysplasia usually permit easy differentiation from traumatic dislocation. The neurogenic dislocations, commonly found in neurologically impaired children, share many of the radiologic features of congenital dislocations.

Septic arthritis of the hip is relatively common in infants, and subluxation (Fig. 4-32), or even dislocation, of the affected femoral head is a complication. It has been shown, in some infants with septic arthritis, that the lateral displacement of the femoral shaft is associated with a pathologic fracture through the proximal growth

TABLE 4-2. Causes of Widened Symphysis Pubis

Hypoplasia of pubic bones
 Cleidocranial dysplasia
 Spondyloepiphyseal dysplasia congenita
 Achondrogenesis
 Campomelic dysplasia
 Other syndromes
Congenital separation of symphysis pubis
 Epispadius-extrophy continuum
 Anorectal malformations
Infectious
 Tuberculosis of symphysis pubis, etc.
Traumatic
 Separation of symphysis pubis
Metabolic
 Hyperparathyroidism
Neoplasms
 Tumors of pubic bones
Pregnancy

A slight lateral displacement of the capital femoral epiphysis within the acetabulum is one of the early changes in Legg-Perthes disease and other causes of avascular necrosis of the femoral head. MRI is a proven method of identifying avascular necrosis and differentiating it from traumatic displacements.[15]

Proximal focal femoral deficiency is a congenital partial absence of the proximal end of the femur with shortening of the entire limb.[58] There are four or five varieties, depending on the classification utilized. They vary from a simple shortening of the femur with coxa vara to a complete absence of the proximal femur and hip joint. The more mild types can have a pseudarthrosis in the subtrochanteric region (Fig. 4-49) that should not be mistaken for a fracture.

Congenital coxa vara is a developmental abnormality, occurring when a varus deformity of the femoral neck develops during childhood.[59] Unlike the milder forms of proximal focal femoral deficiency, the limb is normal at birth and there is no overall shortening of the femur. Often a pseudarthrosis develops in the femoral neck (Fig. 4-50) in this condition, which should not be confused with a fracture.

plate.[57] Early in these cases, the acetabulum and femoral head can appear normal and the differentiation between septic arthritis and a traumatic displacement may depend on the clinical history and/or aspiration of the hip joint.

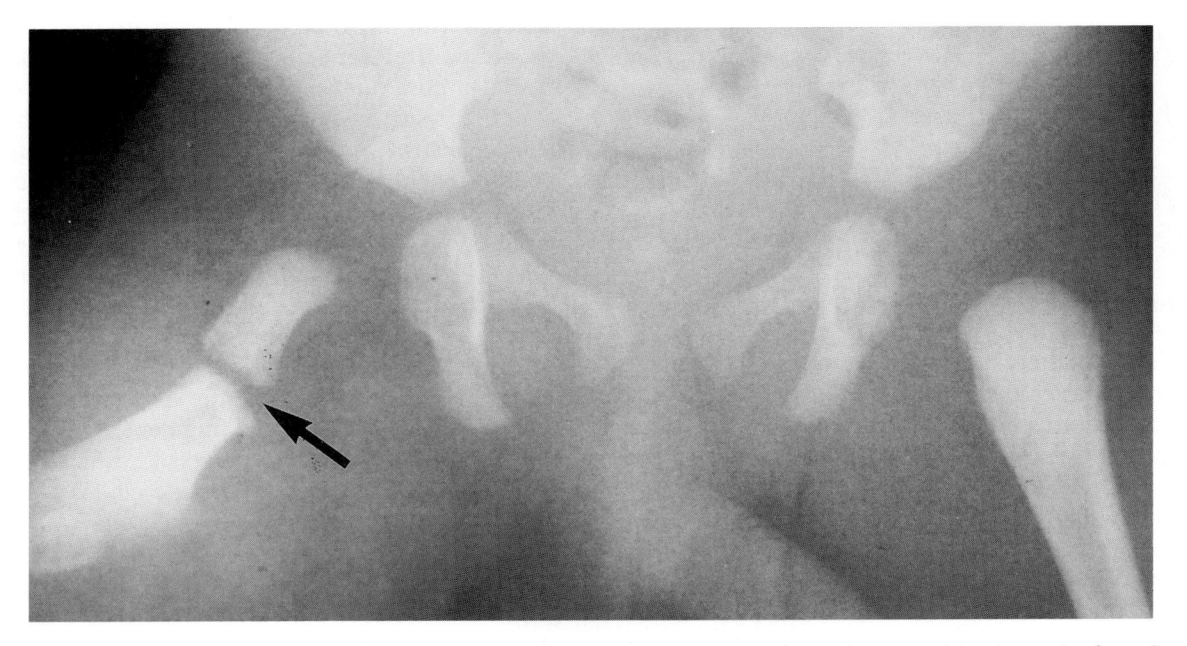

Fig. 4-49. Proximal focal femoral deficiency in a newborn boy. The right femur is short with a hypoplastic and dysplastic proximal end. There is a pseudarthrosis in the subtrochanteric region that could be confused with a birth fracture.

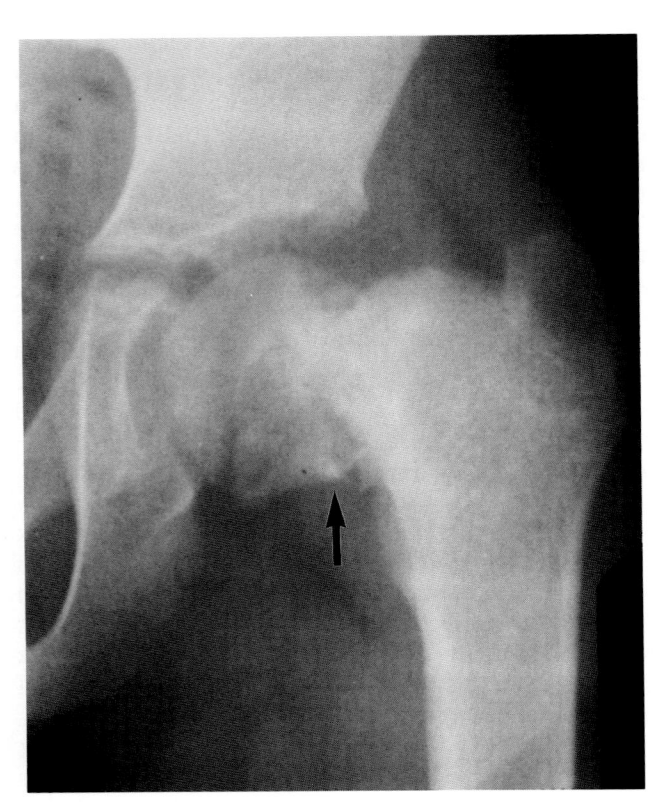

Fig. 4-50. Congenital coxa vara in a 9-year-old girl. The AP radiograph of the left hip shows a varus deformity of the femoral neck with a central defect that could be misconstrued as a fracture. The triangular fragment on the inferior aspect of the femoral neck *(arrow)* is characteristic of congenital coxa vara.

THE FEMUR, KNEE, AND LOWER LEG

Technical Factors in Fracture Diagnosis

The basic radiographic projections for the femur, knee, and lower leg are anteroposterior and lateral views. With knee injuries, intercondylar and stress views may be added to the protocol. The intercondylar view is used to exclude loose fragments in the joint space, while stress views are used to rule out injuries of the medial or lateral collateral ligaments. If a patellar fracture is suspected, tangential views of the patella may be attempted.

The lateral view of the knee should be made as a "true lateral" with the knee slightly flexed. This is important in the evaluation of the quantity of fluid in the knee joint. Knee joint effusions are recognized by distention of the suprapatellar bursa and anterior displacement of the patella. In the case of trauma, the joint effusion is probably a hemarthrosis. The absence of a hemarthrosis lessens the likelihood of a serious acute injury, while its presence increases the chances and should intensify the investigation. For example, a common injury of the child's knee that can be relatively occult is an avulsion of the anterior tibial spine, which is usually associated with a hemarthrosis.

MRI can accurately detect tears in the collateral and cruciate ligaments of the knee.[12] In addition, it can be used to study the integrity of the medial and lateral menisci. If MRI is unavailable or equivocal, arthrography can be used for this purpose.

As stated earlier, fractures of the lower tibia can be associated with fractures of the proximal fibula. For this reason, the radiographic examination of the lower leg should include the knee and ankle joints.

Normal Anatomy and Its Variants That Can Mimic Trauma

There are two normal variants of the femoral shaft that can be confused with trauma. First, it is a common site for the physiologic new bone seen in infants[22] (Fig. 4-23). Second, nutrient vascular channels can be seen penetrating the cortex on the lateral aspect of the femoral shaft and running obliquely away from the knee.

Cortical irregularity is a frequent occurrence on the medial or posterior aspects of the distal femoral metaphysis (Fig. 4-20) in normal older children. It has been called *avulsive cortical irregularity* suggesting that it is an avulsive phenomena, although Keats and Joyce[21] suggest a developmental etiology. It is more likely to be confused with a malignancy than a traumatic lesion. In older children, the margins of the distal femoral epiphysis, particularly the medial aspect, frequently have a ragged, irregular appearance.

The patella normally begins to ossify around 5 to 6 years of age. The primary center of ossification can appear very irregular and even fragmented (Fig. 4-17). In later childhood, accessory centers of ossification can appear, creating a so-called "bipartite patella." These accessory centers are located at the superolateral pole of the patella in 75 percent of cases (Fig. 4-14A), the lateral margin in 20 percent, and the inferior pole in 5 percent[60] (Fig. 4-14B). The variant is bilateral in up to 50 percent of cases and is much more common in males. These normal variants in the patella should not be confused with fractures. Another sesamoid bone, the fabella, is found in the tendon of the gastrocnemious posterior to

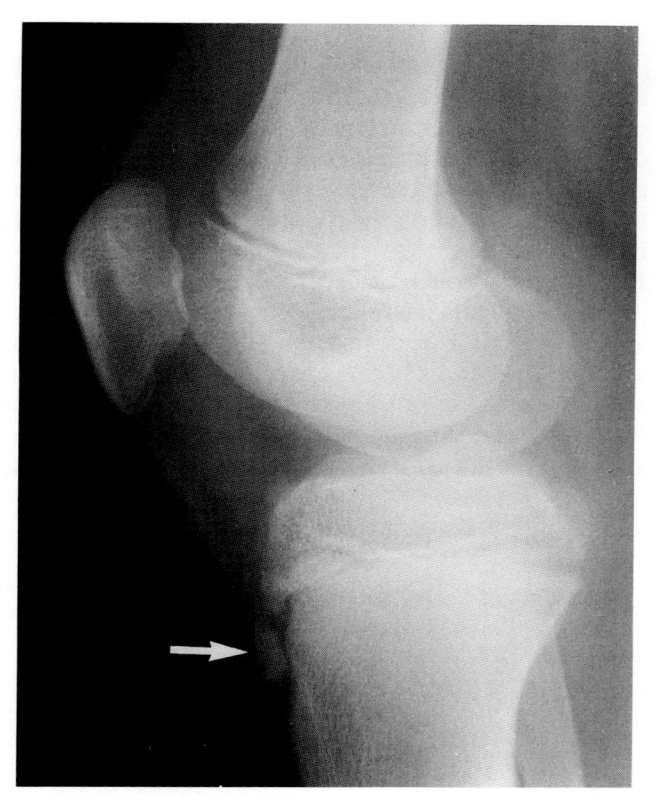

Fig. 4-51. Fragmented secondary center for the tibial tuberosity in a 14-year-old boy. This normal variant could be confused with an avulsion injury.

the knee joint in a minority of children; it should not be confused with a fracture fragment.

The normal secondary center for the tibial tuberosity is often fragmented or irregular in its appearance (Fig. 4-51), making it difficult to exclude an acute avulsion fracture or Osgood-Schlatter's disease.

Nontraumatic Pathology That Can Mimic Trauma

Osgood-Schlatter's disease and osteochondritis dissecans are two pathologic entities associated with the knee that were once attributed to avascular necrosis, but are now believed to be the result of trauma. These issues are discussed elsewhere in this textbook.

Congenital dislocation of the knee can occur but is much less common than that of the hip.[61] Congenital pseudarthrosis of the tibia[62] is a rare disorder of unknown etiology in which there is nonunion of a pathologic fracture through the tibia. The pseudarthrosis is frequently preceded by a congenital anterior bowing, an interosseous cyst, segmental sclerosis, and/or an hourglass constriction involving the affected tibia. There is an association between congenital pseudarthrosis of the tibia and multiple neurofibromatosis. Radiologically, the defect is usually located at the junction of the middle and distal thirds of the tibia (Fig. 4-26). Its margins are frequently tapered and sclerotic, with bowing convex anteriorly.

THE FOOT AND ANKLE

Technical Factors in Trauma Diagnosis

The standard radiographic examination of the ankle for trauma in children is composed of an anteroposterior projection, a lateral projection, and an internal oblique (mortise view) projection. The addition of an external oblique projection to the protocol is optional. Stress views may be employed when a ligamentous injury or Salter-Harris type I growth plate injury is suspected. As was mentioned with the elbow and knee, the lateral view of the ankle must be made as a "true lateral" in order to identify or exclude ankle joint effusions. As with the other joints, an ankle injury without joint fluid is not as serious as one with excess fluid. The presence of an ankle joint effusion is determined by identifying displacement of the periarticular fat planes on the anterior aspect of the joint (teardrop sign).[63]

A fracture through the base of the fifth metatarsal can mimic an injury to the lateral malleolus or ligaments. On this basis, the proximal fifth metatarsal should be evaluated in the course of the ankle study (Fig. 4-3). Some centers do routine foot examinations in conjunction with their ankle studies to avoid this pitfall.

The minimum radiographic examination of the foot should be composed of an anteroposterior, a lateral, and an oblique (dorsiplantar) view. The plantidorsal oblique and detailed lateral views of the toes can be included when necessary. If a fractured calcaneus is suspected, lateral and axial views of the calcaneus should be added. Most fractures of the foot and ankle in children are easily identified on conventional radiography. However, certain articular surfaces, because of their curved surfaces, are not well seen. This is particularly true of the distal tibiofibular articulation, the malleolar articular surfaces, and the intertarsal articulations. Without CT, subtle injuries in these areas can escape detection.[6]

Normal Anatomy and Its Variants That Can Mimic Trauma

Normal anatomic structures and variations of normal anatomy as pitfalls to fracture diagnosis in children are most prevalent in the foot and ankle region. The completely normal "flake apophysis" at the base of the fifth metatarsal (Fig. 4-10A) is frequently misread as a fracture. The growth plate of this apophysis runs parallel to the long axis of the metatarsal, while a fracture ("Jones's" or "Dancer's fracture") traverses the bone (Fig. 4-10B). The distal tibial growth plate can have a wavy configuration, which can create addition linear lucencies, easily mistaken for fracture lines. A common error is the misinterpretation of the almost-closed normal distal fibular growth plate for a fracture. It usually closes slightly later than the adjacent distal tibial growth plate. In addition, there are small ossicles that inhabit the lateral aspect of the distal fibular growth plate (Fig. 4-19) that can mimic the metaphyseal fragments of a Salter-Harris type II growth plate injury.

The medial and lateral malleoli are common sites for accessory centers of ossification (Fig. 4-11), as well as accessory ossicles, namely, the os subtibiale and the os subfibulare. These are two of the many accessory ossicles that can be found in the foot (Fig. 4-18), none of which should be mistaken for fracture fragments. In addition to

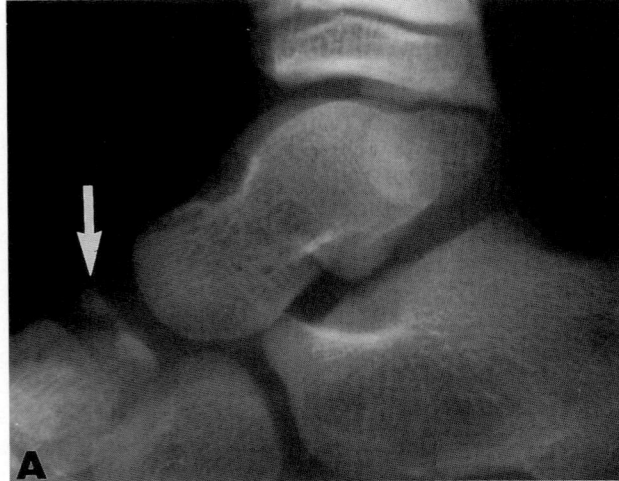

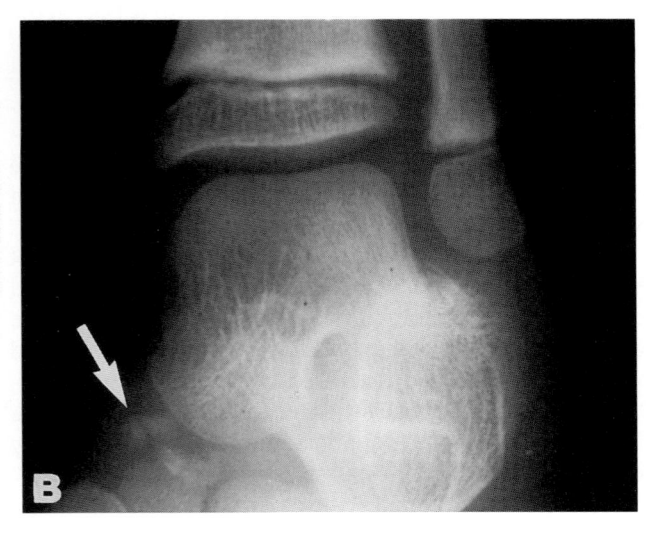

Fig. 4-52. (A & B) Multipartite navicular in a normal 6-year-old boy. This could be mistaken for a fracture or Kohler's disease. The absence of soft tissue swelling will help exclude a recent injury.

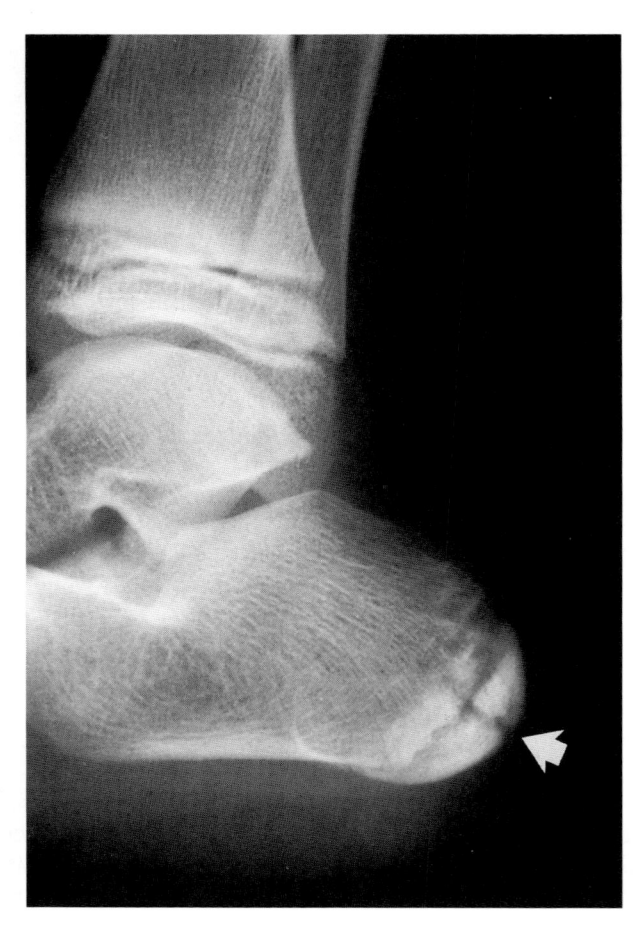

Fig. 4-53. Bipartite secondary center of ossification for the calcaneus in an 11-year-old boy. Note the wavy appearance of the distal tibial growth plate and the overlap of the distal fibular growth plate on the tibial epiphysis. These are other variants that can be confused with fractures.

accessory ossicles, one can encounter accessory sesamoid bones, which will be located primarily adjacent to the heads of the metatarsals. Bipartite centers of ossification are common in the base of the proximal phalanx of the first toe (Fig. 4-16) and tarsal navicular (Fig. 4-52), but less so in the calcaneus (Fig. 4-15) and cuneiforms. The multipartite or fragmented appearance of the secondary center of ossification for the calcaneus (Fig. 4-53) is common pitfall in fracture diagnosis.

In the toes, there is potential confusion created by the growth plates which are usually viewed tangentially creating additional linear lucencies. There also may be incomplete fissures in the metatarsals and phalanges that can mimic fracture lines.

Nontraumatic Pathology That Can Mimic Trauma

Congenital diastasis of the inferior tibiofibular joint is a rare developmental aberration that is present at birth, usually in association with distal tibial dysplasia, talipes equinovarus, and other skeletal anomalies.[64]

REFERENCES

1. Darling DB: Radiography of Infants and Children. 3rd Ed. Charles C Thomas, Springfield, IL, 1979
2. Nelson SW: Some important diagnostic and technical fundamentals in the radiology of trauma, with particular emphasis on skeletal trauma. Radiol Clin North Am 4:241, 1961
3. Ogden JA: Skeletal Injury in the Child. 2nd Ed. WB Saunders, Philadelphia, 1990
4. McCauley RG, Schwartz AM, Leonidas JC et al: Comparison views in extremity injury in children: an efficacy study. Radiology 131:95, 1979
5. Riddlesberger MM: Computed tomography of the musculoskeletal system. Radiol Clin North Am 19:463, 1981
6. Wilkins KE: Changing patterns in the management of fractures in children. Clin Orthop 264:136, 1991
7. Starshak RJ, Crawford CR, Waisman RC, Sty JR: Three-dimensional CT of the pediatric spine. Appl Radiol 18:15, 1989
8. Marzo JM, d'Amato C, Strong M, Gillespie R: Usefulness and accuracy of arthrography in management of lateral humeral condyle fractures in children. J Pediatr Orthop 10:317, 1990
9. Broker FHL, Burbach T: Ultrasonic diagnosis of separation of the proximal humeral epiphysis in the newborn. J Bone Joint Surg [Am] 72:187, 1990
10. Diaz MJ, Hedlund GL: Sonographic diagnosis of traumatic separation of the proximal femoral epiphysis in the neonate. Pediatr Radiol 21:238, 1991
11. Mink JH, Deutsch AL: Occult cartilage and bone injuries of the knee: detection, classification and assessment with MR imaging. Radiology 170:823, 1989
12. Jacobsen HG: Musculoskeletal applications of magnetic resonance imaging. JAMA 262:2420, 1989
13. Park H, Kernek CB, Robb JA: Early scintigraphic findings of occult femoral and tibial fractures in infants. Clin Nucl Med 13:271, 1988
14. Sty JR, Starshak RJ: The role of bone scintigraphy in the evaluation of the suspected abused child. Radiology 146:369, 1983
15. Cohen MD: Pediatric Magnetic Resonance Imaging. WB Saunders, Philadelphia, 1986
16. Mahboubi S: Pediatric Bone Imaging: A Practical Approach. Little, Brown, Boston, 1989
17. Kohler A, Zimmer EA: Borderlands of the Normal and Early Pathologic in Skeletal Roentgenology. 11th Ed. Grune & Stratton, Orlando, FL, 1968
18. Keats TE: An Atlas of Normal Roentgen Variants That May Simulate Disease. 4th Ed. Year Book Medical Publishers, Chicago, 1988
19. Teates CD: Distal radial growth plate remnant simulating fracture. AJR 110:578, 1970
20. Bufkin WJ: The avulsive cortical irregularity. AJR 112:487, 1971
21. Keats TE, Joyce JM: Metaphyseal cortical irregularities in children: a new perspective on a multi-focal growth variant. Skeletal Radiol 12:112, 1984
22. Shopfner CE: Periosteal bone growth in normal infants: a preliminary study. AJR 97:154, 1966
23. Reed MH: Pediatric Skeletal Radiology. Williams & Wilkins, Baltimore, 1992
24. Grewar D: Infantile scurvy. Clin Pediatr 4:82, 1965
25. Solomon A, Rosen E: The aspect of trauma in the bone changes of congenital lues. Pediatr Radiol 3:176, 1975
26. Adams PC, Strand RD, Bresnan MJ, Lucky AW: Kinky hair syndrome: serial study of radiological findings with emphasis on the similarity to the battered child syndrome. Radiology 112:401, 1974
27. Bohrer SP: Bone changes in the extremities in sickle cell anemia. Semin Roentgenol 22:176, 1987
28. Padfield E, Hicken P: Cortical hyperostosis in infants: a radiological study of sixteen patients. Br J Radiol 43:231, 1970
29. Swischuk LE: Differential Diagnosis in Pediatric Radiology. Williams & Wilkins, Baltimore, 1984
30. Schnall SB, King JD, Marrero G: Congenital pseudarthrosis of the clavicle: a review of the literature and surgical results of six cases. J Pediatr Orthop 8:316, 1988
31. Eventov I, Reider-Grosswasser I, Weiss S et al: Cleidocranial dysplasia: a family study. Clin Radiol 30:323, 1979
32. Kirkwood JR, Ozonoff MB, Steinbach HL: Epiphyseal displacement after metaphyseal fracture in renal osteodystrophy. AJR 115:547, 1972

33. Swischuk LE, Hayden CK, Kupfer MC: Significance of intraarticular fluid without visible fracture in children. AJR 142:1261, 1984
34. Mital MA: Congenital radioulnar synostosis and congenital dislocation of the radial head. Orthop Clin North Am 7:375, 1976
35. Kameyama O, Ogawa R: Pseudarthrosis of the radius associated with neurofibromatosis: report of a case and review of the literature. J Pediatr Orthop 10:128, 1990
36. MacEwan DW: Changes due to trauma in the fat plane overlying the pronator quadratus muscle: a radiologic sign. Radiology 82:879, 1964
37. Golding JSR, Blackburne JS: Madelung disease of the wrist and dyschondrosteosis. J Bone Joint Surg [Br] 58:350, 1976
38. Poznanski AK, Pratt GB, Manson G, Weiss L: Clinodactyly, camptodactyly, Kirner's deformity and other crooked fingers. Radiology 93:573, 1969
39. Kattan KR: Two features of the atlas vertebra simulating fractures by tomography. AJR 132:963, 1979
40. Suss RA, Zimmerman RD, Leeds NE: Pseudospread of the atlas: false sign of Jefferson fracture in young children. AJR 140:1079, 1983
41. Jacobsen G, Bleaker HH: Pseudosubluxation of the atlas in children. AJR 82:472, 1959
42. Nanni G, Hudson TM: Posterior ring apophysis of the cervical spine. AJR 139:383, 1982
43. Van Gilder JC, Menenzes AH, Dolan KA: The Craniovertebral Junction and Its Abnormalities. Futura, Mount Kisco, NY, 1987
44. Shapiro R, Robinson F: Anomalies of the craniovertebral border. AJR 127:281, 1976
45. Currarino G: Primary spondylolysis of the axis vertebra (C2) in three children including one with pyknodysostosis. Pediatr Radiol 19:535, 1989
46. Elliott S, Morton RE, Whitelaw RAJ: Atlantoaxial instability in Down's syndrome. Arch Dis Child 63:1484, 1988
47. Tsou PM, Yau A, Hodgson AR: Embryogenesis and prenatal development of congenital vertebral anomalies and their classification. Clin Orthop 152:211, 1980
48. Downey EF, Whiddon SM, Brower AC: Computed tomography of congenital absence of posterior elements in the thoracolumbar spine. Spine 11:68, 1986
49. Fidas A, MacDonald HL, Elton RA et al: Prevalence and patterns of spina bifida occulta in 2707 normal adults. Clin Radiol 38:537, 1987
50. Wertzberger KL, Peterson HA: Acquired spondylolysis and spondylolysthesis in the young child. Spine 5:437, 1980
51. Wilkinson RH, Hall JE: The sclerotic pedicle: tumor or pseudotumor? Radiology 111:683, 1974
52. Sherk HH, Nicholson JT, Nixon JE: Vertebra plana and eosinophilic granuloma of the cervical spine in children. Spine 3:116, 1978
53. Ascani E, Montanaro A: Scheuermann's disease. In Bradford DS, Hensinger RM (eds): The Pediatric Spine. Thieme, New York, 1985
54. Du Lac P, Panuel M, Devred P et al: MRI of disc space infection in infants and children. Pediatr Radiol 20:175, 1990
55. Miller KE, Allen RP, Davis WS: Rib gap defects with micrognathia: the syndrome with rib dysplasia. AJR 114:253, 1972
56. Poznanski AK, Fernbach SK, Berry TE: Bone changes from prostaglandin therapy. Skeletal Radiol 14:20, 1985
57. Kaye JJ, Winchester PH, Freiberger RH: Neonatal septic "dislocation" of the hip: true dislocation or pathological epiphyseal separation? Radiology 114:671, 1975
58. Hillman JS, Mesgarzadeh M, Revesz G et al: Proximal femoral focal deficiency: radiologic analysis of 49 cases. Radiology 165:769, 1987
59. Calhoun JD, Pierret G: Infantile coxa vara. AJR 115:561, 1972
60. Ogden JA, McCarthy SM, Jokl P: The painful bipartite patella. J Pediatr Orthop 2:263, 1982
61. Bensahel H, Dal Monte A, Hjelmstedt A et al: Congenital dislocation of the knee. J Pediatr Orthop 9:174, 1989
62. Paterson D: Congenital pseudarthrosis of the tibia: an overview. Clin Orthop 247:44, 1989
63. Towbin R, Dunbar JS, Towbin J, Clark R: Teardrop sign: plain film recognition of ankle effusion. AJR 134:985, 1980
64. Onimus M, Laurain JM, Picard F: Congenital diastasis of the inferior tibiotalar ligament. J Pediatr Orthop 10:172, 1990

5

Anesthesia for Children's Fractures

William M. Splinter

Pain seldom assists a wound to heal.

Providing safe and effective anesthesia for children with fractures is a daily challenge for orthopaedic surgeons and anesthetists. This chapter includes a description of preanesthetic evaluation, sedation, regional anesthesia, and postoperative concerns, as well as a succinct discussion of general anesthesia of interest to the orthopaedic surgeon who manages children's fractures.

PREANESTHETIC ASSESSMENT AND PREPARATION

The apparently healthy child with a minor fracture requires little assessment, except a good history and physical examination and routine preoperative investigations, such as hemoglobinanalysis and urinalysis. Children with serious or multiple injuries require cautious assessment of their surgical and medical problems. Damage to other organs must be reviewed, and the possible implications for anesthesia must be planned for in advance. Particularly important concerns to the anesthetist are as follows:

1. Major fractures, especially spinal fractures
2. Thoracic trauma
3. Fluid status, especially blood loss
4. Abdominal trauma, including retroperitoneal damage
5. Head injury

Multiple Trauma

Major Limb and Spinal Fractures

Major limb fractures are associated with marked pain, significant blood loss, nerve damage, and embolic phenomena. Anesthetic implications of these problems include decreased gastric emptying (increased risk of aspiration pneumonia), hemodynamic instability, and difficulty with positioning of the patient before and after the induction of anesthesia. It is an understatement to say that spinal fractures are a problem to anesthetists. Unlike adults, children often do not understand the seriousness of an unstable spinal injury. Meticulous, well-planned care should not lead to a deterioration in neurologic status. Careful airway management may include awake intubation, which is stressful to the patient, the anesthetist, and the watching surgeon. Awake intubation is indicated when neurologic assessment after endotracheal intubation is necessary.

Hypotensive anesthesia in the operative treatment of

thoracolumbar fractures has been associated with decreased blood loss and no adverse neurologic sequelae.[1]

Thoracic Trauma

Undetected major thoracic trauma may lead to intraoperative mortality. The anesthetist must be satisfied that there will be no intraoperative disasters because of an undetected pneumothorax, pericardial tamponade, aortic dissection, myocardial contusion, or valvular rupture. A pneumothorax may dramatically increase in size after induction of anesthesia because of the institution of positive pressure ventilation. Also, anesthetic agents, such as nitrous oxide, rapidly diffuse into closed air cavities, such as a pneumothorax, and markedly increase intrathoracic pressure.

Abdominal Trauma

Laceration of abdominal viscera is associated with blood loss, hemodynamic instability, sepsis, decreased organ function (and drug metabolism), acidosis, and decreased gastric emptying (increased risk of aspiration pneumonia). All of these injuries may alter the anesthetist's plan.

Head Injury

The child with a head injury and fracture is another special problem to the anesthetist and surgeon. Head injury has numerous anesthetic implications. The anesthetist should plan to administer drugs that will not have an adverse effect on the central nervous system (CNS) and that will have minimal CNS depressant effects at the end of the anesthetic. In addition, these agents have to be administered in a fashion that will have either a beneficial or a negligible effect on an intracranial lesion. To facilitate the anesthetist's plan, a complete CNS assessment of the traumatized patient is required. The surgical intervention of open fractures may even have to be deferred pending complete assessment of the child with a head injury to prevent further CNS damage. Consultations between the anesthetist, neurosurgeon, and orthopaedic surgeon is the best approach to these patients.

Preexisting Medical Disease

All preexisting medical illnesses are of concern to the anesthetist as well as the orthopaedist administering a local anesthetic. In particular, respiratory disease, cardiac disease, hemoglobinopathies, renal and hepatic disease, and neurologic disease have the greatest adverse impact on the delivery of anesthetic agents.

Respiratory Disease

Respiratory disease is common in children. Many children with fractures will have recently recovered or will be suffering from an upper respiratory viral infection. General anesthesia can augment the adverse effects of a respiratory tract infection by drying the airway, interfering with cilial function, causing atelectasis, and triggering croup. Asthma is an increasingly common respiratory disease encountered in children. Anesthesia may occasionally induce status asthmaticus, which may be fatal. When possible, the respiratory disease should be medically optimized preoperatively. Regional anesthesia is a common approach to the child with significant lung disease. On rare occasions, the respiratory risk of anesthesia/surgery are greater than the benefit of immediate surgery, and anesthesia may be deferred until the respiratory status can be optimized.

Cardiac Disease

Cardiac disease is not as common in children as in adults. Because congenital cardiac disease is often quite complex, each child must be treated individually. Complete medical charts and a recent consultation with a cardiologist are usually of the greatest help to the anesthetist. Occasionally the child with a fracture and coexisting congenital cardiac disease will require in depth preoperative assessment, including electrocardiogram (ECG), echocardiogram, chest radiograph, and cardiology consultation.

Hemoglobinopathies

Hematologic problems are unusual in childhood. Of special significance to anesthesiologists and surgeons is sickle cell trait/disease. Sickling crisis may be triggered by hypothermia, acidosis, and hypoxia, all of which are associated with tourniquet usage. All children of African origin must be screened for sickling before fracture reduction, if there is any possibility of tourniquet usage, which causes limb hypoxia and acidosis and general acidosis upon release of the tourniquet.

The acceptable serum hemoglobin concentration for surgery varies according to each patient. In the past it was believed that a preoperative hemoglobin should be at least 100 g/L. Now, an asymptomatic patient with a known and well-compensated hemoglobin of 75 g/L does not require a preanesthetic transfusion.

Renal and Hepatic Disease

Renal and hepatic disease have marked implications for most anesthetics. The clinician must be aware of the effect these disease processes have on the physiologic status before further stress from anesthesia is induced. Most anesthetic agents are either metabolized or excreted via these organ systems. The pharmacodynamics and pharmacokinetics of many anesthetic drugs will be altered by renal and hepatic disease. For example, many neuromuscular blocking drugs have a markedly prolonged half-life in the presence of renal and/or hepatic disease, toxic metabolites of meperidine accumulate in the presence of renal failure, and lidocaine, diazepam (Valium), and most narcotics depend on the liver for metabolism.

Neurologic Disease

Many neurologic diseases interact with anesthesia. A few examples are as follows:

1. Seizure medications, such as barbiturates, lead to tolerance of sedatives and increase metabolism of many neuromuscular blocking agents.
2. Recently denervated or crushed muscle may release massive amounts of potassium immediately after the administration of succinylcholine.
3. Neuromuscular blockade monitors are not accurate when placed on paralyzed limbs.

Thus, a patient's disease must be described in detail in the preoperative assessment.

Anesthetic History

During routine assessment of children before surgery, a detailed history of any adverse response to general and local anesthesia should be obtained. Generally, such children should be managed by an anesthetist, rather than risk local anesthesia under less than optimal conditions. The anesthetist should be notified immediately of any family history of anesthetic death, malignant hyperthermia, or pseudocholinesterase deficiency. This will allow the anesthetist adequate time for preparation and prevent excessive delays.

Malignant hyperthermia is common among orthopaedic patients. This process is a hypermetabolic state induced by several anesthetic drugs, including succinylcholine, halothane, enflurane, and isoflurane. Initial signs of this hypermetabolic state include hypercarbia, dysrhythmias, and hyperthermia. Initial management of malignant hyperthermia includes discontinuing the triggering agent and treatment with primarily supportive measures (oxygen, active cooling, sodium bicarbonate, respiratory support) and with intravenous dantrolene (initial dose: 1 mg/kg).

Preoperative Fasting

Preoperative fasting prior to anesthesia is a necessity. The appropriate fast results in a minimum amount of gastric contents. A prolonged fast may be in conflict with the surgeon's desire to begin surgery as soon as possible. Each child should be treated individually. The risk of aspiration pneumonia must be compared to the benefit of immediate surgery. After due consideration of both matters, the surgeon and anesthetist should be able to agree as to what is the optimal timing for anesthesia and surgery. Trauma markedly reduces gastric emptying, but the volume of gastric contents decreases inversely with the length of preoperative fast. Delaying fracture reduction may diminish gastric contents, but it will result in increased local swelling, more difficult reduction, and increased risk of infection in open fractures, and may contribute to limb ischemia if the vascular supply has been compromised.

Psychological Preparation

Children and their parents require psychological preparation before anesthesia and surgery. Surgery is a worrisome event in any family. Anxious parents and the child must be reassured and consoled. A brief and concise description of the anesthetic followed by a question and answer session will alleviate most parents' fears. Toddlers may feel like a person trapped in a foreign environment with almost no method of communication, except yelling and crying. School-aged children usually understand the situation and respond to gentle reassurance with properly explained and honest answers to all their questions. Preschool children are somewhere between these two groups and require honest answers, but it may be difficult to adequately explain the situation to them. Children from unusual ethnic backgrounds or dysfunctional families, and children who have undergone repeated hospitalization, often require special attention, including lengthy preoperative reassurance and explanation. Parental presence at the time of induction of general anesthesia is controversial. Investigators have observed both beneficial and detrimental effects from this approach.

Those children who remain excessively anxious, in spite of adequate psychological preparation, require premedication. We have found that oral or intravenous midazolam provides rapid anxiolysis with minimal adverse effects. There are few indications for intramuscular premedication in children. Most anesthetists reserve its use to the large, uncontrollable child who refuses oral or intravenous medication. Often the parents or guardian are the only persons capable of controlling a physically mature, but developmentally delayed child, and their presence may obviate restraint or intramuscular injections.

CONSCIOUS SEDATION

Often the orthopaedic surgeon needs to sedate a child with a fractured limb. Sedation facilitates fracture reduction. With conscious sedation, the child is cooperative, calm, serene, and composed and has an intact airway and other protective reflexes. Sedation to the point of unconsciousness is similar to general anesthesia and should be avoided.

Sedation is achieved with both anxiolytics and narcotics. Each anxiolytic agent and narcotic has particular advantages and disadvantages. A major determinant of the drug(s) chosen is past personal experience. Anxiolytics, such as benzodiazepines, barbiturates, and antihistamines, provide a calming effect, usually amnesia and little respiratory depression, but they are not analgesics. Narcotics provide little sedation and are excellent analgesics, but they are associated with respiratory depression and nausea. Anxiolytics and narcotics appear to work synergistically, resulting in excellent sedation, but on occasion excessive respiratory depression may occur. Nitrous oxide provides analgesia, amnesia, and anxiolysis.[2] A mixture of 50 percent oxygen and 50 percent nitrous oxide is an effective sedative for most children. Occasionally, the sedation from nitrous oxide may be excessive or ineffective.[2]

Rather than discuss a variety of "sedatives," we will discuss the use of only two, morphine and midazolam. Each drug is similar in length of action, onset of action, and dosage. In addition, antagonists (naloxone and flumazenil) exist for both agents. Morphine is widely used by all surgeons and anesthetists. By titrating, every 5 minutes, boluses of 0.05 mg/kg of intravenous morphine, children are safely narcotized after 1 to 3 boluses. Amnesia and marked sedation can be achieved by alternating the morphine with 0.05 mg/kg of intravenous midazolam. (Midazolam is a water-soluble benzodiazepine with a 3- to 4-hour half-life, about twice the potency of diazepam and approximately twice the length of time to onset of action of diazepam.)

Before sedating a child, the parents must consent to the sedation and, if appropriate, the child's assent is obtained. Monitoring is as described in the section on regional anesthesia. Resuscitation equipment must be available. Antagonists must be available and recommended doses are 0.005 to 0.01 mg/kg of naloxone IV and 0.5 mg of flumazenil IV.

GENERAL ANESTHESIA

General anesthesia for emergency fracture reduction carries with it special risks. The most notable is the risk of aspiration pneumonia.[3] Each child must be considered to have a "full stomach." Gastric contents may be decreased by delaying anesthesia. Other options are the decompression of gastric contents with a large-bore gastric tube, the administration of drugs known to enhance gastric emptying, such as metoclopramide,[4] and the neutralization of gastric acid with anticholinergics, such as glycopyrrolate, and antihistamines, such as cimetidine. Only delaying anesthesia and surgery is a commonly practiced method of achieving gastric emptying.

After careful preoperative assessment and the placement of the appropriate monitors, general anesthesia is induced rapidly intravenously after 3 minutes of preoxygenation. Typically induction may be with 4 to 6 mg/kg of sodium thiopentone. Immediately after induction passive gastric reflux should be prevented by gentle pressure on the cricoid cartilage, and a rapid-acting muscle relaxant, succinylcholine, 1 mg/kg, is administered. After endotracheal intubation and confirmation of proper placement of the endotracheal tube, the cricoid pressure is released. The surgeon may begin to examine the patient after the anesthetist has confirmed adequate ventilation and hemodynamic stability, and has begun to administer anesthetic agents for the maintenance of anesthesia. After the fracture has been reduced, the child should be allowed to awaken in the head down, lateral position and should be extubated after the return of all protective reflexes.

TABLE 5-1. Risks of Regional Anesthesia

Block Technique	Local Infection	Toxicity	Nerve Damage	Pneumothorax	Phlebitis	Urinary Retention	Hypotension
Hematoma	x	x					
Intravenous		x			x		
Brachial plexus		x	x	x			x
Nerve		x	x				
Epidural	x	x	x			x	x
Spinal	x		x			x	x
Sympathetic nerve	x	x	x	x	x	x	x

REGIONAL ANESTHESIA

Regional anesthesia for children's fractures may involve a broad spectrum of techniques. Some are relatively simple and safe, while others may be technically very difficult and are associated with significant risk. We will describe the common techniques and appropriate monitoring.

Monitoring

Monitoring of the child undergoing regional anesthesia is critical and vital. Delayed detection of an adverse outcome is unacceptable. Other than very simple techniques, such as digital blocks, monitoring should include electrocardiography (ECG), pulse oximetry, temperature (for prolonged procedures), and an observer. The observer is the key monitor. This person must have the appropriate observational skills such that an adverse effect of the anesthetic technique or an adverse event related to sedation is promptly detected and treated. For major regional anesthetic techniques, such as brachial plexus blockade and epidural blockade, this person is usually an anesthesiologist. For minor techniques, such as hematoma or peripheral nerve block, this person is often a registered nurse. Resuscitation equipment should always be readily available whenever local anesthesia is being used.

Patient Selection

Regional anesthesia should be predicated on the requirements of the surgery and the age and cooperation of the child. It should only be performed in a select group of children who are receptive to such techniques. After hearing appropriate information and with parental guidance, most children over the age of 4 can choose between general and regional anesthesia. Indications for these techniques include significant fears of general anesthesia (which are especially common among teenagers), a family history of malignant hyperthermia, and significant respiratory diseases, such as asthma and cystic fibrosis. We have found that regional anesthesia, among properly prepared children, is a very attractive choice for both parent and child. Items discussed during preparation of the child for a regional anesthetic technique include sedation, the necessity of a needle, and the potential for failure. Contraindications to regional anesthesia are as follows:

1. Lack of parental consent
2. Lack of patient cooperation
3. Bleeding disorder
4. Local infection
5. Neurologic and anatomic anomalies

Risks

There are risks associated with regional anesthesia. These complications vary according to the technique involved and are summarized in Table 5-1. These techniques may cause an adverse effect if the needle is in the wrong place or an inappropriate dosage of local anesthetic agent is used. Overdosage of local anesthetic agents may precipitate seizures, cardiovascular collapse, and death.[5] Rare and usually unavoidable adverse effects include anaphylaxis and vasovagal attacks. Therefore, resuscitation equipment must always be readily available.

Regional Anesthetic Techniques

Local/Hematoma Block

This popular, simple, and safe technique is typically performed by the orthopaedic surgeon before the reduction of uncomplicated, closed forearm fractures.[6-8] It involves the aseptic aspiration of the fracture hematoma and injection of 2 to 6 ml of 1 percent lidocaine into the fracture site. The major problems associated with this technique are the inability to assess the quality of the block in young children, failure of analgesia, no associated muscle relaxation, and the theoretical risk of osteomyelitis. This technique is more successful in teenagers with angulated, distal radial and ulna fractures that only require correction of angulation. It should not be employed for completely overriding fractures where muscle relaxation is essential for fracture reduction. It is seldom an appropriate technique for children under 8 years of age.

Intravenous (Bier) Block

Another popular anesthetic approach to distal limb fractures is intravenous regional anesthesia.[9-17] This technique is much more effective than a local hematoma block.[7] Children over 4 years of age who have simple, unilateral fractures, not involving the elbow or knee, tolerate this anesthetic procedure quite well. Good analgesia is usually achieved in 90 percent of patients. Appropriately trained physicians can safely and adequately perform this anesthetic technique[9] as described in Table 5-2. Physicians who use this technique must be aware of the symptoms and signs of local anesthetic toxicity and the treatment.[13] These include dizziness, circumoral numbness, visual disturbances, and tremors. Severe toxicity results in a loss of consciousness, seizures, and cardiovascular collapse. Young children may be unable to appreciate or adequately verbalize the early symptoms of dizziness, numbness, and visual disturbances. Early symptoms require prompt reinflation of the cuff to prevent further absorption of lidocaine into the systemic circulation, careful monitoring of the child for further progression of the toxicity, and the administration of oxygen. Management of seizures includes resuscitative

TABLE 5-2. Technique for Intravenous Regional Anaesthesia (Bier Block)

1. Patient selection: Cooperative and usually over 4 years of age.
2. Test equipment: The double tourniquet should be an automatic pneumatic device with variable sized cuffs, reinforced hoses, locking connectors, and a check-valve to prevent spontaneous cuff deflation in the event of pressure failure.
3. Establish intravenous access in a nonaffected limb.
4. Sedation with the presence of a parent.
5. Tourniquet is placed on the affected limb.
6. A 24-gauge intravenous catheter is placed in a dorsal vein or the saphenous vein of the affected limb.
7. The affected limb is drained of blood by elevation for 1 to 3 minutes.
8. The tourniquet cuff is inflated to 100 mmHg greater than systolic blood pressure.
9. The affected limb is returned to the horizontal.
10. An iso-osmolar 0.5% lidocaine solution is injected slowly over a minute and to a dose of 3 mg/kg of lidocaine into affected limbs veins via the angiocatheter. (The recommended dose for lidocaine is 1.5–5 mg/kg.[a] We find 3 mg/kg is effective and associated with minimal risk for toxicity, when the block is performed properly.) Satisfactory anesthesia occurs in 5–10 minutes. The angiocatheter is removed and an appropriate dressing applied. (Lidocaine is currently the drug of choice for IV regional anesthesia. Bupivacaine is more cardiotoxic, and prilocaine is associated with methemoglobinemia.)
11. The fracture is reduced and plaster is applied.
12. The cuff is slowly deflated. (The minimum and maximum length of cuff inflation is 20 and 90 minutes, respectively.) The cuff is removed.
13. The cast is extended as appropriate.
14. After observation for 1 hour, the children may be discharged to the care of competent parents.

[a] See refs. 9 to 17.

measures necessitating the management and protection of the airway and the use of intravenous anticonvulsant agents, such as diazepam. The major problems with this technique include (1) lidocaine toxicity due to cuff failure or overdosage and (2) poor analgesia.

Brachial Plexus Block

This approach should be reserved for more complicated fractures, which require operating room facilities. The advantages of this technique include

1. Variable length of action of the block (1 – 12 hours)
2. Muscle relaxation
3. Tourniquet analgesia

Disadvantages include

1. The requirement for the presence of a clinician who is capable of coping with complications
2. The technique is technically demanding and associated with a significant learning curve
3. Increased risk of major adverse effects, such as pneumothorax and nerve damage

There are numerous approaches to brachial plexus blockade, for example, supraclavicular, infraclavicular, intrascalene, and axillary, and each approach has advantages and disadvantages. It has been suggested that the axillary approach, which has a low risk of respiratory complications, is the best method of brachial plexus block in children.[18,19] A continuous anesthetic may be established by inserting a catheter into the brachial plexus via an axillary approach. A description of these techniques is beyond the scope of this chapter.

Digital Nerve Block

Fractured fingers can often be reduced with a digital nerve block.[20] This simple anesthetic technique requires the gentle placement of a small volume (about 0.5 ml) of local anesthetic at the digital nerves in the web space (see Fig. 5-1). The use of small (27- or 30-gauge needles) is tolerated by children if a gentle, patient approach is used.

More extensive fractures involving the hand may require a median nerve, ulnar nerve, and/or dorsal branch of the radial nerve block at the wrist. These nerves are easily blocked with knowledge of basic anatomy.

Ankle Block

Midtarsal ankle block is a safe, efficacious anesthetic for forefoot surgery because of its low risk for toxicity and prolonged anesthesia/analgesia.[28] Five nerves need to be blocked, so this technique should be reserved for children who are an excellent candidate for a regional anesthesia or who have a major contraindication to general anesthesia. Most children will not tolerate the five punctures without sedation unless they possess a very stoical personality. The superficial peroneal nerve and saphenous nerve are blocked by depositing a wheal of local anesthetic in the subcutaneous tissue from the medial to lateral malleolus on the dorsum of the ankle (see Fig. 5-2). The deep peroneal nerve is adjacent to the dorsalis pedis artery, being either lateral or inferior to it at the ankle. It is easily blocked. The sural nerve is

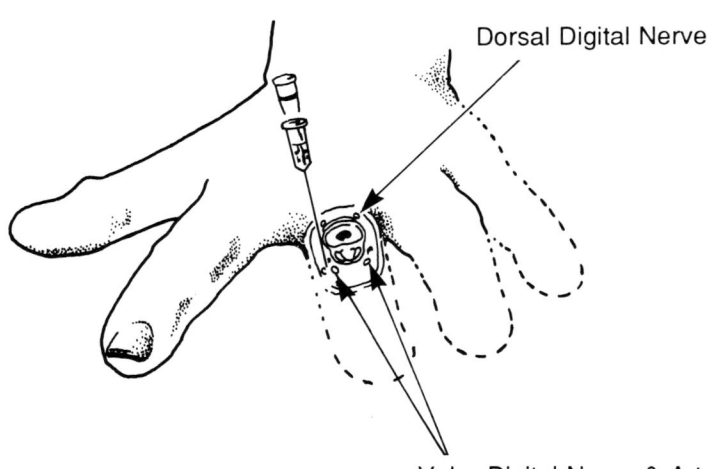

Fig. 5-1. Technique of digital nerve block at base of finger between metacarpal heads.

blocked by a wheal of subcutaneous local anesthetic just posterior to the lateral malleolus. The posterior tibial nerve is blocked by carefully injecting local anesthetic immediately anterior, posterior, and inferior to the posterior tibial artery.

Femoral Nerve Block

The femoral nerve block is a short-onset block useful among children with femoral midshaft fractures.[21-24] These blocks allow simple and comfortable radiography of the femur and closed reduction of the fracture. The injection of 0.5 ml/kg of 1 percent lidocaine adjacent to the femoral nerve at the groin results in a 3-in-1 block of the femoral nerve, lateral femoral cutaneous nerves, and obturator nerves. The needle is inserted just lateral to the femoral artery at the midinguinal point. Typically, a loss of resistance is detected as the needle pops through the fascia lata. If a block of longer duration is required, injection of 2 mg/kg of 0.5 percent bupivacaine should result in a complete 3-in-1 block.

Epidural Block

Epidural block is technically demanding but very effective and rewarding. The technical demands restrict this block to those skilled in its performance and cooperative patients. The rewards exist because the length of blockade and the number and type of nerves blocked may be controlled. This form of regional anesthesia is utilized when requested by the patient with a lower limb fracture and when there is a relative or absolute contraindication to general anesthesia. Examples where epidural anesthesia may be advantageous include patients at risk for malignant hyperthermia and patients with significant lung disease (e.g., severe asthma, cystic fibrosis).

Spinal Block

The indications for spinal block are similar to those for an epidural block. When compared to epidural anesthesia, it is technically easier to perform, but is associated with a clinically significant incidence of headache, is less predictable, and there is little experience in children with this regional anesthetic approach.

Sympathetic Nerve Block

Indications for a block of the sympathetic nervous system include reflex sympathetic dystrophy, which may occur in children after a fracture. It is also indicated in unusual acute situations where the circulation to a limb or portion thereof is compromised and any sympathetic tone present may have an adverse effect. Sympathetic nerve blocks should be performed by experienced physicians. Upper limb sympathetic nerve block is achieved with a stellate ganglion block or intravenous regional

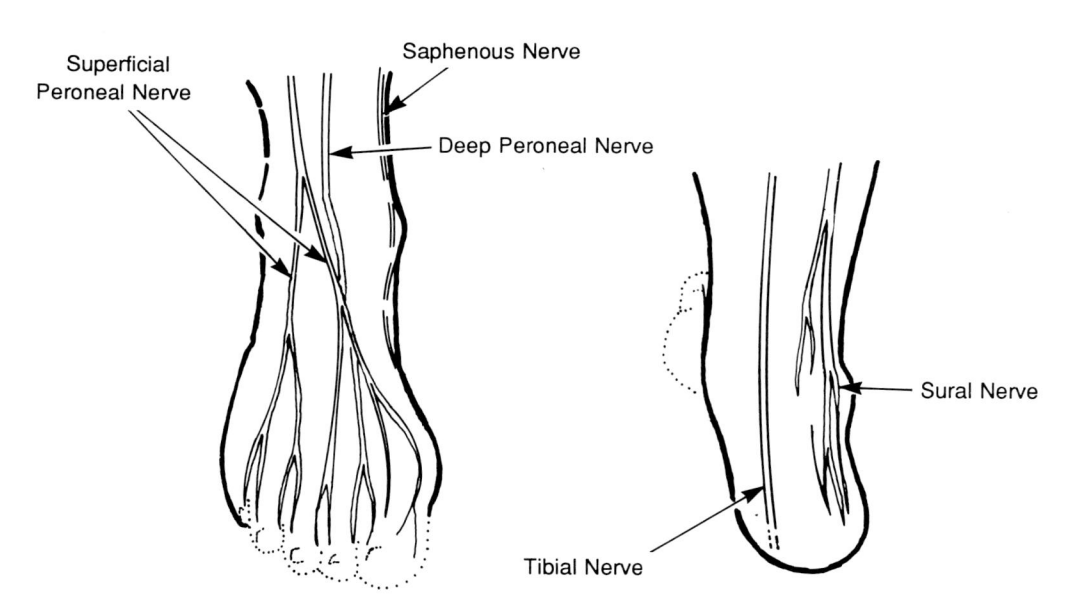

Fig. 5-2. Anatomy and technique of neural blockade for nerves at the ankle.

TABLE 5-3. Pharmacology of Local Anesthetics

Drug	Site of Metabolism	Duration of Action (min)	Potency	Maximum Dose[a] mg/kg	Percent Protein Binding
Lidocaine	Liver	100	1	3–5	64
Bupivacaine	Liver	175	0.25	1.6	96

[a] Maximum dose is for a nonintravenous regional block in a healthy patient. Increase by about 10 to 20 percent, if 1/200,000 epinephrine, is added to the local anesthetic.

guanethidine. Lower limb blockade may be achieved with a lumbar sympathetic block, epidural anesthesia, or with intravenous regional guanethidine.

Pharmacology of Local Anesthetic Drugs

There are only two commonly used local anesthetics in children: lidocaine and bupivacaine. Their pharmacology is briefly described in Table 5-3. Bupivacaine is the more toxic of the two compounds, but it remains a popular agent because its longer half-life is of clinical significance. The addition of 1 in 200,000 epinephrine to a local anesthetic is advantageous because the epinephrine decreases local anesthetic toxicity and prolongs its half-life. Epinephrine should not be used on digits or penile tissue because there is a theoretical risk of vascular compromise due to end-artery vasoconstriction in response to epinephrine.

POSTOPERATIVE CARE (AN ANESTHETIST'S PERSPECTIVE)

Anesthesia interacts with postoperative care. Nausea and vomiting immediately after surgery is typically due to anesthesia. Low doses (25 μg/kg) of droperidol controls most nausea and is associated with minimal adverse effects, such as sedation.

Most fractures are associated with minimal discomfort after reduction and immobilization with a cast. Pain can be assessed in children in a variety of fashions, such as with the modified CHEOPS pain score (Table 5-4), or the Objective Pain Scale.[27] Multiple trauma patients often require aggressive pain management. The physician responsible for this pain control must balance the demand for adequate pain control and the risk of obscuring complications, such as a compartment syndrome. In addition, the physician should know the varied effects of anesthetic agents on postoperative pain. For example, inhalation agents, such as halothane, have minimal effect on pain beyond the recovery room stay, but long-acting narcotics, which were administered as part of the anesthetic, will have an analgesic effect for hours. In addition, a regional anesthetic technique, which was used to supplement a general anesthetic, may have an effect on analgesia for 24 hours.

Occasionally children develop chronic pain syndromes after a fracture. A prompt consultation with an anesthesiologist is indicated if there is a need for a sympathetic nerve block. Early treatment easily controls the sympathetically mediated chronic pain.

TABLE 5-4. Modified CHEOPS Pain Scale

Sign or Symptom	Score
Cry	
No cry	0
Moaning/crying	1
Screaming	2
Facial	
Smiling	0
Composed	1
Grimace	2
Child verbal	
Positive	0
None or other complaint	1
Pain complaint	2
Torso	
Neutral	0
Shifting, tense, upright	1
Restrained	2
Legs	
Neutral	0
Kick, squirm, drawn up	1
Restrained	2
Total	

SUMMARY

A variety of anesthetic approaches to the child with a fracture have been described. Complete preoperative preparation and assessment, plus adequate monitoring have been emphasized. Anesthetic techniques that may be appropriate for use by an orthopaedic surgeon include conscious sedation and simple regional anesthetic techniques.

REFERENCES

1. Ullrich PF, Keene JS, Hogan KJ, Roecker EB: Results of hypotensive anesthesia in operative treatment of thoracolumbar fractures. J Spinal Disord 3:329, 1990
2. Wattenmaker I, Kasser JR, McGravey A: Self-administered nitrous oxide for fracture reduction in children in an emergency room setting. J Orthop Trauma 4:35, 1990
3. Salem MR, Klowden AJ: Anesthesia for pediatric orthopedic surgery. p. 1203. In Gregory GA (ed): Pediatric Anesthesia. 2nd Ed. Churchill Livingstone, New York, 1989
4. Olsson GL, Hallen B: Pharmacological evaluation of the stomach with metoclopramide. Acta Anaesth Scand 26:417, 1982
5. Berde CB: Convulsions associated with pediatric regional anesthesia. Anesth Analg 75:164, 1992
6. Johnson PQ, Noffsinger MA: Haematoma block of distal forearm fractures: is it safe? Orthop Rev 20:977, 1991
7. Cobb AG, Houghton GR: Comparison of local anesthesia infiltration and intravenous regional anesthesia in patients with Colles' fracture. J Bone Joint Surg [Br] 67:845, 1985
8. Case RD: Haematoma block-A safe method of reducing Colles' fractures. Br J Accident Surg 16:469, 1979
9. Olney BW, Lugg PC, Turner PL et al: Outpatient treatment of upper extremity injuries in childhood using intravenous regional anaesthesia. J Pediatr Orthop 8:576, 1988
10. Schiller MG: Intravenous regional anesthesia for closed treatment of fractures and dislocations of the upper extremities. Clin Orth Rel Res 118:25, 1976
11. Lehman WL, Jones WW: Intravenous lidocaine for anesthesia in the lower extremity. J Bone Joint Surg [Am] 66:1056, 1984
12. Gingrich TF: Intravenous regional anesthesia of the upper extremity in children. JAMA 200:135, 1967
13. Turner PL, Batten JB, Hjorth D et al: Intravenous regional anaesthesia for the treatment of upper limb injuries in childhood. Aust N Z J Surg 56:153, 1986
14. Hollingsworth A, Wallace WA, Dabir R et al: Comparison of bupivacaine and prilocaine used in Bier block. Injury: Br J Accident Surg 13:331, 1981
15. Barnes CL, Blasier RD, Dodge BM: Intravenous regional anesthesia: a safe and cost-effective outpatient anesthetic for upper extremity fracture treatment in children. J Pediatr Orthop 11:717, 1991
16. Carrel ED, Eyring EJ: Intravenous regional anesthesia for childhood fractures. J Trauma 11:301, 1971
17. Farrell RG, Swanson SL, Walter JR: Safe and effective IV regional anesthesia for use in the emergency department. Ann Emerg Med 14:288, 1985
18. Haddad RJ, Saer JK, Riordan DC: Percutaneous pinning of displaced supracondylar fractures of the elbow in children. Clin Orthop 71:112, 1970
19. Courtad JG, Reese CA: A case approach: regional anesthesia for the juvenile patient. J Am Assoc Nurse Anesth 51:175, 1983
20. Zachar JB: Management of injuries of the distal phalanx. Surg Clin North Am 64:747, 1984
21. Grossbard GD, Love BRT: Femoral nerve block: a simple and safe method of instant analgesia for femoral shaft fractures in children. Aust N Z J Surg 49:592, 1979
22. Tondare AS, Nadkarni AV: Femoral nerve block for fractured shaft of femur. Can Anaesth Soc J 29:207, 1982
23. Denton JS, Manning MP: Femoral nerve block for femoral shaft fractures in children. J Bone Joint Surg [Br] 70:84, 1988
24. Ronchi L, Rosenbaum D, Athouel A et al: Femoral nerve blockade in children using bupivacaine. Anesthesiology 70:622, 1989
25. Tucker GT, Mather LE: Properties, absorption, and disposition of local anesthetic agents. p. 47. In Cousins MJ, Bridenbaugh PO (eds): Neural Blockade in Clinical Anesthesia and Management of Pain. JB Lippincott, Philadelphia, 1987
26. Sethna NF, Berde CB: Pediatric regional anesthesia. p. 647. In Gregory GA (ed): Pediatric Anesthesia. 2nd Ed. Churchill Livingstone, New York, 1989
27. Berde CB, Anand KS, Sethna NF: Pediatric pain management. p. 679. In Gregory GA (ed): Pediatric Anesthesia. 2nd Ed. Churchill Livingstone, New York, 1989
28. Mineo R, Sharrock NE: Venous levels of lidocaine and bupivacaine after midtarsal ankle block. Reg Anesth 17:47, 1992

6

Fractures of the Sternum, Scapula, and Ribs

Robert B. Gledhill

> Where all think alike, no one thinks very much.
> WALTER LIPPMAN

FRACTURES OF THE STERNUM

Description and Incidence

Isolated fractures of the sternum are rare and in fact are not discussed in many of the more recent textbooks on fractures.[1-3] The literature suggests that most sternal fractures occur in motor vehicle accidents and are associated with more severe injuries.[4-7] Ostremski and colleagues[5] described an incidence of 3.7 percent with 78 of 2,097 consecutive victims of road traffic accidents suffering sternal fractures. They were most common in seat-belted front-seat passengers involved in head-on collisions. The incidence increased with age and was less frequent in the pediatric population. Sturm and colleagues[6] reviewed the records of 99 patients who suffered sternal fractures over a 20-year period. The patients ranged in age from 5 to 86 years, and most occurred in motor vehicle accidents.

Anatomic Considerations

The sternum is a corticocancellous sandwich containing red marrow and is composed of three parts: (1) the cranial part, or *manubrium;* (2) the middle part, or *body,* and (3) the caudal part, or *xiphoid process.*[8,9] The manubrium has bilateral articulation with the medial ends of each clavicle and a synchondrosis with the costal cartilages of the first rib on each side. The manubrium articulates with the body of the sternum at the sternomanubrial joint, a syndesmosis that allows motion of the sternal body with respiration. The second rib articulates at a notch at the sternomanubrial joint. The body of the sternum is composed of four sternebrae (see the following section on embryology) and has lateral notches for the attachment of the third, fourth, and fifth rib cartilage, with an extra facet on the fourth sternebra for the sixth rib cartilage. The seventh rib cartilage attaches at the body-xiphoid junction. The xiphoid process is thin and flush with the posterior surface of the body so the facets for the seventh costal cartilages lie in front of it (Fig. 6-1A).

Embryology

The sternum develops from bilateral paramedian mesenchymal bars, which chondrify and meet in the median line (Fig. 6-1B). The manubrium is ossified from one to three ossification centers that appear in the fifth month of fetal life. The first and second sternebrae usually ossify from single centers that appear in the fifth or sixth fetal month. The ossification centers for the third

94 / Management of Pediatric Fractures

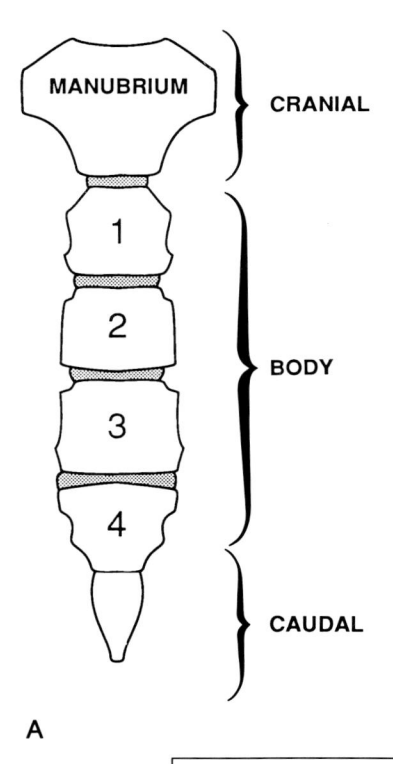

Fig. 6-1. (A) The sternum prior to fusion of the sternebrae is illustrated. The manubrium is cephelad to sternebra 1 and the xyphoid process is caudad to sternebra 4. (B) Development of the sternum. *(A)* The mesoblastic primordia (2 lateral bands and a median rudiment). *(B)* Plate of hyaline cartilage originating from the chondrification and midline fusion of the primordia. *(C)* Appearance of islands of hypertrophied chondroblasts — the future ossification centers. *(D)* Ossification and fusion of the various sternebrae (infant and adult sternum). (Fig. B from: Development of the sternum. In Hensinger RN: Standards in Paediatric Orthopaedics. Raven Press, New York, 1986, with permission.)

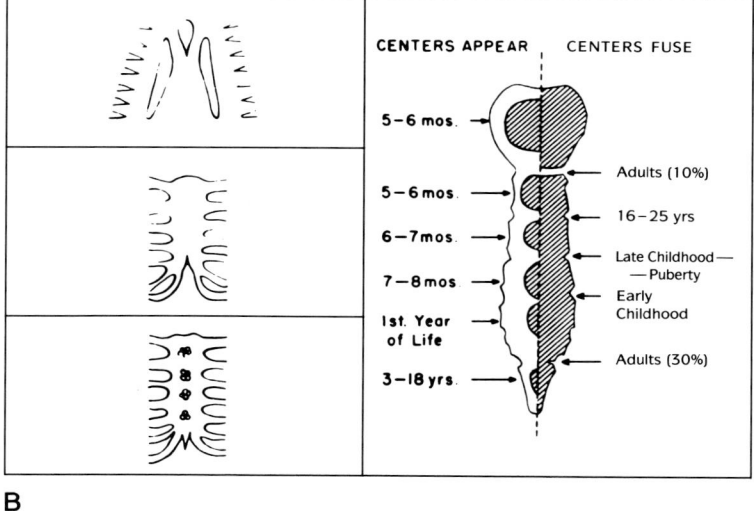

and fourth sternebrae are usually paired and appear at the seventh and eighth fetal month or later, with ossification in general occurring from above downward.

The xiphoid process begins to ossify in the third year or later. Fusions of the sternebrae take place from below upward at the 15th (4 to 3), 20th (3 to 2), and 25th (2 to 1) year, respectively.[8,9] The xiphisternal synchondrosis becomes a synostosis in middle life.[8]

Faulty midline fusion of the paramedian mesenchymal plates may result in defects within the body of the sternum. In adolescence the synchondrosis between sternebrae 1 and 2 may be misinterpreted as a fracture. I have seen two cases of blunt trauma to the sternum in adolescents, which resulted in pain and tenderness in the area of the sternebrae 1-2 synchondrosis for several weeks — presumably undisplaced transsynchondral fractures with healing protracted by the movement of respiration.

Mechanism of Injury

Fractures of the sternum are usually caused by blunt trauma with the vast majority reported in the literature occurring in motor vehicle or road traffic accident.[4-7] The increased incidence with age is probably a reflection of diminishing flexibility of the sternum, sternomanubrial joint and the adjacent costal synchondrosis.[5,6]

Classification

Fractures occurring before sternebral fusion are either through sternebra (Fig. 6-2) or through synchondrosis. Fractures occurring after sternebral fusion can present in the manubrium, body, or xiphoid process. The evolution of ossification and the synchondroses must be kept in mind when looking for fractures of the sternal body to avoid their misinterpretation as fractures. Fractures can, however, occur through the synchondroses prior to fusion and if undisplaced can be clinically suspected and confirmed with bone scan.

Physical Examination

Fractures of the sternum in children are usually associated with massive trauma.[4-7] When associated with minor to moderate direct blunt trauma only, the findings are restricted to the tissues overlying the sternum and the sternum itself. There may or may not be bruising, but there will be tenderness on palpation of the sternum with local pain and on deep breathing.

When associated with massive trauma, the presence of a sternal fracture is an indicator of a frontal contusion and damage to the underlying viscera should be strongly suspected.[4-7] Pelvic, abdominal, and thoracic viscera may be damaged. Injuries to the thoracic viscera are most frequent, and since the sternal injury may be the most easily diagnosed (usually with rib fractures), awareness of probable underlying life-threatening injuries is very important. These include injuries to the aorta, myocardium, trachea, and main bronchi. Aortic and myocardial injury is usually associated with hypovolemic shock, tamponade, and so on, whereas radiographic evidence of subcutaneous emphysema, pneumomediastinum, or pneumothorax suggest the presence of a ruptured trachea or bronchus.[4-7] Concomitant rib and sternum fractures were more often associated with heart ruptures than aortic ruptures in the series by Arajarvi and coworkers[4] on chest injuries in seat-belt wearers.

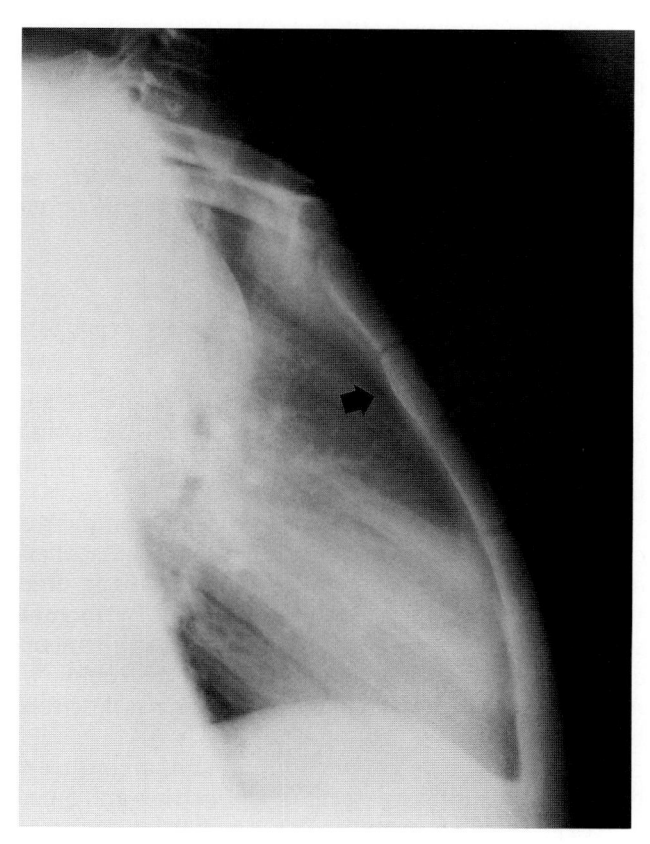

Fig. 6-2. A buckle fracture is seen in the first sternebra in a 2-year-old girl who was involved in a motor vehicle accident. Note the open sternebral synchondroses.

Treatment

In most instances sternal fractures are managed conservatively with rib belt, strapping, time, and analgesics. There is a void in the literature regarding open reduction of sternal fracture. This is probably because fractures that are so displaced as to require open reduction are associated with such severe associated injuries that the patient has not survived. Nonunions, aside from prolonged discomfort, are probably inconsequential. Where repair is indicated, wiring would seem as appropriate as any other technique, since it has been a successful method of closure by cardiovascular surgeons after sternal splitting incisions for many decades.

The management of damage to underlying viscera obviously takes high priority. Detailed management of these injuries is beyond the scope of this chapter but should always be suspected in association with sternal fracture in children.

FRACTURES OF THE SCAPULA

The earliest publication on scapular fractures was in 1805 by Desault.[10] Since that time there have been scattered reports with approximately 60 publications in the last 60 years in the English literature.[11-69]

Most of these have been reports of small numbers of cases or case reports describing fractures of unusual etiology such as avulsion fractures,[10-14] fatigue fractures,[15,16] scapulothoracic dissociation,[17-21] fractures secondary to electrical injury,[22,23] and fractures associated with seizures in patients with osteodystrophy.[24,25] A patient with bilateral scapular fractures was described by Heatley.[26]

Scapular fractures are uncommon and, according to Newell,[27] constitute 1 percent of all fractures and 5 percent of all shoulder fractures. In the pediatric population this incidence is considerably smaller.[27-32]

Two recent publications by McGinnis and Denton,[32] and Ada and Miller[28] present large series with literature reviews and contribute significantly to a better understanding of the management of this uncommon fracture.

Description and Incidence

Scapular fractures are considered by most authors to be an injury of young adult males. In Ada and Miller's[28] series of 113 scapular fractures, the age range was 5 to 75 years, with an average age of 25.9 years. This roughly corresponds with average ages of 27.7 to 43.7 in review of the world literature by McGinnis and colleagues.[32] The average age of McGinnis' own series[32] was 34.7 years. Although scapular fractures are predominantly adult injuries, children are included in most series studied. Infants and children are certainly not precluded from the statistics of motor vehicle injuries, which is the most common cause of this fracture.[27-33]

The male preponderance of 4:1 or greater[28,32] would probably be considerably modified if only the pediatric population under driving age were to be considered.

Anatomic Considerations

The scapula is a flat bone that comprises that shoulder girdle component, which, through its shape and mobility, enhances the flexibility and arc of motion of the upper extremity.[8,9]

It is triangular in shape, has three borders, two surfaces, three angles, a spine running obliquely across the junction of the upper and middle third, and three processes—the acromion, coracoid, and glenoid. The proximal lateral angle is thickened and hollowed out to form an articular surface for the head of the humerus. It has attachments to the clavicle at the acromioclavicular (AC) joint and the coracoclavicular ligaments.

The coracoclavicular ligaments and the AC joint are its least flexible points of scapulothoracic attachment. The rest of the scapula is suspended by muscles. This flexibility, as well as the fact that it is well padded with muscle, both posteriorly and on its costal surfaces, makes it less susceptible to injury than most other bones.

Its relationship with the posterior chest wall and shoulder girdle creates a high association with injuries in these areas, but usually only in the presence of severe trauma.[27-36,70,71]

Embryology

In infancy and childhood the presence of epiphyses and apophyses alter the patterns of injury sustained by adults in any particular bone.[8,9] The zone of hypertrophy adjacent to the zone of provisional calcification creates a "weak plane" not present in the adult bone, so fracture patterns are accordingly modified.

The cartilaginous scapula is ossified from eight or more centers: one in the body, two in the coracoid process, two in the acromion, and one each in the medial border, the inferior angle, and the inferior rim of the glenoid cavity (Fig. 6-3).

Ossification of the middle of the *coracoid process* usually begins in the 1st year with fusion at about the 15th year to the rest of the coracoid. The *subcoracoid center,* which contributes to the upper third of the glenoid, appears at about age 10 and fuses to the rest of the coracoid and the scapula at about age 14 in girls and age 17 in boys. A horseshoe-shaped epiphysis forms at the *lower glenoid rim,* deepening the glenoid cavity. It fuses at about the 20th year. The secondary centers for the *acromion, medial border,* and *inferior angle* also appear around puberty, fusing at about the 20th year (Table 6-1).

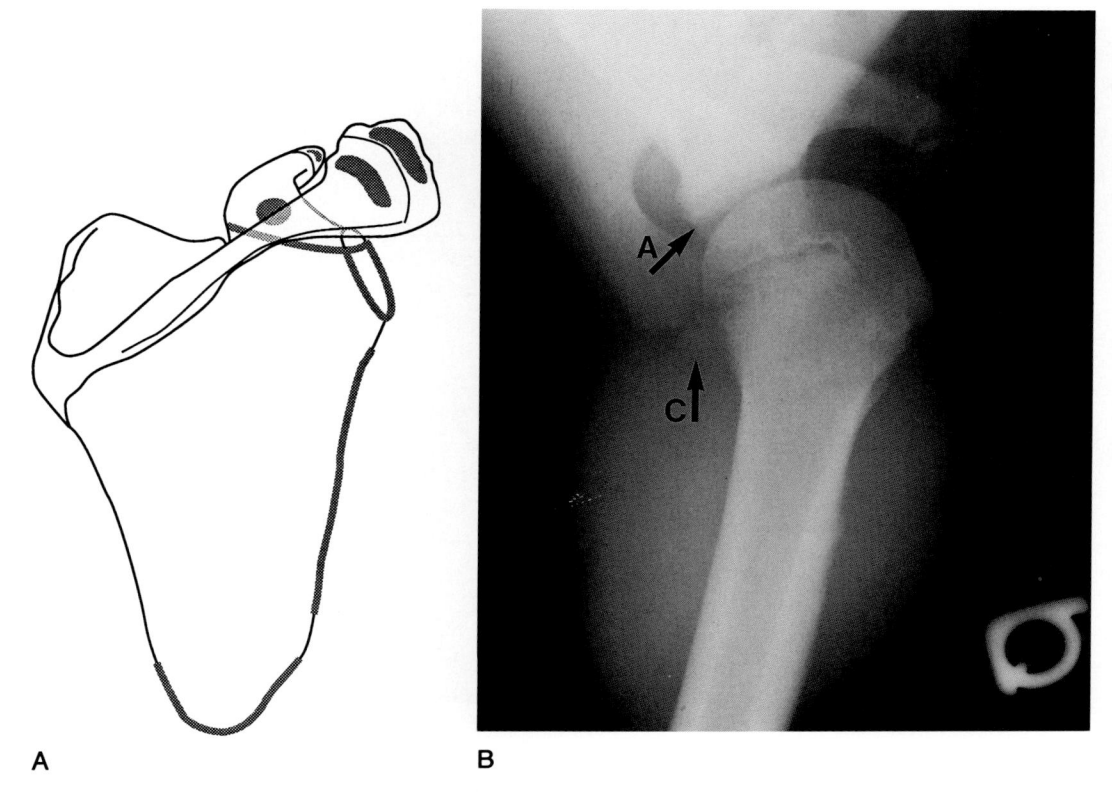

Fig. 6-3. (A) The ossification centers of the scapula. The center for the ossified body is not shown. (B) Axillary view of shoulder joint in a 14-year-old boy. *(A)*, the apophysis of the inferior two-thirds of the glenoid; *(B)*, the apophysis of the coracoid; and *(C)*, the epiphysis of the acromion. *(Figure continues.)*

Mechanism of Injury

Because of its mobility, muscle padding posteriorly and anteriorly, and the resilience of the underlying ribs, the scapula is not easily fractured. Most fractures result from severe trauma: 69 of 116 fractures in the series of Ada and Miller[28] were caused by motor vehicle–pedestrian accidents. Of 8 open fractures in this series, 6 were caused by gunshot wounds. Other series support the role of motor vehicle accidents and include falls from significant heights and crush injuries.[29–36,70,71]

Classification

In their *Handbook of Common Orthopedic Fractures* Kozin and Berlet[1] submit an anatomic classification designating the fractures from 1 to 6 according to site. Hardegger and coworkers[37] modified the classification by including two types of glenoid fractures (rim and fossa) and two types of neck fractures (anatomic and surgical). We will refer to these two types as short vertical and long vertical neck fractures. In 1991, Ada and Miller,[28] on the basis of their series of 116 fractures, again modified the basic anatomic classification by including a horizontal fracture through the neck but did not differentiate rim from glenoid fossa fractures. According to Curtis,[38] rim fractures associated with shoulder instability should be treated differently from fossa fractures of the upper third, so they should be classified separately.

I have proposed a classification (Table 6-2) based on the recommendation of both Hardegger and colleagues[37] and Ada and Miller,[28] in which three types of neck fractures and two types of glenoid fractures are included (Fig. 6-4). The subclassification of coracoid fractures, depending on the presence or absence of AC separation, is based on the etiologic suggestions of Martin-Herrero and colleagues[39] in which they reviewed the world literature and presented seven new cases.

98 / Management of Pediatric Fractures

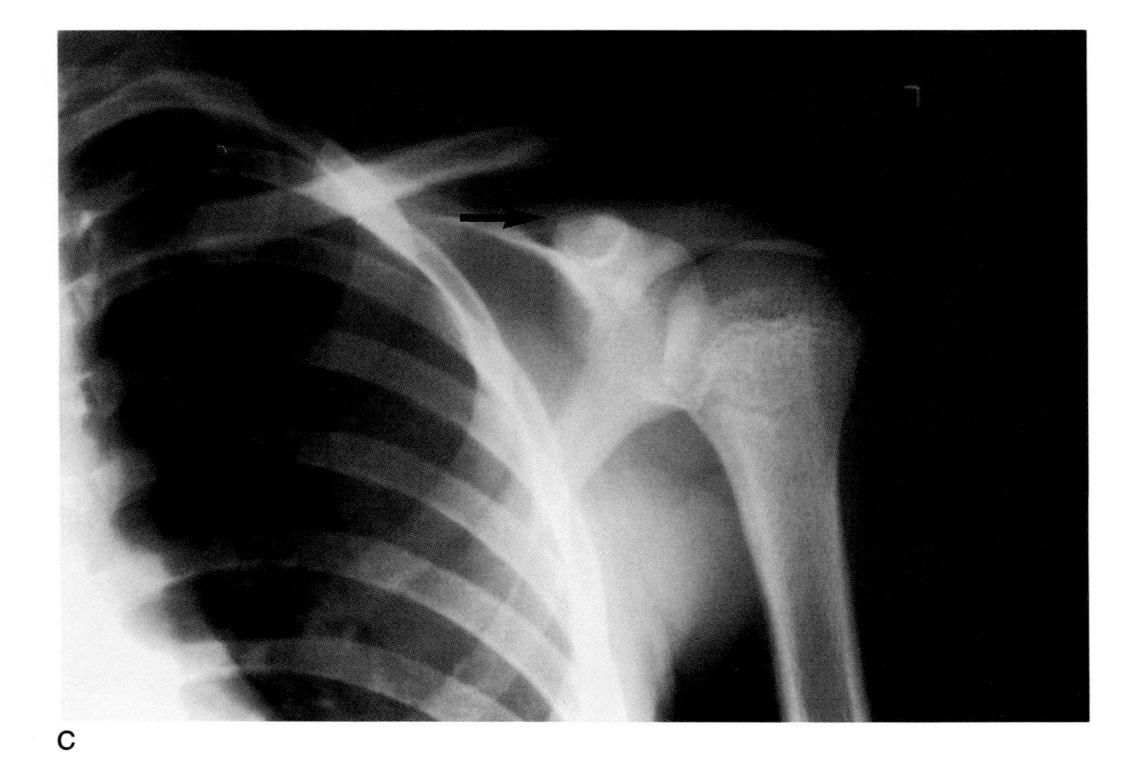

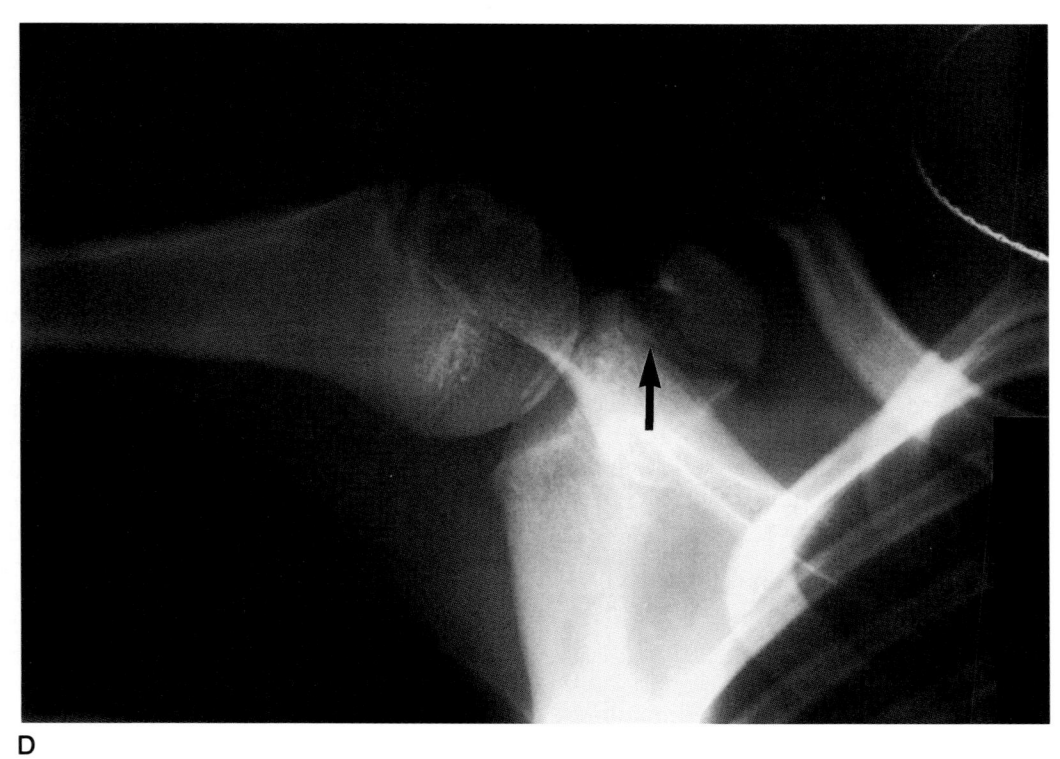

Fig. 6-3 *(Continued).* **(C)** AP view of a 12-year-old boy. The crescentic appearance of the coracoid process might easily be misinterpreted as an avulsion fracture of the coracoid. **(D)** AP view of the scapula clearly shows the subcoracoid physis.

TABLE 6-1. Ossification Centers of the Scapula

Site	No.	Appears: Years (Sex)	Fuses: Years
Body	1	8th fetal week	20
Middle coracoid	1	1	15
Subcoracoid	1	10	15
Acromion	2	13 (F); 15 (M)	20
Medial border	1	13 (F); 15 (M)	20
Inferior angle	1	13 (F); 15 (M)	20
Inferior glenoid	1	13 (F); 15 (M)	20

(Data from Grant[8] and Warwick.[9])

Incidence of Specific Scapular Fractures

McGinnis and Denton[32] reviewed the world literature up to 1989, compiled composite data with respect to the site of the fracture, and compared them with his own and that of Imatani.[30] In 1991 Ada and Miller[28] added another 14 scapular fractures. The breakdown of these studies is outlined in Table 6-3.

Fractures of the body are the most frequent, closely followed by fractures of the neck and glenoid. Fractures of the spine, acromion, and coracoid are less common.

TABLE 6-2. Classification of Scapular Fractures

1. Body
2. Neck
   A. Short vertical (anatomic neck)
   B. Long vertical (surgical neck)
   C. Horizontal
3. Glenoid
   A. Fossa—upper third (through subcoracoid physis)
   B. Fossa—through lower two-thirds
   C. Rim
      (1) Flake
      (2) Large fragment
         i. Shoulder stable
         ii. Shoulder unstable
4. Acromion
5. Spine
6. Coracoid
   (1) Avulsion
   (2) With acromioclavicular dislocation
7. Stress fractures

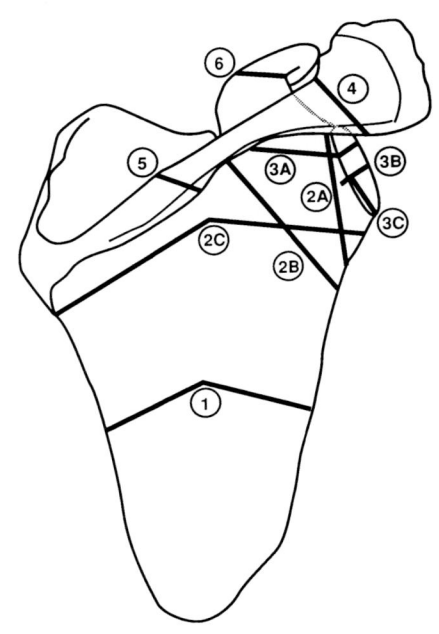

Fig. 6-4. Classification of fracture of the scapula. See Table 6-2 to identify labels.

Diagnosis

Physical Examination

The physical findings will vary according to the site, and mechanism of injury. Isolated avulsion fractures of the coracoid are uncommon,[11,39,40] result from muscular exertion, and the findings usually relate to the region of the coracoid. There is usually minimal swelling, marked tenderness on palpation of the coracoid area, and pain on elbow and/or shoulder flexion. Coracoid fractures from direct trauma may be isolated,[39-46] but they are frequently associated with acromioclavicular separation.[13,39,47-53] In this instance, the trauma is usually direct and the symptoms and signs are referable to the AC joint, with a palpable step and pain with shoulder movement. Coracoid fracture has also been associated with shoulder dislocations.[54,55]

Fractures of the body, spine, acromion, and glenoid are more frequently associated with severe direct trauma, with pain and swelling over the posterior shoulder and upper chest. The differential diagnosis in this situation includes soft tissue contusion, rib fractures, and even spinal injuries. Associated injuries are extensive and are discussed later (Table 6-4).

100 / Management of Pediatric Fractures

TABLE 6-3. Site of Scapular Fractures

Site	McGinnis[32] (%)	Ada[28] (%)	WL[32] (%)
Body	65	35	35–78
Neck	33	27	5–32
Glenoid	23	10	9–26
Spine	13	11	5–15
Acromion	8	12	8–16
Coracoid	13	5	3–13

WL, world literature.
Totals are greater than 100 percent because there are often more than one fracture per scapula.

Radiographic Techniques

When there is a history of major trauma to the shoulder area, fractures of the scapula should be suspected and appropriate radiographs should be taken. Views recommended are an AP 30 degrees antero-oblique view (Fig. 6-5), a lateral Y view (Figs. 6-6 and 6-7), and an AP view with the arm abducted.[28,32] The Y view is so called because the scapular image in this projection is in the shape of a Y, with the V portion being the spine-acromion on one arm of the V and the coracoid on the other. The body forms the vertical arm (Fig. 6-7).

Axillary views are helpful in diagnosing fractures of the acromion.

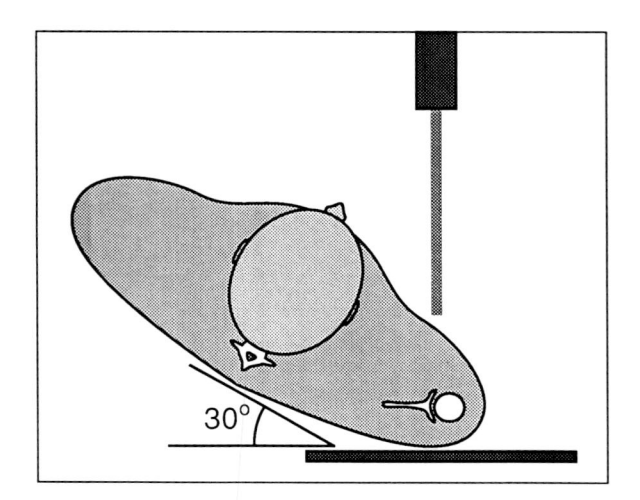

Fig. 6-5. Patient positioning for an AP view of the scapula.

Fractures of the Body

Neer[56] has stated, with respect to fractures of the body of the scapula, that "considerable displacement is compatible with a good result" (Fig. 6-6). This is certainly the general consensus of most authors.[27–33,36,57,71] In the absence of neurologic damage, the response to sling, ice, and graduated range of motion (ROM) exercises is usually excellent. Ada and Miller[28] reported two cases of "snapping scapula" following healing of displaced body fractures.

Treatment

The recommended treatment of displaced scapular fractures is summarized in Table 6-5.

TABLE 6-4. Injuries Associated with Fractured Scapula

Site	Ada[28] (%)	McGinnis[32] (%)
Ribs	>50	51
Pulmonary injuries	37	26
Head injuries	34	28
Clavicle fractures	25	26
Spinal cord injuries	12	NR
Spine fractures	NR	15
Peripheral nerve injuries	3	8

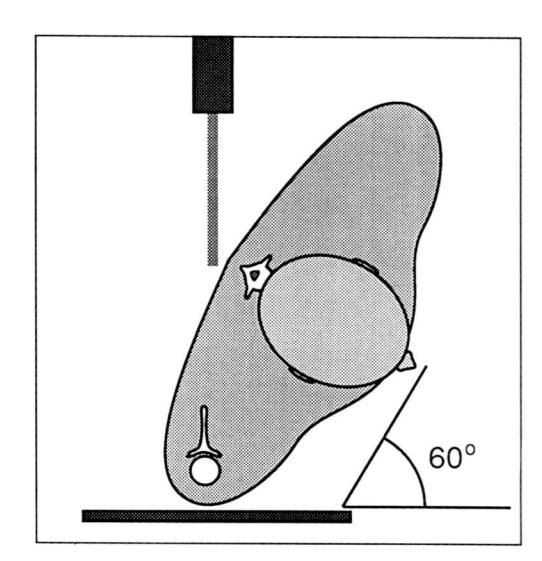

Fig. 6-6. Patient positioning for a true lateral or lateral Y view radiograph of the scapula.

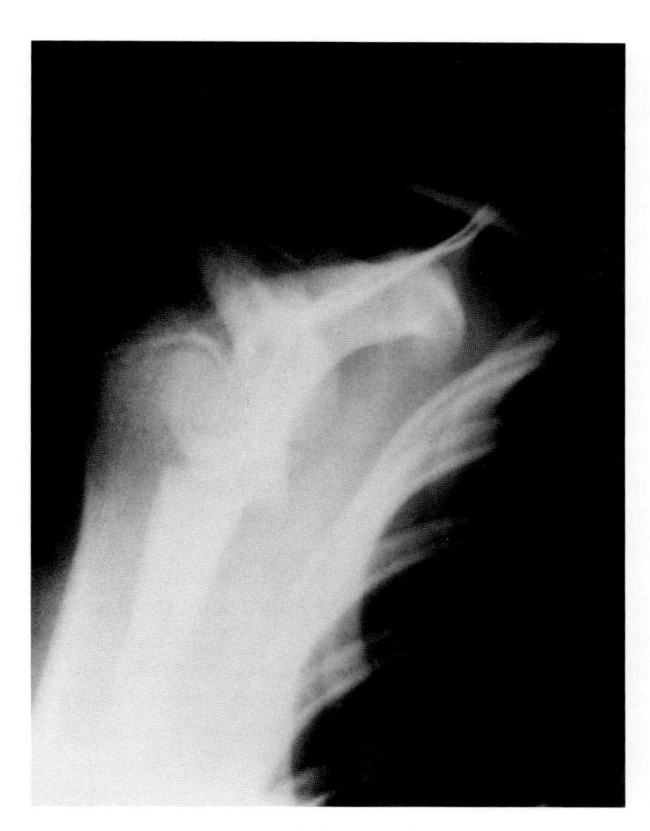

Fig. 6-7. Lateral Y view of the scapula demonstrating a displaced fracture of the body (type 1) of the scapula in a 12-year-old boy.

Fractures of the Neck

The neck is the second most common site of fracture in most series[28,32,58] (Table 6-3; Figs. 6-8 and 6-9). Although McGahan and Rab[31] found no correlation between site of fracture and functional loss, and McLennan and Ungersma[59] claimed full return of function in all scapular fractures, Ada and Miller,[28] in 16 displaced scapular neck fractures, found weakness in 40 percent, pain in 75 percent, decreased range of motion in 20 percent, and "popping" in 25 percent. They feel that these findings were secondary to dysfunction of the rotator cuff. With displacement and angulation of the glenoid, the normal lever arm of the rotator cuff is lost, resulting in decreased mechanical efficiency of the cuff. They also felt that with fractures angulated more than 40 degrees, this dysfunction increased dramatically. Although Neer[56] stated that "the functional results are much better than the x-rays would imply," Armstrong and Van der Spuy[29] reported a high incidence of stiffness in patients with scapular neck fractures.

Hardegger and colleagues[37] treated all displaced fractures of the neck, glenoid, spine, and acromion with open reduction and internal fixation and achieved 79 percent good to excellent results. Because of the high incidence of functional problems with displaced scapular neck fractures, Ada and Miller[28] recommended open reduction and internal fixation (ORIF) for fractures with greater than 40 degrees of angulation or more than 1 cm displacement. They performed all repairs through the Judet posterior approach using AO and ASIF plates and 3.5-mm cortical screws for fixation. The patients were mobilized in the immediate postoperative period, starting with pendulum exercises and progressing as soon as

TABLE 6-5. Recommended Treatment of Displaced Scapular Fractures

Site	Ada[28]	McGahan[31]	McLennan	McGinnis[32]	Hardegger[37]	Curtis[38]	Neer[56]
Body	CONS	CONS	CONS	CONS	ORIF	CONS	CONS
Neck	ORIF >40° >1 cm	CONS	CONS	CONS	ORIF	ORIF	CONS
Glenoid fossa	ORIF	CONS	CONS	CONS?	ORIF	ORIF[a,b]	ORIF[b]
Glenoid rim	ORIF[c]	CONS	CONS	CONS?	ORIF[c]	ORIF[c]	ORIF[c]
Spine	ORIF?	CONS	CONS	CONS	ORIF	CONS	CONS
Acromion	ORIF[d]	CONS	CONS	CONS	ORIF	ORIF[d]	ORIF[e]
Coracoid	CONS	CONS	CONS	CONS	CONS?	CONS	CONS

CONS, conservative; ORIF, open reduction and internal fixation; ?, author's recommendation unclear.
All authors treat all nondisplaced fractures conservatively.
[a] Fractures of upper ¼ fossa treated conservatively.
[b] If fracture dislocation.
[c] If large fragment and dislocation shoulder.
[d] If major displacement.
[e] If subacrominal space compromised.

102 / Management of Pediatric Fractures

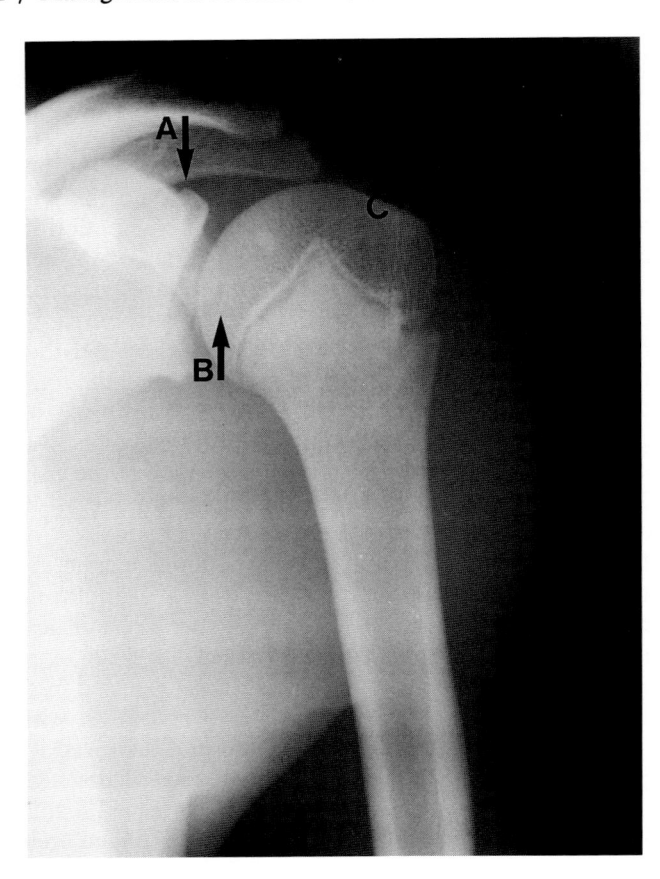

Fig. 6-8. A vertical fracture (type 2a) of the neck of the scapula in a 14-year-old boy. *(A)*. The coracoid *(B)* and acromial *(C)* ossification centers are shown.

discussed elsewhere in this text. Although both McGahan et al.[68] and McLennan and Ungersma,[59] in separate series, claimed that all their patients regained a full ROM regardless of the site of the fracture, Armstrong and Van der Spuy[29] noted that 50 percent of glenoid fractures resulted in markedly restricted and painful shoulder movement. Ada and Miller[28] made similar observations.

Curtis[38] states that fractures through the subcoracoid physis, involving the upper 25 percent of the coracoid, are usually minimally displaced, stable, and respond well to conservative management. Glenoid fractures involving large fagments of the glenoid, are often associated with shoulder dislocation and instability and should be treated by ORIF.[14,28,32,37,56,60] With the high incidence of pain and stiffness reported by Armstrong and Van der Spuy[29] as well as Ada and Miller,[28] this approach seems logical.

For large anterior rim fractures with shoulder instability, Curtis[38] recommends the anterior deltopectoral approach. He splits the subscapularis tendon, retracts it medially, and leaves the capsule as a separate flap. The capsule is incised, and the fracture is reduced and fixed

possible to active and resistive exercises.[28] All patients gained 85 degrees of glenohumeral motion, and none experienced pain at rest or at night.[28]

The results of Hardegger's[37] series and the operated group of Ada and Miller[28] suggest that, when scapular neck fractures are angulated more than 40 degrees or displaced greater than 1 cm, ORIF should be considered. Since severe trauma is often the etiology, the general status of the patient will obviously play a mitigating role in the decision-making regarding the scapula. If surgery is not practical, the results of conservative treatment with early mobilization is also encouraging[31,56,59] (Table 6-5).

Fractures of the Glenoid

With acute shoulder dislocation small flakes of glenoid are often avulsed.[56] The management of this lesion is the management of the acute dislocation and is

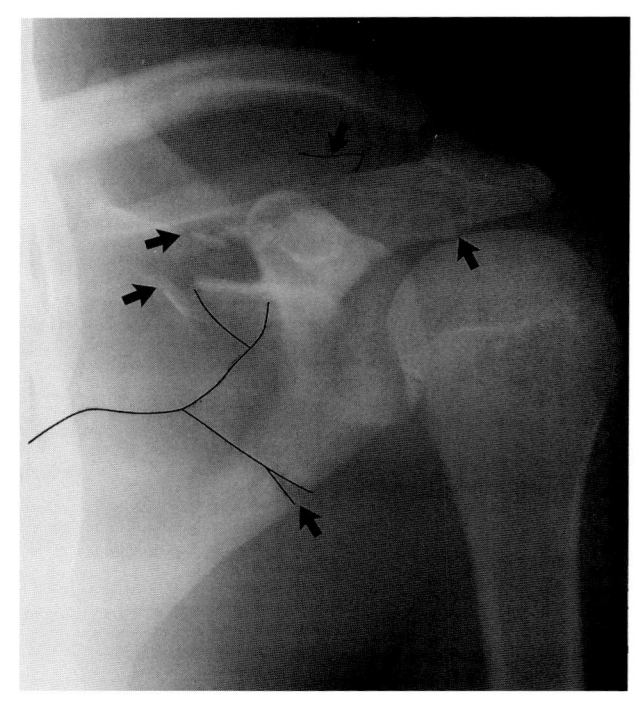

Fig. 6-9. The scapula of a 14-year-old girl struck by an automobile. *Arrows* demonstrate a comminuted fracture of the neck (types 2b and 2c combined) as well as fractures of the acromion (type 4) and the spine (type 5).

with screws or staples. He emphasizes the need to countersink the screw heads and place the staples so that they do not impinge on the humeral head.[38]

For large fractures of the posterior glenoid Ada and Miller[28] recommend the Judet posterior approach to the scapula.

Fractures of the Scapular Spine

Ada and Miller's series[28] contained 10 patients with comminuted spine fractures: 70 percent had pain at rest, 57 percent had night pain, mostly in the subacromial space, and 50 percent had weakness with shoulder abduction. Nevasier[61] referred to this as "pseudorupture of the rotator cuff" and attributed the phenomenon to hemorrhage within the supraspinatus and infraspinatus muscles, resulting in temporary paralysis.

Although most authors recommend conservative treatment for all spine fractures, it would seem that the more severely comminuted ones can be associated with significant long-term disability.[28,61,62] Hardegger and colleagues[37] treated their comminuted and displaced spine fractures surgically and reported 79 percent good to excellent results. Ada and Miller,[28] on the basis of their study, suggested that commuited or severely displaced spine fractures should be considered for ORIF.

The readers are encouraged to read these papers and draw their own conclusions (Table 6-5; Fig. 6-8). It is my impression that the severely displaced spine fractures are best treated with open reduction, especially in the adolescent and young adult where optimum shoulder function is more desirable. Decisions in the older or severely injured patient must be modified accordingly.

Fractures of the Acromion

Most authors recommend conservative treatment for acromion fractures[28,31-33,71] (Table 6-5; Fig. 6-8). Hardegger and colleagues[37] opened and fixed displaced acromion fractures in their series, and Neer[59] recommends open elevation and K-wire fixation if the subcromial space is compromised. Care must be taken not to misdiagnose the acromial physis as a fracture.

Fractures of the Coracoid

Curtis[41] states that isolated fractures of the coracoid can be treated nonoperatively because intact coracoclavicular ligaments, as well as an intact AC joint, hold the base of the coracoid in an acceptably reduced position. Martin-Herrero and coworkers[39] reported seven cases of coracoid fractures. Four cases had associated AC dislocations. Although Neer[56] recommends open reduction of the coracoid fracture and the AC dislocation when they are concurrent, all the cases of Martin-Herrero and coworkers[39] were treated conservatively with excellent results.

Although most authors[28,31-33,36,38,71] concur with nonoperative management of coracoid fractures, open reduction of the coracoid and a concomitant AC separation may be indicated in individuals where maximum function and rapid return to function is critical. Hardegger and colleagues[37] suggest that ORIF of this combination of injuries is indicated when displacement of the coracoid is such that it causes compression of the neurovascular bundle.[37]

Although ORIF is recommended for certain scapular fractures[28,37,63-65] this injury is often associated with massive trauma, making surgical management inappropriate. Under these circumstances it is important and reassuring to note that the results of conservative management of any type of displaced scapular fractures may be excellent.[28,31-33]

Scapulothoracic Dissociation

Scapulothoracic dissociation is a rare entity that has been reported by five authors.[16-20] Morris and Lloyd[19] described a case that occurred in an 8-year-old child. The mechanism in all cases has been severe trauma. The injury is a lateral rotary dislocation of the scapula and upper extremity on the rib cage. The muscular attachments of the scapula are torn and the clavicle is either fractured or the AC joint separated. The major implication in this injury is the potentially life-threatening associated vascular and neural injuries. *All* reported cases have demonstrated occlusion of the subclavian artery as well as severe brachial plexus injury. When this injury is diagnosed, emergency angiography is strongly recommended and the vascular lesion appropriately managed. Neurologic injury is usually on the basis of traction, but appropriate management will vary with the mechanism and site of injury.

Complications

In McGinnis and Denton's series[32] of 39 patients with 40 scapular fractures there were 115 associated injuries, including 20 rib fractures, 11 cerebral contusions, 10 clavicle fractures, 10 severe lacerations, 13 fractures of long bones, and 4 pneumothoraces. Only three patients had no associated injuries[27] (Table 6-4).

In Ada and Miller's series[28] of 113 patients with 148 scapular fractures, 96 percent of the patients had associated injuries, with upper rib fractures being the most common: 37 percent had pulmonary injuries, with hemopneumothorax in 29 percent and pulmonary contusion in 8 percent. Head injuries occurred in 34 percent with 9 skull fractures. Clavicle fractures occurred in 25 percent, 12 percent had spinal cord injury, and 4 patients had brachial plexus injury. Four of six AC separations were associated with coracoid process fractures.[28] This concurs with Martin-Herrero's[39] incidence of four AC separations in seven coracoid fractures.

In McLennan and Ungersma's series,[59] 50 percent of the patients had pneumothorax and of note is the fact that more than half of these developed 24 to 72 hours after the injury.

Other injuries reported in association with scapular fractures include subclavian artery,[34,66] axillary artery,[67] axillary nerve,[31] and suprascapular nerve.[69] Armstrong and Van der Spuy[29] observed a mortality rate of close to 10 percent in patients with scapular fractures.

Late complications include diminished range of shoulder motion, pain, and weakness. These vary with the site of the fracture as previously discussed.

Fractures of the scapula usually imply major trauma, so associated injuries must be carefully looked for. Delayed pneumothorax and pulmonary contusion must be watched for and a 72-hour chest radiograph is recommended.[59]

RIB FRACTURES

Rib fractures in both children and adults are most commonly associated with severe blunt chest trauma.[72-86] Brorsson[87] has shown that rib fracture is "nearly" 11 times higher among the older than in the younger age groups. This study justifies the comment by Harris and Soper[88] that more energy is required to fracture ribs in a child than in an adult. Conversely, the presence of rib fractures in children usually implies very severe trauma,[89] and many authors have studied the implications of the presence of rib fractures on the prognosis of massive chest injuries.[72-77,80,89] Fractures specifically of the first rib have been shown to be associated with a high incidence of visceral injuries and are considered of prognostic significance.[72-75,79,81,83-86,88] Several reports have demonstrated a significant association between first rib fractures and ruptures of the subclavian artery.[90-95]

Fracture of the first rib has also been attributed to violent muscle contractures in activities such as throwing,[96] weight lifting,[97] surfboarding,[98] gymnastics,[99] and rebounding in basketball.[100] Football contact[101] as well as overlarge motorcycle helmets[102,103] have also been reported mechanisms of injury. Although acute first rib fractures are usually associated with violent trauma and multiple injuries, Regoort and Raaymakers[104] reported an isolated first rib fracture in a patient who fell off his bicycle with no secondary vehicle or person contact, and Villa and colleagues[105] reported a patient who suffered from traumatic bilateral fractures of the first rib with no concomitant lesions of bone, viscera, nerve, or vessel.

Stress fractures of the first rib have been associated with a variety of intense physical activities involving the upper extremity.[106-111] The usual explantation is intense repeated contractions of the scalenus anticus and juxtacostal muscles. Mintz and coworkers[111] attributed one case from an exercise machine to overaction of the serratus anterior muscle. I have one patient in whom the cause was prolonged intense coughing. In infancy and early childhood osteogenesis imperfecta[112,113] and child abuse[114-117] are important considerations when rib fractures are diagnosed, especially when the specific traumatic incident is uncertain.

In a study of 50 randomly selected cases of cardiac surgery performed through a midline sternotomy, Curtis and colleagues[118] found six instances of first rib fractures. Suzuki and colleagues[119] reported first rib fracture as well as brachial plexus injury in association with the use of sternotomy incision. Kaye and coworkers[119] described a first rib fracture caused by an automobile shoulder restraint.

Anatomic Considerations

The pleura and lung lie deep to ribs 1 to 10, and this accounts for the most common complications of multiple rib fractures—pneumothorax, hemothorax, and pulmonary contusion.[8,9]

Rupture of the subclavian artery with fractures of the first rib are common.[90-95] The subclavian artery branches off the innominate artery, arches over the first rib between the attachment of the scalenus anticus anteriorly and the scalenus medius posteriorly. It then enters the arm as the axillary artery accompanied by the brachial plexus. Since the origin and termination of the subclavian artery are both distal to the first rib, and since in displaced fractures of the first rib, the tendency will be for the scalenus anticus and scalenus medius to pull the fragments proximally, the subclavian artery is susceptible to stretch and penetration by first rib fragments. In the event of contusion to the base of the neck, it is subject to direct injury, where it lies on the rib.

According to Phillips and colleagues,[94] arterial injury occurs only in displaced first rib fractures, particularly posterior fractures. They feel that the mechanism is downward displacement of the posterior portion of the rib, with upward displacement of the anterior portion, pinching the contents of the thoracic outlet against the clavicle.

As noted, the brachial plexus joins the third part of the subclavian artery after passing between the scalenus anticus and scalenus medius. It is therefore also susceptible to trauma in this area. Since the plexus originates proximal to the first rib, its relationship to it is less intimate than that of the subclavian artery and possibly accounts for the lower incidence of plexus injury. Injury to the brachial plexus still occurs[74,88,94] and must still be ruled out in traumatic first rib fractures. In the series of Phillips and colleagues[94] brachial plexus injury occurred *only* in association with injury to the subclavian artery. On the basis of this, they recommend arteriography if brachial plexus injury occurs with a displaced fracture of the first rib.

Stress and exertional fractures are usually due to the force of the scalene muscles,[96-110] but Mintz and co-workers[111] reported one case in an exercise rower in which the first rib origin of the serratus anterior muscle was implicated.

Unquestionably the intimate relationship of the upper mediastium and major vessels with the first and second ribs, and the extreme trauma usually required to fracture these ribs explains the significance attributed by so many authors of fractures of the first and second ribs to the prognosis in major chest trauma.[72-76,79,81,83-86,88,93,106]

Classification

A classification of rib fractures based on etiology is shown in Table 6-6.

Diagnosis

Physical Examination

Diagnosis of fractures of the lower ribs (3-10) is based on history and physical findings, with pain and tenderness being the major presenting features. In the unconscious patient history of injury is more critical and management is based on overall patient status with the appropriate priorities being attended to.

TABLE 6-6. Classification of Rib Fractures

Traumatic
1. Acute fractures with major trauma
   a. Multiple
      i. Unilateral
      ii. Bilateral
   b. 1st or 1st & 2nd ribs only
      i. Unilateral
      ii. Bilateral
2. Acute fractures minor trauma
   a. Ribs 3-12 (2-12)
   b. Isolated 1st
3. Fractures caused by child abuse
4. Stress fractures
5. Sternotomy

Nontraumatic (Pathologic)
1. Osteogenesis imperfecta
2. Metastasis
3. Others

Diagnosis of isolated fractures of the first and second ribs is usually based on the history of injury. Lorentzen and Movin[106] reviewed 15 cases of isolated first rib fractures and found the mechanism to fall into one of three categories:

1. Direct trauma to the shoulder
2. Sudden violent contraction of juxtacostal muscles
3. A chance finding

In the article by Harris and Soper[88] on pediatric first rib fractures, all six patients had multiple injuries and the mechanism of each was a motor vehicle accident, that is, major trauma. Patients with isolated first rib fractures secondary to muscle contraction present with pain that is deep in the shoulder region or in the base of the neck. Deep inspiration and exertion of the deep neck muscles will generally reproduce the pain. Tenderness may usually be elicited by palpation high in the axilla.[98]

Osteogenesis Imperfecta versus Child Abuse

In infancy and early childhood the suspicion and correct diagnosis of injuries resulting from child abuse are perhaps the most important concern when dealing with pediatric fractures.[121] Failure to diagnose this condition renders the child susceptible to almost certain further abuse and, in some instances, death.[122] Much has been written about injury patterns in child abuse, with rib fractures being perhaps one of the more frequent and telltale injuries[114-117,122] (Fig. 6-10). Kleinman and co-workers[117] have stressed the role of radiographic and histologic study in the postmortem examination of in-

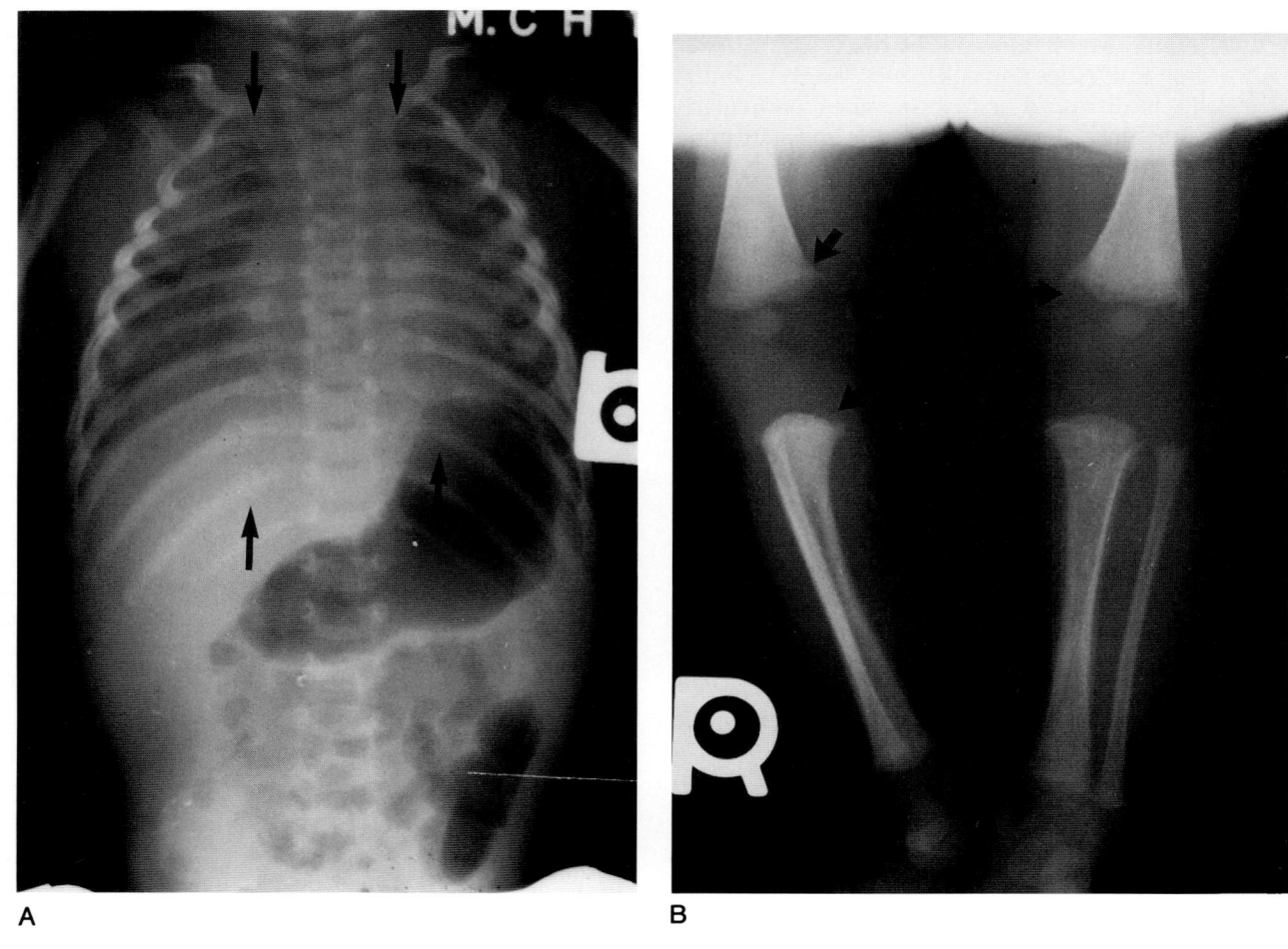

Fig. 6-10. (A) Virtually every rib in this 4-month-old infant has been fractured near the costovertebral junction. (B) Multiple epiphyseal separations in the long bones of the lower extremities of the infant with multiple rib fractures.

fant deaths where child abuse is suspected, and they discuss the detailed investigations that may rule in or out the probability of child abuse. Acute or healing fractures, particularly of the posterior rib arcs[114] (Fig. 6-10A), are an important feature, especially when associated with fresh or healing fractures of the long bones[122] (Fig. 6-10B). Costochondral dislocations may be diagnosed with ultrasound[117] and cystlike lesions of the posterior rib arcs have been described as clues to child abuse[117] (Fig. 6-11).

Although osteogenesis imperfecta congenita is usually easily diagnosed, it is important to entertain this possibility in all neonatal fractures.[112,113–116] Less severe forms of the disease may create a diagnostic dilemma in infancy and childhood,[112] leading to inappropriate accusations and even legal actions. The presence of blue sclerae, bowing of long bones, and a history of easy bruising, may be helpful. The presence of severely carious teeth (dentigenesis imperfecta) may be helpful if osteogenesis imperfecta is suspected. The patterns of fractures in child abuse, however, are generally consistent, and as long as the two diagnoses are entertained, differentiation should not be a major problem.[122]

Treatment

Isolated fractures of the lower ribs without internal injuries may be treated by strapping, rib-belt,[123] local infiltration, or analgesia.

Isolated fractures of the first and/or second ribs from muscle contraction usually respond to conservative

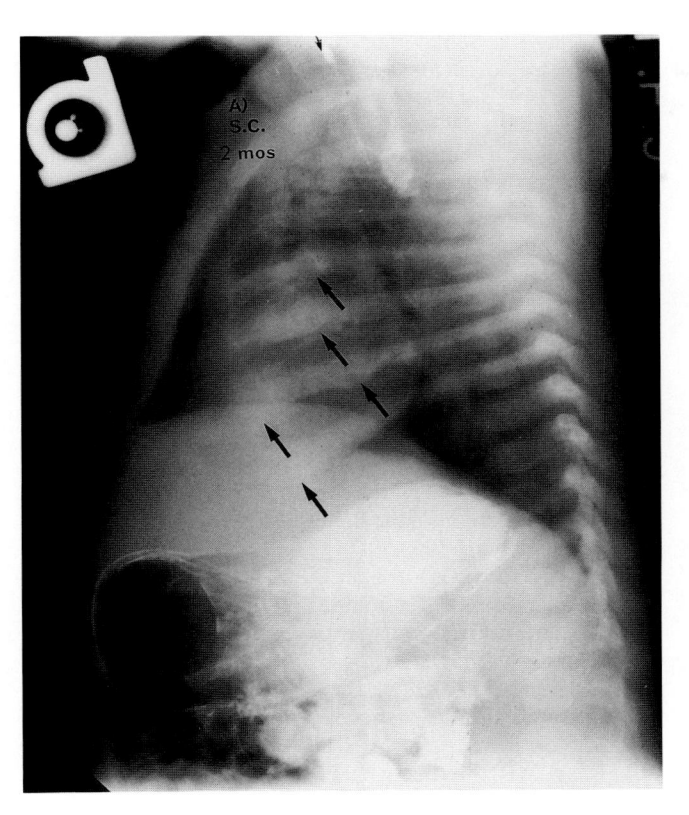

Fig. 6-11. The healed rib fractures in this 2-year-old abused infant create cystlike rib lesions on lateral view of the chest.

treatment and analgesia plus or minus a sling on the involved side. Proffer and colleagues[99] report one fracture in a gymnast that did not heal with conservative management, developed a nonunion with persistent pain, and required transaxillary resection of the involved rib.

When the mechanism of the injury is massive trauma, patient management is centered around those injuries that are life-threatening. The management of flail chest is among those, but is not dealt with in this chapter.

Treatment of pathologic fractures is essentially the same as with nonpathologic fractures, but suspicion of pathology and subsequent diagnosis essential for proper future management.

As with pathologic fractures, rib fractures in children and infants in the absence of a substantive history must provoke suspicion of child abuse. Management of the fractures (which are frequently healed when diagnosed) is less important than the determination of the etiology which, if neglected, may result in the death of the child.

Classification and Complications

In terms of their *complications* rib fractures may be considered in two basic classifications: those associated with major trauma and those not associated with major trauma.

Rib Fractures Not Associated with Major Trauma

Pathologic fractures and child abuse are the principal causes of rib fractures not associated with major trauma. The critical need for diagnosis in these two groups is basic to their management and, in both instances, critical to the future well-being of the child.

The other subgroup in this category is first rib fractures from minor trauma, bicycle fall, violent muscle action, and stress fractures. Even in minor trauma, any first rib fracture should carry the suspicion of subclavian artery or brachial plexus injury. These *complications* have not been reported with first rib fractures from muscle action or in stress fractures.

Rib Fractures Associated with Major Trauma

RIB FRACTURES IN GENERAL: RIBS 1 TO 12

Nakayama and coworkers[89] reviewed the records of 105 children with chest injuries admitted to a level 1 trauma center from 1981 to 1988. Over 50 percent were traffic-related. Rib fractures, usually multiple, were present in 49.5 percent. They found that significant intrathoracic injuries occurred without rib fractures (52 percent) and felt that rib fractures had no effect on the Injury Severity Scale.

Garcia and coworkers,[77] however, looked at the records of 2,080 children with blunt or penetrating trauma admitted to a level 1 pediatric trauma center. Comparing children with and without rib fractures, they found that children with rib fractures had a higher mortality rate. They concluded that the risk of mortality increases with the number of ribs broken and that the combination of multiple rib fractures and head injury was usually fatal.

Lee and associates,[80] on the basis of 105,683 trauma cases, found a significant difference in mortality in children with three or more rib fractures and use this guideline as an indicator for transfer to a level 1 trauma center.

Peclet and associates,[82] looking at thoracic trauma in 2,086 children admitted to a level 1 trauma center, found a mortality rate of 26 percent. Children with multiple rib fractures experienced a mortality rate of 42 percent.

It is apparent from these studies that multiple rib fractures (more than 3) are indeed a marker of severe trauma in children.

FIRST AND SECOND RIB FRACTURES

First and second rib fractures from minor trauma are uncommon. Pierce and colleagues[83] speak of the "special hazards of first rib fractures" and Richardson and colleagues[84] refer to first rib fractures as a "hallmark of severe trauma."

Most authors reporting traumatic first and second rib fractures stress the severity of the trauma usually required to fracture these two ribs[72-77,80-95] and stress the high incidence of associated injury to the subclavian artery[90-95] and brachial plexus.[74,88,94] Several authors discuss the role of arteriography in first rib fractures, with most recommending this study when there is clinical evidence of subclavian tear.[90,92,94,95] Phillips and colleagues[94] recommend arteriography if there is absent pulse, a brachial plexus injury, or a *displaced* first rib fracture.

Of interest are the findings of Livoni and Barcia[93] in 58 patients with fracture of the first and second rib that neither the *site* of the fractures (posterior, lateral, or anterior) nor the *degree of displacement* of the fragments was of value in predicting arterial injury.

In Harris and Soper's[88] series of six pediatric patients ranging in age from 3 to 16, all had multiple injuries, and five required operative intervention.

First and second rib fractures are serious injuries with major implications, the most frequent of which is a tear of the subclavian artery. High suspicion of this injury must be maintained and arteriography performed when clinical findings are suggestive of a major arterial bleed. Brachial plexis injuries must also be looked for, and, when present, they strongly suggest concurrent subclavian artery damage.[94]

REFERENCES

1. Kozin SH, Berlet AC: Handbook of Common Orthopedic Fractures. Medical Surveillance Inc., West Chester, PA, 1989
2. Rang M: Children's Fractures. JB Lippincott, Philadelphia, 1974
3. Rockwood CA Jr, Green DP: Fractures. Vol. 1. JB Lippincott, Philadelphia, 1975
4. Arajarvi E, Santavirta S: Chest injuries sustained in severe traffic accidents by seatbelt wearers. J Trauma 29:37, 1989
5. Ostremski I, Wilde BR, March JL et al: Fracture of the sternum in motor vehicle accidents and its association with mediastinal injury. Injury 21(2):81, 1990
6. Sturm JT, Luxenberg MG, Moudry BM, Perry JF Jr: Does sternal fracture increase the risk for aortic rupture? Ann Thorac Surg 48:697, 1989
7. Unger JM, Schuchmann GG, Grossman JE, Pellett JR: Tears of the trachea and main bronchi caused by blunt trauma: radiologic findings. AJR 153:1175, 1989
8. Grant JCB: Grant's Method of Anatomy. 5th Ed. Williams & Wilkins, Baltimore, 1952
9. Warwick R, Williams PL: Gray's Anatomy. 35th Ed. Longman, Edinburgh, 1973
10. Desault PJ: A Treatise on Fractures, Luxations and Other Affections of the Bones. p. 57. Fry and Kammerer, Philadelphia, 1805
11. Heyse-Moore GH, Stoker DJ: Avulsion fractures of the scapula. Skeletal Radiol 9:27, 1982
12. Houghton GR: Avulsion of the cranial margin of the scapula: a report in two cases. Injury 11:45, 1979
13. Ishizuki M, Yamaura I, Isobe Y et al: Avulsion fracture of the superior order of the scapula. J Bone Joint Surg [Am] 63:820, 1981
14. Rask MR, Steinberg LH: Fracture of the acromion caused by muscle forces: A case report. J Bone Joint Surg [Am] 60:1146, 1978
15. Brower AC, Neff JR, Tillema DA: An unusual scapular stress fracture. AJR 129:519, 1977
16. Sandrock AR: Another sports fatigue fracture: stress fracture of the coracoid process of the scapula. Radiology 117:274, 1975
17. Nettrour LF, Krufky EL, Mueller RE et al: Locked scapula: intrathoracic dislocation of the inferior angle: a case report. J Bone Joint Surg [Am] 54:413, 1972
18. Oreck SL, Burgess A, Levine AM: Traumatic lateral displacement of the scapula: a radiographic sign of neurovascular disruption. J Bone Joint Surg [Am] 66:758, 1984
19. Morris CS, Lloyd T: Case report 642: traumatic scapulothoracic dissociation in a child. Skeletal Radiol 19(8):607, 1990
20. Kelbel JM, Jardon OM, Huurman WW: Scapulothoracic dissociation: a case report. Clin Orthop 209:210, 1986
21. Rubenstein JD, Ebraheim NA, Kellam JF: Traumatic scapulothoracic dissociation. Radiology 157:297, 1985
22. Beswick DR, Morse SD, Barnes AU: Bilateral scapular fractures from low-voltage electrical injury. Ann Emerg Med 11:676, 1982
23. Tarquinio T, Weinstein ME, Virgilio RW: Bilateral scapular fractures from accidental electric shock. J Trauma 19:132, 1979
24. Matthew RE, Cocke TB, D'Ambrosia RD: Scapular frac-

tures secondary to seizures in patients with osteodystrophy. J Bone Joint Surg [Am] 65:850, 1983
25. Peraino RA, Weinman EJ, Schloeder FX: Unusual fractures during convulsions in two patients with renal osteodystrophy. South Med J 70:595, 1977
26. Heatley MD, Breck LW, Higinbotham NL: Bilateral fractures of the scapula. Am J Surg 71:256, 1946
27. Newell ED: Review of over two thousand fractures in past seven years. South Med J 20:644, 1927
28. Ada JR, Miller ME: Scapular fractures: analysis of 113 cases. Clin Orthop 269:174, 1991
29. Armstrong CP, Van der Spuy J: The fractured scapula: importance and management based on a series of 62 patients. Injury 15:324, 1984
30. Imatani RJ: Fractures of the scapula: a review of 53 fractures. J Trauma 15:473, 1975
31. McGahan JP, Rab GT: Fracture of the acromion associated with an axillary nerve deficit: a case report and review of the literature. Clin Orthop Rel Res 147:216, 1980
32. McGinnis M, Denton JR: Fractures of the scapula: a retrospective study of 40 fractured scapulae. J Trauma 29:1488, 1989
33. Findlay RT: Fractures of the scapula. Ann Surg 93:1001, 1931
34. Tomaszek DE: Combined subclavian artery and brachial plexus injuries from blunt upper-extremity trauma. J Trauma 24:161, 1984
35. Wilber MC, Evans EB: Fractures of the scapula. J Bone Joint Surg [Am] 59:358, 1977
36. Zdravkovic D, Damholt VV: Comminuted and severely displaced fractures of the scapula. Acta Orthop Scand 45:60, 1974
37. Hardegger FH, Simpson LA, Weber BG: The operative treatment of scapular fractures. J Bone Joint Surg [Br] 66:725, 1984
38. Curtis RJ Jr: Operative management of children's fractures of the shoulder region. Orthop Clin North Am 21:315, 1990
39. Martin-Herrero T, Rodriguez-Merchan C, Munuera-Martinez L: Fractures of the coracoid process: presentation of seven cases and review of the literature. J Trauma 30:1597, 1990
40. Benton J, Nelson C: Avulsion of the coracoid process in an athlete: report of a case. J Bone Joint Surg [Am] 53:356, 1971
41. Boyer DW: Trapshooter's shoulder: Stress fracture of the coracoid process: case report. J Bone Joint Surg [Am] 57:862, 1975
42. DeRosa GP, Kettelkamp DB: Fracture of the coracoid process of the scapula: case report. J Bone Joint Surg [Am] 59:696, 1977
43. Froimson AI: Fracture of the coracoid process of the scapula. J Bone Joint Surg [Am] 60:710, 1978
44. Germain M, Poilleux F: Fracture de l'apophyse coracoide. Rev Chir Orthop 57:555, 1971
45. Rounds RC: Isolated fracture of the coracoid process. J Bone Joint Surg [Am] 31:662, 1949
46. Wolf AW, Shoji H, Chuinard RG: Unusual fracture of the coracoid process: a case report and the review of the literature. J Bone Joint Surg [Am] 58:423, 1976
47. Bernard TN, Brunet ME, Haddad RJ: Fractured coracoid process in acromioclavicular dislocations: report of four cases and review of the literature. Clin Orthop 175:227, 1983
48. Landoff GA: Eine bisher nicht beschriebene Schadigung am Processus coracoideus. Acta Chir Scand 89:401, 1943
49. Protass JJ, Stampfli FV, Osmer JC: Coracoid process fracture diagnosis in acromioclavicular separation. Radiology 116:61, 1975
50. Smith DM: Coracoid fracture associated with acromioclavicular dislocation: a case report. Clin Orthop 108:165, 1975
51. Urist MR: Complete dislocations of the acromioclavicular joint. J Bone Joint Surg 28:813, 1946
52. Zettas JP, Muchnic PD: Fractures of the coracoid process base in acute acromioclavicular separation. Orthop Rev 5:77, 1976
53. Zilberman Z, Rejovitzky R: Fracture of the coracoid process of the scapula. Injury 13:203, 1981
54. Moseley HF: Shoulder Lesions. 3rd Ed. Churchill Livingstone, Edinburgh, 52:139, 1972
55. Benchetrit E, Friedman B: Fracture of the coracoid process associated with subglenoid dislocation of the shoulder: a case report. J Bone Joint Surg [Am] 61:295, 1979
56. Neer CS II: Fractures about the shoulder. p. 713. In Rockwood CA, Green DP (eds): Fractures. JB Lippincott, Philadelphia, 1984
57. Rowe CR: Fractures of the scapula. Surg Clin North Am 43:1565, 1963
58. Lindholm A, Leven H: Prognosis in fractures of the body and neck of the scapula. Acta Chirurg Scand 140:33, 1974
59. McLennan JG, Ungersma J: Pneumothorax complicating fracture of the scapula. J Bone Joint Surg [Am] 64:598, 1982
60. Kummel BM: Fractures of the glenoid causing chronic dislocation of the shoulder. Clin Orthop 69:189, 1970
61. Nevasier JD: Injuries in and about the shoulder joint. Instr Course Lect 13:187, 1956
62. Nunley RL, Bedini SJ, Sara JB: Paralysis of the shoulder subsequent to a comminuted fracture of the scapula. Phys Ther 40:442, 1960
63. Fischer WR: Fractures of the scapula requiring open reduction. J Bone Joint Surg 21:459, 1939
64. Friedrich B, Winter G: Zur Operativen Therapie von Frakturen der Scapula. Chirurgie 44:37, 1973
65. Izadpanah M: Osteosynthesis in scapular fractures. Arch Orthop Trauma Surg 83:153, 1975
66. Halpern AA, Joseph R, Page J et al: Subclavian artery injury and fracture of the scapula. JAMA 8:19, 1979
67. Stein RE, Bono J, Korn J et al: Axillary artery injury in

closed fracture of the neck of the scapula: a case report. J Trauma 11:528, 1971
68. McGahan JP, Rab GT, Dublin A: Fractures of the scapula. J Trauma 20:880, 1980
69. Edeland HG, Zachrisson BE: Fracture of the scapular notch associated with lesion of the suprascapular nerve. Acta Orthop Scand 46:758, 1975
70. Findlay RT: Fractures of the scapula and ribs. Am J Surg 38:489, 1937
71. Gleich JJ: The fractured scapula: significance and prognosis. Missouri Med 77:24, 1980
72. Albers JE, Rath RK, Glaser RS et al: Severity of intrathoracic injuries associated with first rib fractures. Ann Thorac Surg 6:614, 1982
73. Chen ZH: Clinical significance of first or second rib fracture in closed thoracic injuries (author's translation). Chung Hua Wai Ko Tsa Chih 19:152, 1981
74. Fermanis GG, Deane SA, Fitzgerald PM: The significance of first and second rib fractures. Aust N Z J Surg 55:383, 1985
75. Fordham SD: The significance of first rib fractures. Med Times 105:118, 1977
76. Freedland M, Wilson RF, Bender JS, Levison MA: The management of flail chest injury: factors affecting outcome. J Trauma 30:1460, 1990
77. Garcia VF, Gotschall CS, Eichelberger MR, Bowman LM: Rib fractures in children: a marker of severe trauma. J Trauma 30:695, 1990
78. Garramone RR Jr, Jacobs LM, Sahdey P: An objective method to measure and manage occult pneumothorax. Surg Gynecol Obstet 173:257, 1991
79. Jones D: Bilateral fracture of the first rib with bilateral pneumothorax. Injury 5:255, 1974
80. Lee RB, Bass SM, Morris JA Jr, MacKenzie EJ: Three or more rib fractures as an indicator for transfer to a Level 1 trauma center: a population-based study. J Trauma 30:689, 1990
81. Ou ZK, Cui LS, Zhang QH: Fractures of the first and second rib in chest injuries: report of 97 cases. Chung Hua Wai Ko Tsa Chih 23:227, 254, 1985
82. Peclet MH, Newman KD, Eichelberger MR, Gotschall CS et al: Thoracic trauma in children: an indicator of increased mortality. J Pediatr Surg 25:961, 1990
83. Pierce GR, Maxwell JA, Boggan MD: Special hazards of first rib fractures. J Trauma 15:264, 1975
84. Richardson JD, McElvein RB, Trinkle JK: First rib fracture: a hallmark of severe trauma. Ann Surg 181:251, 1974
85. Theriot BA, Gross BD, Sturrock BD: Isolated fracture of the first rib associated with facial trauma. J Oral Maxillofac Surg 42:610, 1984
86. Yee ES, Thomas AN, Goodman PC: Isolated first rib fracture: clinical significance after blunt chest trauma. Ann Thorac Surg 32:278, 1981
87. Brorsson B: Age and injury severity. Scand J Soc Med 17:287, 1989
88. Harris GJ, Soper RT: Pediatric first rib fractures. J Trauma 30:343, 1990
89. Nakayama DK, Ramenofsky ML, Rowe MI: Chest injuries in childhood. Ann Surg 210:770, 1989
90. Fisher RG, Ward RE, Ben-Menachem Y et al: Arteriography and the fractured first rib: too much for too little? AJR 183:1059, 1982
91. Galbraith NF, Urschel HC Jr, Wood RE et al: Fracture of first rib associated with laceration of subclavian artery. J Thorac Cardiovasc Surg 65:649, 1973
92. Lazrove S, Harley DP, Grinell VS et al: Should all patients with first rib fracture undergo arteriography? J Thorac Cardiovasc Surg 83:532, 1982
93. Livoni JP, Barcia TC: Fracture of the first and second rib: incidence of vascular injury relative to type of fracture. Radiology 145:31, 1982
94. Phillips EH, Rogers WF, Gaspar MR: First rib fractures: incidence of vascular injury and indications for angiography. Surgery 89:42, 1984
95. Poole GV, Myers RT: Morbidity and mortality rates in major blunt trauma to the upper chest. Ann Surg 193:70, 1984
96. Moore RS: Fracture of the first rib: an uncommon throwing injury. Injury 22:149, 1991
97. Mikawa Y, Kobori M: Stress fracture of the first rib in a weightlifter. Arch Orthop Trauma Surg 110:121, 1991
98. Bailey P: Surfer's rib: isolated first rib fracture secondary to indirect trauma. Ann Emerg Med 14:346, 1985
99. Proffer DS, Patton JJ, Jackson DW: Nonunion of a first rib fracture in a gymnast. Am J Sports Med 19:198, 1991
100. Sacchetti AD, Beswick DR, Morse SD: Rebound rib: stress-induced first rib fracture. Ann Emerg Med 12:177, 1983
101. Barrett GR, Shelton WR, Miles JW: First rib fractures in football players. Am J Sports Med 16:674, 1988
102. Hoekstra HJ, Kingma LM: Bilateral first rib fractures induced by integral crash helmets. J Trauma 25:566, 1985
103. Hoekstra HJ, Binnendijk B: Isolated bilateral fracture of the first rib associated with a badly fitting crash helmet. Ned Tijdschr Geneeskd 15:126:899, 1982
104. Regoort M, Raaymakers EL: Fracture of the first rib due to trivial accident. Neg Tijdschr Geneeskd 21:134:819, 1990
105. Villa I, Pessina R, Bonacina P, Gaetani G: Traumatic simultaneous bilateral fracture of the first rib. Chir Ital 37:194, 1985
106. Lorentzen JE, Movin M: Fracture of the first rib. Acta Orthop Scand 47:632, 1976
107. Lankenner PA Jr, Micheli LJ: Stress fracture of the first rib: a case report. J Bone Joint Surg [Am] 67:159, 1985
108. Gurtler R, Pavlov H, Torg JS: Stress fracture of the ipsilateral first rib in a pitcher. Am J Sports Med 13:277, 1985
109. Vinko J, Boros I: Fatigue fracture of the first rib. Orv Hetil 12:128:1455, 1987

110. Rademaker M, Redmond AD, Barber PV: Stress fracture of the first rib. Thorax 38:312, 1983
111. Mintz AC, Albano A, Reisdorff EJ et al: Stress fracture of the first rib serratus anterior tension: an unusual mechanism of injury. Ann Emerg Med 19:411, 1990
112. Patterson CR: Osteogenesis imperfecta and other bone disorders in the differential diagnosis of unexplained fractures. J R Soc Med 83:72, 1990
113. Shapiro JR, Burn VE, Chipman SD et al: Pulmonary hypoplasia and osteogenesis imperfecta type II with defective synthesis of alpha I(1) procollagen. Bone 10:165, 1989
114. Kleinman PK, Blackbourne BD, Marks SC et al: Radiologic contributions to the investigation and prosecution of cases of fatal infant abuse. N Engl J Med 23:320:507, 1989
115. Magid N, Glass T: A "hole in a rib": as a sign of child abuse. Pediatr Radiol 20:334, 1990
116. Rizzolo PJ, Coleman PR: Neonatal rib fracture: birth trauma or child abuse? J Fam Pract 29:561, 1989
117. Smeets AJ, Robben SG, Meradji M: Sonographically detected costo-chondral dislocation in an abused child: a new sonographic sign to the radiological spectrum of child abuse. Pediatr Radiol 20:566, 1990
118. Curtis JA, Libshitz HI, Kalinka MK: Fracture of the first rib as a complication of midline sternotomy. Radiology 115:63, 1975
119. Susuki S, Kikuchi K, Takagi K et al: Brachial plexus injury and fracture of the first rib as complications of median sternotomy. Nippon Kyobu Geka Gakkai Zasshi 38:1459, 1990
120. Kaye RJ, Johnson M, Sproed RP, Nicholson SF: First-rib fractures secondary to shoulder restraints. N Engl J Med 310:1748, 1984
121. Resnik CS: Diagnostic imaging of pediatric skeletal trauma. Radiol Clin North Am 27:1013, 1989
122. Bourget D, Bradford JM: Homicidal parents. Can J Psychiatry 35:233, 1990
123. Quick G: A randomized clinical trial of rib belts for simple fractures. Am J Emerg Med 8:277, 1990

7

Fractures of the Clavicle

John D. Hsu
Colin Fennell

> Technical ability to perform a procedure in not an indicator for the procedure.

Fracture of the clavicle in children is a very common injury and competes with fractures of the distal radius as the most frequently seen fracture in children. Over 60 percent of clavicular fractures are seen in children less than 10 years of age.

Fractures of the clavicle are generally classified in the following manner: (1) outer end, (2) shaft (midclavicular), and (3) medial end. Over 90 percent of the fractures occur along the shaft. A small percentage occur on the outer end, and even a smaller percentage occur on the medial end. The latter can occasionally be confused with a sternoclavicular dislocation.

Confusion may occasionally arise between an acute injury and nontraumatic or congenital entities such as congenital pseudarthroses of the clavicle. Results of the treatment of these developmental clavicular abnormalities can be quite disappointing, and most need no treatment at all.

DEVELOPMENT AND ANATOMIC CONSIDERATIONS

The clavicle is the first fetal bone to ossify with two (some authors state one)[1] primary ossification centers appearing in the seventh week. Growth continues by intramembranous ossification from this primary ossification center up to the fifth year. Secondary ossification centers appear both medially and laterally in the teenage years with the medial center providing about 80 percent of the overall length of the clavicle. The secondary centers are the last of all bones to fuse, with fusion occurring in the early to middle twenties.

The clavicle functions as the primary osseous support or strut for the scapula and humerus. It is attached medially to the thorax by the sternoclavicular ligaments and laterally to the scapula by the acromioclavicular ligaments. In addition, the scapula is suspended from the clavicle by the coracoclavicular ligaments and the deltopectoral fascia. The clavicle has the insertion of the sternocleidomastoid muscle medially and the trapezius, deltoid, and subclavius laterally. The bone itself is more tubular medially and forms a flattened bone laterally. It has been suggested that the central third of the clavicle is most susceptible to fracture because of the relative paucity of muscular coverage and because of stress localization in the transition from the lateral concave shape to the medial convex shape.[2] The ligament and muscle attachments are responsible for the typical deformity seen in fractures of the middle third of the clavicle. The medial fragment is always elevated due to the unopposed pull of the sternocleidomastoid muscle while the lateral fragment is held in place by the coracoclavicular ligament attachments (Fig. 7-1).

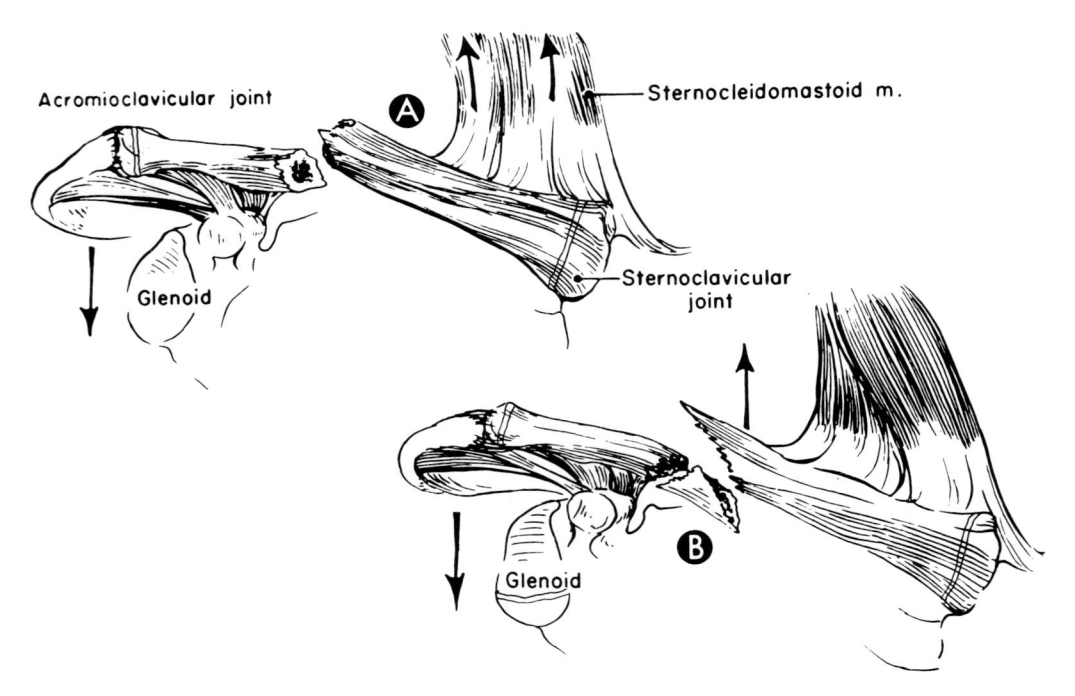

Fig. 7-1. **(A)** Simple transverse fracture. Medial fragment is pulled superiorly by the sternocleidomastoid muscle. The lateral fragment is tethered in place by the coracoclavicular ligaments. **(B)** Comminuted fracture with floating segment. The periosteum remains intact and clavicle heals with widening at fracture site. (Modified from Cave EF (ed): Fractures and Other Injuries. Year Book Medical Publishers, Chicago, 1958, with permission.)

MECHANISM OF INJURY

Birth injuries have most frequently been ascribed to problems with shoulder dystocia or macrosomia[3] and possibly forceps deliveries resulting in a traumatic delivery with a resultant fracture of the clavicle. Another study by Joseph and Rosenfeld[4] has suggested, however, that there are indeed a large number of occult fractures that occur in what are otherwise normal deliveries. In older children the more usually described mechanism for injury has been of a fall on an outstretched hand with indirect trauma to the clavicle. A prospective study by Stanley and colleagues,[5] however, has shown that the vast majority of individuals have sustained fracture to the clavicle through a direct fall on the shoulder.

The increased use of high-speed recreational vehicles by children, such as all-terrain vehicles or snowmobiles, and increased participation in high-energy sports, such as gymnastics and football, result in high-velocity trauma-producing fractures that do not follow classical patterns. Frequently there is significant comminution of the clavicle fracture with associated injuries and complications. These are of great concern to an orthopaedic surgeon treating children or adolescents, especially those with multiple trauma. In multiple trauma the clavicle fracture is often ignored, while more life- and limb-threatening injuries are managed. Fortunately, the child is usually nursed supine, resulting in reduction of the clavicle fracture due to the weight of the shoulders. This can be accentuated in more severely displaced clavicular fractures by inserting a rolled towel between the shoulder blades to increase the traction effect of the shoulders.

BIRTH FRACTURES

Fractures in newborns have been widely quoted[5] to occur in approximately 0.5 percent of all live births. A recent prospective study,[4] which looked carefully at follow-up of newborns, found clavicular fractures occurred in approximately 3 percent of all live births, with 83 percent of the fractures being occult.

Neonates with complete clavicle fracture will present with a mass or pain with movement of the affected arm and associated with pseudoparalysis of the arm. The pseudoparalysis can be best demonstrated with the Moro reflex, resulting in a unilateral loss of arm motion on the Moro reflex. The differential diagnosis of the pseudoparalysis includes fracture of the proximal humeral physis, brachial plexus injury, infection of the shoulder region and rarely dislocation of the shoulder. On physical examination the infant will show tenderness and swelling over the midclavicle with crepitation being present if there is a complete fracture of the clavicle. Undisplaced greenstick fractures of the clavicle can

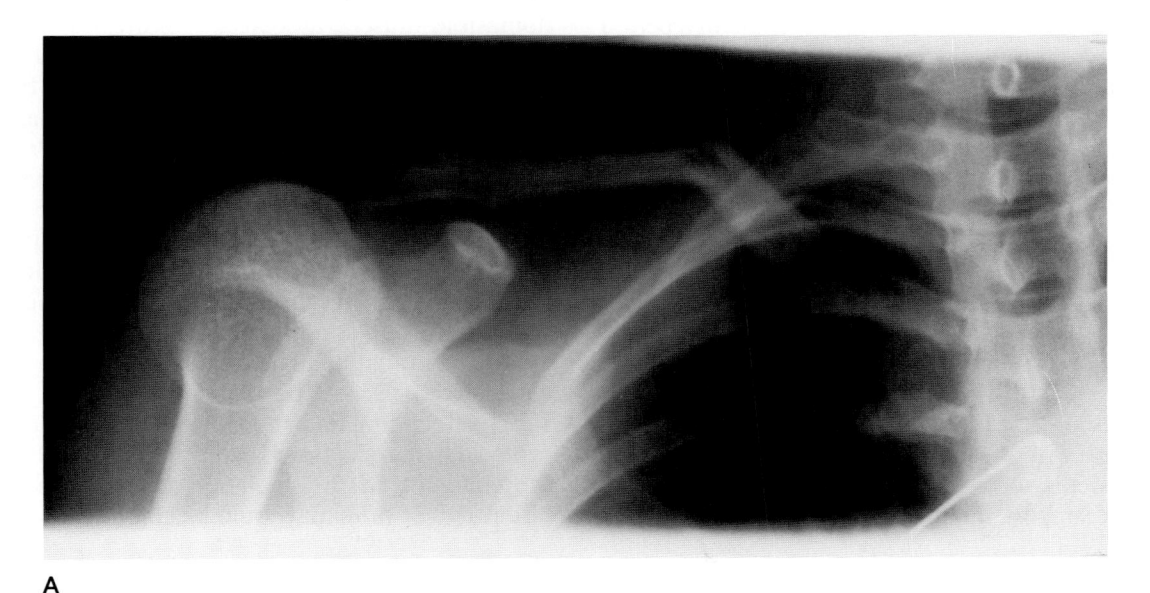

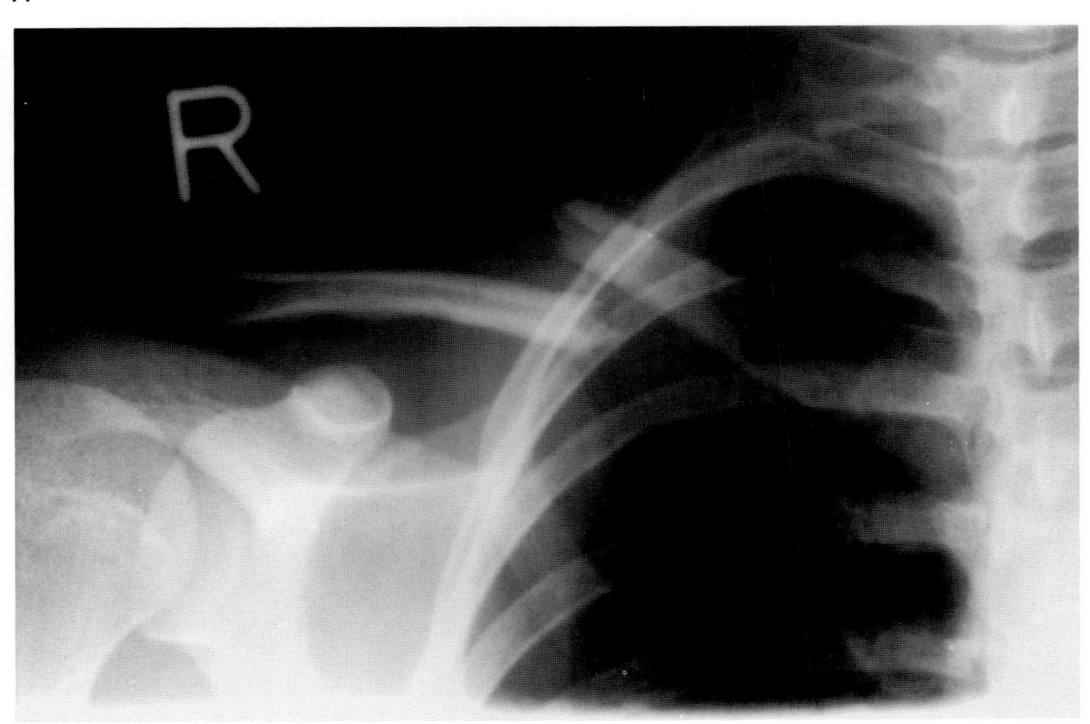

Fig. 7-2. (A) Greenstick fracture of clavicle with angulation. (B) Classical fracture of midshaft clavicle with medial fragment elevated by the pull of the sternomastoid muscles.

often be detected by an increase in the intensity of the cry on clavicular palpation.

The majority of newborn clavicle fractures are relatively asymptomatic and not diagnosed until the callus becomes palpable in the later healing stages. The symptomatic newborn can be managed most easily just with a swathe holding the affected limb to the trunk for a period of 7 to 10 days, during which adequate healing will occur to then allow movement.

Parents need to be assured that the fracture is not serious and the bony callus mass will remodel and disappear spontaneously over the course of a few months.

MIDCLAVICULAR SHAFT FRACTURES

In young children, greenstick fractures are most common and heal without any significant complication (Fig. 7-2). A clavicular or figure-of-eight strap should be applied to give support and maintain comfort (Fig. 7-3). In older children a complete fracture is generally seen with separation of the fracture fragments. The lateral fragment is displaced forward and downward. The displacement is usually caused by the weight of the limb and attachments of the coracoclavicular ligaments. The medial fragment is usually pulled upward by the sternocleidomastoid muscle. Displaced fractures can be reduced by extending the shoulder backward and applying a clavicular strap with appropriate padding in the axilla. Gradual tightening of this strap should occur as swelling subsides or the bandage stretches or loosens. Precautions should be given to the family to check the circulation of the hand, to observe for swelling and abnormal sensation to the fingers. Occasionally, a manipulation is required for massive displacement, but caution should be exercised because of the proximity of the brachial plexus, subclavian vein, and the pleura.

Postmanipulation, the reduction of the fractured clavicle can usually be maintained with a clavicular strap. Overriding and moderate angulation can be accepted. Open reduction is rarely indicated. The younger the child the more angulation that can be accepted. "Tenting" of the skin should be corrected, however, as

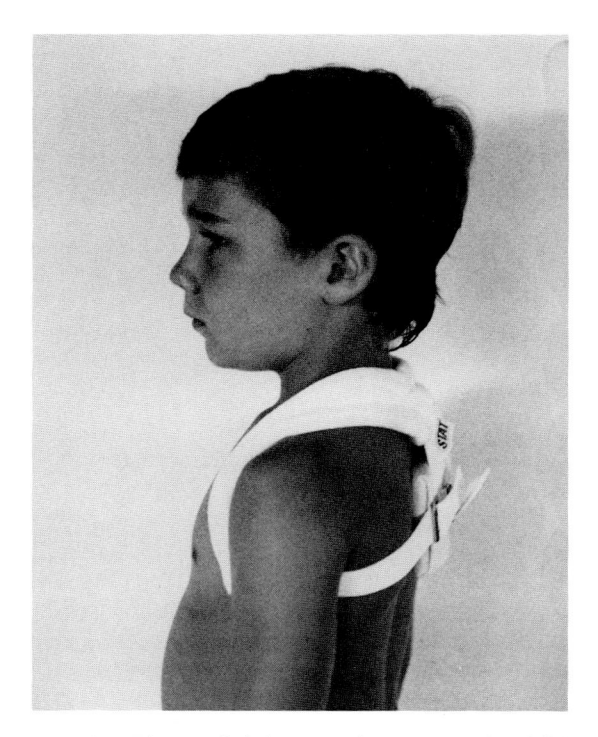

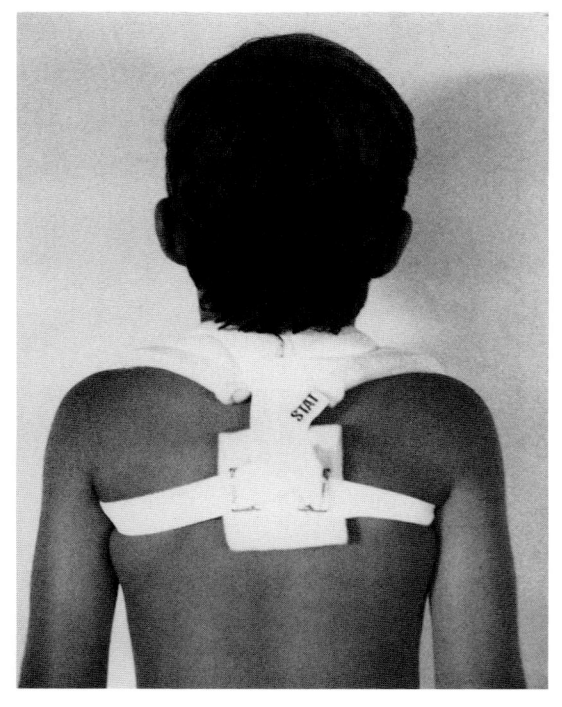

Fig. 7-3. Figure-of-eight strapping retracts the child's shoulder minimizes fragment motion. Displacement of the fragments is reduced and the child is more comfortable. A sling can be used in conjunction for the initial 3 to 4 days.

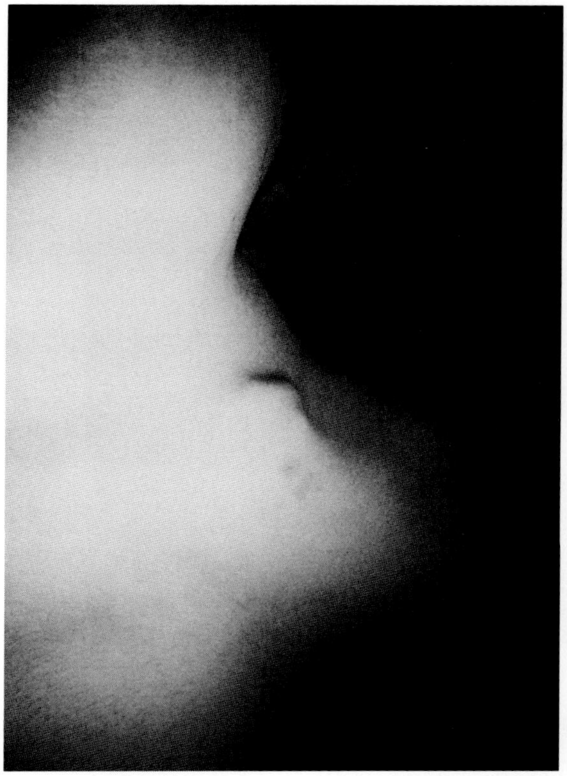

Fractures of the Clavicle / 117

fractured clavicle. Reduction of the fracture by local manipulation with strapping and positioning is usually possible and best accomplished with the patient seated and arms held up and supported by an assistant. If a bone spicule is resulting in skin erosion, excision of the spicule may be necessary. Internal fixation is not necessary and should not be used. The soft tissue and periosteum can be repaired and the clavicle allowed to heal with a clavicular strap or sling used for support for a duration of 3 weeks.

Fig. 7-4. Tenting of the skin by the elevated medial fragment can result in an open fracture and an ugly cosmetically unacceptable malunion. This should be reduced under local anesthesia and held in a clavicular strap or figure-of-eight cast.

this may result in skin necrosis and conversion of the closed fracture to an open one (Fig. 7-4).

MIDCLAVICULAR SEGMENTAL FRACTURE (Z FRACTURE)

In the older child, particularly the adolescent teenager, extreme trauma can produce a midclavicular segmental fracture. This is the Z type of midclavicular fracture. The middle third fracture is comminuted and can be severely angulated (Fig. 7-5). Occasionally, the skin is tented and breached. The fractures are generally caused by motorcycle or motor vehicle accidents and sports injuries, falls from bicycles and falls from heights. These children are initially extremely disabled with pain and an inability to raise the arm and a tilting of the whole body to the affected side in an attempt to decrease the pull on the

FRACTURES OF THE MEDIAL END OF THE CLAVICLE

Medial fractures of the clavicle are rare. The injuries are usually Salter-Harris type I or II epiphyseal fractures and are commonly misdiagnosed as anterior sternoclavicular dislocations. Injury to the medial clavicle can be diagnosed by the tenderness and swelling on palpation. Radiographic confirmation is aided by a 35-degree cephalad clavicle view and can be seen most clearly on computed tomography (CT) scan, though this is rarely indicated. Because internal fixation is fraught with danger in this region these injuries are best treated nonoperatively with an explanation given to parents about the cosmetic protuberance that will persist for a year or so.

FRACTURES OF THE LATERAL END OF THE CLAVICLE

Fractures of the lateral end of the clavicle have been classified as to their location compared to the coracoclavicular ligaments,[2] the implication being that certain lateral fractures are more prone to result in nonunion. Children's clavicles are fortunately blessed by a thick periosteum to which the coracoclavicular ligaments remain attached (Fig. 7-6). The periosteal sleeve is capable of regenerating a new clavicle to fill in the displaced segment of bone, and the outcome is typically very acceptable both functionally and cosmetically. Nonoperative treatment remains the standard for management of this injury. Fractures of the lateral third left untreated have produced "double clavicles" where the displaced periosteal sleeve produces a new bone and the original lateral clavicle resorbs with time. These lateral fractures can produce a painful lump on the outer aspect of the

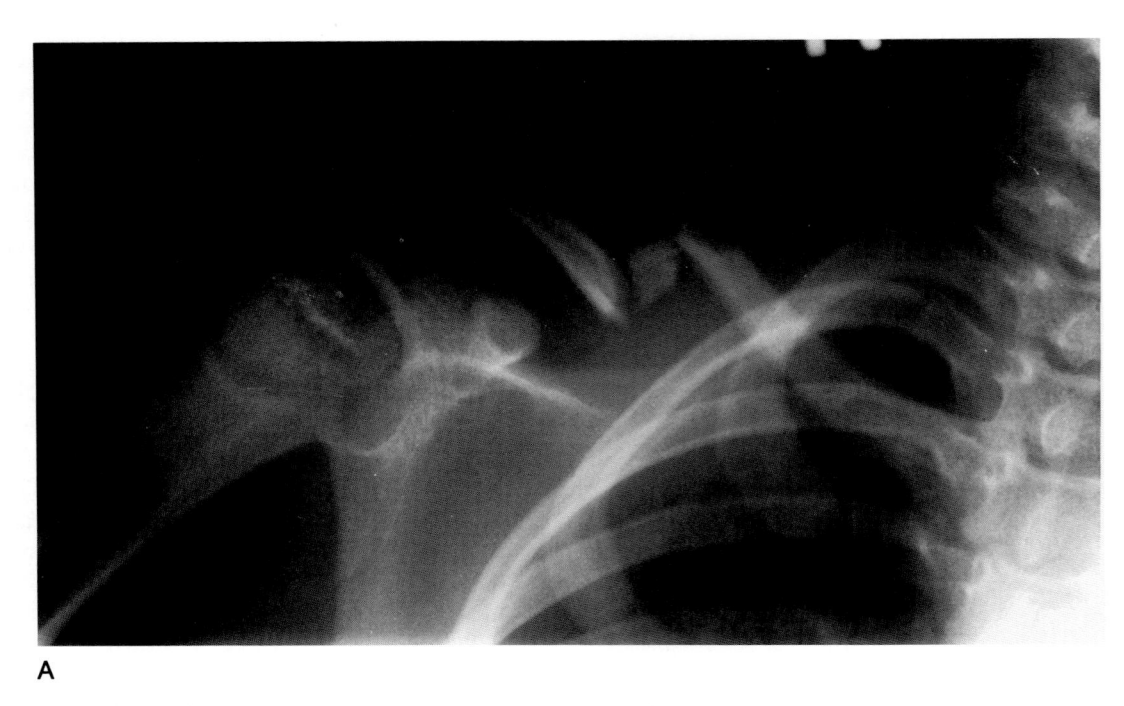

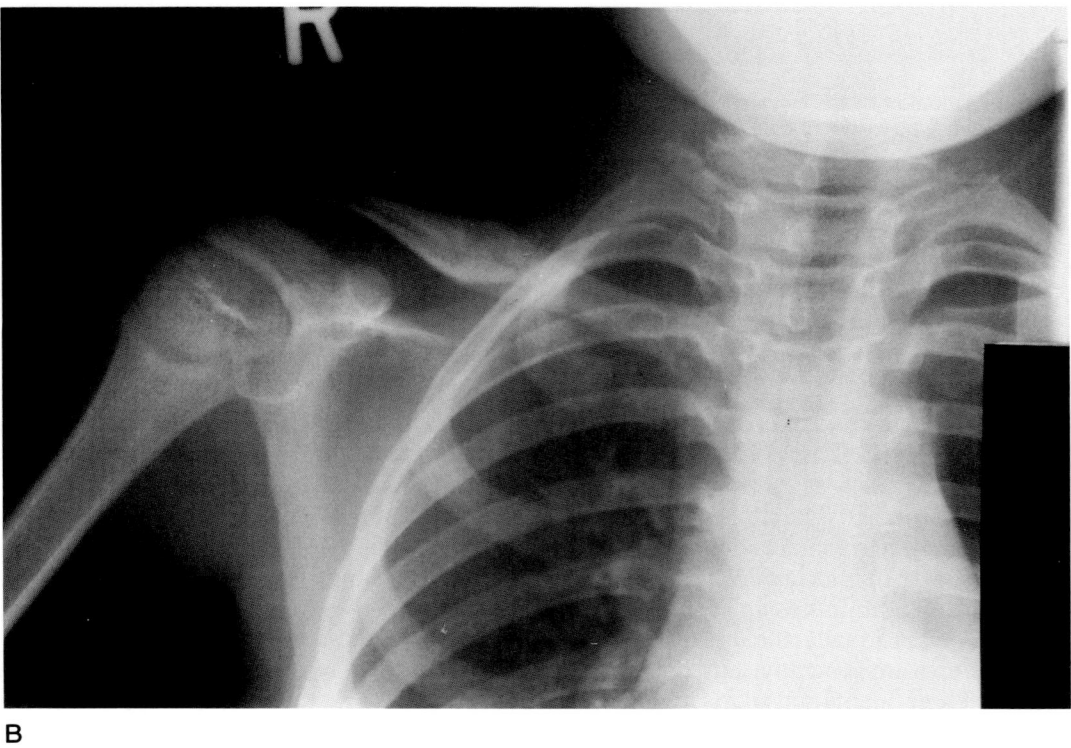

Fig. 7-5. **(A)** Segmental or Z fracture of the clavicle in a 10-year-old boy injured in a snowmobile accident. **(B)** The fragment has become incorporated into the callus generated by in the intact periosteal sleeve.

Fractures of the Clavicle / 119

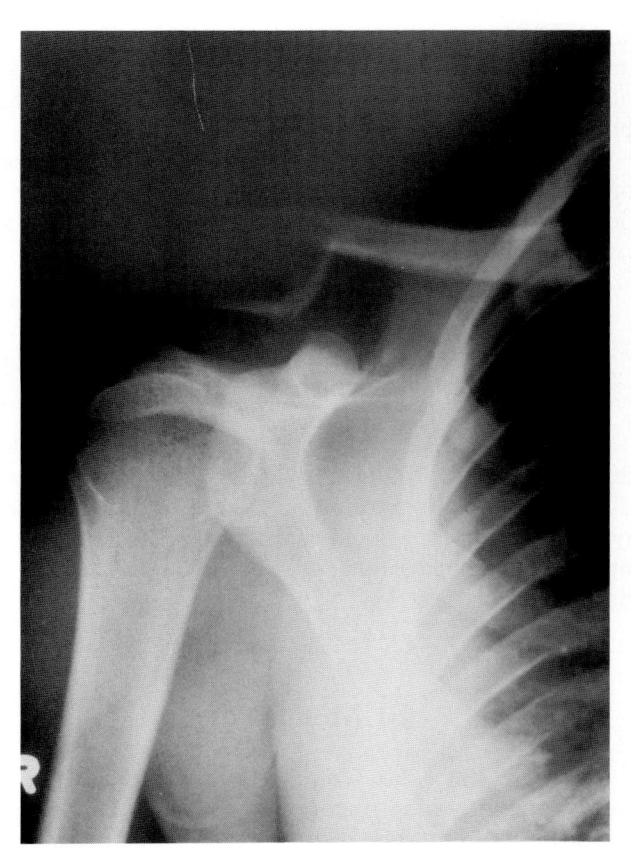

Fig. 7-6. Fracture of the outer clavicle illustrating the periosteal sleeve remaining attached to the coracoclavicular ligaments.

clavicle and can sometimes be confused with an acromioclavicle separation[6] (see Ch. 8).

CLAVICULAR FRACTURE IN HEAD TRAUMA PATIENTS

Clavicular fracture in head-injured children represents a concern in that they may be overlooked while more threatening injuries are addressed. A study by Wilkes and Hoffer[7] showed that of 499 children admitted to Rancho Los Amigos Medical Center for rehabilitation over a 15-year interval, 35 (7 percent) sustained a clavicle fracture. Two-thirds of the children were male and the most common cause of injury was a motor vehicle accident. There were many associated injuries in addition to the head injuries. The majority of the fractures were midshaft and healed without incident.

SURGICAL TREATMENT

Indications for open reduction of clavicular fractures in children are exceedingly uncommon. These include open fractures, fractures with vascular compromise, and grossly displaced fractures that are irreducible with closed techniques. If internal fixation is required, plating with a small fragment set is preferable to pins due to the high incidence of pin migration in the clavicle.

Open fractures require debridement, irrigation, closed reduction without internal fixation, and secondary closure with appropriate antibiotic coverage. The rare fracture with demonstrable vascular complications such as an expanding hematoma or an ischemic limb necessitates open reduction and fixation of the clavicle as part of the management of the vascular injury. Venous occlusion producing edema of the arm has been successfully managed by a closed reduction with towel clips to reduce the pressure on the subclavian vein.[8]

COMPLICATIONS

The majority of fractures of the clavicle in children heal without any complications, and fractures of the clavicle readily remodel so completely that the outcome is ultimately acceptable both functionally and cosmetically.

Nonunion

Nonunion of the clavicle is rarely seen even in adult fractures of the clavicle and is extremely uncommon in children.[9] Nonunion in a child must be differentiated from congenital pseudarthrosis, cleidocranial dysostosis, and neurofibromatosis. Nonunion of the clavicle is most likely to occur in the older child or young adolescent and is best managed by internal fixation and bone grafting.[10,11–13,14]

Brachial Plexus Injury

Neurologic injuries in association with clavicle fractures can either occur acutely at the time of the injury at which time the brachial plexus can be damaged or there can be a chronic plexus impingement secondary to hypertrophy of callus.[15,16] Plexus injuries require careful documentation to determine the location of the defect and in teenagers with plexus impingement it may be necessary to reduce the malunion, or resect the fracture callus.

Vascular Injury

Vascular injury can occur to either the subclavian artery or vein and penetration of either can lead to life-threatening hemorrhage. Occlusion of the artery can cause distal ischemia, which also requires surgical intervention. Occlusion of the subclavian vein can sometimes be managed by closed reduction of the fracture to reduce the pressure that is occurring from the displaced clavicle.[8] Occult injury to the underlining vasculature has been known to produce false aneurysms and emboli that may present on a delayed basis.

Pneumothorax

Pneumothorax can occur as a result of displaced clavicular fractures and should be looked for on radiographs of the chest. Standard treatment of both the clavicle fracture and the pneumothorax usually produce satisfactory results.

Other Complications

Other rare complications that can occur secondary to clavicular fractures include reflex dystrophy which has been reported to respond well to stellate ganglion blocks[17] and plastic bowing of the clavicle which does not appear to have any significant clinical consequence.[18] Goddard has reported on concomitant atlantoaxial rotatory subluxation which may have been instigated by an associated clavicle fracture.[19]

CONDITIONS MIMICKING CLAVICULAR FRACTURE

Congenital Pseudarthrosis

Congenital pseudarthrosis was first described in 1910.[20] It is typically right-sided but has been rarely found on the left side in association with dextrocardia. Congenital clavicular pseudarthrosis is rarely bilateral.[21,22] The defect is typically between the lateral and middle third of the clavicle and on examination the medial fragment can be found to be pulled upward and forward and the lateral fragment to be pulled upward and backward along with a thickening of the ends of the bones. The involved shoulder is typically lower than the other, and the medial border of the scapula will be more prominent. The deformity is progressive with time.

The radiologic appearance shows a characteristic lack of continuity in the middle of the clavicle without evidence of reactive bone secondary to fracture which distinguishes it from a nonunion.

Cleidocranial Dysostosis and Neurofibromatosis

Cleidocranial dysostosis typically has bilateral clavicle defects along with other bony deformities that help to distinguish it from a nonunion. Neurofibromatosis has typical neurofibromas and café au lait spots along with other skeletal changes that help to distinguish it from a nonunion.

SUMMARY

Midshaft clavicular fractures represent one of the most frequently seen fractures in children. Those that are displaced should be treated closed with a clavicular strap and almost all heal satisfactorily. We have noticed more and more special types of fractures, including Z fractures and fractures on both the medial and lateral end of the clavicle with increasing trauma. These clavicular fractures need to be recognized and selective treatment applied. Operative reduction is rarely indicated in children. Complications can occur but are uncommon in the pediatric age group.

REFERENCES

1. Fawcett J: The development and ossification of the human clavicle. J Anat 47:225, 1913
2. Dameron TB, Rockwood CA: Fractures of the shaft of the clavicle. p. 608. In Rockwood CA, Wilkins KE (eds): Fractures in Children. JB Lippincott, Philadelphia, 1984
3. Oppenheim WL, Davis A, Growdon WA: Clavicle fractures in the newborn. Clin Orthop 250:176, 1990
4. Joseph PR, Rosenfeld W: Clavicular fractures in neonates. Am J Dis Child 144:165, 1990
5. Stanley D, Trowbridge EA, Norris SA: Mechanism of clavicle fracture. J Bone Joint Surg [Br] 70:461, 1988
6. Ogden JA: Distal clavicular physeal injury. Clin Orthop 188:68, 1984

7. Wilkes JA, Hoffer MM: Clavicle fractures in head injured children. J Orthop Trauma 1:55, 1987
8. Mital MA, Aufranc OE: Venous occlusion following greenstick fracture of clavicle. JAMA 206:1301, 1969
9. Nogi J, Heckman JD, Hakala M et al: Nonunion of clavicle in a child. Clin Orthop 110:19, 1975
10. Jupiter JB, Leffert RD: Nonunion of the clavicle. J Bone Joint Surg [Am] 69:753, 1987
11. Neer CS: Nonunion of the clavicle. JAMA 172:1006, 1960
12. Pyper JB: Nonunion of fractures of the clavicle. Injury 268:9, 1978
13. Manske DJ, Szabo RM: Operative treatment of mid-shaft clavicular non-unions. J Bone Joint Surg [Am] 67:1367, 1985
14. Wilkins RM, Johnston RM: Ununited fractures of the clavicle. J Bone Joint Surg [Am] 65:773, 1983
15. Miller DS, Boswick JA: Lesions of the brachial plexus associated with fractures of the clavicle. Clin Orthop 64:144, 1969
16. Howard FM, Shafer SJ: Injuries to the clavicle with neuromuscular complications. J Bone Joint Surg [Am] 47:1335, 1965
17. Ivey M, Britt M, Johnston RV: Reflex sympathetic dystrophy after clavicle fracture. J Trauma 31:276, 1991
18. Bowen AD: Plastic bowing of the clavicle in children. J Bone Joint Surg [Am] 65:403, 1985
19. Goddard NJ, Stabler J, Albert JS: Atlanto-axial rotatory fixation and fracture of the clavicle. J Bone Joint Surg [Br] 72B:72, 1990
20. Fitzwilliams DC: Hereditary craniocleido dysostosis. Lancet 2:1466, 1910
21. Lloyd-Roberts GC, Apley AG, Wen R: Reflections upon the aetiology of congenital pseudoarthosis of the clavicle. J Bone Joint Surg [Br] 57:24, 1975
22. Russo MT, Maffulli N: Bilateral congenital pseudarthroses of the clavicle. Arch Orthop Trauma Surg 109:177, 1990

8

Dislocations and Pseudodislocations of the Clavicle

Pierre Mercier

The decision is more important than the incision.

DISLOCATION OF THE MEDIAL END OF THE CLAVICLE

Description and Incidence

Dislocation of the medial end of the clavicle is a rare injury. It is reported to account for 1 percent of clavicular injuries in children[1] and 6 percent of all clavicular fractures.[2] From a review of 1,603 injuries of the shoulder girdle, Cave reported a 3 percent incidence of sternoclavicular lesions.[3] In the literature the youngest child reported was 7 months old.[4] Most appear to occur between the ages of 10 and 25.[5]

Anatomic Considerations

The majority of children with apparent dislocation of the medial end of the clavicle have Salter-Harris type I or II fracture-separations through the medial physis.[6,7] The epiphysis remains in its anatomic location while the metaphysis is displaced out of its periosteal tube. True sternoclavicular dislocations in children have been reported,[8] but such lesions are uncommon in the skeletally immature.

The clavicle begins ossification by the fifth week of gestation.[9,10] It is the first long bone to ossify, but its medial epiphysis does not appear before 18 to 20 years of age. In addition, the medial physis, which accounts for 80 percent of the growth of the clavicle, does not fuse until age 23 to 25.[9,10] These factors explain why many of these injuries are misinterpreted as sternoclavicular dislocations, since the growth plate remains open until early adulthood, and the epiphysis is not visible on radiographs until late adolescence.

The sternoclavicular joint is incongruous when one compares the small articular surface of the sternum with its large clavicular counterpart. The joint is diarthrodial; the presence of a disc compensates for this incongruity and provides some stability. The articular disc is convex-concave in shape and is attached to the anterior and posterior capsule of the joint and inferiorly to the synchondral junction of the first rib to the sternum[11] (Fig. 8-1).

The ligaments that stabilize the joint are the costoclavicular (rhomboid), the interclavicular and capsular ligaments. The costoclavicular ligament arises from the upper surface of the first rib and its synchondral junction with the sternum and attaches to the underside of the medial end of the clavicle. It opposes the pull of the

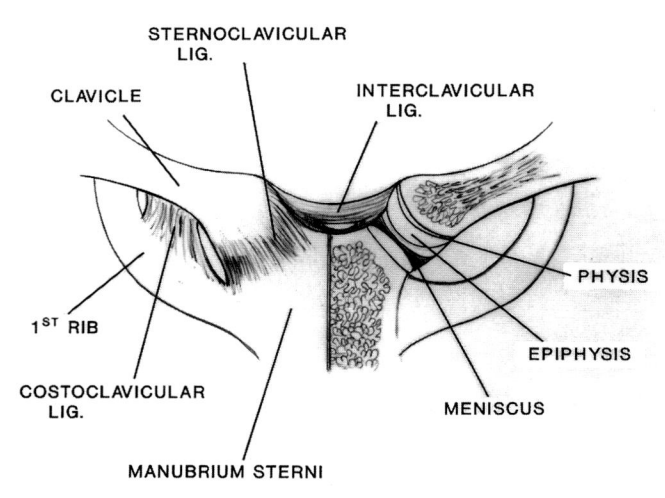

Fig. 8-1. Anatomic representation of the medial end of the clavicle with relations to the sternum and ligamentous structures.

sternocleidomastoid muscle.[11] In cases of dislocation of the medial end of the clavicle in children, when the epiphysis remains in place and the clavicle is displaced through a tear in the periosteum, the costoclavicular ligament is probably intact retaining the periosteal sleeve in place (Fig. 8-2).

The interclavicular ligament connects the superior aspect of each medial end of the clavicles, and it assists in maintaining the shoulders up (poise).[12] The capsular ligaments run from the manubrium sterni to the medial epiphysis of the clavicle. The anterior capsular ligaments are stronger and resist downward displacement of the shoulders. The interclavicular and capsular ligaments provide stability to the medial clavicular epiphysis, while the physis is extracapsular and more likely to be injured (Fig. 8-1).

Of significant importance are the structures lying posterior to the joint, as they could be injured by a posterior displacement of the clavicle. The sternothyroid and sternohyoid muscles are in close proximity to the posterior capsule and provide some protection to the vessels with the omohyoid and clavipectoral fasciae.[12] Behind lie the innominate artery and vein, the phrenic and vagus nerves, the internal jugular vein, the trachea and the esophagus. These structures can be compressed or lacerated by the medial metaphysis of the clavicle. Awareness of the proximity of these structures is essential in detecting associated lesions and for the surgeon who will attempt an open reduction of a posterior dislocation (seldom necessary in children).

The sternoclavicular joint is quite mobile. It allows for rotation and elevation of the clavicle to occur with scapular movement during shoulder motion. This degree of mobility is significant and explains why K-wires migrate so frequently when used to stabilize this joint.

Mechanism of Injury

Displacement of the medial end of the clavicle can occur from a direct or indirect force.[12,13] Anterior displacement is more common[14] and is usually caused by a force applied to the anterior aspect of the shoulder while

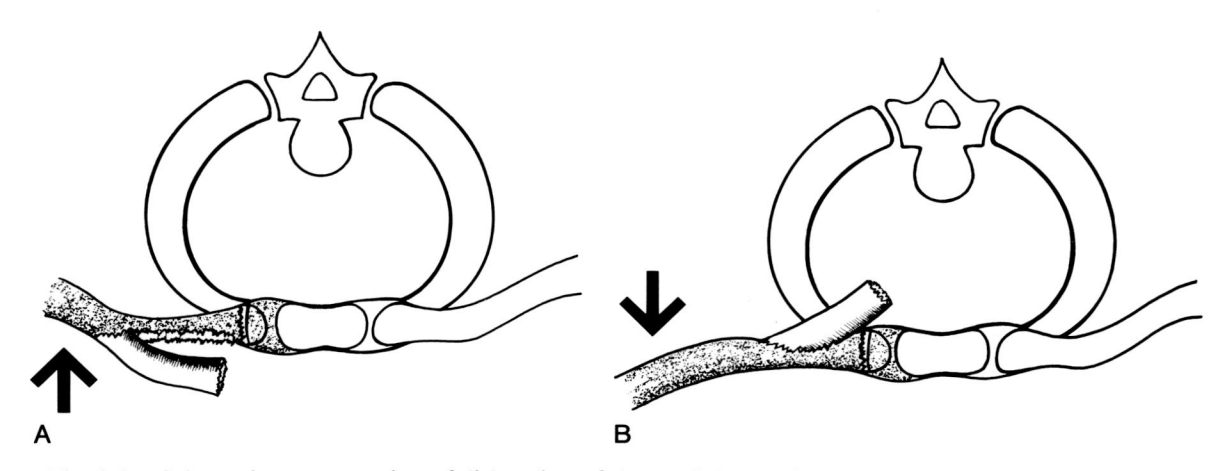

Fig. 8-2. Schematic representation of dislocation of the medial end of the clavicle in children. **(A)** Anterior displacement is usually caused by an indirect force applied anteriorly to the shoulder. **(B)** Posterior displacement is caused by a direct blow to the medial clavicle or by an indirect force applied on the posterior aspect of the shoulder.

the arm is in abduction (Fig. 8-2A). The shoulder is rolled posteriorly levering the medial end of the clavicle out of its sternal attachment. Such a mechanism can be the result of a motor vehicle accident, a fall at play, or, in the case of adolescents, during a piling-on while playing football. It has also been reported to result from a sudden pull on the arm with the shoulder in extension and abduction.[15]

Posterior displacement can occur from a direct blow to the medial end of the clavicle or more often from an indirect force applied to the posterolateral aspect of the shoulder rolling it forward.[16] The clavicle is driven inward by the push of the shoulder (Fig. 8-2B). This mechanism occurs when a child is lying on his side while another child falls onto his shoulder, therefore applying considerable force. As the clavicle is the only resistance to the stress applied, it fractures at the physis. The epiphysis remains in its anatomic location, but the metaphysis and shaft are pushed inward and posteriorly into the mediastinum. A similar mechanism can be reproduced during a piling-on at football or from crushing injuries of motor vehicle accidents.[17]

Classification

Types

True sternoclavicular joint dislocations in children, although reported,[8] are considered rare. Displacement occurs usually through the physis or the medial shaft of the clavicle[7,16,17] (Fig. 8-2).

Displacement

The degree of displacement has led to a classification of such injuries in adults according to the amount of ligament damage. In children; since the injury occurs through the physis, it can be described as displaced or undisplaced.

Direction

The medial end of the clavicle is displaced either anteriorly or posteriorly.

Physical Examination

With anterior or posterior displacement of the medial end of the clavicle there is local point tenderness and swelling. The child supports and guards the injured limb, the shoulder is pulled forward, and the neck is often flexed to the side of the injury.[1]

Anterior displacement can sometimes be apparent at inspection or by palpation, but considerable swelling can mask the prominence, and it is often difficult to determine the direction of the displacement. One can notice the loss of normal contours of the neck.

With posterior displacement of the medial end of the clavicle a depression can sometimes be seen[16] at the joint before the onset of swelling. The superior border of the manubrium sterni becomes easily palpable.[12] Should the degree of displacement be severe, signs of compression on vital structures will become apparent: dyspnea, dysphagia, diminished radial pulse, venous engorgement, weakness or paresthesias of the upper extremity.[15] These signs should be looked for by the examiner, as the situation can become life-threatening. Appropriate management requires early detection and assessment of the injury.

Diagnosis

Plain radiographs of anteroposterior (AP) views of the sternoclavicular joint are difficult to interpret because of the superposition of various structures. A true lateral view of the joint is not possible to obtain. Rockwood[12] has developed and proposed the so-called "serendipity view" for better assessment of the joint. This view is taken with the patient in dorsal decubitus with the cassette under his shoulders and neck. The x-ray tube is angulated 40 degrees cephalad and centered over both sternoclavicular joints. The projection on the film will show the displaced clavicle to be riding higher or superiorly in relation to the manubrium sterni in case of anterior dislocation. Conversely, a posterior dislocation will project the clavicle to ride inferiorly to the sternum.

Other methods have also been proposed by Heinig[13] and Hobbs[18] to obtain adequate views of the joint from plain radiographs. Tomography can also help to assess the direction of the displacement and to differentiate a true dislocation of the joint from a fracture of the medial end of the clavicle.

Computed tomography (CT) scan has now become the best tool to grade the degree of posterior displacement of the medial clavicle and its relationship to the underlying structures. A view of both joints should be obtained for comparison. It can also help in differentiating a fracture from a true dislocation.[19]

Management

As most injuries to the medial end of the clavicle occur through the physis, a significant amount of remodeling can be expected even in late adolescence. Therefore nonoperative management is the rule for anterior displacements and posterior displacements without sign of compression in children. It is emphasized that in cases of posterior displacement the situation can become life-threatening, and a very detailed and accurate assessment is essential.[15] One should look for signs of airway obstruction, pneumothorax, vascular compromise of the limb, and nerve impairment. Adequate radiographs and CT scans should be obtained, and an arteriogram may be indicated after consultation with a vascular or thoracic surgeon. If the airway is compromised, early intubation may be necessary and manual abduction of the involved shoulder combined with in-line traction on the limb will help reduce the encroachment of the medial clavicle on the trachea (Fig. 8-3).

Technique of Closed Reduction

Anterior Dislocation

Local anesthesia may be used with a cooperative teenager, but general anesthesia is preferable for a child. A bolster or a towel rolled 3 to 4 in. thick is inserted between the scapulae with the child in dorsal decubitus. Bilateral shoulder pressure is applied by an assistant, and the medial part of the clavicle is reduced by manually pushing it into place.[1] Grasping the medial end of the clavicle with a towel clip may give better control for the reduction. The reduction is often stable, and it is maintained with the help of a figure-of-8 harness. A sling can also be used in addition to the harness to support the limb and limit shoulder abduction for the first week or two. The harness is maintained in place for a total of 3 to 4 weeks. Should the reduction be unstable or lost, the displacement should be accepted as considerable bone remodeling can be expected. Percutaneous K-wire fixation should be avoided because of the dangers of pin migration.

Posterior Dislocation

In cases of severe displacement with vascular or airway compromise the reduction should be carried out as an emergency procedure after appropriate assessment and consultations. General anesthesia is used, and the patient is positioned in dorsal decubitus with a sandbag or a rolled towel between the shoulder blades. Two methods of closed reduction can be utilized.

Abduction Method: The upper extremity is brought into abduction, and axial traction is applied on the limb as the shoulder is gradually extended in an attempt to lever the medial part of the clavicle anteriorly. Direct pressure is also applied anteriorly over the shoulder. The medial end of the clavicle can be grasped to pull it forward with the fingers or percutaneously with a sterile towel clip, after disinfection of the skin.

Adduction Method: Direct pressure is applied on both shoulders by an assistant while axial traction is exerted on the upper extremity with the shoulder in adduction.

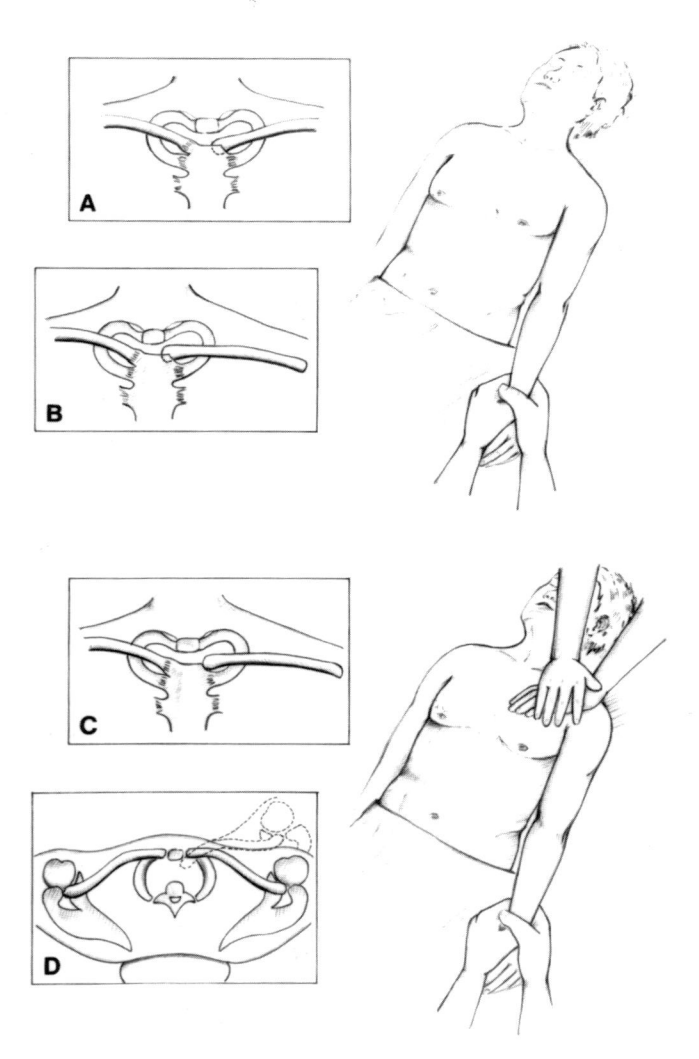

Fig. 8-3. Closed reduction of a retrosternal dislocation of the medial end of the clavicle by the adduction method. **(A & B)** Axial traction is applied to the upper extremity to bring the medial end of the clavicle superiorly. **(C & D)** Then a downward pressure is applied by an assistant onto the shoulder to lever the medial end of the clavicle into place.

The medial end of the clavicle is levered superiorly over the first rib into position (Fig. 8-3). Again grasping the medial end of the clavicle with a towel clip improves the leverage and facilitates reduction. This method was reported by Buckerfield and Castle[5] to be effective when the abduction method has failed or in cases that are 3 to 4 days old.

Postreduction immobilization is as described for anterior displacements. Should the reduction fail or be lost after reduction, and if no sign of compression is present the displacement can be accepted in a child as remodeling will correct the deformity. The use of fixation with K-wires is to be condemned, as the risk of pin migration is significant. Vascular, pulmonary, and tracheal injuries, and even death have been reported as a result of pins migrating from the sternoclavicular joint.

Technique of Open Reduction

The only indication for open reduction of a sternoclavicular dislocation in a child is in the case of a severe posterior displacement, unreducible by closed methods, with compression on vital structures by the medial end of the clavicle. Assistance by a thoracic surgeon is recommended. The area is prepped and draped including a free-arm drape technique should traction and manipulation be necessary during the procedure. The incision is carried superiorly to the medial end of the clavicle extending medially and inferiorly over the joint. The technique consists of soft tissues dissection around the proximal end of the clavicle while preserving as much of the anterior ligaments as possible to maintain some stability. A periosteal elevator can be used to pry the clavicle into place. The periosteal tube is then sutured and a No. 0 Mersilene suture can be passed through drill holes in the epiphysis and metaphysis for added stability.

Once again the use of K-wires is to be discouraged for fear of migration.

Complications

The complications reported as a result of sternoclavicular dislocations are mainly related to the retrosternal displacement of the medial end of the clavicle. Injuries or compression of vital structures have been reported to occur in 25 percent of cases.[20] These range from lesions to the major arteries, veins, and nerves of the area to injuries to the viscera such as lung perforation and pneumothorax, compression, laceration or necrosis of the esophagus and trachea, tracheoesophageal fistula, and death.

Iatrogenic complications are also well documented and are mainly related to the use of K-wires for fixation. Migration of these pins to the heart,[21] pulmonary artery,[22] innominate artery, and aorta[23,24] were reported and even death has occurred as a result of the use of K-wires for fixation of the sternoclavicular joint.

Complications directly related to the skeletal injury appear to be rare, as bone remodeling will correct the local deformity considerably. Similarly joint instability as a result of this injury is not reported as a problem in the growing skeleton. Recurrence may occur in children with excessive ligamentous laxity due to stretching of the sternoclavicular ligaments. Children with spasticity such as cerebral palsy may also experience a redislocation. Even in the adult population, sternoclavicular instability is often not symptomatic and can be dealt with by resection of the medial end of the clavicle.

DISLOCATION OF THE OUTER END OF THE CLAVICLE

Description and Incidence

Injuries to the outer end of the clavicle in children[1] are most often fractures rather than true dislocations.[1,25,26] Havranek[27] reported that 3.8 percent of all clavicular

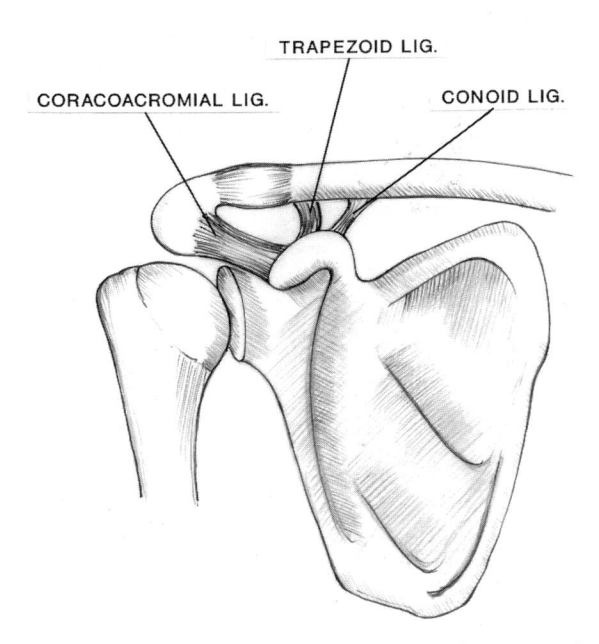

Fig. 8-4. Anatomic representation of the distal end of the clavicle with relations to the shoulder and ligamentous structures.

128 / Management of Pediatric Fractures

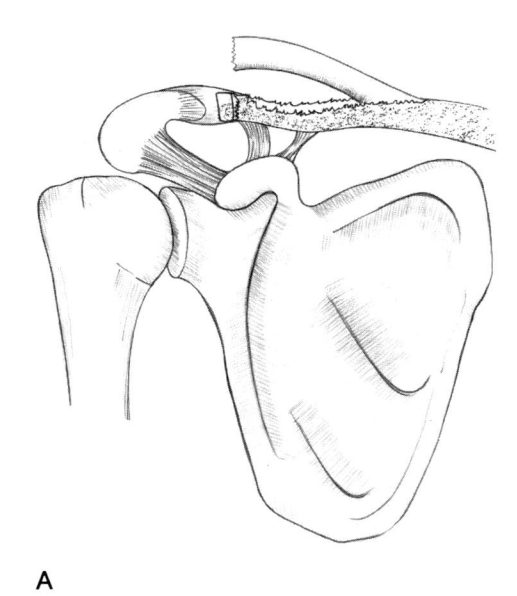

Fig. 8-5. **(A)** Pseudodislocation of the distal end of the clavicle with superior displacement in children. The epiphysis and physis are retained in their anatomic location while the medial fragment is stripped through a tear in the periosteum. **(B)** Sleeve fracture of outer clavicle at time of injury illustrating a thin wisp of subchondral bone. *(Figure continues.)*

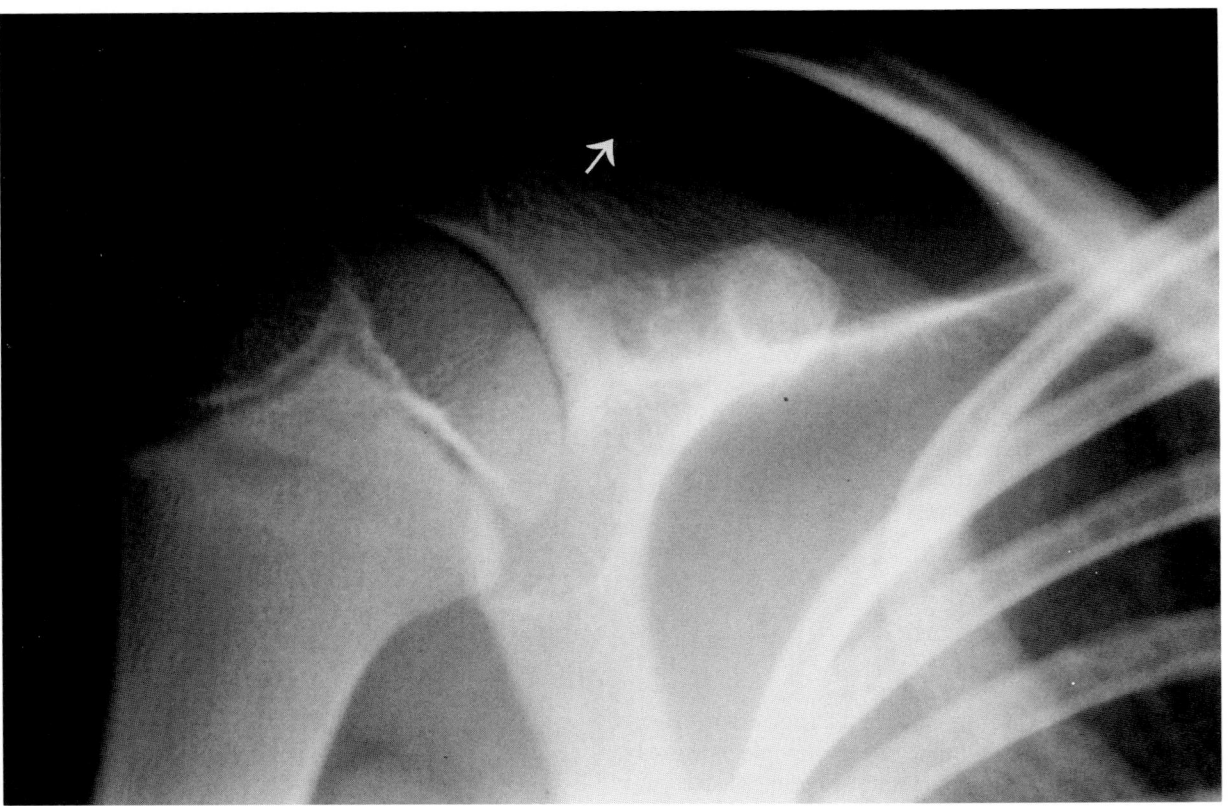

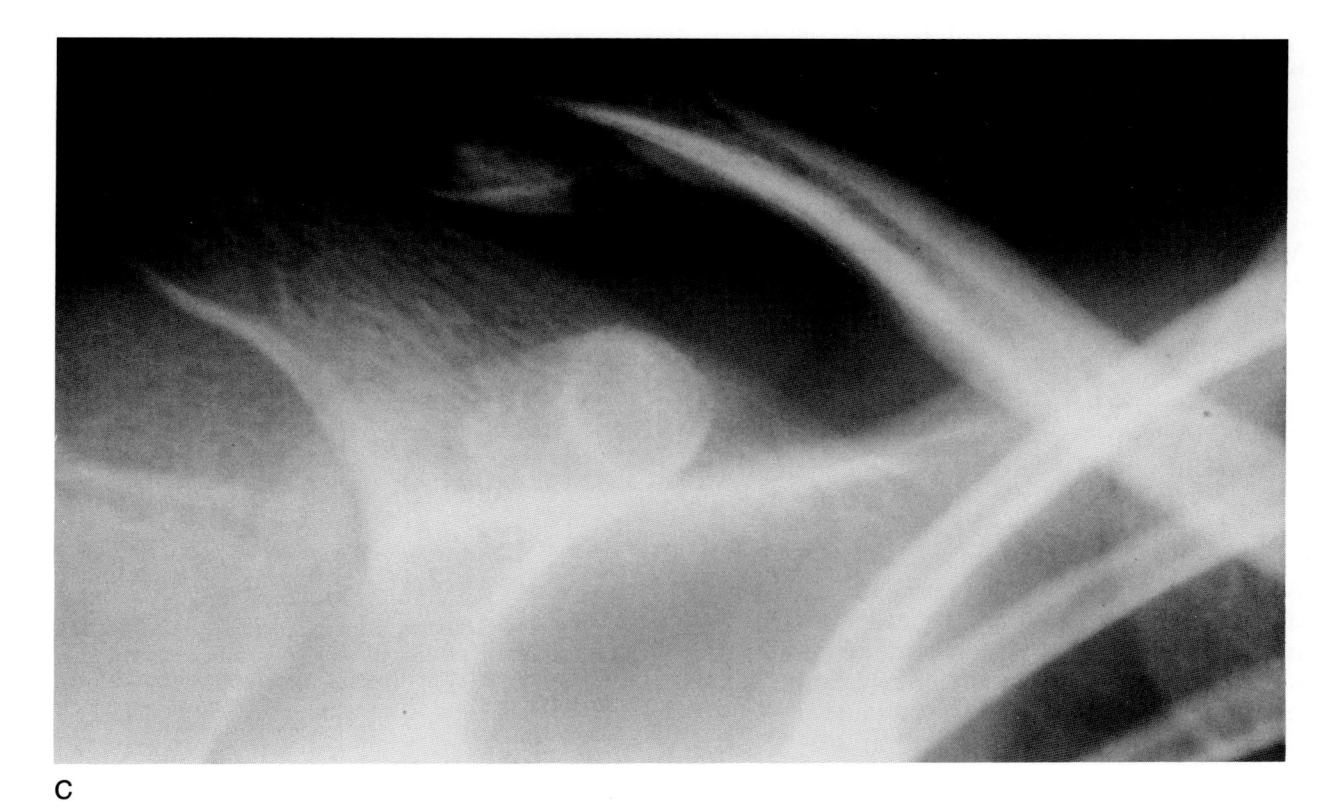

Fig. 8-5 *(Continued).* **(C)** Two weeks later following strapping with periosteal sleeve new bone formation.

fractures seen at their hospital involved the distal physis. Cave[28] reported that 12 percent of dislocations about the shoulder in adults occur at the acromioclavicular joint and Rowe[29] found 50 acromioclavicular lesions out of 1,603 shoulder injuries. The injury is more common in boys and occurs more often on the dominant side. Eidman and colleagues[30] reported a high incidence of complete displacement in adolescents but the injury was seen also to occur in all age groups, including neonates.

Anatomic Considerations

The acromioclavicular joint connects the lateral end of the clavicle to the medial end of the acromion. De Palma[11] describes the joint to be filled with a fibrocartilaginous bridge under the age of 2 years. The joint cavity appears around age 3½, and hyaline cartilage covers the bone ends until age 17. The joint is diarthrodial with an articular disc dividing the cavity. The disc is often partial or meniscoid.

The acromioclavicular ligaments reinforce the thin and weak articular capsule. They run from the medial border of the acromion to the clavicular epiphysis. The superior acromioclavicular ligament is strongest. They provide stability to the joint in the horizontal plane as their sectioning in cadaver experiments did not lead to superior displacement of the clavicle[1] (Fig. 8-4).

The stability of the acromioclavicular joint is greatly improved by the presence of the coracoclavicular ligaments. These are the true suspensory ligaments of the upper extremity and provide the strongest restraint to vertical displacement of the distal clavicle and downward sag of the scapula.[31] The conoid is cone-shaped; the apex attaches on the posteromedial side of the coracoid, while the base is fixed to the conoid tubercule on the posterior undersurface of the clavicle. The trapezoid is anterior and lateral to the conoid ligament. It attaches on the coracoid just behind the origin of the pectoralis minor tendon and reaches the clavicle to a line that extends anteriorly and laterally of the conoid tubercule. In children these coracoclavicular ligaments are very strong and seldom rupture.

According to Ogden[26] the distal clavicular physis contributes 20 to 30 percent of the growth of the clavicle. The epiphysis is thin and resembles the epiphysis of distal phalanges. This epiphysis appears and fuses late at about age 19. It is often not visible on radiographs. Bone remodeling can therefore be expected after physeal injuries even in late adolescence.

Most injuries to the distal end of the clavicle in children occur through the physis.[1,25-27] The epiphysis is maintained in place by the acromioclavicular ligaments, while the medial portion of the clavicle is displaced through a longitudinal tear in the periosteum. The clavicle is stripped out of the periosteal tube like a banana out of its skin (Fig. 8-5). The coracoclavicular ligaments are usually left intact with their attachment to the clavicular periosteum. At times the coracoid process may fracture and allow the superior displacement of the outer clavicle.[1,11,30-32]

Anatomic structures in close proximity to the joint include the brachial plexus and the axillary artery and vein as they run under the pectoralis minor muscle. The acromiothoracic artery passes in front of this muscle after piercing the costocoracoid membrane.

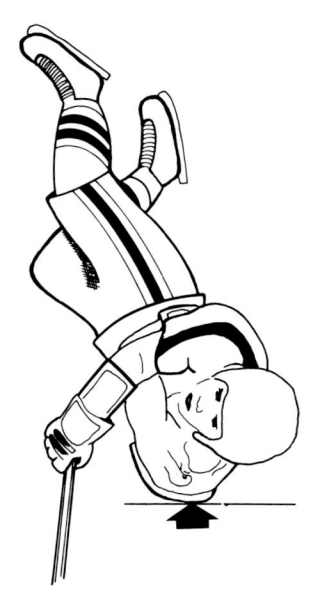

Fig. 8-6. A fall directly on the shoulder usually results in an acromioclavicular dislocation in the adult, but in a child the clavicle fractures either through the distal epiphyseal plate or through the shaft.

Mechanism of Injury

Rockwood and Young[33] state that a fall on the point of the shoulder is the most common mechanism of acromioclavicular injuries. They also describe an indirect mechanism caused by a strong pull on the upper extremity. In children the injury has been reported to occur from birth trauma, child abuse, falls, and vehicular accidents.[26,27] Adolescents and young adults often sustain the injury during sports and athletic activities, especially football or hockey (Fig. 8-6).

As the shoulder is driven inferiorly by a force applied from above a sequence of events will lead to the complete disruption of the acromioclavicular joint. In adults the superior acromioclavicular ligament ruptures first, but in children, because of the strong ligamentous attachments to the epiphysis, the clavicle fractures at or near the physis. With additional force the lateral end of the medial clavicular fragment tears the superior aspect of the periosteum.[25-27] The clavicle is strongly maintained in position at the sternoclavicular joint by the interclavicular ligament, which prevents its downward displacement. As the scapula is further pushed inferiorly the periosteal tear will lengthen and the clavicle is gradually peeled of its periosteal tube. The coracoclavicular ligaments are usually left intact with their attachments to the periosteum (Fig. 8-7).

With downward displacement of the scapula, the clavicle is usually left in place, but it can also migrate superiorly, inferiorly, or posteriorly. The inferior displacement of the clavicle is caused by a direct blow on its lateral aspect from above while the shoulder is in abduction. Posterior displacement is caused by a direct force pushing its outer clavicular end into the mass of the trapezius muscle.[33]

Classification

The classification of acromioclavicular injuries is based on the amount of tissue damage and the direction of displacement of the scapula and clavicle. Rockwood[1] adapted his classification of such injuries for children in relation to their anatomic differences (Fig. 8-7).

Type 1: Mild sprain of the acromioclavicular joint. The periosteum is intact.

Type 2: Partial tear in the periosteum with instability and widening of the acromioclavicular joint. No increase in the coracoclavicular distance.

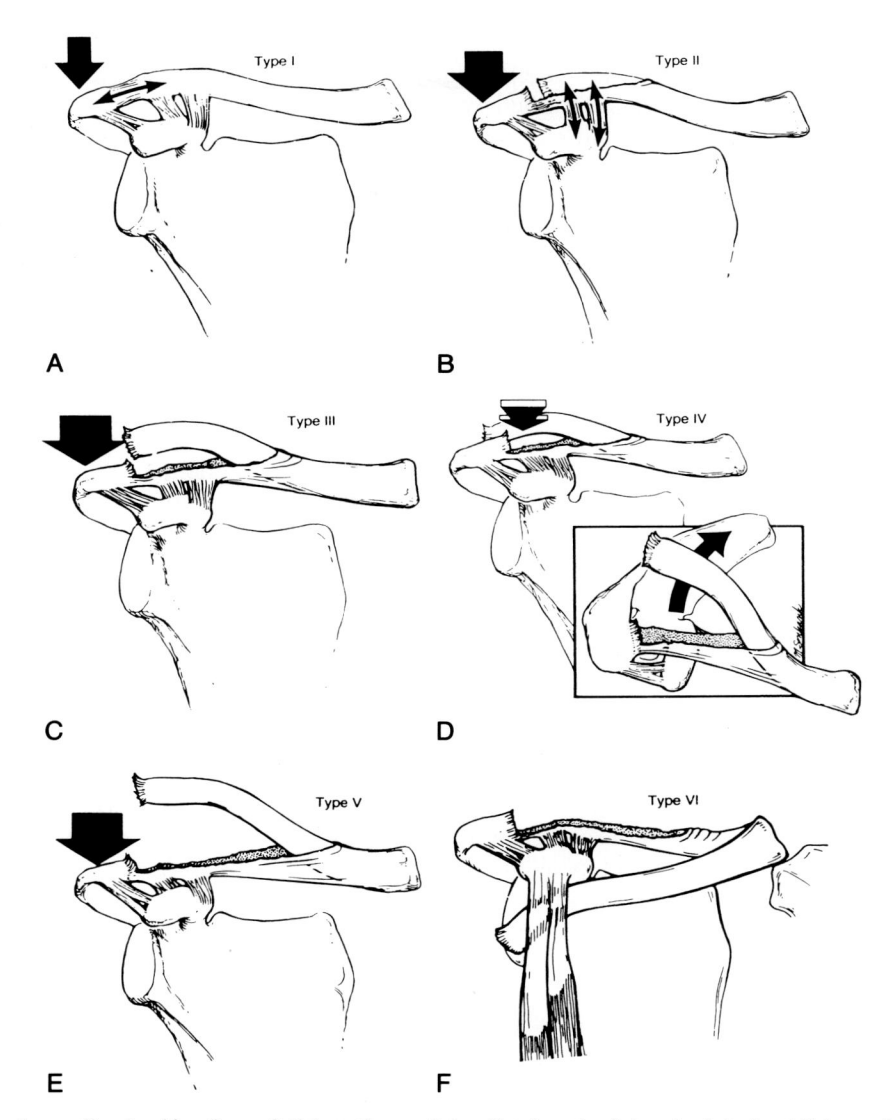

Fig. 8-7. Rockwood's classification of dislocations of the distal end of the clavicle in children. (See text for description). (From Rockwood,[1] with permission.)

Type 3: Large periosteal tear with gross instability of the distal clavicle. The coracoclavicular distance is increased by 25 to 100 percent.

Type 4: Large periosteal tear with posterior displacement of the distal clavicle into the trapezius muscle. Some widening of the acromioclavicular distance but minimum increase in the coracoclavicular space.

Type 5: Complete periosteal tear with severe superior displacement of the distal clavicle. Split of deltoid and trapezius muscle fibers and wide increase of coracoclavicular distance by more than 100 percent.

Type 6: Inferior displacement of the distal clavicle under the coracoid.

Physical Examination

For Rockwood's types 1 and 2 injuries the acromioclavicular joint is found to be tender and swollen. There is no significant deformity or instability of the distal clavicle. In type 3 injuries the deformity is more obvious with prominence of the outer clavicle. Swelling and pain are more severe and there may be local bruising. These children will support their injured limbs under the elbow.

For type 4 injuries the displacement can be masked by the amount of swelling and is often best visualized when seen from above by the examiner standing behind the patient. In cases of type 5 injuries the deformity and pain are severe, and the clavicle can be seen tenting the skin.

Type 6 injuries will also give considerable pain and swelling. Motion of the shoulder is greatly reduced and the acromion is prominent. The distal clavicle is not palpable and paresthesias of the upper extremity can be present.

Diagnosis

Adequate visualization of the acromioclavicular joint and the distal end of the clavicle necessitates a lower radiographic exposure than for the shoulder joint. A 10- to 15-degree cephalic tilt of the x-ray beam is suggested for the AP view.[1]

In type 1 injuries radiographs are essentially normal. The acromioclavicular distance may be widened in type 2 lesions, but the coracoclavicular distance is not increased.

Stress views in the AP plane can be obtained to differentiate type 2 from type 3 injuries. With the child standing in a relaxed position, 5- to 10-pound weights are strapped to the wrists according to age. An AP projection of both shoulders is taken for comparison. The coracoclavicular distance is compared between both sides and is usually found to be normal in types 1 and 2 injuries while it will be increased from 25 to 100 percent in type 3 lesions (Fig. 8-8).

The posterior displacement of the clavicle in type 4 injuries is best seen on the lateral axillary projection, which could also reveal a fracture. Severe superior displacement of the clavicle is easily recognized from AP view on plain films in type 5 injuries; the coracoclavicular distance increased by over 100 percent. In type 6 lesions the clavicle is found to be located under the coracoid.

A fracture of the coracoid process can be demonstrated by the Stryker Notch technique—an AP view of the shoulder is taken with the patient's hand resting on top of his head.[1]

Treatment

Since displacement of the distal clavicle in children occurs through the growth plate, a significant amount of remodeling can be expected.

Types 1 and 2 injuries are usually treated by conservative means. Analgesics and ice packs are prescribed and the limb is immobilized with a protective sling until the pain subsides. Early mobilization and isometric exercises are advocated, but the shoulder should be protected from strenuous exercises and further trauma for 4 to 6 weeks to prevent extension of the damage.

For type 3 injuries in children under the age of 15 the same regimen can be applied, as bone remodeling will improve the local deformity. In teenagers over 15 years of age the necessity of a reduction is as controversial as in adults with this injury and the best treatment is still being debated. Most type 3 injuries treated nonoperatively will do well, but individuals involved in strenuous daily activities may experience discomfort and fatigue after a few hours of heavy manual work. The indication for reduction in adolescents over 15 years of age therefore appears to be based on their future career expectations and their athletic activities. Those who will likely put a significant demand on their shoulder may benefit from a reduction.

Reduction of the distal clavicle can be accomplished by closed or operative means:

Closed Reduction: Many devices have been described but most use the principle of the Kenny Howard harness, which applies direct inferior pressure on top of the displaced distal clavicle while supporting the upper extremity under the elbow (Figs. 8-9 and 8-10). The disadvantage of such devices comes from their poor tolerance by the child and from skin irritation on the superior aspect of the shoulder by the superior pad.

Open Reduction: A straplike incision in Langer's line is used beginning 1-inch posterior to the distal clavicle, extending anteriorly 1-inch medial to the tip of the clavicle to reach a point 1-inch medial to the coracoid pro-

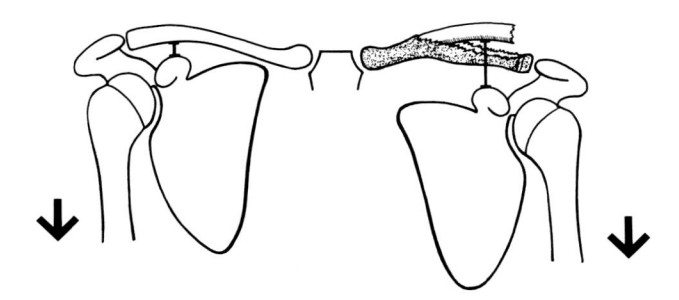

Fig. 8-8. Schematic representation based on an AP view of both shoulders with weights strapped to the wrists to demonstrate an increase in the coracoclavicular distance on the injured side.

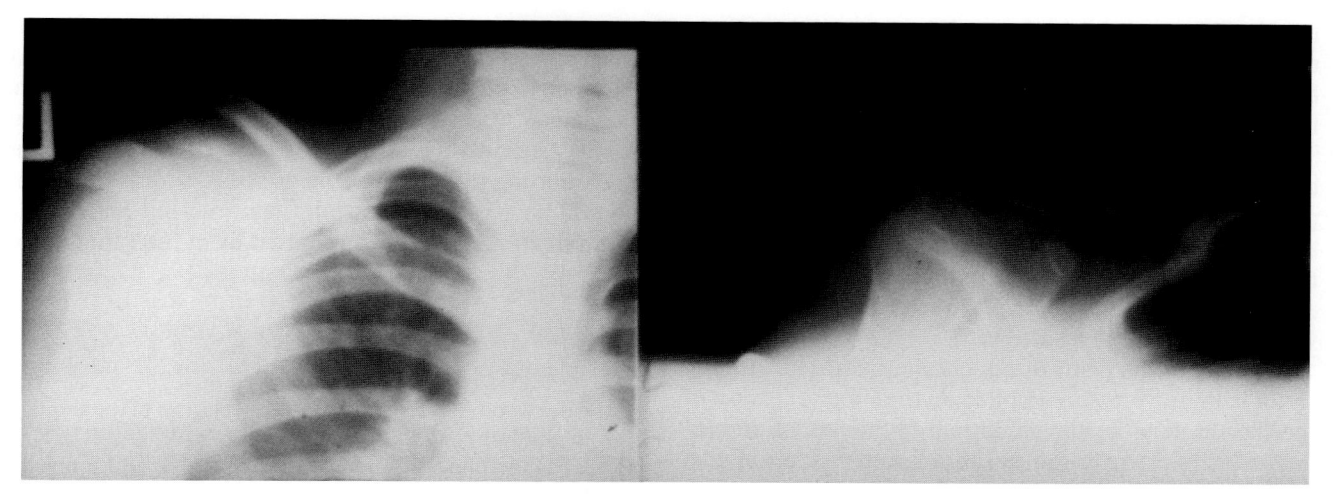

Fig. 8-9. Sleeve fracture and pseudodislocation of distal end of clavicle illustrating reduction with strapping.

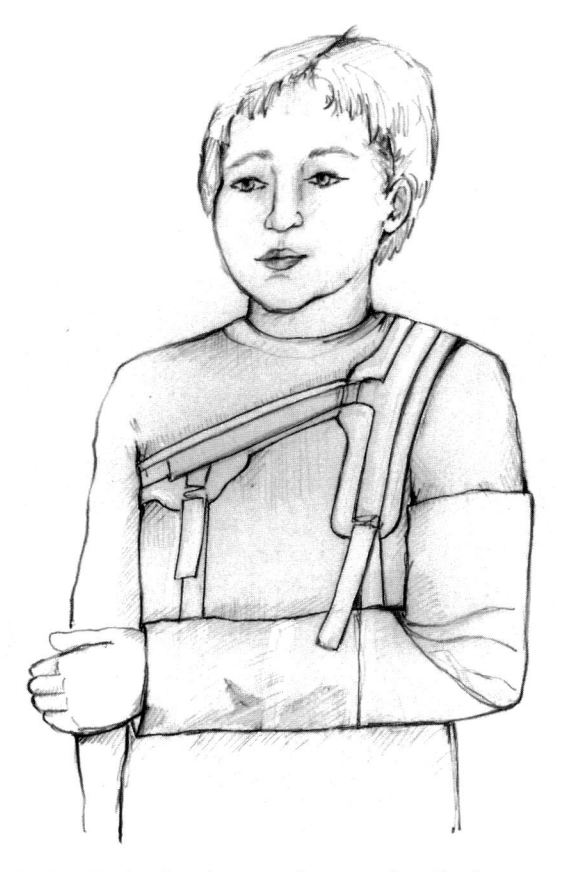

Fig. 8-10. Reduction harness for superior displacement of the distal clavicle. The superior strap applies a downward pressure onto the displaced clavicular fragment while the scapula is prevented to sag by supporting the limb under the elbow.

cess. The distal clavicle is exposed and reduced to its anatomic location. The periosteal tube is strongly sutured over the outer clavicle as well as the torn or detached fibers of the deltoid and trapezius muscles. For added stability, some authors[26-28] recommend threaded K-wires or Steinmann's pins through the acromioclavicular joint. These should be bent distally to prevent migration and are removed at 4 to 6 weeks after the injury. Others suggest the use of a temporary coracoclavicular screw.[1] Splitting the muscle fibers of the deltoid will give adequate exposure to the coracoid for insertion of the screw.

Types 4, 5, and 6 injuries should be reduced because of the amount of pain experienced by the patient and the severity of the displacement. A closed reduction under anesthesia can be attempted, but an open reduction may be necessary. The same surgical principles apply as for the reduction of a type 3 injury. For type 4 lesions the distal clavicle needs to be mobilized from the trapezius muscle mass and from under the coracoid in type 6 lesions.

Complications

Complications from the injury itself are uncommon in children. Paresthesias of the upper extremity in type 6 lesions were reported,[34] but cleared after reduction. Calcification of the coracoclavicular ligaments were noticed in 14 of 25 patients in the series of Eidman and colleagues,[30] but the phenomenon did not interfere with the results. Havranek[27] mentions that 7 of his 9 patients treated by nonoperative means had a residual local deformity.

Ogden[26] reported on a case of duplication of the clavicle after displacement of the distal clavicle through a physeal injury. He suggested that the phenomenon could be explained by the periosteal tube filling in with new bone while the clavicle was left displaced superiorly. Because of the residual deformity the displaced distal clavicular portion was resected.

Complications from nonoperative treatment usually result from the pressure applied on the superior aspect of the shoulder by the clavicular pad of the reduction harness. Local skin irritation, abrasions, and ulcerations can occur.

Operative procedures also carry their own risks. Wound infections, osteomyelitis, the presence of a scar, and the need for implant removal. Pins from the acromioclavicular joint were reported to have migrated to the lung, spinal cord,[35] carotid sheath,[36] pleural cavity,[37] subclavian artery, and aorta. These complications can be prevented by the use of threaded pins and by bending them at the point of insertion.

SUMMARY

Dislocations of the clavicle occur in children with a frequency comparable to that of the adult population. The outer end of the clavicle is involved far more frequently than its medial end. In both situations the injury tends to occur through the growth plate with displacement of the clavicular fragment through a rent in the periosteal tube. This pattern of injury is unique to children and true dislocations of the sternoclavicular or acromioclavicular joints in the growing skeleton are rare. The lesion usually heals rapidly with filling of the periosteal tube with new bone and significant remodeling of the displaced clavicular fragment. Most injuries can be treated by conservative means with good results.

Severe retrosternal displacement of the medial end of the clavicule can be life-threatening by compression of vital structures. Early assessment of the injury is essential, and appropriate management requires rapid intervention to reduce the displacement of the clavicle. Vascular and airway lesions are frequently associated with this injury and should be recognized and dealt with in conjunction with appropriate consultants.[38]

Displacement of the distal end of the clavicle can most often be treated by closed means. Only the most severe displacements will require open reduction.

When open reduction of the medial or distal end of the clavicle is necessary, it is often possible to obtain adequate stability by suturing the periosteum and surrounding soft tissues. The use of K-wires for fixation should be avoided if possible, as numerous and serious complications have been reported from their migration.

REFERENCES

1. Rockwood CA: Fractures and dislocations of the shoulder in children. p. 880. In Rockwood CA, Wilkins KE, King RE: Fractures in Children. 3rd Ed. Vol. 3. JB Lippincott, Philadelphia, 1991
2. Rowe CR, Marble HC: Sternoclavicular dislocations. In Cave EF (ed): Fractures and Other Injuries. Year Book Medical Publishers, Chicago, 1958
3. Cave EF: Fractures and Other Injuries. Year Book Medical Publishers, Chicago, 1958
4. Wheeler ME, Laaveg SJ, Sprague BL: S-C joint disruptions in an infant. Clin Orthop 139:68, 1979
5. Buckerfield CT, Castle ME: Acute traumatic dislocation of the clavicule. J Bone Joint Surg [Am] 66:379, 1984
6. Brooks AL, Henning GD: Injury to the proximal clavicular epiphysis. J Bone Joint Surg [Am] 54:1347, 1972
7. Denham RH Jr, Dingley AF Jr: Epiphyseal separation of the medial end of the clavicle. J Bone Joint Surg [Am] 49:1179, 1967
8. Lunseth PA, Chapman KW, Frankel VH: Surgical treatment of chronic dislocation of the sternoclavicular joint. J Bone Joint Surg [Br] 57:193, 1975
9. Grant JBC: Method of Anatomy. 7th Ed. Williams & Wilkins, Baltimore, 1965
10. Goss CM: Gray's Anatomy of the Human Body. 28th Ed. p. 324. Lea & Febiger, Philadelphia, 1966
11. De Palma AF: Surgical anatomy of acromioclavicular and sternoclavicular joints. Surg Clin North Am 43:1541, 1963
12. Rockwood CA: Disorders of the sternoclavicular joint. p. 479. In Rockwood CA, Matsen FA (eds): The Shoulder. Vol. 1. WB Saunders, Philadelphia, 1990
13. Heinig CF: Retrosternal dislocation of the clavicle: early recognition, x-ray diagnosis and management. J Bone Joint Surg [Am] 50:830, 1968
14. Nettles JL, Linscheid R: Sternoclavicular dislocations. J Trauma 8:158, 1968
15. Winter J, Sterner S, Maurer S et al: Retrosternal epiphyseal disruption of medial clavicle: case and review in children. J Emerg Med 7:9, 1989
16. Salesnick HF, Jablon M, Frank C, Post M: Retrosternal dislocation of the clavicle. J Bone Joint Surg [Am] 66:287, 1984

17. Simurda MA: Retrosternal dislocation of the clavicle: a report of four cases and a method of repair. Can J Surg 11:487, 1968
18. Hobbs DW: Sternoclavicular joint: a new axial radiographic view. Radiology 90:801, 1968
19. Levinsohn ME, Bunnel WP, Yuan HA: Computed tomography in the diagnosis of dislocations of the sternoclavicular joint. Clin Orthop 140:12, 1979
20. Worman LW, Leagus C: Intrathoracic injury following retrosternal dislocation of the clavicle. J Trauma 7:416, 1967
21. Schechter DC, Gilbert L: Injuries of the heart and great vessels due to pins and needles. Thorax 24:246, 1969
22. Leonard JW, Gilford RW: Migration of a Kirschner wire from the clavicle into pulmonary artery. Am J Cardiol 16:598, 1965
23. Norback I, Markula H: Migration of Kirschner pin from clavicle into ascending aorta. Acta Chir Scand 151:177, 1985
24. Salvatore JE: Sternoclavicular joint dislocation. Clin Orthop 58:51, 1968
25. Falstie-Jensen S, Mikkelsen P: Pseudodislocation of the acromioclavicular joint. J Bone Joint Surg [Br] 64:368, 1982
26. Ogden JA: Distal clavicular injuries. Clin Orthop Rel Res 188:68, 1984
27. Havranek P: Injuries to the distal clavicular physis in children. J Pediatr Orthop 9:213, 1989
28. Thomas CB, Friedman RJ: Ipsilateral sternoclavicular dislocation and clavicle fracture. J Orthop Trauma 3:335, 1989
29. Rowe CR: An atlas of anatomy and treatment of midclavicular fractures. Clin Orthop 58:29, 1968
30. Eidman DK, Siff SJ, Tullos HS: Acromioclavicular lesions in children. Am J Sports Med 9:150, 1981
31. Cadenat FM: The treatment of dislocations and fractures of the outer end of the clavicle. Int Clin 1:145, 1917
32. Taga I, Yoneda M, Ono K: Epiphyseal separation of the coracoid process associated with acromioclavicular sprain. Clin Orthop Rel Res 207:138, 1986
33. Rockwood CA, Young CD: Disorders of the acromioclavicular joint. p. 420. In Rockwood CA, Matsen FA (eds): The Shoulder. Vol. 1. WB Saunders, Philadelphia, 1990
34. Gerber C, Rockwood CA: Subcoracoid dislocation of the lateral end of the clavicle: a report of three cases. J Bone Joint Surg [Am] 69:924, 1987
35. Norrel H, Llewellyn RC: Migration of a treaded Steinmann pin from an acromioclavicular joint into the spinal canal: a case report. J Bone Joint Surg [Am] 47:1024, 1965
36. Lindsey RW, Gutowski WT: The migration of a broken pin following fixation of the acromioclavicular joint: a case report and review of the literature. Orthopedics 9:413, 1986
37. Eaton R, Serletti J: Computed axial tomography: a method of locating Steinmann pin migration: a case report. Orthopedics 4:1357, 1981
38. Hardy JRW: Complex clavicular injury in childhood. J Bone Joint Surgery [Br] 74:154, 1991

SUGGESTED READINGS

Asher MA: Dislocation of the upper extremity in children. Orthop Clin North Am 7:583, 1976

Curtis RJ: Operative management of children's fractures of the shoulder region. Orthop Clin North Am 21:315, 1990

De Jong KP, Kaulesar Sukul DMKS: Anterior sternoclavicular dislocation: a long term follow-up study. J Orthop Trauma 4:420, 1990

Kennedy JC: Retrosternal dislocation of the clavicle. J Bone Joint Surg [Br] 31:74, 1949

Leighton RS, Burh AJ, Sinclair AM: Posterior sternoclavicular dislocations. Can J Surg 29:104, 1986

Lemire L, Rosman M: Sternoclavicular epiphyseal separation with adjacent clavicular fracture. J Pediatr Orthop 4:118, 1984

Levinsohn EM, Bunnel WP, Yuan HA: Computed tomography in the diagnosis of dislocations of the sternoclavicular joint. Clin Orthop Rel Res 140:12, 1979

Nevasier JS: Injuries of the clavicle and its articulations. Orthop Clin North Am 11:233, 1980

Rogers LF: The radiography of epiphyseal injuries. Radiology 96:289, 1970

9

Fractures of the Proximal Humerus and Humeral Shaft

Robert F. Martin

> Luck in orthopaedic surgery is what happens when preparation meets opportunity.

FRACTURES OF THE PROXIMAL HUMERUS

Description and Incidence

Proximal humeral epiphyseal fractures comprise approximately 3 percent of epiphyseal injuries.[1,2] They are generally Salter-Harris type I (16 percent) or II (84 percent) in configuration.[2-4] They may occur in all ages from birth to skeletal maturity, although the incidence is higher in the 8- to 16-year age group.[1,4-6]

Anatomic Considerations

The proximal humeral epiphysis is spherical and the most mobile articulation in the human skeleton. The physis is concave inferiorly, somewhat tent-shaped, with the apex posterior and medial to center.

There are three ossification centers. The central appears between 4 and 6 months, the greater tuberosity by 3 years, and the lesser tuberosity by 5 years. They coalesce to one center by 6 to 7 years and are not known to separate due to injury. The physis closes at about 19 years.[1,5] The periosteum is thick posteriorly.[5,7]

In proximal epiphyseal separations or metaphyseal fractures, the pectoralis major pulls the metaphysis anteriorly and medially. Teres minor, infraspinatus, and subscapularis hold the epiphysis in slight flexion, abduction, and external rotation, but generally these muscle forces neutralize each other, and the proximal fragment remains relatively neutral (Fig. 9-1).

Mechanisms of Injury

Due to the shape of the physis and strong posterior periosteum, the metaphysis is difficult to displace posteriorly, but displaces anteriorly with ease. Various mechanisms of injury have been described, according to Williams,[8] who has done a detailed anatomic analysis of the subject. There are six mechanisms of fracturing the proximal humerus in children (Table 9-1).

A direct blow generally causes a metaphyseal fracture rather than one through the physis. Obstetrical difficulty with shoulder dystocia may lead to type I physeal injury. The shearing force on the physis results in separation through the zone of hypertrophic cartilage.[9] The germinal cells are usually not damaged in this fracture pattern. However, in some cases, additional physeal injury

138 / Management of Pediatric Fractures

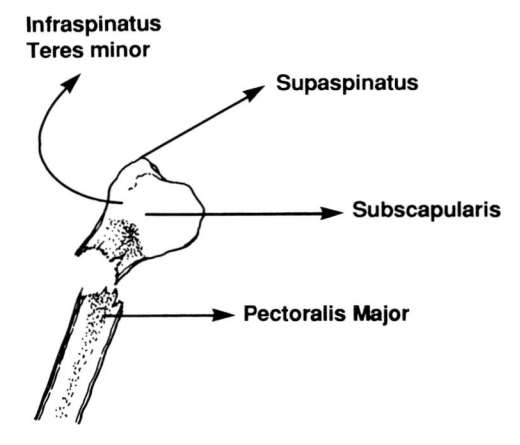

Fig. 9-1. In proximal epiphyseal separation or metaphyseal fractures, the posterior periosteum acts as a hinge. The pectoralis major pulls the metaphysis anteriorly and medially. Teres minor, infraspinatus, and subscapularis hold the epiphysis in slight flexion, abduction, and external rotation.

from metaphyseal impingement does occur with partial growth arrest being more common than is usually appreciated.[1,4,5] In older children, a metaphyseal fragment remains attached to the posterior medial epiphysis. The fracture remains stable until sufficient displacement occurs to rupture through anterior periosteum. Instability thereafter is much greater with the increased periosteal stripping.[5]

Classification

Proximal humeral epiphyseal separations are either Salter-Harris type I (16 percent) or II (84 percent).[2] They may be further divided into degrees of displacement[1] (Table 9-2).

TABLE 9-1. Mechanisms of Fracture

1. Pure extension
2. Pure flexion
3. Forced extension with lateral rotation
4. Forced extension with medial rotation
5. Forced flexion with lateral rotation
6. Forced flexion with medial rotation

TABLE 9-2. Classification of Proximal Humeral Physeal Separations

Grade I:	to 5 mm displacement
Graded II:	to $\frac{1}{3}$ humeral shaft
Grade III:	to $\frac{2}{3}$ humeral shaft
Grade IV:	greater than $\frac{2}{3}$, including total separation
Grade III and IV have varying degrees of angulation	

Physical Examination

Fracture of the proximal humerus is associated with swelling and localized tenderness of the entire shoulder area. The upper arm is adducted and extended. The end of the metaphyseal fragment is usually prominent anteriorly and laterally. The arm may be slightly shortened. Neurovascular injury is uncommon.

Differential Diagnosis

Anterior dislocation of the shoulder is differentiated by the classical clinical findings of external rotation and fixed abduction of the arm and confirmed radiologically. Due to the relative weakness of the physis, failure of the growth plate occurs before dislocation, hence dislocation is less common than physeal fracture in children. In the newborn infant, brachial plexus injury may be suspected because of pseudoparalysis of the arm that may occur with the fracture. There may, however, be an associated brachial plexus injury, which must be differentiated by careful repeated clinical assessment.

Radiologic Examination

Positioning of the arm is difficult due to pain, so that standard lateral views may not be possible (Fig. 9-2). Anteroposterior (AP) and oblique views will usually provide the diagnosis. In the AP views, displacement may not be as evident as in the lateral view (Fig. 9-3). In newborn infants, however, diagnosis may not be possible with plain radiographs because of the lack of ossification centers in the proximal fragment. Strong clinical suspicion warrants an arthrogram for confirmation.

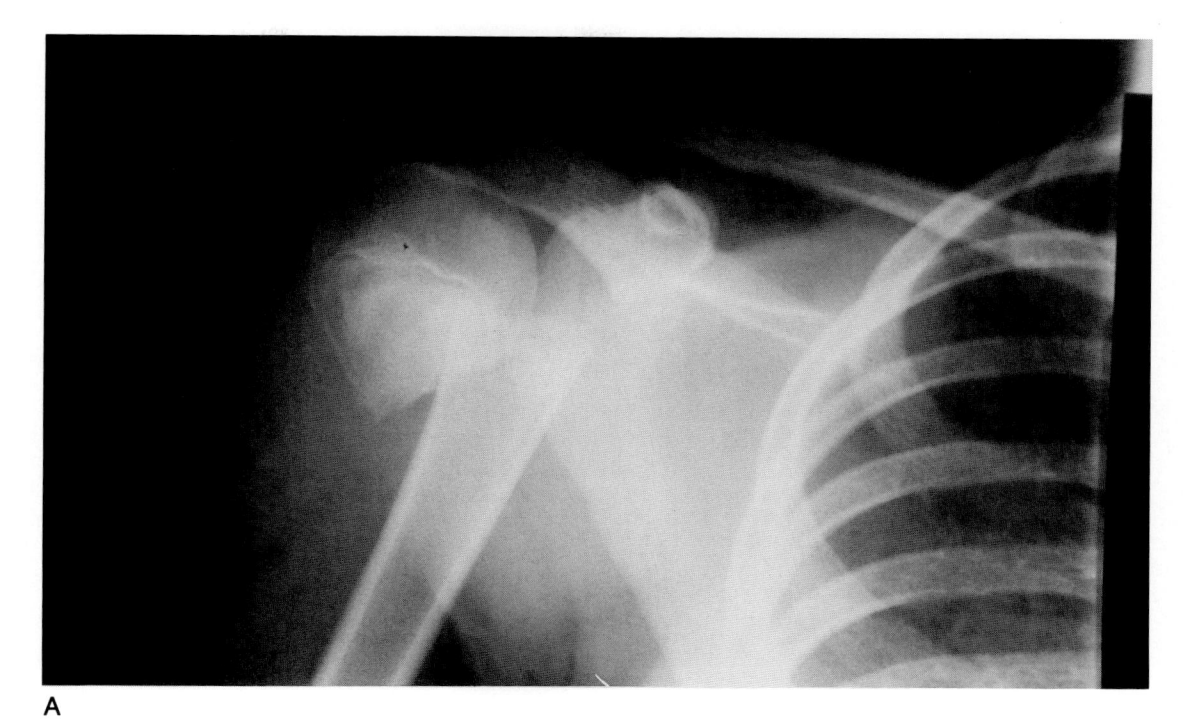

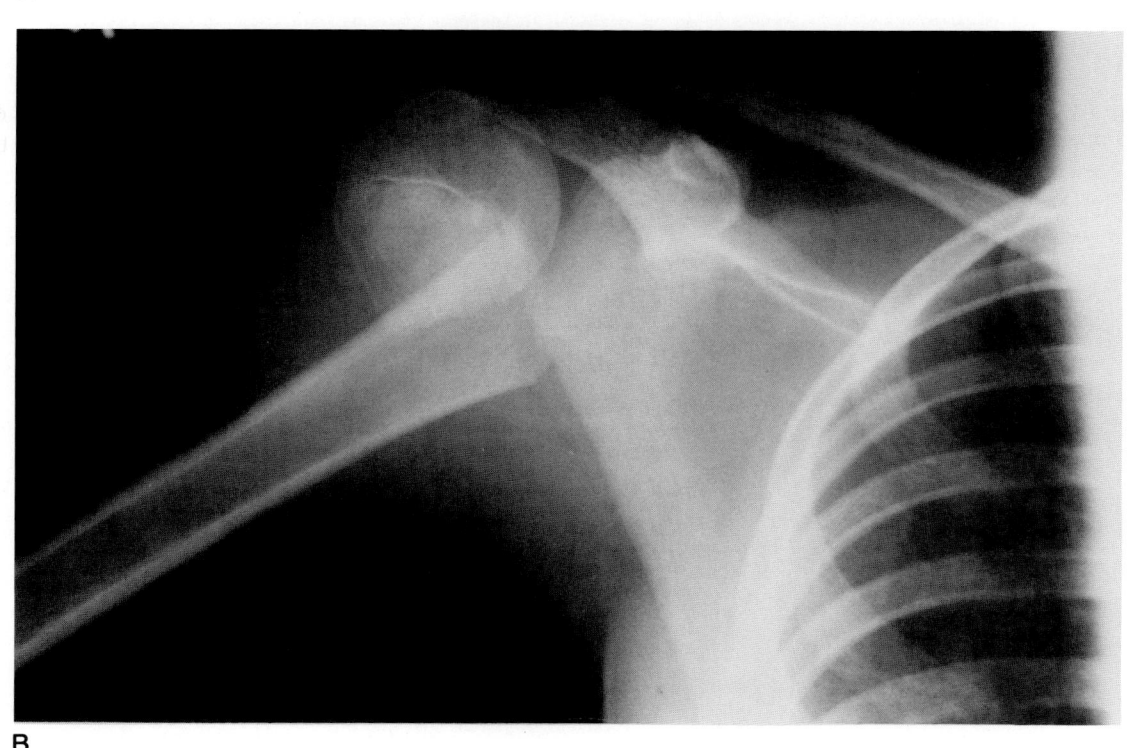

Fig. 9-2. (A) Fracture of the neck of the proximal humerus with complete displacement of the metaphyseal fragment sustained in a fall from a horse. (B) An injudicious attempt by the radiology technician to obtain an abduction view of the unsplinted extremity. All fractures should be immobilized before the patient is sent for radiographs to minimize this type of unnecessary trauma.

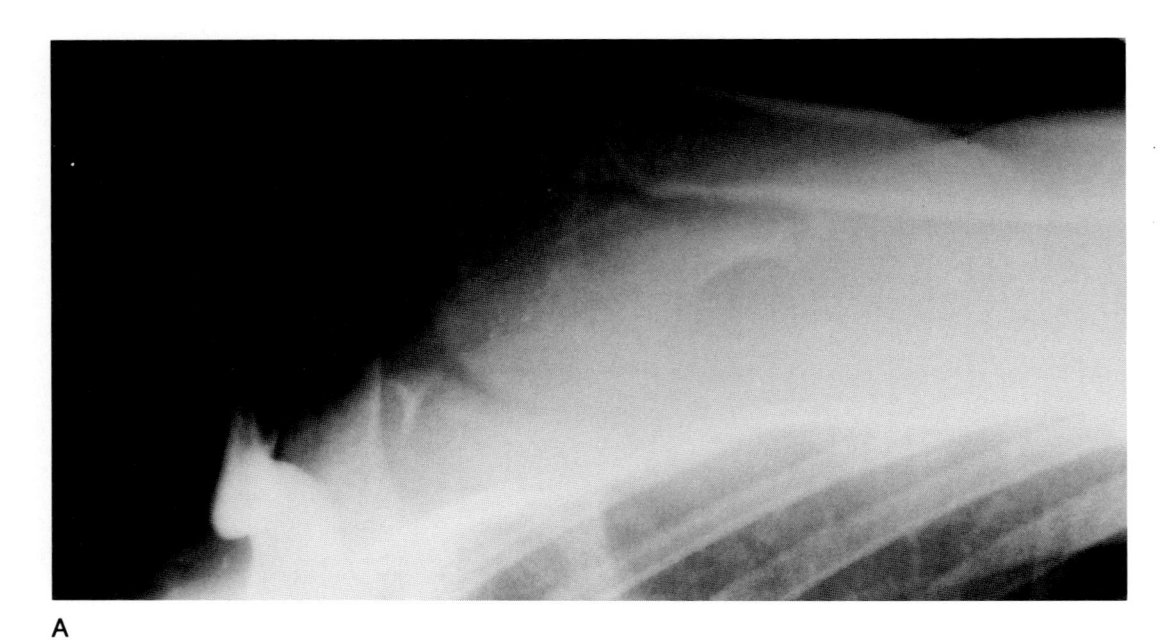

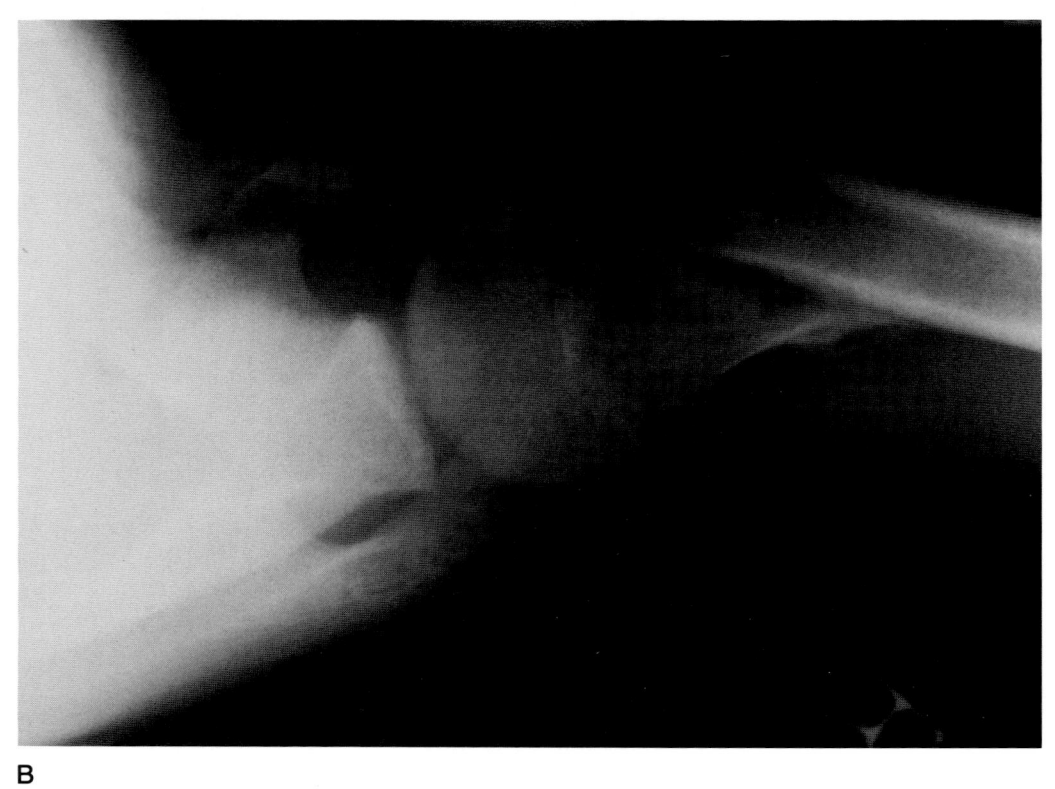

Fig. 9-3. (A) Anteroposterior view of proximal humeral fracture in a 14-year-old girl. (B) Lateral view of same fracture via axillary view.

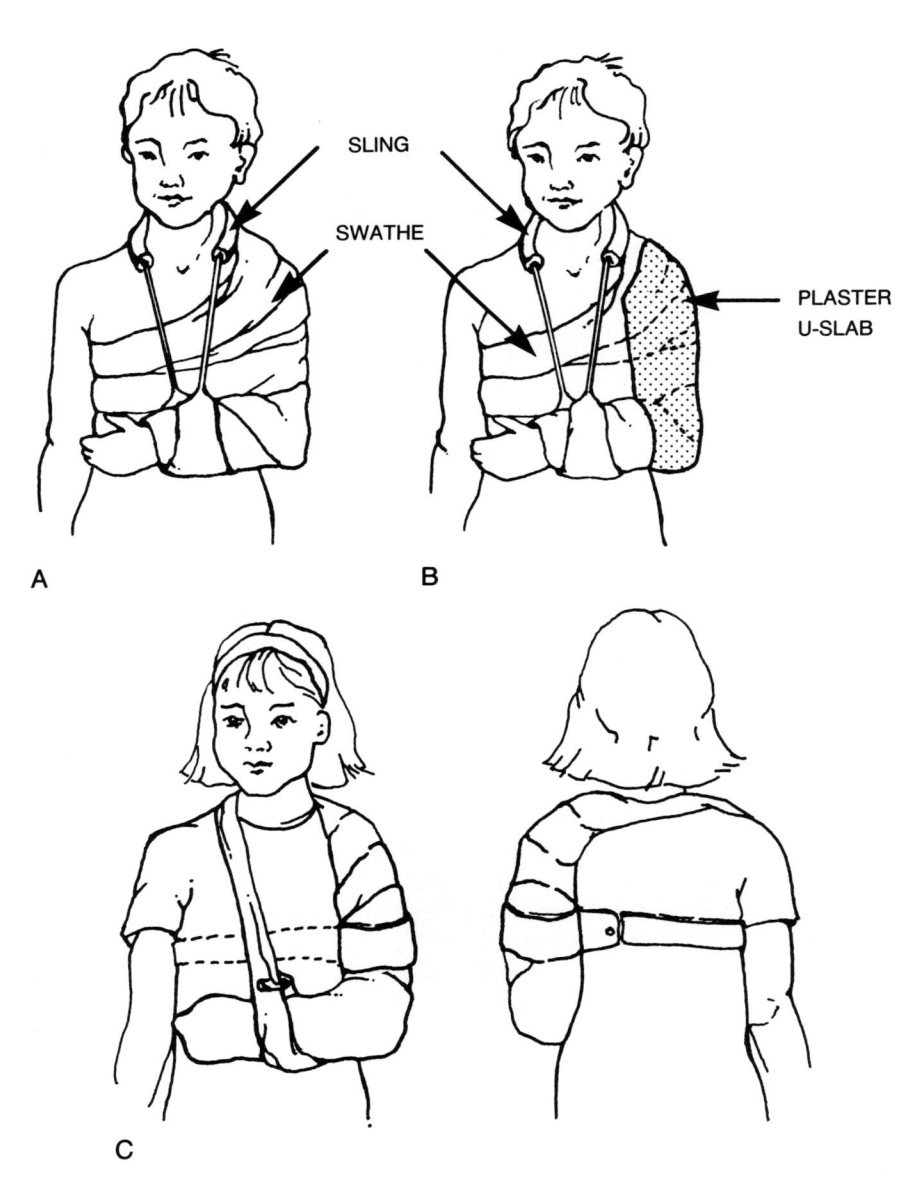

Fig. 9-4. Methods of immobilization. **(A)** Sling and swathe. **(B)** Sling and swathe with plaster U splint. **(C)** Stockinette velpeau. *(Figure continues.)*

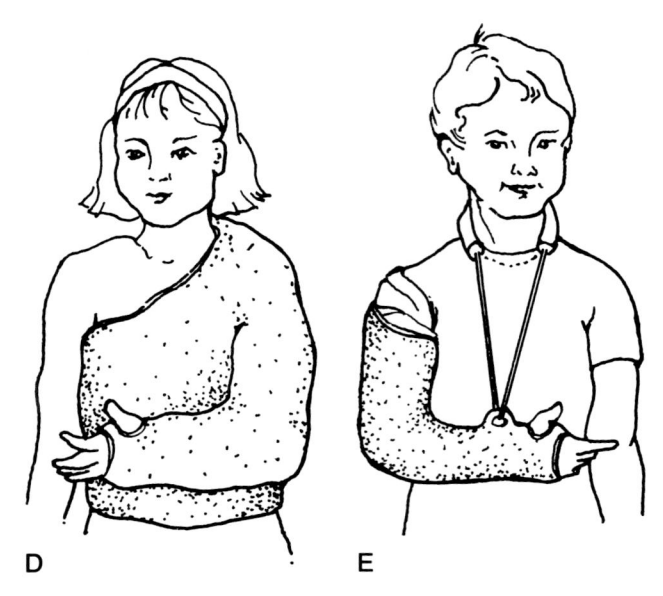

Fig. 9-4 *(Continued).* (D) Plaster thoracobrachial box. (E) Hanging cast.

Treatment Indications

The majority of these fractures require no reduction. Controversy continues regarding reduction of grades III and IV injuries. Open reduction is necessary only for complicated cases. All grades I and II fractures in all age groups may be treated with simple immobilization. Depending on the expected compliance, this may consist of a stockinette sling, a simple sling and swathe, or reinforcing the sling and swathe with plaster to make a thoracobrachial box, which is not as unstable nor easy to remove (Fig. 9-4). At 3 weeks, early movement may be started with progression to full motion as tolerated.

Grade III injuries may be treated in the same way, except in cases of severe angulation in the older child where there is not enough time for satisfactory remodeling, that is, girls 13 years or older and boys 15 years or older. Grade IV injuries generally require closed reduction.

Reduction may be achieved by gentle manipulation under general anesthesia. The patient is positioned so that intraoperative radiography is possible—on a radiolucent table, a frame or backboard, leaving the shoulder girdle free. If a shoulder spica is to be applied, positioning should be such that the cast may be applied without changing position, in which case an orthopaedic frame or backboard are best. If it is expected that a shoulder spica will be required, it is simpler to apply the body portion of the cast prior to the anesthesia, with the patient standing upright. Gentle abduction, flexion, and external rotation while applying traction will utilize the intact posteromedial periosteal hinge and generally will result in an adequate reduction, but it need not be absolutely anatomic. Failure of attempted closed reduction may require a review of the radiographs to deduce the exact mechanism of injury. Reduction may then be achieved by reversing this mechanism (Fig. 9-5).

Radiographs will determine in which position the reduction is stable. Usually it is necessary to maintain moderate flexion and abduction and occasionally extreme abduction. Stability in moderate abduction is suitable for shoulder spica immobilization. The need for extreme abduction necessitates a statue of liberty cast (Fig. 9-6). This can result in brachial plexus traction and paralysis for several weeks. It is better to avoid this method of immobilization and secure stability with percutaneous crossed K-wires instead. K-wires may be removed in 3 weeks (Fig. 9-7).

An alternative method of closed reduction is by traction, using a percutaneous olecranon wire and traction bow, an olecranon traction screw, or skin traction on the extended arm. The arm is then placed in traction in a position of flexion, external rotation and abduction (Fig. 9-8). The fracture position is monitored by radiographs, and in 2 to 3 weeks removed from traction, placed in a sling for an additional week, and then started on graduated activity.

Open reduction is rarely required. In the event of an irreducible complete displacement or the interposition of the biceps tendon, open reduction may be indicated.

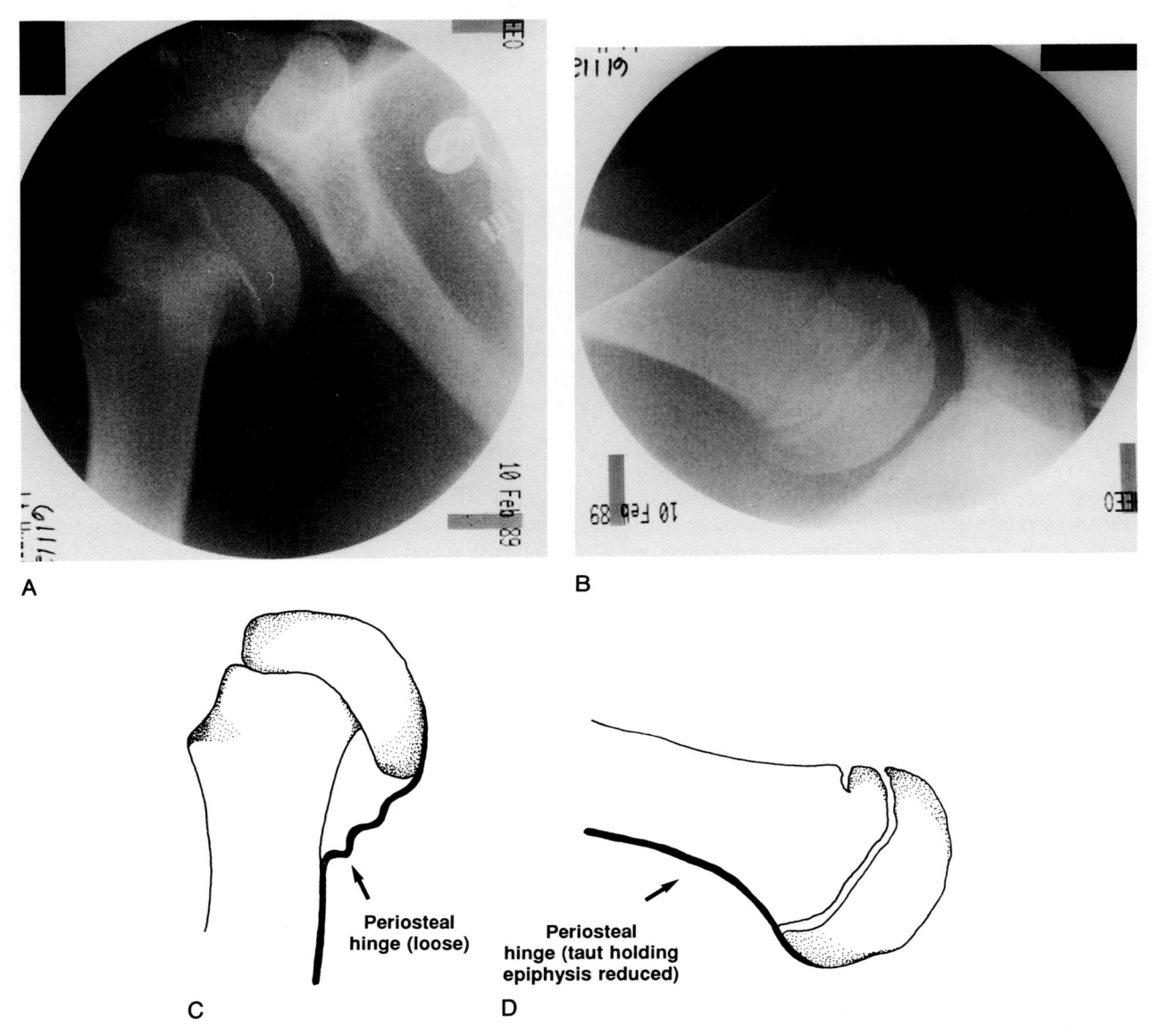

Fig. 9-5. **(A&B)** Technique of reduction using the intact medial periosteal hinge. Abduction of the arm tightens the hinge and creates a fulcrum to gently lever the metaphysis onto the head, which is also stabilized by the pull of the taut periosteum. **(C&D)** The periosteal hinge concept *diagramatically.*

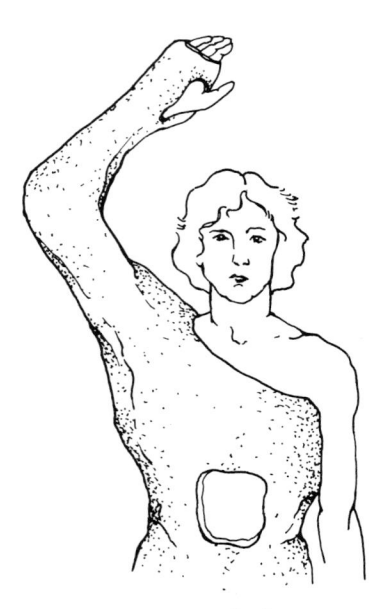

Fig. 9-6. Statue of Liberty cast.

Multiple system trauma may also be an indication, in order to facilitate general care. The resultant scar is a significant cosmetic blemish, which is much less acceptable than a mild anterior bump which usually remodels in a year or two.

Complications

Varus Angulation

Depending on the age of the child and degree of initial displacement, some residual varus is acceptable. In most cases remodeling is dramatic and varus is not a problem as 70 to 80 percent of humeral growth occurs at this physis (Fig. 9-9). Minor degrees of varus are compensated for by the excellent mobility of the shoulder. A physeal growth arrest due to severe compression of the physis may lead to premature medial physeal closure and varus[10] (Fig. 9-10).

Humeral Shortening

Growth arrest and shortening up to 4 cm has been reported[1,4,5] in 9 to 10 percent of grades I and II fractures, and in 30 to 40 percent of grades III and IV proximal humeral fractures. In all series, the degree of shortening was independent of the method of treatment, but more common with more severe displacement.[11] About 75 percent of growth occurs at the proximal physis before age 2, 85 percent at age 8, and 90 percent by age 11. This accounts for the excellent remodeling, but also indicates the susceptibility of the upper humerus to growth disturbance in the event of physeal injury at younger ages (Fig. 9-11). No reported series of proximal humeral physeal fractures has shown overgrowth as a complication of this injury.

Limitation of Motion

Most children regain full shoulder motion despite the grade of injury. Older children with severe displacement may have mild residual restriction of rotation.[5,12] The return of functional shoulder motion may take a number of months. Although most children easily regain full shoulder motion without aggressive physiotherapy, for the older teenager physiotherapy consultation and treatment may be helpful.

Neurologic Injury

The axillary nerve may undergo stretching or contusion and result in transient loss of deltoid function. This is unusual and is more commonly encountered in dislocation of the shoulder, an uncommon event in children. There may be associated brachial plexus injury in humeral birth fractures.

Vascular Injury

Brachial artery disruption has been reported,[4] requiring arterial reconstruction. Vascular injury is very unusual, because of the anteromedial position of the neurovascular bundle relative to the proximal humeral epiphysis, which protects it from the usual anterolateral displacement of the metaphyseal fragment.

METAPHYSEAL FRACTURES OF THE HUMERUS

Description and Incidence

Fractures of the metaphyseal area are reported to occur in two-thirds of proximal humeral fractures in children.[2] They usually occur at a younger age than physeal injuries. They *are parallel to* the line of the physis in 90 percent of injuries and are transverse in 10 percent. Incomplete fractures have a torus or buckle fracture pat-

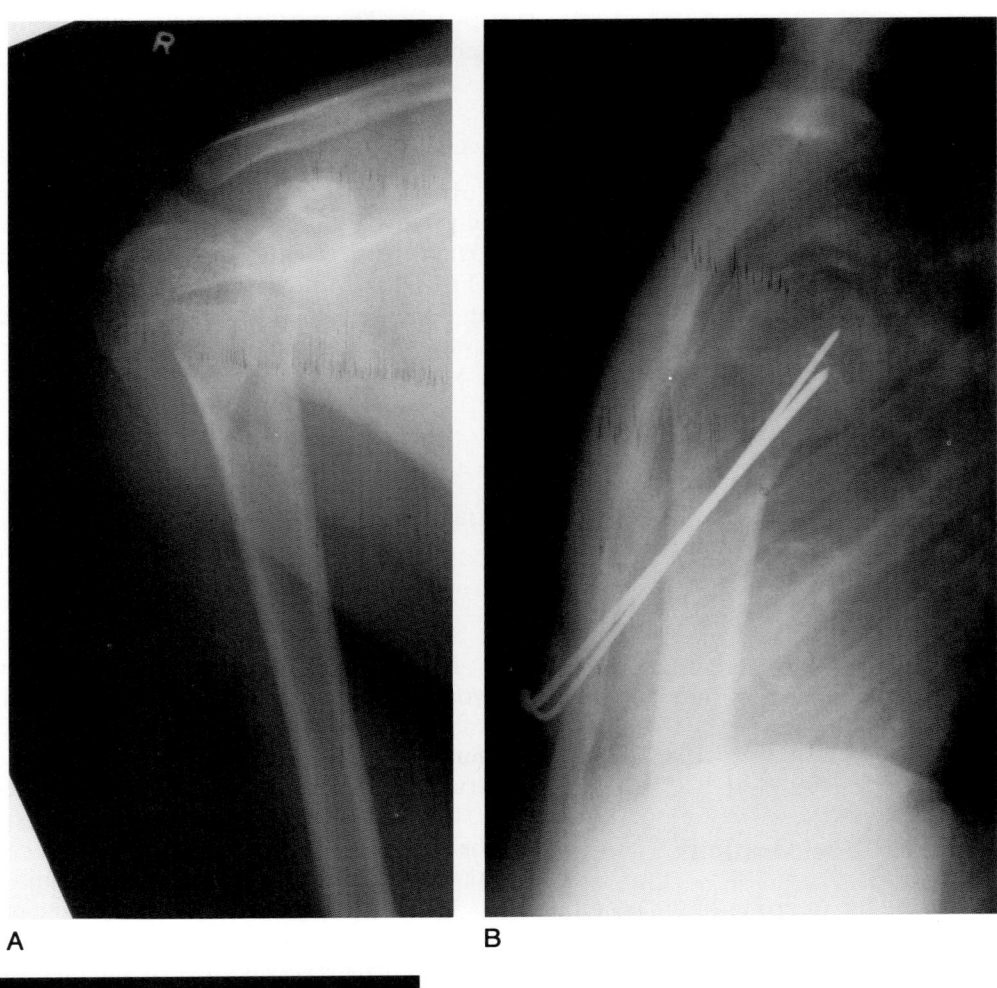

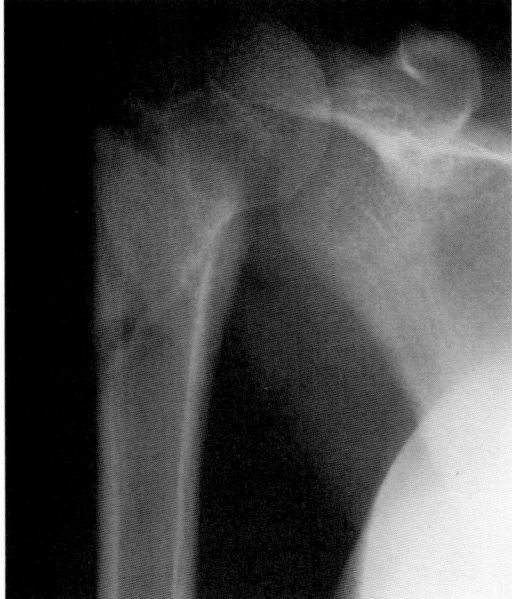

Fig. 9-7. (A) Type II fracture of proximal humerus that was extremely unstable. (B) Stabilization of the fracture with two percutaneous Kirschner wires. (C) Fracture 4 weeks later following pin removal in the clinic.

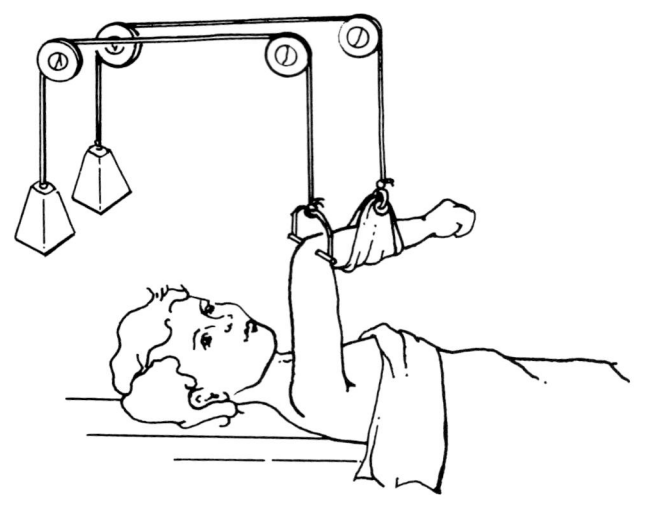

Fig. 9-8. Olecranon pin traction to maintain reduction of humerus.

tern (Fig. 9-12). Completely displaced fractures may have intrusion of the shaft fragment into the deltoid muscle and require open reduction.[7]

Anatomic Considerations

Fractures occur above the insertion of the pectoralis major. The proximal fragment is slightly abducted and externally rotated by the supraspinatus and rotator cuff muscles. The pectoralis major pulls the metaphysis anteriorly and medially (Fig. 9-1).

Mechanism of Injury

In normal bone, metaphyseal humeral fracture is usually due to trauma of considerable force and the fracture pattern is frequently associated with multiple trauma[2] (Fig. 9-13). Minor forces may cause pathologic fractures in bone weakened by such lesions as unicameral bone cysts, which are common in this area (Fig. 9-14).

Classification

The classification of proximal metaphyseal humeral fractures is shown in Table 9-3.

Physical Examination

Physical examination will reveal a painful shoulder. In young children localization of the actual fracture site may be difficult, necessitating radiography of the entire humerus. Completely displaced fractures may have intrusion of the shaft fragment into the deltoid muscle.

The differential diagnosis includes a physeal fracture or the rare shoulder dislocation, which can be differentiated by physical examination and radiographs.

Radiologically, the physis on oblique projection may be mistaken for a fracture. The proximal humeral growth plate is very undulated and may appear at differ-

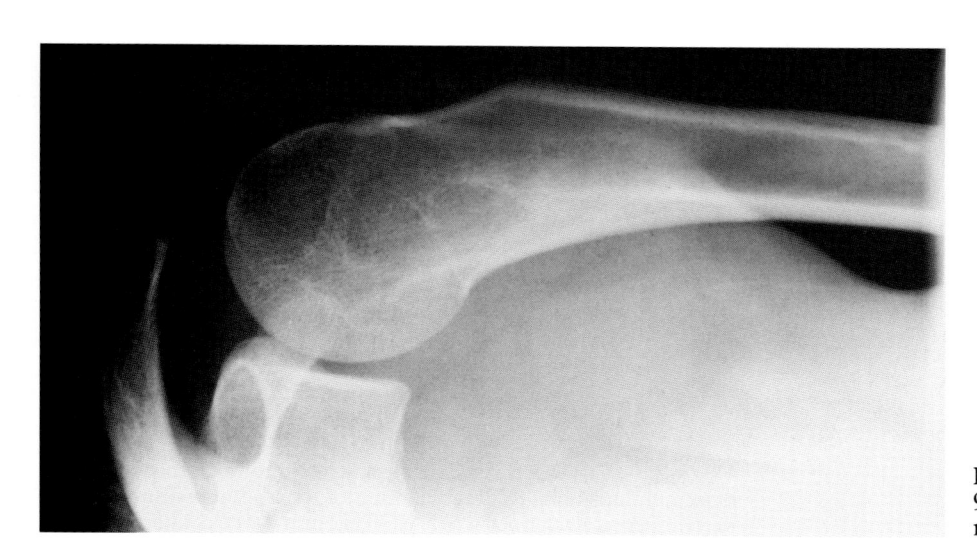

Fig. 9-9. Same fracture as in Figure 9-2 showing excellent remodeling 9 months after fracture.

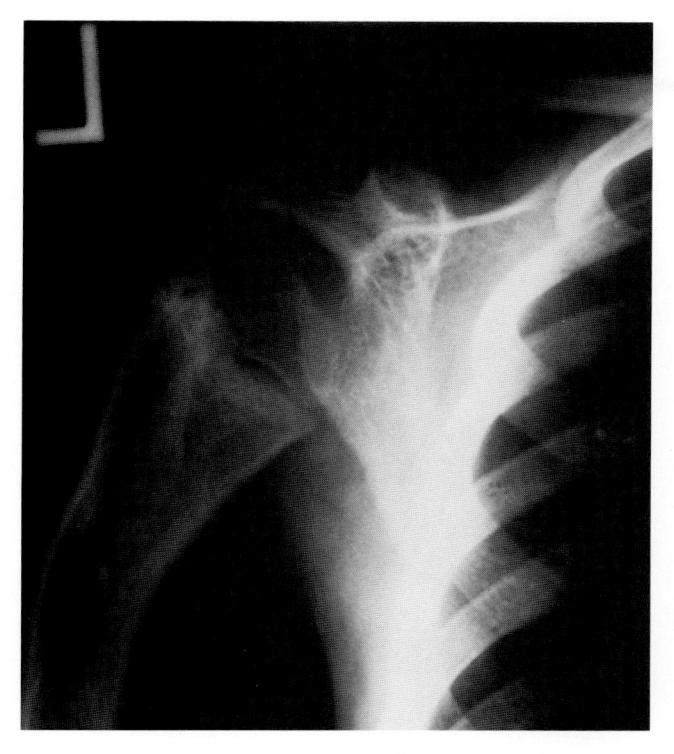

Fig. 9-10. Physeal growth arrest of the proximal humerus secondary to a displaced epiphyseal fracture due to child abuse at age 2 years.

ent levels resulting in two distinct physeal lines, one of which is often misinterpreted as a fracture (Fig. 9-15).

Treatment

Most of these fractures require only simple immobilization. Closed reduction may be indicated in the severely angulated fracture in the older child. Closed reduction is best performed under general anaesthesia with gentle abduction, flexion, and external rotation, with gentle traction. Operative reduction will be necessary if the bone is impaled in muscle and cannot be reduced, or in open fractures. Once reduced, the fracture is usually stable and can be immobilized in a sling and swathe, thoracobrachial box or stockinette sling (Fig. 9-4).

Severe deformity in the adolescent approaching the end of growth will also require open reduction. Prognosis for remodeling is excellent, so that considerable displacement and angulation are acceptable unless the adolescent is within a year of skeletal maturity (Fig. 9-16). Results do not appear to be influenced by treatment, so there appears to be no advantage to open operative intervention,[2] in children with 2 years or more of growth remaining. Slight drift of the fracture into some varus is not uncommon and does not warrant closed or open reduction (Fig. 9-17).

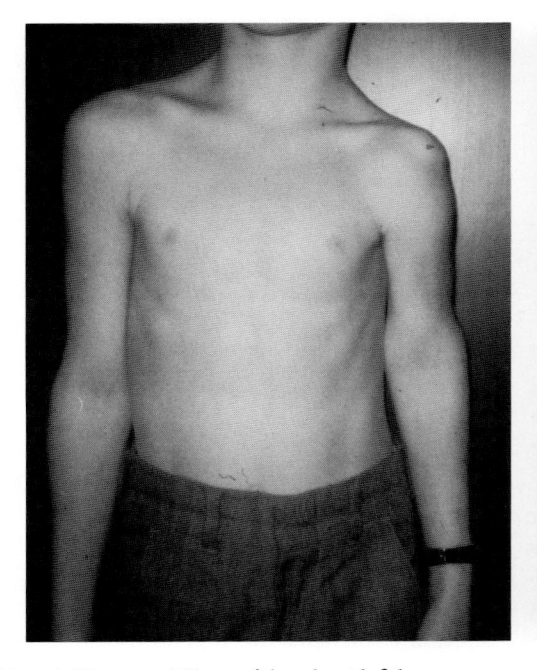

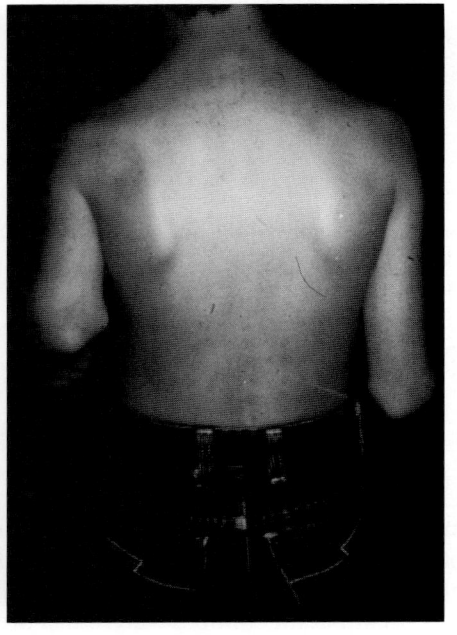

Fig. 9-11. A 10-year-old boy with a short left humerus secondary to a proximal humeral growth arrest as a result of child abuse.

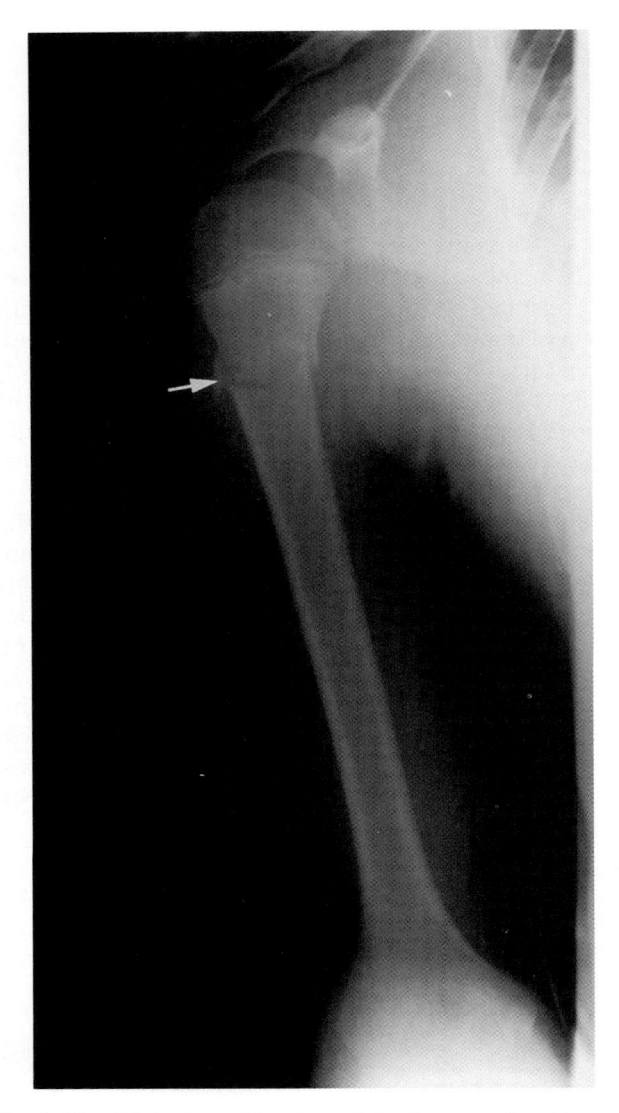

Fig. 9-12. Metaphyseal fracture of the humerus in a 7-year-old child due to a fall from a height.

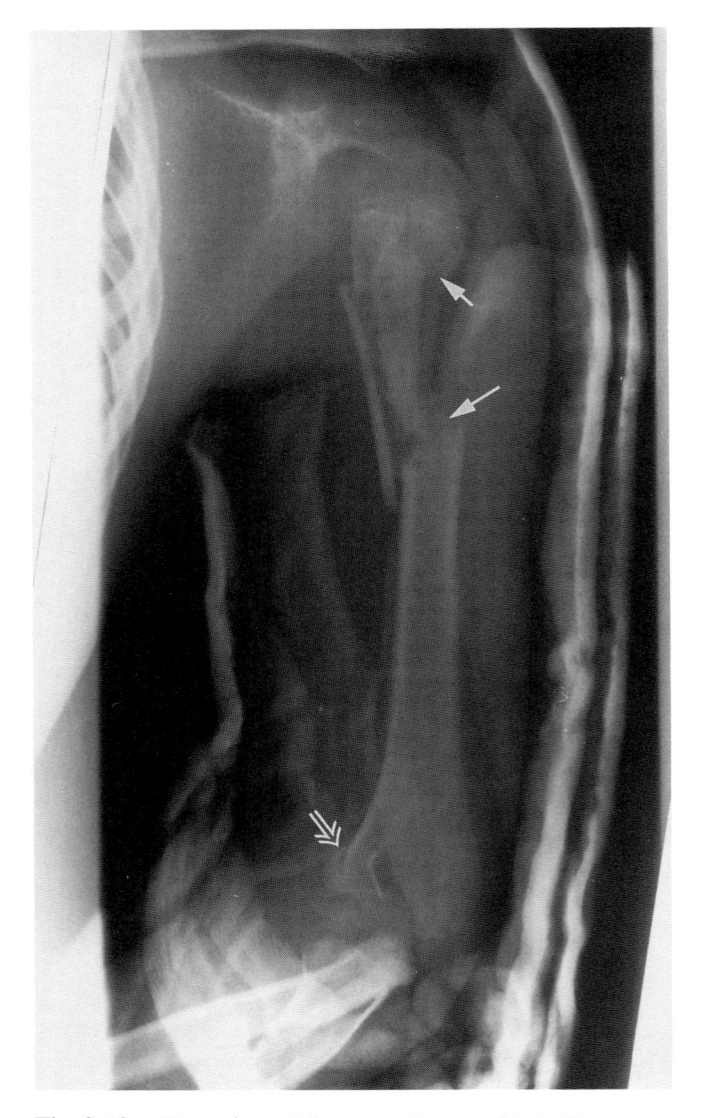

Fig. 9-13. Comminuted fracture of upper third of humerus in a 7-year-old boy struck by a car while riding a snowmobile. Note concomitant fracture of the medial condyle of the humerus.

Complications

Due to the close proximity of the physis, premature growth arrest may result from internal fixation. No fixation other than smooth Kirschner wires should be allowed to transgress the physis. Refracture is occasionally encountered in very exuberant children who return prematurely to the same activities that engendered the initial fracture. Sports activities should be discouraged until 6 weeks postinjury.

FRACTURE OF THE SHAFT OF HUMERUS

Description and Incidence

Shaft fractures are less common in children than in adults. They occur in all age groups and may occur in association with difficult deliveries in the newborn. They are the most common birth fracture after fracture of the

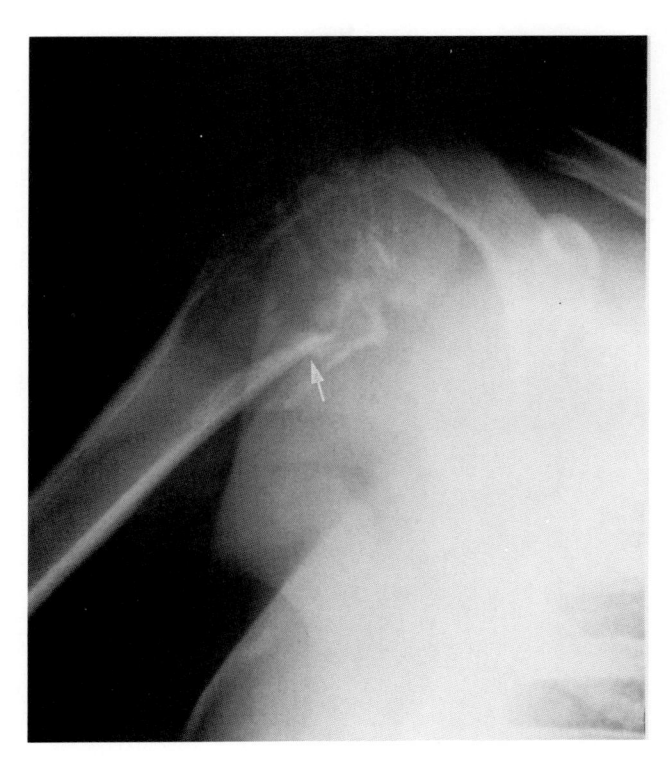

Fractures of the Proximal Humerus and Humeral Shaft / 149

TABLE 9-3. Classification of Proximal Metaphyseal Humeral Fractures

Skin
  Closed
  Open
Bone
  Normal bone
  Pathologic bone
Pattern
  Greenstick, torus
  Complete
    Parallel to physis
    Transverse
Position
  Displaced
  Undisplaced
  Angulated
Forces
  High velocity
  Low velocity
Other injuries
  Isolated
  Associated trauma

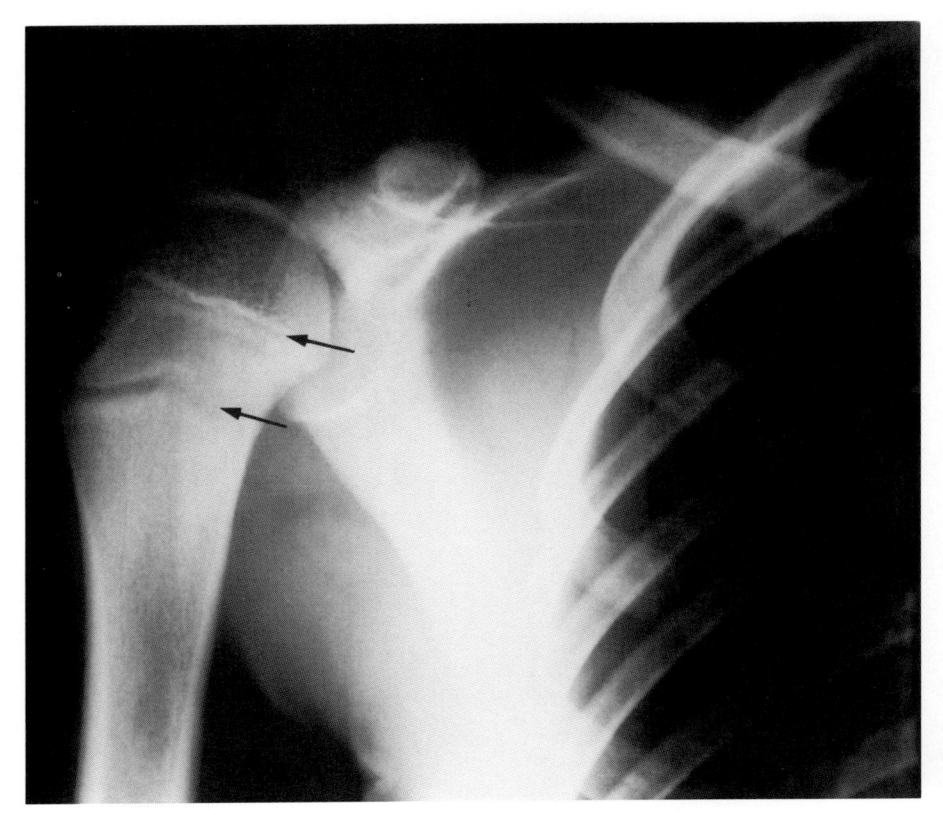

Fig. 9-14. Pathologic fracture through unicameral bone cyst.

Fig. 9-15. Pseudofracture of the proximal humerus. The physis is seen at two different levels.

Fig. 9-16. (A) A completely displaced metaphyseal fracture in a 12-year-old boy that is (B) treated in a hanging cast with no change in alignment but with (C) abundant callus and (D) complete remodeling a year later.

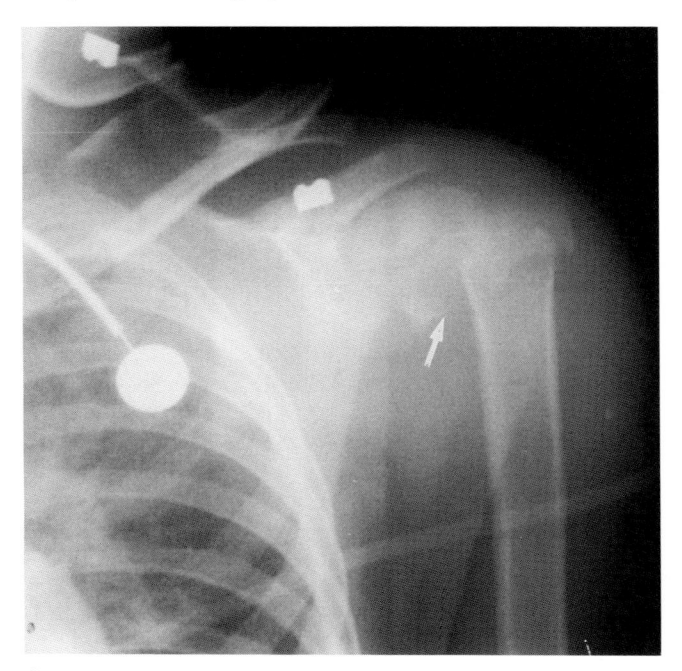

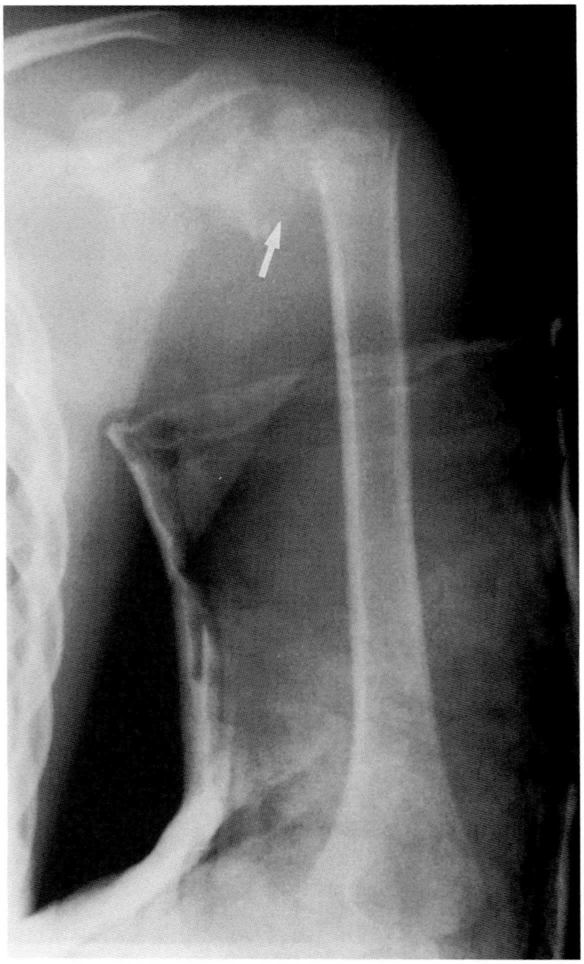

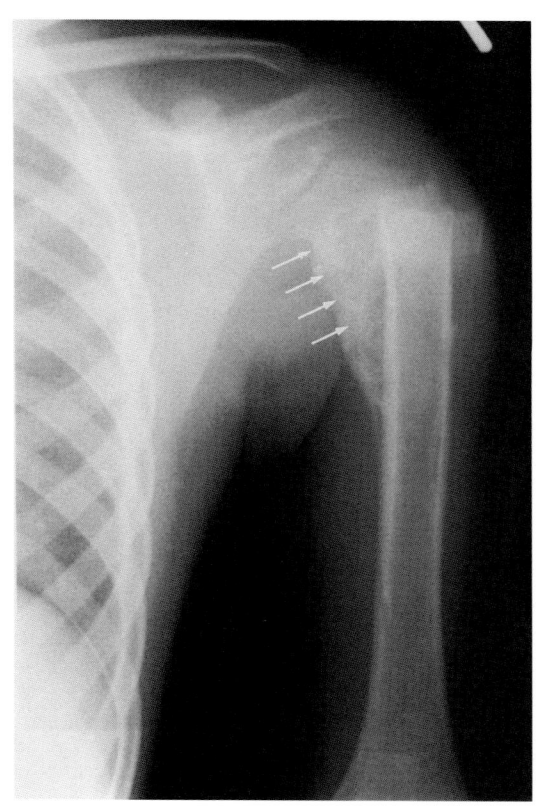

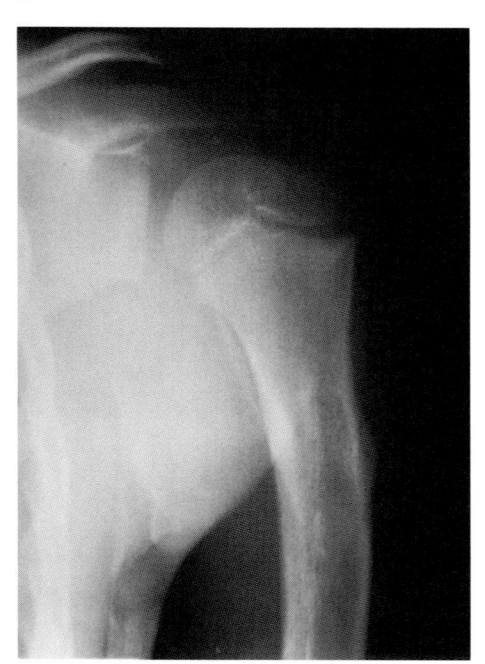

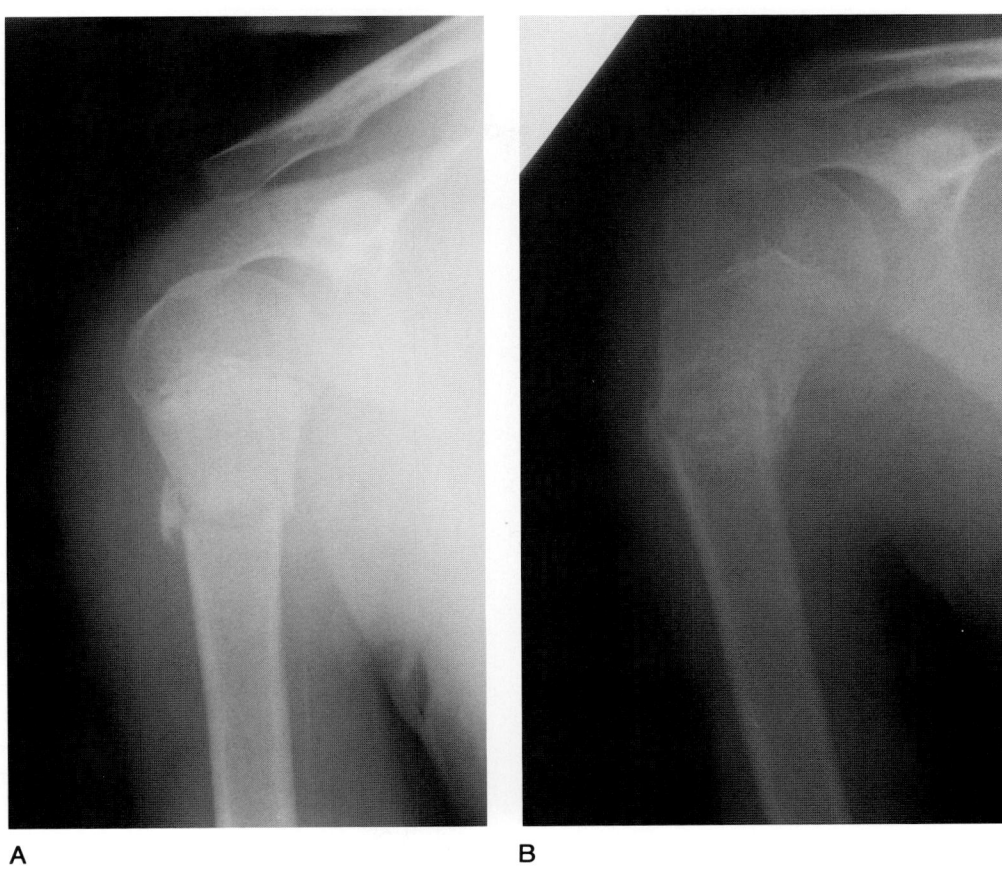

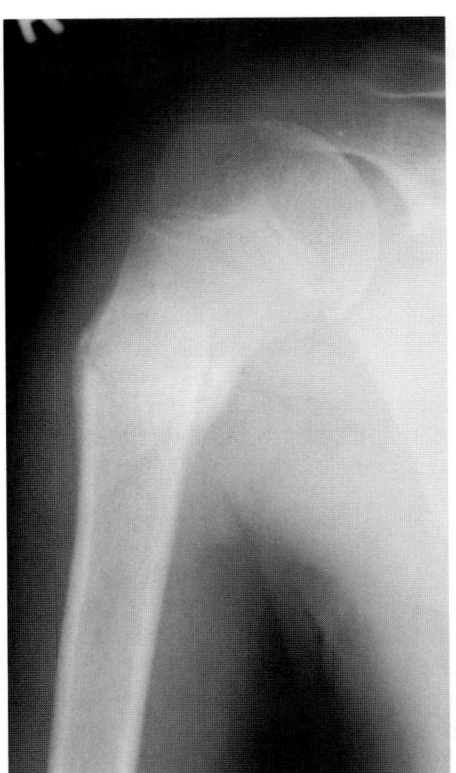

Fig. 9-17. (A) Metaphyseal fracture of the proximal humerus sustained in a fall while downhill skiing in a 13-year-old boy. (B) After 3 weeks in a Velpeau dressing and sugar tong cast. (C) The fracture at 6 weeks shows good callus formation and slight varus drift, which is quite acceptable and causes no limitation of shoulder motion.

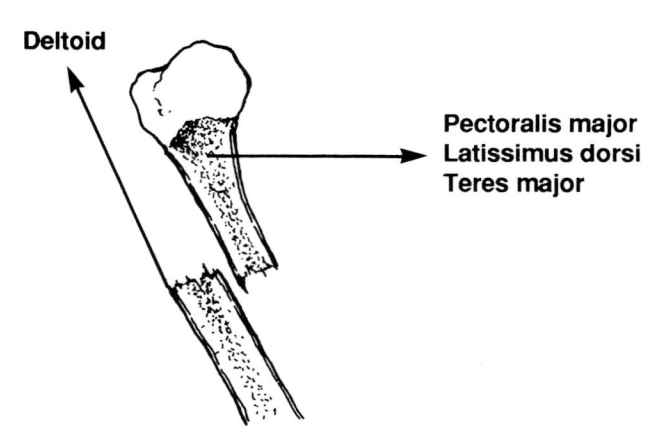

Fig. 9-18. Fracture between the pectoralis major and the deltoid—the proximal fragment is adducted by the pectoralis major, latissimus dorsi, and teres major.

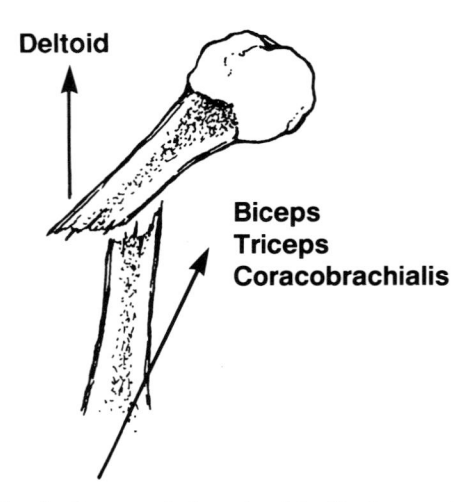

Fig. 9-19. In fractures below the deltoid, the proximal fragment is abducted by the deltoid, while the distal fragment is pulled upward by the coracobrachialis, biceps, and triceps.

clavicle. Generally, birth fractures are complete and significantly angulated. Children involved in contact and throwing sports, or recreational vehicle use, are particularly susceptible to humeral shaft fractures.

Anatomic Considerations

The muscles of the upper arm influence deformity, which depends on the level of fracture. Between the pectoralis major and the deltoid, the proximal fragment is adducted by the pectoralis major, latissimus dorsi, and teres major and the distal fragment is pulled outward and upward by the deltoid (Fig. 9-18). Below the deltoid, the proximal fragment is abducted by the deltoid, while the distal fragment is pulled upward by the coracobrachialis, biceps, and triceps (Fig. 9-19).

Mechanism of Injury

Humeral birth fractures usually occur in difficult breech deliveries during extraction of the extended arms, in delivery of stiff extremities, as in arthrogryposis, or in traction on the axilla in shoulder dystocia (Fig. 9-20). Such fractures are often necessary to allow delivery. These fractures may be transverse or spiral. The amount of deformity will depend on the level of the fracture, but remodeling corrects all residual deformities. Direct blows may produce a transverse fracture or comminution. Forces are often violent and may be associated with other fractures (Fig. 9-21). Longitudinal forces associated with torsion, such as falling on the elbow or outstretched hand, will produce oblique or spiral patterns of fractures.

Multiple fractures, especially in younger children, should alert one to the possibility of child abuse. Fracture of the humerus in a young child or infant is always secondary to considerable force and seldom occurs from minor falls or getting an extremity caught in the crib rungs (Fig. 9-22). Twisting injuries result in spiral fractures with much less force, as in throwing sports, but twisting injuries may also be associated with great force (Fig. 9-21). Pathologic fractures may occur through lytic lesions in cysts and tumors (Fig. 9-23).

Classification

Classification need not be complex, but a number of differentiating factors should be considered in order to aid in management decisions (Table 9-4).

Physical Examination

The arm will, in most cases, be painful to move, swollen, bruised, and tender. Deformity will give some clue as to the level of the lesion. Careful neurologic and vascular assessment is important, especially in the newborn and in the unconscious patient. Whether or not skin is broken and the degree of associated soft tissue trauma

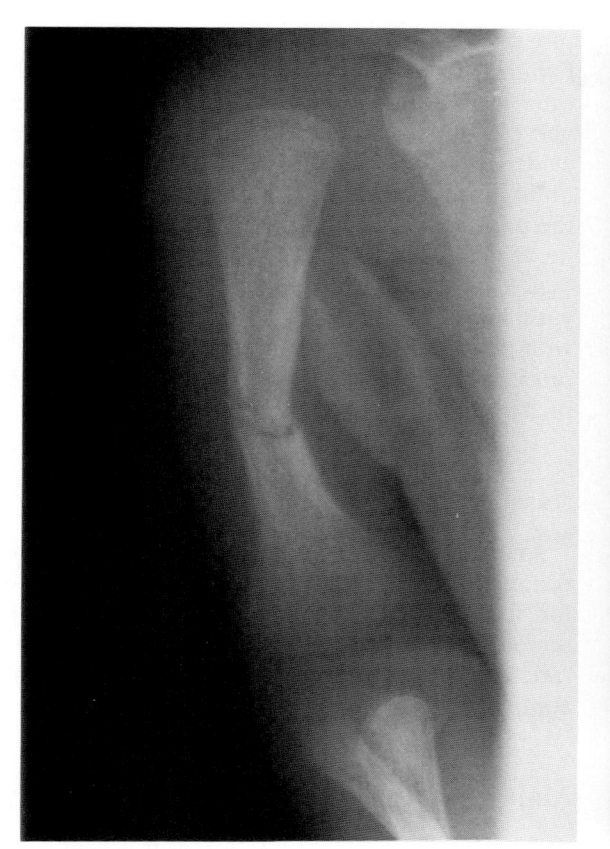

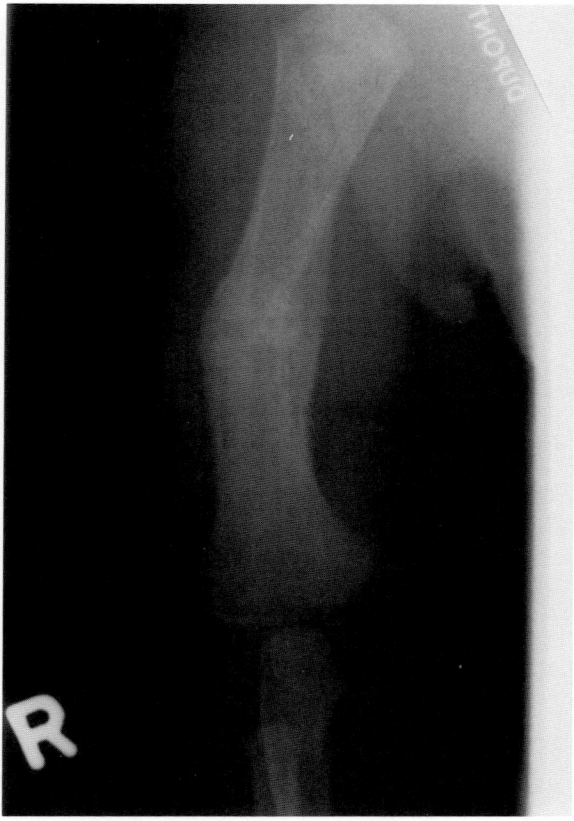

Fig. 9-20. Birth fracture in an infant with arthrogryposis, resulting in difficult delivery. Healing occurs rapidly with abundant callus in 10 days.

should be determined and all findings recorded early in the emergency department.

Radiologic Examination

The level and pattern of fracture can be confirmed radiographically. Care should be taken in splinting the arm and in avoiding unnecessary rotation during radiography.

Treatment

In birth fractures, a simple padded splint may be strapped to the upper arm and the entire limb immobilized in a sling and swathe for 3 weeks (Fig. 9-4A). In other young children, the sling and swathe should be reinforced with plaster to make a thoracobrachial box (Fig. 9-4C). Alternatively, elasticized adhesive may be used to reinforce the sling and swathe. About 6 weeks of immobilization is necessary. Older children and adolescents may need a hanging cast to correct the deformity; however, hanging casts are not suitable if the level of fracture corresponds to the upper limit of the cast because of the deforming effect of the proximal cast. In most instances a plaster U splint with a sling and swathe or stockinette sling are preferable (Fig. 9-4B,D,E). Severe displacement and instability can be treated by olecranon pin traction (Fig. 9-8).

Open reduction should be considered if there are associated multiple fractures, particularly in the same limb, or multiple system trauma has been sustained. Flexible intramedullary nails or Rush rods, with early removal at 6 to 8 weeks, are best. In severe open wounds requiring frequent attention, external fixators are preferable. These are suitable until the open wounds have been closed or covered with skin graft. Prolonged use of external fixators is undesirable because of risk of nonunion and pin tract infection.

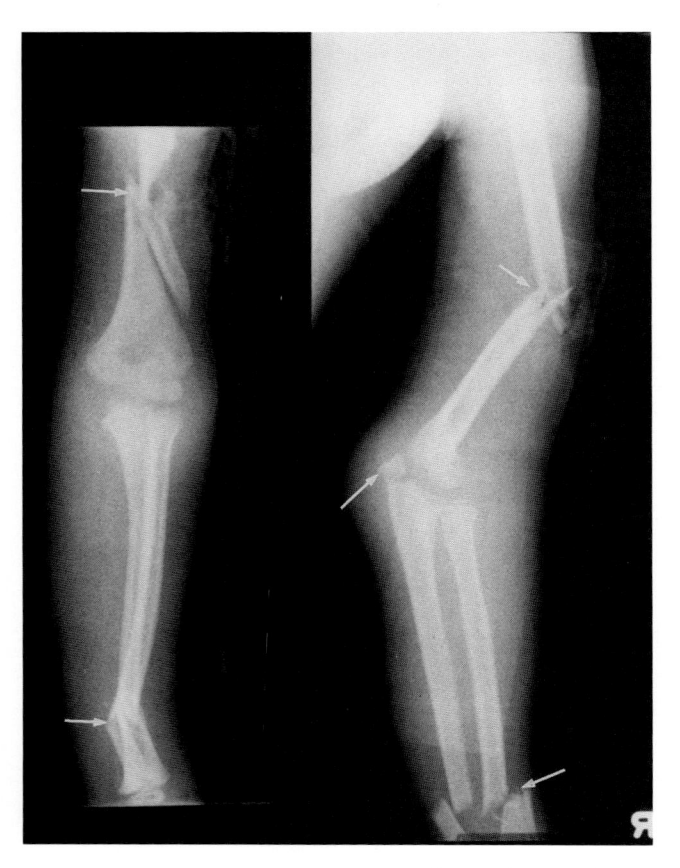

Fig. 9-21. An 8-year-old boy caught his arm in machinery, resulting in a "floating elbow" with fractures of humerus and forearm.

After early callus formation at about 3 to 4 weeks, removal of external fixators and use of external immobilization with a sling and swathe or cast is recommended. If one anticipates the need for more prolonged fracture fixation, and external immobilization is not possible because of other factors, such as chest trauma, open reduction with intramedullary or plate fixation may be considered. Converting external pin fixator to internal fixation carries a risk of deep infection and is best avoided.

Complications

Radial Nerve Injury

The radial nerve is particularly vulnerable in lower third fractures and has been entrapped in the fracture line[13] or in the callus[14] (Fig. 9-24). Nerve deficit at fracture onset should be observed and will usually recover. Failure to show any recovery within fracture healing time justifies electromyographic (EMG) examination, nerve conduction tests, and exploration if there is no evidence of nerve regeneration. Gradual recovery requires ongoing observation, wrist and finger splinting in the position of function, and physiotherapy. If a radial nerve deficit occurs after fracture manipulation, immediate exploration is necessary. Nerve transection is rare with a closed injury. Radial nerve deficit in association with penetrating wounds necessitates immediate exploration of the radial nerve at the time of wound debridement.

Vascular Injury

Arterial injury is unusual, but the precautions of repeated examination of distal circulation and assessment for forearm compartment syndrome should be observed. Should there be vascular occlusion, early exploration and repair within a few hours is essential, as is compartmental decompression.

Malunion

Angular deformity of 20 degrees is acceptable in the middle and distal one-third, while in the proximal third 30 degrees is acceptable and will remodel with growth. The closer the fracture is to the proximal humeral epiphysis and the more growth remaining, the better the remodeling potential. Distal and middle one-third angulation corrects poorly, since only 20 percent of humeral growth occurs at the distal humeral physis.

Malrotation is generally not a problem, but excessive external rotation of the proximal fragment and internal rotation of the distal fragment may result in anteversion and a predisposition to dislocation of the shoulder. This may require a corrective rotation osteotomy (Fig. 9-25).

Overgrowth

The average humeral fracture will overgrow approximately 1 cm.[10] This should be considered when allowing overriding of fragments. Patients should be warned of the possibility of overgrowth; however, in contradistinction to the lower extremity, moderate upper limb length inequality is seldom a functional or cosmetic disability.

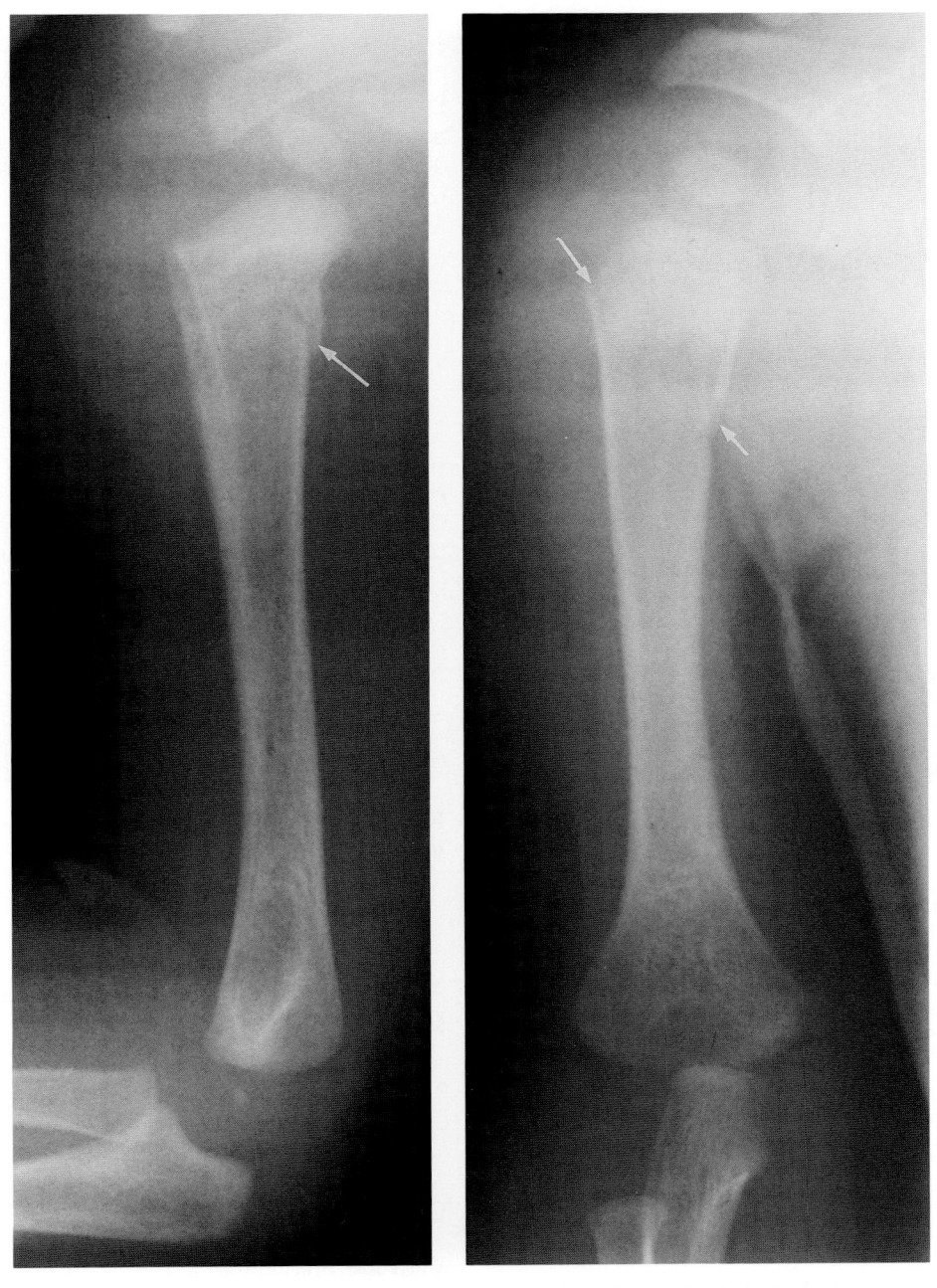

Fig. 9-22. An undisplaced fracture of the proximal humerus in a 6-month-old infant who presented with a history of not using the arm for the past 24 hours. Since fractures of the humerus in children require considerable force an investigation was instituted and child abuse by a babysitter was ultimately revealed.

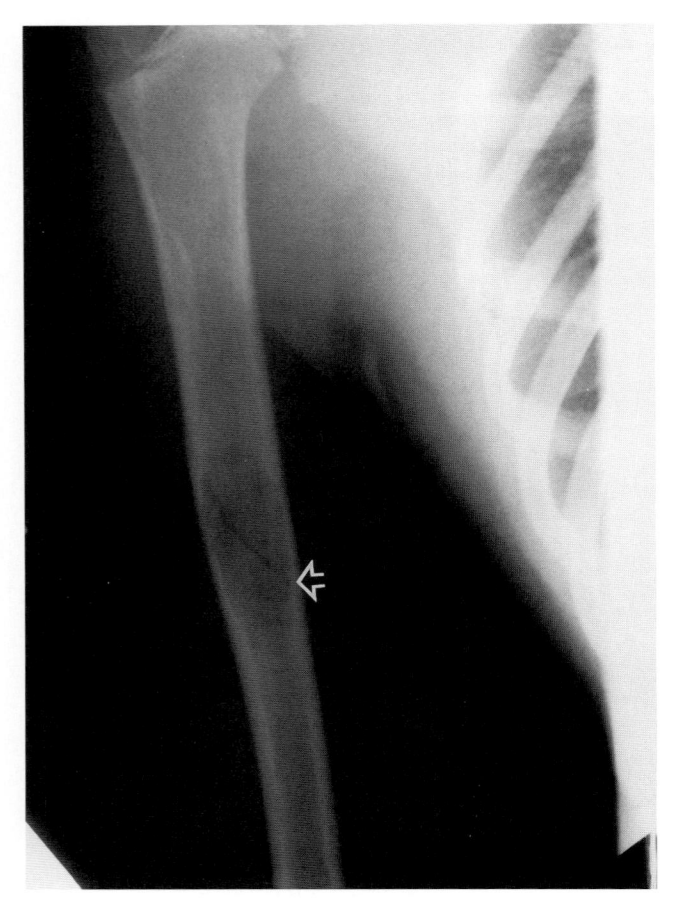

Fig. 9-23. Pathologic fracture through an eosinophilic granuloma.

Fig. 9-24. A spiral fracture in a 16-year-old girl with radial nerve entrapment—the Holstein fracture.

TABLE 9-4. Classification of Fractures of the Humerus

Skin
  Closed
  Open
Bone
  Normal bone
  Pathologic bone
Pattern
  Greenstick
  Transverse
  Oblique
  Spiral
  Comminuted
Forces
  High velocity
  Low velocity
Other injuries
  Isolated
  Associated trauma

Nonunion seldom occurs in children unless there is severe soft tissue trauma or infection.

SUMMARY

In general, fractures of the proximal humerus and shaft are predictable and seldom complicated. Reduction is generally unnecessary, or can be accomplished by reversing the deforming forces when indicated. Exceptional circumstances will require operative intervention. Even when angular and rotational deformities or growth disturbances occur, they are usually not of cosmetic or functional significance and often correct with growth.

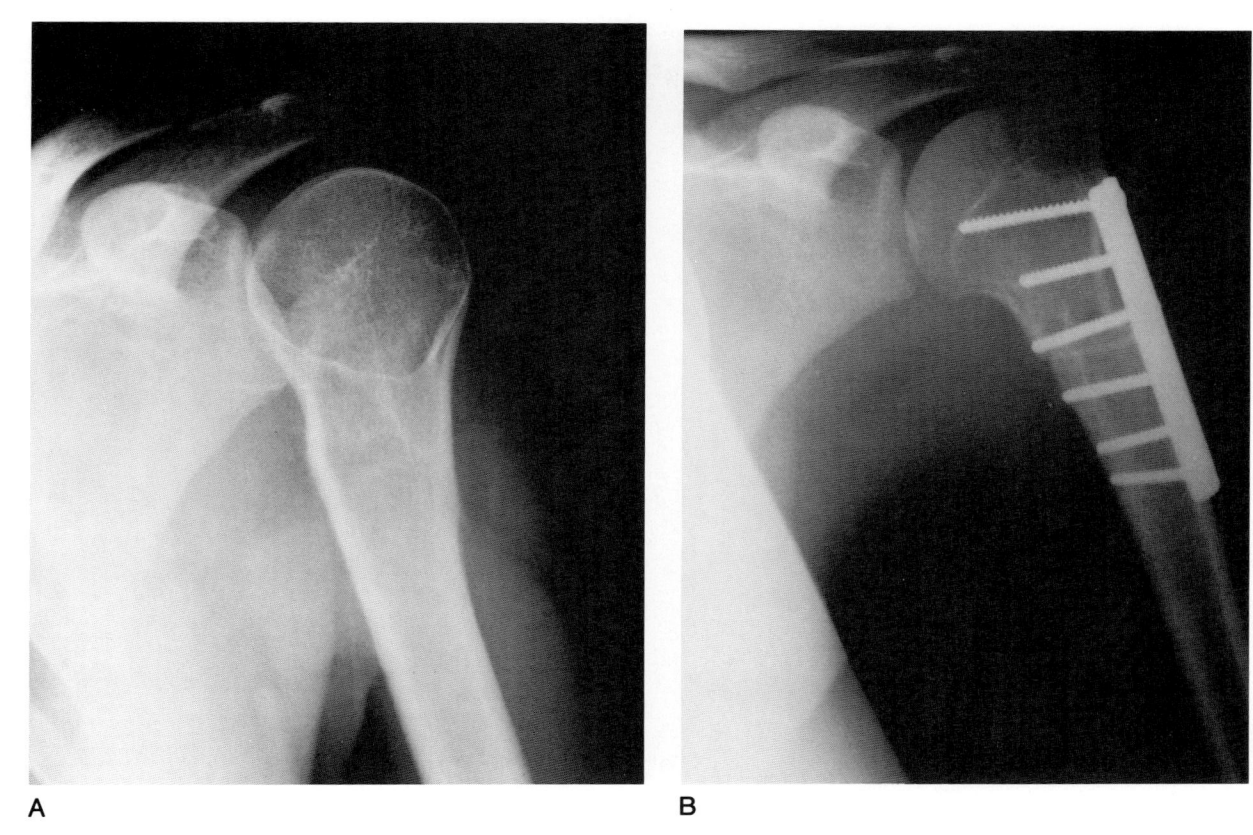

Fig. 9-25. (A) Rotational deformity resulting in recurring subluxation during rotation, (B) treated by derotation osteotomy.

REFERENCES

1. Neer CS, Horwitz BS: Fractures of the proximal humeral epiphyseal plate. Clin Orthop 41:24, 1965
2. Kohler R, Trilland JM: Fracture and fracture separation of the proximal humerus in children: report of 136 cases. J Pediatr Orthop 3:326, 1983
3. Salter RB, Harris WR: Injuries involving the epiphyseal plate. J Bone Joint Surg [Am] 45:587, 1963
4. Eaxter MP, Wiley JJ: Fractures of the proximal humeral epiphysis. J Bone Joint Surg [Br] 68:570, 1968
5. Dameron TB Jr, Reibel DB: Fractures involving the proximal humeral epiphyseal plate. J Bone Joint Surg [Am] 51:289, 1969
6. Fraser RL, Haliburton RA, Barber JR: Displaced epiphyseal fractures of the proximal humerus. Can J Surg 10:427, 1967
7. Rang Mercer: Children's Fractures. 2nd Ed. JB Lippincott, Philadelphia, 1982
8. Williams DJ: The mechanisms producing fracture-separation of the proximal humeral epiphysis. J Bone Joint Surg [Br] 63:102, 1981
9. Harris WR, Martin RF, Tile M: Transplantation of epiphyseal plates: an experimental study. J Bone Joint Surg [Am] 47:897, 1965
10. Ogden JA: Skeletal Injury in the Child. 2nd Ed. WB Saunders, Philadelphia, 1990
11. Pritchett JW: Growth plate activity in the upper extremity. Clin Orthop 268:235, 1991
12. Ciernik IJ, Meier L, Hollinger A: Humeral mobility after treatment with hanging cast. J Trauma 31:230, 1991
13. Holstein A, Lewis GB: Fractures of the humerus with radial nerve paralysis. J Bone Joint Surg [Am] 45:1382, 1963
14. Macnicol MF: Roentgenographic evidence of median-nerve entrapment in a greenstick humeral fracture: a case report. J Bone Joint Surg [Am] 60:998, 1978

10

Dislocations of the Shoulder

R. Baxter Willis
Robert D. Galpin

> We should know on who's shoulders we stand.
> —Jason Hannah

DESCRIPTION AND INCIDENCE

Dislocation of the glenohumeral joint in children is extremely rare. Rowe,[1] in his classic article on shoulder dislocation, revealed that 8 of 500 patients were under age 10 and a further 99 were between ages 10 and 20. It is not clear from this article the exact number of patients who had open epiphyses at the time of treatment. Apart from isolated case reports there are few reported series on this topic in the medical literature.[2-5]

ANATOMIC CONSIDERATIONS

Proximal Humerus

There are three ossification centers in the proximal humerus, one each for the head, greater tuberosity, and lesser tuberosity. The ossification center for the head appears by the sixth month, that for the greater tuberosity by the third year, and that for the lesser tuberosity by the fifth year. The ossification centers for the tuberosities coalesce during the fifth year and fuse with the center for the head during the seventh year. Obliteration of the proximal humeral physis is extremely variable, occurring as early as 14 years in females and as late as 19 years in males.[6]

Glenohumeral Joint

The shoulder joint is inherently unstable, likened to a golf ball sitting on a tee with the large head of the humerus articulating against the small and shallow glenoid fossa. This relationship allows for remarkable ranges of motion in every direction at the expense of stability of the joint. The average vertical dimension of the surface of the adult humeral head is 48 mm (25-mm radius of curvature) with an average transverse diameter of 45 mm (22-mm radius of curvature). These measurements contrast sharply with the glenoid fossa in the adult, which measures 35 mm in its vertical dimension and 25 mm in its transverse dimension.[6]

The capsule of the shoulder has about twice the surface area of the humeral head. The capsule extends from the glenoid neck and labrum to the anatomic neck of the humerus. On the medial side of the humerus the capsule extends distally for about 1 cm and actually attaches distal to the proximal humeral physis.

MECHANISM OF INJURY

The mechanism of traumatic dislocation and subluxation of the shoulder parallels the mechanism seen in adults. Traumatic dislocations are associated with severe injuries including severe falls on to an outstretched hand, and forced abduction and external rotation injuries during contact sports.[1,5-9]

CLASSIFICATION

The classification of shoulder instability may be according to the degree of instability (dislocation or subluxation), the time relationship or circumstances of the instability (acute, chronic, recurrent, involuntary), and the cause of the instability (traumatic or nontraumatic). Rockwood,[3] in his treatise on shoulder instability, proposed a classification specifically for children (Table 10-1). He used two broad categories based on whether the instability was considered traumatic or atraumatic in origin. Of 44 cases, 8 were traumatic and 36 had atraumatic dislocations of the shoulder. Wagner and Lyne[9] reported on 9 children with traumatic instability, 80 percent of whom had recurrent dislocations.

PHYSICAL EXAMINATION

Traumatic Dislocations

A child with a traumatic anterior dislocation presents with the arm held in slight abduction and external rotation as in the adult. The shoulder has a squared-off appearance rather than the normal rounded contour. Any attempt to passively or actively move the shoulder results in increased pain.

A child with a traumatic posterior dislocation would also resemble the similar situation in the adult. The arm is held markedly adducted and internally rotated with the forearm held across the abdomen. There is a flattening across the anterior aspect of the shoulder while the humeral head may be palpable posteriorly.

The rare situation of luxatio erecta occurs usually during a difficult delivery. The arm assumes an overhead position in full abduction and external rotation. The humeral head is locked inferiorly to the glenoid through a rent in the anteroinferior capsule.[10]

Atraumatic Dislocations

Atraumatic dislocations may occur voluntarily or involuntarily. The hallmark of these dislocations is the lack of pain associated with them. The patient usually learns to subluxate or dislocate the glenohumeral joint with a trick maneuver. With time the shoulder will begin to dislocate with involuntary movements such as raising the arm overhead or carrying heavy objects. The involuntary dislocations are usually anterior at first, but the joint capsule may become so stretched that eventually the dislocations will be multidirectional (i.e., anterior, posterior, and inferior).

Physical examination of the child complaining of instability of the shoulder requires reproduction of the provocative symptoms of subluxation and documentation of the amount of passive translation between the humeral head and glenoid fossa.

Glenohumeral Translation

The test for glenohumeral translation should be carried out in both the supine and sitting position. The scapula is held with one of the examiner's hands, and the other hand grasps the humeral head between the thumb and fingers. The humeral head is "loaded" against the glenoid fossa and then translated anteriorly. The amount of translation is recorded by using this load and shift test to ascertain if there is significant pathologic translation when compared to the opposite side (see Fig. 10-1). Translation in both anterior and posterior directions is performed in this way, and inferior translation is ascertained by grasping the patient's elbow and pulling the humerus in an inferior direction. While carrying out this maneuver the area below the acromion is observed

TABLE 10-1. Classification of Dislocations of the Glenohumeral Joint in Children

Traumatic Dislocation
 As result of true traumatic force, proximal humerus may displace anteriorly, posteriorly, or inferiorly
 May occur at birth or later as a result of injury to brachial plexus or central nervous system
Atraumatic Dislocation—Voluntary or Involuntary
 Occurs from a number of nontraumatic causes
 Congenital abnormalities or deficiencies
 Hereditary joint laxity problems—Ehlers-Danlos syndrome
 Developmental joint laxity problems
 Emotional and psychiatric disturbances
 Other

(From Dameron and Rockwood,[3] with permission.)

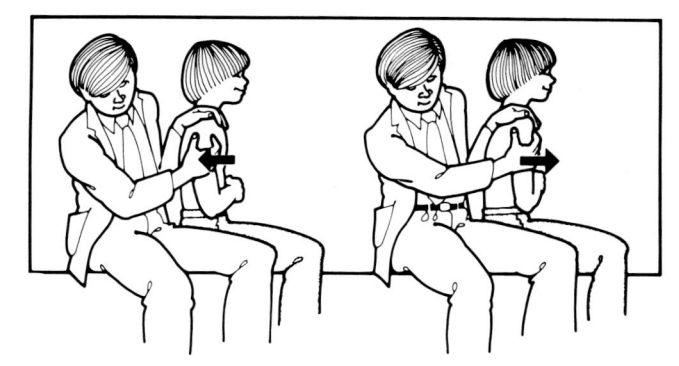

Fig. 10-1. The drawer test for anteroposterior instability. The examiner, seated next to the patient, uses one hand to grasp the humeral head to translate it anteriorly and posteriorly, while stabilizing the scapula with the opposite hand and forearm. (Modified from Curtis RJ Jr, Rockwood CA: Fractures and dislocations of the shoulder in children. p. 991. In Rockwood CA Jr, Matsen FA III (eds): The Shoulder. WB Saunders, Philadelphia, 1990, with permission.)

for the development of a depression known as a "sulcus sign" (see Figs. 10-2 and 10-3).

Apprehension Tests

It is important to document the direction of glenohumeral instability and to confirm it by provocative stress tests. For anterior subluxation or dislocation, the arm is abducted and externally rotated. With the thumb of one hand pushing from behind and the fingers of the same hand anterior to the humerus to protect the patient from a sudden episode of instability, increasing external rotation force and anterior force (thumb of one hand) is applied.

The patient may look apprehensive and protect his shoulder by grabbing the examiner's hand or volunteering that his shoulder is about to come out. The test should be carried out in both the sitting and supine positions.

Posterior instability is usually a more difficult diagnostic challenge. The instability is usually recurrent subluxation rather than true dislocation, and therefore pain is not a major feature. Therefore true apprehension does not occur.

The posterior instability usually occurs in a position of adduction, forward elevation, and internal rotation. The patient can often duplicate the instability by muscular control, and the examiner should try to duplicate this in various arm positions.

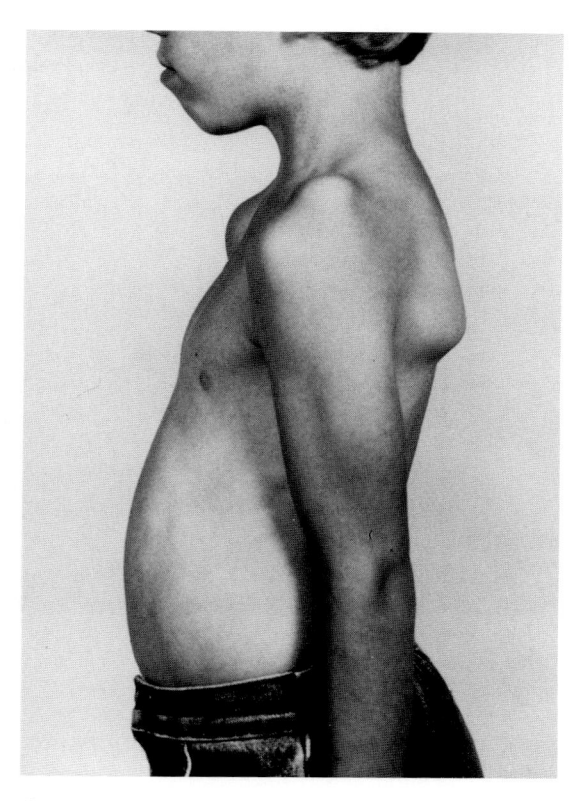

Fig. 10-2. Lateral view of patient with voluntary, atraumatic instability of left shoulder demonstrating "sulcus" sign.

Radiographic Examination

For suspected glenohumeral instability the recommended radiographs are a true anteroposterior view and an axillary lateral or true lateral scapular view (see Fig. 10-4). Modified lateral axillary views and CT scans may also prove to be beneficial. The classical Hill-Sachs lesion or impression fracture may be appreciated on the posterolateral aspect of the humeral head. Calcification near the anterior inferior rim of the glenoid fossa is indicative of a Bankart lesion with stripping of the capsule from its bony attachment.

Differential Diagnosis

Depending on the age of the child and presentation of symptoms the differential diagnosis may include trauma to adjacent structures, (i.e., clavicle, acromioclavicular joint, proximal humeral fracture), sepsis, including septic arthritis and osteomyelitis, congenital problems, in-

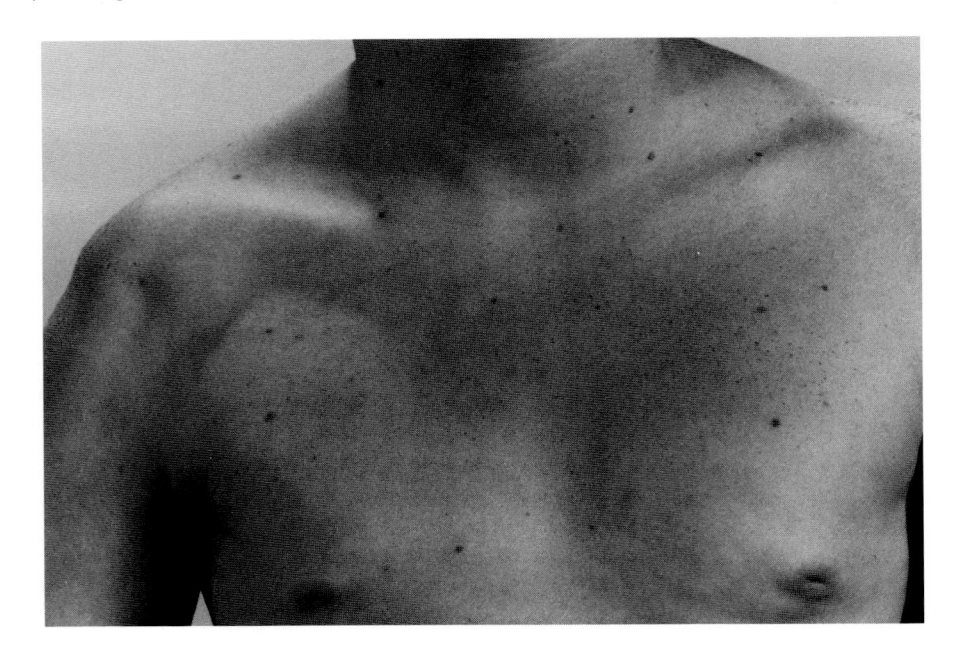

Fig. 10-3. AP view of patient with voluntary, atraumatic instability of right shoulder demonstrating "sulcus" sign.

cluding birth fracture, brachial plexus injury, and, finally, tumors or tumorlike processes.

A careful history and physical examination including appropriate radiographs will usually pinpoint the correct diagnosis.

TREATMENT INDICATIONS

Closed Methods

Closed methods of treatment are indicated in acute traumatic glenohumeral dislocations. Reduction of anterior dislocations can usually be achieved by applying traction on the abducted and flexed arm after appropriate analgesia/anesthesia. As traction is applied longitudinally, a gentle rotation force may be added (alternating internal and external rotation), as well as lateral traction on the proximal humerus and increasing abduction of the shoulder.

Postreduction radiographs are performed to ensure adequacy of the reduction and to detect any occult fractures of the glenoid or proximal humerus. The neurovascular status is always checked before and after a reduction.

For first-time dislocations, the arm is immobilized in a position of adduction and internal rotation with a combination sling and swathe bandage or Velpeau dressing. Immobilization is continued for 3 to 4 weeks, and then rehabilitation is commenced vigorously.

The recurrence rate for anterior glenohumeral dislocations is extremely high in children and adolescents. Recurrence rates of 50 percent and higher have been reported by several different authors despite appropriate immobilization.[11] Dameron and Rockwood[3] reported a recurrence rate of 50 percent. Wagner and Lyne,[9] 80 percent and Rowe and Sakellarides,[12] up to 100 percent.

For recurrent dislocations, we advocate a period of rest (3 to 5 days) in a simple sling until the patient is comfortable, followed by aggressive rehabilitation.

Rehabilitation should commence in the first few weeks in the form of isometric exercise for the internal and external rotators. Following removal of the immobilization, vigorous strengthening of all muscle groups is encouraged.

Recurrent instability of the glenohumeral joint may be amenable to improvement with a vigorous conservative exercise program. There are documented cases of anterior and posterior subluxation in competitive athletes which have responded to a specific muscle training regimen to strengthen the internal rotators for anterior subluxation and the external rotators for posterior subluxation.

Despite excellent conservative management, a high percentage of patients with acute traumatic dislocations and nontraumatic dislocations will continue to experience instability.

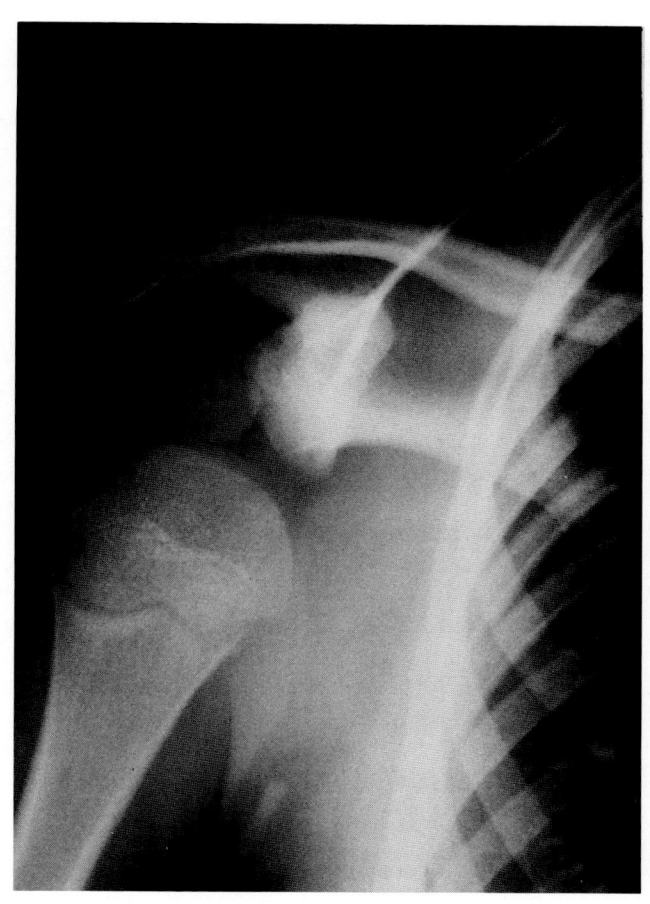

Fig. 10-4. AP view of shoulder of patient seen in Figure 10-3, demonstrating inferior subluxation of humeral head.

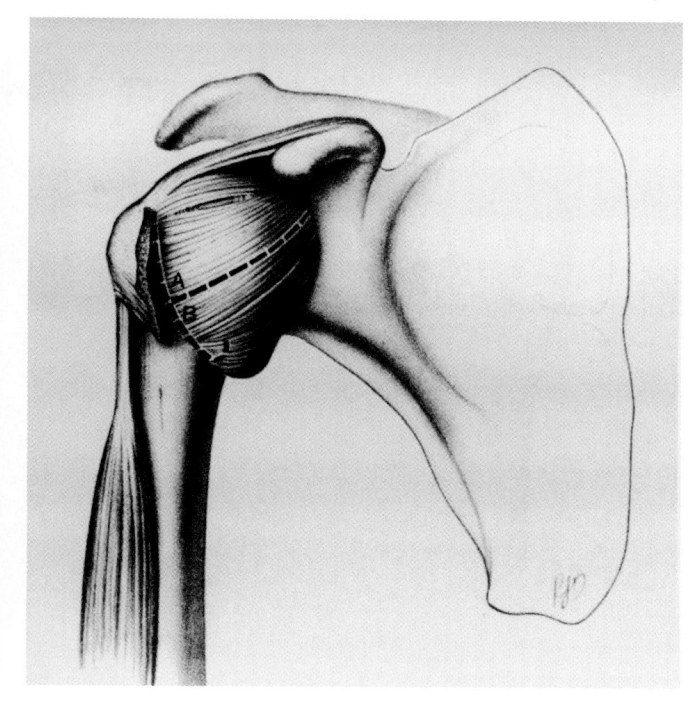

Fig. 10-5. T-shaped incision in capsule in preparation for inferior capsular shift. (From Neer CS: Shoulder Reconstruction. WB Saunders, Philadelphia, 1990, with permission.)

Open Methods

Open surgical techniques are reserved for children with failure of prolonged conservative treatment after a documented traumatic cause, or with irreducible acute dislocations. Surgical treatment of recurrent atraumatic instability is universally a failure.[13,14]

Irreducible acute dislocations may be congenital or acquired. In one case of a child with luxatio erecta an anterior approach was used with release of the anterior inferior capsule.[10] The humeral head could not be reduced until the deltoid was partially released as well. Irreducible acquired dislocations can be treated surgically by an anterior approach with release of the subscapularis and anterior capsule. Surgical repair involves plication of both the capsule and subscapularis after open reduction of the humeral head.

Open methods of surgical repair for recurrent anterior dislocation are many and varied. Surgery should only be considered after a vigorous rehabilitation regimen for at least 6 to 12 months has failed. Some involve repair or reattachment of the anterior capsule and glenoid labrum,[15] others involve detaching and plicating the anterior capsule and/or subscapularis to limit external rotation, or,[7] if part of the glenoid rim is deficient, a bone block is placed on the anterior glenoid rim.[16]

In children with open physes, the approach recommended by Neer[17,18] or Rockwood and colleagues[6] has considerable merit. Both Neer and Rockwood employ a capsular shift reconstruction method with repair of any Bankart lesion. The capsular shift technique is similar to the technique of capsulorrhaphy for congenital dislocation of the hip. The redundant portion of the capsule is "shifted" to eliminate redundancy anteriorly and inferiorly (see Figs. 10-5 and 10-6).

For recurrent posterior dislocation a similar posterior approach with plication or elimination of capsular redundancy is employed.[16] The use of screws or staples about the shoulder joint is to be avoided because of reported complications.[19]

Children with atraumatic voluntary dislocations should not be considered as surgical candidates and re-

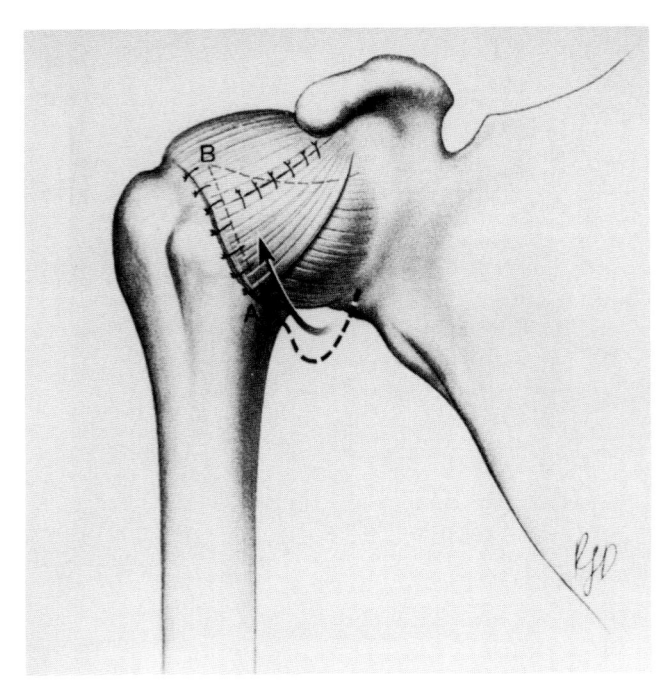

Fig. 10-6. Diagram of capsule after inferior capsular shift. After preparing the posterior, inferior, and anterior humeral neck, the lower flap is brought upward reducing the joint volume and eliminating redundant capsule. The upper flap is sutured over the lower one for further reinforcement. (From Neer CS: Shoulder Reconstruction. WB Saunders, Philadelphia, 1990, with permission.)

quire a careful psychological and physical rehabilitation program.[13,14]

COMPLICATIONS

The axillary nerve is not uncommonly injured in a traumatic anterior glenohumeral dislocation. Careful motor examination of the deltoid and teres minor muscles and sensory examination along the lateral border of the upper arm is mandatory prior to and after reduction of the shoulder.

A complete neurologic examination should always be performed to rule out any associated brachial plexus injury.

Careful and strict attention to surgical detail should avoid the complications of injury to the axillary and musculocutaneous nerves, which have been reported in surgical procedures for recurrent anterior dislocation.[20,21]

Most nerve injuries following anterior dislocation of the shoulder are neuroproxias and will recover with rest and time.

THE SHOULDER IN OBSTETRICAL BRACHIAL PLEXUS PALSY

The incidence of congenital brachial plexus palsy ranges from 0.25 to 2.60 per 1,000 live births.[22-24] In the upper lesions (Erb's palsy), the muscles innervated by the fifth and sixth cervical roots are involved. Specifically, the deltoid, supraspinatus, infraspinatus, and teres minor are weak or paralyzed, resulting in an inability to abduct and externally rotate the arm. Paralysis or weakness of the biceps, brachialis, and supinator results in an inability to flex the elbow and supinate the forearm.

The most common form of obstetrical brachial plexus palsy involves all the nerve roots (C5 through T1). As a consequence the hand and wrist are involved as well as the shoulder and elbow. Isolated involvement of the seventh, eighth and first thoracic nerve roots (Klumpke's palsy) results in a position of supination of the forearm, dorsiflexion of the wrist and flexion contracture of the fingers.

Shoulder contractures and subluxation in congenital brachial plexus palsy occur due to the shortening of subscapularis, teres major, and latissimus dorsi, resulting in the shoulder being held in adduction, internal rotation, and slight forward flexion. With time, the contractures lead to bony deformities, including retroversion of the humeral head and posterior subluxation of the shoulder. The acromion bends anteriorly and inferiorly over the front of the retroverted humeral head and this deformity increases with age and the degree of posterior subluxation. The pull of the unopposed coracobrachialis results in an elongated coracoid process.

Prognosis

The incidence of spontaneous recovery is difficult to determine because of the wide variation in results Tada reported in the literature. Figures range from 7 percent to an incredible 95 percent complete recovery.[24-26] A study by Tada and coworkers[27] revealed that 70 percent of patients with myelographic evidence of root avulsion has significant sensory recovery, and 33 percent had useful motor recovery.

Nonoperative Treatment

Treatment for upper root lesions involves stretching of those muscles that potentially may become contracted. The parents are taught to stabilize the scapula against the thorax so true glenohumeral motion is realized. These exercises should continue until the child is old enough to carry out active exercises with the parents and therapist. The use of splints and braces to place the shoulder in a position of abduction and external rotation is historic now with no recent recommendations for their use in the literature.[28,29]

Operative Treatment

Operative treatment may be subdivided into three distinct types: There are proponents of primary repair of the nerve root lesion in the neonate especially in those cases with little chance of recovery.[30] The second group of operative procedures are aimed at correction of both soft tissue and bony deformity.[31] The third group of procedures involves musculotendinous transfers to augment or replace weakened or paralyzed muscles.[31,32]

For those children with significant internal rotation deformity, the shoulder capsule may be released anteriorly by sectioning the subscapularis, and pectoralis major (the Sever procedure).[26] Others believe the internal rotation deformity is best managed by an osteotomy of the humerus above the deltoid insertion with external rotation of the distal fragment, enough to allow the hand to move to the mouth (30 to 45 degrees of external rotation).[33,34] The osteotomy is fixed with a four-hold compression plate.

The third group of operative procedures involve transfers to facilitate external rotation and abduction of the shoulder. The L'Episcopo procedure involves transfers of the teres major and latissimus dorsi to the posterior aspect of the humerus to promote external rotation.[35] There have been many modifications to the L'Episcopo procedure since its original description in 1934. Aston[36] reviewed the Texas Scottish Rite experience with congenital brachial plexus palsy and found the best results were those with a combined anterior release and tendon transfer (Sever-L'Episcopo procedure).

Others have tried to provide abductor function by transferring the trapezius after elongating it with a fascial tube to the proximal humerus or transferring the latissimus dorsi and teres major into the rotator cuff. Hoffer and coworkers[37] reported a 64 percent increase in active abduction and 45 percent increase in active external rotation.

SUMMARY

The overall incidence of shoulder dislocation in children is small. However, the recurrence rate after traumatic dislocations is extremely high. It is vitally important to determine whether the dislocation is traumatic or atraumatic for the surgical treatment of recurrent traumatic dislocation is most often successful, while surgery for atraumatic recurrences is universally doomed to failure.

REFERENCES

1. Rowe CR: Prognosis in dislocation of the shoulder. J Bone Joint Surg [Am] 38:957, 1956
2. Asher MA: Dislocations of the upper extremity in children. Orthop Clin North Am 7:583, 1976
3. Dameron TB, Rockwood CA: Part 2: Subluxations and dislocations of the glenohumeral joint. In Rockwood CA, Green DP (eds): Fractures. 2nd Ed. Vol. 3. JB Lippincott, Philadelphia, 1984
4. Foster WS, Ford TB, Dreg D: Isolated posterior shoulder dislocation in a child. Am J Sports Med 13:198, 1985
5. Heck CC: Anterior dislocation of the glenohumeral joint in a child. J Trauma 21:174, 1981
6. Matsen FA III, Thomas SC, Rockwood CA Jr: Anterior glenohumeral instability. In Rockwood CA, Matsen FA III (eds): The Shoulder. Vol. 1. WB Saunders, Philadelphia, 1990
7. Magnuson PB, Stack JK: Recurrent dislocation of the shoulder. JAMA 123:889, 1943
8. Rowe CR: Anterior dislocation of the shoulder: prognosis and treatment. Surg Clin North Am 43:1609, 1963
9. Wagner KT, Lyne ED: Adolescent and traumatic dislocations of the shoulder with open epiphyses. J Pediatr Orthop 3:61, 1983
10. Laskin RS, Sedlin ED: Luxatio erecta in infancy. Clin Orthop 80:126, 1971
11. Simonet WT, Cofield RH: Prognosis in anterior shoulder dislocation. Am J Sports Med 12:19, 1984
12. Rowe CR, Sakellarides HT: Factors related to recurrences of anterior dislocation of the shoulder. Clin Orthop 20:40, 1961
13. Lawhon SM, Peoples AB, McEwen GD: Voluntary dislocation of the shoulder. J Pediatr Orthop 2:590, 1982
14. Rowe CR, Pierce DS, Clark JG: Voluntary dislocation of the shoulder. J Bone Joint Surg [Am] 55:445, 1973
15. Bankart ASB: The pathology and treatment of recurrent dislocation of the shoulder joint. Br J Surg 26:23, 1939
16. Barry TP, Lomardo SJ, Kerlan RK et al: The coracoid transfer for recurrent anterior instability of the shoulder in adolescents. J Bone Joint Surg [Am] 67:383, 1985
17. Neer CS II: Involuntary inferior and multidirectional in-

17. stability of the shoulder: etiology, recognition and treatment. Instr Course Lect 34:232, 1985
18. Neer CS II, Foster CR: Inferior capsular shift for involuntary inferior and multidirectional instability of the shoulder: a preliminary report. J Bone Joint Surg [Am] 62:897, 1980
19. Zuckerman JD, Matsen FA: Complications about the glenohumeral joint related to the use of screws and staples. J Bone Joint Surg [Am] 66:175, 1984
20. Back FR, O'Brien SJ, Warren RF, Leighton M: An unusual neurological complication of the Bristow procedure: a case report. J Bone Joint Surg [Am] 70:458, 1988
21. Richards RR, Hudson AR, Bertoia JT et al: Injury to the brachial plexus during Putti Platt and Bristow procedures: a report of eight cases. Am J Sports Med 15:374, 1987
22. Greenwald AE, Schute PC, and Shively JL: Brachial plexus birth palsy: a ten-year report on the incidence and prognosis. J Pediatr Orthop 4:689, 1984
23. Hardy AE: Birth injuries of the brachial plexus and incidence and prognosis. J Bone Joint Surg [Br] 63:98, 1981
24. Specht EE: Brachial plexus palsy in the newborn: incidence and prognosis. Clin Orthop 110:32, 1975
25. Rubin A: Birth injuries: incidence, mechanism and end results. Obstet Gynecol 23:218, 1964
26. Sever JW: Obstetrical paralysis. Surg Gynecol Obstet 44:547, 1927
27. Tada K, Tsuyuguchi Y, Kawai H: Birth palsy: natural recovery course and combined root avulsion. J Pediatr Orthop 4:279, 1984
28. Brown KLB: Review of obstetrical palsies, nonoperative treatment. p. 499. In Terzis JK (ed): Microreconstruction of nerve injuries. WB Saunders, Philadelphia, 1987
29. Leffert R: Brachial plexus injuries. In: Congenital Brachial Palsy. Churchill Livingstone, New York, 1985
30. Kawabata H, Masada K, Tsuyuguchi Y et al: Early microsurgical reconstruction in birth palsy. Clin Orthop 215:233, 1987
31. Wilkins KE: Special problems with the child's shoulder. p. 1033. In Matsen FA III, Rockwood CA Jr. (eds): The Shoulder. Vol. 2. WB Saunders, Philadelphia, 1990
32. Wickstrom J, Haslam ET, Hutchinson RH: The surgical management of residual deformities of the shoulder following birth injuries of the brachial plexus. J Bone Joint Surg [Am] 37:27, 1955
33. Blount WP, Zuegr RC: Drilling osteoclasis for upper extremity deformity. Orthop Rev 7:53, 1978
34. Goddard NJ, Fixsen JA: Rotation osteotomy of the humerus for birth injuries of the brachial plexus. J Bone Joint Surg [Br] 66:257, 1984
35. L'Episcopo JB: Tendon transplantation in obstetrical paralysis. Am J Surg 25:122, 1934
36. Aston JW: Brachial plexus birth palsy. Orthopedics 2:544, 1979
37. Hoffer MM, Wickenden R, Roper B: Brachial plexus birth palsies: results of tendon transfers to the rotator cuff. J Bone Joint Surg [Am] 60:691, 1978

11

Supracondylar Fractures of the Humerus

William McIntyre

> God grant you in orthopaedic surgery and in the common ways of life, sound common sense.
>
> —HPH GALLOWAY

DESCRIPTION AND INCIDENCE

The supracondylar fracture is a fracture in the supracondylar region of the distal humerus through the region of the coronoid and olecranon fossae. It is the most common fracture about the elbow in children. Most occur in the first decade with a peak incidence around age 6 years. The left arm is reported to be fractured up to twice as often as the right even in left-handed individuals.[1,2]

Elbow hyperextension and relatively weak upper extremity muscles are predisposing factors in producing this fracture in the skeletally immature. Children falling on their outstretched arms will be more likely to lock their elbows in hyperextension rather than rely on weak muscles to ease them down in flexion.

The thinner bone of the supracondylar area both in the lateral and medial ridges, and in the central coronoid and olecranon fossae, combine to produce a structurally weaker area of the distal humerus.

ANATOMIC CONSIDERATIONS

There is a variable anterior tilt of the ossified capitellum as seen on the lateral radiographic view (the lateral humerocapitellar angle). With any elbow injury it is often advisable to obtain radiographs of the opposite elbow for comparison. The lateral humerocapitellar angle can vary from 25 to 70 degrees, with most in the 35- to 40-degree range.

All three major nerves median, radial, and ulnar, as well as the brachial artery running with the median nerve, are vulnerable to injury in the type 3 displaced fractures (especially type 3b) (Table 11-1).

It is the proximal shaft metaphyseal fragment that penetrates the soft tissues (usually the brachialis anteriorly) that produces the greatest damage. The falling body weight of the child predisposes to this penetration and falls from heights are more prone to result in associated soft tissue injury. When there is a posteromedially displaced distal fragment the proximal shaft fragment penetrates anterolaterally placing the radial nerve at greater risk for injury. With the posterolaterally displaced distal fragment the median nerve and brachial artery are at greater risk from the penetrating proximal shaft fragment. The ulnar nerve is more at risk with the rarer anteriorly displaced distal fragment.

DIAGNOSTIC FEATURES

The Periosteal Hinge

The periosteum is torn on the side where the shaft comes to rest, and is intact on the side to which the distal fragment displaces. The "closed" side of the fracture

TABLE 11-1. Classification of Supracondylar Fractures in Children

Type	Displacement	Tilt
1a	No displacement	<5° retrotilt No medial or lateral fracture gap
1b	No displacement	≤15°–20° retrotilt ≤1 mm medial or lateral fracture gap
2a	Displacement 0–2 mm on AP or lateral radiographic views	Retrotilt >15°–20° And/or >1 mm medial or lateral fracture gap And/or impaction of medial or lateral bone on the "closed" side
2b	Straight or rotatory displacement of 2–15 mm, but still some fracture contact	Variable tilt
3a	Complete loss of fracture contact and ≤20 mm overlap, or rotatory displacement >15 mm with one side fracture contact	Variable tilt
3b	Wide displacement with soft tissue gap between bone ends And/or >2 cm overlap And/or rotatory displacement >15 mm with no fracture contact	Variable tilt

refers to the side with the intact periosteum. The "open" side of the fracture refers to the side where the periosteum is disrupted. Frequently, there is an element of medial or lateral displacement along with posterior displacement so that the periosteum is more intact posteromedially or posterolaterally. One can sometimes surmise this from the initial radiograph but can be deceived in the fully displaced fracture.

The position of the forearm in pronation or supination during reduction in many fractures will stabilize the reduction thus minimizing excessive varus or valgus tilt.[3,4] It depends mainly on the direction of the initial force and where the periosteal sleeve remains intact. With a medially displaced distal fragment the periosteum is intact on the medial side. As the forearm is pronated the medial collateral ligament is tightened, pulling the distal fragment down medially and tightening the periosteal hinge to stabilize the reduction preventing varus tilt, and closing up the lateral gap.

Varus or Valgus Tilt

The fracture that has buckling (crush) of the medial or lateral supracondylar ridges has the potential to tilt into varus or valgus. The minimally displaced fracture where the fracture line is visible on one side and not the other as seen on the anterior view (Fig. 11-1) already has some slight varus or valgus tilt, which has the potential to increase if the fracture is not securely stabilized. This can usually be accomplished by pronating or supinating the forearm to counteract the tilt. Hence in Figure 11-1 the forearm should be supinated to prevent further valgus tilt and to close the medial gap. It must be emphasized that the distal fragment only exerts correction of the varus or valgus tilt after the forearm has reached the *maximum* range of pronation or supination.

Carrying Angle

The carrying angle in children varies; often less in the young and increasing to an average of 15 degrees of valgus at maturity, but in a given individual it may vary from 0 to 25 degrees. The carrying angle tends to favor varus tilt, medial redisplacement, and medial rotation through the force of gravity on the immobilized arm. Those fractures that were initially displaced posteromedially are therefore more prone to redisplacement after closed reduction than those fractures that were initially displaced posterolaterally. The opposite elbow should always be examined to determine the child's normal carrying angle. If the initial carrying angle was 20 to 25 degrees, a loss of 10 degrees would not be as visible as a

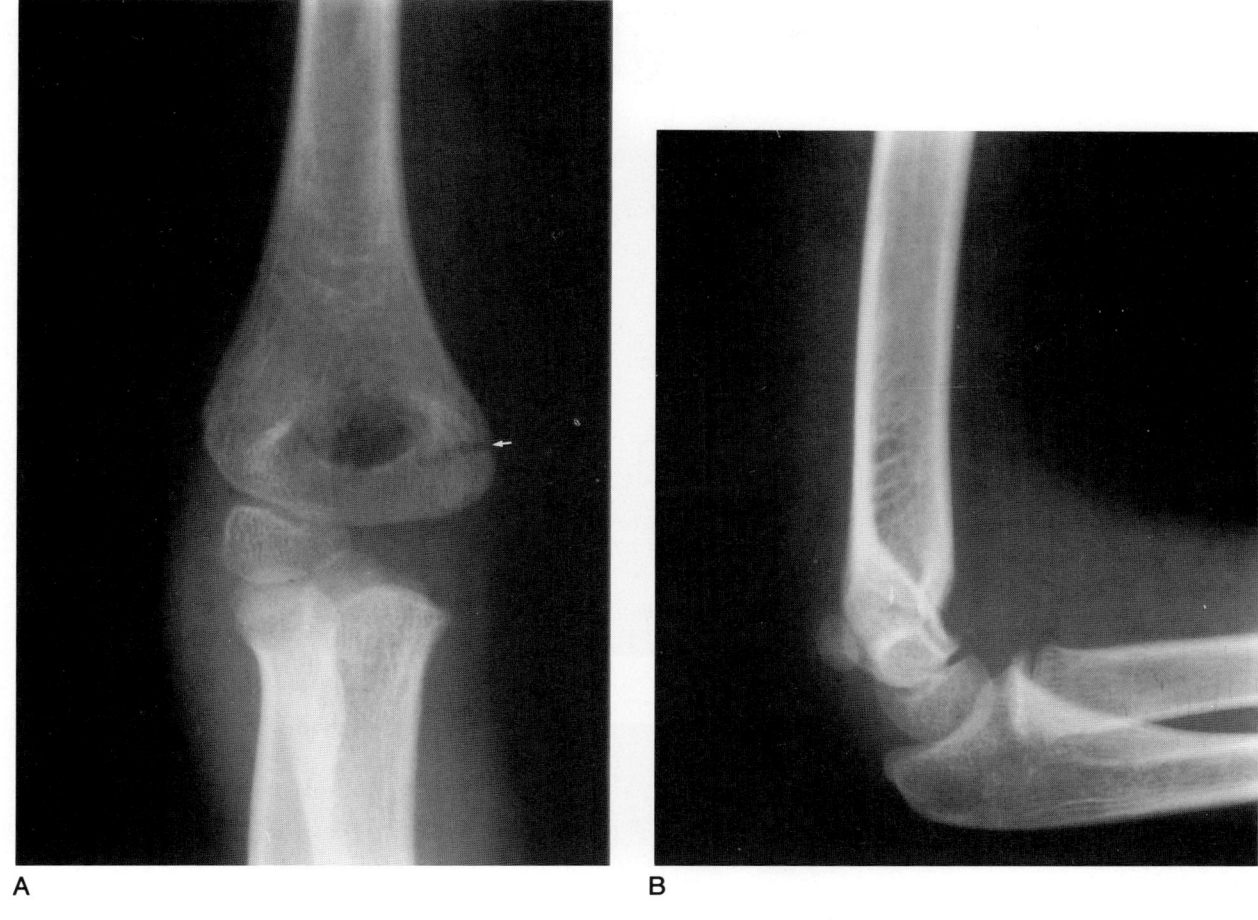

Fig. 11-1. (A) A minimally displaced type 1b fracture with the fracture visible on the "open" medial side. (B) The lateral shows the fracture anterior with only 5 to 10 degrees of retrotilt of the distal fragment.

loss of 10 degrees from an initial carrying angle of 0 to 5 degrees.

Radiologic Measurements

The radiologic anatomy that needs to be considered in evaluating fragment tilt and displacement include the following:

1. The anterior humeral line: This is a line drawn along the anterior humeral shaft and intersecting the middle to posterior one-third of the capitellar ossification center.[5] This will detect posterior tilt or displacement, but will not distinguish between the two (Fig. 11-2).

2. The lateral humerocapitellar angle: This is the angle of anterior tilt of the capitellum as determined on a lateral view by a line along the flat proximal edge of the capitellar ossification center, and a transverse line perpendicular to the shaft. This angle is usually about 35 to 40 degrees, but may vary from 25 to 65 degrees, the higher angles being in younger children, emphasizing the need to have a radiograph of the other elbow for comparison (Fig. 11-3).

On anteroposterior (AP) radiographic views Baumann's angle (Fig. 11-4) can be useful and several authors have indicated that this is helpful in the acute management as well as in follow-up.[2,6,7-9] This angle is formed by a line drawn along the distal capitellar metaphysis and the transverse line that is perpendicular to the

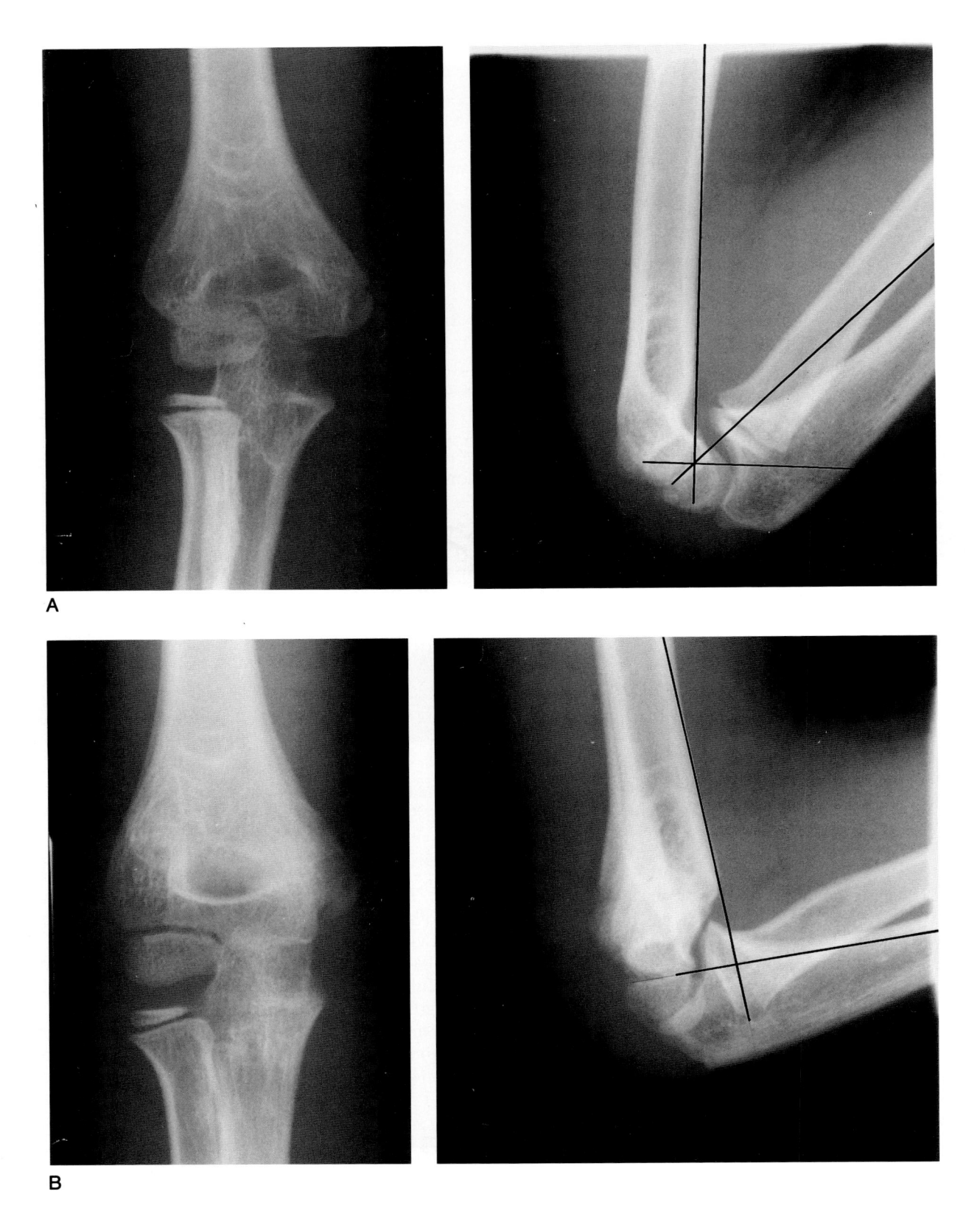

Fig. 11-2. **(A)** The normal anterior humeral line intersects the middle to posterior one-third of the capitellum. On this patient the humerocapitellar angle is 45 degrees (if the shaft above were used it would be 50 degrees). **(B)** The opposite elbow 3 months following a fracture that healed in retrotilt of 45 degrees, with the anterior humeral line well in front of the capitellum, and the humerocapitellar angle of 0 degrees.

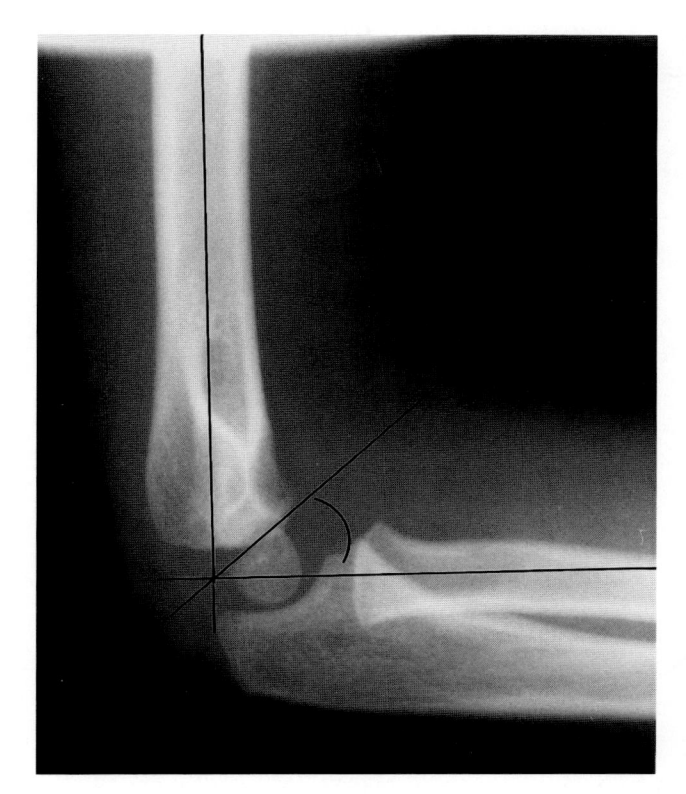

Fig. 11-3. The humerocapitellar angle measuring from the midhumerus—in this patient 40 degrees.

shaft. This usually subtends an angle of 10 to 20 degrees. It has been mentioned that this Baumann's angle is calculated on a radiograph taken perpendicular to the *humerus*, not tilted to be parallel to the capitellar physis.[10]

With all of these radiologic measurements the best reference for the achievement of an adequate reduction is the child's other elbow.[8,7] It is surprising how often the capitellum will be retrotilted 15 to 30 degrees and be interpreted as "undisplaced" if the angles are not measured on the radiograph of the uninjured extremity.

MECHANISM OF INJURY

The most common mechanism of injury is a fall on the outstretched hand with the elbow locked in hyperextension. In this position, the olecranon levers within the olecranon fossa creating a stress concentration at the supracondylar area posteriorly, while the tight anterior capsular structures help to lever the condyles into a posterior tilting and/or displacing position.[10]

This mechanism is more likely to be present in falls backward where there is greater likelihood of landing in the hyperextended position as occurred in the twin girls illustrated in Figure 11-5. Direct falls onto the elbow, usually from a height, result in anteriorly displaced supracondylar fractures of the humerus.

CLASSIFICATION

Supracondylar fractures are generally classified into extension-type fractures (95 to 98 percent) (Fig. 11-6) and flexion-type fractures (2 to 5 percent) (Fig. 11-7). We agree with the broad classification into three types as suggested by Gartland[11] and Wilkins,[12] but would subdivide these into "a" and "b" categories. The subcategories would then facilitate the appropriate management decision.

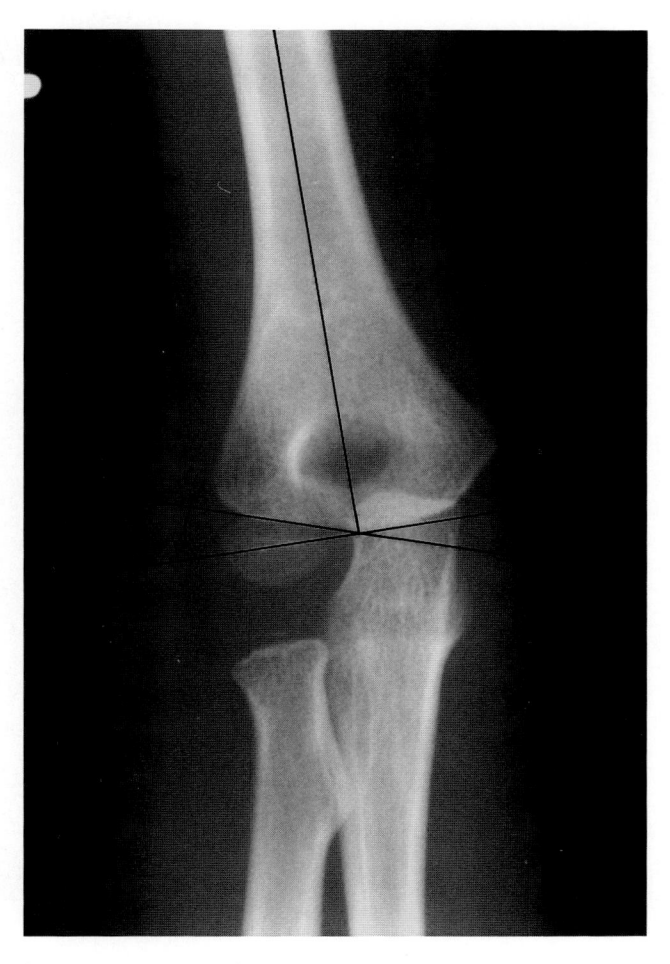

Fig. 11-4. Normal side Baumann's angle (here 18 degrees). The normal side should again be used as reference for similar placement of lines.

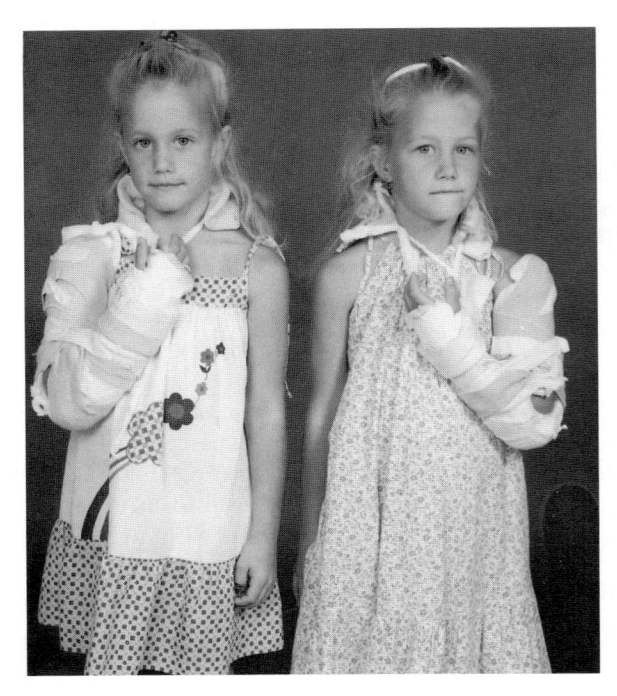

Fig. 11-5. Twins with identical type 3b posterolaterally displaced supracondylar fractures, treated by closed reduction and cast splint in full supination. The posterior splint is from hand to above shoulder. The forearm and hand are circularized to maintain maximum pronation or supination with an access hole for the radial pulse. The bandage at the elbow can be cut to allow for swelling and the cerclage tape from forearm to arm maintains flexion at the elbow. A nonstretch collar-cuff provides forward pull on the distal fragment.

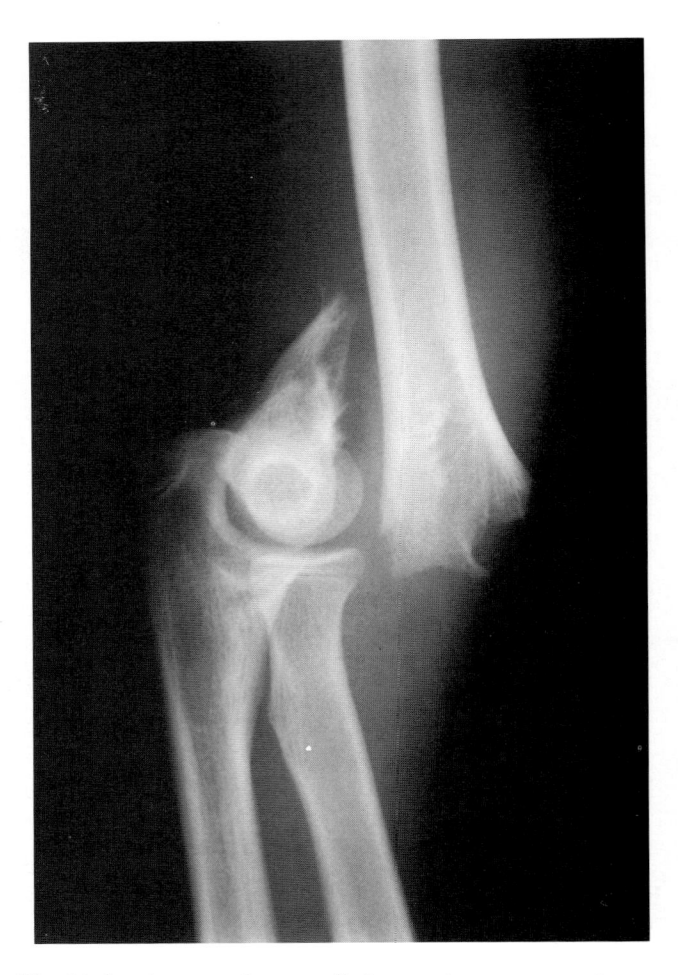

Fig. 11-6. An extension type 3b fracture in a teenager with an unstable oblique fracture pattern.

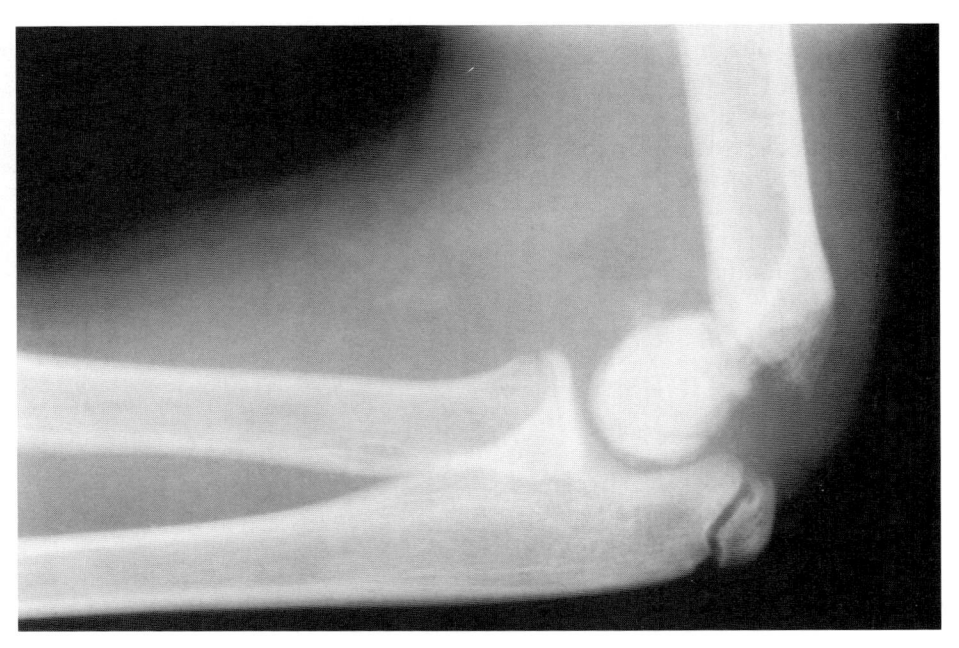

Fig. 11-7. A flexion type 2b fracture.

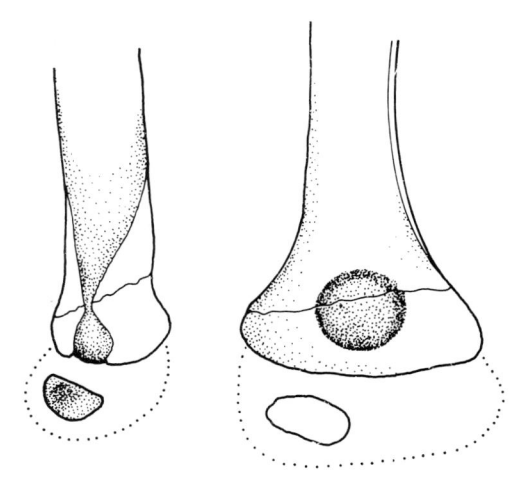

Fig. 11-8. Type 1a fracture essentially undisplaced and less than 5 degrees tilt on the lateral.

Using the terms *tilt* (rather than angulation) and *displacement* the following principles apply:

1. There can be tilt of the distal fragment posterior, anterior, medial (varus) or lateral (valgus).
2. There can be displacement in any of those four directions as well.
3. There can be axial rotation of the distal fragment in a medial (internal) or lateral (external) direction.

The residual malrotation after reduction is also important, not for the alteration of rotation of the humerus, but as it predisposes to varus or valgus tilt.[8,13] The greater the rotation the less contact between the two thin surfaces of the humeral fragments, and a teeter-totter effect occurs, which often results in the distal fragment slipping into varus and, less commonly, valgus.

This classification is described for the more common posteriorly displaced fractures but would equally apply in reverse for the anteriorly displaced fractures (Table 11-1).

Type 1a

Type 1a fractures (Fig. 11-8) are completely undisplaced with under 5 degrees of tilt on the lateral view, and no medial or lateral fracture gap visible on the AP view. They may be only detectable by clinical tenderness. If initial radiographs show no fracture, the "fat-pad sign" may indicate the possible presence of a fracture (Fig. 11-15).

Type 1b

Type 1b fractures (Fig. 11-9) demonstrate no displacement on the AP and lateral views. On the lateral view there is a mild tilt of less than 15 to 20 degrees loss of humerocapitellar angle; and on the AP view less than 1 mm of fracture gap, medial or lateral, on the "open" side of the fracture. There is *no* impaction (buckling) of supracondylar bone on the "closed" side of the fracture.

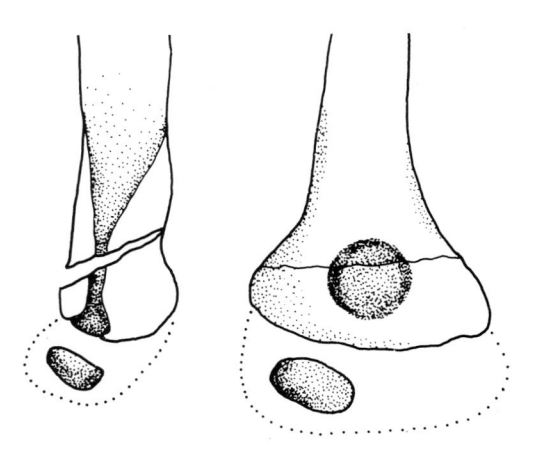

Fig. 11-9. A type 1b fracture no displacement, less than 15 to 20 degrees tilt on the lateral, and 1 mm or less of medial or lateral fracture gap.

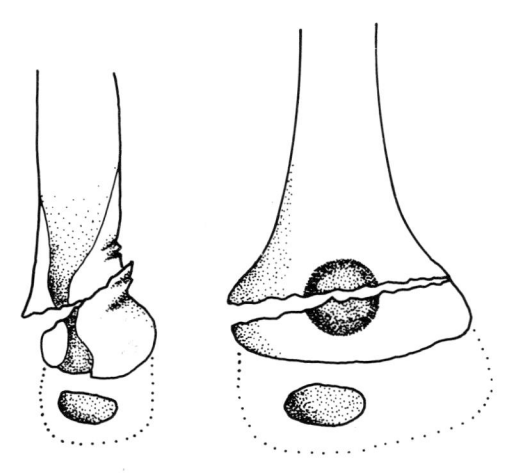

Fig. 11-10. A type 2a fracture, which has slight displacement up to 2 mm and/or moderate retrotilt over 15 to 20 degrees and/or medial or lateral fracture gap over 1 mm and/or impaction of bone on the "closed" side.

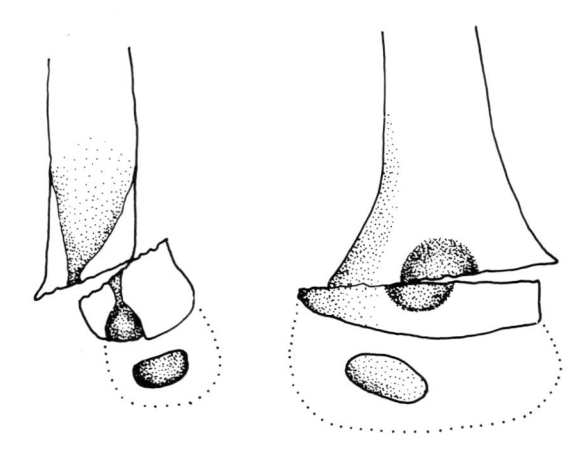

Fig. 11-11. A type 2b fracture with displacement of 2 to 15 mm, and usually with moderate tilt on AP or lateral views.

Type 2a

Type 2a supracondylar fractures (Fig. 11-10) may have displacement of up to 2 mm on AP or lateral view, and/or moderate retrotilt of over 15 to 20 degrees on the lateral film; and/or *on the anteroposterior radiographic view* a varus or valgus *tilt* with greater than 1 mm lateral or medial gap, and/or impaction of medial or lateral supracondylar bone on the "closed" side.

Type 2b

Type 2b fractures (Fig. 11-11) have a straight or rotatory displacement of 2 to 15 mm on AP or lateral views but still some fracture surface contact; and usually with a moderate tilt on the lateral and/or AP views.

Type 3a

Type 3a fractures (Fig. 11-12) demonstrate a full loss of fracture surface contact but still retain some bone contact. There is an overlap of up to 20 mm, or rotatory displacement over 15 mm with some fracture contact on one side. There may be a variable tilt on the AP and/or lateral radiographic views.

Type 3b

Type 3b fractures (Fig. 11-13) exhibit a wide displacement with (soft tissue) space between bone ends and/or over 2 cm of overlap, and/or rotatory displacement over 15 mm without any fracture contact.

Treatment Decisions

The reasons for subclassifying the three fracture types is to encourage the treating surgeon to look more critically at the radiographs and treat more vigorously those with a greater potential to develop a malunion even with "minimal" displacement (types 1b and 2a), and to very carefully deal with those that have a greater potential for neurovascular compromise.

The truly undisplaced type 1a fracture does not need treatment in terms of reduction but just protection against reinjury.

Type 1b might remodel satisfactorily untreated, but some of these may worsen during immobilization and

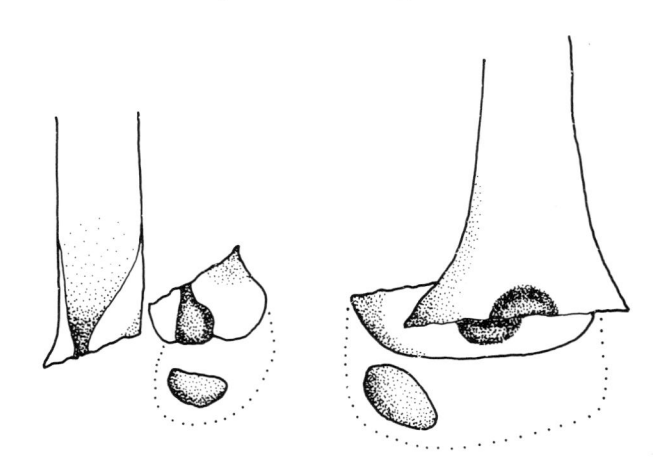

Fig. 11-12. A type 3a fracture with full loss of fracture surface contact and overlap up to 20 mm, or rotatory displacement over 15 mm with fracture contact on one side.

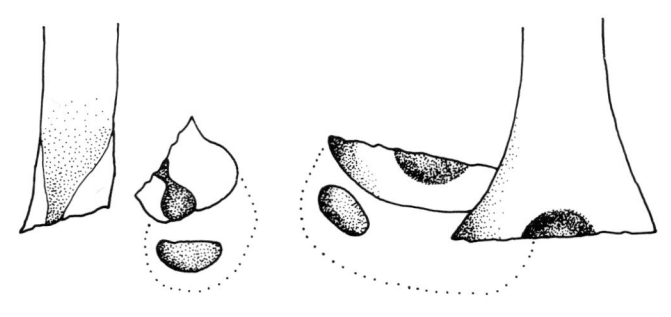

Fig. 11-13. A type 3b fracture with full loss of bone contact (space for soft tissue trapping between bone ends) and/or over 2 cm overlap, and/or over 15 mm rotatory displacement, without fracture contact.

become more like type 2a and end up with a malunion. Appropriate positioning in a cast splint would minimize this.

Types 2a and 2b should have a closed reduction, preferably under anesthesia with image intensifier assessment of position and stability and the effect of pronation and supination. Some type 2b fractures may need pinning.

Types 3a and 3b fractures all need reduction, some closed with pinning and others possibly open with pinning. Because of the greater potential for soft tissue interposition with type 3b fractures, the indications for open reduction with these fractures is greater.

PHYSICAL EXAMINATION

Because of the frequency of neurovascular compromise with the supracondylar fracture of the humerus it is important to perform an accurate neurovascular examination, and when possible a *quantitative* comparison to the normal side.

The status of the radial pulse must be documented on arrival in the emergency department, and monitored following any position or splinting change. An absent pulse should initiate expeditious management.

An obviously deformed elbow should be splinted before the child is sent to the radiography department to minimize chances of further damage to vital structures. Specific instructions should be given to the x-ray technician to take a "shoot through" lateral and not to rotate the arm for the lateral view.

The sensory function in a child should always be compared to the normal side. The young child may state he or she can feel touch when there is a partial sensory deficit, but frequently can identify a difference between the two sides, when the same finger on each hand is touched simultaneously. Motor function should be documented in a quantitative fashion for individual nerve function and range of active motion of the fingers. It is helpful to retest the neurovascular status immediately before treatment as it is not uncommon for the findings to worsen between initial arrival and treatment. Swelling of the elbow region may be extensive even in the mildly displaced fractures.

Focal ecchymosis or skin puckering is usually an indication of a markedly displaced type 3b fracture.

Doppler assessment of the radial pulse may be helpful for the difficult to palpate or absent pulse, and it may be of some help to trace the brachial pulse anterior or posterior to the shaft fragment in type 3b fractures. The position of prereduction splinting should usually be between 30 and 45 degrees flexion to relax the anterior structures of the elbow.

Excess flexion may kink the neurovascular structures and excess extension might stretch them over the sharp shaft fragment. A recheck of the radial pulse after splinting will ensure that the splinting position has not made it worse.

Differential Diagnosis

A posterolateral dislocation of the elbow can produce a deformity similar to a displaced supracondylar fracture.

Many of the other fractures about the elbow also have to be ruled out by appropriate radiographic assessment. These would include T-condylar, lateral condylar (Salter-Harris type IV), medial condylar (Salter-Harris type IV), transcondylar (epiphyseal) (Salter-Harris types I and II).

Less often, fractures below the elbow, such as the radial neck or olecranon, may have a similar appearance to a supracondylar fracture and in rare instances may coexist with a supracondylar fracture.

Concomitant fractures in the forearm do sometimes occur (Fig. 11-14) and the double injury would necessitate greater care in management to minimize chances of neurovascular compromise from the enhanced swelling potential. Percutaneous pinning of the supracondylar fracture would be strongly indicated so that the elbow need not be flexed acutely.

TREATMENT

There has been no uniformity of opinion concerning the ideal method of treatment of displaced supracondylar fractures. Treatment modalities recommended include no reduction and immobilization, closed reduction and plaster immobilization,[14-21] closed reduction

176 / Management of Pediatric Fractures

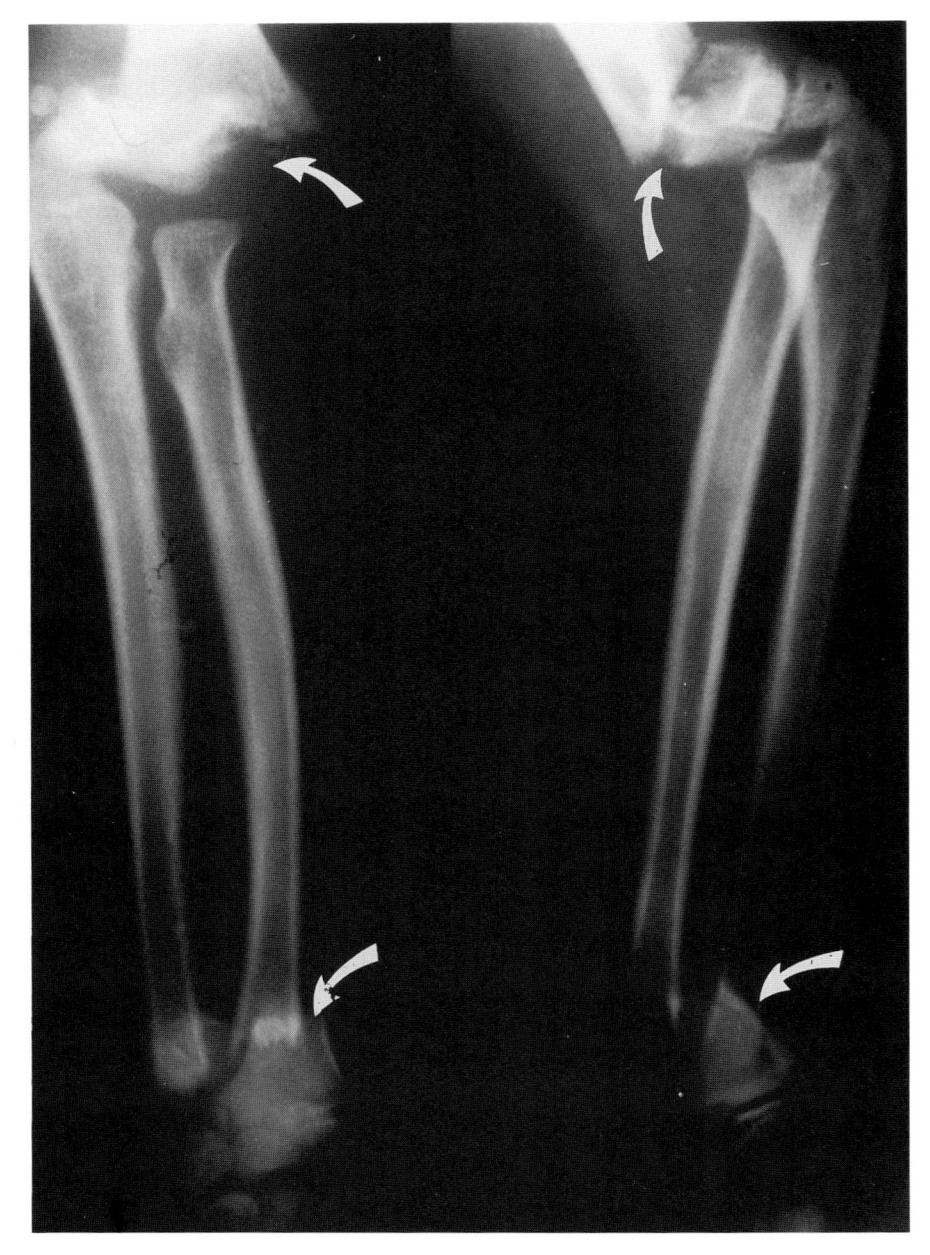

Fig. 11-14. A supracondylar fracture of the humerus with distal radius and ulna fracture in a 6-year-old who fell from a play structure.

and percutaneous pinning,[2,7,8,12,19–26] open reduction and internal fixation,[12,14,19,27–29] and occasionally the use of traction.[14,17,19,24,30–36]

It is often beneficial to compare the fractured elbow with the normal side to properly classify the fracture and follow appropriate principles of management. It is critical at all stages of the initial treatment and early follow-up to monitor the radial pulse, as well as the sensory and motor function of all three major nerves, especially in the type 3b fractures.

Supracondylar Cast-Splint

With the potential for further swelling in even the minimally displaced or tilted supracondylar fractures a circular cast about the elbow should be avoided.

With most of the methods of treatment, continuous immobilization is required for only the first 3 weeks. Following this, a removable splint can be used for protection during activities until the child regains confidence in the elbow, and bone healing is more complete, allowing removal for frequent supervised *active* mobilization to minimize stiffness.

The preferred immobilization technique for any fracture that is closed reduced or has a potential to displace should (1) allow access to the radial pulse, (2) allow for swelling anterior to the elbow, (3) allow for adjustability of the elbow flexion (toward elbow extension if the pulse is decreased and toward more flexion as swelling diminishes), and (4) control maximum pronation or supination position. A plaster analogous to a cast-splint can fulfill this role reasonably well (Fig. 11-5).

After reduction, the assistant maintains a finger on the radial pulse, cast padding is wrapped on the forearm and hand and a long-arm posterior splint (3-in.) is lined with padding and is applied from the hand to *above* the shoulder. This is wrapped with a 2-in. plaster around the hand, wrist, and lower half of the forearm with the appropriate maximum pronation or supination. The finger on the pulse ensures subsequent pulse access as the cast is applied around it. A flexible gauze bandage is firmly wrapped from below elbow to above shoulder to mold the upper part of the splint. An elastic bandage is added over the gauze after the first 24 to 48 hours. The gauze is frequently split at the anterior elbow, and sometimes at the axilla.

Flexion is maintained by a cerclage of 1-in. tape around the back half of the upper arm and circumferential around the forearm cast component. This can easily be adjusted for further flexing or extending the elbow as required by the associated elbow swelling. If medial rotation is to be avoided, an elastic bandage loosely swathing the upper arm to the chest with a soft bolster attached to the medial forearm can minimize internal rotation forces. A nonstretchable collar-cuff should be applied from the wrist to the neck to keep the splint pulled forward on the posterior distal humerus if a less stable fracture is treated without pin fixation.

Management Plans for the Supracondylar Fracture Types 1 and 2

The treatment must be tailored to the fracture type.

Type 1a

A type 1a fracture (Fig. 11-15) is undisplaced and effectively not tilted. A posterior splint in 90 degrees of flexion in neutral pronation-supination for 3 weeks, fol-

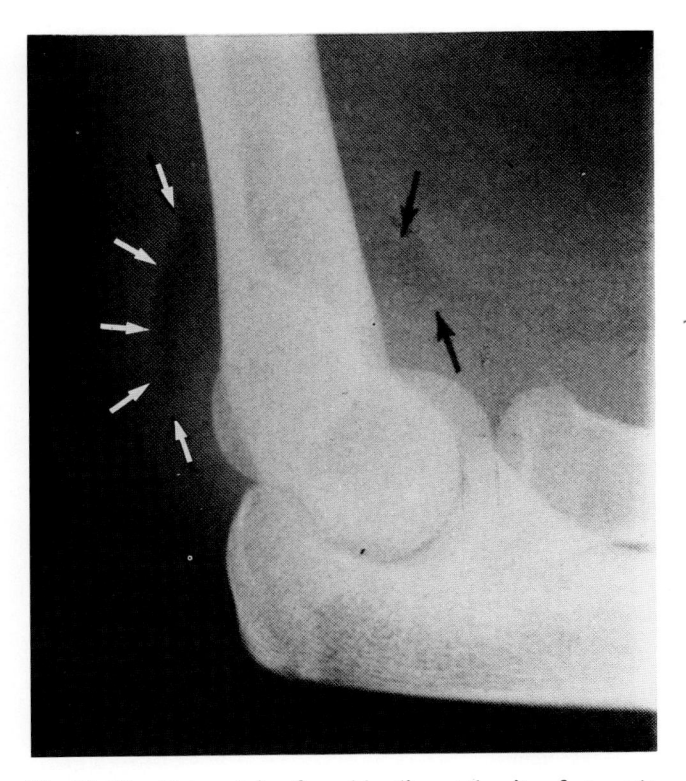

Fig. 11-15. Fat-pad sign from bleeding at the site of a type 1a fracture.

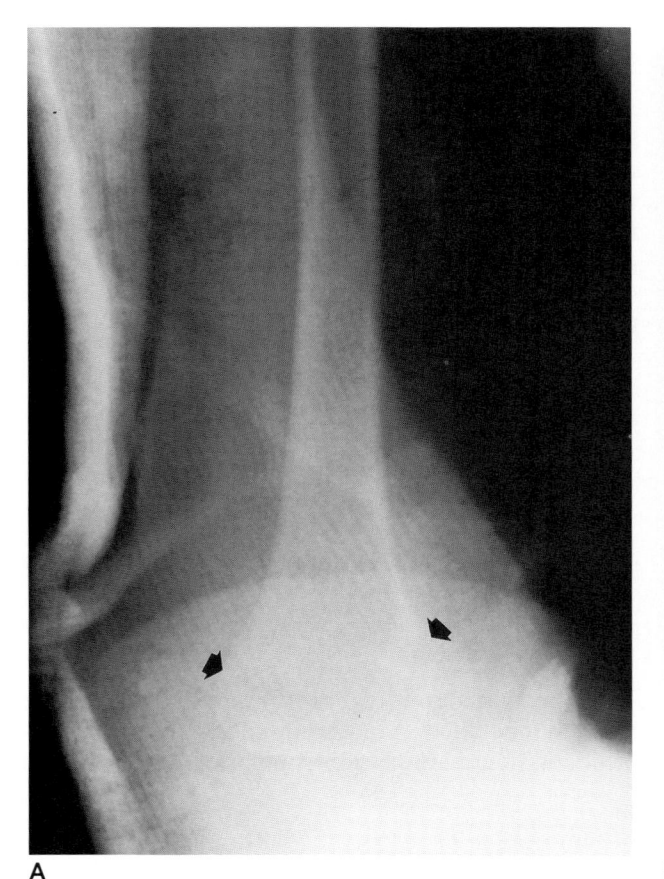

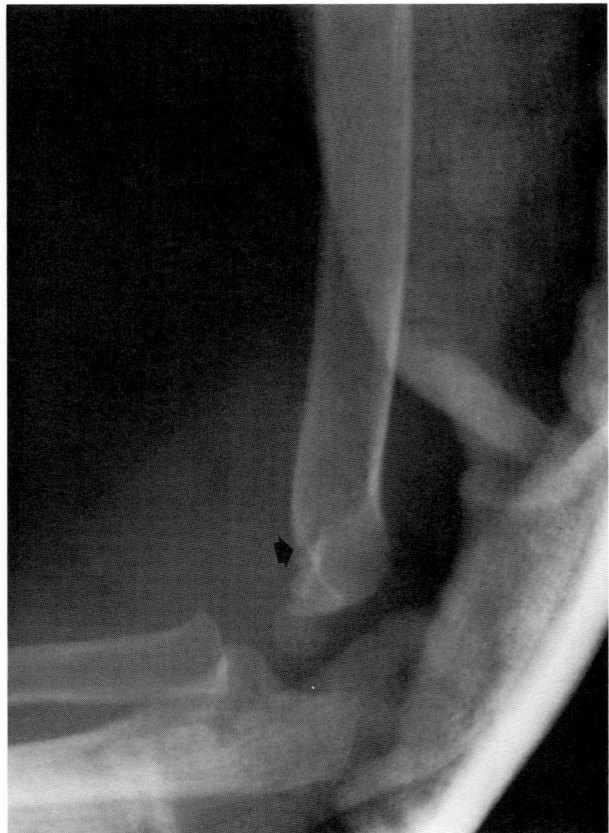

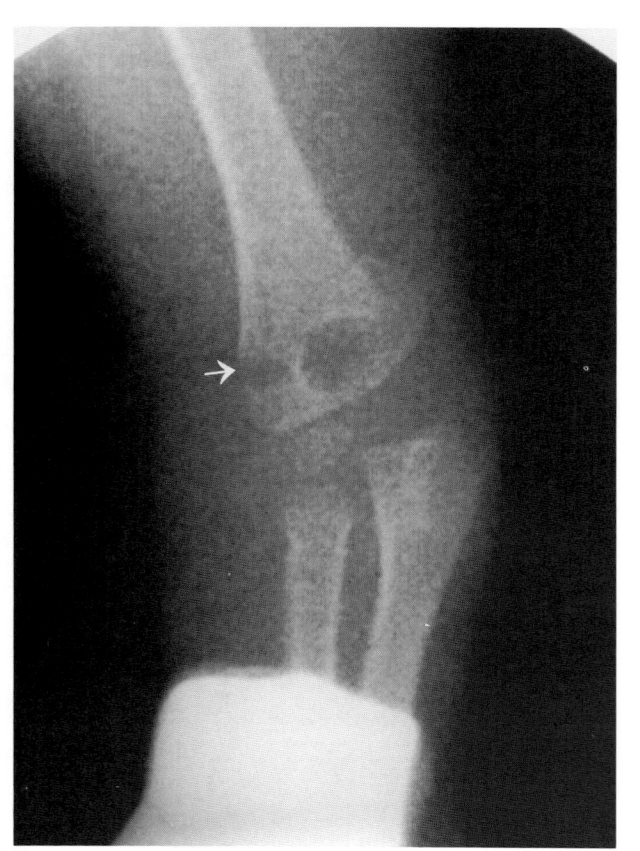

Fig. 11-16. (A) "Minimally" displaced AP view as seen through plaster splint. Note slight fracture gap laterally and a question of some impaction medially. (B) Lateral of the same "minimally" displaced fracture humerocapitellar angle measured 22 degrees. It could pass as a type 1b fracture with less than 15 to 20 degrees of retrotilt if the AP view was interpreted as undisplaced or "minimally" displaced. (C) On examination under anesthesia full supination showed lateral fracture gap opening coupled with medial overlap and impaction. *(Figure continues.)*

D   E

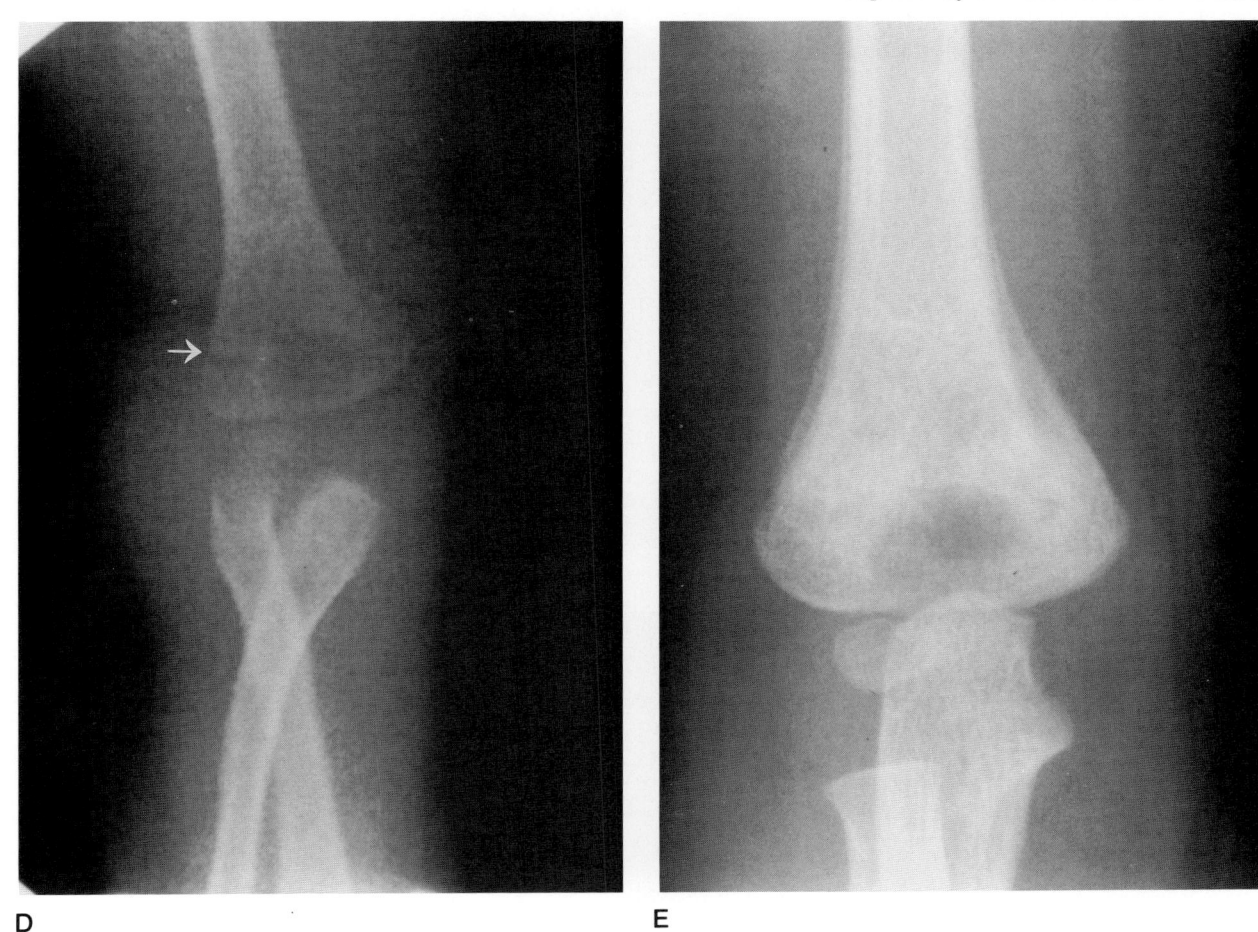

Fig. 11-16 *(Continued).* **(D)** Full pronation is shown to close up the lateral gap and improve the medial impaction. **(E)** Healing at 6 weeks shows the greater periosteal new bone medially. There is also some decrease in Baumann's angle. Pronation alone was used here with an acceptable result, but with the medial comminution and impaction, the fulcrum for closing the open lateral side by pronation has been damaged, and a better result might have been achieved if pins had been used. This is the type of case that, if not treated in pronation, would have healed in an unacceptable degree of cubitus varus.

lowed by mobilization and splinting for activities for a further 2 to 3 weeks as necessary is all that is indicated.

Type 1b

Type 1b fractures (Fig. 11-1AB) are undisplaced, but are retrotilted up to 15 to 20 degrees and may have a medial or lateral fracture gap of less than 1 mm. Some of these minimally tilted fractures have the ability to tilt further, especially into varus (Fig. 11-16). These should be managed with the long-arm combination cast-splint previously described, maintaining the appropriate pronation or supination to close the fracture gap (pronation to close a lateral gap and supination to close a medial gap).

Initial flexion should be as far as comfort allows with maintenance of a strong pulse (usually to 90 to 110 degrees). Over the following 5 to 10 days further flexion in the cast-splint is possible, gradually to about 130 degrees maintaining flexion with cerclage tape and continuing to monitor the pulse.

Type 2a

Closed reduction under general anesthesia is recommended for type 2a with appropriate testing of the pronation and supination effect on the fracture (Fig. 11-17).

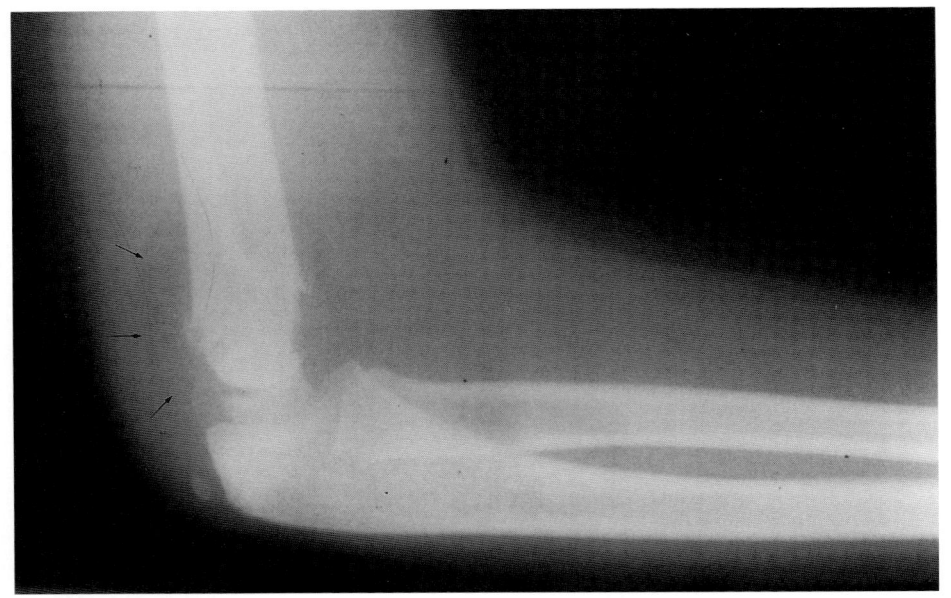

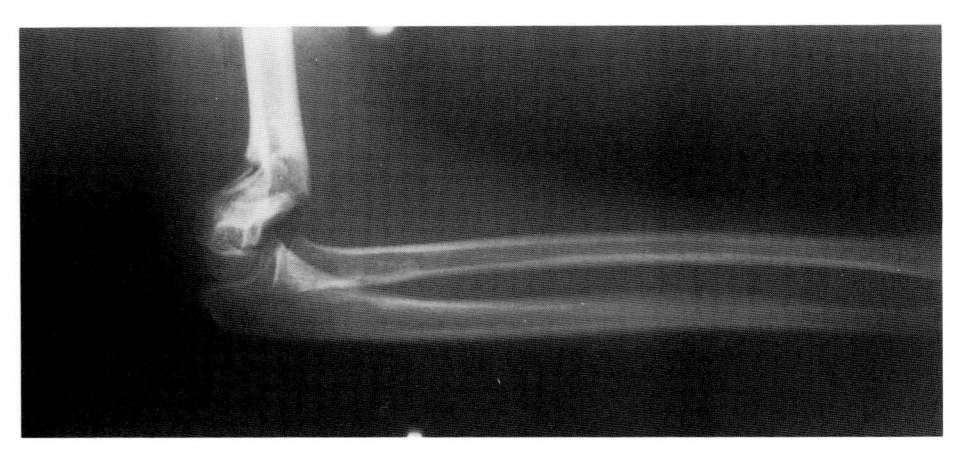

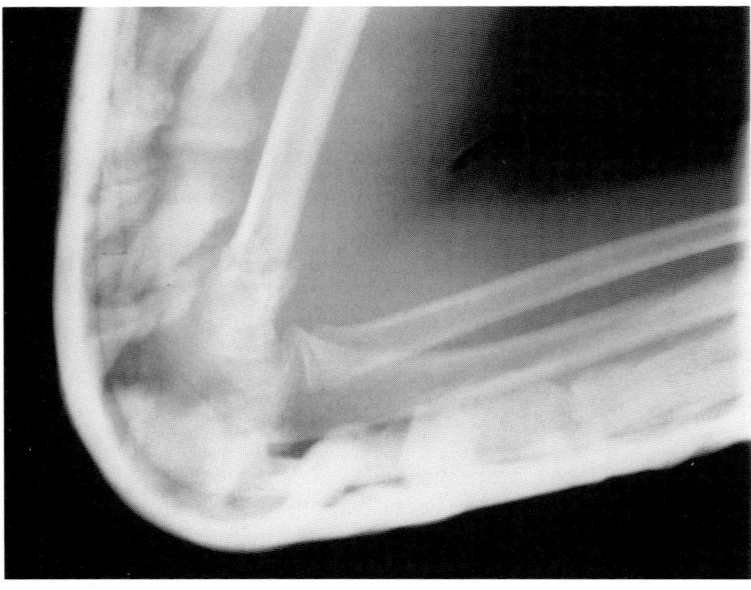

Fig. 11-17. **(A)** A type 2a fracture. This lateral view shows the fat pad sign with humerocapitellar angle demonstrating about 25 degrees of retrotilt, and 1 to 2 mm of retrodisplacement. If this were coupled with any varus or valgus tilt on AP view it probably should be reduced under relaxation with image intensifier assessment of the effects of pronation and supination. **(B)** A type 2a fracture with more significant tilt-displacement is about 2 mm (borderline for type 2b). **(C)** Following closed reduction humerocapitellar angle is restored to an acceptable degree.

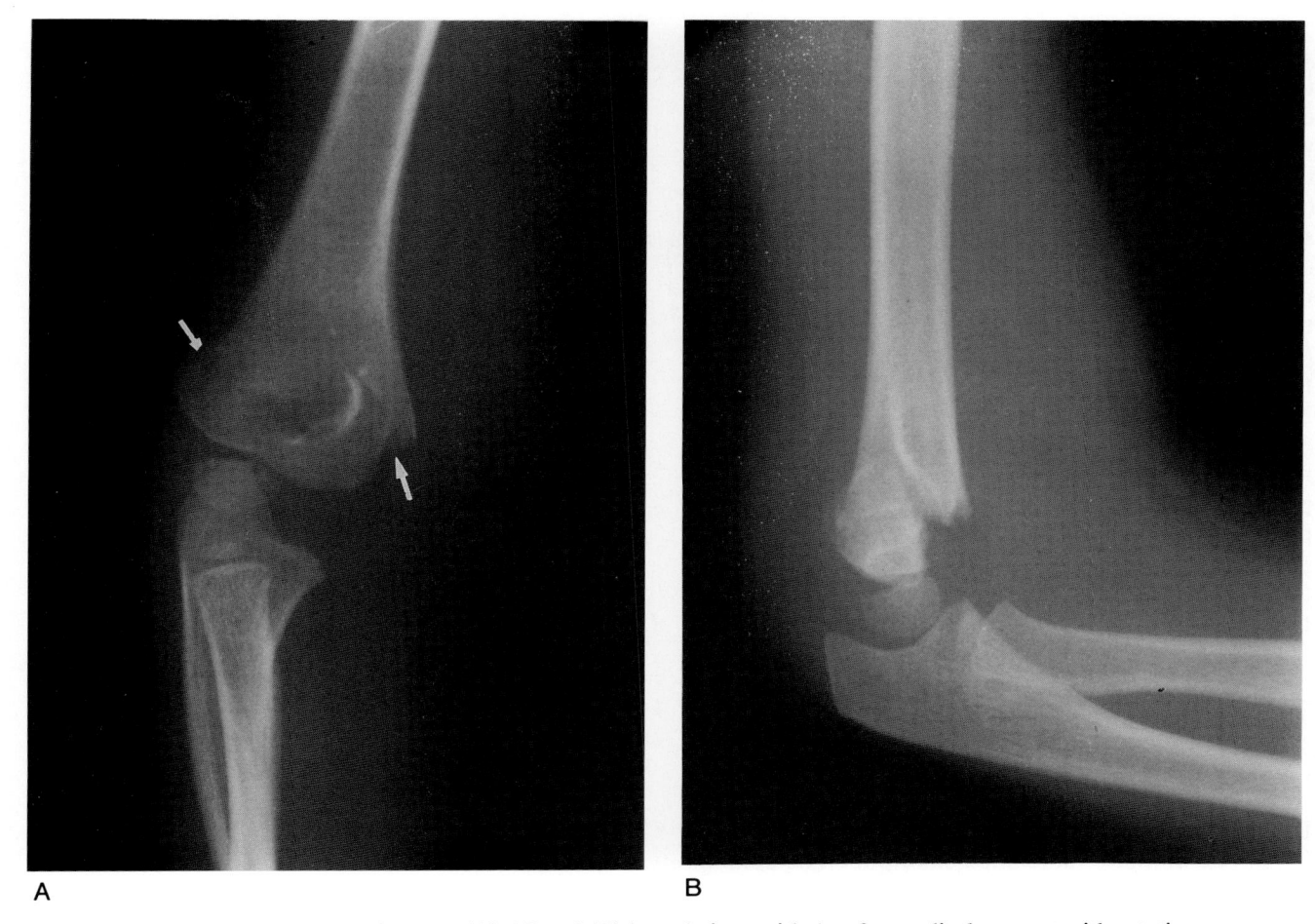

Fig. 11-18. A type 2b fracture. **(A)** AP and **(B)** lateral views with 4 to 8 mm displacement with rotation.

If there is bone buckling and shortening, particularly on the medial side, consideration for percutaneous pinning to prevent varus tilt should be entertained, as pronation alone might not be able to prevent varus tilt of the distal fragment. A single lateral pin might suffice to lock the "open" side of the fracture.

Type 2b

Treatment for type 2b may be closed reduction and immobilization with the cast-splint *as long as the fracture is stable* ie the fracture line relatively transverse, an anatomic reduction, no medial impaction, and the pulse preserved to allow 120 degrees of flexion (Fig. 11-18). It is helpful to flex the elbow until the pulse diminishes or disappears (the pulse obliteration angle), and then back down about 5 degrees from that point.

If this stable reduction cannot be obtained (and often swelling will not allow safe flexion to 120°) then percutaneous pinning should be carried out.

Closed Reduction Technique

Closed reduction should be initiated by longitudinal traction on the forearm with the elbow maintained in 30 to 40 degrees flexion to relax the anterior soft tissue structures. The traction should be in the line of the humerus, and a posteriorly directed force may be applied on the anterior humerus to control the proximal fragment.

The image intensifier should be positioned with the C-arm running parallel to the operation table so that it can be rotated for a lateral view, rather than rotating the child's arm when reduction may be incomplete, and vital soft tissue structures still at risk.

The pulse should be monitored by palpation (and, when indicated by Doppler) before reduction, after traction, and *before* flexion. If the pulse is absent initially and does not return with traction, or if the pulse disappears with traction, or the hand turns white with traction; then the brachial artery (and possibly median nerve) may be caught directly or indirectly in the fracture. The elbow should not be forcibly flexed, nor rotated for lateral radiography, and consideration should be given to open management. If circumstances are not suitable for open reduction some form of skeletal olecranon traction (modified Dunlop's) might be considered, providing there is good collateral circulation to the forearm and hand.

With displaced fractures the intact posterior periosteum needs to be relaxed to reduce the horizontal displacement of the distal fragment. This can be achieved by one person maintaining longitudinal traction on the partially flexed forearm, while the other operator applies thumbs to either side of the fracture site posteriorly controlling displacement while allowing the distal fragment to retrotilt. Medial or lateral displacement and posterior displacement should be corrected before flexing. Care should be taken to avoid anterior pressure over the distal end of the proximal shaft fragment to minimize increasing the damage to the vulnerable neurovascular structures. Only after displacement is corrected should gentle flexion until mild resistance is felt be carried out. A recheck lateral image radiograph should then be done to see if the displaced component is corrected completely. If incomplete, with thumbs posterior to block redisplacement, the distal fragment is allowed to tilt back while traction and posterior thumb pressure on the distal fragment are repeated. Sometimes pressure needs to be more medial or lateral if the radiograph shows residual malrotation. Medial or lateral displacements should also be reduced with the distal fragment retrotilted to relax the periosteal sleeve.

Once the fracture is reduced, the image intensifier can be rotated into the AP position—the AP alignment is checked, with 15-degree internal and external rotated views, to better visualize the supracondylar ridges.

Whether the fracture position will be stabilized by pronation or supination in supracondylar fractures can sometimes be inferred from the initial posteromedial or posterolateral displacement on the radiograph. However, this can be more accurately tested by placing the now reduced flexed elbow on the image intensifier in the AP mode with a small bolster, such as a sponge behind the distal fragment to give forward pressure, as a lead-gloved hand applies a downward force to the midhumerus anteriorly. This will maintain reduction while the elbow is extended below 90 degrees for a clearer radiograph of the supracondylar fracture line. Under fluoroscopy the forearm can be pronated maximally and supinated maximally (using the wrist and not the hand) to see whether the location of the periosteal hinge allows the fracture line to open up medially on pronation or laterally on supination.

If there is impaction or comminution on the hinged or "closed" side, or incomplete rotatory reduction, or a very oblique fracture line; the distal fragment may tilt by overlapping of the bone fragments on the "closed" side with or without opening up on the "open" side of the fracture line.[4,37]

Treatment of Type 3 Fractures

These are the fractures that have the highest incidence of neurovascular complications. Because of greater soft tissue disruption there is more instability after reduction. The obliquity of the fracture line, is not always well demonstrated on initial radiographs: but is better visualized on postreduction lateral views.

One should always consider where the periosteal sleeve is still intact both for achieving reduction and for determining what influence pronation and supination as well as flexion will have on the stability of the reduction. This is useful to consider even for those cases that are to be pinned for maintenance of a more accurate anatomic position while pinning; as well as for those that might be treated without pinning. Frequently, swelling will not allow flexion to 120 degrees without compromising the radial pulse.

In a type 3a (Fig. 11-19) fracture where there is still bone contact a closed reduction can be attempted as previously described. Sometimes it may be possible to achieve a stable anatomic reduction. If it is a transverse fracture, the appropriate pronation or supination can be selected, and the elbow flexed to 120 degrees without loss of pulse[8,17]; then closed management may be possible without pinning. More commonly, with excess swelling, 120 degrees of flexion is not possible without a risk of vascular compromise, and percutaneous pinning is indicated.

As with the type II fractures if there is any medial supracondylar bone impaction associated with a medial displacement tendency, a lateral pinning should be considered to close the "open" side of the fracture, thus lessening the tendency of varus tilt. More unstable fractures usually require two-pin fixation.

In type 3a fractures where malrotation is the main displacement, there is always concern that vital soft tissues might be trapped behind the humeral shaft spike

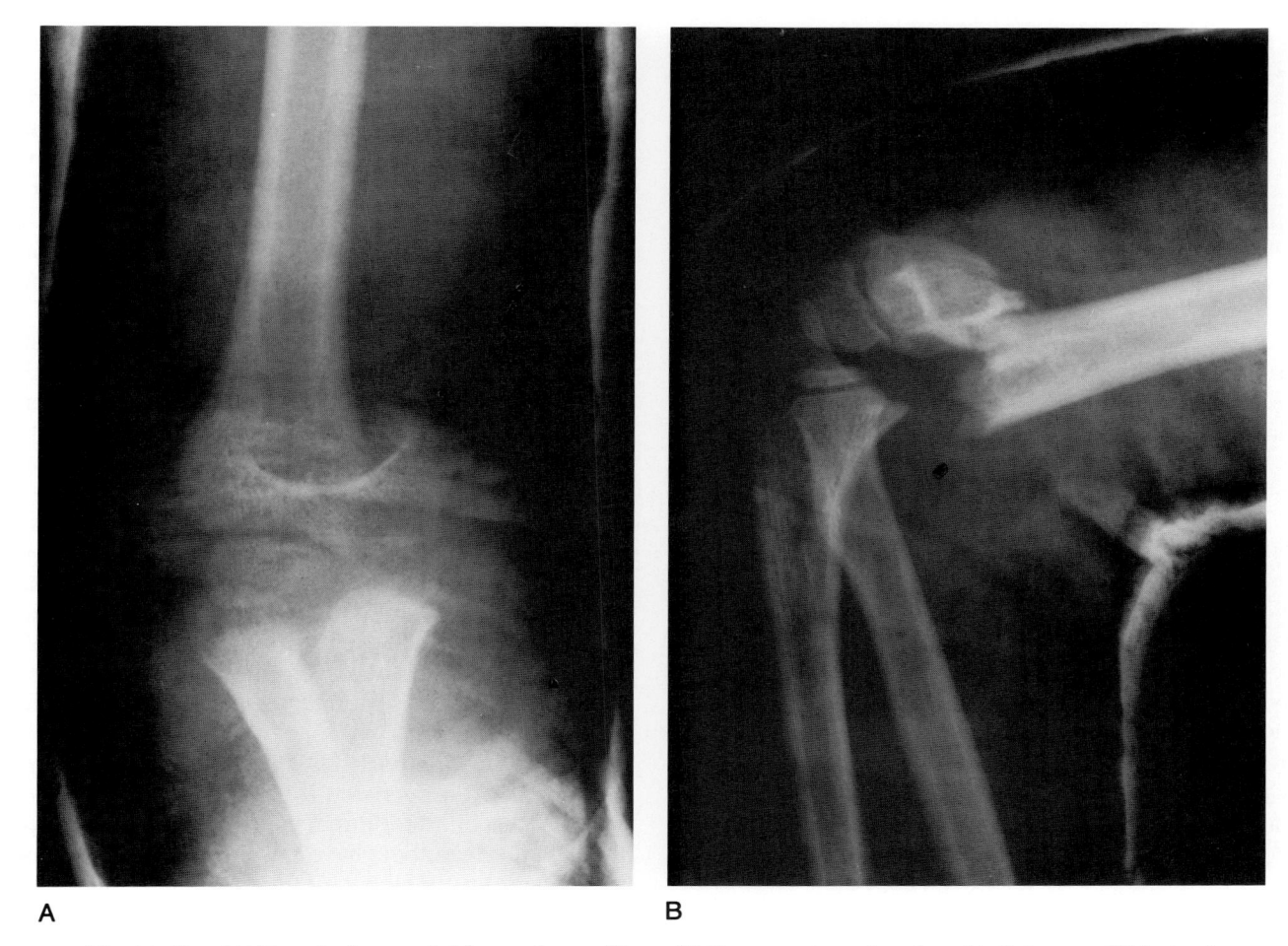

Fig. 11-19. (A) Type 3a fracture left in overlap position with Baumann's angle reduced to 0 degrees. (B) Lateral showing overlap position that was accepted with resultant varus.

during closed reduction. Partial fracture surface contact would imply that perhaps there was not as much displacement at the time of injury when compared to type 3b fractures.

Type 3b fractures (Fig. 11-20) have definite soft tissue interposed between the bone ends, and therefore have a higher risk of having neurovascular complications either initially or with reduction attempts. For reduction of these type 3b fractures, longitudinal traction with the elbow partially flexed as previously described may effect a partial and sometimes complete reduction.

In this fracture type it is most important that the elbow *not* be flexed more than 45 to 60 degrees until lateral views on radiographs taken by rotating the image intensifier (rather than the patient's arm) document adequate reduction. Once the fracture is reduced, external rotation of the arm for a lateral view can be performed.

However, if the fracture is oblique or the reduction is incomplete, rotation of the arm may redisplace the fracture and the C-arm should be rotated rather than the patient's arm.

If the pulse is absent initially, disappears with traction, and/or does not return with traction, this fracture should be considered for open exploration.

Open Reduction of Supracondylar Fractures

If an open reduction is necessary, these fractures should be exposed through the "open" side, that is, the side to which the metaphyseal shaft fragment has displaced, as this is where the artery and/or nerve or other

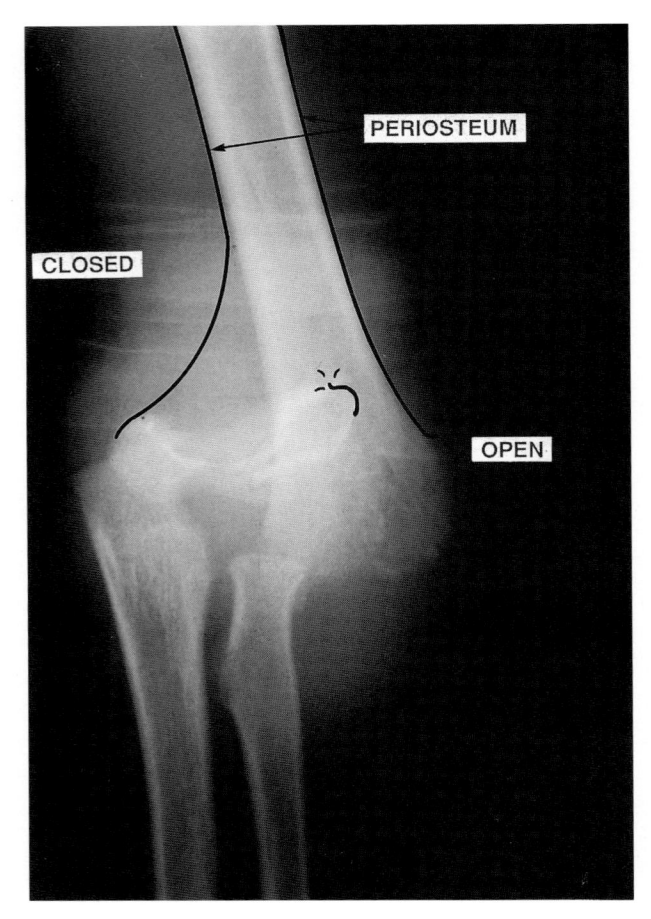

Fig. 11-20. Wide displacement of type 3b fracture putting soft tissues at risk of injury from the fracture and possibly from the reduction. Closed reduction is more safely achieved by working with the periosteal hinge. Open reduction may be necessary.

soft tissue structures such as periosteum[12] may be encountered and removed from the fracture site.

There has historically been a reluctance on the part of orthopaedic surgeons to explore supracondylar fractures with an absent pulse, but there have been more authors recently recommending direct exploration of these cases,[2,12,19] and we would concur.

A vascular surgeon could be contacted to be on stand by for the rare case where more significant brachial artery damage is anticipated. There is, however, no need to delay exploration to perform an angiogram as it can be done at the time of exploration if necessary, but it is rarely helpful.[19,38]

In our experience, in most instances the pulse will return once the obstructing cause is carefully corrected surgically, providing there has not been repeated forceful closed reduction attempts that may have damaged the artery. A careful open reduction is less traumatic to vital structures than a forceful closed reduction.

The best operative approach for these fractures with vascular compromise is directly anteromedially[12] along the course of the brachial artery and median nerve. Sometimes the shaft has buttonholed through the brachialis muscle, at other times it has widely transected this muscle. The shaft fragment, when displaced anteromedially (distal fragment posterolateral), places the brachial artery and median nerve at greater risk.

The anterolaterally displaced shaft fragment (distal fragment posteromedial) is more likely to compromise the radial nerve.[12] If this is not reducible, then a lateral approach would be indicated on the "open" side of the fracture. There have been more reports in the literature of permanent deficits of the radial nerve than median or ulnar, some with radial nerve transection in type 3b fractures. Lateral displacement of the shaft with absent radial nerve function should be treated similarly with earlier consideration for open reduction. If partial fracture apposition is not achieved with traction alone, forceful reduction should be avoided, especially if soft tissue is interposed or there is a radial nerve deficit before reduction.

A posterior approach has been advocated by some authors, but this approach is through the intact periosteum, and is blind for direct viewing of the anterior pathology. Some authors have suggested there is a greater subsequent loss of elbow motion using this approach.[12]

It is recommended that these cases treated by open reduction be internally fixed with two pins, although some might be stable enough with a single pin on the "open" side if the fracture is transverse and anatomically stable.

Percutaneous Pinning

There have been numerous variations of pinning techniques recommended for supracondylar fractures. The most stable construct is with medial and lateral epicondylar pins through the supracondylar ridges and into but not through the opposite cortices.[39] This technique should be considered when the most unstable fracture circumstances are encountered, such as in (1) oblique fracture line (Fig. 11-21) (2) widely displaced fracture (more soft tissue disruption), and (3) medial column impaction or other comminution.

The ulnar nerve is always a concern with the insertion of the medial pin. Some ulnar nerve pareses have been reported,[41] but to date nerve deficits in these reported cases have been transient.

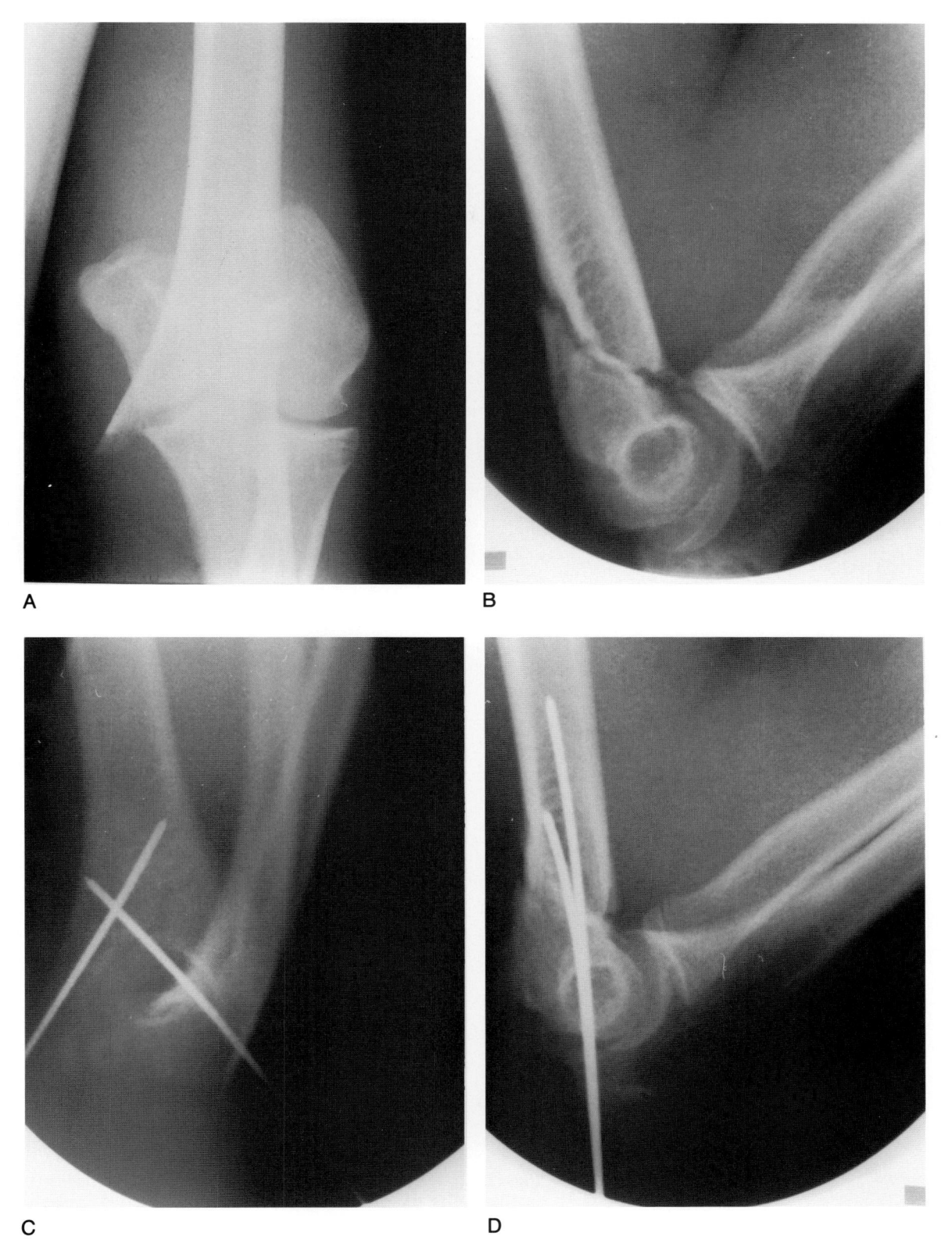

Fig. 11-21. **(A)** Marked displacement with overlap type 3b with a sharp medial shaft spike. **(B)** Lateral view following closed reduction demonstrates an oblique fracture line that would contribute to instability of this reduction. **(C)** Internal fixation with medial and lateral pins on AP view. **(D)** Medial and lateral pins on lateral view.

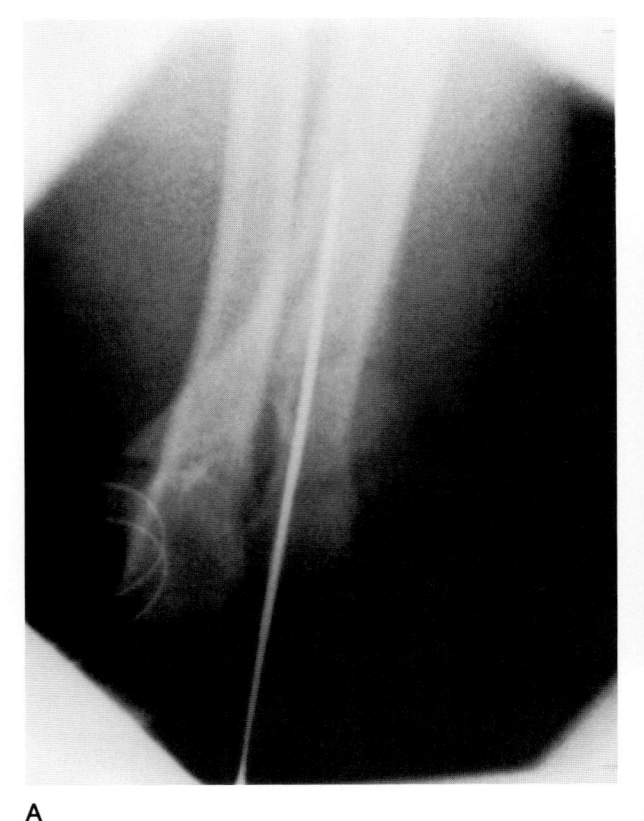

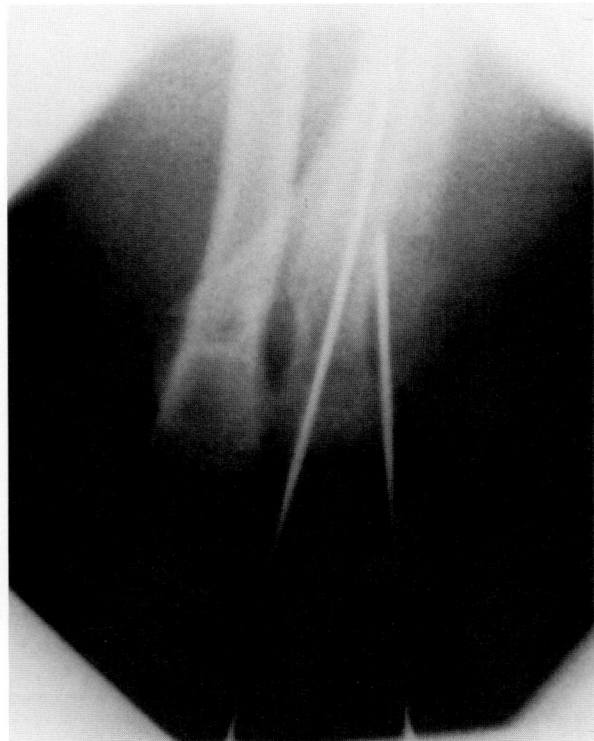

Fig. 11-22. (A) First of two lateral pins inserted transarticular just lateral to the olecranon. (B) Second pin inserted in the lateral epicondyle AP. (C) Lateral view showing good reduction with about 2 mm residual posterior displacement.

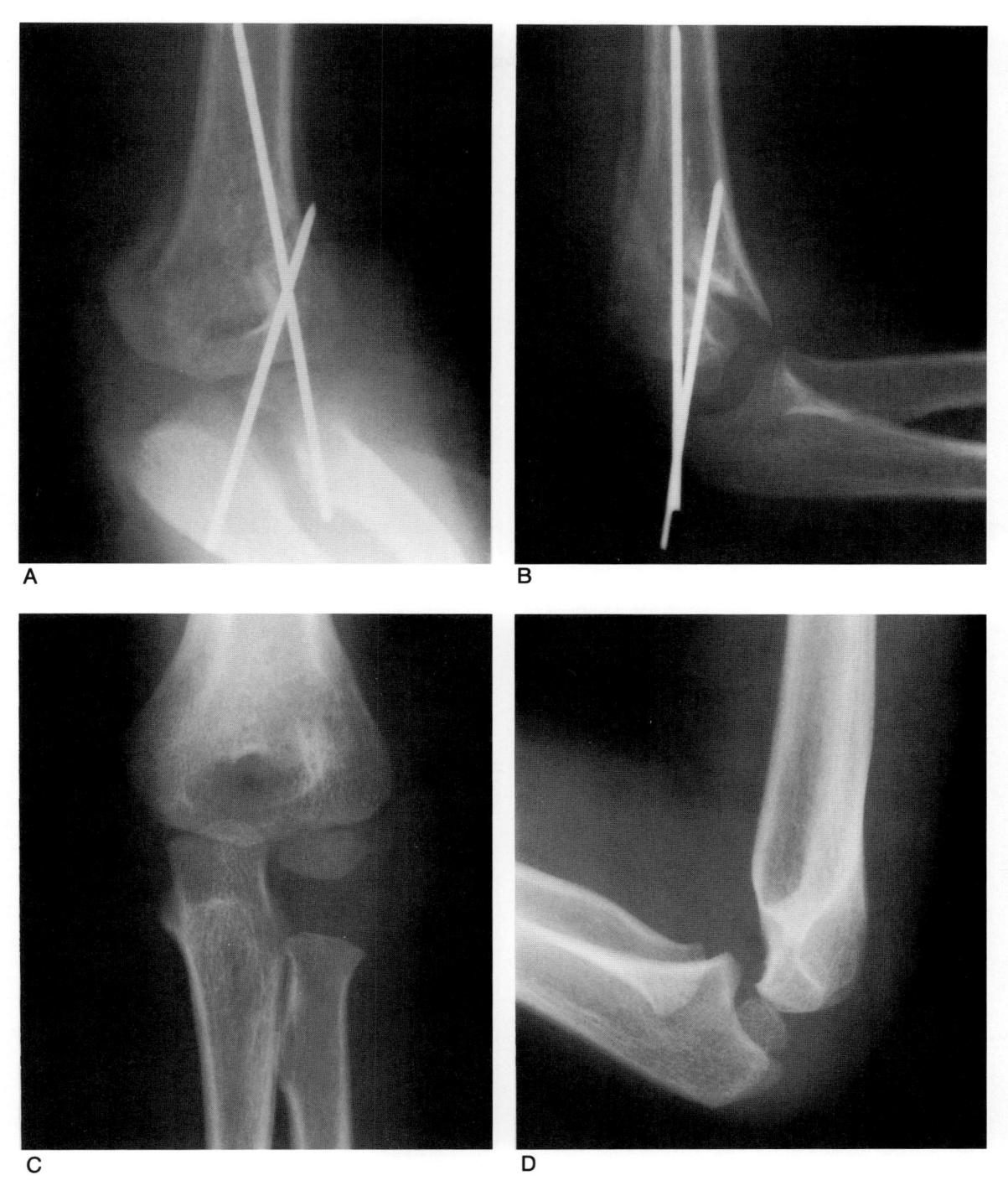

Fig. 11-23. (A) AP view of a different patient 3 weeks postreduction with two lateral pins crossing at the fracture level. This allowed rotation of the medial side. (B) Lateral view showing the medial rotation of the distal fragment revealing the medial shaft fragment anterior. This is an oblique (unstable) fracture pattern and a medial and lateral pinning would have been more secure. (C) Despite the malrotation the remodeling 9 months postfracture reveals only a 5-degree decrease in Baumann's angle. (D) A normal humerocapitellar angle on the lateral view. Although the anterior spike had remodeled, this was maximum flexion at 120 degrees.

188 / Management of Pediatric Fractures

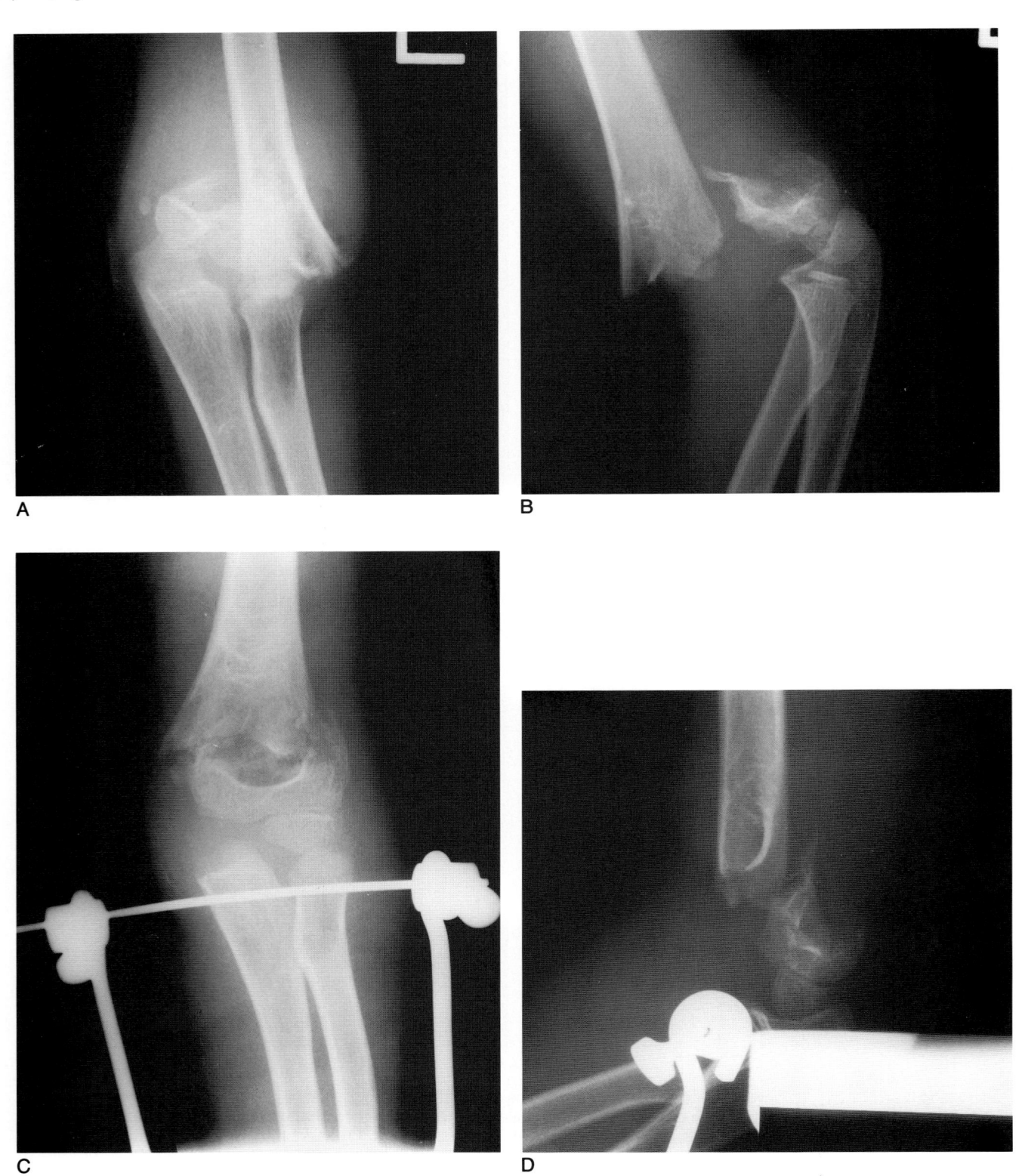

Fig. 11-24. **(A&B)** A type 3b supracondylar fracture that was received late from a remote area with marked swelling. **(C&D)** This was treated in skeletal traction achieving partial reduction to bayonet position. *(Figure continues.)*

E F

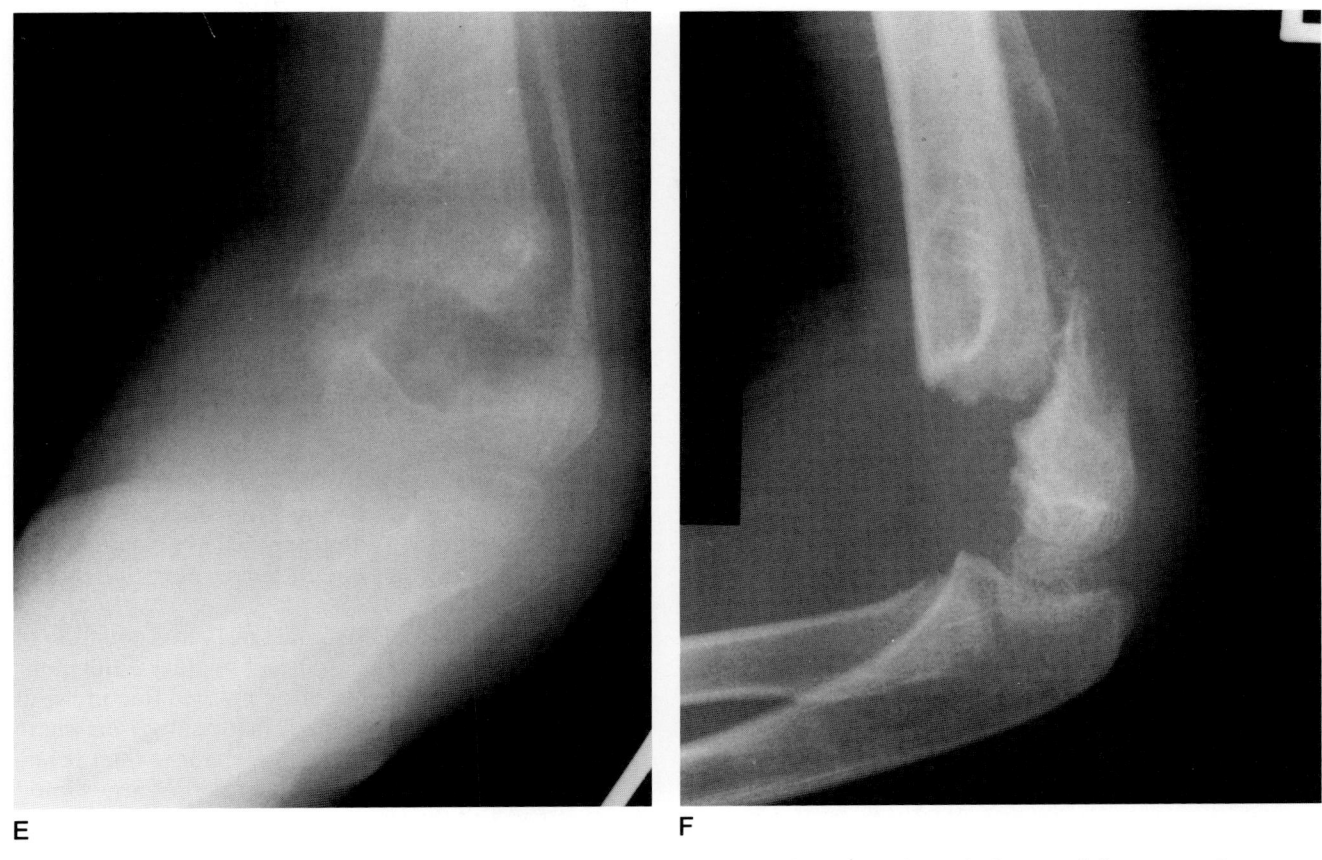

Fig. 11-24 *(Continued).* **(E&F)** Early healing, perhaps some loss of Baumann's angle, but a satisfactory result was achieved. Usually a posteriorly directed force (a sling around the upper arm) is necessary to restore the humerocapitellar angle on the lateral view.

Only smooth pins should be used. If there is difficulty palpating the medial epicondyle, a small incision with blunt dissection and the use of a drill guide facilitates localization of the medial epicondyle. Displacing the nerve posteriorly during pinning may be of assistance, especially if the pinning is done in acute flexion.

The entrance point for the pin should be more anterior on the medial epicondyle. The elbow should not be flexed above 70 to 80 degrees during immobilization to avoid bringing a mobile ulnar nerve against the pin by increased flexion.

A single lateral pin might occasionally create enough stability if the lateral side is the "open" side and the fracture is of the more stable type but usually the insertion of two pins is preferable.

Until recently, we have been reluctant to use the medial pin because of concern for the ulnar nerve, and have more commonly used two lateral pins. The first is inserted transarticularly just lateral to the olecranon (Fig. 11-22A) and the second through the lateral epicondyle (Fig. 11-22B&C). Other variations of insertion of two lateral pins have been recommended.[7,8]

This method is not as stable as the medial and lateral pin technique but is more stable than a single lateral pin, or two pins in the lateral epicondyle. If two lateral pins are used they should cross the fracture line at some distance apart to provide better stability (Fig. 11-23).

We have not had a problem with septic arthritis when these procedures are performed with aseptic technique. The pins are left outside the skin and covered with sterile felt pads, and removed in the outpatient department in about 3 weeks. The elbow is usually maintained in 70 to 80 degrees of flexion.

If medial and lateral pins are employed, a posterior splint is frequently all that is needed for postoperative immobilization.

If only lateral pins are used it is more important to place the forearm in the appropriate pronated or supinated position to reinforce the stability. This is particularly important if the "open" side of the fracture is not pinned.

Traction

Traction as a primary mode of treatment is rarely employed in a modern pediatric orthopaedic setting. If there is delayed treatment with a massively swollen arm with a displaced fracture, traction either overhead or out to the side, can be used as an interim measure, and possibly as definitive treatment (Fig. 11-24).

Skeletal traction with the traction pin or screw inserted in the proximal ulna, has the ability to control varus and valgus tilt,[41] even when there is incomplete reduction. Traction techniques require attention to detail in setting up the traction apparatus and monitoring the arm in traction (Fig. 11-25). Retrotilt of the distal fragment tends to occur more readily with traction.

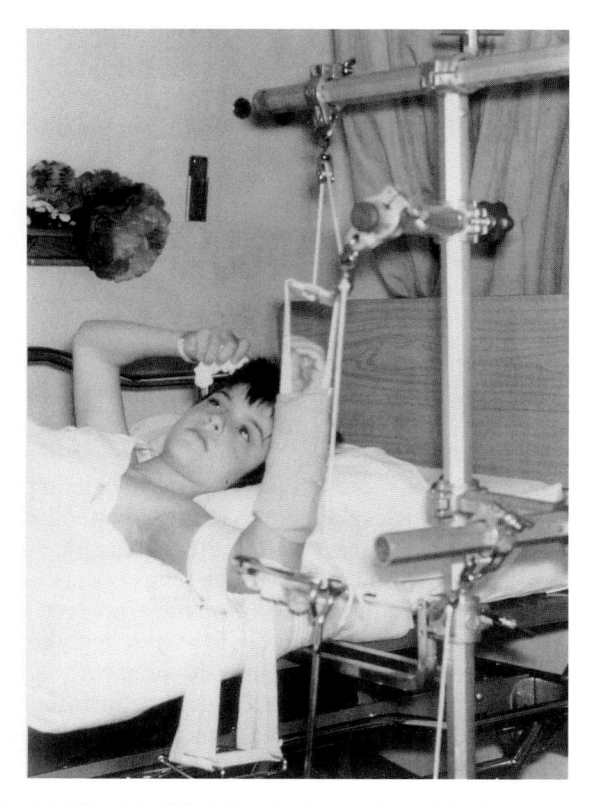

Fig. 11-25. Modified Dunlop's traction with olecranon pin has been an effective form of treatment for supracondylar fractures of the humerus seen late with considerable swelling and the "sausage" arm.

It should be emphasized that many authors have reported a high proportion of good to excellent results with skeletal traction techniques.[14,19,24,30] With hospital cost constraints, traction is not as cost-efficient—about 10 days to 2 weeks in the hospital compared to 24 to 48 hours with most pinned fractures. A recent article by Sutton and colleagues[24] analyzed the differential costs of operative versus traction management, and traction was noted to be a high resource-intensity treatment modality.

Pitfalls in Treatment

1. The child with the absent pulse but adequate circulation, should be considered for open brachial artery exploration, rather than just observation. If the radial pulse is absent by Doppler as well as palpation with an associated inadequate circulation, exploration should be mandatory.

2. It is easy to underestimate the varus potential of some of the minimally displaced fractures. Surgeons should be wary of the minimally displaced fracture with medial supracondylar buckling (shortening) or where medial displacement or tilt is more evident than posterior displacement or tilt. The intact periosteum should be identified and the appropriate pronation and supination used to close the "open" side.

3. The radial pulse should be monitored on arrival in the emergency department and in the operating room before, during, and after reduction. Once reduced, the elbow should be further flexed to demonstrate the pulse obliteration angle (sometimes as little as 90 to 95 degrees) and the immobilization angle ensured to be at least 5 degrees below this pulse obliteration angle. A cast-splint should be utilized that can allow both the continued monitoring of the radial pulse, as well as the adjustability of elbow flexion (Fig. 11-5).

4. A circular cast is not any more stable than the cast-splint demonstrated in Figure 11-5. The circular cast does not allow for observation of swelling or for adjustability of elbow flexion, and usually ends up being a displacing force as the swelling goes down and the cast gets looser, with the top of the cast levering at the midhumerus level.

5. If closed reduction without pinning is elected, a nonstretchable collar-cuff is helpful to maintain the cast-splint pulled forward and minimizes the retrotilt that might tend to occur as swelling diminishes.

6. For medial pinning, appropriate measures need to be taken to minimize risk to the ulnar nerve:

a. Use a smooth small pin *not* threaded.
   b. Pin lateral first for stability with the elbow flexed.
   c. Maintain the appropriate pronation or supination.
   d. Extend the elbow to 90 degrees or straighter.
   e. Manually displace the ulnar nerve posterior while starting the pin somewhat anterior to the midmedial epicondyle.
   f. Do not flex above 70 to 80 degrees during immobilization.

7. Smaller children with "baby fat" may mask the seriousness of the injury initially, and frequently the reduction is more difficult to maintain without pinning.

8. Type 3b fractures (Fig. 11-26) have greater likelihood of vital soft tissue interposition and it is important not to flex the elbow until adequate reduction is achieved by traction alone or traction coupled with posteriorly directed pressure on the anterior humeral shaft. This should be documented by lateral image intensifier views (rotating the C-arm not the patient's arm.)

COMPLICATIONS

Supracondylar fractures are associated with many complications—some early, some delayed or late. The proximal shaft fragment of the fracture is the main culprit in producing many of the early complications.

Early Complications

Neurologic Deficits

The displaced proximal shaft fracture edge may produce median, radial, or ulnar nerve deficit.[2,12,19,42–45] Frequently this is a neuropraxia, not uncommonly an axontemesis (taking several weeks or months to regenerate) and rarely neurotemesis (severance of the nerve). The radial nerve is the most likely to be transected by the fracture.[2,19] About 10 to 15 percent of type 3 displaced supracondylar fractures present with neurologic impairment, most commonly a neuropraxia of the median nerve. Motor deficit is usually in the anterior interosseous distribution, but there is usually some sensory deficit in the median nerve distribution if looked for carefully.

Nerve complications can occur from the pinning whether percutaneous or open.[40] Medial pins can directly traumatize the ulnar nerve at insertion if the pin is placed too far posterior or if the ulnar nerve is subluxable over the medial edge of the medial epicondyle.

Excess flexion of the elbow during pinning may sublux the nerve anteriorly, and excess flexion after pinning may press the nerve against the pin and produce a secondary neuropraxia.

A less common complication of the medial crossed pin is radial nerve palsy from the tip of the pin penetrating the lateral cortex where the radial nerve crosses from posterior to anterior. This was reported recently[40] and should encourage the surgeon not to fully penetrate the lateral cortex with the medial pin.

The ulnar nerve is also at some risk for injury if a horizontal K-wire is used in the olecranon for skeletal traction. Threaded Kirchner wires should not be used in proximity to nerves, and thick felt pads on each side at the skin pin junction will minimize chances that the edge of a traction bow might press on the nerve or skin if the smooth pin used should become loose and slip. The wing-type olecranon screw[33] tends to minimize these problems but has a higher incidence of pull-out.

Vascular Injury

Vascular injury may result from direct brachial artery kinking, contusion, and spasm, and, rarely, an intimal tear or transection is encountered.[2,27,38,46–51] This may precipitate a compartment syndrome and result in Volkmann's ischemic contracture.[19]

All posterolateral (shaft anteromedial) displaced supracondylar fractures should be considered suspect for brachial artery injury, if not primarily then secondarily, with further swelling, handling in radiology, or during reduction. Precautions should be taken to splint early, not rotate the arm for a lateral view, and the limb should be handled carefully in the operating room. Particular concern is needed in type 3b fractures.

Compartment syndromes are the precursor to Volkmann's ischemic contracture. The forearm muscles in supracondylar fractures are not directly involved by the fracture, but potentially secondarily by the vascular compromise to the muscles.

Care should be taken to accurately record the motor and sensory nerve function quantitatively, including the initial assessment. Further loss of motor function should make one suspect vascular impairment. Ordinarily this should be associated with severe pain, but neurologic impairment of sensory (pain) fibers from a contused nerve (e.g., median nerve) might alter the sensation of pain. With further loss of motor function that was

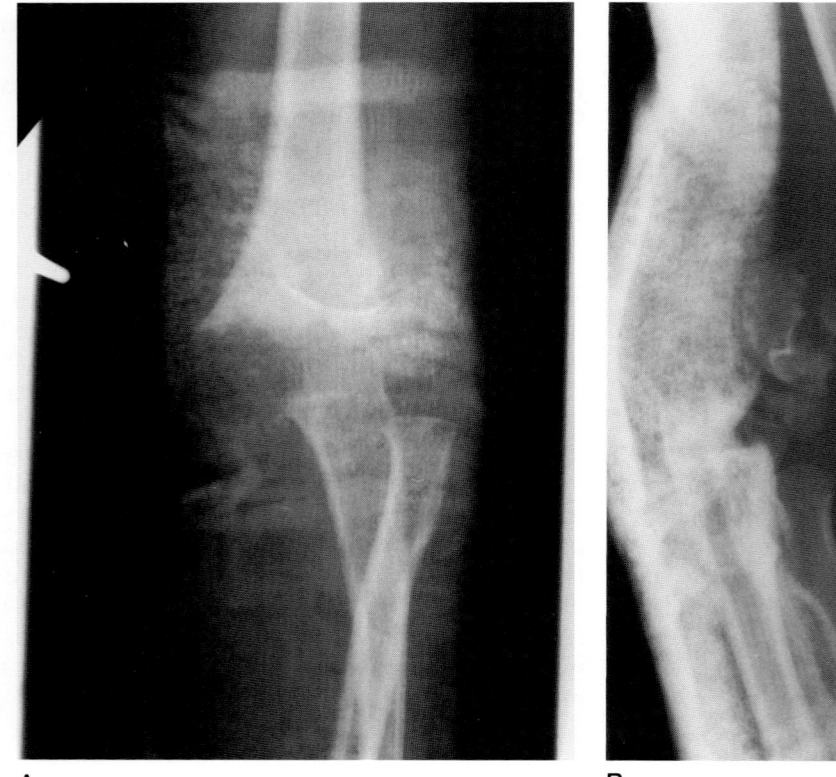

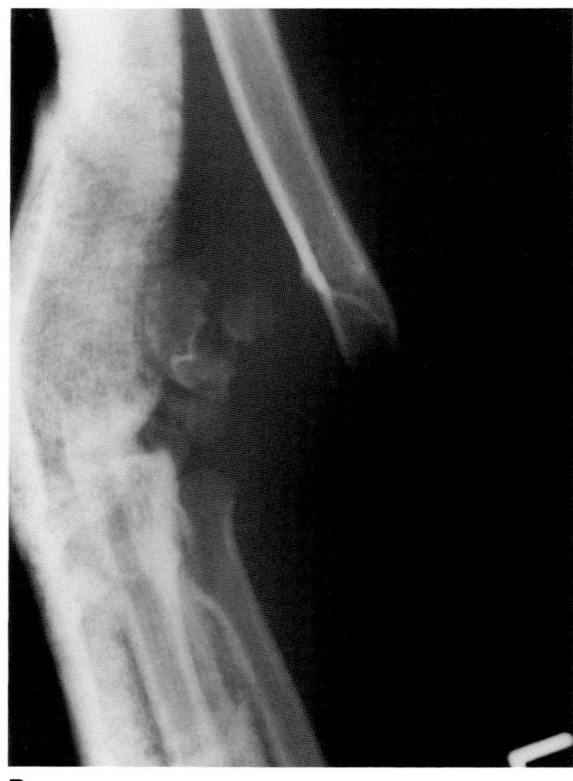

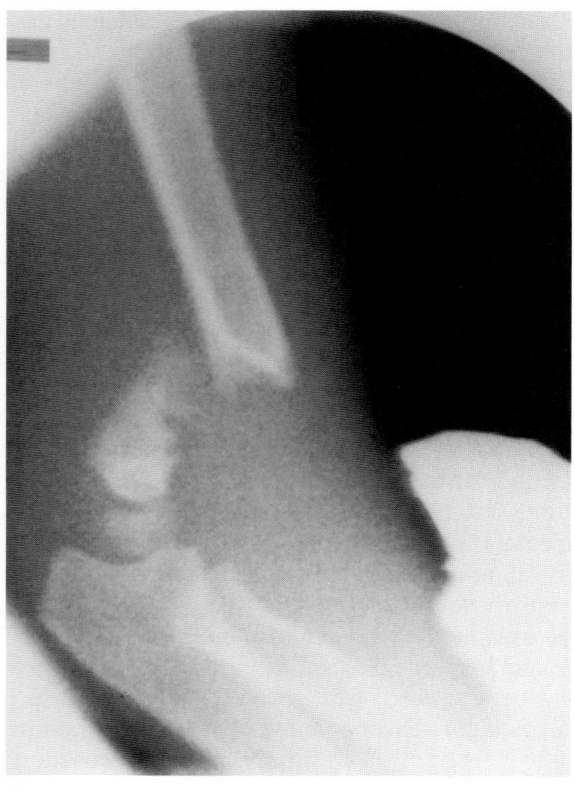

Fig. 11-26. **(A&B)** A type 3b fracture with obvious soft tissue interposition and an absent pulse. **(C)** Still soft tissue interposed after traction. *(Figure continues.)*

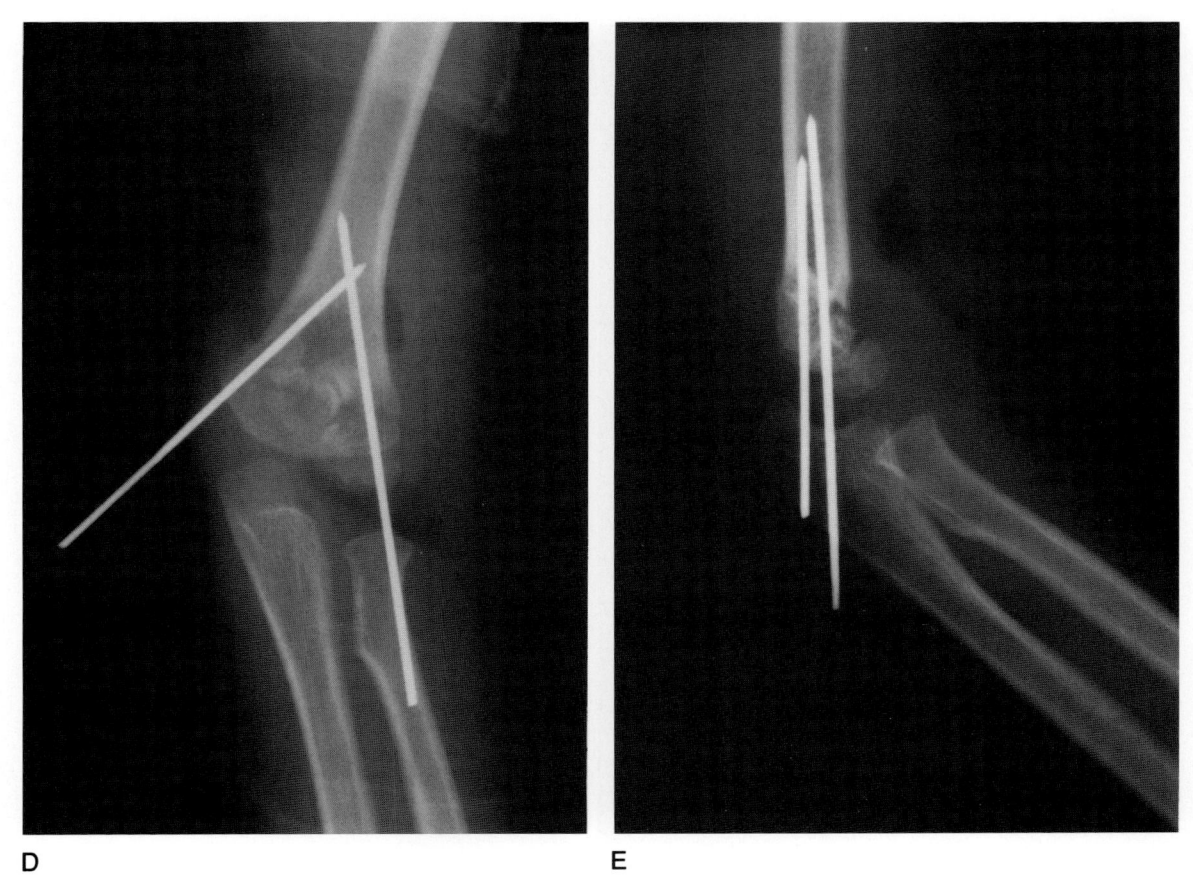

Fig. 11-26 *(Continued).* **(D&E)** AP and lateral views showing medial and lateral crossed pins securing stable near-anatomic position following open reduction via a direct anteromedial approach, with decompression of the brachial artery and median nerve.

present previously one should not assume that the child "won't" move the fingers but that the child "can't" move the fingers. Very small children who cannot cooperate for adequate neurologic assessment make evaluation more difficult and might influence the surgeon to pin more readily. As stated previously, absent radial pulses that do not return should be considered for brachial artery exploration. The elbow should never be placed in the acutely flexed position, as is necessary for closed reduction without pinning.

Infection

With percutaneous pinning there is a risk of infection. The incidence is fortunately low in reported series.[16] Open reduction also can lead to wound infection, and with a deep wound infection can result in increased elbow stiffness.[19]

Late Complications

Neurologic Deficits

Occasionally an increasing neurologic deficit may occur, presumably due to contraction of organizing scar tissue where there has been massive soft tissue damage and swelling.[51,52] This usually spontaneously resolves.

Where there is no neurologic recovery by 5 months (clinically and by electromyography) exploration and neurolysis is advised.[45,52]

Vascular Complications

Forearm claudication with excessive use and cold intolerance may be encountered if there has been significant persistent brachial artery obstruction, and inadequate collateral circulation.

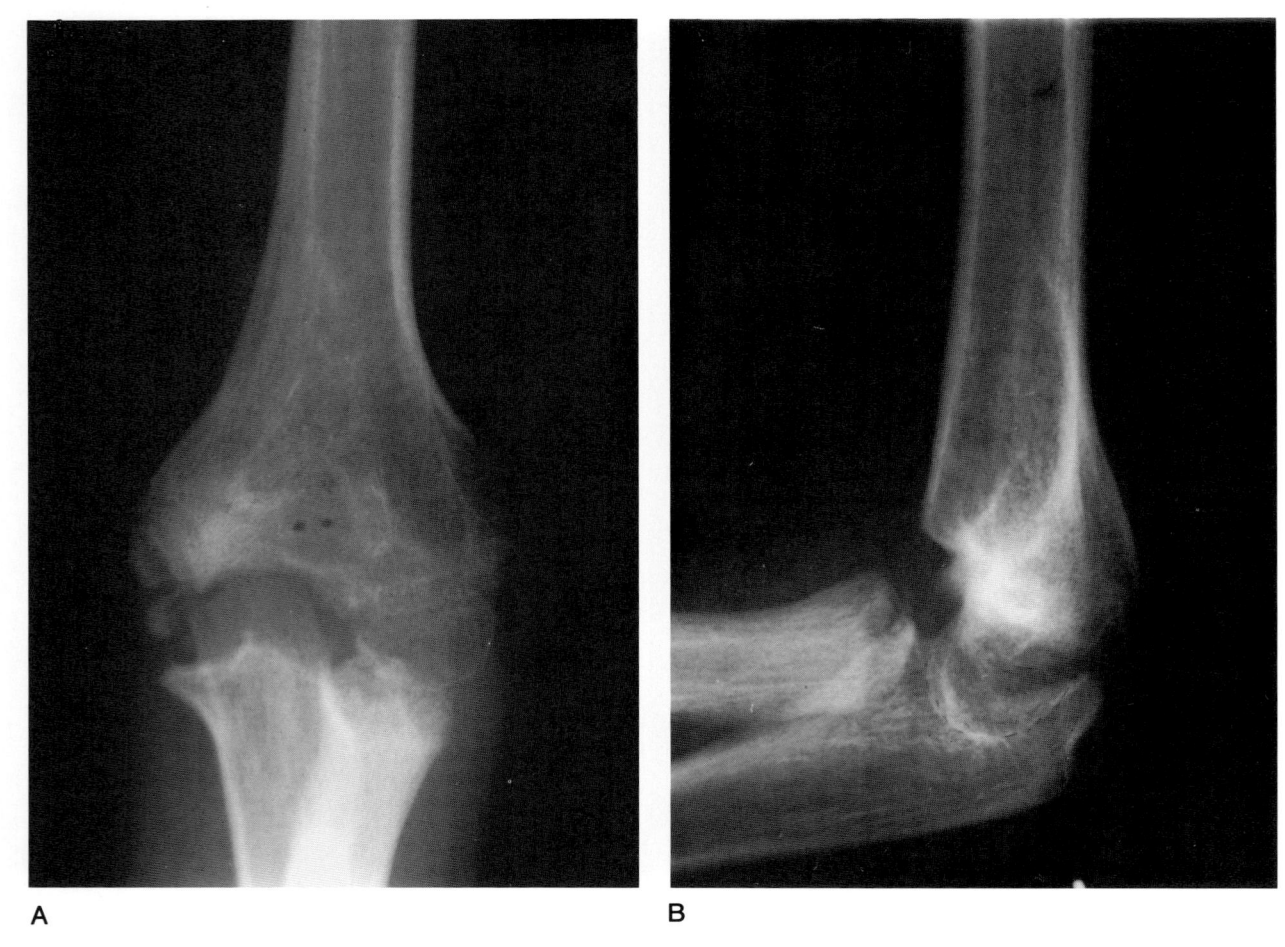

Fig. 11-27. (A&B) Avascular necrosis of the trochlea, 14 months following reduction of a displaced supracondylar fracture.

Avascular Necrosis of Trochlea

Avascular necrosis of the trochlea is a fortunately rare, but serious, complication that occasionally follows supracondylar fractures, as well as medial condyle fractures.

Considering the disruption of soft tissues associated with the markedly displaced supracondylar fracture (type 3b), it is remarkable that avascular necrosis is not seen more often. Presumably there are anatomic variations of the blood supply to the trochlea that predispose to the development of avascular necrosis. Posterior soft tissues should be respected, as the main blood supply to the trochlea is reported to be posterior.[51]

The end result of avascular necrosis of the trochlea is that the olecranon sinks into the avascular trochlea and there is usually marked restriction of motion from the distortion of the articular surface (Fig. 11-27).

Elbow Stiffness

Elbow stiffness, though usually not permanent, can take many months to gradually improve. Early mobilization at 3 weeks usually will minimize this. Parents should be warned that restoration of full elbow range of motion may take several months to achieve. Active exercises are most helpful in regaining elbow motion and passive stretching exercises should be discouraged.

Cubitus Varus

Cubitus varus malunion is the more common and more obvious deformity.[53-55] It is sometimes referred to as "a gunstock" deformity (Fig. 11-28A–C). Cubitus varus deformity has generally been considered to be mainly a cosmetic deformity. We have encountered

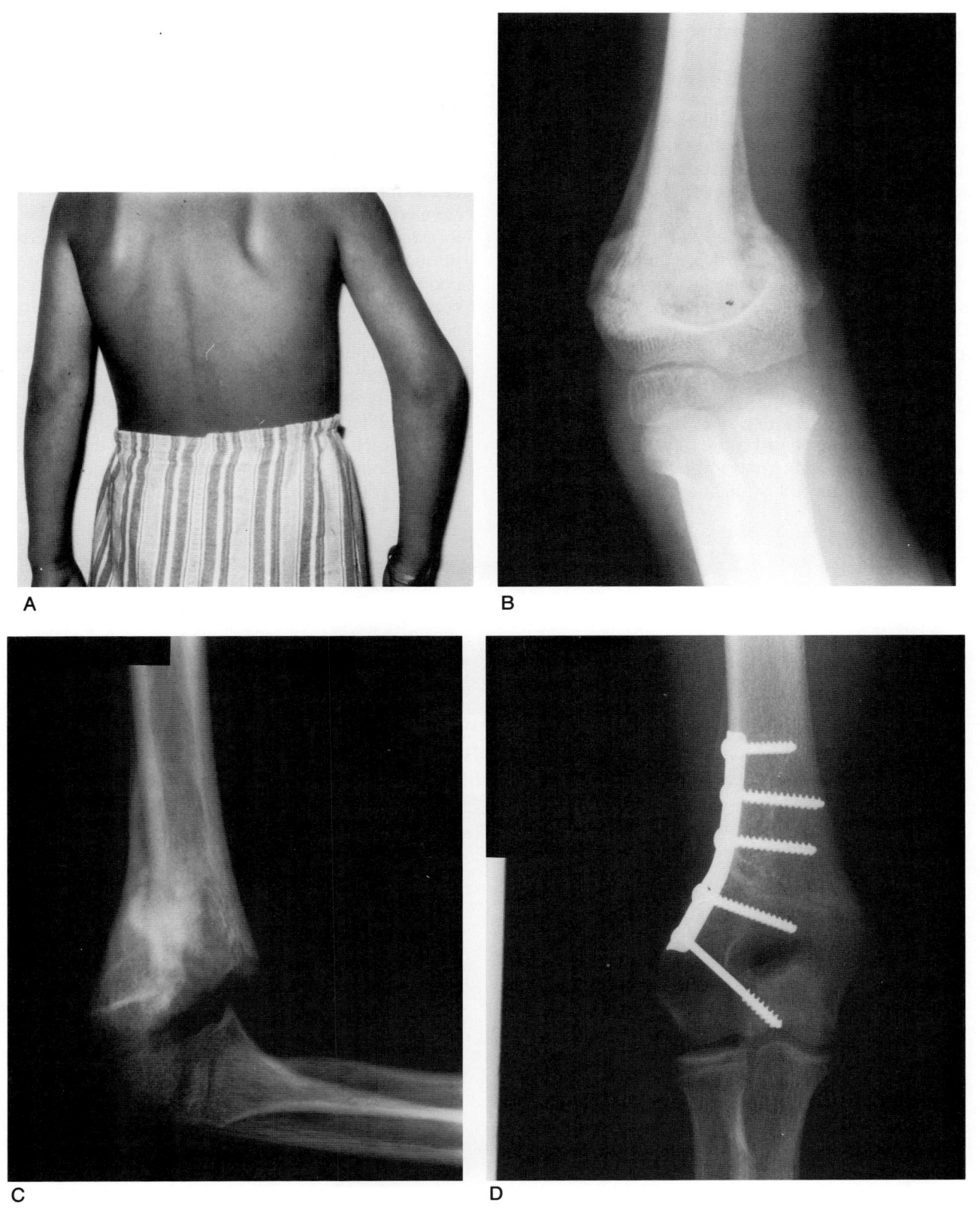

Fig. 11-28. **(A)** A patient with cubitus varus following a supracondylar fracture. **(B&C)** AP and lateral views of a supracondylar fracture with incomplete reduction and about 20 degrees of varus tilt from normal. **(D)** Small plate fixation of a supracondylar lateral closing wedge osteotomy.

fractures of the lateral condyle in elbows with residual varus possibly due to the increased vulnerability of the more exposed lateral condyle. Uchiday[56] from Japan has reported six cases of tardy ulnar nerve palsy in varus deformities of the elbow post supracondylar fracture. It was felt to be due to the trauma to the ulnar nerve from subluxing over the medial epicondyle. Tardy ulnar nerve palsy has more traditionally been associated with cubitus valgus producing a stretch palsy. Functionally, cubitus varus is of minor consequence, as the shoulder accommodates for slight changes in the plane of elbow flexion. The main concern of families is usually the cosmetic appearance.

Hyperextension of the Elbow

Retrotilt malunion can cause increased elbow hyperextension along with some limitation of flexion. The hyperextension tendency might predispose to recurrent supracondylar fractures or dislocations. As a preventive measure against refracture, children can be encouraged to perform regular push-ups—training themselves to stop short of full extension.

Supracondylar osteotomies are sometimes indicated for residual cubitus varus deformity. There have been various descriptions of how these can be performed.[13,57-59] Most agree it is unwise to derotate through the osteotomy site, as this just contributes to poorer bone contact. Rotational malalignment is seldom a problem or a complaint by the child and is compensated for very effectively by shoulder motion.

My preference is a lateral closing wedge osteotomy sloping the proximal cut of the wedge to the medial apex to make both sides of the osteotomy equal length and avoid a lateral step (Fig. 11-29). The medial cortex should be left as an intact hinge, closure of the lateral side can be done with a contoured small plate or crossed K-wires (Fig. 11-28D). If the medial hinge should be-

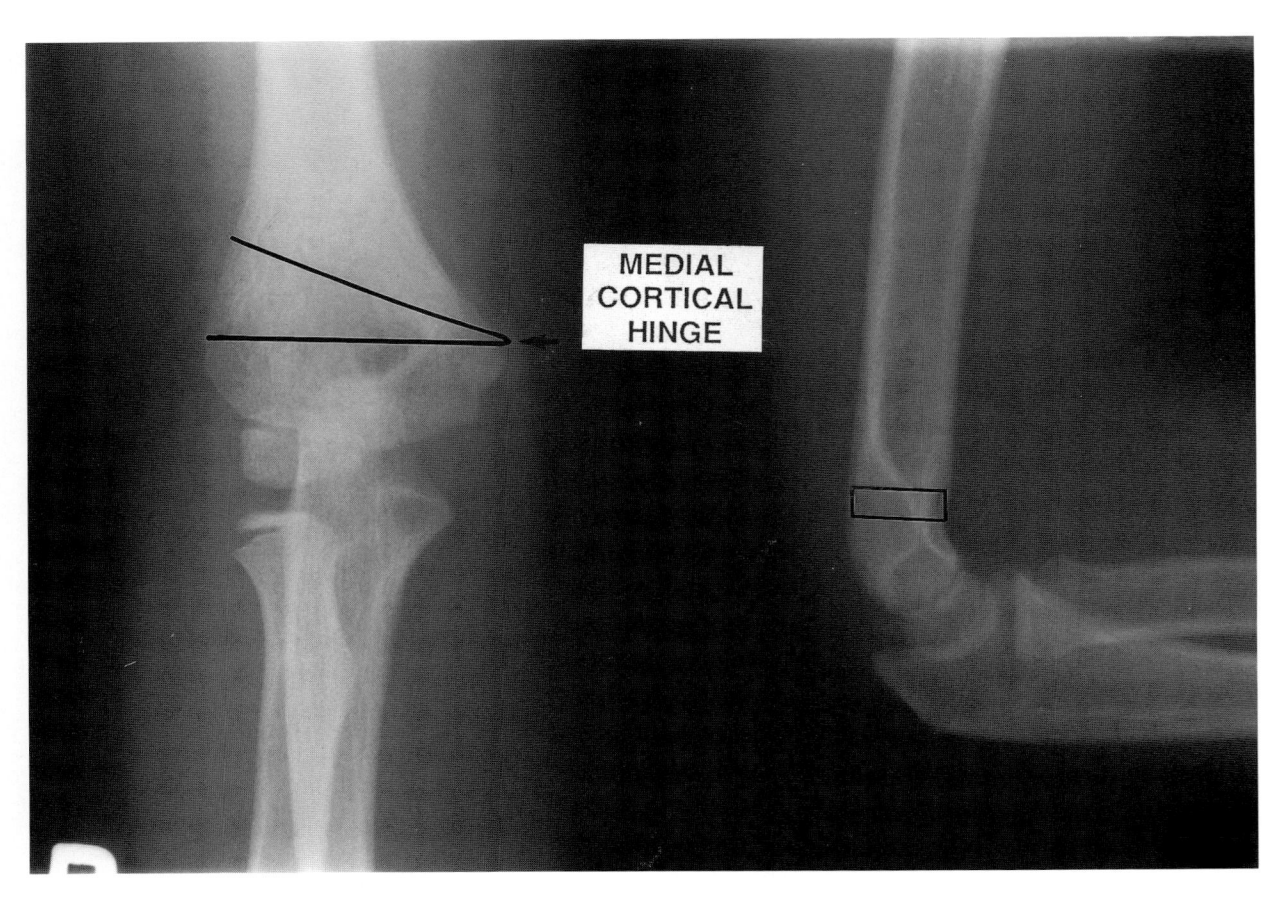

Fig. 11-29. Lateral closing wedge osteotomy of the distal humerus with both cuts being approximately the same length allows a closure with minimal lateral prominence. This can be held with two K-wires or a contoured plate.

come unstable a medial pin could be used to reinstitute the hinge.

This osteotomy is not without complications, particularly of loss of fixation,[60] so that lesser degrees of deformity are best left alone.

SUMMARY

Supracondylar fractures continue to be one of the more challenging fractures to diagnose accurately and treat appropriately. They require accurate assessment of the neurovascular status of the limb at all stages of initial and follow-up management. The classification presented should help with the choice of the optimal method of treatment for the fracture with less risk of neurovascular damage in the early management, and less risk of malunion in the longer term.

REFERENCES

1. Mortensson W, Thonell S: Left-side dominance of upper extremity fracture in children. Acta Orthop Scand 62:154, 1991
2. Mehserle WL, Meehan PL: Treatment of displaced supracondylar fractures of the humerus (type III) with closed reduction and percutaneous crossed pin fixation. J Pediatr Orthop 11:705, 1991
3. Khare, GN, Gautam VK, Kochhar VL, Anand C: Prevention of cubitus varus deformity in supracondylar fractures of the humerus. Br J Accident Surg 22:202, 1991
4. D'Ambrosia RD: Supracondylar fractures of the humerus: prevention of cubitus. J Bone Joint Surg [Am] 54(1):60, 1972
5. Rogers LF, Malave S Jr, White H, Tachdjian MO: Plastic bowing, torus and greenstick supracondylar fractures of the humerus: radiographic clues to obscure fractures of the elbow in children. Radiology 128:145, 1978
6. Gerardi JA, Houkom JA, Mack GR: Treatment of displaced supracondylar fractures of the humerus in children by closed reduction and percutaneous pinning. Orthop Rev 18:1089, 1989
7. Aronson DD, Prager BI: Supracondylar fractures of the humerus in children: a modified technique for closed pinning. Clin Orthop Rel Res 219:174, 1987
8. Kallio PE, Foster BK, Patterson DC: Difficult supracondylar fractures in children analysis of percutaneous pinning technique. J Pediatr Orthop 12:11, 1992
9. Worlock P: Supracondylar fractures of humerus: assessment of cubitus varus by Baumann's angle. J Bone Joint Surg [Br] 68B:755, 1986
10. Rockwood CA, Wilkins KE, King RE: Fractures in Children. 3rd Ed. JB Lippincott, Philadelphia, 1991
11. Gartland JJ: Management of supracondylar fractures of the humerus in children. Surg Gynecol Obstet 109;145, 1959
12. Wilkins KE: The operative management of supracondylar fractures. Orthop Clin North Am 21:269, 1990
13. Wilkins KE: Residuals of elbow trauma in children. Orthop Clin North Am 21:291, 1990
14. Celiker O, Pestilci FI, Tuzuner M: Supracondylar fractures of the humerus in children: analysis of the results in 142 patients. J Orthop Trauma 4:265, 1990
15. Altchek M: Management of displaced extension-type supracondylar fractures of the humerus in children. J Bone Joint Surg [Am] 71:788, 1989
16. Griffin PP: Management of displaced extension-type supracondylar fractures of the humerus in children. [Letter]. J Bone Joint Surg 71:313, 1989
17. Millis MB, Singer IJ, Hall JE: Supracondylar fracture of the humerus in children: further experience with a study in orthopedic decision-making. Clin Orthop Rel Res 188:90, 1984
18. Buhl O, Hellberg S: Displaced supracondylar fractures of the humerus in children. Acta Orthop Scand 53:67, 1982
19. Pirone AM, Graham HK, Krajbich JI: Management of displaced extension-type supracondylar fractures of the humerus in children. J Bone Joint Surg [Am] 70:641, 1988
20. France J, Strong M: Deformity and function in supracondylar fractures of the humerus in children variously treated by closed reduction and splinting, traction, and percutaneous pinning. J Pediatr Orthop 12:494, 1992
21. Eid AM: Reduction of displaced supracondylar fractures of the humerus in children by manipulation in flexion. Acta Orthop Scand 49:391, 1978
22. Gjerloff C, Sojbjerg JO: Percutaneous pinning of supracondylar fractures of the humerus. Acta Orthop Scand 49:597, 1978
23. Flynn JC, Mathews JG, Benoit RL: Blind pinning of displaced supracondylar fractures of the humerus in children. J Bone Joint Surg [Am] 56:263, 1974
24. Sutton WR, Greene WB, Georgopoulos G, Dameron TB Jr: Displaced supracondylar humeral fractures. Clin Orthop Rel Res 278:81, 1992
25. Swensen AL: A treatment of supracondylar fractures of the humerus by Kirschner wire transfixion. J Bone Joint Surg [Am] 30:993, 1948
26. Arino VC, Lluch EE, Ramirez AM, Ferrer J, Rodriguez L, Baixauli F: Percutaneous fixation of supracondylar fractures of the humerus in children. J Bone Joint Surg [Am] 59:914, 1977
27. Danielsson L, Pettersson H: Open reduction and pin fixation of severely displaced supracondylar fractures of the humerus in children. Acta Orthop Scand 15:249, 1980
28. Weiland AJ, Meyer S, Tolo VT, Berg HL, Mueller J: Surgical treatment of displaced supracondylar fractures of the humerus in children: analysis of fifty-two cases followed for five to fifteen years. J Bone Joint Surg [Am] 60:657, 1978
29. Hart GM, Wilson DW, Arden GP: The operative manage-

ment of the difficult supracondylar fracture of the humerus in the child. Injury Br J Accident Surg 9:30, 1977
30. Kramhoft M, Keller IL, Solgaard S: Displaced supracondylar fractures of the humerus in children. Clin Orthop Rel Res 221:215, 1987
31. Worlock Ph, Colton C: Severely displaced supracondylar fractures of the humerus in children: a simple method of treatment. J Pediatr Orthop 7:49, 1987
32. Piggot J, Graham HK, McCoy GF: Supracondylar fractures of the humerus in children: treatment by straight lateral traction. J Bone Joint Surg [Br] 68:577, 1986
33. Palmer EE, Niemann K, Vessely D, Armstrong JH: Supracondylar fracture of the humerus in children. J Bone Joint Surg [Am] 60:653, 1978
34. Lund-Kristensen J, Vibild O: Supracondylar fractures of the humerus in children: a follow-up with particular reference to late results after severely displaced fractures. Acta Orthop Scand 47:375, 1976
35. Merchan ECR: Supracondylar fractures of the humerus in children: treatment by overhead traction. Orthop Rev 21:475, 1992
36. Alburger PO, Weidner PL, Betz RR: Supracondylar fractures of the humerus in children. J Pediatr Orthop 12:12, 1992
37. Arnold JA, Nasca RJ, Nelson CL: Supracondylar fractures of the humerus: the role of dynamic factors in prevention of deformity. J Bone Joint Surg [Am] 59:589, 1977
38. Shaw BA, Kasser JR, Emans JB, Rand FF: Management of vascular injuries without arteriography. J Orthop Trauma 4:25, 1990
39. Hertzenberg JE, Koresd Rang M: Biomechanical testing of pin fixation in pediatric supracondylar elbow fractures. AAOS Meeting presentation, February 1988
40. Royce RD, Outkowsky JP, Kasser JR, Rand FR: Neurological complications after K wire fixation of supracondylar humerus fractures in children. J Pediatr Orthop 11:191, 1991
41. Abraham E, Powers T, Wiott P et al: Experimental Hyperextension supracondylar fractures in monkeys. Clin Orthop 171:309, 1982
42. McGraw JJ, Akbarnia BA, Hanel DP, Keppler L, Burdge RE: Neurological complications resulting from supracondylar fractures of the humerus in children. J Pediatr Orthop 6:647, 1986
43. Moehring HD: Irreducible supracondylar fracture of the humerus complicated by anterior interosseous nerve palsy. Clin Orthop Rel Res 206:228, 1986
44. Ippolito E, Caterini R, Scola E: Supracondylar fractures of the humerus in children: analysis at maturity of fifty-three patients treated conservatively. J Bone Joint Surg [Am] 68:333, 1986
45. Jones ET, Louis DS: Median nerve injuries associated with supracondylar fractures of the humerus in children. Clin Orthop Rel Res 159:181, 1980
46. Clement DA: Assessment of a treatment plan for managing acute vascular complications associated with supracondylar fractures of the humerus in children. J Pediatr Orthop 10:97, 1990
47. Vasli LR: Diagnosis of vascular injury in children with supracondylar fractures of the humerus. Injury Br J Accident Surg 19:11, 1988
48. Karlsson J, Thorsteinsson T, Thorleifsson R, Arnason H: Entrapment of the median nerve and brachial artery after supracondylar fractures of the humerus in children. Arch Orthop Traum Surg 104:389, 1986
49. Kamal AS, Austin RT: Dislocation of the median nerve and brachial artery in supracondylar fractures of the humerus. Injury; Br J Accident Surg 12:161, 1980
50. Reigstad A, Hellum C: Volkmann's ischaemic contracture of the forearm. Injury Br J Accident Surg 12:148, 1980
51. Ogilvie RA, D'Astous JA: A review of 88 supracondylar fractures of the humerus. Presented to the Canadian Orthopedic Resident Meeting, May 1983.
52. Culp RW, Osterman AL, Davidson RS, Skirven T, Bora FW Jr: Neural injuries associated with supracondylar fractures of the humerus in children. J Bone Joint Surg [Am] 72:1211, 1990
53. Dowd GS, Hopcroft PW: Varus deformity in supracondylar fractures of the humerus in children. Injury Br J Accident Surg 10:297, 1979
54. Prietto CA: Supracondylar fractures of the humerus: comparative study of Dunlop's traction versus percutaneous pinning. J Bone Joint Surg [Am] 61:425, 1979
55. Yamamoto I, Ishii S, Usui M et al: Cubitus varus deformity following supracondylar fracture of the humerus. Clin Orthop 201;179, 1985
56. Uchiday Sugioka: Ulnar nerve palsy after supracondylar humerus fracture. Acta Orthop Scand 61:118, 1990
57. Carlson SC, Rossman MA: Cubitus varus a new and simple technique for correction. J Pediatr Orthop 2:199, 1982
58. Derosa GP, Graziano GP: A new osteotomy for cubitus varus. Clin Orthop 236:160, 1988
59. Oppenheim WL, Clader TJ, Smith C et al: Supracondylar humeral osteotomy for traumatic childhood cubitus varus deformity. Clin Orthop 188:34, 1984
60. Labelle H, Bunnell WP, Duhaime M, Poitras B: Cubitus varus deformity following supracondylar fractures of the humerus in children. J Pediatr Orthop 2:539, 1982

12

Transcondylar Fractures of the Distal Humerus

Curtis R. Gruel
J. Andy Sullivan

> You can't depend on your judgment when your imagination is out of focus.
> —MARK TWAIN

DESCRIPTION AND INCIDENCE

A transcondylar fracture of the humerus in a child is a physeal fracture of the entire distal humerus. It may also be called an "epiphyseal separation of the distal humerus" or a "fracture-separation of the distal humeral epiphysis." In his 1902 monograph on elbow injuries in children, Frederic Cotton[1] remarked, "In the days before the advent of the X-ray accurate distinctions were possible only in compound cases; at this time many epiphyseal separations were reported; today there are apparently less of them." This injury was once thought to be rare, but is now encountered relatively frequently, and is probably more common than is recognized even today,[2,3] since many are still misdiagnosed as either elbow dislocations or lateral condyle fractures.

The true incidence of this injury is not known. Wilkins[3] has stated that he sees about two or three new cases per year. de Jager and Hoffman[4] estimated that about the same number are seen at Cape Town Red Cross Children's Hospital. Rogers and Rockwood[5] reported seeing five cases in 16 months. McIntyre and colleagues[6] saw 12 patients over a 10-year period in Ottawa.

ANATOMIC CONSIDERATIONS

Transcondylar fractures propagate through the physis of the distal humerus, often with a lateral metaphyseal fragment. Based on arthrographic findings in six cases, Mizuno and coworkers[7] maintain that these are extracapsular supracondylar fractures. They often occur before the capitellum ossifies,[8] accounting for some of the confusion with elbow dislocation. Until about age 6 to 7 years in girls and 8 to 9 years in boys, the epiphysis extends across to include the physis of the medial epicondyle. Thus, fractures in this age group often involve the medial epicondyle, which travels with the distal fragment.[3] After this age, the epiphysis involves only the physes of the medial and lateral condyles.

The distal epiphysis comprises a larger volume of the distal humerus in younger children. Also, in older children the physis assumes a V-shaped configuration, thus mechanically protecting the physis from injury.[9] This probably explains why most of these fractures occur before the age of 6 to 7 years.

These fractures extend through a thicker portion of the distal humerus than do supracondylar fractures. Some authors feel that this affords greater stability to the fracture after closed reduction, and lessens the risk of cubitus varus.[2,3,10] Mauer and colleagues[11] dissected the elbow of a child who died shortly after sustaining a transcondylar fracture during delivery. They found that the posterior and medial periosteum was intact. This supports the notion that immobilization in flexion and pronation will confer stability on the fracture.

Blood vessels cross the physis to supply the medial crista of the trochlea, making it susceptible to avascular necrosis following these fractures. This probably explains the occasional fishtail appearance seen following these injuries[3]

MECHANISM OF INJURY

The mechanism of injury in these fractures is really unknown. Wilkins[3] suspects that it may vary among different age groups. He postulates that rotatory shear forces are responsible for producing these fractures in infants and younger children and that hyperextension forces are more likely in older children. Dameron[10] was unable to produce supracondylar fractures by forceful manipulation of the elbow in eight stillborns, producing epiphyseal separations instead. He noted that a dorsally directed force seemed to be most effective. Siffert[12] produced the fracture in two stillborns, one with hyperextension, the other with a backward thrust on the forearm with the elbow flexed 90 degrees. Cotton[1] said that the fracture could be "readily produced" in the newborn by hyperextension, adduction, abduction, or a forward thrust from behind. He found that a backward thrust with the arm flexed produced a supracondylar fracture in a 6-year-old.

Clinically, this fracture is usually the result of a fall on the hand or elbow[1,4,5,13,14] Holda and colleagues[13] felt that the common mechanism was probably a varus and posteriorly directed force, which often resulted in an avulsion of the lateral condyle by the common extensor origin. Cotton[1] stated that open transcondylar fractures

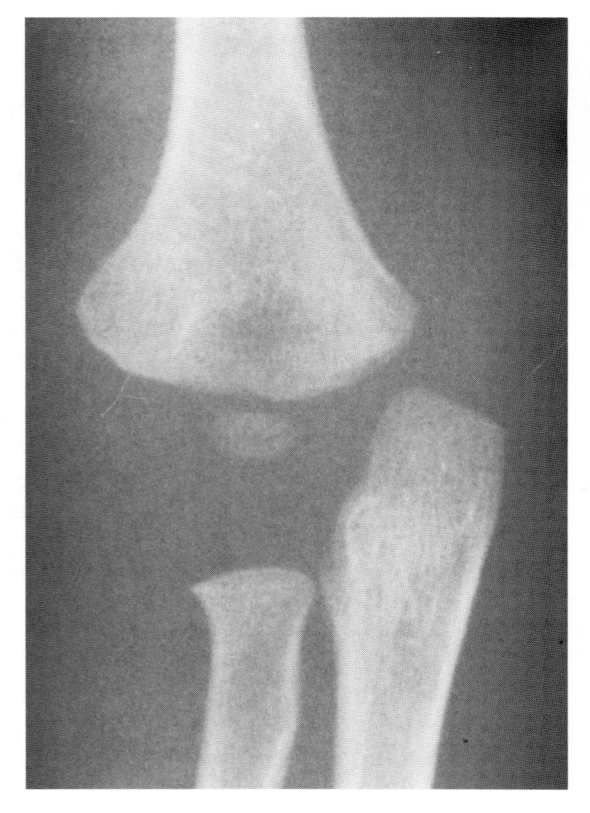

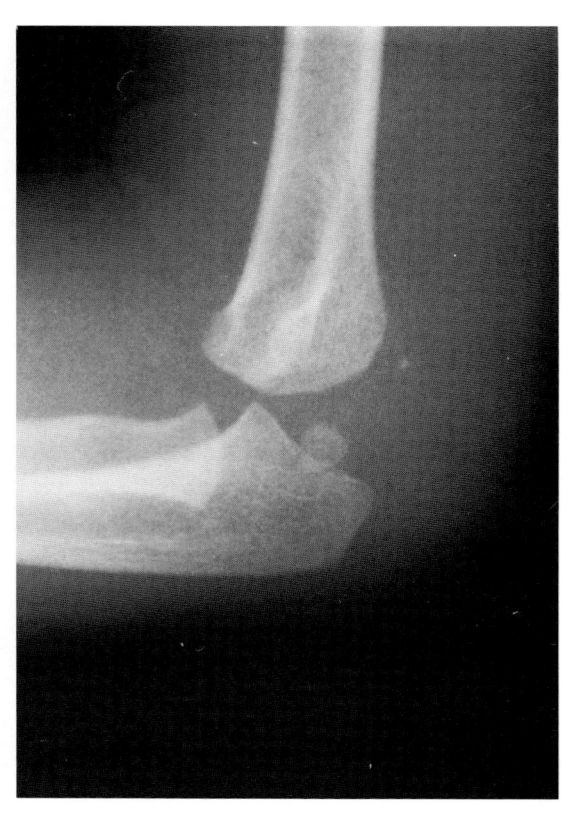

Fig. 12-1. Group A transcondylar fracture in a 2-year-old child resulting from child abuse. Note that the capitellum aligns with the radius on both views.

were more common in the past, often produced by a wagonwheel crushing the child's arm. de Jager and Hoffman[4] mentioned that some of their patients were injured in motor vehicle accidents.

Lifting or pulling an infant by the forearm might produce this fracture.[5,15] Many authors have noted the association of this injury with child abuse.[2-4,10,15-18]

Another common source of this fracture is a birth injury. There is commonly a history of traumatic delivery, and an unusual presentation, such as footling breech, transverse lie, or shoulder dystocia.[2-4,10-12,15,19-23]

CLASSIFICATION

Most authors[2,3,6] classify these injuries into three groups as described by DeLee and colleagues.[17] Group A fractures occur in the newborn to 9-month-old, and are characterized by the lack of a capitellar ossification center and no metaphyseal (Thurston-Holland[24]) fragment (Fig.12-1). Group B includes infants from 7 months to 3 years old, in whom a capitellar ossification center is present; a Thurston-Holland fragment is very small or lacking (Fig. 12-2). Group C fractures occur in children from 3 to 7 years old, and have a well-developed capitellar ossification center and a large metaphyseal fragment[17] (Fig. 12-3)

There are other unusual variants of this fracture that occur occasionally. Cothay[25] described a fracture that involved the medial epicondyle and the medial two-thirds of the trochlea. Grantham and Tietjen[26] reported a patient who had a transcondylar fracture in association with an elbow dislocation.

PHYSICAL EXAMINATION

Most authors note that swelling, hypermobility, and crepitus are found in patients with this fracture.[7,15,17,19,23] In a newborn or infant, one may find paresis of the

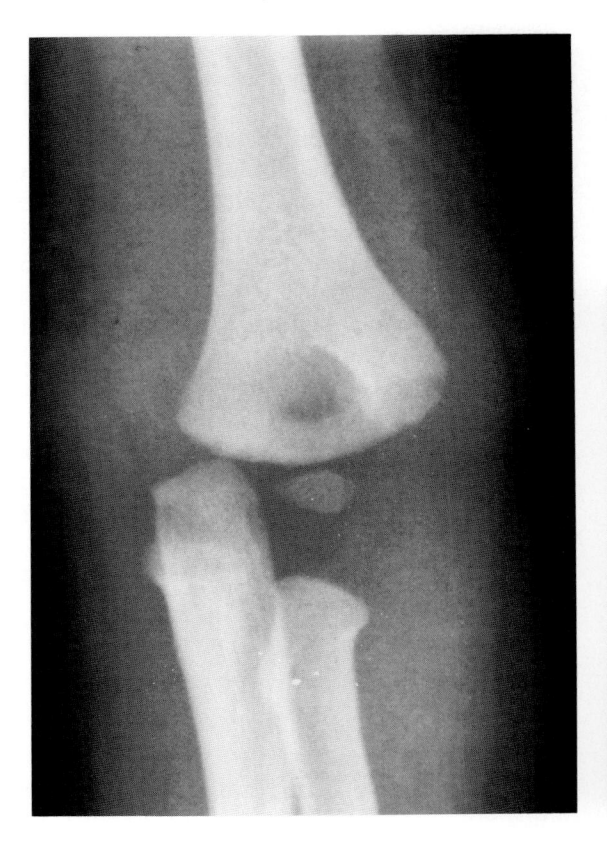

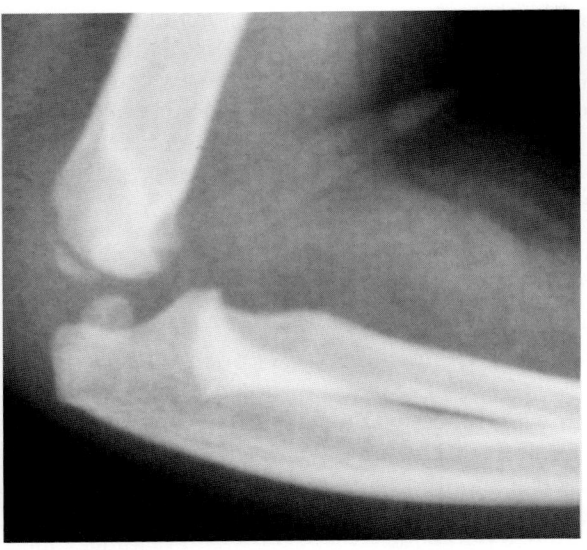

Fig. 12-2. Group B transcondylar fracture in a 9-month-old infant from child abuse. Note the small metaphyseal fragment, seen best on the lateral view.

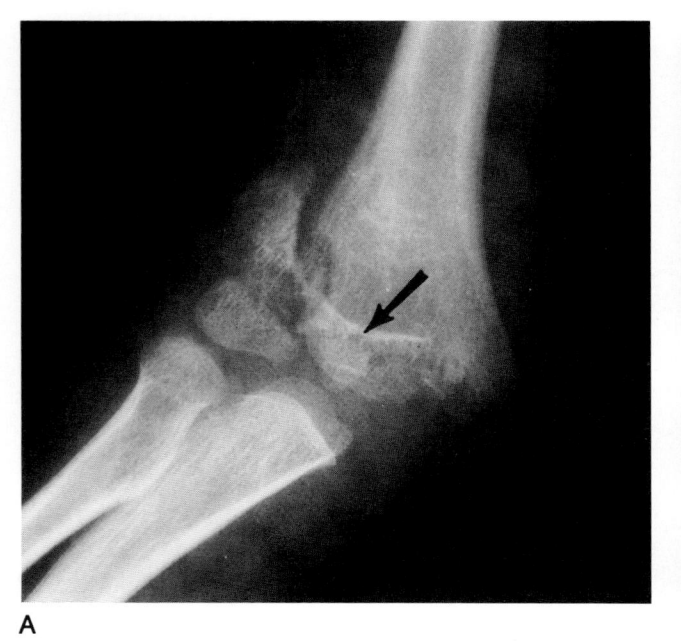

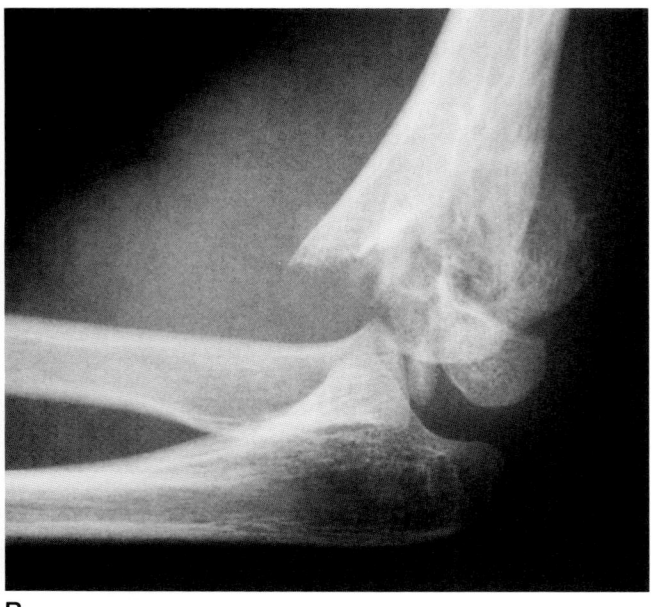

Fig. 12-3. (A & B) Group C transcondylar fracture in a 7-year-old child who fell. Note the large metaphyseal fragment. The arrow indicates a Werenskiold fragment. In this case the displacement is lateral, which is unusual.

extremity, but a normal grasp.[15] There is a particular type of "muffled crepitus," which is due to contact between the cartilage surfaces of the fracture, as opposed to the usual grating felt in bony supracondylar fractures.[3,5,10,12,15,17,18,20,21] The deformity is above the elbow, rather than in the elbow joint.[15] The medial and lateral epicondyles normally form an equilateral triangle with the olecranon. This relationship is maintained in a transcondylar fracture, and the three structures move together.[3,5,12,15-17,20,23] In a dislocation they would move independently. One may note foreshortening of the distance from the acromion to the olecranon.[21] However, all of these findings may be difficult to appreciate in a swollen newborn elbow.[3,7,19-21,27]

DIFFERENTIAL DIAGNOSIS

Transcondylar fractures are often missed initially.[4,6,7,13,17,25] DeLee and coworkers[17] had eight patients in whom there was a delay to diagnosis of 1 to 6 days. Similarly, McIntyre and coworkers[6] found a delay of 1 day to 1 month in 5 of his 12 patients.

These fractures are most commonly confused with dislocation of the elbow.[2-5,7,8,14-16,19-21,27,28] DeJager and Hoffman[4] observed that a dislocation of the elbow had never been reported in a child under age 4. Rang[18] stated that elbow dislocations unaccompanied by fracture are rare in children, and wondered if "an infant's elbow ever dislocate(s)".

When a lateral metaphyseal fragment is present, these injuries may be mistaken for lateral condyle fractures.[2-5,7,8,14,16,27,28] If minimally displaced, the distinction may be unimportant. However, if the fragment is widely displaced, the differentiation is an important one, because transcondylar fractures are often successfully treated closed, unlike lateral condyle fractures, which often require open reduction. They also do not have as serious long-term consequences as do neglected lateral condyle fractures[15,27,28] (Fig. 12-4).

A few authors have reported difficulty distinguishing a transcondylar fracture from a supracondylar fracture.[1,19,27] Rang[18] recalls mistaking a few for septic arthritis. Cothay[25] initially thought that a patient with a fracture of the medial two-thirds of the trochlea had a medial epicondyle fracture.

DIAGNOSTIC FEATURES

The keys to recognizing transcondylar fractures are radiographic signs. In evaluating this fracture, as in any pediatric elbow injury, it is advisable to obtain comparison views of the uninjured extremity.[3,5,14,17,28] The most commonly cited finding in transcondylar fractures is

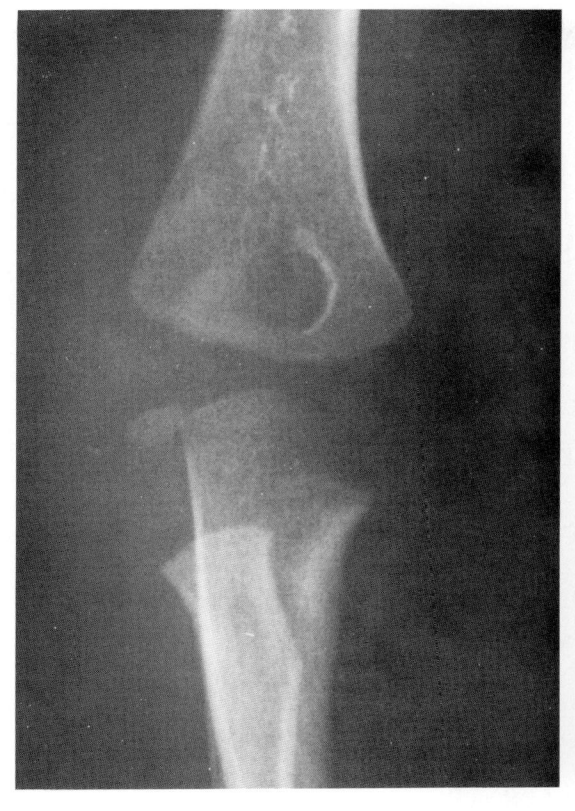

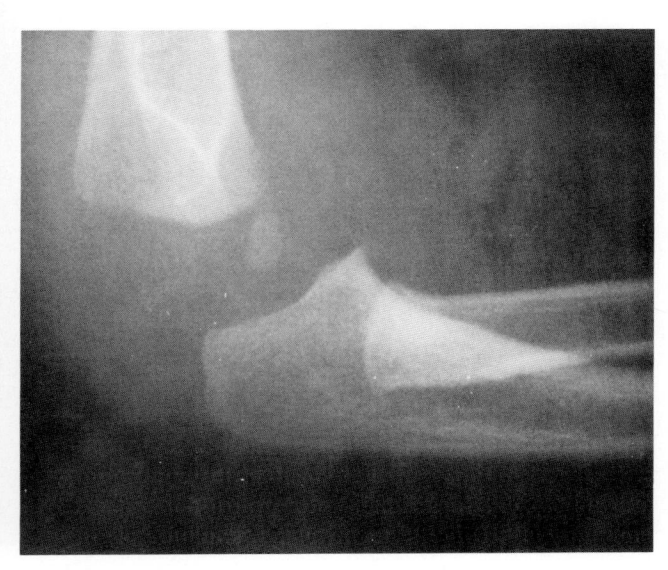

Fig. 12-4. This injury was thought to be a transcondylar fracture, but later proved to be a displaced lateral condyle fracture requiring open reduction. We missed the fact that the capitellum does not align with the radius on the lateral view.

that the radius aligns with the capitellum in all views (Fig. 12-5A&B).[2,3,5,7,10,13,15,17,28-30] In a dislocation this axis is disturbed in both views (Fig. 12-5C). In a lateral condyle fracture, it is usually disrupted in at least one view, as the lateral condyle rotates if there is any significant displacement (Fig. 12-5D). If the radius and ulna maintain their normal alignment, but a fracture is seen, one must consider a supracondylar fracture, a medial epicondyle fracture, or a transcondylar fracture (Fig. 12-5E).[5,13] The displacement in a dislocation or a lateral condyle fracture is often lateral.[17] Transcondylar fractures are almost always displaced medially or posteromedially.[2,3,6,17,19] A lateral condyle fracture usually rotates away from the humerus, hinging anteriorly and opening posteriorly, whereas a transcondylar fracture will tend to hinge posteriorly and open anteriorly[4]

The position of the capitellum itself may be helpful. In a lateral condyle fracture, it changes position with respect to both the humerus and the radius (Figs. 12-4 and 12-5D). In a dislocation, it maintains its relationship to the humerus, but changes with respect to the radius (Fig. 12-5C). In an transcondylar fracture, it changes with respect to the humerus, but maintains its alignment with the radius (Fig. 12-5B)[14]

In infants too young to have an ossified capitellum, some softer signs might be helpful. The radius and the ulna have a normal relationship to each other,[15,17,21,27] but their relationship to the distal humerus is disturbed.[3,15,19] The lateral view shows posterior displacement of the olecranon (or forearm segment).[4,12,16,23] Comparison with the other elbow will reveal a decrease in the gap between the anterior humeral line and the proximal radial metaphysis.[4] The anteroposterior view may show foreshortening of the distance between the humerus and the forearm bones.[12,16,23] There may be a very thin metaphyseal flake (Werenskiold fragment) visible, indicating an epiphyseal fracture (Fig. 12-3A).[5,31] At 7 to 10 days, callus will be seen ensheathing the distal humerus (Fig. 12-6).[17]

Many authors have endorsed the usefulness of arthrography in the evaluation of these injuries, especially in infants.[2-4,7,8,16,19,32,33] Akbarnia and colleagues[8] reported six infants, all of whom had their diagnoses established by arthrography; they felt that the treatment had

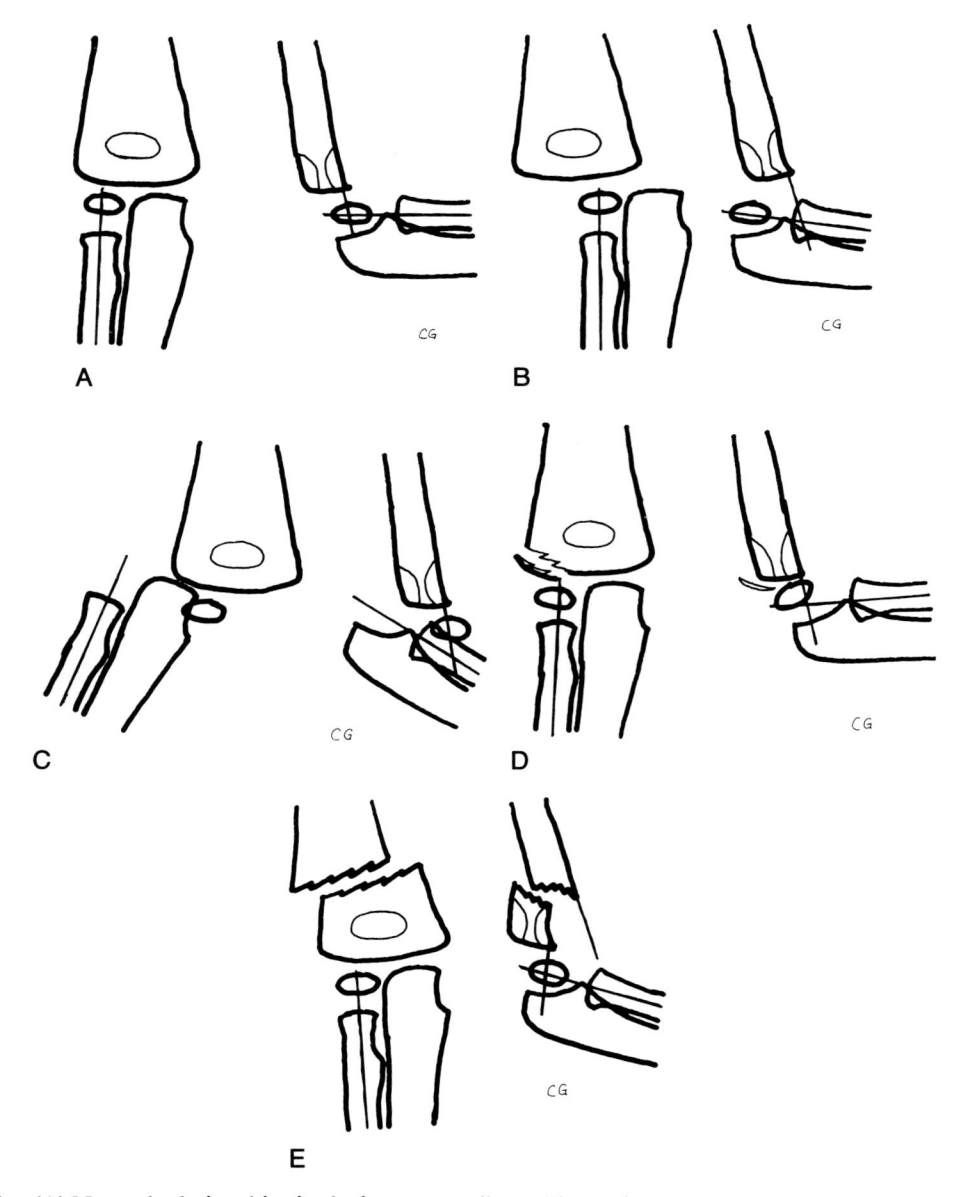

Fig. 12-5. **(A)** Normal relationships in the immature elbow. The capitellum aligns with the proximal radius on both views. Also, the anterior humeral line transects the midportion of the capitellum on the lateral view. **(B)** In a transcondylar fracture, the alignment of the capitellum with the proximal radius is maintained in both projections. However, the relationship between the distal humerus and both the capitellum and the forearm bones is disturbed. **(C)** In a dislocation, the relationship between the capitellum and the distal humerus is preserved, but that between the capitellum and the radius is disrupted. **(D)** In a lateral condyle fracture the relationship between the capitellum and the humerus or between the capitellum and the radius may be disturbed in either view. There is usually a metaphyseal fragment. **(E)** A supracondylar fracture is characterized by a fracture visible in the distal humerus and no disturbance in the relationship between the capitellum and the distal humerus or between the capitellum and the proximal radius.

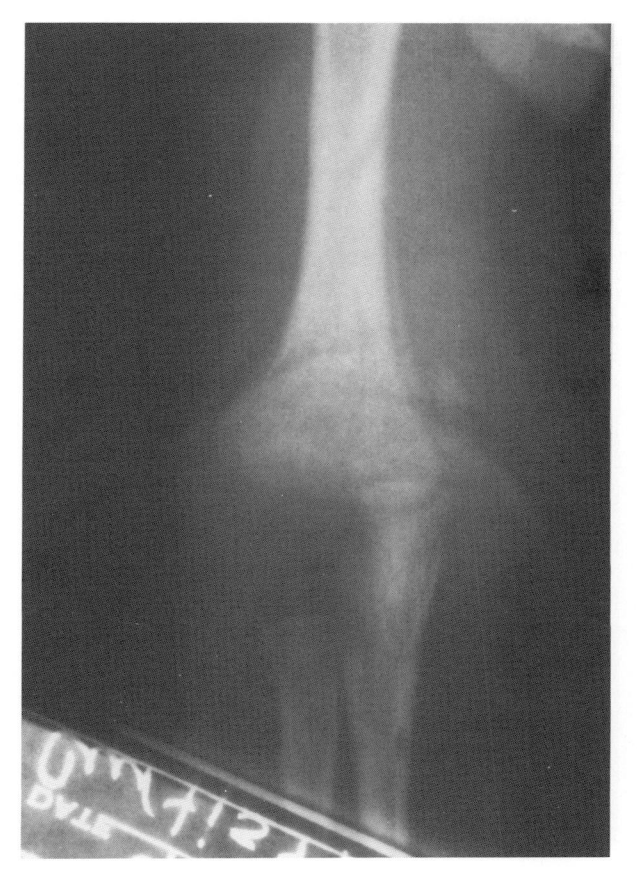

Fig. 12-6. Group A transcondylar fracture in a 5-day-old newborn referred for evaluation of a possible birth palsy. Note the periosteal elevation. She had a history of swelling in the elbow at birth, and was still a little tender.

been significantly affected in five. Yates and Sullivan[33] used arthrography to make the diagnosis in six patients, five of whom had been mistakenly thought to have lateral condyle fractures.

Akbarnia and colleagues[8] recommended instilling 0.5 cc of contrast into the elbow through a lateral approach. Yates and Sullivan[33] found it more helpful to use 1 cc of contrast and 1 cc of air to create a double contrast. They used either a lateral or a posterior approach.

Arthrography can be revealing in several ways. Yates and Sullivan describe obliteration of the coronoid and olecranon fossae by hematoma in supracondylar fractures. They also were able to see an intact articular cartilage surface in epiphyseal separation, as opposed to a lateral condyle fracture, in which the articular surface may be disrupted (Fig. 12-7). The area of dye pooling can define the location of periosteal stripping.[33] Akbarnia and colleagues[8] found that arthrography was most useful in distinguishing a Salter-Harris type I epiphyseal fracture from a dislocation, or a type II fracture from a type IV fracture.

Finally, Dias and colleagues[32] describe using ultrasound to diagnose this injury in the neonate. It is capable of visualizing the cartilaginous distal humerus.

MANAGEMENT

Some authors surmise that many of these fractures are probably missed and heal satisfactorily.[17,32] Ekengren and coworkers[22] noted significant remodeling in some of their patients. McIntyre and associates[6] were of the opinion that these fractures were not disastrous if missed. Wilkins[3] recommended no attempt at reduction if seen after 5 to 6 days; DeLee[17] recommended no reduction after 2 to 3 weeks; and Ogden[2] recommended no reduction after several weeks. However, cubitus varus has been reported with variable frequency following this fracture,[2,4,6,12,17,18] and some recommend that this fracture be treated using the same principles employed with supracondylar fractures.[10,13]

Closed Reduction

Closed reduction followed by splinting in flexion and pronation (because of the usual medial displacement) has been very commonly employed.[2,3,12,16,17,19,20,28–30,34] Ogden[2] advocates reducing the fracture by traction, then gently correcting the medial displacement and varus tilt. He also points out that rotation should be corrected, even though cubitus varus is less common because of the greater surface area at the fracture site. DeJager and Hoffman[4] prefer this treatment for children over age 2 with stable fractures. Wilkins[3] employs this method for infants, and uses a figure-of-eight dressing.

Closed reduction and percutaneous pinning is another acceptable treatment method for this fracture.[2,14,19] DeJager and Hoffman[4] prefer this method for children under age 2, because they encountered greater difficulty evaluating and controlling alignment of the distal fragment in this age group. Peiro and colleagues[14] advise using two pins from the lateral side, because it is so difficult to palpate the medial epicondyle for safe pin placement with these distal fractures (Fig. 12-8). Wilkins[3] uses percutaneous pinning for older infants and young children, and agrees with the use of two lateral pins. He also recommends an arthrogram to better visualize the distal fragment. Whichever method is used,

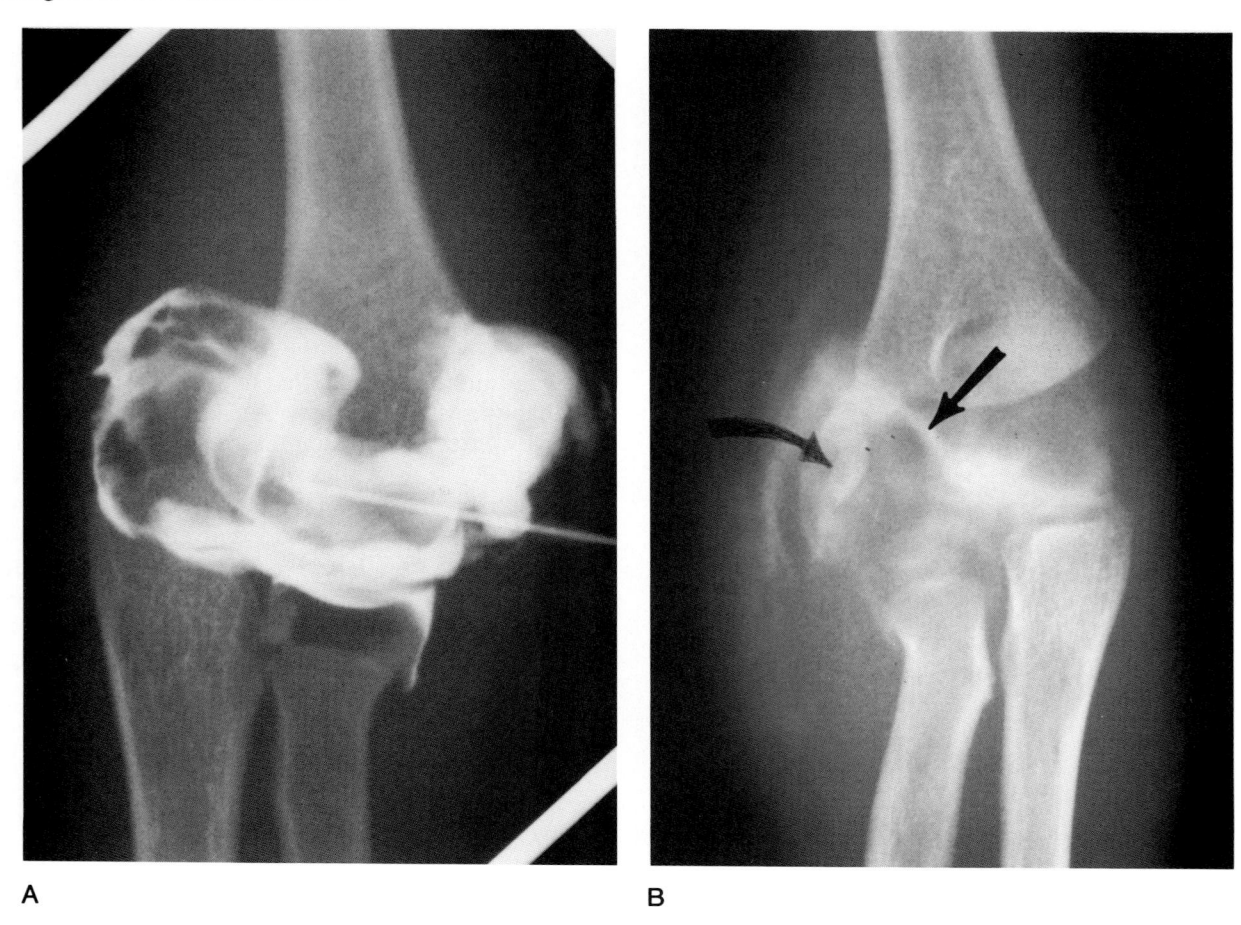

Fig. 12-7. (A) Arthrogram of transcondylar fracture, showing that the articular surface has not been disrupted. (B) Arthrogram of lateral condyle fracture, demonstrating disruption of the articular surface, with dye collecting in the defect *(straight arrow)*. The *curved arrow* indicates the capitellar fragment, which has rotated so that the articular surface points laterally.

several authors urge that the patient be admitted for swelling.[8,17,19,28]

Traction

In the past, traction has been used a great deal to treat this injury. Most of the reports have described the use of Dunlop's traction[16,35,36] It has found its greatest utility in those patients with marked swelling,[2,3,16,17] or a diminished pulse.[28] Another method receiving some attention recently is straight lateral traction.[4,5,18,37] Piggot and colleagues[37] reported this method in the treatment of 98 severely displaced supracondylar fractures, and noted only 4 cases of cubitus varus. They felt that this type of traction afforded better visualization of the distal fragment. DeJager and Hoffman[4] advocate its use in children under 2 with a decreased carrying angle.

Open Reduction

While some authors state that open reduction is not indicated in the treatment of this fracture,[16,17,21,28] others recommend that an accurate reduction be obtained.[6,13] Many do feel that open reduction is indicated in certain situations.[2,3,6,19,20,38] It is occasionally necessary to deal with interposed soft tissues.[19,20,34] McIntyre and colleagues[6] performed one open reduction concurrently with a brachial artery repair. They also opened one elbow in order to verify the diagnosis. Archibald and colleagues[38] reported 79 percent excellent or good results using open

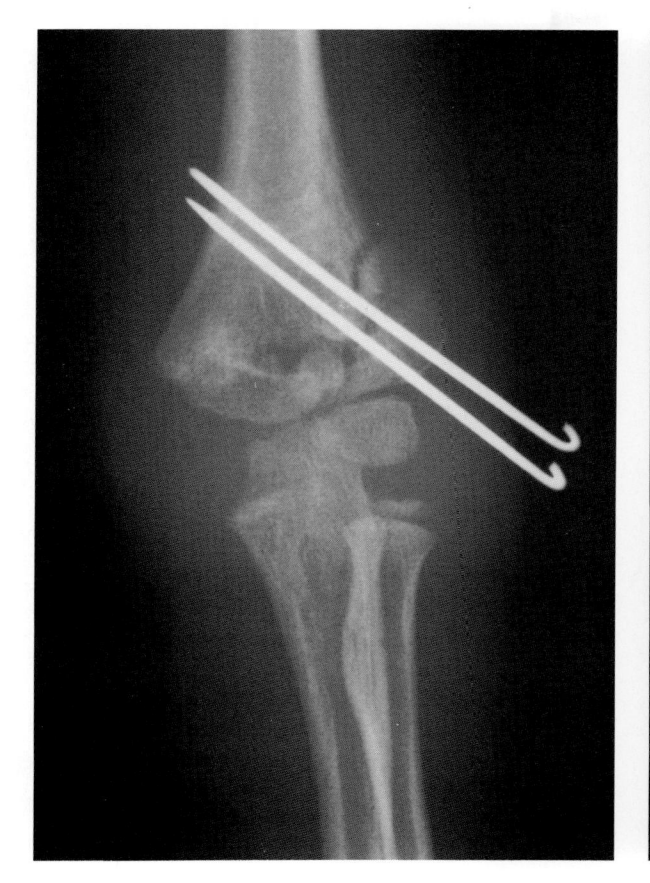

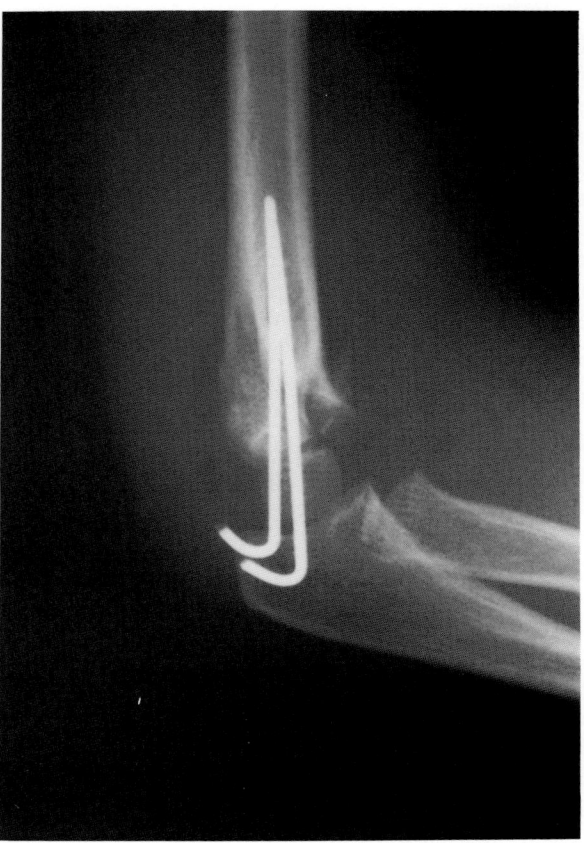

Fig. 12-8. Percutaneous pinning of transcondylar fracture with two laterally placed pins. The small fishtail seen on the lateral view is less than ideal. It blocks flexion for a few months, but usually remodels.

reduction through a medial approach and fixation with 2.4-mm pins placed across the elbow joint. Only one patient out of 34 lost greater than 15 degrees of motion, but 5 had a change in carrying angle of 10 degrees or more, even with this treatment. Finally, one may occasionally be unable to determine with certainty whether the injury is a displaced lateral condyle fracture or a transcondylar fracture, even with an arthrogram. In such a situation, it is probably better to proceed with an open reduction. If the injury is a transcondylar fracture, one may have overtreated it, but the potential for harm is low. If it is a displaced lateral condyle fracture, the open reduction is necessary to avoid significant complications.

Pitfalls of Management

The pitfalls encountered in treating this fracture are largely related to failures in diagnosis. To avoid this requires a high index of suspicion, and the liberal use of comparison views and arthrography. There are also pitfalls related to treatment. The most common complication is cubitus varus, resulting from the failure to obtain or maintain an adequate reduction. This is particularly difficult to do in very young infants, in whom the entire distal fragment may be radiolucent. Here again, arthrography is helpful. Also, percutaneous pinning can add a measure of security.

COMPLICATIONS

The neurovascular complications so frequently seen in supracondylar fractures are "infrequent" in this injury, according to Ogden.[2] Many authors report no neurovascular injuries[3,4,13,14,17] McIntyre and coworkers[6] had one patient who fell from a truck, sustaining a severe distraction injury, resulting in damage to the brachial artery and the brachial plexus.

The most common problem resulting from this injury is cubitus varus.[2,4,6,12,17,18] Ogden[6] stated that it was less common than after supracondylar fractures. Wilkins[3] wrote that it was rare in his experience. DeJager and Hoffman[4] found that 12 of 48 patients in six series had cubitus varus. It was more common under age 2, partly because there was no metaphyseal flake to indicate the position of the distal fragment. They reported that cubitus varus of 5 to 15 degrees occurred in 3 of their own 10 patients, despite the use of open reduction. Baumann's angle was useless in their opinion. DeLee and coworkers[17] found cubitus varus of 5 to 15 degrees in 3 of their 12 patients. All of their patients with cubitus varus were under age 2. Five of the seven patients reported by Holda and coworkers[13] had varus of 10 to 15 degrees. McIntyre and colleagues[6] admitted that 4 of their 12 patients had a loss of carrying angle. Siffert[12] had a 10-degree varus in one of his three patients. Yngve[30] reported a case of cubitus varus requiring osteotomy (Fig. 12-9).

Another fairly frequent complication seen in transcondylar fractures is loss of motion. This can be loss of either flexion or extension. Fortunately, the limitation of motion is seldom more than 10 to 15 degrees, and is seen in about 20 to 50 percent of patients.[4,8,14,17,21,22] de Jager and Hoffman[4] had one patient with a 55-degree flexion contracture, but he was seen late.

Other complications are rare. Ogden[2] states that growth disturbance is a significant complication, but rare. Other authors state that they have not seen it at all.[5,17] Siffert[12] had one patient in whom prominence of the distal end of the humerus was a problem. Wilkins[3] warns of the possibility of developing avascular necrosis of the trochlea, and says that he has had three patients who developed a "fishtail deformity" as a result. Mizuno and coworkers[7] reported one case of nonunion in a patient seen at 3 months.

SUMMARY

Transcondylar fractures are probably more common than we think, but are often not appreciated. They occur as a result of birth injuries, child abuse, and falls on the outstretched hand. They are most frequently mistaken for dislocations and lateral condyle fractures. The most helpful radiographic clue to their diagnosis is that the capitellum aligns with the radius on both views. Arthrography can also be helpful. The treatment is controversial, recommendations ranging from closed reduction to open reduction. These fractures generally do well.

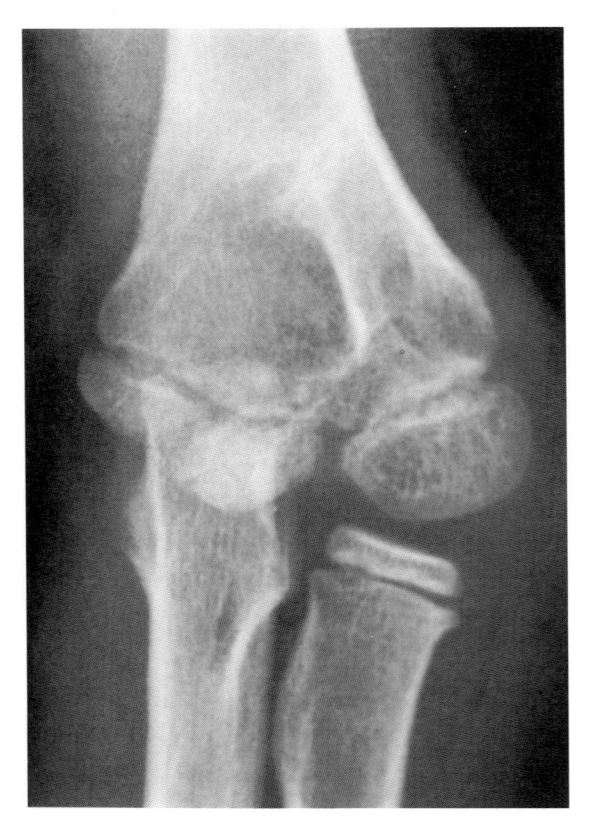

Fig. 12-9. Cubitus varus persisting 7 years after the injury.

The most frequent complications are cubitus varus deformity and mild loss of motion.

REFERENCES

1. Cotton FJ: Elbow fractures in children. Ann Surg 35:75, 1902
2. Ogden JA: Skeletal Injury in the Child. WB Saunders, Philadelphia, 1990
3. Wilkins KE: Fractures and Dislocations of the Elbow Region. In Rockwood CA, Wilkins KE, King RE (eds): Fractures in Children. JB Lippincott, Philadelphia, 1991
4. De Jager LT, Hoffman EB: Fracture-separation of the distal humeral epiphysis. J Bone Joint Surg [Br] 73:143, 1991
5. Rogers LF, Rockwood CA: Separation of the entire distal humeral epiphysis. Radiology 106:393, 1973
6. McIntyre WM, Wiley JJ, Charette RJ: Fracture-separation of the distal humeral epiphysis. Clin Orthop 188:98, 1984
7. Mizuno K, Hirohata K, Kashiwagi D: Fracture-separation

of the distal humeral epiphysis in young children. J Bone Joint Surg [Am] 61:570, 1979
8. Akbarnia BA, Silberstein MJ, Rende RJ et al: Arthrography in the diagnosis of fractures of the distal end of the humerus in infants. J Bone Joint Surg [Am] 68:599, 1986
9. Ashhurst APC: An Anatomical and Surgical Study of Fractures of the Lower End of the Humerus. Lea and Febiger, Philadelphia, 1910
10. Dameron TB: Transverse fractures of the distal humerus in children. Instr Course Lect 30:224, 1981
11. Mauer I, Kolovos D, Loscos R: Epiphyseolysis of the distal humerus in a newborn. Bull Hosp Joint Dis 28:109, 1967
12. Siffert RS: Displacement of the distal humeral epiphysis in the newborn infant. J Bone Joint Surg [Am] 45:165, 1963
13. Holda ME, Manoli A, Lamont RL: Epiphyseal separation of the distal end of the humerus with medial displacement. J Bone Joint Surg [Am] 62:52, 1980
14. Peiro A, Mut T, Aracil J, Martos F: Fracture-separation of the lower humeral epiphysis in young children. Acta Orthop Scand 52:295, 1981
15. Paige ML, Port RB: Separation of the distal humeral epiphysis in the neonate: a combined clinical and roentgenographic diagnosis. Am J Dis Child 139:1203, 1985
16. Chand K: Epiphyseal separation of distal humerus in an infant. J Trauma 14:521, 1974
17. DeLee JC, Wilkins KE, Rogers LF, Rockwood CA: Fracture-separation of the distal humeral epiphysis. J Bone Joint Surg [Am] 62:46, 1980
18. Rang M: Children's Fractures. JB Lippincott, Philadelphia, 1983
19. Barrett WP, Almquist EA, Staheli LT: Fracture separation of the distal humeral physis in the newborn. J Pediatr Orthop 4:617, 1984
20. Berman JM, Weiner DS: Neonatal fracture-separation of the distal humeral chondroepiphysis: a case report. Orthopedics 3:875, 1980
21. Downs DM, Wirth CR: Fracture of the distal humeral chondroepiphysis in the neonate: a case report. Clin Orthop 169:155, 1982
22. Ekengren K, Bergdahl S, Ekstrom G: Birth injuries to the epiphyseal cartilage. Acta Radiol [Diagn] (Stockh) 19:197, 1978
23. Tachdjian MO: Pediatric Orthopedics. WB Saunders, Philadelphia, 1990
24. Holland CT: A radiographical note on injuries to the distal epiphyses of the radius and ulna. Proc R Soc Med 22:695, 1929
25. Cothay DM: Injury to the lower medial epiphysis of the humerus before development of the ossific centre. J Bone Joint Surg [Br] 49:766, 1967
26. Grantham AB, Tietjen R: Transcondylar fracture-dislocation of the elbow. J Bone Joint Surg [Am] 58:1030, 1976
27. Hansen PE, Barnes DA, Tullos HS: Arthrographic diagnosis of an injury pattern in the distal humerus of an infant. J Pediatr Orthop 2:569, 1982
28. Marmor L, Bechtol CO: Fracture separation of the lower humeral epiphysis. J Bone Joint Surg [Am] 42:333, 1960
29. Kaplan SS, Reckling FW: Fracture separation of the lower humeral epiphysis with medial displacement. J Bone Joint Surg [Am] 53:1105 1971
30. Yngve DA: Distal humeral epiphyseal separation. Orthopaedics 8:102, 1985
31. Werenskiold B: A contribution to the roentgen diagnosis of epiphyseal separations. Acta Radiol [Diagn] (Stockh) 8:419, 1927
32. Dias JJ, Lamont AC, Jones JM: Ultrasonic diagnosis of neonatal separation of the distal humeral epiphysis. J Bone Joint Surg [Br] 70:825, 1988
33. Yates C, Sullivan JA: Arthrographic diagnosis of elbow injuries in children. J Pediatr Orthop 7:54, 1987
34. Omer GE, Simmons JM: Fracture of the distal humeral metaphyseal growth plate. South Med J 61:651, 1968
35. Allen PD, Gramse AE: Transcondylar fractures of the humerus treated by Dunlop traction. Am J Surg 67:217, 1945
36. Dunlop J: Transcondylar fractures of the humerus in childhood. J Bone Joint Surg 21:59, 1939
37. Piggot J, Graham HK, McCoy GF: Supracondylar fractures of the humerus in children: treatment by straight lateral traction. J Bone Joint Surg [Br] 68:577, 1986
38. Archibald DAA, Roberts JA, Smith MGH: Transarticular fixation for severely displaced supracondylar fractures in children. J Bone Joint Surg [Br] 73:147, 1991

13

Dislocation of the Elbow and Fractures of the Medial Humeral Epicondyle and Condyle

Walter W. Huurman

> No great advance has ever been made in science, politics or religion without controversy.
> —Lyman Beeches

To clearly appreciate the vagaries of injuries to the medial side of the elbow, a firm grasp of normal anatomy, including embryonic development of the distal humerus, its associated physes, muscles, ligaments, and blood supply is essential.

The distal humerus, shortly after birth until approximately 5 years of age, consists of a single confluent mass of epiphyseal cartilage, which has a single secondary center of ossification. On the metaphyseal margin, it is capped by a single, transverse sinusoidal physis. At this early stage the entire distal humeral epiphysis is intra-articular with the joint capsule attaching just proximal to the physis. Subsequent development is not unlike that of the proximal femur, which, at birth, consists of a single physis underlying the cartilaginous precursor of the femoral head and greater trochanter. The single physis of the distal humerus overlies the lateral condyle, trochlea, medial condyle, and medial epicondyle. With maturation, the medial epicondylar portion of the epiphysis becomes an extra-articular segment, which no longer contributes to longitudinal growth of the bone. The underlying epicondylar growth plate, although nearly continuous with the transhumeral physis, is functionally a separate entity. At this point in time the medial epicondyle is truly an extra-articular apophysis rather than an articular epiphysis (Fig. 13-1). Further justifying its designation as an apophysis, the flexor/pronator muscle mass of the forearm takes a major portion of its origin from the anterior/inferior segment of the epicondyle.[1]

Maturation of the medial condylar process results in development of a groove on its posteromedial surface, which accommodates passage of the ulnar nerve across the posteromedial aspect of the joint. The posterior metaphyseal border of the epicondylar physis forms the medial margin of the groove.

Ossification centers on the medial side of the elbow appear sequentially: the medial epicondyle at approximately age 5, followed by the trochlea at about 8 years of age and olecranon of the ulna shortly thereafter.

The sculpted shape of the distal humeral epiphysis is responsible for some of the consequences seen following fractures in this region. The medialmost margin of the trochlear portion of the distal humeral epiphysis is quite defined as it projects downward from the rather smooth,

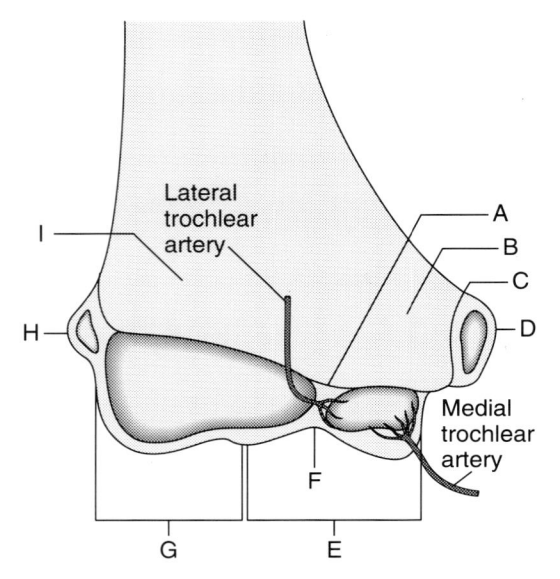

Fig. 13-1. Bony anatomy of the developing distal humerus. *(A)* distal humeral physis; *(B)* medial condyle; *(C)* medial epicondylar physis; *(D)* medial epicondyle; *(E)* trochlea; *(F)* trochlear incisure; *(G)* capitulum; *(E & G)* distal humeral epiphysis; *(H)* lateral epicondyle; *(I)* lateral condyle.

round inferior medial epicondylar surface. The articulating portion of the trochlea is grooved to accommodate the sigmoid prominence of the ulnar articular surface, and on its lateral most margin a second, smaller groove separates it from the capitular portion of the distal humeral epiphysis. Blood to the trochlea comes by way of two small interosseus terminal branches of the recurrent ulnar artery.[2] The medialmost of the two penetrates the medial cartilage of the trochlea, and the lateralmost crosses the physis from the metaphyseal bone entering the lateral margin of the trochlea. This vessel traverses the narrowest portion of the distal humeral epiphysis, which is at the deepest portion of the trochlear incisure (Fig. 13-1). Fractures of the medial condyle, which cross the epiphysis, separate this vessel and may result in avascular necrosis of the lateral portion of the trochlea and a resultant "fishtail" deformity.

FRACTURES OF THE MEDIAL EPICONDYLE

Anatomy

As discussed, the medial epicondyle originates as a portion of the distal humeral epiphysis, contributing to longitudinal humeral growth. By age 2, maturation results in its migration to an extra-articular position juxtaposed to the medial side of the distal humeral metaphysis. At this point, no longer does the epicondyle contribute to longitudinal growth of the humerus, and hence it becomes an apophysis from whose anterior surface the forearm flexor muscles take origin. The proximal end of the joint stabilizing medial ligamentous structures attach to the epicondyle posteroinferiorly.

In most reviews of elbow trauma less than 10 percent of injuries to the elbow involve the medial epicondyle. Blount states that such injuries represent 8 percent of childhood elbow fractures.[3] In several studies there seems to be a rather high prevalence of boys (up to 80 percent)[4] sustaining this injury as compared to girls. Despite the infrequency of medial epicondylar injuries, at the child's elbow only supracondylar and lateral condylar fractures occur more frequently.

Mechanism of Injury

Fracture of the medial epicondyle usually occurs as a result of a fall on the outstretched arm with the elbow extended and the wrist dorsiflexed[5] (Fig. 13-2). The protective reflexes stimulated by this posture causes the flexor/pronator muscle mass to contract, avulsing the epicondyle from its attachment to the medial metaphysis.[6] This detachment can take the form of a Salter-Harris type I fracture, in which the entire apophysis is detached through its physis (Fig. 13-3), a Salter-Harris type II fracture when a portion of the medial metaphysis remains attached to the apophyseal/physeal fragment, or a fracture in which only a portion of the apophysis is avulsed (Fig. 13-4).

The normal mild valgus alignment of the extended forearm enhances the valgus-induced stress on the elbow and concentration of the forces will further disrupt the medial supporting soft tissues. If the force continues after anteromedial soft tissue supporting structures of the joint are disrupted, the joint opens and lateral subluxation of the olecranon and radial head from the trochlea and capitellum occurs. The avulsed epicondylar fragment, with the elbow in valgus and medial capsule disrupted, may be pulled intra-articularly; at the conclusion of the fall the elbow tends to resume normal alignment. The epicondyle, at this point, has been either extruded from or entrapped within the joint (Fig. 13-5).

The ulnar nerve, lying in its groove on the posteromedial aspect of the humeral condyle, is subjected to an elongation force with progressive elbow valgus.[7] It may,

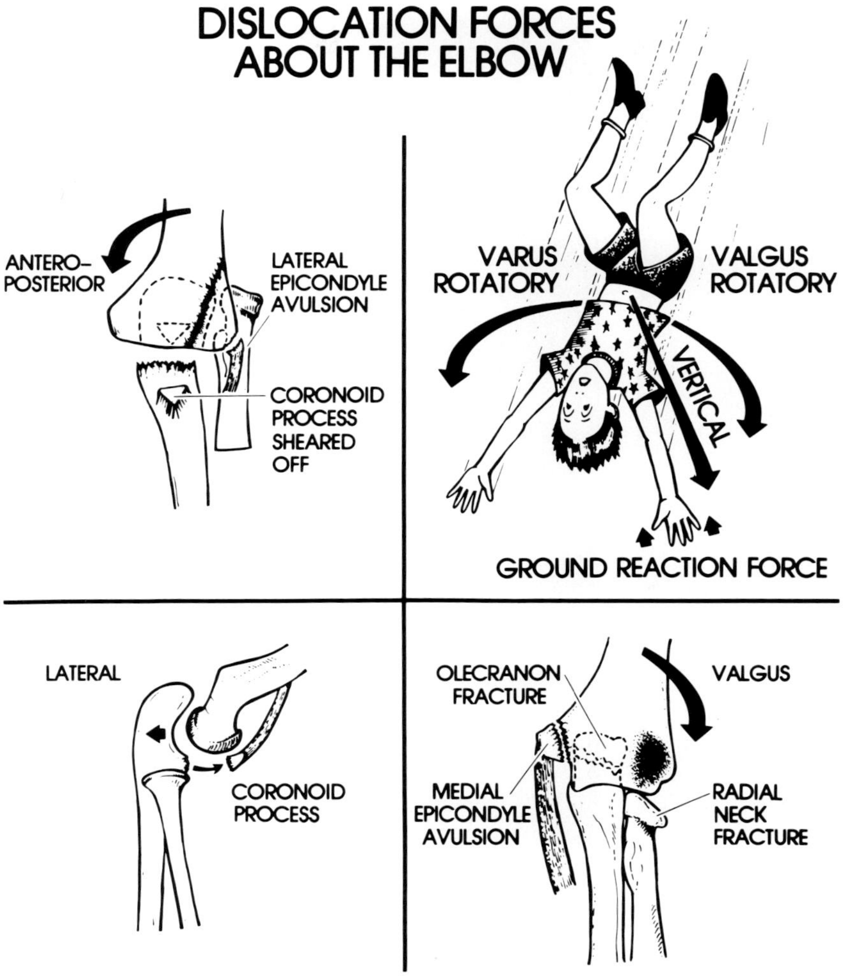

Fig. 13-2. Fracture patterns about the elbow secondary to varus or valgus forces. (From Letts RM: Dislocations of the elbow in children. In Morrey BF, (ed.): The Elbow and Its Disorders. WB Saunders, Philadelphia, 1985, with permission.)

in fact, slide out of the normal confines of its groove and assume an intra-articular position.

Classification of Injuries to the Medial Epicondyle

In addition to the Salter-Harris classification of physeal fractures, a simple, clinically relevant classification system specific to medial epicondylar fracture has been offered by Rang,[6] shown in Table 13-1. In addition to these four classifications, avulsion of the muscle origin with or without an attached wafer of apophyseal bone may occur. From the clinical standpoint, such avulsion fractures or soft tissue disruptions may be classified along with the Rang type I fractures (Fig. 13-4). It is to this Rang classification that our further discussion of this epicondylar fracture refers.

Radiology

Since the medial epicondyle lies on the posteromedial aspect of the distal humerus, it may be necessary to externally rotate the humerus 10–15 degrees to obtain an anteroposterior view that truly records the relationship of the medial epicondyle to its underlying metaphysis.[8] A true lateral projection of the distal humerus will obscure most of the epicondylar prominence, and hence is of little value as an assessment tool in difficult cases,

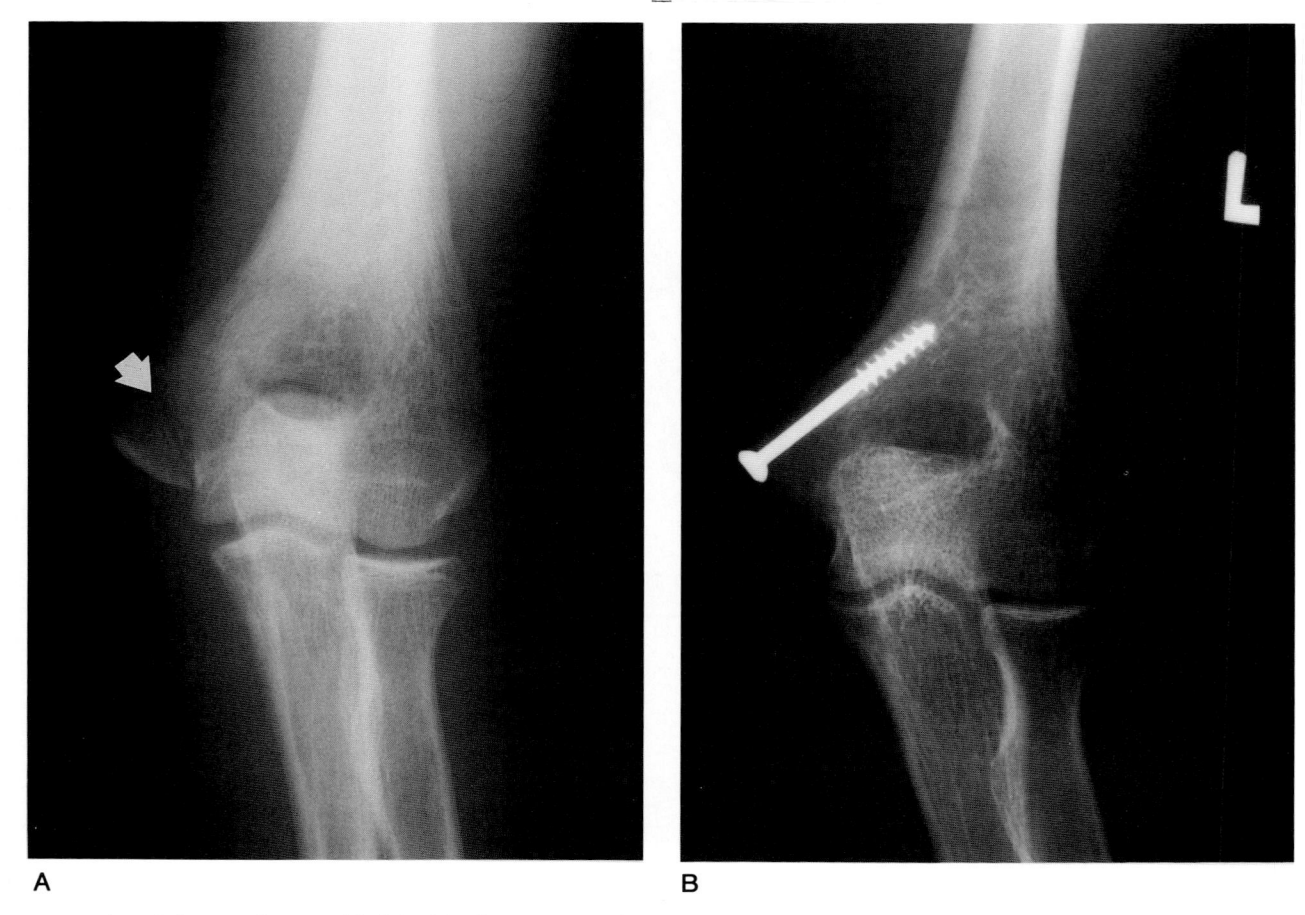

Fig. 13-3. A 13-year-old girl with displaced medial epicondylar fracture, treated with closed reduction and percutaneous screw. **(A)** Fracture fragment displaced inferiorly and rotated. **(B)** Two years post-closed reduction. Note mild overgrowth of the medial epicondyle. (Courtesy of Dr. Paul Esposito.)

unless the epicondyle is anteriorly or posteriorly displaced (Fig. 13-6).

Treatment

Controversy reigns over the need for reduction and fixation. It is unanimously agreed that type I fractures or wafer avulsions of the flexor/pronator origin need only be treated with a brief period (2 weeks) of immobilization. It is also generally agreed that medial epicondylar fragments that are entrapped within the elbow joint as well as those associated with elbow dislocation, require surgical repair.[8–10] It is the moderately displaced type II fracture that has proponents for both surgical and closed treatment methods. Papavisilou[4] joins others[6,11,12] who feel that displacement beyond 2–3 mm may lead to chronic elbow instability and therefore recommend reduction and internal fixation for all but the very minimally displaced fragment (Fig. 13-7). Others have found little problem with simple immobilization.[8,9,13] Support for closed treatment is provided by a long-term follow up review of 56 medial epicondyle fractures treated without reduction. Josefsson and Danielsson[14] espoused nonoperative treatment after reviewing these cases some 35 years after injury. It is worthy to note that 60 percent of their cases failed to develop bony union and a significant 21 percent had residual symptoms; the symptoms, however, were seemingly unrelated to presence or absence of a pseudarthrosis.

Similarly, because they found no long-term difference between 7 patients treated operatively and 12 others nonoperatively, Bernstein and colleagues[9] felt the only indication for surgery was a type III or IV fracture in

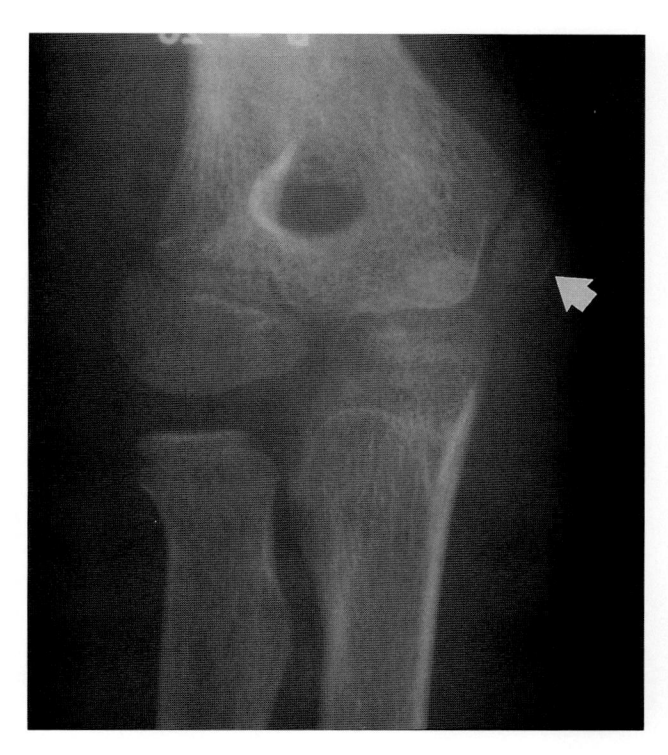

Fig. 13-4. Avulsion of the forearm flexor origin, carrying with it a wafer of medial epicondyle.

which the epicondylar fragment could not be manipulatively extruded from the elbow joint.

Another consideration which at times influences treatment is ulnar nerve symptomatology.[15] Some earlier authors felt that open reduction should be routinely accompanied by anterior transfer of the ulnar nerve, particularly if prereduction physical examination demonstrates any evidence of sensory or motor compromise.[3,16] Close association of the posteromedial condylar groove, which accommodates passage of the ulnar nerve across the joint, to the medial epicondylar base, predisposes the nerve to trauma during an event that results in epicondylar fracture. Damage to the nerve may be due either to direct contusion or stretching.

Author's Preferred Method of Treatment

Advances in surgical technique as well as instrumentation improvement over the past decade have redefined the constitution of a satisfactory treatment result for many fractures, including those of the medial humeral epicondyle. Intraoperative fluoroscopy, powered instrumentation, cannulated screws, and modern anesthetic techniques have decreased morbidity and facilitated performance of reduction and fixation. Hence it is my practice to treat without internal fixation only those fractures that are displaced less than 2 mm at the time of injury and remain undisplaced during the subsequent 2 or 3 weeks of immobilization. All other fractures of the epicondyle tend to be reduced and rigidly fixed under general anesthesia.

Type I Fractures

Immobilization in a long-arm cast is recommended with the elbow at 90 degrees of flexion, the forearm slightly pronated, and the wrist in moderate flexion. This should be maintained for 2 or 3 weeks, then changed to a simple sling for 1 week. A radiograph of the distal humerus at 3 and 8 days after casting should be obtained to assure that no change in fragment position due to muscle forces has occurred. In order to obtain a clear anteroposterior view of the epicondyle, the arm should be externally rotated 10 degrees and the x-ray tube tilted distally 15 degrees. After sling removal, the child is allowed to return to activities slowly (over 2 or 3 weeks) and a final radiograph obtained 6 weeks following injury. Since longitudinal growth is not affected, long-term follow-up is usually unnecessary.

Type II Fractures

When the fragment is displaced (Fig. 13-8), more than 2 mm but not entrapped within the joint, reduction and fixation serve to promote bony union, protect against late instability, and permit early motion to enhance return of full flexion/extension.

On occasion, the displaced epicondylar fragment may be manipulated into a position of anatomic reduction by flexing the elbow, flexing the wrist, and "urging" the epicondyle into position with one's fingers. If swelling is not too great and soft tissues are not interposed, reduction by this method can frequently be accomplished.

Using the image intensifier, a single .062 Kirschner wire is then drilled through the manually reduced epicondylar fragment into the metaphysis. If necessary, once the epicondyle is engaged, the K-wire may be used to further manipulate the fragment into better position. Firm fixation is mandatory, and hence a second divergent wire is inserted or a single, cannulated screw placed over the already stabilizing K-wire (Fig. 13-3). I prefer to leave the pins protruding extracutaneously in order that they may be removed in the office; they are bent 90 degrees at the skin, using a large needle driver to stabilize

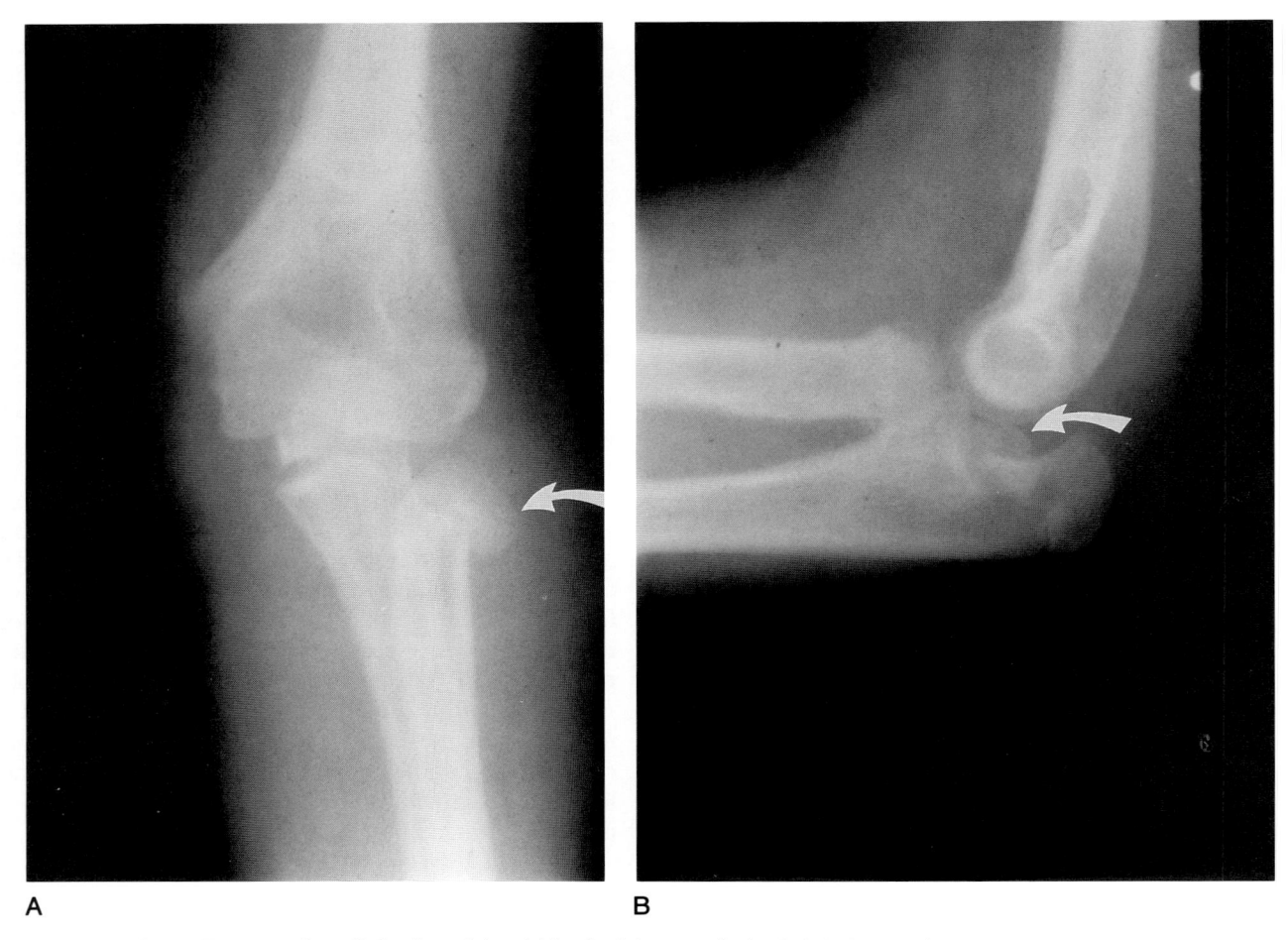

Fig. 13-5. Entrapped medial epicondyle within the joint seen in both **(A)** the AP view and **(B)** the lateral view. Note the fracture of the radial neck seen best in the AP view due to the valgus force that also avulsed the medial epicondyle.

the pin while the drill and chuck act as an instrument to create the 90-degree bend. The pins are cut, padded with orthopaedic felt, and incorporated within the cast.

Postoperatively the cast is left in place for 4 weeks and both cast and pins removed at the same time. Gradual return to activity over the ensuing 3 weeks should promote return of motion, although full motion may not be realized for several months.

Above all, the physician is cautioned to avoid use of physical therapy modalities or passive exercises. I have shared the experience of others that even well intended, "gentle" therapy may result in permanent stiffness.

If closed manipulation is unsuccessful in effecting a near-anatomic reduction, a lateral curved incision 3 cm in length centered over the epicondylar metaphysis is made. Identification or stripping of specific muscle origins requiring meddlesome dissection is to be avoided. The incision usually leads directly to the fracture site,

and a special effort to dissect out the ulnar nerve is usually unnecessary. After gently cleansing the soft tissues and bone ends of clotted blood, the epicondyle, which is consistently rotated 90–180 degrees, may be grasped with forceps and gently reduced into its bed. Again, with the assistance of fluoroscopy, the fragment is fixed rigidly either with a single small, cannulated screw or two divergent K-wires. After wound closure, care is much the same as in the percutaneously pinned/screwed fracture. Occasionally overgrowth of the medial epicondyle will result in a protrusion, which may take a couple of years to remodel out.

Type III Fractures

Any fragment entrapped within the medial elbow joint must be removed. On occasion, manipulation of the semiflexed elbow into valgus will pull the epicondy-

TABLE 13-1. Rang's Classification of Medial Epicondylar Fractures

I. Minimally displaced (less than 2 mm)
II. Moderately displaced (with and without rotation)
III. Markedly displaced and occupying a position within the elbow joint, trapped between the articular groove of the ulna and trochlea
IV. Displaced and accompanied by posterolateral dislocation of the elbow

lar fragment toward the joint's medial margin. At this point, extension and supination of the elbow, with extension of the wrist, may sufficiently pull on the attached muscle origin to extract the fragment through the torn anteromedial capsule. Once extra-articular, manipulative reduction and percutaneous pinning may be attempted if no evidence of retained intra-articular fragments is noted (Fig. 13-9). If unsuccessful, open reduction and fixation as noted earlier is recommended.

It must be remembered that in both types III and IV (those associated with elbow dislocation) injuries, the ulnar nerve is often traumatized. Although routine transposition of the nerve anteriorly is not necessary, open reduction to visualize the nerve and avoid further trauma, is recommended.

Postoperative treatment after reduction of the incarcerated fragment is similar to the other types: immobilization is continued for 4 weeks, at which time both the cast and pins are removed and gentle active motion begun.

Type IV Fractures

As in type III fractures, those associated with posterolateral elbow dislocation result in ulnar nerve compromise in up to 50 percent of cases (Fig. 13-10). Closed reduction of the dislocation has reportedly resulted in the nerve actually being entrapped within the joint. Following closed reduction of the dislocation, open reduction and fixation of the epicondylar fragment is carried

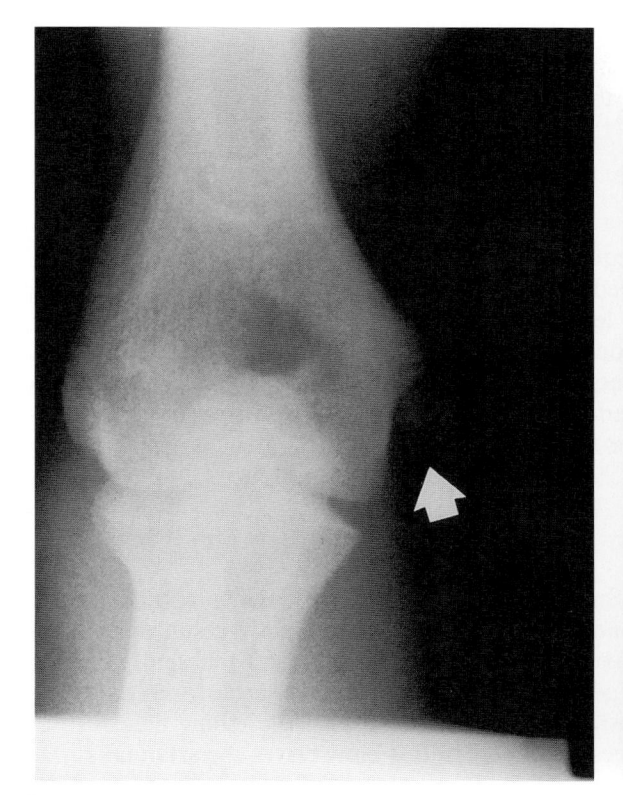

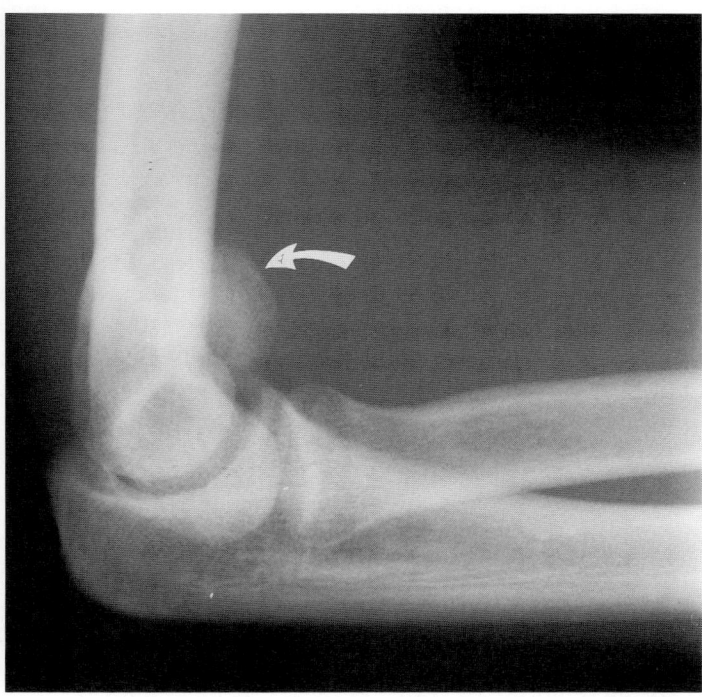

Fig. 13-6. (A) Fracture of the epicondyle in a 15-year-old hockey player which appears relatively undisplaced in the AP view. (B) Anterior displacement seen in the lateral view of the elbow indicating a need for open reduction.

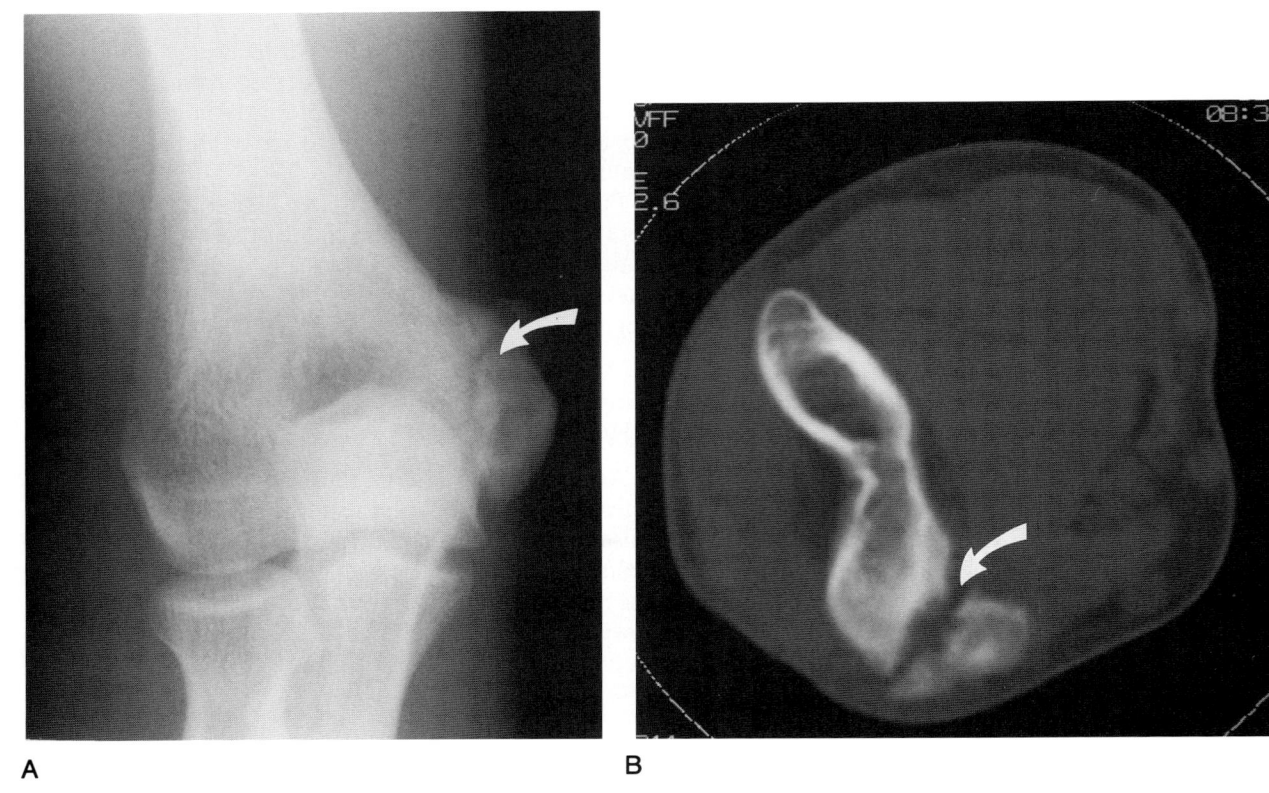

Fig. 13-7. (A) Nonunion of medial epicondyle initially displaced 2 or 3 mm and treated nonoperatively. (B) CT scan illustrating nonunion 14 months after injury. This 16-year-old is complaining of pain during sports and has lost the last 15 degrees of extension of the elbow.

out. The ulnar nerve at this point should be explored and its normal anatomic routing assured. It is not necessary or advisable to attempt repair of the elbow capsule, since stability is restored when the epicondyle and its attached medial ligamentous structures are returned to their normal position. Neither is it necessary to acutely transpose the ulnar nerve, the vast majority of neuropraxia symptoms resolve spontaneously without surgical transposition.

THE MEDIAL HUMERAL CONDYLE

Incidence

So uncommon are fractures of the medial condyle, Ingersoll[17] denied that such injuries occur. They are of such rarity that Kilfoyle[18] reports a "once in a lifetime" frequency. Nonetheless, the true incidence has been cited at 1 to 2 percent of elbow fractures.[19-22] Although at least one such fracture has been reported in a 6-month-old boy,[23] most series give an age range of 3 to 12 years with an average of 9 to 10 years.[19,24,25] Again boys seem to have a higher rate of occurrence than girls for this fracture.

Mechanism of Injury

Similar to fractures of the medial epicondyle, medial condylar fractures most frequently result from a fall. Two specific mechanisms are most frequently reported by victims; in the first instance, a blow directly to the posterior proximal ulna with the elbow flexed 90 degrees. The force of this blow drives the articular surface of the olecranon into the trochlear incisure as a wedge, splitting off the medial condyle.[24] The second proposed mechanism is similar to that which results in medial

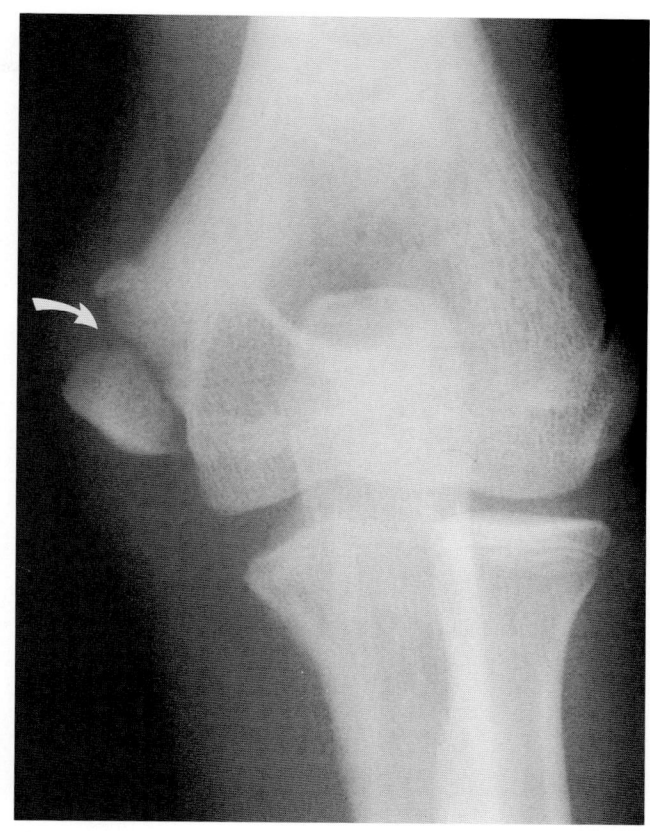

Fig. 13-8. A 13-year-old boy with type II medial epicondylar fracture. **(A)** Epicondylar fragment displaced inferiorly and rotated. Elbow was unstable to valgus stress. **(B)** Fixation using non-parallel Kirschner wires.

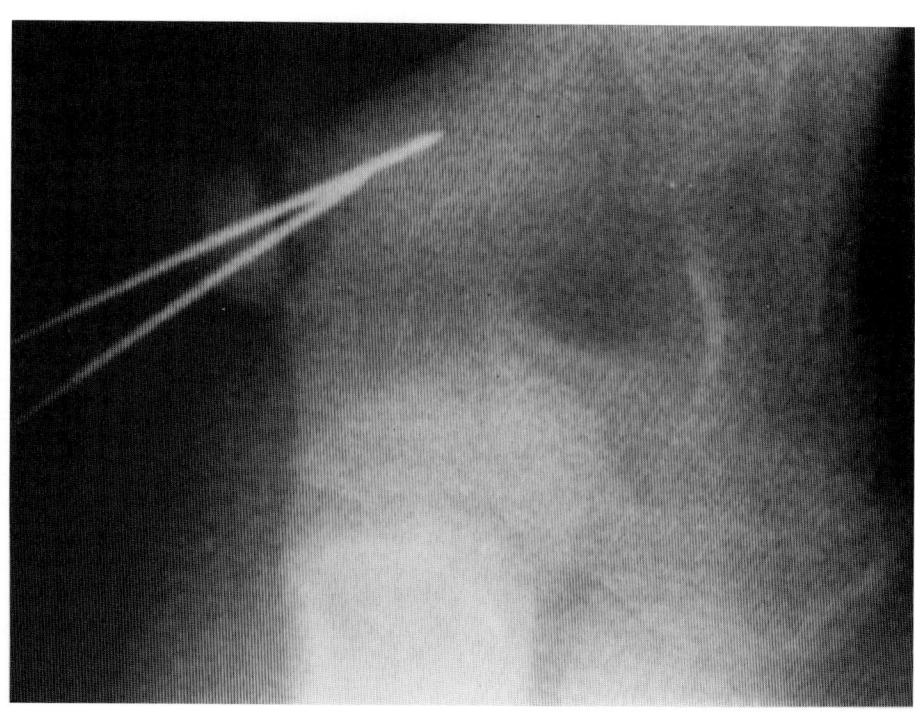

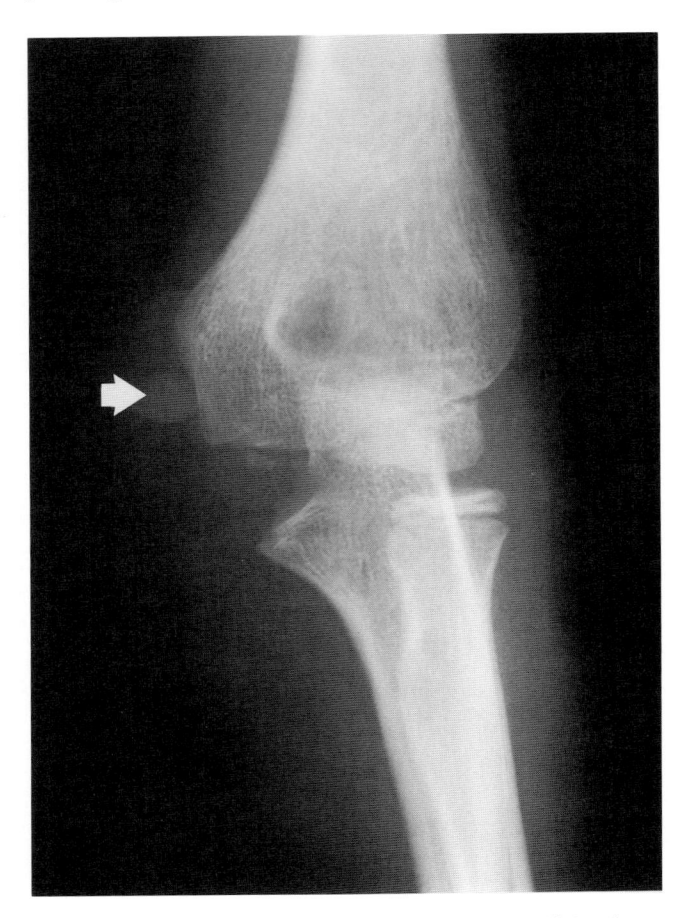

Fig. 13-9. A 10-year-old boy with displaced medial epicondylar avulsion and valgus instability. Open reduction should be accompanied by joint inspection to assure irregularities noted on the radiograph are trochlear centers of ossification and not loose fragments retained with the joint.

epicondylar fractures—a fall on the outstretched upper extremity with the elbow extended and supinated, the wrist dorsiflexed. Avulsion of the medial condyle results from contraction of the forearm flexors and increased valgus stress on the extended elbow (Fig. 13-11).

Classification of Medial Condylar Fractures

Because the fracture line crosses the distal humeral physis separating a portion of both distal humeral epiphysis as well as metaphysis, these are Salter-Harris type IV fractures. As such, potential for growth abnormality as well as loss of articular surface integrity exists. Kilfoyle[18] described three types of medial condylar fractures (Fig. 13-12):

Type I: An incomplete disruption of the medial metaphyseal cortex with the fracture line failing to cross the physis.
Type II: Extension of the type I across the physis, through the epiphysis, and entering the joint at the trochlear incisura.
Type III: Similar to type II, but the condylar fragment is rotated anteriorly, distally, and displaced inferiorly by pull of the flexor muscles, which arise from the medial epicondyle.

The fracture line routinely is oblique, beginning at the supraepicondylar region of the medial metaphyseal cortex and coursing distally and laterally. It crosses the physis, epiphysis, and articular cartilage terminating (in type II and type III) in the joint. Milch[26] described two points of fracture line entry into the joint: the trochlear incisura (his type I) and the capitulotrochlear groove (type II) (Fig. 13-13). Wilkins[22] feels that the Milch type I is most common in children, and it would seem reasonable that, since the wedging force of the ulna is directed into the depth of the trochlear incisura during a fall on the flexed elbow, this most common mechanism would result in such a fracture pattern.

Radiology

Fractures of the medial condyle may be difficult to diagnose radiographically in the very young. Prior to ossification of the medial epicondyle (age 5 years) or trochlea (age 7 years) only visualization of a metaphyseal wafer may serve as a clue to the true nature of the injury (Fig. 13-14). Any injury prior to secondary center ossification, which is accompanied by a great deal of swelling and potential medial instability, deserves further in depth investigation.[20] Although magnetic resonance imaging (MRI) evaluation has been suggested, heavy sedation or general anesthesia would be required to accomplish such a study. An arthrogram performed in the surgical suite under general anesthesia and accompanied by fluoroscopic stress testing is more practical and allows the surgeon to proceed directly with operative treatment when required. A positive arthrogram will demonstrate extra-articular extravasation of contrast material along

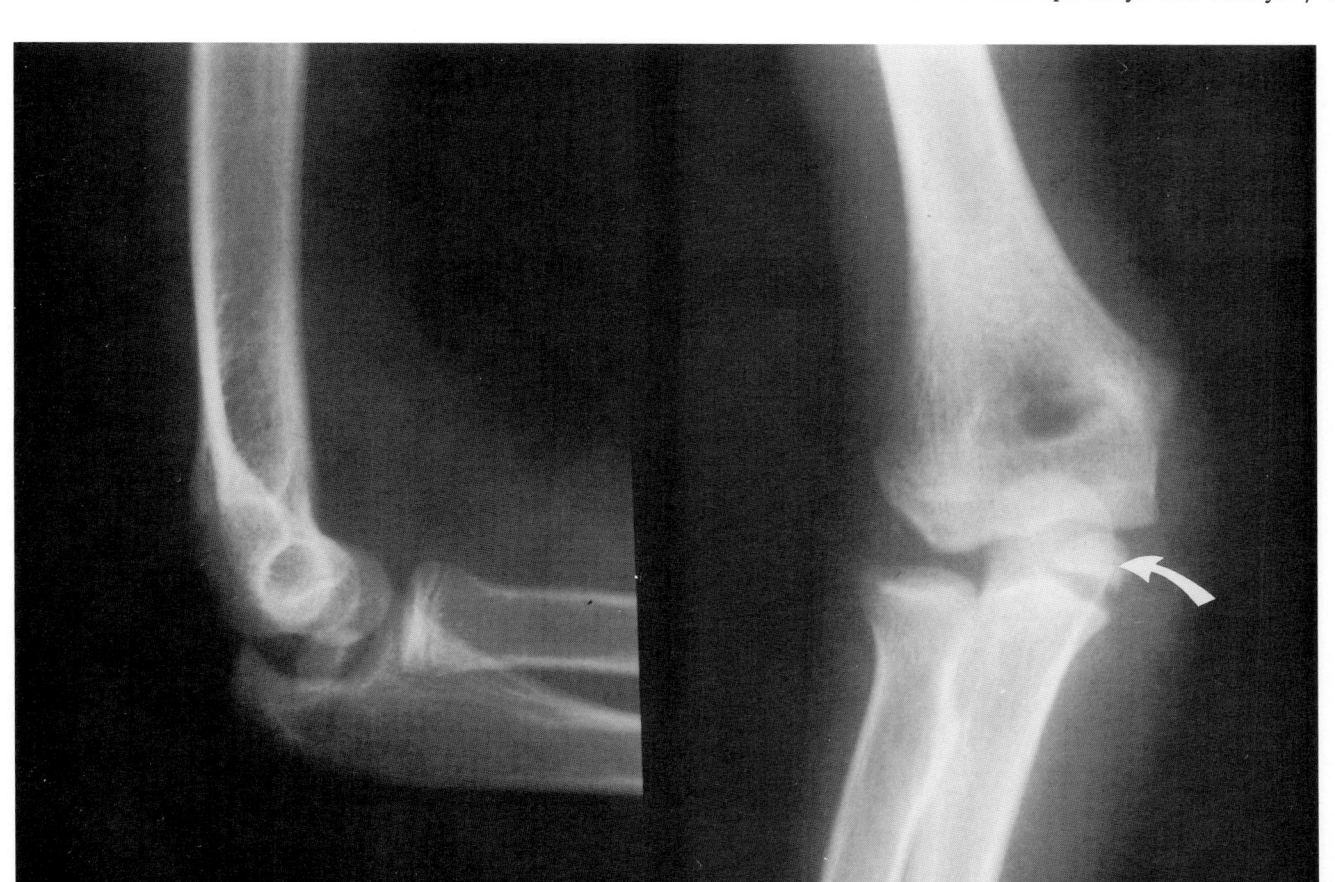

Fig. 13-10. A 14-year-old boy with medial epicondyle avulsed and entrapped within a posterolaterally dislocated elbow. Open reduction and internal fixation resulted in normal function.

the fracture line, while a negative study outlines an intact distal humeral articular surface (Fig. 13-15).

Treatment

Little dispute exists regarding the appropriate approach to treatment, hence my preference follows that common to virtually all experienced orthopaedists treating these injuries.

Type I Fractures

Since these fractures do not cross the physis, nor involve articular cartilage, the elbow need only be immobilized until the child can comfortably and safely use the extremity. Immobilization in a long-arm cast with the elbow flexed 90 degrees for 3 weeks will result in sufficient healing to permit return to normal activities.

Type II Fractures

Close evaluation of the type II injury is necessary to assure that migration of the condylar fragment has not and will not occur. Nonunion of these fractures is only occasionally a problem and hence, so long as the position of the condyle is anatomic, treatment by simple immobilization as in the type I injury is usually sufficient. Due to the intra-articular nature of the fracture, however, immobilization should probably be continued for 4 to 5 weeks. During the early period of casting, it is important

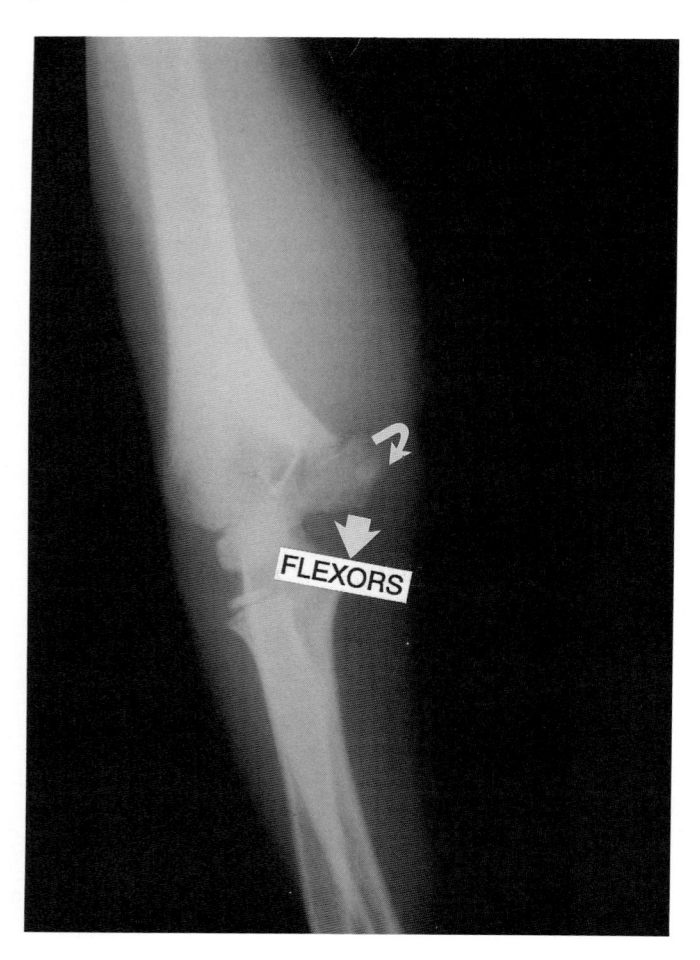

Fig. 13-11. Avulsion of medial condyle displaced by pull of forearm flexor musculature.

to obtain one or two intermittent radiographic studies to ensure that no shifting of the fragment has occurred.

Type III Injuries

As a Salter-Harris type IV fracture, anatomic reduction is mandatory in order to provide the best environment for a satisfactory result. It is highly unlikely that an acceptable reduction can be maintained without rigid internal fixation, hence any displaced medial condylar fracture, regardless of the degree of displacement, should be treated operatively.

It may be possible to anatomically reduce the fracture with manipulation. Flexion of the elbow and wrist flexion relaxes the ligamentous and muscular soft tissues attached to the medial condylar fragment, enhancing digital manipulation. In my experience, sufficient soft tissue trauma has occurred to cause interposition of disrupted muscles/ligament, preventing bony apposition. If, however, anatomic closed reduction is accomplished, percutaneous pinning using two divergent .026 unthreaded Kirschner wires should be satisfactory. One must remember the ulnar nerve and ensure normal prereduction sensory and motor function prior to accepting closed treatment. Injury to the nerve is not common with these fractures and when present is the result primarily of a stretch neuropraxia.[27] Directing the percutaneous pins away from the condylar groove accommodating the nerve is mandatory. Immobilization in a long-arm cast for 4 to 5 weeks with both pins and cast removed at that time (providing radiographs leave no concern for delayed union) should be followed by gradual return to activity. One must again remember to avoid the use of physical therapy in injuries to the child's elbow, active motion alone will minimize long-term stiffness.

In most cases, open reduction of the type III fracture is necessary. Through a posteromedial incision the fracture and ulnar nerve are approached and the nerve protected from iatrogenic injury. Anatomic reduction of the fragment should be followed by rigid internal fixation; either with two divergent K-wires or bone screws (Fig. 13-16). Because of the physeal involvement and therefore a desire to remove any fixation device, I prefer two smooth, externalized K-wires as in medial epicondylar fractures.

Postoperatively, the child should be immobilized for 4 to 5 weeks in a long-arm cast with the elbow flexed 90 degrees and the wrist neutral. At least one radiograph should be performed at 7 to 10 days postreduction to ensure that satisfactory position has been maintained.

Complications

Loss of Motion

Restricted motion is perhaps the most common postinjury problem.[19,25,28] If passive therapy is avoided, loss of significant motion should be minimal. However, as in other elbow injuries, it may be several months before improvement is maximized. Even at this point, loss of the terminal 15–20 degrees of extension is common; this degree of extension loss is usually clinically insignificant.

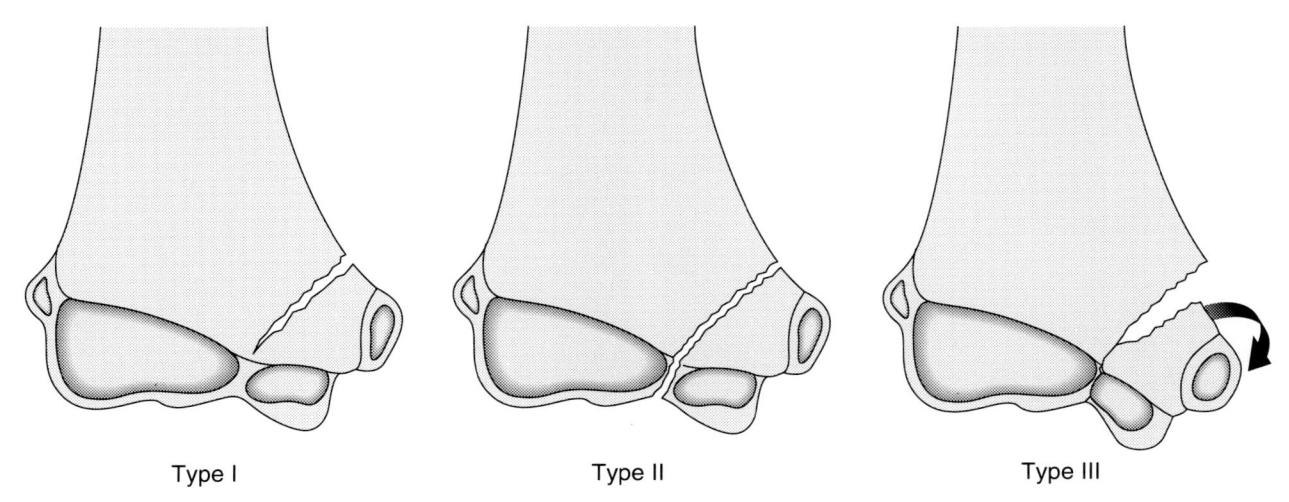

Fig. 13-12. Three types of medial condylar fractures. (Adapted from Kilfoyle,[18] with permission.)

Nonunion

Failure of the fracture to unite is less of a problem on the medial side of the elbow than on the lateral. Although nonunion can occur, rigid internal fixation will help guard against this eventuality[6,25] (Fig. 13-14). When reduction is maintained by periosteally suturing the fragment into position or use of a single K-wire, nonunion is more common. Early union should be ensured prior to discontinuing external mobilization — up to 6 weeks in a cast may be required, especially in older individuals. One must balance the risk of nonunion with an inevitable increased risk of motion loss.

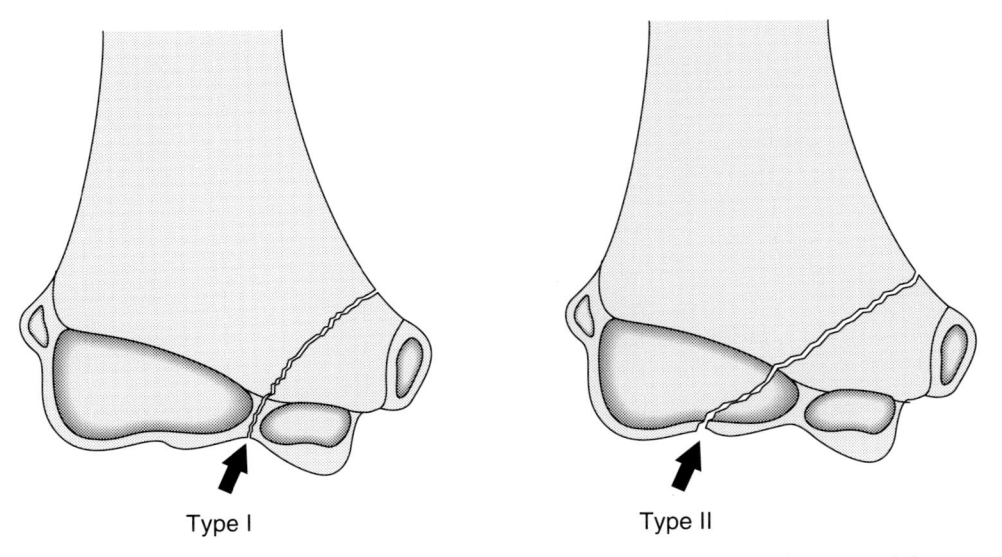

Fig. 13-13. Milch classification of medial condylar fractures. **(A)** Type I: fracture line enters joint at trochlear incisura. **(B)** Type II: fracture crosses entering joint at groove between capitulum and trochlea. (Adapted from Milch,[26] with permission.)

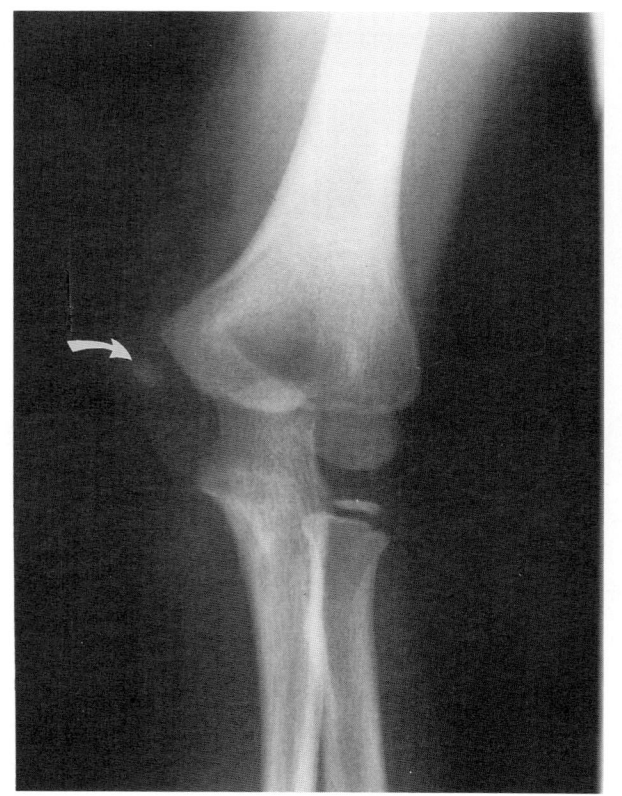

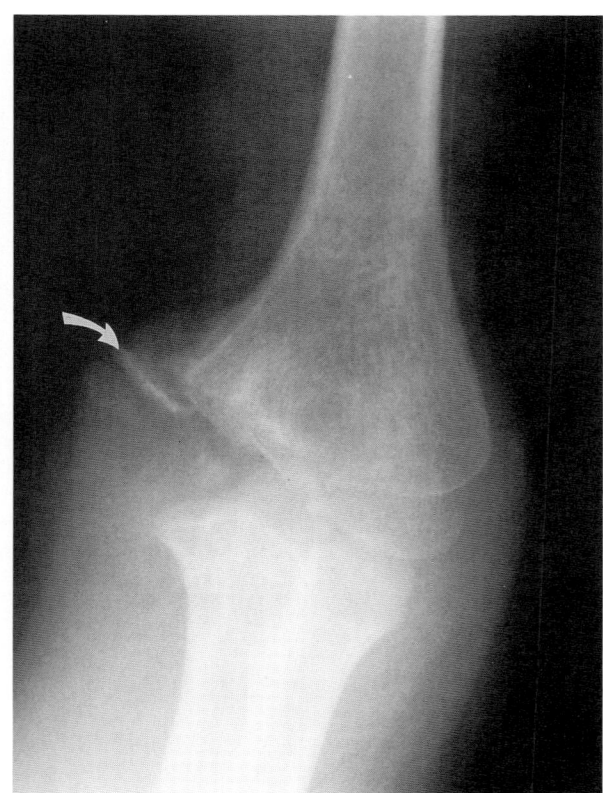

Fig. 13-14. An 8-year-old boy fell on elbow and initial radiograph **(A)** showed slight displacement of the medial epicondyle. This was splinted for 2 weeks and physiotherapy prescribed. **(B)** Radiograph several months later shows ossification of the unrecognized cartilaginous fragment of the medial condyle. **(C)** Two years later size of original cartilaginous fragment involving whole medial condyle is evident and has gone on to a nonunion.

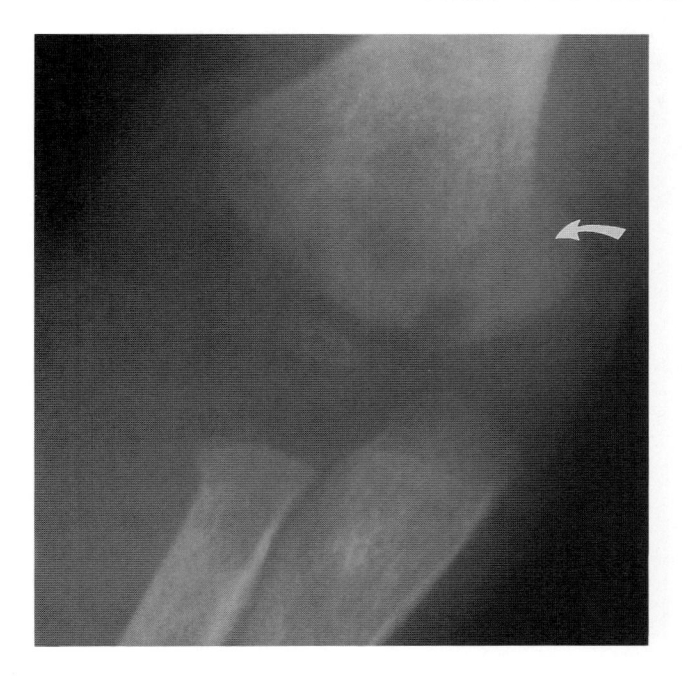

Fig. 13-15. A presumed fracture of the medial condyle in an 8-month-old boy. Medial displacement of the proximal radius and ulna with normal capitular-radial relationship identifies this as a Salter-Harris II fracture of the distal humerus; the medial condyle is the Thurston-Holland fragment.

Avascular Necrosis

Blood supply to the trochlea is via two nonanastomosing intraosseous vessels (Fig. 13-1). The medial portion is supplied by a small artery entering the epiphysis through the nonarticular medial cartilage; nutrition to the lateral portion of the trochlea and potentially the medial capitellum arrives via a vessel that traverses the physis from the metaphyseal bone. A medial condylar fracture may disrupt this latter vessel, leading to avascular necrosis of the central epiphysis and a "fishtail" growth deformity. Fortunately, such deformity is usually of little clinical consequence (Fig. 13-17). If the area of involvement is large, restriction of elbow motion may be severe (Fig. 13-18).

Of greater clinical significance is loss of blood supply to both lateral and medial trochlea as may occur if extensive dissection is used to attain operative reduction. Delayed surgical intervention may require extensive dissection to attain reduction and result in avascular necrosis, leading to cubitus varus. Late osteotomy may be necessary to correct the cosmetic deformity.

Overgrowth

On either the medial or lateral side of the elbow overgrowth often occurs in response to injury. A medial condylar fracture may stimulate overgrowth to a moderate degree. Rarely does this lead to functional impairment, and parents should be advised early on that a mild degree of medial prominence will be an inevitable result of the injury to the medial condyle or epicondyle (Fig. 13-19).

DISLOCATION OF THE ELBOW

Incidence

Elbow dislocation in children, is relatively common among injuries to this joint, although often not appreciated, as many are reduced spontaneously. It occurs more frequently than medial condylar fractures, comprising 3 to 6 percent of all elbow injuries.[29,30] Although elbow dislocations do occur in all age groups, they are more frequent in children and, according to Pollen,[31] are the most common dislocation of childhood. Although the injury has been reported in infancy,[5,32] it is more frequently an injury of older children. Again, boys seems to be more subject to elbow dislocation than girls by a factor of at least 2:1.

Anatomy

There are three articulations that make up the elbow joint:

1. *Radiocapitular joint:* The radial articulation with the capitellum is formed as a shallow ball and socket.
2. *Ulna–trochlear joint:* The semilunar incisura of the trochlea envelopes a central coronoid ridge located in the trochlear notch of the ulna.
3. *Proximal radioulnar joint:* The head of the radius rotates during pronation and supination in a matching groove on the lateral side of the proximal ulna.

These bony articular relationships provide a modicum of elbow stability; the medial and lateral collateral ligaments as well as the anterior and posterior joint capsule are responsible for the majority of elbow constraint.[33] The medial collateral ligaments consist of an anterior band connecting the anterior epicondyle to the medial coronoid, the anterior portion of this band is taut in extension and the posterior portion taut in flexion; a posterior band leads from the inferior medial epicondyle

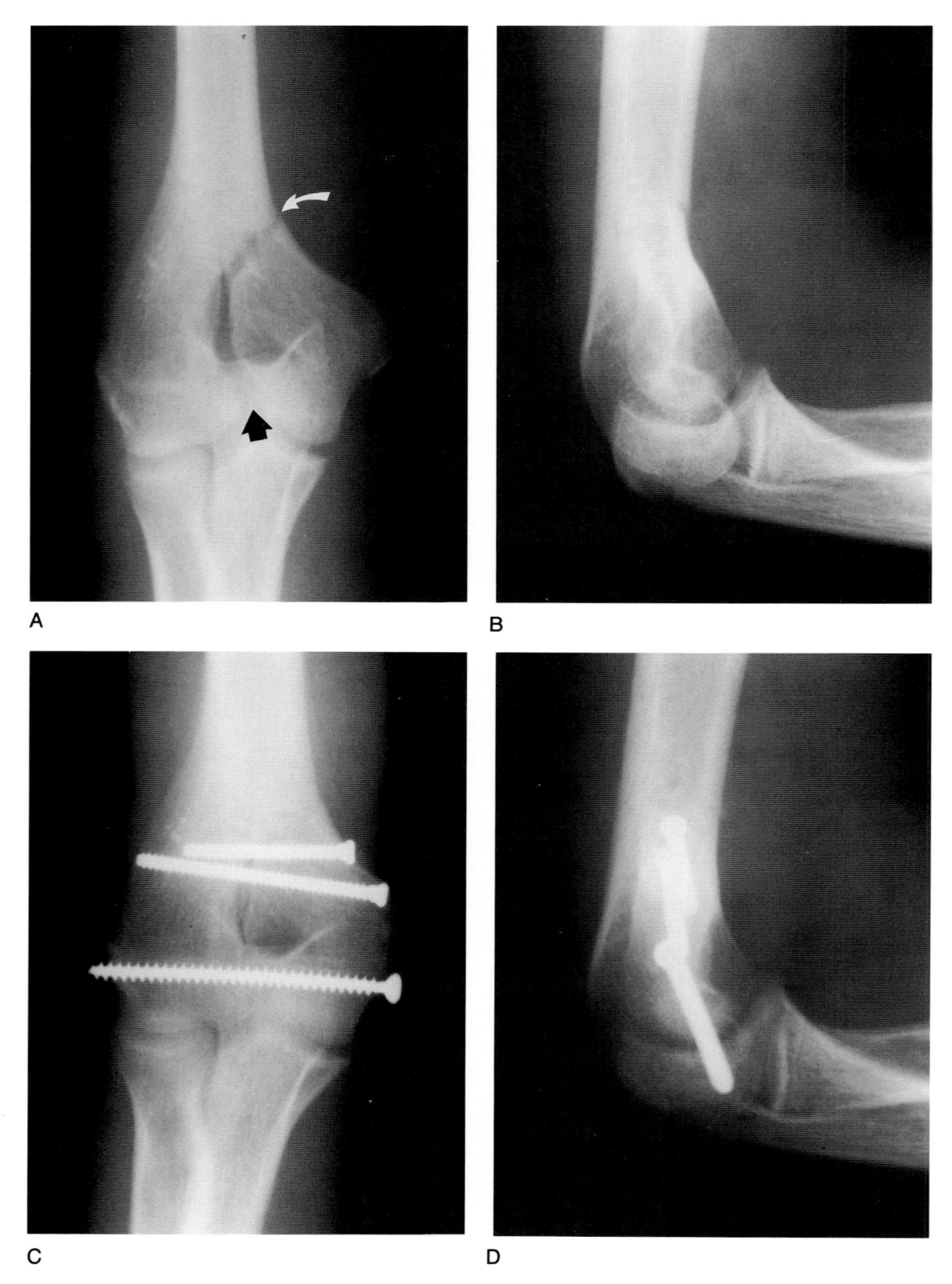

Fig. 13-16. 13-year-old boy with type I medial condylar fracture. **(A)** AP view; fracture enters joint at trochlear incisura. **(B)** Lateral view. **(C)** AP view after open reduction and fixation with cannulated screws. **(D)** Lateral view postoperatively. (Courtesy of W.W. Beckett, M.D.)

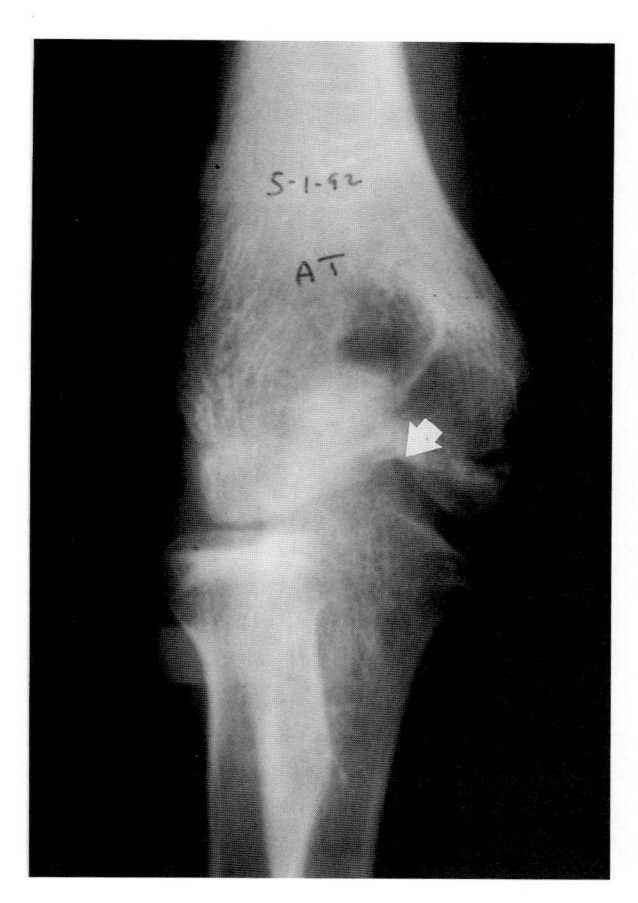

Fig. 13-17. Avascular necrosis of central epiphysis (lateral portion of trochlea) creating "fishtail deformity."

to the mid medial margin of the ulnar-trochlear notch; this band is taut in flexion. Oblique fibers connect the base of the anterior and posterior bands (Fig. 13-20). Lateral support is provided by (1) the radial collateral ligament extending from the lateral humeral condyle to the lateral trochlear notch of the ulna, and (2) the annular ligament coursing from the lateral trochlear notch around the radial neck to the lateral aspect of the coronoid process (Fig. 13-21). The olecranon fossa of the posterior distal humerus accepts the olecranon when the elbow is extended, providing medial lateral stability. Shallower radial and ulnar fossae of the anterior distal humerus accept the proximal end of these bones when the elbow is flexed (Fig. 13-22A & B).

In addition to the bony relationship and mediolateral ligamentous constraints, the forearm muscle origins play a role in stabilizing the elbow, particularly medially where the strong forearm muscles arise. Schwab and colleagues[33] designate these muscular origins as the first line of defense against valgus stress.

Mechanism of the Two Most Common Types of Dislocation

As in other injuries to the medial elbow, dislocations usually result from a fall on the outstretched arm, in this instance with the supinated elbow in near full extension and the wrist dorsiflexed.[34] The type of dislocation depends upon direction of forces transmitted through the olecranon and radial head to the bony and soft tissue restraints (Figs. 13-21 and 13-22). With the elbow in near full extension or hyperextended, a distraction force is transmitted to the anterior and medial soft tissues. The coronoid is compressed against the trochlea and continued valgus stress will avulse the medial collateral ligament, with or without the medial epicondyle attached. The acute medial instability resulting from loss of ulnar collateral ligament complex integrity allows the coronoid of the olecranon to slide around the trochlea posterolaterally; articular continuity between the radial head and capitellum is also lost. The proximal ends of the radius and ulna will then come to lie posterior and lateral to their normal humeral articulations; when the medial epicondyle is avulsed, it trails the medial collateral ligament and lies beneath the midportion of the distal humeral articular surface. The anterior and posteromedial portions of the joint capsules are disrupted to a variable degree. Because the distal portion of brachialis muscle has very little tendinous tissue, its muscle fibers are disrupted, and the distal humerus comes to lie anterior to the proximal radius and ulna within these torn fibers. The pronator teres is then located posterior to the medial humeral articular surface (Fig. 13-23).

Other Types of Dislocations

On rare occasions the extended elbow is pronated rather than supinated during a fall, and as a result, the axial force transmitted drives the ulna medially on the trochlea and the radius laterally on the capitellum. The interosseus soft tissues, including annular ligament, interosseus membrane, and, on occasion, the collateral ligaments, are ruptured. The proximal radioulnar articulation is disrupted and the distal humerus forced between the two forearm bones. This transverse divergent type of elbow dislocation is much less common than the posterior or posterolateral type.[35,36] Similarly, anterior elbow dislocation occurs so infrequently in children as to

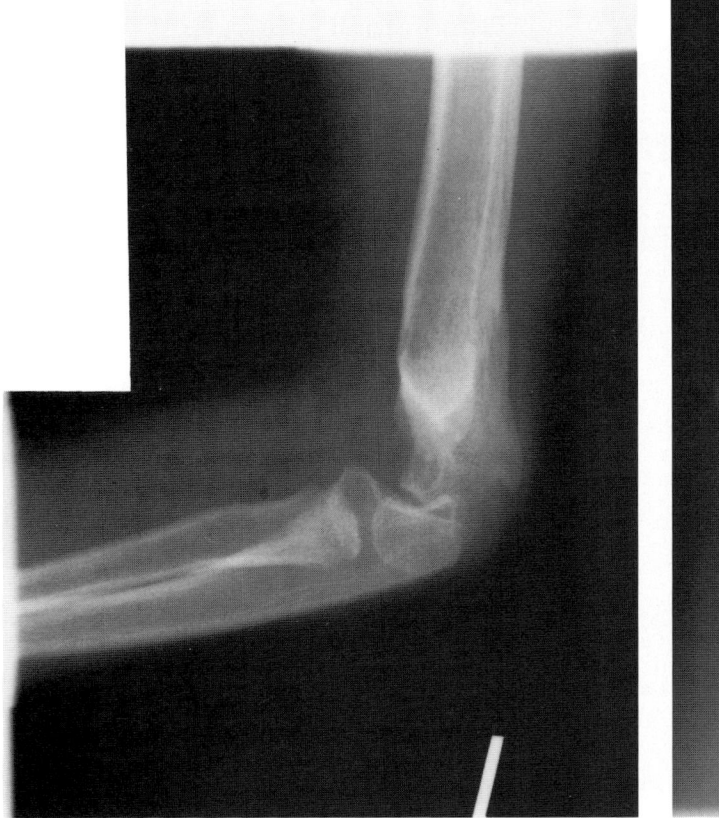

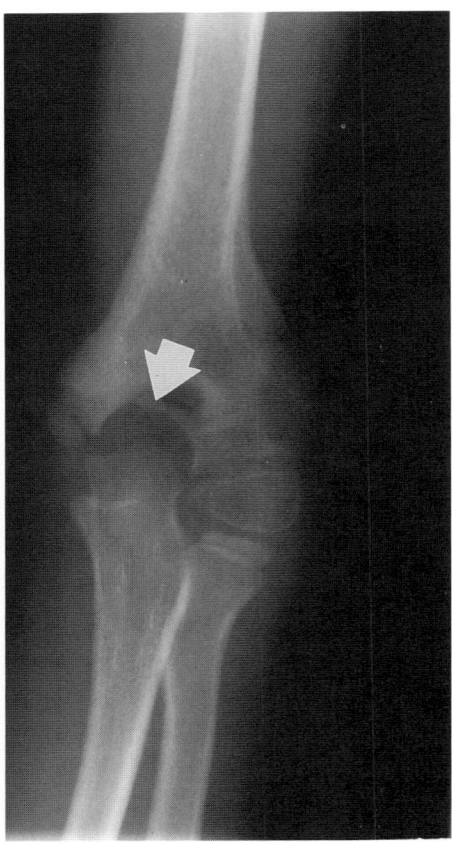

Fig. 13-18. Severe avascular necrosis of trochlea following open reduction of medial condylar fracture. This 10-year-old boy had marked restriction of flexion and extension. (Courtesy of R. Mervyn Letts, M.D.)

be noted only in occasional incidental case reports. Pure medial or lateral dislocations of the elbow joint do not appear to occur in children.

Neurovascular Considerations

In virtually all cases of posterior or posterolateral dislocation, the median nerve and brachial artery are tented over the distal humerus and lie immediately under the anterior skin. Some disruption of the ulnar collateral vessels routinely occurs, leading to significant bleeding into the soft tissues. Further damage to the arterial trunk will result in vascular compromise to the forearm and hand. The median nerve is subjected to stretch, and symptoms of distal sensory or motor dysfunction may be present. Less commonly, the ulnar nerve is subjected to a stretch neuropraxia.[37] Quite obviously, in open posterior dislocations these structures are placed at higher risk to severe damage.

Treatment

The anteroposterior and lateral radiographs of the elbow splinted in mild flexion should be carefully examined prior to any reduction maneuver in an attempt to identify loose bony fragments (Fig. 13-24). Evidence of medial epicondylar avulsion warns the treating physician that residual long-term instability may be a problem.[33] A careful neurovascular evaluation of the forearm and hand is mandatory with particular attention to peripheral sensation as well as distal radial and ulnar pulses.

Reduction of a simple elbow dislocation can usually be carried out under sedation and analgesia. In certain circumstances (hyperexcitable child and/or parents, in-

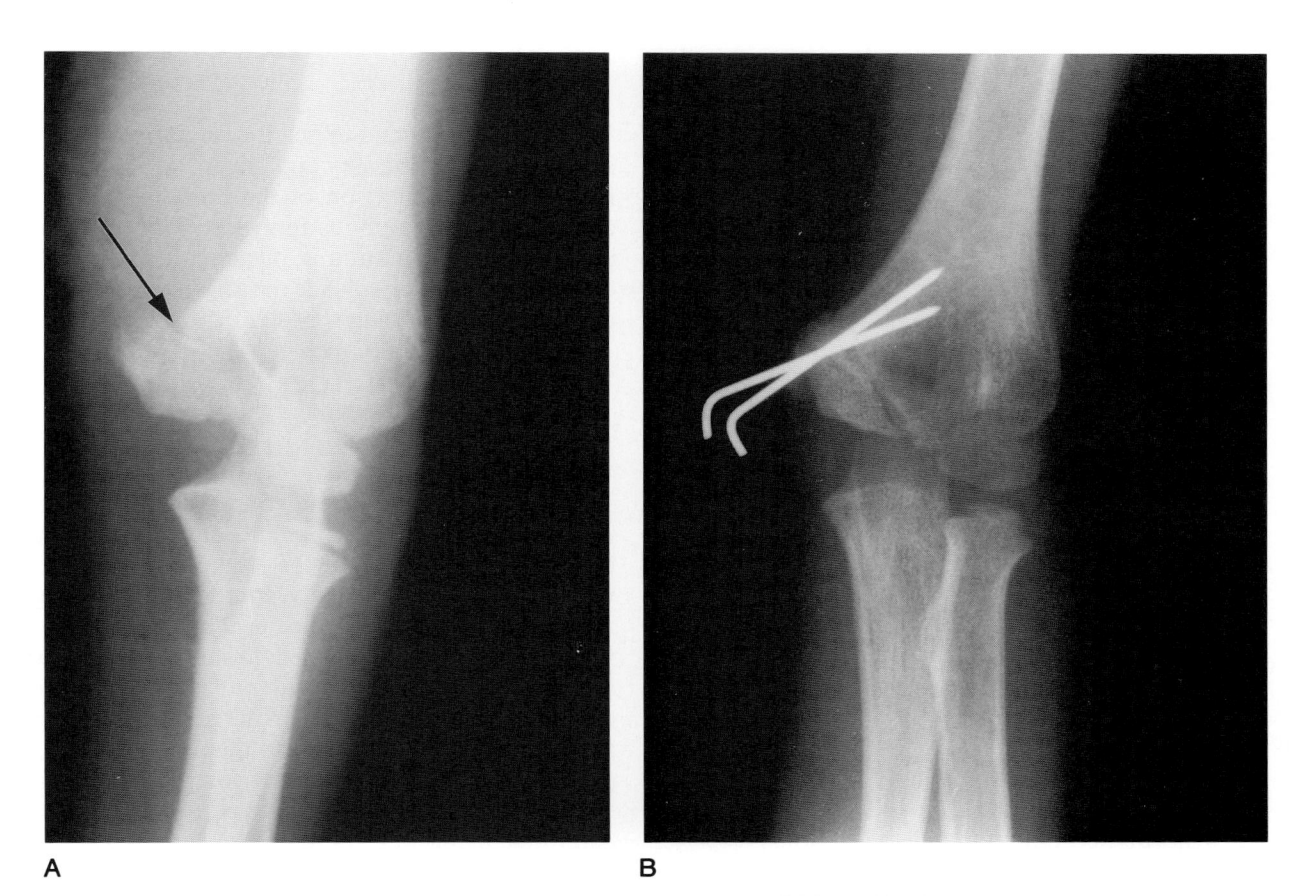

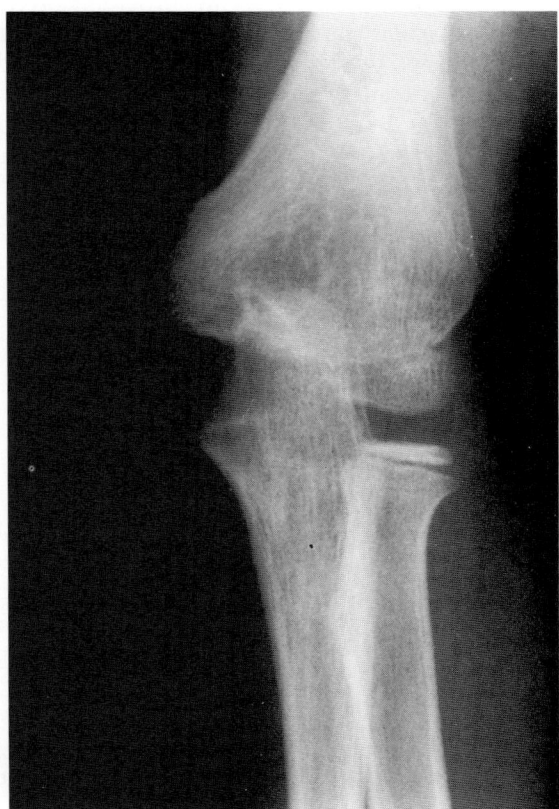

Fig. 13-19. (A) Fracture of medial condyle sustained in an 8-year-old boy in a fall off his bicycle. (B) This was reduced and pinned with two K-wires. (C) Two years later there is some overgrowth but a full range of motion of the elbow.

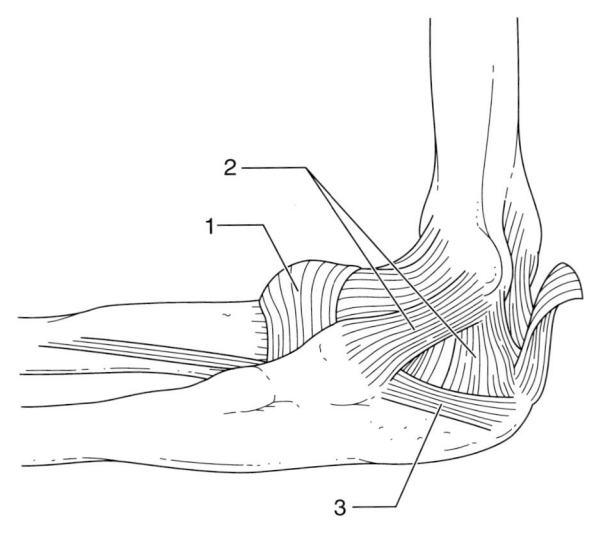

Fig. 13-20. Ligaments as viewed from medial side of elbow. *(1)* Annular ligament; *(2)* medial collateral ligament, anterior and posterior bands; *(3)* medial collateral ligament, oblique fibers.

ability to adequately obtain muscle relaxation, etc.) general anesthesia is preferable. If open treatment to restore stability is likely to be necessary and providing prereduction neurovascular status is intact, reduction under anesthesia followed by fixation of the avulsed epicondylar fragment is indicated.

Wilkins[22] has described "puller" and "pusher" methods of reduction, citing advocates of both approaches.[22]

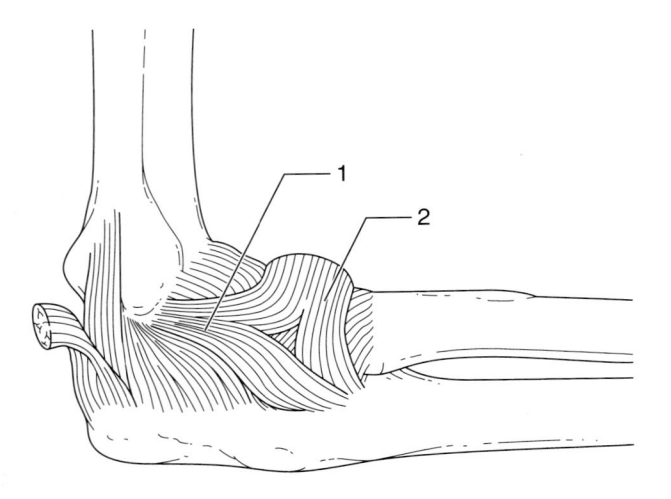

Fig. 13-21. Ligaments as viewed from the lateral side of the elbow. *(1)* Radial collateral ligament; *(2)* annular ligament.

The "puller" will tend to flex the forearm to 70 degrees and distract the elbow by applying force to the anterior forearm in the direction of the humeral longitudinal axis. The "pusher" groups apply force posteriorly on the olecranon with the thumbs, pushing the proximal ulna distally and anteriorly, while the fingers wrap around the distal humerus, pulling it posteriorly (Fig. 13-25).

Author's Preferred Method

A combination of the puller and pusher technique is utilized. With the sedated patient lying supine, the arm is brought over the edge of the emergency room gurney with the shoulder abducted to approximately 60 degrees. A sling of felt is laid over the distal one-third of the arm with a weight hanger attached. Distal traction is applied to the semiflexed forearm with one hand, while the second hand stabilizes the wrist. After about 30 seconds, an assistant adds 5 lb of weight to the weight hanger, thus pulling the distal humerus posteriorly. Medial or lateral subluxation is manually corrected, followed by slight additional extension to unlock the coronoid tip. These maneuvers are followed by elbow flexion. If this manipulation is carried out while applying a moderate distractive force, reduction of the dislocation will result; the elbow is then further flexed to 90 degrees.

Postreduction neurovascular function should be carefully assessed, and the elbow immobilized in oblique medial/lateral splints, which will not radiographically obscure the distal humerus. Careful radiographic studies are obtained, again looking for bony fragments as well as checking adequacy of reduction. Immobilization at 90 degrees of flexion is continued for 2 or 3 weeks and the limb is then place in a forearm sling. The sling permits further flexion, pronation and supination but blocks extension and is used for an additional week. The elbow should be examined within a few day of cast/splint removal to ensure continued adequacy of reduction.

Following simple dislocation and closed reduction, significant long-term sequelae are uncommon.[38-40] Despite the usual extensive soft tissue damage, the majority of patients do very well. A persistent mild decrease in extension is common but encountered less frequently in children than adults who sustain posterior dislocation. Radiographic evidence of mild osteoarthritic changes are also common but, again, are usually not a source of difficulty. On occasion, however, significant problems in the immediate postreduction period are present and must be addressed.

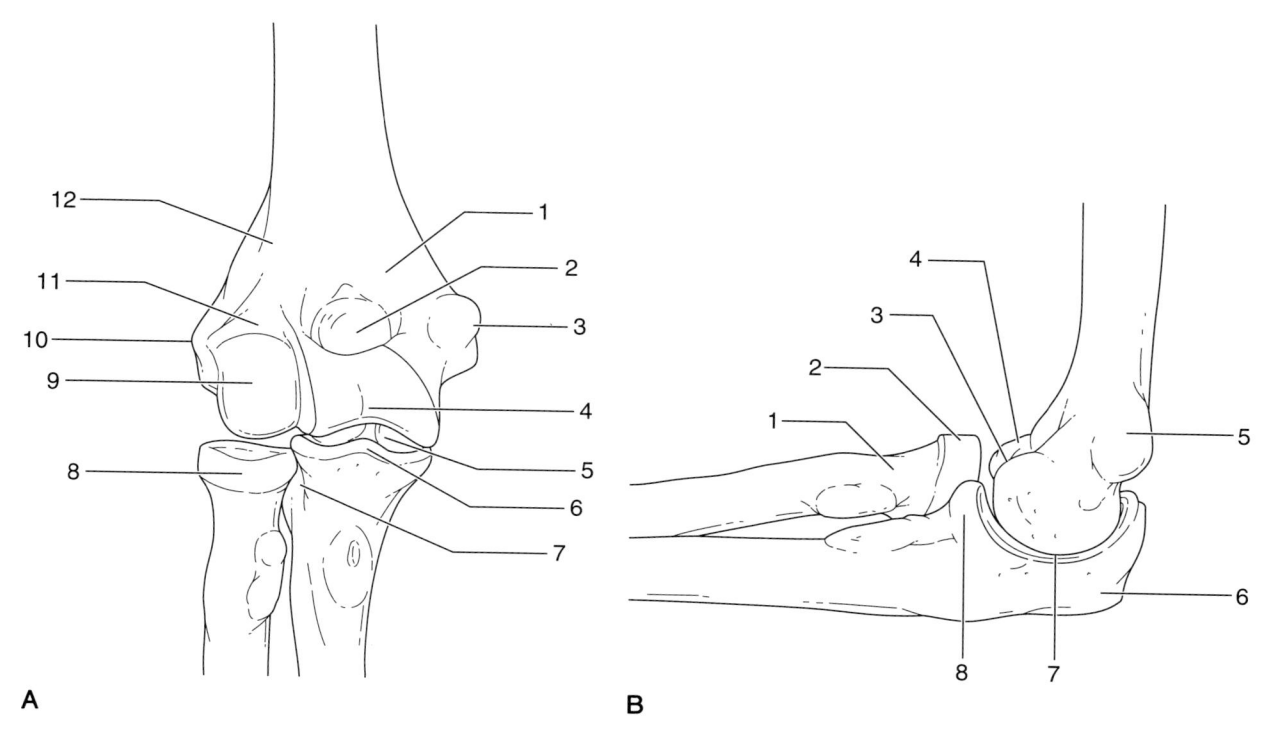

Fig. 13-22. (A) Anterior view of the extended bony elbow. *(1)*, Medial condyle; *(2)*, coronoid fossa; *(3)*, medial epicondyle; *(4)*, trochlear incisura; *(5)*, coronoid ridge; *(6)*, coronoid process; *(7)*, radial notch of ulna; *(8)*, radial head; *(9)*, capitulum; *(10)*, lateral epicondyle; *(11)*, radial fossa; *(12)*, lateral condyle. **(B)** View of the medial elbow bony elements. *(1)*, Neck of radius; *(2)*, radial head; *(3)*, trochlea; *(4)*, capitulum; *(5)*, medial epicondyle; *(6)*, olecranon; *(7)*, trochlear notch of ulna; *(8)*, coronoid process.

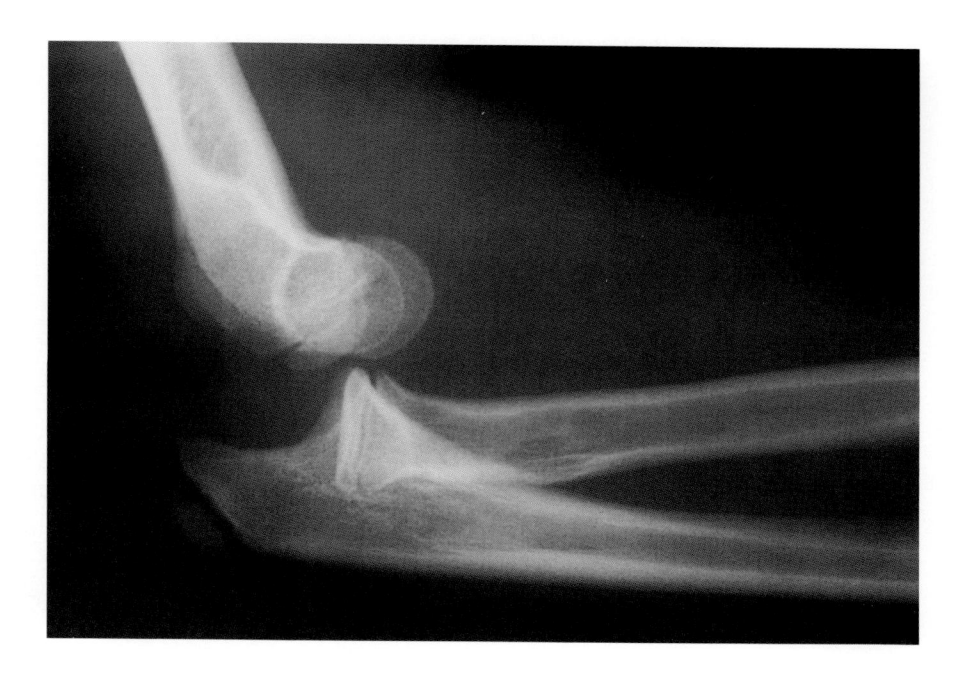

Fig. 13-23. Posterior elbow dislocation without evidence of fracture in a 13-year-old boy.

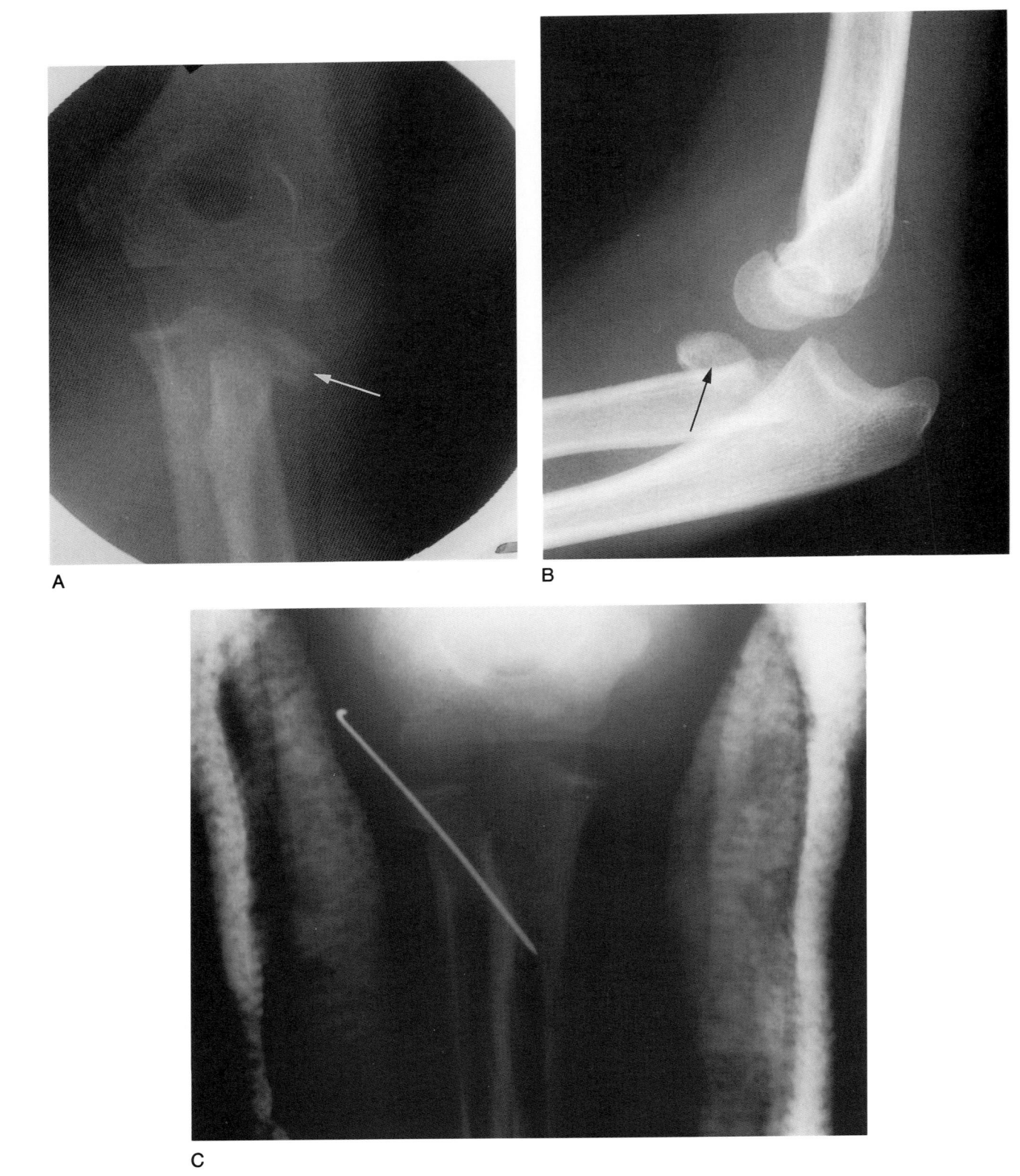

Fig. 13-24. Posterior dislocation of the elbow with displaced radial neck fracture in a 9-year-old girl. **(A&B)** Initial anteroposterior and lateral radiographs. **(C)** Postreduction pinning with a single K-wire. *(Figure continues.)*

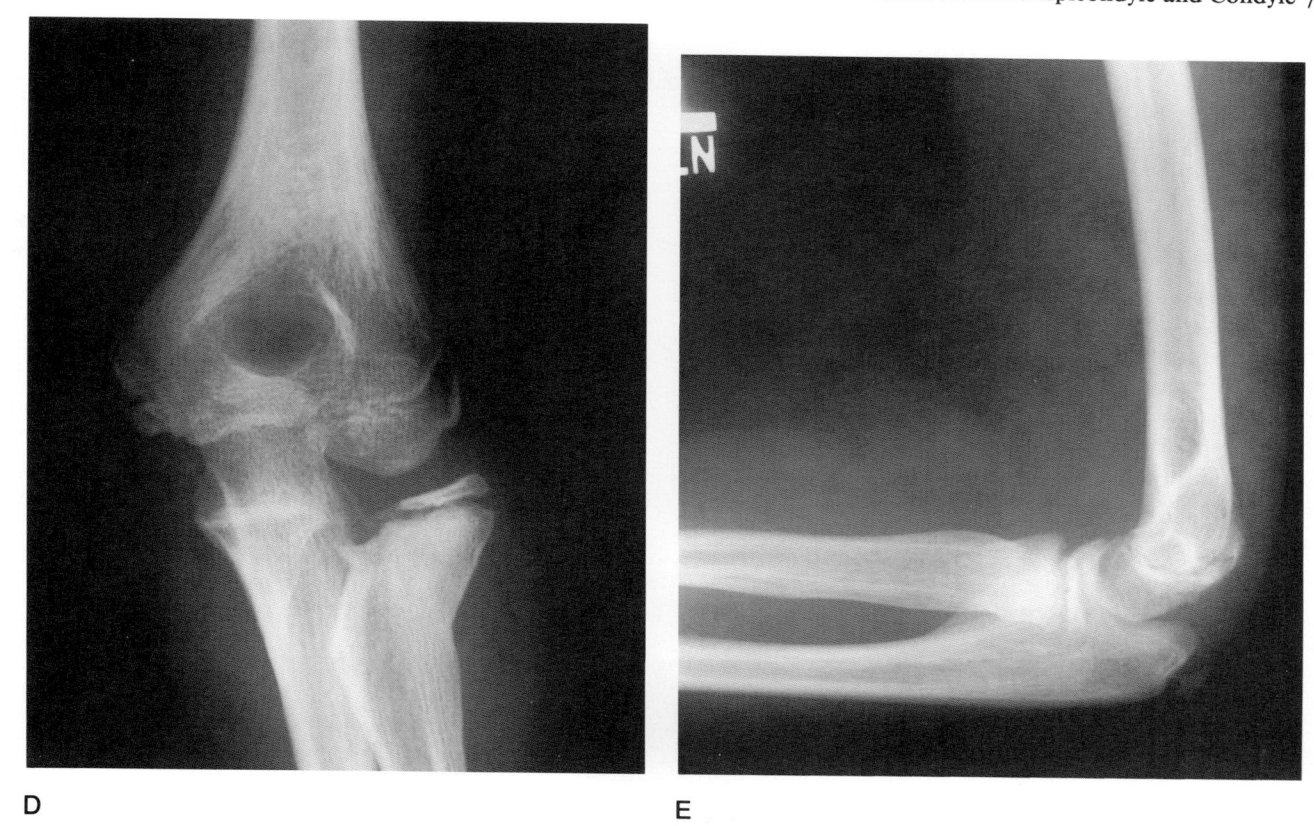

Dislocation of the Elbow and Fractures of the Medial Humeral Epicondyle and Condyle / 233

Fig. 13-24 *(Continued).* **(D&E)** 12 months after injury, flexion-extension are full, supination is limited by 20 degrees.

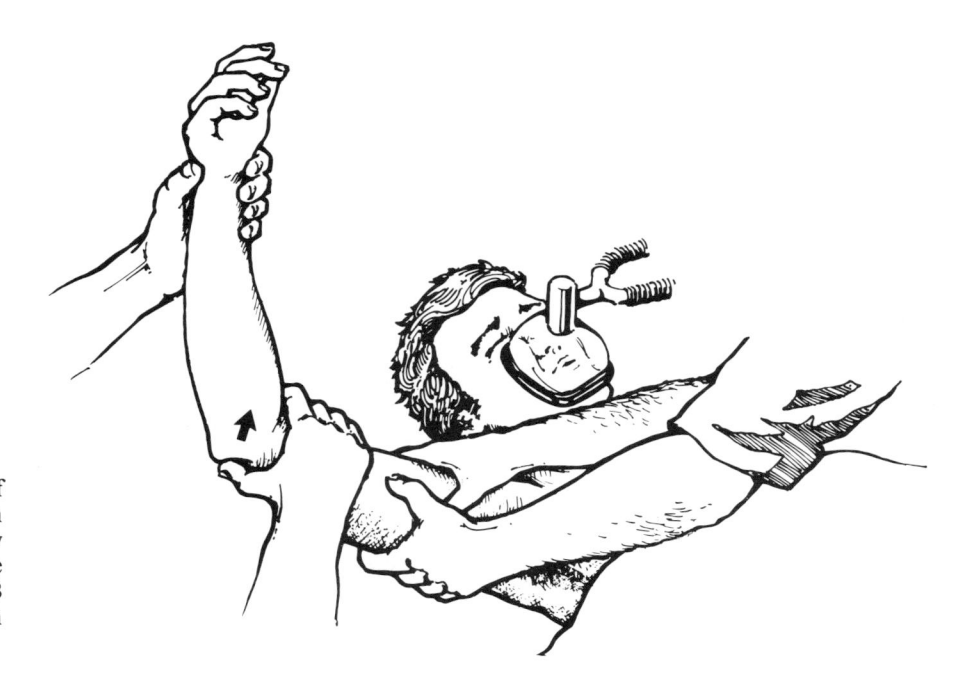

Fig. 13-25. The Pusher method of elbow dislocation reduction. (From Letts RM: Dislocations of the elbow in children. In Morrey BF (ed): The Elbow and Its Disorders. WB Saunders, Philadelphia, 1985, with permission.)

Complications

A medial epicondyle entrapped within the joint must be surgically removed.[38,39,41] If the epicondyle remains displaced following reduction of the dislocation, open reduction and fixation of the fragment as discussed under medial epicondylar fractures is advocated[12] (Fig. 13-10).

The identification of an osteochondral flap of ulnar articular surface, which has been turned back on itself during reduction, has been reported.[42,43] In such cases the postreduction lateral radiographic view may appear normal; however, passive motion causes crepitus. Plain tomography with contrast may assist in the diagnosis.[44] Open lateral or medial arthrotomy to return the fragment to normal alignment in its bed is required; a lateral approach avoids risk to the ulnar nerve.[43]

Neurovascular Injuries

Repeated, careful neurovascular examinations postreduction are necessary to promptly uncover evidence of neurovascular compromise. Postreduction entrapment of the median nerve between the trochlea and olecranon can occur if lateral displacement is not corrected prior to anatomic reduction of the radial ulnar complex, or the elbow is hyperextended during the reduction maneuver.[45-48] When the nerve is entrapped, postreduction radiographs are usually normal. Unless median nerve compromise is discovered early, entrapment can result in weakness of thumb and index finger flexion and sensory deficit in the median nerve distribution. Persistent displacement can result in formation of a groove at the posterior base of the medial epicondyle, which will be visible as two parallel sclerotic lines on the AP radio-

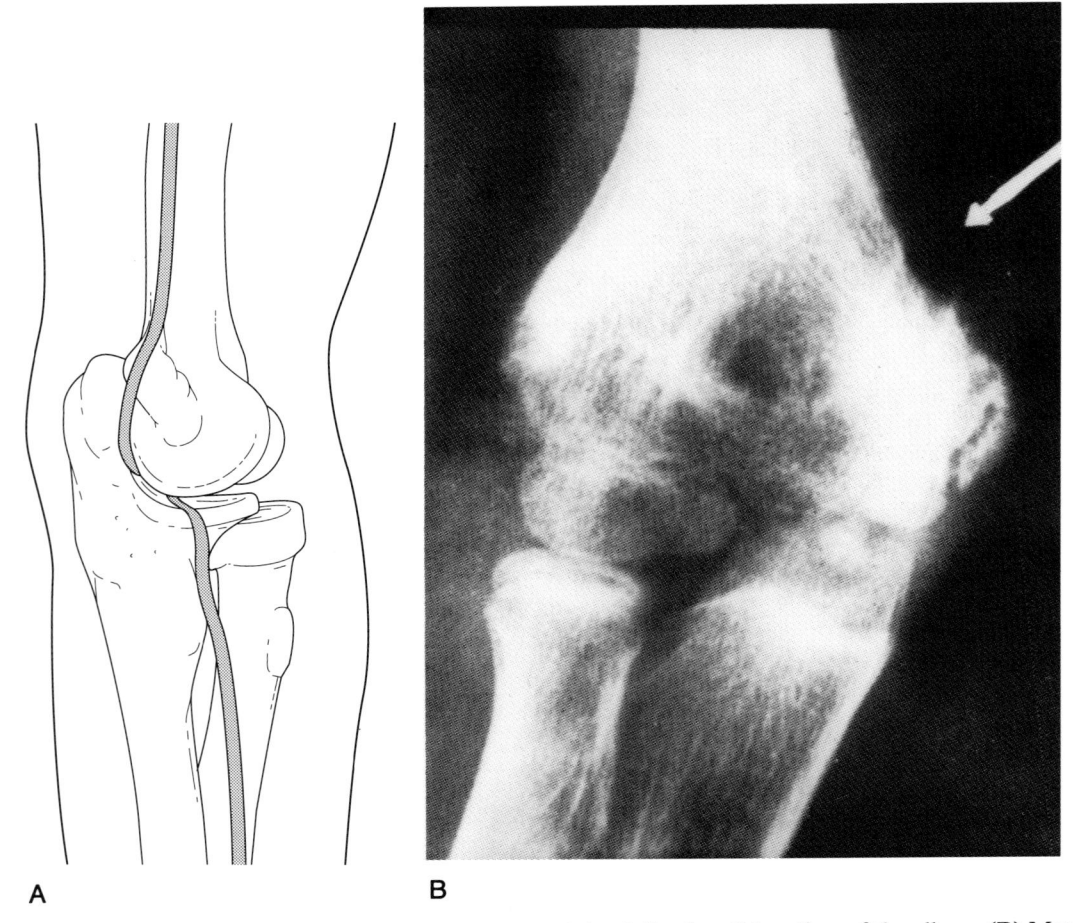

Fig. 13-26. (A) Median nerve entrapment in the elbow joint following dislocation of the elbow. (B) Matev's sign, notching of the medial humerus from the taut median nerve. (Figure B from Matev,[49] with permission.)

graphic view[49] (Mateu's sign) (Fig. 13-26). These radiographic findings together with electromyographic confirmation of a median nerve lesion at the level of the elbow combine to confirm the diagnosis. Surgical extraction of the nerve from the joint may be accomplished by osteotomizing the medial epicondyle or carefully rongeuring open the bony tunnel overlying the nerve, thus allowing it to come forward into normal position.

Trauma to the ulnar nerve, with the exception of neuropraxias associated with combined medial epicondyle avulsion and elbow dislocation, occurs less often than median nerve trauma.[37] The majority of ulnar nerve injuries spontaneously resolve following treatment of the medial epicondylar apophyseal displacement.[38,50] Anterior transfer of the nerve does not seem to be routinely required, being reserved for the those cases in which dysfunction remains unimproved for 3 months postreduction.

Recurrent Dislocation

Recurrent dislocation is a problem seen only on rare occasions in children. Usually it is encountered in an adult who had sustained an initial elbow dislocation during the later years of adolescence. A few case reports are present in the literature, the largest series being that of Osborne and Cotterill.[51] Failure of the posterolateral capsule to reattach to the humerus following closed reduction is the presumed primary etiology of the problem. As repeated episodes of redislocation occur, both the coronoid and anterior portion of the radial head become attenuated, further promoting instability and redislocation.[50,52] Treatment in children should be aimed at strengthening the anterior musculature to prevent hyperextension. Exercise may be accompanied by a temporary extension block splint, which is used for 3 or 4 months[53] (Fig. 13-27). If redislocation occurs following this nonoperative approach, reconstruction of the posterolateral ligamentous complex has been uniformly satisfactory.[51,52,54]

Unreduced Dislocations

Reports reviewing chronic dislocation of the elbow paint a mixed prognostic picture for return of useful motion. If the dislocation has been present less than 3 months, open reduction through a posterior approach is reasonable.[22] Naidoo,[55] in reviewing 23 patients with chronic dislocations noted that 5 were in patients under 16 years of age. All were treated with open reduction through a posterior approach, and in short-term follow-up total flexion/extension motion ranged from 45 to 115 degrees. Fowles and colleagues[56] described an average preoperative range of motion of 13 degrees in 12 children treated surgically for dislocations of 3 to 156 weeks duration. Postoperatively, the average motion totaled 50 degrees; however, included in this average were two patients whose dislocation had been present a year or more and in whom restoration of motion was minimal. Periarticular calcification was commonly noted and occasionally interfered with function. In a report of 11 patients with neglected posterior elbow dislocations, 5 of whom were below or just at skeletal maturity, Arafiles[57] reported postoperative flexion/extension motion varying from 55 to 105 degrees. In his series, the medial collateral ligament was reconstructed using tendon graft and, to provide additional stability, a portion of tendon was routed through the joint to act as an elbow cruciate ligament. Ainsworth and Avlicino[58] were pleased with a resultant 70 to 110-degree arc of flexion/extension in a 13-year-old following surgery for a posterior dislocation present for 1 year (preoperative motion 0 to 45 degrees).[58] This would seem to indicate that limited results are to be expected when treating a neglected elbow dislocation in a child. In this age group, restoration of a stable, painless joint with modest motion in a functional arc is preferred to a joint stuck in a nonfunctional position.

Heterotopic Calcification

In nearly one-third of cases, some element of periarticular calcification occurs.[39,40] Because the brachialis muscle is frequently torn at the time of injury, actual myositis ossificans occurs anterior to the joint capsule. In order to minimize this potential, gentle reduction and avoidance of passive rehabilitative stretching are paramount. There is little documented evidence that the current trend to use passive range of motion devices is appropriate for injuries of the child's elbow; it may have the potential of doing more harm than good in this age group.

The Pulled Elbow

The pulled elbow is often erroneously referred to as a dislocation of the elbow or radial head. This is simply a subluxation of the radial head inferiorly into the annular ligament. It occurs primarily in children under the age of 2 but occasionally can be seen in children up to the age of 5 or 6. In young children, the ligamentous structures are very lax and resilient and with a longitudinal pull on the arm, the head of the radius can become lodged within the

236 / Management of Pediatric Fractures

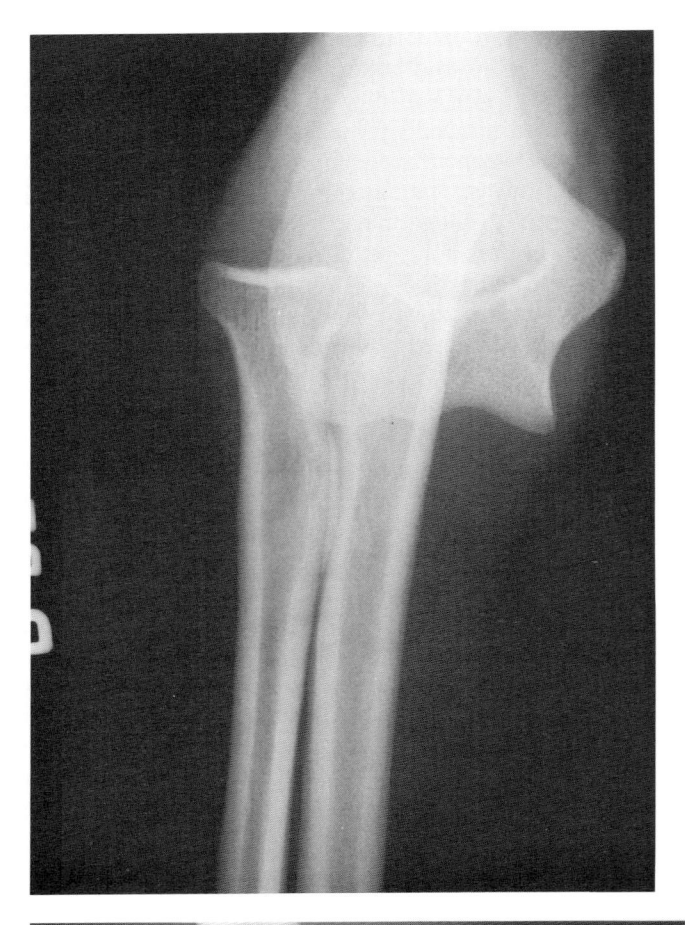

Fig. 13-27. Recurrent posterolateral elbow dislocation in a 15-year-old gymnast. Dislocations began at age 9. Treated with closed reduction, 3 weeks of immobilization and active exercise, she has been dislocation free for 6 years.

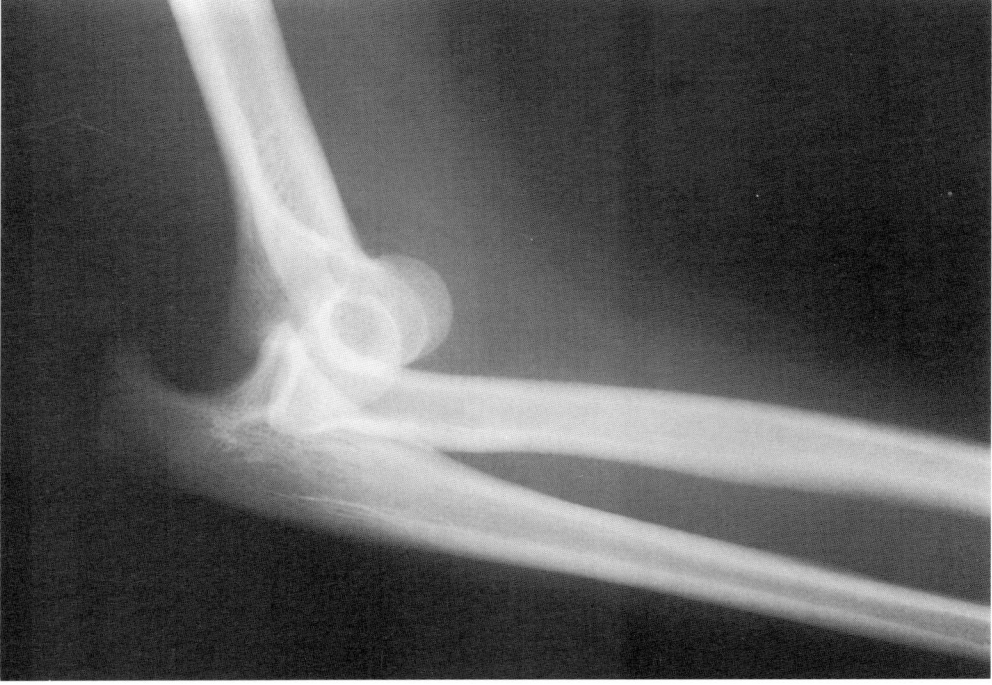

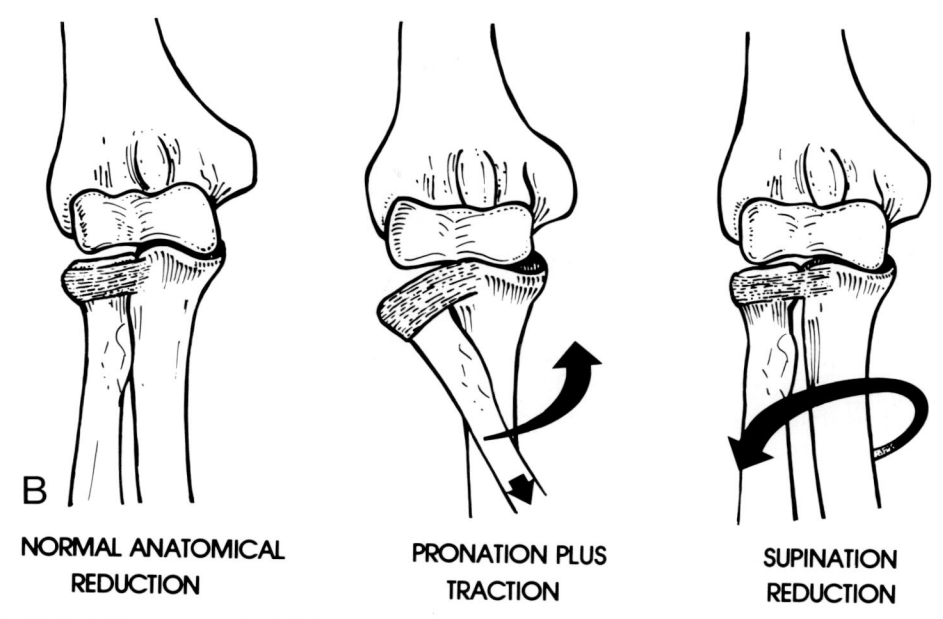

NORMAL ANATOMICAL REDUCTION   **PRONATION PLUS TRACTION**   **SUPINATION REDUCTION**

Fig. 13-28. Pulled elbow occurs in children under 3 years of age secondary to a traction injury with the forearm pronated. A supination maneuver is usually successful in relocating the head of the radius snugly above the annular ligament. (From Letts RM: Dislocation of the elbow in children. In Morrey BF (ed): The Elbow and Its Disorders. WB Saunders, Philadelphia, 1985, with permission.)

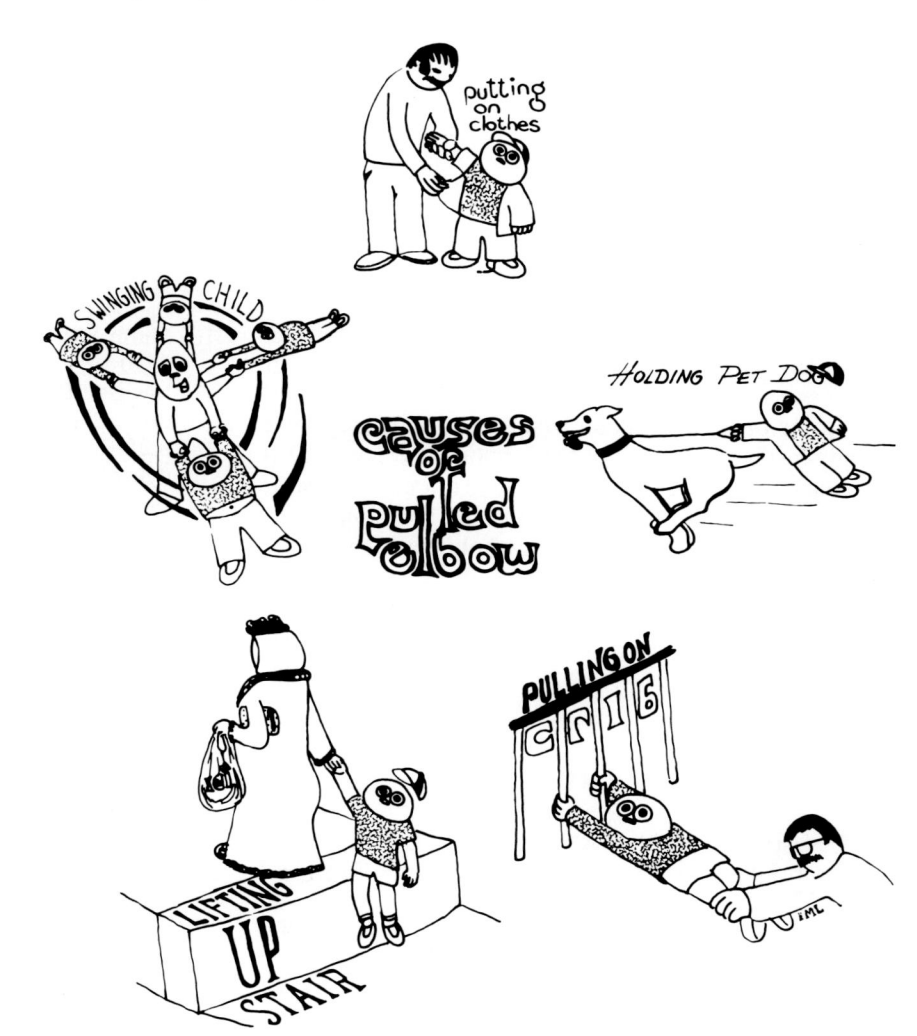

Fig. 13-29. Common causes of pulled elbow in children under 4 years of age. (From Letts RM: Dislocation of the elbow in children. In Morrey BF (ed): The Elbow and Its Disorders. WB Saunders, Philadelphia, 1985, with permission.)

annular ligament (Fig. 13-28). The child usually presents with the arm in pronation and with pain and apprehension, since minor degrees of pronation or supination creates spasm in the annular ligament and results in considerable pain and discomfort. Occasionally, in older children, the proximal rim of the annular ligament will actually be torn.

Reduction is usually accomplished by a quick deft supination maneuver, and if the hand is placed over the lateral aspect of the elbow, a small click can often be palpated as the radial head slips out of annular ligament. The child will often have almost instant relief, although if the annular ligament has been torn, there may be residual pain and tenderness for several days and immobilization of the elbow in a splint is indicated for comfort.

Children who are especially prone to this injury due to the anatomy of their annular ligament and generalized laxity requires special care in the family to avoid any situation where traction on the arm will occur (Fig. 13-29). As the child grows older, the radial head becomes a little larger and the annular ligament stronger and with less laxity. For this reason, a pulled elbow is uncommon over the age of 3 years, hence the syndrome is usually self-limited.

SUMMARY

In summary, elbow dislocation in children has a good prognosis when treatment is prompt and gentle. Diagnosis is usually evident clinically, but radiographs to document the direction of dislocation and presence or absence of associated fractures are mandatory. Signs and symptoms of neurovascular insult may be present and usually resolve following reduction; however, persistent vascular compromise requires surgical attention. In simple dislocations, closed reduction under sedation or anesthesia, followed by 3 weeks of immobilization with the elbow at 90 degrees of flexion, provides satisfactory results. Dislocations associated with fractures, however, more commonly require open reduction, and a persistent mild loss of motion is not uncommon in this group.

REFERENCES

1. Silberstein MJ, Brodeur AE, Graviss ER, Luisiri A: Some vagaries of the medial epicondyle. J Bone Joint Surg [Am] 63:524, 1981
2. Haraldsson S: Osteochondrosis deformans juvenalis capituli hueri including investigation of the intraosseous vasculature in the distal humerus. Acta Orthop Scand Suppl:38, 1959
3. Blount WP: Fractures in Children. Williams & Wilkins, Baltimore, 1955
4. Papavasiliou VA: Fracture separation of the medial epicondylar epiphysis of the elbow joint. Clin Orthop 171:171, 1982
5. Letts RM: Dislocations about the elbow in children. 2nd Ed. In Morrey B, ed. The Elbow and Its Disorders. WB Saunders, Philadelphia, 1993
6. Rang M: Children's Fractures. 2nd Ed. JB Lippincott, Philadelphia, 1983
7. Royce SG, Burke D: Ulna neuropathy after elbow injuries in childhood. Pediatr Orthop 10:495, 1990
8. Dias JJ, Johnson GV, Hoskinson J, Sulalman K: Management of severely displaced medial epicondyle fractures. J Orthop Trauma 1:59, 1987
9. Bernstein SM, King JD, Sanderson RA: Fractures of the medial epicondyle of the humerus. Contemp Orthop 3:637, 1981
10. Fowles JV, Kassab MT, Moula T: Untreated intra-articular entrapment of the medial humeral epicondyle. J Bone Joint Surg [Br] 66:562, 1984
11. Hines RF, Herndon WA, Evans JP: Operative treatment of medial epicondylar fractures in children. Clin Orthop 223:170, 1987
12. Wood GW, Tullos JS: Elbow instability and medial epicondyle fractures. Am J Sports Med 5:23, 1977
13. Smith FM: Surgery of the Elbow. 2nd Ed. WB Saunders, Philadelphia, 1972
14. Josefsson PO, Danielsson LG: Epicondylar elbow fractures in children. Acta Orthop Scand 57:313, 1986
15. Higgs S: Fractures of the internal epicondyle of the humerus. Br Med J 2:666, 1936
16. Smith FM: Medial epicondyle injuries. JAMA 172:396, 1950
17. Ingersoll RR: Fractures of the humeral condyles in children. Clin Orthop 41:32, 1965
18. Kilfoyle RM: Fractures of the medial condyle and epicondyle of the elbow in children. Clin Orthop 41:43, 1965
19. Bensahel H, Csukonyl Z, Badelon O, Badaoul S: Fractures of the medial condyle of the humerus in children. J Pediatr Orthop 6:430, 1986
20. Fowles MB, Kassab MT: Displaced fractures of the medial humeral condyle in children. J Bone Joint Surg [Am] 62:1159, 1980
21. Papavasiliou V, Nenopoulos S, Venturis T: Fractures of the medial condyle of the humerus in childhood. J Pediatr Orthop 7:421, 1987
22. Wilkins KE: Fractures and dislocations of the elbow region. p. 457. In Rockwood CA, Wilkins KE, King RE, eds. Fractures in Children. Vol. 3. JB Lippincott, Philadelphia, 1984
23. De Boeck H, Casteleyn PP, Opdecam P: Fracture of the medial humeral condyle. J Bone Joint Surg[Am] 69:1442, 1987
24. Chacha PB: Fractures of the medial condyle of the hu-

24. [continued] merus with rotational displacement: report of two cases. J Bone Joint Surg [Am] 52:1453, 1970
25. El Ghawabi MH: Fracture of the medial condyle of the humerus. J Bone Joint Surg [Am] 57:677, 1975
26. Milch H: Fracture and fracture dislocations of the humeral condyles. J Trauma 4:592, 1964
27. Royle SG, Burice D: Ulna neuropathy after elbow injuries in children. J Pediatr Orthop 10:495, 1990
28. Hanspal RS: Injury to the medial humeral condyle in a child reviewed after 18 years. J Bone Joint Surg [Br] 67:638, 1985
29. Blount W: Fractures in Children. Williams & Wilkins, Baltimore, 1954
30. Henrikson B: Supracondylar fractures of the humerus in children. Acta Chir Scand, suppl. 369, 1966
31. Pollen AG: Fractures and Dislocations in Children. Churchill Livingstone, Edinburgh, 1973
32. Neviaser JS, Wickstrom JK: Dislocation of the elbow: a retrospective study of 115 patients. South Med J 70:172, 1977
33. Schwab GH, Bennett JB, Woods GW, Tullos JS: Biomechanics of elbow instability: the role of the medial collateral ligament. Clin Orthop 146:42, 1980
34. Asher MA: Dislocations of the upper extremity in childhood. Orthop Clin North Am 7:583, 1976
35. DeLee JL: Transverse divergent dislocation of the elbow in a child. J Bone Joint Surg [Am] 63:322, 1981
36. Holbrook J, Green NE: Divergent pediatric elbow dislocation. Clin Orthop 234:73, 1988
37. Royce SG, Burice O: Ulna neuropathy after elbow injury in children. J Pediatr Orthop 10:495, 1990
38. Carlioz H, Abols Y: Posterior dislocation of the elbow in children. J Pediatr Orthop 4:8, 1984
39. Fowles JV, Slimane N, Kassab MT: Elbow dislocations with avulsion of the medial humeral epicondyle. J Bone Joint Surg [Br] 72:102, 1990
40. Joseffson PO, Johnell O, Gentz CP: Long term sequelae of simple dislocation of the elbow. J Bone Joint Surg [Am] 66:927, 1984
41. Tachdjian MO: Pediatric Orthopaedics. WB Saunders, Philadelphia, 1972
42. Blasier RD: Intra-articular flap fracture of the olecranon in a child. J Bone Joint Surg [Am] 71:945, 1989
43. Blamoutier A, Klaue K, Damsin JP, Carlioz H: Osteochondral fractures of the glenoid fossa of the ulna in children: review of four cases. J Pediatr Orthop 11:638, 1991
44. Yates C, Sullivan AJ: Arthrographic diagnosis of elbow injuries in childhood. J Pediatr Orthop 7:54, 1987
45. Green NE: Entrapment of the median nerve following elbow dislocation. J Pediatr Orthop 3:384, 1983
46. Hallett J: Entrapment of the median nerve after dislocation of the elbow. J Bone Joint Surg [Br] 63:408, 1981
47. Pritchett JW: Entrapment of the median nerve after dislocation of the elbow. J Pediatr Orthop 4:752, 1974
48. St. Clair Strange FG: Entrapment of the median nerve after dislocation of the elbow. J Bone Joint Surg [Br] 64:224, 1982
49. Matev I: A radiological sign of entrapment of the median nerve in the elbow joint after posterior dislocation. J Bone Joint Surg [Br] 58:353, 1976
50. Trias A, Comeau Y: Recurrent dislocation of the elbow in children. Clin Orthop 100:74, 1974
51. Osborne G, Cotterill P: Recurrent dislocation of the elbow. J Bone Joint Surg [Br] 48:340, 1966
52. Hassmann GL, Brunn F, Neer CS: Recurrent dislocation of the elbow. J Bone Joint Surg [Am] 57:1080, 1975
53. Herring JA, Sullivan JA: Recurrent dislocation of the elbow. J Pediatr Orthop 9:483, 1989
54. Symeonides PP, Paschaloglou C, Starou Z, Pangalides TH: Recurrent dislocation of the elbow. J Bone Joint Surg [Am] 57:1084, 1975
55. Naidoo KS: Unreduced posterior dislocations of the elbow. J Bone Joint Surg [Br] 64:603, 1982
56. Fowles JV, Kassab MT, Dovak M, Kassab S: Untreated posterior dislocation of the elbow in children. J Bone Joint Surg [Am] 66:921, 1984
57. Arafiles RP: Neglected posterior dislocations of the elbow. J Bone Joint Surg [Br] 69:199, 1987
58. Ainsworth SR, Avlicino PL: Chronic posterolateral dislocation of the elbow in a child. Orthopaedics 16:212, 1993

14

Lateral Condylar Fractures of the Humerus

William McIntyre

> The greatest attribute is the ability to recognize ability.
> —E. Hubbard

DESCRIPTION AND INCIDENCE

Fractures of the lateral condyle of the humerus account for about 10 to 15 percent of fractures about the elbow.[1-3] They tend to occur in the same age group as supracondylar fracture with an average age of about 6 years. They are also one of the easiest fractures to miss because there is frequently so little metaphyseal bone involved with much of the fracture line extending through the cartilage of the epiphysis and the physis (Fig. 14-1).

ANATOMIC CONSIDERATIONS

The classical lateral condyle fracture is a Salter-Harris type IV fracture traversing metaphysis, physis, and the epiphysis.[4-6] Frequently the metaphyseal fragment consists of only a thin sliver of bone barely visible radiographically with the rest of the fracture line involving physeal cartilage (Fig. 14-1), traversing the epiphysis to exit in the joint usually at the cartilaginous midtrochlea.

Dallek and Jungbluth[7] in the German literature have studied the microarchitecture of the distal humeral epiphyseal cartilage and found bundles of collagen sloping from proximal capitellum to distal midtrochlea. They have proposed that the architecture of these collagen fibers predispose the child to the typical lateral condyle fracture.

The inexperienced viewer may call this a lateral epicondyle fracture, not recognizing the much more extensive intra-articular extension of the fracture as well as the fact that the lateral epicondyle does not ossify until later.

MECHANISM OF INJURY

A fracture commencing laterally over the distal metaphysis is the most common fracture pattern produced by a varus force, usually from a fall on the outstretched arm. This was well described in 1975 by Jakob and colleagues,[8] who, in cadaver studies, found that the classical articular hinge-type fracture could be consistently reproduced by a varus force in full supination and extension. Experimentally, they also found that they could not produce a free fragment with a varus force alone. With the varus force applied, they could open the lateral fracture as much as 2 or 3 cm only to have it return to less than a 5-mm gap when the arm was realigned. They further found that they had to cut the articular hinge with a scalpel to produce a free fragment that would in turn allow horizontal displacement.

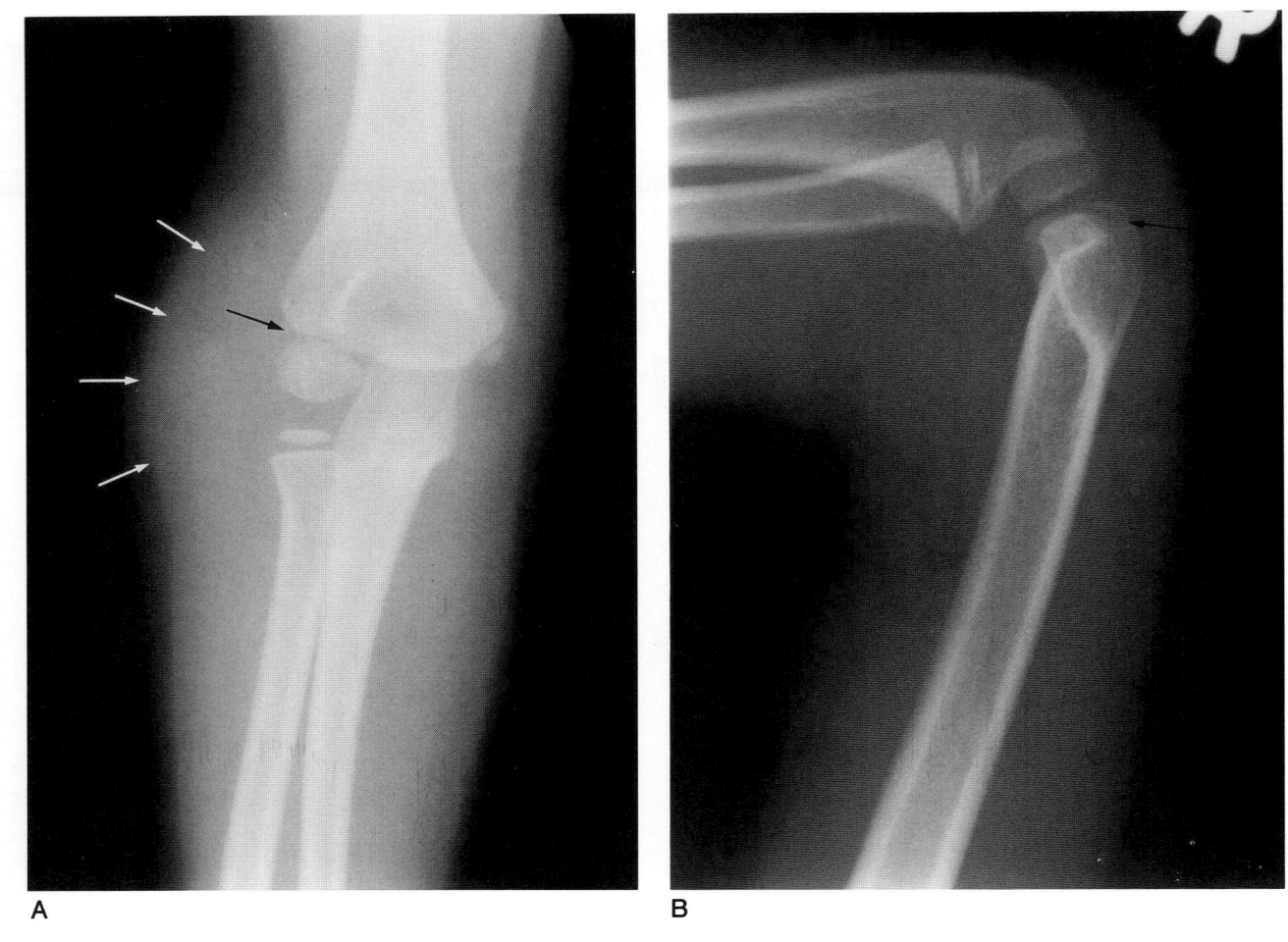

Fig. 14-1. **(A)** Anteroposterior view of a small metaphyseal fragment. Note the localized marked lateral soft tissue swelling. **(B)** Lateral view showing the fracture line more clearly. The metaphyseal fragment is more posterolateral. The fracture appears to be "minimally" displaced.

A fracture of the olecranon (Fig. 14-2) is sometimes seen in association with a lateral condyle fracture.[8,9] The olecranon fracture is usually gapped open on the lateral surface. This double injury was produced by Jakob and colleagues[8] by a varus force with the elbow locked in full extension and supination. In such a varus mechanism the last structure to fracture is the humeral articular surface (Fig. 14-3), and in fractures with lesser force the articular cartilage may remain intact in hinge fashion with wedge-shaped lateral fracture gaps of up to 4 or 5 mm or more on initial radiographs.

It has been found in previous studies[8,10] that if there is horizontal displacement of over 1 mm, it is probable that the articular hinge is no longer intact. Such a fracture is likely to require open reduction and pinning. With displaced complete fractures, the lateral condyle becomes a very mobile unstable fragment, and may be malrotated over 90 degrees in both coronal and sagittal planes. A second mechanism of fracture production can occur by an axial loading force through the radial head to the capitellum. This may shear the articular cartilage closer to the capitellar trochlear junction (Fig. 14-4).

The work of Jakob and colleagues[8] indicated that there is difficulty producing a complete articular surface fracture with a pure varus force. This would suggest that axial and varus loading are the mechanisms involved in producing a fully displaced unstable fragment. If the mechanism were mainly axial loading, this may on occasion leave the lateral soft tissues at least partially intact, in the presence of a complete fracture that could be

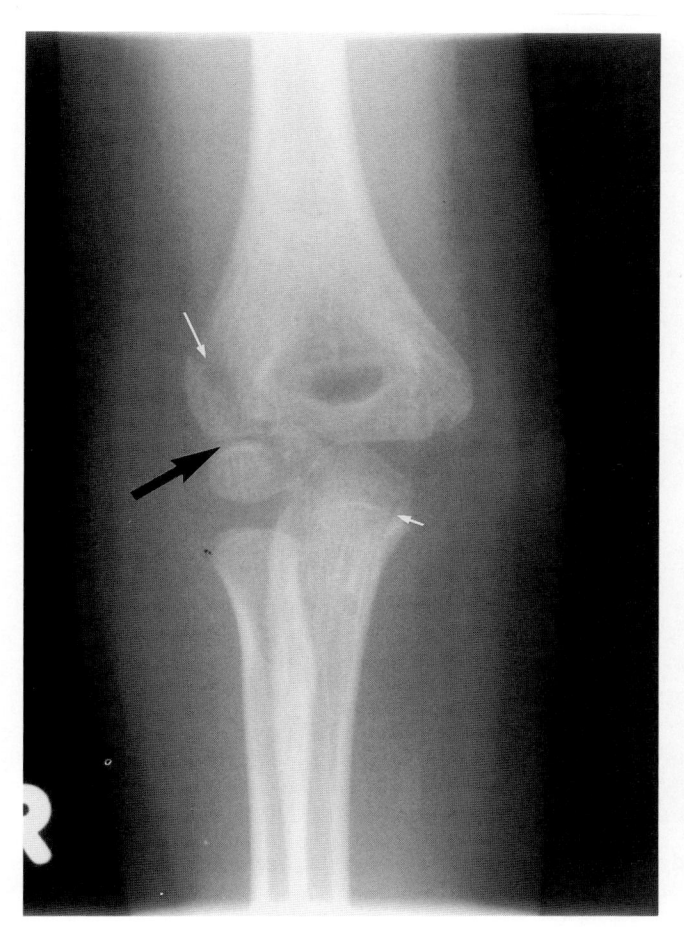

Fig. 14-2. A lateral condyle fracture with associated olecranon fracture, produced by a varus force on the fully extended elbow.

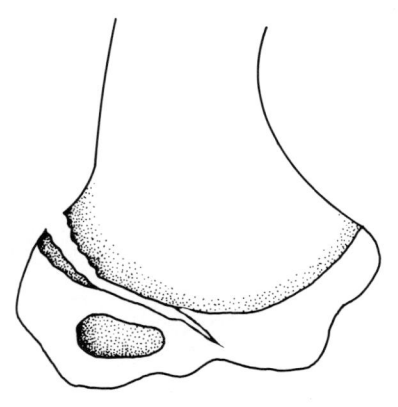

Fig. 14-3. The more common Milch type II fracture, the most common fracture pattern encountered.

missed and possibly go on to nonunion.[8,11-13] The fracture gap in this circumstance is often parallel rather than wedge-shaped (Fig. 14-4).

With the varus force mechanism or a combination of axial load and varus force the lateral periosteum may be peeled off the lateral cortex above the horizontal exit of the fracture line. This can sometimes peel off a layer of bone with the periosteum and interfere with the interpretation of the degree of horizontal displacement (the fragment appearing more displaced than it really is).

It is common for the metaphyseal fracture line to extend higher posteriorly, which has prompted Peterson to call this configuration the *triplane fracture* of the elbow.[14,15] Such a triplane configuration might imply a shearing or perhaps a lateral rotation force on the capitellum. A fall on the somewhat flexed elbow and pronated forearm might allow more loading via the radial head on the capitellum. A hyperextending force along with varus and axial loading might produce the same result. The interosseous membrane between the radius and ulna is taut in supination, allowing an axial force on the radius to be transmitted to the ulna; however, in pronation this interosseous membrane is lax, allowing greater transmission of load to the capitellum rather than to the ulna (a similar mechanism to that demonstrated for an isolated radial head dislocation).[16]

With the more displaced fractures (Fig. 14-5), there can be a fracture dislocation with potential ulnar-humeral instability. Greater instability would exist if there is disruption of the medial collateral ligament of the elbow, allowing greater lateral drift of the ulna. In the pure varus injury there may be medial subluxation or rarely dislocation of the ulnar-humeral joint.

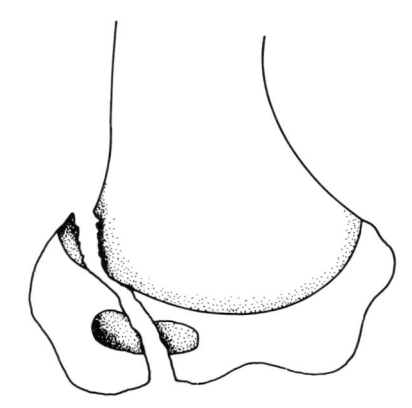

Fig. 14-4. A Milch type I fracture traversing the capitellar ossification center (note the parallel gap), a complete fracture. This would be a displacement type 3b fracture requiring open repair.

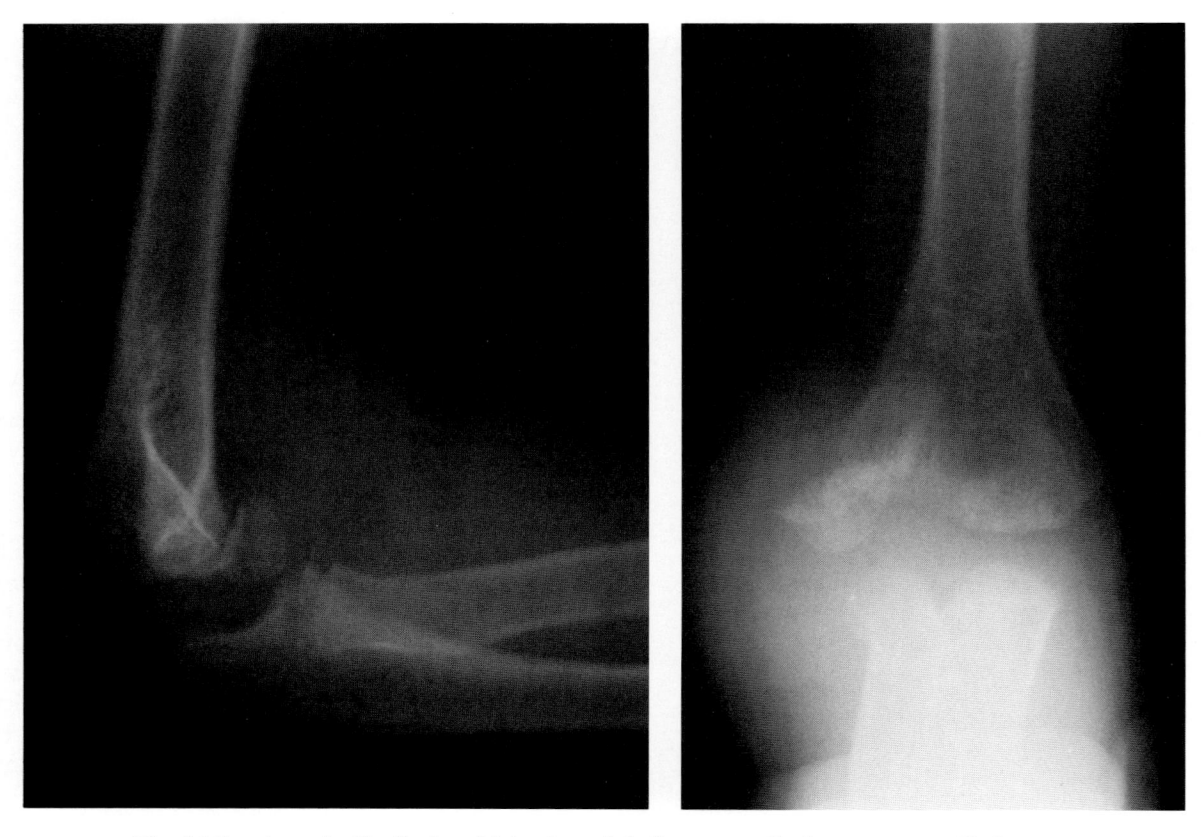

Fig. 14-5. A markedly displaced lateral condyle fracture, a displacement type 3b fracture.

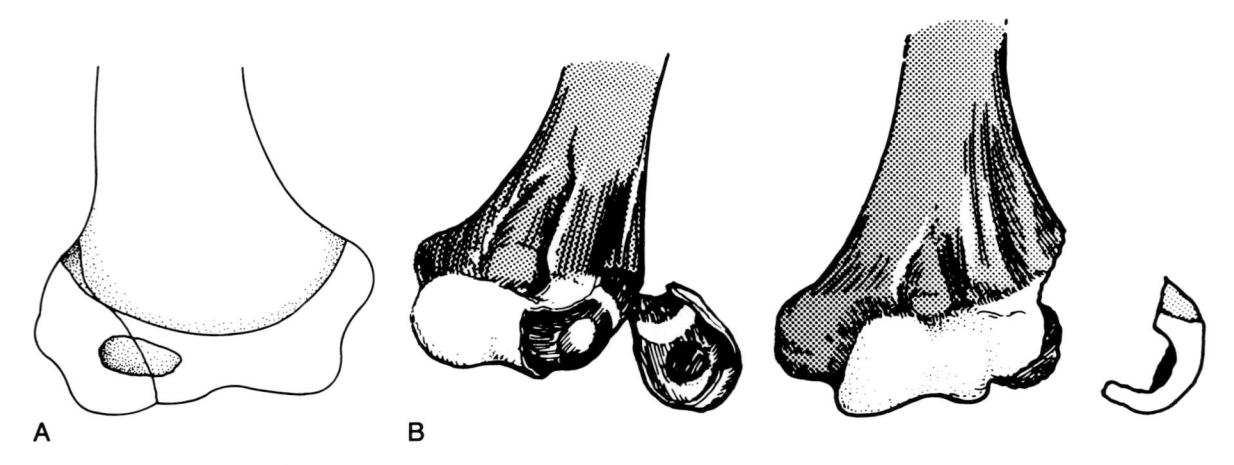

Fig. 14-6. **(A)** A Milch type I fracture undisplaced. The articular end of this fracture line is usually at the junction of the medial edge of the capitellum and the trochlea. **(B)** A variant of a Milch I fracture occasionally seen in children. Articular cartilage sleeve fracture of the lateral humeral condyle capitellum. (Figure B from Agins and Marcus,[19] with permission.)

Because these fractures can be caused by a varus force, they can also be produced by a traction injury, such as in physical child abuse. This traction mechanism is more likely to produce a type I (or II) Salter-Harris fracture with classically medial displacement, which, in the very young, is easy to miss and has a higher correlation to child abuse[1] (see Ch. 12).

CLASSIFICATIONS

Fracture Site

Classification according to the site of the fracture is as follows[17,18]:

1. Milch type I, traversing the capitellar ossification center (Fig. 14-6)
2. Milch type II, missing the capitellar ossification center and extending into the midtrochlea (Fig. 14-7)

The majority of lateral condyle fractures are of the Milch type II variety.[8]

It should be noted that the capitellar ossification center extends medially into the lateral trochlea so that Milch type I fractures usually extend to the medial edge of the capitellar articular surface. Those fractures that miss the ossification center (Milch type II) extend into the midtrochlea. This is the reason for the greater potential for lateral subluxation of the olecranon in displaced Milch type II fractures (Fig. 14-8), especially if the medial ligament is stretched or torn.

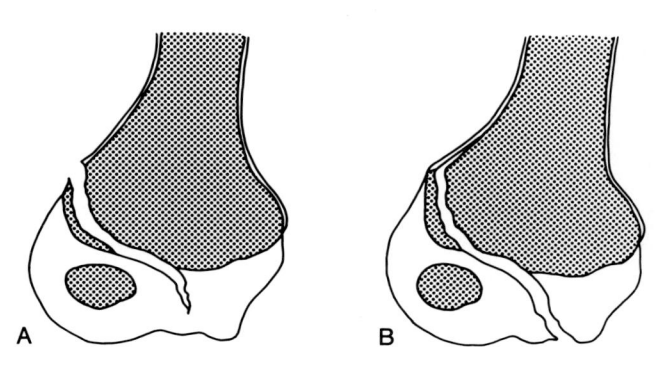

Fig. 14-7. (A) The "articular cartilage" hinge and (B) the "soft tissue" hinge in a Milch type II fracture. The fracture line missing the capitellar ossification center and extending to the midtrochlea. Figure A with the intact articular hinge would be displacement type 2 or 3a depending on the size of the gap at the lateral bone margin. Figure B with horizontal displacement and disrupted articular hinge would be displacement type 3b likely requiring open reduction. (From McIntyre and Lawton,[10] with permission.)

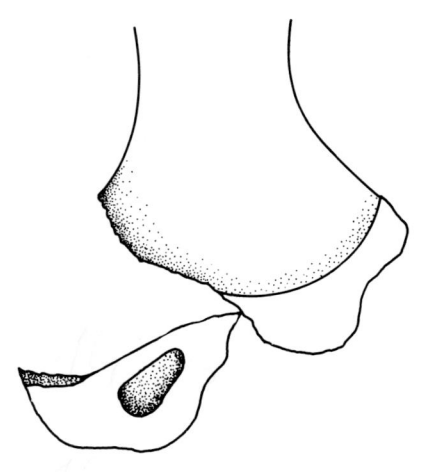

Fig. 14-8. A diagram of a Milch type II fully displaced fracture as in Figure 14-5. This would be a type 3b in the displacement classification and requires open reduction with fixation.

Another atypical Milch type I fracture involves the lateral margin of the capitellar ossification center. A variation of this was described in 1984 by Agins and Marcus[19] as a sleeve fracture of the lateral condyle. In spite of a thin sliver of lateral bone radiologically, the fracture involved 75 percent of the articular surface of the capitellum (Fig. 14-6B).

Degree of Displacement

In the classification according to the degree of displacement, the term *vertical gap* is the distance between lateral (or posterior) fracture margins measured perpendicular to the fracture surfaces; and the term *horizontal displacement* is the overlap of the metaphyseal fragment beyond the line of the lateral (or posterior) metaphyseal surface.[10] The classification system is as follows:

Type 1: Vertical gap less than 1 mm, and no horizontal displacement
Type 2: Wedge shaped vertical gap up to 2 mm, but horizontal displacement less than 1 mm
Type 3a: Wedge shaped vertical gap of over 2 mm, but horizontal displacement still under 1 mm (articular hinge possibly intact)
Type 3b: More significantly displaced with articular hinge not intact

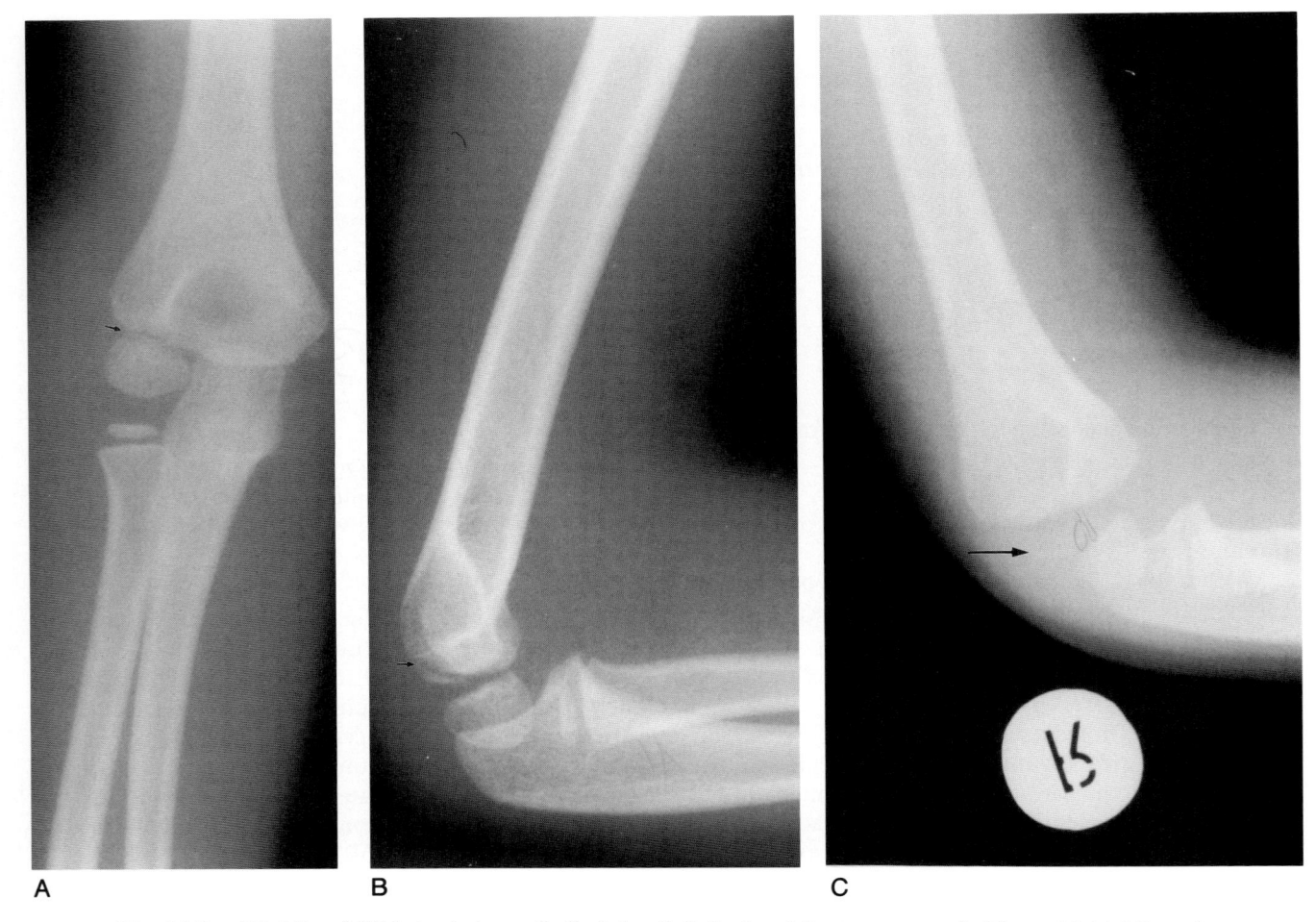

Fig. 14-9. (A) AP and (B) lateral views of a "minimally" displaced fracture as seen in Figure 14-1A&B, again note the marked lateral soft tissue swelling. This could pass as displacement type 1. (C) An oblique view taken on the same day as Figures A&B with the fracture opening up in a parallel gap over 5 mm. This is a displacement type 3b fracture and would require open repair.

There is horizontal displacement over 1 mm. This could be a small fracture gap that is often *parallel* rather than *wedge-shaped,* and may appear to be minimally displaced (Fig. 14-9A,B) or more obviously displaced (Fig. 14-9C).

PHYSICAL EXAMINATION AND RADIOGRAPHIC APPEARANCE

With fractures that are undisplaced the actual fracture line may not be visible, but a "fat-pad sign" may be present as well as soft tissue swelling. The diagnosis is often made on clinical grounds, with lateral supracondylar ridge tenderness and absent tenderness over the medial supracondylar ridge. As with undisplaced supracondylar fractures, subsequent radiographs may show healing periosteal new bone revealing the previously clinically diagnosed fracture.

When there is marked localized lateral elbow swelling clinically and radiographically, one should suspect that there may be an unstable lateral condyle fracture, even if on initial films the fracture is deemed to be minimally displaced (Fig. 14-9A,B). As with other significant elbow injuries there will be guarding of movement that will vary with the child and the fracture displacement. Neu-

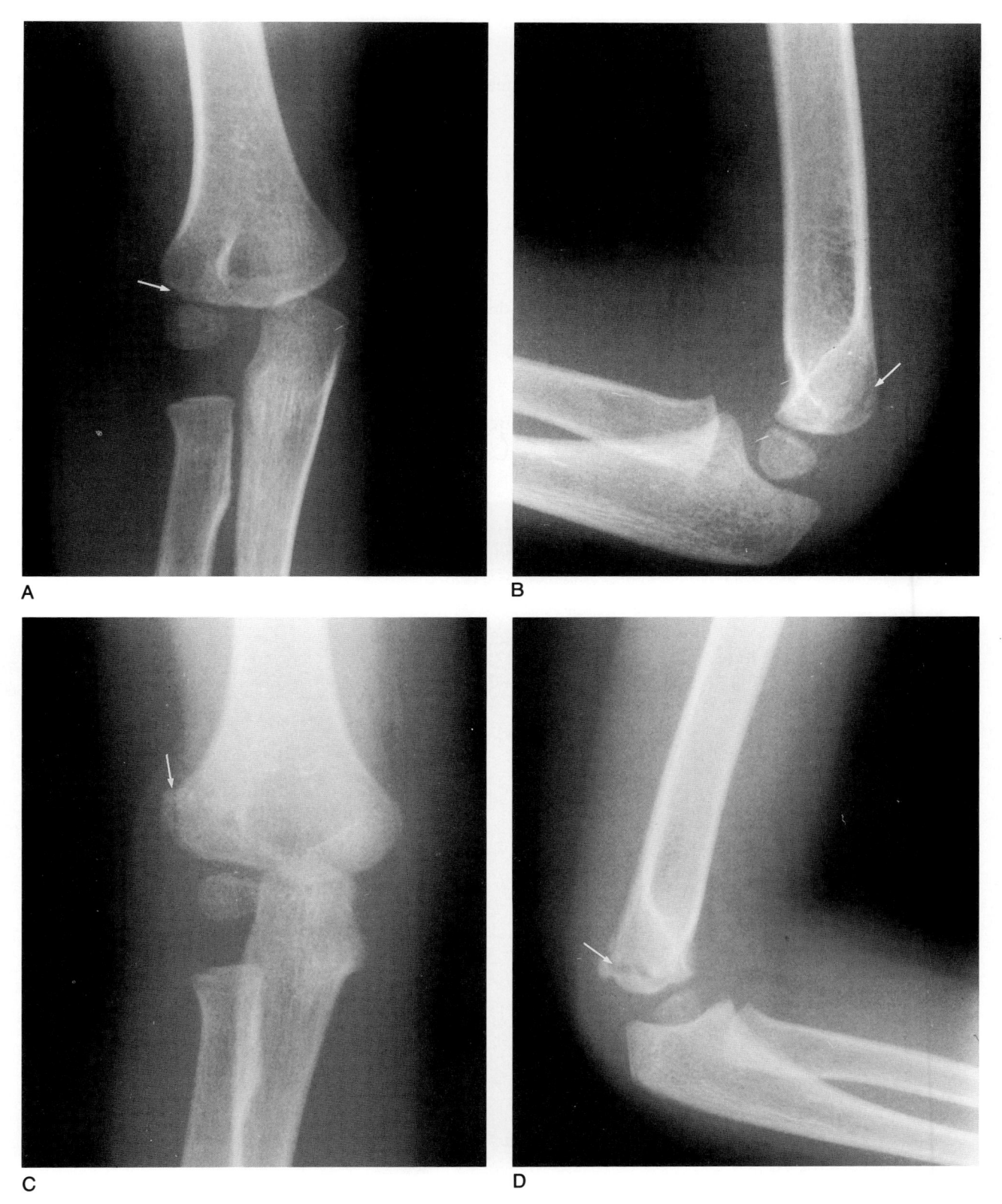

Fig. 14-10. (A) Initial AP view with only a small lateral sliver of metaphyseal bone involved undisplaced type 1. (B) Initial lateral radiograph showing again a larger posterior dimension to the metaphyseal fragment, again undisplaced. (C) AP and (D) lateral views 3 weeks following fracture demonstrating the fracture line resorption and new bone forming at the lateral and posterior margins.

248 / Management of Pediatric Fractures

rovascular compromise is fortunately rare as an early finding.

DIFFERENTIAL DIAGNOSIS

The main differential diagnoses include

1. Any of the other elbow dislocations or fracture dislocations
2. Supracondylar fractures
3. Rarer T condylar fractures
4. Medial condyle fractures
5. Distal humeral transcondylar epiphyseal fractures

TREATMENT INDICATIONS

All clinically or radiologically diagnosed lateral condyle fractures should be followed closely with recheck radiographs *out of the plaster splint,* at 1 and 2 weeks postinjury. Active elbow mobilization is initiated at 3 to 4 weeks postfracture.

Nonoperative Management

Completely undisplaced type 1 fractures (Fig. 14-10) and those deemed to be minimally displaced, that is, those type 2 fractures that have an intact articular hinge (Fig. 14-11) (with less than 1 mm of horizontal displace-

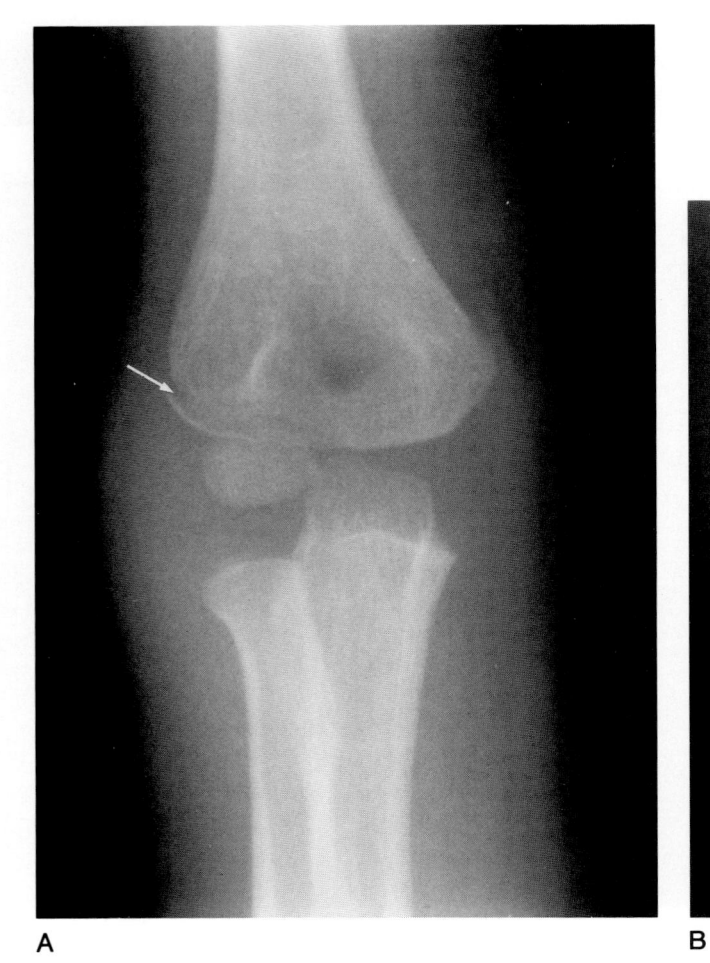

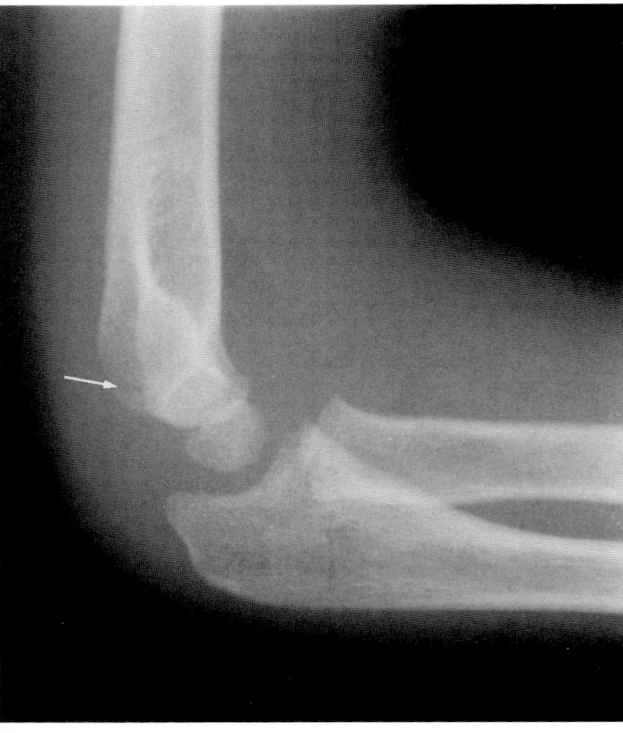

Fig. 14-11. (A) AP view of displacement type 2 fracture demonstrating a wedge-shaped gap, open laterally less than 2 mm. No horizontal displacement is present. (B) Lateral view showing no horizontal displacement. The fracture line again being higher posterior.

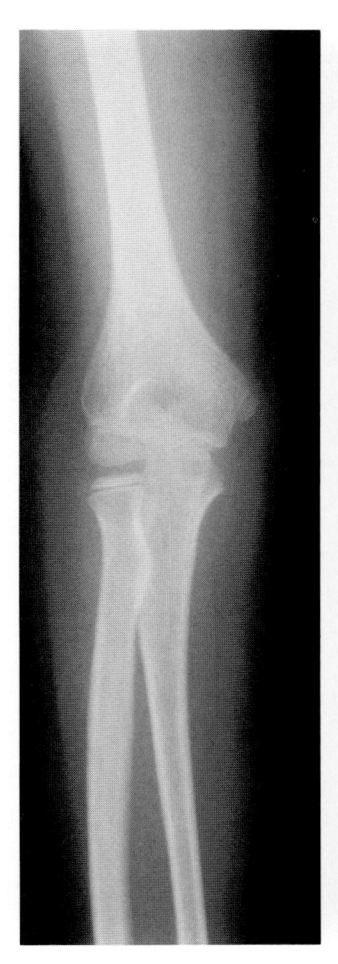

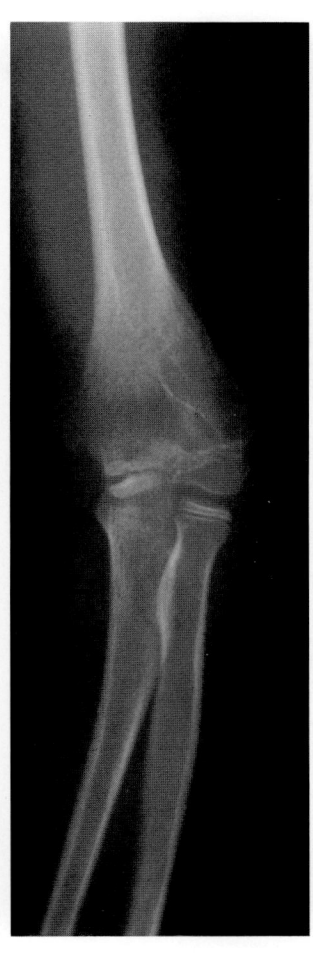

Fig. 14-12. AP view of both arms after three fractures of the left lateral condyle treated nonoperatively with subsequent healing in significant varus.

ment and less than 2 mm of vertical gap), should be treated in a long-arm posterior plaster splint. The post-fracture routine with radiographs taken with the splint removed should be followed. Active range of motion is commenced at 3 to 4 weeks with removable protective splinting for play activities until 6 weeks or solid radiologic union. A full range of elbow motion should ordinarily be obtained by 6 to 12 weeks, although, as in any elbow trauma, the occasional child may take a longer period of time to regain full preinjury elbow motion.

Some authors have indicated the need to immobilize lateral condyle fractures for more prolonged periods of 6 to 12 weeks.[12] These fractures need to be followed until there is radiologic solid union, but most elbows can be mobilized carefully at 3 to 4 weeks. This does not usually compromise their healing, and minimizes chances of stiffness.

When there is lateral gapping of the fracture some decrease in the valgus carrying angle can be expected partly from the varus angulation at the time of injury and partly from lateral overgrowth of the capitellum. This is rarely more than 5 to 10 degrees for an individual fracture with less than 2 mm vertical gap.[20-23] and would only be obvious in a child who had a small carrying angle prior to the fracture (e.g., 0 degrees).

With a 2- to 3-mm lateral fracture gap the contralateral carrying angle should be assessed. If the fracture has significantly altered the carrying angle by the production of a varus displacement, reduction should be performed. If not, the arm can be casted and the fracture monitored closely.

We have treated a child (with a neuromotor disorder associated with frequent falls) who had three consecutive gap-type lateral condyle fractures: the first, essentially undisplaced, was a type I fracture, the second, 4 weeks later, was a type 2 fracture with 2 mm of lateral gap, and the third, 3 months later, was a type 3a fracture with over 3 mm of gap. He was treated nonoperatively each time and healed, but with significant cubitus varus (differing by 25 degrees from the other side) (Fig. 14-12).

We have treated several other children where cubitus varus after a supracondylar fracture was followed by a lateral condyle fracture. The varus residual deformity might have predisposed them to the varus type of reinjury. Others have also reported cases of repeat lateral condyle fractures.[10,21,24,25]

Operative Management

For type 3a fractures (that have less than 1 mm of horizontal displacement, but more than 2 mm of wedge-shaped vertical gap) one should consider operative management (Fig. 14-13). On image intensifier examination under general anesthetic, if the fracture behaves like a "hinge" fracture and closes anatomically when a valgus force is applied, then percutaneous smooth pin fixation through the lateral condyle (1 or 2 pins) are recommended to maintain reduction.[23] If a closed reduction without pin fixation is carried out, it is very difficult to maintain, as gravity tends to cause the fracture to fall into a more varus (less valgus) position. If the closed reduction is not anatomic, then open reduction should be undertaken.

If there is horizontal displacement of over 1 mm (Fig. 14-9C) it is unlikely that the articular hinge is intact. Fully displaced and rotated lateral condyle fractures are generally more obvious and not likely to be missed (Fig. 14-5).

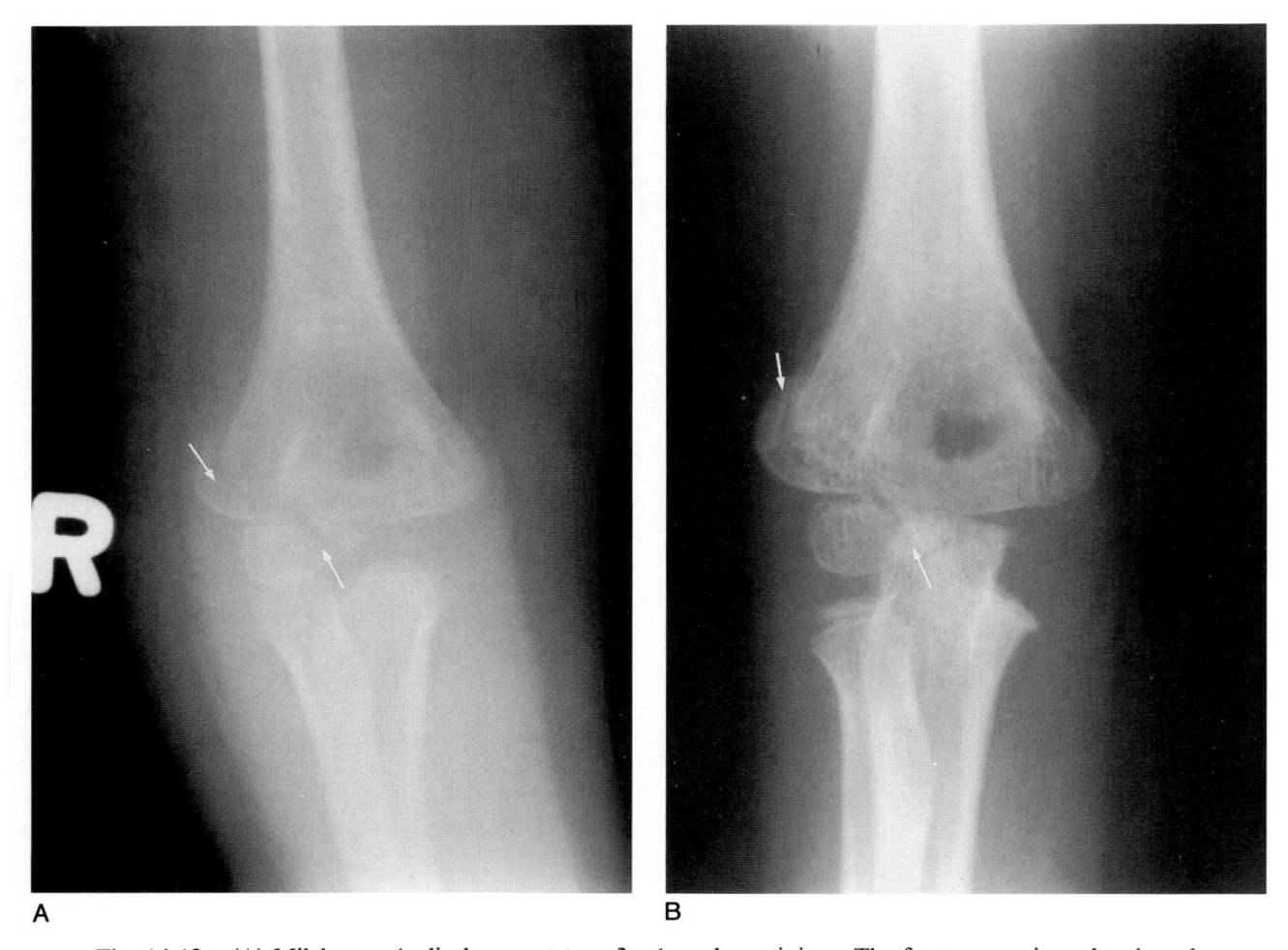

Fig. 14-13. (A) Milch type 1, displacement type 3a, 1 week postinjury. The fracture gap is wedge-shaped, suggesting the articular cartilage may be intact. There is apparently greater than 1 mm of horizontal displacement, but this is from a "peeling off" of some metaphyseal cortex above the main fracture line. (B) This view illustrates the same fracture healing at 4.5 weeks. Some varus is likely, and this fracture would have been better handled by closed reduction and percutaneous pinning.

With these type 3b fractures, closed reduction with or without pinning, should not be undertaken, as there is usually rotation in two planes that can be difficult to interpret even with the fracture open. Where there is only a thin sliver of metaphyseal bone on the condyle fragment, radiographic interpretation of the adequacy of reduction can be misleading. The lateral ossified edge may appear to match the metaphysis when the radiolucent articular cartilage end of the fracture in the mid-trochlea is still malrotated.

Several authors have reported on the value of elbow arthrography.[26-29] Earlier reports concentrated on its use in the younger child where the distal humerus was unossified and found it assisted in the diagnosis and management. It was particularly helpful in distinguishing Salter-Harris types I and II distal humeral epiphyseal injuries from lateral condyle fractures. In 1987 Yates and Sullivan[29] advocated double-contrast studies using small (0.5 to 1 ml), equal amounts of air and dye to line the cartilage surfaces, but not obscure the pathology. A more recent study by Marzo and coworkers[28] outlined the use of arthrography specifically for lateral condyle fractures. All of these authors concur that arthrography is a useful and accurate procedure particularly in the very young child.

Type 3b fractures (Figs. 14-5 and 14-9) should be

open-reduced, with care being taken not to strip soft tissues along the growth plate or over the lateral condyle, particularly posterior. Use of a headlight is helpful to visualize the articular cartilage congruity through the "keyhole" visibility after reduction. To control rotation, two smooth K-wires should be inserted to cross the fracture at some distance apart to hold the reduction.

Even with open surgery, obtaining anatomic reduction of the unstable (type 3b) lateral condyle fracture can be difficult. The reduction requires gentle and not forceful fragment handling. The arm should not be medially rotated, as this tends to pull the lateral condyle anteriorly. The peeled-off lateral periosteum frequently makes it difficult to use the lateral surface to interpret an anatomic reduction. Finger control of the biplane rotation tendency of the condyle is often as effective as clamps until a first smooth K-wire is inserted. The position should then be rechecked with particular reference to the anteromedial fracture line, which can be visualized with a small retractor and a headlight. A minimal release of anterior muscle may be necessary to achieve this view. The periosteum and perichondrium should not be further dissected from the condyle fragment. A second smooth K-wire is inserted for rotatory control (Fig. 14-14).

The pin ends can be left outside the skin, supported with sterile felt pads, for easy pin removal about 3 to 4 weeks postinsertion. Gentle *active* range of motion exercises are then begun with the arm out of a removable splint. In the first 3 weeks a posterior plaster splint can be used rather than a circular cast, as the pin fixation usually provides adequate stability.

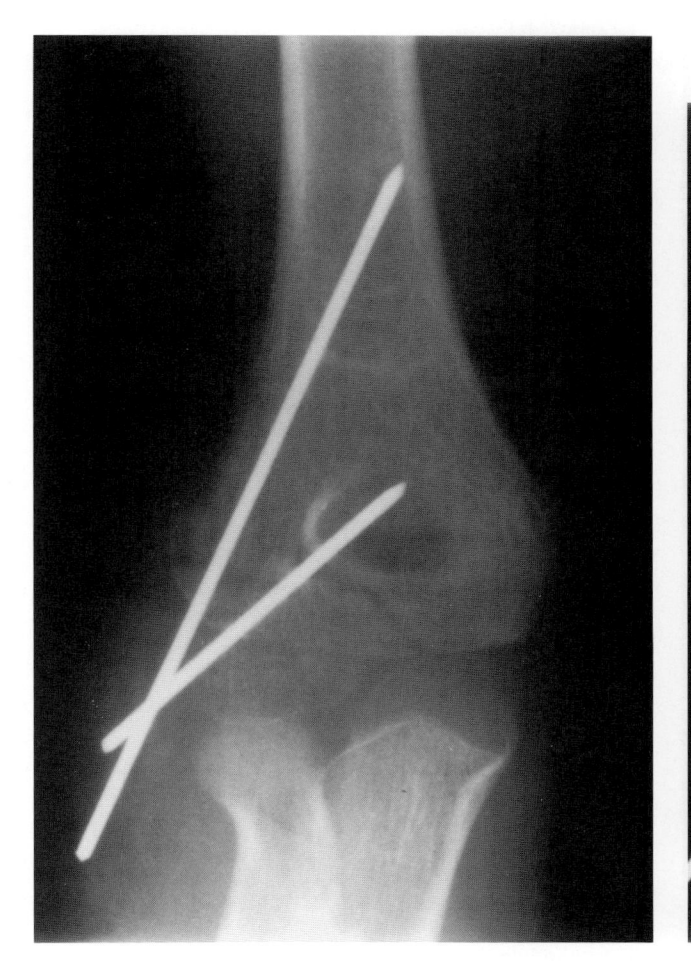

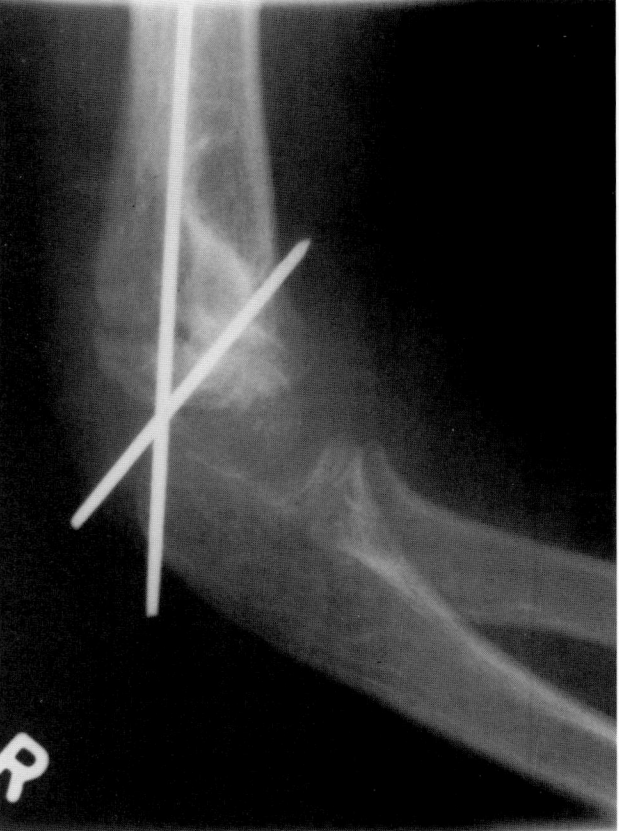

Fig. 14-14. Two-pin fixation. The anteriorly directed pin is in too far. The pin points are best embedded in, but not through the opposite cortex. The pin ends may be left outside the skin for easy removal at 3 to 4 weeks.

PITFALLS OF MANAGEMENT

Diagnostic Pitfall

The lateral condyle fracture of the humerus is easily missed,[2,12,25,30] especially in the very young child where there is only a small sliver of metaphyseal bone on the distal fragment (Fig. 14-15).

Operative Decision-Making

The other difficulty after the fracture is identified is trying to decide whether a fracture is stable enough to be managed closed or whether it needs pin fixation to stabilize it. Some series[31] report a high percentage (80–90 percent) of lateral condyle fractures requiring open reduction. This may reflect differences in referral patterns with undisplaced fractures probably not being referred by the primary care physician. Our experience with lateral condyle fractures indicates that about half can be managed closed, the remainder requiring reduction with pin fixation.[8,10] About 10 percent of those initially managed closed went on to further displacement, and required open reduction and two-pin fixation. Only a few could be treated by closed reduction and pinning. Several children with an intact articular hinge fracture went on to heal in unacceptable varus (Figs. 14-12 and 14-13), and, in retrospect, should have been closed reduced and percutaneously pinned.

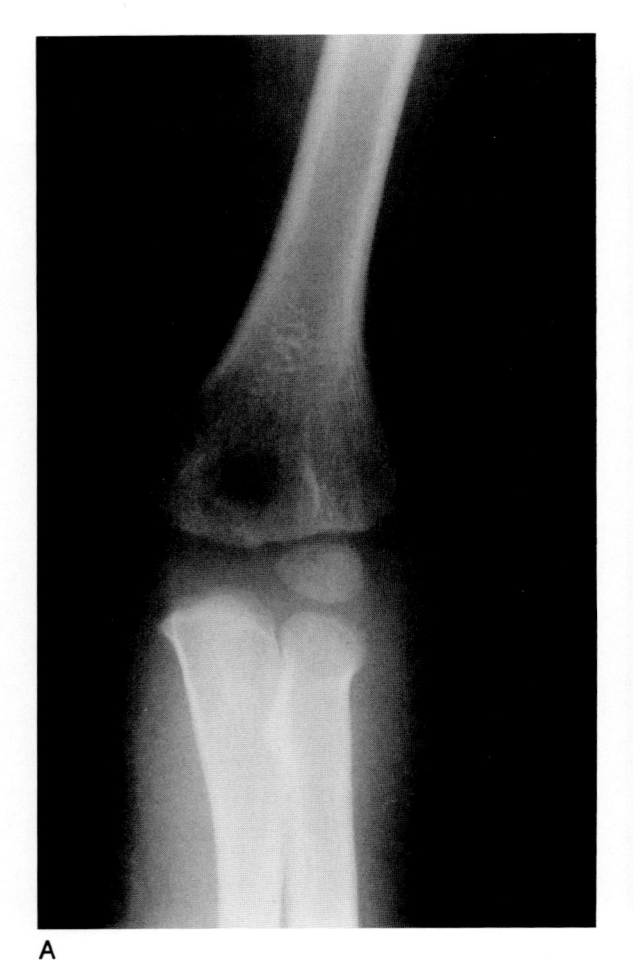

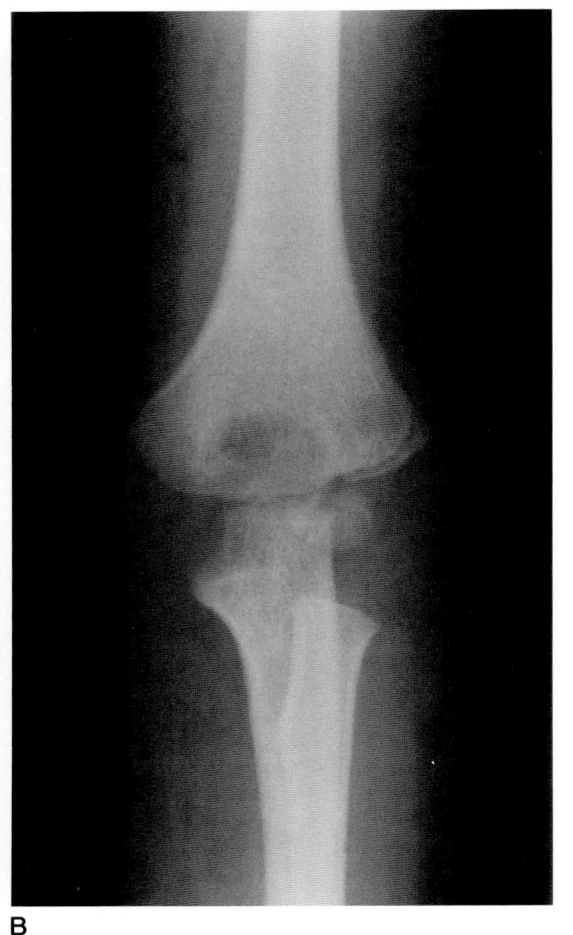

Fig. 14-15. (A) A minimally displaced fracture of the lateral condyle that is difficult to identify and unfortunately frequently missed by those not familiar with this subtle fracture. (B) One month later the fracture is more clearly visible with the development of fracture callus.

A fully free and unstable fragment should be suspected when there is horizontal displacement of greater than 1 mm, especially with a parallel gap (Fig. 14-9). Open reduction with pin fixation is recommended in such cases. It is not advisable to try to percutaneously pin these type 3b complete fractures.

COMPLICATIONS

Nonunion

The earlier literature recommended to avoid operative intervention for lateral condyles that were delayed in diagnosis after 3 or more weeks.[3,8,15,31] More recent experience has suggested that if care is taken not to strip the lateral condyle of its soft tissues, delayed operative management is possible and advisable.[9,12,22,23,36] We concur with this latter approach, especially for the nonunion that is in relatively good position, with a metaphyseal fragment that is large enough to fix to the humeral metaphysis; care being taken to preserve the vascular soft tissue attachments to the lateral condyle, especially posteriorly.[22,37]

The operative treatment is technically complex, but some form of fixation with or without bone graft can frequently result in union of metaphysis of the lateral condyle fragment to the main shaft fragment, with retention of physeal growth.

For the high-riding nonunion (Fig. 14-16) reduction may be limited and should not be done at the expense of devascularizing the condylar fragment. In such cases, treatment of the residual valgus with a more proximal varus osteotomy and/or anterior transposition of the ulnar nerve may be indicated.[9,36]

Figure 14-17 is illustrative of a 5-year-old girl who had an unstable lateral condylar fracture with a small metaphyseal sliver of bone that was missed by emergency officers at two different hospitals, the child presenting 2 years later with a nonunion and complete ulnar nerve palsy.

Since introducing the policy of reradiographing suspected lateral condyle fractures *out of plaster* at 1 and 2 weeks following injury, we have not experienced a nonunion of the lateral condyle. Displacement of the condylar fragment that predisposes to nonunion can be identified early, and, although the open reduction may be delayed 1 or 2 weeks, uneventful healing has been the rule.

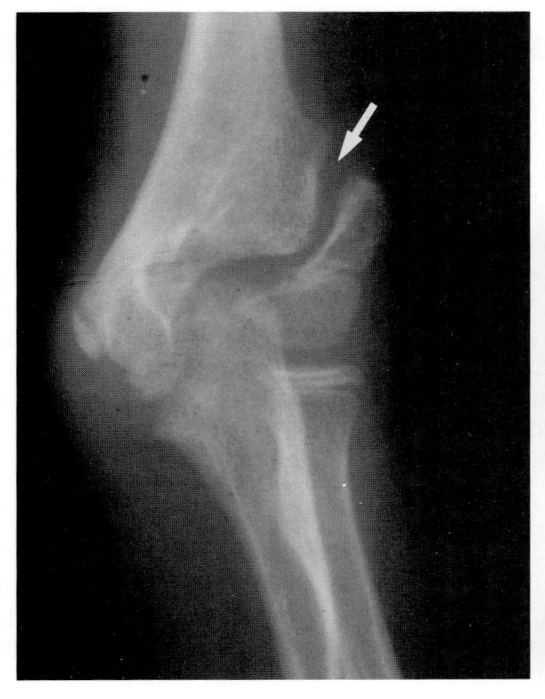

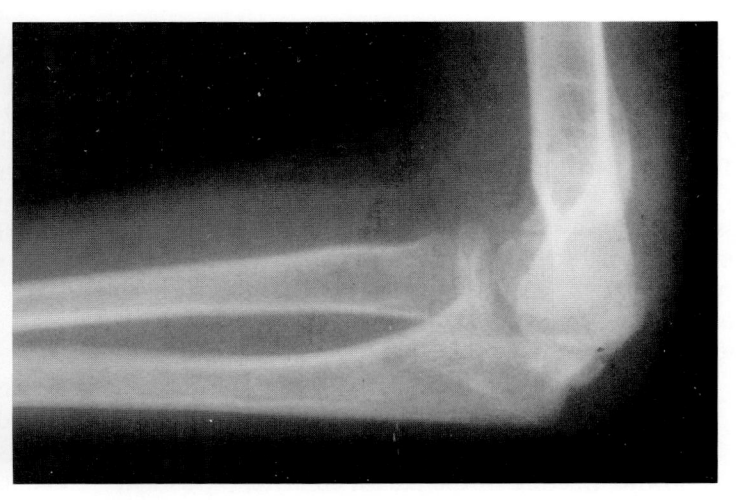

Fig. 14-16. Nonunion of the lateral condyle with established pseudoarthrosis and proximal drift of the fragment. This child would have high risk of developing tardy ulnar nerve palsy.

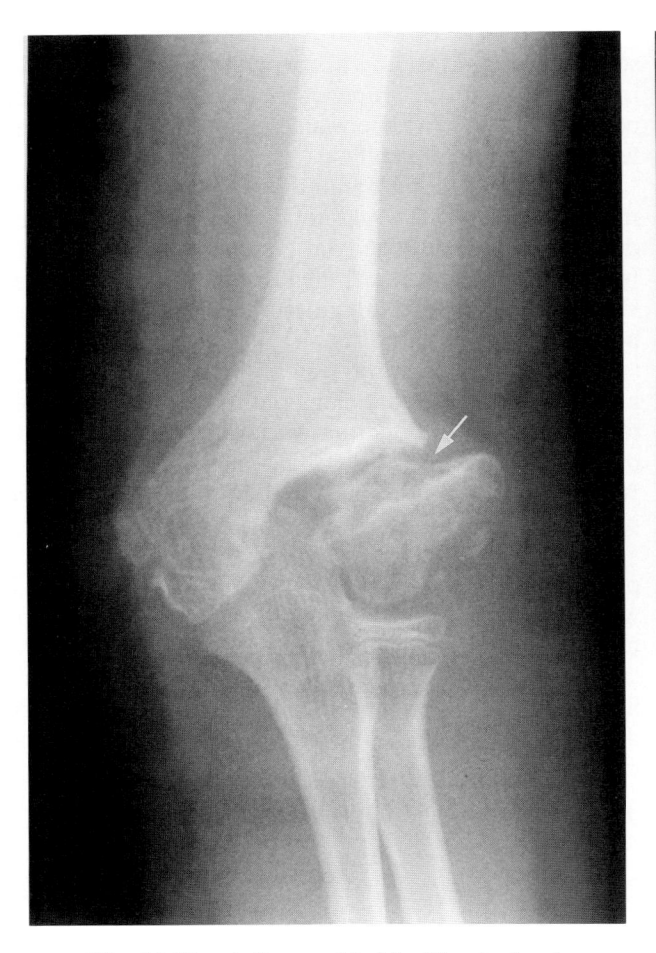

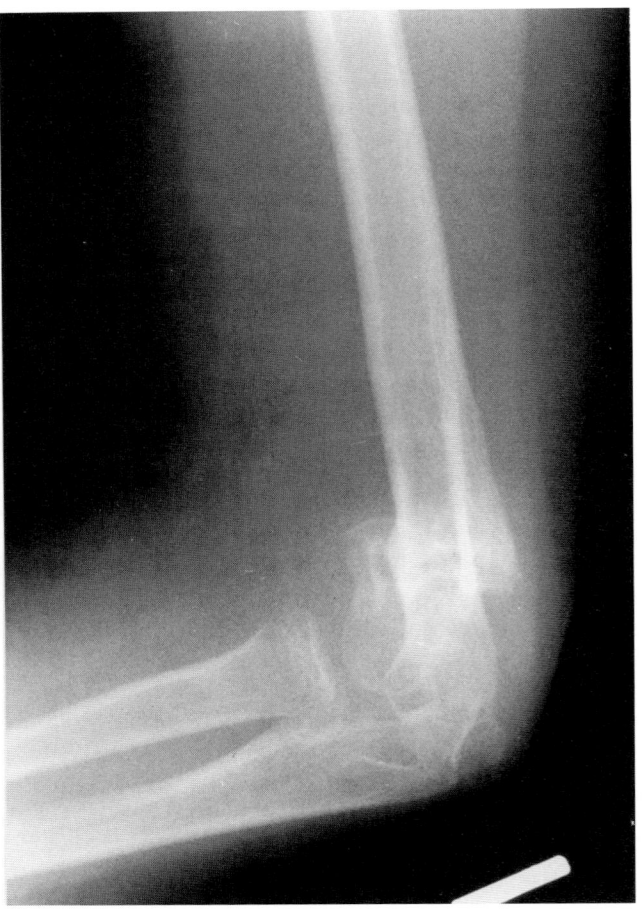

Fig. 14-17. A 7-year-old girl with a tardy ulnar nerve palsy secondary to a long-established nonunion of the lateral condyle and valgus deformity of the elbow.

Delayed Union

Delayed union (over 6 to 8 weeks) has been identified by many authors.[12,31] If the fragment is in good position and stable (i.e., not mobile at the fracture site), this may be observed with the expectation of healing in most cases.[31] If, however, there are signs of motion at the fracture site, fragment movement on serial radiographs, stress radiographs, or arthrograms, there is greater likelihood of this going on to nonunion, and surgical treatment should be undertaken.

Malunion

Following fracture of the lateral condyle,[21,23] fishtail deformity (Fig. 14-18) of the distal humerus may be encountered. It is a tenting of the central humeral epiphysis, presumably from partial growth interference at the medial end of the fracture (the lateral trochlear ridge). We would agree with Rutherford,[21] who found that 9 of 10 cases with this deformity were due to a malreduction, the fracture gap being over 2 mm. This deformity usually did not result in any clinical problem and did not appear to influence the carrying angle.

Physeal Arrest

Frank growth arrest of the lateral condyle, though reported,[15,21,25] is very rare. It results in progressive cubitus valgus, depending on how much physeal growth remained. The extensive cartilage formation of the condyles at the age that these fractures occur is presumably more forgiving in mild malunions, rarely allowing a

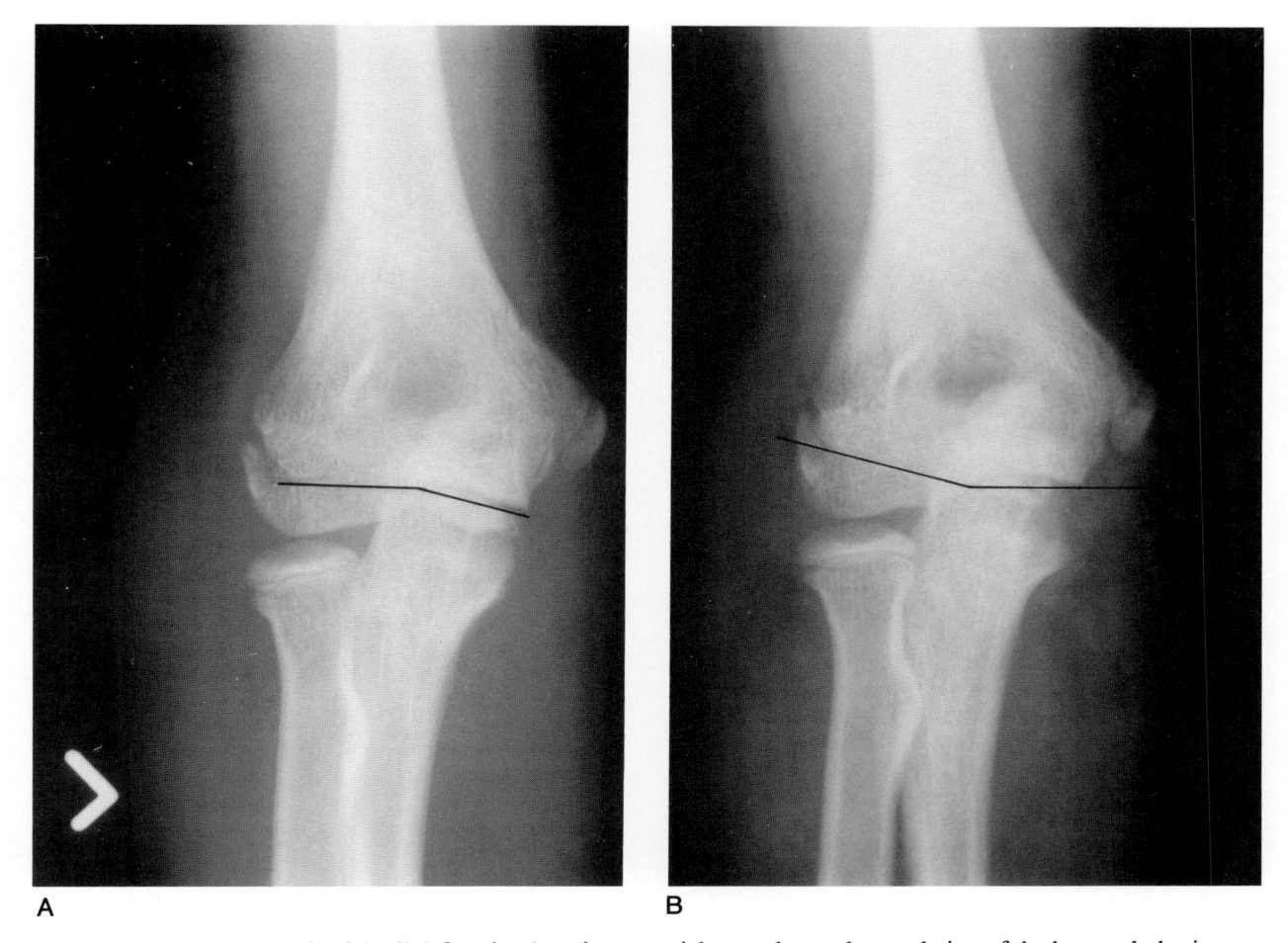

Fig. 14-18. (A) A mild fishtail deformity denoting a partial central growth retardation of the humeral physis. Note the central tenting of the metaphyseal-physeal margin compared with the normal side (B).

bony bridge to form. The more displaced fractures that might ordinarily be expected to go on to a bridge-type malunion, more often go on to a nonunion, which generally allows physeal growth to continue in both fragments.

Prominence of the Lateral Condyle

Lateral humeral condyle prominence (Fig. 14-19) is a common finding (40 to 50 percent) at follow-up after healing of displaced fractures of the lateral condyle, presumably due to lateral epicondyle overgrowth.[15,23] This prominence may be accentuated in those with some varus overgrowth. Although it is often noticed by the family as a cosmetic bump, it does not affect elbow function, and no treatment is usually necessary.

Varus Deformity

Varus deformity has been mentioned in relation to closed management, but mild varus (or simply less valgus) deformity is a common sequel to lateral condyle fractures treated operatively or non operatively.[23,25] The varus is, however, seldom more than 5 degrees, as compared to the contralateral normal carrying angle, and seldom requires treatment.

Tardy Ulnar Nerve Palsy

The undiagnosed lateral condyle fracture that is a completely separate fragment can occasionally be missed, or mistaken for a stable fracture (Fig. 14-9). These are prone to develop a nonunion[8,11,12,15,32] rather

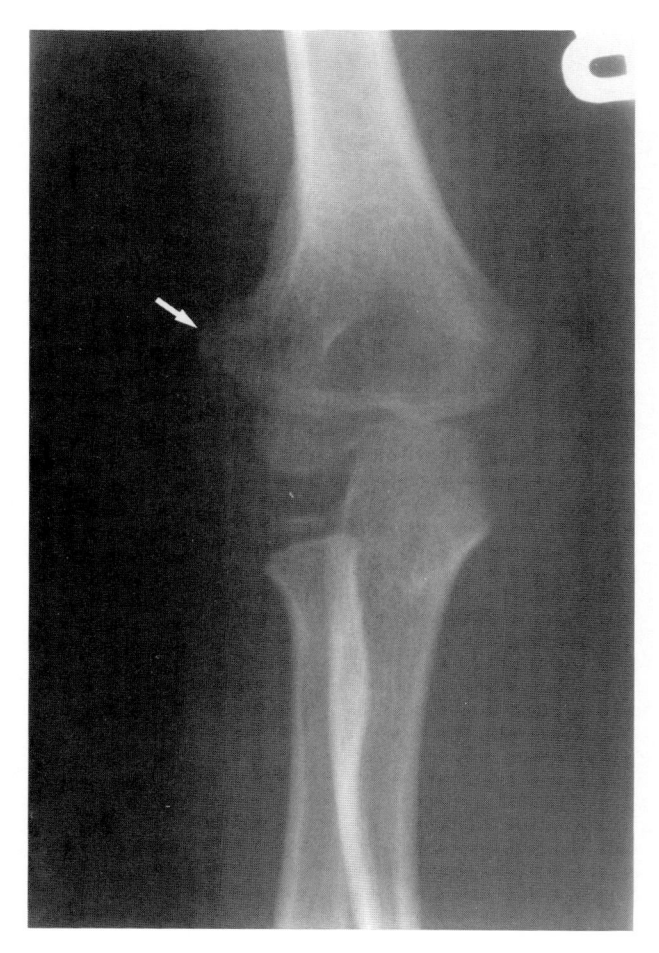

Fig. 14-19. Lateral bone overgrowth following a lateral condyle fracture commonly seen at follow-up.

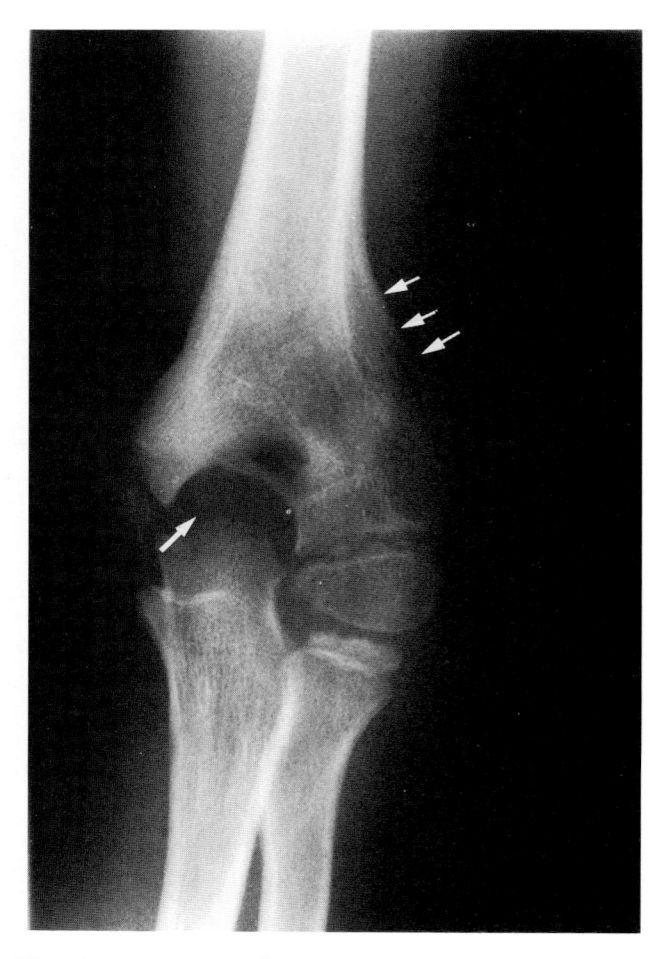

Fig. 14-20. AP view of avascular necrosis of the trochlea developed in an 8-year-old boy who sustained a lateral condylar fracture of the humerus 18 months earlier. (Note the residual periosteal ossification of the lateral humerus.)

than a malunion. Such nonunions often have a tendency to progressive valgus, with resultant tardy ulnar nerve palsy.[15,31,33-35] The literature reports an average of 22 years following injury as the time interval for development of the ulnar nerve palsy. This was reinforced by the report of Holmes and Hall[33] who found only five tardy ulnar nerve palsies at Boston Children's Hospital between 1945 and 1976, and only one of these was a lateral condyle fracture. However, this is not universal and we have seen one young child with tardy ulnar nerve palsy who developed it within 2 years of a fracture that went on to a high-riding unstable nonunion.

Part of this valgus may occur secondary to interference with physeal growth of the lateral humeral physis, but a major component is due to erosion of bone at the fracture site from continued excess motion with gradual proximal migration of the lateral condyle. The fracture surfaces and articular surfaces lose their congruity, making late nonunion repair difficult, especially in high-riding nonunions.

Avascular Necrosis of the Capitellum

In the literature, avascular necrosis of the capitellum is almost always secondary to late repair of a nonunion. The excess stripping of soft tissue attachments to the lateral condyle fragment required to achieve union results in an interference with the blood supply of the capitellum.[8,15,23,31] Rarely, trochlear avascular necrosis can complicate lateral condyle fracture,[24] but it is more commonly encountered secondary to supracondylar and medial condyle fractures (Fig. 14-20).

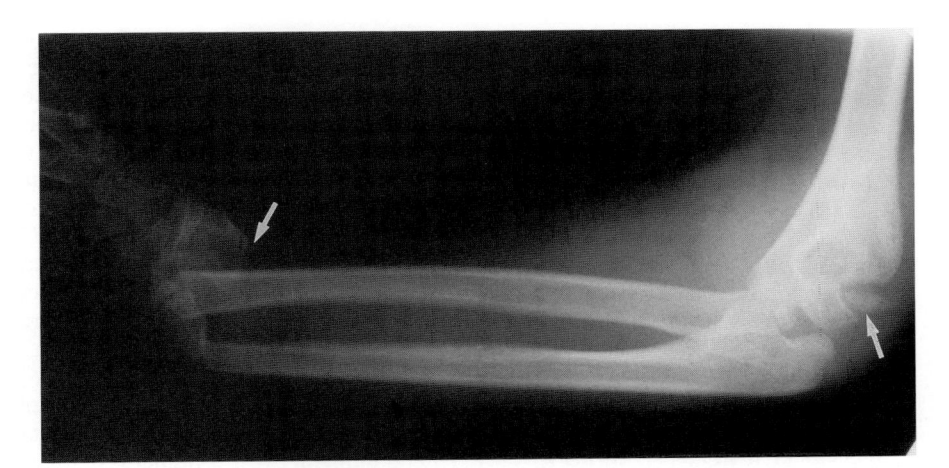

Fig. 14-21. A displaced distal radius and ulna fracture along with a displaced lateral condyle fracture. There should be greater concern for the consequences of swelling with these double level fractures.

Late Degenerative Arthritis

Degenerative changes as a sequel to lateral condyle fracture have occasionally been reported[25] and would be more likely to follow the distortion of joint associated with avascular necrosis or nonunion.

Infection

Infection has been rarely reported following open reduction of lateral condylar fractures, but when it occurs it has a greater potential to produce elbow stiffness,[23] and early elbow motion should be encouraged.

Associated Fractures

Like supracondylar fractures, lateral condyle fractures can occasionally be associated with distal radius and ulna fractures (Fig. 14-21). With two levels of injury in the same extremity the associated swelling may be more severe, and the potential for vascular compromise (compartment syndrome) or carpal tunnel syndrome is greater. Closed reduction of the distal radius and ulna may be accomplished first, especially if there is marked displacement.

SUMMARY

The lateral condyle fracture is one of the most easily misdiagnosed fractures about the elbow. Careful inspection of the radiographic vertical gap and the horizontal displacement should give more information to distinguish between stable and unstable fractures. The degree of localized soft tissue swelling laterally often reflects the severity of the initial fracture displacement. Even with these precautions, first impressions can be deceiving, and careful follow-up with radiographs *out of the plaster splint* at 1 and 2 weeks following fracture will pick up those unstable fractures that were missed initially. If the fracture is unstable enough to alter position from being radiographed out of a splint, then it should be treated operatively with pinning.

Consideration should be given to closed reduction and percutaneous pinning of those wedge-shaped "gap" fractures where the articular hinge is intact, and the gap opening is over 2 mm. Reduction and pinning should also be considered for those with less gap if the carrying angle is in less valgus than normal, especially if there is associated clinical evidence of marked lateral swelling, indicative that the fracture may have hinged open much more at the time of original injury. A stress radiograph under anesthesia and/or arthrogram might help with decision-making[14,18,34] in those cases where the diagnosis is less certain.

REFERENCES

1. Rockwood CA, Wilkins KE, King RE: Fractures in Children. 3rd Ed. JB Lippincott, Philadelphia, 1991
2. Ogden JA: Skeletal Injury in the Child. p. 399. 2nd Ed. WB Saunders, Philadelphia, 1990
3. Blount WP: Fractures of the lateral condyle of the humerus. p. 43. In Fractures in Children. Williams & Wilkins, Baltimore, 1954

4. Salter RB, Harris WR: Injuries involving the epiphyseal plate. J Bone Joint Surg [Am] 45:587, 1963
5. Salter RB, Harris WR: Classification of epiphyseal injuries. p. 97. In Uhthoff HK, Wiley JJ (eds): Behaviour of the Growth Plate. Raven Press, New York, 1988
6. Ogden JA: Skeletal growth mechanism injury patterns. p. 85. In Uhthoff HK, Wiley JJ (eds): Behaviour of the Growth Plate. Raven Press, New York, 1988
7. Dallek M, Jungbluth KH: Histomorphological studies on the development of the radial condyle fracture of the humerus in the growth years. [In German]. J Unfall Chir. 16:57, 1990
8. Jakob R, Fowles J, Rang M, Kassab M: Observations concerning fractures of the lateral humeral condyle in children. J Bone Joint Surg [Br] 57:430, 1975
9. Badelon O, Bensahel H, Mazda K, Vie P: Lateral humeral condylar fractures in children: a report of 47 cases. J Pediatr Orthop 8:31, 1988
10. McIntyre WMJ, Lawton LJ: Fractures of the lateral condyle of the humerus: Management. p. 175. In Uhthoff HK, Wiley JJ (eds): Behavior of the Growth Plate. Raven Press, New York, 1988
11. Flynn JC, Richards JF: Nonunion of minimally displaced fractures of the lateral condyle of the humerus in children. J Bone Joint Surg [Am] 53:1096, 1971
12. Flynn JC, Richards JF Jr, Saltzman RT: Prevention and treatment of non-union of slightly displaced fractures of the lateral humeral condyle in children. J Bone Joint Surg [Am] 57:1087, 1975
13. Fontanetta P, MacKenzie DA, Rossman M: Missed, maluniting and malunited fractures of the lateral humeral condyle in children. J Trauma 18:329, 1978
14. Peterson H: Triplane fracture of the distal humeral epiphysis. J Pediatr Orthop 3:81, 1983
15. Wadsworth TG: Injuries of the capitular (lateral humeral condylar) epiphysis. Clin Orthop 85:127, 1972
16. Wiley JJ, Pegginton J, Horwich JP: Traumatic dislocation of the radius at the elbow. J Bone Joint Surg [Br] 56:501, 1974
17. Milch H: Treatment of humeral cubitus valgus. Orthop Clin North Am 6:120, 1955
18. Milch H: Fractures of the external humeral condyle. JAMA 160:641, 1956
19. Agins HJ, Marcus NW: Articular cartilage sleeve fracture of the lateral humeral condyle capitellum: a previously undescribed entity. J Pediatr Orthop 4:620, 1984
20. So YC, Fang D, Leong JB, Bong SC: Varus deformity following lateral humeral condylar fx in children. J Pediatr Orthop 5:569, 1985
21. Rutherford A: Fractures of the lateral humeral condyle in children. J Bone Joint Surg [Am] 67:851, 1985
22. Wilkins KE: Residuals of elbow trauma in children. Orthop Clin North Am 21:291, 1990
23. Foster DE, Sullivan JA, Gross RH: Lateral humeral condylar fractures in children. J Pediatr Orthop 5:16, 1985
24. Herring JA: Lateral condylar fracture of the elbow. J Pediatr Orthop 6:724, 1986
25. Morin BM, Poitras BP, Labelle H, Fassier F: Fractures of the lateral humeral condyle: long term results following early open reduction. p. 183. In Uhthoff HK, Wiley JJ (eds): Behaviour of the Growth Plate. Raven Press, New York, 1988
26. Akbarnia BA, Solberstein MJ, Rende RJ et al: Arthrography in the diagnosis of fractures of the distal end of the humerus in infants. J Bone Joint Surg [Am] 68:599, 1986
27. Hansen PE, Barnes DA, Tullos HS: Case report: arthrographic diagnosis of an injury pattern in the distal humerus of an infant. J Pediatr Orthop 2:569, 1982
28. Marzo JM, D'Amato C, Strong M, Gillespie R: Usefulness and accuracy of arthrography in management of lateral humeral condyle fractures in children. J Pediatr Orthop 10:317, 1990
29. Yates C, Sullivan JA: Arthrographic diagnosis of elbow injuries in children. J Pediatr Orthop 7:54, 1987
30. Attarian DE: Lateral condyle fractures: missed diagnosis in pediatric elbow injuries. J Military Med 155:433, 1990
31. Hardacre J, Nahigian S, Froimson A, Brown J: Fractures of the lateral condyle of the humerus in children. J Bone Joint Surg [Am] 53:1083, 1971
32. Jeffrey CC: Nonunion of the epiphysis of the lateral condyle of the humerus. J Bone Joint Surg [Br] 40:396, 1958
33. Holmes JC, Hall JE: Tardy ulnar nerve palsy in children. Clin Orthop Rel Res 135:128, 1978
34. Smith FM: An eighty-four year follow-up on a patient with ununited fracture of the lateral condyle of the humerus. J Bone Joint Surg [Am] 55:378, 1973
35. Gay JR, Love JG: Diagnosis and treatment of tardy paralysis of the ulnar nerve: based on a study of 100 cases. J Bone Joint Surg 29:1087, 1947
36. Roye DP, Bini SA, Infosino A: Late surgical treatment of lateral condylar fractures in children. J Pediatr Orthop 11:195, 1991
37. Harroldsson S: On osteochondrosis deformans juvenilis capituli humeri including investigation of intra-osseous vasculature in distal humerus. Acta Orthop Scand, suppl 38:1, 1959

15

Olecranon and Coronoid Fractures

R. Dale Blasier

> As scarce as truth is, the supply has always been in excess of the demand.
> —Josh Billings

DESCRIPTION AND INCIDENCE

Fractures of the bony olecranon are not uncommon. The incidence has been estimated at between 5 and 14 percent of all children's elbow fractures seen in the emergency department.[1-5] Injuries to the olecranon physis are much more unusual[6] and are thought to represent 0.7 percent of all physeal injuries.[7] Fractures of the coronoid process in children occur primarily in association with elbow dislocation and are much more uncommon. Of fractures seen around the elbow in children presenting to the emergency department, the incidence of coronoid fractures has been estimated at between less than 1 percent to 3 percent,[2,4] which is in contradistinction to the adult coronoid, which is injured in up to 15 percent of elbow dislocations.[8]

ANATOMIC CONSIDERATIONS

Structural Characteristics

There are two functional prominences of the proximal ulna. These are the olecranon and coronoid, spanned by the glenoid notch, which provides a smooth surface for coapting with the trochlea (Fig. 15-1). The glenoid articulates with the trochlea and allows flexion and extension at the elbow. The proximal ulna also articulates with the head of the radius through an extension of the joint laterally. The radial head is tightly constrained to the capitellum and the ulnar articular surfaces. The annular ligament stabilizes the proximal radial metaphysis against the proximal shaft of the ulna and the ulnar articular extension.[9]

As in most joints, ligaments help to add stability above that provided by the bony congruency of the joint itself. Whereas there is a medial collateral ligament complex, there is no true lateral collateral ligament of the elbow.[10] The lateral ligament arises from the lateral epicondyle and inserts on the annular ligament (Fig. 15-2). The medial collateral ligament complex is formed of the anterior oblique ligament, posterior oblique ligament, and the transverse ligament, which is nonfunctional.[10] The anterior oblique ligament is band-shaped and thick and runs from the undersurface of the medial epicondyle to the medial aspect of the ulna just below the coronoid process.[10] It is taut throughout flexion and extension and is the major medial joint stabilizer to valgus stress when the elbow is flexed (Fig. 15-3). The posterior oblique ligament is taut in flexion, lax in extension, and is not a major elbow stabilizer.[10] There is inherent bony stability of the elbow in extension. With the elbow extended, even without the anterior oblique ligament, the olecranon

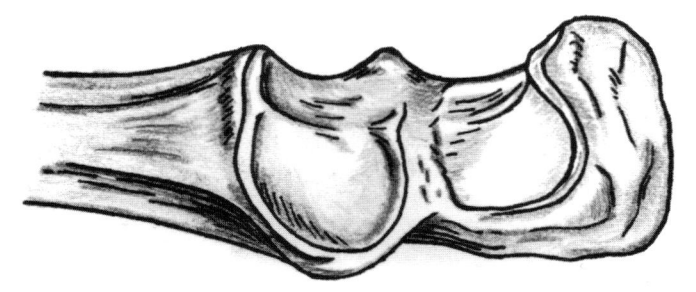

Fig. 15-1. Anterior view of the glenoid fossa of proximal ulna. The olecranon is most prominent anteriorly and proximally. The glenoid fossa itself is ridged in the middle for articulation with the trochlea. Distally and anteriorly, the fossa ends at the peak of the coronoid. There is an articulation laterally at the left for the radial head. (Drawing by S. D. Temple, M.D.)

process locks into the olecranon fossa, thus resisting valgus stress. In flexion, the process disengages from the fossa and valgus instability is possible.[10] Varus stress is resisted by the lateral ligament complex, which runs from the lateral epicondyle to the annular ligament, by the linear crest of the glenoid gliding in the grooved trochlea, and by the natural cubitus valgus about the elbow.

Anteroposterior elbow stability depends on an intact coronoid process and anterior oblique ligament. The olecranon provides very little resistance to anterior in-

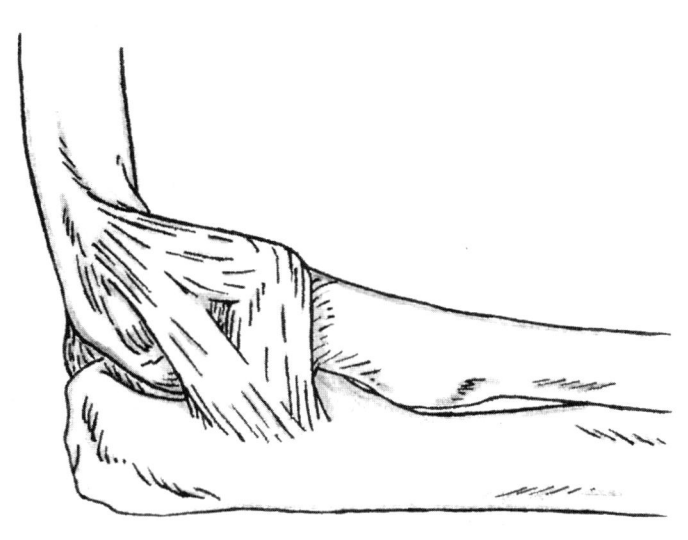

Fig. 15-2. The lateral ligament complex. The lateral ligament is not a true collateral ligament. It arises from the lateral epicondyle and inserts on the annular ligament, which restricts the proximal radius. (Drawing by S. D. Temple, M.D.)

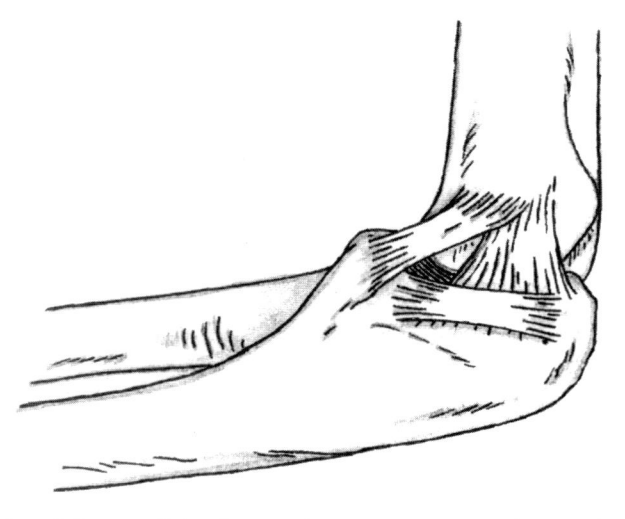

Fig. 15-3. Medial collateral ligament complex. The anterior oblique ligament runs from the undersurface of the medial epicondyle to the medial aspect of the ulna just below the coronoid process. The posterior oblique ligament runs from the undersurface of the medial epicondyle to the proximal medial ulna. The transverse ligament spans the medial aspect of the glenoid fossa of the olecranon and is nonfunctional. (Drawing by S. D. Temple, M.D.)

stability at the elbow. If the anterior oblique ligament is absent, the elbow is unstable to valgus stress even if the olecranon process is retained.[10]

The elbow joint provides a range of motion from full extension (0 degrees) to flexion of 150 degrees. Due to the lateral tilt of the joint surfaces, in full flexion the elbow is in varus and gradually angulates into valgus in full extension.[10] Pronation and supination are enabled by allowing the radial head to rotate as it is constrained to the capitellar and ulnar articular surfaces by the annular ligament.

Developmental Characteristics

Embryologically at 5 weeks, there appears a mesenchymal condensation that includes the radius and ulna, which are indistinguishable from each other. At 6 weeks, the radius and ulna form an anlage of cartilage surrounded by perichondrium, which is continuous with the humerus above and the wrist below. At 8 weeks, the cartilaginous anlage is well-defined. The olecranon and coronoid processes are formed. The capsular ligaments

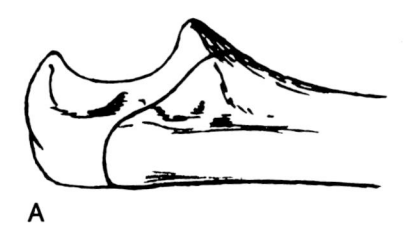

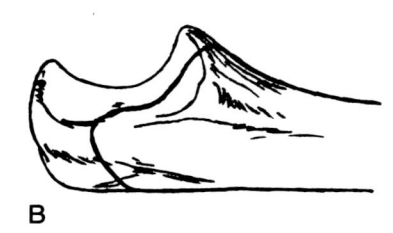

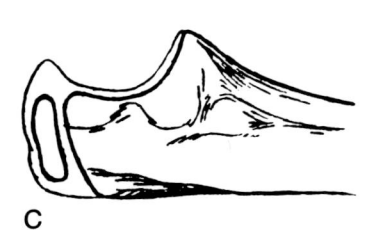

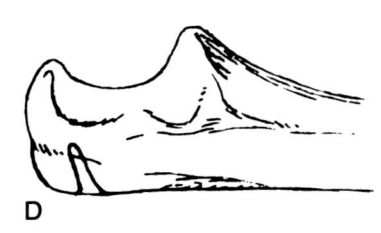

Fig. 15-4. Radiographic features of the olecranon apophysis. **(A)** In the immature elbow, the olecranon appears stubby and round in lateral view. **(B)** Just prior to appearance of the olecranon ossification center, the ossified olecranon develops a straight distinct sclerotic border. **(C)** With further maturity, the epiphyseal center appears and enlarges. Less of the cartilaginous epiphysis is lucent on radiograph. **(D)** The olecranon physis closes from anterior to posterior just prior to maturity and the remaining physis may be mistaken for a fracture line. (Drawing by S. D. Temple, M.D.)

are formed, but there is no true joint cavity. Ossification of the body of the ulna begins, but the proximal and distal epiphyses are not yet seen. The elbow joint cavity forms next and is well developed by birth.[11]

In the immature elbow,[12] the olecranon is stubby and well founded as visualized on radiographs (Fig. 15-4). The major olecranon ossification center lies within the tip of the olecranon and is enveloped by the triceps insertion.[6,43] The epiphysis of the proximal ulna is the only traction epiphysis that contributes to the length of the long bone as well as representing a major portion of its articular surface.[7,13] The proximal ulnar physis contributes 20 percent of the longitudinal growth of the forearm.[7] Shortly before the epiphysis ossifies in the olecranon, a sclerotic metaphyseal line occurs.[6,7] The secondary ossification center of the olecranon does not appear until the ninth or tenth year.[12] Its age of appearance has been described as from age 8 to age 11 or 12.[4,6,7,11,12,14] It fuses at around age 14,[6,7,12,14] although it has been reported to close as late as age 16 to 20.[11] The secondary ossification center, which appears in the olecranon at about age 8 or 9, may be single or multipartite.[12] When bipartite, the accessory center, is located near the tip of the olecranon.[6,9,11,12,15] No secondary ossification center appears in the coronoid.[6] Rarely, a patella cubiti may occur, which is a sesamoid bone located in the triceps tendon.[9,16,17] It may represent an unfused ossification center or may be of traumatic origin.[18]

Prior to fusion of the physis, there may be a surprisingly large space between the ossifying epiphysis and the metaphysis,[7,12] which can be mistaken for an epiphyseal separation on radiographs. As the epiphyseal center matures, sclerosis of the subchondral bone occurs both in the metaphysis and the bony epiphysis.[12] With advancing age, the physis, which originates proximally, may migrate to the center of the joint space beneath the trochlea.[12] This is the so-called "wandering physeal line of the olecranon." The epiphysis may contribute significantly to the articular surface of the glenoid notch.[12]

With further maturity, the physis comes to run from anterior to posterior and can be mistaken for fracture line entering the joint.[12] Closure of the olecranon physis occurs from the joint side posteriorly,[11] so that at about age 13, the anterior portion of the physis is closed and the posterior portion is open and represented by a thin radiolucent line on radiographs[11] (Fig. 15-4). It has a well-defined sclerotic margin not like that of an acute fracture.[9,12] The olecranon physis fuses between 14 and 20,[6,7,11,12,14] although it may occasionally persist into adulthood.[12] In the immature elbow, the physis extends up to the area of the coronoid process. With maturity, the growth plate becomes more horizontal. The cartilage extending up to the coronoid becomes articular only and does not contribute to physeal bone growth.[6]

MECHANISM OF INJURY

Fractures of the olecranon may occur as a result of several different mechanisms: in extension, as in a fall on an outstretched hand, in flexion, as in a fall on the flexed elbow, or as a result of a direct blow or penetrating wound to the elbow. They can also occur by means of triceps avulsion, or in association with elbow dislocation.

Coronoid fractures have been reported to occur by avulsion of the brachialis muscle; however, the more likely mechanism is that it is sheared off by the trochlea in association with posterior dislocation of the elbow.

Unique Features of the Child's Elbow

The child's olecranon is unique in that the bone is much more trabecular in the metaphyseal area[9] than the adult olecranon which tends to be more cortical. In the child, the articular and epiphyseal cartilage are much thicker than in the adult predisposing to osteochondral fractures.[9] The transversely oriented subchondral bone of the metaphysis tends to fracture into the metaphysis rather than into the physis, thus accounting for the rarity of physeal injuries of the olecranon in children.[9] Due to the mechanics of the elbow, when fractures occur distal to the insertion of the triceps mechanism, additional displacement of the fracture fragments may occur as a result of triceps pull.[9]

The relative ligamentous laxity of the child's elbow frequently allows hyperextension producing fracture patterns that are rarely seen in less flexible adult elbows.[19] Stress fracture has been observed through the olecranon growth plate in the adolescent baseball pitcher.[14]

Fractures of the Olecranon

Extension Injuries

The majority of fractures about the olecranon in children occur with the elbow in extension. With the elbow extended, the olecranon is locked in the olecranon fossa of the distal humerus. When varus or valgus stress is applied to the forearm, the deforming force is concentrated in the proximal ulnar metaphysis.[6,9,20-26] This usually results in a greenstick fracture of the olecranon, often with longitudinal multiple fracture lines extending distal to the coronoid.[6] The valgus injury pattern typically causes an apex medial fracture of the proximal ulna

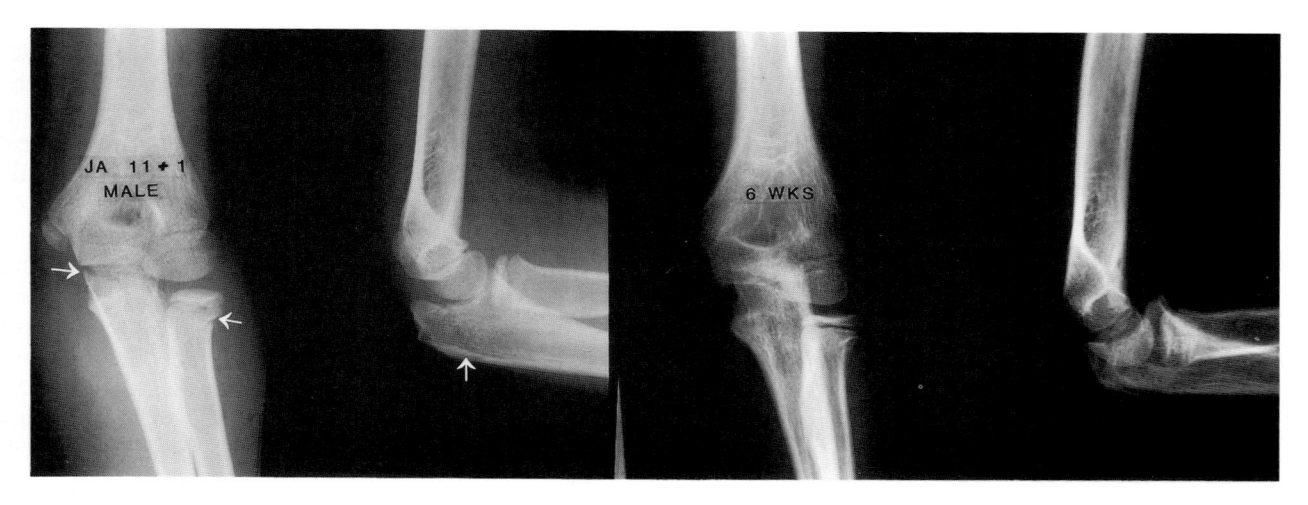

Fig. 15-5. An 11-year, 1-month-old boy sustained a valgus metaphyseal fracture of the proximal ulna with a radial neck fracture. Closed reduction was obtained. The elbow was immobilized for 3 weeks. At 2 months follow-up, elbow function was excellent.

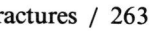

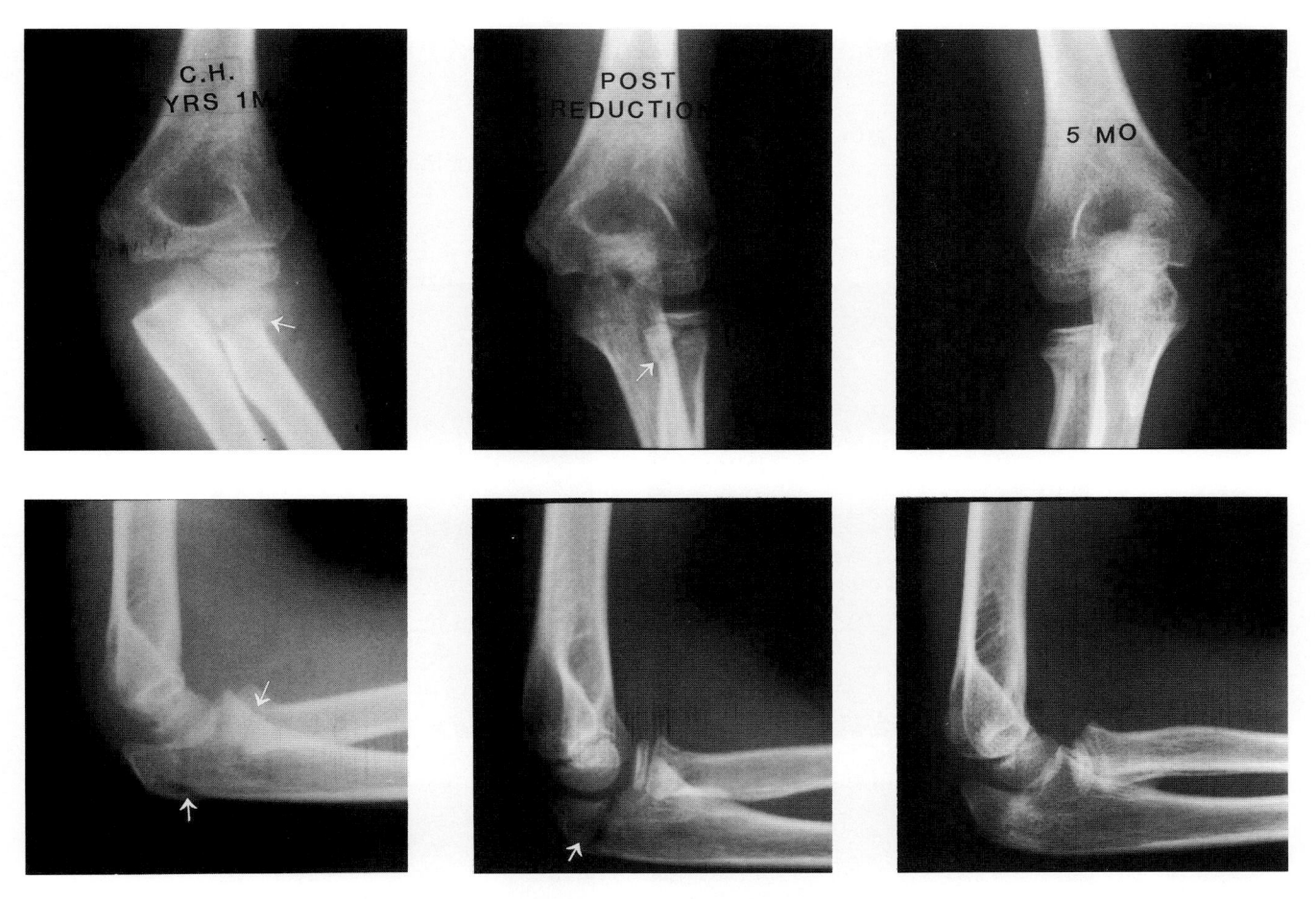

Fig. 15-6. A 10-year, 1-month-old girl sustained a valgus greenstick fracture of the proximal ulna with radial neck fracture. Closed reduction was performed, followed by 3 weeks of immobilization. There was full range of motion at 5 months follow-up.

with associated lateral compressive fracture of the radial head or neck and sometimes an epicondyle avulsion medially[6] (Figs. 15-5 to 15-8). A varus stress may produce an apex lateral proximal ulnar fracture with partial or total lateral dislocation of the radial head (type III Monteggia injury)[22] (Figs. 15-9 and 15-10). This injury can be associated with posterior interosseus nerve palsy.[6] The ulnar fracture occurs at the level of the superior radioulnar joint.[22]

Whenever the radial head dislocates in association with a proximal ulnar injury, the direction of angulation of the ulna is the *same* as the direction of the dislocation of the radial head.[24] The most common proposed cause for the extension injury is a fall on the outstretched hand, with the forearm supinated as if the child were falling backward.[24,25] Hume[23] felt that when the olecranon is fractured in extension, the radial head is dislocated forward by concomitant pronation of the forearm. It is impossible to fracture and angulate the proximal ulna without a concomitant fracture or dislocation of the proximal radius.[26]

Flexion Injuries

Fractures of the olecranon may occur as a flexion injury. This injury is usually the result of resisting a fall on the outstretched hand with the elbow flexed. The strong pull of the triceps resists the fall and fractures the olecranon across the fulcrum provided by the humeral troch-

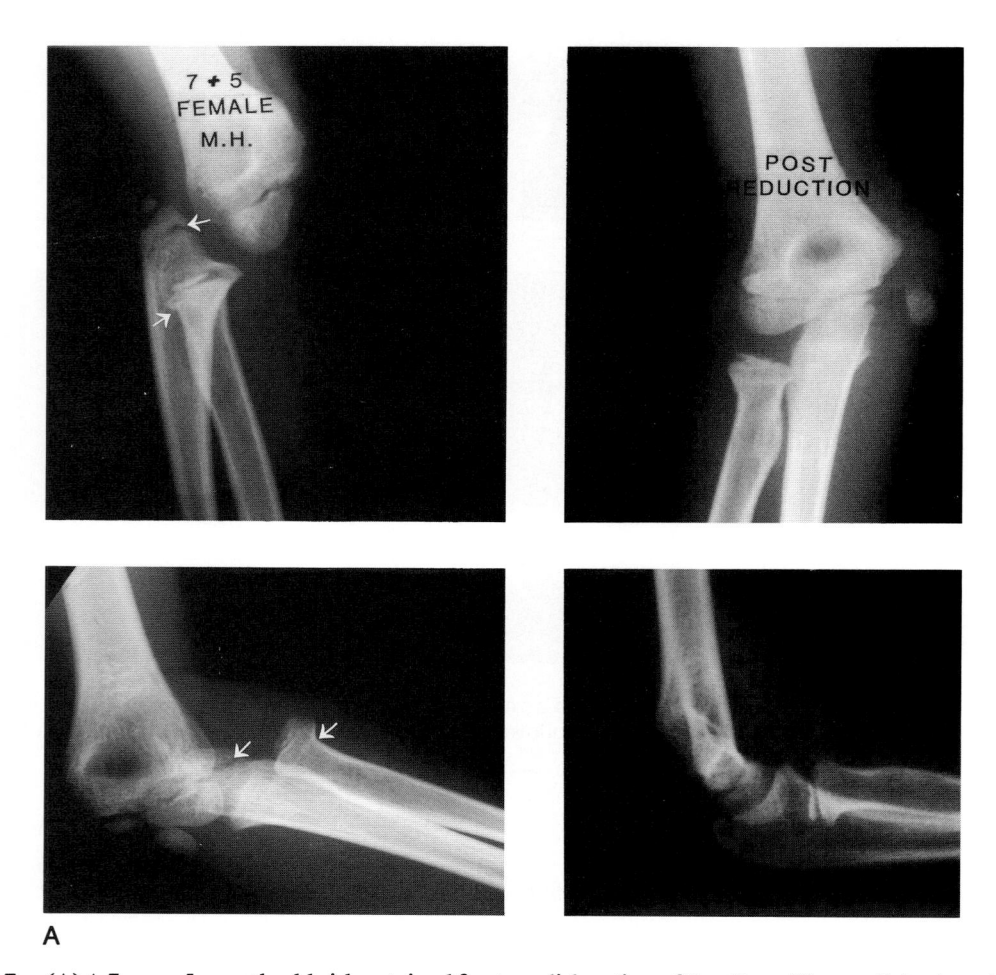

Fig. 15-7. (A) A 7-year, 5-month-old girl sustained fracture dislocation of the elbow. The medial epicondyle was avulsed. There was an undisplaced fracture of the radial neck as well as the olecranon metaphysis. Closed reduction was obtained, but the joint was unstable medially and there was wide displacement of the medial epicondyle. *(Figure continues.)*

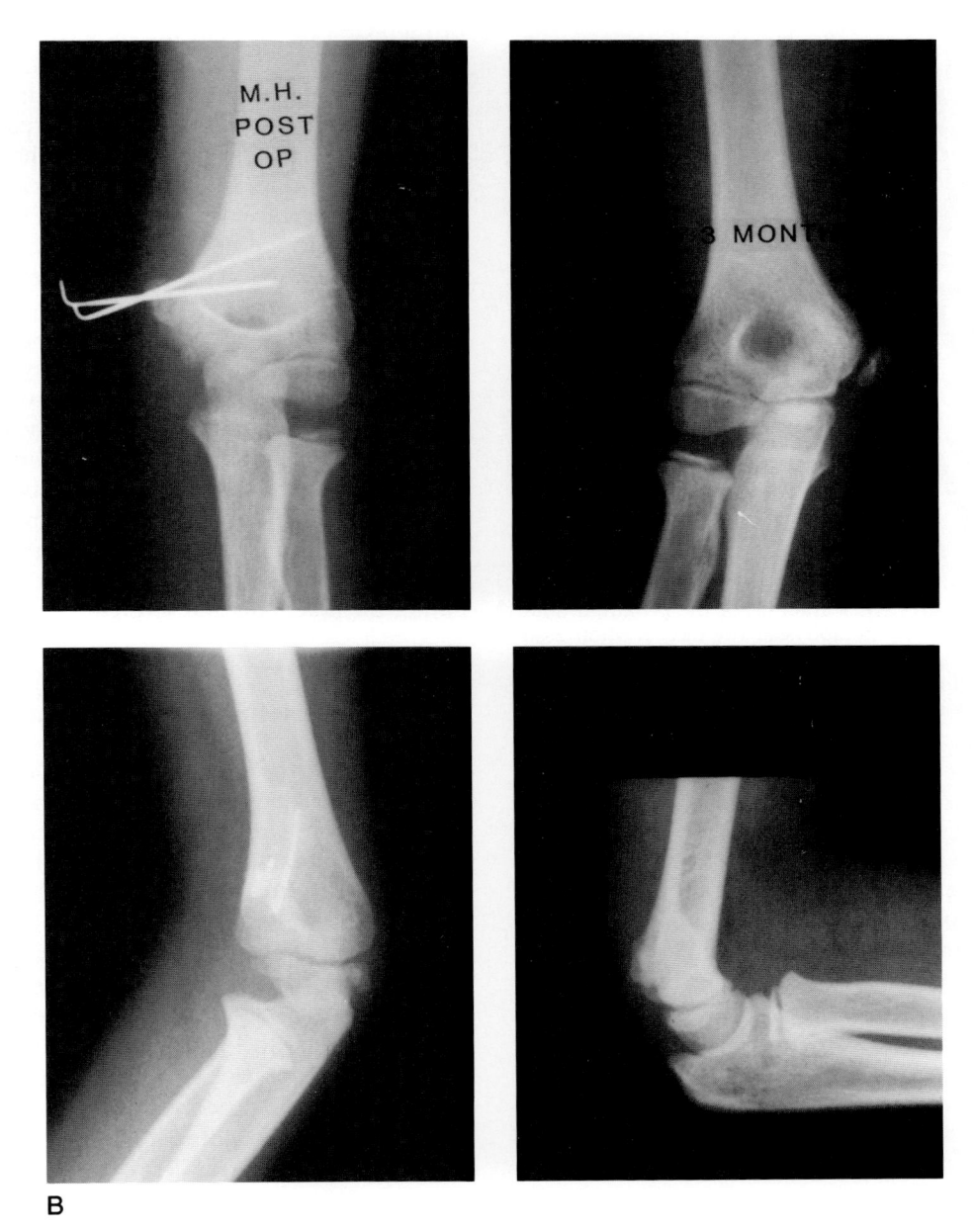

Fig. 15-7 *(Continued).* **(B)** The medial epicondyle was openly reduced and fixed with pins. The elbow was immobilized for 3 weeks, followed by active range of motion of the extremity. At 3 months, healing was complete with minimal loss of motion.

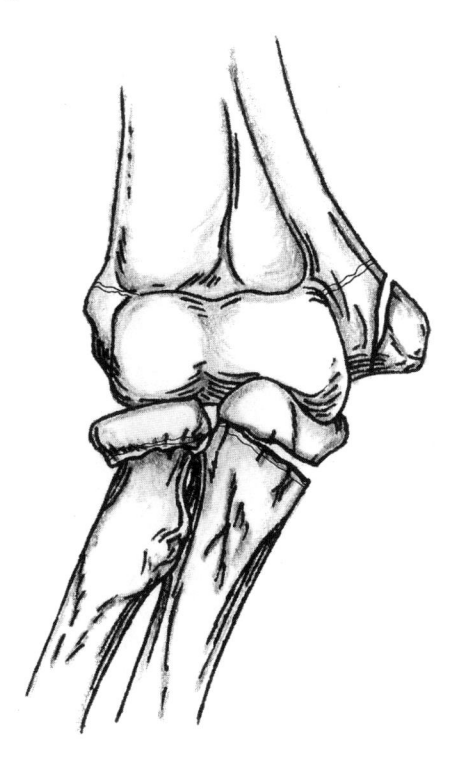

Fig. 15-8. Valgus greenstick fracture of the proximal ulnar metaphysis. The valgus metaphyseal fracture is often associated with an impacted fracture of the radial head or neck. It may or may not involve an avulsion fracture of the medial epicondyle. (Drawing by S. D. Temple, M.D.)

lea. Flexion-type injuries can also occur as a result of a direct blow to the tip of the bony olecranon posterior to the distal humerus.[2,4,6,9,27] In Newell's series,[44] 20 of 33 olecranon fractures resulted from a direct blow to the elbow with the fall.[44] Avulsion fractures may occur through epiphysis or metaphysis. A fracture analogous to the patellar sleeve fracture has been described about the elbow involving the proximal cartilaginous olecranon in association with a small metaphyseal fragment.[9] In flexion injuries, tension in the olecranon causes the fracture of the posterior cortex of the olecranon (Fig. 15-11). The fracture tends to occur perpendicular to the long axis of the ulna[2,6] and usually extends to the articular surface of the semilunar notch.[6] Flexion injuries may disrupt the extensor mechanism as traction applied by the triceps tends to separate the fragments.[3,21] For this reason, flexion injuries can require open reduction and internal fixation to restore extensor continuity. On the other hand, separation may be resisted in some cases by the intact triceps expansion.[2,6]

Direct Trauma

Fractures that occur as a result of a direct blow or hockey stick injury distal to the olecranon tip, often result in comminution but are less likely to result in disruption of the extensor mechanism, as soft tissues and periosteum tend to remain intact (Figs. 15-12 to 15-14).

Fractures of the olecranon may occur in shear.[28,41] By this mechanism, the distal ulna is sheared from the proximal ulna along a line just anterior to the distal humerus (Figs. 15-15 and 15-16). This usually occurs as a result of a direct blow to the posterior surface of the ulna at a level just anterior to the humeral condyles. This produces a bending or shear force across the olecranon. Tension forces occur anteriorly.[6] The integrity of the proximal radioulnar joint is maintained, but the distal fragment is displaced anteriorly.[6] This injury may occur with the elbow flexed or extended. The fracture line may be transverse or oblique. This is clearly distinguishable from the more common flexion injury in which the proximal olecranon is displaced proximally. The proximal olecranon is not displaced proximally in the shear injury as the thick posterior periosteum is intact.[6] The distal fragment is probably displaced anteriorly by the pull of the brachialis and biceps.

Fractures of the Coronoid

Fractures of the coronoid occur in older children[8,14] (Fig. 15-17). Commonly, the coronoid is fractured in association with posterior dislocation of the elbow.[6,8,15,26,29] Fractures of the coronoid can be caused by abutment of the trochlea during forcible displacement of the proximal end of the ulna during dislocation.[8] Osteochondral fractures of the glenoid fossa of the ulna can occur as a result of a posterior dislocation of the ulna.[29,30] In posterior dislocation, the trochlea of the humerus is dislocated distal to the coronoid. During spontaneous reduction, it snaps back down and the trochlea meets the tip of the coronoid process and may peel the cartilage off its articular slope bending it back proximally as an osteochondral flap[29,30] (Fig. 15-18).

CLASSIFICATION

There are numerous factors that need to be taken into account when classifying fractures of the olecranon. Fractures can be physeal or extraphyseal. They can be articular or nonarticular. Fractures can occur as avul-

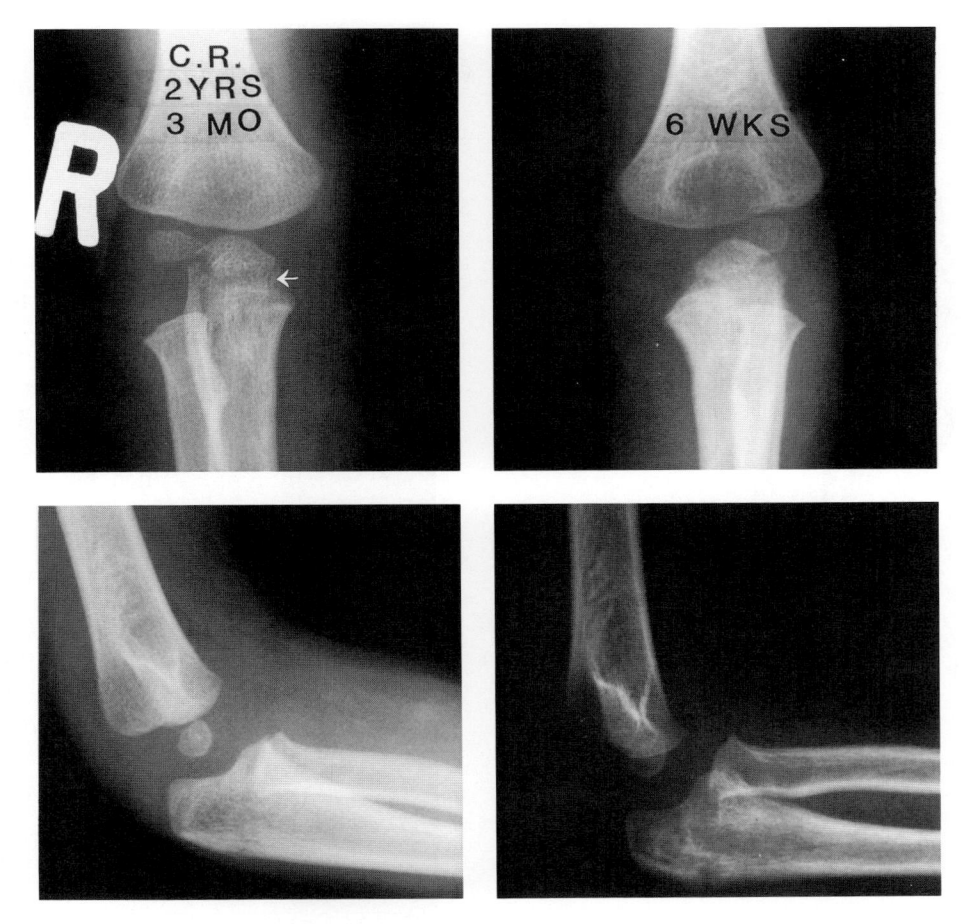

Fig. 15-9. A 27-month-old boy fell on outstretched arm and sustained varus metaphyseal fracture of the proximal ulnar metaphysis. The radial head was not displaced. After 3 weeks of immobilization, full motion was allowed. Functional results at 6 weeks were normal.

sion or direct blow injuries. They can be complete or incomplete, displaced or undisplaced, comminuted or simple. Olecranon fractures can also be classified as penetrating, hockey stick, or stress injuries.

Physeal injuries have been classified by Graham and Kiernan.[20] There are two types: Type I is a purely epiphyseal fracture that is transverse and occurs primarily in young patients. Type II is an epiphyseal fracture with a metaphyseal fragment that occurs in older children.[20] Poland found that the proximal epiphyseal fragment tends to include the coronoid process in the type II fracture.[47]

Papavasiliou and colleagues[31] have separated olecranon fractures into two groups. Group A is intra-articular and may be displaced or undisplaced. Group B fractures are greenstick fractures which involve the metaphyseal olecranon in older children. Papavasiliou and colleagues[31] believe that the thicker cartilage in the younger children protects these fractures from displacement. Canale[20] and Graves at the Campbell Clinic classified olecranon fractures into three types: type I fractures are displaced less than 5 mm, type II displaced greater than 5 mm, and type III are open fractures.

Wilkins[6] has developed a thoughtful classification of olecranon fractures. He separates them into epiphyseal types, including the purely epiphyseal type and the epiphyseal with metaphyseal fragment that occurs in the older child. The second major category is that of metaphyseal fractures, which he divides into Group A flexion injuries, Group B extension injuries—subtype I valgus and subtype II varus—and Group C injuries, which occur in shear.

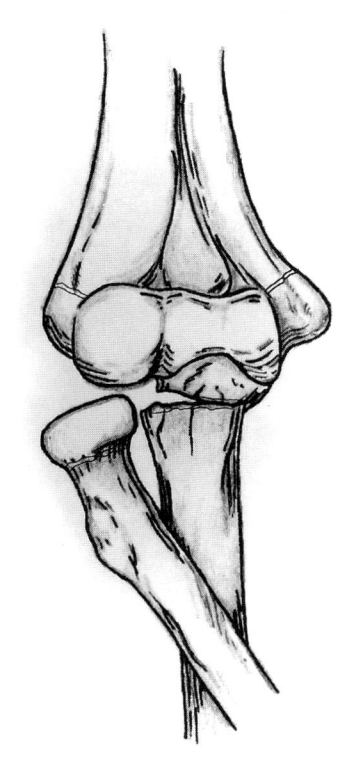

Fig. 15-10. Varus greenstick fracture of the proximal ulna. With the varus greenstick fracture there is often a lateral radial head dislocation in association. This injury may place the radial nerve at risk. (Drawing by S. D. Temple, M.D.)

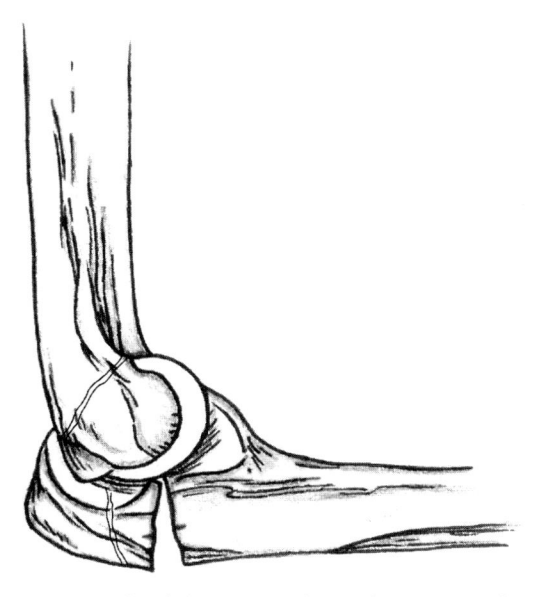

Fig. 15-11. Flexion injury occurs in tension over the fulcrum provided by the humeral condyles. (Drawing by S. D. Temple, M.D.)

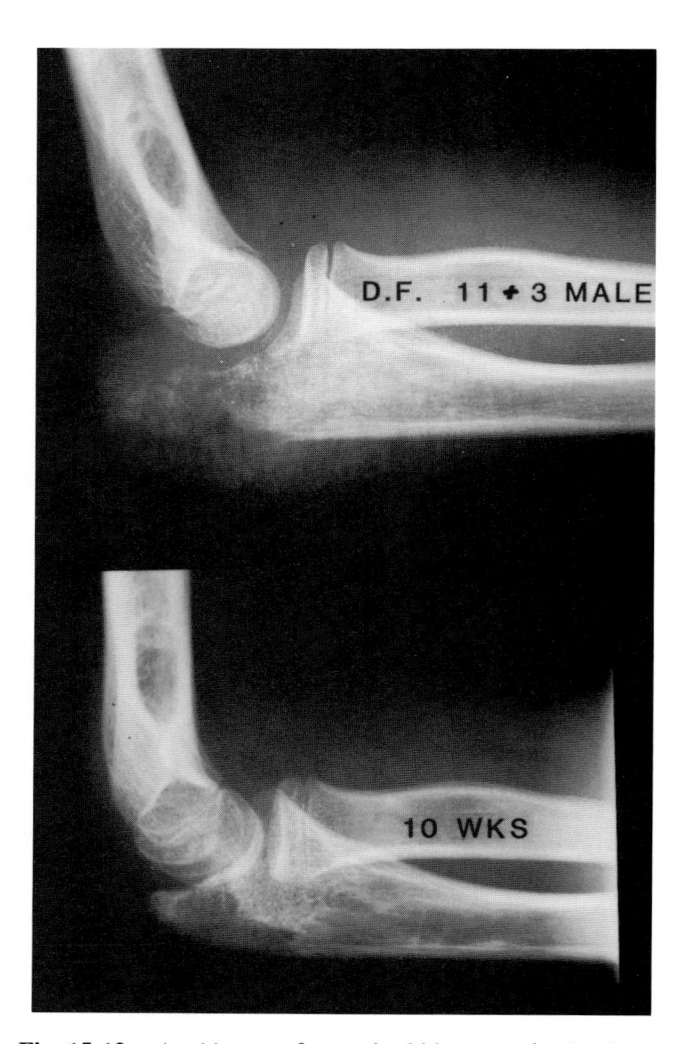

Fig. 15-12. An 11-year-, 3-month-old boy sustained a shotgun blast that grazed the left elbow. The proximal olecranon metaphysis was shattered, but extensor continuity was maintained by the intact medial and lateral periosteum. The wound was irrigated and debrided in the operating room and underwent delayed primary closure using the redundant skin about the elbow. Fracture consolidation was achieved after 3 weeks of immobilization. At 2 months follow-up, elbow function was essentially normal. No evidence of growth derangement was noted by that time.

Other types of fractures that have been described include the greenstick fracture of proximal ulna fracture with radial head dislocation[22,25] and osteochondral fracture of the olecranon.[29]

We have found the most useful classification of olecranon fractures to include six categories expanding upon those developed by Wilkins; these are shown in Table 15-1.

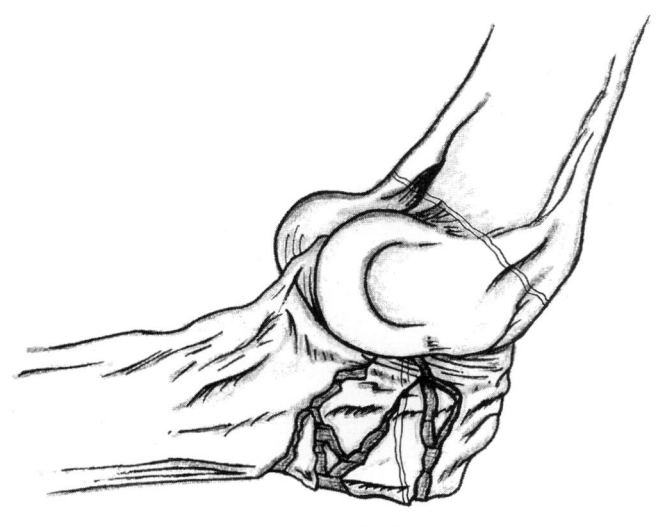

Fig. 15-13. Fracture as a result of a direct blow may be comminuted, but the intact periosteal sleeve prevents gross displacement. (Drawing by S. D. Temple, M.D.)

TABLE 15-1. Classification of Pediatric Olecranon Fractures

1. Physeal fractures
2. Metaphyseal fractures
   A. Flexion
   B. Extension
   C. Shear
3. Intra-articular fractures associated with dislocations of the elbow
4. Extensor avulsion fractures
5. Direct blow fractures
6. Stress fractures

Physeal Fractures

The physeal fractures can be divided into two types: purely epiphyseal or Salter-Harris type I fracture and the epiphyseal with metaphyseal fragment with the so-called Salter-Harris type II type fracture[6,7,20] (Fig. 15-19). Like most epiphyseal fractures these tend to have a good prognosis for healing. However, physeal

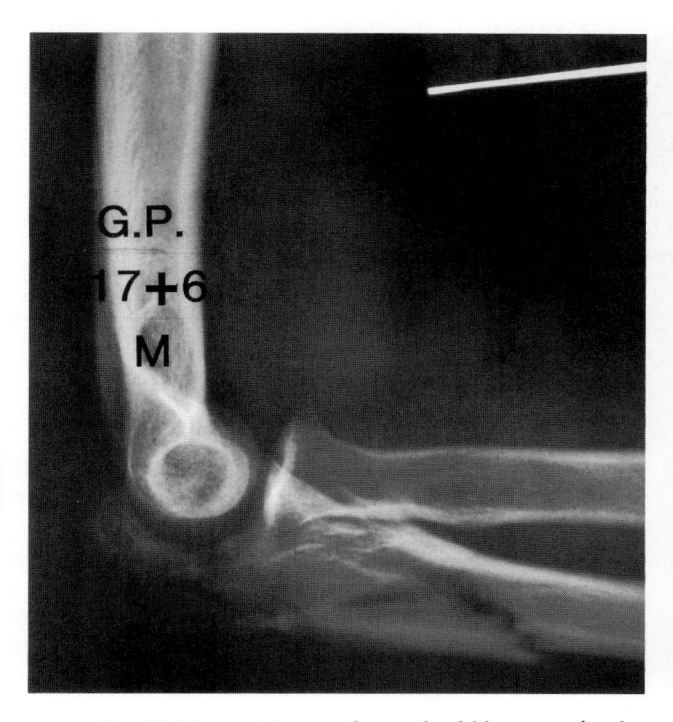

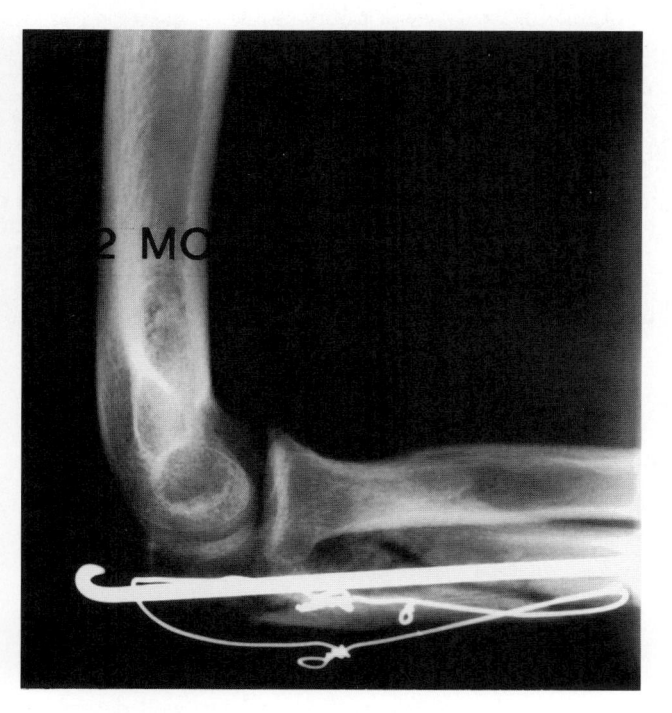

Fig. 15-14. A 17-year, 6-month-old boy sustained a comminuted fracture of the proximal ulna in association with multiple other injuries. Rigid internal fixation was attempted at open reduction but was not possible due to severe comminution. An intramedullary Rush rod was placed with tension band wiring to restore extensor continuity. At 2 months follow-up, the fracture was solidly healed. There was mild loss of elbow flexion and extension.

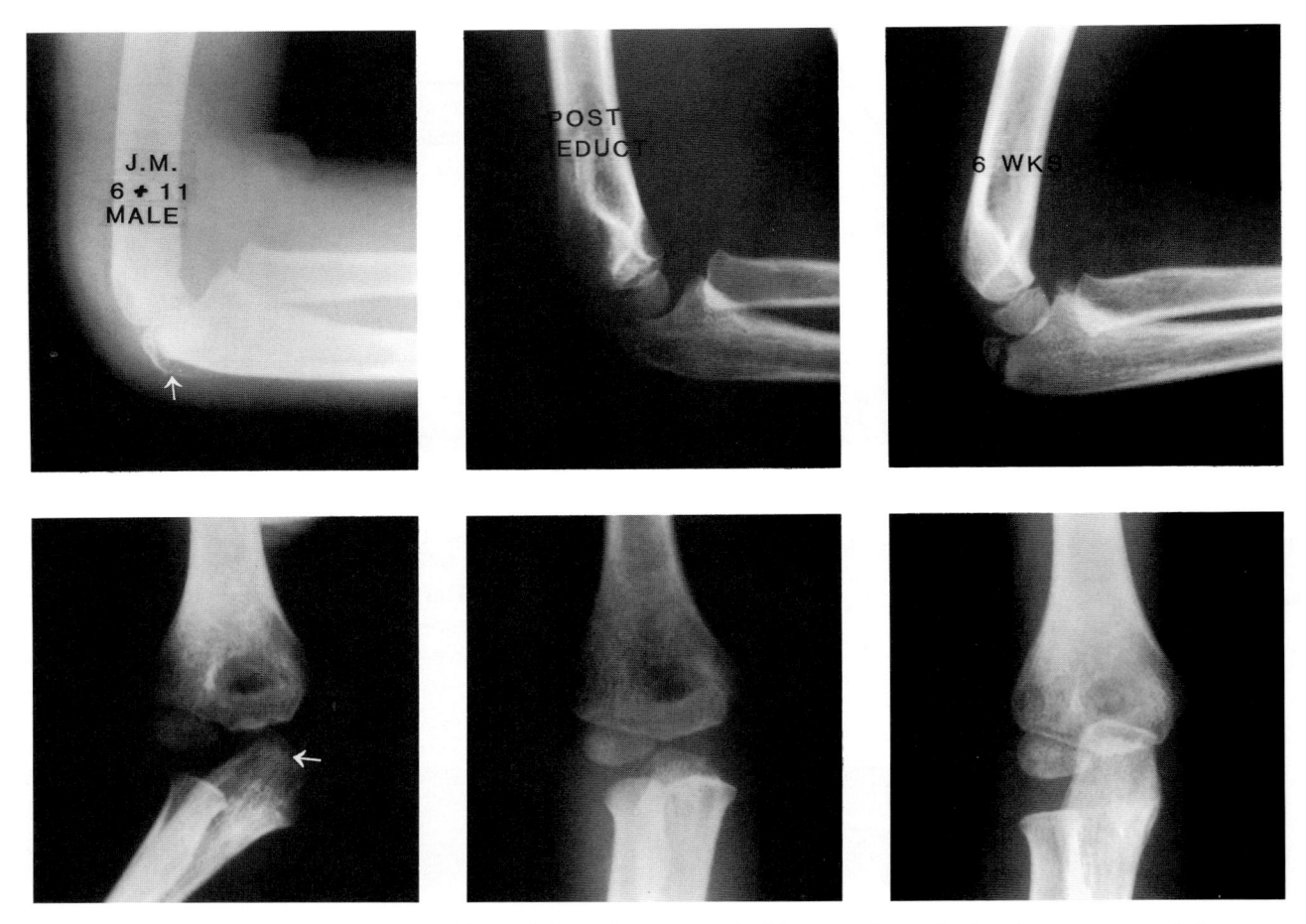

Fig. 15-15. A 6-year, 11-month-old boy fell on the outstretched hand and sustained a shear fracture of the proximal ulna with anterior dislocation of the ulna and proximal radius. Closed reduction was obtained in the emergency room. The elbow was immobilized for 3 weeks, followed by active use. The functional results at 6 weeks were excellent.

fractures can be displaced, separating into the joint, and care must be taken to make sure that the joint surface is congruous.

Metaphyseal Fractures

The metaphyseal fractures have been well described by Wilkins.[6] His Group A fractures occur as a result of a flexion force (Fig. 15-11). The flexion fracture occurs posteriorly in tension as a result of bending across the intact humeral condyles. Fracture results in the midportion of the olecranon. This can occur as a result of a direct blow to the posterior olecranon or in resisting a fall on the outstretched hand with the elbow in flexion. This fracture tends to be intraarticular.[6]

Wilkins' Group B metaphyseal extension injuries occur with the elbow in full extension. The olecranon process is locked in the olecranon fossa of the distal humerus. With the elbow locked, the forearm is subjected to further varus or valgus stress. This stress is concentrated in the metaphysis of the proximal ulna where fracture occurs, often in association with injury of the radial head or neck. In the more common valgus pattern (Fig. 15-8), the child may fall with the forearm in supination, resulting in a valgus greenstick fracture of the proximal ulna with associated compression injury of

Intra-articular Fractures

The third type of olecranon fracture is the intra-articular free fragment which may occur in conjunction with elbow dislocation. The source may be an osteoarticular fragment of the olecranon glenoid fossa[29,30] (Fig. 15-18A) an avulsion fragment of the olecranon apophysis[32] (Fig. 15-18B), or a fracture of the coronoid tip.[29] These tend to have a poorer prognosis than fractures not associated with dislocation as there is greater capsule tearing, bleeding, and a propensity toward stiffness due to the more extensive injury. Neurovascular injuries are more likely to occur in association with dislocation.

Extensor Avulsion Fracture

Unlike the purely flexion injury that causes fracturing across the fulcrum provided by the humeral condyles, the extensor avulsion injury can occur at any level in the olecranon (Fig. 15-20). This is the result of the strong pull of the triceps against the fixed distal forearm usually resisting a fall toward the ground with the elbow in flexion. These fractures are usually displaced and tend to require open reduction and internal fixation to restore elbow extensor continuity.

Direct Blow Fracture

Fractures occurring as a result of direct trauma or penetrating injury often are comminuted but not displaced due to the intact periosteal sleeve. These have a good prognosis for healing with simple immobilization and are not well amenable to internal fixation due to comminution (Fig. 15-13).

Stress Fractures

Stress fracture can occur as a result of repetitive forced extension of elbow as in throwing activity. Stress fractures do not displace and respond rapidly to removal of the inciting stress. These are less common in children under 12 years, since the Little League regulations have limited the innings a pitcher is allowed to play.

Open Fractures

Open fractures of the olecranon in children are rare and are not usually widely displaced. They tend to be metaphyseal and result from direct blow to the olecranon.

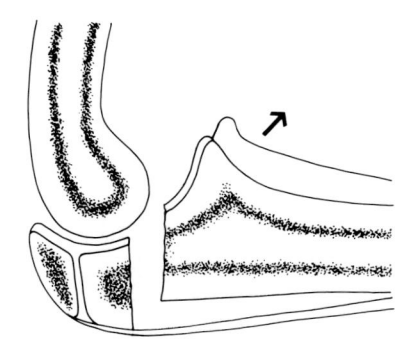

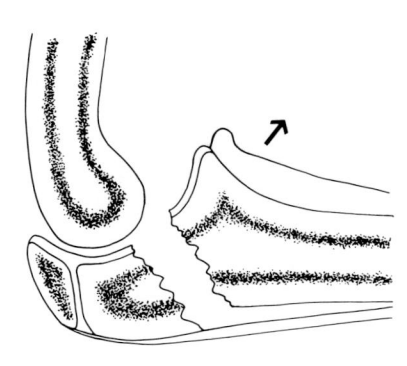

Fig. 15-16. Shear injury occurs as the ulna distal to humeral condyles is displaced anteriorly. Intact posterior periosteal hinge prevents proximal migration of proximal fragment. (Drawing by Tish O'Neil, M.D.)

the radial neck, or there may be avulsion of the medial epicondylar apophysis.[6]

If the elbow fails in varus (Fig. 15-10), there will be a varus greenstick fracture of the proximal ulna in association with lateral dislocation of the radial head (type III Monteggia lesion).

Wilkins' Group C fracture of the metaphysis involves a shearing injury (Figs. 15-15 and 15-16). This occurs as a result of a blow to the proximal ulna just in front of the humeral condyles resulting in shearing of the proximal ulna through metaphyseal bone.[6] Generally, the proximal radioulnar joint is intact and the radial head will displace in the same direction as the distal ulnar fragment. Displacement is usually anteriorly, however, Newman has described a case in which the shear force was directed medially with associated radial neck fracture.[48]

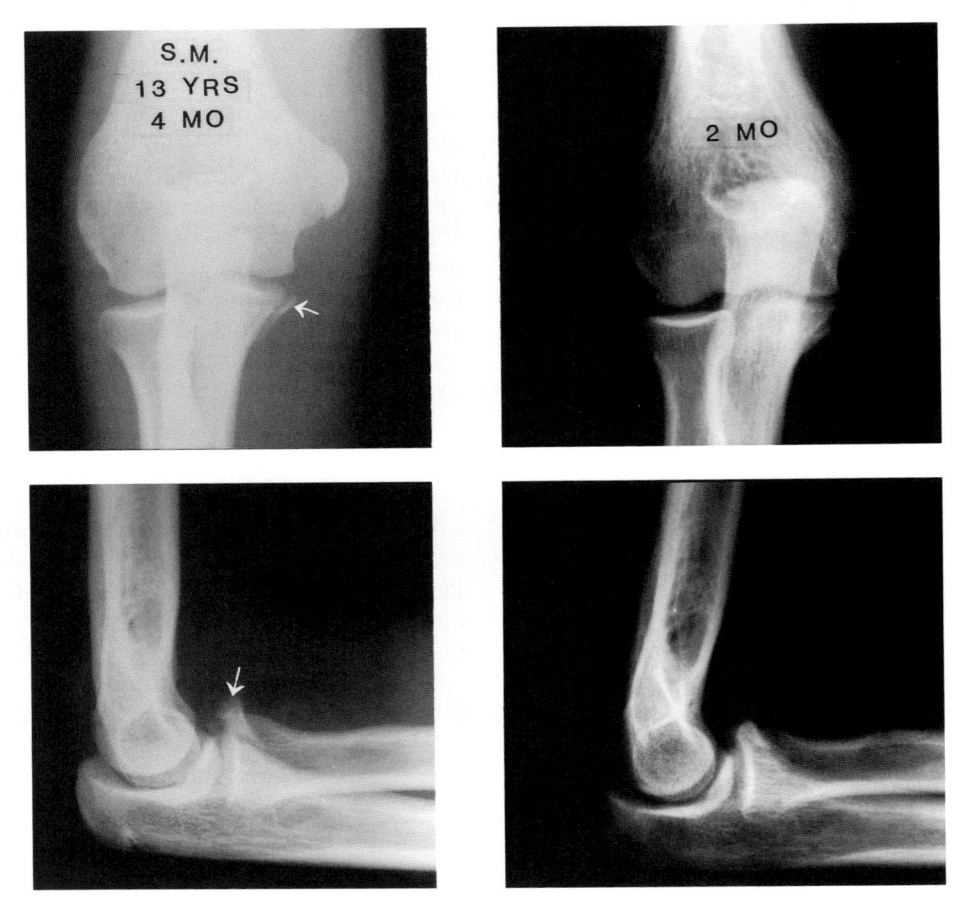

Fig. 15-17. A 13-year, 4-month-old girl with minimally displaced fracture of coronoid process. The fracture was treated with 3 weeks of immobilization followed by active range of motion exercises. Functional result at 2 months was normal.

PHYSICAL EXAMINATION

Most often the child will present to the emergency department with a history of having fallen and injured the elbow. Little other information will be available unless the incident was witnessed by a friend or parent. Typically, the child will have subjective pain, swelling, and loss of motion. There may or may not be associated deformity. Occasionally there will be the history that the elbow dislocated and popped back into place. The child is sometimes able to remember a snap or pop at the time of injury.

Observation of the injured elbow will usually reveal swelling at the fracture site, although in undisplaced fractures the elbow may appear normal.

Palpation of the elbow will reveal tenderness along the physis or metaphysis depending upon the location of the fracture site. There will be tenderness along the medial joint line after dislocation with spontaneous reduction or there may be tenderness along the radial head laterally or anteriorly if it is dislocated.[23] If the elbow is not too swollen, the dislocated radial head will appear prominent compared to the opposite normal side.

In avulsion-type injuries or flexion injuries with separation of the proximal fragment, there may be a palpable defect in the extensor mechanism.[20] The proximal fragment can be displaced by the pull of the triceps mechanism up into the distal posterior upper arm.[28]

Active range of motion testing of the elbow usually reveals a pseudoparalysis or refusal of the child to move

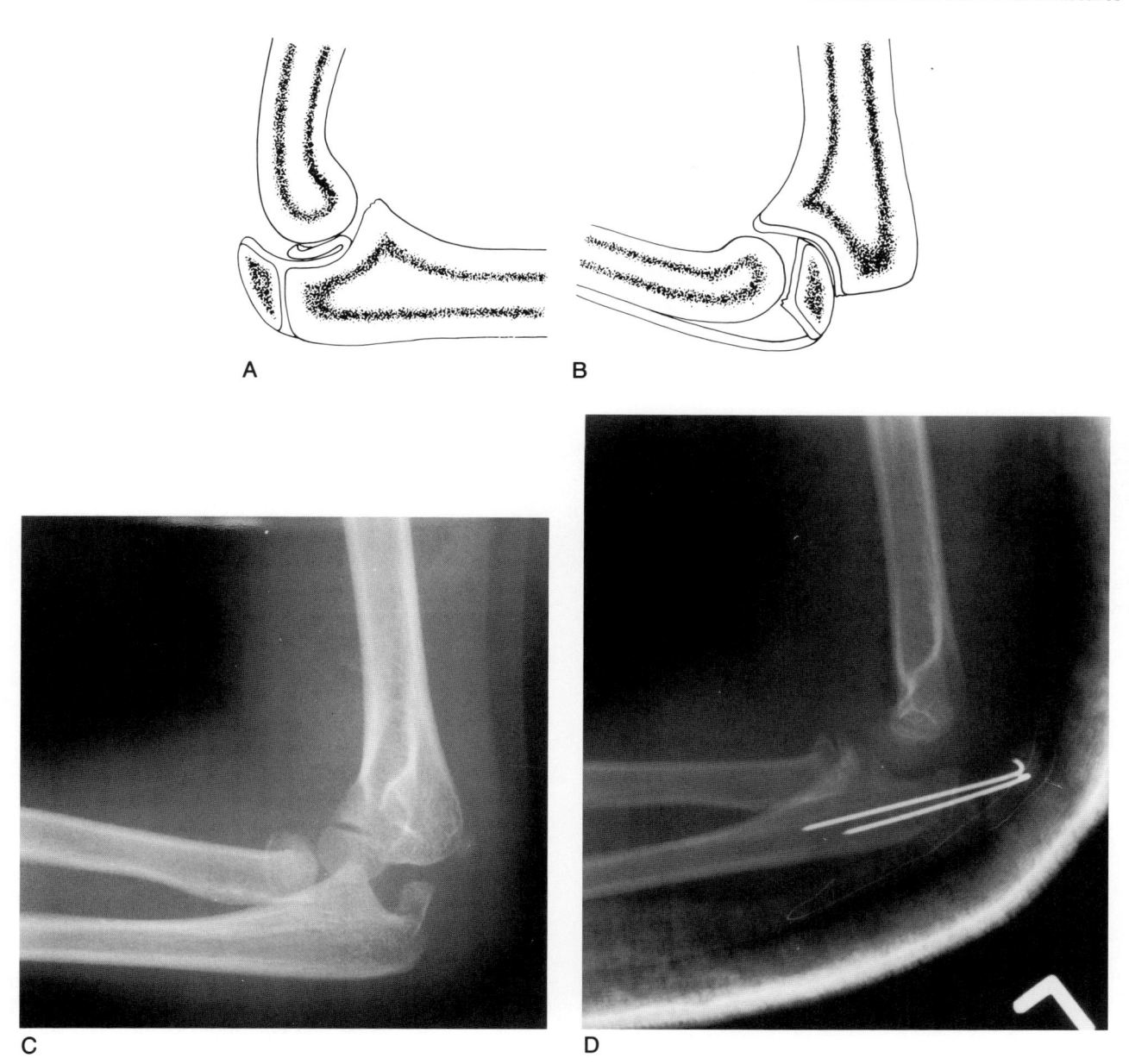

Fig. 15-18. **(A)** Intra-articular flap fracture of the glenoid fossa. A flap of cartilage with subchondral bone may be turned posteriorly such that it folds back upon itself during spontaneous reduction of a posterior elbow dislocation. **(B)** Intra-articular apophyseal avulsion. Olecranon tip is avulsed and comes to lie within humeral ulnar joint. (Drawing by Tish O'Neil.) **(C)** Valgus injury to elbow with type II fracture radial neck and intra-articular avulsion fracture of olecranon. **(D)** Postreduction of radial head and olecranon fractures.

the painful extremity. When the extensor mechanism is disrupted, there may be inability to actively extend the elbow against gravity or resistance.

Varus/valgus instability testing may reveal instability after extension type injuries and in spontaneously reduced dislocations. Wilkins[20] recommends flexion of the elbow to determine stability of olecranon fractures, although children may find these stress tests to be too painful. Intra-articular injection of lidocaine may alleviate the discomfort and enable stability testing, but careful neurovascular examination must be undertaken first.

Nerve and vascular injuries are distinctly unusual in olecranon fractures but may occur in association with fracture dislocations. Compartment syndrome must always be ruled out.

DIFFERENTIAL DIAGNOSIS

The most important considerations in the differential diagnosis of olecranon and coronoid fractures are as follows:

1. Making a correct diagnosis in the presence of undisplaced fracture
2. Ruling out pseudofracture, which is a problem due to the unusual ossification pattern of the proximal ulna

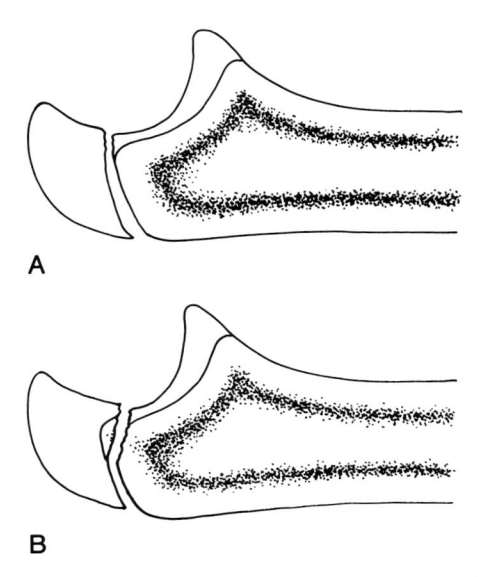

Fig. 15-19. Cartilaginous epiphysis may be avulsed from metaphysis: **(A)** without a fragment of bone (type I) or **(B)** with a fragment of bone (type II). (Drawing by Tish O'Neil.)

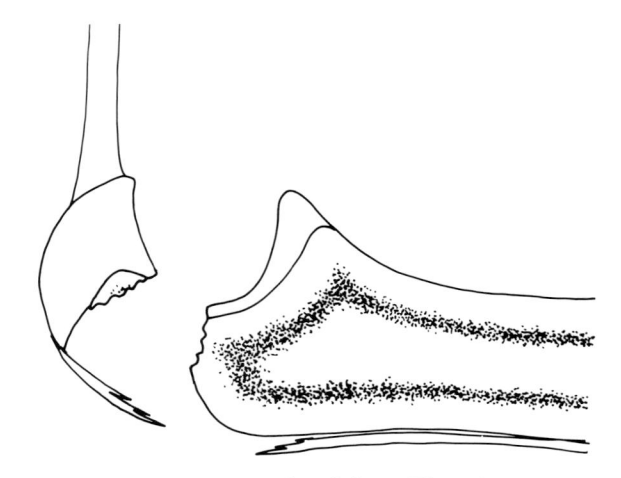

Fig. 15-20. Extensor avulsion injury. The triceps extensor mechanism of the elbow may avulse the insertion of the triceps with a sleeve of periosteum with or without a fragment of metaphyseal bone. The cartilaginous epiphysis is usually included with the displaced fragment. If displacement is wide, extensor discontinuity can be assumed. (Drawing by Tish O'Neil.)

3. Recognizing associated injuries such as intra-articular fractures, spontaneously reduced dislocations and disruption of the extensor mechanism.

Knowledge of the radiographic anatomy, frequent fracture patterns, and the use of special tests may be useful.

The diagnosis is usually obvious on a plain lateral radiograph of the injured elbow. Injuries can, however, be difficult to assess radiographically because the ossification centers may be primarily cartilaginous and not visible on routine radiographs.[33] Absence of soft tissue swelling and joint effusion is almost incompatible with fracture of the olecranon entering the joint space.[9] If there is a positive fat-pad sign and the physeal line extends into the joint, comparison radiographs with the opposite elbow may be indicated.[9]

Interpretation of the radiographs may be a challenge. As mentioned in the section of anatomy, radiographs of maturing ulna are prone to misinterpretation due to three reasons:

1. Just prior to ossification of the olecranon epiphysis, a straight sclerotic edge develops in the associated metaphysis and the proximal part of the ulna. This may simulate a fracture.
2. Ossification of the olecranon begins in two or more centers that commonly fuse with each other before

fusing with the parent bone and may be separated widely from the metaphysis in the early stages, again simulating a displaced fracture.
3. The physis of the olecranon frequently migrates distally into the joint and may simulate a fracture line.[12] At maturity, the sclerotic margin at the site of physeal fusion may persist being mistaken for a fracture.[20]

ARTHROGRAPHY OF THE ELBOW

In younger children a so-called "chip" fracture may represent a separation of a large (radiolucent) epiphysis of the olecranon with associated metaphyseal avulsion.[6,9] Arthrogram may help to delineate the nature of the fracture.

Arthrography is recommended in the skeletally immature patient when the diagnosis is in doubt.[33] Arthrography can be performed usefully in the emergency room in the radiographic suite or in the operating room. Sedation may be appropriate for the anxious child outside the operating room. The elbow is sterilely prepped. Arthrocentesis is performed by posterolateral puncture using a small-diameter needle. Fluid is aspirated and its character is noted. A contrast agent such as Conray (Malinckrodt Chemical, St. Louis, Missouri) and air, 1 ml of each is injected into the elbow. A half dose is used for children less than age 2.[33] Anteroposterior, lateral, and oblique radiographs are taken of the elbow. This technique is most useful in young children with cartilaginous epiphyses about the elbow in whom the diagnosis of fracture is strongly suspected on the basis of clinical grounds, but is unproven on the basis of plain radiographs.

Unusual lesions have been shown to occur. Congenital pseudoarthrosis[40] and patella cubiti must be ruled out.[9,23] Associated injury must always be ruled out. Intra-articular fractures are known to occur with elbow dislocation and may be difficult to discover on plain films alone. Plain tomography, computed tomography, arthrography, and magnetic resonance imaging may be helpful. Osteochondral fracture of the glenoid fossa of the ulna can occur.[29,30] This is most reliably diagnosed with conventional sagittal tomography.[29] If fracture occurs in the coronoid process, the radial head may obscure the coronoid on plain film views. In this case, oblique views may be necessary to visualize the fracture.

When fracture involves the proximal ulnar metaphysis, the radial head, neck, or shaft[42] should be examined carefully for associated injury. The direction of displacement of the proximal radius will be the same as the apex of the ulnar fracture. Fracture of the olecranon may be associated with fracture of the distal end of the radius and ulna.[4]

Stress testing may be appropriate in evaluating the injured child who is adequately anesthetized. This will help to determine the presence of joint laxity after elbow dislocation or the presence of an unstable olecranon fracture in elbow flexion, as the intact triceps pulls the fragment proximally.

TREATMENT

The overall goals of fracture treatment of the proximal ulna are similar to those in any joint. Restoration of a smooth articular surface in any fracture which enters the joint is essential. The olecranon provides an important part of the extensor mechanism of the elbow and this continuity must be maintained. Fractures about the olecranon often involve the physis and attention must be given to restoring the functional integrity of the physis to prevent growth arrest or deformity. Proximal radioulnar joint continuity must also be maintained to allow free pronation and supination of the forearm.

Methods

Fractures of the olecranon and coronoid are amenable both to operative and nonoperative methods of treatment. If the fracture is undisplaced or easily reducible, only, simple immobilization is indicated (Fig. 15-21). For fractures which are undisplaced and stable in flexion, a well-molded long-arm cast in 90 degrees of flexion is the most convenient method of treatment. In general, we recommend that the treatment duration be no longer than 3 weeks as the elbow joint, even in children, may develop restricted motion. In fractures that appear to be unstable in flexion, it may be appropriate to place a long-arm cast in some degree of extension to prevent distraction of the fragments by the intact pull of the triceps. We have found, however, that the use of an extension cast about the elbow is more of a hardship to the child than the flexion cast because the extension cast is more difficult to suspend from the sling, and it is harder to rest on a desk or table in a sitting position. The hand on the casted side is more easily usable in the elbow-flexed position both during casting and during that period of time after cast removal when full motion is not yet restored.

Surgical treatment is reserved for those cases (1)

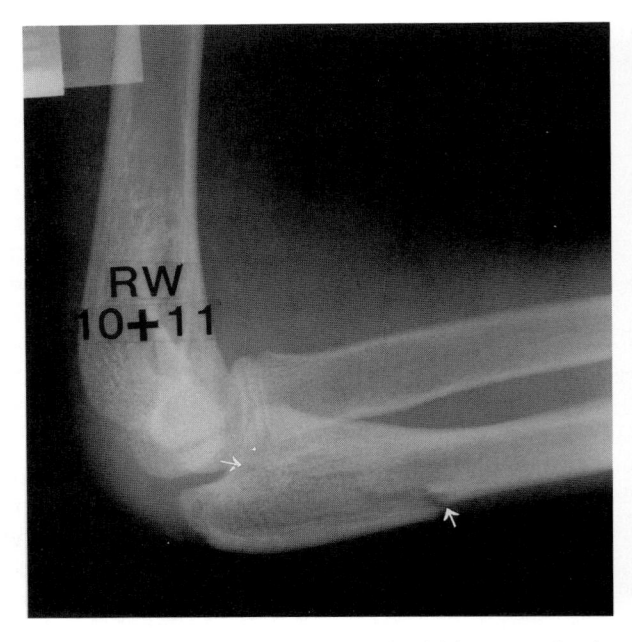

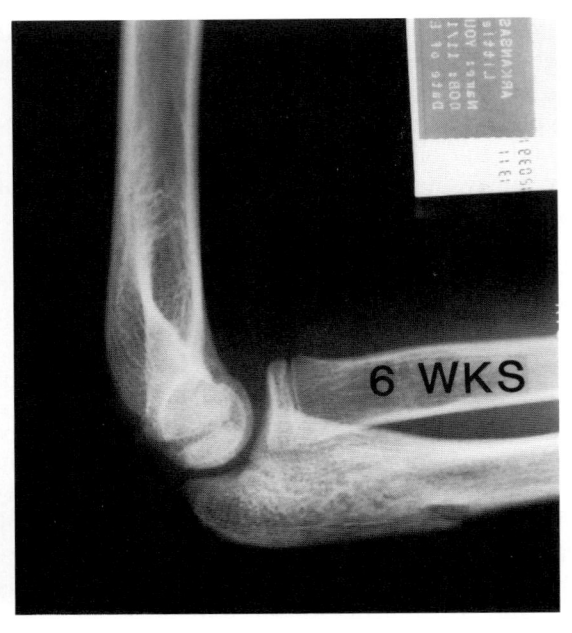

Fig. 15-21. A 10-year, 11-month-old boy sustained multiple injuries, including an oblique intra-articular fracture of the left elbow. The fracture was treated with 3 weeks of immobilization followed by range of motion. The elbow function was essentially normal at 3 months follow-up.

with articular incongruity, (2) discontinuity of the extensor mechanism, (3) irreducible displacement of the physis, (4) proximal radioulnar joint disruption, (5) propensity for stiffness or (6) a risk of impaired fracture healing.

When an operation is required, we recommend a general anesthetic with the patient placed supine on the operating room table, although others have recommended a prone positioning.[21] A dorsal S-shaped incision should be made just lateral to the olecranon tip. For transverse-type fracture lines or physeal injuries, we recommend the use of tension band as described by Weber.[49] The fragments first should be reduced and fixed with two axial Kirschner pins. The wires should be parallel to allow compression of the fragments. A figure-of-eight wire should then be placed around the pins and through the triceps aponeurosis connecting to a hole drilled transversely through the proximal ulnar metaphysis. The figure-of-eight wire should be tight and of adequate thickness to assure strong fixation. The proximal ends of the Kirschner pins should be bent round and pushed beneath the triceps aponeurosis to prevent late prominence (Fig. 15-22).

When there is an oblique fracture line that can be crossed with a screw without violating the physis, it is appropriate to use screw fixation, which provides intrafragmentary compression. The screw should be long enough to engage the far cortex[34] (Fig. 15-23). The head of the screw should abut the proximal cortex, and consideration should be given to the use of a washer if the bone quality is poor. The threads must not distract the fracture line. Tension band wiring is more reliable fixation in maintaining reduction than the use of an intrafragmentary screw.[34] This advantage is however offset by the higher incidence of local complications related to subcutaneous wires.[34] The recommended approach for internal fixation of the proximal ulna is posterior medial.[35,36]

When there is an associated osteochondral fracture, the surgical approach to the elbow is dependent upon which side of the elbow joint is involved. The use of a lateral hockey stick incision[29] may allow access to the lateral side of the joint and a view of the radial side of the ulnar glenoid fossa without damaging the ulnar nerve or muscle insertion.[29] An anterior approach may be used for fixing a coronoid fracture.[8] If an osteochondral fracture does not appear to be approachable by the anterolateral means, then it may be appropriate to approach from medially. It is necessary to protect the ulnar nerve and take down the medial epicondyle to access the joint.

The use of absorbable pins and suture material to create a tension band fixation for fracture of the proximal ulna may be useful, as it will alleviate the necessity

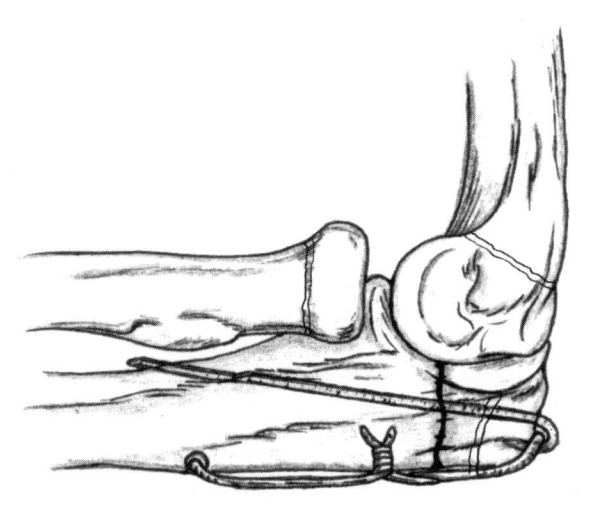

Fig. 15-22. Tension band wiring as described by Weber. Kirschner wires must be parallel. (Drawing by S. D. Temple, M.D.)

for a second operation to remove hardware. However, we believe that this method does not give as rigid fixation as the use of metallic pins and wires, hence it would be mandatory to supplement this fixation with external immobilization for at least 3 to 4 weeks to allow preliminary healing of the fracture before initiating free range of motion. Treatment of a large series of olecranon fractures with absorbable fixation has not yet been described.

Specific Fracture Types

Physeal Injuries

Physeal injuries of the proximal ulna are Salter-Harris type I or II. Usually they are undisplaced. Treatment for this type of injury is immobilization for 3 weeks in a long-arm cast followed by range of motion exercises. As the triceps mechanism will be intact and has the potential to displace the fragment, a follow-up radiograph should be obtained 1 week after application of the cast.

In a displaced fracture, the elbow should be radiographed in extension to see if reduction of the fragments can be achieved. If so, then application of a cast in extension is appropriate. This is more inconvenient for the patient and does require some time after cast removal to regain full flexion of the elbow. In cases that are grossly displaced and unreducible by closed means, it is appropriate to pursue operative technique. This can be done by a posterior approach, using tension band wiring.[6] Threaded screws may be used but should not cross the physis.

Metaphyseal Fractures

FLEXION INJURIES

Flexion metaphyseal injuries often enter the humeral ulnar joint. If undisplaced, closed treatment is recommended.[2,6,7,9,20,37] The use of a collar and cuff has been suggested. However, a long-arm cast provides better protection for the tender elbow and can prevent inadvertent displacement by sudden forced movement.

Displaced flexion fractures need to be treated operatively. Guidelines for displacement have ranged from 2 mm[7] to 5 mm.[20] We choose to operate on flexion injuries that have greater then 4 mm of displacement through metaphyseal bone or greater than 2 mm of stepoff in the joint surface. Operative fixation of the olecranon is generally successful.[2,6,7,9,11,20,34,37,45] Following fixation, it is wise to immobilize the elbow for a week to allow time for wound healing. If fixation is rigid, as in tension band wiring, then motion may be started after that time. If the fixation is nonrigid, we recommend a 3-week course of casting prior to mobilizing the elbow.

Pitfalls. Unlike in the adult where the proximal fragment of olecranon may be excised and the extensor mechanism reattached, this is not feasible in the child due to the presence of the growth plate.

METAPHYSEAL EXTENSION INJURIES

Metaphyseal extension injuries usually involve an oblique fracture of the metaphysis angulated into varus or valgus. The fractures often are greenstick and may be

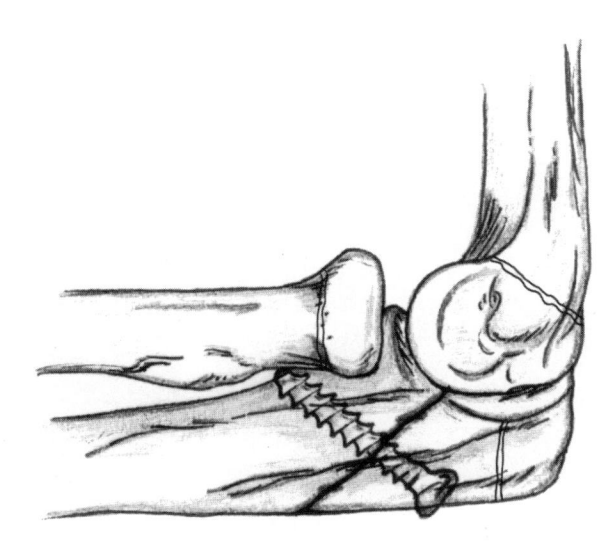

Fig. 15-23. Intrafragmentary screw can be used in oblique fractures in which physis can be avoided. (Drawing by S. D. Temple, M.D.)

difficult to reduce. Attention must be given to congruous reduction of the radiocapitellar joint. These fractures do not generally involve the physis.

Initial treatment of choice is closed reduction of the fracture and immobilization.[3,6,9,20-22,26,37] We perform this maneuver under an intravenous regional anesthesia or intravenous sedation in the emergency room or, if necessary, under a general anesthesia in the operating room. The reduction maneuver involves extending the elbow fully to lock the olecranon into the fossa of the distal humerus and then correcting the varus or valgus deformity (Fig. 15-6).

In the case of the varus greenstick fracture, an attempt should be made to overcorrect the deformity as it has been reported by Zimmerman[21] that the varus deformity has a tendency to recur. Following reduction, the elbow should be immobilized for 3 weeks in 90 degrees or more of flexion with the forearm fully supinated in order to stabilize the radial head.

Operative treatment may be necessary[6,9,20,21,37,39] if there are greater than 4 mm of metaphyseal displacement, if there is greater than 2 mm of articular stepoff, or if angulation cannot be corrected enough to allow relocation of the radial head (Fig. 15-24). Suitable fixation is by tension band wiring or intrafragmentary screw fixation, if the physis can be avoided.

Pitfalls. There are several pitfalls that can occur with the metaphyseal extension fracture. After varus greenstick fracture, reangulation may occur as documented by Zimmermann.[6] As a result, the radial head may sublux laterally. Reconstruction using the Belle-Tawse procedure in conjunction with an osteotomy of the proximal ulna is indicated if this complication occurs. Care must

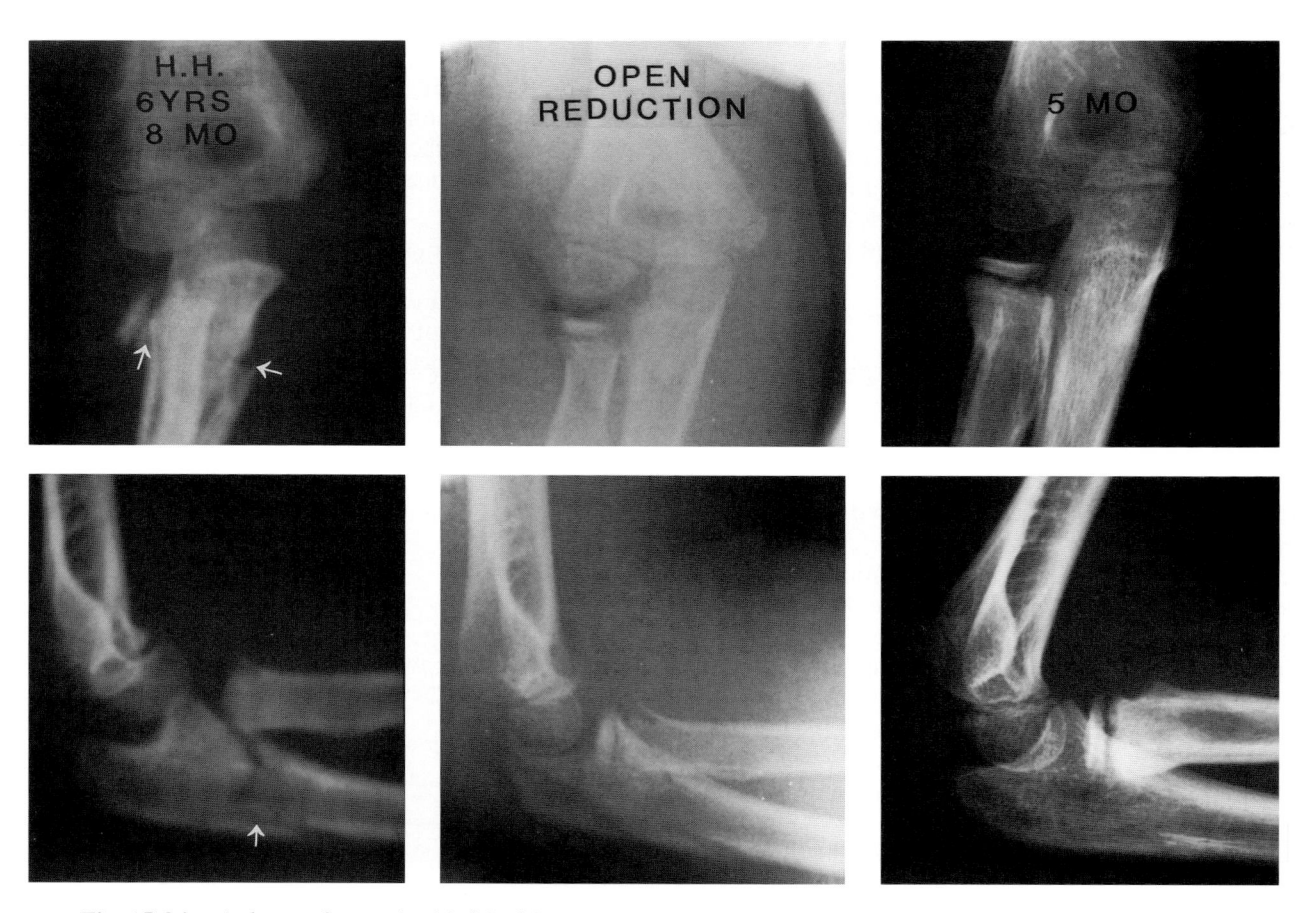

Fig. 15-24. A 6-year, 8-month-old girl with valgus greenstick fracture of proximal ulna and fracture of radial neck. Closed reduction was not possible. The radial neck was openly reduced in the operating room and the valgus greenstick was corrected by osteoclasis. Healing was excellent at 5 months postoperative.

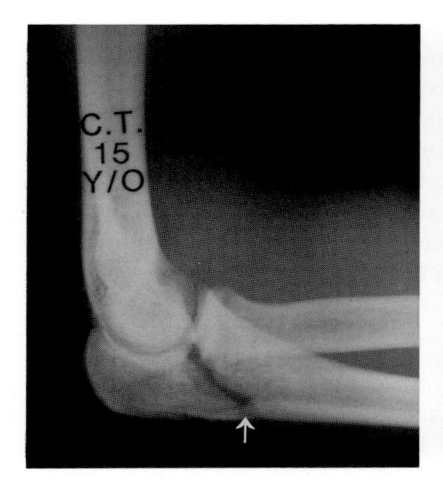

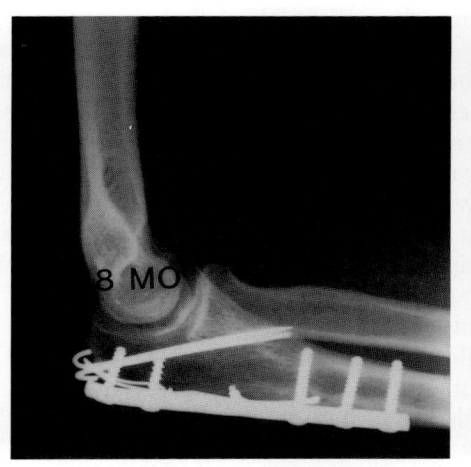

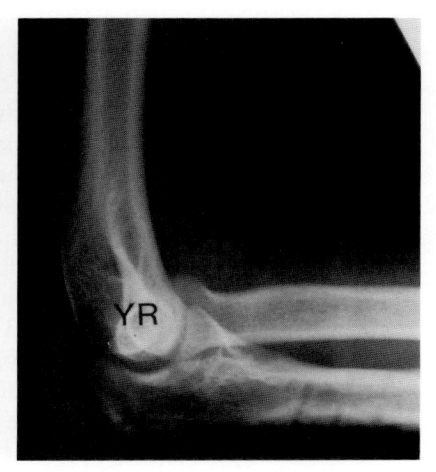

Fig. 15-25. A 15-year-old boy had intra-articular olecranon fracture. The fracture was treated with open reduction and internal fixation with intramedullary pins, tension band wiring, and a DCP plate. The patient recovered with full function of the elbow and had uneventful hardware removal at 1 year after injury.

be taken to ensure that the varus angulation is corrected or even overcorrected at the time of initial treatment. Parents must be warned of the possibility of recurrence of the deformity.

Associated elbow injuries must be searched for diligently. The radial head can be dislocated even with an undisplaced olecranon fracture.[23] One-fifth of all olecranon fractures will be associated with other injuries, frequently a fracture of the medial epicondyle.[5] Fractures of the proximal ulna have also been associated with fractures at the wrist.[25]

METAPHYSEAL SHEAR INJURIES

Metaphyseal shear injuries tend to occur with fracturing perpendicular to the shaft of the ulna, just anterior to the humeral condyles. Oblique fracture may occur from anterior proximal to posterior distal ulna. These are usually displaced anteriorly; however, they can be displaced medially.[6] Reduction is achieved by traction and direct manipulation of the distal fragment posteriorly or medially back into approximation with the proximal fragment. The reduction is maintained by hyperflexion of the elbow.[6] This provides compression across the fracture site in conjunction with the intact posterior periosteum.[6]

Alternatively, prolonged overhead traction with the child lying supine creates a posteriorly directed reducing force to the anteriorly displaced distal fragments.[26] In the event that the fracture is irreducible or unstable due to tearing of the posterior periosteum, then open reduction and internal fixation with tension band wiring is indicated (Fig. 15-25). If the fracture is oblique, then fixation with intrafragmentary screw perpendicular to the fracture line may be successful as described by Zimmermann.[21]

Pitfalls. In the anterior shear injury, the radial head may be dislocated anteriorly. Attention must be given to reduction of the radiocapitellar joint as well as the proximal radioulnar joint.

Intra-Articular Fractures of the Proximal Ulna Occurring as a Result of Dislocation

The common articular fractures of the proximal ulna occurring after dislocation are fracture of the coronoid process, osteoarticular fracture of the glenoid fossa, and fracture avulsion of the olecranon apophysis (Fig. 12-18). Other nonulnar intra-articular fractures must be ruled out, such as a displaced medial epicondylar fragment. Small fractures of the coronoid process can be treated by immobilization of the elbow in flexion for 3 weeks followed by active range of motion exercises.[6] Coronoid fracture may require open reduction and internal fixation. Indications include (1) displacement of a large fracture fragment that would allow recurrent dislocation,[8,36] (2) a displaced fragment that appears to lie between the humerus and ulna[8,26] and (3) a fragment that blocks full flexion.[8] The operative approach for these rare indications can be from anterior with screw fixation from anterior to posterior[8] or medially taking down the medial epicondyle with screw fixation from posterior to anterior.[36]

An osteochondral flap fracture of the glenoid fossa of the proximal ulna can be approached using a lateral hockey stick incision, which avoids damaging nerve and muscle origins. If the fracture is on the medial side of the fossa, it may be necessary to take down the medial epicondyle to approach the medial joint while protecting the ulnar nerve. The osteochondral flap is usually stable once repositioned, but may be held in place with a drop in fibrin glue.[29] Immobilization for 3 weeks followed by active range of motion is adequate follow-up treatment.

Intra-articular entrapment of a displaced olecranon fracture has been described.[32] Some degree of humeral ulnar dislocation must be necessary to allow this to occur. This lesion is amenable to open reduction from posterior, with replacement of the fragment and fixation by tension band wiring (Fig. 15-18).

Pitfalls. Elbow dislocation without fracture in the child's elbow is rare.[4] Whenever there is a history of dislocation or there is considerable swelling and tenderness suggesting a dislocation, it is appropriate to look for an associated fracture. It should be kept in mind with reduced dislocations that, even though the fracture may appear to be undisplaced or minor, there is still considerable soft tissue damage to the capsule, muscle, ligament, and even nerve. For this reason, the prognosis for fracture associated with dislocation is more guarded than for fracture without dislocation.[46] Parents must be warned with regard to these potential problems.

Extensor Avulsion Injuries

Extensor avulsion can involve a large or small portion of the triceps insertion. A periosteal sleeve may be avulsed analogous to the periosteal sleeve fracture of the patella. Typically these injuries are displaced and require operative fixation to restore extensor continuity. This can be performed through a posterior approach with suture of the torn aponeurosis with or without the use of Kirschner pins and tension band wiring.

Direct-Blow Fracture

These fractures tend to be comminuted due to shattering of the bone as a result of a blow. In these fractures, the periosteal sleeve often remains intact and the fragments are not widely displaced. Treatment with simple immobilization should provide a good result. If the fracture is displaced causing disruption of the articular surface or disruption of the extensor mechanism, then open reduction and internal fixation may be necessary. Due to the comminution, these fractures are very difficult to stabilize (Fig. 15-14). For this reason, we recommend minimal internal fixation, such as the use of a rush rod or a tension band wire, giving just enough fixation to restore the articular surface or to restore extensor continuity without attempting to rigidly fixate all fragments.

Stress Fractures

Stress fracture occurs as a result of chronic, repetitive, forceful extension movements of the forearm as in throwing sports. In general, stress fracture will respond to simple abstinence from the throwing activity or enforced rest in a splint or a cast. Nonunion of a stress fracture has been described[14] which required an operative fixation and bone grafting. Fortunately, this complication is rare.

Open Fractures

Open fracture of the olecranon occurs as a result of direct or penetrating trauma to the elbow. Management is by irrigation and debridement under a suitable anesthetic. If the fracture is clearly undisplaced and stable after wound toilet, simple cast immobilization may be appropriate. If the fracture is seen to communicate with the joint surface, then open reduction, exposure of the joint, and thorough irrigation and debridement is necessary followed by fixation with screws or tension band wiring. Postoperatively, immobilization should be used until wound healing is complete. If there is a small to moderate skin defect, closure is achieved by approximation of the redundant skin about the elbow.

COMPLICATIONS OF OLECRANON FRACTURES

Vascular and Neurologic Injuries

Fractures about the coronoid and olecranon tend to have few complications. Neurologic and vascular injuries are rare, except in association with dislocations.[38] Although a potential exists for physeal arrest, growth derangement is unusual in association with these fractures, though olecranon overgrowth may occasionally be an annoyance.

Nonunion

Olecranon nonunion has been described,[6,9,14,21] although this is unusual. Satisfactory treatment includes bone grafting with rigid internal fixation. Nonunion has occurred after open reduction and internal fixation of an ulnar fracture with catgut suture.[38] Nonunion has been described in a displaced coronoid fracture.[6] Satisfactory treatment would include excision of the fragment if small or operative repair with bone grafting is of significant size.

Joint Stiffness

As with all injuries about the elbow, there is a tendency for the elbow to lose motion as a result both of the fracture itself and treatment. Stiffness or loss of range of motion is worse if there is associated soft tissue injury.[20,21,38] Loss of pronation and supination is likely to occur when there is luxation of the radial head in association with an upper ulnar fracture.[3,25] Ankylosis has been described after upper radioulnar joint injury with complete loss of pronation and supination.[24]

Persistent or Increasing Varus Deformity

Zimmerman[21] has reported that after metaphyseal varus extension fracture, varus deformity may persist or increase with fracture healing. This may lead to late subluxation of the radial head and require operative osteotomy of the ulna.[21,24]

Myositis Ossificans

Unlike the adult, heterotopic ossification after elbow injury is unusual in children, although it has been described to occur anterior to a displaced radial head.[23] Operative excision to improve motion may be necessary once the heterotopic bone has matured.

SUMMARY

Injuries of the proximal ulna are common in children. Fractures of the olecranon occur frequently. Fractures of the coronoid occur rarely, usually in association with elbow dislocation. The olecranon and coronoid help to form the glenoid fossa of the proximal ulna, which is crucial to the stability of the joint. Due to the peculiar pattern of ossification of the cartilaginous model of the proximal ulna, interpretation of radiographs may be difficult for those unfamiliar with the ossification pattern. In younger children with injuries about the elbow in which there is a large amount of cartilage present, there is a tendency to under diagnose injuries. In older children in whom the ossified epiphyses have appeared, there is a tendency to overdiagnose fractures due to the peculiar appearance of the ossification centers. Olecranon fractures occur by a variety of mechanisms, most frequently as a result of resisting a fall on the outstretched hand. Injuries can also occur as a result of a direct blow, in association with dislocation, and or as a repetitive stress injury. Special tests including computed tomography scans, tomograms, magnetic resonance imaging, and arthrography may be indicated to arrive at the correct diagnosis.

The overall goals for treatment involve maintaining a smooth articular surface, ensuring extensor continuity, maintaining integrity of the physis, ensuring union, and maintaining a functional range of motion. The majority of these injuries can be treated closed. Operative techniques may be necessary to achieve the overall goals of treatment. Complications are unusual.

REFERENCES

1. Lichtenberg RP: A study of 2,532 fractures in children. Am J Surg 87:330, 1954
2. Wilson PD: Fractures and dislocations in the region of the elbow. Surg Gynecol Obstet 477:335, 1933
3. Fahey JJ: Fractures of the elbow in children. Instr Course Lect 17:13, 1960
4. Maylahn DJ, Fahey JJ: Fractures of the elbow in children. JAMA 166:220, 1958
5. Landin LA, Danielsson LG: Elbow fractures in children: an epidemiological analysis of 589 cases. Acta Orthop Scand 57:309, 1986
6. Wilkins KE: Fractures and dislocations of the elbow region. p. 363. In Rockwood CA, Jr, Wilkins KE, King RE (eds): Fractures in Children. Vol. 3. JB Lippincott, Philadelphia, 1984
7. Petersen HA: Physeal fractures. p. 233. In Morrey BF (ed): The Elbow and Its Disorders. WB Saunders, Philadelphia, 1985
8. Selesnick FH, Dolitsky B, Haskell, SS: Fracture of the coronoid process requiring open reduction with internal fixation. J Bone Joint Surg [Am] 66:1304, 1984
9. Ogden JA: Radius and ulna. p. 451. In: Skeletal Injury in the Child. 2nd Ed. WB Saunders, Philadelphia, 1990

10. Tullos HS, Schwab G, Bennett JB, Woods GW: Factors influencing elbow instability. AAOS Instr Course Lect 30:185, 1981
11. Grantham SA, Kiernan HA: Displaced olecranon fracture in children. J Trauma 15:197, 1975
12. Silberstein MJ, Brodeus AE, Graviss ER, Luisiri A: Some vagaries of the olecranon. J Bone Joint Surg [Am] 63:722, 1981
13. Parsons FG: Observations on traction epiphyses. J Anat Physiol 38:248, 1903–1904
14. Torg JS, Moyer RA: Non-union of a stress fracture through the olecranon epiphyseal plate observed in an adolescent baseball pitcher. J Bone Joint Surg [Am] 59:264, 1977
15. Ogden JA: Elbow. p. 426. In: Skeletal Injury in the Child. 2nd Ed. WB Saunders, Philadelphia, 1990
16. Van Demark RE, Anderson TR: Fractured patella cubiti: report of a case with pathologic findings. Clin Orthop 53:131, 1967
17. Levine MA: Patella cubiti. J Bone Joint Surg [Am] 32:686, 1950
18. Zeitlin A: The traumatic origin of accessory bones at the elbow. J Bone Joint Surg 17:933, 1935
19. Wadström J, Kinast C, Pfeiffer K: Anatomical variations of the semilunar notch in elbow dislocations. Arch Orthop Trauma Surg 105:313, 1986
20. Canale ST: Metaphyseal and epiphyseal olecranon fractures. p. 981. In Canale ST, Beaty JH (eds): Operative Pediatric Orthopaedics. Mosby Year Book, St. Louis, 1991
21. Zimmerman H: Fractures of the elbow. p. 166. In Weber BG, Brunner Ch, Freuler F (eds): Treatment of Fractures in Children and Adolescents. Springer-Verlag, New York, 1980
22. Beddow FH, Corkery PH: Lateral dislocation of the radiohumeral joint with greenstick fracture of the upper end of the ulna. J Bone Joint Surg [Br] 42:782, 1960
23. Hume AC: Anterior dislocation of the head of the radius associated with undisplaced fracture of the olecranon in children. J Bone Joint Surg [Br] 39:508, 1957
24. Wright PR: Greenstick fracture of the upper end of the ulna with dislocation of the radio-humeral joint or displacement of the superior radial epiphysis. J Bone Joint Surg [Br] 45:727, 1963
25. Theodorou SD: Dislocation of the head of the radius associated with fracture of the upper end of the ulna in children. J Bone Joint Surg [Br] 51:700, 1969
26. Smith FM: Children's elbow injuries: fractures and dislocations. Clin Orthop 50:7, 1967
27. Gartsman GM, Sculco TP, Otis JC: Operative treatment of olecranon fractures. J Bone Joint Surg [Am] 63:718, 1981
28. Schweitzer G: Bilateral avulsion fractures of olecranon apophyses. Arch Orthop Trauma Surg 107:181, 1988
29. Blamoutier A, Klaue K, Damsin JP, Carlioz H: Osteochondral fractures of the glenoid fossa of the ulna in children: review of four cases. J Pediatr Orthop 11:638, 1991
30. Blasier RD: Intra-articular flap fracture of the olecranon in a child. J Bone Joint Surg [Am] 71:945, 1989
31. Papavasiliou VA, Beslikas TA, Nenopoulos S: Isolated fractures of the olecranon in children. Injury 18:100, 1987
32. An HS, Loder RT: Intraarticular entrapment of a displaced olecranon fracture: a case report. Orthopaedics 12:289, 1989
33. Yates C, Sullivan JA: Arthrographic diagnosis of elbow injuries in children. J Pediatr Orthop 7:54, 1987
34. Helm RH, Hornby R, Miller SWM: The complications of surgical treatment of displaced fractures of the olecranon. Injury 18:48, 1987
35. Taylor TKF, Scham SM: A posteromedial approach to the proximal end of the ulna for the internal fixation of olecranon fractures. J Trauma 9:594, 1969
36. Heim U: Forearm and hand/mini-implants. p. 453. In Müller ME, Allgöwer M, Schneider R, Willenegger H (eds): Manual of Internal Fixation. 3rd Ed. Springer-Verlag, New York, 1991
37. Tachdjian MO: Fractures of the olecranon. p. 3145. In: Pediatric Orthopaedics. Vol. 4. 2nd Ed. WB Saunders, Philadelphia, 1990
38. Matthews JG: Fractures of the olecranon in children. Injury 12:207, 1980
39. Rang M: Fractures of the olecranon. p. 190. In: Children's Fractures. 2nd Ed. JB Lippincott, Philadelphia, 1983
40. Burge P: Bilateral congenital pseudoarthrosis of the olecranon. J Bone Joint Surg [Br] 69:460, 1987
41. Guerra A, Innao V: Transolecranal dislocations. Halian J Orthop Trauma 8:175, 1982
42. Suprock MD, Lubahn JD: Olecranon fracture with ipsilateral closed radial shaft fracture in a child with open epiphysis. Orthopaedics 13:463, 1990
43. Porteous CJ: The olecranon epiphyses. J Anat 94:286, 1960
44. Newell RLM: Olecranon fractures in children. Injury 7:33, 1975
45. Sharrard WJW: Fractures of the olecranon. p. 1551. In: Pediatric Orthopaedics and Fractures. Vol. 2. 2nd Ed. Blackwell Scientific Publications, London, 1979
46. Josefsson PO, Gentz CF, Johnell O, Wendeberg B: Dislocations of the elbow and intraarticular fractures. Clin Orthop 246:126, 1989
47. Poland J: A Practical Treatise on Traumatic Separation of the Epiphyses. Smith, Elder and Co., London, 1898.
48. Newman JH: Displaced radial neck fractures in children. Injury 9:114, 1977.
49. Müller ME, Allgöwer M, Schneider R, Willenegger H (eds): Manual of Internal Fixation. 3rd Ed. Springer-Verlag, New York, 1991.

16

Fractures of the Capitellum

R. Mervyn Letts
Kevin Rumball

> In orthopaedic surgery errors of omission are more common than errors of commission.

DESCRIPTION AND INCIDENCE

Fractures of the capitellum humeri are uncommon at any age but are particularly rare in children. This is reflected in the few reports that exist in the literature concerning capitellar fractures in children. However, the fractures are important, since a failure to recognize the injury and treat it appropriately can lead to permanent elbow disability.

The fracture is usually a shear type of injury produced by impaction of the radial head. Recognition of this fracture in children is difficult due to the large cartilaginous component of the capitellum. The fracture is often confused with the more common type IV lateral humeral condylar fracture. The capitellar fracture is really an osteochondral fracture with the fragment being entirely intra-articular and not involving the physis of the distal humerus. It has been sporadically reported, since two cases were described in 1841 by Sir Astley Cooper.[1] Capitellar fractures have not been described in children under 10 years of age. Fractures of the lateral condyle are much more common in these younger children. This may be related to the smaller size and weaker strength of the radial head in younger children being unable to shear off a large portion of the capitellum.[2-6] Alternatively, the large cartilaginous component of the capitellum at this age may simply absorb the energy, thus preventing an osteochondral fracture.[7-10]

Fractures of the capitellum are usually seen in teenagers near skeletal maturity when the capitellum is nearly completely ossified.[2-4,6]

ANATOMIC CONSIDERATIONS

The capitellum is the articular portion of the lateral condyle of the distal humerus. The term *capitellum* is derived from Latin and means "a small head" (Fig. 16-1). The articular surface extends well anteriorly and inferiorly (Fig. 16-2). The radial head articulates on the anterior surface when the elbow is in flexion and on its inferior surface when the elbow is in extension.

The capitellum is the first epiphyseal center of the elbow to ossify. This occurs by the age of 2 years and generally is more rapid in girls, in whom it may appear as early as 6 months of age. The ossific nucleus of the capitellum will extend into the lateral ridge of the trochlea, hence the occasional involvement of a small portion of this ridge with the capitellar fragment.[8,10,11] The capitellum, lateral epicondyle, and trochlea fuse to form a common epiphyseal center. By around 14 years of age in

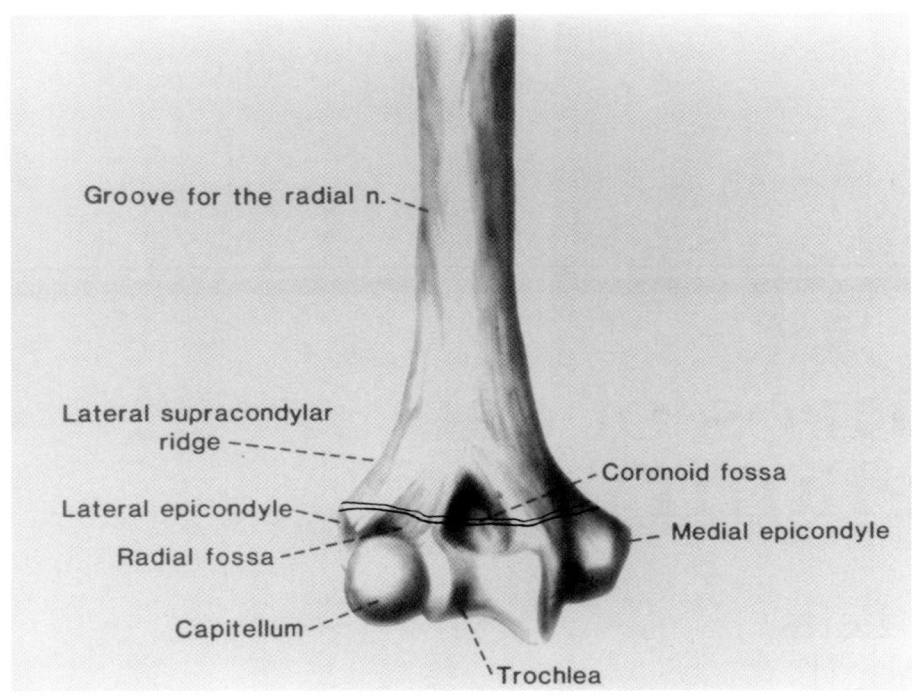

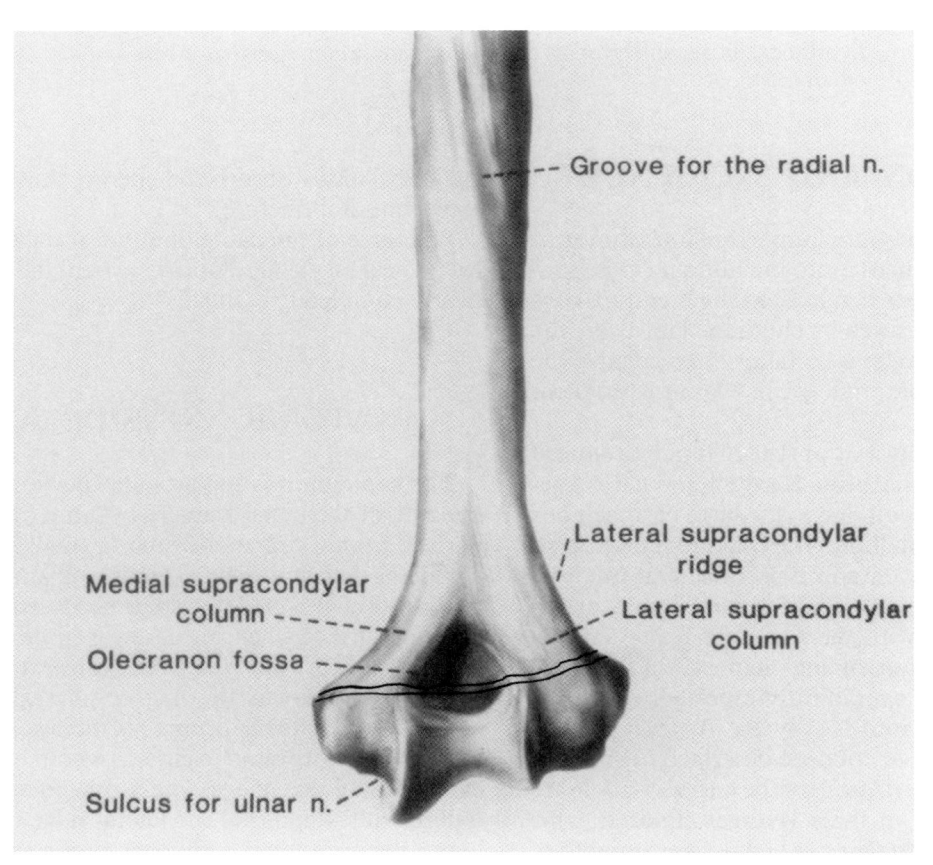

Fig. 16-1. Bony landmarks of **(A)** anterior and **(B)** posterior aspects of distal humerus. (Modified from Morrey BF: The Elbow and Its Disorders. p. 20. WB Saunders, Philadelphia, 1993. By permission of Mayo Foundation.)

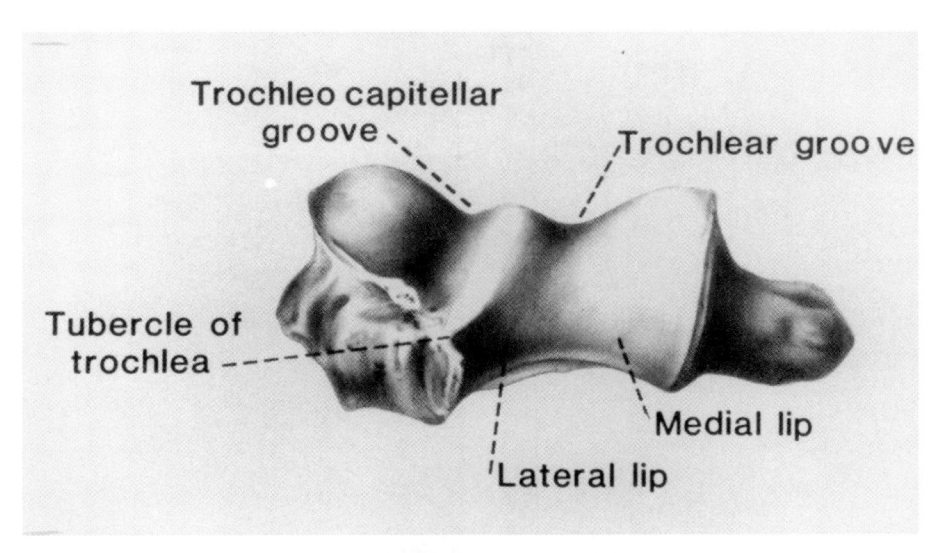

Fig. 16-2. Axial view of the distal humerus illustrating the anterior position of the capitellum and the trochlea capitellar groove separating the trochlea from the capitellum. (From Morrey BF: The Elbow and Its Disorders. p. 24. WB Saunders, Philadelphia, 1993. By permission of Mayo Foundation.)

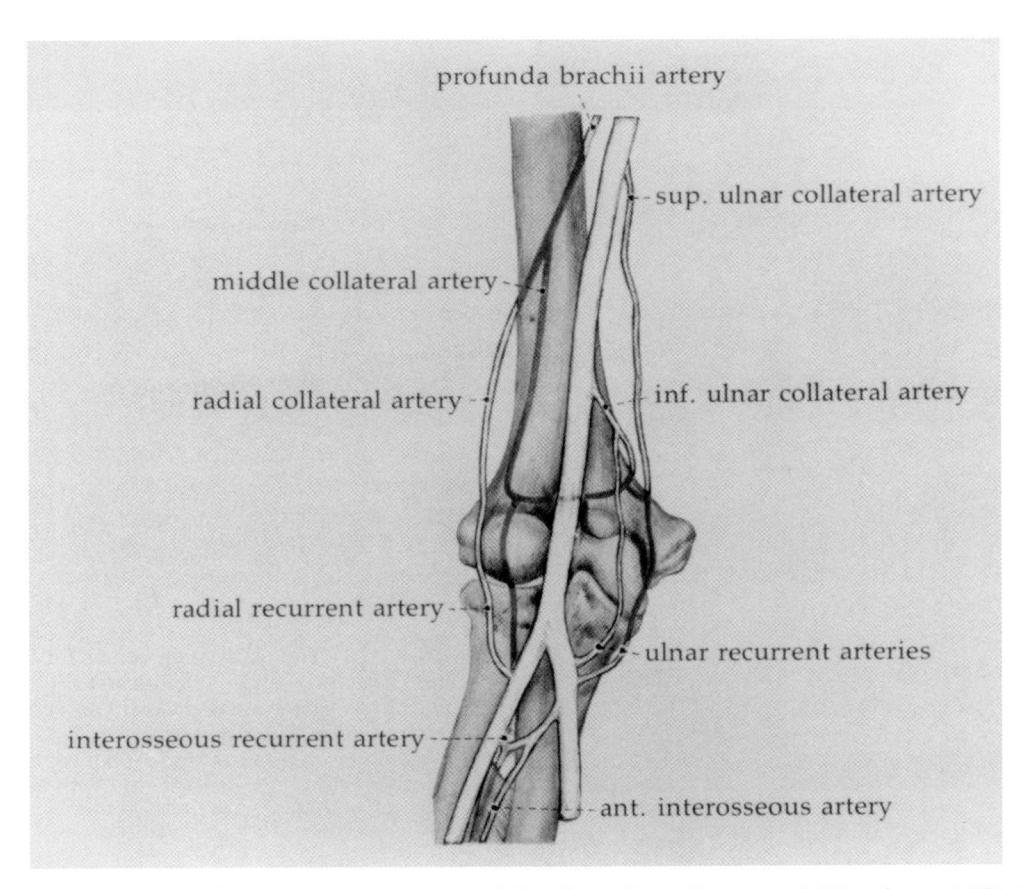

Fig. 16-3. Anterior arterial vascular network around the elbow. (From Langman J, Woerdeman MW: Atlas of Medical Anatomy. WB Saunders, Philadelphia, 1976, with permission.)

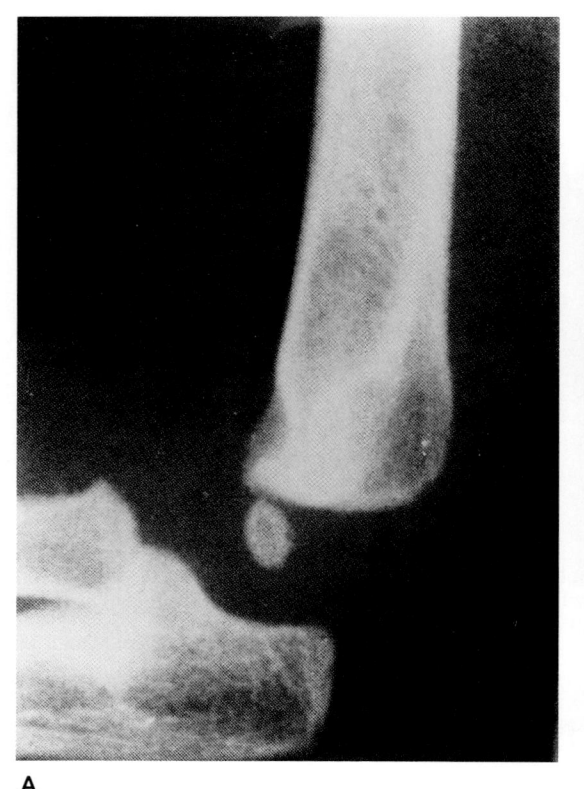

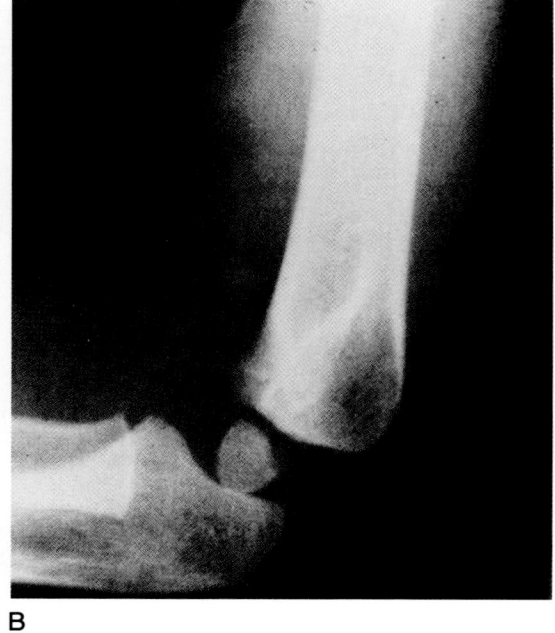

Fig. 16-4. (A) The ossification center for the capitellum is situated anteriorly and is frequently "tilted" downward. (B) The physis separation of the ossifying capitellum from the humerus is often wider posteriorly. (C) As the child grows older, the physis narrows anteriorly, but continues to be wider posteriorly. (From Silberstein et al.,[11] with permission.)

boys and 12 years in girls, this has usually fused with the distal humerus. Since the capitellum often unites with the trochlea and lateral epicondyle before uniting with the humerus, this may account for the fractures of the capitellum occurring predominantly in teenagers.[12]

The capitellum is supplied by end blood vessels, which arise from the inferior ulnar collateral artery (Fig. 16-3). These cross the olecranon fossa posteriorly to enter the lateral condyle and then traverse the ossific nucleus of the capitellum. These vessels are disrupted with a complete capitellar fracture, thus predisposing the fragmented capitellum to avascular necrosis. Studies of elbow stability by Dushuttle and colleagues[13] have demonstrated that the capitellum does not contribute significantly to elbow stability.

In young children, the capitellar ossification center is located anteriorly, which gives it a normal tilted position, sometimes misinterpreted as capitellar displacement. With further ossification of the capitellum, there develops a widening of the physis posteriorly, which again may be misinterpreted as an epiphyseal separation[11] (Fig. 16-4). Silberstein and colleagues[11] have pointed out that on the true lateral radiographic view, two dense lines outlining the olecranon (position line) and coronoid fossas (anterior line) are seen to form a "teardrop." If the anterior coronoid line is projected downward, it just touches the anterior border of the capitellar ossific center. Significant deviation of the capitellum from this line is suggestive of displacement (Fig. 16-5).

The humeral shaft line, a line drawn along the anterior border of the humerus and projected down through the elbow joint, normally passes through the posterior half of the ossific nucleus of the capitellum (Fig. 16-5). This line may be useful in detecting subtle displacements of the capitellum, especially when compared to the contralateral humeral line in the normal elbow. These radiologic signs are probably more useful in detecting subtle supracondylar or transcondylar fractures than isolated capitellar displacement, since the capitellum alone is seldom injured at these younger ages. Silberstein and co-workers[11] has also pointed out that the angle described by the intersection of the coronoid and humeral-shaft line encompasses most of the ossified capitellum at any

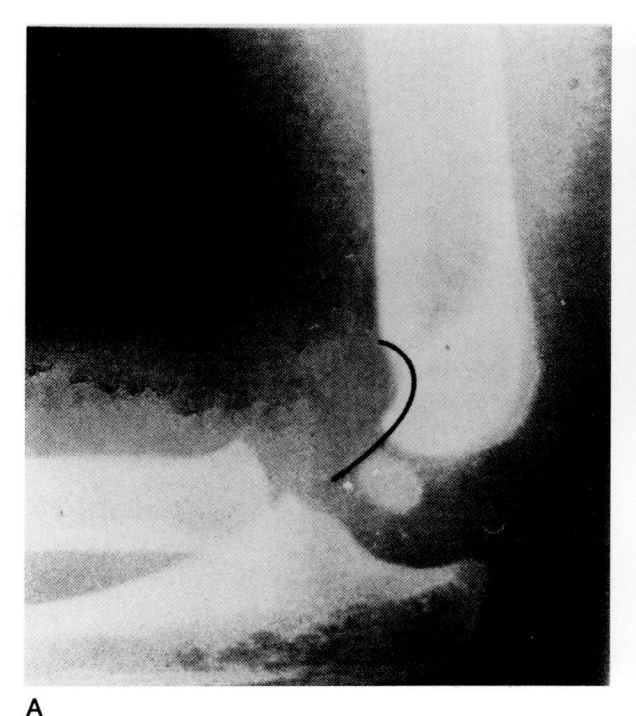

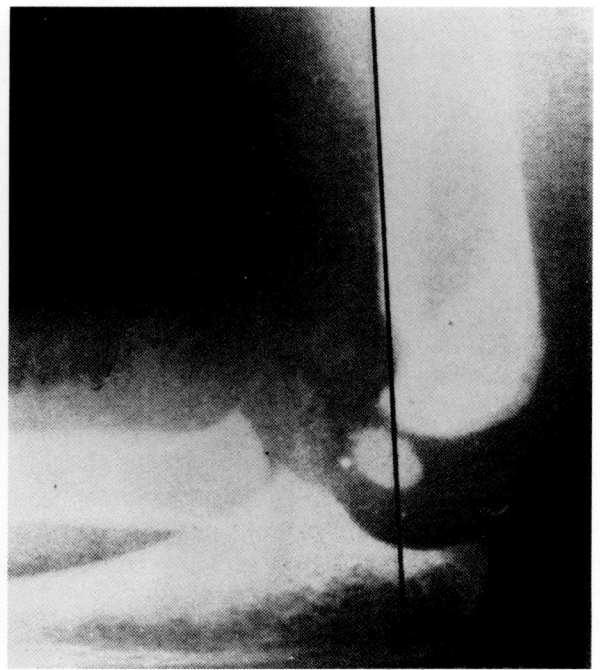

Fig. 16-5. **(A)** Continued downward, the curved coronoid line either just touches or projects just anteriorly to the developing capitellum. **(B)** On a true lateral radiographic view, continuation of the humeral-shaft line will normally project through the posterior half of the developing capitellum. (From Silberstein et al.,[11] with permission.)

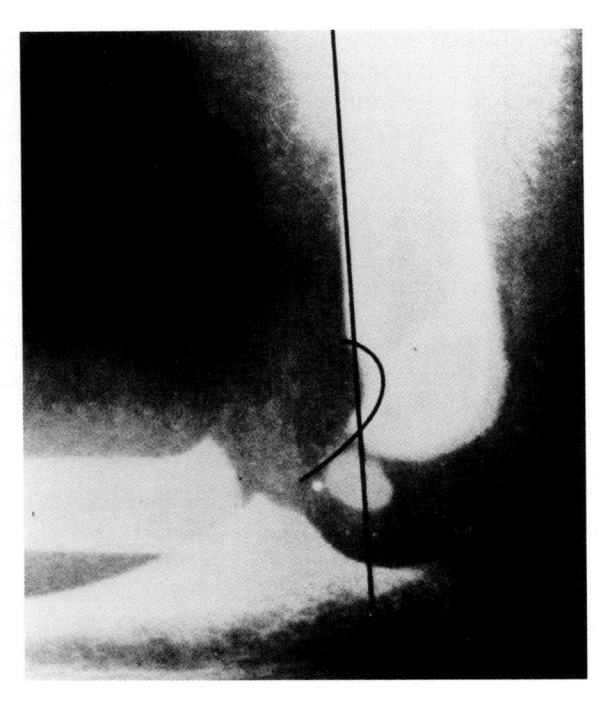

Fig. 16-6. The coronoid line and the humeral-shaft line describe an angle within which normally lies most of the ossified portion of the capitellum. (From Silberstein et al.,[11] with permission.)

age. This may be more useful in detecting small displacements of isolated capitellar fragments (Fig. 16-6).

MECHANISM OF INJURY

The fracture generally occurs after a fall on the outstretched hand. Forces are transmitted through the radial head, which shears off all or part of the capitellum with a pistonlike action. The more extended the elbow, the larger the capitellar fragment (Fig. 16-7). Cubitus recurvatum may be a factor that predisposes to this fracture pattern. Concomitant fractures of the radial head have been reported in adults,[9] but these are not common in children, probably due to the cushioning effect of the larger cartilaginous component of the head in children.

In adults, tears of the medial collateral ligament of the elbow have been reported in conjunction with the fracture of the capitellum,[13] but this has not been reported in children where the ligaments are much stronger than the surrounding osseous structures. The sheared-off segment of the capitellum, often involving the lip of the trochlea, is forced anterosuperiorly into the radial fossa.

Because the fracture plane is coronal, the radiologic appearance in the anterior posterior view is often confusing and may in fact appear almost normal (Fig. 16-8). It is the lateral radiographic view that is most helpful in identifying the free capitellar fragment lying in the radial fossa.

CLASSIFICATION

Two distinct fracture patterns have been observed in children. The following classification is useful for both treatment and prognosis (Fig. 16-9).

Type I: A complete fracture of the capitellum, which frequently includes the lateral third of the trochlea. This is the most common fracture pattern seen in children.

Type II: A partial or slice fracture of the capitellum, comprised mainly of articular cartilage with only a thin margin of subchondral bone. This type of fracture is a "decortication" of the capitellum.

PHYSICAL EXAMINATION

The physical findings often include tenderness localized to the anterolateral side of the distal humerus, an elbow effusion and the elbow held in slight flexion, which enlarges the joint cavity, thus reducing the intraarticular pressure and pain. A large fragment may be palpable anteriorly. Forearm rotation is usually not limited. In children, the elbow cannot be properly examined until the child is anesthesized. At this time, a mechanical block to flexion will be encountered in type I fractures. The proximal radius and medial epicondyle should be examined for associated injuries.[9]

DIFFERENTIAL DIAGNOSIS

Elbow injuries are very common in children. The capitellum has a normal anterior inclination on the lateral radiograph and its physeal line is usually wider posteriorly[11] (Fig. 16-4). This may be misinterpreted as an epiphyseal separation and, if in doubt, comparison radiographs of the opposite elbow are advisable.

A fracture of the lateral condyle may be confused with a fracture of the capitellum.[8,10] This is a type IV physeal fracture with the capitellum often comprising a major

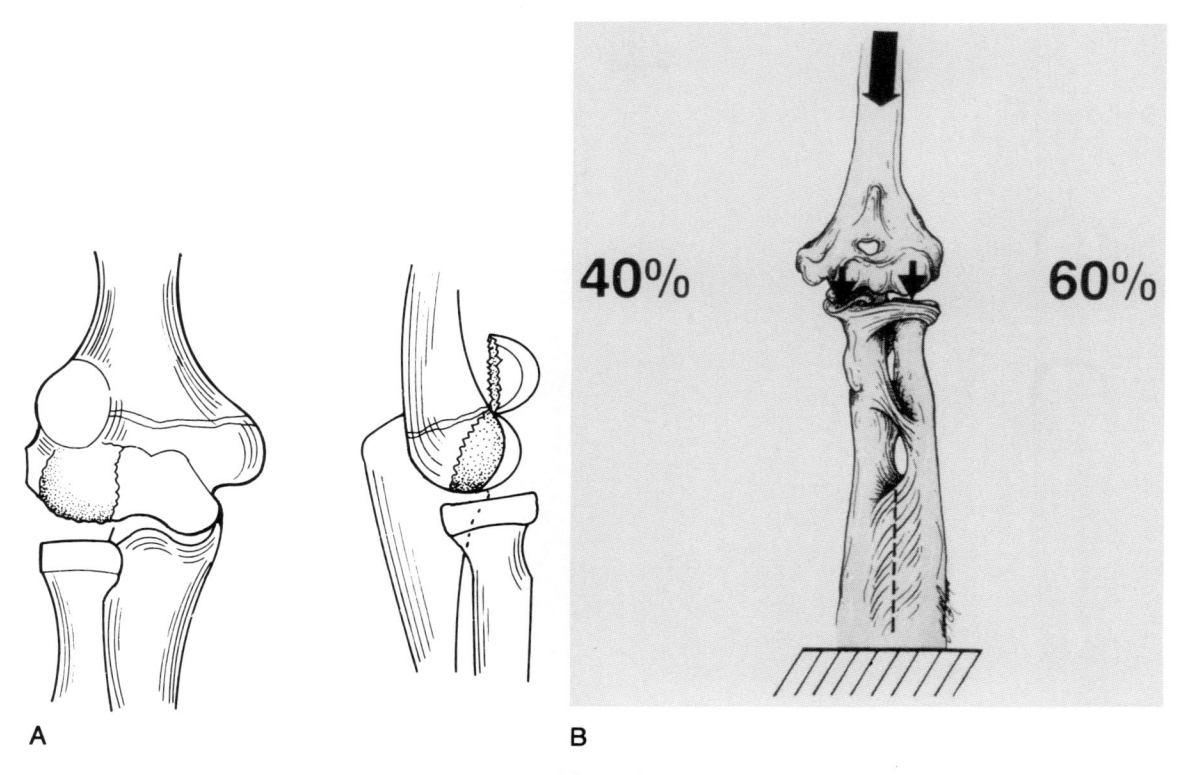

Fig. 16-7. (A) The more extended the elbow at impact the larger the capitellar fragment that is sheared off by the radial head. (B) The force exerted through the elbow in a fall on the outstretched arm is greater on the lateral side explaining the more frequent fracturing of the capitellum and lateral condyle than the medial condyle. (Figure B from Morrey BF: The Elbow and Its Disorders. p. 68. WB Saunders, Philadelphia, 1993. By permission of Mayo Foundation.)

portion of the fragment. The associated metaphyseal fragment of the humerus and the involvement of the entire capitellum within the fracture line are the distinguishing hallmarks of the type IV physeal injury (see Ch. 14).

A displaced type 1 fracture of the capitellum may not be obvious on the anteroposterior radiographs. The outline of the distal humerus is well preserved, and the fracture fragment may not be seen against the overlapping background of the distal humerus. A good lateral radiographic view is usually diagnostic. The capitellar fragment usually lies anterior and proximal to the distal humerus. In skeletally immature children, extension of the fracture into the non ossified trochlea will not be appreciated.

The findings of a minimally displaced type I fracture of the capitellum are subtle and include a displaced fatpad, a slight step at the fracture and a break in the coronoid line.

Small slice fractures of the capitellum may be hidden and require oblique views to be visualized radiographically. A displaced fracture of the coronoid process or flap fracture of the olecranon may mimic a type II fracture of the capitellum, especially if it has become entrapped in the elbow joint.[14]

TREATMENT

Fractures of the capitellum represent such a small proportion of elbow injuries in children that little has been published concerning their optimal treatment and prognosis.

There has been considerable controversy in the adult orthopaedic literature regarding the best method for the treatment of capitellar fractures.[12,13,15] Open reduction with internal fixation and excision of the fragment have been the two most commonly recommended methods, with excision being preferred by most authors. The advocates of early excision have shown no evidence of

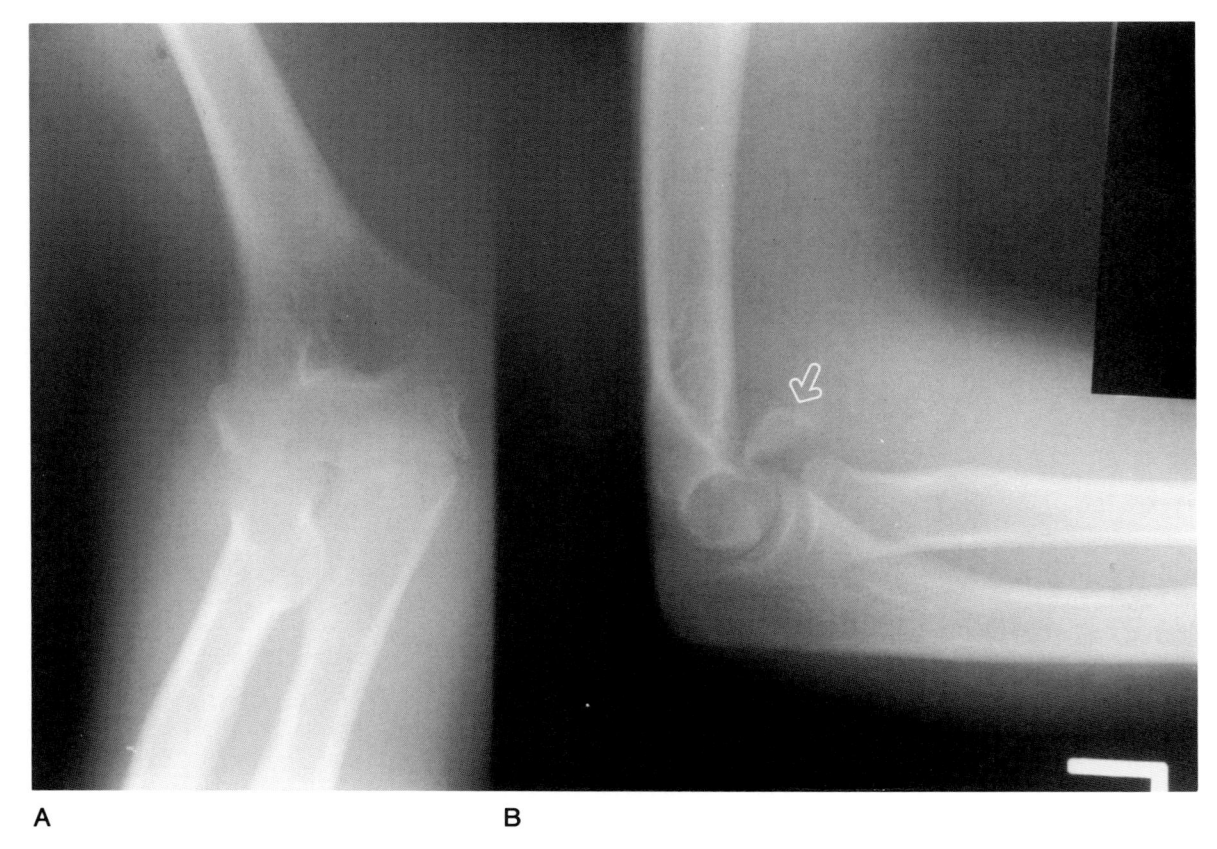

Fig. 16-8. Fracture of the capitellum in a 12-year-old girl illustrating the near-normal appearance of the AP radiograph in (**A**) and the capitellar fragment readily visible in the radial fossa (**B**).

valgus instability of the elbow resulting from the excision of the large capitellar fragment. They have emphasized that excision is a simple procedure and early motion of the elbow can be instituted.[2] In children, however, it would seem that open reduction and internal fixation, although difficult, is certainly the most physiologic. Replacing the fragment also avoids a large area of raw bone, which Watson-Jones[16] felt predisposed to adhesions and limitation of elbow motion. In children, the danger of avascular necrosis of the fragment is less than in the adult elbow.

We would favor treatment being individualized, taking into consideration the type of fracture, the presence or absence of comminution and associated elbow injuries, and the length of time from injury to treatment. Large fragments should be put back with open reduction and internal fixation and smaller comminuted fragments removed. Capitellar fractures that have been missed and not treated for 2 to 3 weeks should probably be removed rather than replaced.

Closed reduction has been accomplished by traction to the supinated forearm and then flexing the arm to 90 degrees and at the same time, applying direct pressure over the fragment. Few clinicians have found this to be a successful method. Closed reduction by a percutaneous probe under image intensification has also been described.[17] However, restoration of joint congruity is difficult to judge, the chances of displacement in children are high and immobilization for periods of greater than 3 to 4 weeks predisposes to elbow stiffness. The literature and our personal experience are not supportive of closed reduction, with most reports documenting loss of reduction and restricted elbow motion.

Open reduction and internal fixation allows restoration of joint congruity and avoids leaving a large raw surface of bone. However, internal fixation of the capitellar fragment is difficult. This is primarily because the fragment may be composed entirely of cartilage, thus maintaining a reduction with a screw may be impossible without damaging the articular surface. The use of bone pegs has been tried with poor results.[15] Biodegradable pin fixation of some elbow fractures has been success-

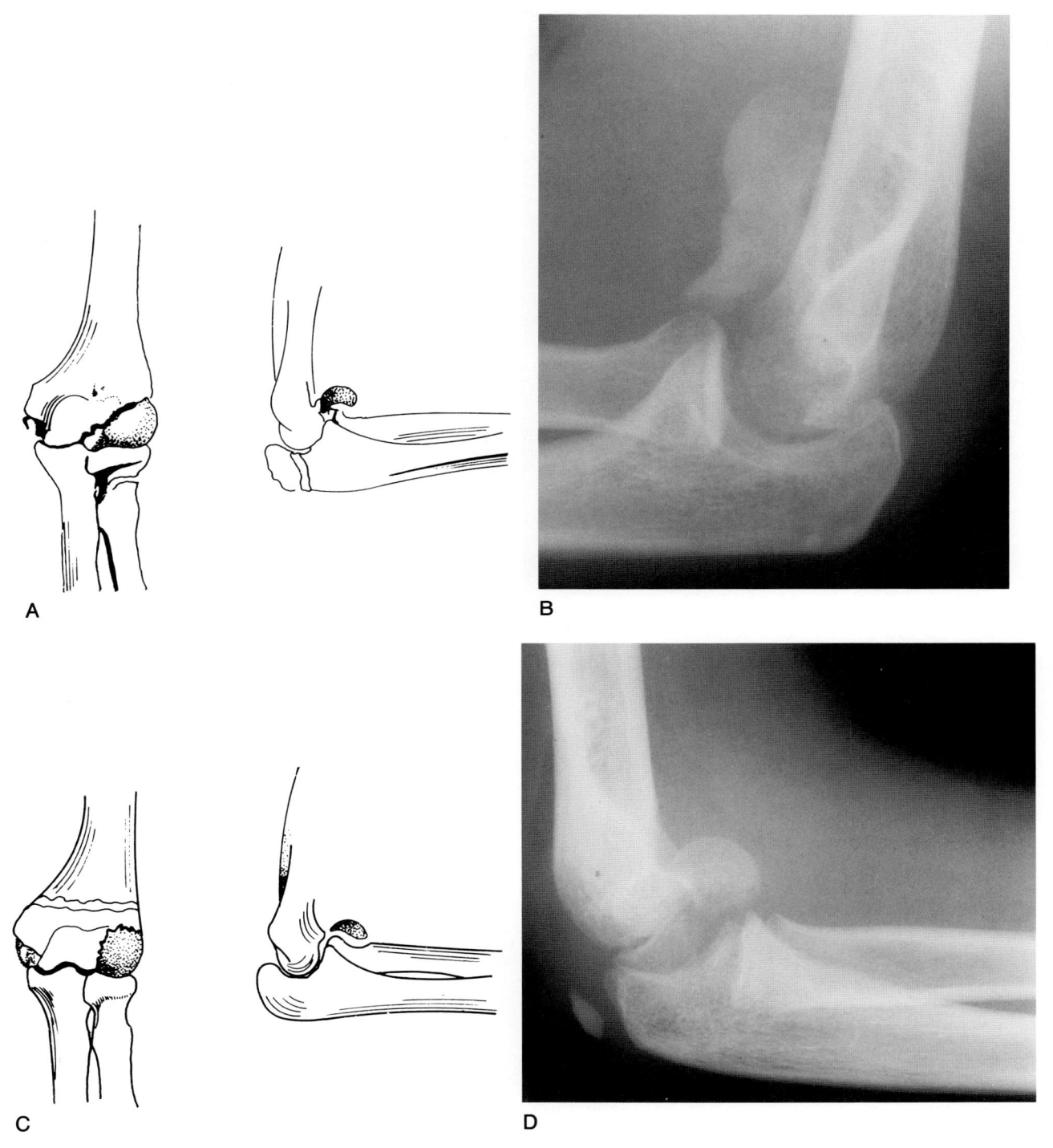

Fig. 16-9. Fractures of the capitellum in children. **(A&B)** Type I includes capitellum and portion of trochlea. **(C&D)** Type II is a slice fracture of only the capitellum.

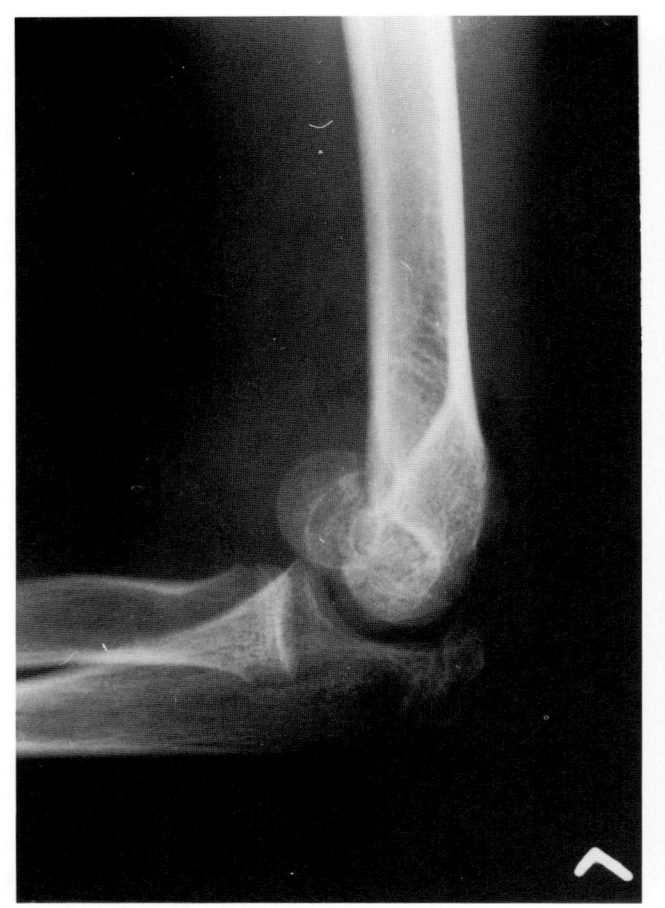

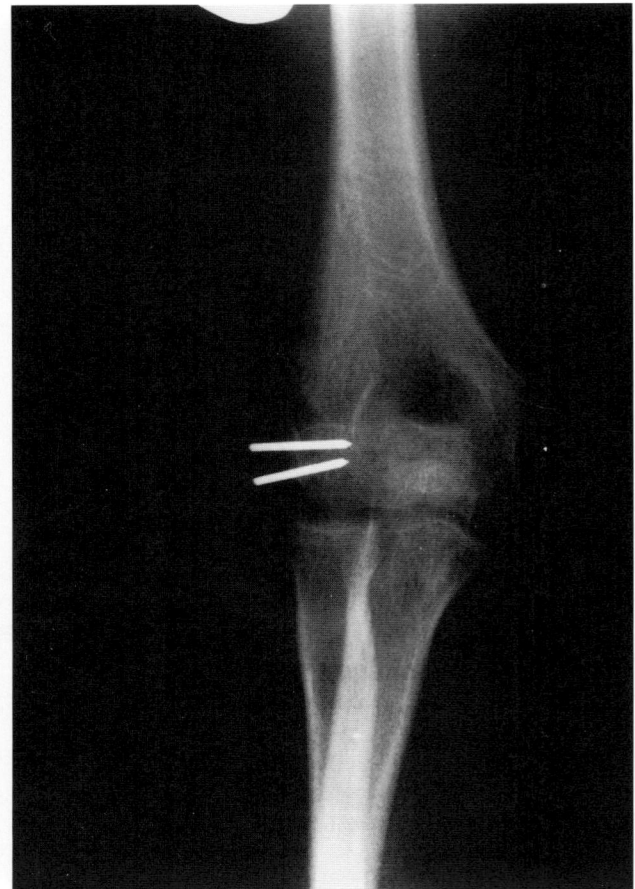

Fig. 16-10. **(A)** Type I fracture of the capitellum in a 12-year-old girl treated with open reduction and pinning in a postero-anterior direction **(B&C).** (Courtesy of Dr. Bill McIntyre, Children's Hospital of Eastern Ontario.)

fully described but not in capitellar fractures.[18] This technique may be an option for smaller capitellar fragments.[19] The use of K-wires to transfix the fracture in an anatomic position while the fracture is healing is a standard technique utilized in other pediatric fractures with little danger of growth arrest should the pin cross the physis. In some instances, it may be easier to insert the K-wire posteriorly through the distal humerus to transfix the capitellar fragment anteriorly. This technique also facilitates subsequent removal of the pins. We have employed this technique with success in four children and feel it is the type of internal fixation that can be recommended as being safe and effective for either type I or II fractures of the capitellum (Fig. 16-10). The use of the Herbert screw[6] or small canulated lag screw is another option available that has been successfully employed in small-fragment fixation, but is technically more difficult in a large, soft, cartilaginous fragment.

Postoperatively early protected motion following 3 to 4 weeks of plaster immobilization is appropriate postpinning or for undisplaced fractures.

Excision of the capitellar fragment is a simple and definitive procedure with a short postoperative immobilization period. Fowles has reported excellent short term results in two children, 14 and 15 years of age.[2] If excision is considered it must be ensured that the medial collateral ligament be maintained intact to prevent valgus instability[13] and elbow motion initiated within 10 days.

Excision of small fragments is recommended by most authors. Our only experience is in a 12-year-old girl who has had an excellent result at 4 years following excision of a small capitellar fragment. Johansson and colleagues[4] reported only a fair result at 1 year following similar treatment in a 12-year-old girl. In this case, the defect measured over 2.5 cm. These limited data suggest that, with significant defects, cartilage preservation by fragment replacement is preferable. Fibrin sealant has been recently recommended as a good alternative to traditional osteosynthesis techniques in these fractures [19] but we have no personal experience with this technique in the elbow.

COMPLICATIONS

As with all elbow injuries it is important to advise parents when their child is first seen that this is an intra-articular injury thus prone to residual limitation of elbow motion postoperatively. The possible complication of avascular necrosis in the retained fragment is less common in children than in adults. Cartilage damage either from the initial trauma or avascular necrosis may predispose to degenerative arthritis. Early diagnosis with replacement of large fragments by K-wire fixation and early elbow mobilization will avoid the major complication of elbow stiffness and boney blocks to flexion.

SUMMARY

Fractures of the capitellum are not common in children. However, the nature of the injury requires early optimal treatment for a successful long-term outcome. Treatment should be individualized taking into consideration the type of fracture, associated elbow injuries, skeletal maturity of the patient, and technical abilities of the surgeon. Large fragments should be anatomically replaced and internally fixed with Kirschner wires. Small fragments should be removed. Early active elbow motion following these procedures usually ensures a good result.

REFERENCES

1. Cooper, Sir A: Fracture of the external condyle of the humerus. p. 508. In Lee, AC (ed): A Treatise on Dislocations and Fractures of the Joints. Vol. I. Joseph Butler, London, 1841
2. Fowles JV, Kossob MT: Fracture of the capitellum humeri: treatment by excision. J Bone Joint Surg [Am] 56:794, 1974
3. Granthem SA, Norris TR, Bush DC: Isolated fracture of the humeral capitellum. Clin Orthop 161:262, 1981
4. Johansson J, Rosman M: Fracture of the capitellum humeri in children: a rare injury often misdiagnosed. Clin Orthop 146:157, 1980
5. Lensinger O, Mare K: Fracture of the capitellum humeri. Acta Orthop Scand 52:39, 1981
6. Liberman N, Kota T, Howard CB et al: Fixation of the capitellar fractures with the Herbert screw. Acta Orthop Trauma Surg 110:155, 1991
7. Rockwood CA Jr, Wilkins KE, King RE: Fractures in Children. 3rd Ed. JB Lippincott, Philadelphia, 1991
8. Agins HA, Marcus NW: Articular cartilage sleeve fracture of the lateral humeral condyle capitellum: a previously described entity. J Pediatr Orthop 4:620, 1984
9. Ward WG, Nunley JA: Concomitant fractures of the capitellum and radial head. J Orthop Trauma 2:110, 1988
10. Alvarez E, Patel MR, Nimberg G, Pearlman HS: Fracture of the capitellum humeri. J Bone Joint Surg [Am] 57:1093, 1975

11. Silberstein MJ, Brodeur AE, Graviss ER: Some vagaries of the capitellum. J Bone Joint Surg [Am] 61:244, 1979
12. Collert S: Surgical management of fracture of the capitellum humeri. Acta Orthop Scand 48:603, 1977
13. Dushuttle RP, Coyle MD, Zawadsky JP et al: Fractures of the capitellum. J Trauma 25:317, 1985
14. Blasier RD: Intra-articular flap fracture of the olecranon in a child. J Bone Joint Surg [Am] 71:945, 1989
15. Rhodin Rolf: On the treatment of fracture of the capitellum. Acta Clin Scand 86:475, 1942
16. Watson-Jones R: Fractures and Joint Injuries. 5th Ed. p. 609. Williams & Wilkens, Baltimore, 1976
17. Yuan-Zhang M, Chun-Bo Z, Tai-Len Z et al: Percutaneous probe reduction of frontal fractures of the humeral capitellum. Clin Orthop 183:17, 1984
18. Hope PG, Williamson DM, Coates CJ, Cole WG: Biodegradable pin fixation of elbow fractures in children. J Bone Joint Surg [Br] 73:965, 1991
19. Plaga BR, Royster RM, Donigian AM et al: Fixation of osteochondral fractures in rabbit knees. J Bone Joint Surg [Br] 74:292, 1992
20. Scapinelli R: Treatment of fractures of the humeral capitellum using fibrin sealant. Acta Orthop Trauma Surg 109:235, 1990

17

Monteggia and Galeazzi Fractures

R. Mervyn Letts

> Those of you who think you know it all are very annoying to those of us who do!
> —Ian MacNab

The Monteggia and the Galeazzi fractures were initially described in adults where the injuries are fairly easily recognized and treated in most instances by open reduction. In children, these fractures are seldom of the classic variety and frequently are variations of the standard classifications. This is primarily due to the presence of adjacent growth plates and an increased ligamentous laxity and flexible bone structure that are present in the skeletally immature.

THE PEDIATRIC MONTEGGIA FRACTURE-DISLOCATION

The Monteggia injury is uncommon in children in its classic form but when the equivalent injuries are included it is by no means a rare fracture. Although the true incidence of Monteggia fracture-dislocations is not well documented, it is more common than has been generally appreciated. The Monteggia fracture complex was first documented in 1814 by Giovanni Monteggia.[1,2] The classic fracture was traditionally described as a fracture of the ulna in the proximal third with a dislocation of the radius, either anteriorly or posteriorly. Few publications appeared regarding this fracture until Cunningham[3] in 1934 emphasized its importance, and in 1940 Speed and Boyd[4,5] emphasized treatment and noted the poor results of the missed Monteggia fracture dislocation. Until recently, few authors addressed the "unique equivalent" injuries that create the same injury, although with different fracture patterns. In 1962 Bado[6] addressed some of the equivalent injuries but did not include them in his classification of Monteggia fractures.

Mechanism of Injury

Hyperextension at the elbow joint is the most common cause of the Monteggia fracture dislocation in children.[7] This results in an anterior dislocation of the radial head and a fracture of the ulna with anterior angulation. Hyperpronation of the forearm is another mechanism resulting in the Monteggia injury due to a levering of the proximal radius anteriorly combined with an increased mechanical advantage of the contracting biceps and a stronger pull on the radius by the bicipital tendon as the bicipital tuberosity is more posterior in hyperpronation.[8] This predisposes to anterior dislocation of the radius. This mechanism is less significant in younger children as the force generated by the biceps is less than in adults, and the mechanism is probably operative only in older children (Fig. 17-1). A direct blow over the arm raised in

296 / Management of Pediatric Fractures

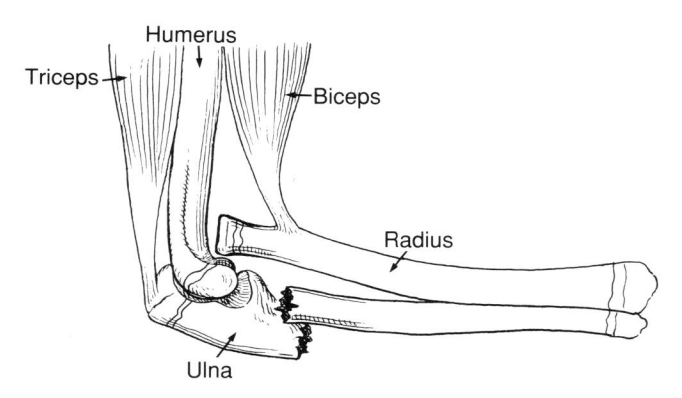

Fig. 17-1. The Monteggia fracture dislocation. The biceps pulls the radius anteriorly. The triceps pulls the ulnar olecranon fragment (U) posteriorly. (Modified from Caffey J: Pediatric X-ray Diagnosis. 6th Ed. p. 1098. Year Book Medical Publishers, Chicago, 1972.)

protection will produce a Monteggia lesion, and this is a mechanism sometimes seen in adolescent athletes engaged in sports such as hockey and lacrosse.[9]

The forearm bones in children also have considerable inherent elasticity, which may allow the radial head and neck to slip under the annular ligament as both the radial and ulnar shaft bends. In this injury the child will present with an isolated dislocation of the radial head without the usual concomitant fracture of the ulna[10,11] (Figs. 17-2 and 17-3).

Classification

Standard classifications of the Monteggia fracture complex in the adults do not take into consideration the equivalent injuries frequently encountered in children (Fig. 17-4). Although the Bado classification[12] can be applied to the more classic Monteggia lesions that occur in children, many of the so-called equivalent lesions will

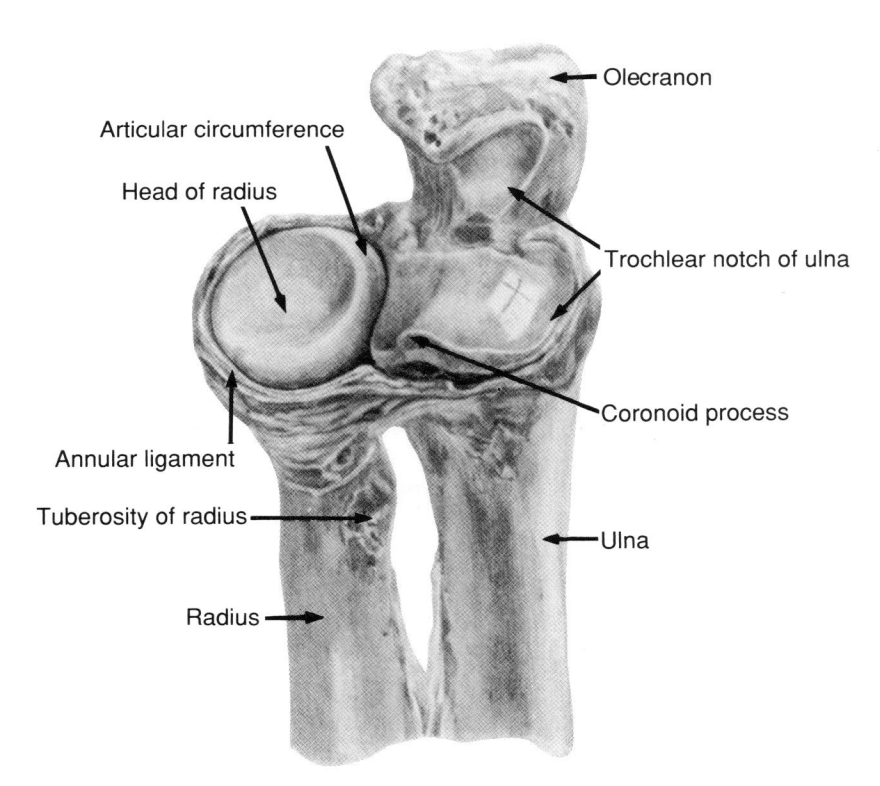

Fig. 17-2. Relationship of annular ligament to the neck and head of the radius. (From Langman J, Woerdeman MW: Atlas of Medical Anatomy. WB Saunders, Philadelphia, 1976, with permission.)

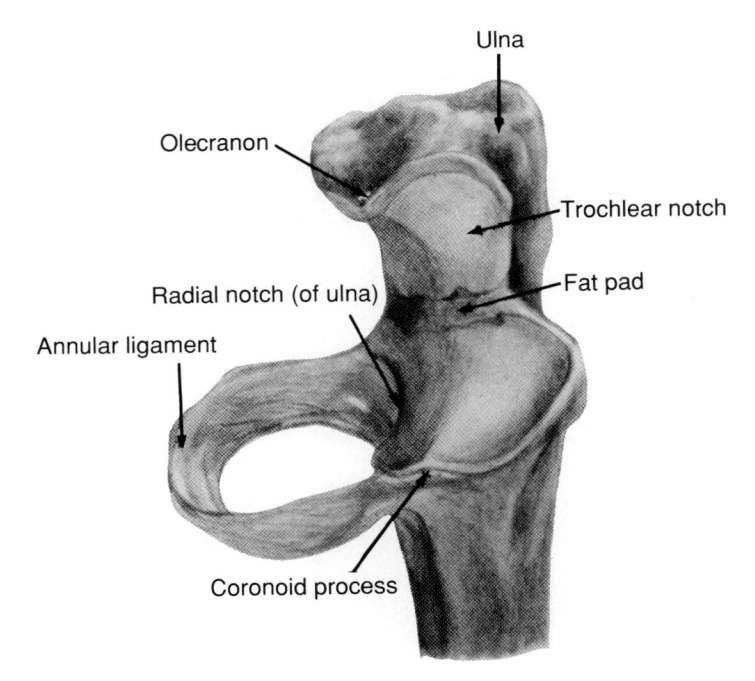

Fig. 17-3. Attachments of the annular ligament to the ulna. (From Langman J, Woerdeman MW: Atlas of Medical Anatomy. WB Saunders, Philadelphia, 1976, with permission.)

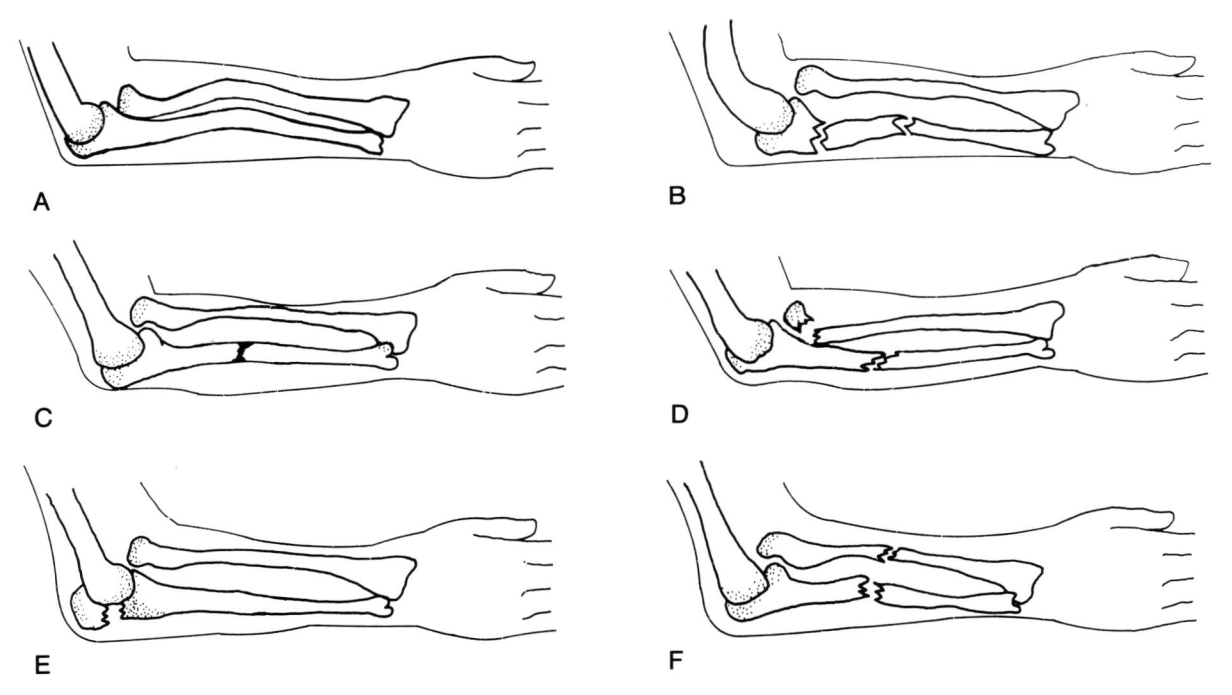

Fig. 17-4. Monteggia equivalent injuries that may be encountered in children. **(A)** Bowing of radius and ulna with dislocation of radial head. **(B)** Fracture of olecranon plus shaft of ulna with radial head dislocation. **(C)** Bowing of radius and ulna with greenstick fracture of ulna and anterior dislocation of radial head. **(D)** Fracture of ulna with fracture of neck of radius and dislocation of radial head fragment. **(E)** Fracture of olecranon with dislocation of radial head. **(F)** Fracture of shaft of both radius and ulna with dislocation of the radial head.

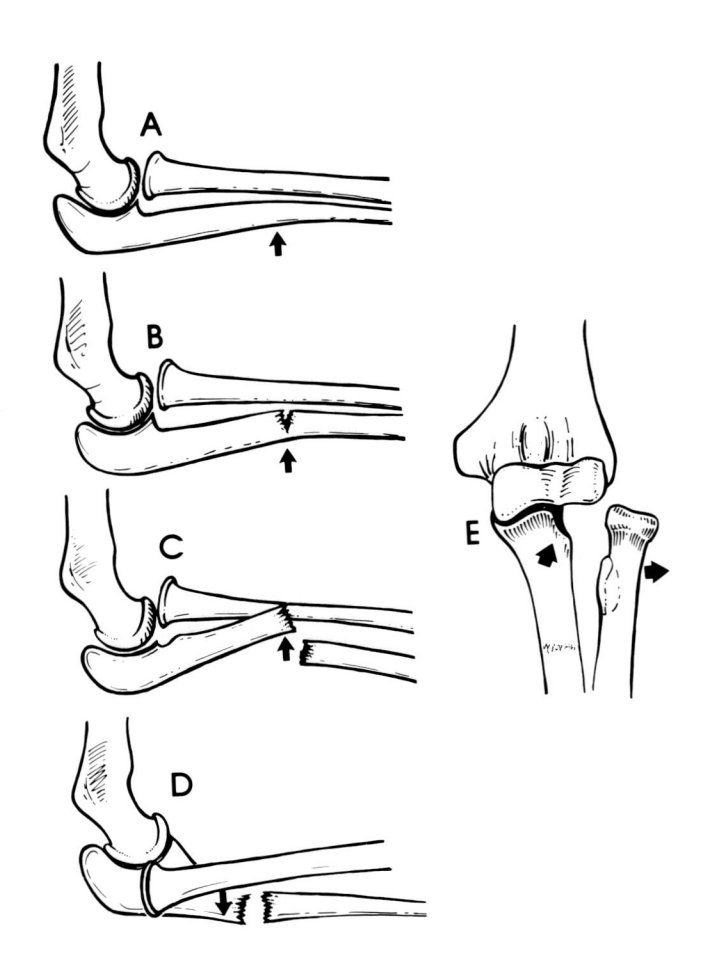

Fig. 17-5. Classification of Monteggia fractures in children — types A–E. (From Letts et al.,[7] with permission.)

be missed. To emphasize the differences in the configuration of the injury in childhood a classification has been devised to include dislocation of the radial head associated with variations secondary to the elasticity of the forearm bones in childhood[7,13] (Fig. 17-5). The most common types of Monteggia fracture dislocations are anterior dislocation of the radial head and lateral dislocation of the radial head associated with ulnar fracture or bending (Fig. 17-6). Ulnar fractures may occur at any level in children, even through the olecranon, and all should be classified as a Monteggia injury, since the principles of treatment are the same.

Types of Monteggia-Equivalent Lesions

As illustrated in the classification outlined in Figure 17-5 the commonest type of equivalent lesions are associated with anterior dislocation of the head of the radius and ulnar bending with no visible fracture or with a greenstick fracture (Fig. 17-7). Other variations, however, do occur, one being the fracture of the olecranon with or without a fracture of the ulnar shaft and a dislocation of the radial head (Fig. 17-8). Fracture of the ulna with fracture of the radial neck and dislocation of the radial head fragment is an unusual Monteggia equivalent injury but one that usually requires an open reduction of the head of the radius to avoid malunion and continued growth of the radial neck and head in a lateral direction.

Various combinations and permutations of these fractures can be sustained in the pediatric age group as illustrated in Figure 17-4. All are related to the inherent elasticity that the radius and ulna possess at this age and the amount of bend that these bones may undergo before fracturing.[14] The radius may bend to the extent that the head and neck of the radius slip underneath the annular ligament, or the ligament may become detached along one of its ulnar borders, resulting in an apparent "isolated" dislocation of the radial head.

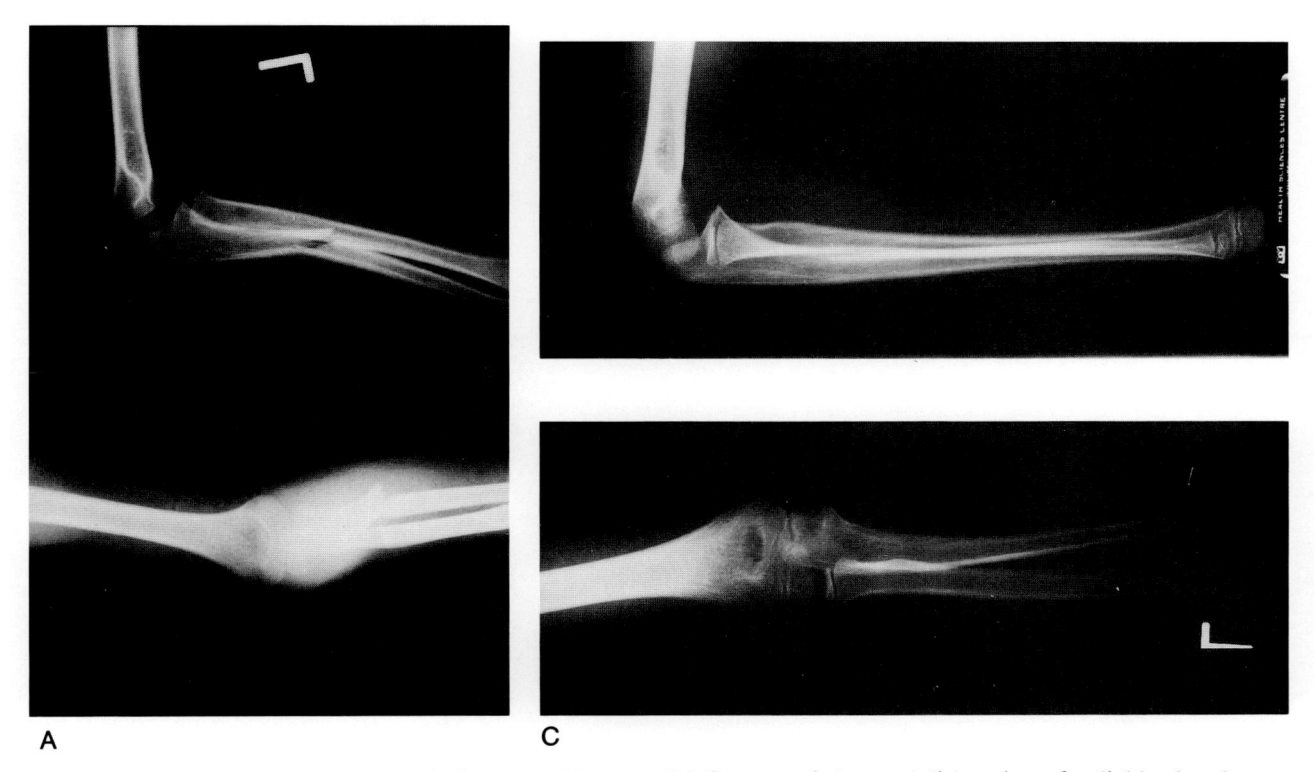

Fig. 17-6. (A) Type B Monteggia fracture with greenstick fracture of ulna and dislocation of radial heal and (B&C) following a closed reduction and 5 weeks immobilization.

Clinical Course

A classic appearance of the Monteggia fracture-dislocation in children is as illustrated in Figure 17-9. The radial head is usually seen tenting the skin, especially when it is displaced laterally. The fracture of the ulna is also usually quite obvious. The presence of an isolated fracture of the ulna no matter where in the shaft it is located should always prompt careful evaluation of the radial head. A mental line drawn through the shaft and neck of the radius should always intercept the capitellum in all views taken (Fig.17-10). If it does not, dislocation of the radial head should be suspected. A complete fracture of the ulna is not a prerequisite for an associated radial head dislocation in children, as the ulna may simply bend or sustain a minor greenstick fracture. Disruption of the forearm parallelogram occurs as a result of this ulnar bend, as well as an associated radial shaft bend and a slippage of the radial head out from under the annular ligament. The apex of the ulnar bend or angulation will always be in the direction of the radial head dislocation. Adequate radiographs must be obtained in both the anteroposterior (AP) and lateral planes to ensure that the pediatric Monteggia-equivalent lesions will not be missed (Fig.17-11).

Treatment

Most of the various types of fracture-dislocations of the Monteggia variety can be treated by closed manipulation in the pediatric age group. Straightening the angulated ulna will often result in the radial head reducing spontaneously but if not, pressure over the dislocated radial head will usually result in a stable reduction (Fig. 17-12). It is important that the stability of the reduction of radial head be maintained by flexion of the elbow to more than 90 degrees (Fig. 17-13). Keeping the forearm in supination assists in minimizing the pull of the biceps. In the less-common type D Monteggia fracture, with posterior dislocation of the head, stability must be achieved by extension and *not* flexion of the elbow.

Provided the radial head is well reduced angulation of the ulna up to 15 degrees can be accepted and will remodel out satisfactorily over the next year. If the ulna

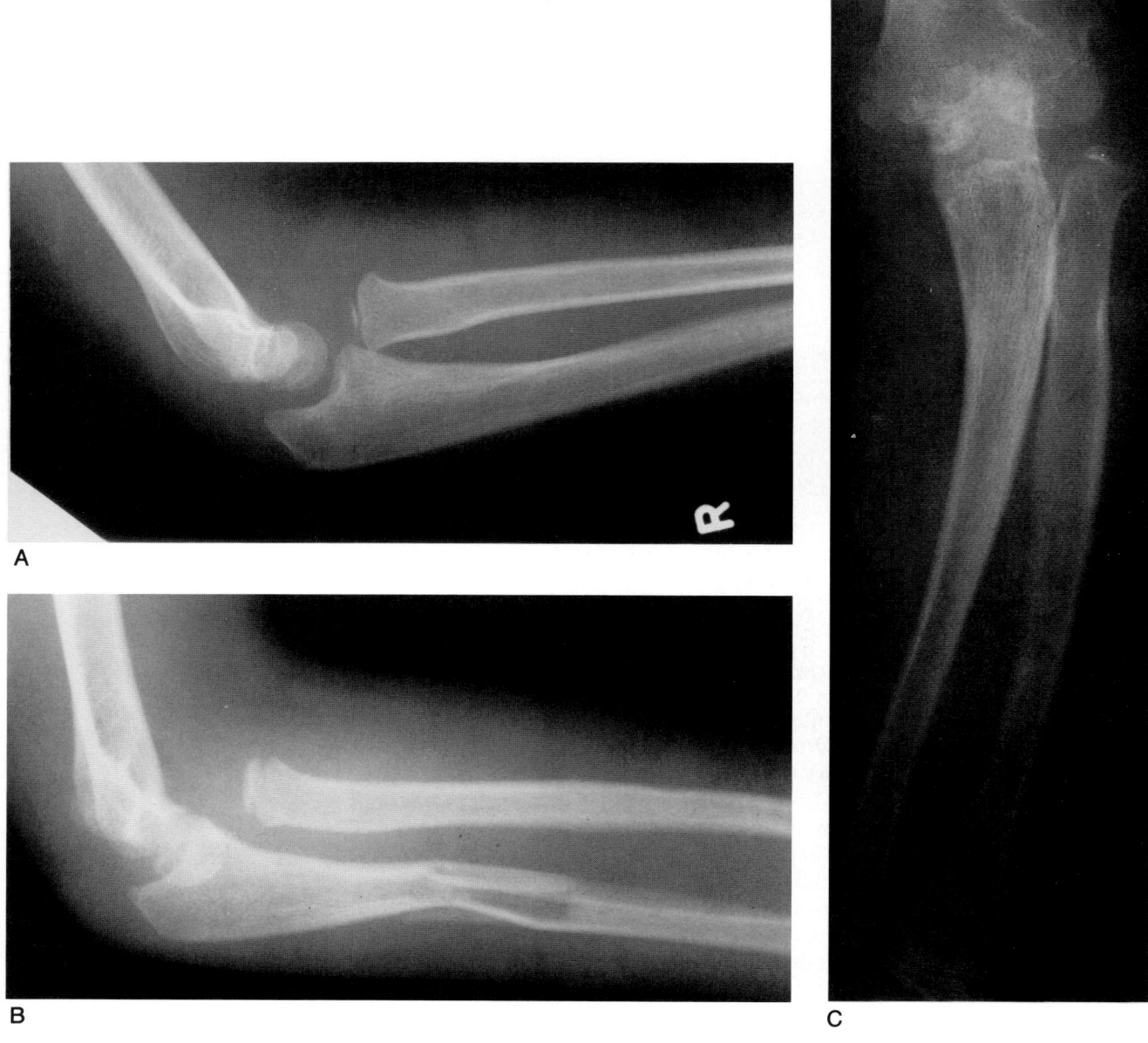

Fig. 17-7. (A) Anterior bowing of the ulna with anterior dislocation of the radial head. (B) Greenstick fracture of the ulna with anterior dislocation of the radial head. (C) Type A Monteggia equivalent fracture illustrating a bowed ulna with lateral dislocation of the head of the radius in a 6-year-old girl who fell off a play structure.

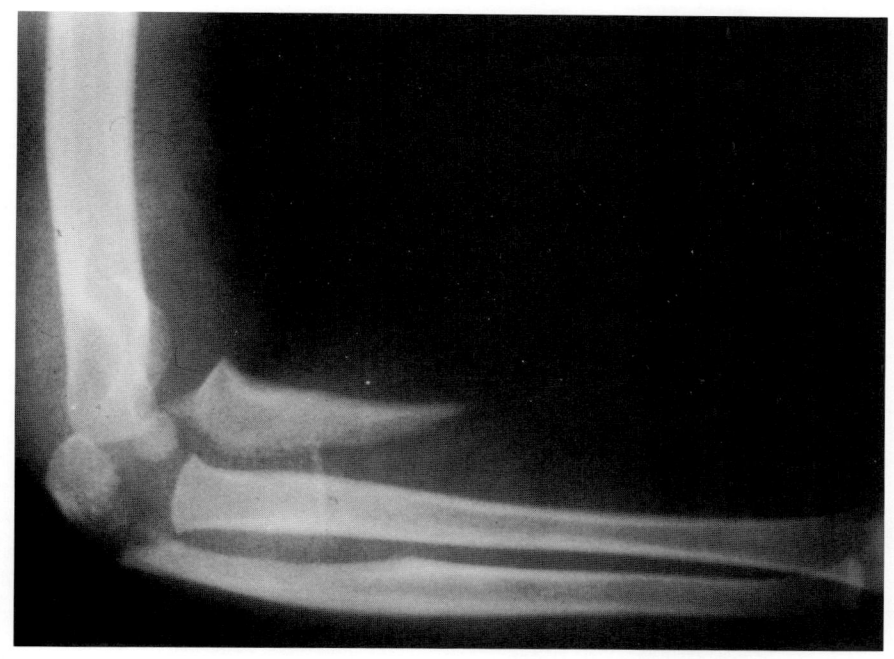

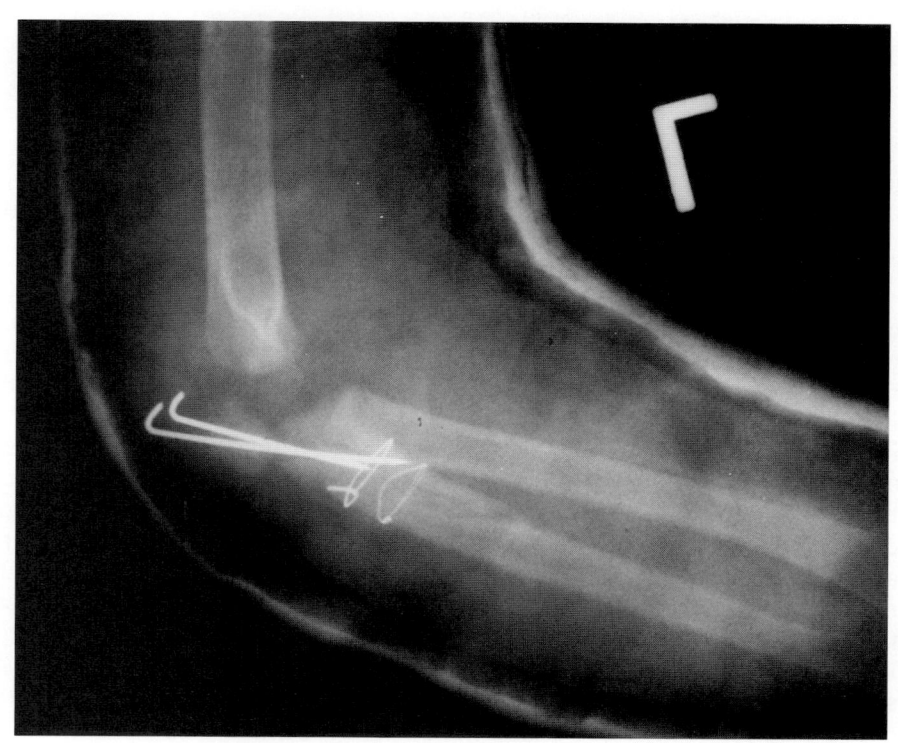

Fig. 17-8. (A) Monteggia equivalent fracture in a 5-year-old girl whose arm was caught under a closing garage door. An olecranon fracture and proximal ulnar fracture has occurred with a posterior dislocation of the radial head. (B) The ulna was reduced and internally fixed with K-wires and cerclage wires. The radial head is now reduced.

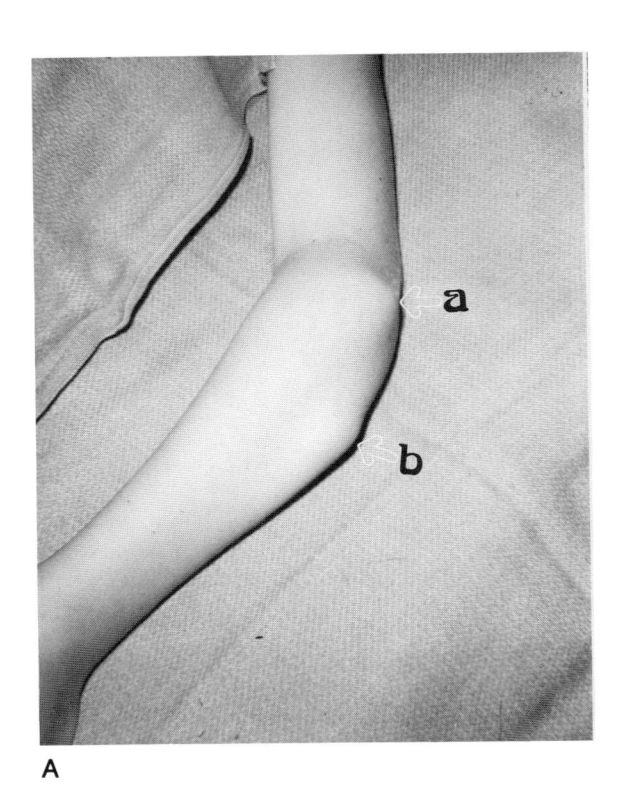

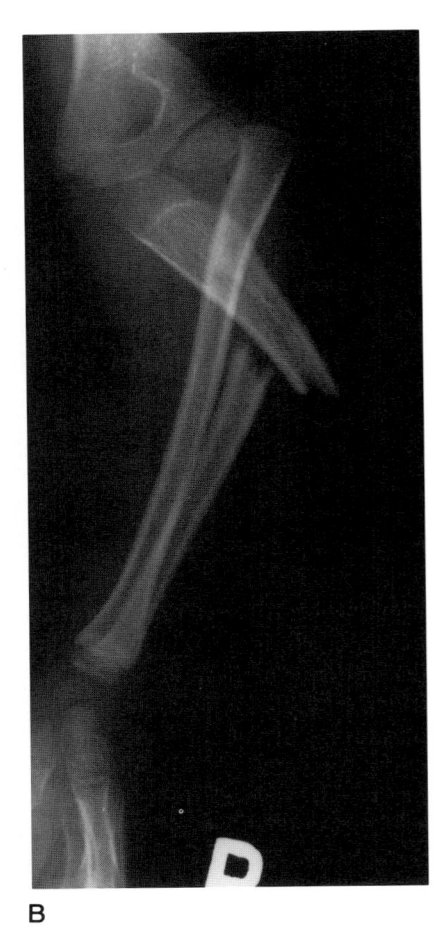

Fig. 17-9. (A) Clinical appearance of a type E Monteggia fracture-dislocation. The laterally dislocated head of radius *(a)* and the angulated fracture of the ulna *(b)* can be seen. (B) Radiographic appearance of the same arm.

cannot be adequately reduced to allow a radial head reduction, an open reduction of the ulna may be rarely required and alignment can often be achieved with an intramedullary pin (Fig. 17-14). If the radial head is still irreducible in spite of bringing the ulna into normal alignment a supination-pronation maneuver may facilitate repositioning of the annular ligament, which is seldom completely torn off but often detached usually at its anterior attachment to the ulna. If the radial head remains irreducible an open reduction is necessary through a posterolateral Kocher incision and the annular ligament reapproximated to the radial neck. Occasionally, internal fixation of the radial neck will be required due to marked instability or a fracture through the radial neck. It is best to internally fix the radius to the ulna with a Kirschner wire rather than trying to maintain the reduction by a wire inserted through the capitellum and into the radial head (Fig. 17-15). This type of fixation results in micromovement of the elbow and fatiguing of the pin with breakage requiring a more formal elbow arthrotomy to remove the broken fragments. Immobilization of the elbow for 4 weeks ensures adequate healing of the annular ligament and stability of the radial head. In older children and adolescents, immobilization will be required for 6 weeks to allow the ulnar fracture to heal, but the last 2 weeks can usually be accomplished with a below-elbow or Munster type of cast to allow elbow motion (Fig. 17-16).

In children most Monteggia injuries recognized and treated early go on to a good long-term result. Some long-term reviews of Monteggia fractures in children have indicated minor degrees of loss of flexion and some hyperextension possibly related to the mechanism of injury.[7,15-17] Increased epiphyseal maturation on the ef-

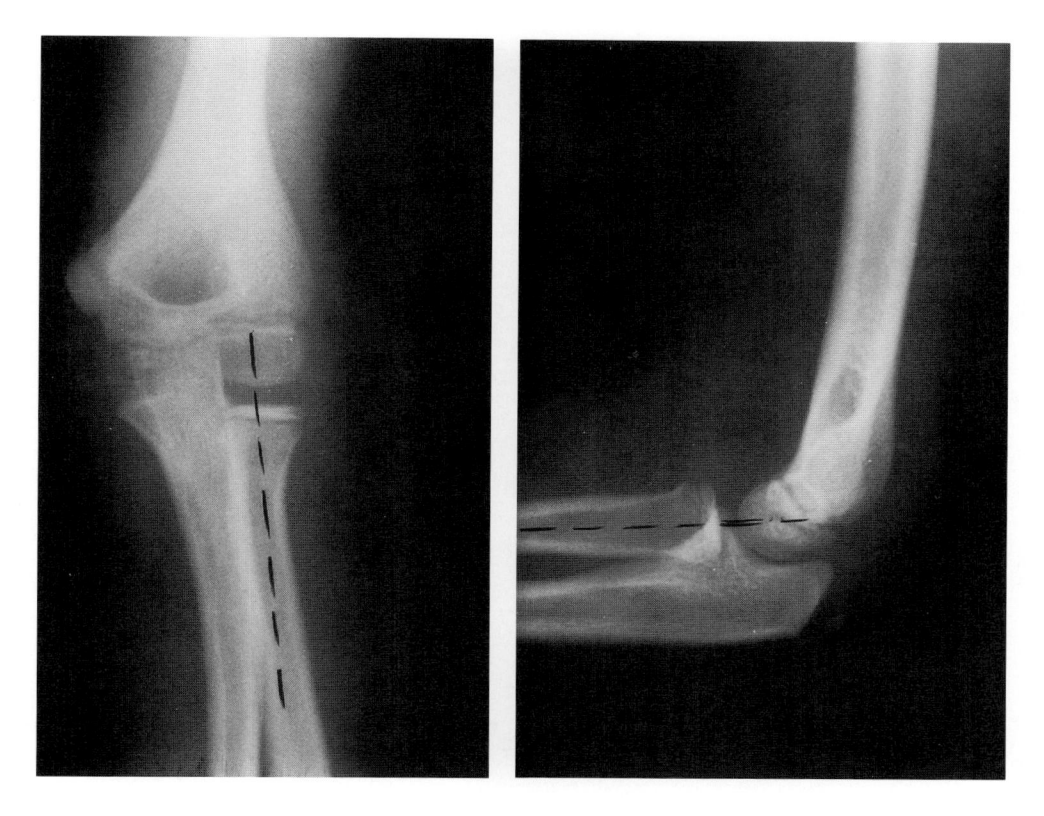

Fig. 17-10. In all elbow injuries in children a mental line should be drawn through the proximal shaft of the radius and it should always intersect the capitellum in every radiographic view.

fected side has been noted but has had no effect on elbow function.[16] Mild radial head subluxation has been noted in some children subsequent to the Monteggia fracture-dislocation but this is usually of a minor degree measuring from 3 to 6 mm. This does not seem to affect elbow joint motion and may actually be related to an eccentric development of the ossific nucleus of the radial head after injury rather than true subluxation[18] (Fig. 17-17).

The "Missed Monteggia Lesion"

Unfortunately the Monteggia fracture-dislocation, especially in children, is frequently misinterpreted as a simple ulnar fracture and the dislocation of the radial head may be unappreciated by clinicians not familiar with this complex fracture.[19-21] Fortunately most films are read by experienced radiologists and the lesion may be picked up a week to 10 days later. At this point the fracture can be treated as if it were an acute injury and the result is still usually quite satisfactory. In some instances, however, the dislocated radial head may not be identified for months or even years after the initial injury has occurred. There may even be some controversy as to whether the dislocated radial head is congenital or developmental rather than traumatic. The contour of the radial head in this instance is usually very helpful with the congenital lesion having a convex appearance to the head, whereas the more recently dislocated radial head usually has a typical concave appearance. In the younger child this may be less reliable due to the large cartilaginous component of the radial head and neck (Fig. 17-18).

Children with undiagnosed Monteggia lesions presenting after 3 weeks will usually require an open reduction of the radial head. It is probably worthwhile to attempt a closed reduction up to 6 or 8 weeks postinjury; however, once the radial head has been out of joint for longer than 3 or 4 weeks, the annular ligament becomes fibrotic and matted together, preventing an adequate reduction. In children a persistent angulation of the ulna can usually be straightened by a closed reduction up to 6

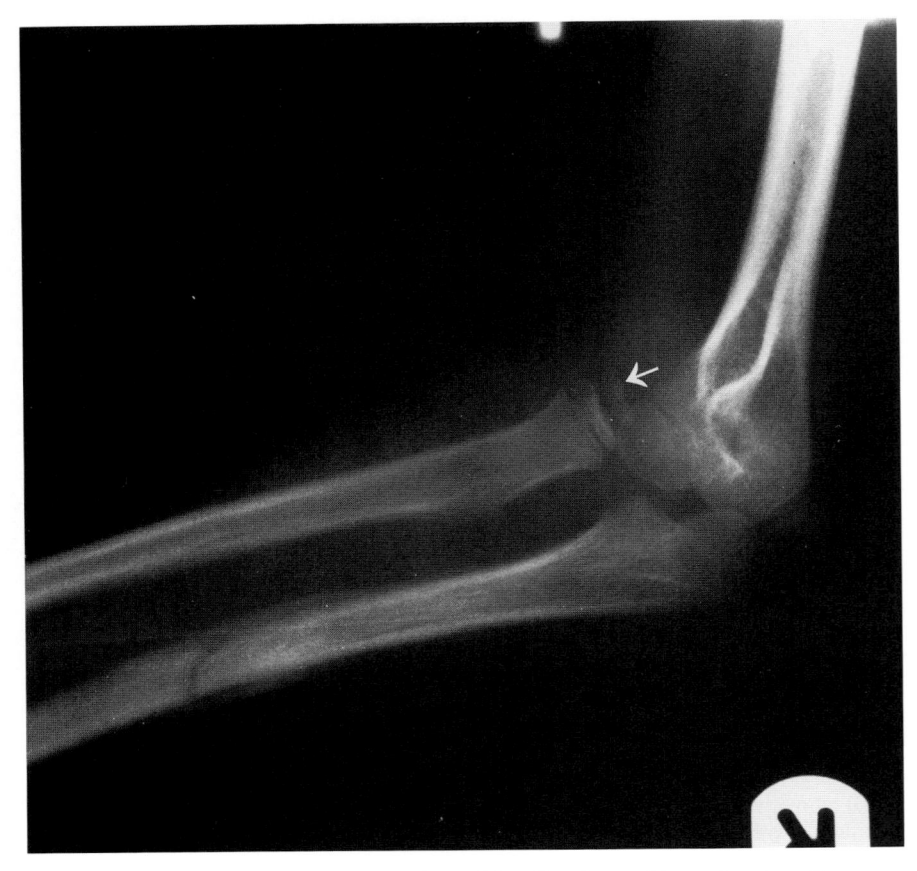

Fig. 17-11. "Missed" Monteggia fracture-dislocation with callus formation at the ulnar fracture and persistent dislocation of the radial head. The *arrow* points to a loose fragment — the coronoid process of the ulna — suggesting a probable dislocation of the entire elbow at the moment of impact.

to 8 weeks postinjury. After that time an ulnar osteotomy is usually necessary. Straightening the ulna frequently provides sufficient lengthening to allow radial head reduction. If not, a lengthening of the ulna may be necessary.

Fascial Reconstruction of the Annular Ligament

In neglected Monteggia injuries seen later than 3 to 4 weeks it may be necessary to provide a reconstruction of the annular ligament in order to maintain the radial head reduction. The reduction of the radial head may have to be facilitated with an osteoclasis or formal osteotomy of the ulna if there has been considerable bending or shortening of the ulna and union is solid. This in effect will lengthen the ulna and allow the radial head to be reduced. The techniques that can be used to reconstruct the annular ligament are (1) triceps fascial reconstruction and (2) forearm fascial reconstruction. Both techniques are essentially the same, other than the fact that either the triceps tendon or the overlying forearm fascia is utilized to reconstitute the annular ligaments in the second technique (Fig. 17-19).

TRICEPS ANNULAR LIGAMENT
RECONSTRUCTION

The technique of triceps annular ligament reconstruction was described by Lloyd-Roberts and Bucknill[11] and popularized by Bell Tause.[22] A posterolateral incision is preferred rather than a posterior incision. which may disorientate the surgeon somewhat to the position of the radial head. The triceps tendon is identified and a long 10-cm strip is removed from the lateral margin ensuring

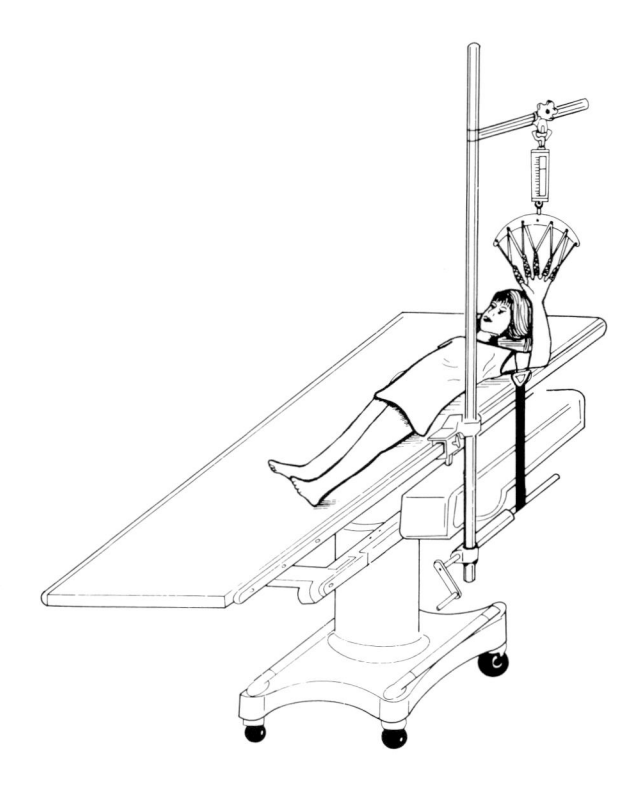

Fig. 17-12. Chinese finger-trap method of forearm traction useful in facilitating closed reduction of fractures of the radius and ulna, including Monteggia fractures and equivalents.

the attachment at the distal ulnar insertion. The tendon is increased in length by continuing the dissection through the periosteum of the ulna to a point opposite the neck of the radius, where it is then passed around the neck and sutured to itself and the ulnar periosteum with enough tension to hold the radial head in place. A Kirschner wire is then passed through the ulna into the radius to assure solid fixation until the tendon has healed (Fig. 17-15). The extremity is kept immobilized in an above elbow cast for 4 weeks at which time the percutaneous K-wire is removed and splinting continued for a further 2 weeks. Gradual mobilization is then begun at 6 weeks. Usually the entire remnant of the annual ligament needs to be removed to allow adequate reduction of the radial head due to the infolding and fibroses that occurs in the residual annual ligament.

Caution must be exercised, however, when exposing the neck of the radius in a child as the normal anatomic guidelines that apply to adult anatomy are not applicable in the smaller arm (Fig. 17-20). The radial nerve may only be a fingerbreadth below the head of the radius rather than the classic three fingerbreadths that is often used as a standard of measurement for locating the radial nerve in adults.

FOREARM FASCIAL RECONSTRUCTION OF THE ANNULAR LIGAMENT

This technique was described by Boyd[4,23] and is more applicable in the teenager rather than the younger child. A thinner fascial envelope exists in the younger child around the forearm muscles. A strip of fascia is dissected off the forearm muscles but left attached to the proximal ulnar attachment. The length of this fascial strip should be about 10 cm × 2 cm. It is passed under the neck of the radius proximal to the tuberosity and distal to the radial notch of the ulna, and is brought around and fastened to itself with nonabsorbable sutures (Fig. 17-19). Care should be taken to ensure that the length of this fascial strip is adequate. Cross radioulnar pin fixation for 4 weeks is recommended with active mobilization of the elbow at 6 weeks.

Long-Standing Untreated Monteggia Fracture-Dislocations

Long-standing Monteggia fracture-dislocations of more than 3 months will present major reconstructive surgical problems and each case needs to be assessed on

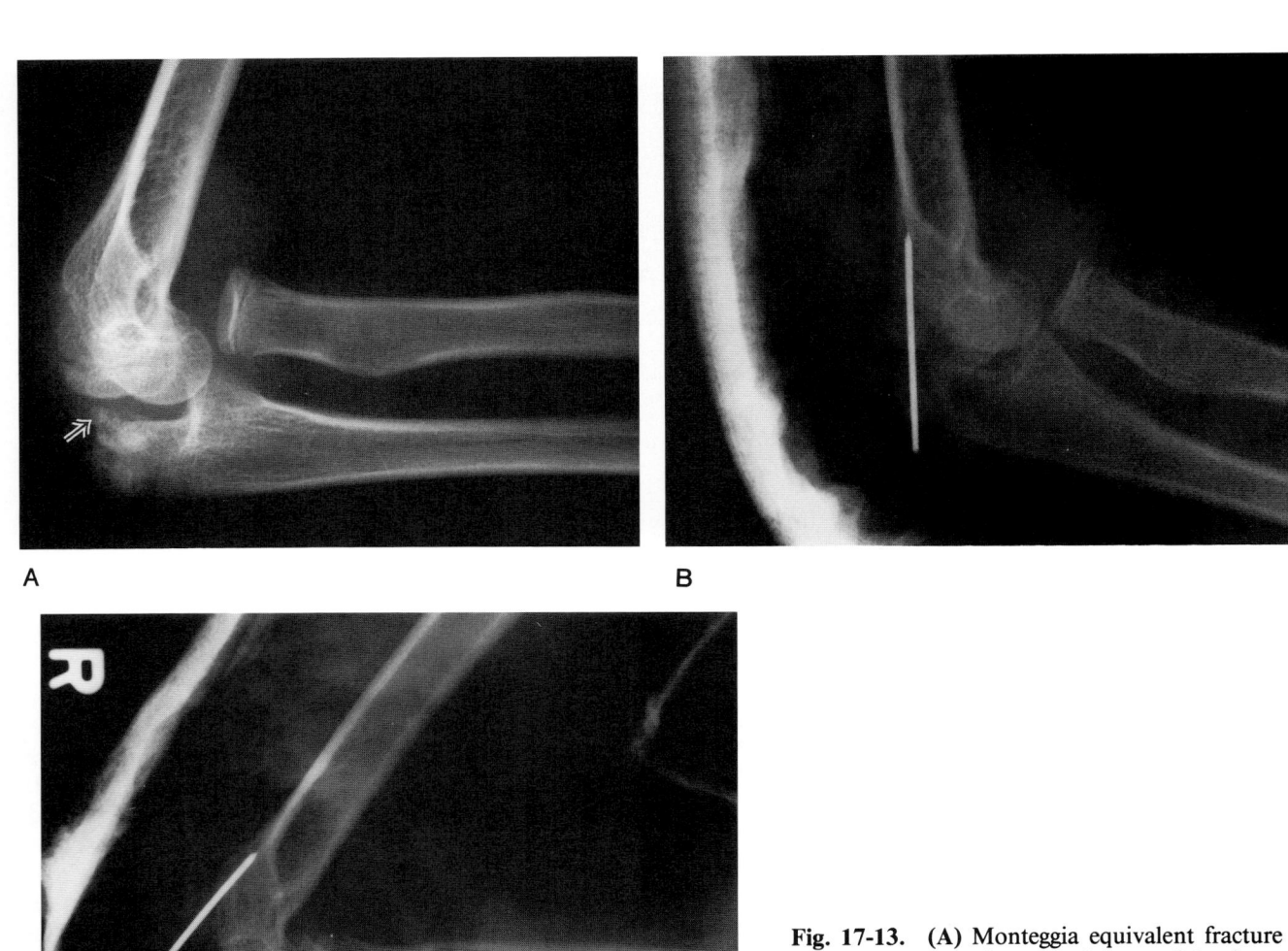

Fig. 17-13. (A) Monteggia equivalent fracture with an associated fracture of the medial epicondyle that was trapped in the joint. (B) The initial reduction of the radial head was lost as there is too much extension of the elbow. (C) This has been corrected by flexing the elbow to 105 degrees with a normal capitellar-radial head alignment. (Case contributed by Dr William MacIntyre, Children's Hospital of Eastern Ontario, Ottawa, Canada.)

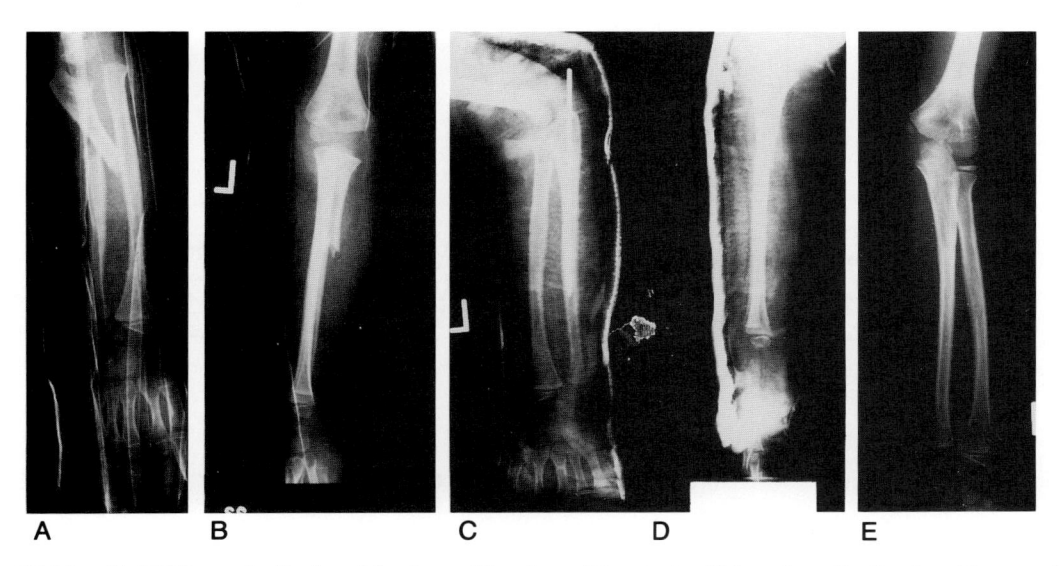

Fig. 17-14. **(A&B)** Severely displaced fracture of the ulna with anterior dislocation of radius in a 10-year-old boy in whom closed reduction could not be maintained. **(C)** An intramedullary small steinman pin held the ulna and secondarily the radial head, nicely reduced. **(D&C)** The appearance of the forearm and elbow following removal of the ulnar pin 2 months later.

its own merits. In these situations, it will usually be necessary to perform an osteotomy of the ulna to allow for some lengthening to facilitate reduction of the radial head.[24,25] A reconstructive procedure will also need to be done for the annular ligaments to hold the radial head in place once it has been reduced. Many children function very well with a dislocation of the radial head, and, in spite of a disconcerting radiograph, have a very functional range of motion of the elbow. In these situations it may be more pragmatic to accept the deformity and remove the radial head if it becomes a cosmetic or functional problem at skeletal maturity. The laterally dislocated radial head is often more of a problem in this regard and creates a rather grotesque swelling in the elbow as well pain in adolescence when the radial head becomes quite large and protuberant.[17,26] The younger the child when first seen with a long-standing dislocation of the radial head secondary to a Monteggia lesion, the better the long-term prognosis following an open reduction. The radial head should not be excised in a child, since this will further aggravate the shortening of the radius by eliminating the proximal radial physis which contributes about 30 percent of the final radial length. Great care should be taken in assessing children with long-standing dislocation of the radial head secondary to a neglected Monteggia fracture and the temptation to treat the radiograph rather than the child should be resisted. If there is pain or a grotesque appearance when the child is near skeletal maturity, the radial head can always be removed at that time. Attempts to reduce a long-standing dislocation of the radial head by shortening the radius or lengthening the ulna combined with reconstructing the annular ligament should be reserved for those children who are having significant disability occasioned by the radial head dislocation.

Complications

In most children, provided the Monteggia fracture is identified early, the complication rate from this fracture dislocation will be minimal. The most major complication is not recognizing it as a Monteggia fracture treating the injury as a simple forearm fracture.

Redislocation of the Radial Head

Redislocation of the radial head seldom occurs if the ulnar fracture is out to length and adequate reduction of the head at the time of the injury has been achieved. Care must be taken to flex the elbow past 90 degrees to stabilize the radial head reduction. If the elbow is kept at less than 90 degrees flexion the radial head has a tendency to redislocate most probably as a result of the increased mechanical advantage of the biceps. If this should happen, a rereduction is required immediately and empha-

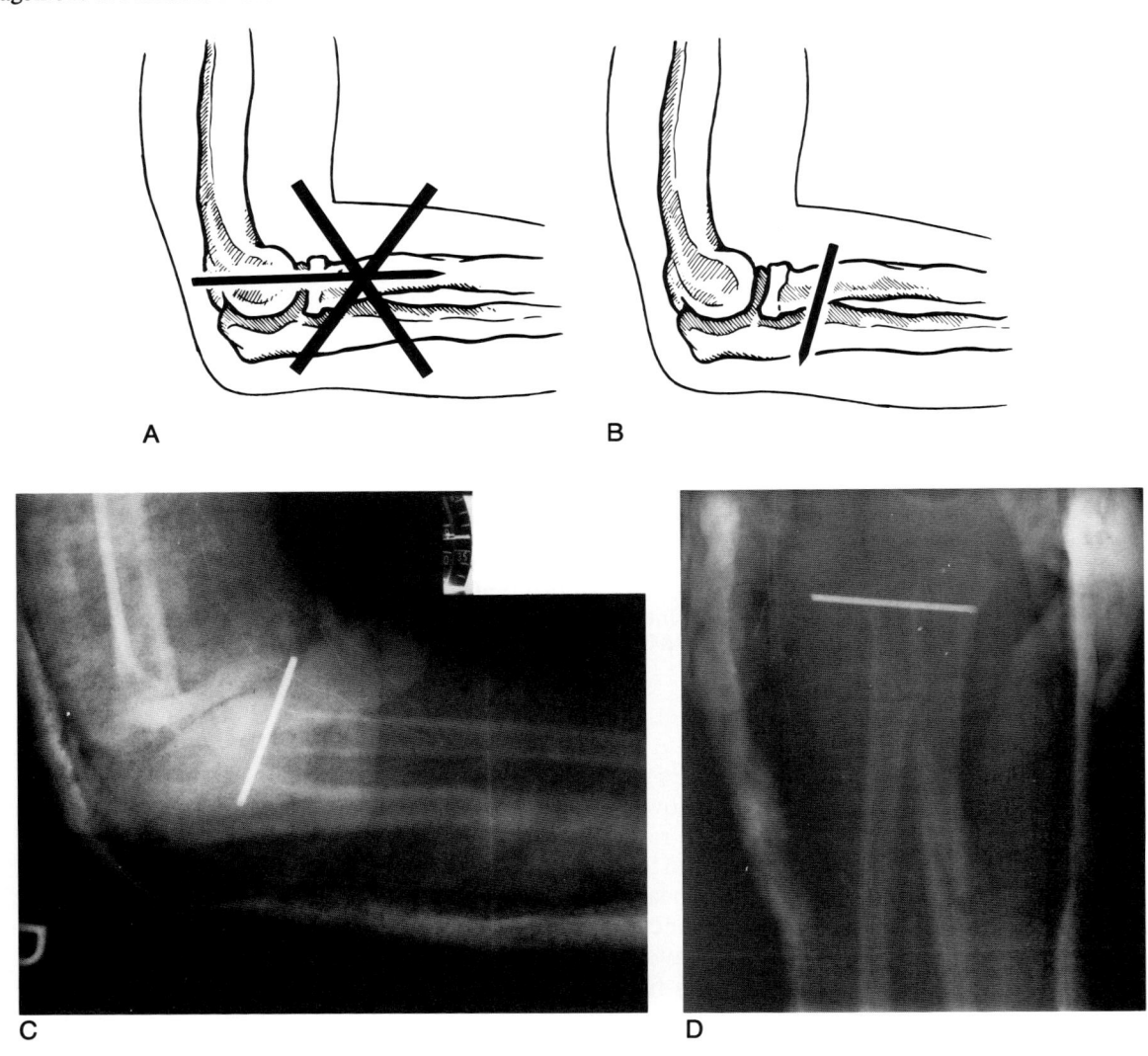

Fig. 17-15. (A) Not recommended and (B) preferred methods for maintaining radial head reduction in the Monteggia fracture-dislocation with persistent radial head dislocation. (C&D) Radiologic appearance after fixation. (From Letts et al.[7] with permission.)

sizes the need to follow the Monteggia injury carefully during the first 2 weeks with weekly radiographs, especially in the lateral projection.

Persistent Subluxation of the Radial Head

Persistent subluxation of the radial head can be identified in about 10 percent of Monteggia injuries in long-term follow-up. This is usually not a serious problem and may be related to hypertrophy of the head that is sometimes seen secondary to the enhanced blood supply in the region of the elbow joint engendered by this injury (Fig. 17-17). Not only is the maturation of the epiphyseal plates increased following Monteggia fractures in children, but there is also sometimes an eccentric development of the radial head ossific nucleus possibly due to a partial growth arrest of the physis from the contusion sustained at the moment of impact. Usually this does not require any treatment with elbow function being normal and this becomes more a radiologic curiosity. If there is significant radial head subluxation that is impeding flexion significantly a decision may have to be made as to whether an annular ligament reconstruction would be in the child's best interest to try and maintain congruity with the capitellum, thus pre-

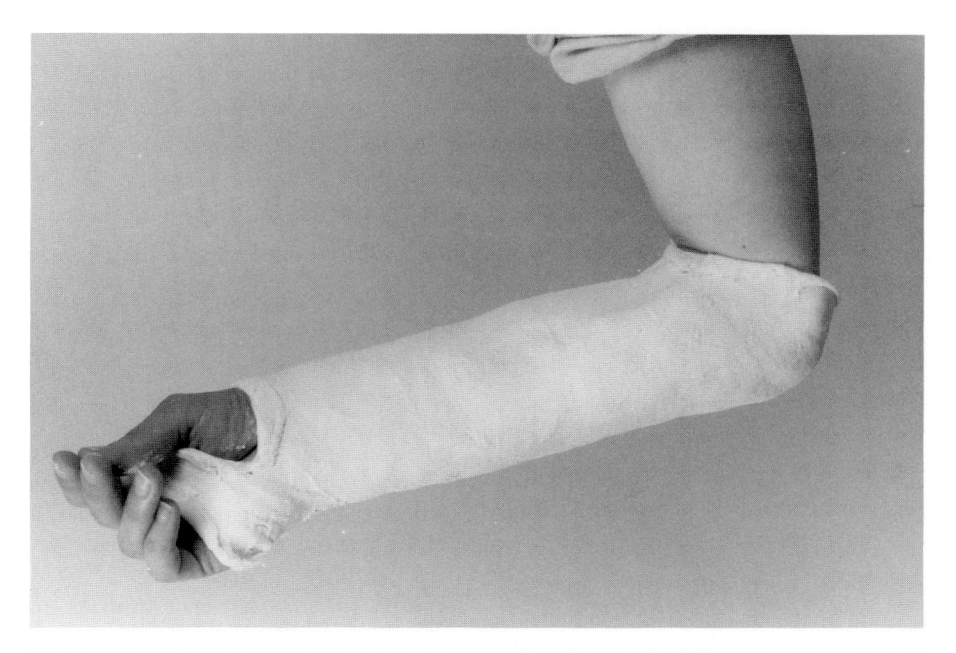

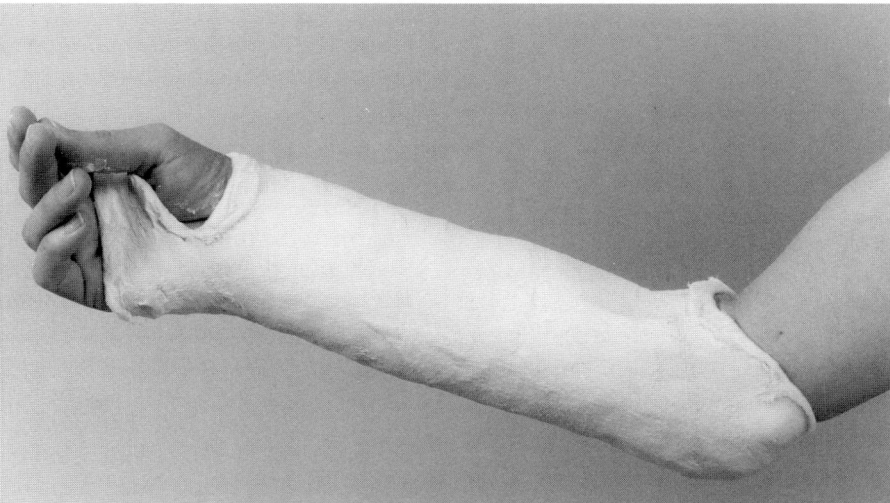

Fig. 17-16. The "Munster" cast allows early elbow motion but provides support for the fractured ulna.

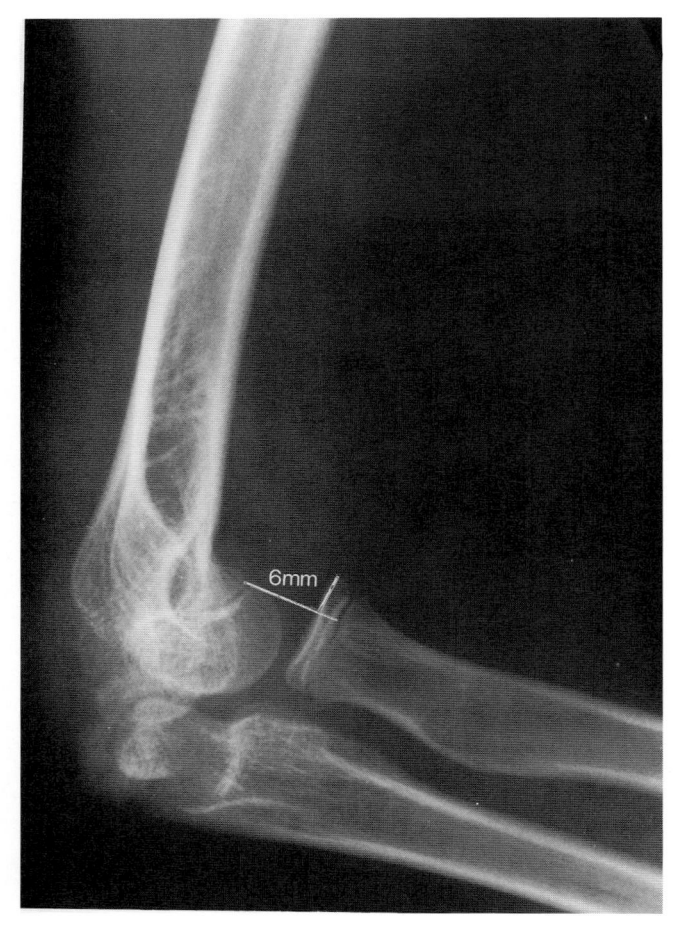

Fig. 17-17. Mild radial head subluxation (<6 mm) has little effect on elbow joint motion.

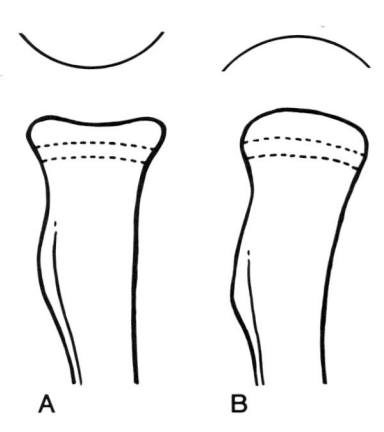

Fig. 17-18. (A) Head of radius has a normal concave appearance which becomes convex when it has been out of joint for several years (B) (From Letts.[13] By permission of Mayo Foundation.)

venting future articular degeneration.[27] In this instance, the radial head relationship to the capitellum should be assessed with a magnetic resonance imaging scan (MRI) and/or an arthrogram of the elbow. If there is significant hypertrophy of the radial head it may not be possible to simply reduce it and reconstruct the annular ligament and a shortening osteotomy of the radius may be required.

Nerve Injuries Associated with Monteggia Fracture-Dislocations

The posterior interosseous nerve is most commonly injured nerve in the Monteggia fracture.[28-31] Anterior dislocation of the radial head can result in a stretch injury to the posterior interosseous nerve as it passes posterolaterally around the proximal radius to enter the substance of the supinator muscle mass between the superficial and deep layers (Fig.17-21). Compression of the interosseous nerve may also be aggravated by the fibrous arcade of Frohse, a firm fibrous band at the proximal edge of the supinator muscle. These nerve injuries are usually neuropraxic and most recover by the time the cast is removed. In those nerve injuries that are more severe recovery may be significantly longer, but unless the fracture has occurred in association with a penetrating wound, operative intervention is not recommended until at least 6 months postinjury.

Limitation of Elbow Motion

Most reviews of Monteggia fractures in children have confirmed the minimal limitation of elbow motion that occurs after this injury.[7,16] In older children, there may be a loss of the last 10 degrees of flexion, but the functional range of elbow motion is usually intact. Several reports of hyperextension of the elbow following this injury may be more related to the hyperextension mechanism of the injury rather than to a consequence of the fracture itself. The hyperextension is usually less than 10 degrees and not associated with deleterious effects of elbow function.

Myositis Ossificans

Myositis ossificans is always mentioned as a complication of injuries about the elbow but in my experience is rarely encountered in children. It is usually associated with muscle tearing and hematoma hence in more severe elbow trauma this complication should indeed be con-

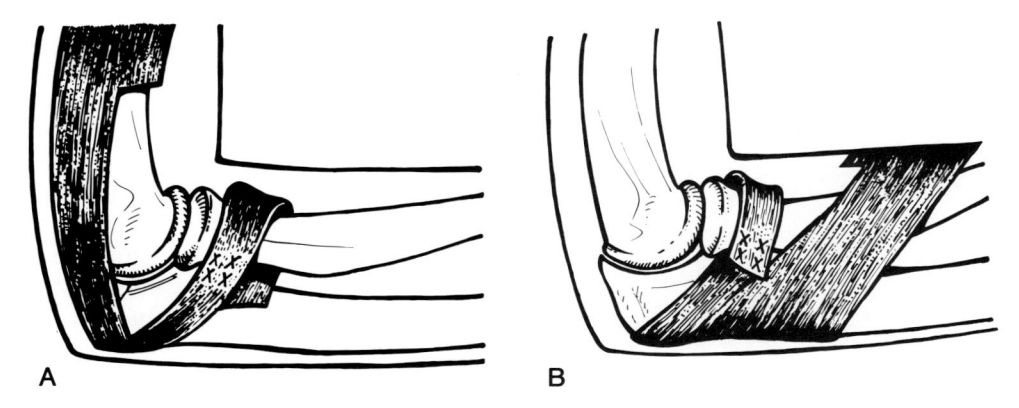

Fig. 17-19. Reconstruction of the annular ligament using the **(A)** triceps transfer (Lloyd Roberts) and **(B)** forearm fascial reconstruction (Boyd). (From Letts.[13] By permission of Mayo Foundation.)

sidered. Early elbow motion assists in minimizing the development of myositis ossificans.

Cross-Union

Cross-union occurs with a higher frequency in Monteggia fractures perhaps due to the proximity between the dislocated radial shaft and the ulnar fragments. If an open reduction is required the risk becomes ever higher (Fig. 17-22).

Associated Fractures of the Elbow

Monteggia fractures may be associated with other fractures in the vicinity of the elbow especially if the child has been subjected to severe trauma such as a fall from a

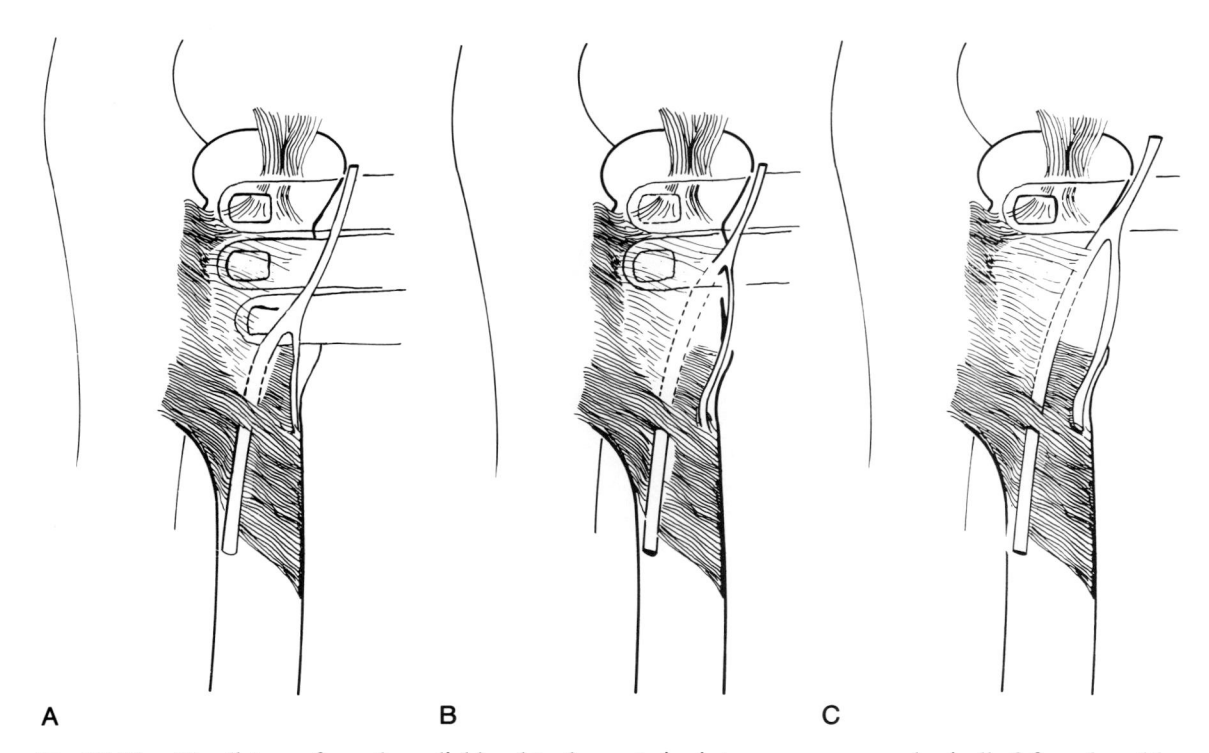

Fig. 17-20. The distance from the radial head to the posterior interosseous nerve, classically 3 fingerbreadths in an adult **(A)** may be only 2 fingerbreadths in preteens **(B)** and only 1 fingerbreadth in children under 6 years of age **(C)**.

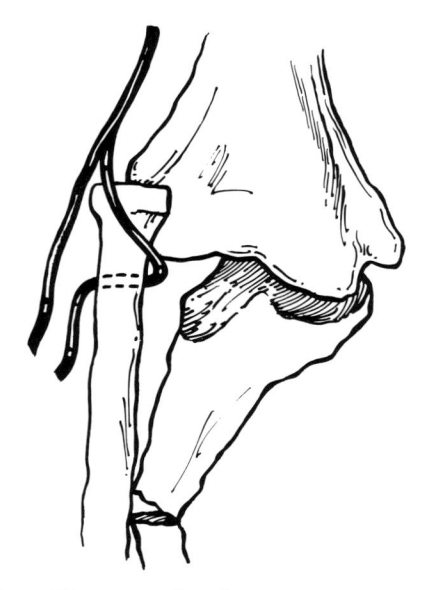

Fig. 17-21. The posterior interosseous nerve may be stretched by a dislocated proximal radius. (From Letts.[13] By permission of Mayo Foundation.)

height or a high-energy machinery or motor vehicle accident (Fig. 17-23). A good rule of thumb to follow in any injury about the elbow joint is to search the elbow region systematically for evidence of fractures of the medial epicondyle, avulsion of the coronoid tip, evidence of intra-articular fragments and associated fractures to the ulna, radial neck, or distal humerus. Obviously the more severe the trauma, the more likelihood that other injury has occurred. Identifying such fractures is more than an academic exercise, since missing an intra-articular fragment for example, may result in more disability than the original Monteggia lesion.

Summary

The Monteggia fracture-dislocation in children, when recognized and treated early, usually has a very good and predictable result. Problems arise if the true nature of the fracture-dislocation is not appreciated and the radial

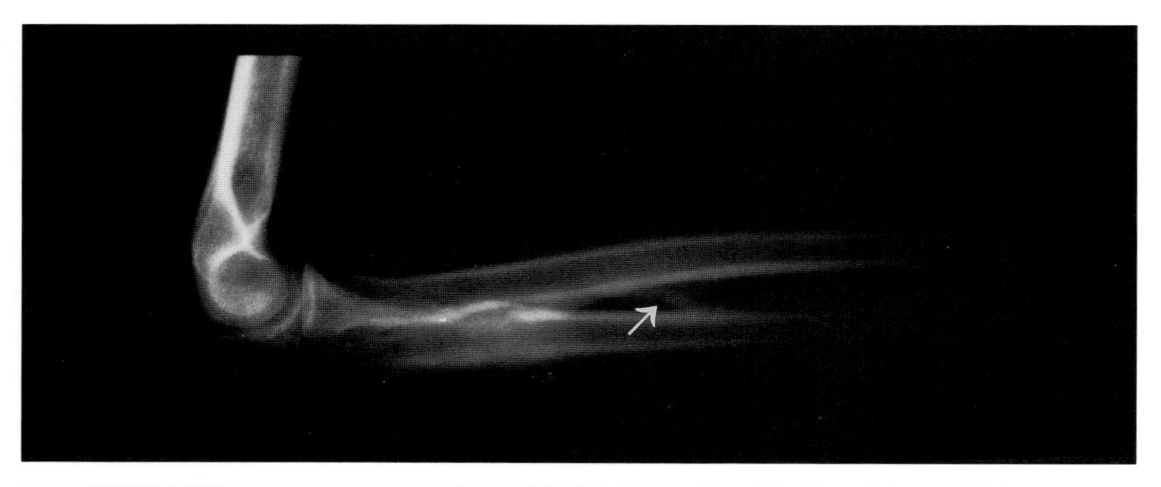

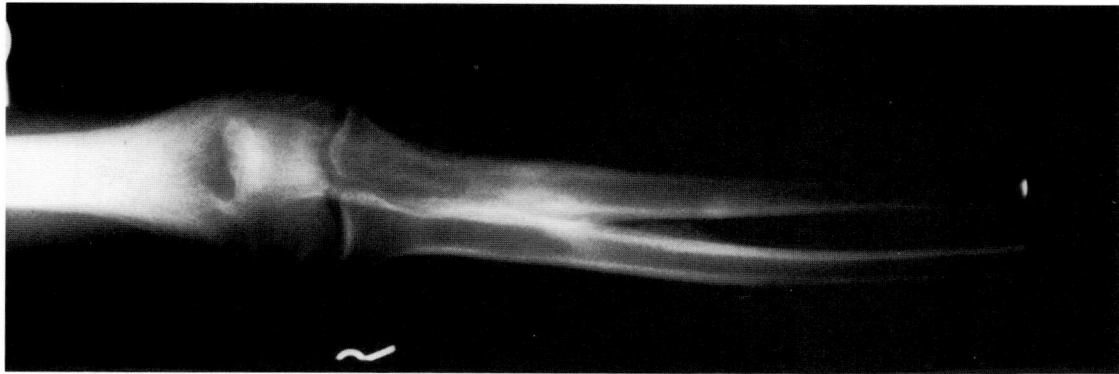

Fig. 17-22. Complication of Monteggia fracture—interosseous ossification leading to cross-union.

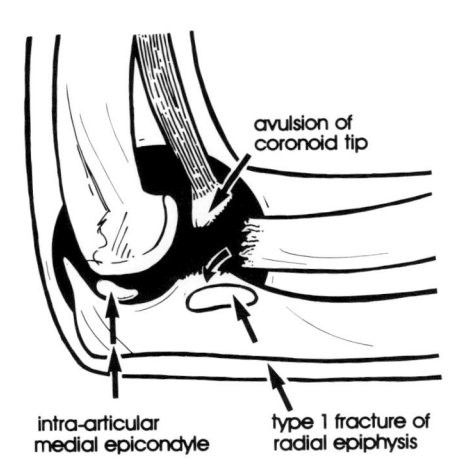

Fig. 17-23. Fractures about the elbow joint which may occur during a Monteggia injury or dislocation of the elbow joint. (From Letts.[13] By permission of Mayo Foundation.)

head dislocation is not dealt with in the initial couple of weeks subsequent to the trauma. In children the Monteggia-equivalent injuries add further confusion to this complex fracture and contribute to the lack of recognition of the seriousness of the injury. When treated immediately few Monteggia fractures in children will require an open reduction, although a closed reduction under a general anesthesia will be required. Students and clinicians dealing with trauma in children should be taught and reminded to always assess the radial head relationship to the capitellum in all forearm fractures, including those about the elbow. If the elbow is carefully examined in any child with a forearm fracture, few Monteggia fracture-dislocations will be missed!

THE GALEAZZI AND GALEAZZI-EQUIVALENT FRACTURES OF THE RADIUS AND ULNA

Description And Incidence

The classic Galeazzi fracture dislocation, although first described in 1822 by Sir Astley Cooper[32] was popularized by a report in 1934 in which the lesion was redescribed by Riccardo Galeazzi.[33,34] The fracture has been traditionally described as a dislocation of the distal ulna with a fracture of the distal third of the radius. The largest in depth study of Galeazzi fractures by Mikic[35] emphasized the higher incidence in the adult age group with only 14 of the patients in his series being children. The apparent low incidence of this fracture pattern in children may be a little factitious due to the omission of so-called equivalent lesions that are so prevalent in the pediatric age group. This is due to the close approximation of the epiphyseal plate at the distal ulna resulting in a similar fracture to the Galeazzi but not the classical lesion originally described (Fig. 17-24). This undoubtedly contributes to the fracture being often misinterpreted in the child, although the forces and displacement are quite analogous to the classic lesion. Very few reviews of Galeazzi fractures in children have been reported, but the unique biomechanics of the distal

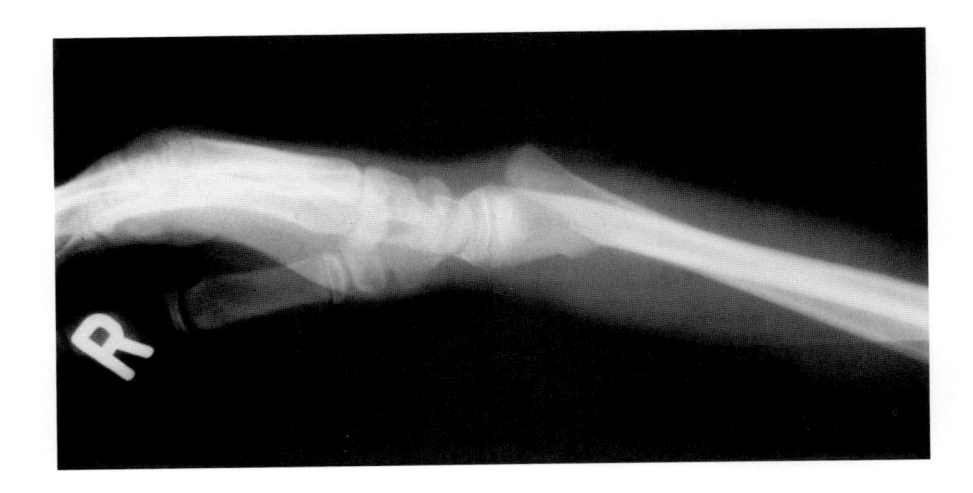

Fig. 17-24. Galeazzi equivalent fracture in a 13-year-old girl illustrating a type I physeal injury of the ulna, with the ulnar metaphysis displaced dorsally and the epiphysis held in place by the radioulnar ligamentous complex.

radioulnar joint due to the presence of the physis has been emphasized by all authors.[36-40]

Anatomy of the Pediatric Distal Radial Ulnar Joint

The distal radioulnar joint in children has considerable inherent mobility. This is due to the generalized ligamentous laxity that is characteristic of children, and it is only in the later teens that the joint ligaments approach their adult stability. This increased laxity may account for the fact that the Galeazzi fracture pattern is less common, the ligaments being more resilient as well as being less likely to rupture. The distal physis of the ulna however poses another area of weakness in children. The surrounding ulnar collateral ligaments are much stronger than the adjacent physis thus the biomechanical forces that produce the classic Galeazzi fracture in the adult frequently result in displacement of the distal ulnar epiphysis, the fracture occurring through the physis. The displacement of the metaphyseal shaft of the ulna that occurs in analogous similar to that of the adult Galeazzi lesion.

The ligaments stabilizing the distal radius and ulna are the ulnar collateral ligament, the volar and dorsal carpal ligaments, the pronator quadratus, and a thick triangular fibrocartilage (Fig. 17-25). Because the function of the triangular fibrocartilage is to limit rotational movements of the radius and ulna, it must be ruptured to allow the distal ulnar head to dislocate in the classic Galeazzi fracture pattern. The triangular fibrocartilage ligament can be ruptured by either hyperpronation or hypersupination resulting in a dislocation of the ulnar head. As is characteristic in children the ligaments are much stronger than the adjacent physis, and it is much more common to encounter a type I or type II physeal fracture

Fig. 17-25. The triangular fibrocartilage complex is the major anatomic structure stabilizing the radioulnar joint of the wrist in children.

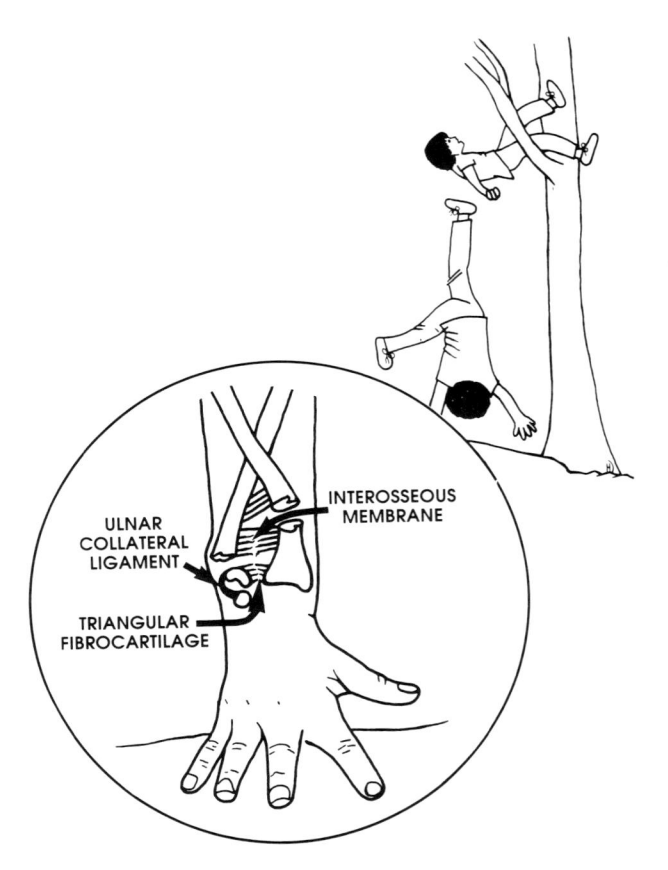

Fig. 17-26. Mechanism of forced pronation in the production of a Galeazzi equivalent fracture resulting in a type I physeal fracture with displacement of the ulnar metaphysis. The ulnar collateral ligaments and triangular fibrocartilage are not torn. The radius fractures volarly in the distal third, the ulnar acting as a fulcrum.

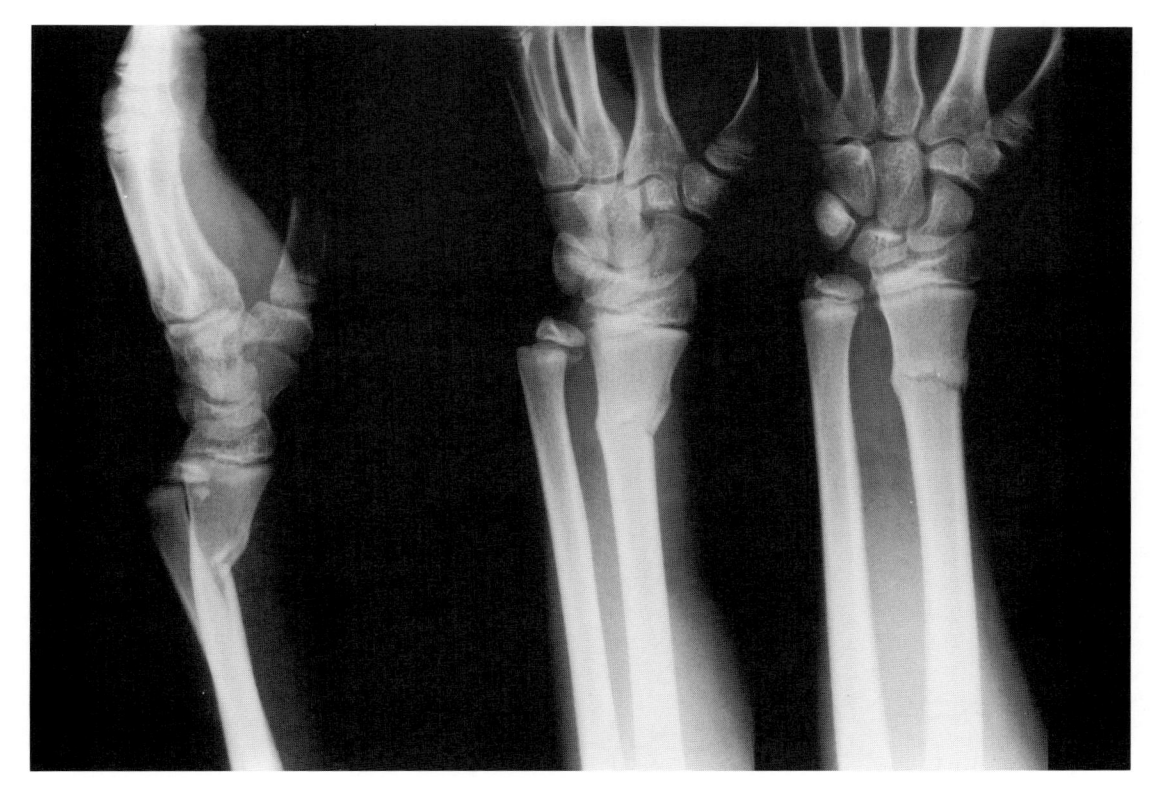

Fig. 17-27. Galeazzi-equivalent fracture type B illustrating an angulated greenstick fracture of the radius and a Salter-Harris type II physeal injury with dorsal displacement of the ulnar metaphyses. (From Letts RM, Rowhani N: J Pediatr Orthop, in press, with permission.)

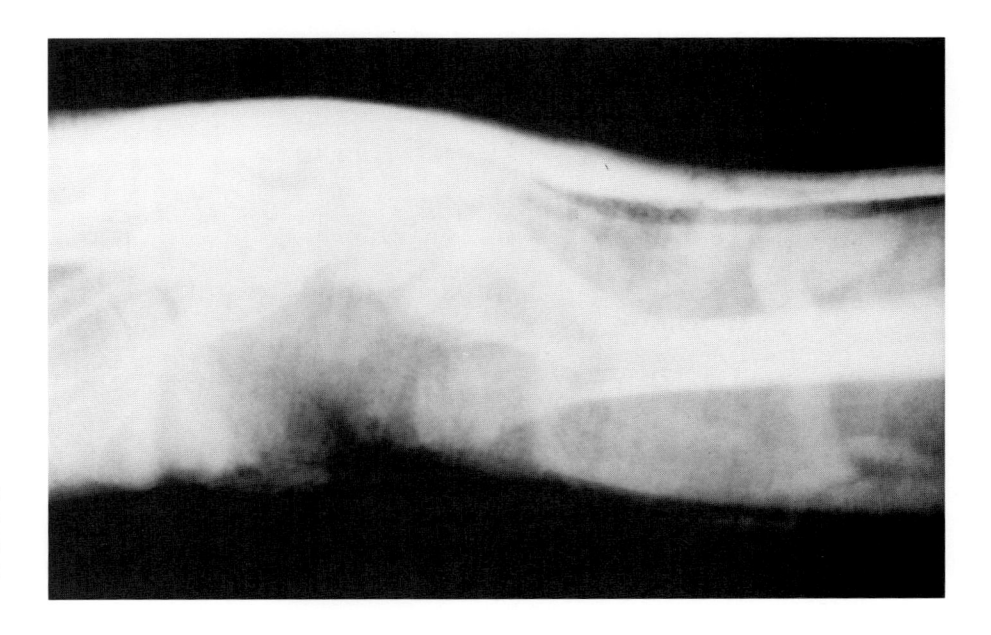

Fig. 17-28. Galeazzi-equivalent fracture type D illustrating an unusual volar displacement of the distal ulna secondary to a hypersupination injury.

of the distal ulna than a rupture of the very thick and much stronger triangular fibrous ligament complex.[41,42]

Mechanism of Injury

As with most pediatric fractures, it is difficult if not impossible to expect a child to accurately describe the mechanism of injury. One common characteristic feature of these fractures in children is a fall from a height (Fig. 17-26). In the laboratory, the Galeazzi fracture pattern can be reproduced by forced pronation as well as forced supination. In a fall from a height the child will characteristically fall on the outstretched hand, usually with the extremity in pronation. Rotation of the entire body on the fixed hand as it strikes the ground can exert considerable torque on the distal radioulnar joint resulting in hyperpronation and a fracture through the ulnar distal physis as well as a volar fracture of the distal radius, the so called Galeazzi equivalent fracture (Fig. 17-27). The ulnar metaphysis is usually dislocated dorsally. Very rarely the ulnar metaphyseal shaft may be dislocated volarly and this may be a rare example of a hypersupination injury[40,43] (Fig. 17-28). The site of the fracture through the radius may vary in children and may involve the metaphysis distally, at the junction of the middle and distal thirds or even the midshaft of the radius. The unusual Essex-Lopresti fracture through the neck of the radius with dislocation of the radioulnar joint appears to be very rare in the pediatric age group.[44] A classification of the Galeazzi and Galeazzi equivalent injuries is illustrated in Figure 17-29 and Table 17-1.

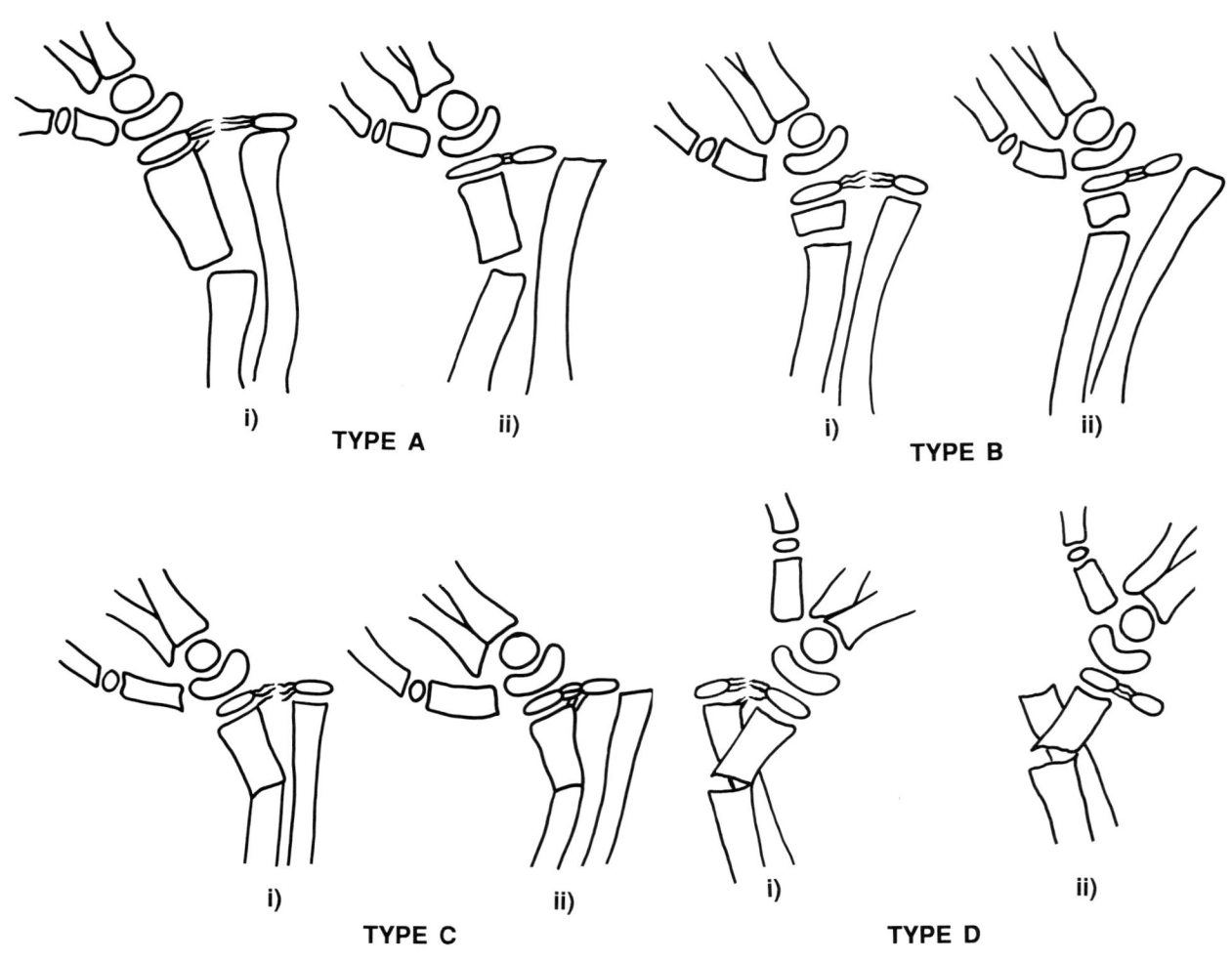

Fig. 17-29. Classification of Galeazzi and Galeazzi equivalent injuries in children. (From Letts RM, Rowhani N: J Pediatr Orthop, in press, with permission.)

TABLE 17-1. Classification of Pediatric Galeazzi Fracture Patterns

Type A	Fracture of the radius at junction of middle and distal thirds with
	  i Dorsal dislocation of distal ulna
	  ii Epiphyseal fracture of distal ulna with dorsal displacement of ulnar metaphysis

Type B	Fracture of the distal third of the radius with
	  i Dorsal dislocation of distal ulna
	  ii Epiphyseal fracture of distal ulna with dorsal displacement of ulnar metaphysis

Type C	Greenstick fracture of radius with dorsal bowing and
	  i Dorsal dislocation of distal ulna
	  ii Epiphyseal fracture of distal ulna displacement of ulnar metaphysis

Type D	Fracture of distal radius with volar bowing
	  i Volar dislocation of distal ulna
	  ii Epiphyseal fracture of distal ulna with volar displacement of ulnar metaphysis

Clinical Appearance

Similar to the Monteggia fracture pattern children with Galeazzi fractures and equivalent injuries are frequently misdiagnosed. This is usually because of a failure to adequately assess the distal ulnar joint in the presence of a fracture of the shaft of the radius. Dislocation of the distal ulna is not always readily obvious simply by inspecting the wrist joint. The dislocated distal ulna may actually have been spontaneously reduced by the time the child reaches the emergency department leaving only the fractured radius obvious on radiologic and clinical inspection. Indeed many of these undetected Galeazzi fracture patterns in children may actually heal uneventfully because of this fact. However, the presence of an isolated fracture of the distal radius especially if there is an angulation or shortening, should always raise the possibility of an injury to the radioulnar joint. The radioulnar should be stressed at the time of reduction of the associated fracture of the radius to detect unrecognized instability. If there is instability at the radioulnar joint, stability of the wrist should be ensured by positioning the extremity in full supination if the ulna appears to dislocate dorsally and full pronation if the dislocation appears to be in the volar direction.

Diagnosis

In the classical appearance of the Galeazzi injury in children whether it is due to a ligamentous rupture at the radioulnar joint or a physeal injury of the distal ulna, the wrist is swollen and painful. The distal ulna may be very prominent representing dislocation of the ulnar head or the protruding metaphyseal fragment following a physeal fracture of the distal ulna. The angulated or displaced fracture of the radius will be the most obvious deformity. Mikic[35] has described fractures of both bones of the forearm associated with dislocation of the distal radial ulnar joint in adults. This Galeazzi fracture pattern has not been reported in children.

The radiographic appearance of this fracture in children may indicate a complete fracture of the distal radius or a greenstick angulated fracture. The distal ulnar physis may exhibit a type I or type II physeal fracture or there may be widening of the growth plate indicating the possibility of a type I physeal injury that is undisplaced or has relocated following the trauma. The integrity of the distal radioulnar joint can usually be ascertained by stressing the joint at the time of reduction of the radial fracture. The use of arthrography of the radioulnar joint has been recommended to diagnose uncertain clinical instability.[45,46] Rupture of the triangular fibrocartilage is indicated by the passage of contrast medium from the wrist into the inferior radioulnar joint. This technique is

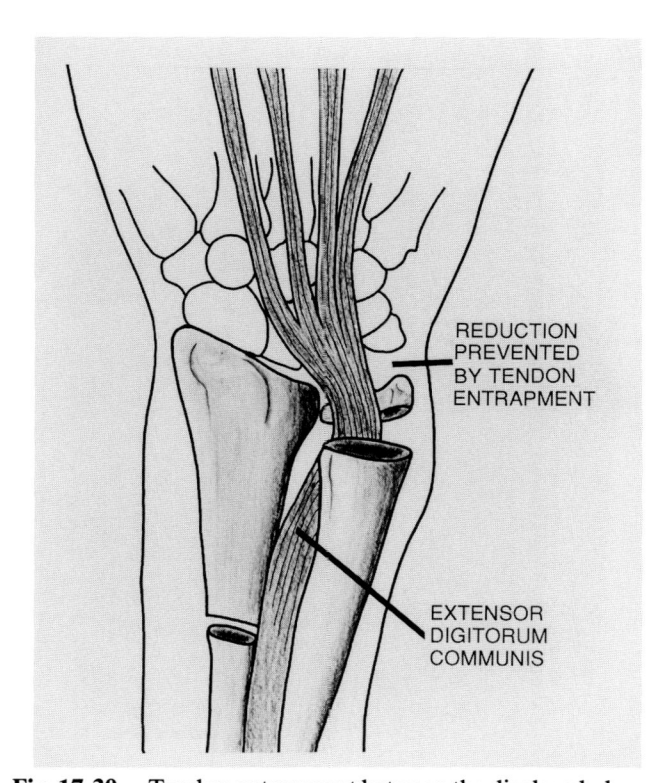

Fig. 17-30. Tendon entrapment between the displaced ulnar epiphysis and the metaphysis should be suspected when a reduction of the distal ulna cannot be obtained by closed reduction. Tendons trapped are usually the flexor carpi ulnaris and/or the extensor digitorium communis.

said to be of more value in children as perforations of the triangular fiber cartilage occurs from degenerative changes in older individuals.[47] However, in the vast majority of children, clinical evaluation of the stability of the radioulnar joint should provide the diagnosis without having to resort to arthrographic techniques. A true lateral radiograph of wrist is essential in detecting displacement of the ulna either dorsally or volarly. Oblique views and anterior/posterior views of the wrist may mask the displacement of the distal ulna.

Treatment

In contradistinction to the adult Galeazzi fracture, most such injuries in children can be treated by closed reduction. Reducing the angulated radial fracture and ensuring reduction of the radioulnar joint or the distal ulnar physis is usually accomplished with minimal difficulty under a general anesthesia. If the distal radioulnar joint cannot be reduced or if the physis of the distal ulna cannot be anatomically restored entrapment of the extensor tendons between the displaced metaphysis and the epiphysis should be suspected[48-51] (Fig. 17-30). This will necessitate an open reduction in order to free the tendons and reduce the physeal injury. If the distal ulna is displaced dorsally as is the usual case the forearm should be kept in full supination with an above-elbow cast. If there is volar displacement of the ulnar head, the radioulnar joint will be more stable in full pronation. It is essential to hold the reduction in an above-elbow rather than a below-elbow cast to avoid the displacing forces of supination/pronation. Healing is complete within 6 weeks and internal fixation is usually not required. In the rare instance of instability of the radial ulnar joint in spite of placing the extremity in full supination the radius and ulna can be held by cross K-wires inserted

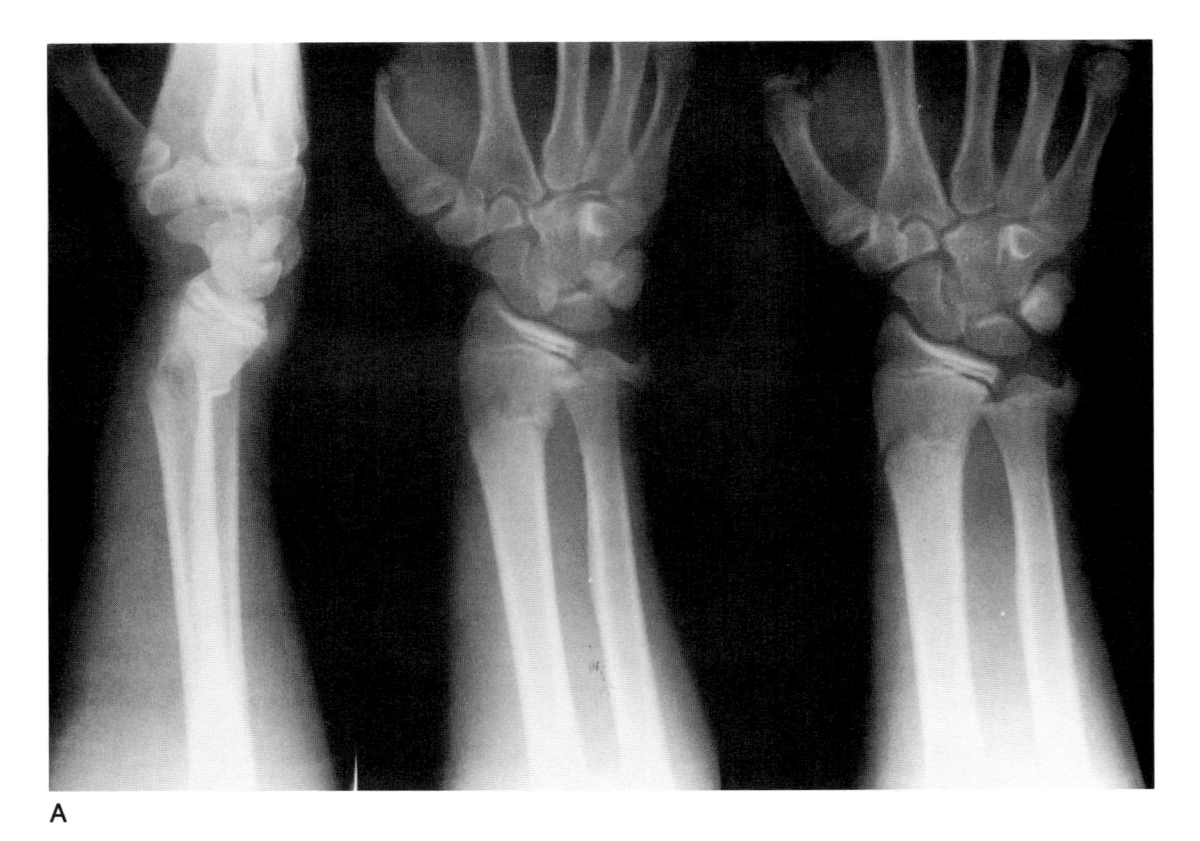

Fig. 17-31. (A) This 13-year-old boy fell from his bicycle sustaining a pediatric Galeazzi equivalent injury that could not be reduced. Open reduction revealed the flexor carpi ulnaris and extensors blocking the reduction. *(Figure continues.)*

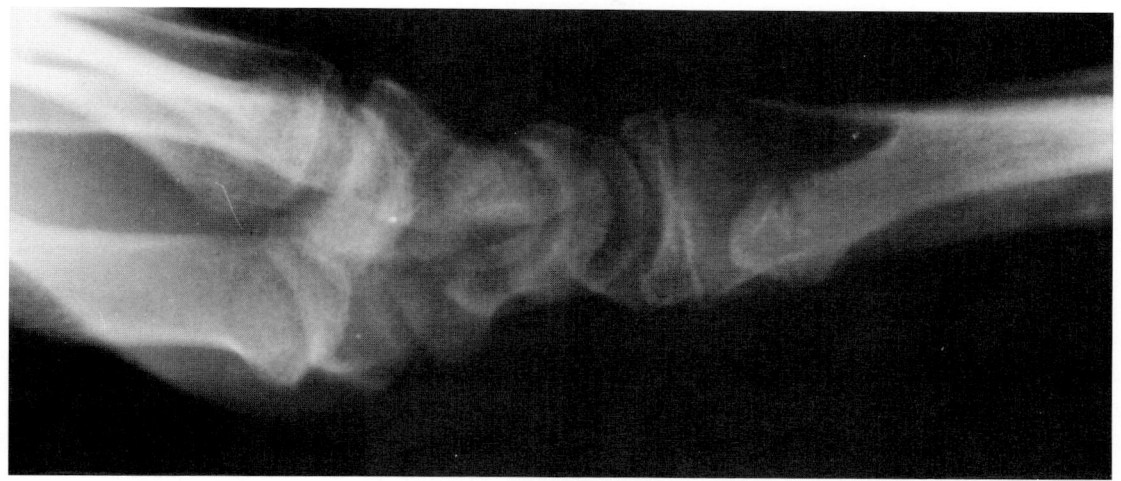

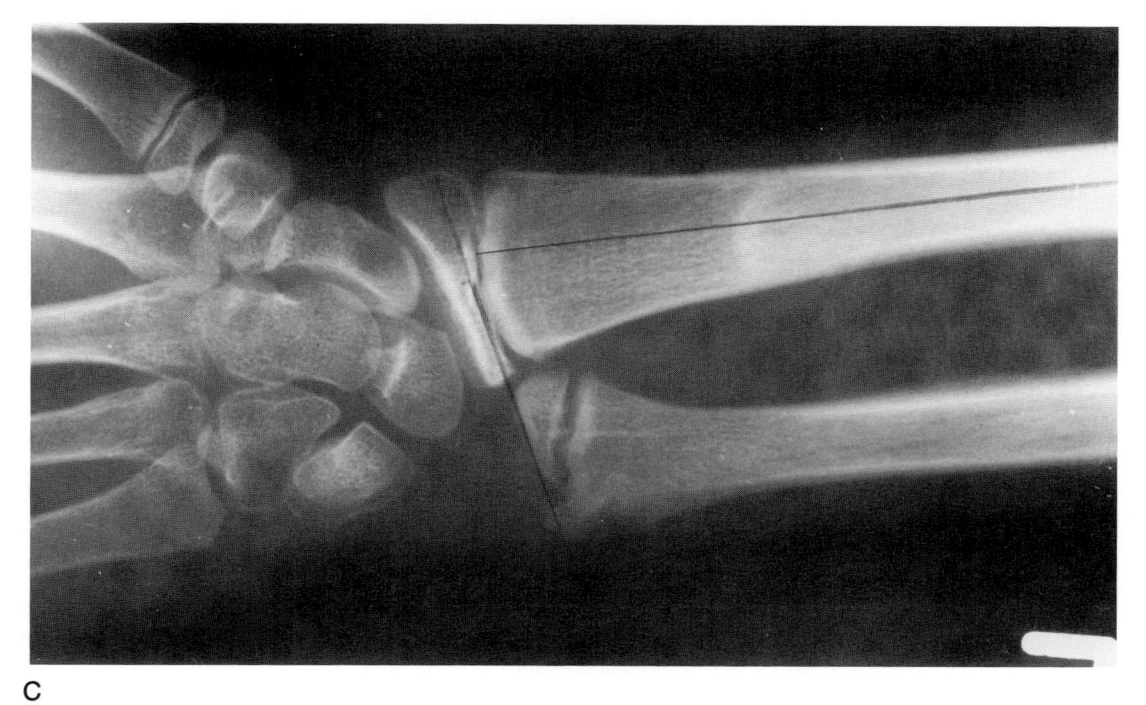

Fig. 17-31 *(Continued).* **(B)** At 5 months a physeal arrest of the distal ulna is obvious. **(C)** At 3 years postfracture an ulnar minus deformity has developed.

percutaneously. Rarely the radius may require internal fixation as is usually necessary in the adult injury.[52,53]

Complications

Treatment of the Galeazzi fracture pattern in children both classic and equivalent injuries usually results in good healing with no residual deformity. If, however, the fracture has not been recognized as a Galeazzi injury and the radioulnar joint remains unreduced, prominence of distal ulna is an annoying and painful complication. In younger children this may improve with time and further growth and development of the wrist joint. In teenagers, however, the dislocated distal ulna may be a cosmetic and a functional disability necessitating a radioulnar tenodesis or resection of the distal prominent ulna at skeletal maturity.[54,55]

Failure to reduce the distal ulnar physeal fracture due to entrapped tendons will result in a physeal growth arrest of the distal ulna and depending on the age of the child considerable shortening of the ulna[56] (Fig. 17-31).

Summary

Pediatric Galeazzi- and Galeazzi-equivalent fractures need to be appreciated by the clinician in order to provide optimum treatment, thus ensuring good reduction of the displaced distal ulna as well as reduction of the fractured radius. The fracture may appear rather innocuous, since the radius may only be bowed at the fracture site and the displacement of the distal ulnar fracture or dislocation may not be readily apparent in routine radiographs. Careful clinical examination of the wrist will almost always confirm the presence of this fracture pattern. Treatment by closed reduction is usually successful with the forearm position in full supination with an above elbow cast. The Galeazzi equivalent injury in children requires the same management as the classic Galeazzi fracture.

REFERENCES

1. Monteggia GB: Instituzione Chirurgiche. Presso Guiseppe and Maspero, Milan, 1813–16
2. Peltier LF: Fractures: A History and Iconography of Their Treatment. Norman Publishing, San Francisco, 1990
3. Cunningham SR: Fracture of the ulna with dislocation of head of radius. J Bone Joint Surg 16:351, 1934
4. Boyd HS: Surgical exposure of ulna and proximal 3rd of radius through one incision. Surg Gynecol Obstet 71:86, 1940
5. Speed JS, Boyd HB: Treatment of fractures of ulna with dislocation of the head of the radius (Monteggia fracture) JAMA 115:1699, 1940
6. Bado JL: The Monteggia Lesion. Charles C Thomas, Springfield, IL, 1962
7. Letts M, Locht R, Weins J: Monteggia fracture dislocations in children. J Bone Joint Surg [Br] 67:724, 1985
8. Evans EM: Pronation injuries of the forearm with special reference to the anterior Monteggia lesion fracture. J Bone Joint Surg 31B:578, 1949
9. Tompkins DG: The anterior Monteggia fracture: observations on ideology and treatment. J Bone Joint Surg [Am] 53:1109, 1971
10. Stelling FH, Cote RH: Traumatic Dislocation of Head of Radius in Children. JAMA 160:723, 1956
11. Lloyd-Roberts TC, Bucknill TM: Anterior dislocation of the radial head in children: aetiology, common natural history and management. J Bone Joint Surg [Br] 59:402, 1977
12. Bado JL: The Monteggia lesion. Clin Orthop 50:71, 1967
13. Letts RM: Dislocations of the elbow in children. In Morrey BF (ed): The Elbow and Its Disorders. WB Saunders, New York, 1985
14. Salter RB: Textbook of Disorders and Injuries of the Musculoskeletal System. Williams & Wilkins, Baltimore, 1970
15. Bruce AT, Harvey Jr JP, Wilson Jr JC: Monteggia fractures. J Bone Joint Surg [Am] 56:1563, 1974
16. Wiley JJ, Galey JP: Monteggia injuries in children. J Bone Joint Surg [Br] 67:728, 1985
17. Peiro A, Andres F, Fernandez-Esteve F: Acute Monteggia lesions in children. J Bone Joint Surg [Am] 59:92, 1977
18. Friedman L, Luck K, Leong JCY: Radial head reduction after a missed Monteggia fracture. J Bone Joint Surg [Br] 70:846, 1988
19. Stoll TM, Willis RB, Patterson DC: Treatment of the missed Monteggia fracture in the child. J Bone Joint Surg [Br] 74:436, 1992
20. Dormans JP, Rang M: The problems of Monteggia fracture dislocations in children. Orthop Clin North Am 21:251, 1990
21. Kalamchi A: Monteggia fracture dislocation in children: late treatment in two cases. J Bone Joint Surg [Am] 68:615, 1986
22. Bell Tause AJF: The treatment of malunited anterior Monteggia fractures in children. J Bone Joint Surg [Br] 47:718, 1965
23. Boyd HB, Boals JC: The Monteggia lesion: a review of 159 cases. Clin Orthop 66:94, 1969
24. Hurst LC, Dubrow EN: Surgical treatment of symptomatic chronic radial head dislocation: a neglected Monteggia fracture. J Pediatr Orthop 3:227, 1983
25. Fowles JV, Sliman N, Kassab MT: The Monteggia lesion in children. J Bone Joint Surg [Am] 65:1276, 1983
26. Mullick F: The lateral Monteggia fracture. J Bone Joint Surg [Am] 59:543, 1977

27. Bell SN, Morrey BF, Bianco AJ: Chronic posterior subluxation and dislocation of the radial head. J Bone Joint Surg [Am] 73:392, 1991
28. Spar I: A neurologic complication following Monteggia fracture. Clin Orthop 122:207, 1977
29. Spinner M, Freundlich BD, Teicher J: Posterior intraosseous nerve palsy as a complication of Monteggia fractures in children. Clin Orthop 58:141, 1968
30. Stein F, Grabias SL, Deffer PA: Nerve injuries complicating Monteggia lesions. J Bone Joint Surg [Am] 53:1432, 1971
31. Olney BW, Menelaus MB: Monteggia and equivalent lesions in childhood. J Pediatr Orthop 9:219 1989
32. Cooper Sir A: A Treatise on Dislocations and on Fractures of the Joints. 5th Ed. Longman, London, 1826
33. Galeazzi R: Di una particolare sindrome traumatica dello scheletro del-avambracci. Atti Mem Soc Lomb Chir 2:12, 1934
34. Reckling FW, Peltier LF: Riccardo Galeazzi and Galeazzi's fracture. Surgery 58:453, 1964
35. Mikic ZDJ: Galezzi fracture-dislocations. J Bone Joint Surg [Am] 57:1071, 1975
36. Campbell RM Jr: Fractures and dislocations of the hand and wrist region. Orthop Clin North Am 20:237, 1990
37. Kraus B, Horne G: Galeazzi fractures. J Trauma 25:1093, 1985
38. Lanfried MJ, Stenclik M, Susi JC: Variant of Galeazzi fracture dislocation in children. J Pediatr Orthop 11:332, 1991
39. Hughston JC: Fractures of the distal radial shaft: mistakes in management. J Bone Joint Surg [Am] 39:249, 1957
40. Ogden JA: Skeletal Injury in the Child. 2nd Ed. p. 521. WB Saunders, Philadelphia, 1990
41. Reckling FW: Unstable fracture-dislocations of the forearm. J Bone Joint Surg [Am] 64:861, 1982
42. Bowers WH: The distal radioulnar joint in operative hand surgery. p. 195. In Green DP (ed): Operative Hand Surgery. Churchill Livingstone, New York, 1988
43. Moore TM, Klein JP, Patzkis MJ, Harvey JP: Results of compression-plating of closed Galeazzi fractures. J Bone Joint Surg [Am] 67:1015, 1985
44. Essex-Lopresti P: Fractures of the radial head with distal radio-ulnar dislocation. J Bone Joint Surg [Br] 33:244, 1957
45. Mikic Z: 2D arthrography of the wrist joint: an experimental study. J Bone Joint Surg [Am] 66:371, 1984
46. Walsh HPJ, McLaren CAN, Owen R: Galeazzi fractures in children. J Bone Joint Surg [Br] 69:730, 1987
47. Mikic ZD: Age changes in the triangular fibrocartilage of the wrist joint. J Anat 126:367, 1978
48. Biyani A, Bhan S: Dual extensor tendon entrapment in Galeazzi fracture dislocation: a case report. J Trauma 29:1295, 1989
49. Karlsson J, Appelguist R: Irreducible fractures of the wrist in a child: entrapment of the extensor tendons. Acta Orthop Scand 58:280, 1987
50. Itoh Y, Horirichi Y, Takahashi M, Uchinishi K, Yabe Y: Extensor tendon involvement in Smith's and Galeazzi's fractures. J Hand Surg [Am] 12:535 1987
51. Paley D, McMurty RY, Murray JF: Dorsal dislocation of the ulnar styloid and extensor carpi ulnaris tendon into the distal radioulnar joint: the empty sulcus sign. J Hand Surg [Am] 12:1029, 1987
52. Mohan K, Gupta AK, Sharma J, Singh AK, Jain AK: Internal fixation in 50 cases of Galeazzi fracture. Acta Orthop Scand 59:314, 1988
53. Reckling C: Fracture-dislocation. Arch Surg 96:1002, 1968
54. Rockwood C, Wilkins K, King R: Fractures in Children. p. 356. JB Lippincott, Philadelphia, 1984
55. Linscheid RL: Biomechanics of the distal radioulnar joint. Clin Orthop 275:46, 1992
56. Nelson OA, Buchanan JR, Harrison CS: Distal ulnar growth arrest. J Hand Surg [Am] 9:164, 1991

18

Fractures of the Midshaft Radius and Ulna

Charles T. Price

> Neoideophobia (fear of new ideas) affects humans worldwide.
> —IAN STEVENSON

DESCRIPTION AND INCIDENCE

Fractures of the forearm shaft in children differ considerably from those in adults. Closed treatment is preferred in children, but reduction and maintenance of position can be difficult. Healing occurs rapidly in children and nonunion is rare. One or both bones may be broken and the fractures can be complete, greenstick, or plastically deformed. Treatment differs for each of these types of fractures. Treatment may also vary depending upon the age of the child and location of the fracture. Many complications can occur, but the most common concerns are residual deformity and loss of forearm rotation.

Fractures of the radius constitute approximately 40 percent of all childhood skeletal injuries.[1-3] Approximately 80 percent of radius fractures are in the distal third, 15 percent are in the middle third, and 5 percent are in the proximal third.[3-6] Fractures of the forearm shaft account for 6 to 10 percent of all pediatric fractures.[1,2]

ANATOMY

The radius is a curved bone with rotational joints at either end. The axis of pronation and supination is oblique passing approximately from the radial head to the ulnar head.[7] The fibers of the interosseous membrane pass obliquely from distal on the ulna to proximal on the radius. These fibers are most relaxed in supination and tighten in pronation.[8-10]

The principal muscles of pronation are the pronator teres inserting into the middle third of the radius and the pronator quadratus inserting into the distal fourth. The supinating muscles insert proximally on the radius and are primarily the biceps brachii and the supinator.[7] Thus, complete fractures of the proximal shaft will usually allow the proximal fragments to rest in supination. With middle and distal shaft fractures the proximal fragments usually rest in neutral or slightly supinated position. Evans[11] plotted the rotational position of the proximal radius in 50 fractures of the forearm shaft (Fig. 18-1). All were in neutral or supination. The distal third fractures were in neutral to 30 degrees of supination, while the middle third fractures varied from neutral to full supination. None were in pronation.

Greenstick fractures behave differently than complete fractures because there is an intact cortex and periosteal hinge that can be utilized to obtain reduction. Rotational deformity of greenstick fractures is primarily due to the mechanism of injury rather than being caused by unrestrained muscle pull.

Shaft fractures in the distal third have the best prognosis for recovery of motion and remodeling.[3,12-14] The anatomic reasons for this observation are unclear. Per-

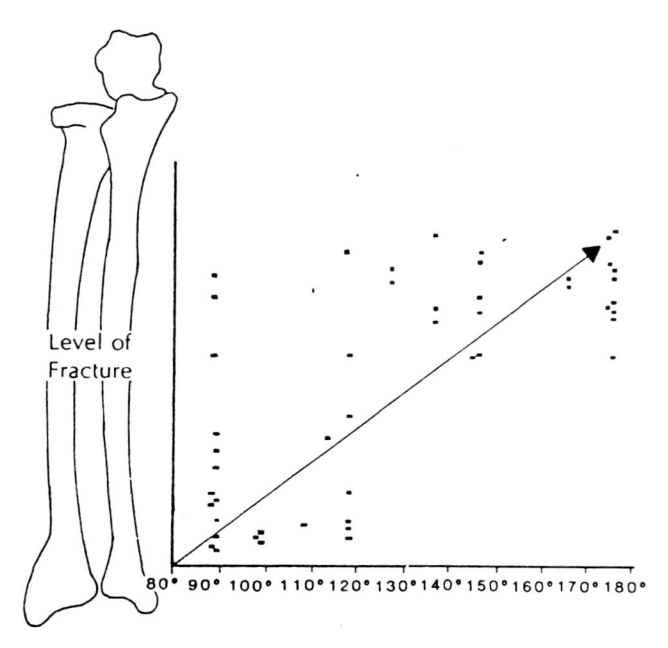

Fig. 18-1. The rotational position of the proximal radius in 50 cases of complete fracture. Each dot represents one case. Note that all are in neutral or supination. (From Evans,[11] with permission.)

haps it is because the interosseous membrane is widest in the distal third of the shaft. Also, the distal radius and ulna contribute 75 to 80 percent of the total growth of the forearm.[15] This may contribute to more rapid remodeling.[16] Younger, Tredwell, and Mackenzie[17] have proposed axis deviation as a predictor of fracture outcome. They defined axis deviation as the distance that the apex of the deformity was displaced from the normal axis. This calculation utilized both angulation and fracture position in its determination. Thus, a distal fracture angulated 15 percent would produce less axis deviation than a midshaft fracture angulated 15 degrees. This anatomic observation has not been tested for proximal fractures and needs to be confirmed by other authors, but it could explain why distal fractures have a better prognosis than midshaft fractures.

MECHANISM OF INJURY

The majority of these fractures occur as the result of indirect trauma from a fall as the child is trying to protect himself with the outstretched hand. As a result of this mechanism, upper extremity fracture in children are twice as common on the left side as they are on the right.[18] Distal fractures are usually caused by indirect trauma.

Direct trauma by a blow to the forearm is more likely to result in a midshaft fracture. Direct trauma is often implicated in dislaced or open fractures. Proximal fractures have complex mechanisms of injury similar to elbow injuries.[3] Tredwell and colleagues[19] have noted that the location of forearm fractures tends to move distally with increasing age.

Evans,[11] Rang,[20] and others[21,22] have emphasized that greenstick fractures sustained with the forearm in supination will result in volar angulation deformity. A greenstick fracture sustained with the forearm in pronation will cause dorsal angulation deformity (Fig. 18-2). This is an important consideration for the reduction of greenstick fractures.

Plastic deformation with bowing of the radius or ulna can occur in children as a result of axial compression. The bones of children are more porous and flexible than adults resulting in a larger zone of plastic deformation on the stress-strain curve.[23] Chamay[24] produced bowing deformities of the dog ulna in vivo and in vitro. Histologic studies demonstrated microfractures from the medullary cavity through the concave cortex with fracture lines oriented approximately 30 degrees to the long axis. Subperiosteal hemorrhage was not observed with plastic deformation.

CLASSIFICATION

A specific classification system for forearm fractures has not been described. These fractures are usually described by their anatomic characteristics of location, angular deformity or amount of cortical disruption. Treatment principles are influenced primarily by the amount of cortical disruption. Therefore the treatment section of this chapter will classify forearm fractures as complete, greenstick, or plastic deformation.

PHYSICAL EXAMINATION

The deformed, painful extremity usually makes the diagnosis readily apparent. However, soft tissue swelling may obscure mild to moderate deformity. It is helpful to

Fractures of the Midshaft Radius and Ulna / 325

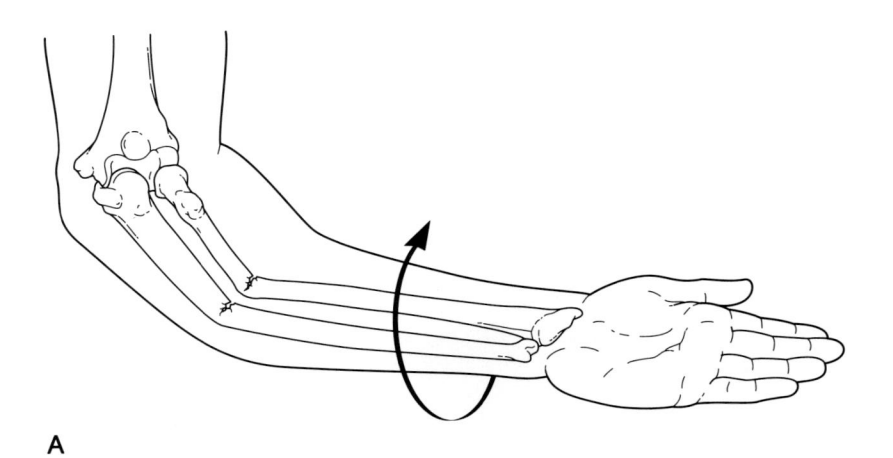

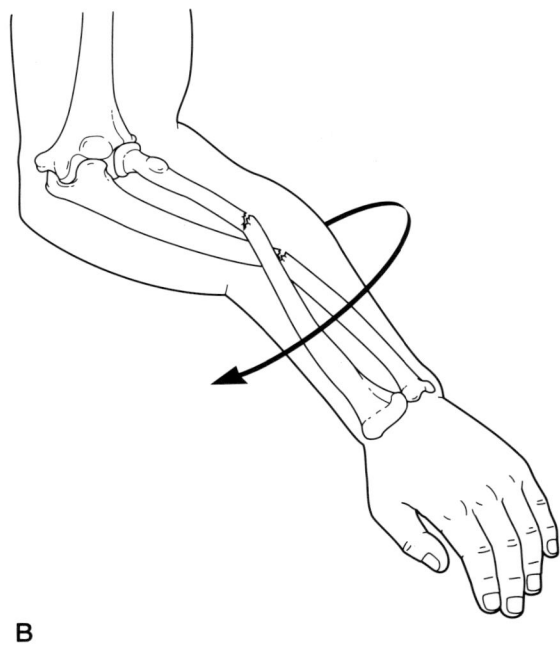

Fig. 18-2. (A) Volar angulation greenstick fracture results from supination injury. (B) Dorsal angulation greenstick fracture results from pronation injury.

obtain a history regarding the appearance of the arm immediately after the accident. If the child or accompanying adult indicate that the arm was immediately crooked, then a reduction is usually advisable.

Acute bowing from plastic deformation can be deceptive because swelling is minimal and pain is usually moderate. The degree of deformity should be assessed clinically to determine the need for reduction. Particular attention should be given to limitation of active pronation and supination. Children with mild plastic deformation will actively pronate and supinate through a functional arc of motion, approximately 120 degrees, indicating that reduction is unnecessary.

Careful neurocirculatory assessment is essential. Rare complications of Volkmann's ischemic contracture or postreduction nerve entrapment are more appropriately managed if the neurovascular status was clearly documented at the time of the initial examination.

DIFFERENTIAL DIAGNOSIS

Anterior-posterior and lateral radiographs are essential. These are best obtained by placing the forearm in as much supination as tolerated and using the distal humerus as a reference point for determining the anterior-posterior and lateral projections. These radiographs should include the elbow and the wrist on both views. One must always consider the possibility of Monteggia or Galeazzi fracture even when both bones are fractured (Fig. 18-3). Pathologic fractures should be suspected when there has been minimal trauma. Child abuse should be considered for children under the age of 3 years or when the history of trauma is inconsistent.

Proper treatment depends upon differentiating complete fractures, greenstick fractures and plastic deformation. The next section will address the management of each of these types of forearm fractures.

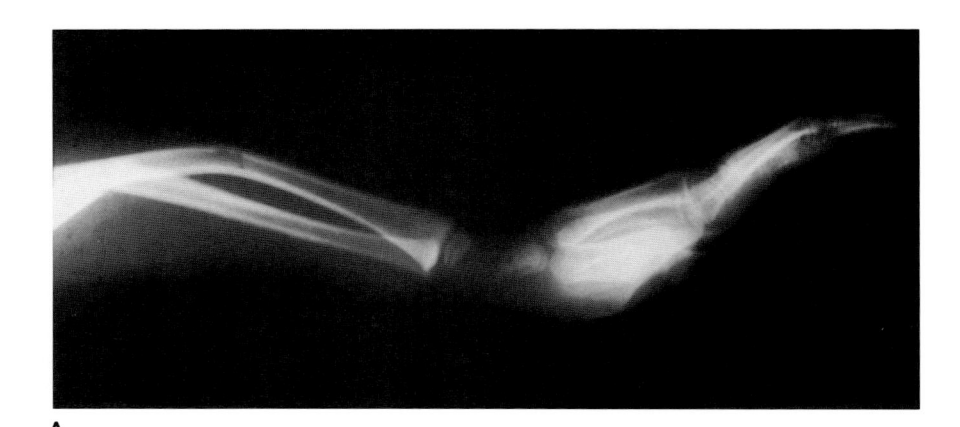

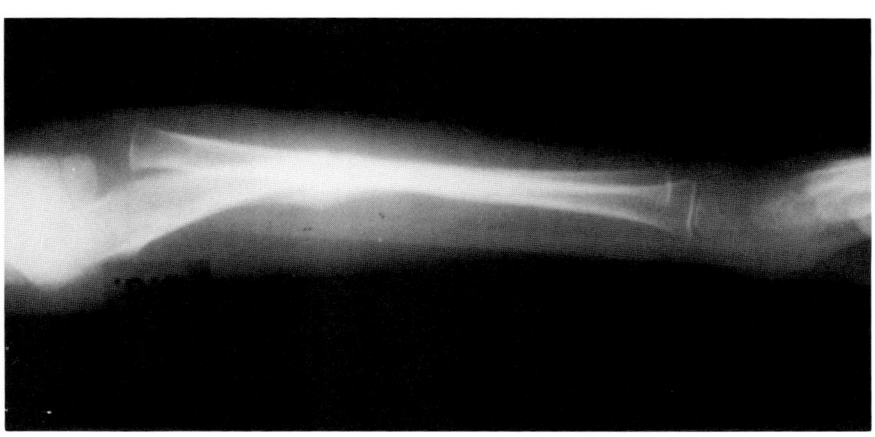

Fig. 18-3. (A) A 4-years, 8-month-old child sustained both bone forearm fracture. (B) At time of union the diagnosis of Monteggia fracture-dislocation was evident.

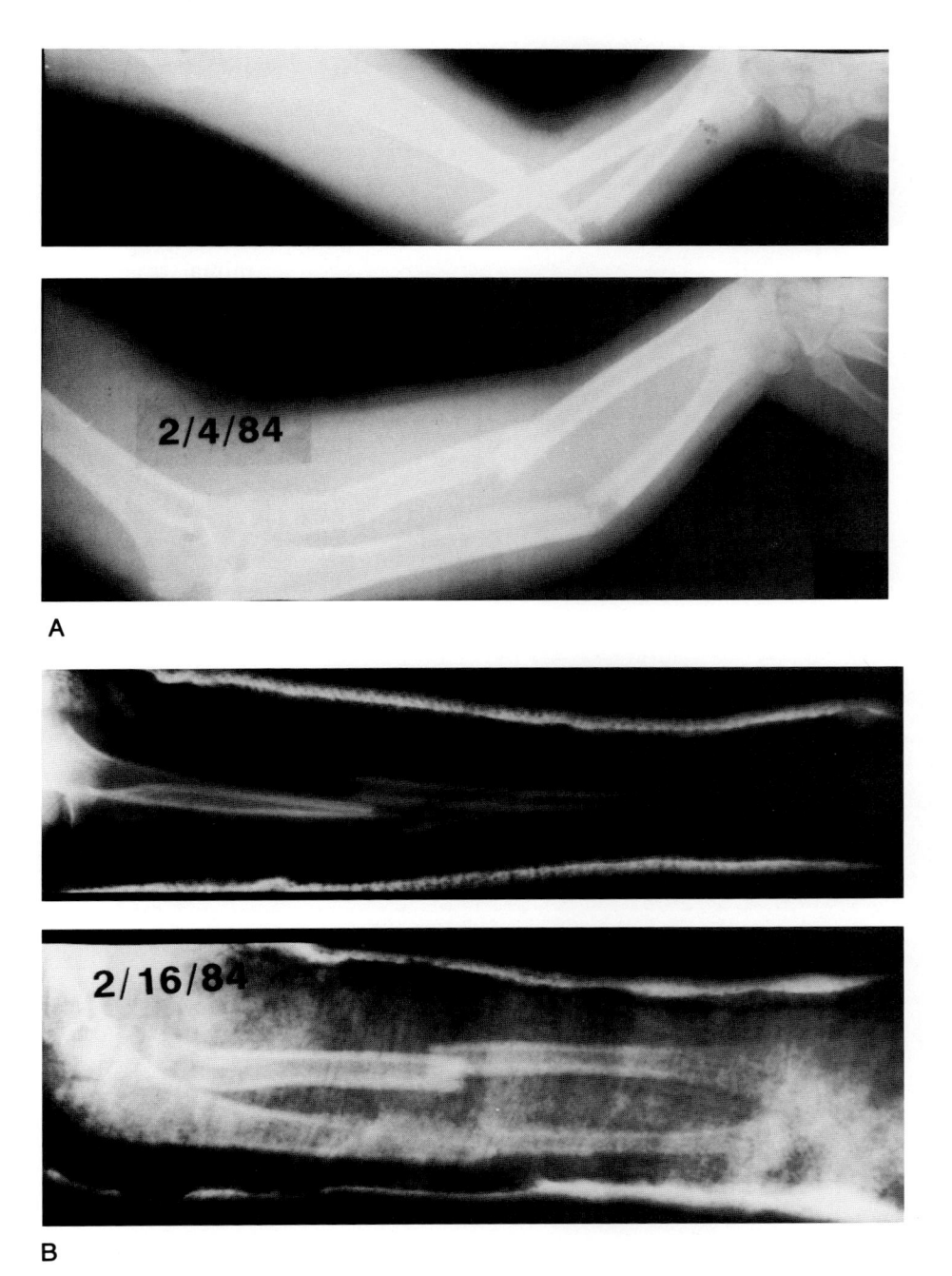

Fig. 18-4. (A) A 10 year, 5 month-old-girl sustained severe midshaft fracture right forearm. (B) Acceptable alignment 12 days after injury. *(Figure continues.)*

328 / Management of Pediatric Fractures

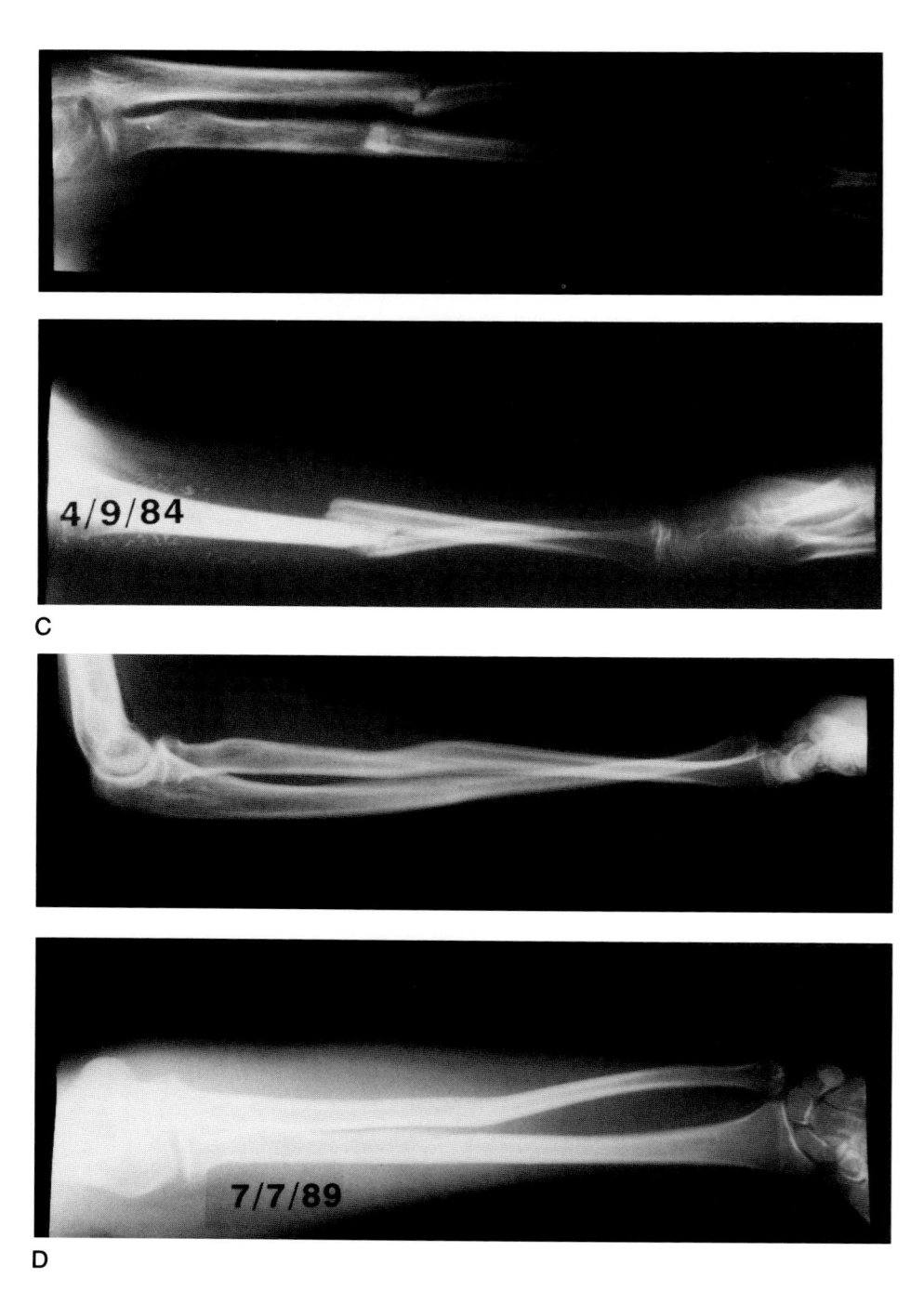

Fig. 18-4 *(Continued).* **(C)** Fracture at time of union. **(D)** Incomplete remodeling 5 years after injury. *(Figure continues.)*

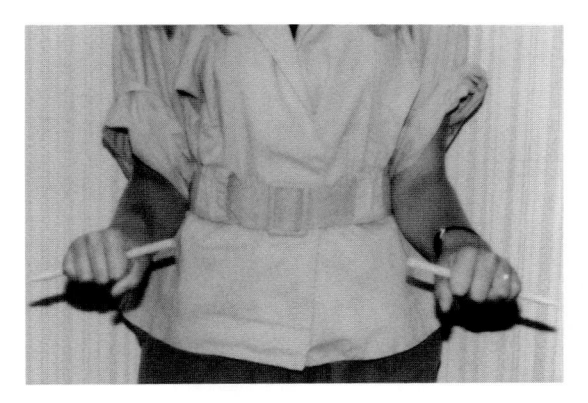

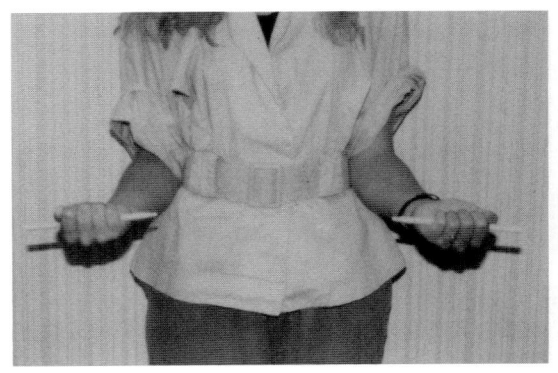

Fig. 18-4 *(Continued).* **(E)** Clinical appearance 5 years after injury.

TABLE 18-1. Guidelines for Acceptable Alignment of Forearm Shaft Fractures

Age <9 years
   Complete displacement
   Angulation 15°
   Malrotation 45°

Age 9–14 years (girls) or 9–16 years (boys)
   Distal shaft
      Complete displacement
      Angulation 15°
      Malrotation 30°
   Proximal shaft
      Complete displacement
      Angulation 10°
      Malrotation 30°

TREATMENT

Complete Shaft Fractures

Indications

The primary goals of treatment are to obtain satisfactory cosmetic appearance and restore full pronation and supination. Factors more frequently associated with poor results are proximal third fractures, age older than 12 years, and significant angular deformity.[13,14,25,26] Fortunately, forearm fractures in children are very forgiving. Most authors have noted excellent cosmesis and function even in the presence of moderate malunion (Fig. 18-4).[12,14,27-29] In children there is poor correlation between residual angular deformity and final range of pronation and supination.[12,13] In spite of these observations, significant angulation should not be accepted (Fig. 18-5). One should strive for anatomic alignment by closed reduction but we have used the following guidelines for acceptable alignment (Table 18-1). For children age 8 years or younger, one may accept complete displacement, angulation up to 15 degrees, and malrotation up to 45 degrees. For girls age 9 to 14 years or boys 9 to 16 years old distal fractures have a better prognosis than proximal shaft fractures, therefore distal fractures may be treated closed in the presence of complete displacement, up to 15 degrees angulation, and 30 degrees malrotation. Proximal shaft fractures in the older age group will have a satisfactory result with complete displacement, up to 10 degrees angulation and 30 degrees malrotation.

Closed Methods

General anesthesia is preferred for reduction of complete forearm shaft fractures. Regional anesthesia or narcotic and sedative hypnotics may suffice, but muscle relaxation is better under general anesthesia. Also, several reduction attempts may be required due to fracture instability. This is facilitated by general anesthesia.

If an initial attempt at closed reduction is unsuccessful, traction should be applied with finger traps (Fig. 18-6). The fingers should be taped to protect the skin before suspending the arm. Around 10 to 15 pounds of countertraction is applied through a strap over the upper arm. Time should be allowed for gradual distraction. This technique also allows the forearm to seek the correct rotational position spontaneously. Further manipulation with the arm in traction may permit end-to-end apposition but this is not necessary. Complete overriding may be accepted as long as angulation and rotation are within the acceptable range.

The rotational alignment can be assessed by several methods. The first method is to compare the bone diameter, shape, and alignment at the fracture site, but this can be misleading. Another method is to obtain a com-

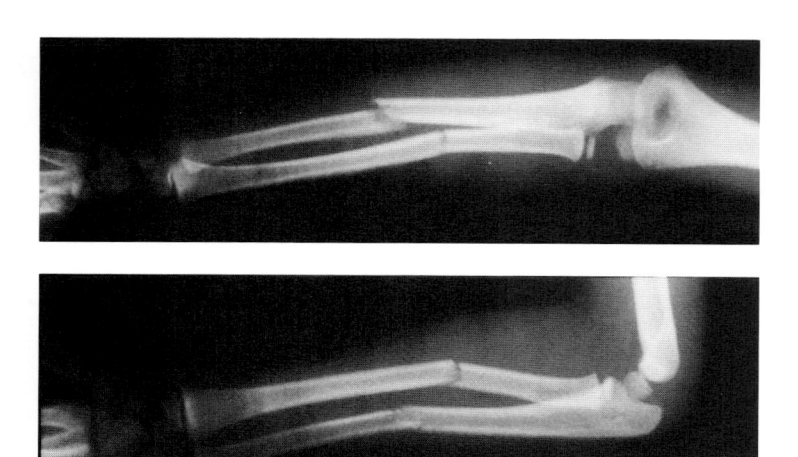

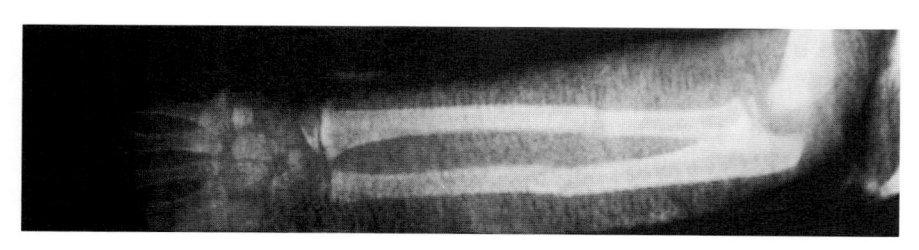

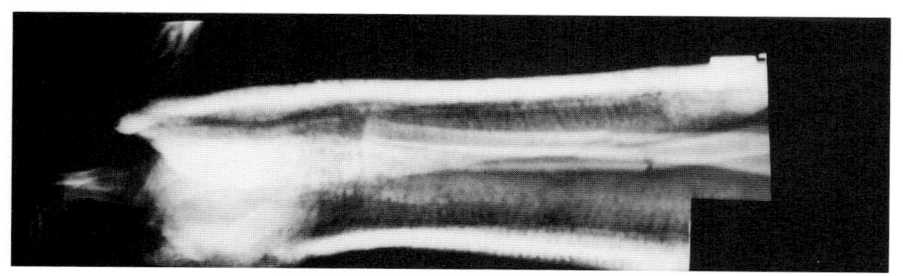

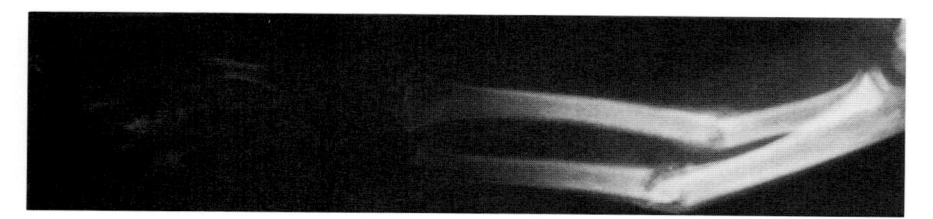

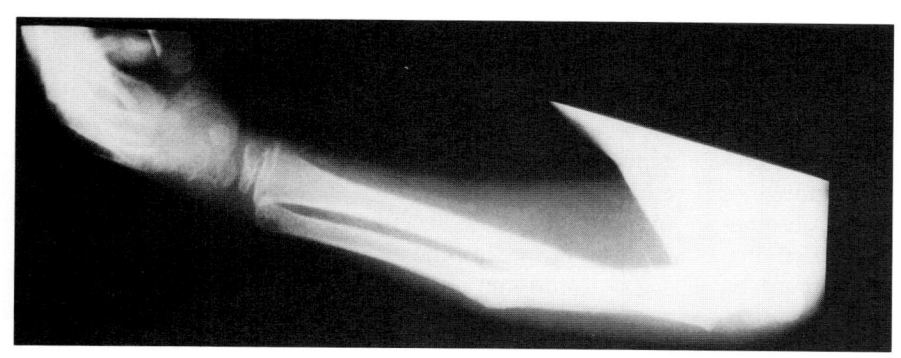

Fig. 18-5. (A) Radiograph of 6-year, 1-month-old male who sustained complete both bone forearm fracture. (B) At 7 days after reduction and plaster immobilization. No follow-up radiographs were obtained until cast removal. (C) Cast removal 6 weeks postinjury. *(Figure continues.)*

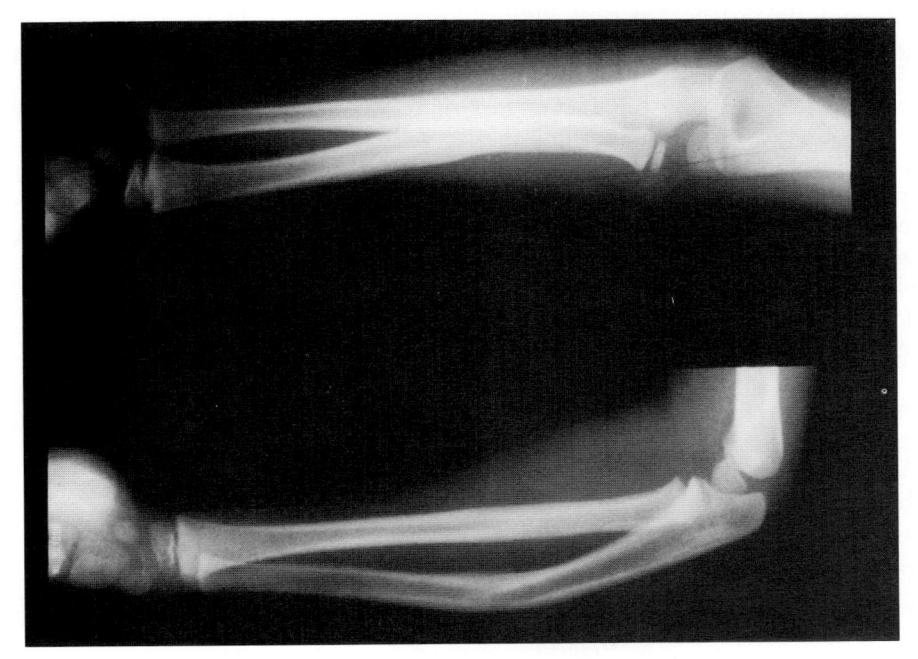

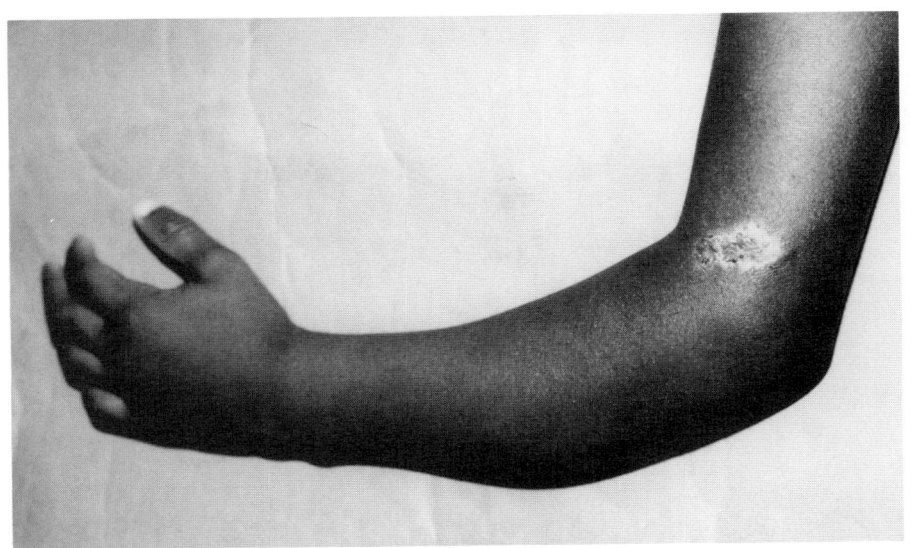

Fig. 18-5 *(Continued).* **(D&E)** At 8 months after fracture, child lacks 60 degrees of supination.

parison radiograph of the opposite forearm in the same position of pronation-supination. Creasman, Zaleske, and Ehrlich[25] have published a series of radiographs of a normal forearm taken in varying degrees of rotation. A very useful method for assessing rotation uses the position of the radial tuberosity and was described by Mervyn Evans[30] in 1945. A "tuberosity view" (Fig. 18-7) is obtained as an anteroposterior radiograph of the proximal forearm with the tube angled cephalad 20 degrees. In this view the radial tuberosity points in the direction opposite the thumb and is on the opposite side of the radius from the styloid process. Evans[11,30] observed that all complete forearm fractures should be immobilized in some degree of supination to maintain proper rotational alignment (Fig. 18-1). Others have noted that some distal shaft fractures may require varying degrees of pronation for reduction.[27,31,32] It is our opinion that pronation is rarely required for reduction of complete shaft fractures. Davis and Green[21] also cautioned against pronation of shaft fractures.

Stable reduction is usually maintained with the elbow flexed to 90 degrees although proximal fractures may be more stable with the elbow in extension.[33]

Once an acceptable closed reduction has been achieved, the arm is immobilized in a well-padded double sugar-tong splint or bivalved long arm cast. The cast should be molded into an oval in an attempt to preserve the interosseous space (Fig. 18-8). Traction is released after the plaster has hardened and radiographs are repeated.

Follow-up radiographs are made 10 to 14 days after the initial reduction. By this time some of the swelling has subsided and the patient is comfortable enough to permit application of a new long-arm cast. Minor corrections of angular deformity can be made at this time without sedation by gently molding the new cast. Significant loss of reduction requires remanipulation under anesthesia. Voto and coworkers[34] found significant redisplacement in 7 percent of forearm fractures but reported that remanipulation provides an effective means of management. For most completely displaced forearm fractures, 6 to 8 weeks of immobilization is sufficient.

Open Methods

Open reduction of complete forearm shaft fractures is occasionally indicated in children.[14,19,35-40] Some of the indications are:

1. Irreducible fracture due to soft tissue interposition
2. Refractures with significant deformity
3. Fracture shortly before skeletal maturity
4. Innability to maintain an acceptable closed reduction

The techniques for operative management of forearm fracture have included pins and plaster,[41] fixation with plates and screws[36,38,42,43] and (Fig. 18-9) intramedullary nailing.[35,37,44,45] Intramedullary nailing with supplemental casting is probably superior to compression plates in children. Less dissection is required for insertion of intramedullary nails, removal is simple, and refracture is less likely than with compression plates.

The technique of closed intramedullary nailing of forearm fractures in children has been described by Lascombes and colleagues[35] and also by Verstreken and colleagues.[44]

Under general anesthesia the patient is placed with the arm on a radiolucent side table. The fracture is partially reduced. The bone that is easiest to reduce is fixed first (Fig. 18-10).

Blunt ended nails of 1.5 and 2.5 mm diameter are prepared by precurving the nail so the apex of the curve will lie at the level of the fracture. A 5-mm tip is bent at an angle of 30 to 45 degrees. This bent tip aids in inser-

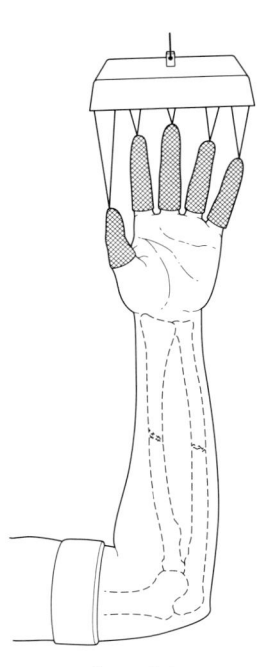

Fig. 18-6. Finger trap traction with 10–15 lb of countertraction facilitates reduction.

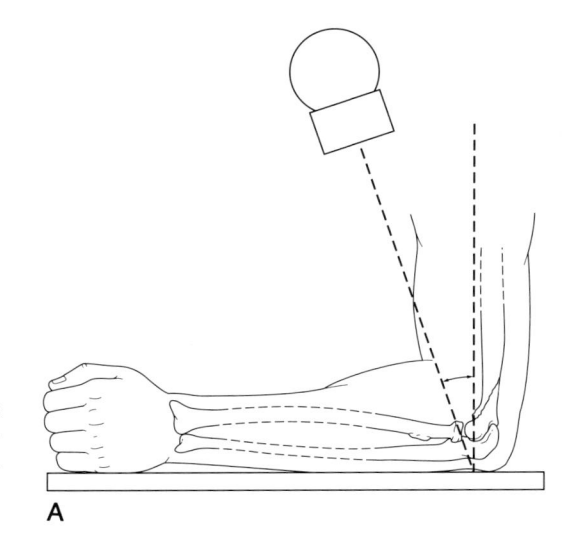

Fig. 18-7. **(A)** The "tuberosity view" is obtained with the x-ray tube angled cephalad 20 degrees. **(B)** The radial tuberosity points in the opposite direction from the thumb. (From Evans,[11] with permission.)

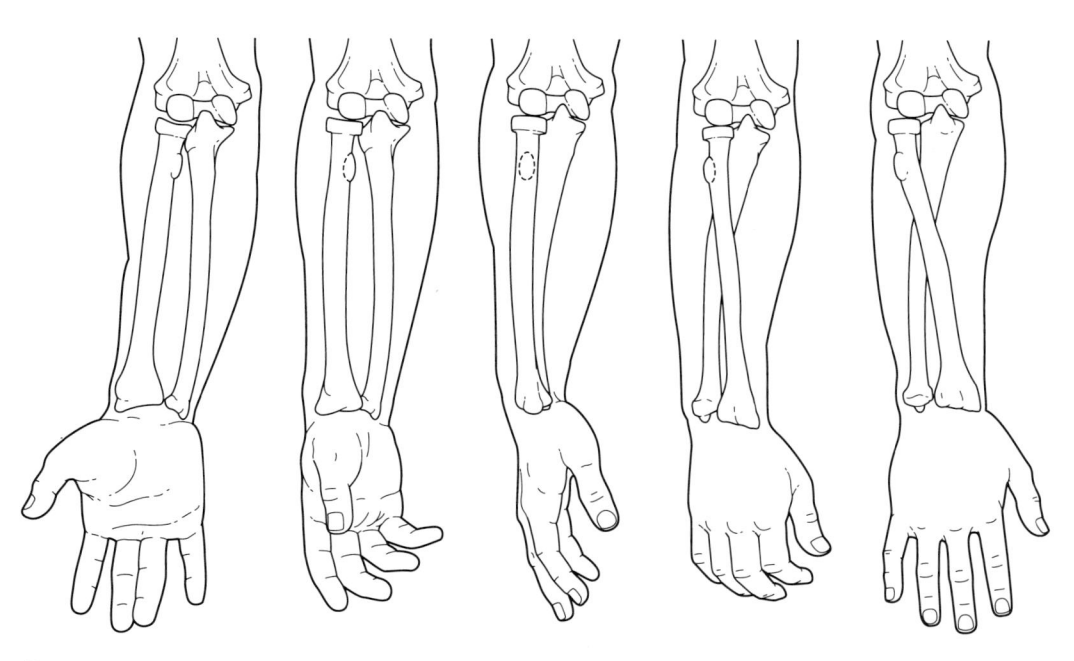

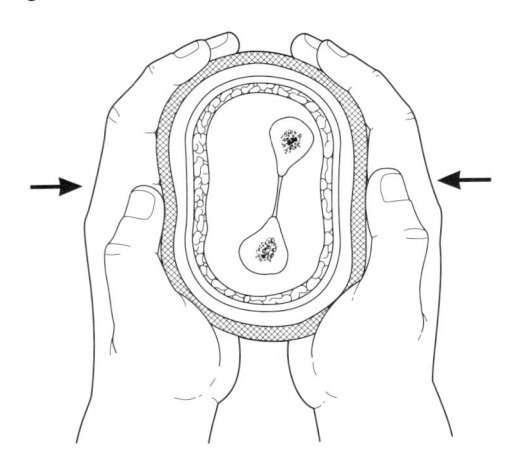

Fig. 18-8. Following reduction, the plaster should be molded into an oval in order to preserve the interosseous space. Arrows indicate gentle compression.

tion and avoids penetration of the opposite cortex during advancement of the nail.

The distal radial metaphysis is approached through a 1-cm incision on the lateral side just proximal to the physeal plate. The radial vein and nerve are protected. An oblique hole is drilled through the lateral cortex at a 45-degree angle. A nail is introduced into the hole and worked proximally through the medullary canal until the tip is close to the fracture site. The fracture is reduced and the proximal fragment is engaged with the bent tip. The nail is advanced to the proximal metaphysis. Minor adjustments in reduction can be performed by rotating the nail. The protruding portion of the nail is then bent 90 degrees at the entry hole and cut off with 5 mm protruding to permit later extraction.

The ulna may be approached proximally through the olecranon apophysis. An incision on the lateral side is used in order to avoid the ulnar nerve. The distal ulnar metaphysis may also be used as an entry point and is preferred by Verstreken.[35,44]

Intramedullary nailing may provide enough stability to permit early range of motion.[35,44,46] However, a brief period of plaster immobilization seems advisable in children. The nails are removed 3 to 12 months after operation.

External fixation can be usefully employed in open fractures of the radius and ulna or where there has been severe associated soft tissue and skin trauma (Fig. 18-11). Care must be taken to use smaller pediatric fixators to avoid iatrogenic fracturing of the radius and ulna from large pins.

Greenstick Fractures

Indications for Reduction

The indications for reduction of greenstick fractures are similar to those for complete fractures (Table 18-1). The clinical appearance of a forearm at the time of injury also provides a gauge regarding the need for reduction.

Closed Methods

It is essential to understand that greenstick forearm fractures have significant rotational deformity (Fig. 18-2). Several authors advocate breaking the intact cortex and immobilizing the forearm in neutral rotation with a long-arm cast.[5,47] However, in 1951 Evans[11] wrote a classic paper in which he observed that correcting the rotational deformity will correct the angulation simultaneously without the necessity of fracturing the opposite cortex. This has been confirmed by Rang[20] and others.[21,32] Gruber[48] noted that incomplete greenstick fractures may have delayed consolidation and advocated fracturing the opposite cortex in order to prevent refracture. It is our opinion that completion of a greenstick fracture is not necessary for reduction but may decrease the risk of refracture.

Reduction of greenstick fractures should be obtained by supinating the forearm if the angulation is dorsal. The forearm should be reduced in pronation if the angulation is volar (Fig. 18-12). Postoperative management is the same as closed treatment of complete fractures. However, an incomplete greenstick fracture should be splinted for several weeks after cast removal to prevent refracture.

Open Methods

Open methods are rarely indicated for greenstick fractures. Exploration is occasionally indicated if one suspects tendon or nerve entrapment in the reduced fracture.[49-51]

Plastic Deformation

Traumatic plastic deformation of the forearm bones in children was first reported by Borden[52,53] in 1974 (Fig. 18-13). Several reports since then have emphasized the difficulties of diagnosis and treatment.[54-59] The need for reduction is best determined by the clinical examina-

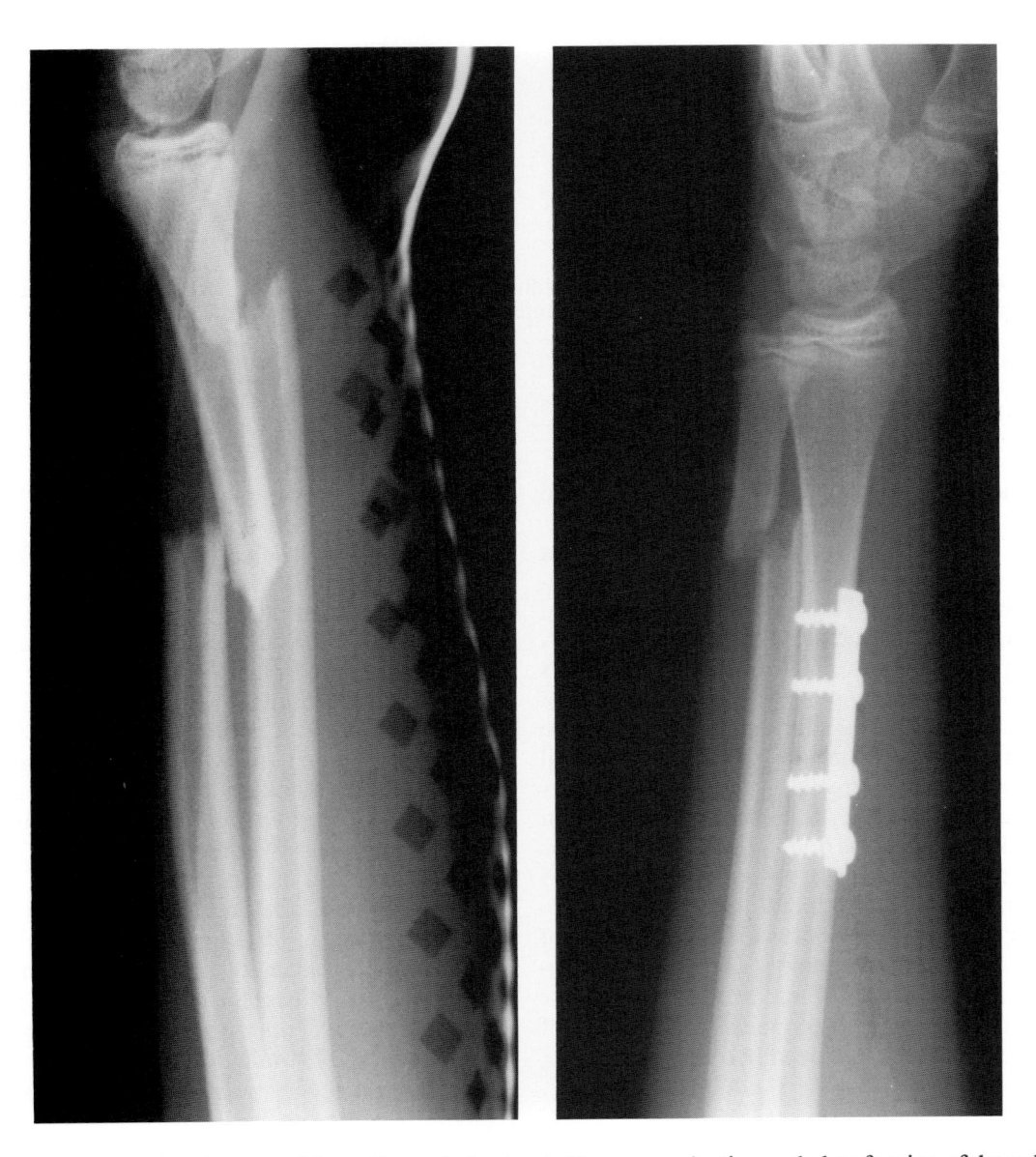

Fig. 18-9. Irreducible fracture of the radius and ulna treated by open reduction and plate fixation of the radius only to preserve the interosseous space.

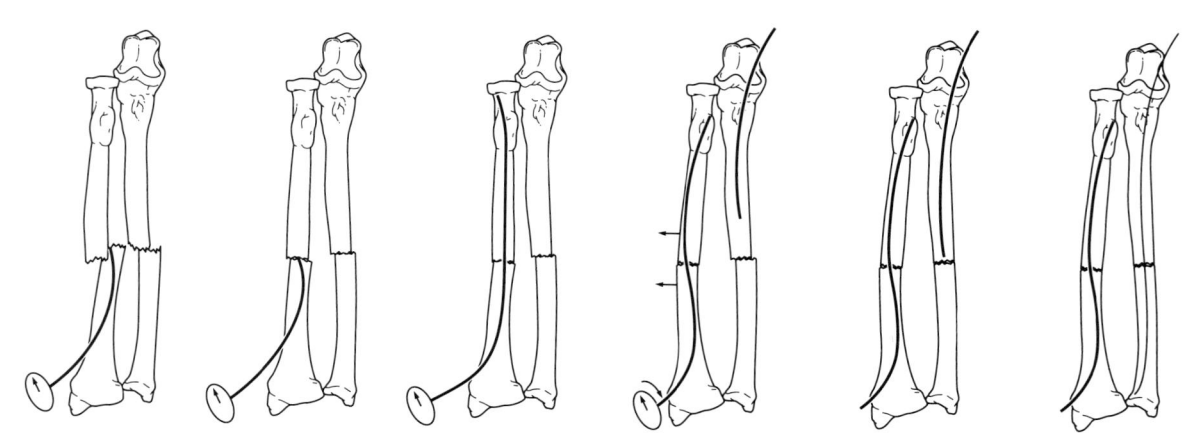

Fig. 18-10. Technique of elastic intramedullary nailing: Introduction of radial nail, reduction and manipulation of fracture, rotation of nail, ulnar nailing. (Adapted from Lascombes et al.,[35] with permission.)

tion. Cosmetic deformity with restricted rotation should be reduced.

Reduction is difficult to obtain and maintain unless the technique of Sanders and Heckman[54] is used. General anesthesia is required. The apex of the bow is placed over a fulcrum such as a sandbag (Fig. 18-14). Considerable force equaling 100 to 150 percent of the child's weight is applied gradually to the metaphyseal ends of the forearm. Pressure over the epiphysis should be avoided. This must be sustained for several minutes until the deformity gradually corrects. Occasionally, it is necessary to completely fracture one or both bones to obtain reduction. When one bone is fractured and the other has plastic deformation, it is necessary to correct the bowed bone before reducing the fractured one.

Adequate reduction is demonstrated by restoration of full pronation and supination under anesthesia. A long-arm cast is applied with the forearm supinated for correction of dorsal bowing or pronated for correction of volar bowing. The cast is removed in 6 to 8 weeks.

COMPLICATIONS

Malunion

Some fractures will heal with deformity or loss of motion regardless of careful management. Remodeling potential depends upon the age of the child, the distance of the fracture from the epiphyseal plate and the amount of angulation.[14,16,31] However, the degree of remodeling is unpredictable particularly in children older than 11 years.[12-14,16]

Several authors[12-14,27,28] have noted that there is poor correlation with limitation of motion and varying degrees of angulation (Fig. 18-15). Cadaver studies have shown that residual angulation of 10 degrees does not significantly limit forearm rotation.[60-62] Matthews and colleagues[60] noted that 20 degrees of angulation only restricted pronation-supination by 30 percent. Tarr and colleagues[61] observed that soft tissue scarring and interosseous tension may be important factors in restriction of forearm rotation. This is evidenced by the fact that some cases with anatomic alignment will have loss of forearm rotation.[12,28] Morrey and coworkers[63] found that only 50 degrees of pronation, and 50 degrees of supination were necessary for most activities of daily living. Some patients with only 60 degrees of pronation or 60 degrees of supination may be unaware of loss of motion,[12] thus correction of malunion is rarely indicated unless there is more than 45 to 60 degrees loss of forearm rotation.

Blackburn and associates[64] recommended correction of malunited forearm fractures by drill osteoclasis through a small incision. In 4 of their 15 cases an intramedullary Rush pin was used to secure the ulna, but most were treated with plaster immobilization only. Full range of motion was regained by 11 patients. Linscheid and Trousdale[65] reported 25 corrective osteotomies for

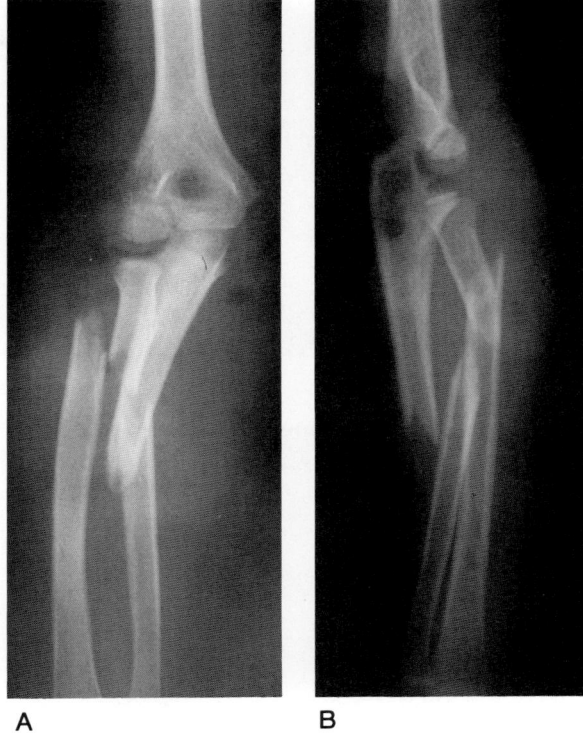

Fig. 18-11. **(A&B)** Open fractures of the proximal radius and ulna in an 8-year-old boy subsequent to being struck by a car while riding his bicycle. **(C)** Management of the fractures and open wound with an external fixator. **(D)** Radiographs at age 15 illustrating the excellent remodeling with no loss of pronation or supination.

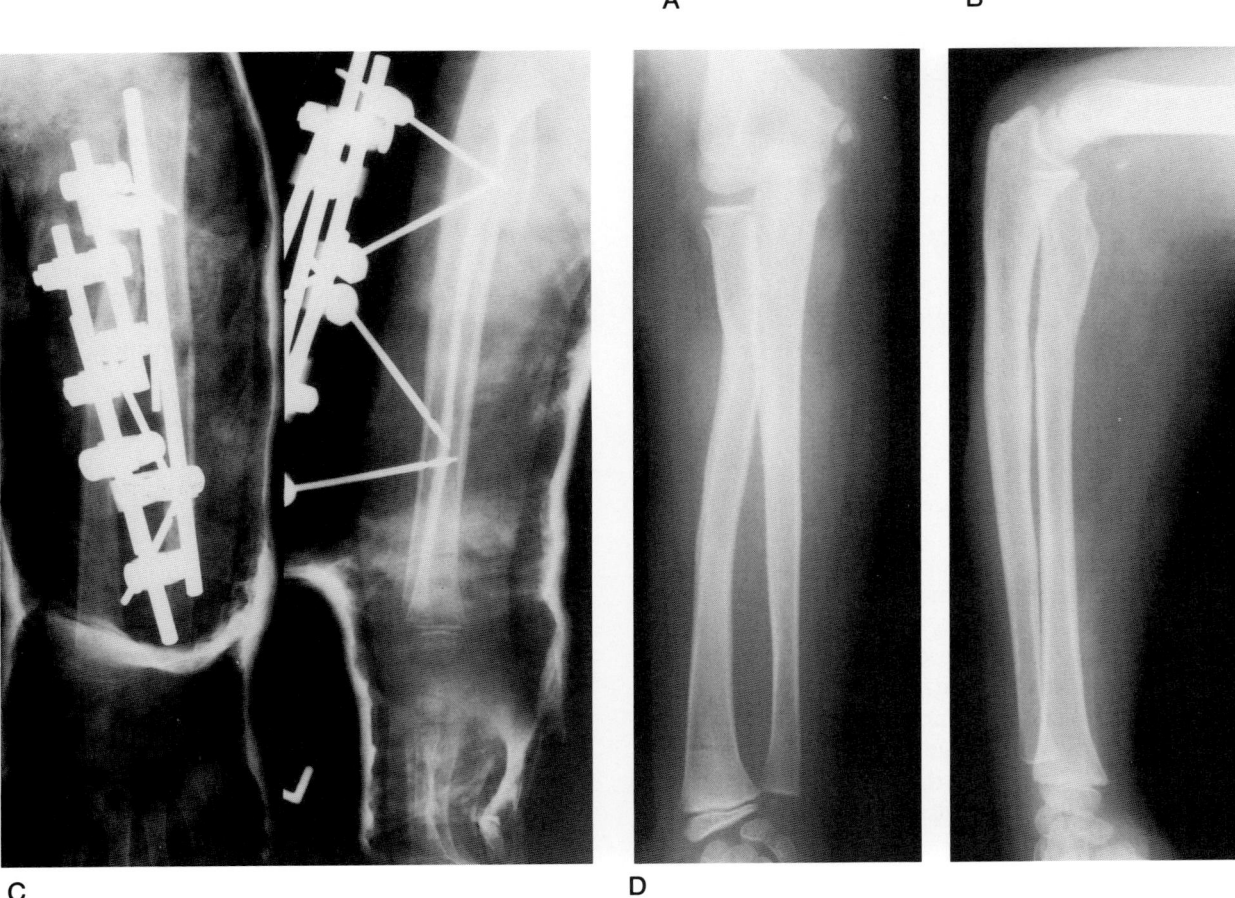

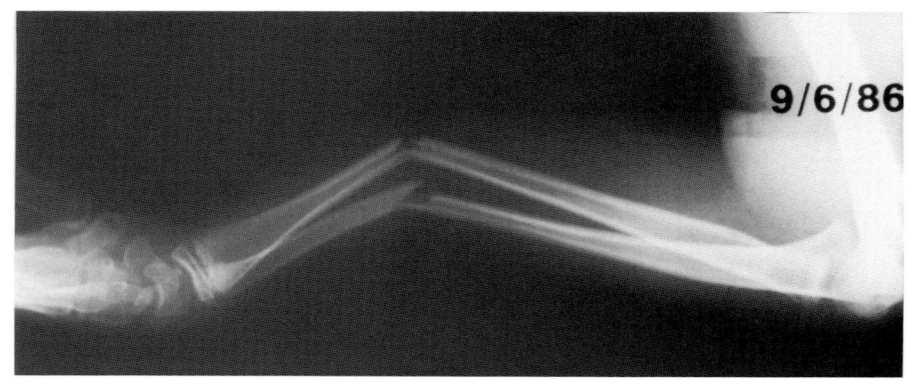

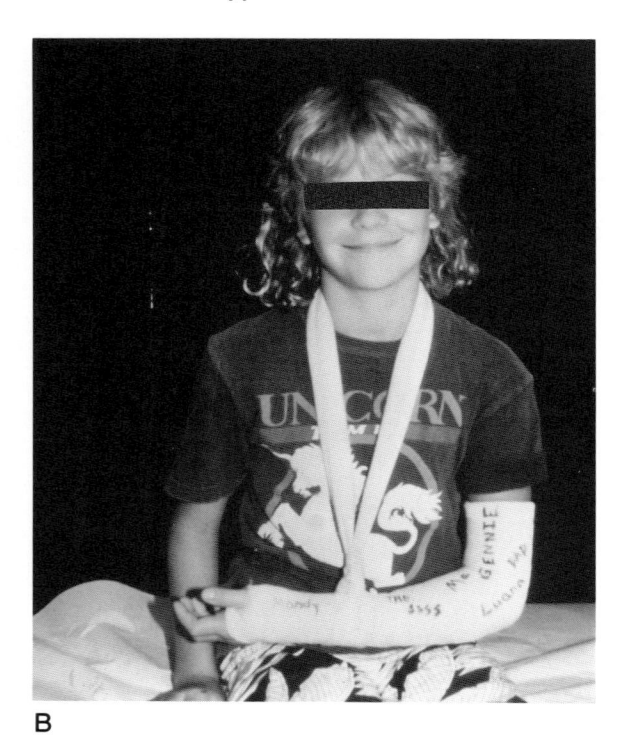

Fig. 18-12. **(A)** Volar angulated greenstick fractures should be reduced in pronation. A 12-year, 8-month-old girl sustained a volar angulated greenstick forearm fracture. **(B)** The fracture was inappropriately immobilized in supination. *(Figure continues.)*

forearm malunions. They noted better results in those patients treated within 12 months of the initial fracture.

In our opinion, corrective osteotomy is rarely indicated for malunited forearm fractures. From 6 to 12 months of observation is warranted to determine the potential for recovery of range of motion and remodeling. Osteotomy is indicated if loss of forearm rotation is greater than 60 degrees after this period of observation.

Refracture

The most likely site of recurrent fracture in children is the forearm. All other areas are rarely involved.[40] Greenstick fractures have a higher rate of recurrence than complete fractures.[48] This increased incidence cannot be explained on the basis of inadequate immobilization or incomplete reduction. Gruber[48] has postulated that the unbroken cortex prevents contact healing of the fractured cortex and results in a weak union. Gruber[48] advo-

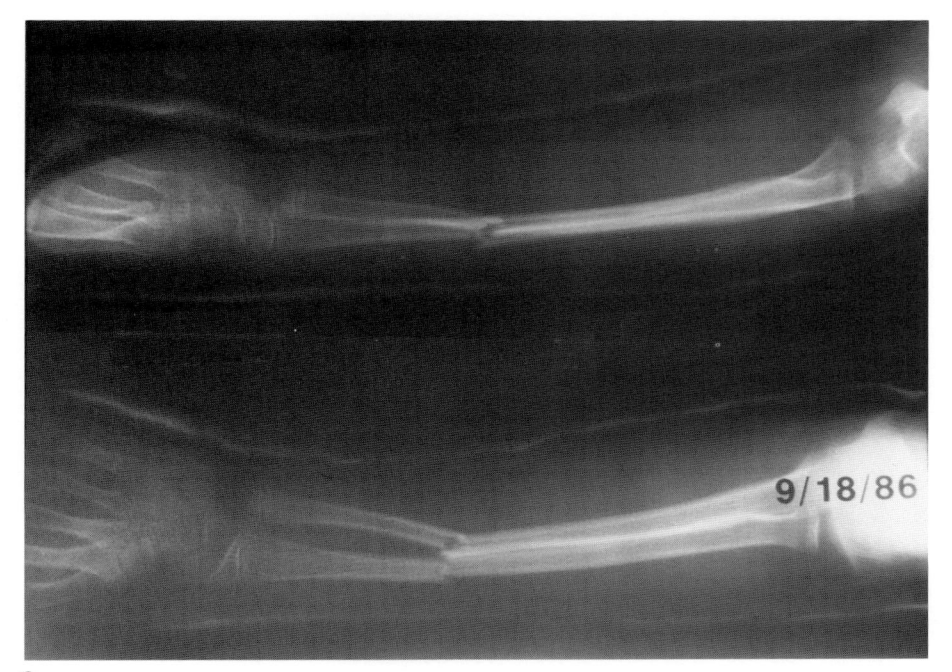

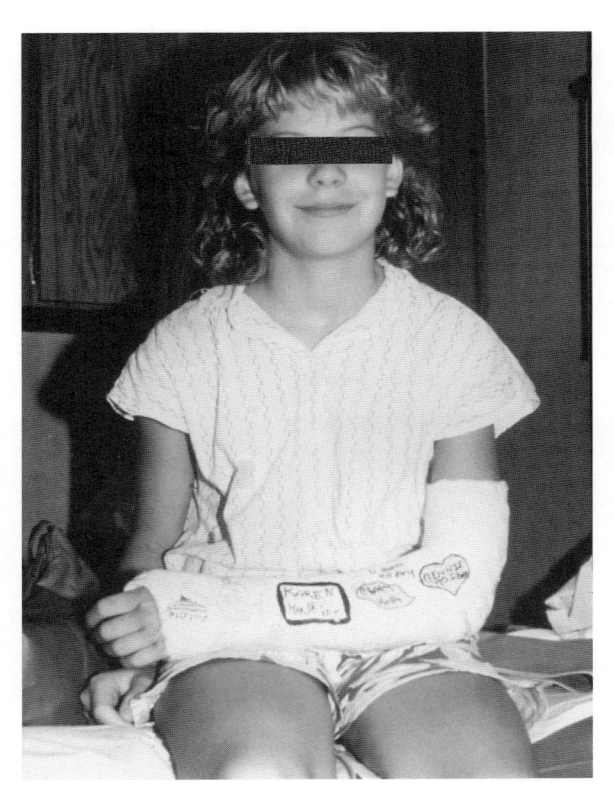

Fig. 18-12 *(Continued).* **(C)** At time of reduction with forearm in supination. **(D)** Under general anesthesia the forearm was placed in slight pronation and a cast was reapplied. *(Figure continues.)*

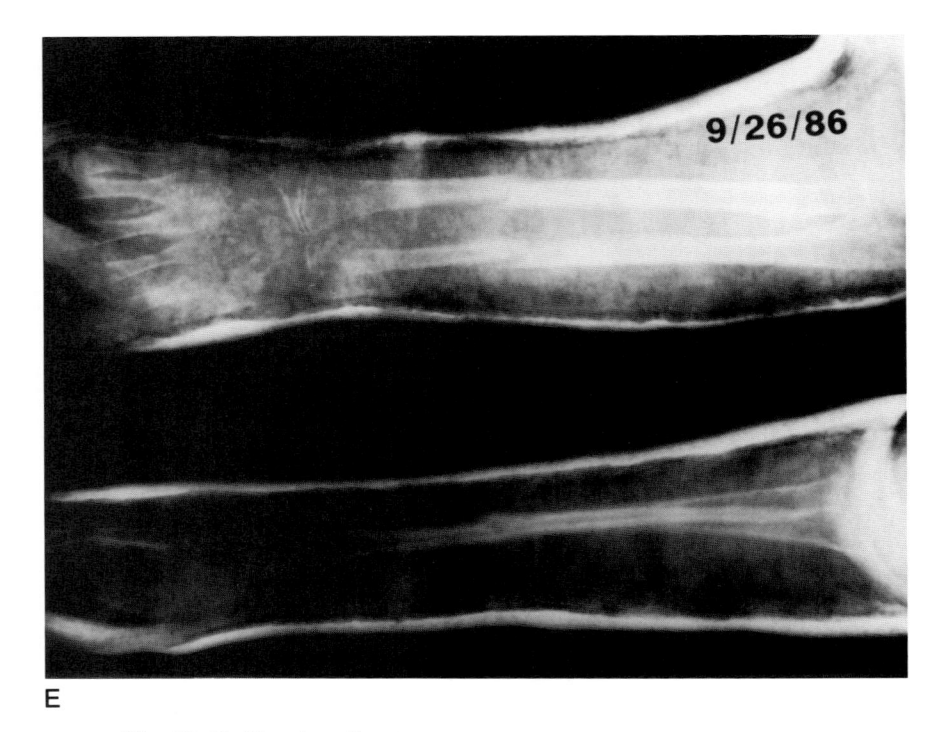

Fig. 18-12 *(Continued).* **(E)** Improved reduction with pronation.

cated fracturing the intact cortex during reduction of greenstick fractures to prevent fracture recurrence.

Occasionally, a refracture converts a minor deformity into an unacceptable one. Reduction of a refracture and maintenance of reduction can be quite difficult. Open reduction with internal fixation is indicated if deformity is significant.[22,40]

Synostosis

Synostosis following fractures of the forearm shaft are very rare in children. Vince and Miller[66] reported four cases and noted that all previous reports of cross-unions involved the proximal radius and ulna rather than the shaft. Severe trauma was implicated in each case.

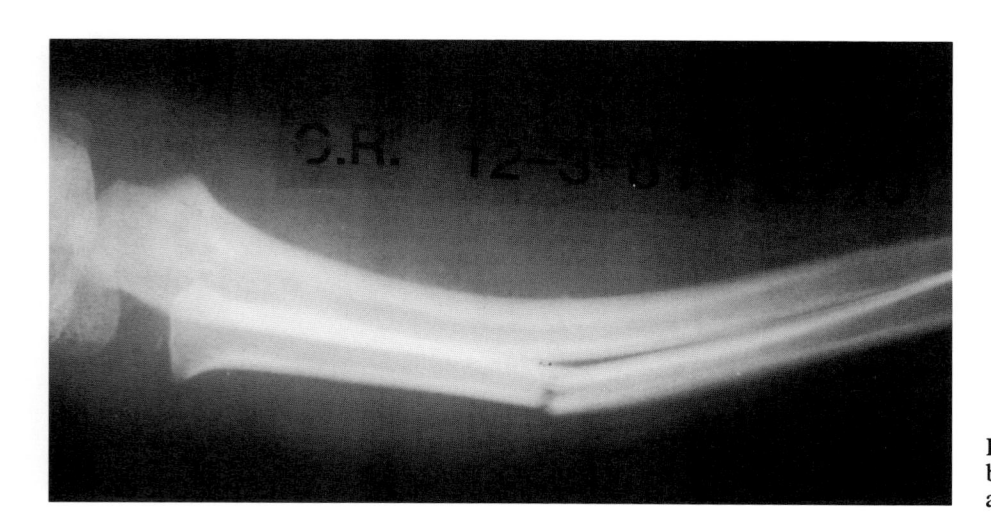

Fig. 18-13. A 6-year, 10-month-old boy with greenstick fracture of radius and plastic deformation of the ulna.

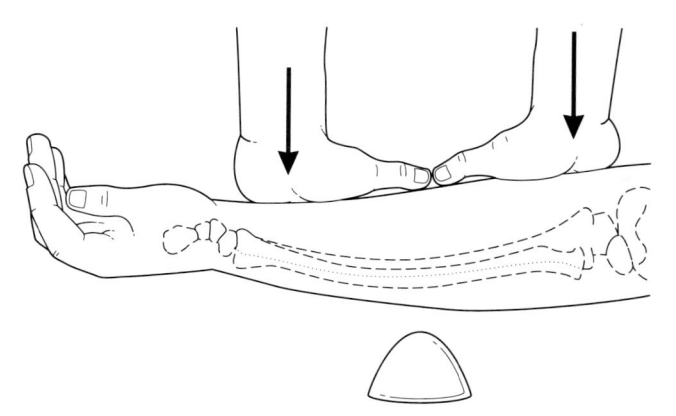

Fig. 18-14. Method of reduction of plastic deformation fracture. Gradual sustained pressure is required. Arrows indicate direction of applied force. (Adapted from Sanders and Heckman,[54] with permission.)

Resection of a diaphyseal posttraumatic synostosis may result in some improvement of forearm rotation.[66-69] An interval of 1 year between injury and excision of the cross-union is recommended. Fat or Silastic should be interposed between the bones after resection is complete.

Nerve Injury

Fractures of the shaft of the radius and ulna are occasionally associated with neurologic injury. The median nerve and the anterior interosseous nerve are most likely to be damaged. Nerve entrapment in complete and greenstick fractures has been reported.[39,50,51,70]

A meticulous physical examination before and after reduction is important in formulating a plan of management. Observation is warranted for 2 to 3 months. Electromyography (EMG) should then be performed if there is no clinical evidence of recovery. Evidence of reservation on EMG justifies further observation. Complete denervation 2 to 3 months after injury warrants exploration.

Other Complications

Rare complications such as tendon entrapment, compartment syndrome, and gas gangrene (Fig. 18-16) have also been reported following forearm fractures in children.[49,71,72] The generally benign nature of pediatric forearm fractures may create a false sense of security for the orthopaedic surgeon. Any deviation from a normally smooth course should arouse suspicion. Osseous complications of forearm fractures are often correctible, but soft tissue complications may be permanent.

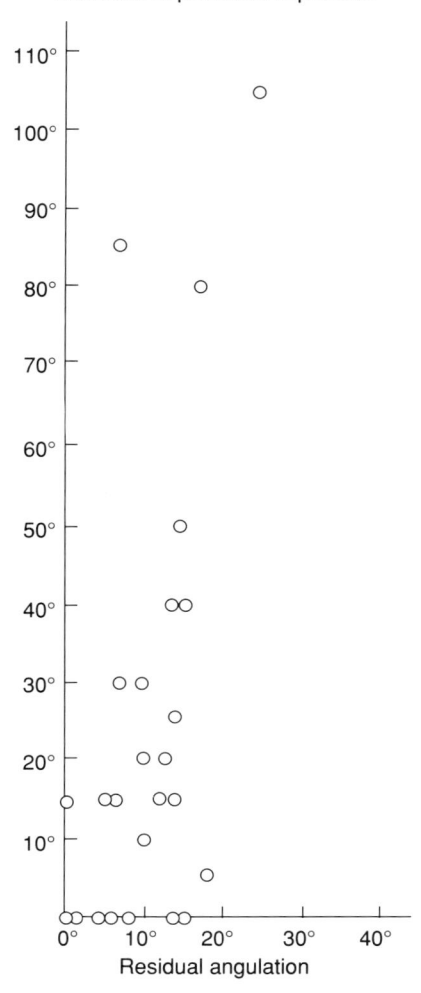

Fig. 18-15. Poor correlation exists between late residual angulation and limitation of pronation-supination. (Adapted from Hogstrom et al.,[13] with permission.)

SUMMARY

Fractures of the shaft of the radius and ulna account for 6 to 10 percent of all childhood fractures. Forearm fractures in children may be complete, greenstick or plastically deformed. Treatment varies with the type and location of the fracture, and the age of child. Closed

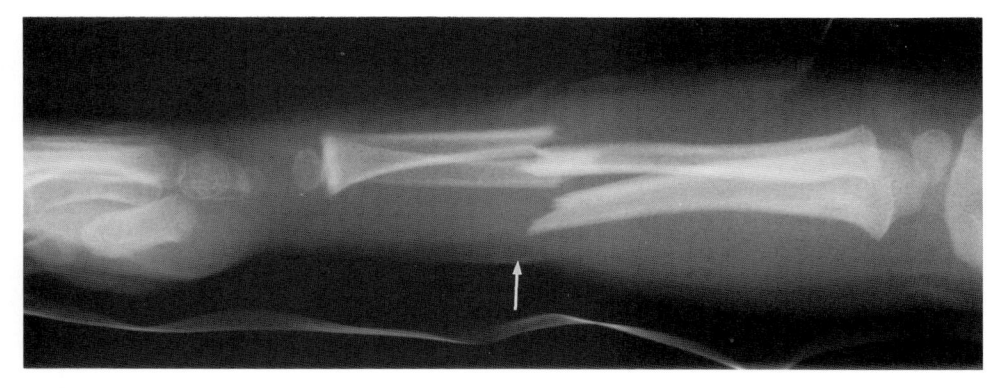

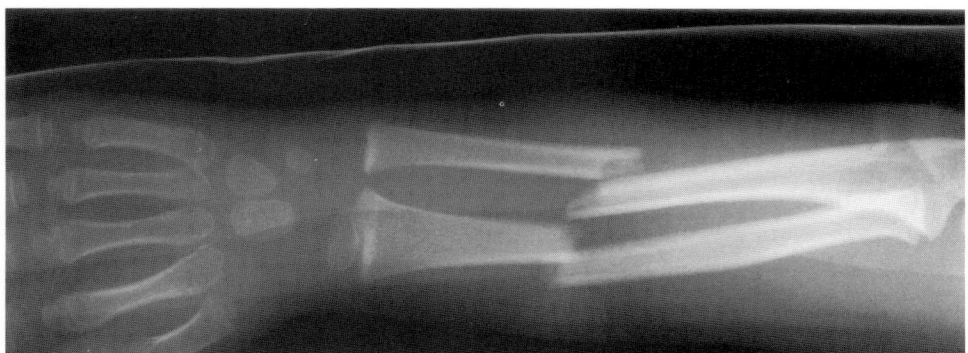

Fig. 18-16. An open fracture of the radius and ulna. The proximal ulnar fragment has penetrated the volar aspect of the forearm *(arrow)*. Although the puncture wound is minute, it means the bone end has been contaminated and an open debridement of the bone end is mandatory to avoid severe complications such as gas gangrene.

reduction is the initial treatment in most cases. Open reduction with flexible intramedullary nailing is indicated when satisfactory alignment can not be maintained, when the child is near skeletal maturity, or in the case of refracture with significant deformity.

Correct rotational alignment is essential for reduction. The radial tuberosity may be used as a guide to the rotational position of the proximal fragment. The thumb should point in approximately the opposite direction from the radial tuberosity. Complete fractures of the shaft are generally reduced in a position ranging from neutral to full supination. Pronation is rarely required.

Greenstick fractures behave differently from complete fractures. Volar angulated greenstick fractures should be reduced by pronating the forearm. Dorsally angulated greenstick fractures require supination for reduction. It is not necessary to complete the greenstick fracture to obtain alignment, but completing the fracture may reduce the risk of refracture.

Plastic deformation or traumatic bowing occurs when microfractures develop as a result of axial loading. Significant plastic deformation should be treated under general anesthesia by applying sustained corrective forces continuously for 2 to 3 minutes.

Significant complications of forearm fractures are uncommon. Malunion may occur, but it correlates poorly with limitation of motion. In most cases, 10 to 15 degrees of angulation and complete displacement can be accepted. More severe malunions may require corrective osteotomy if deformity and restriction of motion persist for 6 to 12 months. More serious complications such as synostosis, nerve injury, and compartment syndrome are rare but should not be overlooked in the management of forearm fractures.

REFERENCES

1. Mann DC, Rajmaira S: Distribution of physeal and nonphyseal fractures in 2,650 long-bone fractures in children aged 0–16 years. J Pediatr Orthop 10:713, 1990
2. Worlock P, Stower M: Fracture patterns in Nottingham children. J Pediatr Orthop 6:656, 1986
3. Gandhi RK, Wilson P, Mason Brown JJ, Macleod W: Spontaneous correction of deformity following fractures of the forearm in children. Br J Surg 50:5, 1962
4. Blount WP: Fractures in children. Robert E. Krieger Publishing, Huntington, NY, 1977

5. Blount WP, Schaefer AA, Johnson JH: Fractures of the forearm in children. JAMA 120:111, 1942
6. Thorndike A, Jr, Dimmler CL, Jr: Fractures of the forearm and elbow in children: an analysis of three hundred and sixty-four consecutive cases. N Engl J Med 225:475, 1941
7. Goss CM: Gray's anatomy of the human body. 28th Ed. Lea & Febiger, Philadelphia, 1966
8. Hughston JC: Fractures of the forearm: anatomical considerations. J Bone Joint Surg [Am] 44:1664, 1962
9. Glatzer RL, Perlman RD, Michaels G, Matles A: Fractures of both bones of the distal forearm in children. Bull Hosp Joint Dis 28:14, 1967
10. Patrick J: A study of supination and pronation, with especial reference to the treatment of forearm fractures. J Bone Joint Surg 28:737, 1946
11. Evans EM: Fractures of the radius and ulna. J Bone Joint Surg [Br] 33:548, 1951
12. Price CT, Scott DS, Kurzner M, Flynn JC: Malunited forearm fractures in children. J Pediatr Orthop 10:705, 1990
13. Hogstrom H, Nilsson BE, Willner S: Correction with growth following diaphyseal forearm fracture. Acta Orthop Scand 47:299, 1976
14. Fuller DJ, McCullough CJ: Malunited fractures of the forearm in children. J Bone Joint Surg [Br] 64:364, 1982
15. Digby KH: The measurement of diaphysial growth in proximal and distal directions. J Anat Physiol 50:187, 1915
16. Vittas D, Larsen E, Torp-Pedersen S: Angular remodeling of midshaft forearm fractures in children. Clin Orthop 265:261, 1991
17. Younger ASE, Tredwell SJ, Mackenzie WG: Axis deviation as a predictor of fracture outcome, abstracted. 9th Combined Meeting of the Orthopedic Association of the English Speaking World, 1992, Toronto, Ontario, Canada, June 12–26, 1992
18. Mortensson W, Thonell S: Left-side dominance of upper extremity fracture in children. Acta Orthop Scand 62:154, 1991
19. Tredwell SJ, Van Peteghem K, Clough M: Pattern of forearm fractures in children. J Pediatr Orthop 4:604, 1984
20. Rang M: Children's fractures. 2nd Ed. JB Lippincott, Philadelphia, 1983
21. Davis DR, Green DP: Forearm fractures in children. Clin Orthop 120:172, 1976
22. King RE: Fractures of the shafts of the radius and ulna. p. 415. In: Rockwood CA, Wilkins KE, King RE (eds): Fractures in Children. 3rd Ed. JB Lippincott, Philadelphia, 1991
23. Currey JD, Butler G: The mechanical properties of bone tissue in children. J Bone Joint Surg [Am] 57:810, 1975
24. Chamay A: Mechanical and morphological aspects of experimental overload and fatigue in bone. J Biomech 3:263, 1970
25. Creasman C, Zaleske DJ, Ehrlich MG: Analyzing forearm fracture in children: the more subtle signs of impeding problems. Clin Orthop 188:40, 1984
26. Roberts JA: Angulation of the radius in children's fractures. J Bone Joint Surg [Br] 68:751, 1986
27. Daruwalla JS: A study of radioulnar movements following fractures of the forearm in children. Clin Orthop 139:114, 1979
28. Nilsson BE, Obrant K: The range of motion following fracture of the shaft of the forearm in children. Acta Orthop Scand 48:600, 1977
29. Onne L, Sandblom PH: Late results in fractures of the fore-arm in children. Acta Chir Scand 98:549, 1949
30. Evans EM: Rotational deformity in the treatment of fractures of both bones of the forearm. J Bone Joint Surg 27:373, 1945
31. Blount WP: Forearm fractures in children. Clin Orthop 51:93, 1967
32. Fernandez DL: Conservative treatment of forearm fractures in children. p. 158. In Chapchal G (ed): Fractures in children. Thieme, New York, 1981
33. Gainor JW, Hardy JH III: Forearm fractures treated in extension: immobilization of fractures of the proximal both bones of the forearm in children. J Trauma 9:167, 1969
34. Voto SJ, Weiner DS, Leighley B: Redisplacement after closed reduction of forearm fractures in children. J Pediatr Orthop 10:79, 1990
35. Lascombes P, Prevot J, Ligier JN et al: Elastic stable intramedullary nailing in forearm shaft fractures in children: 85 cases. J Pediatr Orthop 10:167, 1990
36. Nielsen AB, Simonsen O: Displaced forearm fractures in children treated with AO plates. Injury 15:393, 1984
37. Kay S, Smith C, Oppenheim WL: Both-bone midshaft forearm fractures in children. J Pediatr Orthop 6:306, 1986
38. Spiegel PG, Mast JW: Internal and external fixation of fractures in children. Orthop Clin North Am 11:405, 1980
39. Gainor BJ, Olson S: Combined engrapment of the median and anterior interosseous nerves in a pediatric both-bone forearm fracture. J Orthop Trauma 4:197, 1990
40. Arunachalam VSP, Griffiths JC: Fracture recurrence in children. Injury 7:37, 1976
41. Voto SJ, Weiner DS, Leighley B: Use of pins and plaster in the treatment of unstable pediatric forearm fractures. J Pediatr Orthop 10:85, 1990
42. Alpar EK, Thompson K, Owen R, Taylor JF: Midshaft fractures of forearm bones in children. Injury 13:153, 1981
43. Vainionpaa S, Bostman O, Patiala H, Rokkanen P: Internal fixation of forearm fractures in children. Acta Orthop Scand 58:121, 1987
44. Verstreken L, Delronge G, Lamoureux J: Shaft forearm fractures in children: intramedullary nailing with immediate motion: a preliminary report. J Pediatr Orthop 8:450, 1988
45. Gyrtrup HJ, Fosse L: The use of Kirschner wires in diaphyseal fractures of the forearm. Acta Orthop Belg 55:86, 1989
46. Ono M, Bechtold JE, Merkow RL et al: Rotational stabil-

ity of diaphyseal fractures of the radius and ulna fixed with rush pins and/or fracture bracing. Clin Orthop 240:238, 1989
47. Hughston JC: Fractures of the forearm in children. J Bone Joint Surg 44A:1678, 1962
48. Gruber R: The problem of the relapse fracture of the forearm in children. p. 154. In Chapchal G (ed): Fractures in children. Thieme, New York, 1981
49. Kolkman KA, van Niekerk JL, Rieu PN, Festen C: A complicated forearm greenstick fracture: case report. J Trauma 32:116, 1992
50. Genelin F, Karlbauer AF, Gasperschitz F: Greenstick fracture of the forearm with median nerve entrapment. J Emerg Med 6:381, 1988
51. Wolfe JS, Eyring EJ: Median-nerve entrapment within a greenstick fracture. J Bone Joint Surg [Am] 56:1270, 1974
52. Borden S IV: Traumatic bowing of the forearm in children. J Bone Joint Surg [Am] 56:611, 1974
53. Borden S IV: Roentgen recognition of acute plastic bowing of the forearm in children. AJR 125:524, 1975
54. Sanders WE, Heckman JD: Traumatic plastic deformation of the radius and ulna. Clin Orthop 188:58, 1984
55. Nimityongskul P, Anderson LD, Sri P: Plastic deformation of the forearm: a review and case reports. J Trauma 31:1678, 1991
56. Crowe JE, Swischuk LE: Acute bowing fractures of the forearm in children: a frequently missed injury. AJR 128:981, 1977
57. Rydholm U, Nilsson JE: Traumatic bowing of the forearm: a case report. Clin Orthop 139:121, 1979
58. Miller JH, Osterkamp JA: Scintigraphy in acute plastic bowing of the forearm. Radiology 142:742, 1982
59. Komara JS, Kottamasu L, Kottamasu SR: Acute plastic bowing fractures in children. Ann Emerg Med 15:585, 1986
60. Matthews LS, Kaufer H, Garver DF, Sonstegard DA: The effect on supination-pronation of angular malalignment of fractures of both bones of the forearm. J Bone Joint Surg [Am] 64:14, 1982
61. Tarr RR, Garfinkel AI, Sarmiento A: The effects of angular and rotational deformities of both bones of the forearm. J Bone Joint Surg [Am] 66:65, 1984
62. Sarmiento A, Ebramzadeh E, Brys D, Tarr R: Angular deformities and forearm function. J Orthop Res 10:121, 1992
63. Morey BF, Askew LJ, An KN, Chao EY: A biomechanical study of normal functional elbow motion. J Bone Joint Surg [Am] 63:872, 1981
64. Blackburn N, Ziv I, Rang M: Correction of the malunited forearm fracture. Clin Orthop 188:54, 1984
65. Linscheid RL, Trousdale RT: Surgical treatment of forearm malunions, abstracted. Ninth Combined Meeting of the Orthopedic Association of the English-Speaking World, Toronto, Ontario, Canada, June 21–26, 1992
66. Vince KG, Miller JE: Cross-union complicating fracture of the forearm. J Bone Joint Surg [Am] 69:654, 1987
67. Failla JM, Amadio PC, Morrey BF: Post-traumatic proximal radio-ulnar synostosis. J Bone Joint Surg [Am] 71:1208, 1989
68. Watson FM, Jr, Eaton RG: Post-traumatic radio-ulnar synostosis. J Trauma 18:467, 1978
69. Yong-Hing K, Tchang SPK: Traumatic radio-ulnar synostosis treated by excision and a free fat transplant. J Bone Joint Surg [Br] 65:433, 1983
70. Geissler WB, Fernandez DL, Graca R: Anterior interosseous nerve palsy complicating a forearm fracture in a child. J Hand Surg 15A:44, 1990
71. Royle SG: Compartment syndrome following forearm fracture in children. Injury 21:73, 1990
72. Fee NF, Dobranski A, Bisla RS: Gas gangrene complicating open forearm fractures. J Bone Joint Surg [Am] 59:135, 1977

19

Fractures of the Distal Radius and Ulna

Louis J. Lawton

A problem forseen is half avoided.

DESCRIPTION AND INCIDENCE

Fractures of the distal radius and ulna are the most common fractures encountered in children.[1-7] Landin[1] analyzed 8,682 fractures in children in Sweden. Fractures of the distal radius and ulna represented 22.7 percent of all fractures. Physeal injuries of the distal radius represented 41 percent of all physeal injuries. The peak incidence in boys was age 13 to 14, in girls age 9 to 10. The ratio of boys to girls was 1.6:1. Beekman[2] studied 2,094 fractures of long bones in children. Of these, 45 percent occurred in the radius and ulna, 82 percent of which occurred in the distal forearm. He also found that separation of the distal radial epiphysis was the commonest physeal injury.

As the child matures, there is a trend for fractures of the forearm to migrate distally.[8,9] Fractures of the shaft occur more frequently in the preadolescent age group, with distal physeal injuries tending to occur in adolescence.[3,4,8-11] The increase in fractures of the distal radius may be just due to an increase in sports activity occurring during adolescence. Bailey and colleagues[11] correlated the incidence of distal forearm fractures with peak velocity of growth in height in boys and girls. They concurred with the theory that there is a dissociation between bone growth and bone mineralization during the adolescent growth spurt that leads to a period of relative bone fragility prior to skeletal maturity.

Among fractures involving the distal radial epiphysis, Salter-Harris type II fractures are the most commonly seen, with type I injuries the next most frequently encountered. Type III and type IV injuries are rarely sustained at the distal radial physis.[12-14] Fractures of the radius and ulna in children are frequently, but inappropriately, labeled as "Colles fractures" by clinicians inexperienced in pediatric fracture management. The adult Colles fractures differ in most respects, including anatomy, bone structure, fracture pattern, and healing. Intra-articular fracture and nonunion are rarely problems in children, but are frequently encountered in the Colles fracture. Neurovascular complications or malunion with loss of range of motion are seldom seen in fractures of the distal radius and ulna in the pediatric age group but are more commonly associated with the adult Colles fracture.

ANATOMIC CONSIDERATIONS

The ossific nucleus of the distal radial epiphysis appears at about 10 months of age in girls, 12 months in boys. The ossific nucleus of the distal ulnar epiphysis appears at about 7 years in boys and 5½ years in girls.[15] Cessation of growth in the distal radial and ulnar physis occurs at age 19 in boys and age 17 in girls.[15] The distal

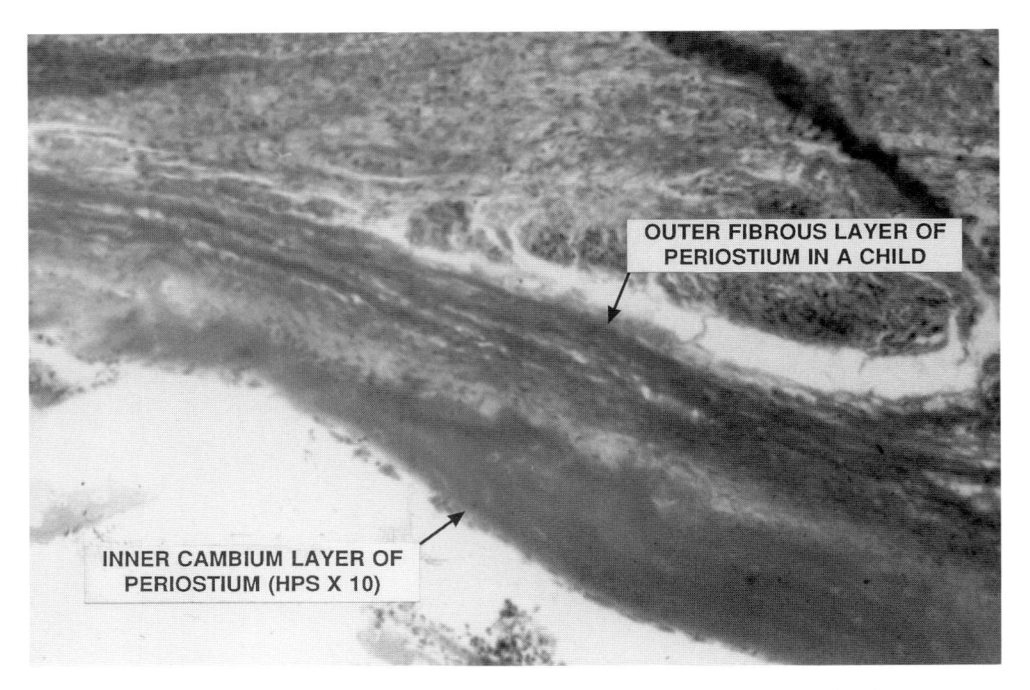

Fig. 19-1. Photomicrograph of periosteum in the child, showing a thick active layer of periosteum. The layer is strong and has great osteogenic potential.

radial and distal ulnar physes contribute 75 to 80 percent of the growth of the forearm and 40 percent of the overall longitudinal growth of the upper extremity.[12]

Because immature bone is more porous, and therefore less brittle, than adult bone, it can buckle more readily. Buckle fractures are therefore very common in children, especially at the distal radius and ulna. The strength of soft tissues relative to bone in the child influences fracture pattern and assists with treatment. Fractures of the physis and metaphysis are common, but dislocations of the wrist and of the distal radioulnar joint are rare, due to the relatively stronger ligaments.

The strong periosteum in a child tends to tear on the tension side of a displaced or angulated fracture, remaining intact on the compression side. Subsequent reduction of the fracture utilizes the intact periosteum to guide the reduction and then aid with maintaining it, as the cast is molded against the fracture (Fig. 19-1).

The distal radioulnar joint is a pivot joint. As the forearm moves from pronation to supination, the radius rotates around the ulna. The relative lengths of the radius and ulna must be maintained to allow normal wrist function in all planes of motion. Restoration of this anatomy after a fracture is desirable.[16]

Fortunately, the distal radius and ulna have a great capacity to remodel, especially in the younger child. Within limits, significant amounts of angular malalignment will remodel in the child's distal radius. Rotational malalignment however does not remodel well. A certain degree of complacency has existed in the past concerning the treatment of these fractures; however, persistent angulation over 15 to 20 degrees may result in significant malunion, producing a cosmetic and to a lesser extent a functional disability. In spite of the potential for considerable remodeling of fractures of the distal radius and ulna, an anatomic reduction should be pursued in those with initial angulation exceeding 15 to 20 degrees.[4]

MECHANISM OF INJURY

The commonest mechanism of injury in fractures of the distal radius and ulna is a fall on the outstretched hand. The amount and direction of the force determines the fracture pattern. A direct axial load of lower magnitude will cause compression of one cortex (a buckle fracture). If a significant angular force is added, the opposite cortex will fail in tension, creating a complete fracture (Fig. 19-2). With higher angular forces, displacement occurs. Dorsal displacement results when the hand strikes the ground with the wrist extended. Volar dis-

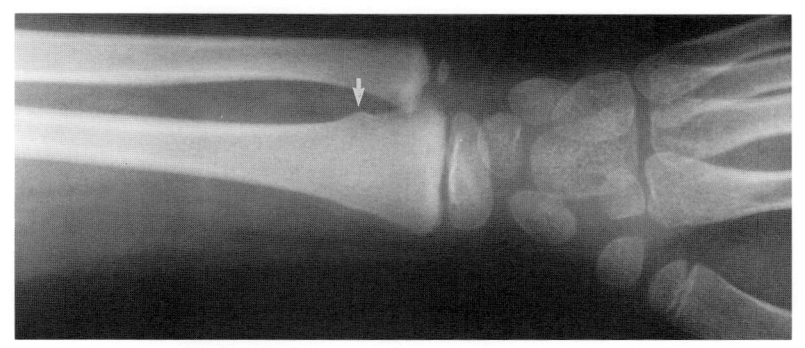

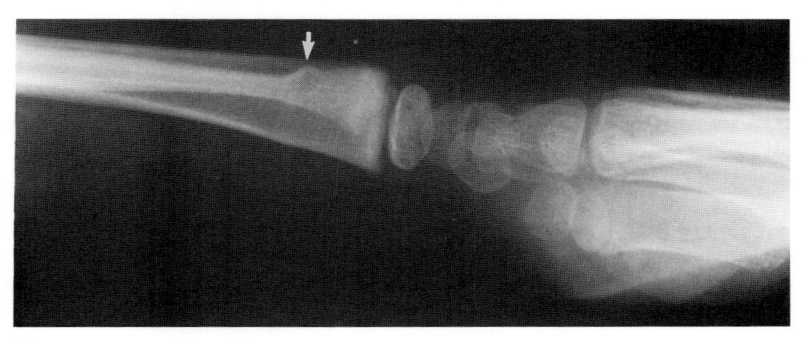

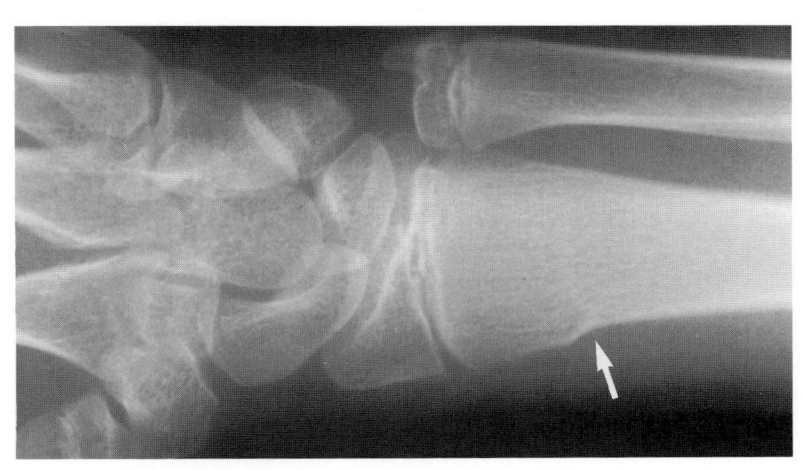

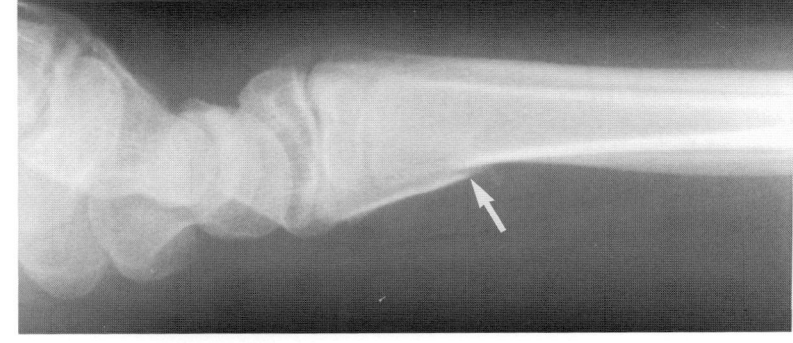

Fig. 19-2. (A&B) Buckle or "torus" fracture of distal radius which always occurs in the thinner metaphyseal cortex. (C&D) Buckling of dorsolateral cortex of the distal radial metaphysis *(arrow)* with (D) failure of the volar cortex.

TABLE 19-1. Classification

Metaphyseal
    Buckle (torus)
    Greenstick
    Complete
Physeal
    Salter-Harris types I to V
Special fractures
    Open
    Pathologic

placement occurs if the wrist is flexed. It is not clear why metaphyseal injuries occur in some children, while physeal injuries occur in others.

CLASSIFICATION

A classification of fractures of the distal radius and ulna is shown in Table 19-1.

Buckle (Torus) Fracture

The buckle fracture is essentially a compression fracture of one cortex, with the opposite cortex remaining intact. It is probably the commonest fracture of the distal forearm. Usually the dorsal cortex is compressed. This fracture is inherently stable (Fig. 19-2A & B). Buckle fractures of the ulna are also inherently stable, but if associated with a more complex fracture of the radius, the treatment of the radial fracture takes precedence.

Greenstick Fracture

Similar to a buckle fracture, the greenstick fracture results when the child's plastic forearm bones respond to an angular force with buckling of the cortex on the compression side and cracking of the cortex on the tension side. It is inherently stable, but significant deformity usually requires correction (Fig. 19-3).

Complete Fractures

When forces are sufficient, complete failure of the bone occurs. Typically, complete fractures are angulated, or displaced or both, and require reduction (Fig. 19-4).

Physeal Fractures

Physeal injuries usually involve the radius. Ulnar involvement is not common. Salter-Harris type I fractures are relatively common. An undisplaced Salter-Harris

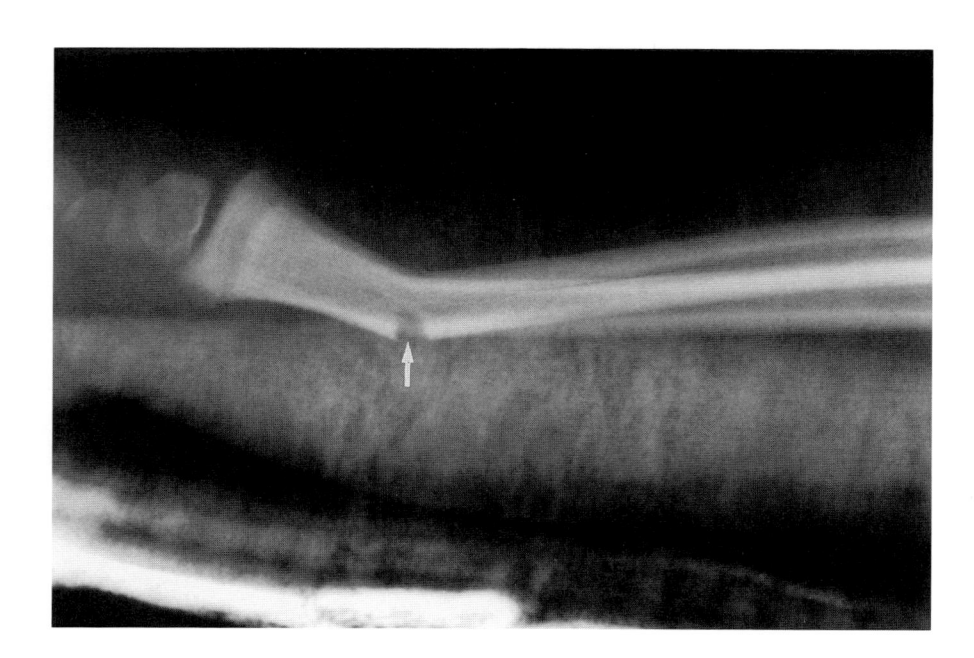

Fig. 19-3. Greenstick fracture. The dorsal cortex is still in continuity.

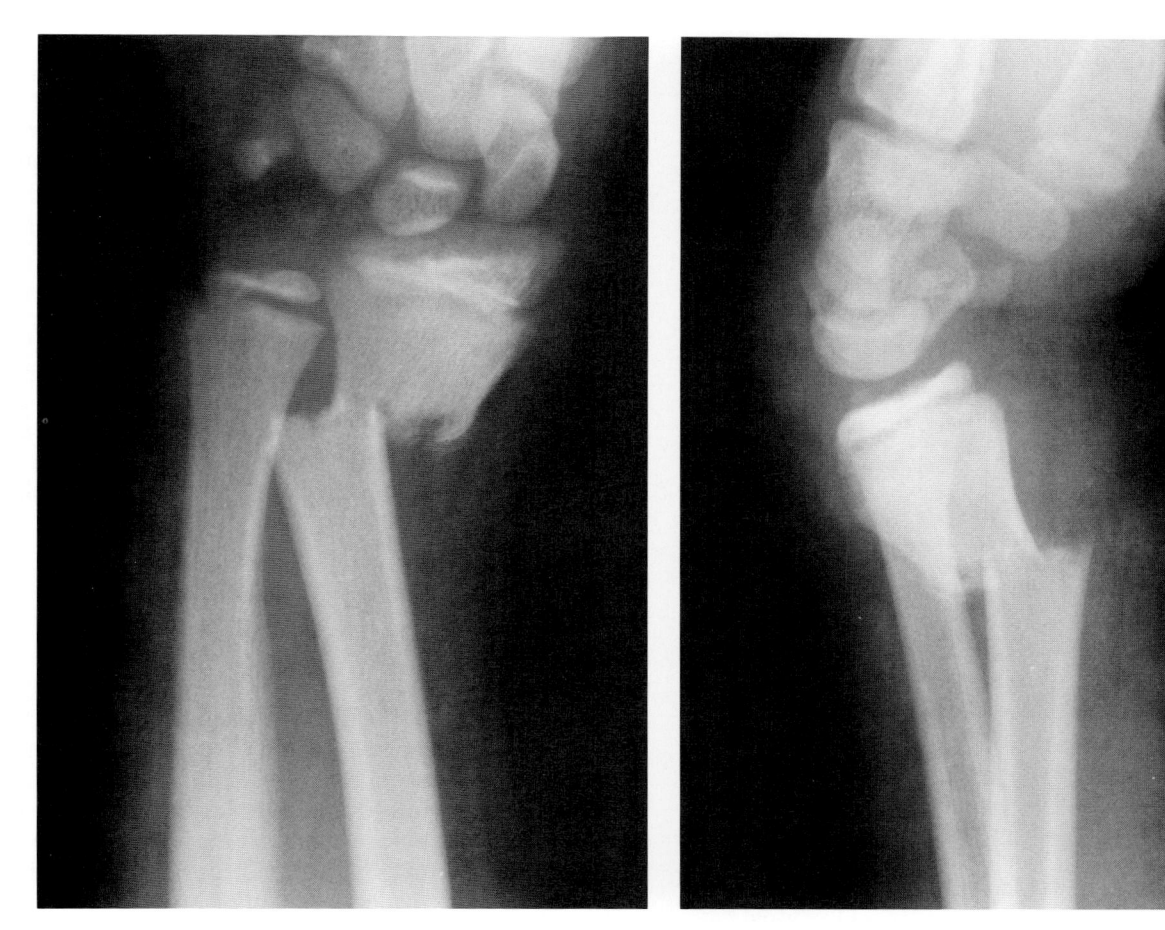

Fig. 19-4. Complete fracture. The radial metaphysis has failed completely. The ulna has sustained a probable undisplaced type I physeal fracture suggested by the widening of the growth plate.

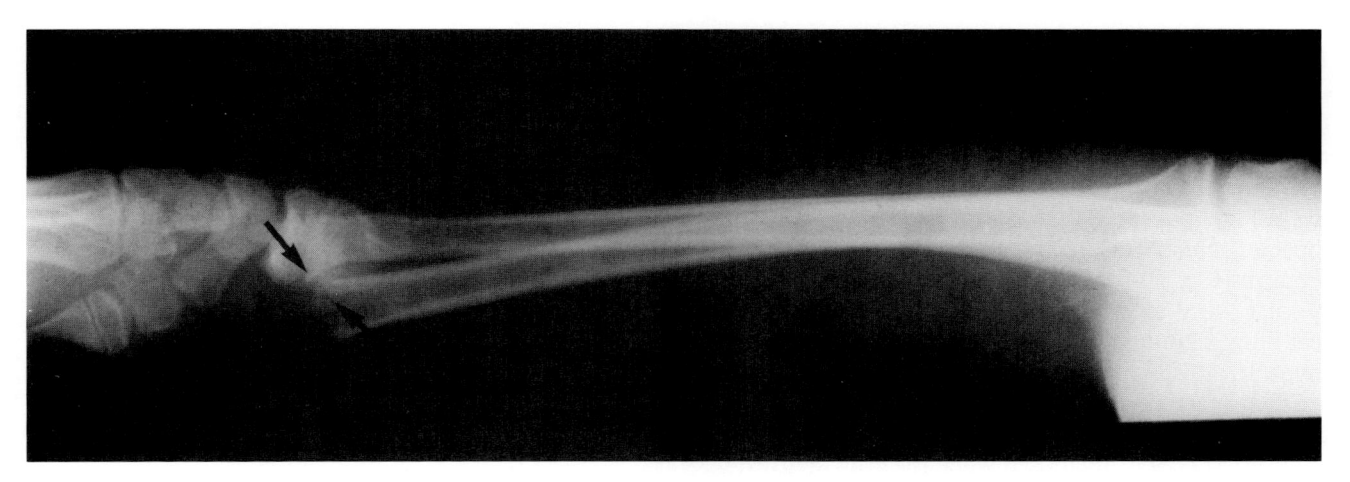

Fig. 19-5. Salter-Harris type II fracture. Arrows point to the area of possible impaction of the metaphysis into the physis. Growth plate damage can occur at the initial injury or after injudicious manipulation of the fracture.

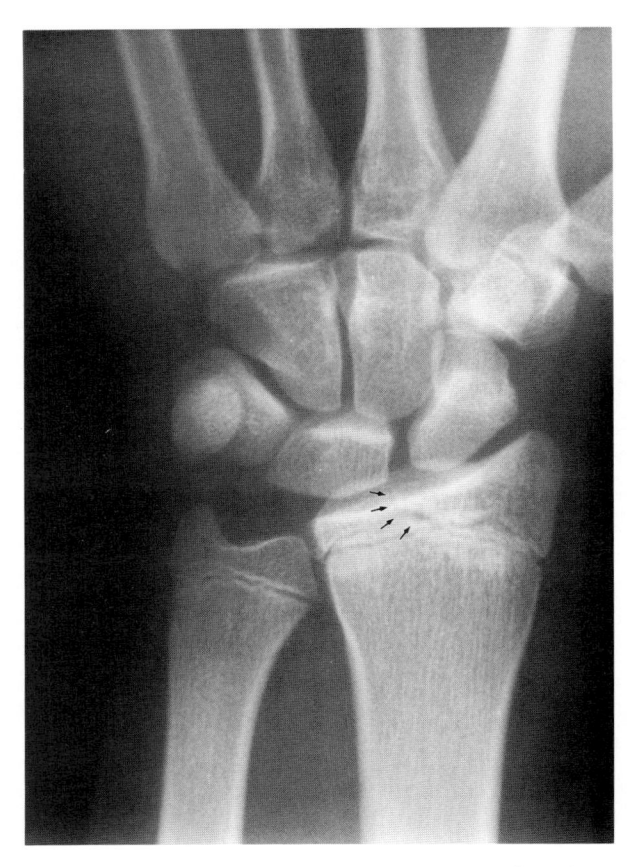

Fig. 19-6. Type III fracture of distal radial epiphysis sustained in a fall on the outstretched hand in a 14-year-old boy.

type I fracture may require a clinical diagnosis. Local tenderness at the physis in the absence of wrist tenderness may differentiate from a wrist sprain. The radiograph may be normal, or there may only be slight widening of the physis. Salter-Harris type II fractures are the commonest of the physeal injuries of the distal forearm (Fig. 19-5). Usually the metaphyseal fragment is dorsal, as is any associated displacement. The periosteal hinge is intact on the side of the metaphyseal fragment.

Salter-Harris types III and IV injuries are rare in the distal forearm (Fig. 19-6). Salter-Harris type V injuries are retrospectively diagnosed when the growth arrest becomes evident. Growth arrests are rare, and usually related to Salter-Harris type II injuries.

Open Fractures

Open fractures are not uncommon in the distal forearm. Even a small hole in the skin represents an open fracture, and requires full treatment as an open fracture (see the section "Pitfalls," later in this chapter).

Pathologic Fractures

Any condition that causes mechanical weakening of the bone may predispose to fracture. The weakening may occur due to generalized bone fragility (i.e., osteogenesis imperfecta, osteomalacia), or localized bone fragility (i.e., benign or malignant tumor, previous fracture, infection). Pathologic mechanisms of injury, as in child abuse, must also be considered.

PHYSICAL EXAMINATION

The child typically presents with a painful, swollen wrist. The classic deformity is that of a dinner fork, caused by the dorsal displacement of the distal fragment (Fig. 19-7). A reversed dinner fork deformity may result if the distal fragment is displaced volarward. The initial assessment includes examination of the rest of the upper extremity for other sites of possible injury. Examine the elbow for possible associated radial head dislocation (Monteggia lesion) or elbow fractures. The neurologic and vascular status of the hand should be assessed.

The sensory and motor functions of the radial, ulnar, and median nerves are assessed individually. The pulses are usually not palpable due to local tenderness. Capillary filling of the nail beds, and finger color, temperature, and neurologic function should be assessed. The forearm compartments should be gently palpated to examine for abnormal swelling that may cause or result from compartment syndrome.

The children are invariably fearful, with motion of the wrist causing discomfort; therefore it helps to play games with the child, in order to elicit signs. The skin should be carefully inspected, since even a small puncture converts the fracture to an open injury requiring open exploration. Once the examination is complete, the limb should be splinted before taking radiographs.

Immediate splinting is preferable because it gives immediate relief for the child. Splintage rarely obscures radiographic detail sufficiently to prevent accurate diagnosis. If this should occur, a second radiograph, unsplinted and supervised by the physician, is optimal.

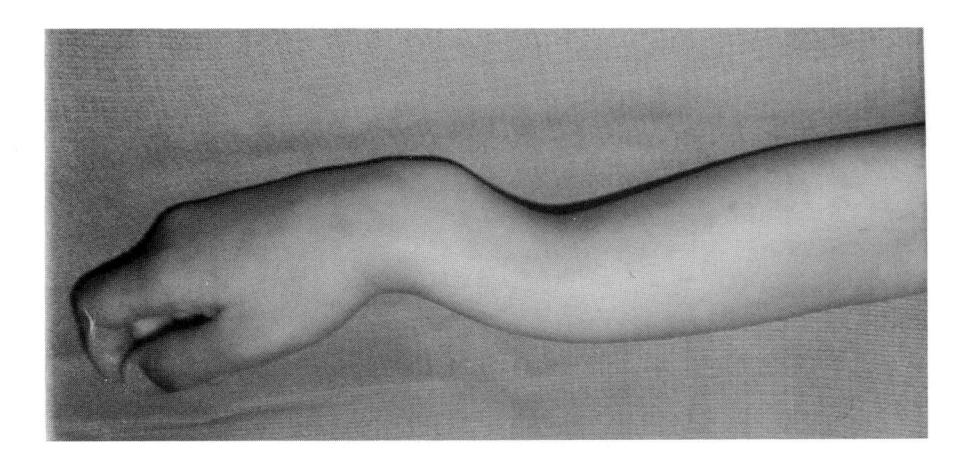

Fig. 19-7. Classic "dinner-fork" deformity of a fracture of the distal radius and ulna in a 7-year-old child.

DIFFERENTIAL DIAGNOSIS

The diagnosis is usually clear from the history, physical examination, and radiographs. A careful history of the precise mode of injury is important. It may give clues about the severity of the injury to the arm, alerting the physician to consider other relevant aspects (i.e., concomitant injuries, child abuse, open fracture, future growth arrest). Standard anteroposterior (AP) and lateral views of the injured wrist are radiographically recorded. If other areas of the upper extremity are symptomatic, they should also have radiographs. Possible injuries may include variants of Galeazzi or Monteggia lesions. Concomitant scaphoid fracture has been described.[17,18]

Some conditions that may cause pathologic fractures include leukemia, primary bone tumors, or tumorlike conditions, osteomyelitis, or septic arthritis, metabolic conditions, child abuse, and osteogenesis imperfecta.

TREATMENT INDICATIONS

Closed Methods

Anesthetic Considerations

Fractures that are minimally displaced or angulated without displacement can usually be treated by using intravenous sedation. A narcotic agent will give pain relief, and a benzodiazepine may be added for muscle relaxation and general sedation of the patient. Full precautions for possible respiratory suppression should be taken (see Ch. 5).

Completely displaced fractures of the metaphysis require complete anesthesia of the arm, either by regional anesthetic (brachial plexus block), intravenous block,[19] or general anesthetic. Complete muscle relaxation in the reduction of physeal fractures will also minimize the danger of growth plate trauma secondary to the reduction.

There is controversy about the usage of hematoma blocks in growth plate fractures. Although not reported, there is a theoretical risk of infection, which could cause a major growth arrest. Other anesthetic modalities are readily available that avoid this potential complication and are more acceptable to the child.

Metaphyseal Fractures

BUCKLE FRACTURES

Below-elbow casting, with the wrist in a neutral position, for 2 to 4 weeks, is sufficient depending on the age of the child. This mainly provides comfort and protects the child from converting an innocuous fracture into a more serious displaced fracture.

GREENSTICK FRACTURES

Some authors advocate conversion of the greenstick fracture to a complete fracture,[20,21] by manipulation of the fragments under suitable analgesia. Others prefer to manipulate to reduce an angulation but do not complete the fracture. If the fracture is a supination injury, with volar angulation, the forearm is rotated into full pronation and cast in this position to correct the deformity.[21,22] If the greenstick fracture is a pronation injury, with dor-

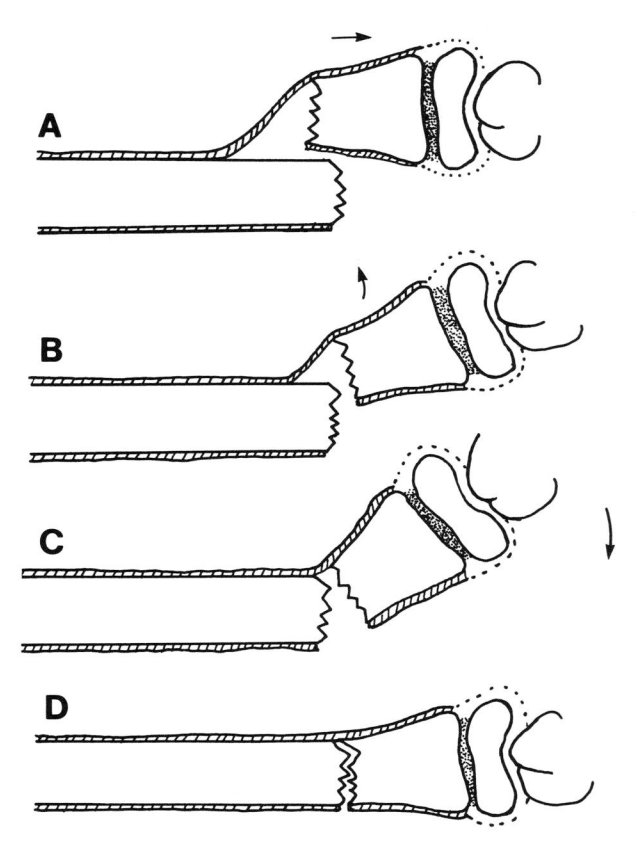

Fig. 19-8. Steps in the reduction of distal radial metaphyseal fracture using the periosteal hinge. See text.

sal angulation, then the fracture is manipulated and cast in supination. Beware of the so-called greenstick or buckle fracture of the distal radius, which is in fact a complete fracture (Fig. 19-2C&D). It has a small crack in the volar surface, making it a complete, potentially unstable fracture. It should be reduced, if necessary, and placed in a well-moulded cast. Failure to do so may result in loss of position that presents later as a malunion.

COMPLETE FRACTURES

Adequate relaxation of forearm musculature is required for reduction of a displaced fracture of the distal radius and/or ulna and general anesthesia is recommended. Reduction maneuvers use the intact periosteal hinge on the concavity of the fracture to effect and maintain reduction. Image intensifier fluoroscopic control is recommended to monitor the manipulation and confirm an adequate reduction (Fig. 19-8).

Manipulation of the fracture begins with longitudinal traction, to bring the fracture ends out to length (Fig. 19-8A). Once the fracture surfaces are opposing, the deformity is increased (Fig. 19-8B). The fragments are gently angulated, and the distal fragment is gently translated, to eliminate displacement (Fig. 19-8C). The fracture is then closed without force (Fig. 19-8D). Gravity can be used to hold the reduction while check radiographs are taken in the AP plane. Force should only be required for the initial distraction. Once the fragments are out to length, the rest of the manipulation can be easily performed with minimal force in young children, although in teenagers both thumbs may be needed to push the distal fragment forward and down.

The wrist should be cast in neutral to mild flexion and neutral rotation with molding over the distal fragment. Forced flexion of the wrist in the so-called Cotton position should be avoided. Severely pronating or supinating these fractures may cause angulation or displacement. Careful observation for cast tightness or compartment syndrome is required for the initial 12 to 24 hours. The arm should be moderately elevated. Ice packs around the cast may help to minimize swelling. Healing is usually complete in 6 to 8 weeks.

An above-elbow cast is recommended to minimize pronation/supination force. An initial below-elbow cast for these fractures has been recommended and used successfully by some experienced clinicians[23] but must be very meticulously molded and applied. Since elbow stiffness is not a major concern or complication at this age, an above-elbow cast is recommended until early callus formation provides some fracture stability. Check radiographs should be taken at 1- and 2-week intervals because of the possibility of loss of reduction in the cast[24] (Fig. 19-9). After 2 or 3 weeks the cast may be converted to a below-elbow cast, for patient convenience.

Physeal Injuries

Displaced Salter-Harris type I or II fractures are usually easily reduced if the concept of the periosteal hinge is appreciated (Fig. 19-10). Radiographic control during the reduction is recommended. Initial longitudinal traction brings the fracture fragments out to length (Fig. 19-10A). The distal fragment is then angulated in the direction of the deformity using the periosteal hinge (Fig. 19-10B) and then gently translated, to eliminate displacement (Fig. 19-10C). The position is verified by radiographs. An above-elbow cast is applied with the forearm pronated if the displacement was dorsal, and supinated if the displacement was volar (Fig. 19-11). At 2

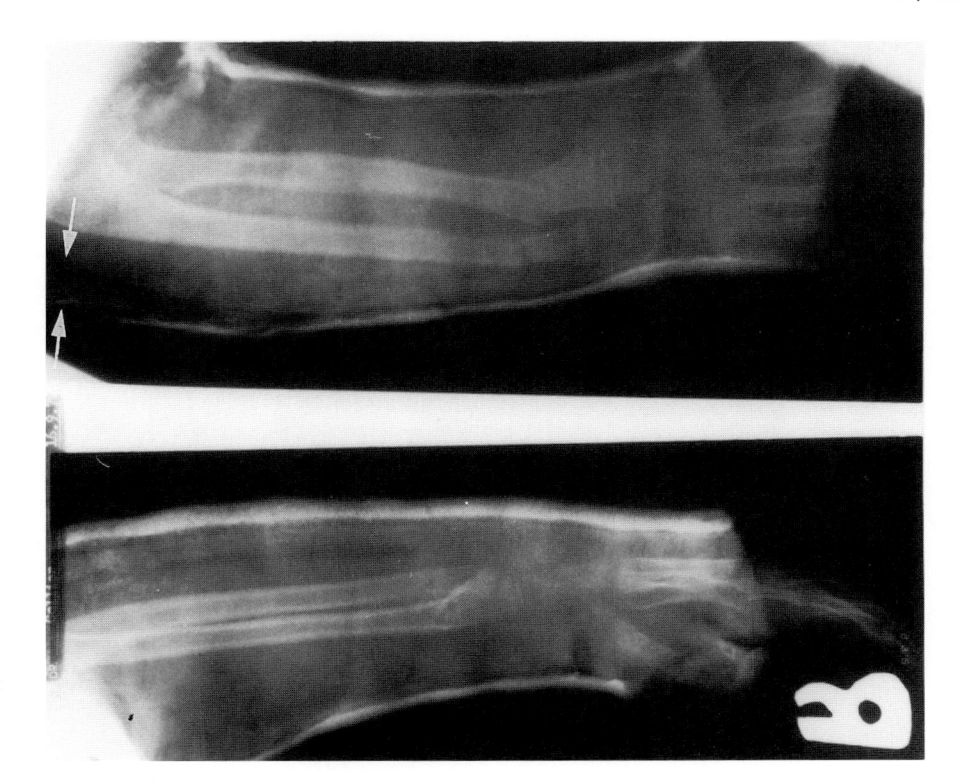

Fig. 19-9. Loss of reduction of the fractured distal radius and ulna due to the cast becoming loose as the swelling subsides. The cast then slips down the arm resulting in angulation of the previously well reduced fracture. In small children, tincture of benzoin applied to the upper arm may prevent this slippage.

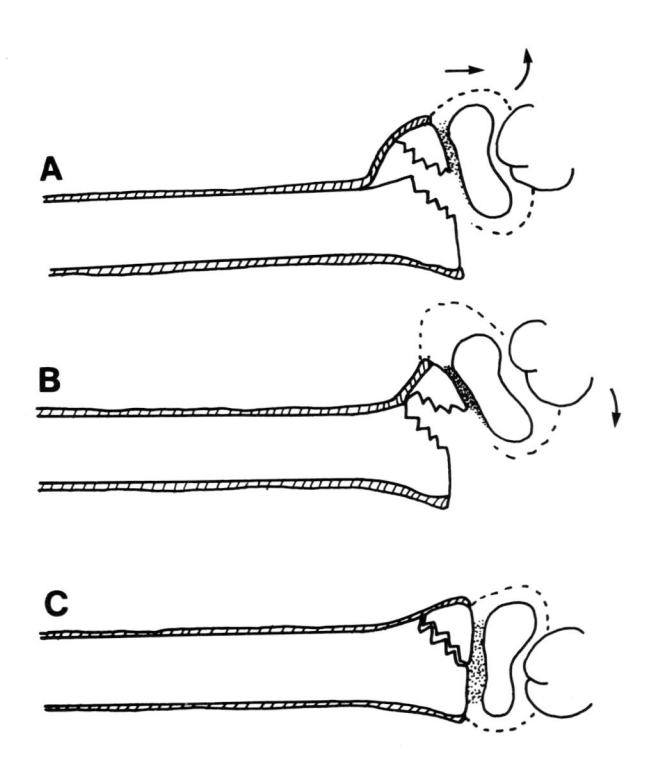

Fig. 19-10. Reduction of Salter-Harris type II fracture of the distal radius working with the periosteal hinge. See text.

weeks the cast may be changed to a below-elbow cast, for the convenience of the child. The physeal fracture is typically healed at about 5 weeks.

Analgesia or anesthesia will be required to accomplish the reduction. Although an anatomic reduction is desirable and strived for, a 50 percent apposition of the physis is compatible with a good long-term result and avoids several remanipulations, which may cause traumatic injury to the plate itself.

Repeated manipulations of physeal injuries are not warranted. Growth plate injuries tend to heal much more rapidly than fractures through bone. It is preferable to avoid forceful manipulations, which would be required after 5 to 10 days postinjury, as damage to the growth plate may be inflicted.[25-28] The remodeling potential of the distal radius is significant even in the adolescent. Therefore, the window for safe reduction of physeal fractures of the distal radius is a maximum of 5 days.

Salter-Harris types III, IV, and V injuries are rare but serious.[12,14] In a displaced Salter-Harris type III or IV fracture, reduction may be achieved by closed methods, but percutaneous pinning with smooth K-wires is recommended to ensure maintenance of reduction. An anatomic reduction of the joint surfaces and physis is re-

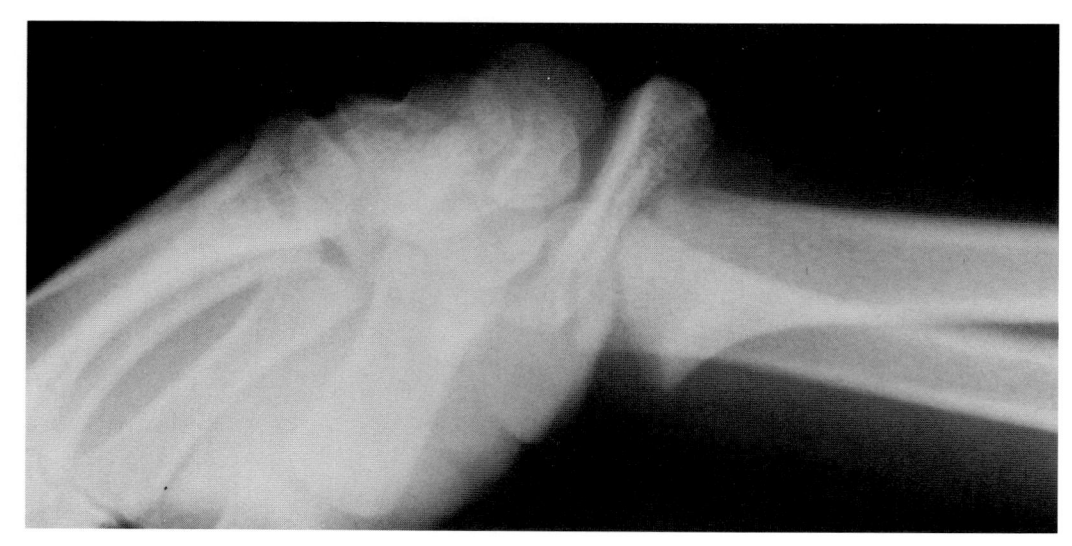

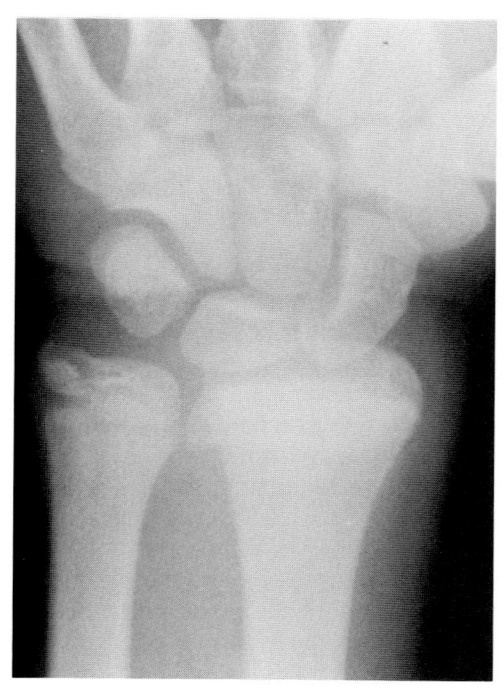

Fig. 19-11. **(A)** Type I physeal fracture with typical dorsal displacement on lateral view. **(B)** The AP view demonstrates apparent radial shortening and probable undisplaced type I fracture of the ulnar physis suggested by the widened physis. *(Figure continues.)*

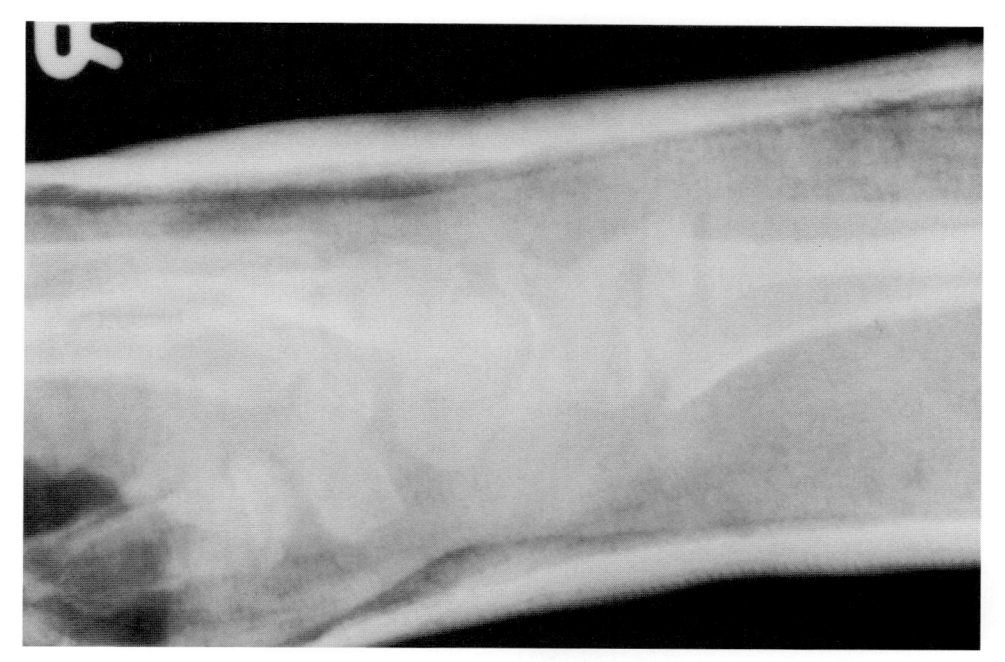

C

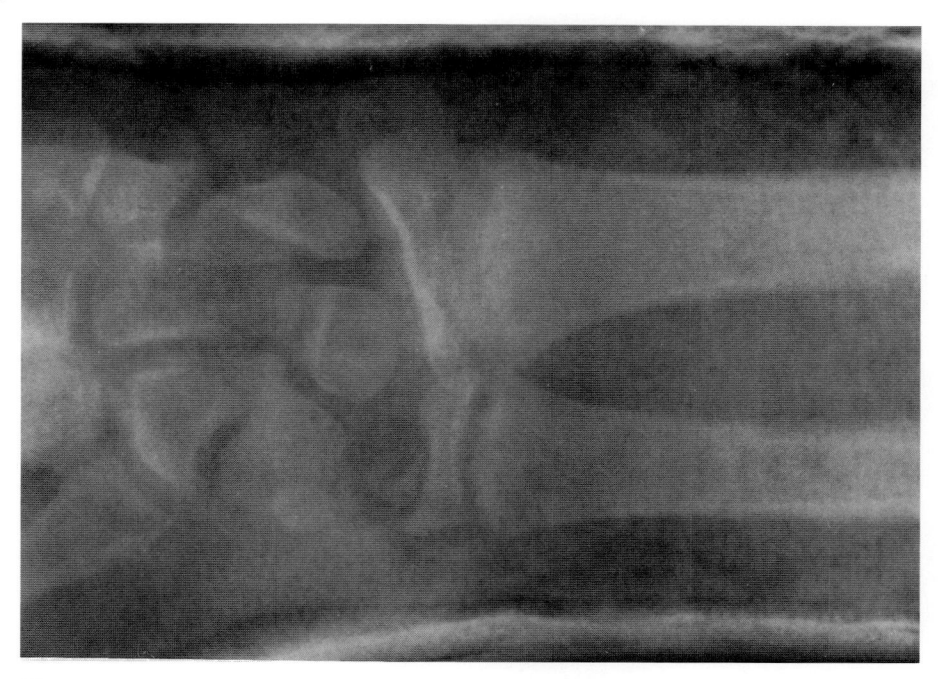

D

Fig. 19-11 *(Continued).* **(C&D)** Postreduction.

356 / Management of Pediatric Fractures

quired, and if this cannot be achieved by closed techniques, an open reduction must be accomplished.

Open Methods

Anesthetic Considerations

Open reduction of the distal radius or ulna generally requires general anesthesia. In a very cooperative child or teenager regional anesthesia is an option, using a brachial plexus block (see Ch. 5).

Open Reduction

Open reduction is rarely required for fractures of the distal radius and ulna in children.[14,20,29,30] Reduction is usually easily obtained and maintained by closed methods. Generally, 20 percent displacement and up to 20 degrees of angulation of a metaphyseal fracture is acceptable if the growth plate is still open.[31-36] With physeal separations, up to 50 percent displacement can be expected to remodel in children under 6 years, but such displacements should not be electively accepted, due to the abnormal appearance of the wrist, which persists

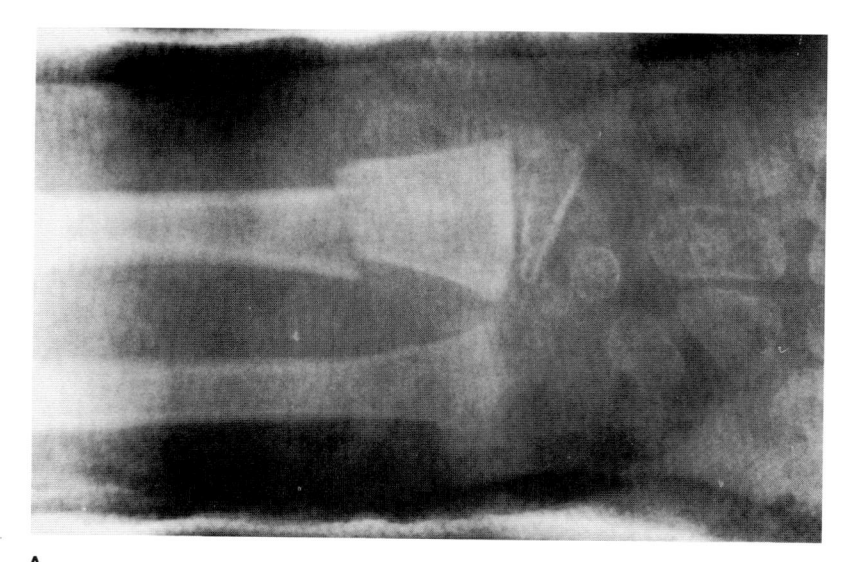

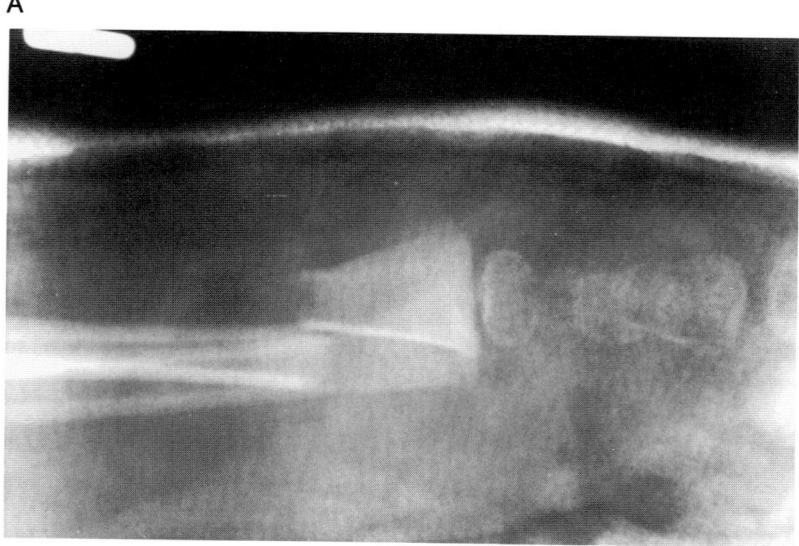

Fig. 19-12. (A&B) Displaced fracture of the distal radius, after failed attempt at anatomic reduction. Alignment was adequate, so bayonet apposition was accepted. *(Figure continues.)*

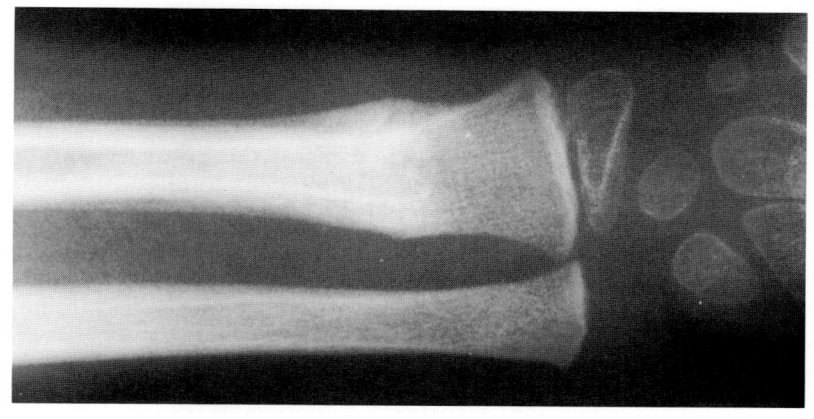

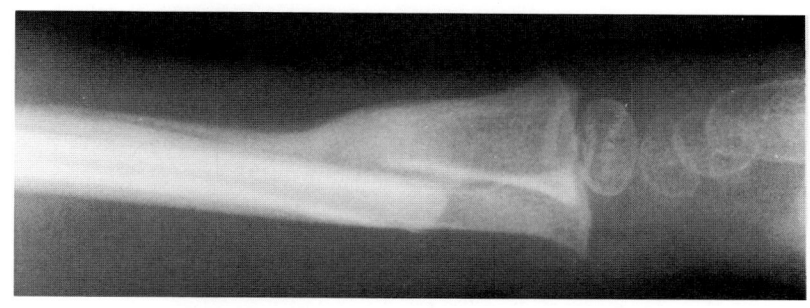

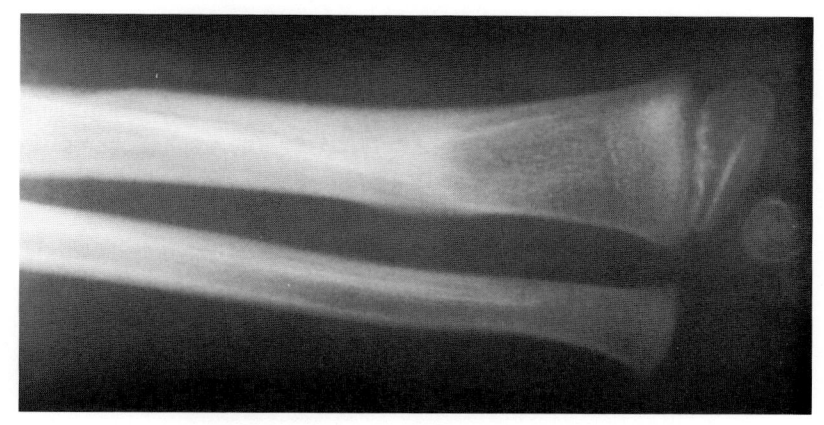

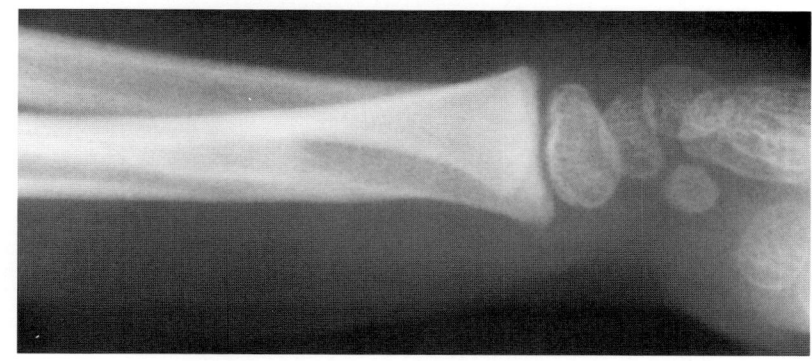

Fig. 19-12 *(Continued).* **(C&D)** Initial healing of the fracture with initial remodeling apparent. **(E&F)** Extensive remodeling is evident. The patient had full range of motion, and normal function.

until several years of remodeling has occurred. If a physeal displacement of 40 to 50 percent has eluded good orthopaedic management and the child presents late, the malunion can be accepted without proceeding to an open reduction or osteotomy, and ultimately remodeling will correct the deformity over several years growth (Fig. 19-12).

Open Fractures

Open fractures should be treated according to the standard principles of debridement, appropriate antibiotic coverage, tetanus prophylaxis and fracture immobilization. Grades 1 and 2 wounds can be treated in plaster, with windows cut to monitor the wounds. Grade 3 fractures can be treated with external fixators, or percutaneous K-wire fixation of the radius supplemented by a cast, depending on the extent of the wound.

Irreducible Fractures

Rarely a fracture of the distal radius may prove irreducible by closed manipulation. This usually occurs in teenagers close to skeletal maturity. A long oblique fracture, with long spikes opposing, may prevent closed reduction, necessitating operative exposure of the fragments. The subsequent reduction may prove stable enough to be held in cast only. Alternatively, the fragments may be internally fixed with smooth K-wires, supplemented by a cast. Rarely are plates and screws required for pediatric distal radius and ulna fractures.[37]

Case reports exist describing irreducibility due to entrapped structures, usually as the result of physeal injuries. Infolded periosteum has been implicated in preventing reduction in physeal separations of the distal radius[37] and the distal ulna.[1] Entrapped extensor tendons have also prevented closed reduction of distal radial[39] and distal ulnar[40] separations (see Ch. 17). The median nerve and flexor policis longus have been trapped in a physeal fracture-dislocation of the distal radioulnar joint.[41] The median nerve has also been caught in a greenstick fracture of the radius.[42] Surgical removal of the entrapped structures was required in each case. These are rare occurrences but must be considered if closed reduction is unsuccessful in any fracture of the distal radius and ulna in children.

Segmental Fractures

Segmental fractures of the radius and ulna may necessitate internal fixation of one or both fractures. The distal radius and ulna are usually adequately treated with a closed reduction supplemented by a smooth percutaneous K-wire. Once this fracture has been stabilized a closed reduction of the more proximal fracture of the radius and ulna is facilitated. An external fixator may sometimes prove useful in this situation, especially if there are associated skin wounds.

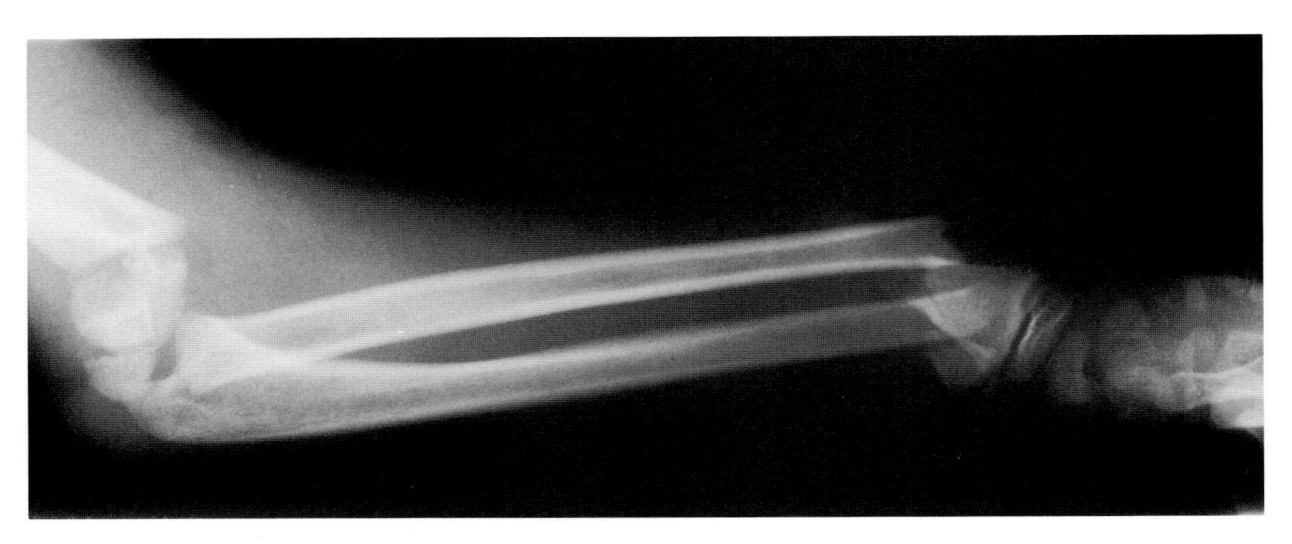

Fig. 19-13. The so called "floating elbow" can result from a fracture of the distal radius and ulna associated with a fracture of the humerus.

Segmental fractures involving the forearm and the humerus (floating elbow) also occur (Fig. 19-13). Treatment may require fixation of one or both of the fractures, especially if the humerus fracture is a displaced fracture of the medial epicondyle, the lateral condyle, or the supracondylar region. Percutaneous K-wire pinning of the humeral injuries is usually indicated with internal fixation of the distal radial and ulnar injuries optional.

Head-Injured Patient

Operative stabilization of fractures may be required in an unconscious but moving patient. Cast immobilization is usually sufficient, but on occasion the patient may require internal or external fixation to maintain control of the fracture fragments. Percutaneous pinning of the fracture fragments following a closed reduction is a simple way to ensure a stable reduction and avoid displacement due to muscle spasm or excessive movement of the limb.

Pitfalls

THE PUNCTURE WOUND

A tiny puncture wound is never an innocuous injury. Gas gangrene may occur if these wounds are neglected. Four of five cases of gas gangrene described by Fee and colleagues[43] were in children with small puncture wounds overlying forearm fractures. Typically, there will be a 1-mm hole in the skin with a small amount of dark blood oozing from it. Skin is highly distensible and such a wound could represent a complete exiting of the bone through the skin with rereduction of the bone underneath the skin, taking significant amounts of the environment back into the wound. It demands all the respect accorded to any open fracture, with opening of the wound, direct inspection of the bone ends, and complete cleansing and debridement. Subsequent manipulative reduction without internal fixation is usually adequate. On occasion, the fracture may be unstable because of the soft tissue injuries. The fracture may be stabilized by a smooth K-wire inserted percutaneously. The forearm is then supported in an above-elbow cast.

REPEAT REDUCTIONS

Repeat reduction of physeal injury is contraindicated after 5 to 10 days. Repeated manipulation may lead to growth arrest.[28] Complete remodeling can be anticipated in fractures displaced as much as 50 percent in children under 6 years and up to 30 percent displacement will usually remodel satisfactorily in older children after several years. Osteotomy to correct deformity should be deferred for 2 or 3 years unless the displacement is massive and interfering substantially with wrist function (Fig. 19-12).

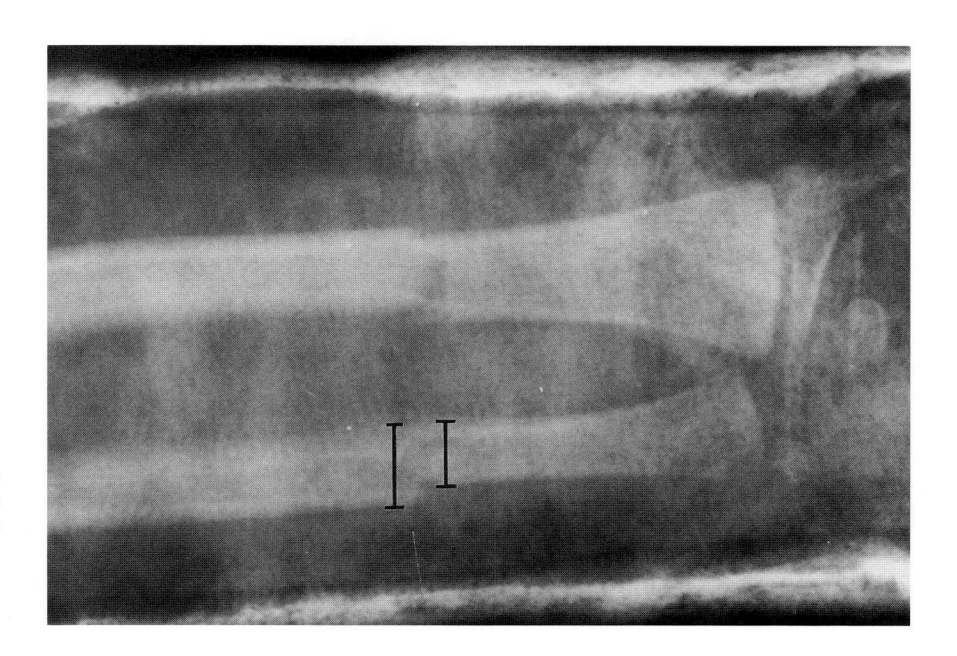

Fig. 19-14. Rotational mismatch of ulna. The width at the fracture site of the distal ulna is less than the width of the proximal ulna. The diameters should be equal on either side of the fracture.

POSITION IN CAST

Evans put forth the concept of treating greenstick fractures of the distal radius in pronation for volarly angulated fractures and supination for dorsally angulated fractures. This presupposes that the greenstick fracture is still intact. Using the same treatment rationale for complete fractures of the distal radius and ulna may cause a rotational malalignment. With complete fractures of the distal radius and ulna neutral rotation is recommended.[20] The radius is oval in cross section; thus rotation may be verified by measuring the diameter of the radius on either side of the fracture. Differing widths indicate malrotation, which should be corrected (Fig. 19-14).

As most fractures of the distal radius and ulna are dorsally displaced, casting in slight (15 degrees) flexion of the wrist is usually satisfactory to keep slight tension on the dorsal periosteal hinge. There is no reason to flex the wrist any more, as it does not add to the stability of the reduction but may predispose to compression of the carpal tunnel (the so-called Cotton position).

COMPLICATIONS

Neurologic Injury

Nerve injury is not common in fractures of the distal radius and ulna in children. The nerve most at risk is the median secondary to ischemia after a vascular insult or direct trauma from a displaced fragment or poorly molded cast. The most commonly encountered type of nerve injury is a neurapraxia, which is usually transient.

Vascular Injury

Direct trauma to the radial or ulnar artery is rare (Fig. 19-15). However, compartment syndrome as a result of fractures in this area has been described.[5,44] D'Astous[5] found that compartment syndrome was not an uncommon sequela of distal radius and ulna fracture. Treatment is by the usual, well-established principles of compartment syndrome management (see Ch. 64).

If a child exhibits signs of impending compartment syndrome, all encircling casting must be split. If relief is not achieved by splinting the cast, then fasciotomy must be performed. Both dorsal and volar compartment pressures should be measured and fasciotomy performed in involved compartments. Internal fixation of the fracture with a smooth K-wire will facilitate maintaining the re-

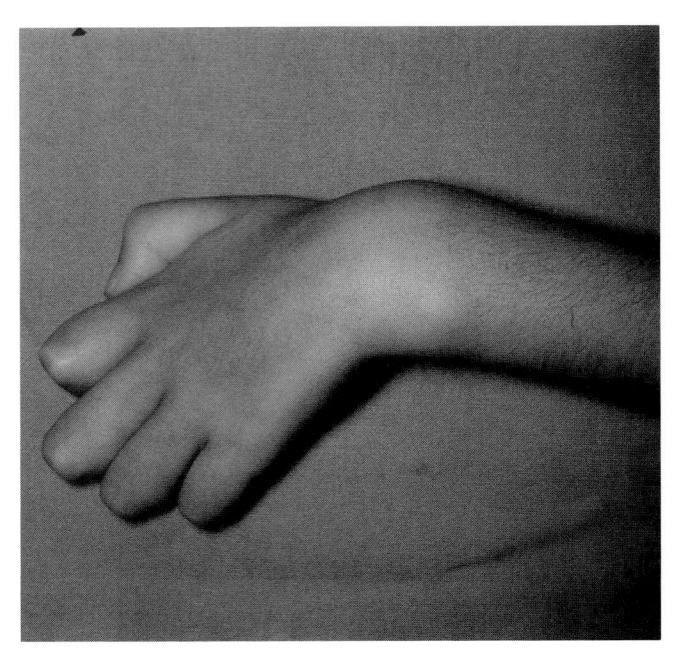

Fig. 19-15. Volkmann's ischemic contracture may occur in association with fractures of the distal radius and ulna. The same vigilance regarding circulatory integrity should be exercised for fractures of the radius and ulna as for supracondylar fractures of the distal humerus.

duction. Alternatively, an external fixator may be useful to assist with subsequent wound management.

Malunion

Malreduction of the fracture is the commonest complication. There is some disagreement about what represents an acceptable amount of malposition in the growing child (Fig. 19-12). Generally speaking up to 30 degrees of metaphyseal or epiphyseal angulation of the radius on the lateral radiographic view will remodel in children under 10 and up to 20 degrees in older children.[31,32,45] Remodeling will be much more efficient in a younger child, when the deformity is in the same plane of wrist motion and in growth plate injuries. However, even in an older child a surprising amount of remodeling can occur. Approximately 50 percent of displacement of a metaphyseal or a physeal fracture can remodel providing the alignment is correct. However, anatomic reductions are more stable and the chances of a further loss of position of the fragments are much less with a better initial reduction. If the fracture has started to heal, repeated attempts at manipulation are likely to cause fur-

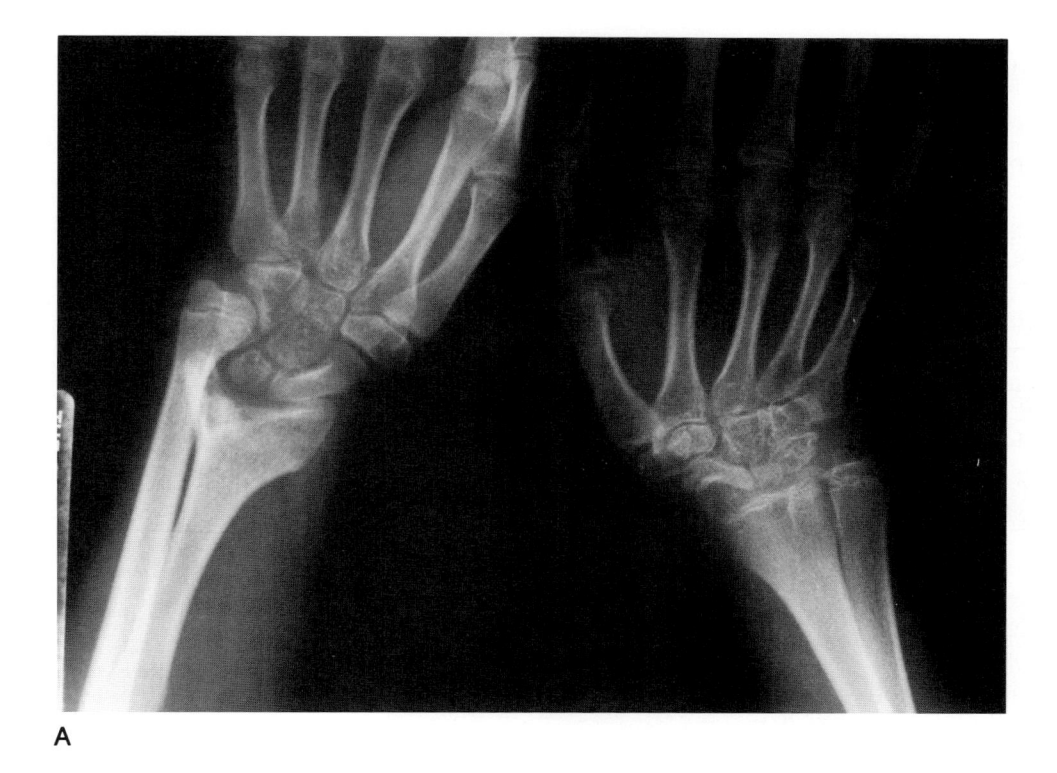

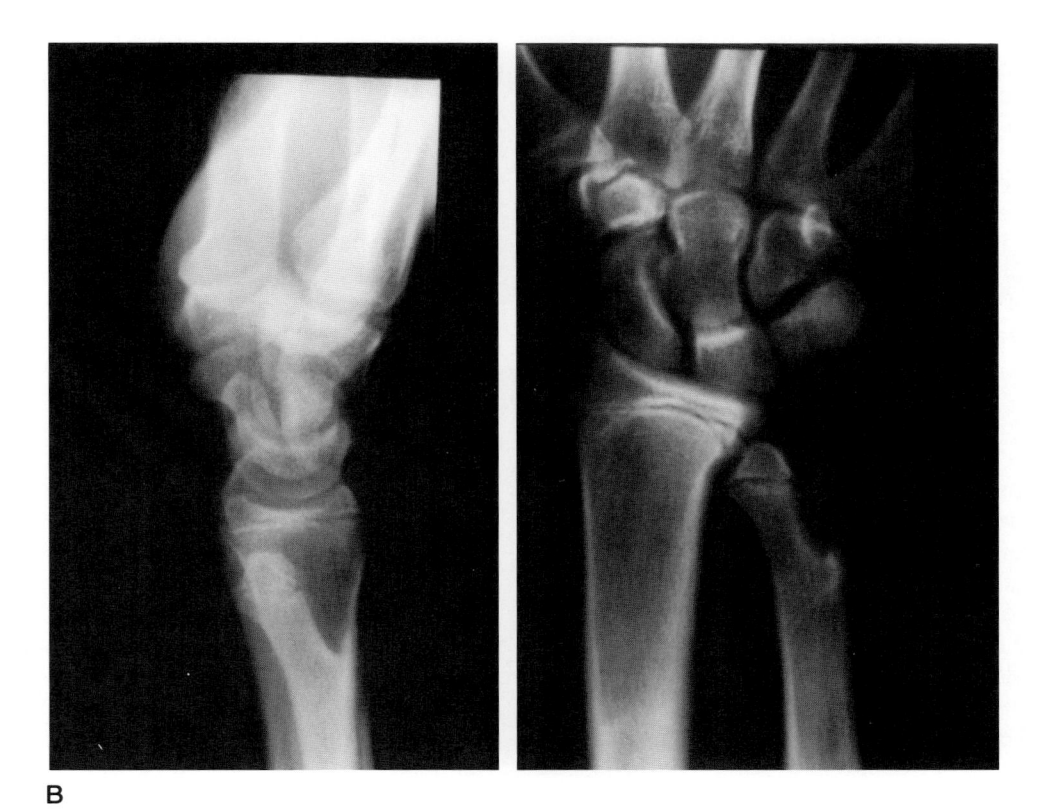

Fig. 19-16. (A) Growth arrest of the distal radius. (B) Growth arrest of the distal ulna. Both these physeal injuries result in altered wrist mechanics and predispose to future osteoarthritis of the wrist joint.

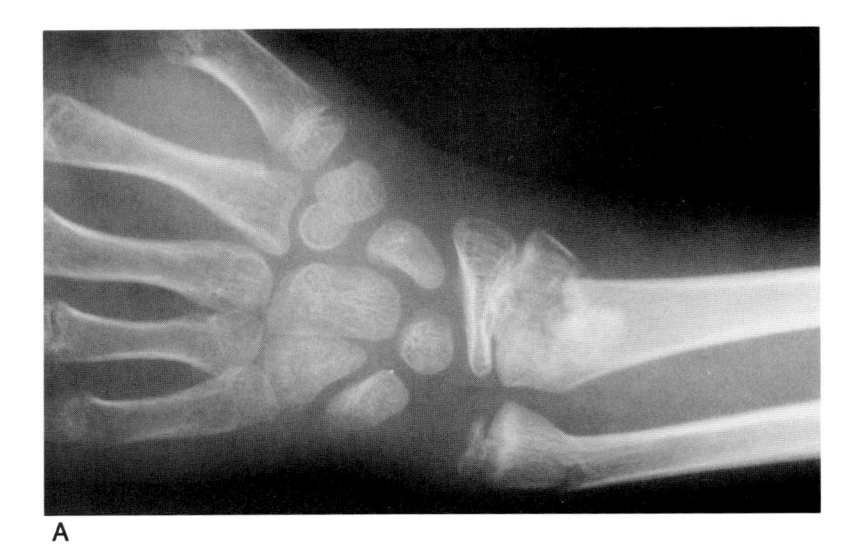

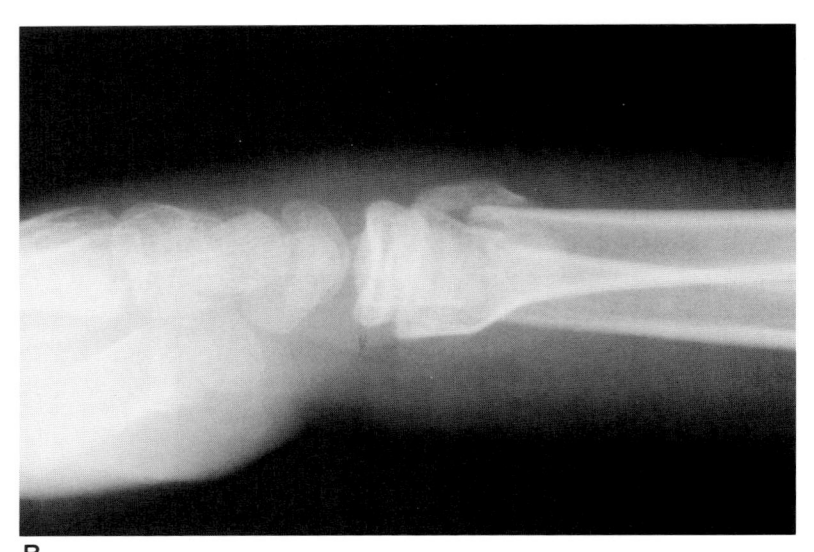

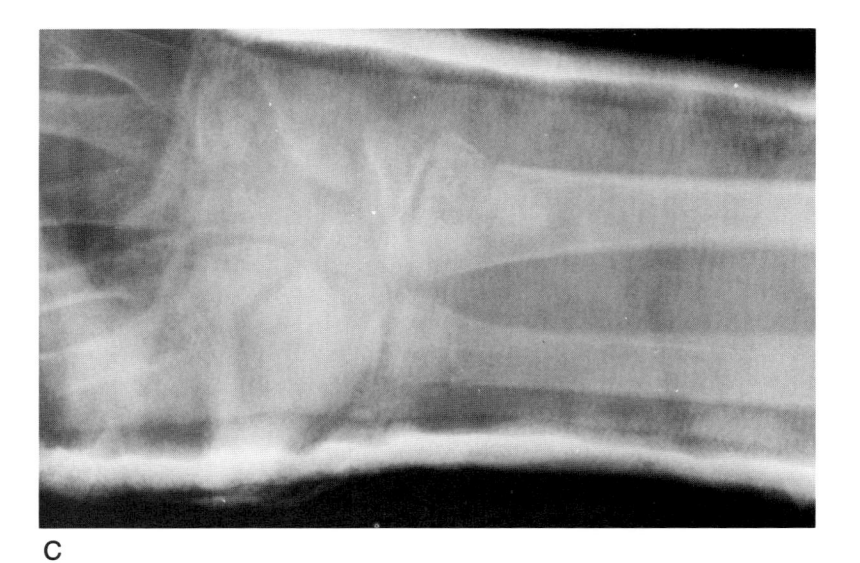

Fig. 19-17. **(A&B)** Eleven-year-old boy who fell off a dirt bike onto his outstretched arm sustaining a Salter-Harris type II fracture with comminution of the distal radius and a metaphyseal greenstick fracture in the distal ulna. **(C&D)** Closed reduction was achieved without difficulty. Immobilization was maintained for six weeks. At six months the growth arrest was apparent. *(Figure continues.)*

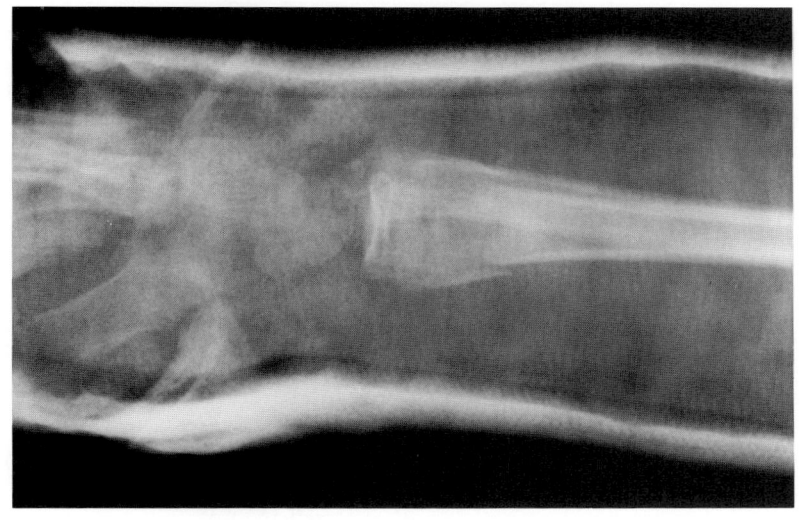

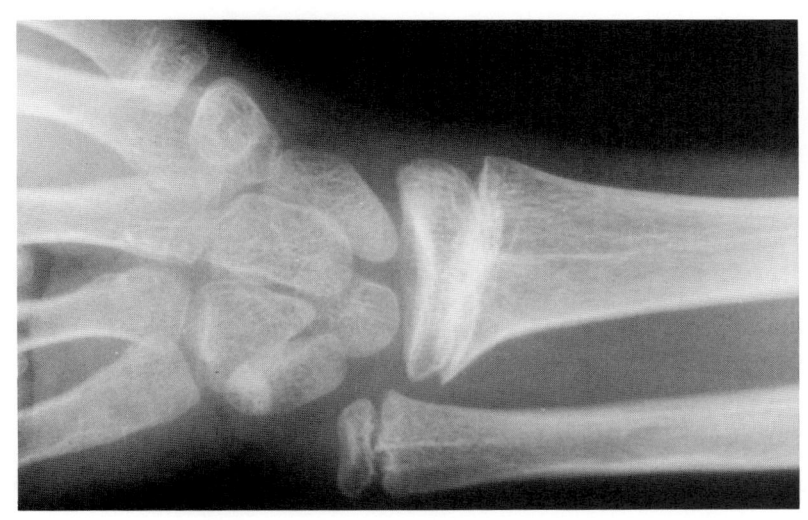

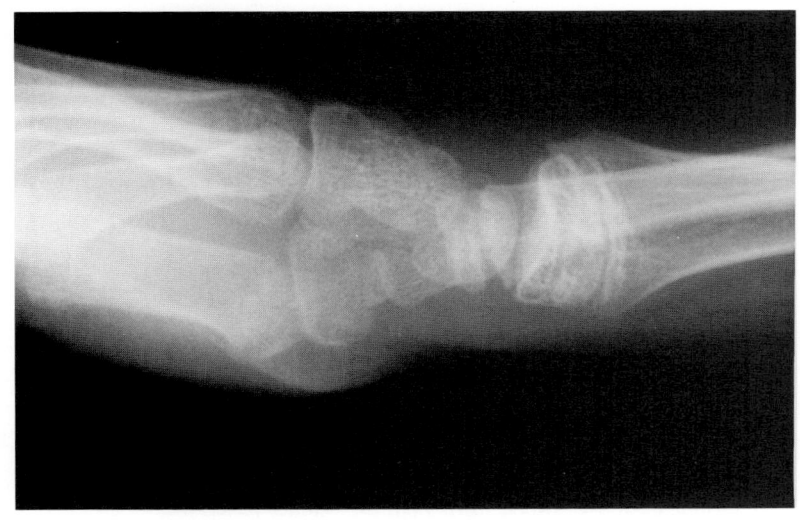

Fig. 19-17 *(Continued).* **(E&F)** Two and a half years later there is marked shortening of the radius indicative of a combined type II and type V injury to the physis.

ther physeal damage and possible growth arrest of the distal radius. In the case of a healed, malunited fracture, it is preferable to observe the child's extremity for several years until remodeling is complete. Osteotomy may then be performed if significant deformity or interference in wrist function persists.

If an established malunion should occur and persist, osteotomy of the radius may be performed. Blackburn and colleagues[30] described a method of percutaneous drill osteoclasis, which is reliable in shaft and metaphyseal malunions. The bones are pierced with several drill holes and then closed osteoclasis is performed. Cast immobilization is sufficient. No internal fixation is required. A physeal malunion may require a more formal open osteotomy and reduction with internal fixation.

Growth Arrest of the Radius

Lee and colleagues[28] reviewed 10 cases of distal radial growth arrest, which were caused by either compression of the growth plate at the time of injury (Fig. 19-5), or by repeated forceful manipulations. He recommended avoiding repeat manipulations if the fracture was 50 percent opposed and the alignment satisfactory. Abram and Thompson[46] described a child in whom a physeal arrest of the distal radial growth plate occurred in association with a torus fracture of the distal radius. The interference with growth was unrecognized until several years later. This may have been a type V injury to the physis, which often occurs in association with other fractures and is usually secondary to higher velocity injury such as falls from heights or motor vehicle accidents (Figs. 19-16 and 19-17).

Treatment of a growth arrest of the distal radius may require an epiphyseodesis of the distal ulna if significant malalignment of the distal radial joint surface has occurred. Resection of a bar if less than 30 percent of the physeal surface should be considered. Corrective osteotomies of the radius may also be required for associated deformity. Zehntner and coworkers[47] described a corrective radial osteotomy using a trapezoidal tricortical graft to correct multiplanar deformity of the distal radius (Fig. 19-18).

Lengthening of the radius using the newer concepts of callotasis via the Ilizarov or Orthofix techniques should be considered if the physeal arrest has occurred at a young age, resulting in considerable radial shortening.

Growth Arrest of Distal Ulna

Trauma to the physis of the distal ulna may rarely cause a growth arrest, resulting in varying patterns of ulnar shortening and associated progressive radial deformity[48,49] (Fig. 19-16B). Physeal arrest may sometimes occur in the absence of apparent physeal injury at the time of initial injury.[49] Patients tend to complain of the deformity, but symptoms or functional deficits seem to be unusual. Described treatments have included ulnar lengthening, radial osteotomies, radial stapling and epiphyseodesis, in various combinations.[48,49]

Goltz felt that ulnar physeal injury was less common

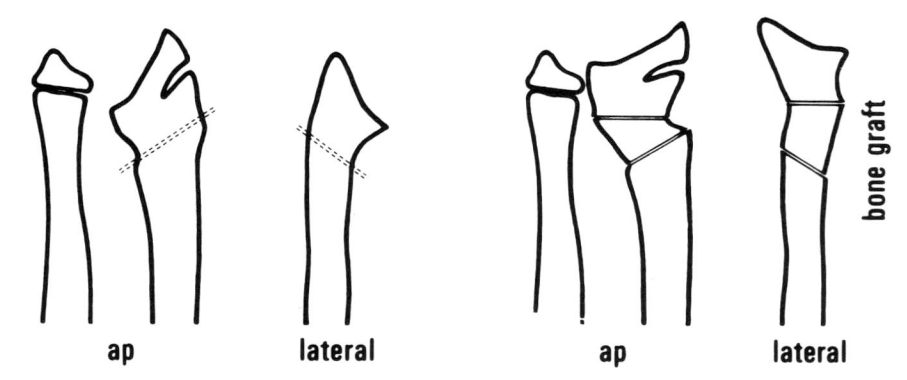

Fig. 19-18. Osteotomy of distal radius to correct deformity secondary to a growth arrest plus lengthening with bone graft. (Modified from Zehntner et al.[47])

than styloid fracture, due to the anatomy of the distal radioulnar joint. The styloid tends to be avulsed by the triangular fibrocartilage, whereas the physis is protected by the cushioning of the fibrocartilage (see Ch. 17).

Refracture

Refracture is not common in the distal radius and ulna but occasionally occurs in hyperactive children who following cast removal immediately return to the type of activity that produced the initial injury!

Cross-Union

Cross-union is rarely seen in distal radius and ulna fractures in spite of the intimate proximity of the bones at this level.[24]

Nonunion

Nonunion of fractures of the distal radius and ulna are very unusual. One should suspect additional pathology such as neurofibromatosis or osteomyelitis.[50,51]

MISINTERPRETATION OF FRACTURE PATHOLOGY

In children, several other disease processes can be misinterpreted as a routine fracture of the distal radius and ulna. These include physeal and periosteal changes secondary to rickets (Fig. 19-19), leukemia, scurvy, child abuse, and prostaglandin infusion (Fig. 19-20), to name a few. As with any fracture in children, the overall health status of the child must be appraised, including a good social history.

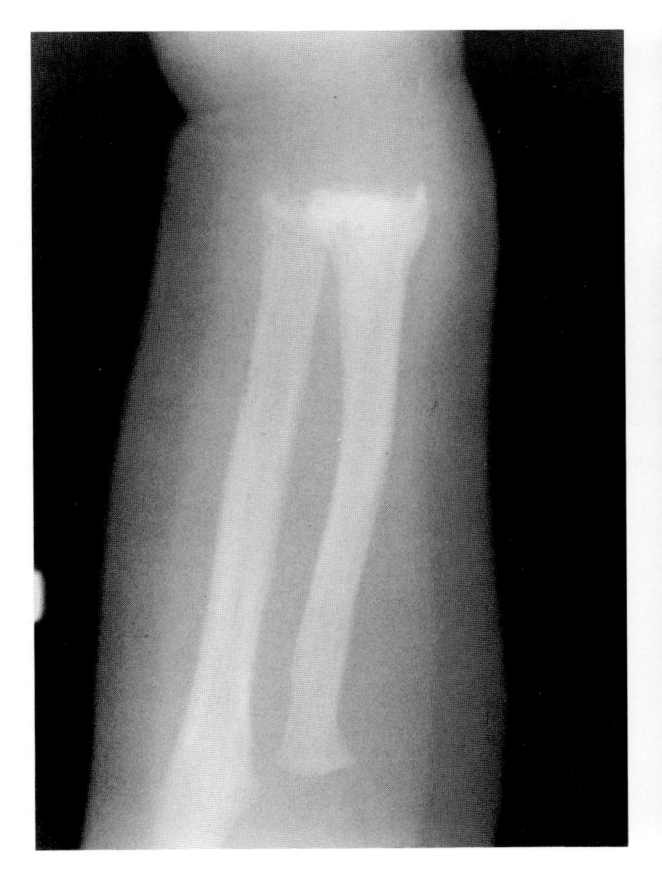

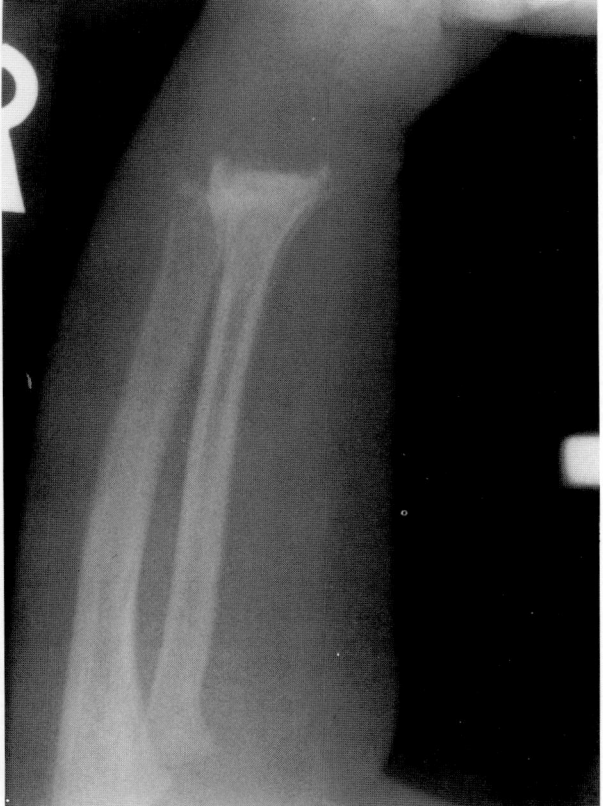

Fig. 19-19. A 4-month-old child with enlarged slightly tender wrists illustrating some periosteal elevation and fragmentation of the distal radius and ulna that was initially misinterpreted as secondary to trauma. This is consistent with the osseous changes of dietary rickets.

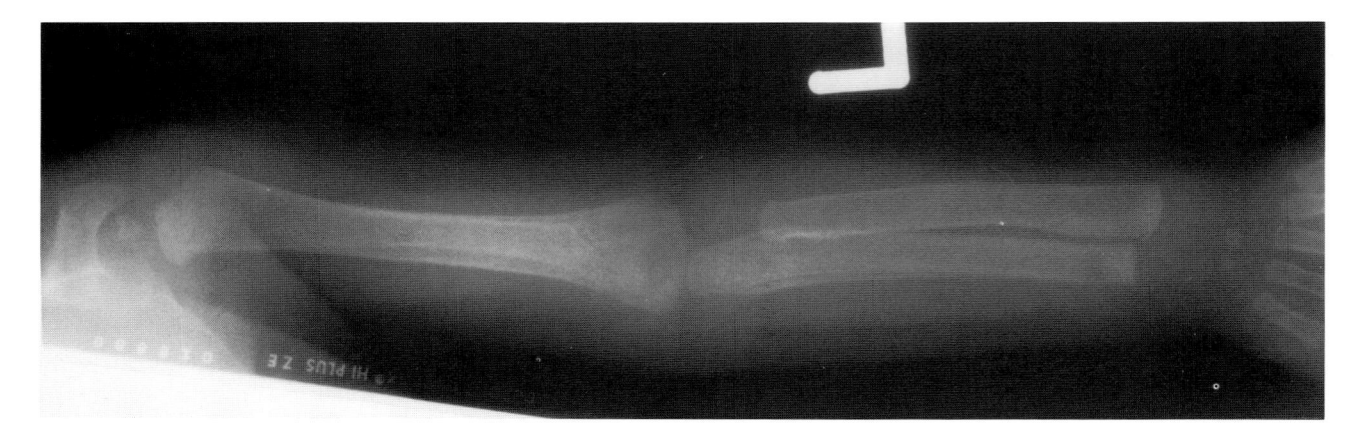

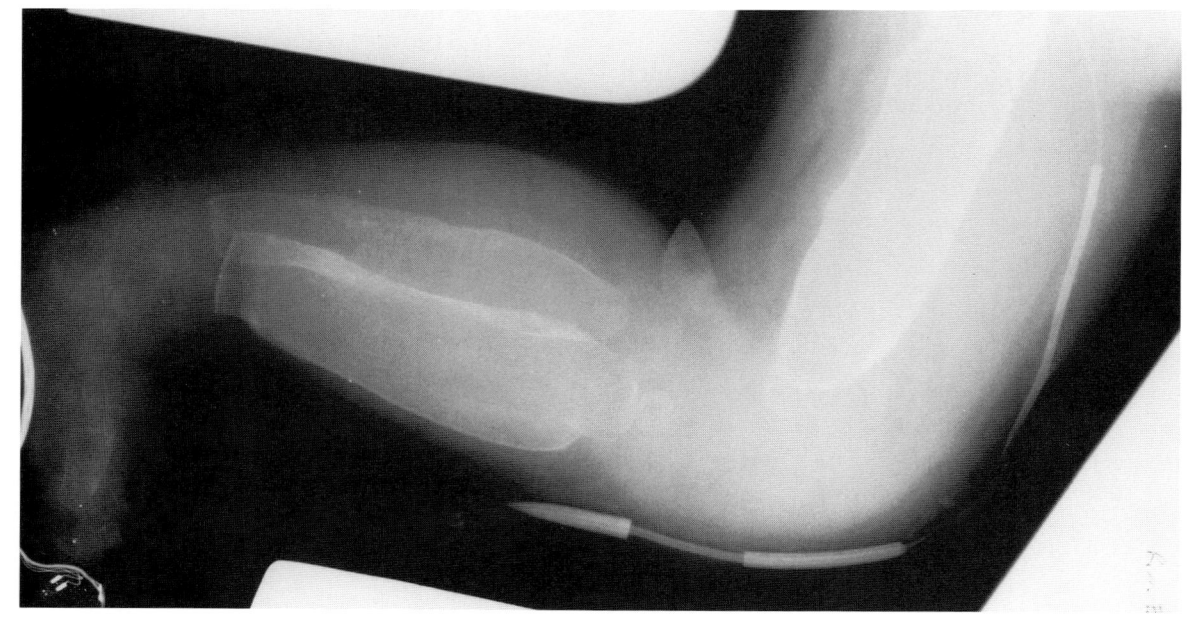

Fig. 19-20. Two infants with periosteal elevation secondary to prostaglandin E infusion for ductal dependent congenital heart disease.

SUMMARY

Fractures of the distal radius and ulna are the most common fractures encountered in children. Fortunately, these fractures are very forgiving in that significant amounts of displacement and angulation will remodel and lead to excellent results. However, an accurate anatomic reduction should always be the goal if it is achievable to avoid further unacceptable displacement as well as prolonged cosmetic deformity engendering parental anxiety. Complications are seldom encountered but physeal arrests do occur but tend to result in low morbidity unless very severe or sustained at a young age.

REFERENCES

1. Landin LA: Fracture patterns in children. Acta Orthop Scand, suppl 54:202, 1983
2. Beekman F, Sullivan JE: Some observations on fractures of long bones in children. Am J Surg 51:722, 1941
3. Thomas EM, Tuson KWR, Browne PSH: Fractures of the radius and ulna in children. Injury 7:120, 1975

4. Skillern PG: Complete fracture of the lower third of the radius in childhood, with greenstick fracture of the ulna. Ann Surg 61:209, 1915
5. D'Astous JL, Martin D: A review of compartment syndromes at the Children's Hospital of Eastern Ontario 1976–1988. Orthop Trans 15:112, 1991
6. Blount WP: Fractures in Children. Williams & Wilkins, Baltimore, 1955
7. Sharrard WJW: Paediatric Orthopedics and Fractures. 2nd Ed. Blackwell Scientific Publications, Oxford, 1979
8. Tredwell SJ, Van Peteghem K, Clough M: Pattern of forearm fractures in children. J Pediatr Orthop 4:604, 1984
9. Alexander CG: Effect of growth rate on the strength of the growth plate-shaft junction. Skeletal Radiol 1:67, 1976
10. Davis DR, Green DP: Forearm fractures in children. Clin Orthop 120:172, 1976
11. Bailey DA, Wedge JH, McCulloch RG et al: Epidemiology of fractures of the distal end of the radius in children as associated with growth. J Bone Joint Surg [Am] 71:1225, 1989
12. Ogden JA: Skeletal Injury in the Child. Lea & Febiger, Philadelphia, 1982
13. Salter RB, Harris WR: Injuries involving the epiphyseal plate. J Bone Joint Surg [Am] 45:587, 1963
14. Canale ST: Fractures and dislocations in children. p. 1067. In Crenshaw AH (ed): Campbell's Operative Orthopedics. 8th Ed. Mosby-Year Book, St. Louis, 1992
15. Greulich WW, Pyle SI: Radiographic Atlas of Skeletal Development of the Hand and Wrist. Stanford University Press, Stanford, CA, 1950
16. Creasman C, Zaleske DJ, Ehrlich MG: Analyzing forearm fractures in children. Clin Orthop 188:40, 1984
17. Albert MC, Barre PS: A scaphoid fracture associated with a displaced distal radial fracture in a child. Clin Orthop 240:232, 1989
18. Greene WB, Anderson WJ: Simultaneous fracture of the scaphoid and radius in a child. J Pediatr Orthop 2:191, 1982
19. Olney BW, Lugg PC, Turner PL et al: Outpatient treatment of upper extremity injuries in childhood using intravenous regional anaesthesia. J Pediatr Orthop 8:576, 1988
20. Rang M: Children's Fractures. 2nd Ed. JB Lippincott, Philadelphia, 1983
21. Evans EM: Fractures of the radius and ulna. J Bone Joint Surg [Br] 33:548, 1951
22. O'Brien ET: Fractures of the hand and wrist region. In Rockwood CA, Wilkins KE, King RE (eds): Fractures in Children. 3rd Ed. Vol. 3. JB Lippincott, Philadelphia, 1991
23. Chess DG, Hyndman JC, Leahey JL: Short arm plaster for pediatric distal forearm fractures. J Bone Joint Surg [Br] 69:506, 1987
24. Vince KG, Miller JE: Cross-union complicating fracture of the forearm. II. Children. J Bone Joint Surg [Am] 69:654, 1987
25. Bragdon RA: Fractures of the distal radial epiphysis. Clin Orthop 41:59, 1965
26. Aitken AP: The end results of the fractured distal radial epiphysis. J Bone Joint Surg 17:302, 1935
27. Aitken AP: Further observations on the fractured distal radial epiphysis. J Bone Joint Surg 17:922, 1935
28. Lee BS, Esterhai JL, Das M: Fracture of the distal radial epiphysis. Clin Orthop 185:90, 1984
29. Thompson GH, Wilber JH, Marcus RE: Internal fixation of fractures in children and adolescents. Clin Orthop 188:10, 1984
30. Blackburn N, Ziv I, Rang M: Correction of the malunited forearm fracture. Clin Orthop 188:55, 1984
31. Fuller DJ, McCullough CJ: Malunited fractures of the forearm in children. J Bone Joint Surg [Br] 64:364, 1982
32. Gandhi RK, Wilson P, Mason Brown JJ et al: Spontaneous correction of deformity following fractures of the forearm in children. Br J Surg 50:5, 1962
33. Larsen E, Vittas D, Torp-Pedersen S: Remodeling of angulated distal forearm fractures in children. Clin Orthop 237:190, 1988
34. Price CT, Scott DS, Kurzner ME, Flynn JC: Malunited forearm fractures in children. J Pediatr Orthop 10:705, 1990
35. Roberts JA: Angulation of the radius in children's fractures. J Bone Joint Surg [Br] 68:751, 1986
36. Voto SJ, Weiner DS, Leighley B: Redisplacement after closed reduction of forearm fractures in children. J Pediatr Orthop 10:79, 1990
37. Voto SJ, Weiner DS, Leighley B: Use of pins and plaster in the treatment of unstable pediatric forearm fractures. J Pediatr Orthop 10:85, 1990
38. Lesko PD, Georgis T, Slabaugh P: Irreducible Salter-Harris type II fracture of the distal radial epiphysis. J Pediatr Orthop 7:719, 1987
39. Karlsson J, Appelqvist R: Irreducible fracture of the wrist in a child. Acta Orthop Scand 58:280, 1987
40. Evans DL, Stauber M, Frykman GK: Irreducible epiphyseal plate fracture of the distal ulna due to interposition of the extensor carpi ulnaris tendon: a case report. Clin Orthop 251:162, 1990
41. Sumner JM, Khuri SM: Entrapment of the median nerve and flexor pollicis longus tendon in an epiphyseal fracture-dislocation of the distal radioulnar joint: a case report. J Hand Surg [Am] 9:711, 1984
42. Wolfe JS, Eyring EJ: Median-nerve entrapment within a greenstick fracture. J Bone Joint Surg [Am] 56:1270, 1974
43. Fee NF, Dobranski A, Bisla RS: Gas gangrene complicating open forearm fractures. J Bone Joint Surg [Am] 59:135, 1977
44. Santoro V, Mara J: Compartmental syndrome complicating Salter-Harris type II distal radius fracture. Clin Orthop 233:226, 1988
45. Friberg KSI: Remodeling after distal forearm fractures in children. Acta Orthop Scand 50:537, 1979
46. Abram LJ, Thompson GH: Deformity after premature

closure of the distal radial physis following a torus fracture with a physeal compression injury. J Bone Joint Surg [Am] 69:1450, 1987
47. Zehntner MK, Jakob RP, McGanity PLJ: Growth disturbance of the distal radial epiphysis after trauma: operative treatment by corrective radial osteotomy: case report. J Pediatr Orthop 10:411, 1990
48. Nelson OA, Buchanan JR, Harrison CS: Distal ulnar growth arrest. J Hand Surg 9:164, 1984
49. Golz RJ, Grogan DP, Greene TL et al: Distal ulnar physeal injury. J Pediatr Orthop 11:318, 1991
50. Kameyama O, Ogawa R: Pseudarthrosis of the radius associated with neurofibromatosis: report of a case and review of the literature. J Pediatr Orthop 10:128, 1990
51. Bell D: Congenital forearm pseudarthrosis: report of six cases and review of the literature. J Pediatr Orthop 9:438, 1989

20

Fractures of the Radial Head and Neck

Gerhard N. Kiefer

Innovation is the daughter of necessity.

Radial head and neck fractures in children represent approximately 10 to 20 percent of all injuries involving the proximal radius.[1-3] This equates to 1 to 2 percent of all fractures in children.[4] A fracture of either the neck or physis is involved in 90 percent of these cases. The average age of occurrence in most series is from 9 to 10 years, with a range from 4 to 14 years of age.[4-6] Although there is no sex difference in the occurrence rate,[8] this injury occurs approximately 2 years earlier in girls than in boys, as expected, based on skeletal maturity. There is no difference in right or left extremity involvement.[6] Fractures of the radial head are very rare in the pediatric age group.

ANATOMIC CONSIDERATIONS

The symptoms associated with this injury vary, depending upon the magnitude of the injury sustained. Medical treatment may be delayed for several days because of trivial initial symptoms. Localized swelling and pain are usually present and related to distension of the elbow joint by the hemarthrosis. There can be an absence of a significant hemarthrosis because of joint capsule disruption or extracapsular involvement of the radius. On occasion, the pain may be referred to the wrist region. This discomfort is aggravated by forearm supination and pronation, with only minor discomfort associated with elbow flexion-extension movements.

At 4 years of age, the radial head and neck assume adult contours and proportion.[8] Ossification of the epiphysis begins with a small flat osseous nucleus, usually not visualized before 5 years of age. This ossification nucleus may be bipartite or spherical. Although some angulation of the radial head as compared to the radial shaft is normally present (Fig. 20-1), the central line of the proximal metaphysis of the radius and the midpoint of the radial head bisects the center of the capitellum (Fig. 20-2).

The orbicular ligament originates from the radial side of the ulna and surrounds the radial neck. The arc of motion of the radial head and neck preclude ligamentous attachment to bone. However, the radial collateral ligament is confluent with the orbicular ligament. The articular joint capsule arises from the proximal third of the radial neck and protrudes distally under the orbicular ligament to form a pouch. Thus a large portion of the radial neck is extracapsular and does not create an intra-articular effusion if injured. Hence the traditional "fat-pad sign" may be negative if the fracture occurs in the extracapsular portion of the radial neck.[9]

The biomechanics of the proximal radioulnar joint are unique. The axis of rotation is seen to be within in the

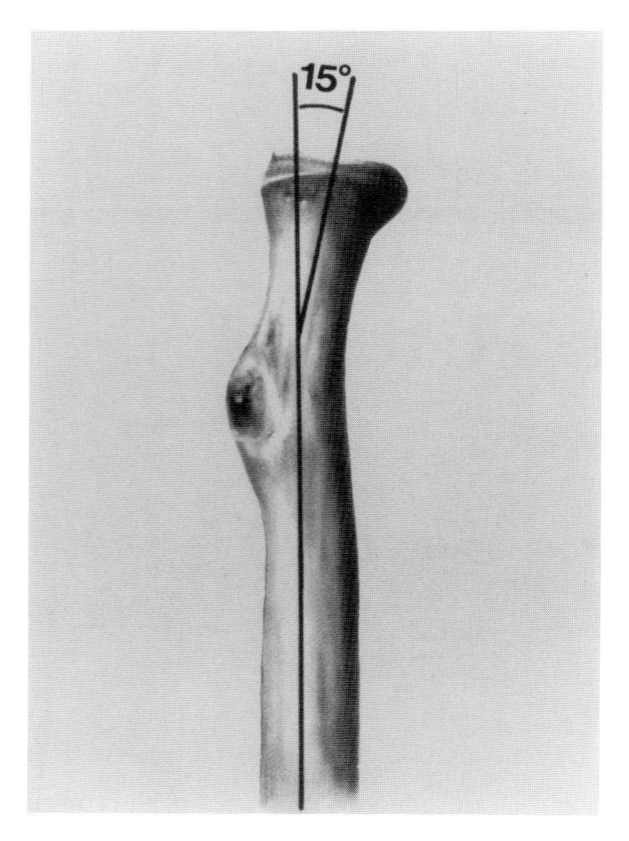

Fig. 20-1. The neck of the radius is angulated 15 degrees to the long axis of the proximal radius. (From Morrey BF. The Elbow and Its Disorders. p. 16. WB Saunders, Philadelphia, 1985. By permission of Mayo Foundation.)

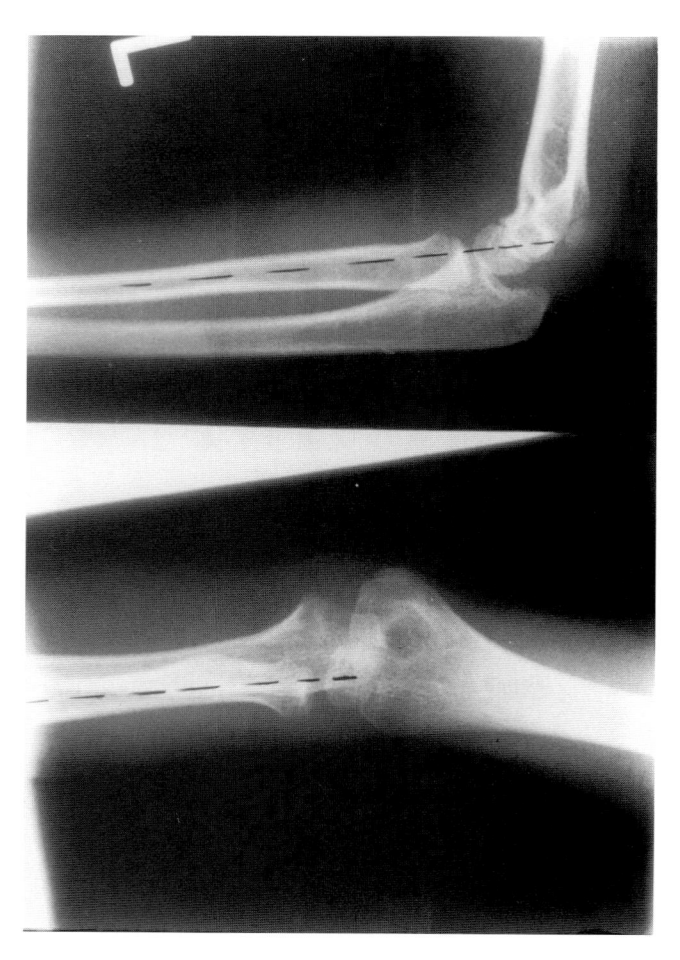

Fig. 20-2. Radiocapitellar line. A line through the shaft of the radius should intersect the capitellum in every radiographic view of the elbow joint.

center of the radial neck. Therefore the offset radial head results in "rotation with cam effect."[10] This cam effect causes the radial head to circumscribe an exact circle within the proximal radioulnar joint. Any change in the center of the radial head from its alignment with the center of the radius of the neck alters the arc of rotation of the head. Therefore, a translocation deformity will limit rotation of the forearm by disrupting the congruity of this proximal radioulnar joint.

MECHANISM OF INJURY

These fractures require a major force to be applied across the radial head, usually as the result of a fall on an outstretched arm. The mechanical forces are then transmitted to the radial neck, which sustains the fracture because of the weaker metaphyseal bone or growth plate. The physical attitude of the outstretched elbow results in a valgus injury because of the normal anatomic carrying angle of the elbow. The degree of flexion and extension determines associated injuries of the ulna. If the olecranon is keyed into the olecranon fossa in full extension, the ulna is locked into position. This results in a fracture of the radial neck and ipsilateral olecranon. In flexion the olecranon and ulna permit movement within the olecranon fossa. This play in movement permits absorption of force without fracture. The degree of force and displacement determines the location of the ipsilateral ulnar fracture (Fig. 20-3).

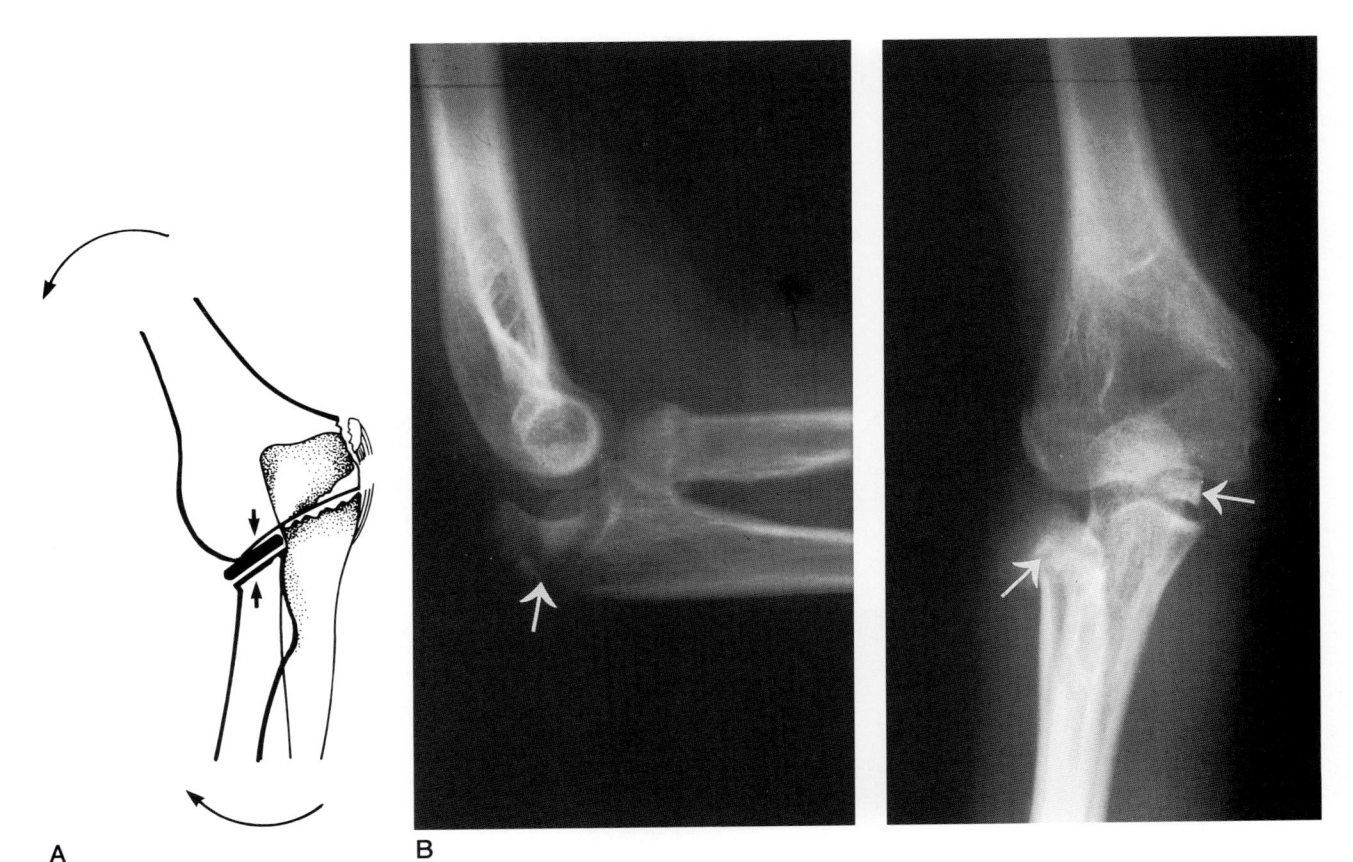

Fig. 20-3. (A) Valgus high-energy force, as in a fall from a height, may result in a triad of fractures, including the olecranon and medial epicondyle, as well as the radial neck. (B) A 6-year-old child who fell out of a tree exhibits the triad with the medial epicondyle seen trapped within the elbow joint.

Additional rotational forces can occur in a very young child. This most commonly results in subluxation of the radial head (pulled elbow syndrome). However, if the force is applied in a supination vector, rather than in pronation, a torsional radial neck may occur. Arthrography and examination under anesthesia may be required to diagnose this injury in this age group but is seldom necessary, as the fracture is usually innocuous, healing with short-term (2 weeks) immobilization.

Dislocation of the elbow joint can result in associated ipsilateral fractures of the radial head, either at the time of dislocation or upon reduction.[11] The radial head is usually entrapped within the elbow joint, requiring open arthrotomy with pinning of the radial head fragment to the neck. These may result in a late angular deformity of the radial neck (Fig. 20-4). Articular cartilage injuries have been known to result in osteochondritis dissecans or lytic lesions of the radial head.

CLASSIFICATION

Radial head and neck fractures have been classified by a variety of authors. Jeffrey[2] was the first to recognize the two major mechanisms of injury. His first group of valgus injuries were further subclassified into three subtypes based upon the degree of angulation.[8] The injuries were classified by Newman[12] into five fracture patterns based upon the mechanism of injury. Wilkins[13] subsequently combined the classifications of Jeffrey and Newman into three groups: Group I, involving primary displacement of the radial head, encompasses the majority of proximal radial injuries; Group II involves the fractures resulting in displacement of the radial neck and the rare stress injuries are grouped into Group III. The classification is illustrated in Figure 20-5.

O'Brien's[8] classification of results dependent upon the degree of residual angulation of the radial head contin-

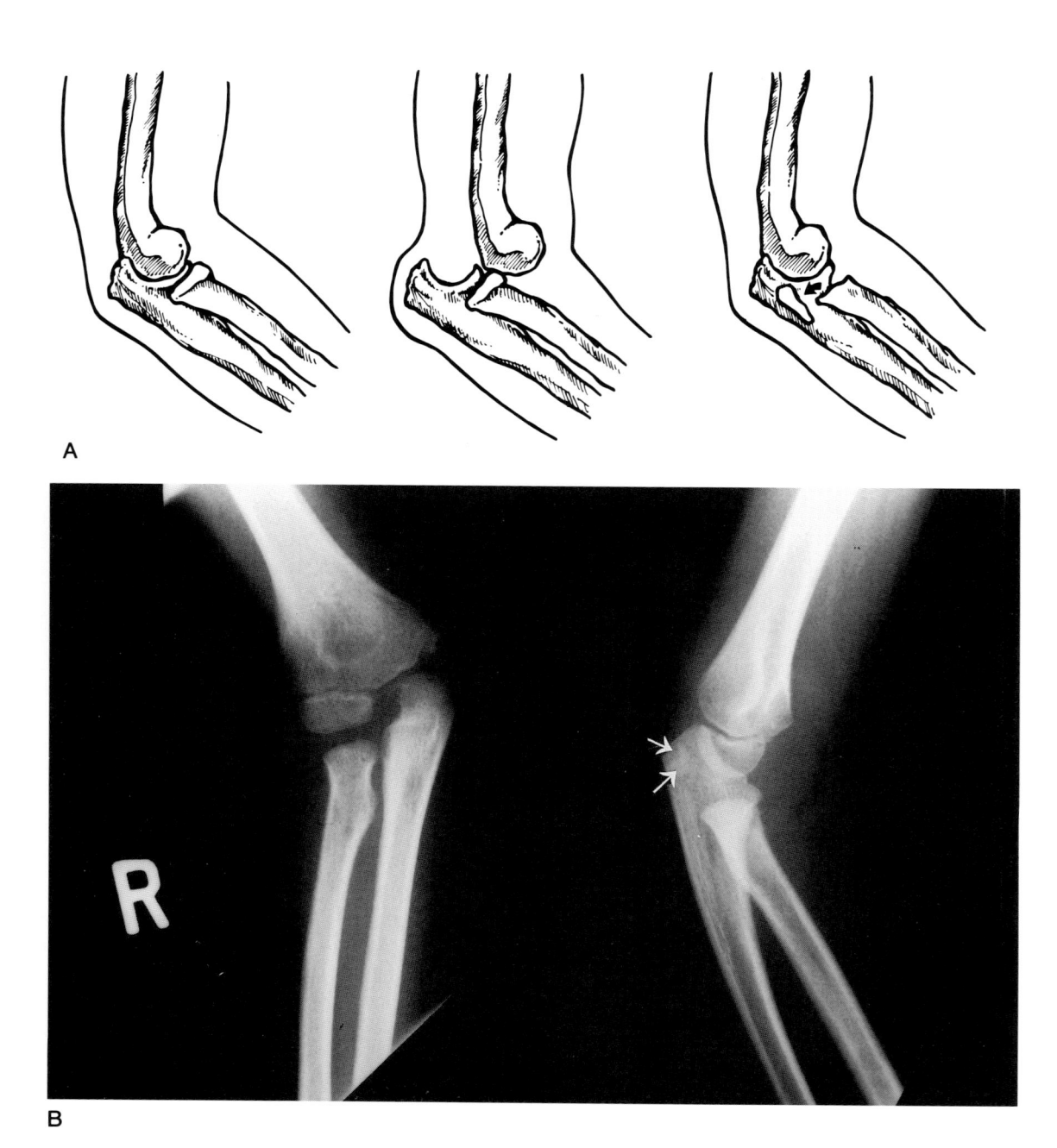

Fig. 20-4. **(A)** The head of radius may be sheared off and remain within the elbow joint as the radius and ulna relocates from their dislocated position. **(B)** Intra-articular fragment of the radial head in a 6-year-old with a small radial head ossific center ossified, and **(C)** in a 10-year-old during an attempt to reduce a dislocated elbow. (Figure A from Letts RM: Dislocations of the elbow in children. In Morrey BF (ed): The Elbow and Its Disorders. p. 281. WB Saunders, Philadelphia, 1985. By permission of Mayo Foundation.) *(Figure continues.)*

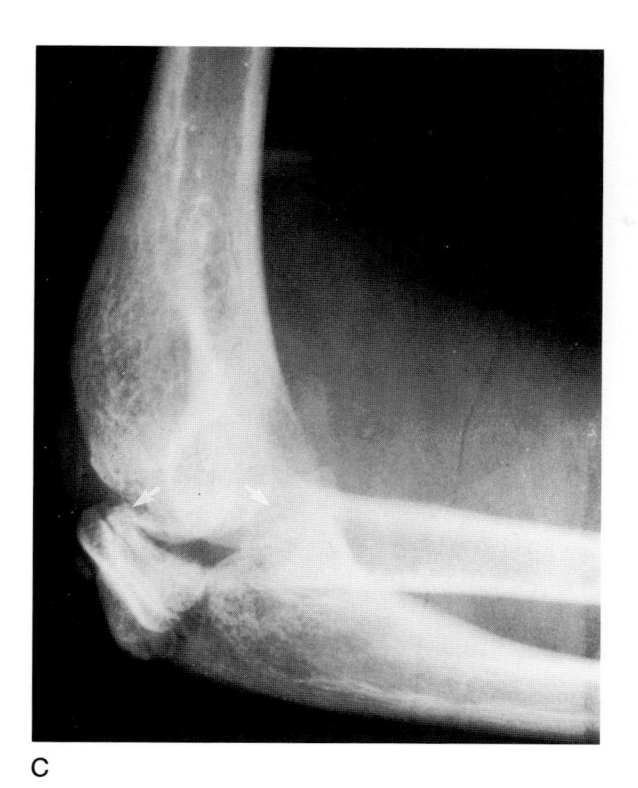

Fig. 20-4 *(Continued).* **(C)**

ues to be the most clinically reliable and useful grouping.[8-10,13]

PHYSICAL EXAMINATION

Because of minimal initial symptoms, diagnosis of a fractured neck of radius is frequently delayed. Elbow pain and restricted arc of motion may result from the initial injury, followed by progressive swelling and distention of the elbow. Passive forearm supination and pronation results in increased discomfort. Elbow flexion and extension may not be significantly limited. Occasionally the pain is referred to the wrist. When this occurs, pressure over the proximal forearm will accentuate the wrist pain. In addition, the degree of force may occasionally cause wrist fractures including scaphoid fractures, which can mask ipsilateral proximal forearm discomfort.

DIFFERENTIAL DIAGNOSIS

These injuries may occasionally be mistaken for a subluxation of the head of the radius. However, the mechanism of injury and history should permit differentiation from a pulled elbow "or nursemaid's elbow." The history is critical for this clinical distinction.

Dislocation of the head of the radius must also be considered in light of the limitation of range of motion and occasional excessive swelling which can occur. Ligamentous laxity has been implicated as facilitating this injury. Hence the most frequent age of dislocation is around 7 years, at which time the associated soft tissue laxity is felt to be at its peak. Associated ipsilateral ulnar fractures must be ruled out in order to assure that a variant of the Monteggia fracture dislocation is not present (see Ch. 17).

Following careful clinical evaluation, radiographic studies should permit visualization and diagnosis of the fracture.

RADIOGRAPHIC EXAMINATION

The fracture is usually easily visualized on one or both of the anteroposterior or lateral radiographs. Radiographs in both supination and pronation are occasionally necessary to verify the fracture site (Fig. 20-6).

If an elbow cannot be extended because of patient discomfort, then adaptations of the anteroposterior radiograph may be required to allow adequate examination. The initial radiograph should be obtained with the x-ray beam perpendicular to the distal humerus. A second radiograph with the beam perpendicular to the proximal radius will permit complete examination of the elbow.

In minimally displaced fractures oblique views of the proximal radius may be required. Greenspan and Norman[14,15] have recommended a special radiocapitellar view to project the radial head anterior to the coronoid process. These authors recommend this radiograph if full supination and pronation radiographs are unattainable because of discomfort.

It is important to recognize that the radial head and metaphysis should be aligned with the center of the capitellum in all views irrespective of orientation or obliquity (Fig. 20-2). If the radial epiphysis is ossified, the displacement of the radial head can be readily detected. Prior to its ossification, however, difficulty may be en-

Group I: Primary Displacement of the Radial Head.

Valgus Fractures

Type A — Salter Harris Type I and II injuries

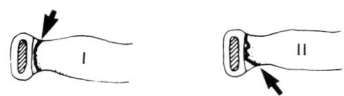

Type B — Salter Harris Type IV injuries

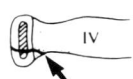

Type C — Fractures involving only the proximal radial metaphysis

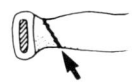

Elbow Fracture - Dislocations

Type D — Reduction Injuries

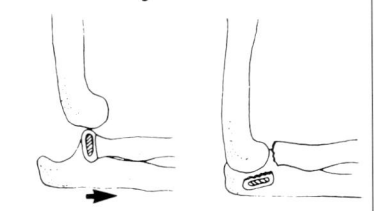

Type E — Dislocation Injuries

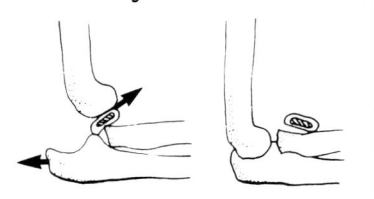

Group II: Primary Displacement of the Radial Neck.

A. Angular Injuries (Monteggia Type III Variant)

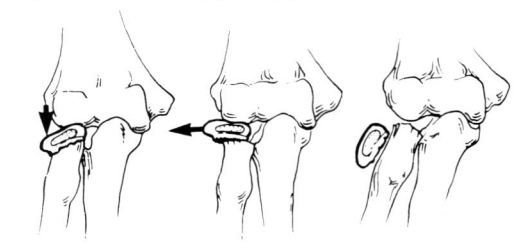

B. Torsional Injuries

Group III:

A. Osteochondritis Dissecans of the Radial Head.
B. Physeal Injuries with Neck Angulation.

Fig. 20-5. Classification of radial head and neck fractures in children.

---

countered in determining the degree of displacement of the radial head without an arthrogram or MRI.

In the preossification stage, a radial epiphyseal fracture may demonstrate a loss of smoothness of the metaphyseal margin. Displacement of the anterior and posterior fat-pads are not always reliable signs of injury. These may not be displaced with occult fractures of the radial neck or physis. Intraoperative arthrography may be necessary to determine displacement of the unossified radial head.

TREATMENT INDICATIONS

The indications for treatment relate to the fracture location, degree of displacement, ipsilateral injuries, the time elapsed since injury, and the age of the patient.

The natural history of radial neck fractures in children have demonstrated very satisfactory results with up to 30 degrees of angulation.[1,2,5,8,12,16] Fractures with 30 to 45 degrees of angulation exhibit a minimal residual loss of supination and pronation, prompting many authors to suggest only cast immobilization for children less than

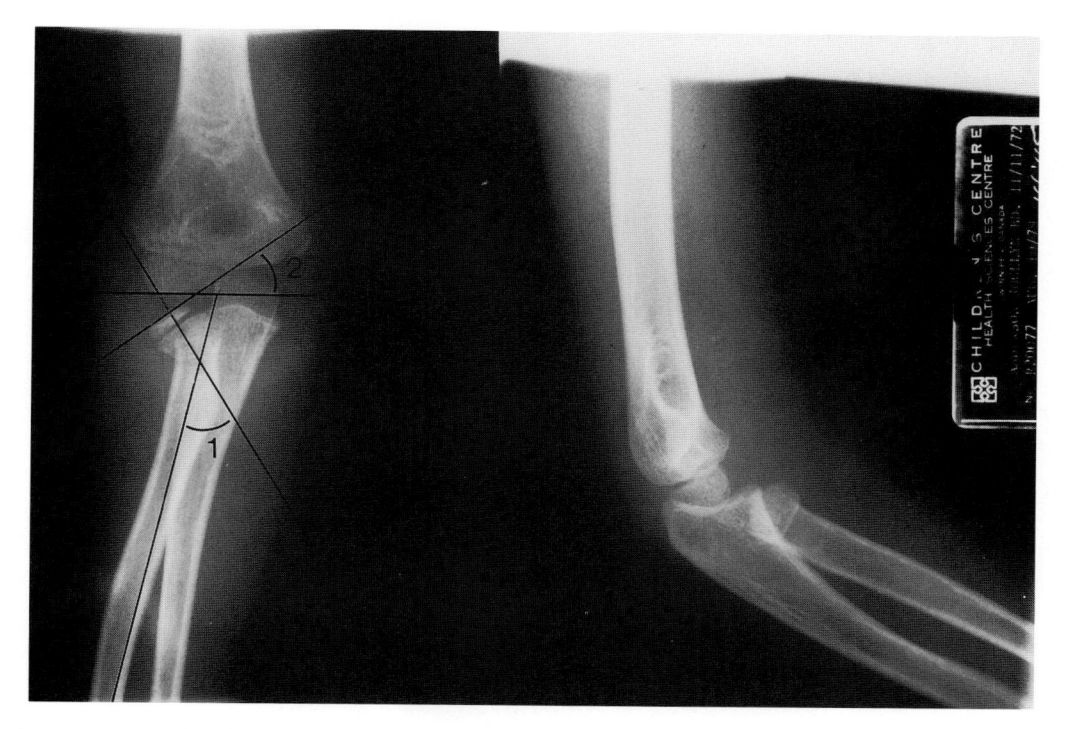

Fig. 20-6. An angulated fracture of the radial neck in a 7-year-old girl injured in a fall from monkey bars. The degree of angulation can be calculated by *(1)* measuring the intersection of a line drawn through the neck of the radius and one drawn through the center of the displaced head and neck, or by *(2)* measuring the intersection of a line drawn parallel with the articular surface of the displaced radial head and a horizontal line tangential to the capitellum representing the position of the normal radial head articular surface. Whichever technique is used, it should be consistently employed for assessment in a particular patient.

10 years of age. Spontaneous remodeling of some residual neck deformity will occur with growth (Fig. 20-7). A closed reduction may be warranted for older children with angulation exceeding 30 degrees. Those requiring no reduction can be managed by simple immobilization utilizing either a posterior splint, an above-elbow cast, or a simple collar and cuff sling. Early range of motion is initiated at 10 and 21 days. Aspiration of the intra-articular hematoma is not necessary, since the improved comfort provided by this technique is questionable.

The incidence of poor outcome following unreduced proximal radial head and neck fractures is as high as 50 percent when severely displaced fractures are considered. Overall the incidence of poor results with limitation of motion varies from 15 to 33 percent, depending upon the literature review.[5,16,17] It is essential to discuss with the parents the potential for a poor result prior to initiating treatment. The older the child, in association with an ipsilateral fracture, the greater the probability of significant limitation of motion. Functional improvement following fracture care is evident up to 6 months following the injury. Thereafter, little improvement in function can be anticipated.[5]

Closed reduction of these fractures can be performed by manipulation under fluoroscopic control. Radial neck fractures angulated in excess of 45 degrees warrant reduction. Fractures with angulation up to 60 degrees can often be reduced to an acceptable position utilizing the following technique. Under general anesthetic, with adequate relaxation, the surgical assistant holds the arm proximal to the elbow joint. The assistant must provide a medial buttress over the distal humerus in order to allow a varus stress to be administered by the surgeon utilizing the distal humerus as the fulcrum. With the supposition that the orbicular ligament will stabilize the proximal fracture fragment the surgeon proceeds to supinate the forearm while applying distal traction. This maneuver will relax the supinators and biceps muscles. Thereafter, a varus force is applied medially across the elbow to overcome the ulnar deviation of the distal fragment.

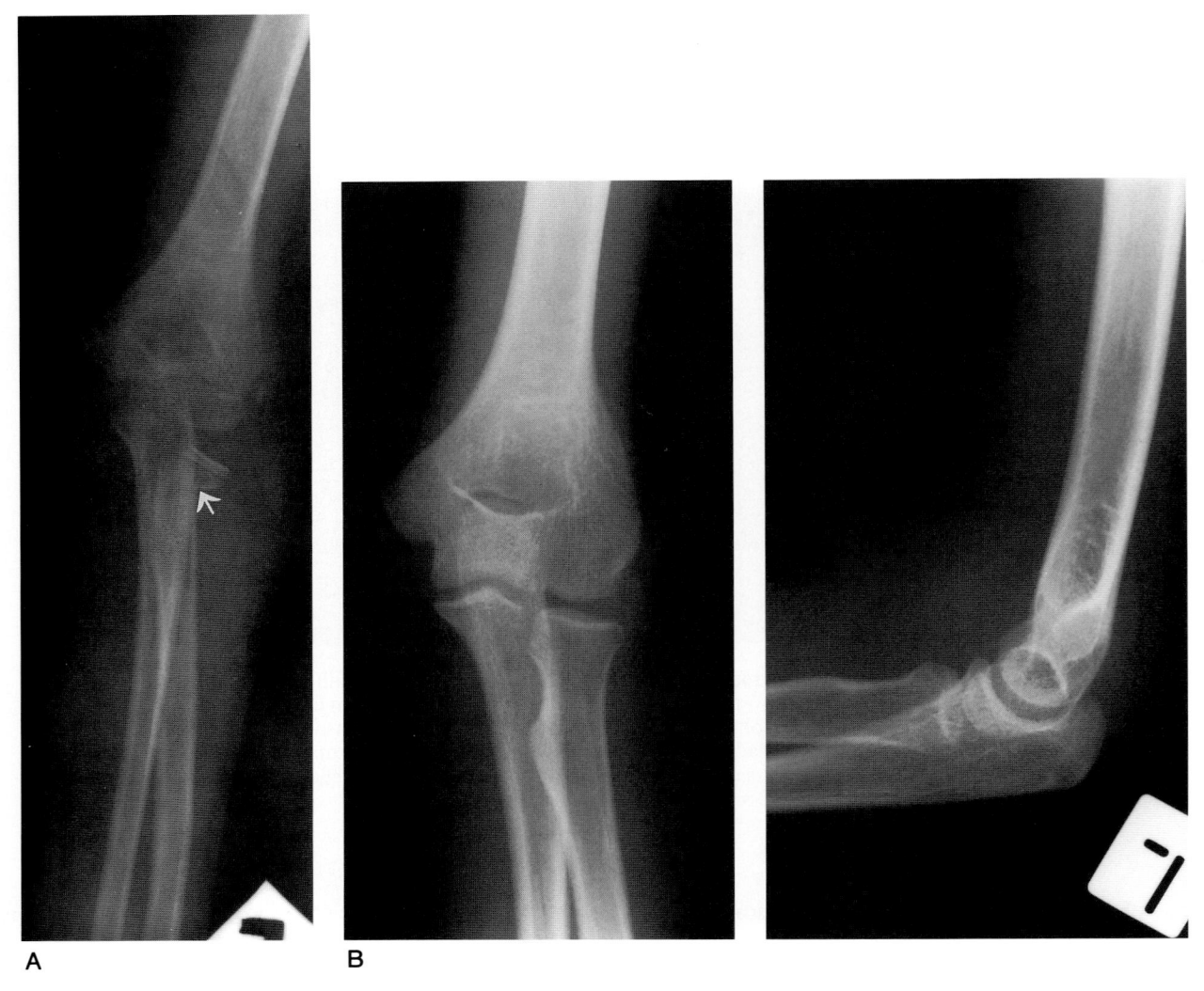

Fig. 20-7. (A) Radial neck fracture sustained at age 10 years. (B) Spontaneous remodeling on follow-up seen 4 years later.

This maneuver should align the distal fragment with the proximal fragment. Concurrently, a varus force is applied with the surgeon's thumb directly over the radial head.[2] This varus force will facilitate manipulation of the radial head into the open radiocapitellar joint space. It is important to remember that the tilt of the radial head can be anterior or posterior, depending on the position of the forearm at the time of injury.

Jeffrey[2] recommended the forearm be rotated until maximal tilt of the proximal fragment is clinically evident and palpated laterally. Confirmation of the direction of maximal tilt should be confirmed with fluoroscopic control. Digital pressure thereafter over the radial head should permit manipulation into a position of reduction.

Intraoperative radiographs permit confirmation of the direction of maximum tilt of the displaced radial head and neck fragment. When the radiographic beam is perpendicular to the maximal fracture angulation, the radial head is seen to be an oblong or rectangular shape.[2] When the radiograph is not perpendicular to the plane of fracture angulation the radial head often appears to be oval or circular in shape.[2]

The fracture reduction is usually not detected clinically. Occasionally a previously irreducible radial neck fracture is found to have spontaneously reduced follow-

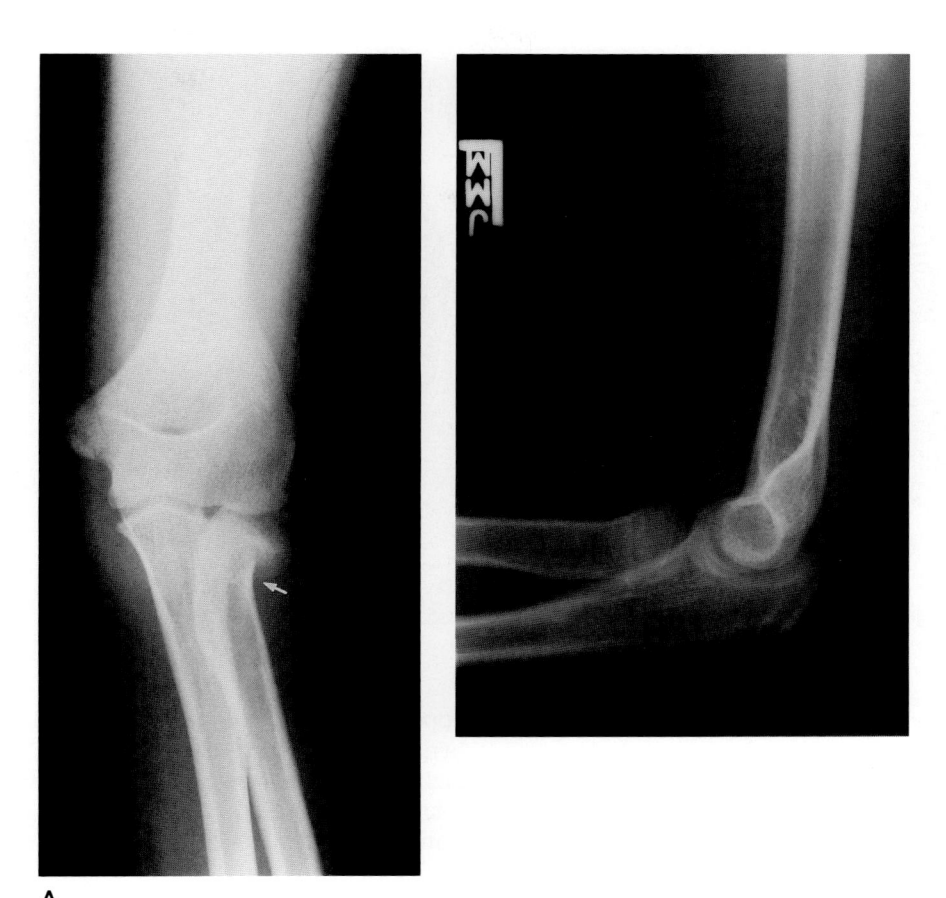

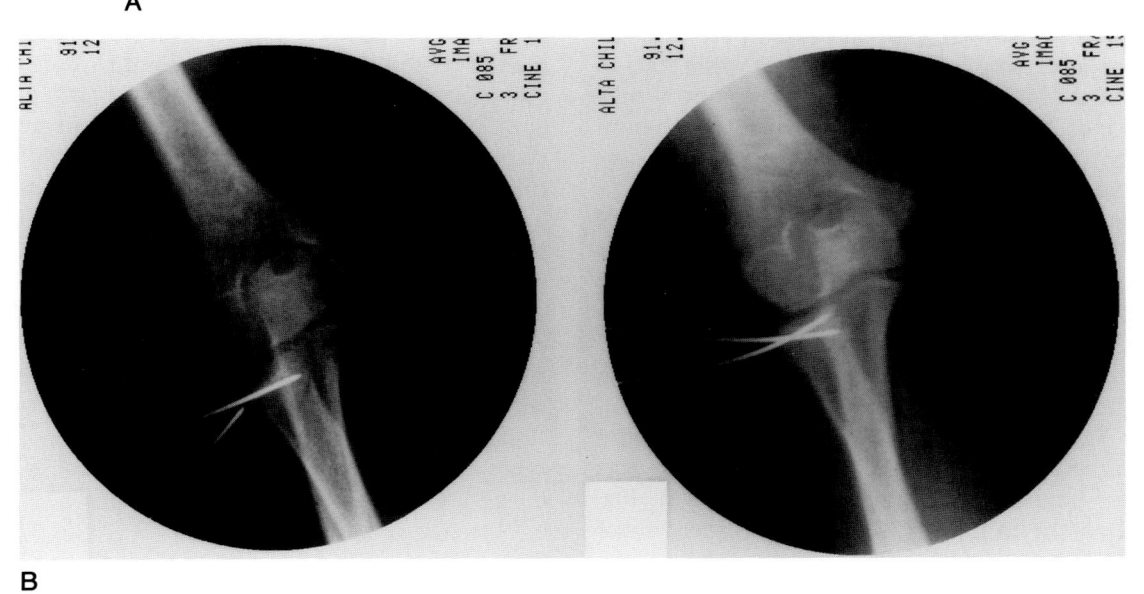

Fig. 20-8. Percutaneous pin reduction technique. **(A)** A 14-year-old male with left displaced radial neck fracture, which could not be adequately manipulated by closed reduction. **(B)** Percutaneous pin insertion into radial head, followed by reduction. *(Figure continues.)*

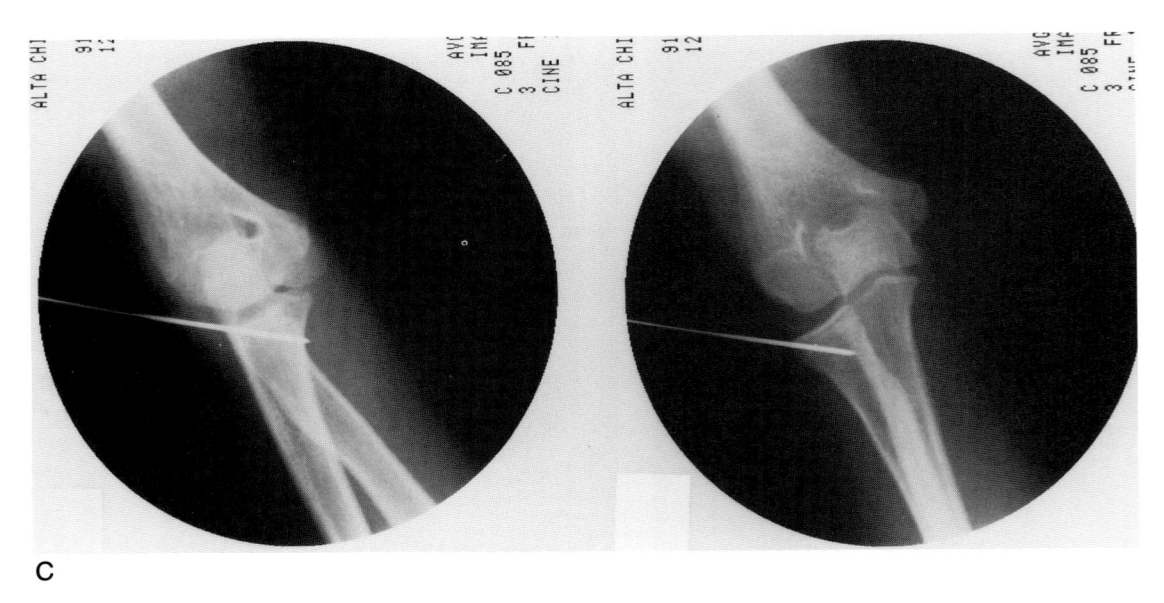

Fig. 20-8 *(Continued).* **(C)** Fracture site transfixion by single cross-wire technique.

ing Esmarch bandage limb exsanguination in preparation for an open reduction.

An alternative to closed manipulation in extension involves flexing the elbow to 90 to 100 degrees.[18] Thereafter, the surgeon's thumb is pressed against the inferior surface of the radial head as the forearm is gradually pronated from initial full supination. Following this maneuvre, it is imperative to obtain anteroposterior, lateral, and oblique radiographs of the elbow while placing the forearm in both supination and pronation positions. Although most fractures are stable following reduction, redisplacement is a concern, especially if the initial angulation was in excess of 60 degrees.

When closed reduction with residual angulation of less than 30 to 45 degrees cannot be obtained then percutaneous repositioning of the radial head with a smooth pin is advocated.[19,20] Under image intensification, a smooth Kirschner wire is placed either proximal or distal to the proximal radial physis. One or two 1.6-mm smooth Kirschner wires can be placed under direct visualization. These pins then provide sufficient control to permit manipulation of the radial head and leverage of the fracture fragment into an acceptable position (Fig. 20-8). Given the initial degree of displacement these fractures may require transfixion.

If these techniques prove to be inadequate, then open reduction should be considered. Surgical intervention has resulted in significant loss of motion when performed beyond 7 to 10 days postinjury. Fracture alignment with less than 45 degrees of residual angulation appears to result in a more functional outcome. Steinberg and coworkers[5] demonstrated the results of moderately displaced fractures (30 to 45 degrees) treated operatively to be equal to the results of those treated nonoperatively. Severely displaced fractures achieved good results in only 50 percent of the cases. The lateral Kocher approach along the distal lateral humeral condyle between anconeus and the extensor carpi ulnaris muscle permits exposure of the joint capsule of the radiocapitellar joint. Pronation of the forearm during this approach allows the posterior interosseous nerve to be displaced medially away from the operative field. The rule of thumb of not incising further than 2 fingerbreadths (3 cm) below the radial head in order to avoid injury to the posterior interosseous nerve must be modified to one or one and a half fingers (1 to 2 cm) in small children. Debris and torn annular ligament should be removed. The fracture should be reduced gently and fixation secured with suture or K-wire. When the annular ligament is torn simple approximation is indicated.

FIXATION TECHNIQUES

Fracture stability must be adequately assessed at the time of closed or open reduction. Several authors believe that simple open reduction is all that is required. Wedge and Robertson[10] found that fractures without internal fixation exhibited a greater number of good results. Historical recommendations of transcapitellar pin transfixion has resulted in multiple complications related to pin breakage due to fatigue failures of the metal, even when the limb is immobilized with a cast.[13,17] This technique should be discouraged.

The technique advocated involves placement of a smooth pin obliquely across the fracture site into the radial head. This can be either in a proximal to distal or distal to proximal direction. These pins are subsequently removed upon documentation of early fracture union. Occasionally radial head displacement cannot be maintained without transfixion of the proximal radius to the ulna.

Transverse radioulnar transfixion requires minimal dissection. In addition, the smooth Kirschner wire should be placed without multiple transgressions of the soft tissue. Proximal radioulnar synostosis is a potential rare complication. Alternative techniques reported in the literature include the utilization of a bone peg, mini-transfixion plate, and the use of flexible intermedullary fixation in a retrograde fashion to maintain reduction of this fracture pattern.[5,6,13,21]

PRINCIPLES OF POSTOPERATIVE MANAGEMENT

Postoperatively, the elbow is splinted with a posterior splint in a position of neutral forearm rotation or mild pronation with 90 degrees of elbow flexion. This splint is maintained and removed only for pin site and wound care if necessary. My personal preference involves the use of a 2 × 2 gauze with Betadine ointment dressing over top of the protruding pin. This is removed at 3 weeks to allow removal of pin without supplemental anesthesia. In children over age 12 fracture fixation is maintained for 4 weeks prior to its removal.

Thereafter, the posterior splint is continued intermittently for a total of 8 weeks. In the 3- to 8-week interval postinjury, early active range of motion is encouraged by recommending bath time activities as well as household chores, such as dishwashing, with the splint being worn only to school.

Physiotherapy is usually not necessary in the initial 12 weeks postinjury. If a child is not improving active range of motion by 12 weeks, then active assisted and active range of motion exercises are prescribed and supervised in a physiotherapy setting. Physiotherapy for patients under age 12 has not been necessary. Forearm supination and pronation range does not significantly improve following the initial 6- to 8-month interval postinjury.[5] Elbow flexion and extension will improve for 12 to 18 months postinjury.

TREATMENT PITFALLS

Since nonoperative treatment has in the past demonstrated minimal disability, one must be attentive to the patient's range of motion. Loss of motion can occur despite an anatomic reduction of these fractures. It is important to emphasize function over radiographic appearance. Fractures with displacement of less than 45 degrees must be carefully examined to document residual loss of supination and pronation. If angulation is greater than 30 degrees, then treatment may be indicated.

In the child with a painful proximal radial head and neck injury under age 5, arthrography may be indicated if the ossification of the proximal fragment is inadequate to determine fracture position.

Following the aforementioned technique of closed reduction, radiographic correction to less than 45 degrees of residual angulation may be acceptable, depending upon the arc of motion. Proximal radial head and neck fractures should be aggressively assessed in terms of translocation as well as angulation. Fractures with translocation require a more aggressive approach in order to attain an acceptable result. If passive range of supination and pronation is in excess of 60 degrees in either direction, the reduction can be accepted.

If closed reduction cannot be accomplished with digital pressure in full elbow extension; then the technique advocated by Kaufman[18] in flexion with pronation may be useful. Failure of these two techniques prompts the use of either an Ace bandage or Esmarch for wrapping and exsanguination of the extremity. My personal experience and the literature have confirmed reduction of an angulated radial neck being accomplished by this technique.

Failure of closed methods should result in an attempt at a semiclosed reduction utilizing the percutaneous pin technique previously described. Placement of these pins requires image intensification. Injury to the posterior interosseous nerve can be avoided if the pin is inserted posteriorly or posterolaterally with the forearm pronated.

Transcapitellar fixation pins should be avoided because of their high complication rate. Ideally a small transfixion pin placed obliquely through a separate stab incision is preferable to maintain reduction of the fracture.

Early range of elbow motion is encouraged, using active exercises. Household activities, particularly dishwashing, are beneficial and assists in the distraction of the child during the acquisition of functional range of motion.

COMPLICATIONS

A significant incidence of imperfect results and complications has been reported. If these fractures are associated with other injuries or dislocation then the frequency of problems are increased. Rang[22] describes the predisposition to poor results as being a lesson of "persistence with closed techniques prior to open reduction."

Loss of Motion

Despite anatomic reduction, loss of motion in the forearm may occur.[5] Loss of forearm pronation is most common. This is compensated for by shoulder and elbow positioning. Flexion and extension are rarely limited to a significant degree. Ipsilateral soft tissue and osseous injuries have a significant influence on functional motion. In addition to fibrous adhesions, joint incongruity may result in late posttraumatic osteoarthropathy.

Premature Physeal Closure

Premature physeal closure has been reported in many series but does not appear to significantly affect functional outcome.[1,5,8,10,12,17] Radial limb length discrepancy of less than 5 mm was inconsequential, with the exception of the rare incidence of severe cubitus valgus. The cubitus valgus attitude does not usually affect functional outcome and has minimal cosmetic deformity.

Proximal Radioulnar Synostosis

Although an uncommon complication, proximal radioulnar synostosis is the most serious sequela following this injury.[1,12] Although the synostosis can occur after manipulative closed therapy, it is most often seen in fractures with severe displacement and operative intervention. Delayed treatment beyond 5 days postinjury results in an increased incidence. This bony union may also result in a cubitus varus (Fig. 20-9).

Myositis Ossificans

Heterotopic ossification of soft tissue is one of the more troublesome complications known to occur.[16] Open reduction is the most common mode of treatment resulting in this complication. This may be seen to some extent in almost a third of all cases. Although usually limited to the supinator muscle, it often results in minimal long-term sequelae.

Nonunion of the Radial Neck

Nonunion of the radial neck is an uncommon complication that has been described in children.[10] Union eventually occurs. Both poor and satisfactory elbow function have been documented in the literature following this complication.

Osteonecrosis of the Radial Head

Osteonecrosis of the radial head is a rare complication that has been described in severely displaced fractures.[12] In each instance, operative intervention with poor results were implicated. Minimal degrees of osteonecrosis are often radiographically detected, but rarely result in functional loss. If residual joint stiffness occurs, then excisional arthroplasty excision may be indicated at skeletal maturity (Fig. 20-10).

Alteration of Upper Limb Alignment

The carrying angle of the involved elbow is not significantly altered unless there is a significant radioulnar synostosis or loss of fracture reduction.[5] An increase in carrying angle does not appear to result in a functional deficit. Jones found an overall increase of approximately 10 degrees when compared to the uninjured side.[21]

Neurovascular Complications

Vascular injuries have not been reported with isolated injuries of the proximal radial head and neck. Partial ulnar nerve injuries and posterior interosseus nerve in-

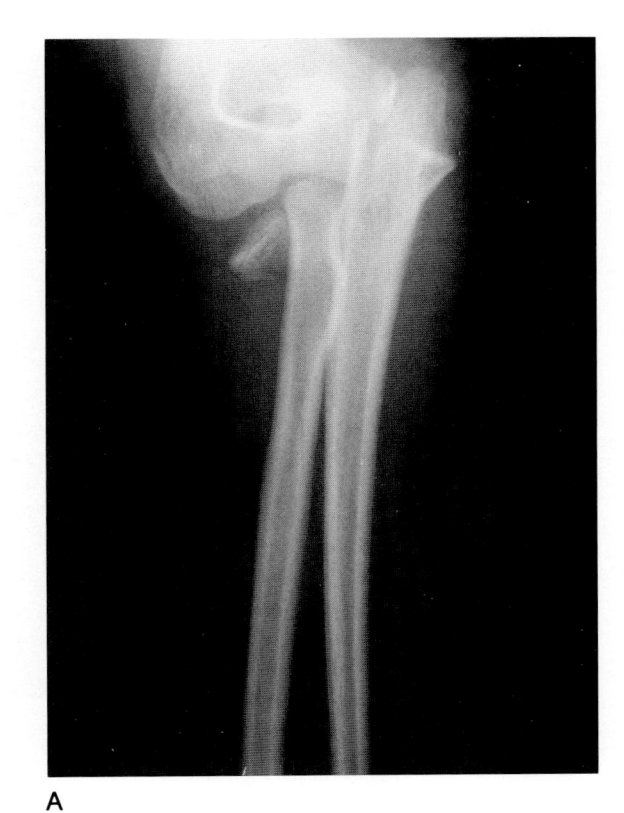

Fig. 20-9. **(A)** Displaced fracture of the radial neck. **(B)** Reduced by manipulation and closed reduction. **(C)** Cross-union between the proximal radius and ulna developed over the ensuing 2 months. (Courtesy of Dr. Jacques D'Astous, Children's Hospital of Eastern Ontario, Ottawa, Canada.)

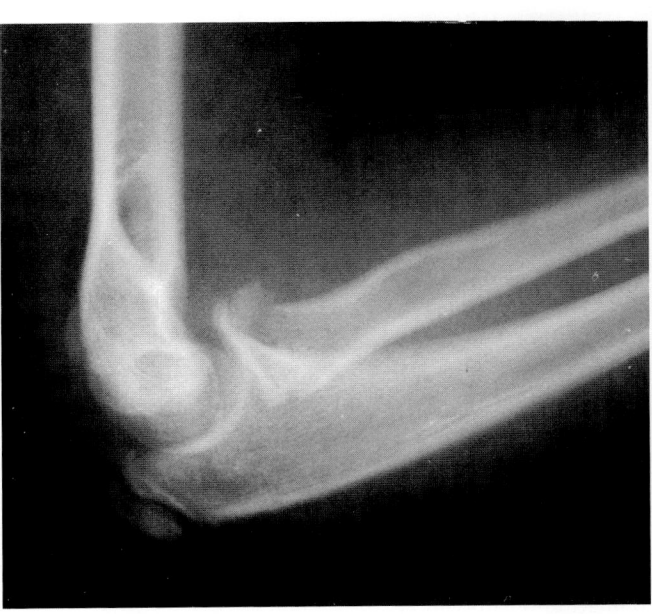

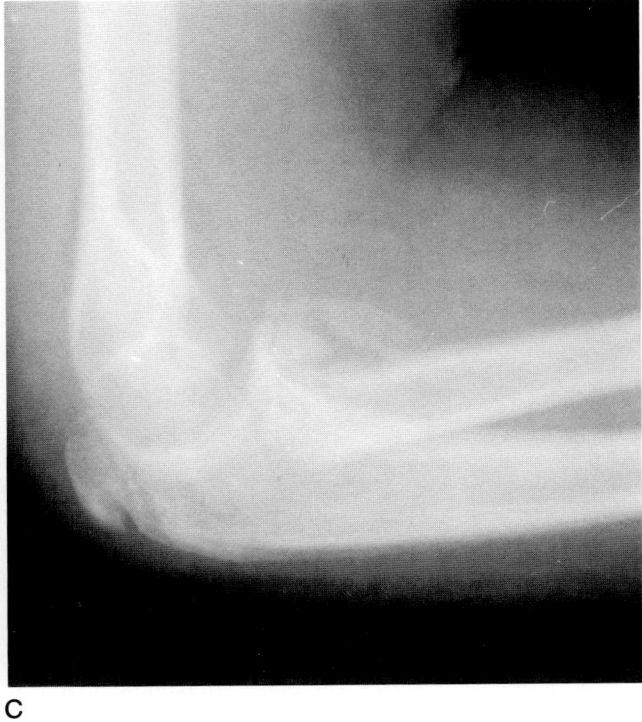

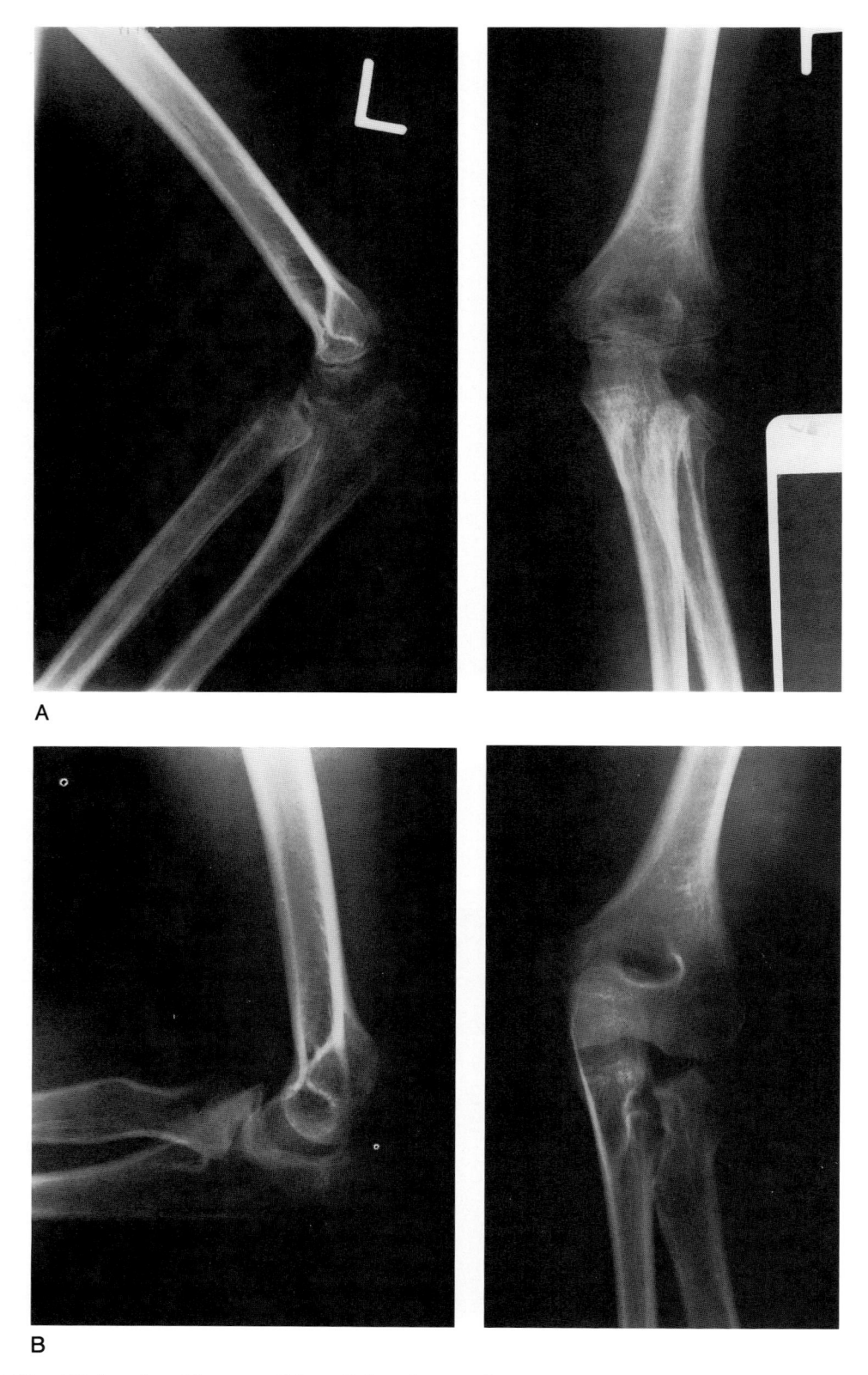

Fig. 20-10. (A) Angulated fracture of the radial neck at age 7 years was accepted. (B) Subsequent joint incongruity 4 years later has resulted in painful crepitus with limitation of supination contributed to by the partial avascular necrosis of the radial head.

juries have been reported as a direct result of the injury.[16] Operative misadventure can result in injury to the posterior interosseus nerve at time of surgical treatment.

Misdiagnosis

Before age 5 in the preosseous phase these injuries may be difficult to diagnose.[13] Contralateral radiographs may be necessary if unusual ossification centers are seen following an elbow injury. Arthrography is occasionally indicated as a diagnostic tool.

Protruberance of Radial Head

If the angulation of the neck recurs due to inadequate maintenance of reduction, the growth of the radial head will be directed laterally, resulting in an increasing protruberance of the radial head. This may cause both a cosmetic and a functional disability at skeletal maturity, necessitating radial head excision.

Forearm Compartment Syndrome

Although uncommon, volar compartment syndrome can occur in children with a nondisplaced radial head or neck fracture without associated crushing, high energy, or soft tissue trauma.[23] The possibility of increased compartmental pressure should always be kept in mind, in spite of the innocuous appearance of the proximal radial fracture. As with any compartment syndrome, early recognition of the signs and symptoms will prevent the late disabling sequelae.

SUMMARY

Although children primarily injure the radial neck, radial head fractures in association with or without a dislocation may also occasionally occur. The majority of these injuries are due to a valgus force applied to an outstretched elbow. It is important to recognize ipsilateral fractures around the elbow in order to adequately treat and prevent long-term functional impairment. The classification of fracture outcome based upon the degree of residual radial head angulation continues to be the mainstay of therapeutic decision-making. Accurate diagnosis and fastidious treatment techniques in which functional outcome is the primary objective will result in minimal long-term disability.

REFERENCES

1. Gastion SR, Smith FM, Boab OD: Epiphyseal injuries of the radial head and neck. Am J Surg 85:266, 1953
2. Jeffrey CC: Fractures of the head of the radius in children. J Bone Joint Surg [Br] 32:314, 1950
3. Murray RC: Fracture of the head and neck of the radius. Br J Surg 28:106, 1940
4. Landin LA: Fracture patterns in children. Acta Orthop Scand [Suppl] 54, 1983
5. Steinberg EL, Golomb D, Salama R, Weintroub S: Radial head and neck fractures in children. J Pediatr Orthop 8:35, 1988
6. Tibone JE, Stoltz M: Fracture of the radial head and neck in children. J Bone Joint Surg [Am] 63:100, 1981
7. DeSault DJ: A treatise on fractures, luxations and other affections of bones. Kimber and Conrad, Philadelphia, 1811
8. O'Brien PI: Injuries involving the radial epiphysis. Clin Orthop 41:51, 1965
9. Silberstein MJ, Brodeur AE, Graviss ER: Some vagaries of the radial head and neck. J Bone Joint Surg [Am] 64:1153, 1982
10. Wedge JH, Robertson DE: Displaced fractures of the neck of the radius. J Bone Joint Surg [Br] 64:256, 1982
11. Ward WT, Williams JJ: Radial neck fracture complicating closed reduction of a posterior elbow dislocation in a child: case report. J Trauma 31:1686, 1991
12. Newman JH: Displaced radial neck fractures in children. Injury 9:114, 1977
13. Wilkins KE: Fractures and dislocations of the elbow region. p. III:509. In Rockwood CJ, Wilkins KE, King RE (ed): Fractures in Children. 3rd Ed. Vol. 3. JB Lippincott, Philadelphia, 1991
14. Greenspan A, Norman A: The radial head-capitellum view: useful technique in elbow trauma. AJR 138:1186, 1982
15. Greenspan A, Norman A, Rosen H: Radial head-capitellum view in elbow trauma: clinical application and radiographic-anatomic correlation. AJR 143:355, 1984
16. Vahvanen V: Fracture of the radial neck in children. Acta Orthop Scand 49:32, 1978
17. Fowles JV, Kassab MT: Observations concerning radial neck fractures in children. J Pediatr Orthop 6:51, 1986
18. Kaufman B, Rinott MG, Tanzman M: Closed reduction of fractures of the proximal radius in children. J Bone Joint Surg [Br] 71:66, 1989
19. Feray C: Methode originale de reduction "peu sanglante"

des fractures graves de la tete radiale chez l'enfant. Presse Med 77:2155, 1969
20. Pesudo JV, Aracil J, Barcelo M: Leverage method in displaced fractures of the radial neck in children. Clin Orthop 169:215, 1982
21. Jones ERW, Esah M: Displaced fracture of the neck of the radius in children. J Bone Joint Surg [Br] 53:429, 1971
22. Rang M: The Elbow in Children's Fractures. 2nd Ed. JP Lippincott, Philadelphia, 1986
23. Scott SA, Peters CL: Forearm compartment syndrome as a complication of minimally displaced radial head and neck fractures in children. Presented at the annual meeting of the Pediatric Orthopedic Society of North America, Newport, Rhode Island, May 6–9, 1992

21

Fractures of the Carpal Bones

R. Mervyn Letts
Geoff Dervin

> An increasing worship of an instrument for it's own sake sometimes leads to enslavement by it.
> —David Seegal

DESCRIPTION AND INCIDENCE

Carpal fractures are relatively uncommon in the skeletally immature wrist. The predominant cartilaginous nature of the carpus serves to dissipate the energy of axial loading and minimize fracturing. This explains the frequency of distal forearm metaphyseal and physeal injuries with falls on the outstretched hand by the child. The corollary holds that carpal fractures usually result from direct trauma or significant loading injuries that are often associated with other contiguous fractures in the forearm. The epidemiology of fractures of the carpus in children has not been well studied. In most large reviews of pediatric fractures, fractures of the carpus comprise less than 2 percent. This figure may be much lower than in reality, since many so-called "wrist sprains" are minor avulsion injuries of the carpus often involving the triquetrum or scaphoid and often misdiagnosed.

EMBRYOLOGY

An understanding of the embryology and development of the carpus is helpful in appreciating the common fracture patterns. The carpus develops from a condensation of mesenchyme from the upper limb bud, that appears at about 26 days gestation. By 44 days, most of the carpus has begun to chondrify, and at 10 months, all intercarpal joints are well developed.[1-5] The carpus, cartilaginous at birth, begins to ossify according to a fairly defined sequence as depicted in Table 21-1. Some variation is seen with respect to the scaphoid, trapezium, and trapezoid. Most carpal bone ossification patterns are eccentric, which can make injury interpretation difficult (Fig. 21-1). This is particularly true of the scaphoid, whose ossification begins in the distal pole and proceeds proximally. Karion[5] reported on an occult osteochondral fracture of the scaphoid, which ultimately progressed to nonunion and avascular necrosis of the proximal pole in a 3-year-old child. At birth, the carpal bones are entirely cartilaginous. The ossification begins with the capitate at about 3 months of age and concludes with the pisiform at about 8 years of age. Failure in differentiation of the individual carpal bones during embryologic development results in congenital fusions. Such coalitions may result in later confusion in the interpretation of the injured carpus in a child. These fusions are more common in syndromes such as arthrogryposis, dystrophic dwarfism, otopalatal digital syndrome, Holt-Oram syndrome, and Turner syndrome. Although many combinations of coalitions have been described,

TABLE 21-1. Onset of Carpal Ossification (Months)

	Boys		Girls	
	Mean	SD	Mean	SD
Capitate	2.9	1.7	2.5	1.8
Hamate	4.2	2.7	3.1	2.2
Triquetrum	29.5	16.2	26.6	14.0
Lunate	43.5	14.7	36.1	17.3
Scaphoid	69.6	15.4	53.7	13.8
Trapezium	72.0	16.1	51.8	12.3
Trapezoid	72.7	18.4	51.6	16.4
Pisiform	94.6	13.1	120.0	12.1

(Modified from Light,[2] with permission.)

the most common is the lunate-triquetral coalition, followed by capitate-hamate, pisiform-triquetral, and trapezium-trapezoid coalition. The incidence is much higher in the black population[6] (Fig. 21-2).

The confusion in the interpretation of fractures in children arises particularly in those fusions that are not always radiologically complete. This is particularly common in lunate-triquetral coalitions.

BIPARTITE CARPAL BONES

Carpal bones can also be bipartite, which also can confuse the radiographic interpretation and be misinterpreted as a fracture. The scaphoid is the most common carpal bone that develops as a congenital bipartite struc-

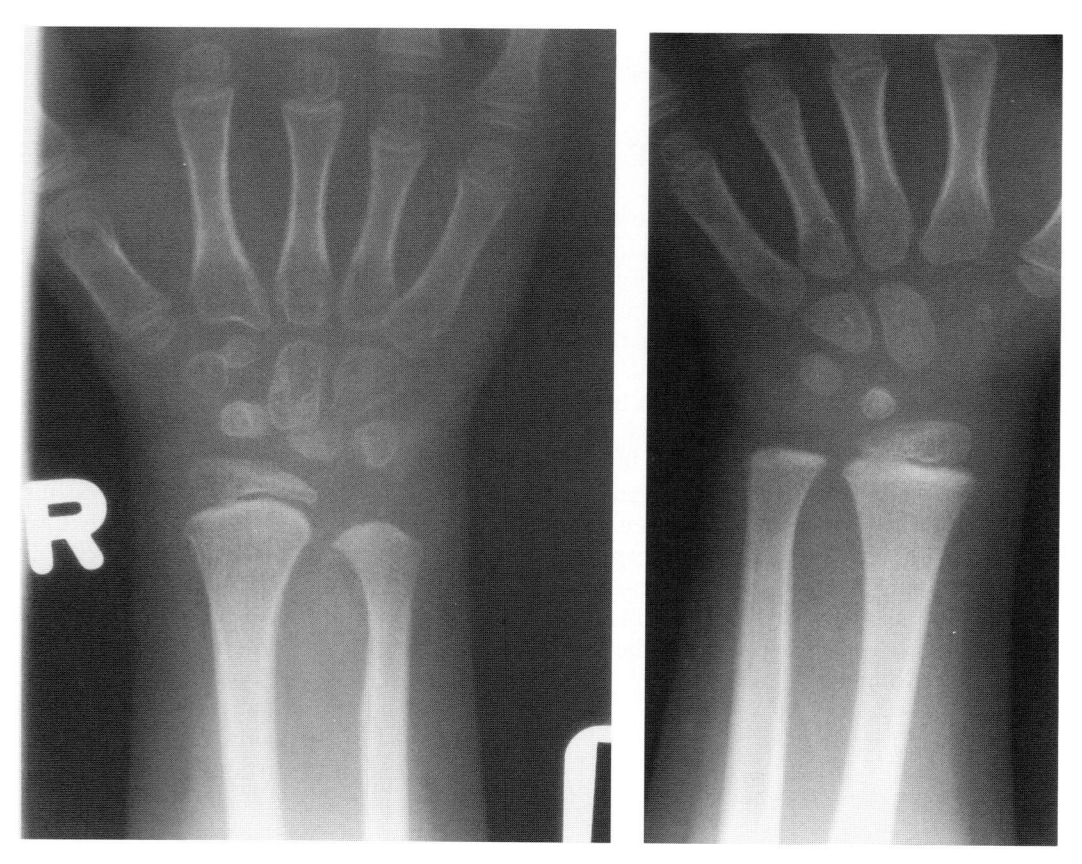

Fig. 21-1. The right and left wrist of a 4½-year-old girl taken at same time. Note the much greater maturation and carpal ossification of the right wrist as compared to the left. In carpal injuries in children, a comparison view of the uninjured wrist may be helpful.

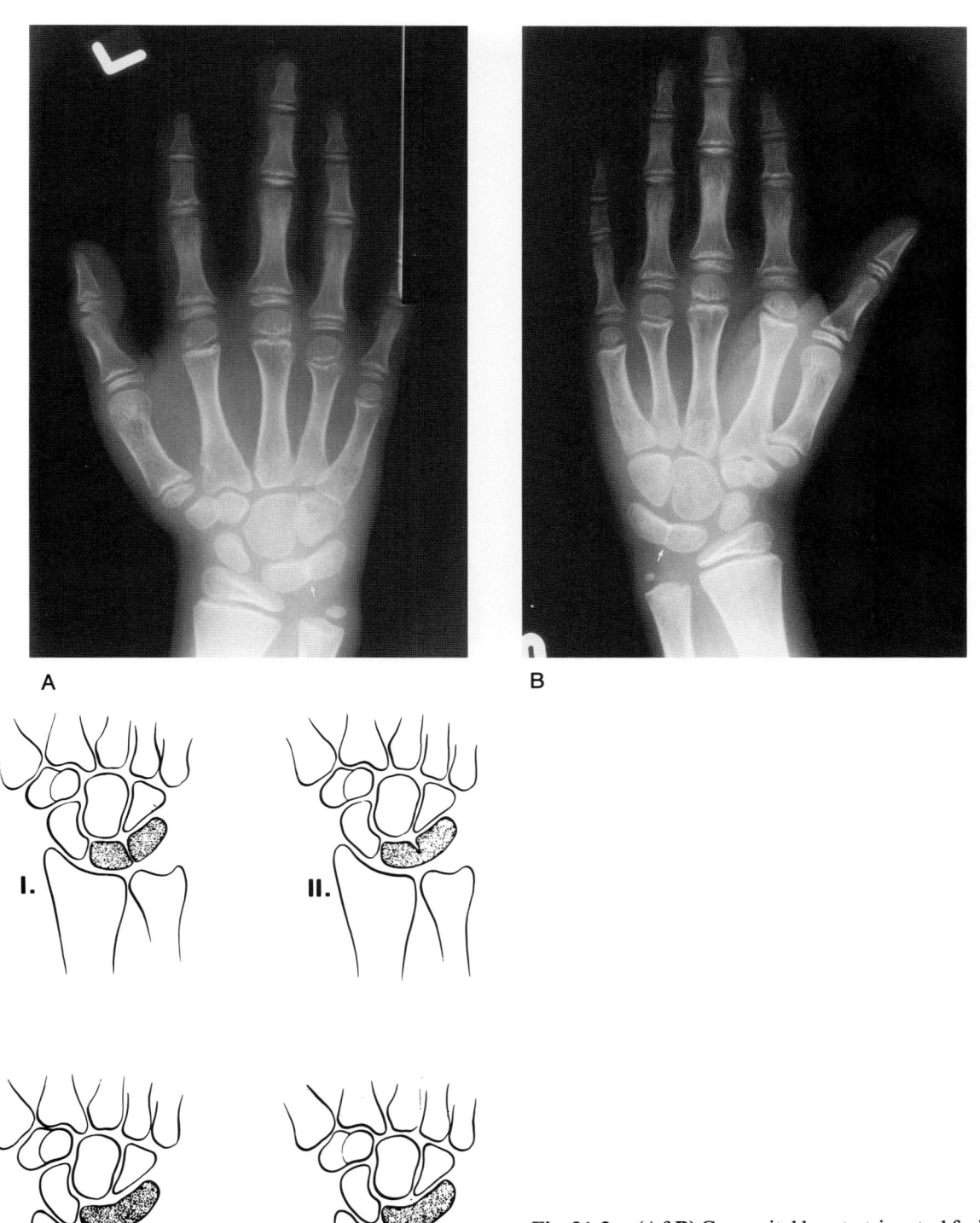

Fig. 21-2. **(A&B)** Congenital lunate-triquetral fusion in both wrists in a 10-year-old boy who sustained a type I injury to his left distal radius revealing the congenital carpal anomaly. (Courtesy of Dr. Tim Carey, Children's Hospital, Ottawa.) **(C)** Lunate-triquetral coalition classified by degree of fusion. (Fig. C from Simmons,[8] with permission.)

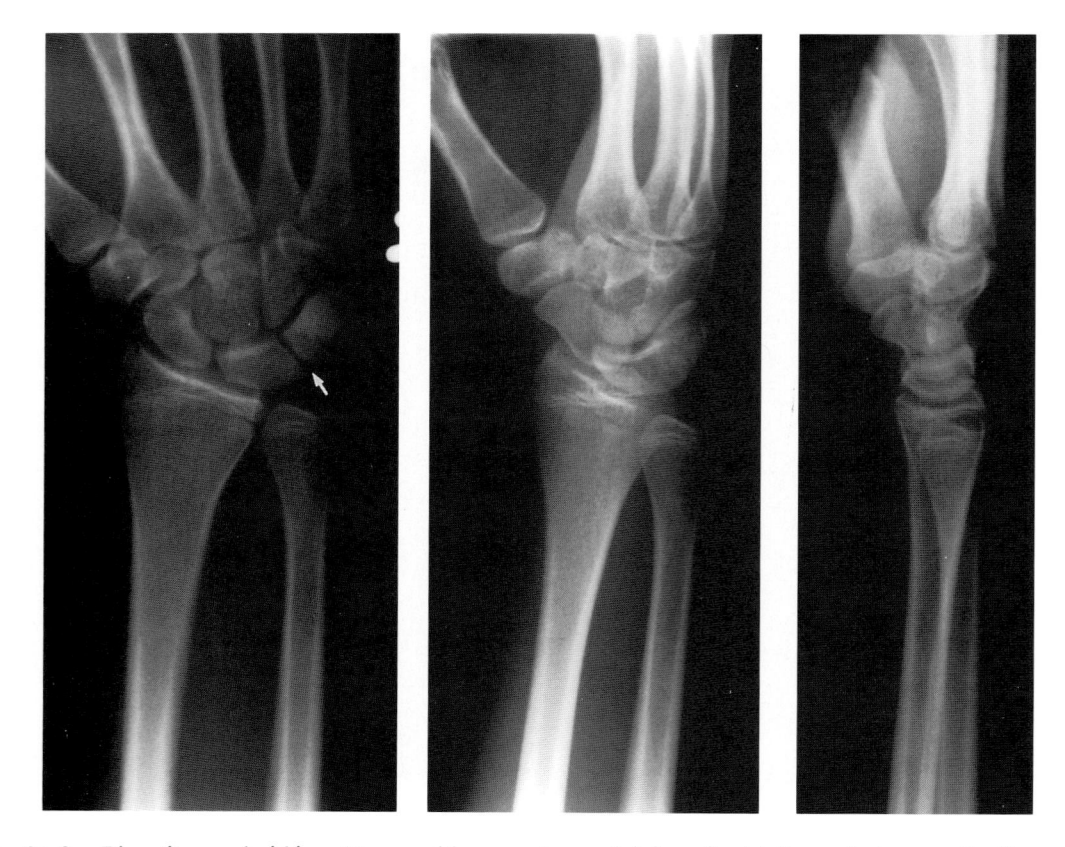

Fig. 21-3. Bipartite scaphoid in a 15-year-old gymnast complaining of wrist discomfort on vaults. No previous history of a wrist injury and margins are smooth and well separated.

ture. The criteria for making a diagnosis of a bipartite scaphoid is as follows[6] (Fig. 21-3):

1. Absence of history of trauma
2. Presence of bilateral scaphoid bipartition
3. Equal size and density of both ossicles
4. Absence of any sign of degenerative changes in the radioscaphoid articulation
5. Clear space between the fragments with smooth edges at the joint surfaces

ACCESSORY CARPAL BONES

Accessory bones about the wrist can also cause confusion and be misinterpreted as avulsed fractures. The most common accessory carpal bones are the os centrale, os triangulare, and os styloideum.[7]

The os centrale is a dorsal ossicle that forms between the scaphoid, capitate and trapezoid. The ossicle fuses with the dorsal distal ulnar side of the scaphoid usually before birth. The os triangulare also is seen only in the embryo and its location varies somewhat from the ulnar side of the radius to the ulnar styloid.

The os styloideum is the only potentially symptomatic ossicle. Its location dorsally between trapezoid, capitate and second and third metacarpals results in fusion to the third metacarpal styloid process, and it may become symptomatic as a carpal boss[8,9] (Fig. 21-4).

MECHANISM OF INJURY

A fall on the outstretched dorsiflexed hand is the most common mechanism of injury to the child's wrist. Buckle fractures of the wrist usually occur in infants and

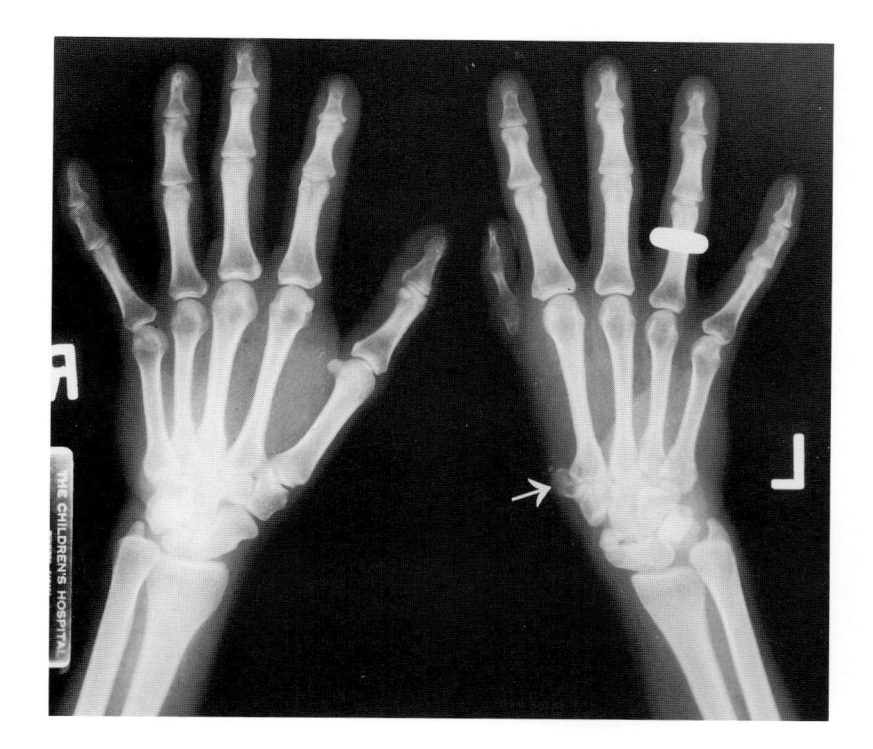

Fig. 21-4. Accessory carpal bone in an 18-year-old girl with the Holt Oram syndrome with hypoplasia of the radial ray on the left associated with a hypoplastic scaphoid compared to the normal right side. This type of scaphoid is susceptible to fracturing and fragmentation, so-called Preiser's disease of the scaphoid.

preschoolers, while metaphyseal on physeal injuries of the distal radius and ulna are more characteristic of older children. Adolescents seem most prone to carpal injuries as ossification has replaced the protective cartilaginous buffer around the carpal bones. Nevertheless, distal radius fractures still account for the large majority of injuries sustained in a fall on the outstretched hand, even in the adolescent age group. Mussbichler[10] recorded that only 2.9 percent of hand and wrist fractures in children less than 15 years of age involved the scaphoid. Although intercarpal ligamentous injuries are being recognized with increasing frequency in the adult population, they are extremely rare in children. This is related to the overall increased strength of ligamentous attachments relative to the adjacent growth plate and subchondral bone. Thus it is far more common for the force to be dissipated, resulting in a type I fracture of the distal radius or a ligamentous avulsion of the carpus. Scapholunate dissociation as an example is extremely rare in children, even though it may appear to be present due to the eccentrically placed ossific nucleus of the scaphoid and lunate giving a false impression of an abnormally wide scapholunate interval.[11]

Direct blows to the carpus usually associated with sports activities such as hockey, lacrosse, or the martial arts can also result in carpal bone fracture in the adolescent.

SCAPHOID FRACTURES

The scaphoid is the most frequently fractured carpal bone in both children and adults. The peak age of scaphoid fracturing is between 15 and 35. Most of the pediatric fractures to the scaphoid occur in children between 11 and 15. Fractures of the scaphoid in younger children have been reported but are uncommon. Christodoulon and Colton[12] have calculated the incidence of fractures of the scaphoid prior to skeletal maturity as comprising 0.34 percent of all fractures in children and 0.45 percent of children's upper limb fractures. It is probable that the more resilient cartilaginous carpus of the child under 10 years old protects the scaphoid, and when fractures do occur at this age, it usually follows considerable trauma to the carpus.[12-14] Under these circumstances, adjacent carpal fractures can also occur, the most common associated carpal bone fracture being the capitate.[15]

Scaphoid fractures in children are uniquely different from adults with a vast majority — almost 90 percent — occurring in the distal third and, of these, 44 percent are of the avulsion variety, usually involving the tubercle (Fig. 21-5). The ossific nucleus of the scaphoid appears at an average of 4 years, 5 months in girls and 5 years, 10 months in boys. The ossification center expands eccen-

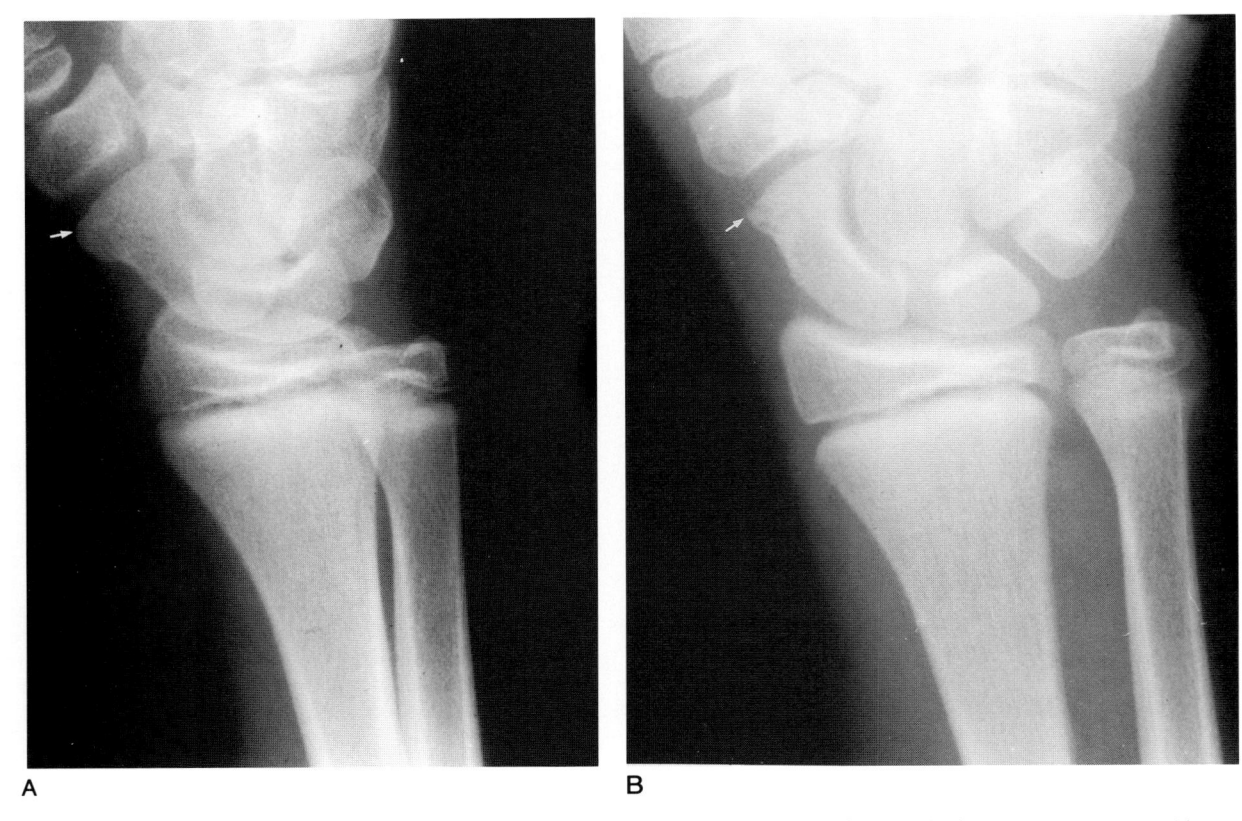

Fig. 21-5. Fracture of the scaphoid tubercle are the most common types of scaphoid fractures encountered in children. **(A)** Oblique view illustrating fractured tubercle. **(B)** AP view of wrist demonstrating tubercle fracture.

trically, centrifugally until ossification is complete between 13 and 15 years of age (Fig. 21-6). During its development, the scaphoid is covered by both articular cartilage and a circumferential epiphyseal plate. With the onset of skeletal maturity, the epiphyseal cartilage disappears leaving only articular cartilage. The changes in the cartilaginous composition of the maturing scaphoid are paralleled by changes in its vulnerability to fracture.

Site of Scaphoid Fractures

The site of the scaphoid fracture in children is different from the typical waist fracture in adults, being more frequent in the distal third of the scaphoid and tubercle. In a large review of 100 pediatric scaphoid fractures by Mussbichler,[10] 52 involved avulsions of the dorsal radial aspect of the distal pole. Similarly, Christodouleu and Colton[12] reported that 33 of 63 fractured scaphoids in children occurred in the distal third and only 15 in the waist. Cockshott[16] theorized that combined dorsiflexion, ulnar deviation, and pronation of the wrist predisposes to avulsion of the distal tubercle. He speculated that the more recently ossified scaphoid cartilage was vulnerable to this particular type of injury, being avulsed by the strong ligamentous attachment of the radioscaphoid and scaphotrapezial joint capsule. Whether there exists a true radial collateral ligament to the scaphoid is controversial.[17,18]

The prevalence of this avulsion type of fracture pattern in the immature scaphoid is not inconsistent with the behavior of strong ligamentous attachments to immature bone in other parts of the developing skeleton, such as the attachment of the anterior cruciate or avulsion injuries associated with the patella or ankle joint.[19] The blood supply to the scaphoid is not compromised by such avulsion injuries (Fig. 21-7).

Preiser's Disease of the Scaphoid

Preiser's disease is an uncommon syndrome associated with radial ray hypoplasia resulting in a hypoplastic thumb and scaphoid. If there is good hand function and grip strength, very high compressive loads are generated across the radiocarpal and intercarpal joints. The small hypoplastic scaphoid cannot withstand these forces and may fracture with fragmentation. The hypoplastic scaphoid is also peculiarly vulnerable to ischemic necrosis and may cause considerable pain and disability following fatigue fracturing[2] (Fig. 21-4).

Bipartite Scaphoid

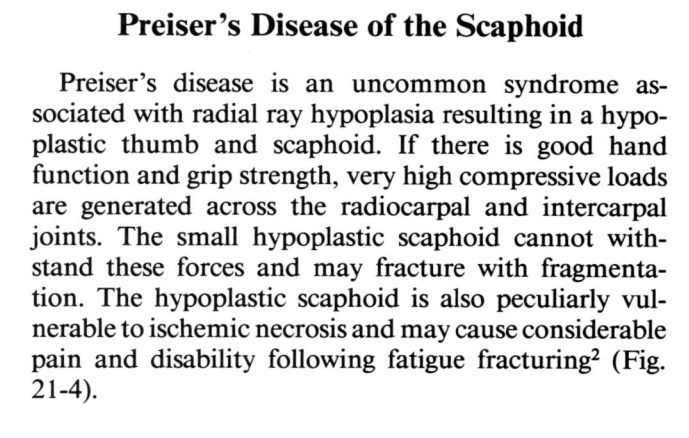

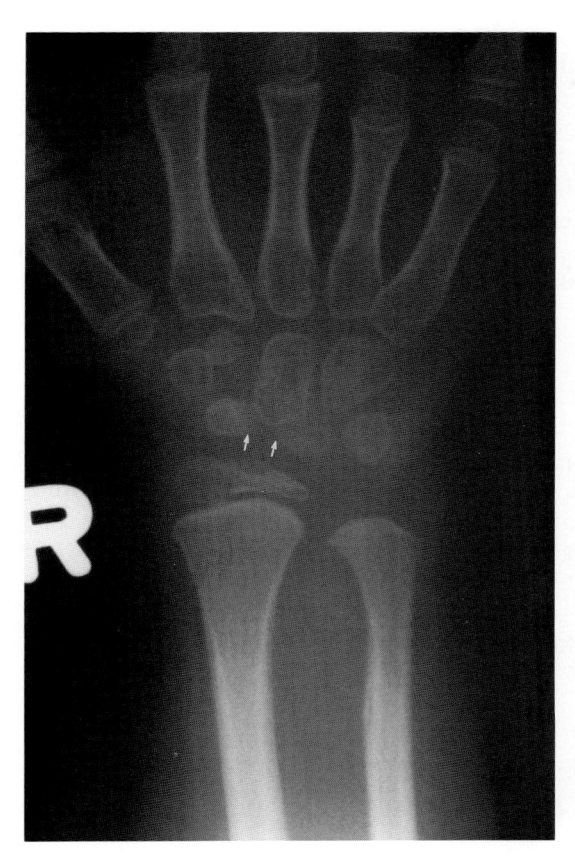

The existence of the bipartite scaphoid is controversial. Although the scaphoid may occasionally ossify from multiple scaphoid ossification centers, it is very difficult to prove in a given instance that an apparent bipartite scaphoid is not a previous nonunion of an old fracture (Fig. 21-3). The essential role of the scaphoid in the biomechanics of wrist motion would predispose the bipartite scaphoid to degenerative arthritis in the same manner as a traumatic nonunion at the same site. From a pragmatic point of view "bipartite" scaphoid should be assumed to be of traumatic origin and observed accordingly.[6,20]

Fig. 21-6. Eccentric ossification of the scaphoid in young children, illustrated here in a 4-year-old child, can lead to misinterpretation of a scapholunate dissociation due to the normal widened gap between the lunate and scaphoid.

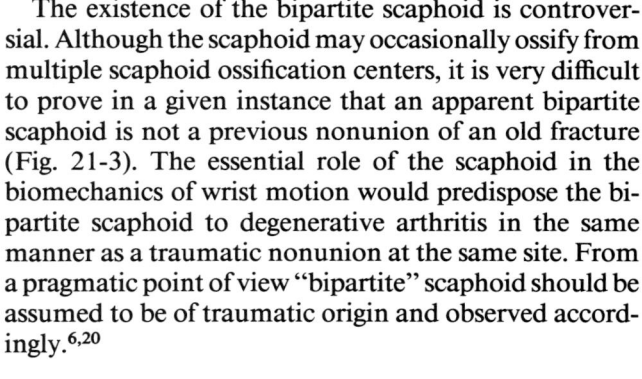

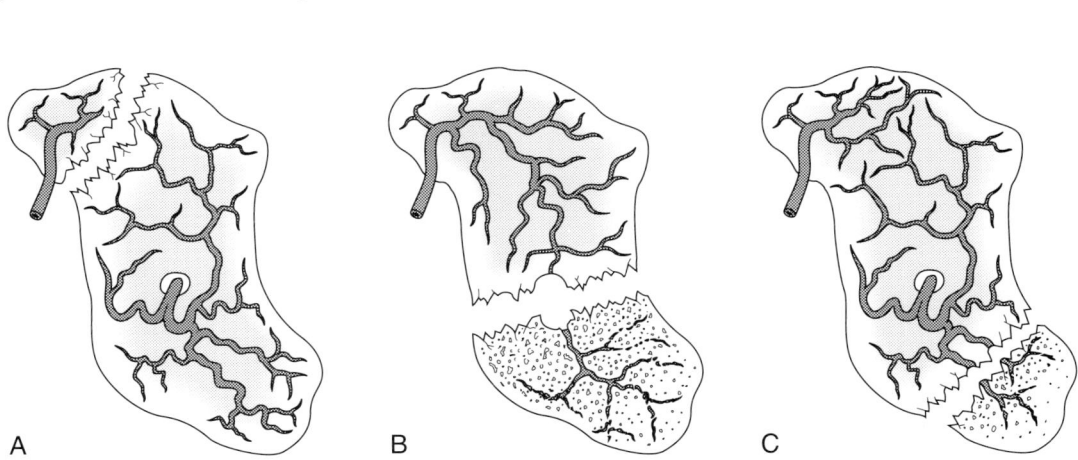

Fig. 21-7. Schematic drawing of the different types of breaks in relation to arterial circulation in scaphoid fractures. **(A)** Fracture between the two sources of arterial blood with good prognosis because each fragment has a satisfactory arterial supply. **(B&C)** Fractures at the central and proximal levels in which the blood supply of the proximal segment is impaired or lost. (Adapted from Cave EF: Injuries to the carpal bones. p. 376. In: Fractures and Other Injuries. Year Book Medical Publishers, Chicago, 1958, with permission.)

Distal Avulsion Fractures

Distal avulsion fractures of the scaphoid are the commonest type of scaphoid fracture seen in children. The incidence may well be much lower than reported, since some of these injuries undoubtedly are dismissed as "wrist sprains." The pathogenesis of this avulsion injury is extension of the wrist combined with ulnar deviation and pronation. The avulsing ligament has been stated to be the radial collateral ligament or the capsular fibrous attachment of the radial scaphoid. There is debate about the entity of a radial collateral ligament; however, Taleisnick described the radial collateral ligament as originating from the volar margin of the styloid process and inserting into the tuberosity of the scaphoid and the walls of the flexor carpi radialis tendon.[9] Whatever the anatomic name of the ligament attaching to the tuberosity of the scaphoid, it, like most other ligaments in children, is much stronger and well attached by Sharpey's fibers to the subchondral bone resulting in avulsion of the tuberosity rather than rupture of the ligament, which probably occurs in the similar adult injury. Radiologic recognition of the avulsed scaphoid tuberosity may be difficult. Magnification techniques with 0.1-mm focus may be helpful as well as several projections (Fig. 21-8). Cockshott[16] has recommended a tangential lateral oblique supination view to deliniate the avulsed tuberosity. The avulsion flakes from the scaphoid are pure lateral avulsions. Treatment with plaster immobilization for 6 weeks is almost always effective, with nonunion being rare.

Treatment

Scaphoid fractures usually heal with plaster immobilization in a thumb spica in 6 to 8 weeks.[21] Extending the cast to the tip of the phalanx of the thumb and ensuring that the child can pinch thumb to forefinger while the cast is setting will ensure both a good immobilization of the scaphoid and a hand that will be functional for the child in school (Fig. 21-9). The distal avulsion fractures

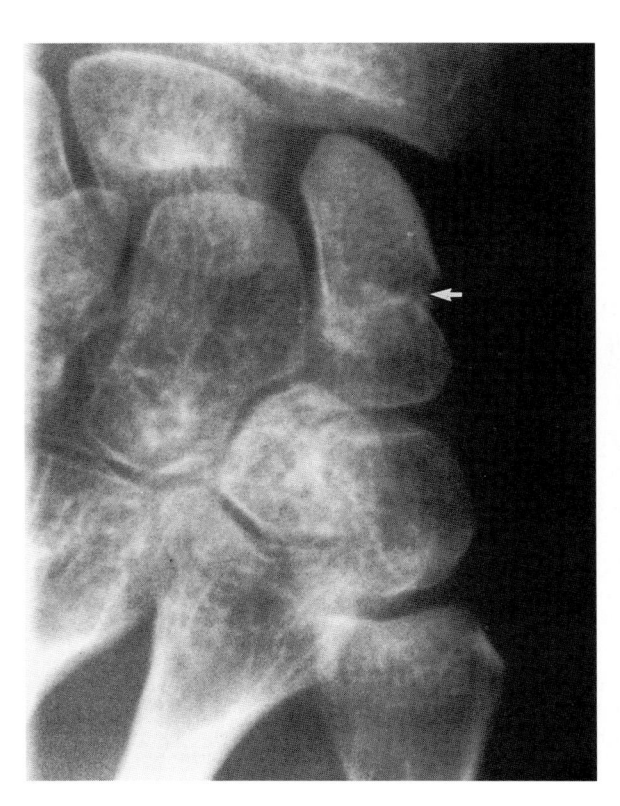

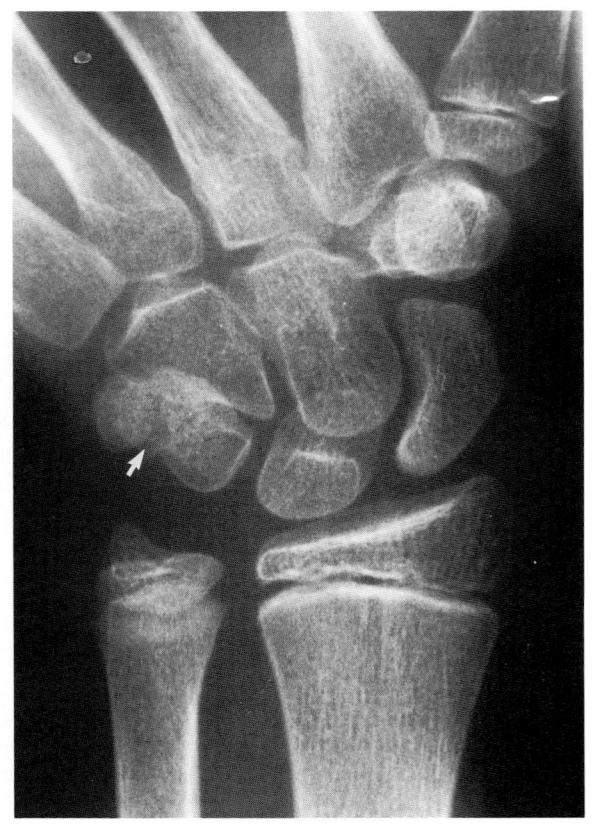

Fig. 21-8. Magnified radiographic views are helpful in identifying carpal fractures.

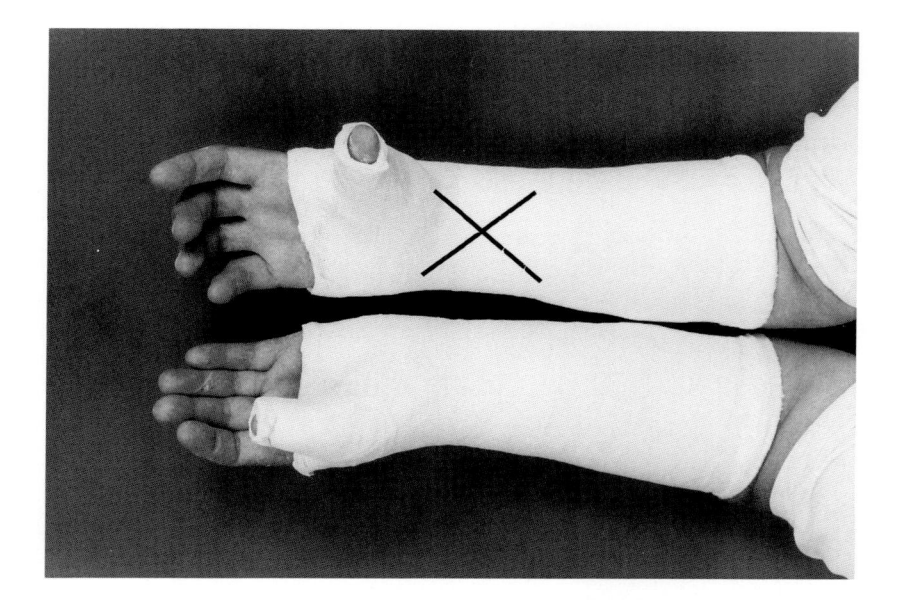

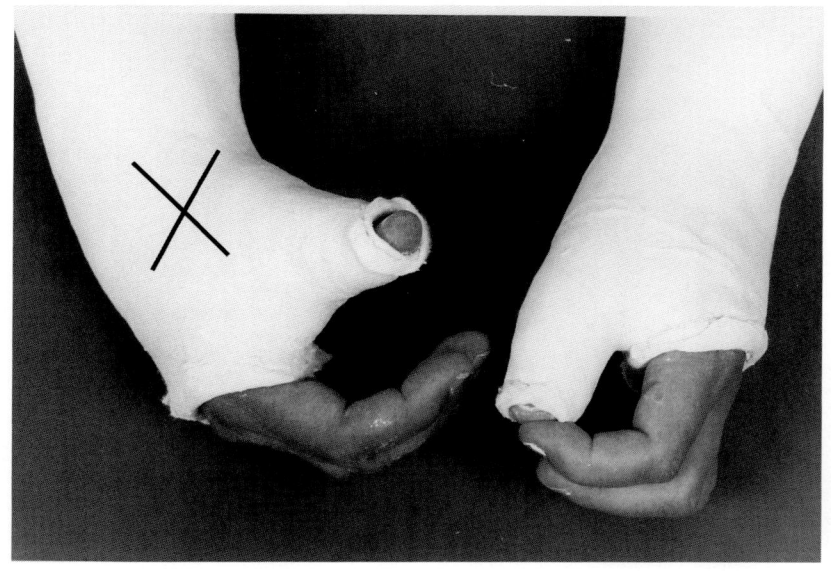

Fig. 21-9. The correct method of applying a scaphoid cast facilitates pinch. The incorrect position of the thumb in extension does not allow the child to pinch thus prevents writing in school.

of the scaphoid heal almost universally with this treatment. These avulsion fractures do not have a compromised blood supply, since the major blood supply to the scaphoid enters via the distal dorsal ridge of the scaphoid. As most pediatric fractures of the scaphoid occur in the region of the distal pole rather than through the waist, nonunion of fractures in this portion of the scaphoid are extremely rare. In scaphoid fractures in children that have not been recognized and are seen late, a longer period of immobilization may be necessary to achieve union.

Nonunion of the Scaphoid

Scaphoid nonunion in children does occur in association with fractures through the waist of the scaphoid in a manner similar to adults.[22-24] It is more frequently encountered if the scaphoid fracture has been initially missed and treatment is started several weeks after the injury (Fig. 21-10). A period of 10 to 12 weeks of immobilization in a below elbow thumb spica cast should be a prerequisite to declaring a scaphoid nonunion. Some authors have advocated prolonged immobilization even

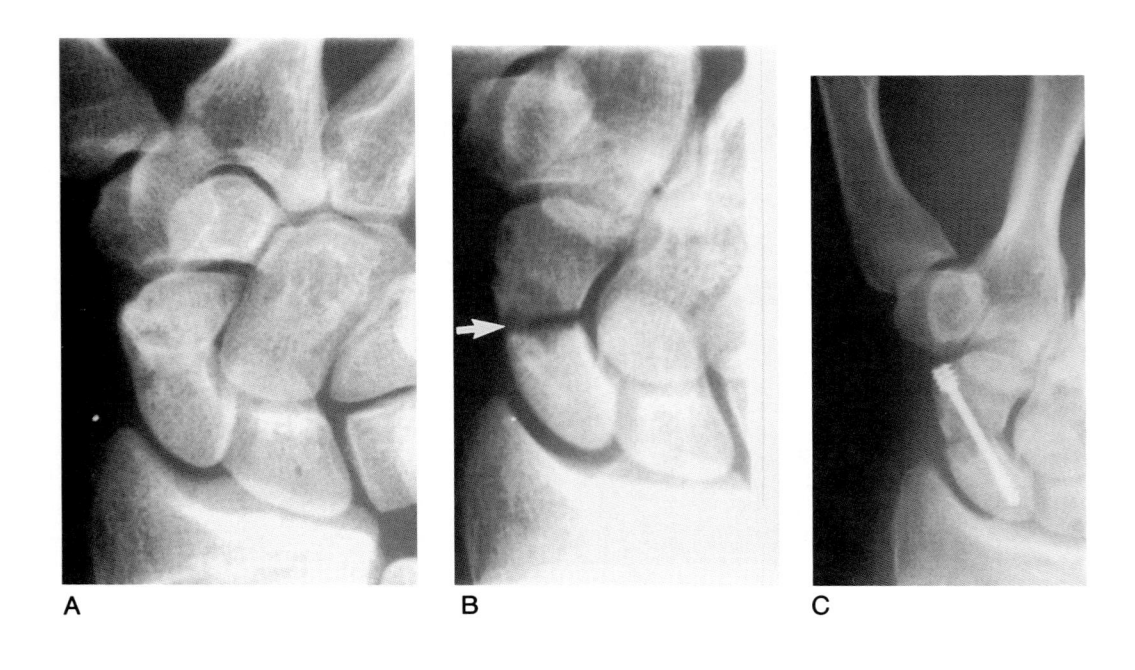

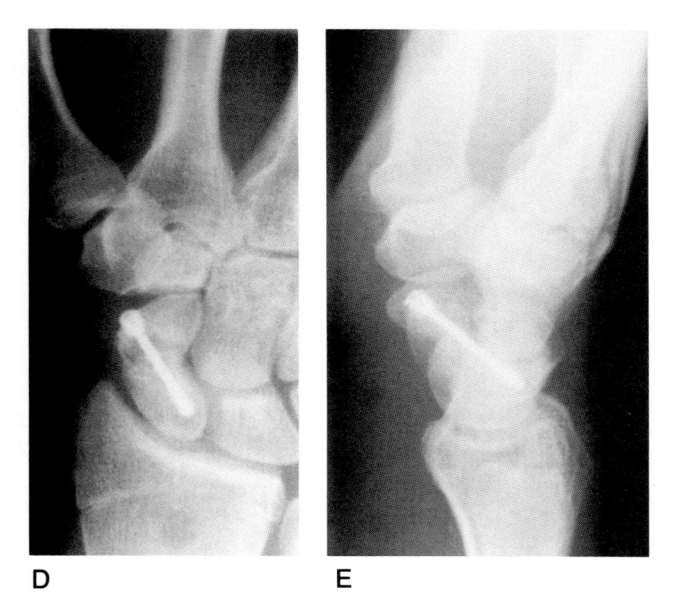

Fig. 21-10. (A&B) Nonunion of the scaphoid in a 14-year-old boy. Treatment with immobilization in a cast for 3 months was unsuccessful in achieving union. (C–E) Open reduction with bone grafting and internal fixation with a Herbert screw was successful in achieving union. (Case courtesy of Dr. Jay Jarvis, CHEO, Ottawa.)

in established nonunions as a method of treatment and have reported success.[19,21] Many children who develop scaphoid nonunions, may be relatively asymptomatic for several years following the injury. Symptoms usually occur when the wrist is subjected to stress such as tennis, golf, or work-related activities. It is doubtful that any child with a scaphoid nonunion will continue to be asymptomatic, and all will be predisposed to the development of future osteoarthritis. It would therefore seem appropriate to ensure a union in all scaphoid nonunions prior to skeletal maturity. The role of electrical stimulation in attaining union of the scaphoid is somewhat controversial but seems to have been successful in some reported cases. Compliance with external stimulation

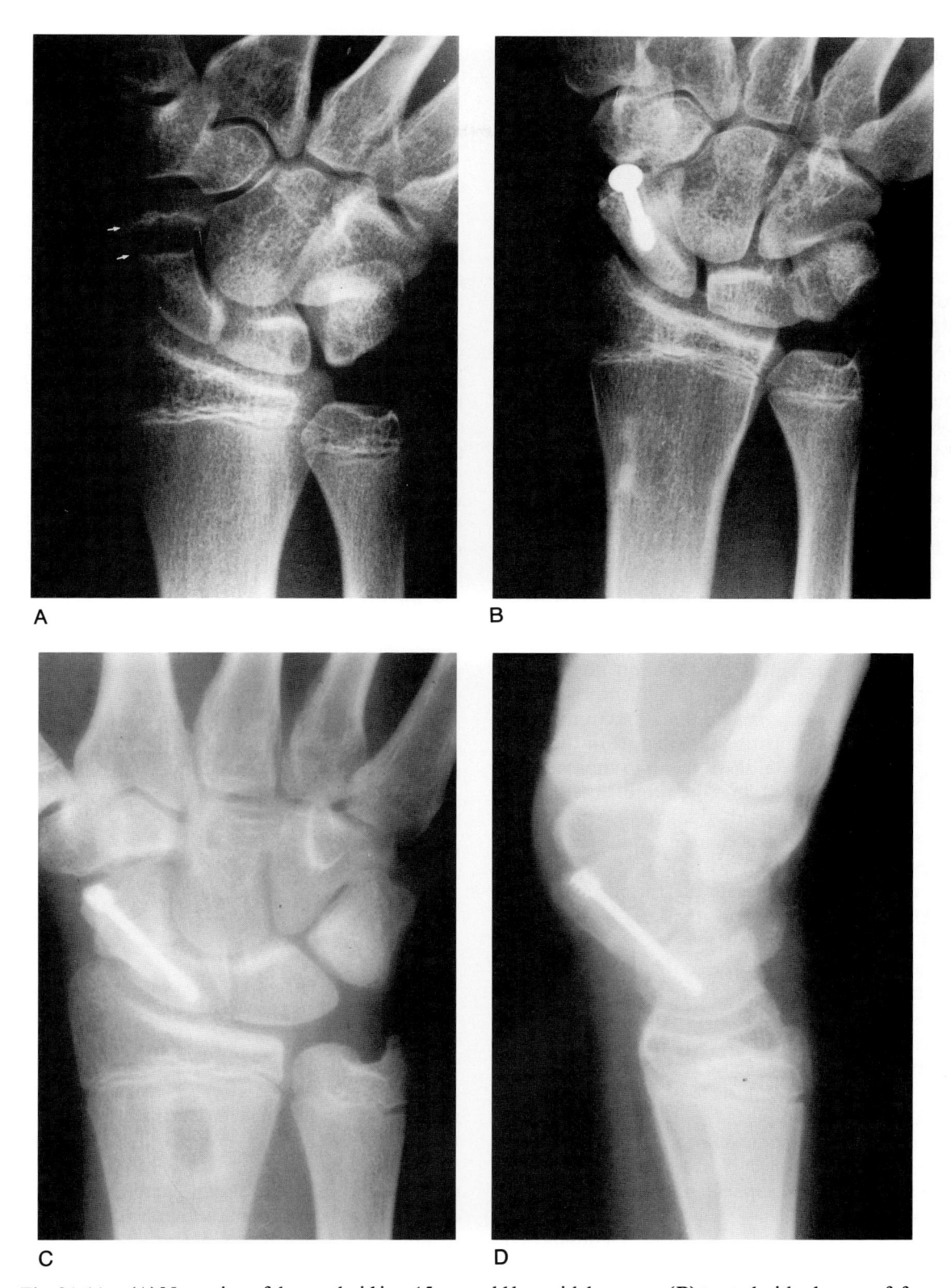

Fig. 21-11. **(A)** Nonunion of the scaphoid in a 15-year-old boy with large gap; **(B)** treated with a bone graft from the radius and a compression screw to achieve union. **(C&D)** Nonunion of fracture scaphoid in a 13-year-old boy treated with bone graft from the radial metaphysis and internal fixation with a Herbert screw. (Case courtesy of Dr. Tim Carey, Children's Hospital, Ottawa, Canada.)

devices can be a problem in this age group. Ischemic necrosis of the proximal pole of the scaphoid rarely occurs in children but is not unknown.[25,26]

Bone Grafting and Internal Fixation

In established nonunion bone grafting of the scaphoid through a volar Russe approach is recommended with internal fixation, using a compression screw (Fig. 21-11A&B) or a Herbert screw (Fig. 21-11C&D) in conjunction with the graft.[27,28] The success rate using this technique is very high in nonunions of the scaphoid in the adolescent age group. It is recommended that the bone graft be taken from the adjacent distal radius proximal to the epiphyseal plate, as it is convenient and just as efficacious as graft from the iliac crest. The Russe approach volarly to the scaphoid is simple and safe, providing the radial artery is palpated prior to inflating the tourniquet to ensure its location. The wrist joint begins at approximately the *proximal* wrist crease. The wrist capsule should always be incised longitudinally and never transversely, as a transverse incision severs the volar radiocarpal ligaments. In adolescent nonunions, the site of the nonunion may be difficult to ascertain. Radial deviation of the wrist and distal traction on the thumb will assist in delineating the fracture or the nonunion site. Although it would be difficult to approach the wrong carpal bone through this incision if there is any question, a radiograph should be taken to confirm the scaphoid bone. The sclerotic margins of the nonunion should be curetted preferably with nonpowered instruments. A trough should be made for the corticocancellous graft from the radius, and it should be locked in place and impacted. A Herbert screw or a small compression screw can be added for further stability. If the scaphoid has begun to heal and there is a fibrous union, part of this should be left intact to provide stability to the fracture fragments and only a portion of the fracture surface curetted and grafted. The graft should always be placed on the nonarticular surface of the scaphoid.

The results of the few reported series on scaphoid nonunions in children using autogenous bone grafting have been excellent.[22,23] Internal fixation with Kirschner wires and compression screws has also received support in the literature.

Controversy exists concerning the immobilization of the carpal scaphoid as to whether a long-arm or a short-arm cast is required. The results from the few studies in the literature concerning treatment of carpal scaphoid fractures in children appear to be inconclusive, with some authors reporting good results with short-arm casts and others with long-arm casts.[31]

Clinical Appearance

The possibility of a fracture of the scaphoid must be kept in mind in the adolescent presenting with a history of a fall on the outstretched hand followed by a persistent wrist pain aggravated by flexion and extension. The characteristic tenderness in the region of the anatomic snuffbox, although a reliable indication of scaphoid injury is not infallible. Initial radiographs frequently will not reveal any obvious fracture in the scaphoid but in a child presenting with these clinical findings immobilization in a short-arm thumb spica cast should be instituted and the child brought back in 7 to 10 days for scaphoid views of the wrist. If no fracture is seen and the symptoms have subsided, immobilization should be discontinued. The telltale fracture line or the presence of an avulsion injury necessitates the continuation of the casting for a further 5 to 6 weeks until union has been achieved. No child should be dismissed from an emergency department with a diagnosis of "a sprained wrist." In most instances, the sprain is simply an undiagnosed fracture. Avascular necrosis of the scaphoid is a rare occurrence in association with other injuries in the environs of the wrist (Fig. 21-12). This undoubtedly reflects a more serious wrist injury than was initially appreciated that resulted in interference with the scaphoid blood supply.

LIGAMENTOUS INJURIES OF THE CARPUS

The ligamentous structure of joints in children is very strong relative to the surrounding epiphyseal plates, subchondral bone, and articular cartilage. Ligaments are attached to subchondral bone through Sharpey's fibers and the attachment is extremely strong. As a result, ligamentous avulsion of a portion of the subchondral bone is much more commonly seen in children, or, if the force is sufficient, the adjacent physes sustains a type I or type II epiphyseal injury. Thus, although intercarpal ligament disruption is being diagnosed with increased frequency in adults, it is very rare in children, and if it does occur, is usually associated with an avulsed subchondral flake fracture. In children, the carpal ligaments are also very elastic and resilient. As a result, there are many more degrees of freedom of motion of the wrist, which tends to

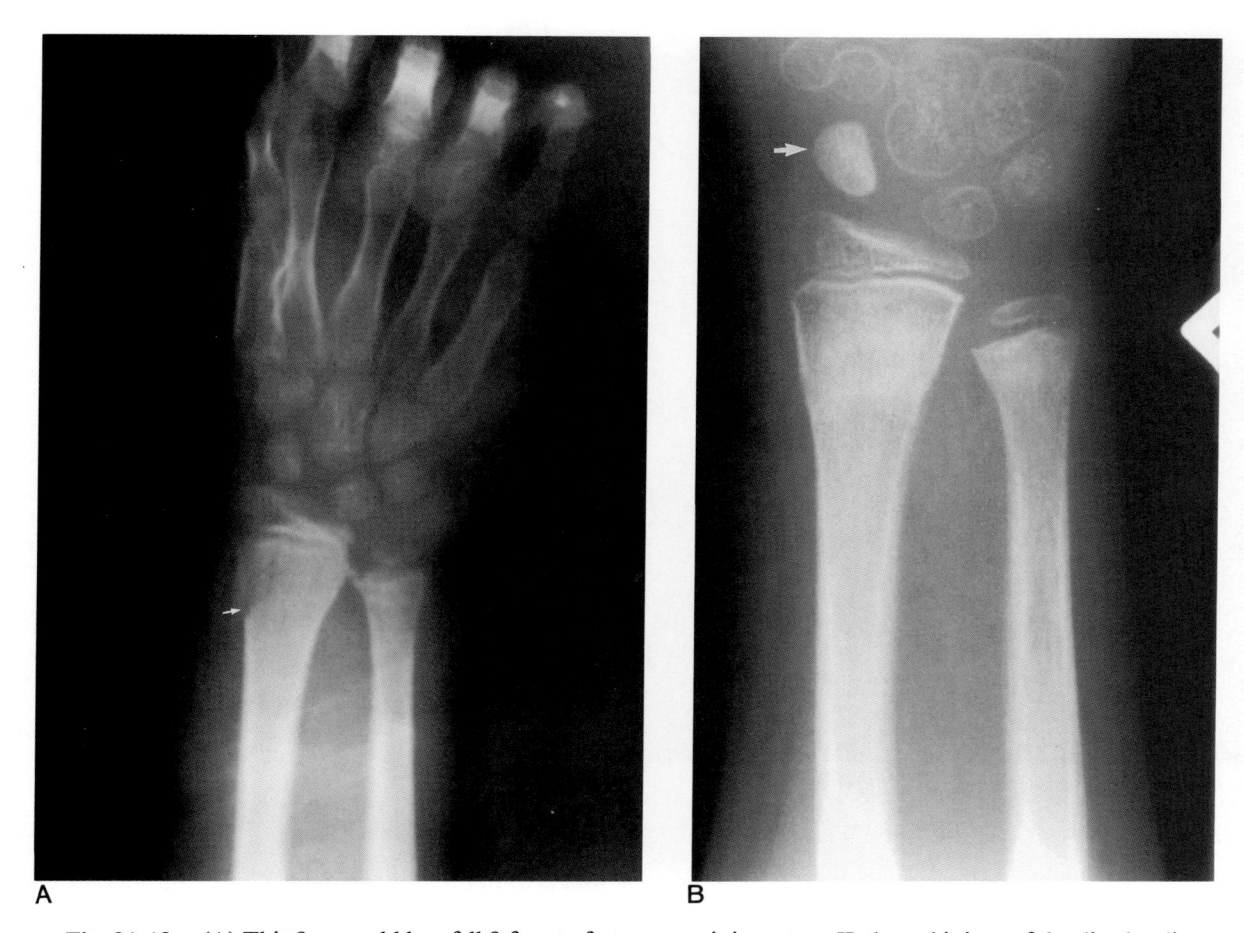

Fig. 21-12. **(A)** This 8-year-old boy fell 8 ft out of a tree sustaining a type II physeal injury of the distal radius. Although the wrist was also a little swollen and tendon this was attributed to the fractured radius. **(B)** At 4 months later the fracture of the radius was healed but wrist pain persisted. A radiograph demonstrated avascular necrosis of the scaphoid. The scapholunate gap is not abnormal in children due to the large lucent cartilaginous component of the scaphoid and lunate.

dissipate some of the force during loading. Recognition of ligamentous carpal injuries in children is extremely difficult and compounded by the eccentric ossification of the scaphoid, which results in the traditional evaluation of the scapholunate gap to be unreliable. After the age of 6 years, the lateral view of the scaphoid usually has sufficient ossification to allow interpretation of the attitude of the scaphoid in a manner similar to the adult wrist. In spite of this, ligamentous injuries to the scaphoid in children are conspicuous by their absence.

Only two reports of scapholunate dissociation in the skeletally immature carpus secondary to ligamentous disruption have been reported.[11,30] If this diagnosis is being entertained, a comparison with the contralateral wrist is mandatory to judge the extent of ossification and the soft tissue scapholunate interval. Watson's test for injury to the scapholunate ligamentous complex should reproduce the pain with passive radial deviation of the wrist if true injury to the scapholunate ligamentous complex has occurred.[31] We personally have never seen this injury in a skeletally immature adolescent.

The shielding of carpal ligaments from major stress primarily is achieved by (1) the dissipation of the energy through metaphyseal or physeal radial fractures, (2) the absorption of such force by the pliable elastic ligaments themselves, and (3) the cushioning effect of the cartilaginous carpus. The pseudodiastasis between the scaphoid

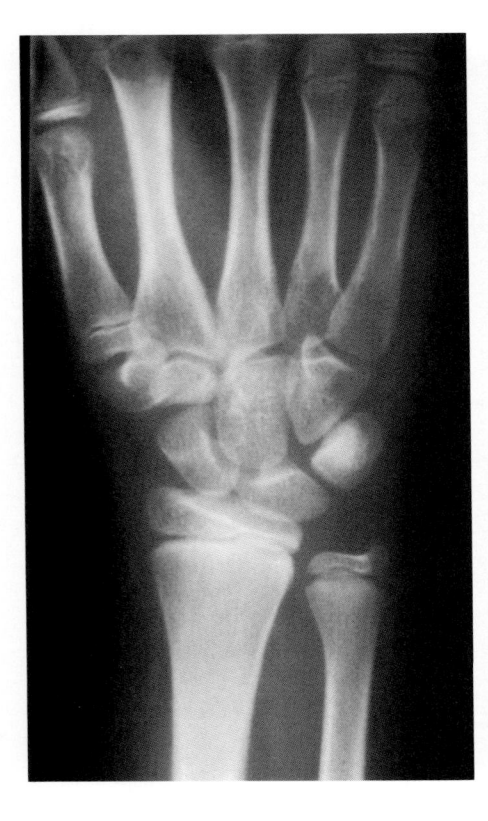

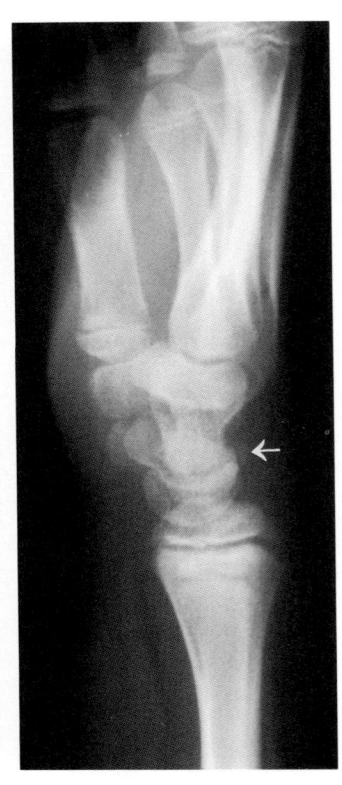

Fig. 21-13. Flake fracture of the triquetrum visible best on the lateral view.

and lunate is usually physiologic secondary to the eccentric ossification of the scaphoid (Fig. 21-6). Comparison with the other wrist can occasionally be a trap; one wrist occasionally being ahead or behind the other in the progression of ossification.

In the adult, the most common pattern of intercarpal instability is dorsal intercalated segment instability (DISI). The radiographic hallmark of this instability is an increased distance between the scaphoid and lunate, or shortening of the scaphoid on the AP view and palmar flexion of the scaphoid and dorsiflexion of the lunate on the lateral view. These measurements are very difficult to perform in young children.

FRACTURES OF THE TRIQUETRUM

The triquetrum is much more commonly injured in children than is generally appreciated. The fracture is rather innocuous and usually heals uneventfully, no matter what the treatment. The fracture itself is usually of the avulsion variety with a very small flake of bone that is difficult to identify on routine radiographs[32] (Fig. 21-13). The triquetrum is the second most common carpal bone to be fractured in children, exceeded only by the scaphoid.[33,34] Although triquetral fractures have been reported to comprise approximately 4 percent of all carpal fractures,[35] the true incidence is probably much higher, as many of these fractures are frequently missed.

Mechanism of Injury

The mechanism of injury of the triquetrum, which is rather protected as part of the midcarpal joint, is a matter of debate.[36,37] Avulsion of a flake of the triquetrum by a ligamentous attachment has been suggested by a number of authors.[38-42] A chisel action of the ulnar styloid process on the dorsum of the triquetrum has been described by Levy and colleagues[34] (Fig. 21-14). To support that concept, it has been found that the ulnar styloid process in patients sustaining a dorsal fracture of the triquetrum is usually larger and more prominent.[43] Thus, impingement of the ulnar styloid process on the dorsum of the triquetrum during strong forced dorsiflexion and ulnar deviation of the wrist may shear off a cartilaginous por-

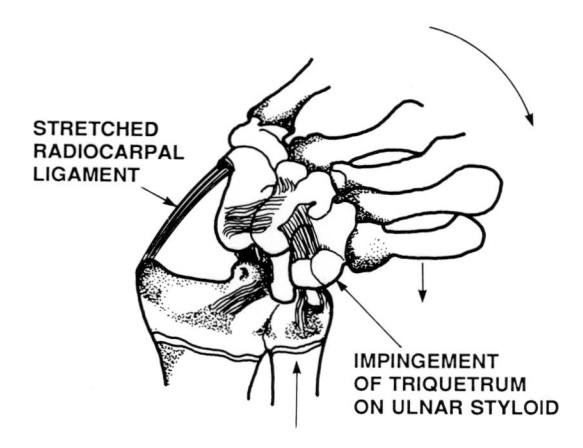

Fig. 21-14. Fracture of the triquetrum may occur by the impingement of the ulnar styloid on the triquetrum resulting in a shear fracture of the carpal bone.

tion of the triquetrum with a small amount of subchondral bone. There is probably not a single common mechanism, and both impaction and avulsion forces may result in triquetral fracturing. Ligamentous avulsion fractures of the triquetrum can occur with the wrist in flexion and radial deviation with the avulsion being caused by the ulnar-triquetral ligament or radiocapitate-triquetral ligament (Fig. 21-15).

Clinical Diagnosis

In children, the small chip or avulsion fractures are much more difficult to see radiographically due to the large cartilaginous component (Fig. 21-13). A classification of pediatric triquetral fractures has been proposed to reflect this cartilaginous predominance in the immature triquetral bone (Fig. 21-16) and is somewhat analogous to the McKeever classification of an avulsion of the tibial attachment of the anterior cruciate. Bryan and Dobbins[33] have postulated that the triquetral fracture may

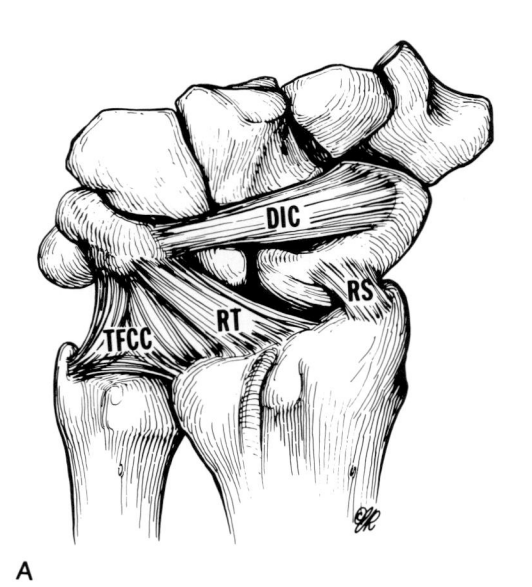

Fig. 21-15. (A) Dorsal carpal ligaments attached to the triquetrum. (B) Volar ligaments of the wrist. *DIC,* dorsal intercarpal ligaments; *TFCC,* triangular fibrocartilage complex; *RT,* radiotriquetral; *RS,* radioscaphoid. *RCL,* radial collateral ligament; *RC,* radiocapitate; *C,* capitate; *T,* triquetrum; *RSL,* radioscapholunate; *ECU sheath,* extensor carpi ulnaris sheath; *UT,* ulnotriquetral; *UL,* ulnolunate; *TFC,* triangular fibrocartilage. (From Palmer AK: Fractures of the distal radius. p. 929. In Green DP (ed): Operative Hand Surgery. 3rd Ed. Churchill Livingstone, New York, 1993. Drawings © Elizabeth Roselius.)

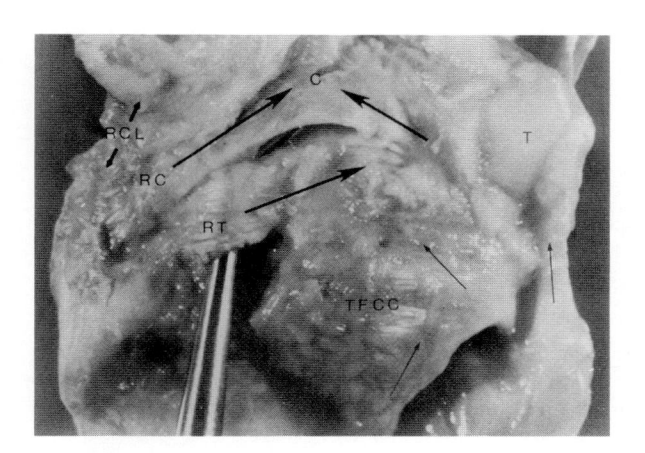

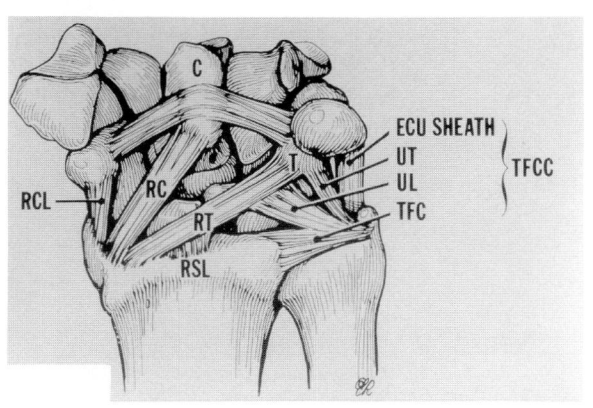

CHISEL OR AVULSION

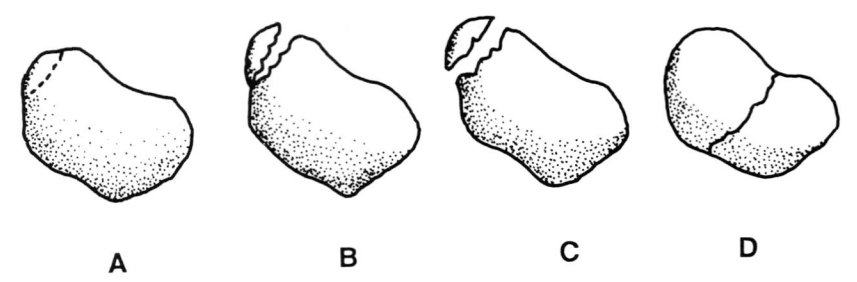

Fig. 21-16. Classification of triquetral fractures in children. **(A)** undisplaced, **(B)** hinged, **(C)** completely avulsed, **(D)** fracture of the body.

result from a fall in which the wrist sustains acute hyperextension and ulnar deviation forces, resulting in the hamate being impinged against the posterior radial projection of the triquetrum and this fragment being sheared off (Fig. 21-17). Similarly, a fall on the volar flexed wrist may result in an avulsion fracture of the triquetrum due to the dorsal radiocarpal ligament attachments. The presence of an ulnar plus wrist together with increased ligamentous laxity that occurs commonly in children's wrists would tend to favor the impingement theory for these fractures of the triquetrum.[44-47] The larger cartilaginous component of the triquetrum in children results in less subchondral bone fracturing with the result that the appearance of the small osseous flake on the radiograph is extremely difficult to visualize. Appreciation of this injury is also difficult clinically unless the possibility of the fracture is kept in mind. Direct pressure over the triquetrum just distal to the ulnar styloid, the so called "triquetral point" will always elicit tenderness in the presence of a triquetral injury. In the presence of this clinical finding and the absence of any obvious fracture on the radiograph, further views are recommended to identify the subchondral flake of bone.[48] Careful radiographic assessment is essential to confirm the diagnosis and should include AP, lateral, and 45 degree oblique projections of the wrist. The oblique view is necessary to orientate the source of the fracture, since the pure lateral view may be misinterpreted and the fracture attributed to the lunate instead of the triquetrum. In some instances, the fragment may even be entirely cartilaginous but in the presence of acute tenderness over the triquetral point and in spite of no subchondral flake of bone being identified on adequate radiographic examination, the child's wrist should still be splinted and treated as a triquetral cartilaginous injury.

Fig. 21-17. Fracture of the body of the triquetrum in a 10-year-old girl who fell from a play structure.

Treatment

Sprains of the wrist are extremely uncommon in children and are usually an unrecognized carpal fracture. A failure to appreciate the possibility of an underlying triquetral fracture will predispose the child to more prolonged morbidity from wrist discomfort and may contribute to the occasional nonunion requiring future excision of the fragment and ligament repair.[33] Three weeks of immobilization in a below-elbow cast appears to be an adequate length of time to allow the triquetral fracture to heal. The more serious fractures through the body of the triquetrum usually from a direct blow is much more obvious and usually ensures adequate treatment with immobilization in a below elbow cast.

CAPITATE FRACTURES

Fractures of the capitate in children are very uncommon and usually result from impingement of the capitate on the dorsal lip of the lunate or of the radius with the wrist in marked dorsiflexion.[2] There is a tendency for the proximal capitate fragment to rotate and its position should be confirmed with good oblique films or computed tomography (Fig. 21-18). The capitate usually heals very well with immobilization of the wrist for 6 weeks in a below elbow cast. The literature contains one instance of capitate nonunion following a crush injury to the wrist in a 12-year-old boy.[49] The central position of the capitate in the carpus protects it from common injury. Anderson[15] has reported on a navicular/capitate fracture in a 13-year-old football player, which went on to union with immobilization. The capitate blood supply depends primarily on a distal to proximal endosteal flow which is jeopardized in proximal fractures. Nonunion of capitate fractures have been reported in children requiring bone graft.[49-51] The capitate is also vulnerable to fracturing from a direct blow to the dorsum, especially of the flexed wrist. The initial fracture of the capitate may be missed, especially since these injuries are often associated with other fractures of the distal radius and ulna or other carpal bones which may be more obvious and take attention away from the capitate itself. The simultaneous fracture of the scaphoid and capitate is very rare but the mechanism of injury described originally by Stein and Seagull[52] and more recently supported

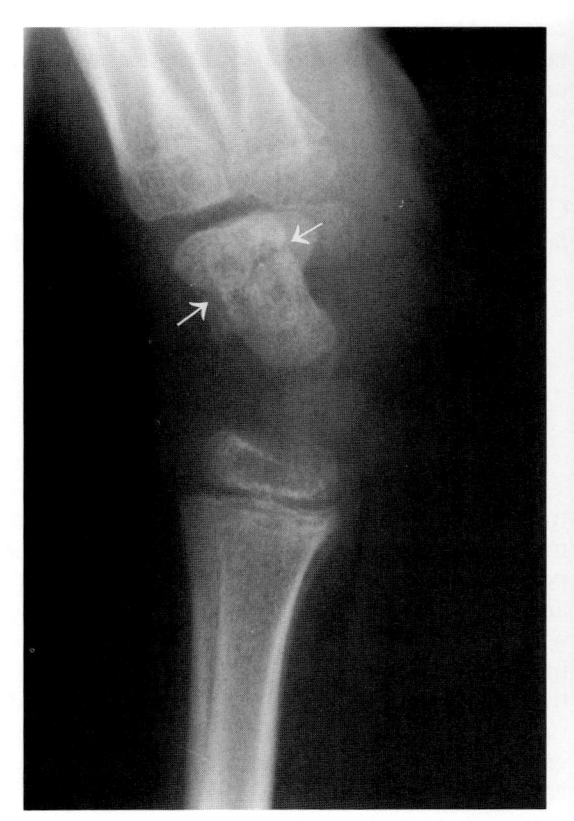

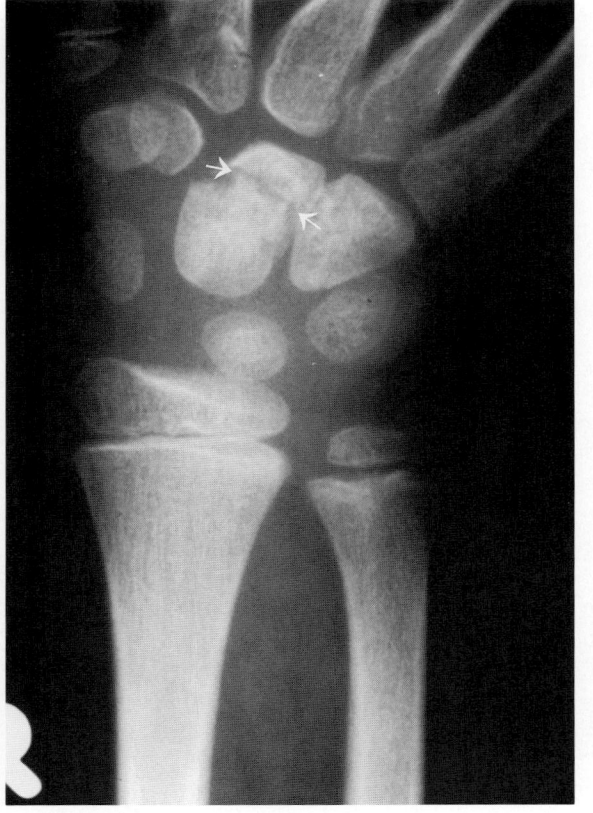

Fig. 21-18. Fracture capitate in a 12-year-old boy who fell off an all-terrain vehicle. Note the rotation of the proximal fragment in the anteroposterior view.

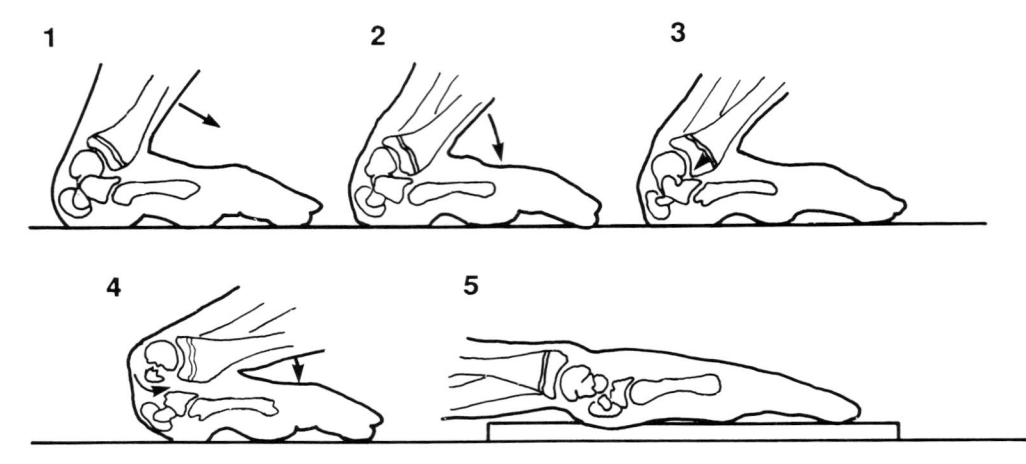

Fig. 21-19. Mechanism of fracture of the capitate and scaphoid due to forced hyperextension of the wrist. (Modified from Stein and Siegel,[52] with permission.)

by Anderson,[15] seems plausible (Fig. 21-19). They postulate that the fractures result from a force transmitted with the wrist in hyperextension. The dorsal cortex of the distal radial articular surface impinges on the waist of the scaphoid causing it first to fracture. As the lunate extends, the capitate migrates dorsally from the lunar concavity. As forceful hyperextension continues, the capitate either dislocates or impinges on the dorsal lunate lip or the dorsal radial lip. The capitate is thus fractured from direct compression against one of these beaked edges and may result in a shearing off at the neck and rotation of as much as 180 degrees on its transverse axis. Concomitant fractures of the distal radius and the capitate may also occur in a similar manner (Fig. 21-20).

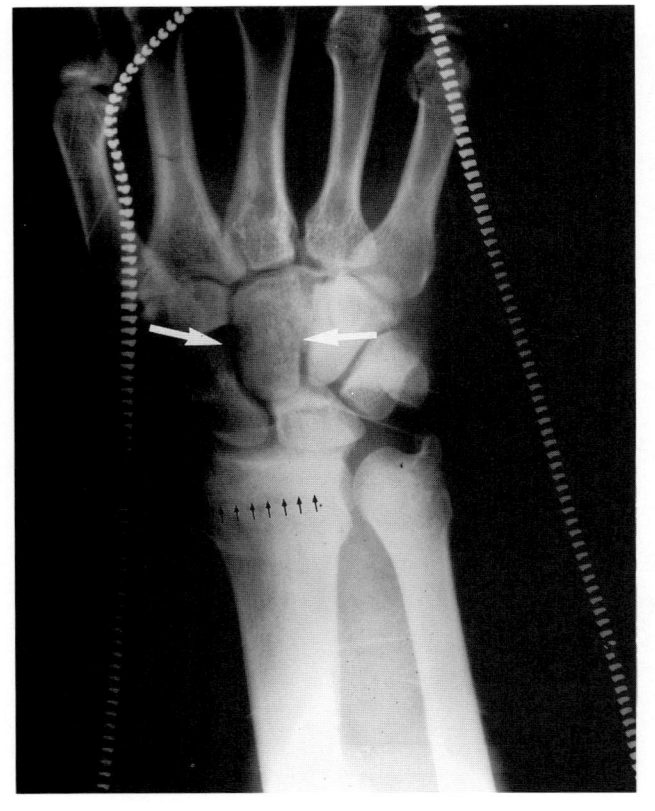

Fig. 21-20. Fracture capitate associated with a fracture of the distal radius.

FRACTURE-DISLOCATIONS

Fracture-dislocations of the wrist in children are extremely uncommon and usually associated with massive trauma. Transscaphoid perilunate dislocation was reported by Peiro[53] in a 10-year-old child who fell 15 feet and by Christodouleu and Colton[12] in a 9-year-old boy who fell from an even greater height. Treatment of such injuries needs to be individualized. Figure 21-21 illustrates a subluxation of the lunate in a 3-year-old girl, a rare form of carpal injury in children. Occasionally severe trauma may predispose to vascular impairment of a carpal bone and result in the development of scaphoid avascular necrosis.

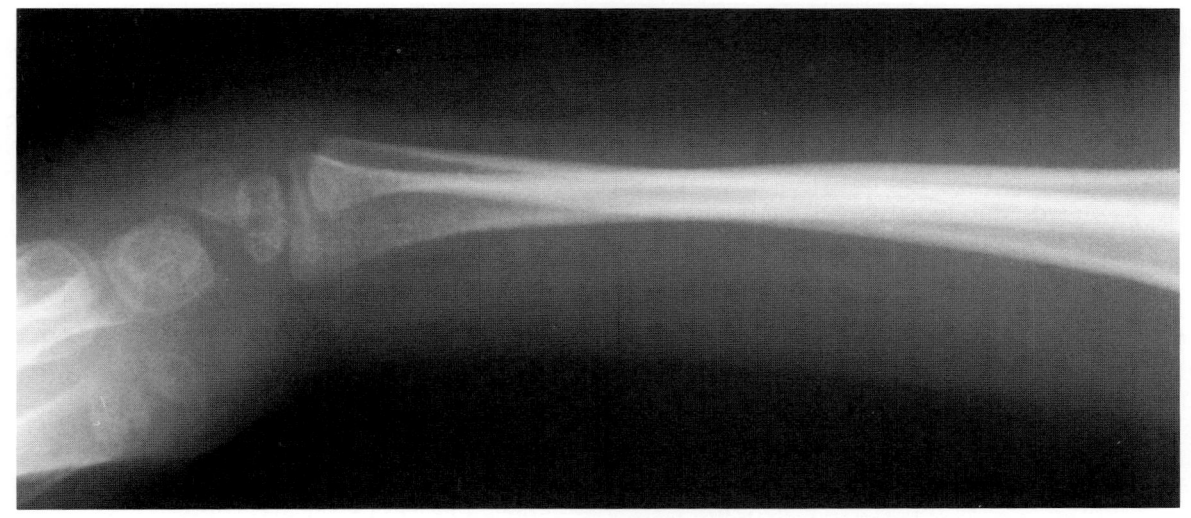

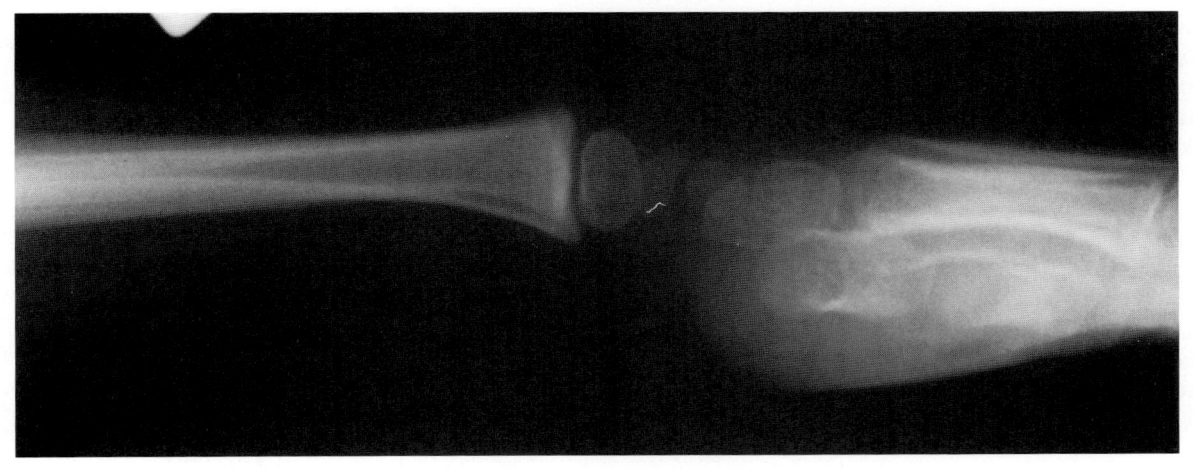

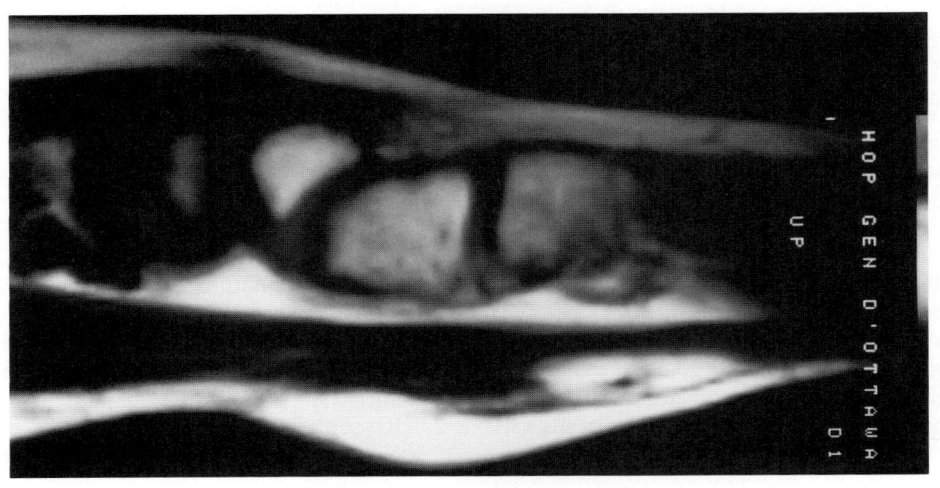

Fig. 21-21. **(A)** Dislocation of the lunate in a 3-year-old girl with no history of trauma—probably a congenital dislocation. **(B)** Left wrist for comparison illustrating normal anatomic position. **(C)** The MRI is a very effective tool in delineating carpal fractures and malformations in children. Here a subluxed position of the lunate is clearly defined.

SUMMARY

Fractures of the carpus in the pediatric age group are uncommon but probably more frequent than are currently diagnosed. Many minor avulsion fractures of the carpus in children are not recognized and continue to be dismissed as wrist sprains. Application of basic physiologic principles that are applied to injuries in other joints must be applied to the wrist in children as well. Ligaments are seldom ruptured in the child and if fracture occurs, it is usually in the adjacent radial physis or an avulsion of subchondral bone by one of the several wrist ligaments. Careful radiologic assessment of the symptomatic wrist in a child is essential to detect subtle fracturing. The most serious long-term disability from injuries to the carpus is fracture nonunion of the waist of the scaphoid especially if the fracture was not initially diagnosed and treated early. Nonunion of fractured scaphoids should be treated aggressively with bone grafting, internal fixation and plaster immobilization for 6 to 8 weeks until union has been obtained. This will avoid future inevitable wrist disability. Triquetral fractures are the second commonest carpal fractures in children. These fractures are difficult to diagnose both radiologically and clinically but should be suspected in any diagnosis of "wrist sprain." Other carpal fractures are much less common in children with the capitate being the third most commonly fractured carpal bone. Fractures of the hamate, trapezium, lunate and pisiform are rarely encountered in children.[54]

REFERENCES

1. Vahvanen V, Westerlund M: Fracture of the carpal scaphoid in children: a clinical and roentgenological study of 108 cases. Acta Orthop Scand 51:907, 1980
2. Light T: Injury to the immature carpus. Hand Clin 4:415, 1988
3. O'Rallihy R, Gardner E: The timing and sequence of events in the development of the limbs in the human embryo. Anat Embryol 148:1, 1975
4. Ogden JA, Grogan DP, Light TR: The postnatal development and growth of the musculoskeletal system. In Albright JA, Brand RA (eds): The Scientific basis of Orthopaedics. 2nd Ed. Appelton & Lange, E. Norwalk, CT, 1987
5. Kauer JMG: Functional anatomy of the wrist. Clin Orthop 149:9, 1980
6. Louis DS, Calhoun TP, Garn SM et al: Congenital bipartite scaphoid: fact or fiction? J Bone Joint Surg [Am] 58:1108, 1976
7. Stuart HC, Pyle SI, Coroni J, Reed RB: Onsets, completions, and spans of ossification in the 29 bone-growth centers of the hand and wrist. Pediatrics 29:237, 1962
8. Simmons BP: Injuries to and developmental deformities of the wrist and carpus. p. 176. In Bora FW Jr (ed): The Pediatric Upper Extremity. WB Saunders, Philadelphia, 1986
9. Taleisnik J: Wrist: anatomy, function and injury. Instr Course Lect 27:61, 1978
10. Mussbichler H: Injuries of the carpal scaphoid in children. Acta Radiol 56:361, 1961
11. Zimmerman NB, Weiland AJ: Scapholunate dissociation in the skeletally immature carpus. J Hand Surg [Am] 15:701, 1990
12. Christodoulou AG, Colton CL: Scaphoid fractures in children. J Pediatr Orthop 6:37, 1986
13. Grundy M: Fractures of the carpal scaphoid in children: a series of eight cases. Br J Surg 56:523, 1969
14. Greene MH, Hadied AM, LaMont RL: Scaphoid fractures in children. J Hand Surg 9A:536, 1984
15. Anderson WJ: Simultaneous fracture of the scaphoid and capitate in a child. J Hand Surg 12:271, 1987
16. Cockshott WP: Distal avulsion fracture of the scaphoid. Br J Radiol 53:1037, 1980
17. Failla JM, Amadio PC: Recognition and treatment of uncommon carpal fractures. Hand Clin 4:469, 1988
18. Smith KL, Harvey FJ, Stalley PD: Nonunion of a pathologic juvenile scaphoid fracture after osteomyelitis. J Hand Surg 16:493, 1991
19. Bloem JJA: Fractures of the carpal scaphoid in a child aged 4. Arch Chir Neerl 23:91, 1971
20. Sherwin JM, Nagel DA, Southwick WO: Bipartite carpal navicular and the diagnostic problem of bone partition: a case report. J Trauma 11:440, 1967
21. Gillman H, Caputo RJ, Carter V et al: Comparison of short and long thumb spica casts for non-displaced fractures of the carpal scaphoid. J Bone Joint Surg [Am] 71:354, 1989
22. Maxted MJ, Owen R: Two cases of non-union of carpal scaphoid fractures in children. Injury 12:441, 1982
23. Southcott R, Rosman MA: Nonunion of carpal scaphoid fractures in children. J Bone Joint Surg [Br] 59:20, 1977
24. Wilson-MacDonald J: Delayed union of the distal scaphoid in a child. J Hand Surg [Am] 12:520, 1987
25. Larson B, Light T, Ogden J: Fracture and ischemic necrosis of the immature scaphoid. J Hand Surg [Am] 12:122, 1987
26. Taleisnik J, Kelly PJ: The extraosseous and intraosseous blood supply of the scaphoid bone. J Bone Joint Surg [Am] 48:1125, 1966
27. Russe O: Fracture of the carpal navicular: diagnosis, nonoperative treatment and operative treatment. J Bone Joint Surg [Am] 42:759, 1960
28. Herbert TJ, Fisher WE: Management of the fractured scaphoid using a new bone screw. J Bone Joint Surg [Br] 66:114, 1984
29. De Boeck H, Van Wellen P, Haentjens P: Nonunion of a

carpal scaphoid fracture in a child. J Orthop Trauma 5:370, 1991
30. Gerard FM: Post traumatic carpal instability in a young child. J Bone Joint Surg [Am] 62:131, 1980
31. Watson K, Ashmead IV D, Makhlouf V: Examination of the scaphoid. J Hand Surg 13A:657, 1988
32. Letts M, Esser D: Fractures of the triquetrum in children. J Pediatr Orthop 13:228, 1993.
33. Bryan RS, Dobyns JH: Fractures of the carpal bones other than lunate and navicular. Clin Orthop Rel Res 149:107, 1980
34. Levy M, Fischel RE, Stern GM, Goldberg I: Chip fractures of the os triquetrum: the mechanism of injury. J Bone Joint Surg [Br] 61:355, 1979
35. Bonnin JG, Greening WP: Fractures of the triquetrum. Br J Surg 31:278, 1944
36. Mayfield JK, Johnson RP, Kilcoyne RF: The ligaments of the human wrist and their functional significance. Anat Rec 186:417, 1976
37. Wioi JP, Dorst JP: Less common fractures and dislocations of the wrist. Radiol Clin North Am 4:261, 1966
38. Bartone NF, Grieco RV: Fractures of the triquetrum. J Bone Joint Surg [Am] 38:353, 1956
39. Borgeskov S, Christiansen B, Kjaer A, Balslev I: Fractures of the carpal bones. Acta Orthop Scand 37:276, 1966
40. De Beer J, Hudson DA: Fractures of the triquetrum. J Hand Surg [Br] 12:52, 1987
41. Durbin FC: Non-union of the triquetrum. J Bone Joint Surg [Br] 32:388, 1988
42. Fairbank TJ: Chip fractures of os triquetrum. Br Med J 2:310, 1942
43. Garcia-Elias M: Dorsal fractures of the triquetrum: avulsion or compression fractures? J Hand Surg [Am] 12:266, 1987
44. Hill NA: Fractures and dislocations of the carpus. Orthop Clin North Am 1:275, 1970
45. Johnson RP: The acutely injured wrist and its residuals. Clin Orthop Rel Res 149:33, 1980
46. Mark LIK: Fractures of the triquetrum. AJR 83:676, 1960
47. Mayfield JK: Mechanism of carpal injuries. Clin Orthop Rel Res 149:45, 1980
48. Thompson JE: Fractures of the carpal navicular and triquetrum bones. Am J Surg 21:214, 1933
49. O'Brien ET: Acute fractures and dislocations of the carpus. Orthop Clin North Am 15:237, 1984
50. Minami M, Yamazaki J, Chisaka N et al: Nonunion of the capitate. J Hand Surg [Am] 12:1091, 1987
51. Rand JA, Linscheid RL, Dobyns JH: Capitate fractures: a long term followup. Clin Orthop 165:209, 1982
52. Stein F, Siegel MW: Naviculo capitate fracture syndrome. J Bone Joint Surg [Am] 51:391, 1969
53. Peiro A, Martos F, Mut T et al: Trans-scaphoid perilunate dislocation in a child. 52:31, 1981
54. Abbitt PL, Riddervold HD: The carpal tunnel view: helpful adjuvant for unrecognized fractures of the carpus. J Skeletal Radiol 16:45, 1987

22

Fractures of the Metacarpals

Timothy P. Carey

> You can't repair a watch in an inkwell.
> —STERLING BUNNELL

DESCRIPTION AND INCIDENCE

Fractures of the metacarpals in children do not usually present major problems in treatment. Injuries to the hands are common, but rarely is the injury severe enough to require operative treatment. As in all children's fractures, the uniqueness of the growing skeleton results in a much different clinical picture than that of an adult. Fracture healing tends to be rapid and predictable in children with little susceptibility to persistent stiffness that can complicate adult fractures. The presence of growth plates is advantageous for remodeling potential, but also leads to unique patterns of injury that must be accurately recognized for appropriate treatment. The presence of the physis also changes the incidence of dislocations in children compared to adults, as the weakness of the growth plate usually results in separation at this level instead of dislocation of the adjacent joint.[1-5]

The incidence of metacarpal injuries is low in infants and young children, but these injuries are very common in the teenage population. The fourth and fifth metacarpal are much more frequently fractured.[6] A seasonal incidence can be noted in northern climates, with certain winter sports, such as skiing, leading to an increase in metacarpophalangeal joint injuries.[7]

ANATOMIC CONSIDERATIONS

The metacarpals are small tubular bones that are unique with an epiphysis at only one end. The thumb metacarpal has the epiphysis located at the proximal end, whereas in the other four metacarpals it is at the distal end. The appearance of the secondary centers of ossification occurs between 12 and 17 months in females and 18 and 27 months in males in the finger metacarpals. The thumb is generally delayed by about 6 months. Fusion of the epiphyses with the metacarpal shaft occurs between 14 and 16 years of age.[8,9] An unusual feature that can be seen occasionally in the thumb metacarpal is the appearance of a *pseudoepiphysis* (Fig. 22-1). This is the development of an apparent secondary ossification center at the distal end of the thumb metacarpal. It is not histologically a true epiphysis, and is of no functional significance, but must be distinguished from a fracture line.[1,10,11] At their proximal end, the metacarpals are firmly anchored to the carpal bones on the radial side of the hand, whereas more motion is present at the carpometacarpal joints on the ulnar border, particularly of the fifth metacarpal. This anatomic arrangement leads to fractures occurring more frequently on the mobile ulnar side of the hand in children and influences the treatment of the metacarpal fractures. The collateral ligament attach-

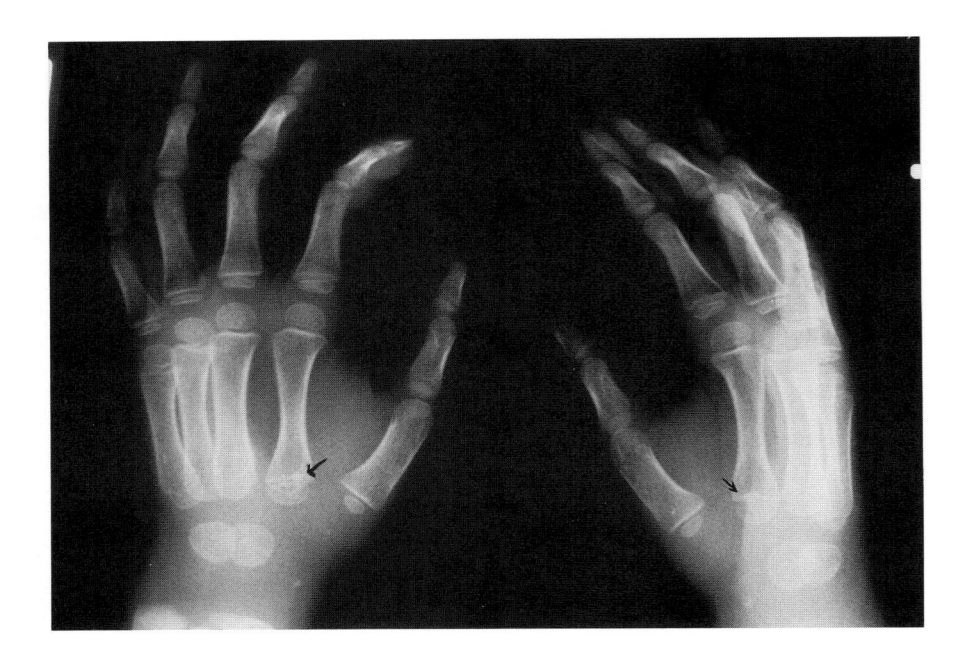

Fig. 22-1. An example of a pseudoepiphysis occurring at the base of the second metacarpal bilaterally.

ments of the metacarpophalangeal joints run from epiphysis to epiphysis predisposing to epiphyseal fracture patterns more commonly at this level than at the interphalangeal joint level.[12,13] The shape of the metacarpal head is "cam"-like, with the radius of rotation increasing as the proximal phalanx moves from extension to flexion. This results in a tightening of the collateral ligament complex with the digit at 90 degrees of flexion at the metacarpophalangeal (MCP) joint. This can be demonstrated clinically with considerable medial and lateral motion occurring at the biaxial ball and socket joint in full extension. With flexion, as the ligaments tighten, this motion disappears. The "position of safety" for hand immobilization is therefore with the MCP joints in flexion, to prevent contractures of the collateral ligaments (Fig. 22-2). This is more important in the treatment of fractures of the skeletally mature hand or in prolonged (greater than 3 weeks) immobilization of the hand. In children, the collateral ligaments seldom contract if immobilized less than 4 weeks. The fact that the collateral ligaments at the MCP joint tighten in flexion can also be utilized in the reduction of fractures. Displaced physeal fractures involving the proximal phalanx, such as the "extra octave fractures," are often difficult to reduce with the fingers in extension because there is considerable mobility at the metacarpophalangeal joints due to the relaxed collateral ligaments. By flexing the finger to 90 degrees, one tightens the collateral ligaments, thereby stabilizing the proximal phalangeal epiphysis at the metacarpophalangeal joint. In this position, one can then medially or laterally deviate the distal segment of the proximal phalanx to reduce the angulation. This is often a more effective technique than using a pencil as a fulcrum between the fingers with the MCP joints in extension.

MECHANISM OF INJURY

Children are by nature very active and exploring, and the tendency to place hands where they "do not belong" results in a high incidence of hand injuries. Fingertip and phalangeal injuries are much more common than severe unstable carpal or metacarpal fractures.[1] The presence of epiphyses and strong resilient ligaments linking the bones leads to a higher incidence of physeal fracture patterns. In spite of this, however, physeal arrest is not a frequent complication.[14,15]

Metacarpal fractures are usually due to a direct blow such as a fall, or hitting an object as in the common "boxer's" fracture of the fifth metacarpal. The second and fifth digits are prone to sudden angular displacements, which can lead to epiphyseal injuries, especially if the displacement is in the mediolateral plane. Excessive displacement in the flexion-extension plane, especially when associated with axial load, usually results in dislocation at the metacarpophalangeal joints. The typical

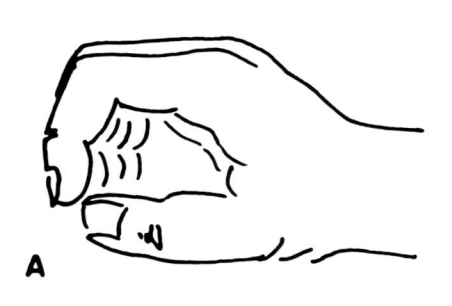

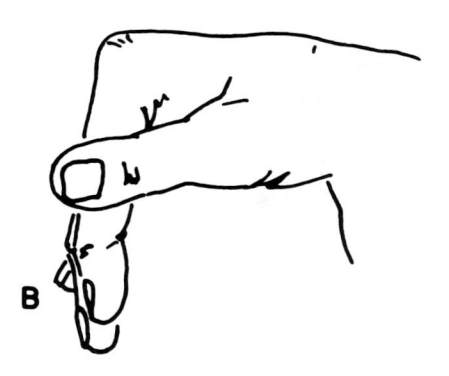

Fig. 22-2. The position of safety for hand immobilization is the intrinsic plus position. (A) Functional hand position. (B) Intrinsic plus position. (From Ogden,[1] with permission.)

mechanism of injury is that of hyperextension, most commonly of the thumb, with a resultant dorsal dislocation. Dislocations of the finger metacarpophalangeal joints are much less common, with the index being the most commonly involved.[6]

Carpometacarpal dislocations are very unusual in children. When seen, they are usually the result of severe trauma and can often have associated fractures of the metacarpals.[16,17]

CLASSIFICATION

Fractures of the metacarpals are usefully classified according to location. Thus, we can consider shaft fractures, physeal fractures, and intra-articular fractures as the major categories. Fractures of the metaphyseal or neck region are seen with enough frequency that they can be accorded a category of their own.

Fractures of the thumb metacarpal are somewhat unique in that the physis lies at the proximal end of the bone. As a result, the majority of fractures occur near the carpometacarpal joint, in contradistinction to the other metacarpals. O'Brien has classified these proximal first metacarpal fractures into four subtypes.[6]

Dislocations of the metacarpophalangeal joints are common, and usually dorsal in direction. The dorsal thumb MCP dislocation should be distinguished from that of the digits, as the former is a frequently seen injury and is usually a simple dislocation, whereas the latter is often a complex, irreducible dislocation (Fig. 22-3). The Farabeuf classification system of incomplete, complete simple, and complete complex, is practical.[18] Incomplete dislocations, as the name implies, occur when the displacement of the phalanx is sufficient to rupture the volar plate, but the collateral ligaments remain intact.

The distinction between the simple and complex forms of the complete dislocation, where there is rupture of the plate and the collateral ligament, lies in whether or not the volar plate has become interposed between the phalanx and the metacarpal head.

The thumb MCP joint is also susceptible to dislocations secondary to a forced abduction of the joint, causing injury to the ulnar collateral ligament complex. The injury can range from a sprain of this ligament, to complete rupture with joint instability. A more common variation in children is an epiphyseal fracture, usually a Salter-Harris type III avulsion of the ulnar portion of the proximal phalangeal epiphysis.[6,14]

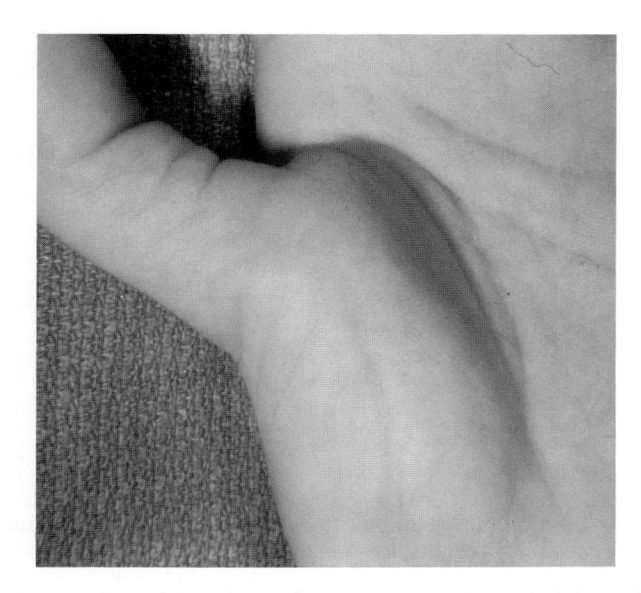

Fig. 22-3. Dislocation of metacarpophalangeal joint of thumb. The palmar prominence is produced by the metacarpal head, the proximal phalanx being dorsally dislocated.

PHYSICAL EXAMINATION

Careful clinical examination of the hand is critical if complications are to be avoided. As in all orthopaedic injuries, the presence of open fractures or neurovascular injury must always be determined immediately. One should keep in mind the mechanism of injury to guide one's examination. Metacarpal fractures, particularly those of the shafts, can result in considerable swelling of the dorsum of the hand, obscuring bony definition. Direct tenderness to palpation is often the most useful sign to localize the affected metacarpal. The common neck fractures also demonstrate considerable swelling, but careful examination can reveal a loss in the normal dorsal prominence of the metacarpal head, particularly when the MCP joints are flexed. Intra-articular and physeal fractures usually have less obvious gross deformities; however, movement of the joint will be exquisitely tender. As in any hand fracture, careful clinical assessment of rotation should be a priority, as even minor degrees of malrotation can result in significant disability.

The most reliable way to assess the rotational alignment of the digits is to assess the alignment of the nail beds. With the fingers extended, one should see coplanar alignment of the nail beds and if malalignment is noted, careful assessment is necessary. A comparison between both hands is often very helpful. If there is any concern about possible rotation of the digits, it is mandatory to assess the alignment of the digits with flexion at the MCP and interphalangeal joints. Any rotation will result in a change in the axis of the joints of the affected digit, and with flexing of the digits there will be a crossing-over of the rotated digit into the path of the adjacent finger (Fig. 22-4). Obviously, this will lead to significant functional impairment and therefore requires immediate correction.

Unreduced dislocations of the metacarpophalangeal joint are usually diagnosed without difficulty. The attitude of the phalanx in relation to the metacarpal often is a useful clue about the type of dislocation, as the simple dorsal dislocation often demonstrates a hyperextension of the phalanx, whereas in the complex type the phalanx is more likely to be dorsally displaced but not angulated, that is, in a bayonet position.[6]

An assessment of ligamentous stability should be performed, especially if the history is consistent with a dislocation that may have already been reduced. The collateral ligaments of the MCP joints are tight in flexion, and so should be stressed in this position. Stress radiographs are occasionally necessary to diagnose complete ligamentous disruption (Fig. 22-5). Volar plate damage can often be revealed by excessive extension on examination.

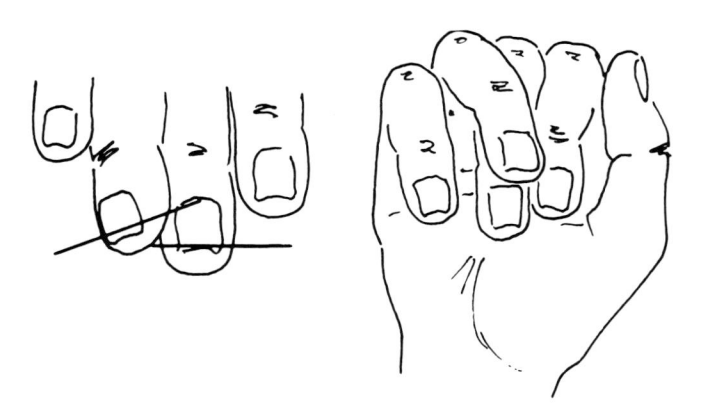

Fig. 22-4. When rotational malalignment is present, viewing the fingers in extension will reveal that the nail beds are not coplanar in alignment. Flexing the finger will reveal the resultant overlap between digits caused by the rotational malalignment. (From Ogden,[1] with permission.)

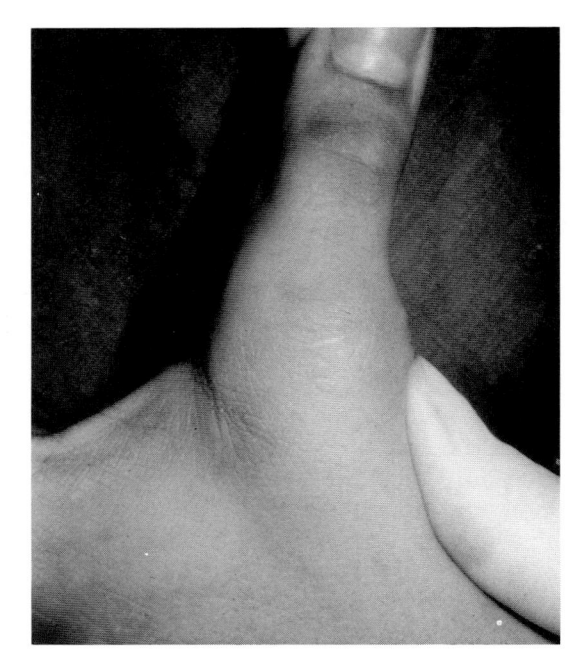

Fig. 22-5. Stressing the first metacarpal phalangeal joint to assess ligamentous stability should be performed with adequate anesthesia and is best performed with the metacarpophalangeal joint held in about 30 degrees of flexion.

DIFFERENTIAL DIAGNOSIS

Most fractures and dislocations of the metacarpals can be diagnosed accurately by history and physical examination. Radiographic examination is necessary to accurately determine the fracture type, and a minimum of two views at 90 degrees to one another are necessary. Due to the overlap of the metacarpals in the lateral view, oblique radiographic views are also recommended. On occasions where a true lateral view is required without overlap, such as the evaluation of intra-articular fractures, tomograms may be useful. The appearance of a pseudoepiphysis can occasionally be misinterpreted as a fracture by the less experienced.

TREATMENT INDICATIONS

The vast majority of metacarpal fractures can be successfully treated with closed methods. Isolated shaft fractures usually demonstrate minimal displacement. The transverse intermetacarpal ligament which runs between the second and fifth metacarpal heads prevents significant shortening of spiral fractures. Neck fractures and type II fractures, if displaced, are usually flexed at the fracture site and can usually be reduced by direct manipulation. Remodeling of metacarpal fractures, especially around the physis, is significant. This fact, plus the increased tolerance of the mobile fourth and fifth metacarpals to moderate angulation, makes these fractures more amenable to closed reduction, and the need for operative

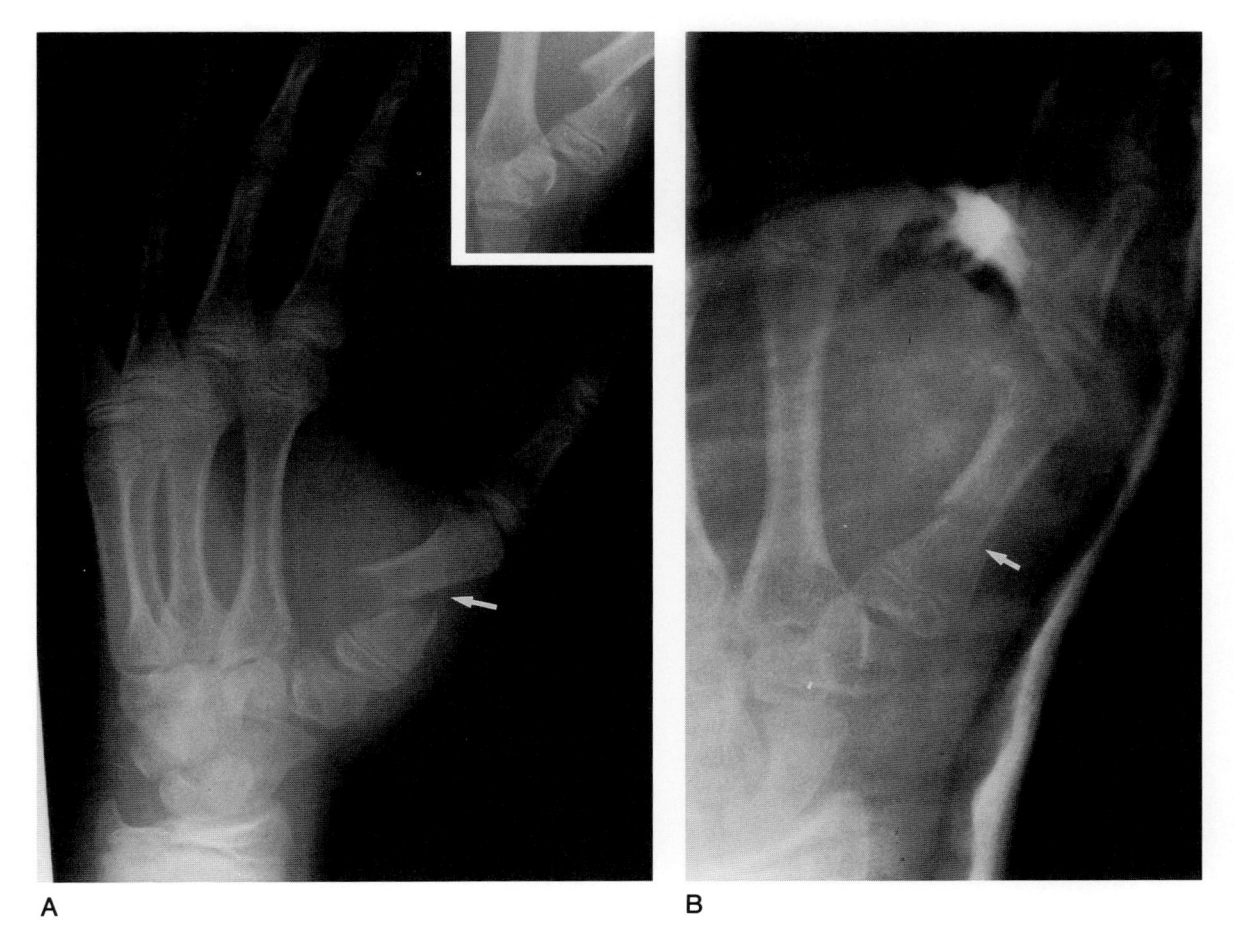

Fig. 22-6. (A) Fracture midshaft thumb metacarpal with typical volar angulation. (B) Post-closed reduction and cast immobilization.

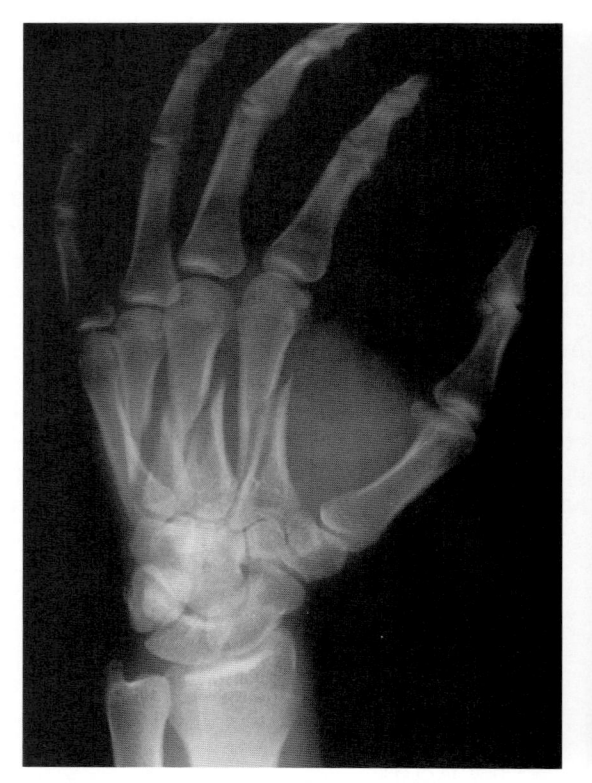

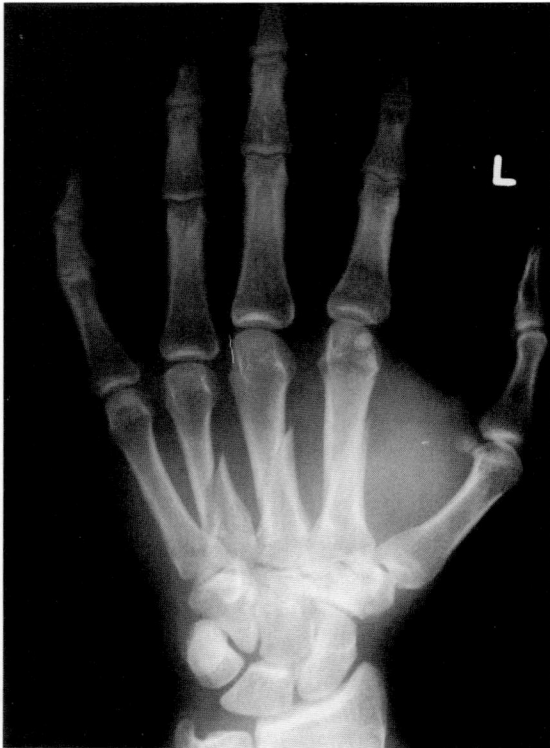

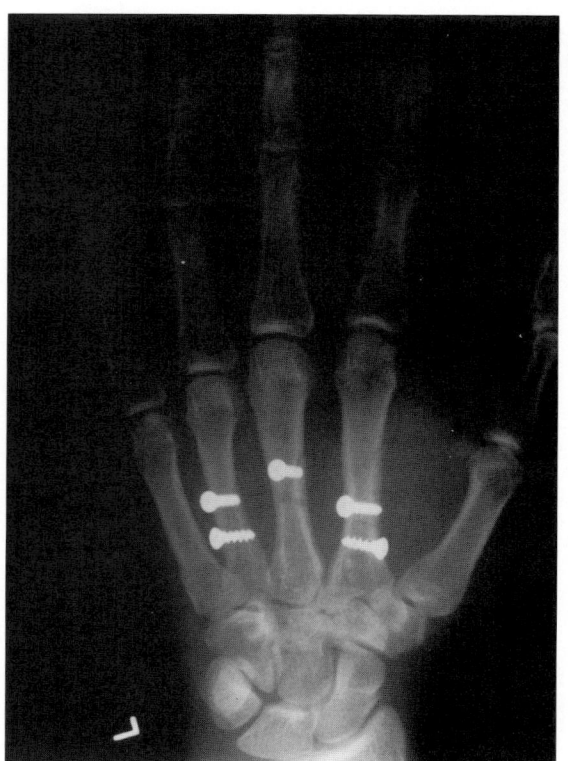

Fig. 22-7. An example of multiple metacarpal shaft fractures internally fixed with multiple small fragment screws in a 14-year-old boy.

treatment of these fractures is rare. Intra-articular fractures will, however, still require accurate reduction, and are the most common indication for operative intervention.[19,20]

Closed reduction of dislocations involving the metacarpals is usually possible. However, complex dislocations are a subgroup that will require operative treatment in most cases.

Metacarpal Shaft Fractures

Shaft fractures can usually be treated by closed manipulation and plaster splinting or casting (Fig. 22-6). Reduction can often be aided by the use of traction applied through "finger traps," especially if there is associated shortening. The cast needs to be accurately molded to provide three-point pressure over the angulated metacarpal shaft, but does not need to immobilize the interphalangeal joints. Care must be taken to keep the metacarpophalangeal joint flexed to at least 60 degrees to minimize stiffness in teenagers. If there is any rotational displacement present, it must be corrected. In this instance, extending the cast down the fingers helps to "buddy-splint" the fingers. The third and fourth metacarpals are less likely to demonstrate significant displacement due to their central "locked-in" position.[1] Immobilization should be continued for 2 to 3 weeks, and activities restricted for an additional couple of weeks including punching "friends."

Unstable shaft fractures occasionally will require operative treatment, especially when there are multiple metacarpal fractures. Unacceptable shortening of a shaft fracture can be treated by percutaneous pinning to an adjacent intact metacarpal with two parallel transverse K-wires.[6] Multiple fractures can be treated by either K-wire fixation or minifragment plates and screws (Fig. 22-7).

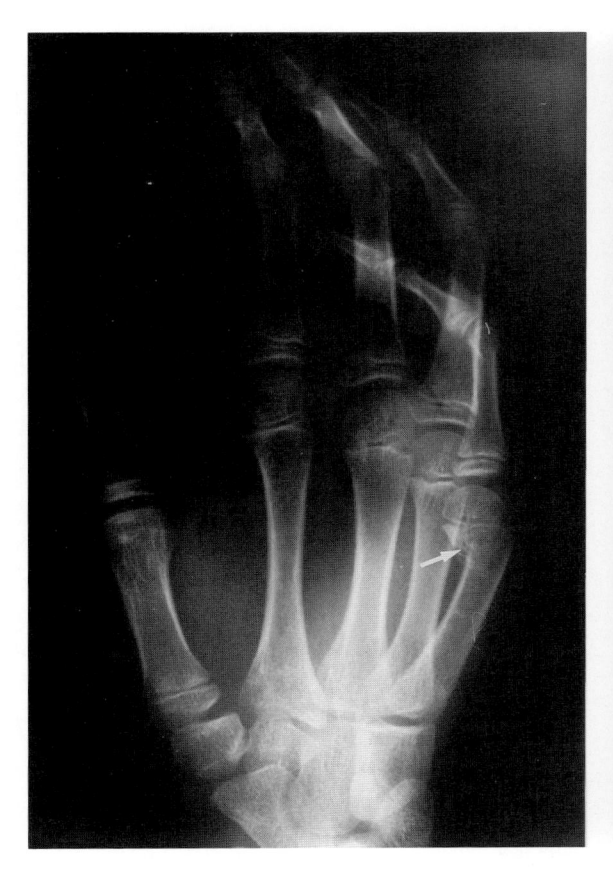

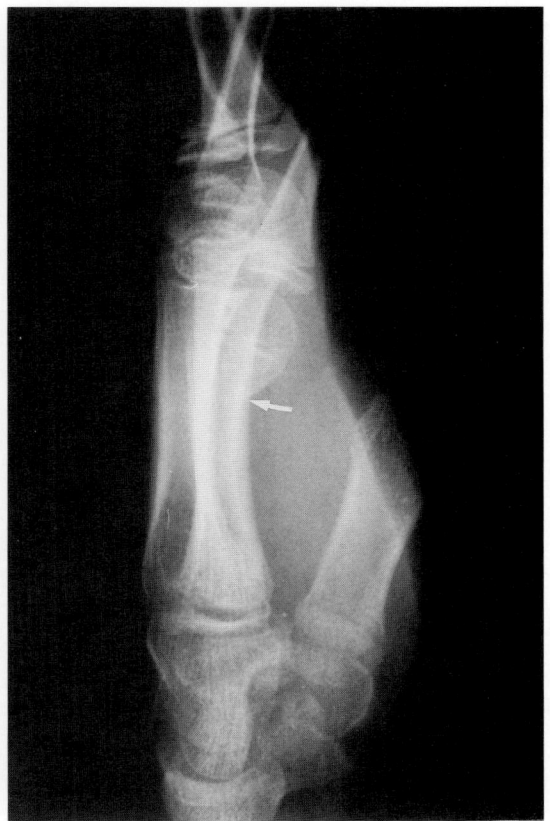

Fig. 22-8. A fracture of the fifth metacarpal neck or so-called Boxer's fracture. This can be a type II fracture in the skeletally immature, but is more often through the metaphyseal region of the bone.

Metacarpal Neck Fractures

Metacarpal neck fractures (both metaphyseal and type II injuries) are best treated by direct manipulation of the displaced distal fragment. The head fragment is easily palpable just distal to the distal palmar crease even in the swollen hand. Pressure directed dorsally usually results in an acceptable reduction in the common "boxer's fracture" of the fifth metacarpal neck (Fig. 22-8). The pressure can be provided directly by the surgeon's digit or indirectly by first flexing the metacarpophalangeal joint and interphalangeal joints to 90 degrees, followed by upward pressure on the flexed digit with dorsal counterpressure.[19,21] Regional anesthesia with a hematoma block or regional nerve block at the wrist is safe and effective. Immobilization should be with a below-elbow cast extending to the tips of the ring and little finger for a period of 3 weeks. Children should be reassessed radiographically after 1 week to ensure reduction has not been lost due to cast loosening as swelling subsides.

Rarely a fracture of the metacarpal neck will be unstable. If an acceptable reduction cannot be maintained with closed methods, percutaneous pinning with crossed K-wires is a useful technique. This is especially important in unstable fractures of the second or third metacarpals, where there is little motion at the carpometacarpal joints to accommodate any residual changes in motion at the MCP joint. Volar displacement of the metacarpal head is particularly annoying in this region, as it often produces a painful palmar protuberance.

Intra-articular Fractures

Intra-articular metacarpal fractures are usually not amenable to closed treatment. If there is any significant displacement, open reduction to accurately restore the joint surfaces is recommended.

The most common indication is usually displaced type III or IV epiphyseal injuries. Open reduction can be performed through a dorsal approach, using K-wire fixation with good results.[2,14,20]

Thumb Metacarpal Fractures

Thumb metacarpal fractures usually involve the proximal end of the bone and have been practically classified by O'Brien into types A through D (Fig. 22-9). The first three types can usually be treated closed, whereas the type D, or pediatric Bennett's fracture, often requires operative treatment (Fig. 22-10).

Direct pressure over the site of angulation at the base

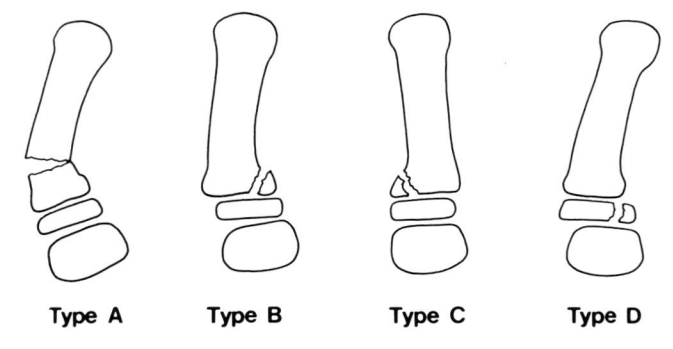

Fig. 22-9. O'Brien's classification of first metacarpal fractures. Type A: a fracture through the proximal metaphysis with adduction of the metacarpal. Type B: a Salter-Harris type II fracture with resultant adduction deformity. Type C: a Salter-Harris type II fracture in the reverse direction with an abduction deformity. Type D: a Salter-Harris type III of the proximal metacarpal epiphysis, or so-called pediatric Bennett's fracture. (From O'Brien,[6] with permission.)

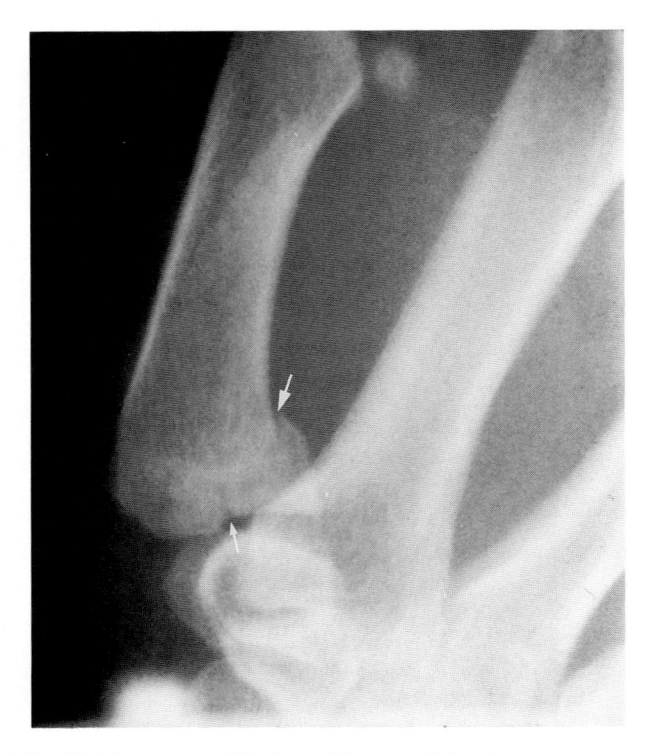

Fig. 22-10. A type III physeal injury of the thumb metacarpal: pseudo-Bennett's fracture typically seen in children. If displaced this fracture requires reduction with K-wire fixation.

of the metacarpal with outward pressure on the head of the metacarpal will usually reduce the common types A and B fractures. Care must be taken that the outward pressure is on the head of the metacarpal for, if it is placed too distally, one ends up hyperextending the MCP joint without effecting a reduction. Type C fractures are more difficult to reduce, and require adduction of the first metacarpal with a radially directed force at the base of the metacarpal. Occasionally the shaft fragment can buttonhole through the periosteum ulnarly preventing reduction. Open reduction of this pattern has been recommended,[1] but the tremendous remodeling potential in this region usually makes it unnecessary.[6,22] Immobilization in a thumb spica cast for 3 to 4 weeks is recommended.

The Pediatric Bennett's Fracture

The pediatric Bennett's fracture (type D), which is a displaced Salter-Harris type III fracture, is a relatively uncommon injury (Fig. 22-10). The ulnar portion of the epiphysis is undisplaced, and the remainder of the epiphysis must be accurately reduced to it and held to prevent joint incongruity. This can be accomplished by a closed reduction and percutaneous pinning[6,23,24] across the carpometacarpal joint, but if there is any question about the accuracy of reduction, open reduction is performed through an L-shaped incision along the radiovolar aspect of the metacarpal. K-wire fixation is supplemented by a thumb spica cast for a 4- to 6-week duration.

Fractures of the first metacarpal neck and head are rare, and are seen only secondary to a direct crushing injury. Treatment principles are the same as those outlined for metacarpals 2-5 neck and head fractures.

Carpometacarpal Fractures-Dislocations

Fractures of the metacarpal base seldom require open reduction, but may occasionally be unstable when associated with a dislocation. Dislocations at the carpometacarpal joint of the thumb are extremely unusual due to the fracture occurring through the weaker adjacent growth plate of the first metacarpal. Fracture-dislocations are usually of the type III variety (pediatric Bennett's fracture) as previously discussed. Dislocations involving the bases of the other four metacarpals are also rare, due to their location and stability of the carpometacarpal joints. Fracture-dislocations are occasionally seen in severe hand trauma, but are also very infrequent. Fractures of the base of the fifth metacarpal can be unstable due to the pull of the extensor carpi ulnaris, analogous to the unstable Bennett's fracture.[25] Closed reduction is usually achieved in these injuries, but if there is residual instability percutaneous pinning is sometimes necessary. In unstable carpometacarpal fracture-dislocations, maintaining the reduction will often require pin fixation of the carpometacarpal joint or alternatively, of the reduced metacarpal shaft to the adjacent shaft.

Dislocations of the Metacarpophalangeal Joints

The Thumb Metacarpal Joint

Dislocations of the metacarpophalangeal joints are not uncommon in children. This may be, in part, attributable to the significant degree of ligamentous laxity seen in many children. The most commonly involved joint is the thumb metacarpophalangeal joint[6] (Fig. 22-11). A fall on an outstretched thumb can often result in a forced abduction causing a subluxation or dislocation of the joint in a radial direction. The ulnar collateral ligament is injured, and in cases where there has not been a dislocation the teenager may sustain a sprain of the ulnar collateral ligament (skier's thumb) or partial avulsion of the ligament attachment. This is a very common injury, particularly in the teenage years and can be simply treated by casting the thumb in neutral position for 3 to 4 weeks.

A complete failure of the ulnar collateral ligamentous complex can occur by either an avulsion of bone from the ulnar aspect of the proximal phalangeal epiphysis (Salter-Harris type III fracture) or by complete failure of the ligament itself. Physeal injury is much more common in the skeletally immature. If there is substantial displacement of the bony fragment, it requires open reduction and internal fixation with K-wire fixation for 3 to 4 weeks.[14,19] When radiographs do not show any bony injury and one suspects a complete avulsion of the ulnar collateral ligament, stress views can be helpful in determining the extent of injury. It is important to remember in performing stress views of the metacarpophalangeal joint that the joint should be tested in about 30 degrees of flexion, as testing the joint in full extension can cause a false negative result due to the intact volar plate stabilizing the joint in extension. Stress radiographs require anesthesia, either by local injection of xylocaine or a pe-

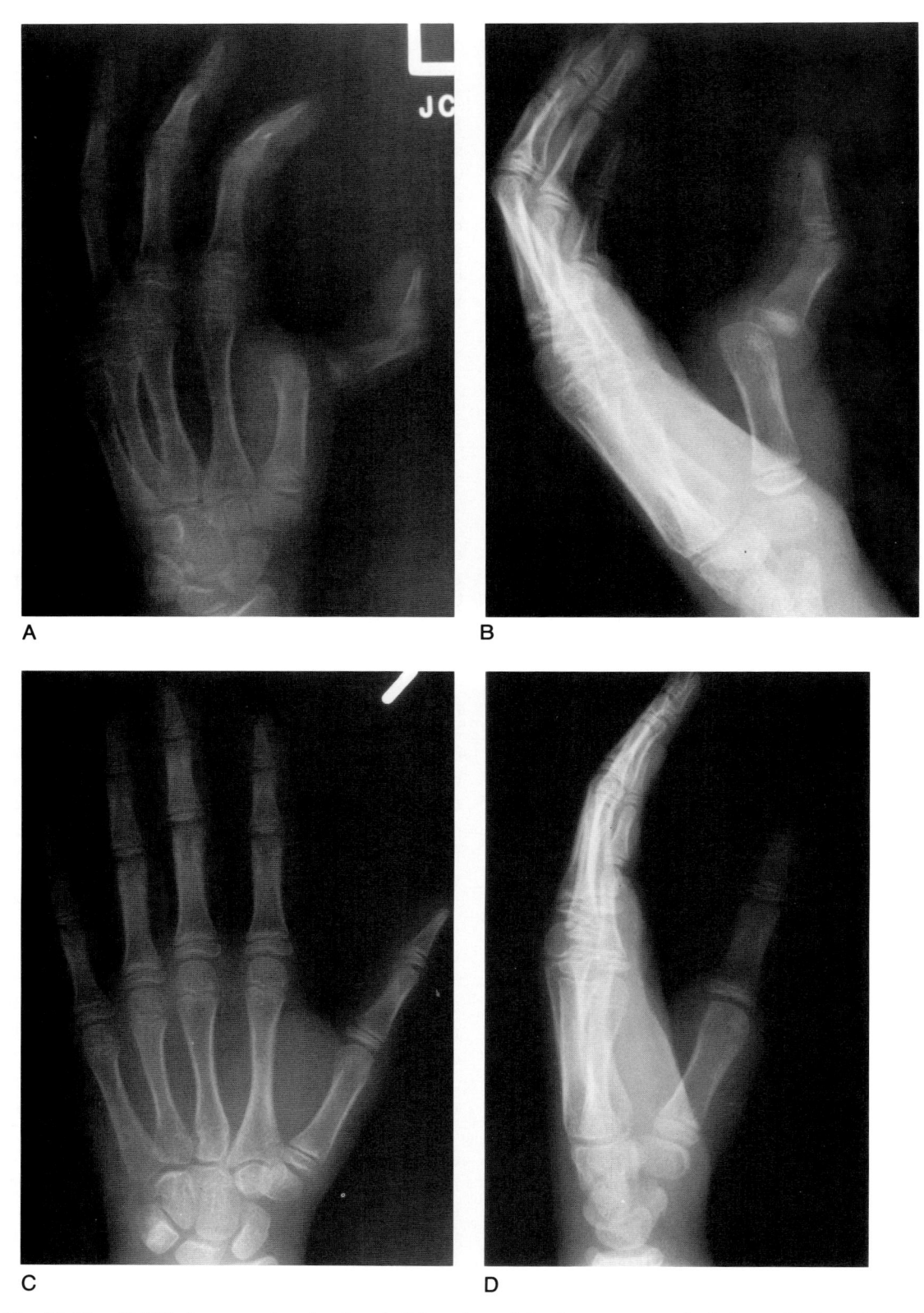

Fig. 22-11. **(A&B)** An example of a dorsal dislocation of the first metacarpal phalangeal joint. Notice the hyperextended attitude of the thumb at the metacarpophalangeal joint. **(C&D)** Postreduction films reveal no associated bony injury.

ripheral nerve block. If the stress views demonstrate radial deviation of the proximal phalanx, measuring 45 degrees or more than the amount seen on the contralateral unaffected side, this suggests complete disruption of the ulnar ligamentous complex. In this situation, it is recommended that operative repair of the ligament be performed, as it can often fold back on itself with prevention of healing by the interposition of the adductor pollicis tendon.[26,27] If stress films demonstrate a partial tear (less than 45 degrees difference between sides) thumb spica cast immobilization should suffice. An important variant injury that can also be appreciated on stress views is the so-called pseudo-gamekeeper's thumb, in which the displacement occurs through a physeal fracture at the base of the proximal phalanx (Salter-Harris type I or type II). If this diagnosis is evident, treatment consists of reduction of the displacement, followed by simple cast immobilization.

Dorsal dislocations of the simple variety can be treated with closed techniques. This is the pattern of injury most commonly seen at the thumb MCP joint, and clinically demonstrates a hyperextended attitude of the proximal phalanx at the MCP joint (Fig. 22-11). Care must be taken to prevent the conversion of a simple dislocation into a complex one, and for this reason traction should not be strongly applied in a longitudinal direction.[28-31] To prevent the volar plate from becoming entrapped, one should first adduct the thumb metacarpal while increasing the hyperextension of the proximal phalanx. The interphalangeal joint is kept extended and light axial pressure is applied to keep the articular surface of the proximal phalanx firmly against the dorsal surface of the metacarpal, thereby preventing any possibility of the volar plate becoming interposed. The phalanx is then "slid" along the dorsum of the metacarpal and around the "corner" of the metacarpal head, and reduction is easily obtained.

Complex Metacarpophalangeal Joint Dislocations

In distinction to the simple dorsal metacarpophalangeal dislocations, complex dorsal dislocations are not usually able to be reduced with closed techniques. This pattern of injury is seen most commonly at the index MCP joint, with a hyperextension injury. Clinically the injury can be suspected by the "bayonet" position of the proximal phalanx relative to the long axis of the metacarpal. Puckering of the skin at the palmar crease is also seen. This dislocation is irreducible due to the interposition of the volar plate between the proximal phalanx and the metacarpal head. With dorsal displacement of the proximal phalanx the plate tears off from its thinner metacarpal attachments and folds up dorsal to the metacarpal head. The head is then lying between the flexor tendons on the ulnar aspect and the lumbrical tendon on the radial aspect. In the case of a first MCP complex dislocation, the metacarpal head is trapped between the flexor pollicis longus and adductor pollicis. Although the volar plate is the structure interposed, the tendon "noose" just described prevents a closed reduction by tightening around the narrow metacarpal neck when traction is applied to the proximal phalanx, thereby making it impossible to position the joint in such a way as to extract the plate. Open reduction is almost always necessary, and extreme caution must be exercised in the approach to the volar aspect of the joint. The digital nerve may be tented over the metacarpal head, and is often the first structure encountered after the skin is incised. A short oblique incision parallel to the proximal and distal palmar creases is recommended for exposure. Often with release of the A-1 pulley, the flexor tendons are relaxed enough to allow reduction of the volar plate, which is extracted using a hook. If this is not successful, an incision of the plate along its radial margin usually suffices.[19]

The dorsal approach has been recommended by some as a safer alternate approach.[32-34] When approached this way, a longitudinal incision in the volar plate is required to allow reduction. This approach does allow easier visualization of any associated osteochondral fractures. Aftertreatment consists of early protected motion with an extension block splint for the first 3 to 4 weeks.

Complex metacarpophalangeal dislocations can also be seen in the fifth digit, and treatment is the same.

COMPLICATIONS

Complications associated with the treatment of metacarpal fractures are usually related to the fracture itself. Neurovascular compromise is not commonly encountered, but can be associated with severe crushing injuries to the hand. The possibility of a compartment syndrome in this situation should always be kept on mind. Malunion with unacceptable shortening or malrotation should be preventable with appropriate treatment as previously outlined. Careful critical appraisal of radiographs is required to avoid unacceptable reductions. Close follow-up of potentially unstable fracture patterns is required to identify early loss of reduction, thus facilitating remedial action. Growth arrest has been reported in a few instances of metacarpal head and neck fractures.[2,20,35] Although this complication is a theoretical concern in any fracture involving the physis, the clinical occurrence in metacarpal and phalangeal fractures is fortunately uncommon.

SUMMARY

Metacarpal fractures in children are fairly forgiving due to their remodeling potential. The common neck and shaft fractures usually do well with simple splinting. An appreciation of potential problems and a recognition of fracture patterns that require more aggressive treatment will ensure that good results will be achieved.

REFERENCES

1. Ogden JA: Skeletal Injury in the Child. 2nd Ed. WB Saunders, Philadelphia, 1990
2. Light TR, Ogden JA: Metacarpal epiphyseal fractures. J Hand Surg [Am] 12:460, 1987
3. Borde J, Lefort J: Injuries of the wrist and hand in children. In Tubiana R (ed): The Hand. Vol. 11. WB Saunders, Philadelphia, 1985
4. Green DP: Hand injuries in children. Pediatr Clin North Am 24:903, 1977
5. Worloch PH, Stower MJ: The incidence of pattern of hand fractures in children. J Hand Surg [Br] 11:198, 1986
6. O'Brien ET: Fractures of the hand and wrist region. In Rockwood CA, Wilkins KE, King RE (eds): Fractures in Children. 3rd Ed. JB Lippincott, Philadelphia, 1991
7. Van Domaekeb BA, Zuirbulis RA: Upper extremity injuries in snow skiers. Am J Sports Med 17:751, 1989
8. Greulich WW, Pyle SI: Radiographic Atlas of Skeletal Development of the Hand and Wrist. 2nd Ed. Stanford University Press, Stanford, CA, 1959
9. Stuart HC, Pyle SI, Cornon J, Reed RB: Onsets, completions and spans of ossification in the 29 bone growth centers of the hand and wrist. Pediatrics 29:237, 1962
10. Caffey J: Pediatric X-ray Diagnosis. 8th Ed. Year Book Medical Publishers, Chicago, 1985
11. Haines RW: The pseudoepiphysis of the first metacarpal in man. J Anat 117:145, 1974
12. Bogumill GP: A morphologic study of the relationship of collateral ligaments to growth plates in the digits. J Hand Surg 8:74, 1983
13. Hankin FM, Janda DH: Tendon and ligament attachments in relationship to growth plates in a child's hand. J Hand Surg [Br] 14B:315, 1989
14. Hastings H II, Simmons BP: Hand fractures in children. Clin Orthop 188:120, 1984
15. Sandzen SC: Growth plate injuries of the wrist and hand. Am Fam Physician 29:153, 1984
16. Hazlett JW: Carpometacarpal dislocations other than the thumb: a report of 11 cases. Can J Surg 11:315, 1968
17. Kleinman WB, Grantham SA: Multiple volar carpometacarpal joint dislocation: case report of traumatic volar dislocation of the medial four carpometacarpal joints in a child and review of the literature. J Hand Surg 3:377, 1978
18. Barnard HL: Dorsal dislocation of the first phalanx of the little finger: reduction by Farabeuf's dorsal incision. Lancet 1:88, 1901
19. Campbell RM: Operative treatment of fractures and dislocations of the hand and wrist region in children. Orthop Clin North Am 21:217, 1990
20. McElfresh EC, Robyns JH: Intra-articular metacarpal head fractures. J Hand Surg 8:383, 1983
21. Jahss SA: Fractures of the metacarpals: a new method of reduction and immobilization. J Bone Joint Surg 20:178, 1938
22. Kleinman WB, Bowers WH: Fractures and ligamentous injuries to the hand. In Bora FW Jr (ed): The Pediatric Upper Extremity Diagnosis and Management. WB Saunders, Philadelphia, 1988
23. Rang M: Children's Fractures. 2nd Ed. JB Lippincott, Philadelphia, 1983
24. Segmuller G, Schonenberger F: Fractures of the hand. In Weber BG, Bruner C, Freuler F (eds): Treatment of Fractures in Children and Adolescents. Springer-Verlag, New York, 1980
25. Sandzen SC: Fracture of the fifth metacarpal resembling Bennett's fracture. Hand 5:49, 1973
26. Stener B: Displacement of the ruptured ulnar collateral ligament of the metacarpophalangeal joint of the thumb: a clinical & anatomical study. J Bone Joint Surg [Br] 44:869, 1962
27. Stener B: Hyperextension injuries of the metacarpophalangeal joint of the thumb—rupture of ligament, fracture of sesanoid bones, rupture of flexor pollicis brevis: an anatomical and clinical study. Acta Chir Scand 125:275, 1963
28. Gilbert A: Dislocation of the metacarpophalangeal joints in children. p. 922. In Tubiana R (ed): The Hand. Vol. 2. WB Saunders, Philadelphia, 1985
29. Green DP, Terry GC: Complex dislocation of the metacarpophalangeal joint. J Bone Joint Surg [Am] 55:1480, 1973
30. Light TR, Ogden JA: Complex dislocation of the index metacarpophalangeal joint in children. J Pediatr Orthop 8:300, 1988
31. McLaughlin HL: Complex "locked" dislocation of the metacarpophalangeal joints. J Trauma 5:83, 1965

32. Bohart PG, Gelberman RH, Vandell RF, Salamon PB: Complex dislocations of the metacarpophalangeal joint: operative reduction by Farabeuf's dorsal incision. Clin Orthop 164:208, 1982
33. Robins RHC: Injuries of the metacarpophalangeal joints. Hand 3:159, 1971
34. Becton JL, Christian JD, Goodwin HN, Jackson JG: A simplified technique for treating the complex dislocation of the index metacarpophalangeal joint. J Bone Joint Surg [Am] 57:698, 1975
35. Brown JE: Epiphyseal growth arrest in a fractured metacarpal. J Bone Joint Surg [Am] 41:494, 1959

23

Fractures and Dislocations of the Phalanges

Timothy P. Carey

Gentleness begets accuracy.

DESCRIPTION AND INCIDENCE

Hand injuries in children present a different spectrum of injury than that seen in adults. Although major crushing injuries and multiple unstable fractures of the hand and wrist are relatively unknown in children, the isolated phalangeal injury is a very common entity in a pediatric orthopaedic practice. A significant proportion of phalangeal fractures tend to be crush injuries to the distal phalanx and fingertip. Physeal injuries are also very common and have been reported to make up almost 40 percent of children's hand fractures in some series.[1-10]

In spite of the relatively common incidence of finger injuries, and the usual good result that occurs secondary to the rapid healing and remodeling potential of children,[11] finger injuries may result in serious permanent disability. Failure to recognize unacceptable reductions or potential complications may result in a permanent functional hand deficit for the child. An awareness of the unique anatomic features of children's phalangeal fractures is necessary to prevent this from occurring.

ANATOMIC CONSIDERATIONS

The presence of the physeal plate and epiphysis in the growing bones of children leads to unique patterns of injury. The phalanges have only one epiphysis, located at the proximal end of the bone, in contrast to the distally located epiphyses of the metacarpals (with the exception of the thumb metacarpal). The proximal epiphysis becomes radiographically apparent in girls between 10 and 15 months of age, and usually fuses by about 14 years of age; in boys, it usually appears between 15 and 24 months of age, with fusion occurring by 16 years of age. The appearance of the epiphysis in the middle and distal phalanges is delayed by about 6 months compared to the proximal phalanx, but fuses at the same time. The development and fusion of the epiphyses of the phalanges is a useful clinical estimation of skeletal maturity, and comparison of hand radiographs with standard atlases is a commonly used technique for determining bone age.[12]

The site of ligamentous attachment on the phalanges prior to skeletal maturity affects the fracture patterns seen. The proximal phalanx has direct attachments of the collateral ligaments to the epiphysis only, whereas in

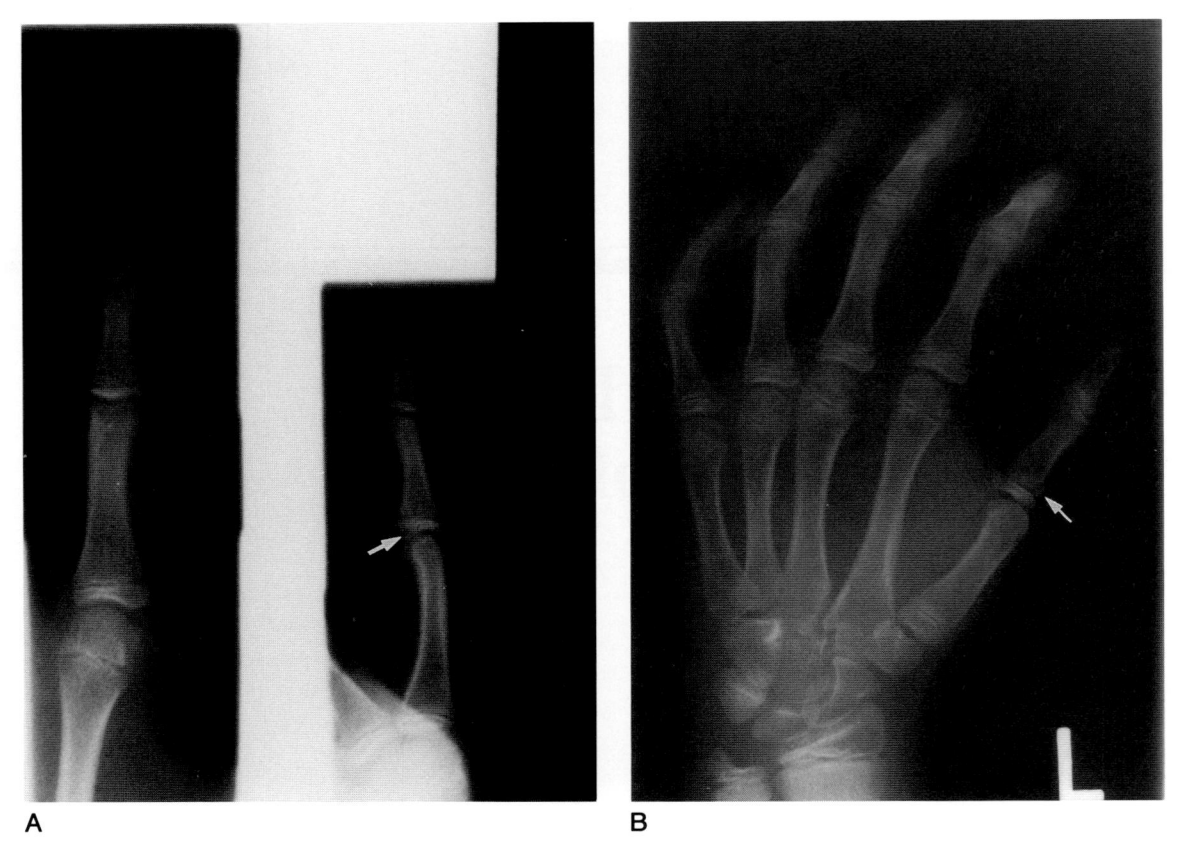

Fig. 23-1. **(A)** Volar plate avulsion fracture of proximal phalanx. This fracture is subtle and usually indicated by a fleck of subchondral bone just anterior to the proximal interphalangeal joint. It is seen only in the lateral or oblique view. **(B)** Many fractures of the phalanges in children are very subtle and indicated only by a small subchondral bone flake or minor metaphyseal avulsion as shown in this undisplaced type II fracture of the proximal phalanx of the thumb in a 7-year-old who fell while skiing.

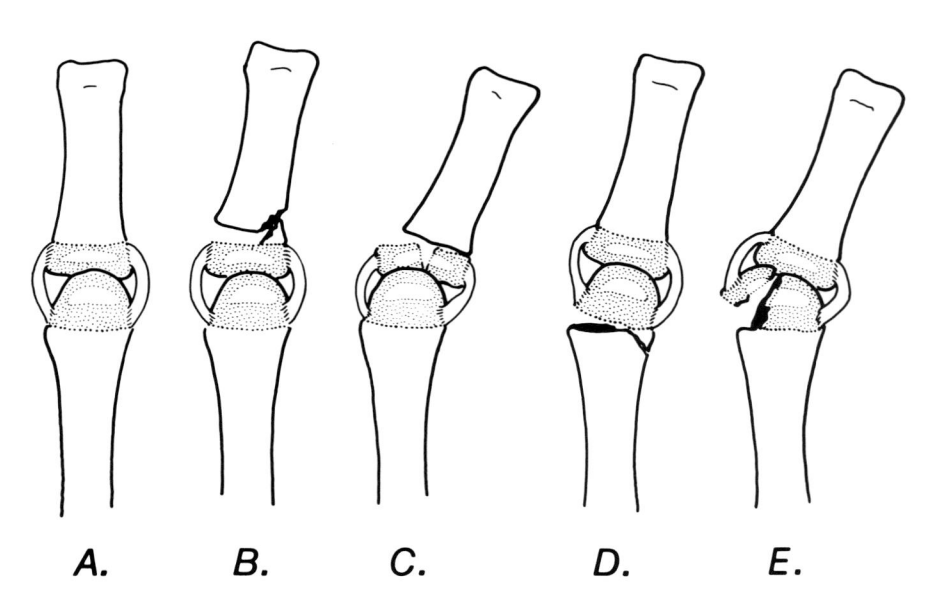

Fig. 23-2. Classification of the patterns of fracture at the metacarpal phalangeal joint. **(A)** Normal anatomy; **(B)** type 2 physeal; **(C)** type 3 physeal; **(D)** type 2 physeal; **(E)** type 3 physeal. The attachments of the collateral ligaments directly to the epiphysis of the metacarpal head and the proximal phalanx result in a frequent occurrence of physeal injury patterns. (Modified from Ogden,[11] with permission.)

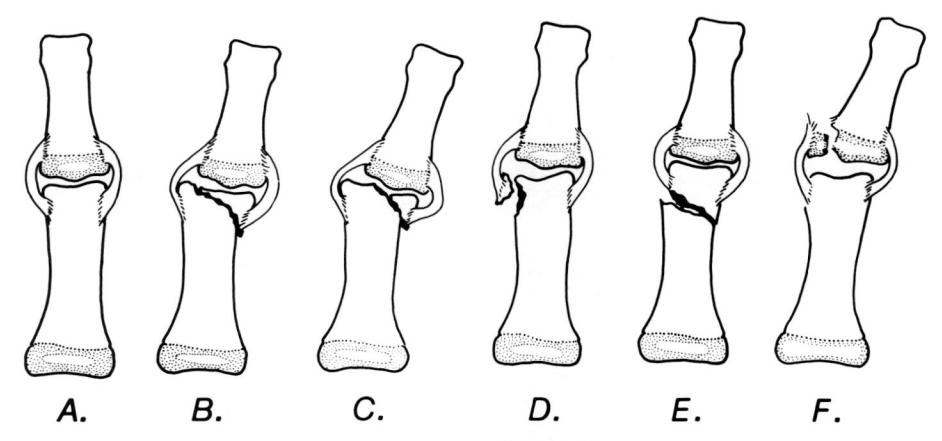

Fig. 23-3. Fracture patterns occurring at the interphalangeal joint. **(A)** Normal anatomy; **(B)** unicondylar; **(C)** partial condylar; **(D)** lateral avulsion; **(E)** bicondylar; **(F)** type 3 physeal. The spanning of the epiphysis and metaphysis by the collateral ligaments results in relative protection of the middle and distal phalangeal physes and resultant increased incidence of avulsion injuries. (Modified from Ogden,[11] with permission.)

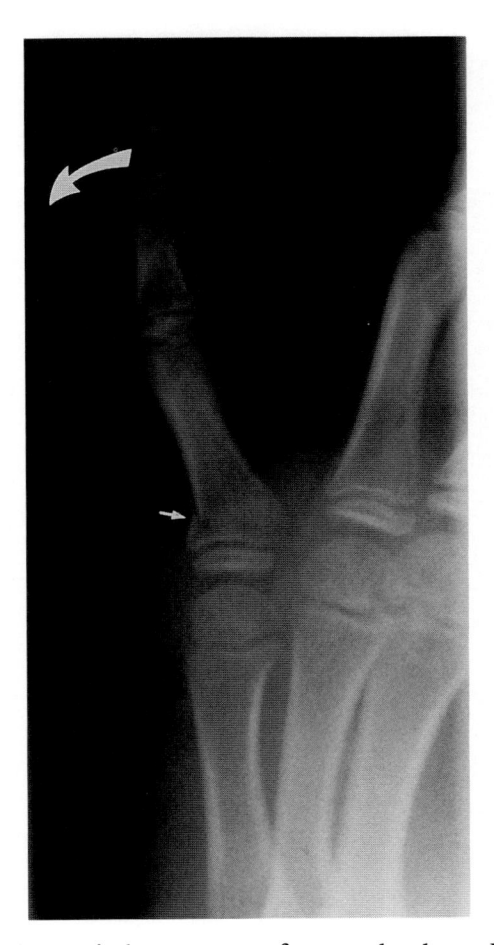

Fig. 23-4. Typical appearance of an angulated type II fracture involving the base of the proximal phalanx of the fifth digit (so-called extra octave fracture).

the middle and distal phalanges the attachment is broader, spanning both the epiphysis and adjacent metaphysis.[13] The volar plate, however, is firmly attached to both the middle and distal phalangeal epiphyses (Fig. 23-1).

Whereas the articulation of the proximal phalanx with the metacarpal is a modified ball and socket joint, the interphalangeal joints are pure hinge joints. The stability of the joint is enhanced by the articular contours. The proximal and middle phalanges have a pair of concentric condyles separated by an intercondylar notch. The corresponding surfaces of the bases of the middle and distal phalanges are broad surfaces with a median ridge. This bony architecture, combined with a strong collateral ligament/volar plate complex, results in a joint well designed to resist rotational and lateral stresses.[11] The strong ligamentous attachments often dictate the type of fracture pattern that will occur depending on the direction and magnitude of the force exerted on the finger[13,14] (Figs. 23-2 and 23-3).

MECHANISM OF INJURY

Mechanisms of injury are often related to the child's age. Toddlers most commonly sustain crush injuries to the distal phalanx, usually due to getting a hand caught in a closing door. As children get older and become more aware, this type of injury is less frequently seen.

As children become more active and involved in play and sports activities, they often get a finger jammed or caught and a very common fracture encountered is the

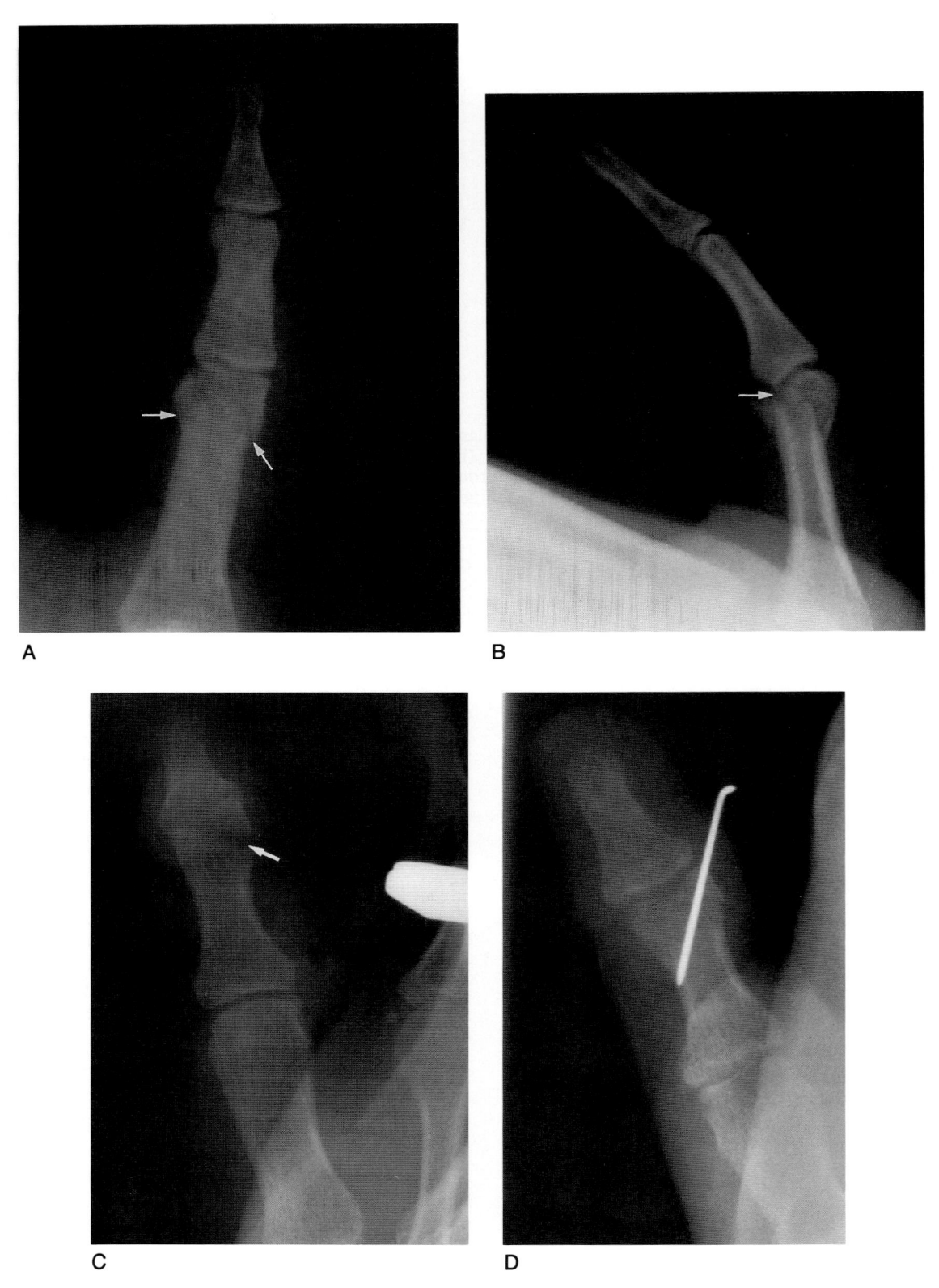

Fig. 23-5. **(A&B)** Condylar fracture of proximal phalanx with dorsal displacement in extension. This is a serious fracture that requires a near-anatomic reduction to preserve motion. **(C)** Condylar fracture of proximal phalanx involving 40 percent of the joint surface in a 15-year-old girl. The physes of the phalanges are the earliest to close and have already fused. **(D)** This type of fracture requires accurate reduction and fixation.

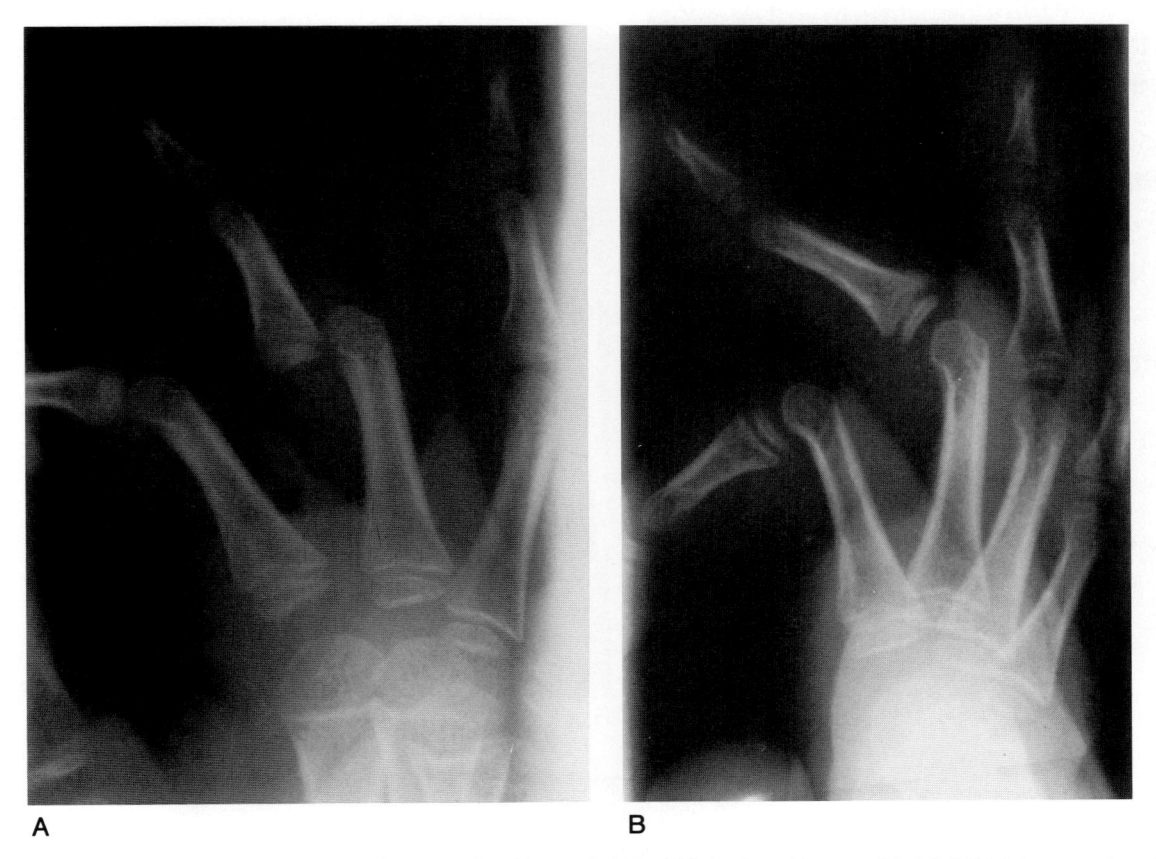

Fig. 23-6. (A) Volar dislocation of the proximal interphalangeal joint in a 4½-year-old girl. (B) This was reduced under mild sedation with traction and volar finger pressure over the base of the middle phalanx.

so-called "extra octave fracture"[15] (Fig. 23-4). This is a Salter-Harris type II fracture of the base of the proximal phalanx of the fifth finger and is so named because of the extreme ulnar deviation that occurs, facetiously making it possible to span two octaves on a piano. Another fracture that is prevalent in the first decade of life is the phalangeal neck fracture. This can be a particularly treacherous fracture, as the head fragment can rotate into extension, causing the volar plate to fold up and get caught in the joint[16] (Fig. 23-5). In the young child, the incompletely ossified condyles of the phalanx can result in this fracture going undetected or the degree of displacement being underestimated, with subsequent poor long-term results.

As children reach their adolescent years and become involved in higher speed and more violent sports, injuries such as a jammed finger can occur. This usually results from direct axial loading of an extended finger, commonly in ball sports such as basketball. The resultant injury can range from simple sprains of the collateral ligaments to frank dislocations of the interphalangeal joints or even a fracture dislocation (Fig. 23-6). Another frequent accompanying injury is an avulsion fracture of the extensor tendon insertion into the dorsal aspect of the distal phalanx. In the adolescent, this often occurs as a Salter-Harris type III injury (Fig. 23-7), whereas in the younger child, it is more commonly a type I or II fracture of the distal phalanx (Fig. 23-8).

Severe mangling or crush injuries of the hand are unusual in the pediatric population, as they are usually due to industrial accidents. In children, they are often secondary to farm machinery accidents.

CLASSIFICATION

Phalangeal fractures are commonly classified on the basis of the location of the injury. Distal phalangeal fractures are unique in that their anatomy predisposes to two

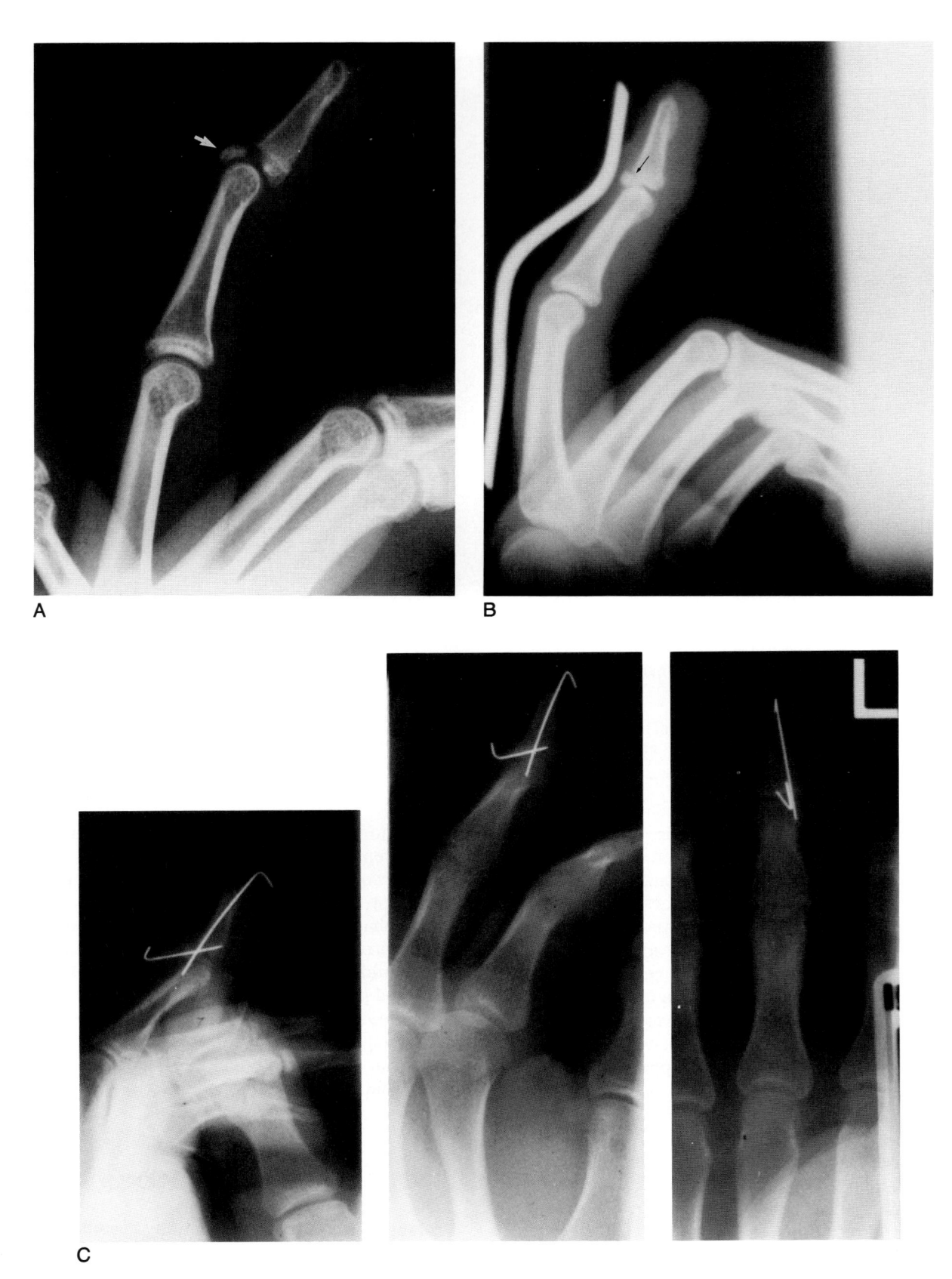

Fig. 23-7. **(A)** An example of a bony mallet finger corresponding to a Salter-Harris type III pattern in a 15-year-old volleyball player. **(B)** Although most can be treated by splinting in extension, if this is not possible, **(C)** K-wire fixation of fragment and the joint in some extension may be indicated.

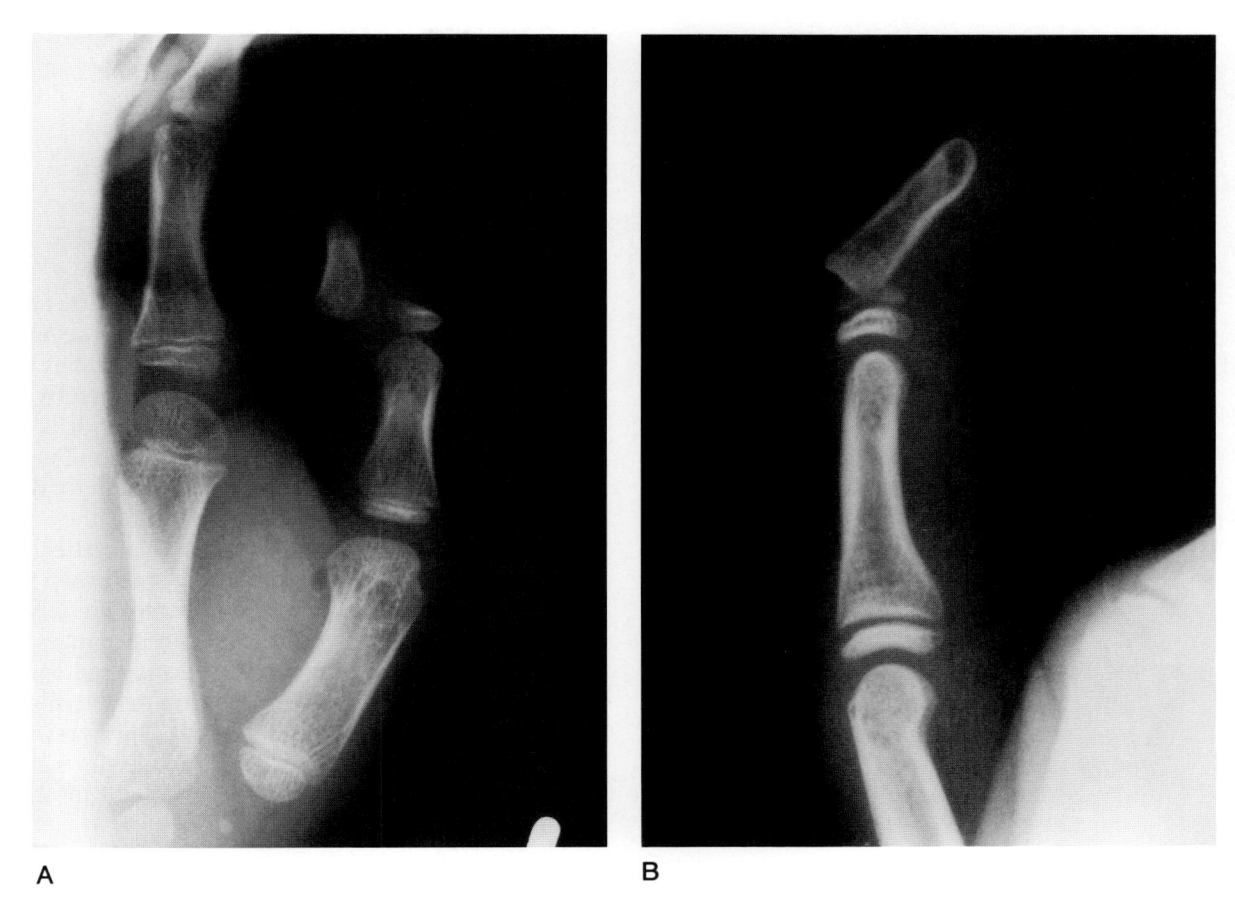

Fig. 23-8. (A) Type I fracture of distal thumb phalanx in a 6-year-old boy. (B) Type II fracture of distal phalanx of index finger in a 10-year-old boy. These fractures usually respond well to closed reduction.

types of fractures. The distal tuft is often involved in crushing-type injuries in which there is usually a stellate-type comminuted fracture not significantly displaced (Fig. 23-9). The second type of distal phalangeal fractures are those involving the physis. These tend to be hyperflexion injuries and result in a flexion deformity through the physeal fracture site. In the skeletally immature, these are Salter-Harris type I or type II injuries and are frequently open. In the teenager, the more common fracture pattern is a Salter-Harris type III with avulsion of the dorsal segment of the epiphysis by the insertion of the extensor tendon (Fig. 23-7).

Proximal and middle phalangeal fractures are grouped similarly depending on the site of the fracture. Articular fractures can be subdivided into epiphyseal fractures or condylar fractures at the nonepiphyseal end (Fig. 23-10). Condylar fractures are described as in the adult with unicondylar and bicondylar fracture patterns occurring, as well as complete comminution of the articular surface. Epiphyseal fractures are best classified using the Salter-Harris classification system.[17] Nonarticular fractures involve the neck, shaft, or the epiphysis, and include Salter-Harris type I or II physeal injuries.

Dislocations are classically described by the direction of displacement of the distal segment relative to the proximal one. Rarely, dislocations can be associated with epiphyseal fractures. Dislocations of the interphalangeal joints are described in this chapter, and metacarpophalangeal joint dislocations are dealt with in the previous chapter on metacarpal fractures.

PHYSICAL EXAMINATION

Clinical examination of the injured hand in the child can be a challenging task. The crying child needs to be calmed down in order to achieve an adequate examina-

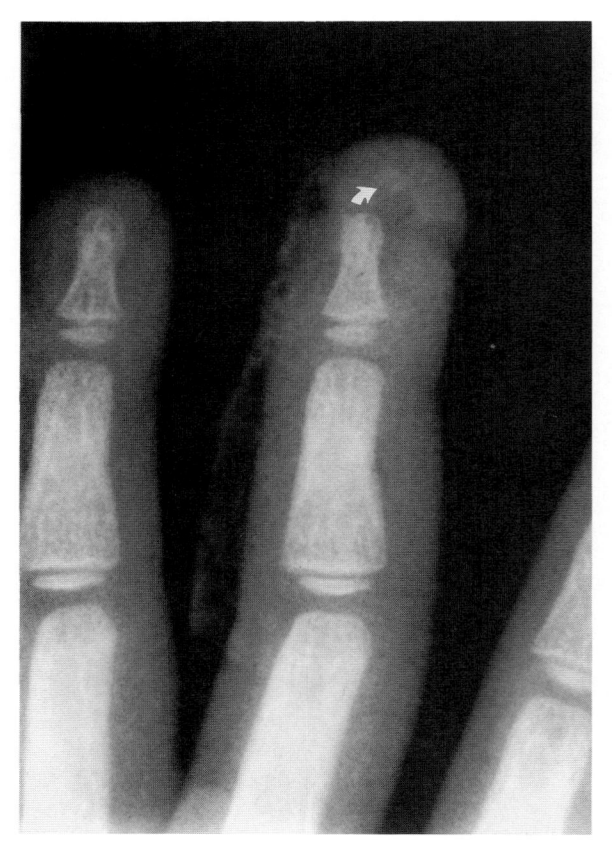

Fig. 23-9. Crush injury of distal phalanx with fracture of the tuft.

tion. Examination of the young infant on the parent's lap may assist in allaying anxiety. Initial examination of the child's normal uninjured hand may be helpful in gaining the child's confidence. Inspection of the fingers for swelling, deformity, and bruising should be performed, with special attention being given to the nail bed and eponychial fold in distal phalangeal injuries to ensure that an open fracture concealed by the fingernail does not go unrecognized. Areas of localized tenderness to palpation (both bony and ligamentous) should be identified. Limitation of motion and joint stability to lateral and hyperextension stresses should be noted. Careful assessment of the rotational alignment of the digit must always be performed, as deformity in this plane can easily be missed. The appearance of the nails is a good indicator, as they should be coplanar or equally aligned in extension. If flexion is possible, rotatory malalignment becomes more apparent (Fig. 23-11).

If a dislocation has occurred, postreduction stability can be tested by having the child actively flex and extend the involved digit. If a near-full range of motion can be performed without redislocation, functional stability is adequate.[18]

DIFFERENTIAL DIAGNOSIS

Most finger injuries are immediately obvious on examination. In the skeletally immature, however, one must be aware that physeal injuries occur preferentially to ligamentous or tendinous avulsions directly from bone.[11] Radiographs should be obtained prior to treatment to ensure that the apparent "dislocation" is not in fact a physeal fracture. Care should be taken to identify small flake fractures on the radiographs as they are indicative of ligamentous avulsions, the cartilagenous fragment being much larger than the small wisp of displaced subchondral bone would indicate (Fig. 23-12).

It is essential that two views of the phalanges at 90 degrees to each other are obtained during radiographic assessment. An overlap of the digits on the lateral radiograph can often obscure displacement. This is especially true in phalangeal neck fractures. Oblique views are also frequently necessary, particularly to evaluate intra-articular injuries with displacement.

The treating physician must also be aware of nontraumatic anomalies that can lead to abnormal radiographic appearances. Angular deformities involving the phalanges, such as Kirner's deformity[19] (Fig. 23-13) or a longitudinal epiphyseal bracket (deltal phalanx) should be recognized on appropriate radiographs.

TREATMENT INDICATIONS

Closed reduction and simple splinting for 2 to 3 weeks is all that is required for the treatment of most children's phalangeal fractures.[11,20] Open techniques are indicated for displaced physeal and articular fractures. Recognition of the fractures that need internal fixation can prevent complications from inadequate closed treatment. In the vast majority of operative cases, Kirschner wire fixation provides a simple and effective method of internal fixation (Fig. 23-7). Regional anesthetic techniques are particularly applicable to phalangeal fractures, both for open and closed treatment in older children. In young or uncooperative children general anesthesia will be necessary for adequate assessment and treatment of the injured digit.

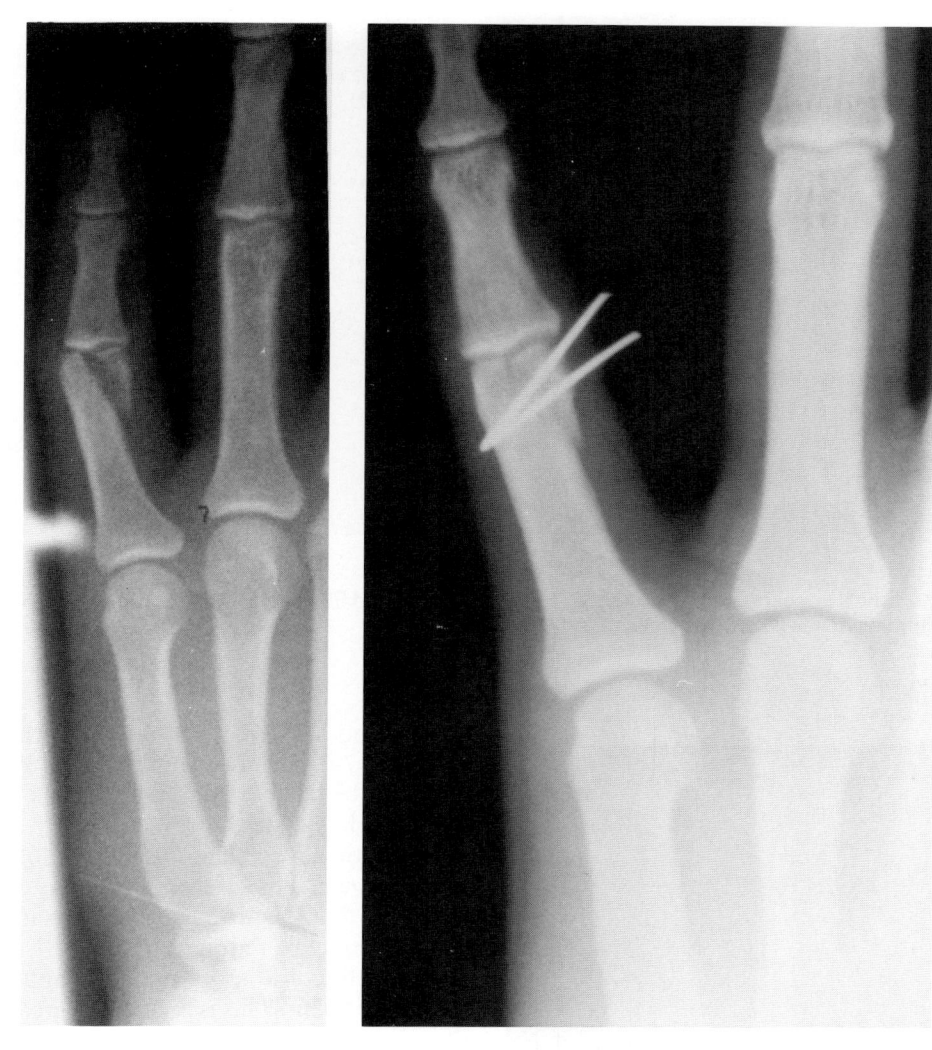

Fig. 23-10. Interphalangeal fracture of the proximal phalanx involving more than 20 percent of the articular surface will require reduction and internal fixation to avoid a large step and drift of the middle phalanx.

Immobilization can usually be achieved with plaster splinting or casting. The activity level of the average child makes the additional protection provided by a plaster cast desirable, even in stable fractures. Metal and plastic splints are usually removed by the child or become loose and ineffective very quickly in children.

Distal Phalangeal Fractures

Distal phalangeal fractures, while very common, are much less prone to complications than middle or proximal phalangeal injuries. The lack of tendons spanning the phalanx, the support of the nail bed and digital pulp, and only one articulation all contribute to this happy situation (Fig. 23-14).

The younger child typically sustains a crush injury to the distal tuft. The bony component of this type of injury is usually insignificant, and treatment should be directed toward the soft tissues. These fractures are often open and demand irrigation and conservative debridement (Fig. 23-15). Often skin that looks to be of tenuous viability will heal well in children.[21-23] Careful attention to the nail bed injury can help prevent a future displeasing cosmetic result. If there appears to be significant disruption of the nail bed, removal of the nail and accurate

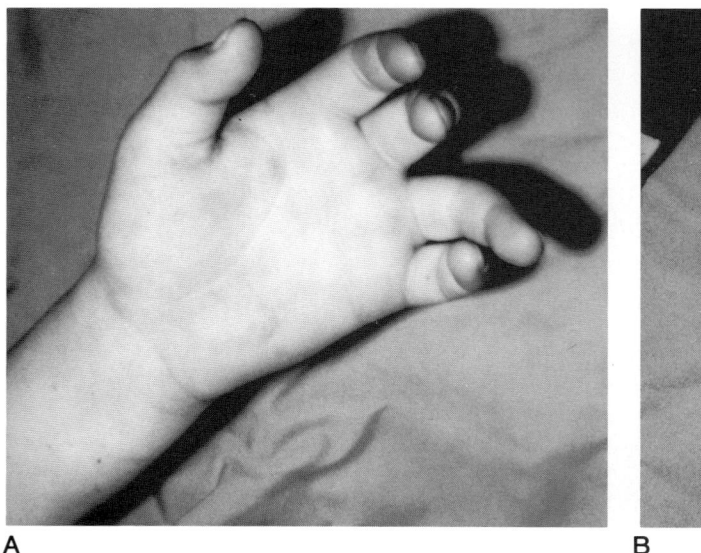

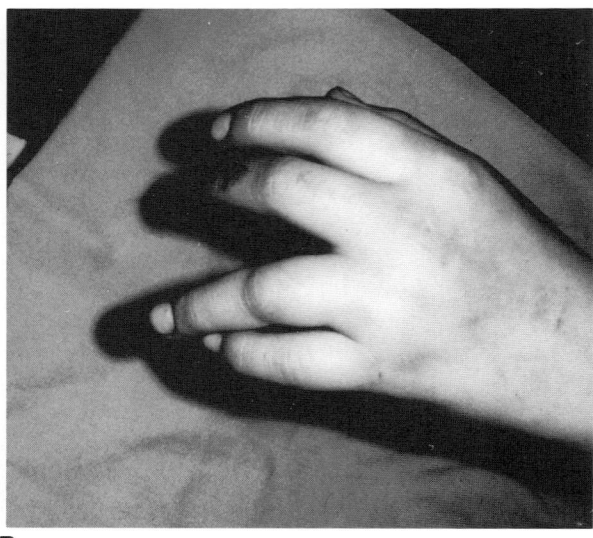

Fig. 23-11. Clinical appearance of an angulated and slightly rotated fracture of the proximal phalanx of the ring finger. **(A)** Palmar view. **(B)** Dorsal view.

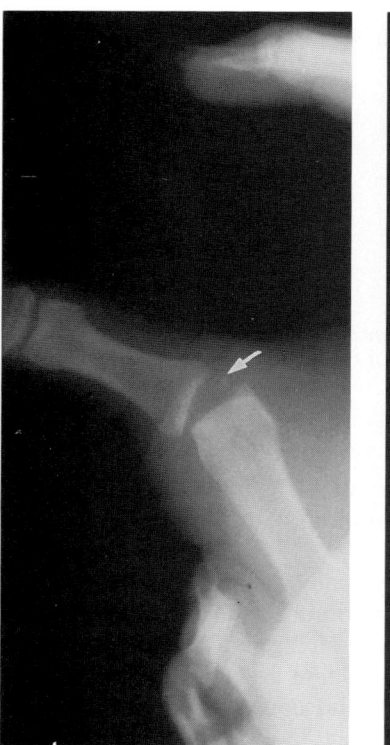

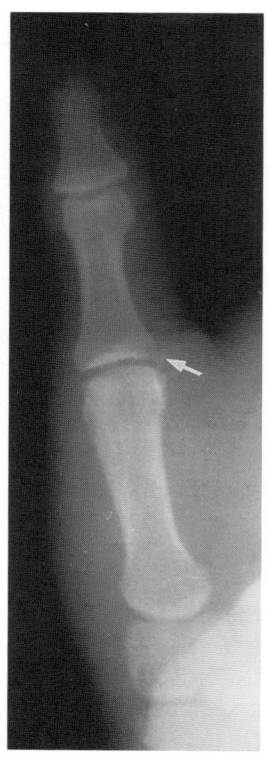

Fig. 23-12. Stress view of a gamekeeper's thumb in a 15-year-old girl who caught her thumb in a ski pole strap. Note the small avulsed bony fragment by the ulnar collateral ligament. This is usual in teenagers rather than the complete rupture of the ligament and facilitates healing.

apposition of the edges of the bed with fine suture, such as 6-0 or 7-0 chromic suture is recommended.[11,24,25] The nail can be trimmed and placed back under the eponychial fold as a stent or, alternatively, a folded piece of petrolatum gauze placed under the folds and across the repaired nail bed. Rarely, the bony injury will be so unstable that longitudinal K-wire fixation to the middle phalanx may be required.[26]

If the fracture is not open, a subungual hematoma may be present. This is a source of great pain, which can be relieved by evacuating the hematoma through a small hole in the nail most practically performed using a hot paper clip. This procedure is a well-established method of treatment,[11] but as in any technique that converts a closed fracture to an open one, there exists a theoretical potential for the development of infection. Care should be taken to ensure that the procedure is done under sterile conditions to minimize this risk.

Volar Avulsion Fractures of the Distal Phalanx

An uncommon fracture of the distal phalanx occasionally is encountered in the form of a type III physeal avulsion fracture due to the contraction of the flexor digitorium profundus against resistance. This occurs, for example, when a finger becomes caught in the back pocket of an opposing football or soccer player as the victim is falling and grasping for support (Fig. 23-16).

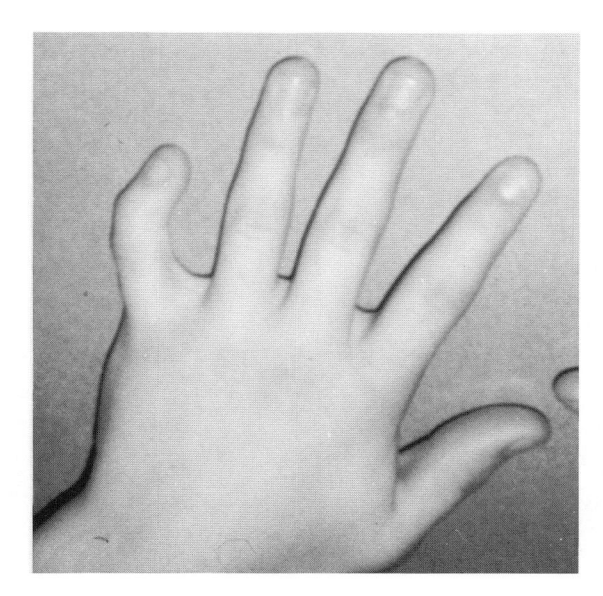

Fig. 23-13. Kirner's deformity of the little finger is sometimes misinterpreted as being the result of previous finger trauma. It is usually bilateral and present in relatives.

Distal Phalangeal Physeal Fractures (The Seymour Fracture)

The other common fracture pattern encountered in the distal phalanx involves the physis. In the preadolescent patient, type I or II fractures are usually seen, with flexion of the distal phalanx in a "mallet finger" position (Fig. 23-8). In the adult, the same mechanism of injury results in avulsion of the extensor tendon insertion. With displacement through the growth plate, the insertion of the extensor tendon into the dorsum of the epiphysis causes it to remain in place, while the pull of the flexor digitorum profoundus, which inserts into the volar aspect of the distal phalangeal metaphysis, flexes the distal part of the phalanx. The most important feature of this fracture pattern is the fact that it is often an open fracture that goes unnoticed. The amount of displacement at the time of injury can result in the metaphysis being displaced dorsally and protruding through the skin

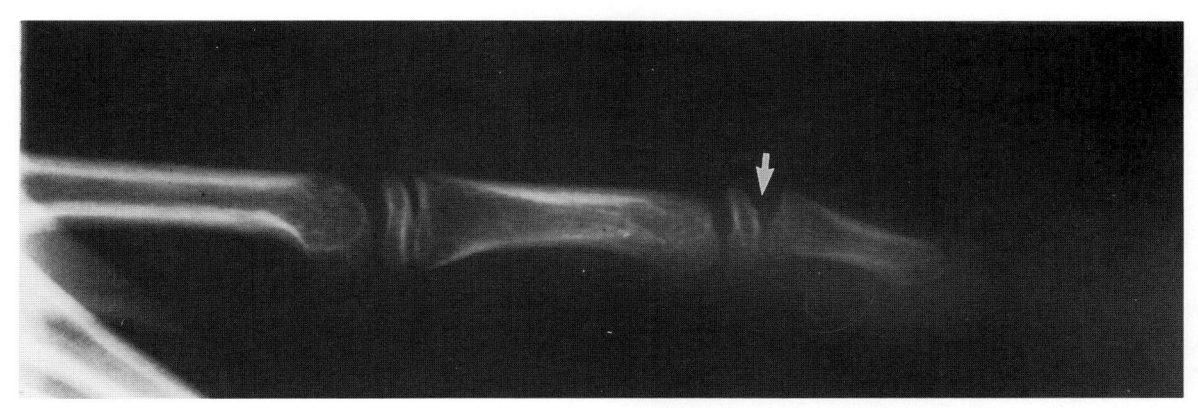

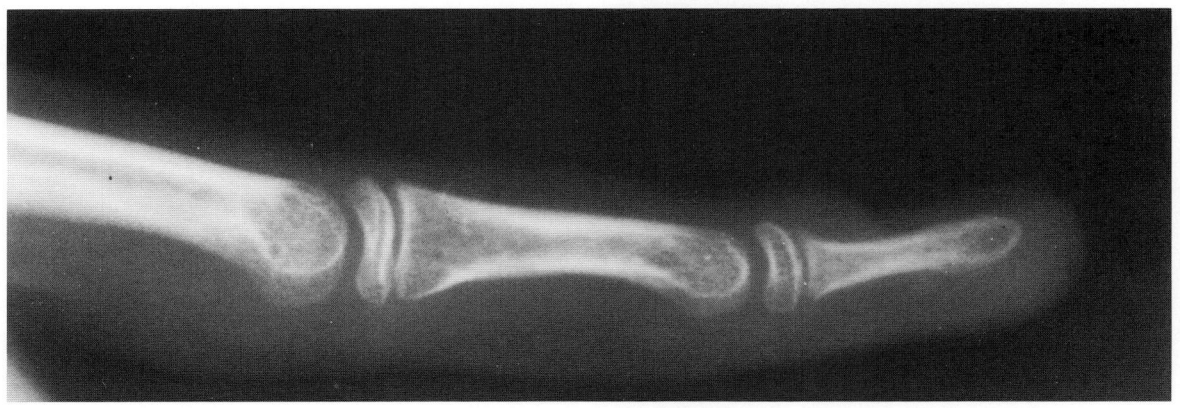

Fig. 23-14. A type I fracture through the distal phalangeal physis (so-called Seymour fracture). **(A)** At time of injury. **(B)** At follow-up there is good alignment with no evidence of growth plate disturbance.

432 / Management of Pediatric Fractures

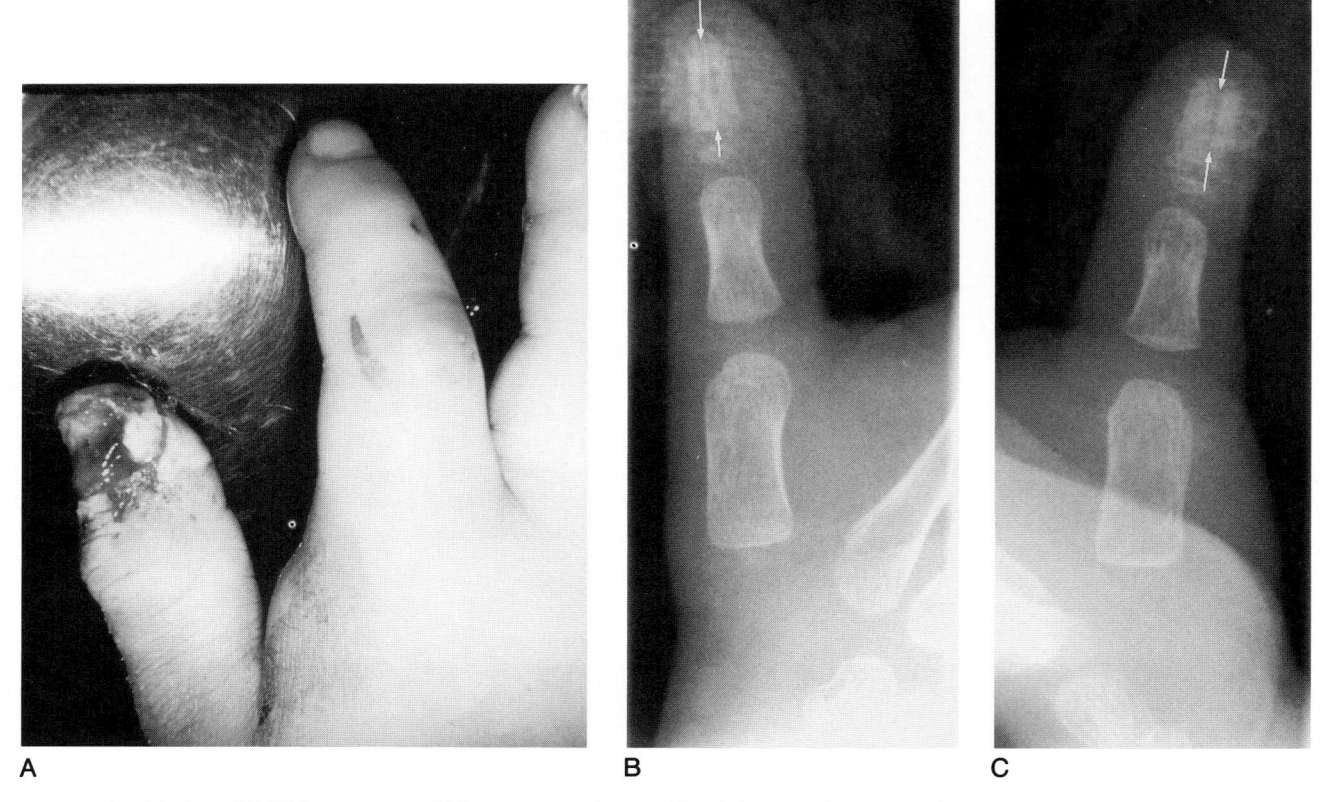

Fig. 23-15. **(A)** This two-year-old boy sustained a crushing injury to his thumb distal phalanx when a window fell on it from a height of 2 ft. **(B&C)** The distal phalanx is split longitudinally in association with a type I physeal injury. The nail was completely avulsed and unusable as a stent.

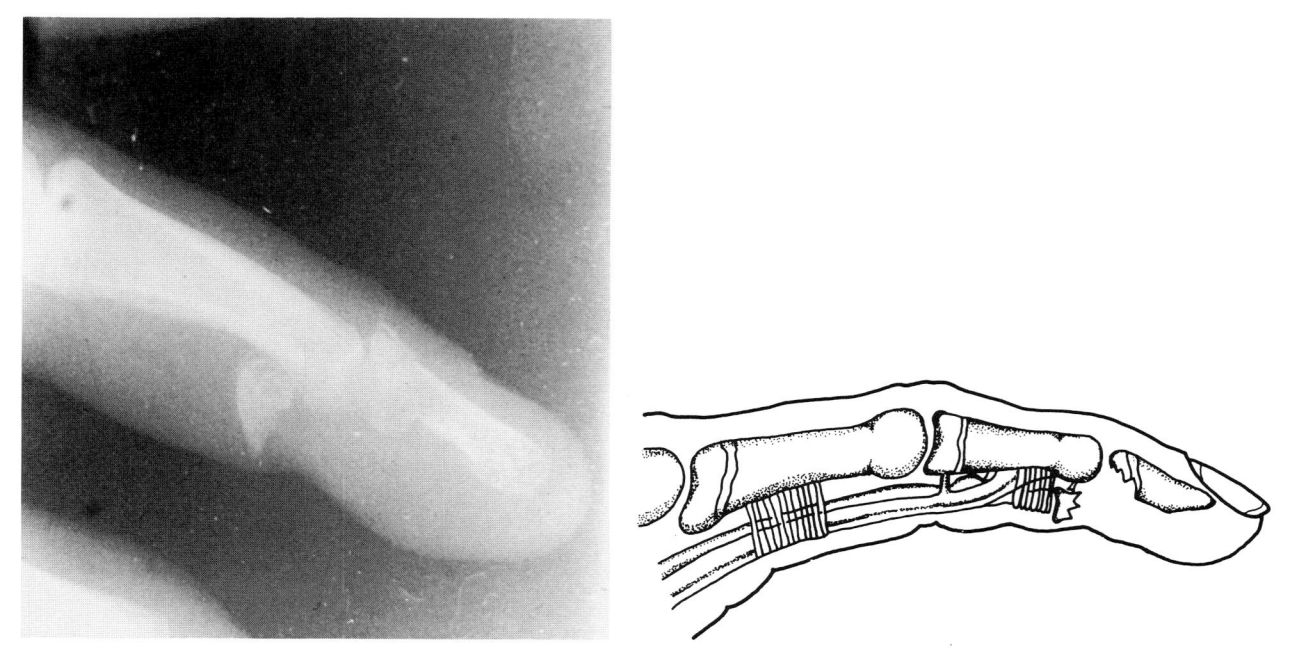

Fig. 23-16. Avulsion of long flexor tendon from base of distal phalanx with associated fracture type III of physis.

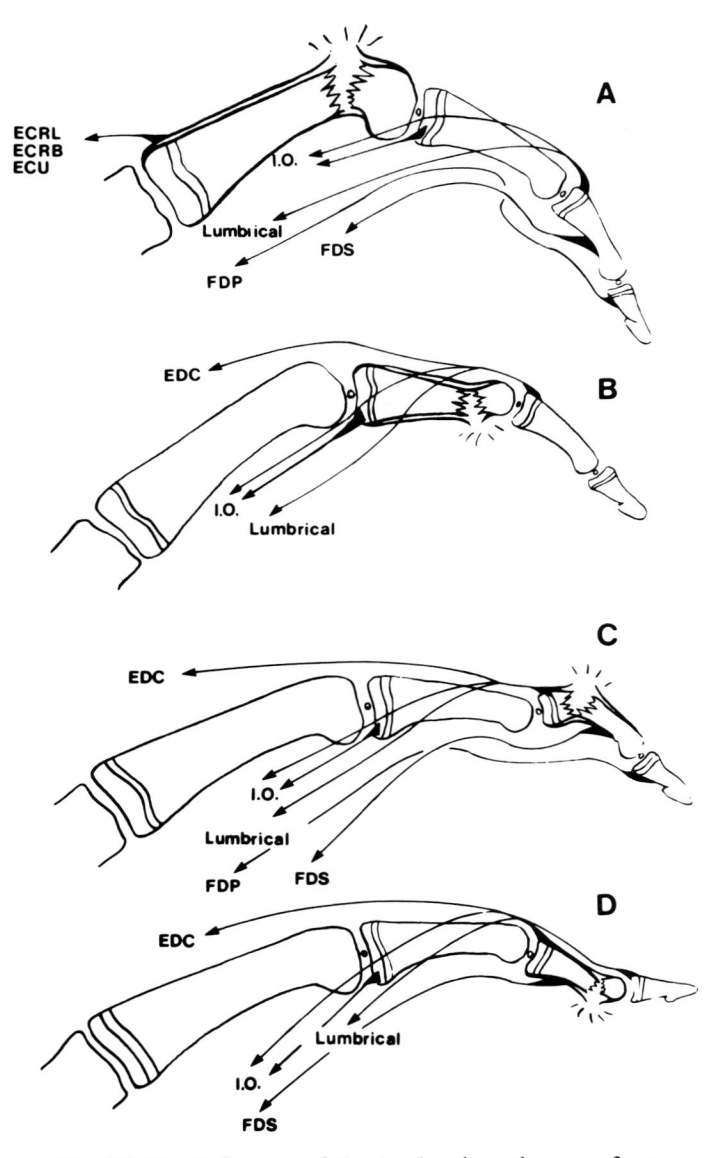

Fractures and Dislocations of the Phalanges / 433

Fig. 23-17. Influence of the tendon insertions on fracture patterns in the digit. **(A)** Fractures of the metacarpal neck tend to angulate dorsally due to the pull of the intrinsics. **(B)** Fractures of the proximal phalanx tend to angulate volarly due to the flexion of the proximal portion by the interossei. **(C)** Fractures of the middle phalanx in the proximal portion tend to angulate dorsally due to extension of the proximal segment via the central slip insertion and flexion of the distal fragment by the superficialis insertion. **(D)** Fractures more distal in the middle phalanx angulate volarly, again, due to the pull of the superficialis insertion along most of the middle of the shaft of the middle phalanx. (From Kleinman WB, Bowers WH: Fractures: ligamentous injuries to the hand. p. 163. In Bora FW Jr (ed): The Pediatric Upper Extremity. WB Saunders, Philadelphia, 1986, with permission.)

at the eponychial fold level. Spontaneous reduction can occur and leave little residual deformity. The only clue to the real nature of the injury is bleeding or protrusion of the base of the nail. Whenever this is present, one must assume an open fracture is present. Failure to recognize and treat it as such can lead to osteomyelitis of the distal phalanx, with resultant destructive changes to both the bone and epiphyseal plate.[27] Treatment of this fracture, the so-called "Seymour" fracture,[28] requires an adequate debridement of the injury prior to reduction. There is some debate as to whether the entire nail needs to be removed for treatment, but certainly the proximal edge often needs to be trimmed to gain exposure to the proximal metaphysis for an adequate irrigation and debridement. Once the wound has been debrided, the fracture can usually be reduced by extension of the distal phalanx and splinting in this position. Retaining at least a portion of the nail assists in the maintenance of stability of this fracture. A short course of oral antibiotics is recommended for 5 to 7 days, and close follow-up is required to ensure that infection does not develop.[15,29]

The Adolescent Mallet Finger

In the adolescent age group, one more often encounters a type III physeal injury, with avulsion of a variable-sized portion of the dorsal aspect of the epiphysis (Fig. 23-7). Clinical appearance is that of an adult "mallet" finger. Treatment consists of a closed reduction with splinting of the distal interphalangeal joint in slight hyperextension with an aluminum splint or plaster. If the fragment remains displaced in this position, open reduction and K-wire fixation will be necessary. Although it has been shown in adults that as long as there is not joint subluxation, internal fixation is not necessary,[26,30,31] the added risk of physeal growth disturbance in the child makes an accurate reduction desirable. Open reduction has been recommended in the presence of joint subluxation or in the case of an incongruous fragment that represents greater than one-third of the articular surface.[26,29,32,33]

Middle Phalangeal Fractures

Proximal and middle phalangeal fractures biomechanically behave similarly. Both bones have the same bony architecture with articulations at both ends, and close apposition of the flexor and extensor mechanisms. The differing insertions of the various tendons influence displacement patterns (Fig. 23-17) depending on the

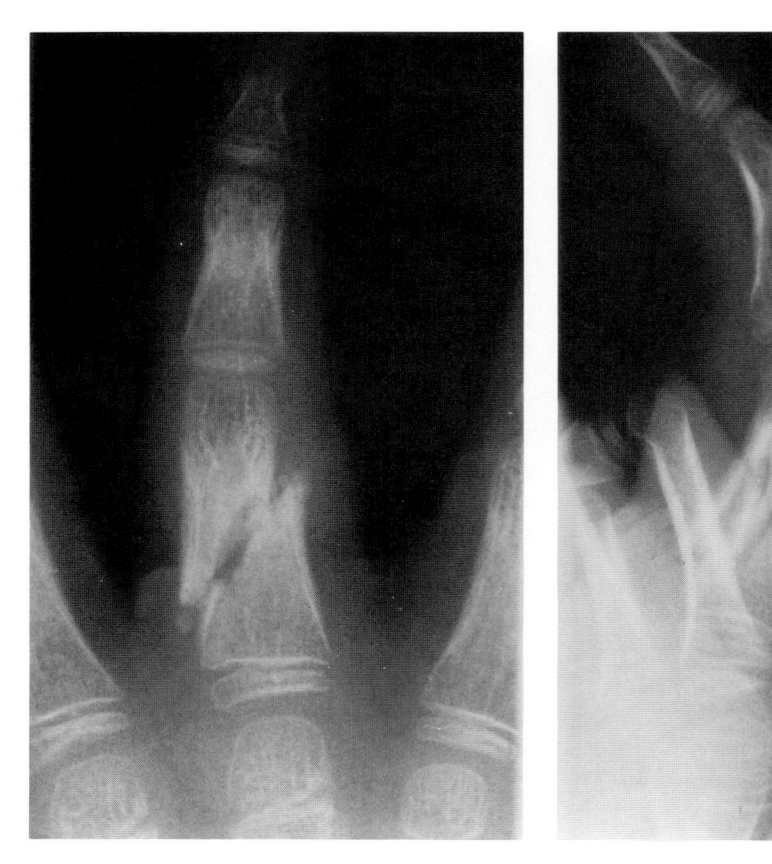

Fig. 23-18. Oblique fracture of proximal phalanx illustrating tendency to volar angulation and shortening. The proximal fragment is pulled volarly by the intrinsic attachment while the distal fragment is shortened and angled volarward by the extensor mechanism.

fracture site. The proximal phalanx tends to develop a volar angulation due to the flexion of the proximal portion by the interossei[11,34] (Fig. 23-18). The middle phalanx can angulate either dorsally or volarly depending on the location of the fracture, and the relative balance between the pull of the central slip on the dorsal side and the superficialis tendon on the volar side.

The middle phalanx is injured less frequently than the proximal phalanx.[29] Fractures of the shaft are often minimally displaced and require only a short 2- to 3-week period of immobilization. Neck fractures, however, can be deceptively difficult to manage. Recognition of the true magnitude of displacement present can be difficult, especially in the young child. Little residual angulation can be accepted in any plane, as the remodeling potential in this area is poor.[11] For this reason, unstable or unreduced fractures often require an open reduction with crossed K-wire fixation (Fig. 23-10).

Fractures at the base of the middle phalanx are usually physeal injuries. Displaced Salter-Harris types I and II fractures are treated by closed reduction and immobilization, whereas types III and IV fractures require anatomic open reduction if there is significant displacement. In contradistinction to the more commonly injured proximal phalanx, less reliance should be placed on the remodeling potential of the middle phalanx in children and one should strive for accurate reductions, especially in the mediolateral plane.[15,29,35]

Proximal Phalangeal Fractures

Type II Physeal Injuries

The most common fractures of the proximal phalanx are those that involve the physis. Twisting or hyperextension injuries result in type II fractures at the base of the phalanges (Fig. 23-19). The typical lateral deviation

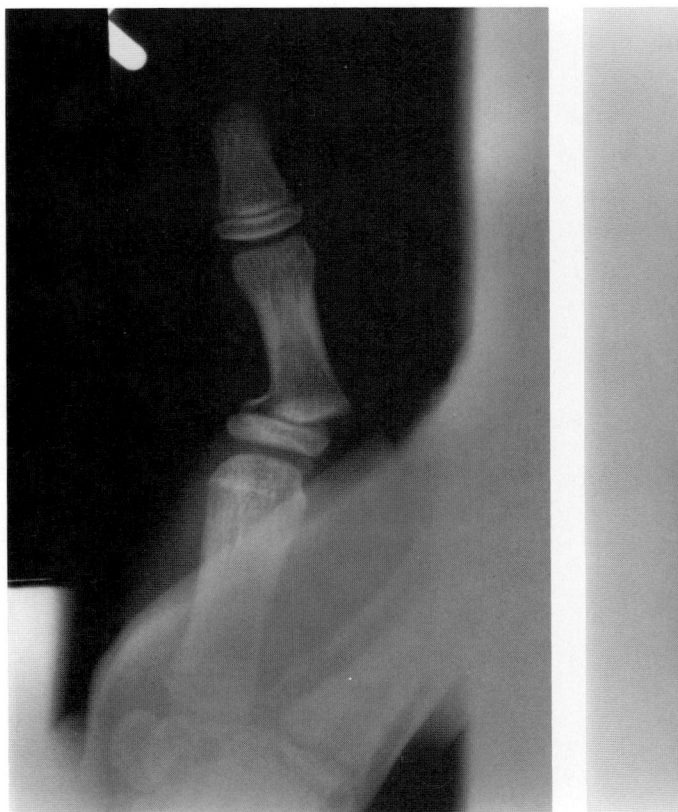

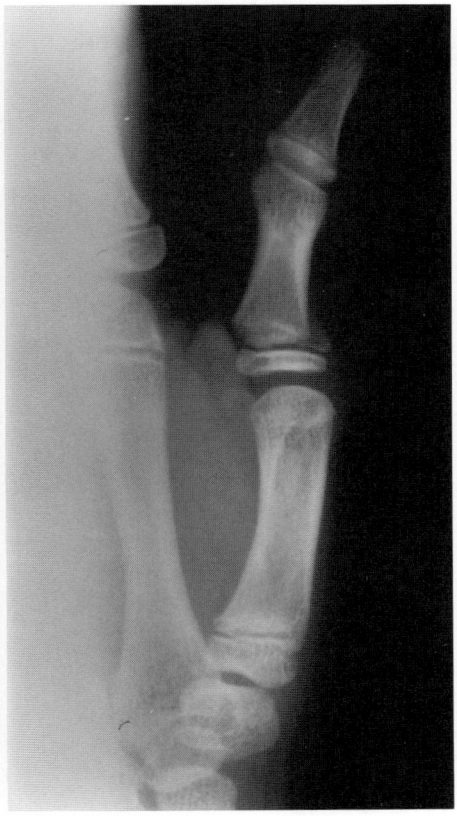

Fig. 23-19. A type II fracture of the physis sustained in an 11-year-old boy in a skiing accident is typical of that in young children with wide physis subjected to severe ulnar strain of the metaphalangeal joint of the thumb. In adults, this mechanism of injury usually would result in rupture of the ulnar collateral ligament—the so-called gamekeeper's thumb.

of the digit, commonly the fifth, has led Rang to dub this the "extra octave fracture" (Fig. 23-4).[15] Interestingly, a close inspection of the radiographs of these fractures often shows that the fracture line starts obliquely at the metaphysis and then traverses the metaphysis just on the edge of the physis, leaving a thin transverse wafer of bone on the metaphyseal side of the plate (a type 2C fracture in Ogden's classification system).[11] Closed reduction of this fracture is usually all that is necessary. Although the use of a pencil in the web space as a fulcrum for reduction of type II fractures of the proximal phalanx is recommended in some texts,[32,36] this places the fulcrum at too distal a position to be effective, as well as being a very painful method of reduction. A simpler method is to flex the metacarpophalangeal joint and then correct the deviation against the taut collateral ligaments.[3,37] Rotation is also easier to assess in this position. Immobilization is usually required for 2 to 3 weeks, splinting the finger against the adjacent digit in the safe position, usually with the additional protection of an ulnar gutter splint.

Types III and IV Physeal Injury of the Proximal Phalanx

Type III fractures are more common in the proximal phalanx than in the middle, and are due to ligamentous avulsion (Fig. 23-20). Any significant displacement implies articular incongruity and must be corrected. Open reduction and pinning of the fragment is often necessary. Type IV fractures are treated in a similar fashion.

Displaced epiphyseal fractures (type II or IV) that cannot be reduced closed are usually approached by a dorsal longitudinal incision, with splitting of the extensor tendon over the proximal phalanx or developing the interval between the central slip and lateral band over the

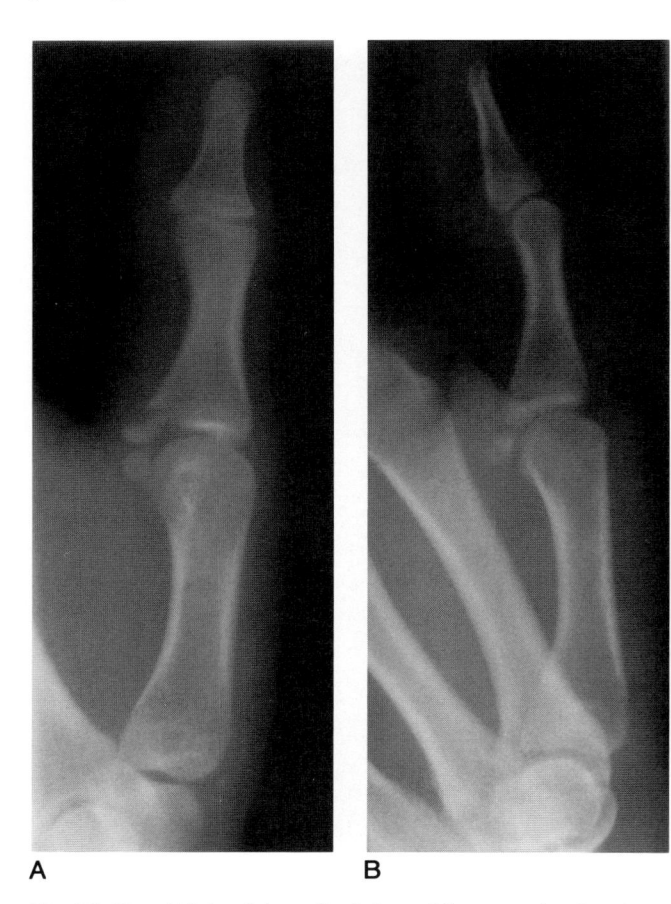

Fig. 23-20. (A) Avulsion of epiphyseal fragment by the ulnar collateral ligament requiring open reduction and internal fixation in a 13-year-old girl. Note the typical early closure of the phalangeal physis relative to the physis of the long bones. The thumb sesamoid in the flexor tendon is well formed and should not be misinterpreted as an avulsed fragment due to its smooth contour. (B) Lateral view of thumb shows no evidence of the fracture, emphasizing the need for several views of the finger in the presences of clinical signs and symptoms of a fracture.

middle phalanx giving exposure to the joint. Small-diameter K-wires (0.028- or 0.035-inch) are recommended to stabilize the fracture fragment, and can be cut off outside the skin for easier removal in 3 to 4 weeks. Protected motion is usually started at 2 weeks.[26]

Fractures of the Shaft

Shaft fractures are less common and often demonstrate a spiral, minimally displaced pattern that merely requires buddy taping to the adjacent finger. As always, accurate rotational alignment must be maintained. Transverse, displaced fractures will require a manipulative reduction and cast immobilization, and, if unstable, crossed percutaneous pinning is a valuable technique. This technique can also be used in unstable spiral fractures, drilling the K-wires parallel to the fracture line in this instance.[26] Traction as a method of dealing with phalangeal fractures in children is not recommended.

Fractures of the Neck of the Phalanx

Fractures of the phalangeal neck region can be deceptively serious injuries (Fig. 23-5). A fracture at this end of the bone should not be mistakenly treated as a metaphyseal fracture with expectations of the great remodeling potential seen at the base of the phalanx. It is not associated with a growth plate and little remodeling can be expected. The typical fracture pattern is a transverse neck fracture with dorsal tilting of the fragment. Problems may be encountered with both the recognition and treatment of this fracture.[1,26,39] Young children may sustain this type of injury while trying to pull their hand out of a closing door. Difficulty in obtaining adequate radiographs, especially lateral views, combined with an uncooperative child can result in significant dorsal displacement going unrecognized.

Entrapment of the volar plate in the joint locking the fragment in 90 degrees of rotation may occur.[9,11] Even when the fracture can be reduced easily, maintenance of reduction can be difficult to achieve and hard to assess radiographically. If doubt persists regarding the adequacy or stability of reduction, percutaneous pinning or open reduction may be required to prevent malunion.[20,26,29,40] Fractures left to heal with residual dorsal displacement result in the volar spike of bone from the shaft, causing a block to flexion of the proximal interphalangeal joint.

Intra-articular Fractures of the Proximal Phalanx

Intra-articular fractures of the proximal ends of the phalanges are by definition epiphyseal injuries, and are described above. At the distal end, fractures of the condyles are occasionally seen, and are treated as in adults, with anatomic reduction and pin fixation required if there is any displacement[29,41,42] (Fig. 23-10). This can often be performed percutaneously. If open reduction is required, a dorsal approach between the central slip and lateral band is used for the proximal phalanx, whereas a midlateral approach to the condyles of the middle phalanx is generally recommended. Two parallel K-wires

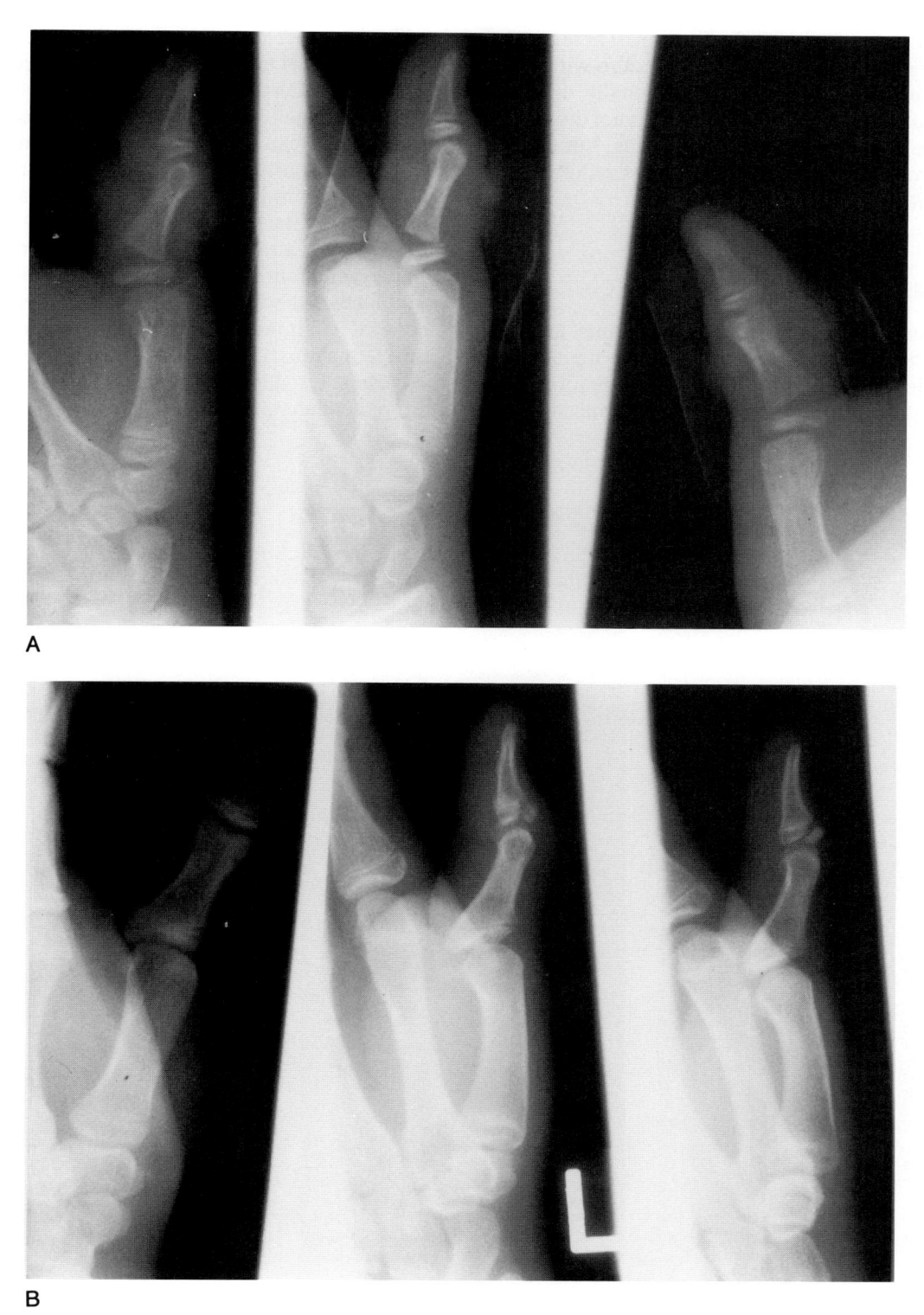

Fig. 23-21. (A) Type I fracture of proximal phalanx in a 6-year-old boy who sustained a crush injury in a car door. (B) Four years later he presented again due to an avulsion of the extensor tendon of the thumb and the physeal arrest subsequent to the previous physeal injury was discovered.

are drilled into the fragment for fixation. These can be cut off under the skin so as not to interfere with early active motion at 7 to 10 days.[29,38] Occasionally, one may see an oblique unicondylar fracture that is not displaced. This may be carefully managed by casting, but careful follow-up must be possible with frequent radiographic reassessment to detect displacement.[42,43]

Dislocations of the Phalanges

Dislocations of the interphalangeal joints are less challenging to deal with than those of the metacarpophalangeal joint (Fig. 23-6). The stable hinge joint construction of the interphalangeal joints is enhanced by the boxlike construct formed by the collateral ligaments and the volar plate. Dislocation occurs more commonly at the proximal interphalangeal joint, and at both joints the direction is usually dorsal. Reduction is easily obtained by slight hyperextension and traction combined with a volar directed push on the distal segment. Prior to reduction, however, radiographs should be obtained to rule out a physeal fracture that could become further displaced by such a maneuver. Rarely, irreducible dislocations are encountered, usually due to interposed soft tissue such as the volar plate or the collateral ligament. Chondral flap injuries have also been reported.[44-46] Obviously, one must open the joint to achieve reduction in these cases. Usually this is combined with repair of the ruptured collateral ligament.

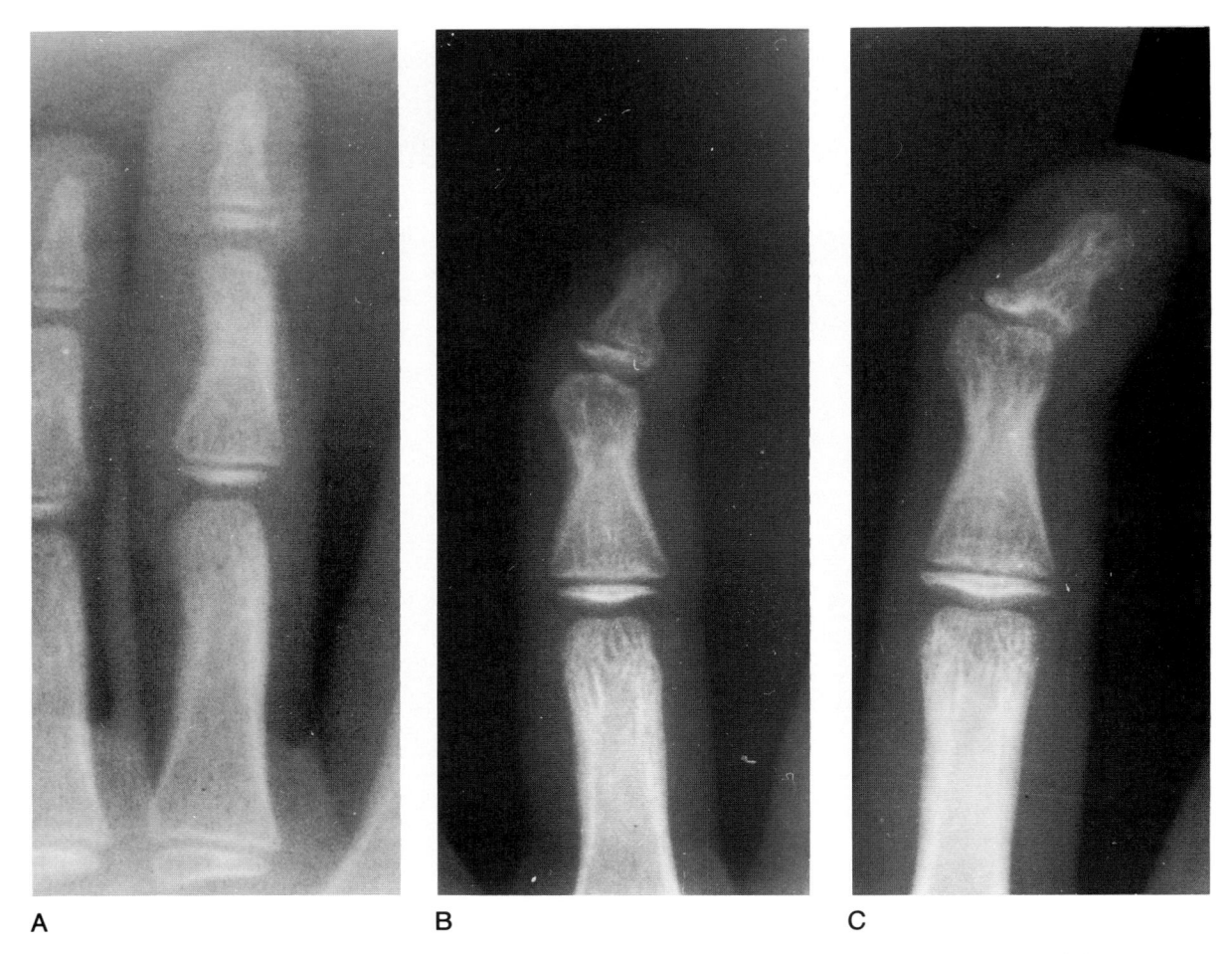

Fig. 23-22. Example of posttraumatic growth arrest. **(A)** Crush injury to distal phalanx with minimal bony injury. **(B)** Development of angular deformity secondary to growth arrest on ulnar aspect of physis. **(C)** Further angulation evident with growth.

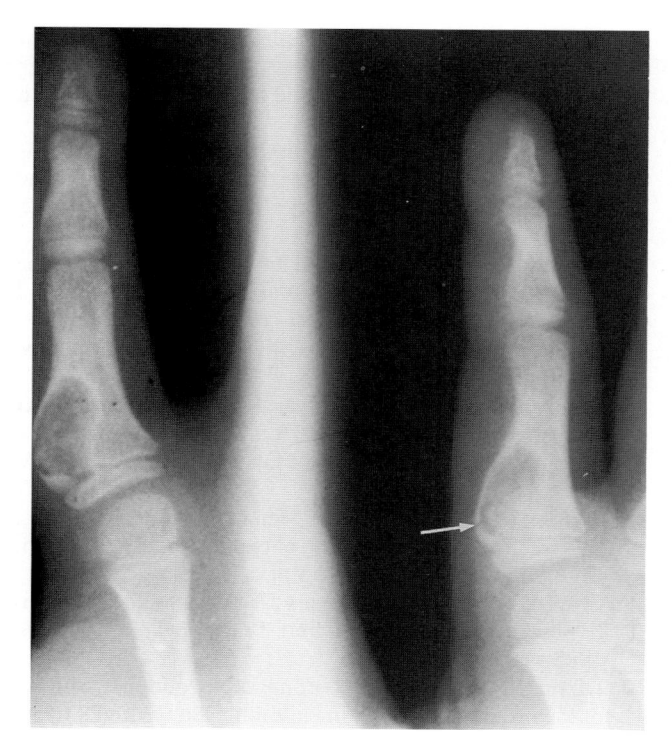

Fig. 23-23. Although uncommon, pathologic fractures do occur in the phalanges of children, most commonly associated with enchondromas.

rare complication in the hand unless the physis has been severely crushed (Fig. 23-21). Problems may be encountered if asymmetrical closure of the growth plate occurs. Further physeal growth leading to a significant angular deformity may then be encountered.[1,39] A complete cessation of growth at a physis can result in shortening of the digit, but this usually does not result in major functional or cosmetic deficits (Fig. 23-22).

Pathologic fractures of the phalanges are uncommon, but when they do occur, they are usually secondary to an enchondroma, the commonest bone tumor seen in the phalanges (Fig. 23-23).

SUMMARY

While it is true that the vast majority of children's phalangeal injuries will heal uneventfully with a brief period of immobilization, the few that do not can result in truly disabling problems and are a major source of parental concern. Recognition of potential problem fractures and timely intervention when necessary can prevent serious future problems from occurring.

COMPLICATIONS

Neurovascular complications are uncommon in phalangeal injuries in children and are only seen in severe open fractures such as partial amputations. The most common complication encountered is malunion.[11,29,47] The growing skeleton allows some improvement in deformities with remodeling, but it must be remembered that the degree of remodeling is by no means predictable and cannot be relied upon to salvage an unacceptable reduction. Rotational malalignment is the most potentially disabling malunion and will not remodel with time (Fig. 23-11). The best way to avoid this complication is to be obsessive about evaluating every phalangeal fracture for malrotation at the outset of treatment.

Articular stiffness and tendon adhesions are not often a major problem in the pediatric population. Parents should be warned that there will likely be several months of periarticular thickening around the joint after a dislocation, and some joint enlargement may be permanent.

With fractures involving the physis, the potential for growth arrest is always a consideration, but luckily it is a

REFERENCES

1. Barton J: Fractures of the phalanges of the hand in children. Hand 11:134, 1979
2. Borde J, Lefort J: Injuries of the wrist and hand in children. In Tubiana R (ed): The Hand. Vol. II. WB Saunders, Philadelphia, 1985
3. Green DP: Hand injuries in children. Pediatr Clin North Am 24:903, 1977
4. Hager DL: Hand injuries in children. Contemp Orthop 4:631, 1982
5. Hastings H II, Simmons BP: Hand fractures in children. Clin Orthop 188:120, 1984
6. Herndon JH: Hand injuries: special considerations in children. Emerg Med Clin North Am 3:405, 1985
7. Landin LA: Fracture patterns in children: analysis of 8682 fractures with special reference to incidence, etiology and secular changes in a Swedish urban population 1950–1979. Acta Orthop Scand, suppl 54:202, 1983
8. Lindsay WK: Hand injuries in children. Clin Plast Surg 3:65, 1976
9. Wood VE: Fractures of the hand in children. Orthop Clin North Am 7:527, 1976
10. Worloch PH, Stower MJ: The incidence and pattern of hand fractures in children. J Hand Surg 11B:198, 1986

11. Ogden JA: Skeletal Injury in the Child. 2nd Ed. WB Saunders, Philadelphia, 1990
12. Greulich WW, Pyle SI: Radiographic Atlas of Skeletal Development of the Hand and Wrist. 2nd Ed. Stanford University Press, Stanford, CA, 1959
13. Bogumill GP: A morphologic study of the relationship of collateral ligaments to growth plates in the digits. J Hand Surg 8:74, 1983
14. Hankin FM, Janda DH: Tendon and ligament attachments in relationship to growth plates in a child's hand. J Hand Surg [Br] 14:315, 1989
15. Rang M: Children's Fractures. 2nd Ed. JB Lippincott, Philadelphia, 1983
16. Wood VE: Fractures of the hand in children. Orthop Clin North Am 7:527, 1976
17. Salter RB, Harris WR: Injuries involving the epiphyseal plate. J Bone Joint Surg [Am] 45:587, 1963
18. Eaton RG: Joint Injuries of the Hand. Charles C Thomas, Springfield, IL, 1971
19. Dykes RG: Kirner's deformity of the little finger. J Bone Joint Surg [Br] 60:58, 1978
20. Leonard MH, Dubravicik P: Management of fractured fingers in the child. Clin Orthop 73:160, 1970
21. Illingworth CM: Trapped fingers and amputated finger tips in children. J Pediatr Surg 9:853, 1974
22. Metcalf W, Whalen WP: Salvage of the injured distal phalanx. Clin Orthop 13:114, 1959
23. Sandzen SC: Management of the acute fingertip injury in the child. Hand 6:190, 1974
24. Ashbell TS, Kleinert HW, Putcha SM: The deformed fingernail: a frequent result of failure to repair nailbed injuries. J Trauma 7:177, 1967
25. Zook EG: Nail bed injuries. Hand Clin 1:701, 1985
26. Campbell RM Jr: Operative treatment of fractures and dislocations of the hand and wrist region in children. Orthop Clin North Am 21:217, 1990
27. Engber WD, Clancy WG: Traumatic avulsion of the fingernail associated with injury to the phalangeal epiphyseal plate. J Bone Joint Surg [Am] 60:713, 1978
28. Seymour N: Juxta-epiphyseal fractures of the terminal phalanx of the finger. J Bone Joint Surg [Br] 48:347, 1966
29. O'Brien ET: Fractures of the hand and wrist region. In Rockwood CA, Wilkins KE, King RE (eds): Fractures in Children. 3rd Ed. JB Lippincott, Philadelphia, 1991
30. Lee MLH: Intra-articular and periarticular fractures of the phalanges. J Bone Joint Surg [Br] 45:103, 1963
31. Wehbe MA, Schneider LH: Mallet fractures. J Bone Joint Surg [Am] 66:658, 1984
32. Wood VE: Fractures of the hand in children. Orthop Clin North Am 7:527, 1976
33. Stark HH, Gainor BJ, Ashworth CR, et al: Operative treatment of intra-articular fractures of the dorsal aspect of the distal phalanx of digits. J Bone Joint Surg [Am] 69:892, 1987
34. Coonrad RW, Pohlman MH: Impacted fractures in the proximal portion of the proximal phalanx of the finger. J Bone Joint Surg [Am] 51:1291, 1969
35. Blount WP: Fractures in Children. Williams & Wilkins, Baltimore, 1955
36. Sandzen SC: Atlas of Wrist and Hand Fractures. PSG Publishers, Littleton, MA, 1979
37. Flatt AE: The Care of Minor Hand Injuries. 3rd Ed. CV Mosby, St. Louis, 1972
38. O'Brien ET: Fractures of the Metacarpals and Phalanges. In Green DP (ed): Operative Hand Surgery. 2nd Ed. Churchill Livingstone, New York, 1988
39. Crick JC, Franco RS, Conners JJ: Fracture about the interphalangeal joints in children. J Orthop Trauma 1:318, 1988
40. Dixon GL, Moon NF: Rotational supracondylar fractures of the proximal phalanx in children. Clin Orthop 83:151, 1972
41. McCue FC, Honner R, Johnson MC and Gieck JH: Athletic injuries of the proximal interphalangeal joint requiring surgical treatment. J Bone Joint Surg [Am] 52:937, 1970
42. Stark HH: Troublesome fractures and dislocations of the hand. Instruct Course Lect 19:130, 1970
43. Bloem JJAM: The treatment and prognosis of uncomplicated dislocated fractures of the metacarpals and phalanges. Arch Chir Neerl 23:55, 1971
44. Whipple TL, Evans JP, Urbaniak JR: Irreducible dislocation of a finger joint in a child. J Bone Joint Surg [Am] 62:832, 1980
45. Blalock HS, Pearce HL, Kleinert H, Kutz J: An instrument designed to help reduce and percutaneously pin fractured phalanges. J Bone Joint Surg [Am] 57:792, 1975
46. Clifford RH: Intramedullary wire fixation of hand fractures. Plast Reconstr Surg 11:366, 1953
47. Bora FW, Ignatius P, Nissenbaum M: The treatment of epiphyseal fractures in the hand. J Bone Joint Surg [Am] 58:286, 1976

24

Nail Bed and Crush Injuries of the Hand

Leslie J. Mintz

> Good judgment comes from experience and experience comes from poor judgment.

DESCRIPTION AND INCIDENCE

Crushing injuries of the hand vary widely in location, mechanism, severity of injury, and as a function of age. Young children often place their hands in places where digits can be crushed or amputated. Older children may incur blast injuries, such as gunshot and explosive wounds, with severe damage to the hand and associated organ system injury.[1] Wringer washers, industrial machinery and farm equipment can cause serious soft tissue and bone injury that may lead to long-term sequela if not properly recognized and treated.[2]

The most common hand injury in children is crushing of the distal phalanx[3-5] (Fig. 24-1). About 50 percent of nail bed injuries have an associated fracture of the distal phalanx (Fig. 24-2). Injury to the nail bed alone is much less frequent than nail or fingertip injuries.[6] Amputation of a digit can occur as a result of a sharp laceration or severe crush injury.[7,8] Under the age of 3, the hand is small and the compressive force is less. Over the age of 7, the child is better able to sense danger and has sufficient strength to pull the arm away. The proximal extent of the injury is inversely proportional to the child's age.[10] Injuries from industrial machinery, although covered with grease, are usually cleaner than farming or lawn mower injuries.[11]

ANATOMIC CONSIDERATIONS

The fingertip is composed of the distal phalanx, the paired digital vessels and nerves, and the flexor and extensor tendons. The perionychium consists of the paronychium (tissue surrounding the nail) and the nail bed (sterile and germinal portion) (Fig. 24-3). The nail sits in the nail fold (proximal depression of nail bed); the nail wall refers to the skin dorsal to the nail fold. The eponychium (cuticle) extends from the nail wall to the dorsum of the nail and the lunula marks the transition between the germinal and sterile matrices[12] (Fig. 24-4). Nail growth occurs at the rate of 0.1 mm per day.[13] If the nail is removed entirely, a delay of 21 days occurs prior to nail regrowth. The nail is abnormal in the first 3 months of regrowth. It is initially thicker, then thinner than usual during this period. Nail growth is slower under the age of 3 (Fig. 24-5).

Damage to the nail bed generally occurs to the middle and distal third, and 50 percent of these injuries involve a distal phalanx or tuft fracture.[6] A subungual hematoma results from bleeding of the germinal or sterile matrix. Laceration of the nail bed refers to any damage to the matrices.[14] In children, fractures of the distal phalanx usually occur through the physis. The nail plate generally remains attached to the nail and is dislocated at its base.

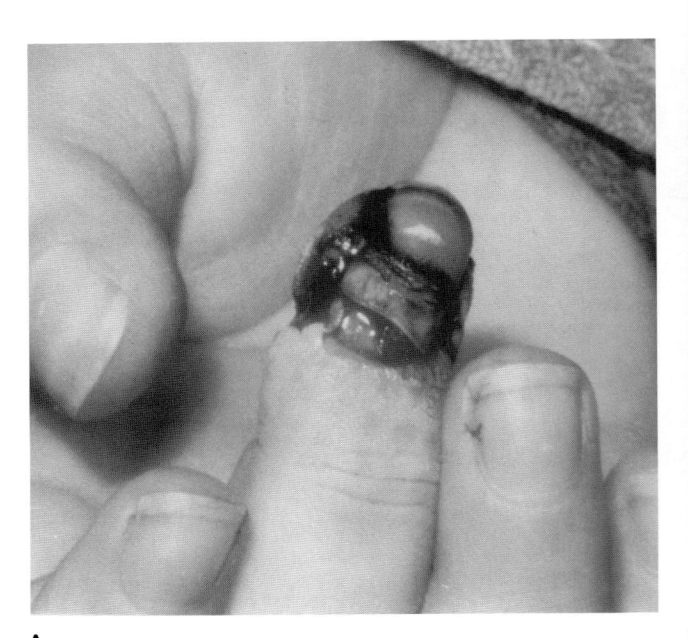

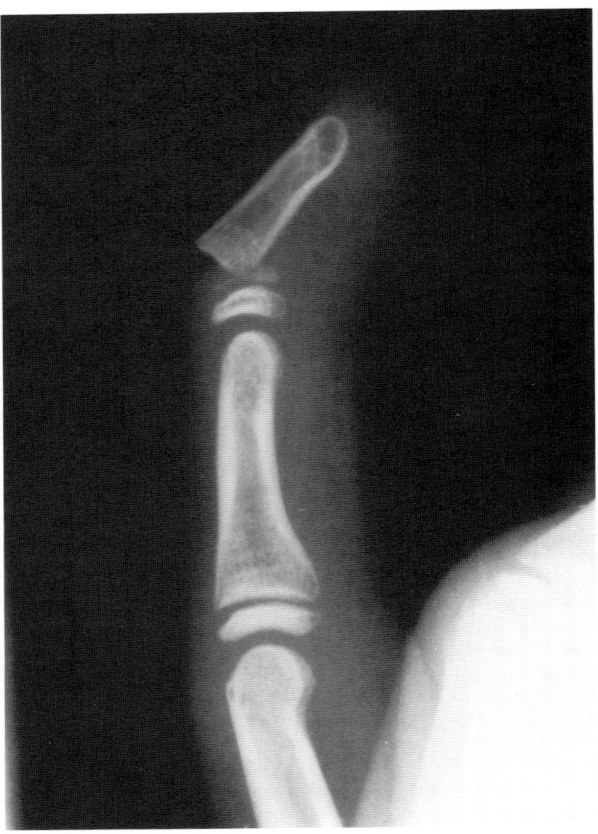

Fig. 24-1. (A) The "car door" fingertip with avulsion of the nail, laceration of the finger and a type I fracture of the distal phalangeal physis (B). This type of injury requires careful reconstruction to preserve the integrity of the nail bed as well as meticulous cleansing of the open fracture. In children, a general anesthesia is usually most practical. (B) The so-called Seymour fracture, a type I or II physeal fracture, which is frequently associated with nail avulsion due to levering of the nail from the nail bed by the displaced metaphyseal base of the distal phalanx (A).

The nail bed is thinnest just above the physis, which accounts for the associated injury with these types of fractures.[2] On a lateral radiograph, the body of the distal phalanx is flexed due to the location of the flexor digitorum profundus insertion. The epiphysis remains extended with the distal fragment dorsally angulated[15] (Fig. 24-6). In crushing injuries of the fingertip, the major damage is to the soft tissues. The tuft fracture that occurs is of little consequence.[16]

MECHANISM OF INJURY

Wringer injuries, first described in 1924, are now uncommon but can be devastating if unrecognized.[17] Injury to the hand itself is generally less relative to the elbow and axillary injury.[18,19] Radiographs of the hand are remarkable for soft tissue swelling, usually without associated fractures,[9] unless the thumb is extended as the hand goes through the wringer (Fig. 24-7). The subcutaneous tissue is separated from the skin with extensive hematoma formation.[20] Subcutaneous crepitation is due to cell wall destruction. It does not indicate bony injury or air beneath the skin.[17] Lawn mowers and other machinery can cause severe mangling injuries of the hand with amputation of the digits.

Crushing or amputation of the fingertips often result from a child's fingers being slammed in a door, being caught in the spokes or between the chains and sprocket of a bicycle.[5,8,21] Fingertips can also be severely lacerated by any sharp object such as galvanized iron fences.[7] It is very important to recognize that crushing or burning of

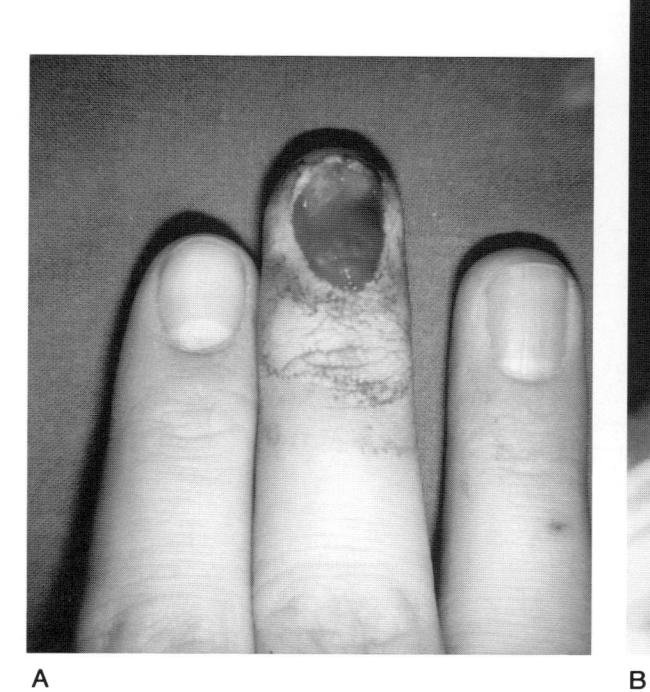

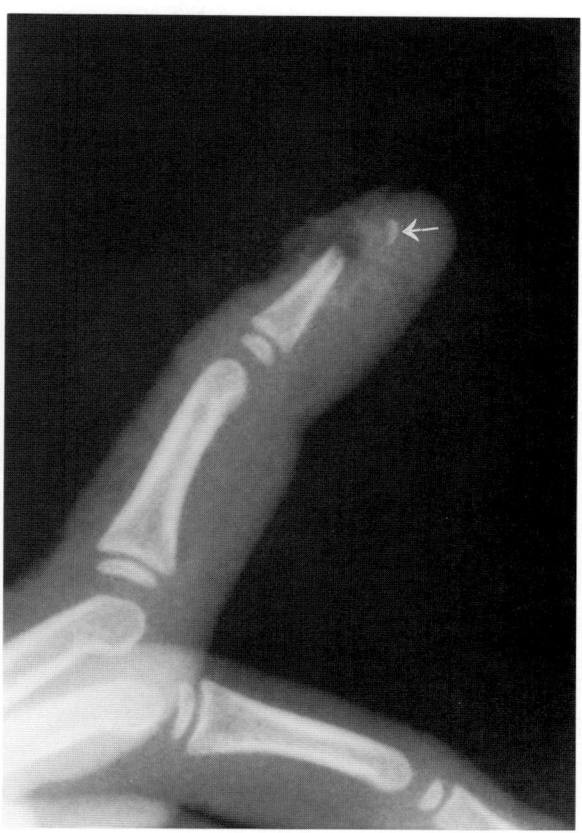

Fig. 24-2. **(A)** Crushed distal phalanx in which the nail has been lost and nail be repaired. **(B)** Fracturing of the distal phalanx is common and frequently open.

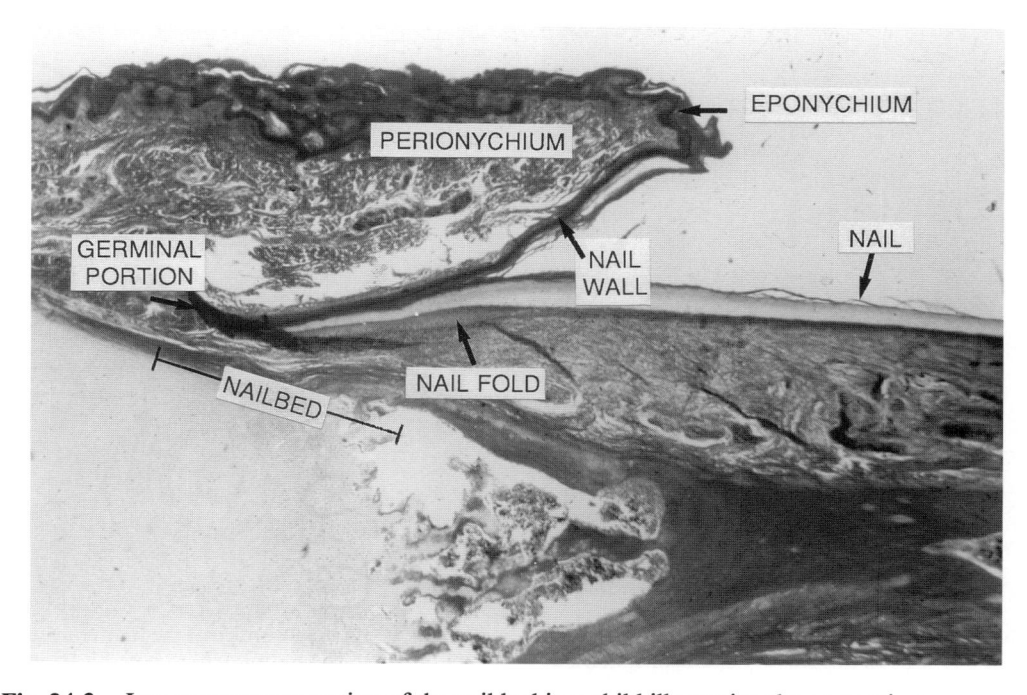

Fig. 24-3. Low-power cross section of the nail bed in a child illustrating the anatomic components.

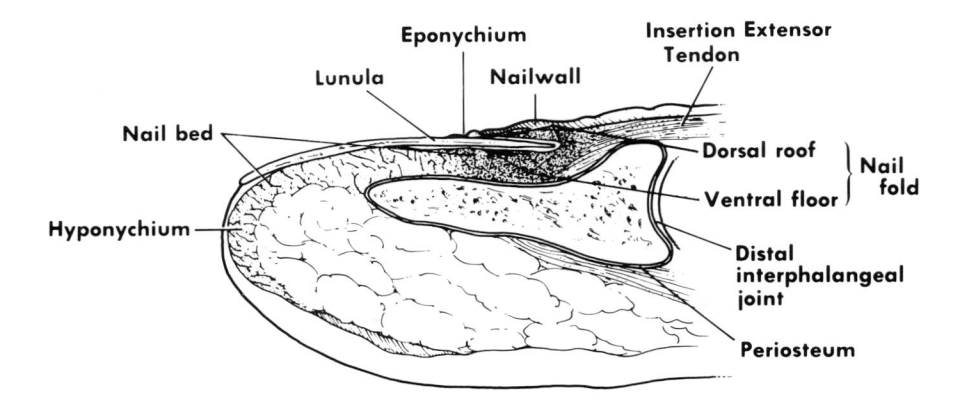

Fig. 24-4. The anatomy of the nail bed shown in sagittal section. (From Zook.[6] © SIU 1985.)

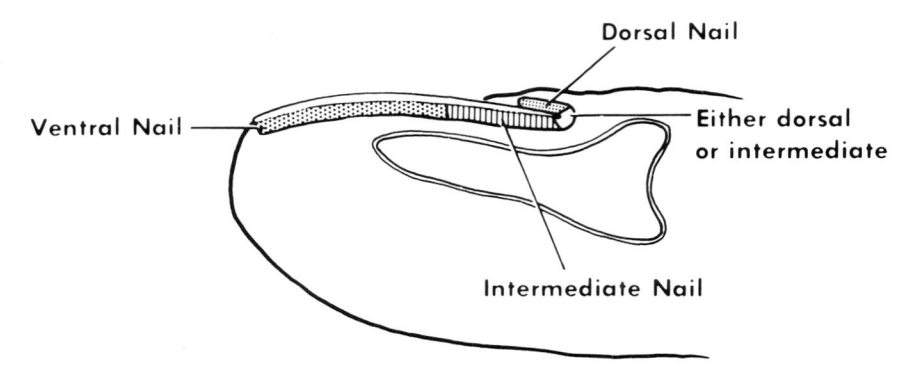

Fig. 24-5. The three areas that contribute to nail production in children. (From Zook[6]. © SIU 1985.)

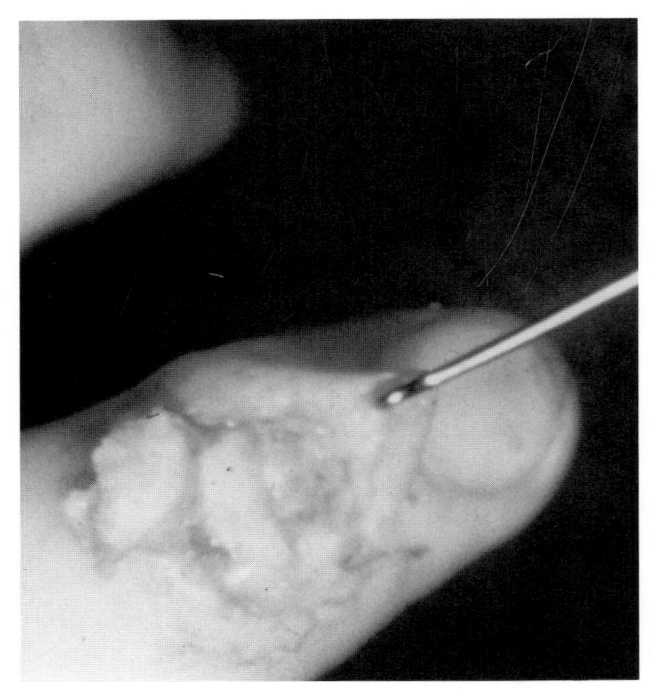

Fig. 24-6. A type I fracture of distal phalangeal physis with displacement of the epiphysis dorsally by extensor tendon attachment. When the overlying skin is disrupted, this is an open fracture and demands debridement.

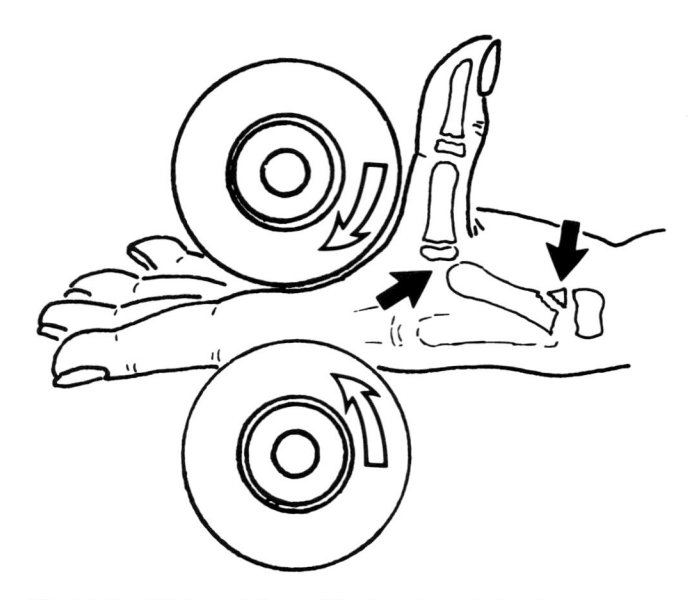

Fig. 24-7. Wringer injury of the hand results in a hyperextension injury to the thumb with a type I fracture of the proximal phalanx physis ulnar collateral ligament disruption associated with a type II injury of the thumb metacarpal.

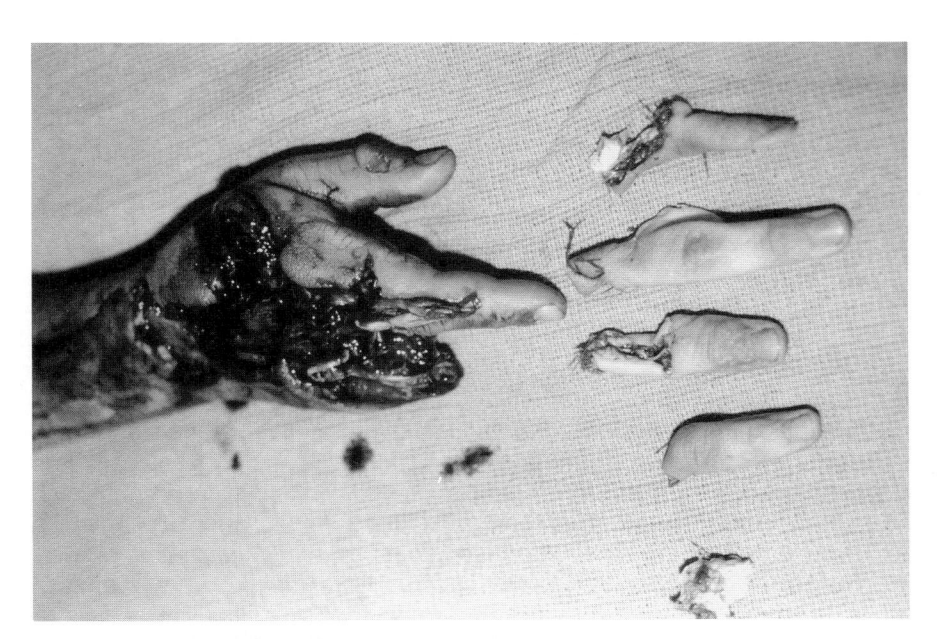

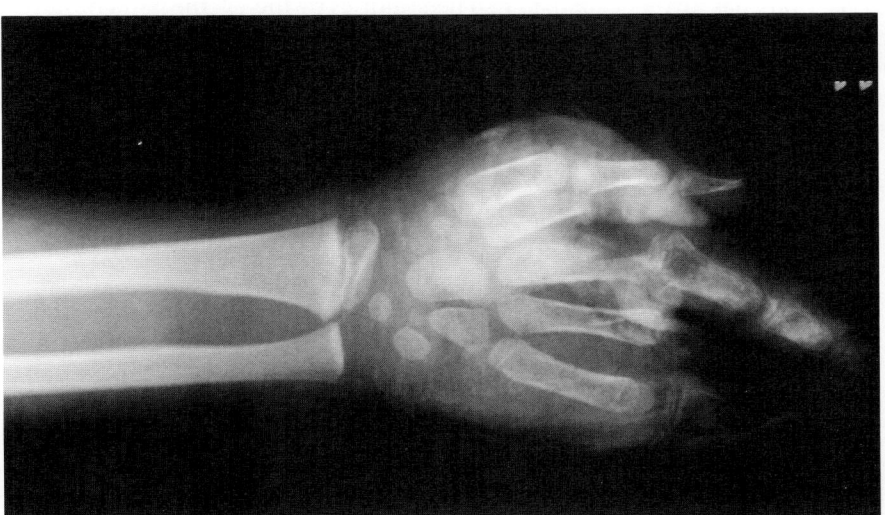

Fig. 24-8. A 6-year-old with severely lacerated hand with multiple fractures and finger amputations secondary to a lawn mower injury. (Courtesy of Dr. William Leighton, Phoenix, AR.)

the hands may also unfortunately be a presentation of child abuse.

Nail bed injuries may be due to local crushing of the nail and bone.[6] This can also result in lacerations of the nail bed by the nail itself. Wringer-type injuries occur when fingertips become trapped between moving rollers.[10,18] This leads to severe compression and abrasions of the hand and upper extremity.

High-velocity gunshot (>2,000 ft/s) or shotgun injuries to the hand cause severe comminution of fracture fragments and extensive soft tissue destruction.[11] In contrast, low-velocity gunshot (<2,000 ft/s) injuries cause little damage to the hand. In explosive injuries (e.g., firecrackers), thermal damage accompanies the soft tissue and bony injuries.[23] Lawn mowers and other farm equipment can severely mangle the hand and amputate digits (Fig. 24-8).

CLASSIFICATION

The classification of fingertip injuries has been described by O'Brien and Zook[6,16] (Table 24-1). No classification system has been developed for severe crushing

TABLE 24-1. Classification of Fingertip Injuries in Children

INCREASING SEVERITY →
1. Subungual hematoma
2. Basal nail avulsion
3. Nail bed laceration
4. Crushing or grinding injury

injuries of the hand. O'Brien has classified fingertip injuries according to increasing injury severity: *first*, a subungual hematoma; *second*, a basal nail avulsion where the nail plate lies atop the nail fold; *third*, a nail bed laceration, either longitudinal or transverse, where the intact nail bed is divided by the lacerated nail; and *fourth*, the most severe, a crushing or grinding injury[16] (Fig. 24-9). Zook has further classified nail bed injuries by the pattern of this injury.[6] Simple linear lacerations result from sharp objects. Stellate or crushing injuries of the nail bed are due to heavy objects. Avulsion injuries occur secondary to heavy sharp objects.

Fractures of the distal phalanx, which are associated with nail bed injuries are usually Salter-Harris type I or II in preadolescents. In adolescents, a Salter-Harris type III fracture can result, resembling the mallet finger injury which occurs in adults.[2] These injuries result from hyperflexion of the distal phalanx (Fig. 24-10).

PHYSICAL EXAMINATION

Assessment of crushing injuries to the hand may be difficult with an awake and crying child. With the child asleep, the hand will rest in a position that allows identification of the tendon injuries.[24,25] The examination should always be performed with the child supine and with adequate lighting. Skin color is an important indicator of circulatory disturbance. A whitish finger indicates arterial compromise; a bluish or purplish finger indicates venous disturbance. It is important to avoid mistaking filth or grease for vascular compromise.[11]

After vascular evaluation, bilateral radiographs (AP and lateral views) should be obtained. When assessing the hand position at rest, look for any abnormality in the normal cascade of the second to fifth digits. Flexor tendon disruptions will cause the digit to rest in relative extension. Dorsal wounds may overlie an extensor mechanism injury. Sensibility testing can be difficult, especially in a crying or very young child. Sharp/dull and two-point discrimination may be unreliable. The presence of severe pain may indicate an impending compartment syndrome, especially in closed, severe crush injuries.

Examination of the fingertip and nail bed is extremely important in physeal fractures of the distal phalanx. Any blood in the nail fold indicates disruption of the nail bed, and an open fracture. Significant swelling and abrasions over the distal interphalangeal joint may indicate complete detachment of the epiphysis.[21]

In wringer-type injuries, there may be severe abrasions on the forearm, or in the elbow or axilla.[10,18] The shearing force of the rollers causes avulsion of the skin from the underlying subcutaneous tissue and subsequent hematoma formation. Ligaments and tendons may also be disrupted.[26] Pain in the forearm may indicate flexor tendon rupture.[27] Avulsion of the thumb and lacerations of the web spaces or thenar and hypothenar eminence may occur as a result of the severe compressive and shear forces.[9,20] Radiographs of the hand are usually negative for fracture (Fig. 24-7).

In mangling injuries, for example, lawn mowers (Fig. 24-8), the injury severity is obvious upon inspection. AP and lateral radiographic views indicate the degree of bony disruption. Blast injuries from low-velocity weapons leave a small entrance wound and a slightly larger

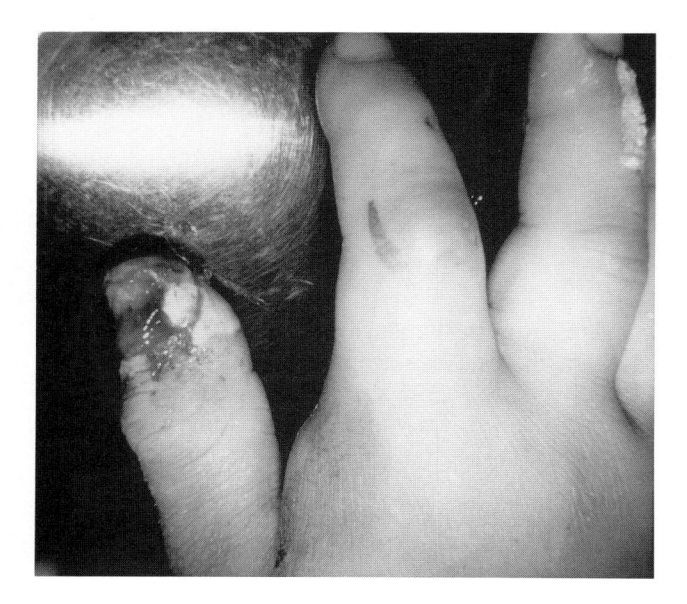

Fig. 24-9. Crush injury of the distal thumb in a 4-year-old boy as a result of being caught in a closing car door—a type IV crush injury.

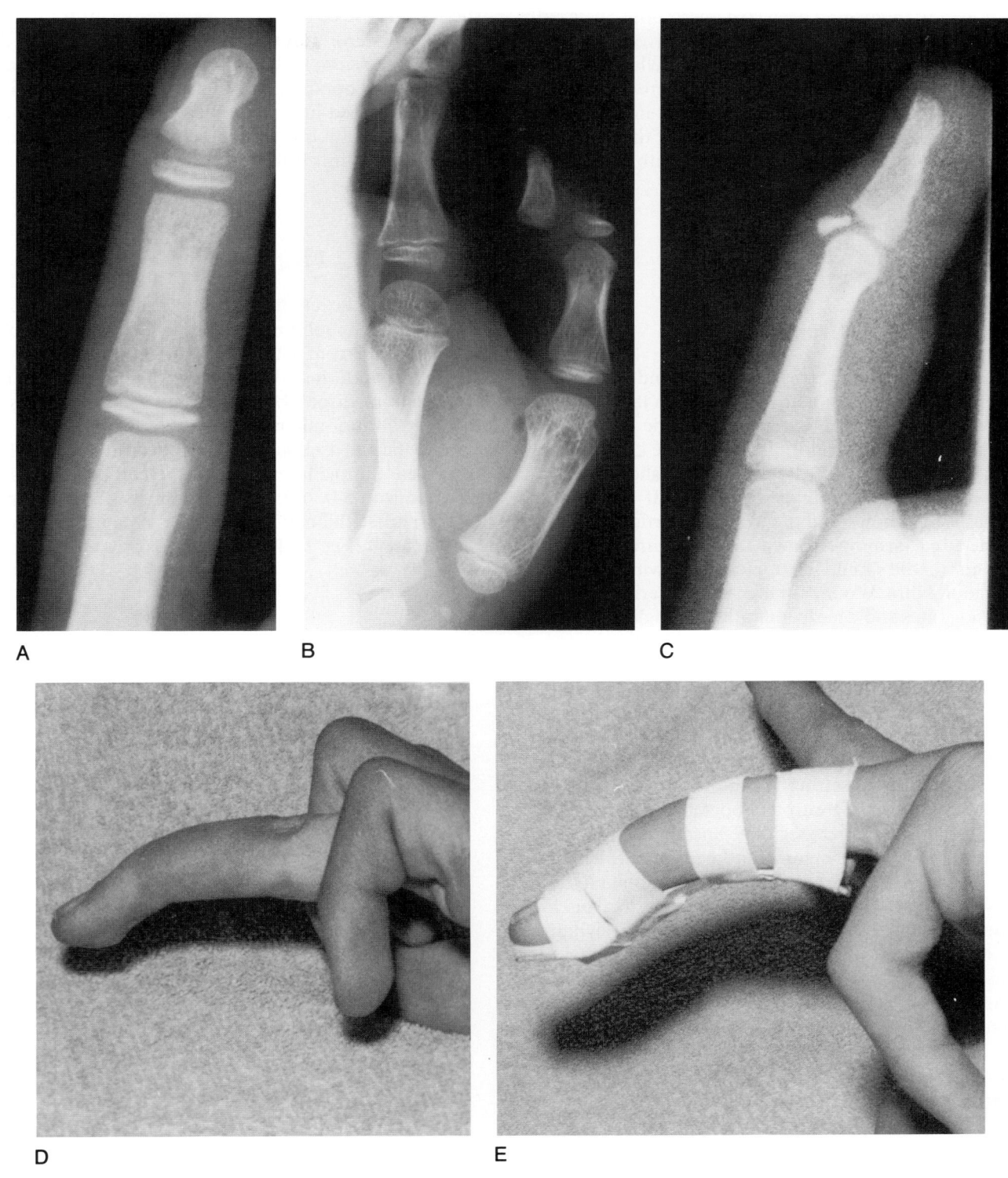

Fig. 24-10. Type I displaced fracture of the distal phalanx of the thumb in a 7-year-old boy secondary to a heavy object falling on the thumb. Note the **(A)** relatively innocuous AP view and **(B)** the marked displacement in the lateral view. **(C)** Avulsion of the extensor tendon involving one-half of the epiphysis—a type III physeal injury. **(D)** Mallet finger secondary to type I fracture of the distal phalanx and **(E)** reduced with volar finger splint.

exit wound, damaging deep structures along their path. In contrast, high-velocity weapons leave a small entrance wound, a large exit wound, and stellate skin lacerations tangential to the exit wound. There is comminution of the fracture fragments, which in turn act as secondary missiles, causing further soft tissue damage. Tendons may be stripped or severed, with shredding of muscle and fascia.[23]

TREATMENT

Crushed Hand

The treatment of any crushing wound to the hand should involve a complete assessment in the emergency department. All open wounds should be cultured and tetanus prophylaxis administered. If the child's immunizations are up to date, tetanus toxoid should be given for obviously contaminated wounds. If the immune status is not known and the wound is particularly worrisome (e.g., farming or lawn mower injuries), then the tetanus toxoid should be supplemented with tetanus immune globulin. Wounds at high risk for serious infection include bites and deep/penetrating, mangling, or crushing injuries with large amounts of devitalized tissue.[11] Antibiotics should be administered after cultures are taken. For most clean wounds, a cephalosporin will suffice. Contaminated wounds require gram-negative and anaerobic microbial coverage.

Although simple wounds may be treated in the emergency department setting, it is best to treat a child with severe injuries in a controlled operating room environment with general or regional anesthesia, tourniquet control, and proper lighting and equipment. Irrigation can be performed with intravenous solution and tubing or with pulsatile lavage.[11,28] It is important to avoid high pressure with pulsatile flow. Debridement of devitalized skin is the most difficult decision. Skin-edge pallor after the tourniquet has been deflated for 5 minutes indicates nonviability. Very little soft tissue in the hand is expendable; thus, it is best to be very conservative initially. Tendons should be debrided only if shredded. Stabilization of fractures with K-wire fixation maintains the integrity of neurovascular repairs and prevents further shortening of damaged soft tissues.

After initial treatment of these injuries, the hand should be placed in a position of function.[5,28] Placing fluffed gauze between the fingers and on the palmar and dorsal surfaces of the hand provides a bulky dressing over which Kling or Kerlix gauze can be wrapped. This should then be covered with a plaster splint (or cast in young children). The wrist should be placed in 15 degrees of extension, and the thumb should be maximally abducted and opposed. The metacarpophalangeal joints should be placed in 45 to 90 degrees of flexion and the interphalangeal joints should be in 10 to 20 degrees of flexion — the "intrinsic plus" position.

Fingertip Injuries

For the less severe fingertip injuries, the treatment is much simpler. Subungual hematomas, which involve less than 25 percent of the nail bed should be treated with sterile preparation of the finger and application of a hot paper clip or disposable electrocautery to the nail surface.[6,14,20] If more than 25 percent of the nail bed is involved, the nail itself should be removed and the nail bed inspected. Simple lacerations of the nail bed should be repaired with 5-0, 6-0, or 7-0 chromic suture. Avulsion of the nail at the nail fold requires repair after formal debridement (Fig. 24-11). If the nail is present and clean,

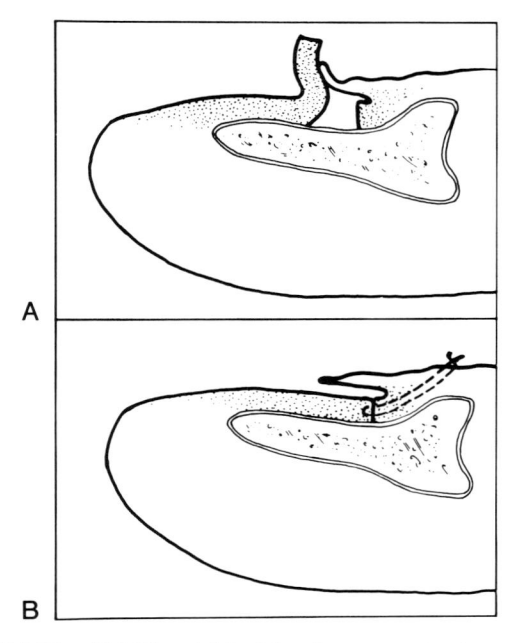

Fig. 24-11. (A) The nail bed has been torn in the proximal nail fold and stripped from the nail fold. (B) A horizontal mattress suture through the nail wall is used to replace the nail bed. The nail is then returned to the nail fold to mold the wound edges. The nail is then returned to the nail fold to mold the wound edges. (From Zook.[6] © SIU 1985.)

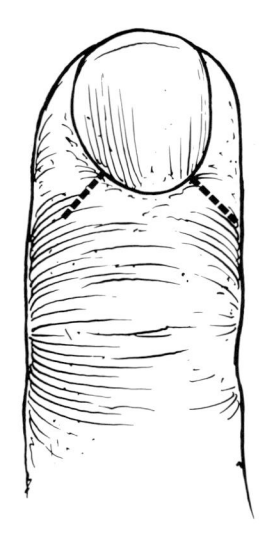

Fig. 24-12. When incisions are made in the eponychium, they should be made at 90-degree angles from the eponychium to prevent deformity. (From Zook,[6] with permission.)

it should be used as a stent. If it is not available, use silicone sheet, Adaptic, Vaseline gauze or foil from the suture package to prevent scar adherence and to maintain the nail fold (Fig. 24-12). In children, the nail bed is often avulsed with the entire nail bed attached. Repair consists of replacement of the entire nail and nail bed as a composite graft. This can be successfully grafted, even to the periosteum of the distal phalanx. The nail should never be left overlapping the skin at the base of the fingernail bed. Stellate lacerations are repaired with the same technique as simple lacerations. Careful attention to aligning fragments of the nail bed is essential to avoid permanent nail bed malformation (Fig. 24-13). Severe crushing or burst injuries may be impossible to repair and should be treated with dressing changes after loose approximation of the fragments.[5,20]

Fingertip Amputation

Amputation of the fingertip should be treated open (dressing changes without closure) in children under the age of 12. Pulp amputations should be reattached in

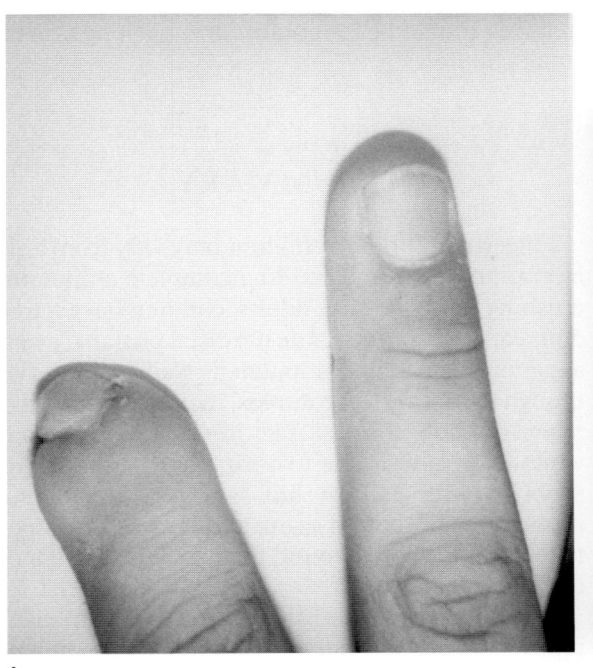

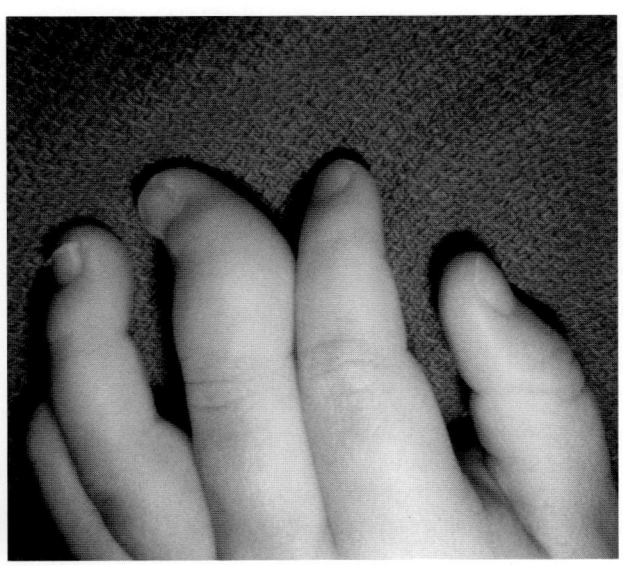

Fig. 24-13. (A) Nail deformation secondary to a crush injury of little finger that was caught in a door slammed shut by a sibling. The nail bed has been permanently damaged. (B) Deformation of the distal phalangeal physis following a crush injury by a car door.

young children as they will frequently survive. Amputation at the level of the middle or proximal phalanx, or in children age 12 or older, should be treated with primary skeletal shortening and closure.[14,24,29,30]

Wringer Injury of the Hand

Children with closed wringer-type injuries should be admitted for observation for compartment syndrome after initial evaluation. After radiographs are obtained, the hand and forearm should be carefully inspected for subcutaneous hematomas. These should be aspirated to prevent skin slough. Xeroform or Vaseline gauze should be applied to the abrasions and a bulky compression dressing, which extends from fingertips to axilla, applied over this. Hourly assessment of neurovascular function should be performed for the next 8 to 12 hours.[9,18-20,31-33] Open-wringer injuries require the addition of tetanus prophylaxis, antibiotics, and conservative operative debridement. Lacerations should be sutured where possible. Repeat debridements may be necessary and split-thickness skin grafts should be performed where the subcutaneous tissue is viable.[10,25,26,33]

Physeal fractures of the distal phalanx associated with nail plate avulsion should be considered open fractures. The fracture bed can be identified by flexing the distal phalanx. The fracture surface should be formally irrigated and debrided to avoid infection. If the nail is attached, the fracture can be easily reduced by hyperextension and a volar splint applied (Fig. 24-10). It is important not to remove the intact nail or instability may result.[2,5,6,35,36] K-wire fixation is usually unnecessary with an intact nail. If the nail is partially or completely avulsed, the attached portion should be removed. Any remaining nail fragment can be used as a stent.[15] Postoperative care includes oral antibiotics for 5 to 7 days and splinting for 4 weeks.

COMPLICATIONS

In closed crush injuries of the hand, failure to recognize an impending compartment syndrome can lead to disastrous consequences. It may be necessary to perform a carpal tunnel release, despite adequate initial treatment. Pain out of proportion to injury severity or increasing narcotic requirements should alert one to this possibility. Persistence of pain after initial treatment may indicate an occult navicular fracture. A navicular view should be repeated in 10 days if initial treatment may indicate an occult navicular fracture. A navicular view should be repeated in 10 days if initial radiographs were negative.[27] Pain present long after a closed crushing injury may indicate the development of reflex sympathetic dystrophy (see Ch. 2).

Open injuries involving bite wounds (animal or human) should *never* be closed or serious infection secondary to *Eikenella corrodens* (human) or *Pasterella multocida* (dog, cat) can result.[11] Children who present themselves for fracture follow-up with nail bed sutures placed in the emergency department should be taken to the operating room for formal irrigation and debridement if an infection of the fingertip has occurred. This will prevent the development of osteomyelitis secondary to an open fracture.[6] K-wiring a physeal fracture of the distal phalanx without formal debridement can also lead to osteomyelitis and/or premature physeal closure.[2,15,21]

Nail bed injuries should have urgent primary reconstruction or a deformed nail will result[38] (Fig. 24-13). Longitudinal nail grooves may also be due to stress, upper extremity ischemia, or direct injury. Transverse grooves are secondary to tourniquets and ischemia of the nail cells.[6,16] In fingertip amputations, a V-Y flap or split thickness skin graft harvested from the forearm should be avoided. Injuries are relatively straightforward to treat but should be immobilized with a long arm cast in small children.[24]

SUMMARY

Fingertip injuries in children may vary from a simple laceration of the nail bed to a complete amputation or crushing injury. Unlike adults, children have a tremendous capacity to regenerate the distal phalanx, even with a significant portion amputated. Nail bed injuries, although appearing less complex, require meticulous early reconstruction. Physeal fractures of the distal phalanx, while relatively simple to treat, can present long-term problems with osteomyelitis or physeal arrest if not appropriately recognized as open fractures. It is important to look for bleeding around the nail fold as a sign of this open injury.

Wringer injuries are less common today but mangling injuries are no less frequent. Simple closed wringer-type injuries require the expertise of a hand surgeon experienced in microvascular surgery. Long-term follow-up and complex reconstruction are usually necessary.

REFERENCES

1. Logan SE, Bunkis J, Walton RJ: Optimum management of hand blast injuries. Int Surg 75:109, 1990
2. Campbell RM: Operative treatment of fractures and dislocations of the hand and wrist region in children. Clin Orthop 21:217, 1990
3. Almquist EE: Hand injuries in children. Pediatr Clin 33:1511, 1986
4. Barton NJ: Fractures of phalanges of the hand in children. Hand 11:134, 1979
5. Wood VE: Fractures of the hand in children. Clin Orthop 7:527, 1976
6. Zook EG: The peronychium. p. 1283. In Green DP: Operative Hand Surgery. 3rd ed. Churchill Livingstone, New York, 1993
7. Griffin PA, Robinson DN: Pediatric hand injuries and the galvanized iron fence. Med J Aust 150:644, 1990
8. Perks AGB, Penny M, Mutimer KL: Finger injuries to children involving exercise bicycles. Med J Aust 155:368, 1991
9. Moseley T, Hardman WW: Treatment of wringer injuries in children. South Med J 58:1372, 1965
10. Allen JE, Beck AR, Jewett TC: Wringer injuries in children. Arch Surg 97:194, 1968
11. Brown PW: Open injuries of the hand. p. 1619. In Green DP: Operative Hand Surgery. 2nd Ed. Churchill Livingstone, New York, 1988
12. Zook EG, Van Beek AL, Russell RC, Beatty ME: Anatomy and physiology of the peronychium: a review of the literature and anatomic study. J Hand Surg 5:528, 1980
13. Baden HP: Regeneration of the nail. Arch Dermatol 91:619, 1965
14. Stevenson TR: Fingertip and nail bed injuries. Clin Orthop 23:149, 1991
15. Engber WD, Glancy WG: Traumatic avulsion of the fingernail associated with injury to the phalangeal epiphyseal plate: a case report. J Bone Joint Surg [Am] 60:713, 1978
16. O'Brien E: Fractures of the hand and wrist region. p. 319. In Rockwood CA: Fractures in Children. 3rd Ed. JB Lippincott, Philadelphia, 1991
17. MacCollum DW: Wringer arm: a report of twenty six cases. N Engl J Med 218:549, 1938
18. Adams JP, Fowler FD: Wringer injuries of the upper extremity: a clinical pathological and experimental study. South Med J 52:798, 1952
19. Posch JL, Weller CN: Mangle and severe wringer injuries of the hand in children. J Bone Joint Surg [Am] 36:57, 1954
20. Green DP: Hand injuries in children. Pediatr Clin 24:903, 1977
21. Savage R: Complete detachment of the epiphysis of the distal phalanx. J Hand Surg [Br] 15:126, 1990
22. Johnson CF: The hand as a target organ in child abuse. Clin Pediatr 29:66, 1990
23. Keinert HE, Williams PJ: Blast injuries of the hand. J Trauma 1:10, 1961
24. Herndon JH: Hand injuries—special considerations in children. Emerg Med Clin 3:405, 1985
25. Posch JL: Injuries to the hand in children. Am J Surg 89:784, 1955
26. Hardin CA, Robinson DW: Coverage problems in the treatment of wringer injuries. J Bone Joint Surg [Am] 36:292, 1954
27. Brown H: Closed crush injuries of the hand and forearm. Clin Orthop 1:253, 1970
28. Carter PR: Crush injury of the upper limb: early and late management. Clin Orthop 14:719, 1984
29. Illingworth CM: Trapped fingers and amputated fingertips in children. J Pediatr Surg 9:853, 1974
30. Rosenthal LJ, Reiner MA, Bleicher MA: Nonoperative management of distal fingertip amputations in children. Pediatrics 64:1, 1979
31. Iritani RI, Silver VE: Wringer injuries of the upper extremity. Surg Gynecol Obstet 113:677, 1961
32. Mason ML, Bell JL: The crushed hand. Clin Orthop 13:84, 1959
33. Poulos E: The open treatment of wringer injuries in children. Am Surg 24:458, 1958
34. Sandzen SC, Oakey RS: Crushing injury of the fingertip. Hand 4:253, 1972
35. Seymour N: Juxta-epiphyseal fractures of the terminal phalanx of the finger. J Bone Joint Surg [Br] 48:347, 1966
36. Kleinert HE, Putcha SM, Ashbell S, Kutz JE: The deformed finger nail: a frequent result of failure to repair nail bed injuries. J Trauma 7:177, 1967

25

Fractures of the Pelvis

Richard E. McCarthy

> The pelvis is a remarkable structure. Through its foramina pass many important nerves and tendons; essential arteries and veins transverse its notches; within its confines lie delicate organs; and under its arch passes all mankind, a notable exception being Julius Caesar.
> —Leonard Peltier

DESCRIPTION AND INCIDENCE

There is no other area of the child's body where a fracture can be associated with such a variety of potential serious injuries as in the pelvis. Rang[1] has characterized the pelvis as a suit of armour "when it is damaged there is much more concern about its contents than the structure itself." Pelvic fractures comprise less than 5 percent of pediatric fractures due to blunt trauma,[2,3] but are frequently associated with severe multiple trauma.

Trauma remains the leading cause of death in children over 1 year of age.[4] With mortality rates in children comparable to those seen in adult pelvic fractures,[2,5,6] it is essential that prompt attention be given to identifying associated injuries when assessing pediatric pelvic fractures in order to establish a definitive diagnosis and to set priorities for care.

ANATOMIC CONSIDERATIONS

The pelvis serves four primary purposes:

1. Protection for nearby urologic, gastrointestinal, genital, and neurologic systems
2. Attachment of truncal and lower extremity muscles and capsular joint structures
3. Support for the spine in the standing and sitting postures
4. The production of blood elements

The junction between the sacrum and the innominate bones are united by the dense fibers of the posterior interosseous ligaments of the sacroiliac joint. Horizontal fibers in the same complex join the posterior superior iliac spine to the posterior sacrum in the midline (Fig. 25-1). Tile[5] has made the analogy between these transverse components acting as the tension struts of a suspension bridge. The pillars of the posterior superior iliac spines are connected to the sacrum via the strong interosseous sacral iliac ligaments, which act as the multiple vertical suspension wires. This is even more true in the child's pelvis, where the pelvic ligamentous structure is much stronger than the adjacent osseous tissue, thus making sacroiliac dislocation a rare event in children. The anterior sacroiliac ligamentous complex is much thinner and weaker. The anterior ligaments join the sacrum and coccyx to the ilium and ischium and resist any external rotation forces on the hemipelvis. These may be torn apart in an "open-book" type of injury. In children, the strength of the pubic symphysis and attachment of the synchondrosis usually prevents diastasis except in very severe trauma, such as a tire passing over the pelvis. In the vertical shear fractures, the ligamentous avulsion of the transverse process of L5 may be the only obvious pelvic fracture seen from the anteroposterior (AP) view

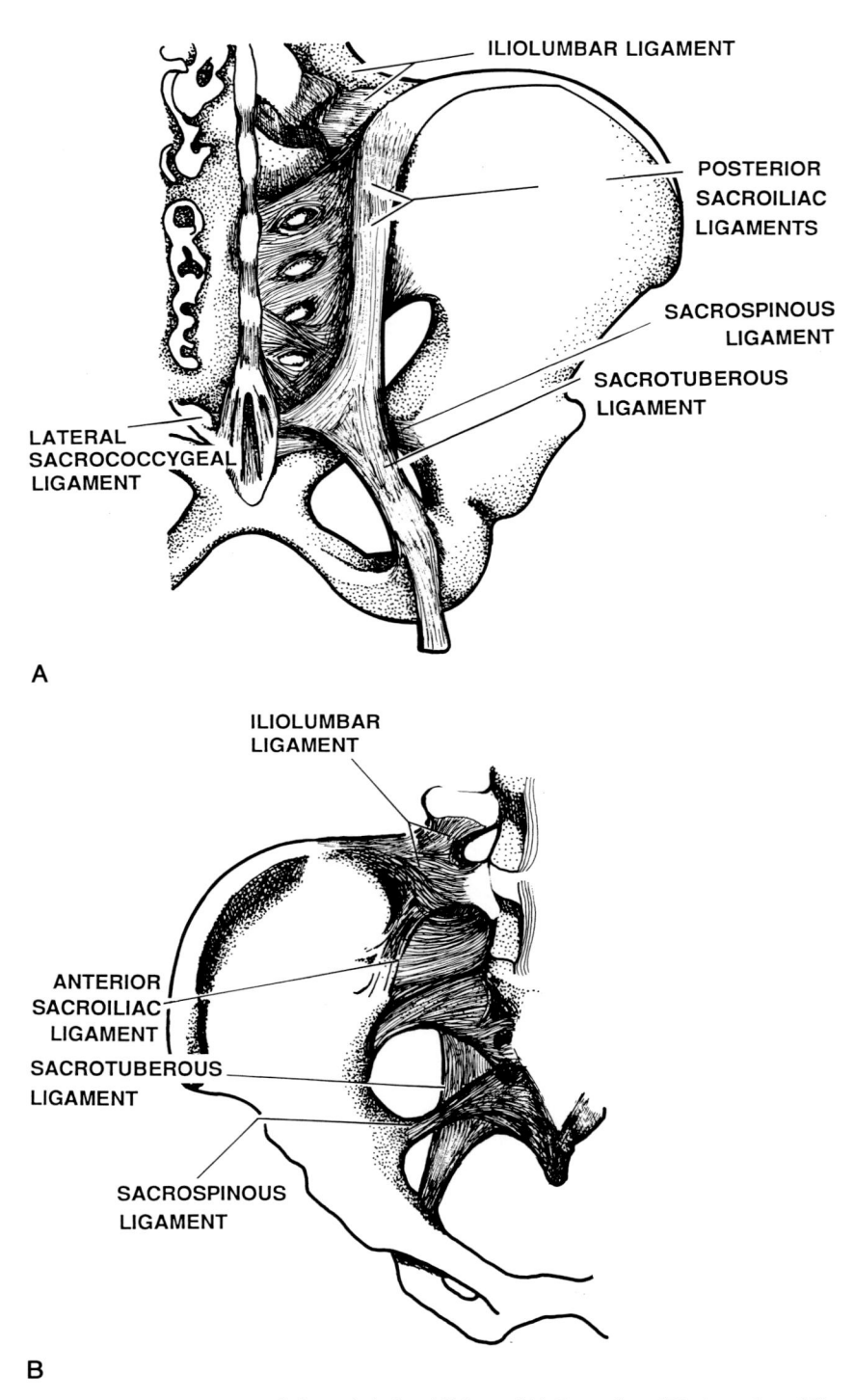

Fig. 25-1. Ligamentous structures of the pelvis in children. **(A)** Posterior. **(B)** Anterior. *(Figure continues.)*

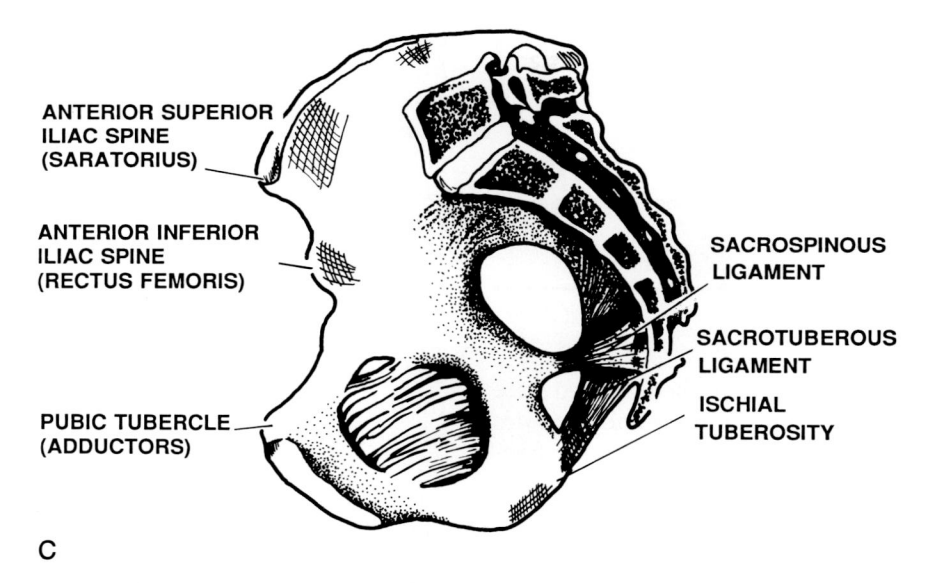

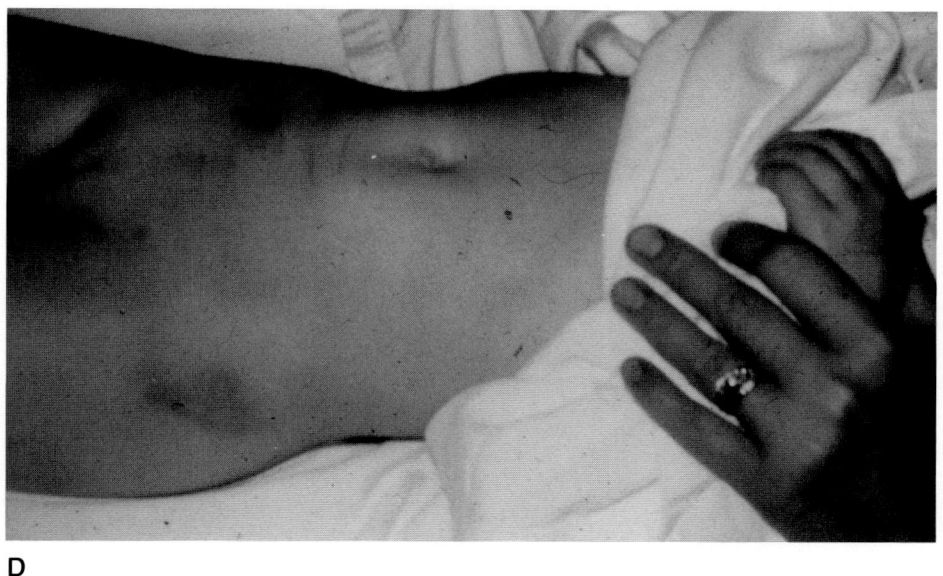

Fig. 25-1 *(Continued).* **(C)** Lateral. **(D)** This 7-year-old girl was run over by her father's tractor. The tire marks can be seen over the lower abdomen. No pelvic fracture was sustained due in part to the flexibility of the immature pelvis and soft ground on which the accident occurred.

on a plain radiograph because of the difficulty in identifying pelvic fractures through the lateral sacral masses. The avulsion occurs due to the iliolumbar ligament connecting the transverse process of L5 and the top of the ilium along the medial wall anteriorly.

The floor of the pelvis is formed by a strong set of muscles connecting the levator ani to the surrounding bony structures. It is also joined anteriorly by the urogenital diaphragm through which the urethra passes. This firmly anchors the urethra, making the urethra distal to this membrane more susceptible to avulsion injuries, such as with a straddle-type fracture. This can be produced by a sudden force applied against the perineum of the male urethra when straddling a motorcycle, motorbike, or snowmobile.[7] On the inside of the urogenital diaphragm, the bladder, in a deflated state, is

456 / Management of Pediatric Fractures

TABLE 25-1. Unique Features of Pediatric Pelvis

Anatomic
   Porous bone (increased haversian canals)
   Cartilage
   Growth plates
Biomechanic
   Increased plasticity (more energy absorption prior to deformation)
   Avulsion fractures
   Triradiate growth injuries
   Potential for remodeling

protected behind the pubis. In a half-filled or filled state it rises precariously above the pubic bone and becomes more susceptible to direct puncture from a bone fragment.[7]

UNIQUE FEATURES OF THE PEDIATRIC PELVIS

The pediatric pelvis has several unique features that distinguish it from its adult counterpart, as shown in Table 25-1. Immature cortical bone in the child is more porous, allowing for plastic deformation and greenstick fractures to occur.[8] The increased number of haversian systems with their osmotically loaded fluid filled canals allow for the major part of this plasticity. The plasticity allows for the absorption of a great deal of force prior to breakage (Fig. 25-1D). This implies that for a given force sufficient to fracture the adult pelvis, the child may sustain only a mild bony deformation. The effect of the traumatic forces upon the abdominal viscera may, however, be the same severity. Plastic deformation coupled with the increased elasticity of the joints in the sacroiliac and symphysis pubis can account for single fractures of the pelvic ring, unique to children.[1,9] The greater volume of cartilage seen in the growing bone, including that around the triradiate cartilage, adds to the buffering capacity for energy absorption and overall fewer numbers of fractures.[10]

While the growing cartilage absorbs energy, it may be injured at the osteochondral junction because of its inherent weakness. Avulsion fractures through an apophysis can occur with athletic injuries in adolescents and fractures extending into the triradiate cartilage or directly crushing the triradiate cartilage also occur.[9,11] Injuries to the triradiate cartilage exemplify the irony in

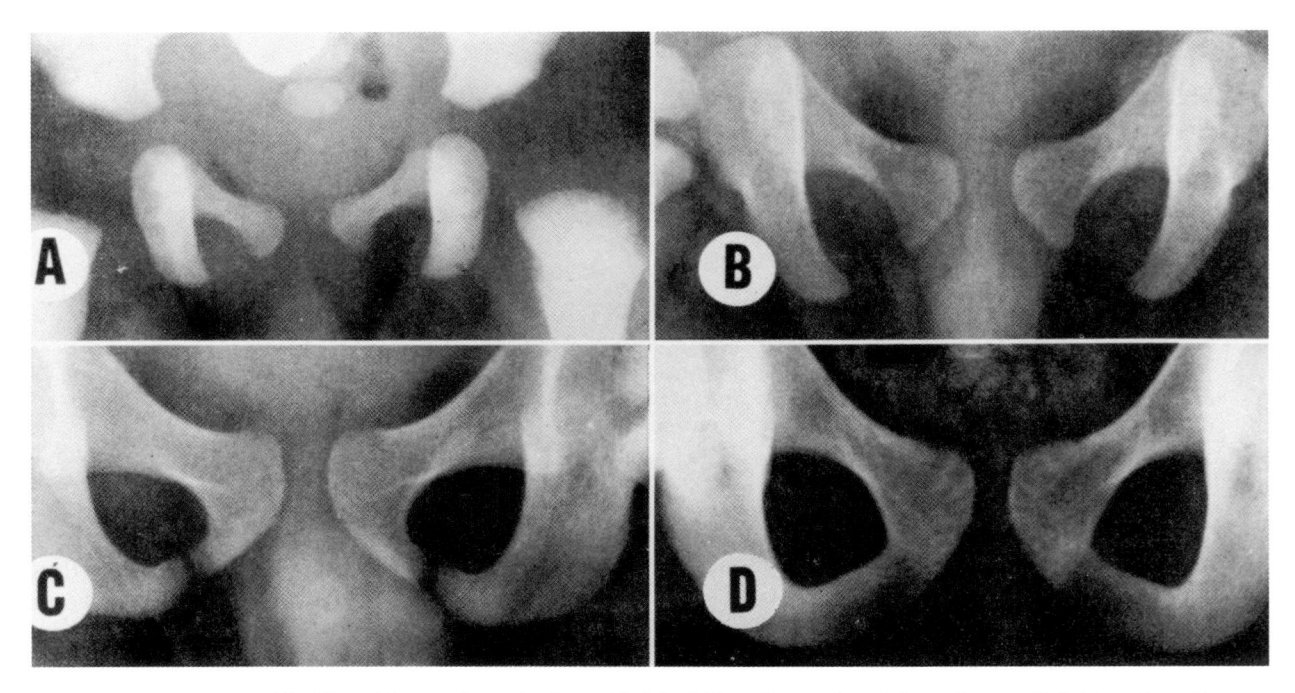

Fig. 25-2. Normal ischiopubic synchrondrosis studied in 549 radiographs of the pelvises of children 2 to 12 years of age. **(A)** 2-day-old infant. **(B)** At 12 months. **(C)** At 2½ years. **(D)** At 6½ years after completed fusion of the ischial and pubic rami. (From Caffey J, Ross SE: The ischiopubic synchrondrosis in healthy children: some normal roentgenologic findings. AJR 76:488, 1956, with permission.)

pediatric pelvic injuries: although the child has a much greater capacity for remodeling of the pelvis after bony injury,[8] injuries to growth areas tend to have long-reaching deleterious effects on the child secondary to poor remodeling. The remodeling that occurs after a bony bridge has formed across the triradiate cartilage can ultimately result in a significantly deformed acetabulum if the injury has occurred under the age of 10 years.[11-14] The growth and development of the pelvis may lead to some confusion on radiographic examination of the pelvis in the child. Familiarity with the patterns of ossification of the pediatric pelvis can help with radiographic diagnoses. The pediatric pelvis consists of three primary ossification centers, the ilium, ischium, and pubis (Fig. 25-2). These three centers join together at the triradiate cartilage and fuse at approximately 16 to 18 years of age.[10] The ischium and pubis meet at the inferior pubic rami, and fusion takes place at approximately 6 to 7 years of age.

Occasionally a swelling occurring bilaterally or unilaterally, may be noted at the ischiopubic junction without symptoms. This synchondrosis may be confused with a stress fracture or a "march" fracture of the inferior pubic arch (Fig. 25-3). The latter is symptomatic and occurs with a history of unusual physical stress.[15] The secondary centers of ossification appear across the tops of the iliac crests progressing laterally to medially from 13 to 15 years in girls and 15 to 17 years in boys. The ischial apophyses appear between 15 and 17 years and fuse between 17 and 19 years, although fusion may be delayed until age 25.[10] There are smaller centers of ossification at the anterior inferior spine, the pubic tubercle, the crest and angle of the pubis, the ischial spines, and the sacrum. Occasionally confusion arises concerning the os acetabuli, which is the epiphysis of the pubis and forms the anterior wall of the acetabulum.[16] This appears within the triradiate cartilage at about age 12, fusing by age 18. At times this appears irregular and can be confused with a fracture of the acetabular rim.[10] These secondary

Fig. 25-3. Inferior pubic synchrondrosis sometimes misinterpreted as a fracture or a tumour.

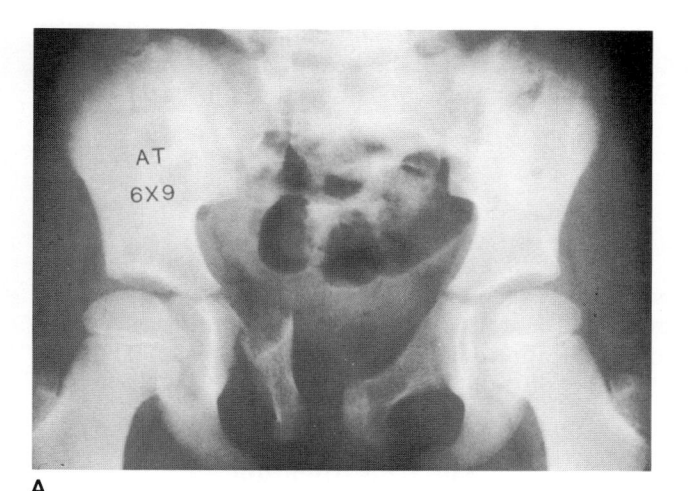

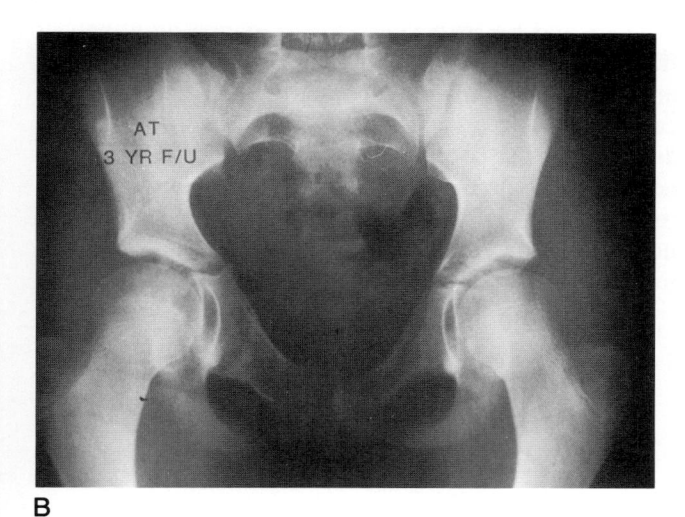

Fig. 25-4. (A) Displaced right pubic ramus fracture in a 6-year-old child. (B) Three years later the ramus has remodeled almost completely and appears only slightly wider than the opposite side.

458 / Management of Pediatric Fractures

TABLE 25-2. Classification of Pelvic Fractures

Type A: Stable
  A1: Fractures of the pelvis not involving the ring
  A2: Stable, minimally displaced fractures of the ring
Type B: Rotationally unstable, vertically stable
  B1: Open book
  B2: Lateral compression—ipsilateral
  B3: Lateral compression—contralateral (bucket handle)
Type C: Rotationally and vertically unstable
  C1: Unilateral
  C2: Bilateral
  C3: Associated with an acetabular fracture

(From Tile,[5] with permission.)

centers should not be misconstrued as avulsion fractures or loose bodies within the hip joint.[9] The potential pitfalls not withstanding, the pediatric pelvis maintains a unique capacity for remodeling after injury (Fig. 25-4).

CLASSIFICATION

To be useful, a classification system should afford the practitioner some guidance concerning immediate treatment, assessment of associated injuries, as well as some indication of long-term outcome. It should be simple and easily applicable to children.

Tile Classification

Tile[65] and his associates have classified *adult* pelvic fractures according to the direction of the impact force and expertly demonstrated each of their classification categories. The primary forces were felt to represent anteroposterior compression, lateral compression, or vertical shear forces. Tile's classification system is shown in Table 25-2. Type A fractures are stable and either do not involve the pelvic ring or have minimal displacement of the ring. Type B fractures are rotationally unstable yet vertically stable and include the subcategories of open-book fractures and lateral compression-type fractures. Type C fractures are rotationally and vertically unstable, including the vertical shear fractures occurring unilaterally or bilaterally. This classification system correlates well with pelvic stability or instability and the necessary treatment of these conditions. However, this system does not seem to be wholly applicable to the younger child or satisfy all of the unique pediatric criteria stated above. It can, however, be applied to pelvic fractures in the teens. Others have described classification systems that tend to be overly inclusive or too simplistic to be useful.[9,10,17,18]

Torode and Zieg Classification

We have found the use of the Torode and Zieg classification, as shown in Table 25-3, to be the most practical[5] for classifying pelvic fractures in younger children.

Type I (avulsion fracture) (Fig. 25-5) includes avulsion injuries through the osteocartilaginous junction of

TABLE 25-3. Torode and Zieg Classification of Fractures

Type	Fractures
I	Avulsion
II	Iliac wing
III	Simple ring (no segmental instability)
IV	Ring disruption

(Adapted from Torode and Zieg,[6] with permission.)

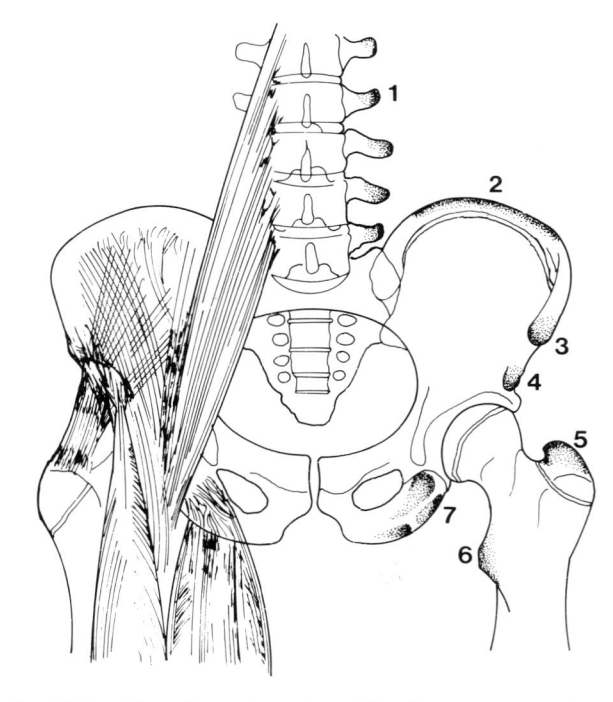

Fig. 25-5. Site of apophyseal avulsion by severe muscle contraction usually against a sudden resistance. *1*, Transverse process apophysis by the iliopsoas origin; *2*, iliac apophysis by the external oblique; *3*, anterior superior spine by the saratorius; *4*, anterior inferior spine by the rectus femorus; *5*, greater trochanter by the abducters; *6*, lesser trochanter by the iliopsoas; *7*, ischial apophysis by the hamstrings.

the secondary centers of ossification. It is usually associated with a sporting injury or sudden contraction of a musculotendinous unit pulling on its site of origin on the immature skeleton. Common sites for this injury are the anterosuperior iliac spine, which provides the origin of the sartorious muscle, the anteroinferior iliac spine the origin for the rectus femoris muscle, and the ischial tuberosity, which is the origin of the hamstring muscles. Relaxation of these muscle attachments in the flexed hip position after avulsion injuries and rest are the treatment of choice, usually with a good result.[6,10,19] Occasionally, an open reduction of a large avulsed fragment of the ischial apophysis may necessitate an open reduction.

Type II (iliac wing fracture) (Fig. 25-6) occurs more commonly in children than adults. This injury is the result of a direct lateral force against the pelvis, producing a vertical or horizontal fracture through the wing of the ilium, often the point of contact of an automobile bumper. The strong periosteum tends to resist more than moderate displacement or inward tilt of the iliac wing. Conservative nonoperative treatment is usually indicated.

Type III (simple pelvic ring fractures) (Fig. 25-7) comprise this group usually with single breaks of the ring. Fractures through the pubic rami or disruptions of the pubic symphysis at the osteocartilaginous junction are the most common type.[3] Displaced fractures may be included in this type if there is no clinical instability of another segment of the pelvis. Torode[6] has pointed out that large diastasis of the symphysis pubis may occur in children with this type of fracture without concomitant instability of the posterior ring through the sacroiliac joints as seen in adults. Presumably this is due to elasticity of the bony pelvis or partial tearing of the anterior sacraliliac joints. Similarly, the sacroiliac joint in the young child may split anteriorly at the bone cartilage

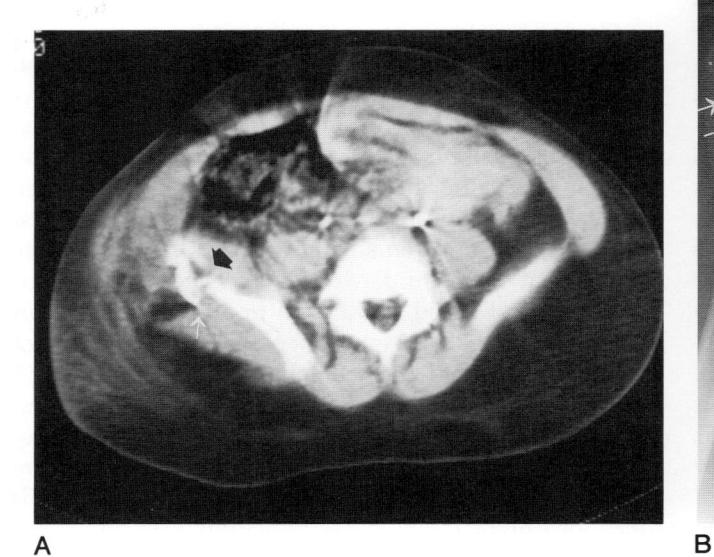

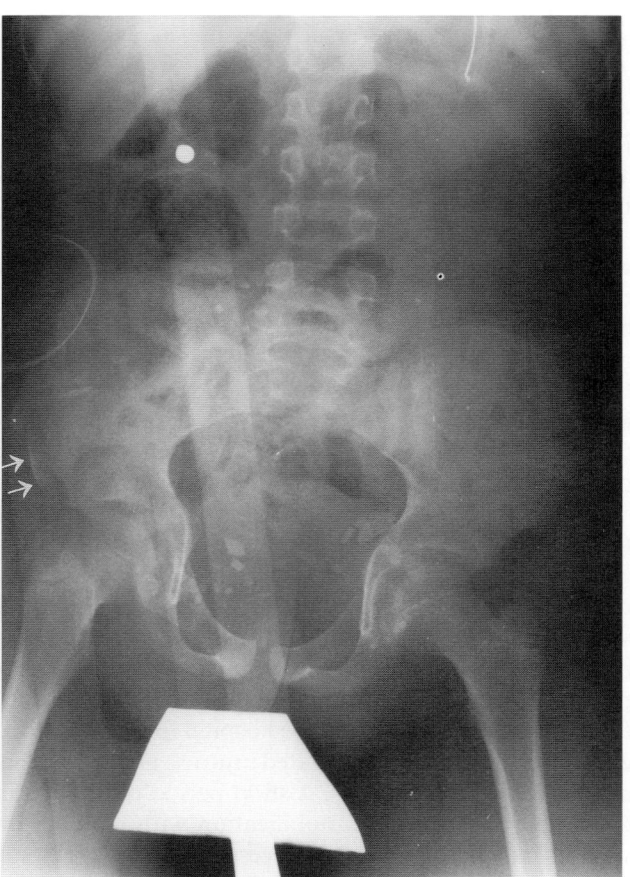

Fig. 25-6. Fracture of wing of ilium seen in **(A)** CT scan and **(B)** on plain film.

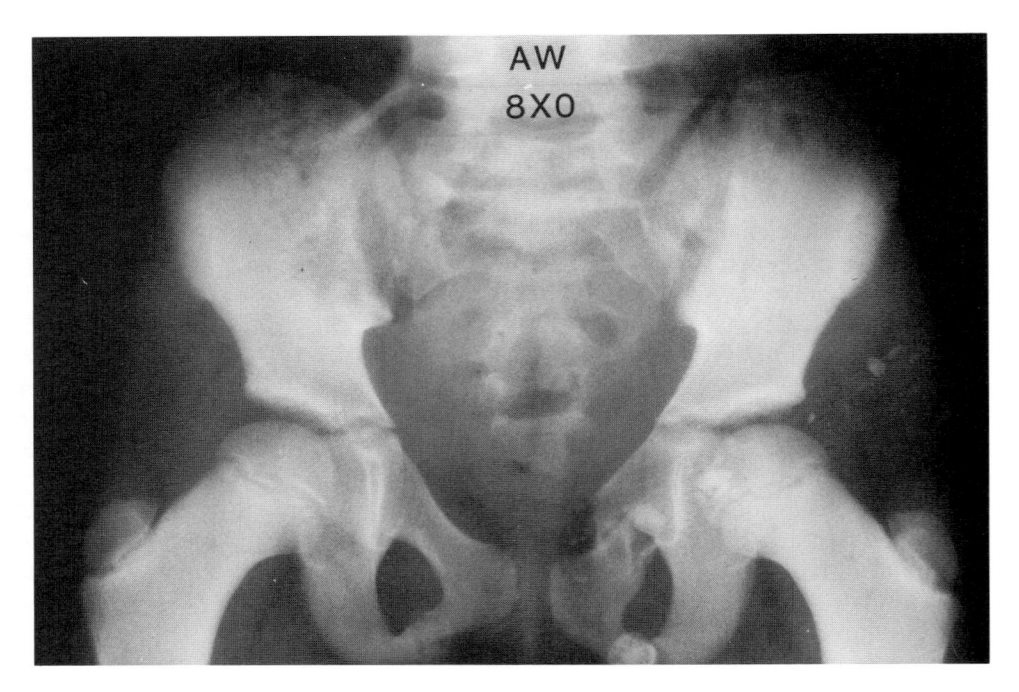

Fig. 25-7. Torade type III fracture through the left superior ramus with no segmental displacement.

interface of the posterior ilium as shown by Ogden.[17] These fractures may also be treated conservatively in most cases.

Type IV fractures include all those ring disruptions with either an unstable segment of the pelvic ring or a major joint disruption (Fig. 25-8). Included in this group are (1) straddle fractures with bilateral pubic rami injuries; (2) the vertical shear injuries (type C) with fractures through the pubic rami in conjunction with sacroiliac joint disruption, sacral fractures, or major iliac fractures[5]; and (3) fractures involving the anterior structures of the pelvic ring, which include the acetabulum.

One of the advantages of this classification system is that it helps one to determine initial care in the emergency department. Type I fractures will generally not require admission to the hospital and may be treated symptomatically with crutches at home. Occasionally bed rest may be indicated in conjunction with this outpatient treatment. Patients with type II and type III fractures should be admitted to the hospital for observation, assessment of possible associated injuries, and treatment of the accompanying ileus. A short period of bed rest is generally indicated, and mobilization with crutches or walkers is all that is generally necessary for this problem. The type IV injuries imply more force exerted upon the pelvis with a higher incidence of associated injuries necessitating the need for hospitalization supervised by a trauma team. These patients are more likely to undergo operative treatment and have the potential for extensive problems from these injuries.

Cryer Classification

Cryer[20] has developed a classification system in adult fractures based upon the initial AP pelvis radiograph seen in the emergency department. His attempts at trying to develop a simple pelvic fracture classification system are based upon the fact that hemorrhage remains the leading cause of death in adults with major pelvic fractures. Although the mortality rate has dropped in the last 20 years, the rate remains steady at 10 percent.[5] He found that unstable pelvic fractures required four or more units of blood transfusion in 50 to 69 percent of patients, and 30 to 49 percent of patients required greater than 10 units of blood. Further he identified that 36 to 55 percent of these patients had intra-abdominal injuries. Instability was defined as more than 0.5 cm of displacement or gap on an AP pelvis radiograph at any fracture site within the pelvic ring anteriorly or posteriorly. His plea for simplistic systems of radiographic classification is well-founded, since most commonly it is nonortho-

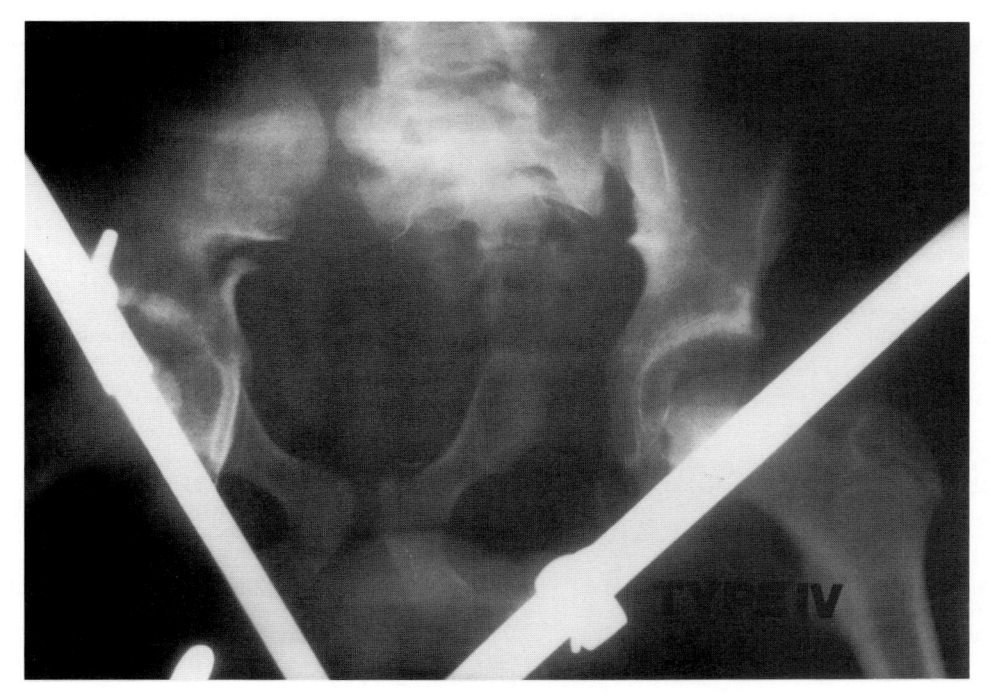

Fig. 25-8. Torade type IV fracture with anterior and posterior ring disruption.

paedists directing the initial management and treatment of these severely traumatized individuals. The extrapolation of this information to the pediatric population seems worthwhile, but needs further study, since blood loss and displacement are less in children due in part to the protection of the thicker and stronger periosteum.

The most practical classification systems and current discussions of pediatric fractures include an injury severity score of some kind. The modified injury severity score (MISS), as shown in Table 25-4, is gaining wider acceptance in helping with the initial assessment of severely injured children.[21,22] Garvin[8] found a high correlation with MISS scores over 20 and long-term disability from pelvis fractures in children.

MECHANISM OF INJURY

The most common cause of pediatric pelvic fractures is motor vehicles striking the young pedestrian on the side of the road or the child crossing into the line of traffic. In most series, this mechanism comprises the majority of patients. Quinby[23] reported 95 percent of his patients were pedestrians, Rang,[1] 90 percent, and Torode,[6] 78 percent. This is in direct contrast to adult series, where 26 to 51 percent of patients sustain injury secondary to motor vehicle-pedestrian accidents.[24] Other than the rare major crush or fall, children as passengers in motor vehicles or on a bicycle or motorcycle constitute the remaining injuries.[3,6,8] In pelvic fractures a male preponderence has been noted in all age groups.[3,24,25]

The majority of children affected are over the age of 10 years,[3,24] Rang has made note of the children under 8 with less "road sense" who are prone to head injuries.[1] In these young patients, the bumper of the car strikes the pelvis with a direct blow and the fender or hood strikes the child's head. This is the mechanism in a high speed injury. With lower speeds the head may be injured as it strikes the ground. A mortality rate of 5 to 14 percent for children's pelvic fractures[2,24,25] is understandable when one considers the severity of injury to the child's head occurring in this common setting of pedestrian-vehicle encounters. The majority of deaths in children occur from the head injury, in direct contrast to the adult population where patients tend to die from hemorrhage or associated abdominal injuries.[20,26] Understanding the mechanism of injury, one can further understand why some series have reported as high as 75 percent of patients as having associated injuries in other organ sys-

TABLE 25-4. The Modified Injury Severity Scale for Rating Multiple Trauma in Children

Body Area	Score on Modified Injury Severity Scale				
	1, Minor	2, Moderate	3, Severe, not life-threatening	4, Severe, life-threatening	5, Critical, survival uncertain
Neural, face, and neck	GCS 13–14 abrasion or contusions of ocular apparatus, vitreous or conjunctival hemorrhage, fractured teeth	GCS 9–12, undisplaced facial fracture Laceration of eye, disfiguring laceration, retinal detachment	GCS 9–12, loss of eye, avulsion of optic nerve Displaced facial fracture "blowout" fracture of orbit	GCS 5–8, bone or soft tissue injury with minor destruction	GCS 4, injuries with airway obstruction
Chest	Muscle ache or chest-wall stiffness	Simple rib or sternal fracture	Multiple rib fractures, hemothorax or pneumothorax, diaphragmatic rupture, pulmonary contusion	Open chest wounds, pneumomediastinum, myocardial contusion	Lacerations, tracheal hemomediastinum, aortic laceration, myocardial laceration or rupture
Abdomen	Muscle ache, seat-belt abrasion	Major abdominal-wall contusion	Contusion of abdominal organs, retroperitoneal hematoma, extraperitoneal, thoracic, or lumbar spine fractures	Minor laceration of abdominal organs, intraperitoneal bladder rupture, spine fractures with paraplegia	Rupture or severe laceration of abdominal vessels or organs
Extremities and pelvic girdle	Minor sprains, simple fractures and dislocations	Open fractures of digits, nondisplaced long-bone or pelvic fractures	Displaced long-bone or multiple hand or foot fractures, single open long-bone fracture, pelvic fractures with displacement, laceration of major nerves or vessels	Multiple closed long-bone fractures, amputation of limbs	Multiple open long-bone fractures

GCS, Glasgow coma scale.
(From Garvin et al.,[8] with permission.)

tems or other parts of the skeleton,[24] with pelvic fractures.

The mechanism of injury for Torode type I fractures is the sudden contracture of the musculotendinous unit as it pulls through its connection to the cartilaginous apophysis, separating the osteocartilaginous junction of the apophysis. As Watts[10] has noted, not uncommonly this occurs when the young adolescent is attempting to emulate the athletic prowess and accomplishments of his or her professional counterpart in that sport. The sudden thrust of force exerted on the relatively weak cartilage produces a painful separation and hemorrhage.

Type II fractures generally occur secondary to a direct lateral force or anterior force on the ilium, such as one might envision happening from a direct blow from a car bumper.

Type III fractures occur from a direct anterior force on the pubis such as might happen with a crush of the pelvis when children are run over by vehicles or with more of a frontal blow from a car in the standing position.

Type IV fractures are associated with disruption of the pelvic ring and are therefore more complex. Straddle fractures can produce this type injury when a motorcycle rider is thrust forward on his vehicle straddling the gas tank after striking a stationary object. A major disruption of the pelvic ring can also occur when severe internal or external rotatory forces come to bear on the hemipelvis, with disruption of the sacroiliac joint and tearing of the sacrotuberous ligaments. With these type of injuries major forces are acting upon the hemipelvis and the adjacent soft tissues. Injuries that involve vertical shear forces or forces through the femoral shaft can produce acetabular fractures with or without dislocation of the hip. Type IV fractures are less common in children, yet comprise the majority of patients with visceral injuries and those with long-term disabilities.

PHYSICAL EXAMINATION AND DIAGNOSIS

In Reichard's[24] series only 25 percent of children had isolated pelvic fractures. The majority of patients with pelvic injuries other than those secondary to athletic

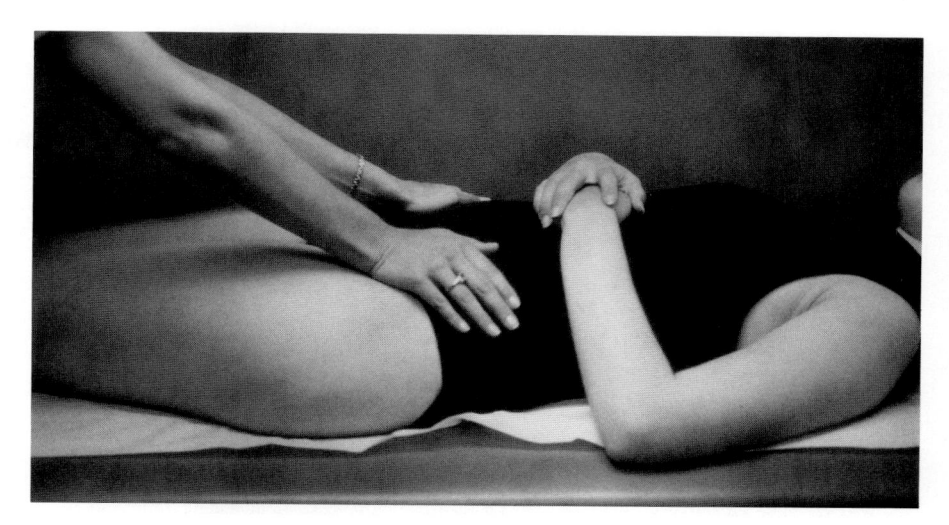

Fig. 25-9. The gapping test for pelvic instability.

avulsions should therefore be carefully assessed by a trauma team. Initial assessment by emergency department personnel should include consultations with pediatric surgeons and orthopaedists; neurosurgeons and urologists should be included wherever injury within their area of expertise is suspected. Careful assessment of the patient's vital signs, including level of oxygenation, blood pressure, and urinary output should be assessed. Close observation and monitoring of vital signs is essential to avoid the regrettable "crash" that occurs all too often in the radiology department due to blood loss. Access intravenous lines and a Foley catheter should be started and appropriate blood studies ordered. Appropriate resuscitation of the severely injured patients should be carried out by the pediatric general surgery service wherever possible. The initial orthopaedic assessment and physical examination should begin with an overall general assessment of the patient looking for associated injuries. Potential spinal injuries, including those of the cervical spine should not be overlooked. Range of motion of all extremities should be checked to identify long bone fractures, joint injuries, burns, lacerations, or punctures. The patient should be rolled over in a logroll fashion to examine the back, looking for any open wounds or penetrating injuries as well as any instability between the spinous processes. While this is being done, lateral compression over the iliac wings will help to determine if there is any instability of the sacroiliac joints or pelvic ring in general. While in the supine position, the gapping test[27] is carried out with the examiners hands applied to the anterosuperior iliac spine and pressure exerted directly downward in an attempt to elicit pain or instability of the pelvis (Fig. 25-9). Pain may also be elicited in the sacroiliac joint by stress exerted through the hemipelvis by lateral rotation of the hip to the extreme in a figure-of-four position with the ankle over the opposite thigh (Fig. 25-10). Pressure is then exerted on the thigh of the flexed leg (Fabere test).

Careful examination of the perineum around the genitalia may demonstrate swelling and early ecchymosis due to disruption of the urogenital diaphragm or hemorrhage from the pubic rami. Manual examination with a gloved hand of the perineum may demonstrate a penetrating injury. Via the rectal examination one may palpate fracture fragments from the sacrum or coccyx or the lateral ischium protruding through or against the rectum. Rectal lacerations occur in approximately 3 percent of patients. Perineal and vaginal lacerations occur in 7 percent of girls with pelvic fractures, most commonly secondary to ischial pubic fragments of bone protruding through the vaginal canal.[24] These will be missed if not specifically examined for and can result in severe sepsis and chronic fistuli.

INVESTIGATION AND RADIOLOGIC ASSESSMENT

Resuscitation of the multiply injured patient should begin prior to leaving the emergency department; this may require blood transfusions. Reichard[24] noted 10 percent of the patients were in hypovolemic shock with a systolic pressure less than 90 mmHg upon admission and blood was administered to 40 percent of their patients at some time during their hospital stay. Of the six

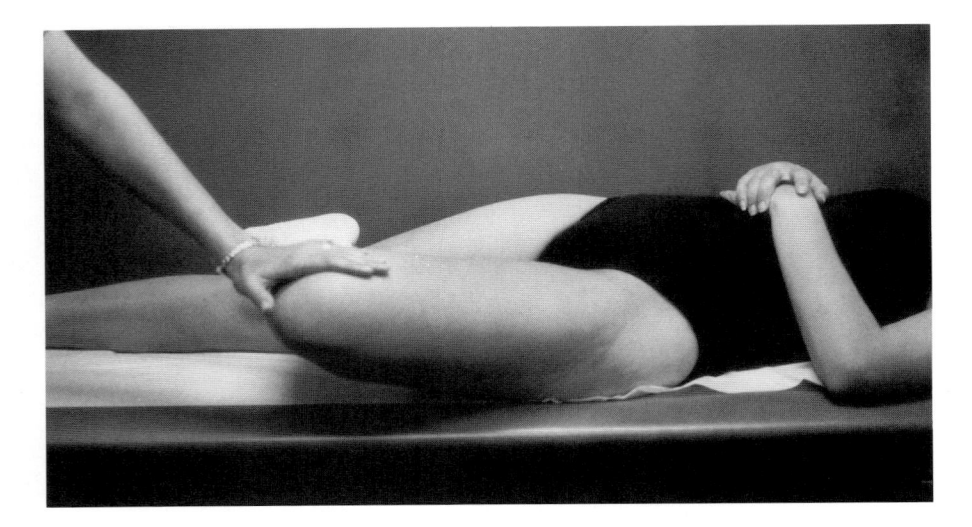

Fig. 25-10. The Fabere test for sacroiliac instability.

patients requiring more than four units of blood, four of them had major intrapelvic arterial disruption. Musmeche[25] noted that 46 percent of children required blood transfusions. The potential need for laporotomy should be assessed. In Reichard's[24] study, 12 percent of patients had laporotomy: 8 had pelvic visceral injuries, 8 had remote intra-abdominal visceral injuries, and only 1 had a negative laporotomy. None of these were done for the purpose of controlling retroperitoneal hemorrhage alone.

Once the patient is stable, x-ray examination can be carried out. It is crucial to perform the x-rays *without* a gonadal shield. Unconscious patients should have at least an AP pelvis as part of their screening to rule out pelvic fractures. When ordering radiographs, it is important to remember that the pelvic ring is seen obliquely on the AP view. This remains, however, a good scout film for initial assessment. At least one further view is necessary for initial assessment (Fig. 25-11). Either the inlet or outlet view can be taken. The inlet or downshot is taken at 30 degrees off the vertical aimed distally to demonstrate the degree of ring disruption. The outlet or "brim" shot is taken at 30 degrees off the vertical aimed proximally to look at those posterior injuries associated with shearing forces.

For stable patients with a type IV injury, and for some patients in type III categories, further radiographic evaluation with computed tomography (CT) scan will give better bony detail than plain films and often identify occult injuries (Fig. 25-12). Where this is not available, Letournel[28] has described a series of oblique films, which can give detailed information to aid in proper diagnosis.

TREATMENT INDICATIONS

Type I Avulsion Fractures

Type I avulsion fractures of the pelvis can be treated on an outpatient basis with crutches, analgesics, and modified activity. Often relaxing the affected muscle with the hip flexed, will relieve pain and minimize displacement of the apophysis. Generally, these fractures unite within 6 weeks sufficiently to form either a solid osseous or fibrous union. These injuries, which should be differentiated from apophysiolysis, are comparable to small, microscopic avulsions of the tendinous attachments to bone and somewhat comparable to Osgood-Schlatter's disease in the knee. These are not associated with history of a single forceful inciting event as with avulsion fractures and should be treated accordingly as a chronic apophysitis.

The avulsion fractures generally respond to conservative management with satisfactory results.[19] However, motion at the site of an inadequate bony or fibrous union may cause chronic pain and can be an indication for surgical intervention. Excision of the poorly united fragment has been reported to provide relief of pain,[29] and, in some rare cases of accomplished athletes, acute reduction and internal fixation of large fragments, such as the ischial apophyseal avulsions, has also been reported with good results.[30] In an age where a high value is placed upon athletic prowess and the desire for college scholarships runs high, the treatment of these injuries in athletes remains controversial. Watts[10] has pointed out that, although a high percentage (68 percent) of these avulsions

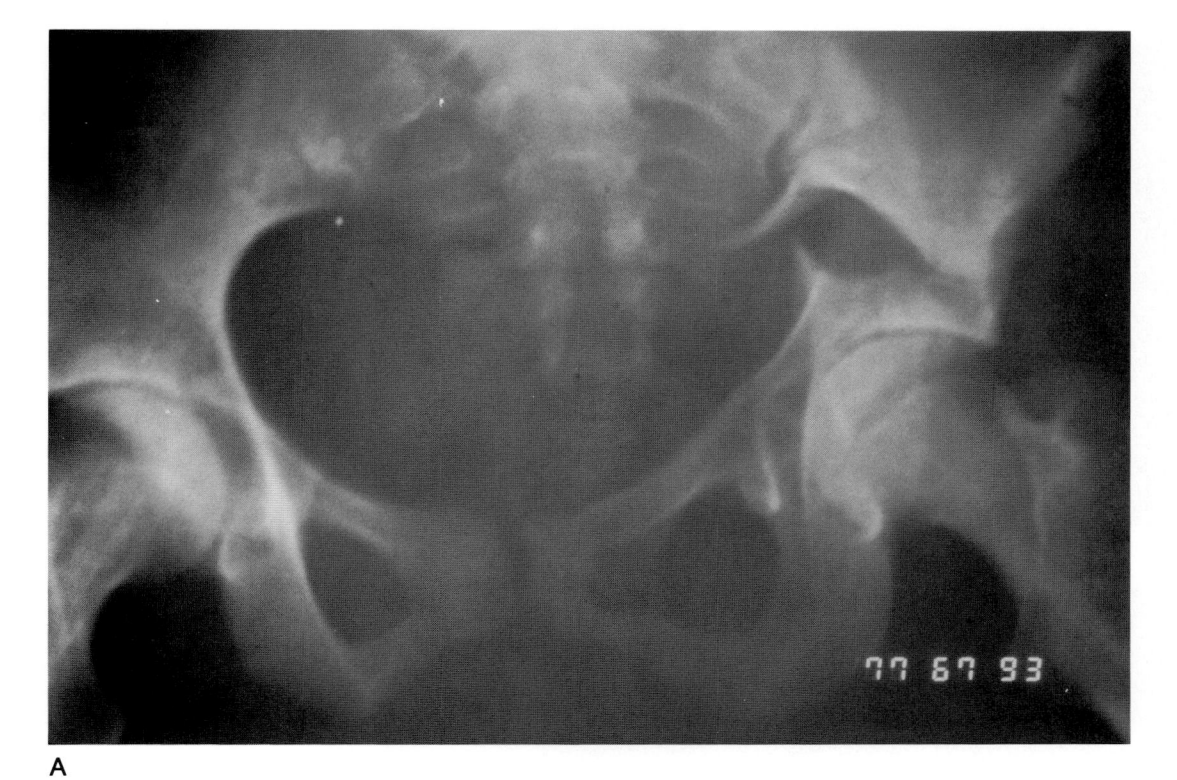

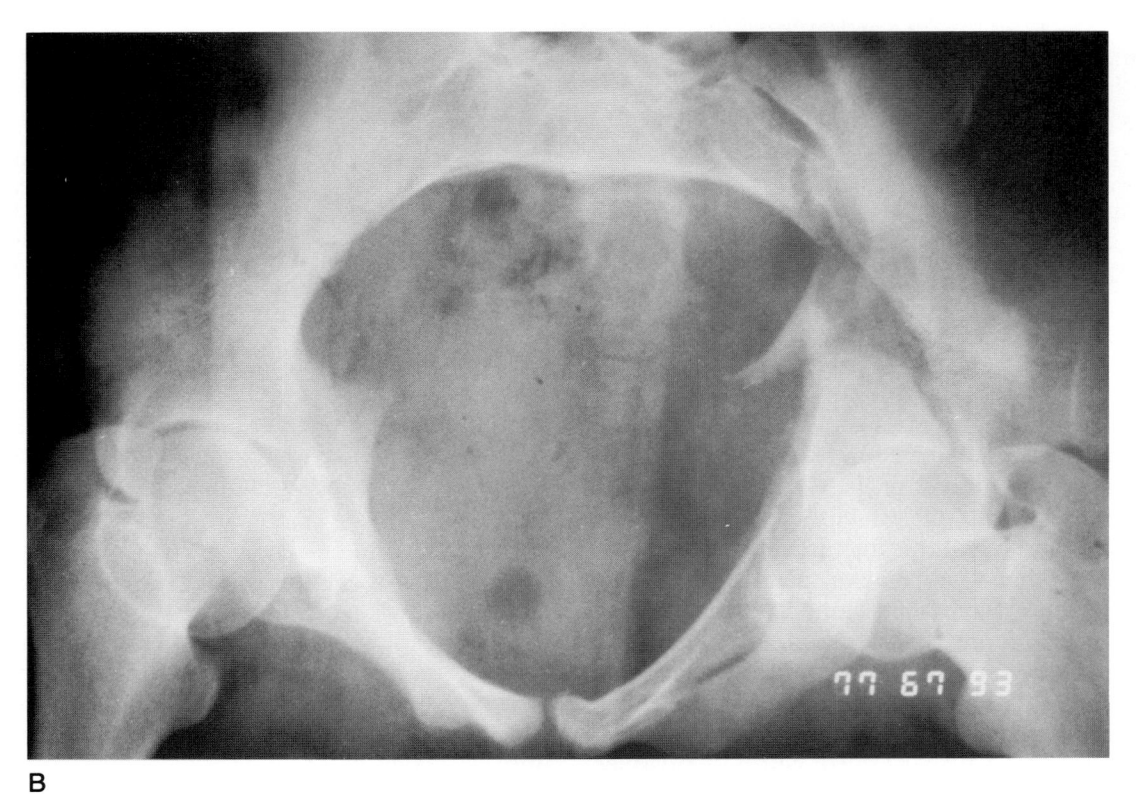

Fig. 25-11. (A) AP view demonstrating fracture of iliac wing. (B) AP inlet view of same fracture illustrating extension of the fracture into the acetabulum.

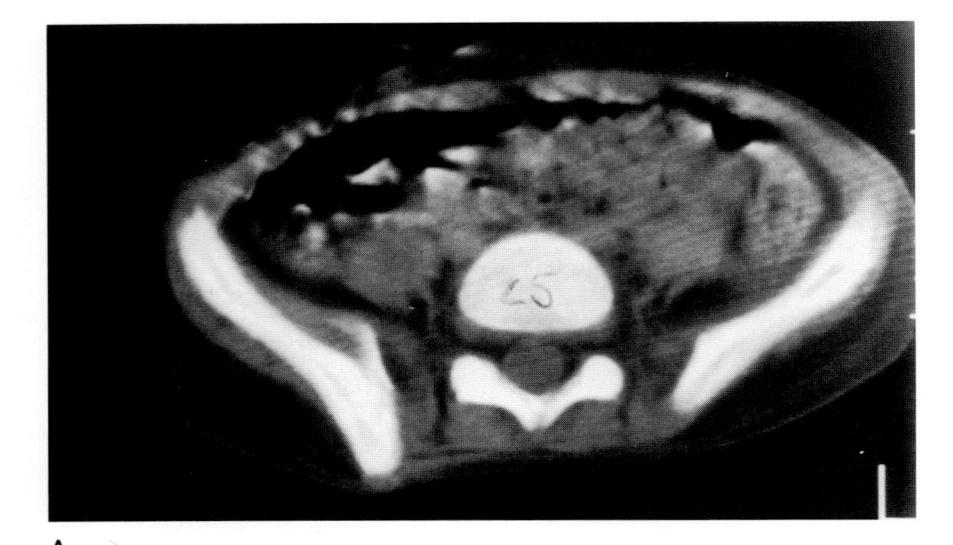

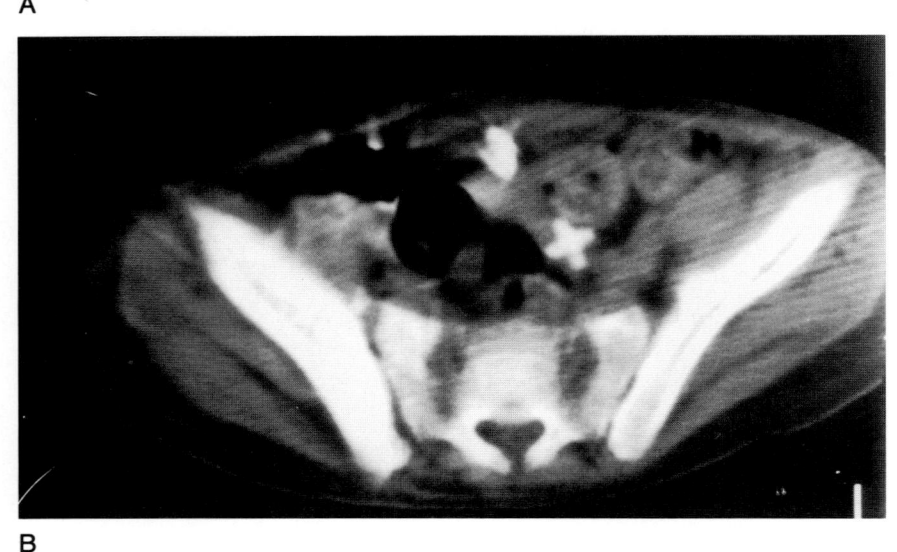

Fig. 25-12. Computed tomography is an excellent imaging technique to confirm pelvic fractures illustrating the **(A)** sacroiliac disruption in this 7-year-old boy, and **(B)** the reduction.

did not unite, the majority had good results. Of 14 cases reported by Watts,[10] 10 treated by late excision and 3 by early reattachment, only 2 of these went on to a solid union. There remains no established proof that the achievement of union of this fracture improves athletic prowess over other nonoperative means. Watts[10] accordingly strongly recommends nonoperative treatment for these injuries. Some consideration might, however, be given to those previously accomplished athletes with marked chronic disability and nonunion with more than 2 cm of displacement.[30-32]

Occasionally the younger athlete with a nonossified apophysis may avulse the cartilaginous attachment with no radiographic evidence to support the diagnosis. Symptomatic treatment is indicated and confirmation with follow-up x-rays later will confirm the diagnosis by periosteal new bone formation.

Type II and Type III Fractures

Type II (iliac wing fractures) and type III fractures (simple ring fractures) should be admitted to the hospital for observation for associated injuries. Such fractures are always indicative of severe trauma. Often the pelvic fracture is treated as an incidental finding. After a short period of bed rest, until comfortable, mobilization with the help of crutches or a walker will restore these children back to normal activities in a short period of time. Canale[9] is careful to point out that one can be fooled by the isolated pubic ramus fracture with significant displacement. Although the pediatric pelvis has greater plasticity and elasticity of the symphysis and sacroiliac joints, there is a limit to the displacement that the pelvic ring can tolerate. If there is wide displacement of a pubic fracture, one should carefully look for a posterior disruption through the sacroiliac joint or sacrum to account for the excessive shift in the ring that has allowed this to occur. Examination of the posterior structures may reveal pain or crepitus and a CT scan may be indicated for accurate diagnosis.

Type II and type III fractures often are associated with an ileus seen early during hospitalization and occasionally requiring nasogastric tube drainage. Pain and discomfort in the abdominal musculature, especially in the area of the iliac wing fracture is to be expected. The majority of the iliac wing fractures are laterally displaced[9] and only rarely is closed manipulation indicated for the grossly displaced iliac wing in a thin individual. Bed rest with the leg abducted will help in the early management by relaxing the abductor muscles pulling on the iliac wing. These fractures all unite without disability. The pubic rami fractures have abundant capacity for remodeling as demonstrated by Garvin[8] (Fig. 25-2). We are not aware of any follow-up studies to look at the birth history in those young women who have sustained pubic or pelvic ring fractures in childhood; therefore, we can probably assume there are no major impediments to vaginal delivery.

Type IV Fractures

Type IV fractures (pelvic ring disruptions and acetabular fractures) are more complex and require a lengthier hospitalization. Treatment of the associated injuries often requires transfusion of blood. Rarely, children with type II fractures require a blood transfusion, but type III and type IV fractures, because of their higher number of associated injuries and violence, account for the greatest number of transfusions.[2,6,24,25] In those children with significant retroperitoneal hemorrhage, some authors have found the use of pediatric pneumatic antishock trousers useful, but this is controversial. The principle behind this treatment is that external pressure will tamponade both arterial and venous bleeding within the pelvis while maintaining a low enough pressure in the trousers to avoid compression of the skin and soft tissues.[33]

The pelvic sling has been employed to minimize motion of the pelvic fracture fragments and secondarily reducing soft tissue trauma and blood loss. This has been found useful for treatment of the rare open-book injuries. Care should be taken to avoid the use of the sling for internal rotation injuries, since they will only further deform the hemipelvis and cause more pain.

The use of an external frame to better immobilize the unstable segments is recommended for children over 10 years of age with marked pelvic disruption and continued hemorrhage.

The use of traction for reduction and maintenance of reduction is most useful for vertical shear fractures. Steinmann pins placed through the supracondylar region of the distal femur pulling against the weight of the patient with the foot of the bed elevated can effectively draw the hemipelvis distally into a reduced position. At times the use of an eyebolt or a similar makeshift traction system through the greater trochanter may be necessary to reduce a fracture-dislocation of the hip associated with acetabular fractures. Two cancellous screws directed into the femoral neck joined by a plate external to the skin will allow for attachment of the traction rope. The trochanteric apophysis should be avoided with traction pins (Fig. 25-13).

For most type IV pediatric fractures, 4 to 6 weeks of bed rest with or without traction will produce a sufficient amount of healing prior to mobilization with a gradual increase in protected weightbearing. During maintenance of traction, the opposite leg can be held with skin traction to maintain a level pelvis. Use of the semi-Fowler position to relax the anterior abdominal musculature is the most comfortable position for bed rest treatment of most pelvic fractures. Rang[1] has noted that 97 percent of children with pelvic fractures need nothing more than bed rest and the avoidance of weightbearing.

Because of the emphasis on shortened hospitalization, consideration could be given to the use of a spica cast for young children after a period of bed rest. This prevents excessive movement of the pelvic fragments and allows for earlier discharge once the associated injuries have been adequately addressed and treated. In 6 to 8 weeks from the time of the fracture, the child can be removed from the cast and given physical therapy for mobilization.

Pelvic External Fixation

Severe crushing injuries to the pelvis can sometimes occur with massive distortion of pelvic anatomy. Life-saving resuscitative measures are necessary to prevent

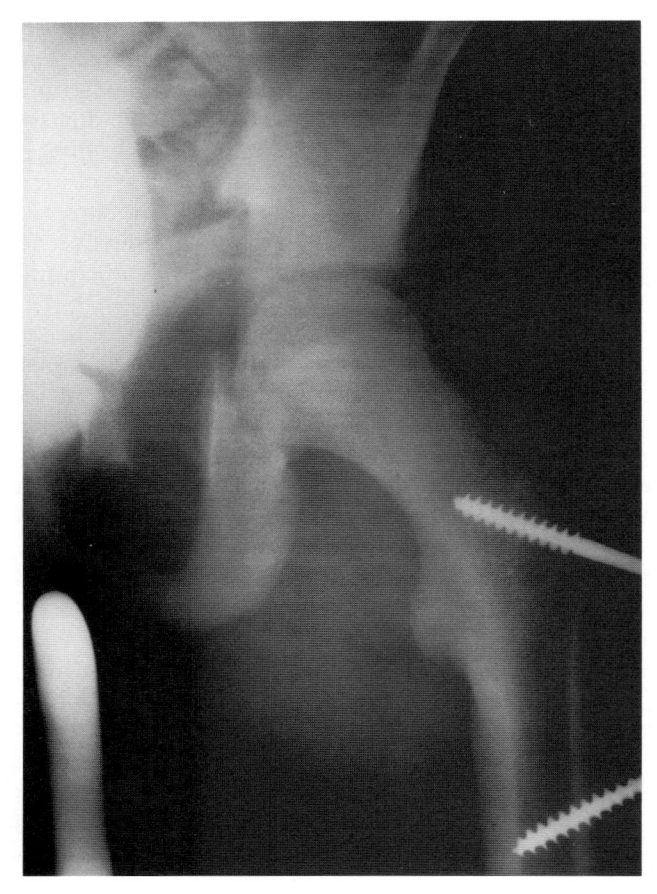

Fig. 25-13. External screw-plate traction device for reduction of central fracture dislocation (plate is outside skin and off x-ray plate).

hypovolemic shock. These injuries are rare in children. Provisional stabilization may be required for pelvic fractures during the resuscitation phase of management to reduce fragment motion and subsequent hemorrhage. These can be safely and quickly achieved with an external fixation frame applied percutaneously in the emergency room in adolescents or at the time of laparotomy in the operating room. Tile[5] has described such a technique utilized to reduce the volume of the pelvis, restore tamponade, and thereby reduce hemorrhage. A simple frame is preferred. Two pins can be placed percutaneously in the ilium, one at the anterior superior spine directed posteriorly and the other over the iliac tubercle aimed approximately 45 degrees to the first pin. The frame is completed in the form of an anterior rectangle. The two pins are joined by vertical bars with a lower horizontal bar joining the two sides of the rectangle. The superior bar is actually two bars joined together with a junction forming an angle with the apex forward to allow for the abdominal contents to protrude forward and also to add stability to the construct (Fig. 25-14). A simple frame cannot fully stabilize the pelvic ring but can allow for the patient to be placed in the upright position for improved ventilation during the acute care phase. This frame is not sufficiently stable for weightbearing, but within 4 to 6 weeks a sufficient amount of healing should have occurred to allow for removal of the frame in most cases.

Closed reduction of pelvic ring displacements with external fixation techniques are difficult and occasionally more definitive reduction of fracture fragments may be necessary. Dabezies[34] has described the use of two threaded compression rods through the posterior iliac spine in order to reduce Malgaine pattern fractures (pubic fractures associated with posterior ring disruptions unilaterally or bilaterally) (Fig. 25-15). These rods are placed under compression through the posterior iliac wings to reduce and hold the sacroiliac joints. This avoids the more risky placement of screws across the iliac wing into the body of the sacrum as described by Matta.[35] Limited experience with the use of external and internal fixation devices in children has been reported in the literature. Alonso[36] and Reff[37] have reported on their limited experience using external fixation devices for complex pediatric polytrauma. Tile[5] has cautioned against the excessive use of open reduction and internal fixation because of the disadvantages of bleeding, infection, and nerve damage. He points out that the ilioinguinal approach as described by Letournel to the femoral neurovascular structures carries with it a greater risk than benefit to the patient.[5]

There is the occasional situation when during intraabdominal surgery for the treatment of abdominal visceral problems, there is some benefit to be derived from the judicious use of hardware. A superior pubic symphysis plate with two screws can reconstruct the symphysis and restore continuity of the pelvic ring. It is simple and easy to insert. The necessity for operative intervention for the pelvic injury in children is rare.

Acetabular Fractures

Acetabular fractures in children and adolescents are uncommon. Consequently, reports of these fractures occurring in children are few and most orthopaedists have a limited experience. Remembering the pliability and elasticity in the pediatric pelvis, one can appreciate that whereas forces coming to bear upon the adult hip joint might shatter the inner acetabular wall, in the child the cartilaginous triradiate cartilage can absorb the high-energy forces with no obvious initial signs of fracture, although the physeal crush may result in a growth arrest[12,38,39] (Fig. 25-16).

Most of the children sustaining acetabular fractures are of a slightly older age group than other pelvic fractures, generally 13 years or above.[38] The majority are associated with high energy motor vehicle trauma and a few from horseback riding. Half of the patients have an associated posterior dislocation of the femoral head.[38]

The mainstay of treatment for acetabular fractures in children as well as adults remains traction. This has persisted in various forms, primarily because of its simplicity and good results in the majority of cases.[10,38,40] It should be noted that because of the cartilaginous nature of the acetabulum, dislocation in the child can occur without an acetabular rim fracture. Chips that do occur are sometimes encased in surrounding cartilage or soft tissue and may spring back into place following reduction. Pre- and postreduction CT scans are very helpful in deciding on the need for a postreduction washout of the joint to eliminate intra-articular fragments that may lead to loose bodies or early degenerative changes[10,41] (Fig. 25-17).

A direct lateral blow through the trochanter can produce a central fracture-dislocation.[40] The goal in treatment of any dislocation of the femoral head is the achievement of reduction within 24 hours of the accident in order to minimize the risk of avascular necrosis.[38,42] The second goal is the maintenance of this reduction in a congruent position. Naturally, the long-term prognosis will depend directly upon the type of fracture sustained, the presence or absence of intra-articular comminuted fragments, the presence or absence of injury to the triradiate cartilage, and the maintenance of the reduction and motion (Fig. 25-18).

Computed tomography can help to determine the amount of bony displacement and the type of acetabular fracture. It has been suggested that the long-term functional results of acetabular fractures in adults were related to the integrity of the superior and posterior articular surfaces of the acetabulum. These are the surfaces that carry most of the body weight and the integrity of these surfaces exerts a major influence on the end result.[40,43] Rowe and Lowell[42] found their best results occurred with fractures involving the anterior aspect of the acetabulum and the poorest results were in fractures affecting the superior articular surface with posterior fractures occupying an intermediate position.

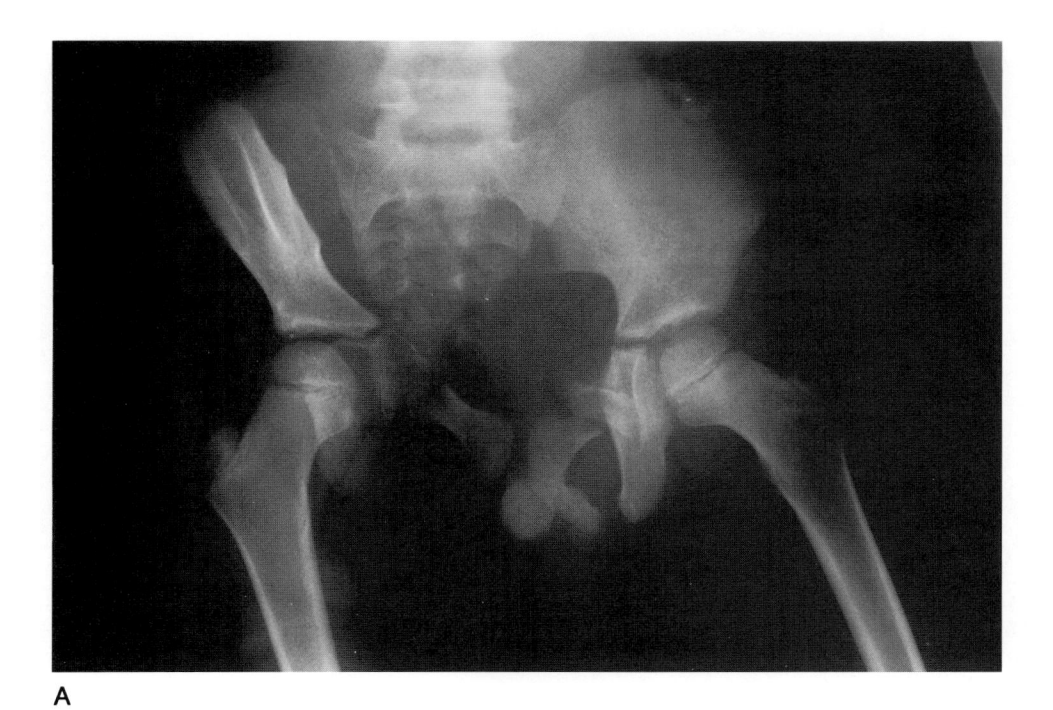

Fig. 25-14. A 7-year-old boy who was run over by a school bus. **(A)** Note that in spite of the tire passing over the pelvis, the symphysis pubis remained intact with the "open-book" phenomenon occurring because of bilateral rami fracturing. The right sacroiliac was however completely disrupted. *(Figure continues.)*

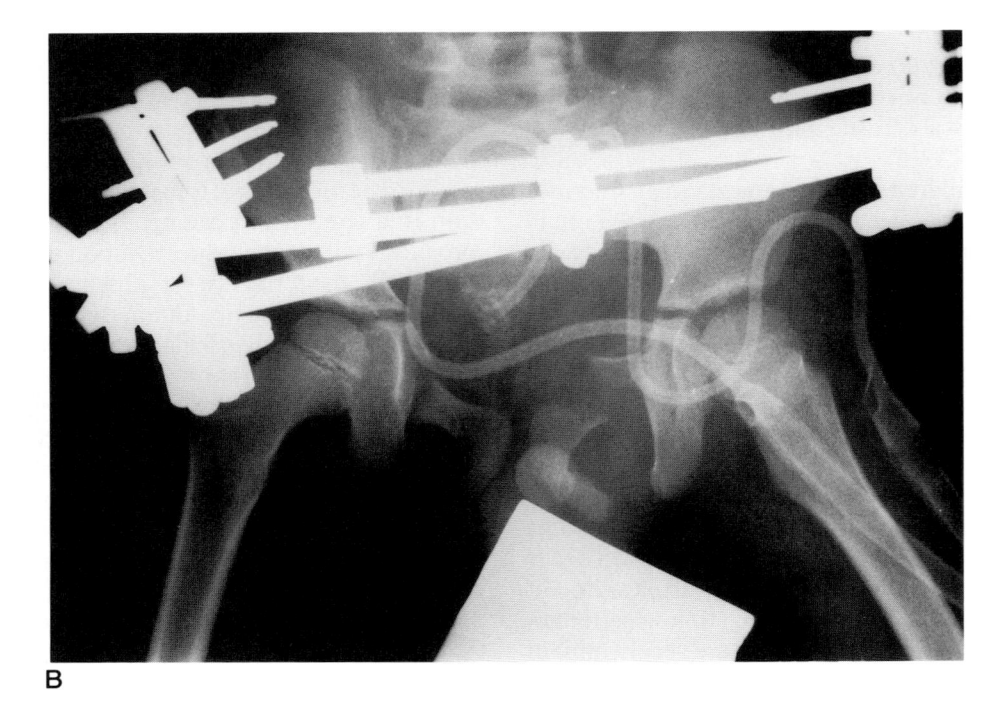

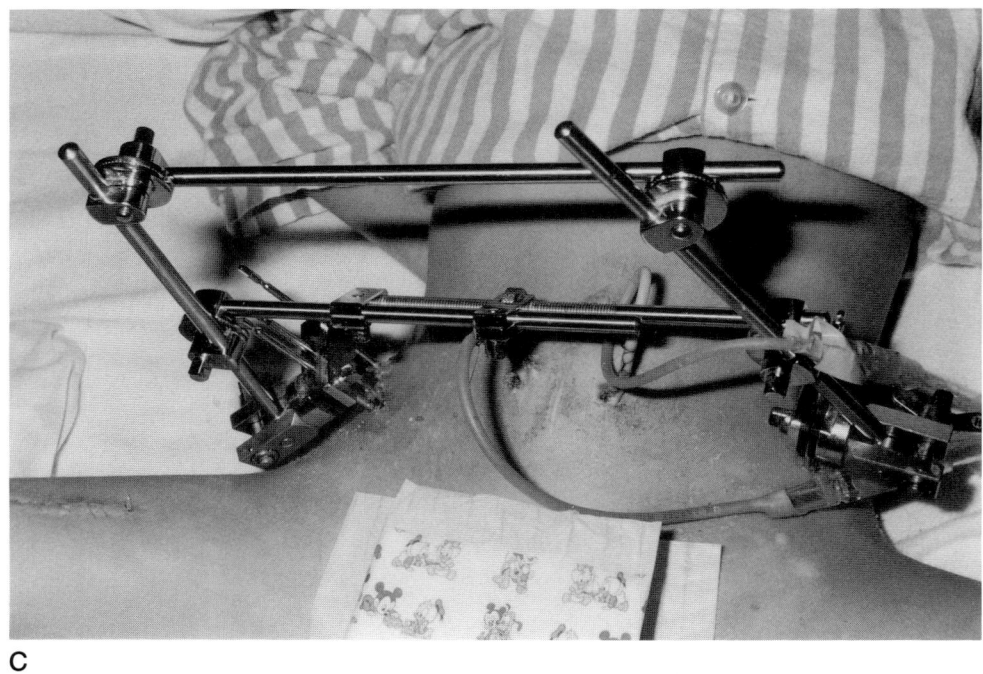

Fig. 25-14 *(Continued).* **(B&C)** The fractures were managed with an external fixator pelvic construct to close the book. This boy had a tear of the posterior urethra and a right L4 to S1 nerve root paresis. (Case contributed by Dr. Jay Jarvis, Children's Hospital of Eastern Ontario.)

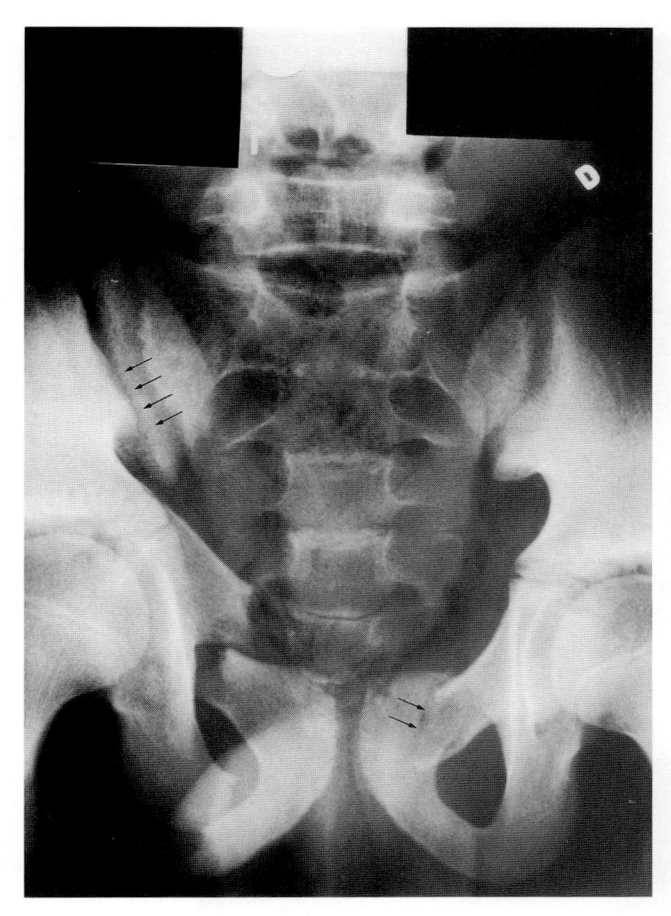

Fig. 25-15. Bilateral fractured rami in straddle-type injury subsequent to a fall from a height. Urethral tearing is common in such injuries. Note disruption of right posterior ring—the sacroiliac joint—the so-called Malgaine fracture.

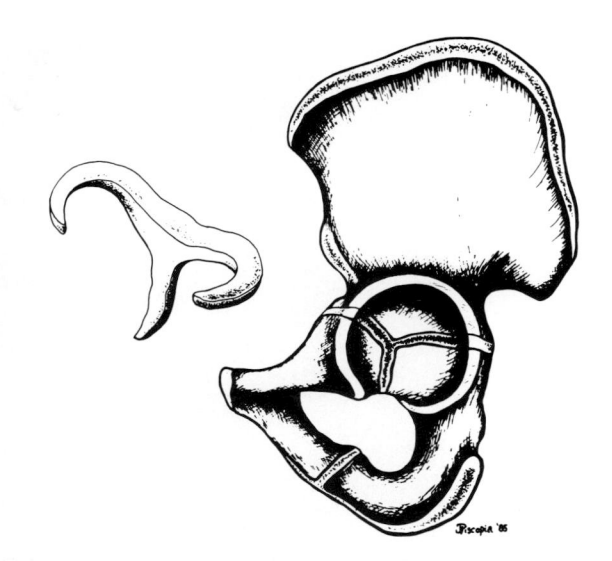

Fig. 25-16. Diagram of the hemipelvis illustrating the three pelvic bones and the limbs of the triradiate cartilage: iliopubic, ilioschial and ischiopubic. (From Scuderi and Bronson,[14] with permission.)

Classification of Acetabular Fractures

Watts[10] identified four types of acetabular fractures in children as shown in Table 25-5. Type I fractures have small chips occurring with dislocation usually in a posterior direction (80 percent of dislocations). Type 2 fractures are linear fractures that occur in association with pelvic fractures without displacement. These are generally stable. Caution must be used, however, when superior dome fractures are present, since displacement may occur with early weightbearing or acetabular dysplasia may development due to triradiate involvement. Type 3 fractures have multiple fragments, which lead to instability. Larger fragments may need open reduction much as in the treatment of adult acetabular fractures. Type 4 fractures occur secondary to a central dislocation of the hip with linear or stellate fractures through the inner wall much as in the adult.

Pennal[40] has classified adult acetabular fractures by a simple system with which most orthopaedists are more familiar and can legitimately be applied to children, since most children with acetabular fractures are adolescents. Type I is a single column fracture occurring either in the anterior (iliopubic) or posterior (ilioischial) column. Type II fractures involve both anterior and posterior columns of the acetabulum with a transverse, oblique, or T-shaped configuration. As one might expect the severity of displacement and comminution directly affects the outcome.

Treatment of Acetabular Fractures

The nonoperative, conservative management of acetabular fractures in children usually consists of early traction to maintain the femoral head in its anatomic position. It is generally discontinued after 3 to 4 weeks and followed by a period of non-weight-bearing physical therapy for 4 to 8 weeks followed by protective weight-bearing with crutches for a total of 10 to 12 weeks from the fracture.[38] There is no reason to promote early weightbearing in children, which may displace fracture fragments.[9] The aim of all treatment is to prevent displacement of the acetabular fragments and in older individuals a prolonged period of nonweightbearing, up to 4

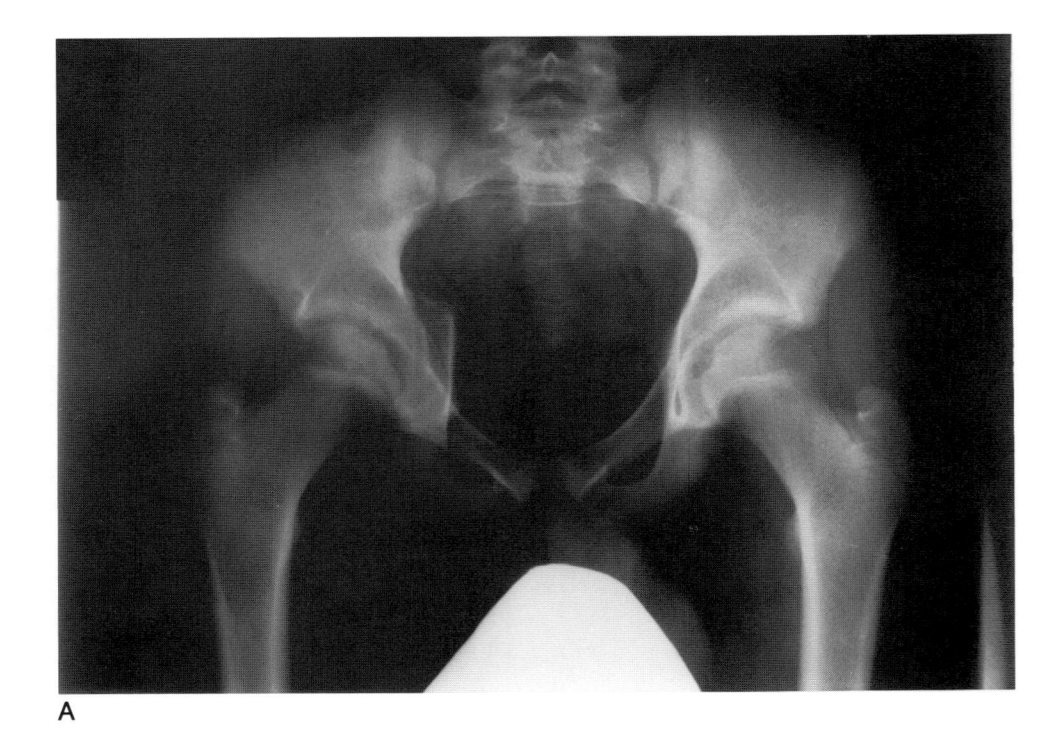

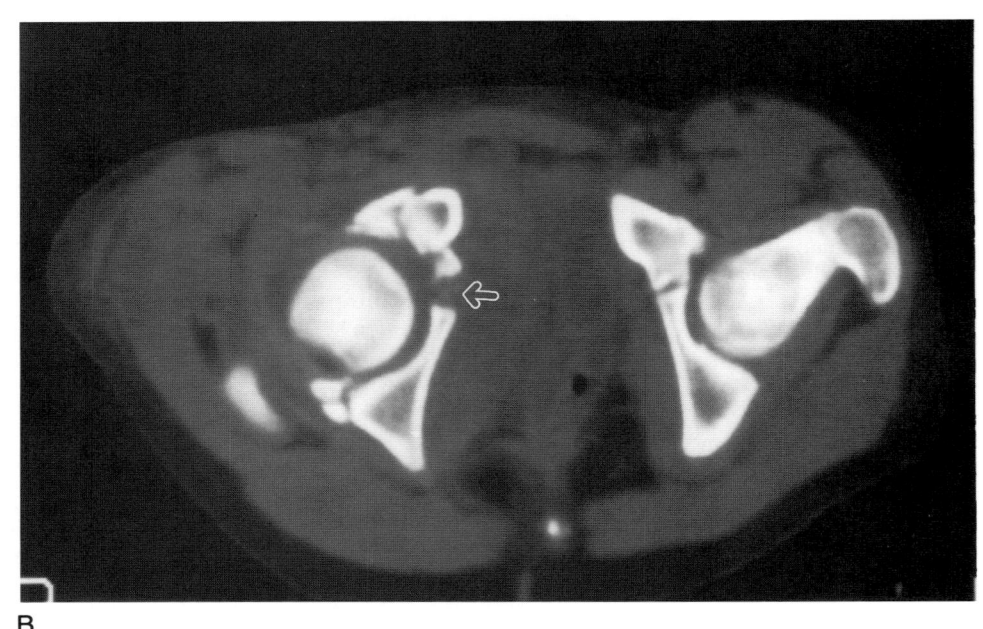

Fig. 25-17. (A) Fracture of the acetabulum in a 14-year-old boy. (B) The CT scan reveals a much clearer image of the extent of involvement of the acetabular fracturing; the involvement of the triradiate cartilage and the presence of any intra-articular loose fragments.

Fractures of the Pelvis / 473

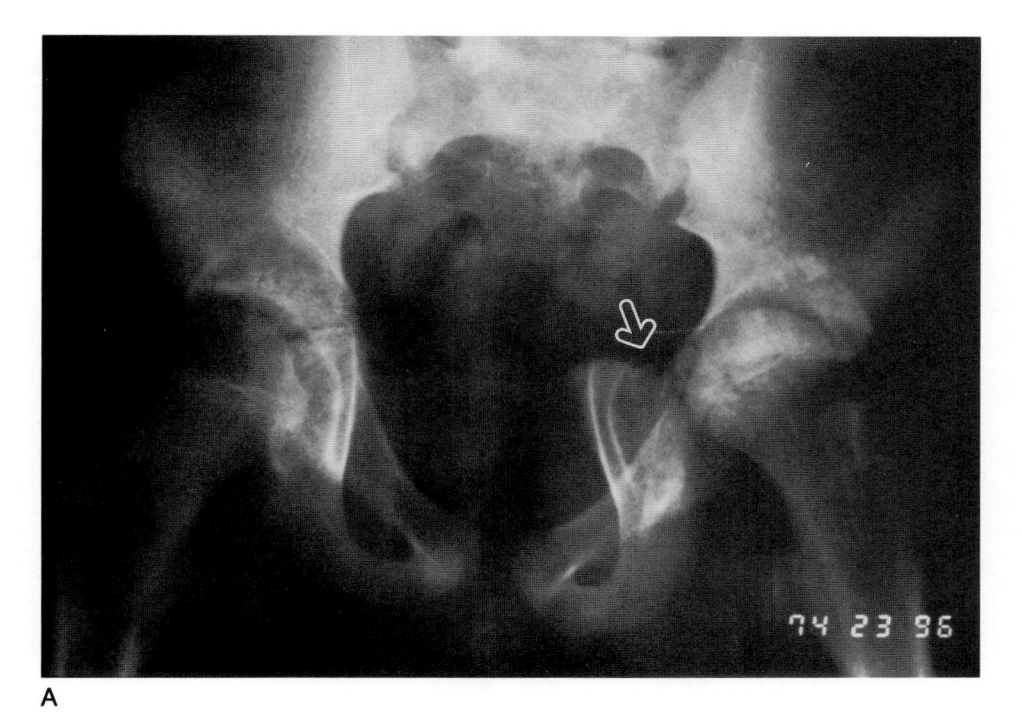

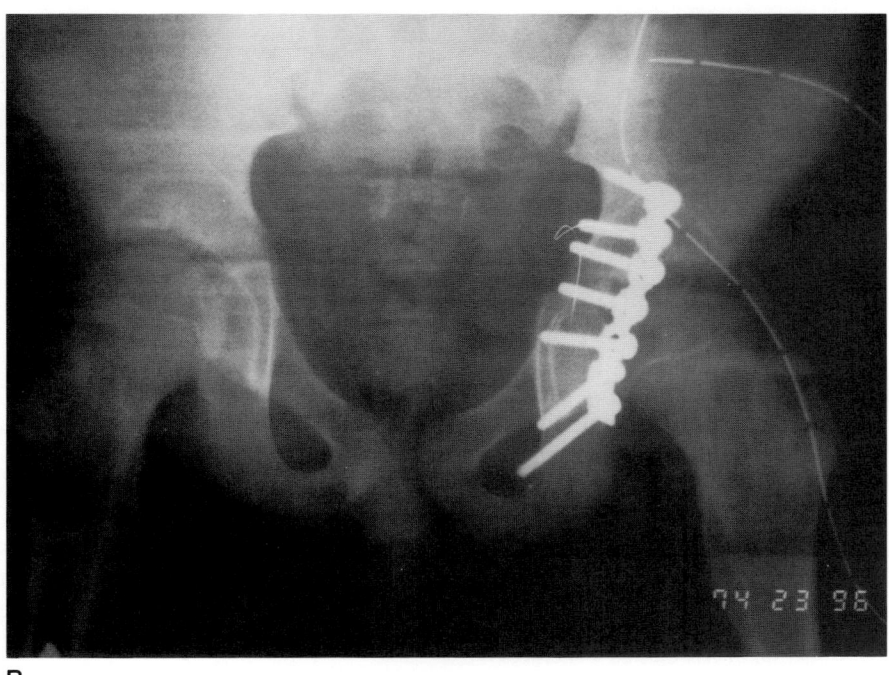

Fig. 25-18. **(A)** Unstable posterior fracture dislocation of hip with significant disruption of posterior column. **(B)** Treated with open reduction and plate fixation. *(Figure continues.)*

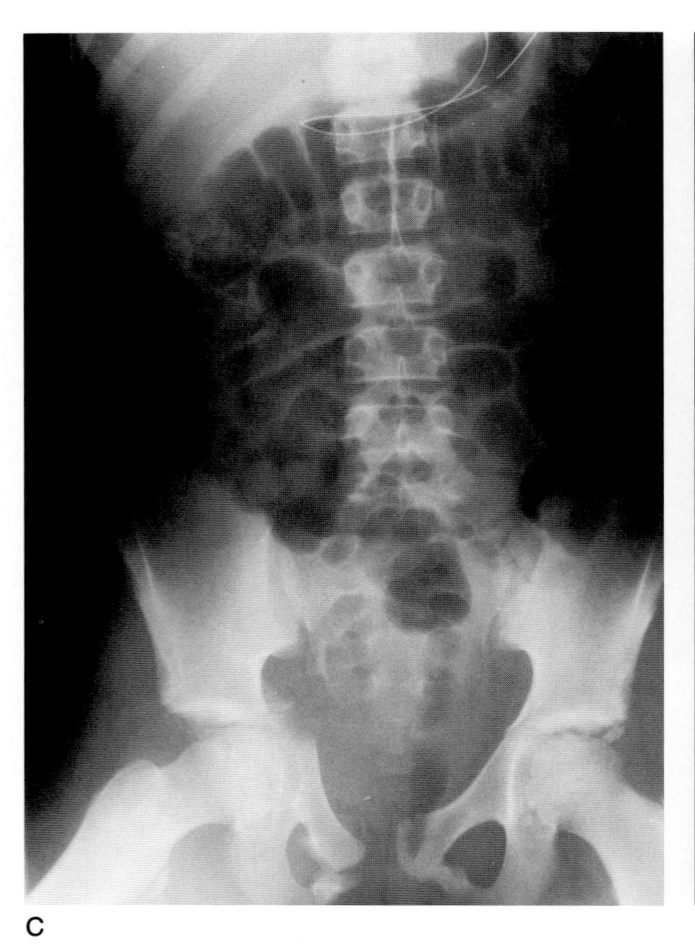

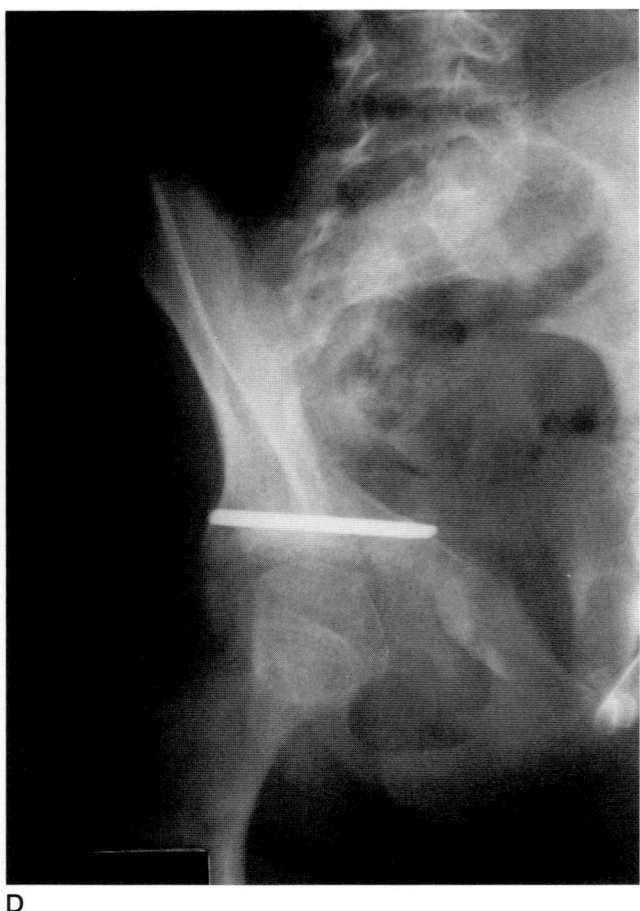

Fig. 25-18 *(Continued).* **(C)** Fracture of right acetobulum with central dislocation of the hip in a 12-yr-old boy. **(D)** Treated with an open reduction and fixation with a threaded pin.

months, has given the best results.[9,43,44] For the older child with large acetabular fragments, especially into the superior dome, weightbearing before 10 weeks is to be discouraged.

Indications for operative intervention as shown in Table 25-6 are: unstable posterior fracture-dislocations (Fig. 25-17), irreducible central fracture-dislocations (Fig. 25-18), the presence of bony fragments within the articular surfaces, and possibly for the reconstruction of the superior weight-bearing dome of the acetabulum where large fragments can be drawn together with cancellous screws. The surgical approaches for these have been well described by Letournel[28] and the ancillary use of malleable plates with screws have been shown to be helpful in the treatment of these fractures in adults.[5,35,44]

Restraint must be exercised when considering surgical options for treatment of acetabular or pelvic fractures in children. Patients whose fractures have less than 2 mm of displacement will generally have good functional and radiographic results. Absolute anatomic restoration is not necessary in children because of their ability to remodel. Incongruency on a postreduction plain radiograph may indicate the presence of loose bodies in the

TABLE 25-5. Classification of Acetabular Fractures

Type 1	Small chips occurring with dislocation
Type 2	Linear fractures that occur in association with pelvic fractures without displacement; generally stable
Type 3	Multiple fragments which lead to instability
Type 4	Fractures secondary to central dislocation of the hip with linear or stellate fractures through the inner wall

(From Watts,[10] with permission.)

TABLE 25-6. Indications for Surgery in Pediatric Acetabular Fractures

1. Unstable posterior fracture-dislocation of hip
2. Irreducible central fracture-dislocation
3. Bone fragments between articular surfaces
4. Reconstruction of weight-bearing dome

joint, which can be confirmed on CT scanning. These should be removed surgically. Adequate reduction and maintenance of reduction must be achieved in central fracture-dislocations, and this sometimes requires surgical intervention. Occasionally posterior acetabular fragments will be large and lead to late instability, which may be prevented by screw or pin fixation. However, results may *still* be unsatisfactory and lead to a poor functional result due to direct cartilage injury.[38]

Triradiate Cartilage Injury

Much has been written about the growth and potential injury to the triradiate cartilage.[12,14,16,39,45] Disruption of the acetabular triradiate cartilage occurs infrequently but may be associated with longterm acetabular dysplasia and subsequent subluxation of the hip. Certainly the earlier the age of the patient at the time of injury, the greater the chance of premature closure of the triradiate cartilage and subsequent acetabular dysplasia. The degree of damage to the triradiate cartilage also appears to be an important variable in predicting the degree of inhibition of growth. As one might expect, the total crush seen in a Salter V fracture has the potential for complete closure of the triradiate cartilage, whereas fractures of a Salter-Harris I or Salter II type may or may not produce a growth arrest (Fig. 25-19). If an osseous bridge forms across the bipolar growth cartilage along the medial wall of the acetabulum and the hemispheric acetabular physeal cartilage remains intact, then lateralization of the femoral head with a shallow acetabulum occurs[39,45] (Fig. 25-20). It has been shown that this is more likely to occur in patients under the age of 10 years and most likely with a type V fracture (Fig. 25-21). This often occurs in association with other pelvic injuries. Only one case of a Salter-Harris type II triradiate fracture has been reported requiring an open reduction due to inability to reduce it closed. No growth arrest was noted at follow-up.[45] If surgical intervention for the treatment of this type of fracture is undertaken, care must be directed toward gentle treatment of the periosteum and perichondrium around the physis so as to prevent the formation of a bony bridge. Late reconstruction of the laterally displaced acetabulum may require the use of a Chiari or other acetabular reconstructive procedures.

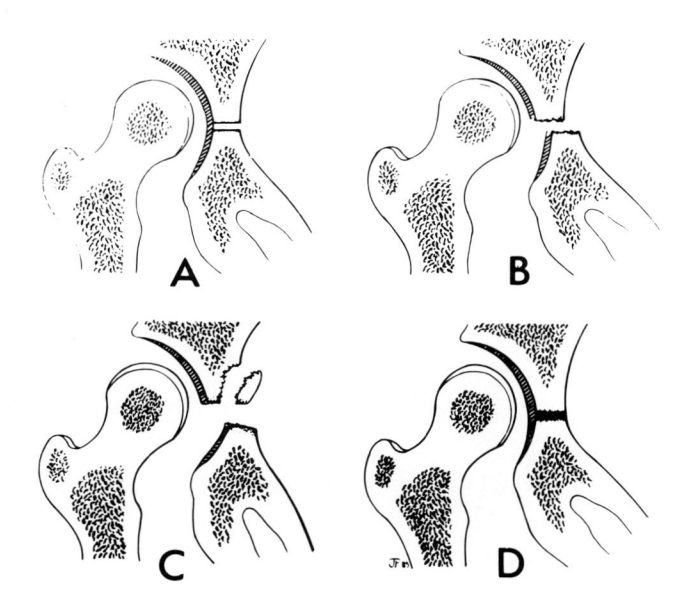

Fig. 25-19. Types of injuries sustained by the triradiate cartilage in children. **(A)** Normal. **(B)** Type I Salter-Harris fracture. **(C)** Type II Salter-Harris fracture. **(D)** Type V Salter-Harris compression fracture. (From Scuderi and Bronson,[14] with permission.)

Pitfalls to Avoid

Misdiagnosis

The initial assessment of the pediatric patient presenting with a pelvic fracture should include an aggressive search for associated injuries. The missed urologic, gastrointestinal, or neurologic injuries could easily lead to both early and late disastrous results. The knight inside his armour must be cared for first, before the fracture. Consequently, an aggressive workup and evaluation of these systems is justified initially and careful monitoring with reexamination is necessary. Hematuria should be evaluated in most instances with an intravenous pyelogram or cystourethrogram.

The avoidance of x-ray shields on the pelvis during the initial films will avoid missing the occult fracture (Fig. 25-21). An understanding of the anatomic growth plates around the pelvis will help in assessing the presence of a true fracture or a synchondrosis, such as the one frequently misdiagnosed at the ischiopubic junction. The

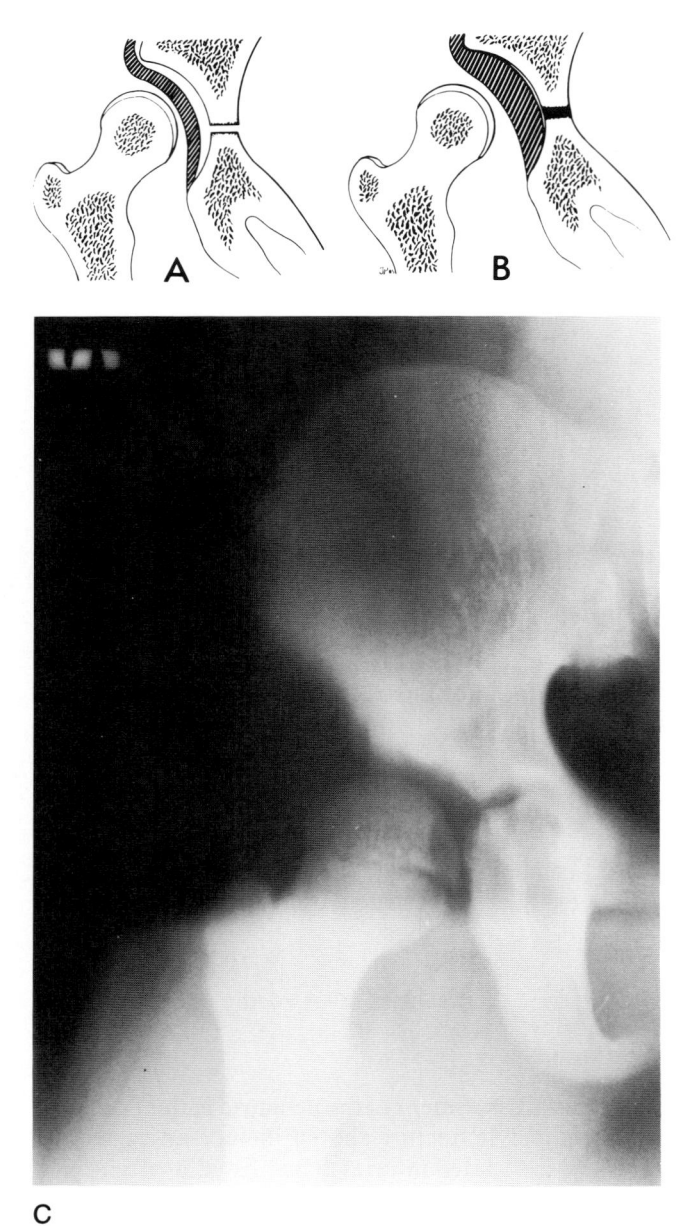

Fig. 25-20. (A) Premature closure of the triradiate cartilage resulting in (B) proliferation of the articular cartilage, thickening of the acetabular floor and a small acetabulum with lateral subluxation of the femoral head. (C) Triradiate cartilage injury has resulted in premature fusion of the physis in this 6-year-old girl, 6 months following a traumatic dislocation of the hip and acetabular fracture. (Figures A&B from Scuderi and Bronson,[14] with permission.)

presence of a completely cartilaginous avulsed apophysis off the ischium may not be visible on plain radiographs until 10 days later but can be suspected on initial clinical examination and a good history. The overuse of a pelvic sling should be avoided, especially where there is internal rotation of the hemipelvis from anterior and posterior disruption of the ring, such as may be seen in type IV fractures.

Careful follow-up is necessary in the treatment of most patients and at times may reveal the presence of associated injuries not previously diagnosed.

Maltreatment

Overtreatment and undertreatment can produce equally unfortunate results. The aggressive use of internal or external fixation around the pediatric pelvis can

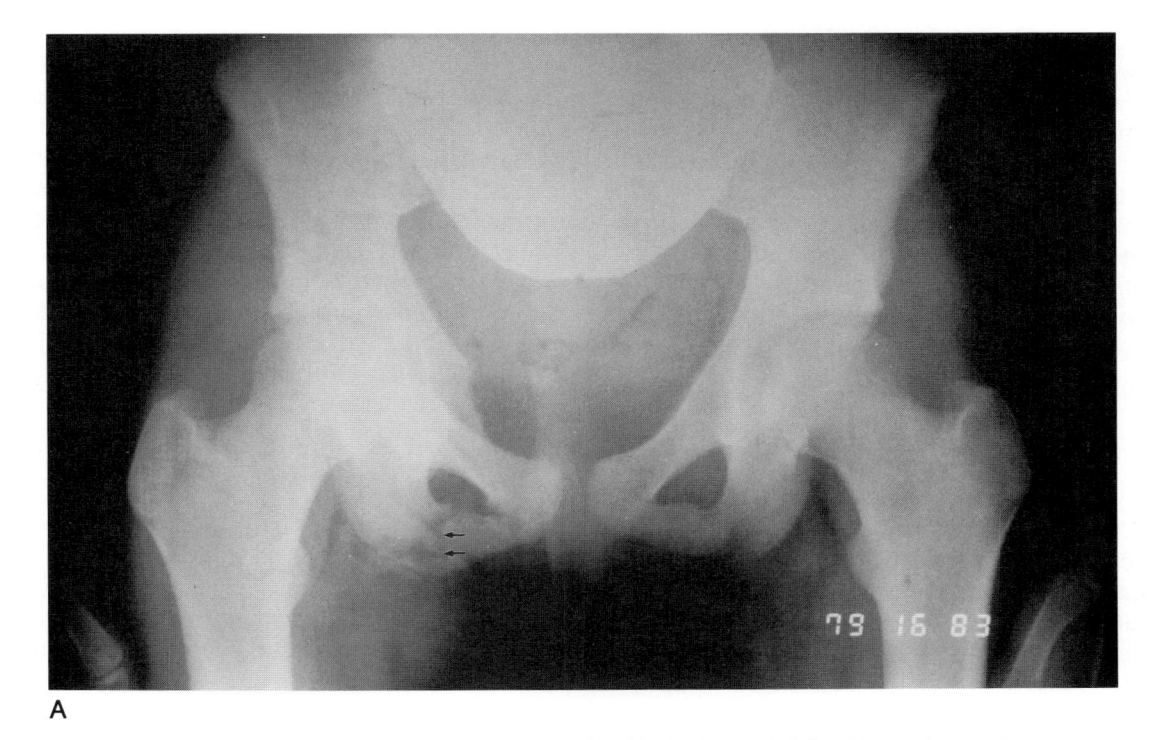

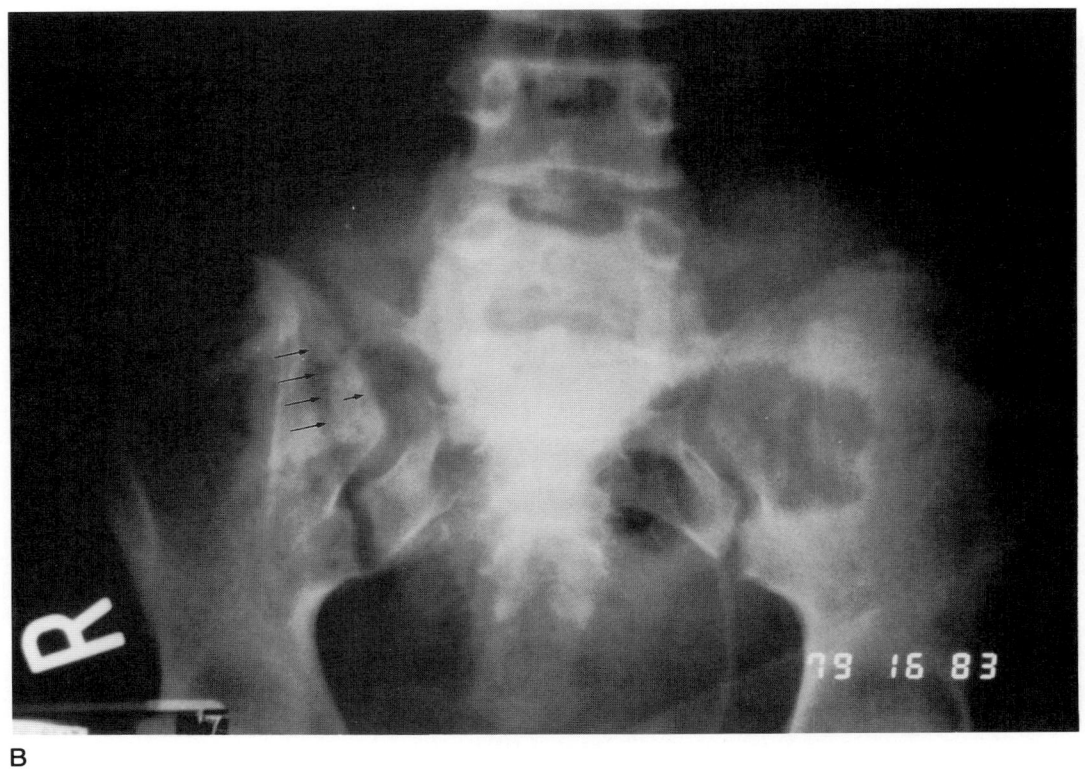

Fig. 25-21. (A) Gonadel shield in place hiding the sacroiliac joint fracture on the right side shown in (B) with shield removed.

lead to an unwarranted incidence of pin tract infection or deep wound infection. Heeg[38] has cautioned us against overuse of surgical intervention in children and has presented an example of treatment of a posterior acetabular fracture with a plate and screws that resulted in extensive heterotopic calcification with a painful, stiff hip. On the other hand, the rare patient with massive hemorrhage may benefit from the application of an external fixation device to improve tamponade and avoid the need for arterial embolization to stem blood loss.

COMPLICATIONS

Neurologic

Complications in this patient population occur primarily from the associated injuries. The high incidence of head trauma has led to the greatest number of deaths in all reported series.[2,3,24,25] A 10 to 11 percent mortality has been attributed to irreversible neurologic injury and only rarely has massive retroperitoneal bleeding been the cause of death in children.[2,3,24,25] Children with severely displaced pelvic fractures especially those associated with a vertical shear injury or a displaced acetabular fracture have a higher incidence of lumbosacral plexus lesions.[5,6] There is a higher incidence of all types of neurologic injuries in type III and type IV fracture groups.[6] The central nervous system injuries are generally diagnosed early, whereas a delay in diagnosis often occurs before identification of peripheral nerve injuries in many patients.[6] Patients with lumbosacral injuries and associated spinal injuries sometimes incur permanent neurologic sequelae and monoplegia.[8]

Urologic

The genitourinary injuries generally occur in association with displaced pubic fractures where there was rupture of the puboprosthatic ligament or the urogenital membrane (Fig. 25-22). Occasionally the bladder is

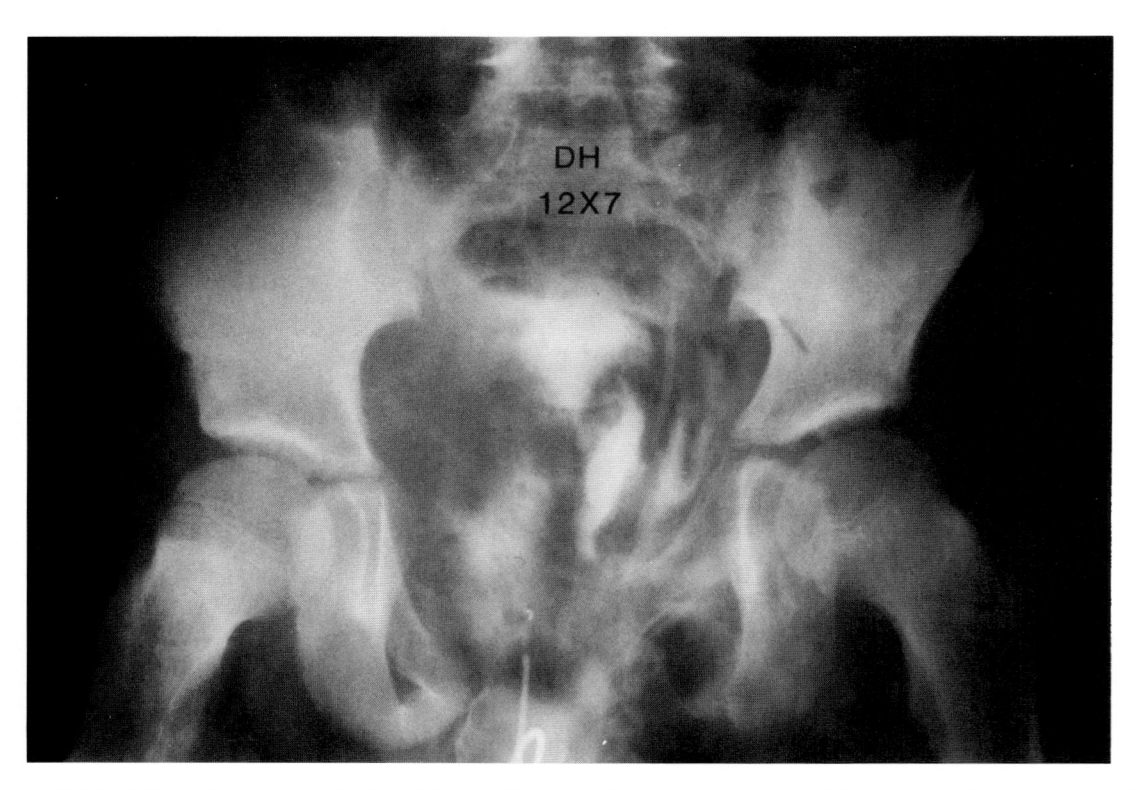

Fig. 25-22. Disruption of symphysis pubis in a 12-year-old motorcyclist resulted in rupture of the bladder and urethra seen on retrograde cystogram with extravasated dye in the pelvis.

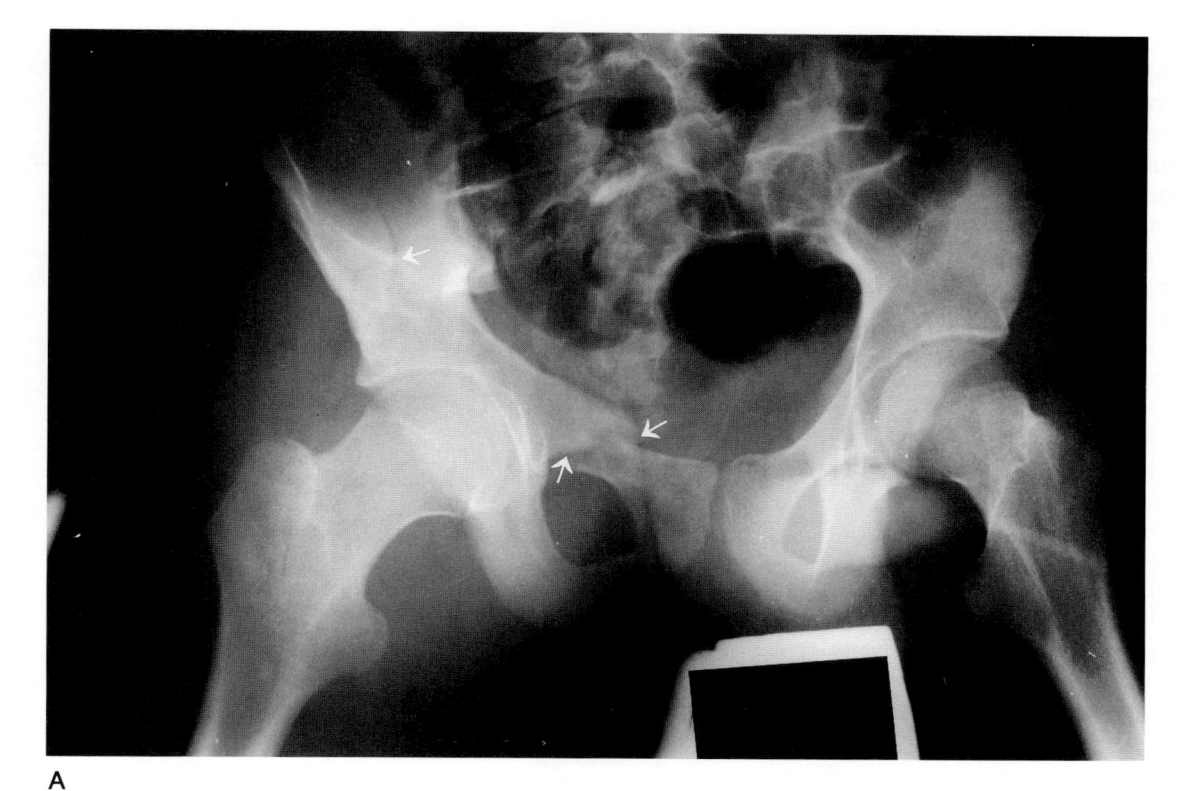

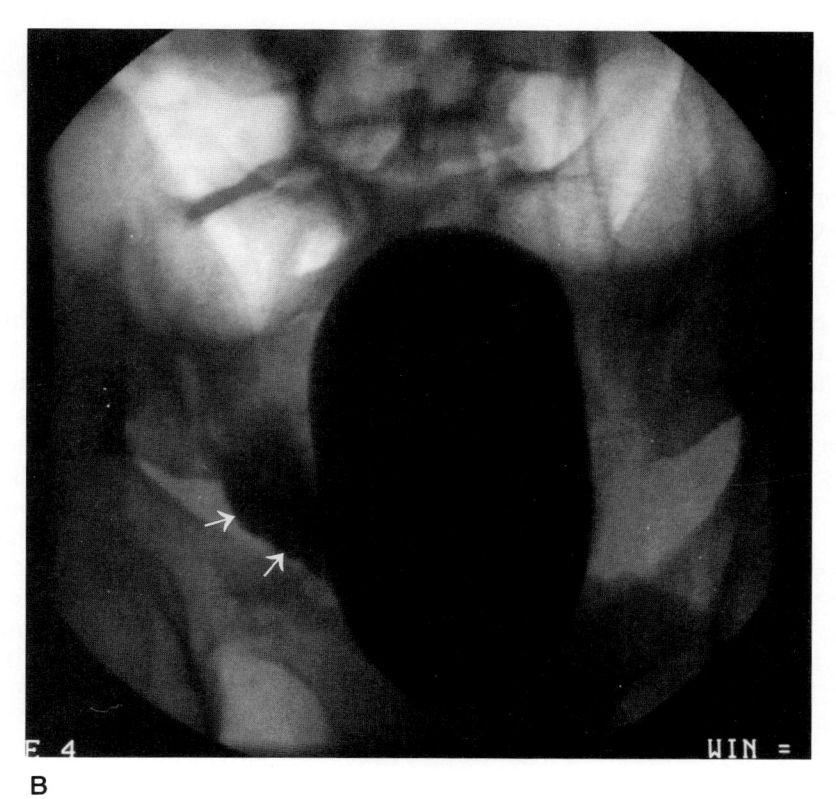

Fig. 25-23. **(A)** Fracture of the right iliac wing and displaced superior ramus fracture in a 15-year-old girl struck by a car. **(B)** The cystogram shows dye leakage confirming a puncture wound of the bladder by the bone fragment of the superior ramus fracture sustained at the moment of impact.

punctured by a direct blow from a bone fragment[3] (Fig. 25-23). Most patients with hematuria, all patients with bladder rupture or vaginal lacerations, and most of the patients with urethral injury were in the type III and type IV fractures.[6] It is not uncommon for patients to have persistent incontinence and long-term problems from these urologic injuries. It has been estimated that the average rate of major lower urinary tract complications is 13 percent. It is essential to rule out urethral or bladder ruptures or tears with a careful work-up. Blood at the urethral meatus suggests urethral disruption and a urethrogram should be done. Urethral catheterization should be left for the urologist if a urethral tear is suspected. Urinalysis is essential with an intravenous pyelogram and/or retrograde cystogram whenever hematuria is encountered.[46]

Abdominal Injuries

Massive hemorrhage is the primary concern with associated abdominal injuries. As has been stated uncontrollable hemorrhage does not occur as frequently in pediatric pelvic fractures.[3,24] Surgical arterial ligation of the hypogastrics is seldom necessary except in rare cases of true significant arterial injury. Arterial embolization, appropriate transfusion, and the judicious use of external fixation devices will allow for control of most hemorrhagic problems due to venous or bone bleeding. Lacerations and injuries to other abdominal organs including kidney, spleen, liver, and pancreas need appropriate surgical attention and treatment.[24,25] We need to continually remind ourselves of the potential for late, delayed appearance of intracapsular splenic injuries as noted by Buckholz.[45] Vaginal and rectal lacerations have occurred from direct puncture by bone fragments and sometimes these are not discovered until late in the course of treatment when infected rectal-vaginal fistulas have developed. Intra-abdominal abscesses and pancreatitis have also been reported as complications of pelvic fractures.[24,25]

Musculoskeletal

The treatment of the concomitant fractures occurring in children with polytrauma is a separate topic and treated elsewhere but fractures of the head and neck region of the femur should be searched for and carefully evaluated as their presence may influence the treatment of the pelvic fracture (Fig. 25-24). The complications of the pelvic fracture itself can be potential or real. The

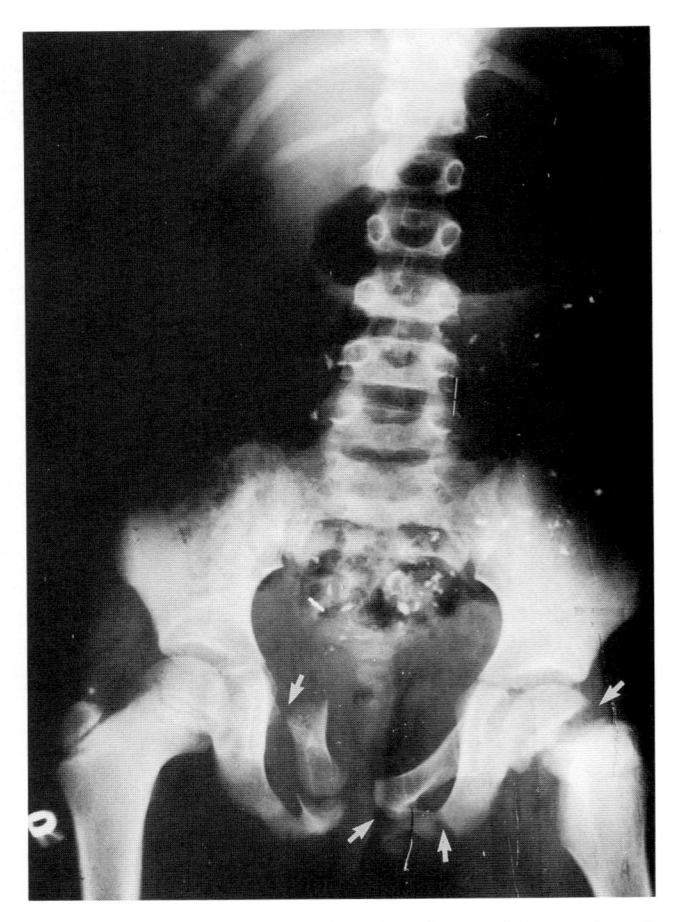

Fig. 25-24. Polytrauma victim with displaced femoral neck fracture in addition to Torode type IV fracture of pelvis.

osseous bridging causing growth arrest that occurs from significant injury to the triradiate cartilage can be identified within the first year following the insult. This has been true in all patients thus far reported and most of them were identified within the first 6 months.[12,45] Whether or not these injuries will go on to a significant lateralization of the hip depends on the age of the child at the time of the injury. Children under the age of 10 years are at greater risk for developing this deformity. Wide diastasis of the pubic symphysis does not commonly occur in the pediatric population nor has this been noted as a complication in follow-up studies. This situation occurs naturally in patients with extrophy of the bladder and lack of union of the symphysis pubis. Nonunion of the bone is rarely a problem in pediatric pelvic fractures. Fibrous unions may occur with avulsion injuries and only occasionally will they cause problems. Malunion is often corrected in the pediatric pelvis by remodeling as growth proceeds. Mild residual deficits from anterior translation of the hemipelvis have been reported as have mild leg-length discrepancies associated with vertical shear fractures, but generally these have not produced significant problems for the patients.[46] It has been recommended by some that where an unstable segment exists in the bony pelvis, the judicious use of external fixators should be applied in children especially where remodeling or bony healing is less likely to occur.[6] Certainly, adolescents have less capacity for remodeling than younger children. In adults, the occurrence of late pain and poor functional outcome has been shown to be adversely related to residual pelvic deformities.[47]

Asymmetry in the anterior ring from displaced pubic fractures will remodel but can remain as a potential obstetrical problem during childbearing years. Displacement of fractures into the articular surface of the hip joint remain as potential problems for the development of degenerative arthritis later in life. Generally, displacements of 2 mm or less are acceptable, but only time and usage will prove this correct.

SUMMARY

The presence of fractures in a child's pelvis should act as a signpost forcing us to look for associated intra-abdominal or perineal injuries. Blood loss is less of a problem in the pediatric pelvis than in the adult setting. Unstable fractures comprise only about one-third of the fractures in children, whereas 50 percent of adult fractures are considered unstable.[3] Acetabular fractures are less common in children and most often can be treated nonoperatively, a general rule which applies to the vast majority of pediatric pelvic fractures. The type I avulsion fractures are generally associated with athletic events and only rarely are they a significant problem. The use of operative intervention for these patients is not common and needs to be individualized. Type II fractures will generally require hospitalization for observation then mobilization with crutches. Type III and type IV fractures require hospitalization and a careful look for associated injuries and treatment appropriate to the particular type of fracture. Reduction of dislocations with traction alone or in conjunction with an operative procedure may be necessary to restore joint congruity and stability. Internal fixation is rarely utilized in children and then with a minimal amount of dissection and hardware in order to minimize potential complications. External fixation may be useful for the initial treatment of pelvic hemorrhage or occasionally for restoration of anatomic alignment.

REFERENCES

1. Rang M: Children's Fractures. 2nd Ed. JB Lippincott, Philadelphia, 1983
2. Bond SJ, Gotschall CS, Eichelberger MR: Predictors of abdominal injury in children with pelvic fractures. J Trauma 31:1169, 1991
3. Reed MH: Pelvic fractures in children. J Can Assoc Radiol 27:255, 1976
4. Peclet MH, Newman KD, Eichelberger MR et al: Thoracic trauma in children: an indicator of increased mortality. J Pediatr Surg 25:961, 1990
5. Tile M: Pelvic ring fractures: should they be fixed? J Bone Joint Surg [Br] 70:1, 1988
6. Torode I, Zieg D: Pelvic fractures in children. J Pediatr Orthop 5:76, 1985
7. Baker WJ, Graf EC: The management of the urinary tract in fractures of the bony pelvis. Instr Course Lect 11:245, 1954
8. Garvin KL, McCarthy RE, Barnes CL, Dodge BM: Pediatric pelvic ring fractures. J Pediatr Orthop 10:577, 1990
9. Canale ST, King RE: Pelvic and hip fractures. p. 991. In Rockwood CA, Wilkins KE, King RE (ed): Fractures in Children. 3rd Ed. JB Lippincott, Philadelphia, 1991
10. Watts HG: Fractures of the pelvis in children. Orthop Clin North Am 7:615, 1976
11. Rodrigues KF: Injury of the acetabular epiphysis. Injury 4:258, 1973
12. Blair W, Hanson C: Traumatic closure of the triradiate cartilage. J Bone Joint Surg [Am] 61:144, 1979
13. Brooks E, Rosman M: Central fracture-dislocation of the hip in a child. J Trauma 28:1590, 1988
14. Scuderi G, Bronson M: Triradiate cartilage injury. Clin Orthop Rel Res 217:179, 1987
15. Selakovich W, Love L: Stress fractures of the pubic ramus. J Bone Joint Surg [Am] 36:573, 1954
16. Ponseti IV: Growth and development of the acetabulum in the normal child. J Bone Joint Surg [Am] 60:575, 1978
17. Ogden JA: Skeletal Injury in the Child. Lea & Febiger, Philadelphia, 1982
18. Key JA, Conwell HE: The Management of Fractures, Dislocations, and Sprains. 5th Ed. CV Mosby, St. Louis, 1951
19. Fernbach SK, Wilkinson RH: Avulsion injuries of the pelvis and proximal femur. AJR 137:581, 1981
20. Cryer HM, Miller FB, Evers BM et al: Pelvic fracture classification: correlation with hemorrhage. J Trauma 28:973, 1988
21. Marcus RE, Mills MF, Thompson GH: Multiple injury in children. J Bone Joint Surg [Am] 65:1290, 1983

22. Mayer T, Matlak ME, Johnson DG, Walker ML: The modified injury severity scale in pediatric multiple trauma patients. J Pediatr Surg 15:719, 1980
23. Quinby WC: Fractures of the pelvis and associated injuries in children. J Pediatr Surg 1:353, 1966
24. Reichard SA, Helikson MA, Shorter N et al: Pelvic fractures in children: a review of 120 patients with a new look at general management. J Pediatr Surg 15:727, 1980
25. Musemeche CA, Fischer RP, Cotler HB, Andrassy RJ: Selective management of pediatric pelvic fractures: a conservative approach. J Pediatr Surg 22:538, 1987
26. Rothenberger DA, Fischer RP, Strate RG et al: The mortality associated with pelvic fractures. Surgery 84:356, 1978
27. Magee DJ: Orthopedic Physical Assessment. WB Saunders, Philadelphia, 1987
28. LeTournel E, Judet R: Fractures of the Acetabulum. Springer-Verlag, New York, 1981
29. Schlonsky J, Olix ML: Functional disability following avulsion fracture of the ischial epiphysis. J Bone Joint Surg [Am] 54:641, 1972
30. Wootton JR, Cross MJ, Holt KW: Avulsion of the ischial apophysis. J Bone Joint Surg [Br] 72:625, 1990
31. Howard FM, Piha RJ: Fractures of the apophyses in adolescent athletes. JAMA 192:842, 1965
32. Martin TA, Pipkin G: Treatment of avulsion of the ischial tuberosity. Clin Orthop Rel Res 10:108, 1957
33. Brunette DD, Fifield G, Ruiz E: Use of pneumatic antishock trousers in the management of pediatric pelvic hemorrhage. Pediatr Emerg Care 3:86, 1987
34. Dabezies EJ, Millet CW, Murphy CP et al: Stabilization of sacroiliac joint disruption with threaded compression rods. Clin Orthop Rel Res 246:165, 1989
35. Matta JM, Saucedo T: Internal fixation of pelvic ring fractures. Clin Orthop Rel Res 242:83, 1989
36. Alonso JE, Horowitz M: Use of the AO/ASIF external fixator in children. J Pediatr Orthop 7:594, 1987
37. Reff RB: The use of external fixation devices in the management of severe lower-extremity trauma and pelvic injuries in children. Clin Orthop Rel Res 188:21, 1984
38. Heeg M, Klasen HJ, Visser JD: Acetabular fractures in children and adolescents. J Bone Joint Surg [Br] 71:418, 1989
39. Gepstein R, Weiss RE, Hallel T: Acetabular dysplasia and hip dislocation after selective premature fusion of the triradiate cartilage. J Bone Joint Surg [Br] 66:334, 1984
40. Pennal GF, Tile M, Waddell JP, Garside H: Pelvic disruption. Clin Orthop Rel Res 151:12, 1980
41. Epstein HC: Posterior fracture-dislocation of the hip: long-term follow-up. J Bone Joint Surg [Am] 56:1103, 1974
42. Rowe CR, Lowell JD: Prognosis of fractures of the acetabulum. J Bone Joint Surg [Am] 43:30, 1961
43. Urist MR: Fractures of the acetabulum: the nature of the traumatic lesion, treatment, and two-year end-results. Ann Surg 127:1150, 1948
44. Tile M: Fractures of the acetabulum. Orthop Clin North Am 11:481, 1980
45. Blair W, Hanson C: Traumatic closure of the triradiate cartilage. J Bone Joint Surg [Am] 61:144, 1979
46. Bryan WJ, Tullos HS: Pediatric pelvic fractures: review of 52 patients. J Trauma 19:799, 1979
47. McLaren AC, Rorabeck CH, Halpenny J: Long-term pain and disability in relation to residual deformity after displaced pelvic ring fractures. Can J Surg 33:492, 1990

26

Fractures of the Hip

Stanley M.K. Chung

> The larger the island of knowledge, the longer the shoreline of wonder.
> —Joseph MacInnis

DESCRIPTION AND INCIDENCE

Hip fractures are uncommon in children. Most orthopedic surgeons will treat no more than three or four in their entire orthopedic career. In childhood, these fractures comprise less than 1 percent of those occurring in adults.[1] Hip fractures in children may occur at all ages, but most frequently occur in the 10 to 12 age group with 60 to 75 percent being in males. Serious complications occur as a result of this injury in nearly 60 percent of children.

ANATOMIC CONSIDERATIONS

Vascular Supply of the Femoral Head and Neck

Avascular necrosis, the most frequent and serious complication, most commonly results from avulsion of arteries and veins on the lateral surface of the femoral neck. These vessels are fixed at one end as they pass through the capsule and at the other end as they pass through the small vascular foramina on their way to supply the interior of the femoral head and neck. Damage may also occur to the extracapsular vascular ring (Figs. 26-1 and 26-2).

The basic arterial pattern to the proximal end of the femur is established at birth and probably persists throughout life. Apparent age-related variations in arterial appearance at the head and neck represent in part changes in the position of the epiphyseal plate, enlargement of the secondary center of ossification, and increases in surface area and volume supplied by the same number of arteries.[2,3]

Of importance are the anatomic relationships between the outer extracapsular arterial ring and surrounding structures, and the ascending cervical arteries as they pass through the capsule, up the femoral neck surface, then branch into intraosseous metaphyseal and epiphyseal branches. Two anastomotic vascular rings provide collateral circulation for the hip: (1) an extracapsular ring formed by the medial and lateral femoral circumflex arteries, and (2) an intracapsular ring at the articular cartilage-neck junction.

The Extracapsular Arterial Ring

The medial and lateral femoral circumflex arteries originate in the femoral triangle and form an extracapsular ring surrounding the base of the femoral neck. The medial, posterior, and lateral ring are a continuation of the medial femoral circumflex artery, while the anterior ring is formed by the lateral femoral circumflex artery (Figs. 26-1 and 26-2).

Most of the arterial supply to the femoral head, neck, and trochanter is provided by the lateral extracapsular ring (an extension of the medial femoral circumflex).

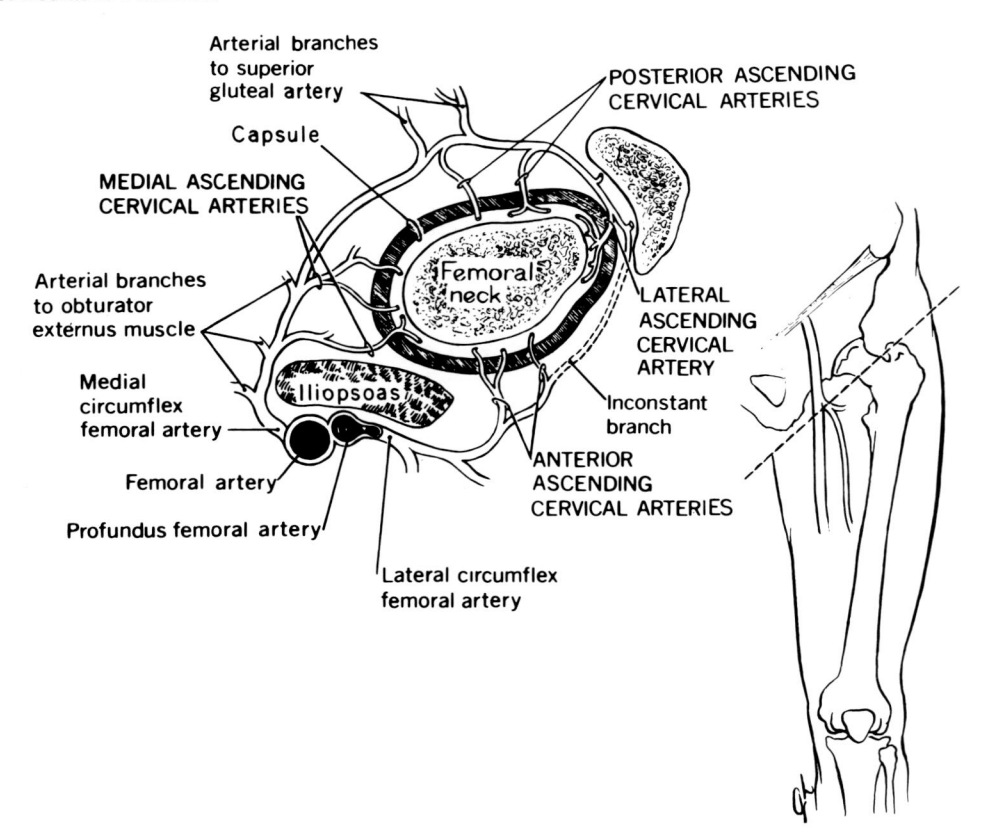

Fig. 26-1. Cross section of the proximal left femur at the base of the neck showing extracapsular ring. Broken lines indicate inconstant connections between anterior and lateral ascending cervical arteries. Note how the single lateral ascending cervical artery branches into multiple arteries after traversing the capsule. (From Chung,[2] with permission.)

LATERAL FEMORAL CIRCUMFLEX ARTERY

The lateral femoral circumflex artery originates from the profunda femoris artery in 90 percent of cases and from the femoral artery in 10 percent. This artery passes anterolateral to the iliopsoas, then divides into several terminal branches that supply the anterior femoral head and neck.

ASCENDING CERVICAL ARTERIES

The ascending cervical arteries, branches of the extracapsular arterial ring, pierce all sides of the capsule along its attachment at the base of the femoral neck. An average of two arteries cross the anterior side, two cross the medial side, 1.4 cross the posterior side, but only 1.1 pierce the lateral capsule.[2,3]

The medial femoral circumflex artery runs adjacent to the posterior capsule and passes obliquely through the lateral capsule in the posterior trochanteric fossa. This single stem artery branches to form many epiphyseal and metaphyseal branches, which are the major supply for the greater trochanter and femoral head and neck during all stages of growth (Fig. 26-1).

The capsule in the trochanteric fossa at the arterial crossing is thick, and the space between the trochanter and capsule is exceedingly narrow, particularly in children less than 8 years old.[2] The important single lateral ascending cervical artery may be compressed or torn as it passes through this very constricted area.

ON THE FEMORAL NECK SURFACE

The ascending cervical branches of the extracapsular arterial ring pierce the joint capsule along its femoral

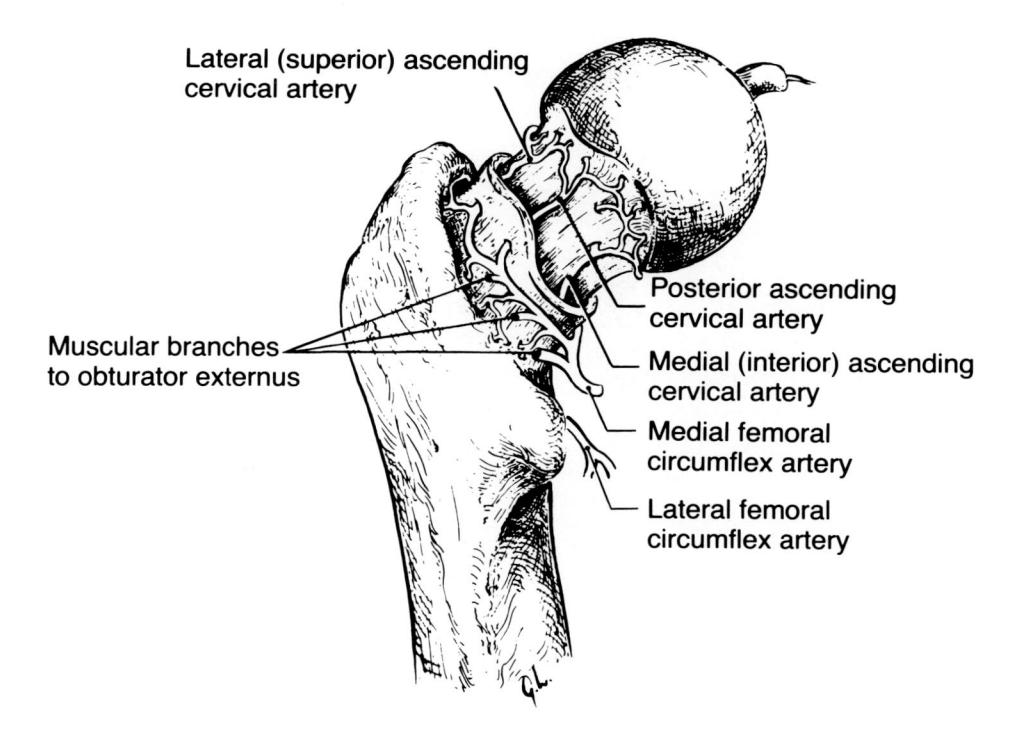

Fig. 26-2. Arterial supply at the posterior femoral neck. Note branches of the medial femoral circumflex pierce the capsule then pass up the femoral neck (the medial, posterior, and lateral cervical ascending arteries). (From Chung,[3] with permission.)

attachment, pass subsynovial, and then branch to supply the epiphysis and metaphysis. The largest number of arteries cross the lateral midneck surface (Fig. 26-2).

Intra-articular Subsynovial Arterial Ring

The four groups of ascending cervical arteries anastomose to form a subsynovial ring on the surface of the femoral neck at the articular cartilage margin in the subcapital sulcus (Fig. 26-2).

Intraosseous Arterial Supply

Arterial Supply to the Metaphysis

Metaphyseal arteries include (1) many small vessels in the bone interior and (2) metaphyseal branches of the lateral ascending cervical artery, which descend vertical to the base of the femoral neck and then turn lateral toward the greater trochanter or medial toward the midneck (Fig. 26-3).

Arterial Supply to the Capital Femoral Epiphysis

Prior to the appearance of the capital secondary ossification center, ascending cervical artery branches pass into the head cartilage and terminate in sinusoidal expansions. Multiple ossification centers may later be present and each center may be supplied by a separate artery.

Barrier Between Epiphyseal and Metaphyseal Blood Supply

The epiphyseal plate is an absolute barrier to blood flow between the epiphysis and ossified metaphysis in children (Fig. 26-3) after 1 year of age. Vessels may cross the epiphyseal plate in infants.

Ligamentum Teres Artery

The ligamentum teres artery supplies one or more large vessels penetrating deeply into the femoral head in 28 percent of children. These arteries may explain why

486 / Management of Pediatric Fractures

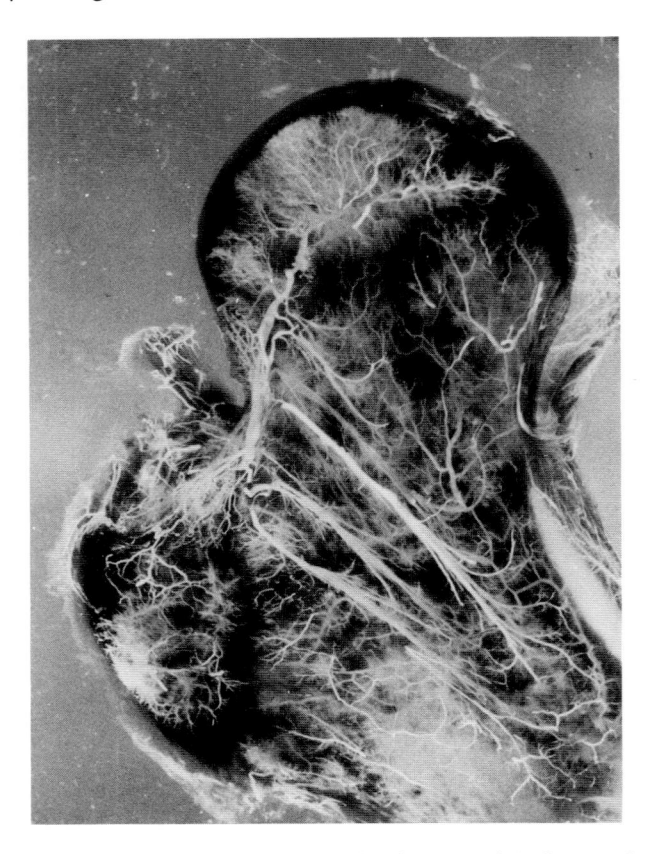

Fig. 26-3. Barium sulfate perfusion from the right femur of a 14-year-old girl. Note that the arteries in the trochanteric notch at the dorsal base of the femoral neck supply the trochanter, femoral neck, and femoral head.

some femoral heads remain viable in severely displaced femoral neck fractures when all femoral neck vessels are probably torn.

Venous Drainage of the Hip

The proximal femur veins have not been studied by perfusion techniques because venous valves prevent the flow of medium injected into the common iliac or femoral veins. The veins have been evaluated by introsseous injection of contrast medium into the femoral head in children.[4,5] The results indicate that the veins parallel arteries in the proximal femur.

Biomechanical Concepts of the Immature Hip

The gradual ossification of the proximal femur, the change in position of the physis, and the decreasing size of the perichondrial ring that surrounds the epiphyseal plate[6] are events that change the mechanical properties of the proximal femur and are thus important factors in determining the outcome in these injuries (Fig. 26-4).

The single physis at birth gradually separates into two physes, one for the femoral head and the other for the greater trochanter (Fig. 26-4). The capital femoral ossification center appears at an average age of 3½ months in girls and 4½ months in boys. The greater trochanter center appears at 2½ years in girls and 3½ years in boys.

Age-related differences in mechanical properties of bone may account for the more frequent hip fractures

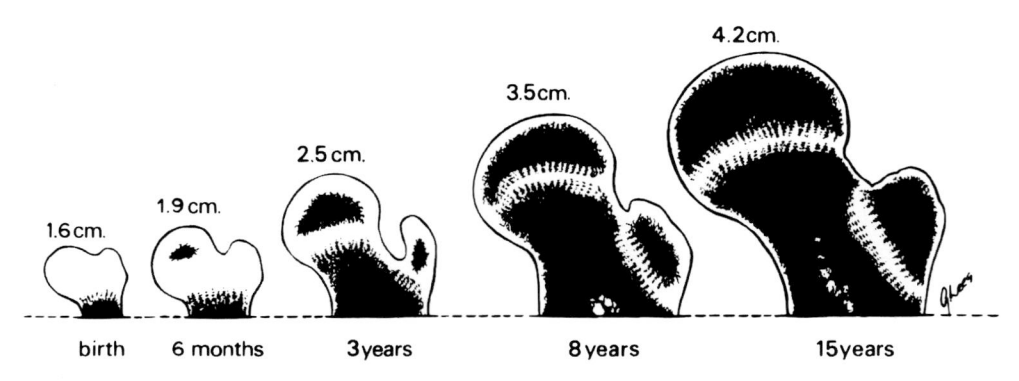

Fig. 26-4. Gradual ossification of the proximal femur is associated with a change of the femoral capital epiphyseal plate from a position below the femoral neck to a level at the junction of the femoral neck and articular cartilage. The perichondrial ring diminishes in size with age.

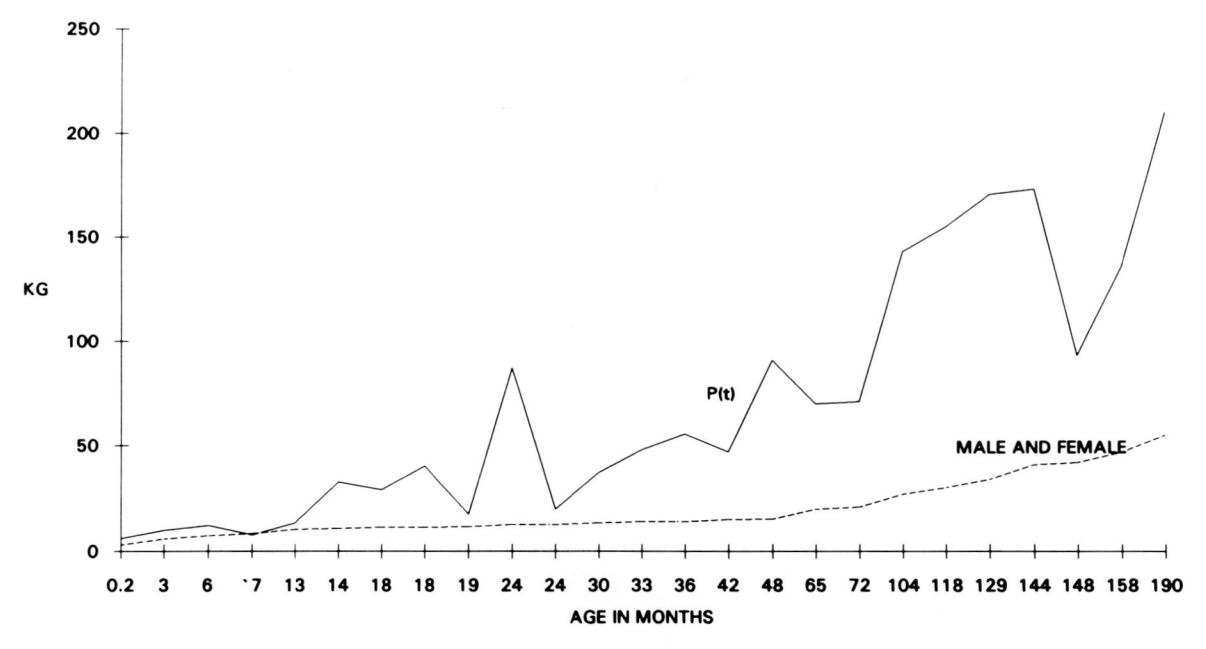

Fig. 26-5. *P(t)* is the load in kilograms which will cause failure of the femoral neck or epiphyseal plate from 5 days to 15 years of age. The *dotted line* represents the average weight of males and females at that age. Note the gradual increasing loads *P(t)* necessary to cause failure as the child matures.

among adults than among children.[7] Cortical bone testing shows that, although children's bones have a lower modulus of elasticity, a lower bending strength, and a lower ash content than adults, the children's bone deflected more and absorbed more energy before breaking and after fracture initiation. The lower ash content of the child's bone may account for its greater plastic deformation.

The proximal femoral specimens from young adults can support 10 to 15 times body weight, while those from elderly subjects support 5 to 7 times body weight.[8] Our studies demonstrated that the femoral neck or epiphyseal plate fails in adolescent specimens at 4 to 5 times body weight, whereas in children under 4 to 5 years old, failure occurs at only 2 to 3 times the body weight[6] (Fig. 26-5).

Although children's bones appear weaker than those of adults by these criteria, other factors may also explain why hip fractures are rare in children: (1) their low center of gravity and the short distances they normally fall, (2) their bone absorbs more energy before breaking,[7] (3) their thick periosteum and perichondrial ring complex protects the femoral neck and epiphyseal plate from fracture[6] (Fig. 26-6), (4) the femoral neck may bend instead of breaking,[6] and (5) their quick reaction time and greater agility. If the normal bone of the femoral neck is compromised, however, by a bone tumor, cyst, or infection, a pathologic fracture may occur with minimal loading.

If a mechanical load is applied by an instron testing machine over the secondary center, either the epiphyseal plate or femoral neck will crack or a greenstick bend will occur.[6] The total load necessary to cause a fracture of the femoral capital epiphysis or femoral neck versus age and the average weight of a child at that age are illustrated in Figure 26-5.[6] Note that the load necessary to cause epiphyseal plate or cervical neck failure increases more rapidly than the average weight of the child. A significant safety factor is thus present as the child matures.

MECHANISM OF HIP FRACTURE IN CHILDREN

In children, hip fractures result from severe trauma, such as a fall from a height or the impact from a moving vehicle. If the hip fractures after a trivial injury, a pathologic fracture should be suspected. Because severe trauma produces hip fractures, abdomen, chest, and head injuries may also be present. Child abuse may be a possible cause in children under 3 or 4 years of age.

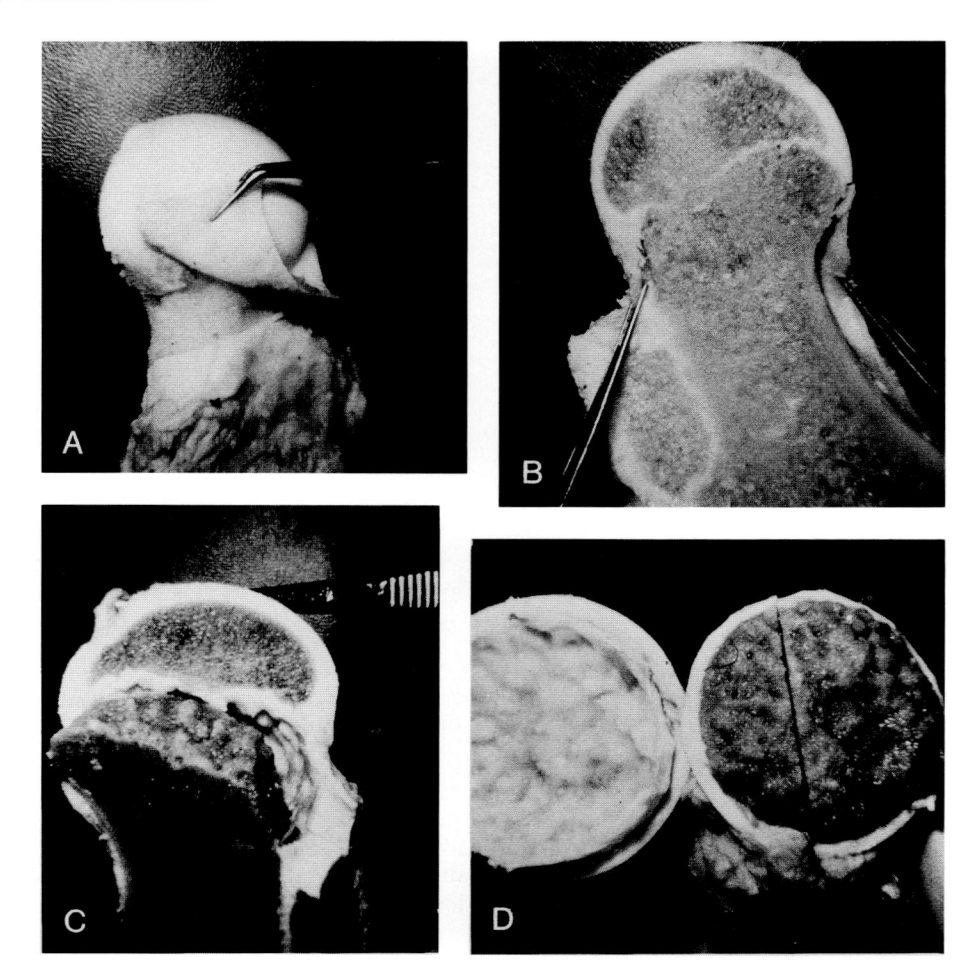

Fig. 26-6. The perichondrial fibrocartilaginous complex in a specimen from a child 10 years, 9 months old. **(A&B)** The thick fibrous layer adjacent to the epiphyseal plate. **(C&D)** The reciprocal pegs of bone and cartilage (mamillary processes). **(D)** The cap formed by the complex which tightly surrounds the metaphysis. (From Chung et al.,[6] with permission.)

TABLE 26-1. Classification of Hip Fracture

Intracapsular	
Type I	Transepiphyseal: acute traumatic separation of previously normal epiphysis (6–11%)
Type II	Transcervical: fracture through the midfemoral neck (47–50%)
Type III	Cervicotrochanteric: fracture through the base of the femoral neck (30–33%)
Extracapsular	
Type IV	Intertrochanteric: fracture from the greater to the lesser trochanter (11–12%)

CLASSIFICATION

A classification of hip fractures is shown in Table 26-1 and Figure 26-7.

The biomechanical properties of bone differ significantly in children, compared to their counterparts in the elderly population. Transcervical fractures are almost never impacted as is commonly seen in osteoporotic adult bone. Transcervical fractures (type II) in children are usually displaced.[10,11]

Rarely, a fracture-dislocation may occur.[12,13] Stress fractures across the femoral neck may also occur in children.[14,15] Occasionally a separation of the capital epiphysis or femoral neck fracture[16] may be associated with an

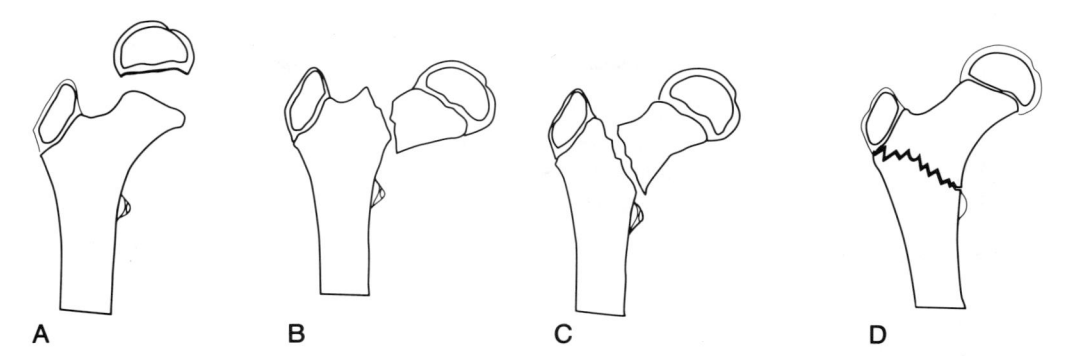

Fig. 26-7. Types of fractures of the hip. **(A)** Type I transepiphyseal. **(B)** Type II transcervical. **(C)** Type III cervicotrochanteric. **(D)** Type IV intertrochanteric.

ipsilateral femoral shaft fracture. Femoral neck fractures have followed pinning of slipped capital femoral epiphysis.[17] The femoral capital epiphyseal plate may fracture at birth[18] (Fig. 26-8). Fracture-separation of the capital femoral epiphysis may occur during attempted closed reduction of a traumatic dislocation of the hip[19] (Fig. 26-9).

PHYSICAL EXAMINATION

The apprehensive child with a hip fracture lies very still, fearful of any passive limb motion and unable to move actively. The affected limb, 1 to 2 cm shorter, is slightly externally rotated, but both the shortening and external rotation deformity is much less than observed in adults with similar fractures. Swelling and anterior hip joint tenderness are present. Active hip motion is impossible. These children usually cannot walk, but occasionally children with undisplaced or stress fractures may exhibit a severe limp and pain with hip motion in all planes.

DIFFERENTIAL DIAGNOSIS

The diagnosis of hip fracture can be confirmed by an anteroposterior and cross-table lateral radiograph. The radiographs should be carefully studied to determine the degree of angulation and the site of the fracture line, and to detect the rare dislocation of the femoral head from the acetabulum. If the child cannot be positioned for a lateral view, several oblique views should be obtained. A technetium 99mdp bone scan, tomogram, or computed tomography (CT) scan will help make the diagnosis of an undisplaced or stress fracture of the femoral neck.

In type I (transepiphyseal separation) injuries there are no prodromal symptoms predating the onset of acute epiphyseal separation (Fig. 26-10) in contrast to the findings in an acute superimposed on chronic slipped epiphysis. These two entities may sometimes be difficult to differentiate (see Ch. 27).

Neonatal epiphysiolysis may occur as a result of birth trauma. The hip is painful with passive motion in contrast to the usually painless congenital dislocated hip. An arthrogram (Fig. 26-8), ultrasound, or CT examination may be required to confirm that the femoral head remains in the acetabulum. Pseudoparalysis may occur in the affected limb. Unfortunately, in children less than 3 years old, abuse may sometimes be a cause to be considered (Fig. 26-10).

In the more common types II, III, and IV fractures there is a history of severe trauma and a painful hip.

Pathologic Fracture

If the hip fracture occurs after a trivial injury, a pathologic condition, such as a bone tumor, osteopetrosis,[20] or Gaucher's disease,[21] may have caused weakening of the bone. The atraumatic history should alert the clinician to investigate the child and hip for a predisposing pathologic condition.

Stress Fractures

Stress fractures do occasionally occur in children with open epiphyseal plates.[14,15,22] They have been reported in athletes[23] and military recruits.[24] These fractures may be

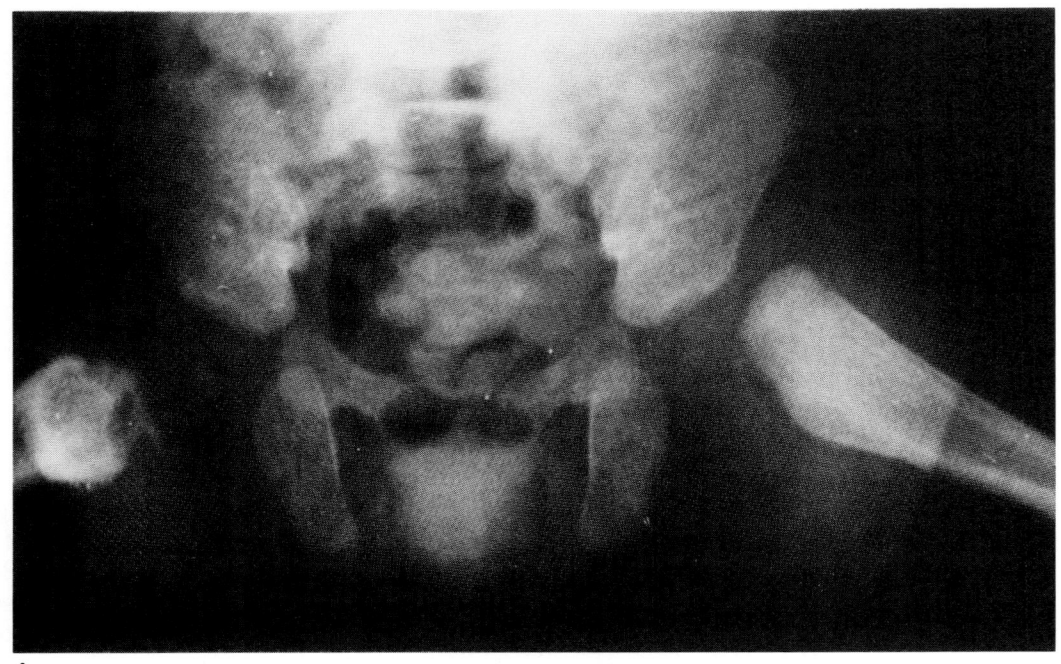

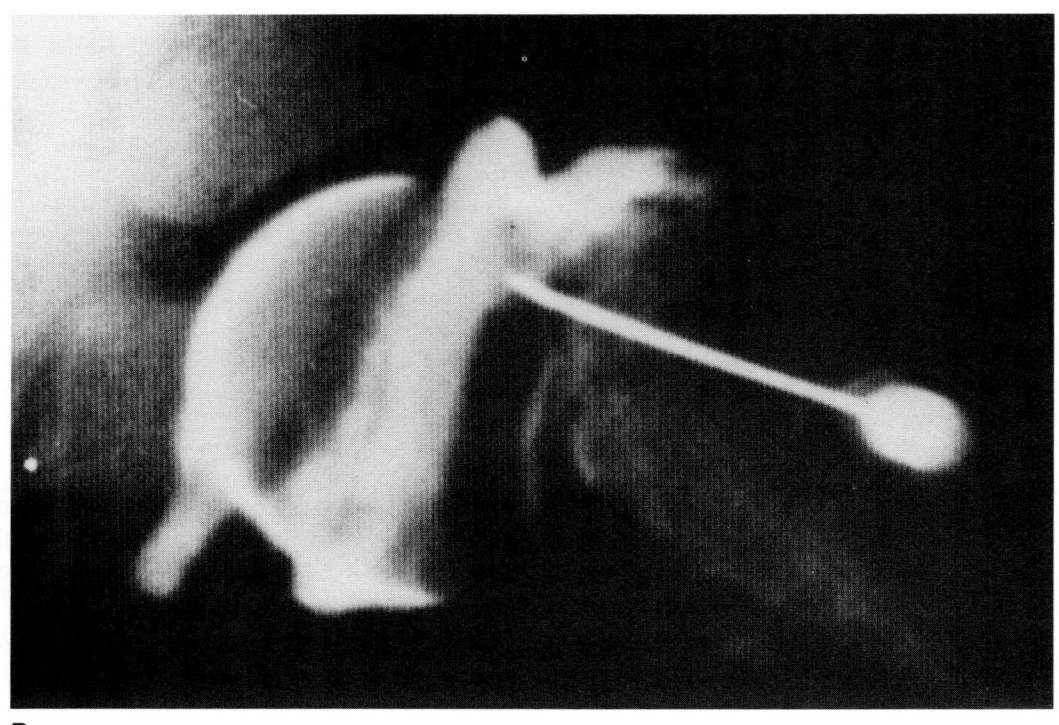

Fig. 26-8. **(A)** Newborn boy with a painful, swollen left hip. The radiograph might be misinterpreted as a congenital dislocation, but the metaphysis is closer to the ilium than in a typical dislocation. Metaphyseal irregularities are present on the right. **(B)** Left hip arthrogram reveals the femoral head within the acetabulum, but the metaphysis displaced lateral. Several months after closed reduction and abduction casting hip motion was normal and painless. (Courtesy Dr. M. Okun. From Chung,[33] with permission.)

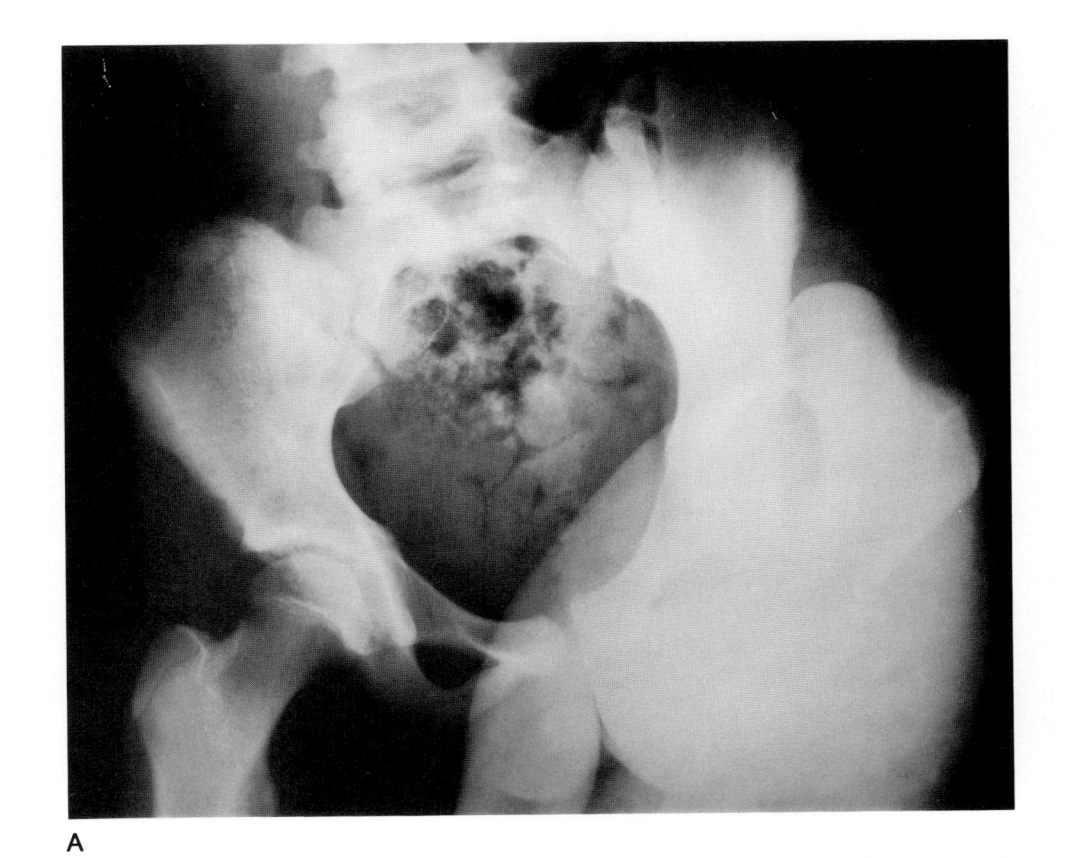

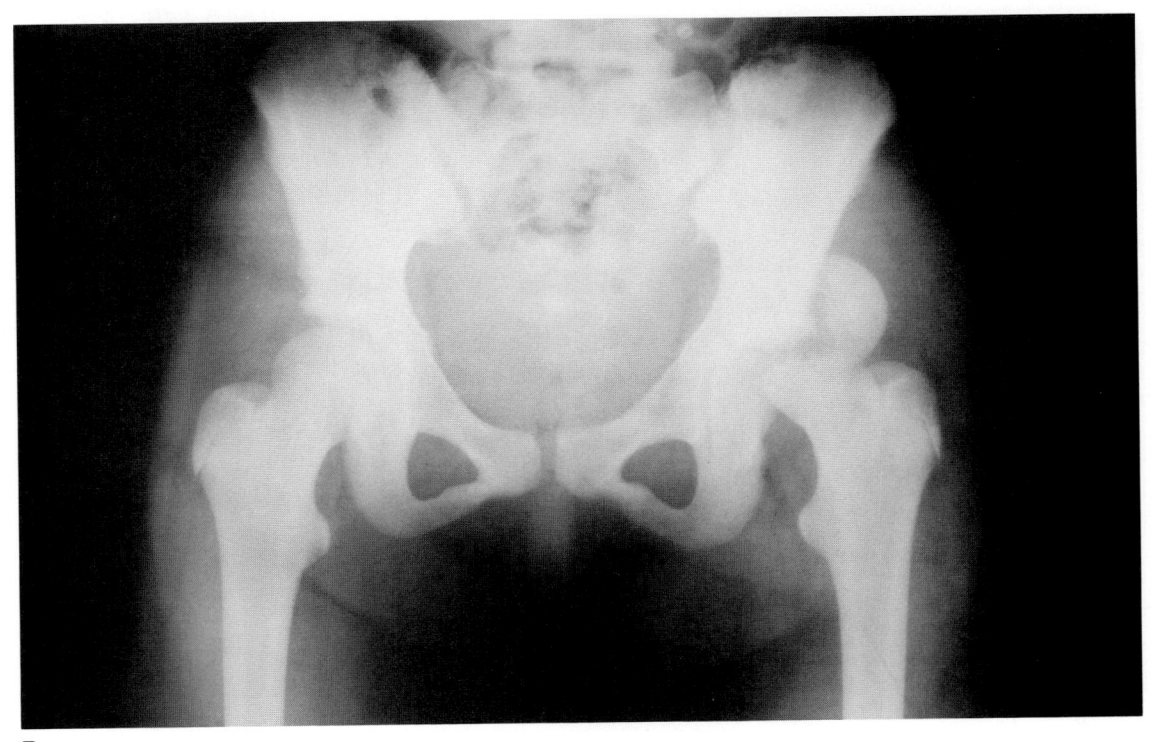

Fig. 26-9. **(A)** A 12-year-old girl sustained a posterior dislocation of her hip in a fall from a tree. **(B)** Five hours later a closed reduction was performed under general anesthesia which resulted in a fracture-separation of the capital femoral epiphysis. *(Figure continues.)*

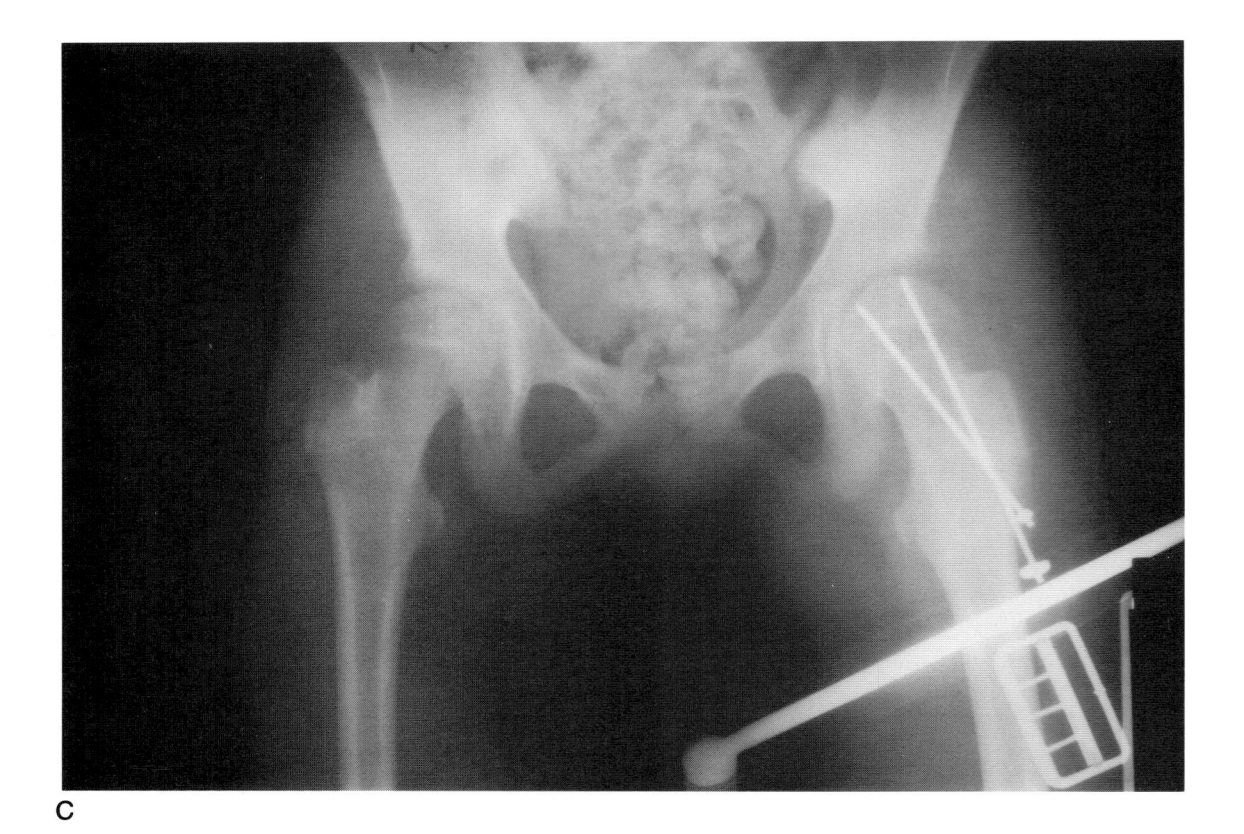

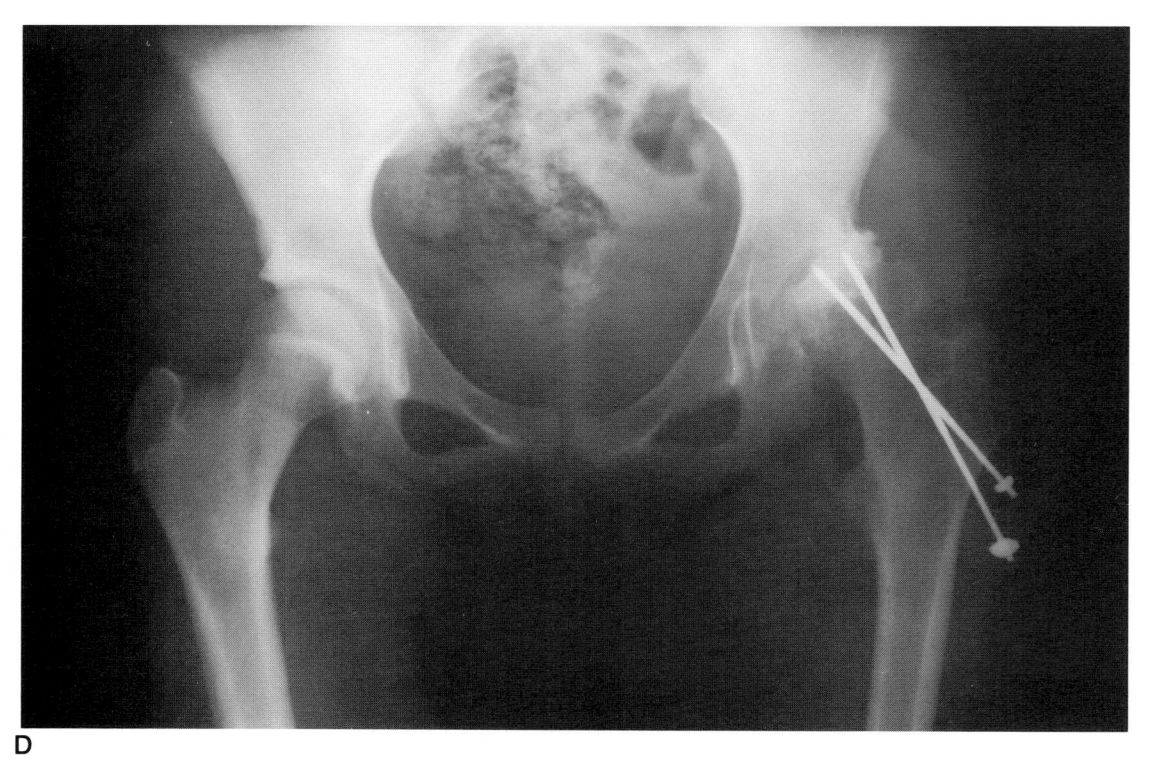

Fig. 26-9 *(Continued).* **(C)** Immediate open reduction through an anterolateral approach was performed. The Salter-Harris type I fracture was reduced and secured with two Moore pins. **(D)** In spite of bed traction for 4 weeks and nonweightbearing on crutches for 9 months, avascular necrosis of the femoral head ensued. (From Fiddian and Grace,[19] with permission.)

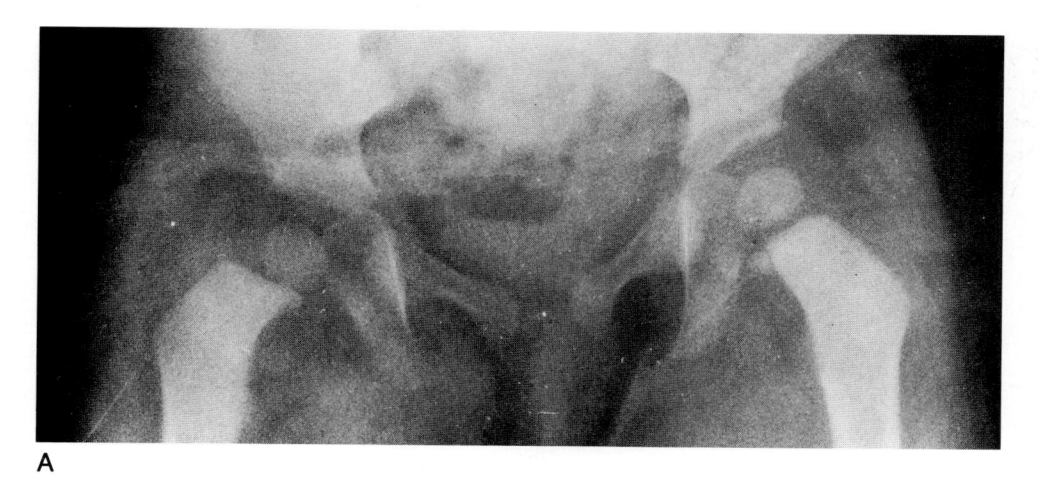

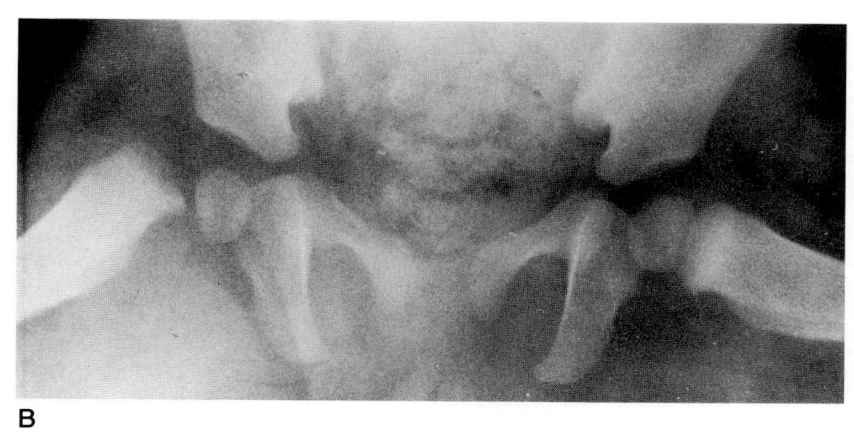

Fig. 26-10. (A) One-year-old girl, suspected child abuse. Right hip on AP view shows slight medial displacement capital femoral epiphysis. Vertical fissure on left side suggests previous trauma. (B) Lateral view shows obvious displacement of the femoral head. *(Figure continues.)*

detected with scintigraphy, especially the frog-leg view.[25] Potentially unstable stress fractures should be initially treated with rigid internal fixation because some of these may displace into a varus position in adolescents or young adults.[24]

TREATMENT

Generally hip fractures in children do not require immediate emergency treatment but should be treated promptly within 24 hours. There are reports that urgent open reduction and pin fixation together with supplemental spica casting in younger children will produce better results than delayed or conservative treatment.[26,27] In the brief period before surgery or casting, place the patient in split Russell traction.

Aspiration of the hip may be done to relieve pain and decrease intra-articular pressure caused by the fracture hematoma. Harper and colleagues[28] have shown that an intracapsular hematoma, in the presence of a damaged intraosseous circulation after an intracapsular fracture, may cause femoral head ischemia, which can be reversed by aspiration of the joint. They recommend that if osteocyte death is to be prevented, aspiration should be performed to relieve tamponade as soon as possible after the fracture.

Type I Intracapsular Fractures

Type I fractures with dislocation of the femoral head should be treated preferably within 6 hours, by open reduction and internal fixation (Fig. 26-9). Avascular

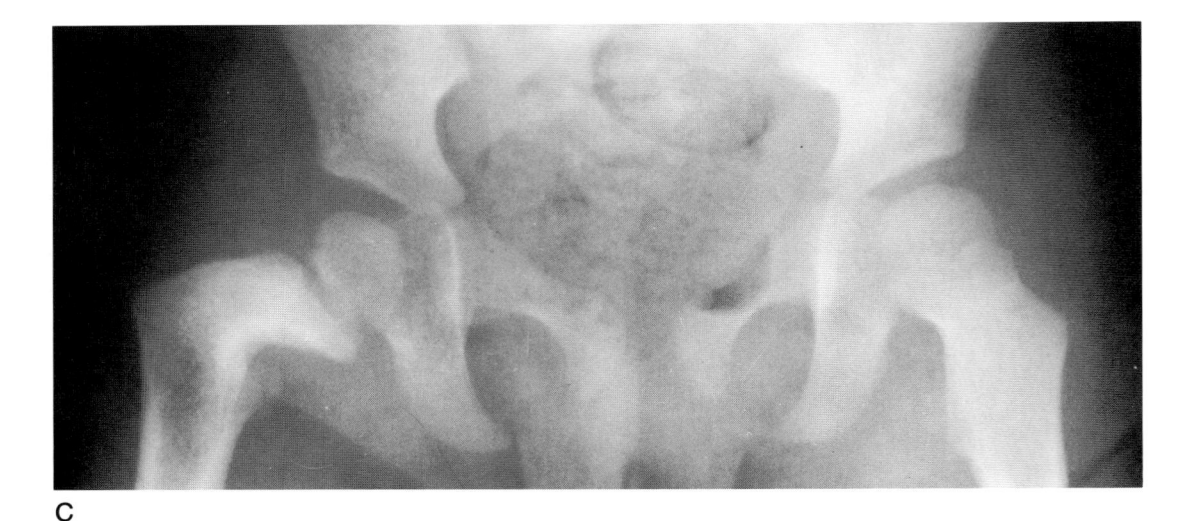

Fig. 26-10 *(Continued).* **(C)** A closed reduction was done and a spica cast applied. Coxa vara and radiodensity of the neck was present 6 months later. **(D)** Two years later the neck-shaft angle had returned to normal, and function was normal.

necrosis may be anticipated in most cases. In patients less than 3 years of age, however, type I fractures treated with gentle closed reduction and immobilization in a spica cast have been reported to have good results[29] (Fig. 26-10). Significant varus will often spontaneously correct, or if not, a valgus osteotomy may be required to correct the neck-shaft angle.[29] Children older than 3 years are best treated with open arthrotomy and internal fixation with pins smooth at the ends (Fig. 26-11) to prevent injury to the epiphyseal plate.

Types II and III Intracapsular Fractures

Intracapsular displaced types II and III fractures are probably best treated with internal fixation because the traction and manipulation necessary to obtain reduction cannot be relied upon to maintain position. Healing in varus and nonunion are also more common in patients treated with traction and casting.[30,31] The fracture may be manipulated by a closed maneuver on a standard fracture table then pinned percutaneously either with

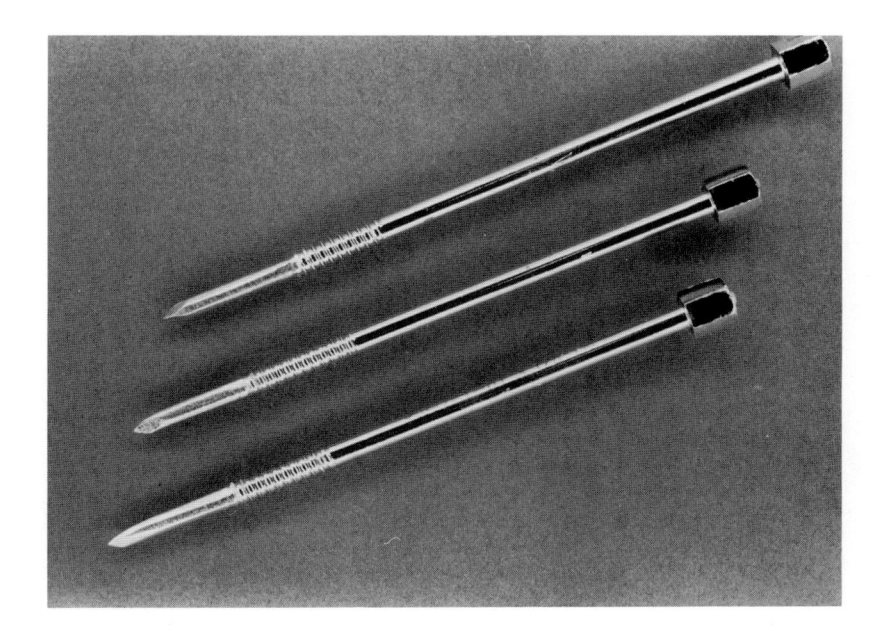

Fig. 26-11. Pins with smooth ends designed for hip pinning in children to allow penetration of growth plate with minimal damage. (Designed by Dr. Ron Monson, Winnipeg Children's Hospital.)

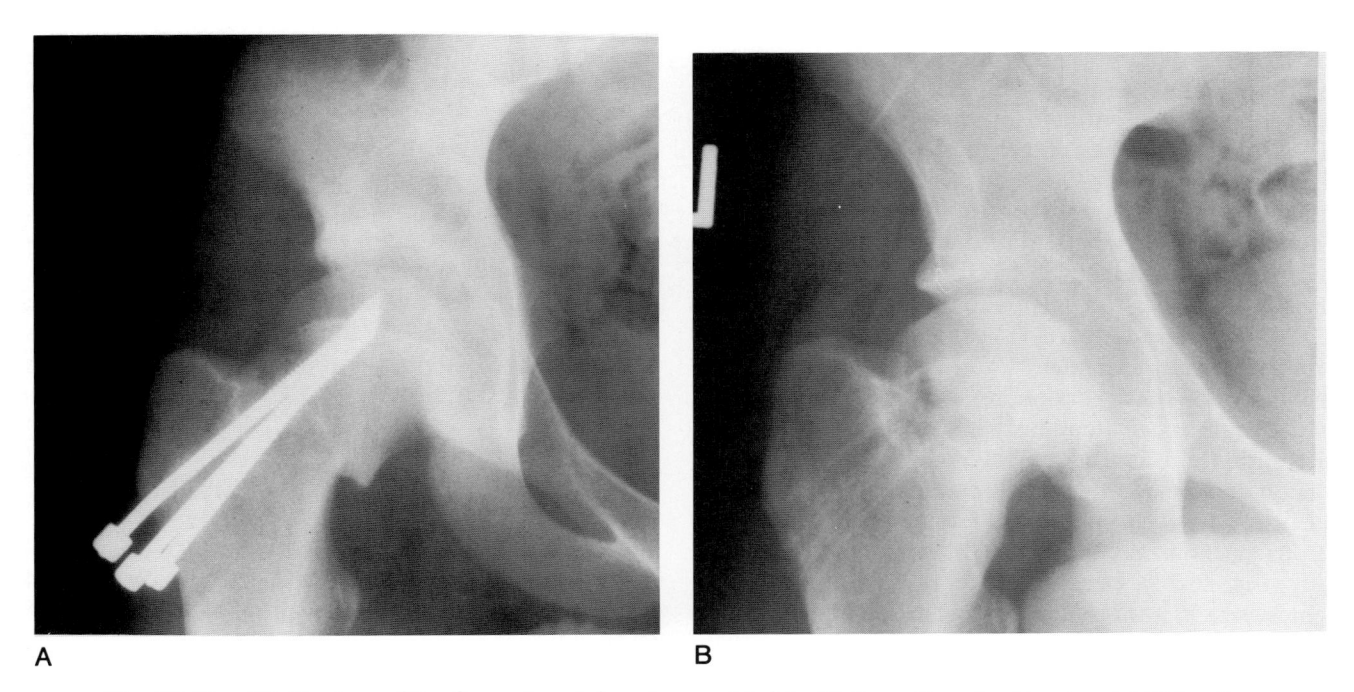

Fig. 26-12. (A) Fracture of the femoral neck in a 5-year-old girl with three Knowles hip pins stabilizing the fracture. Note threaded portion of pins crossing the physis and displacement of 20 percent at the inferior neck. (B) Three years later there is evidence of obvious physeal damage with lateral growth plate arrest resulting in a shortened neck and valgus deformity. (Courtesy of Dr. Ron Monson, Children's Hospital, Winnipeg, Canada.)

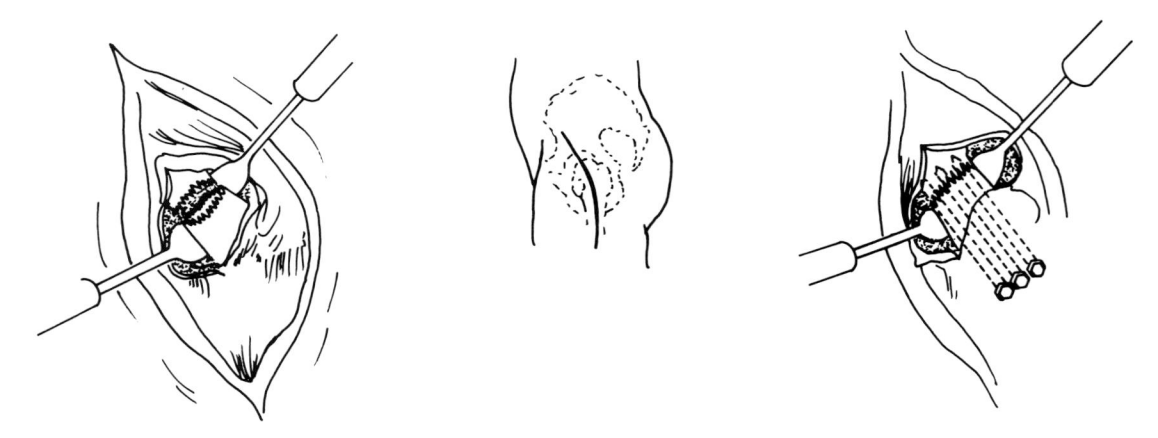

Fig. 26-13. Watson-Jones open arthrotomy technique. The fracture site is exposed, hematoma removed and the fracture reduced anatomically then stabilized with Knowles or other pins. (From Chung,[33] with permission.)

threaded Knowles pins or cannulated screws. Although an anatomic reduction is ideal, most authors state as a general rule, no displacement exceeding 10 or 20 percent of the width of the femoral neck should be accepted[32] (Fig. 26-12).

My preferred method[33,34] (Figs. 26-13 and 26-14) (also advocated by Boitzy[35] and Watson-Jones[36]) is to surgically expose the fracture site, remove the fracture hematoma, reduce the fracture to an anatomic position under direct vision, and then internally fix the fracture with Knowles pins (Figs. 26-13 and 26-14) or cannulated screws. Although some authors indicate that opening the fracture site may not greatly influence the subsequent occurrence of avascular necrosis,[31] we feel that small degrees of malrotation, angulation, translation (Fig. 26-12) or distraction (Fig. 26-15) can usually be corrected when the fracture fragments are reduced under direct vision. Closed manipulation, no matter how gentle, will avulse, tear, or twist tenuously intact vessels at the fracture site. There is undoubtedly a limit to how much torsion and tension the vessels can tolerate before arterial or venous occlusion occurs. Fracture hematoma and serous effusion may be removed through the capsulotomy (Fig. 26-13). Decompression of the joint will prevent increased intra-articular pressure, a potential cause of venous and arterial tamponade. There is evidence that for optimum healing venous drainage must return to normal status.[37] The internal fixation pins should not cross the epiphyseal plate unless the fracture cannot be stabilized without doing so such as in a type I fracture. The child is then placed in a spica cast postoperatively for about 6 weeks.

Pins are usually removed within 12 to 18 months of the injury to prevent bony overgrowth of the pinheads.

Type II undisplaced fractures are inherently unstable and will frequently drift into varus. A type II undisplaced fracture should be internally transfixed initially because the alternative use of spica immobilization is unlikely to prevent the frequently occurring varus deformity. These fractures are more likely to have a nonunion in the older child.[31,38]

Undisplaced type III fractures may be treated with immediate hip spica immobilization.[39] If the fracture displaces in the cast, however, coxa vara may occur (Fig. 26-16), so internal fixation with Knowles pins or cannulated screws may be required. Undisplaced cervicotrochanteric fractures treated with spica immobilization must have at least weekly radiographs to detect any varus displacement. If this angulation occurs, internal fixation must be carried out.

Type IV Extracapsular Fractures

Closed intertrochanteric type IV fractures may be reduced successfully with skin or skeletal traction for 2 to 4 weeks followed by the application of a spica cast.[40] Closed reduction and immediate application of a hip spica cast[39] (Fig. 26-17) has also been successfully employed. Open reduction and internal fixation with methods similar to those used in adults with compression screw and sideplate device that crosses the physis into the femoral head may be indicated in children older than 12 to 14 years. Occasionally, avascular necrosis and premature epiphyseal closure can occur with these fractures.[31]

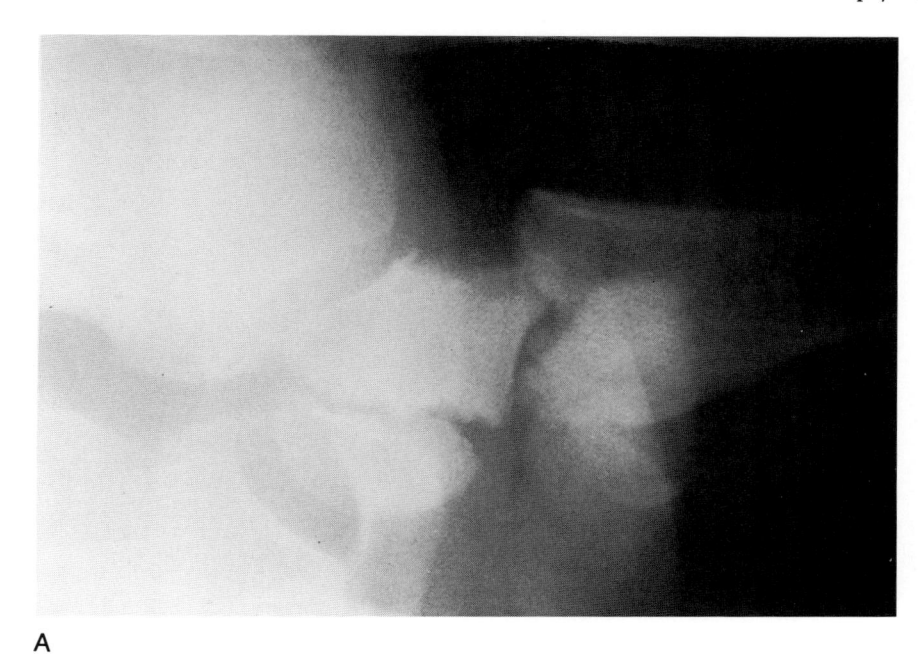

Fig. 26-14. **(A)** A 4-year-old boy struck by an auto sustained a severely displaced transcervical fracture. Both distal and proximal fragments are externally rotated. **(B)** An AP and **(C)** lateral view 4 months after Watson-Jones open anatomic reduction followed by fixation with Knowles pins. *(Figure continues.)*

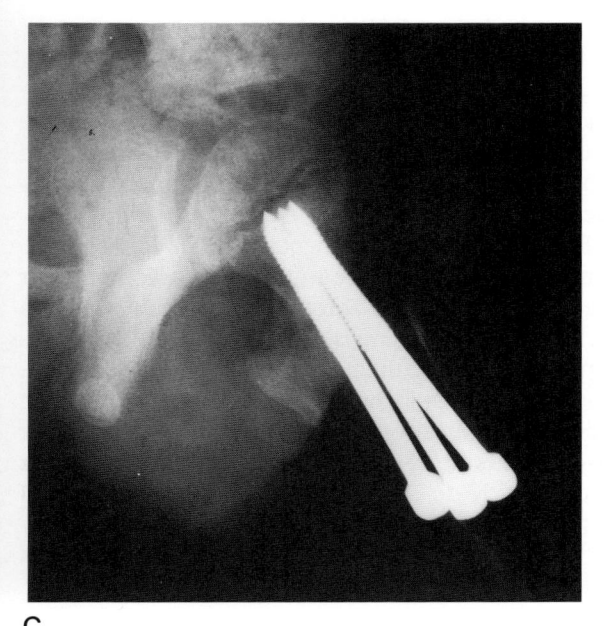

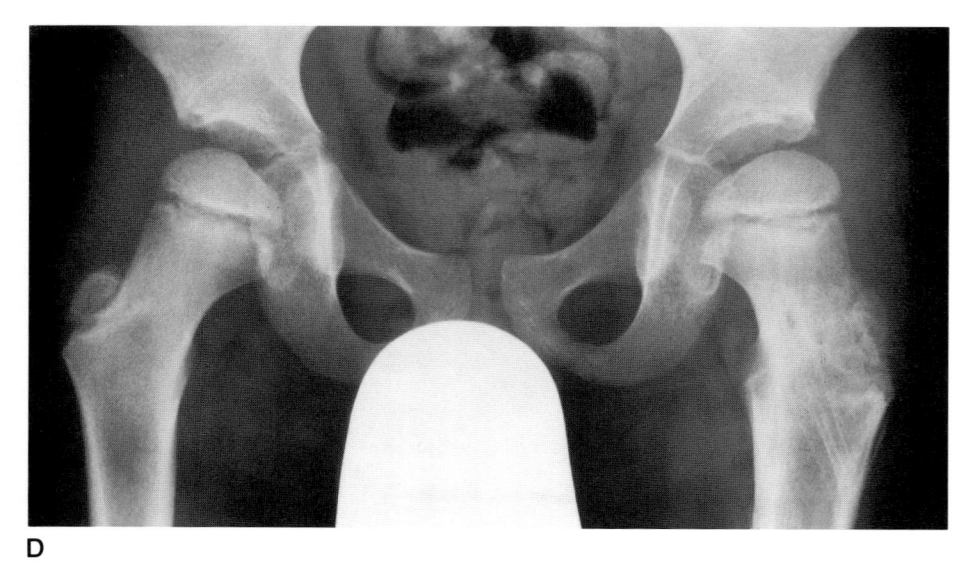

Fig. 26-14 *(Continued).* **(D)** Three years after surgery. The neck and head are slightly wide, but he has excellent function and no sign of avascular changes. (From Chung,[33] with permission.)

Stress Fractures

Potentially unstable transcervical stress fractures in teenagers should be rigidly internally fixed because of the danger of displacement into varus.[24] Early diagnosis and treatment is important, since a delay in diagnosis may lead to extremely poor results.[23]

Technique of Closed Reduction and Pinning

Under general anesthesia, the child is positioned on a fracture table and the hip gently flexed, abducted, and internally rotated until the radiograph or image intensifier reveals a satisfactory, preferably anatomic, reduction. Following this, percutaneous Knowles pins or cannulated screws are introduced, guided by radiographic or image intensifier control across the fracture site from a small 2- to 3-cm lateral incision. This method is particularly useful if the fracture is minimally or nondisplaced. Results by this method, however, are still associated with significant complications of fracture healing. Avascular necrosis occurs in 15 to 58 percent, delayed union or nonunion in 13 to 32 percent, coxa vara in 15 to 54 percent, and premature growth plate fusion in 20 percent,[31,38,42] depending on the type of fracture, degree of displacement and severity of trauma.

Open Arthrotomy Technique

Open anatomic reduction under direct visualization and pinning for displaced fractures after the method of Watson-Jones is my preferred method of treatment[33,35,36] (Figs. 26-13 and 26-14).

The child is anesthetized and placed supine on a fracture table. A modified Smith-Peterson or Watson-Jones approach is used. The incision is started at the anterosuperior iliac spine, extended to the greater trochanter, and then inferiorly 4 to 5 cm. An alternative approach is to use two incisions, an oblique incision over the femoral neck and second lateral incision over the proximal femur. The anterior hip capsule is divided with a T incision. It is important that the transverse limb is made through the capsule at the avascular acetabular margin.

The fracture site is exposed anteriorly, the fracture hematoma removed by suction, and the joint irrigated with saline. The orientation of both fragments, especially the femoral head section, should be carefully assessed. The soft tissue, which carries the blood vessels on the surface of the superior and inferior neck, should be preserved. The serrated fracture fragments are reduced by a thin periosteal elevator back to an anatomic position (Figs. 26-13 and 26-14). At this point it is important not to distract, malrotate, or angulate the fracture fragments (Figs. 26-12 and 26-15).

The hard bone of children is usually not significantly

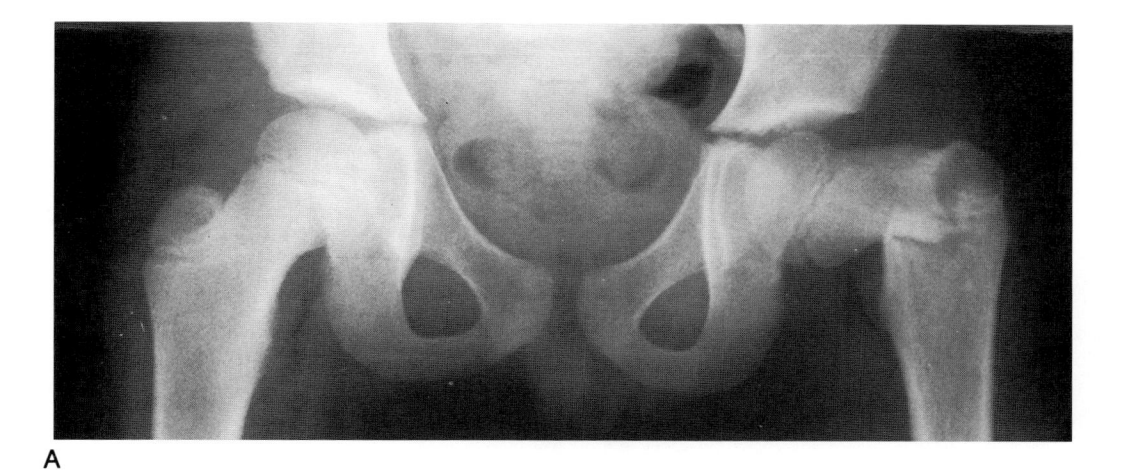

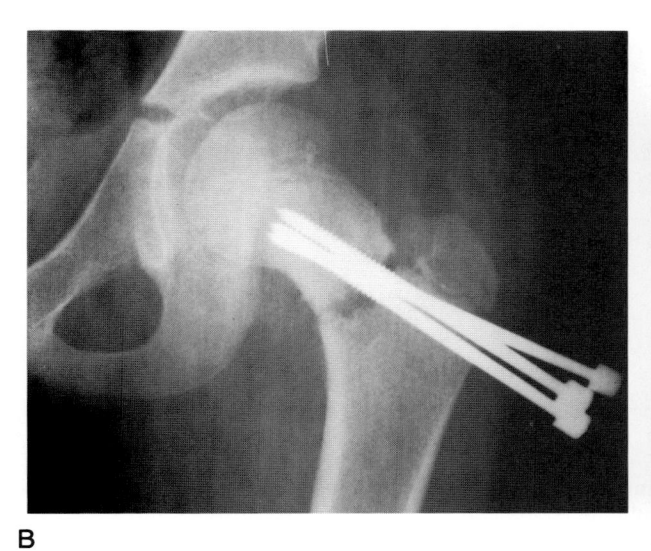

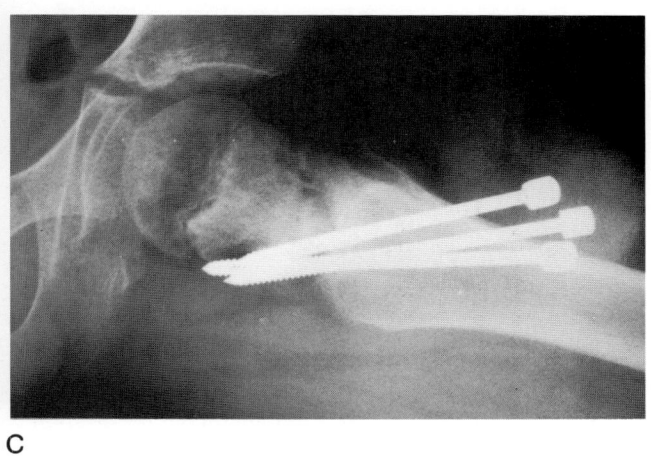

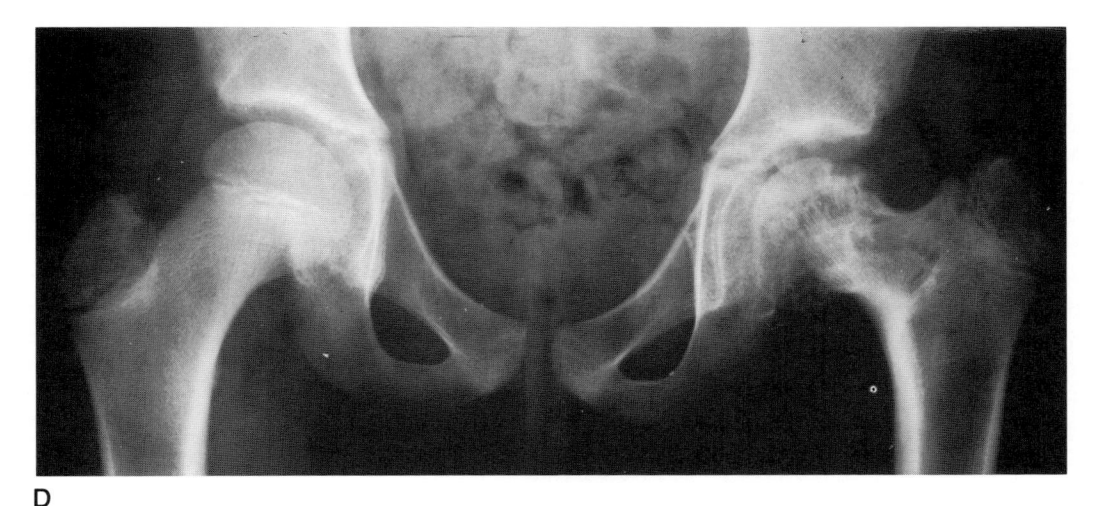

Fig. 26-15. (A) 11-year-old boy struck by an auto while riding his bicycle sustained a cervicotrochanteric fracture. (B) In the AP view fracture is distracted. (C) In the lateral view pins pass outside the posterior neck. (D) 20 months later premature epiphyseal fusion coxa vara, and a short sclerotic neck were seen on the radiograph. Despite the deformity, he had good motion and no disability. A trochanteric epiphysiodesis was performed to stop the trochanter from becoming higher.

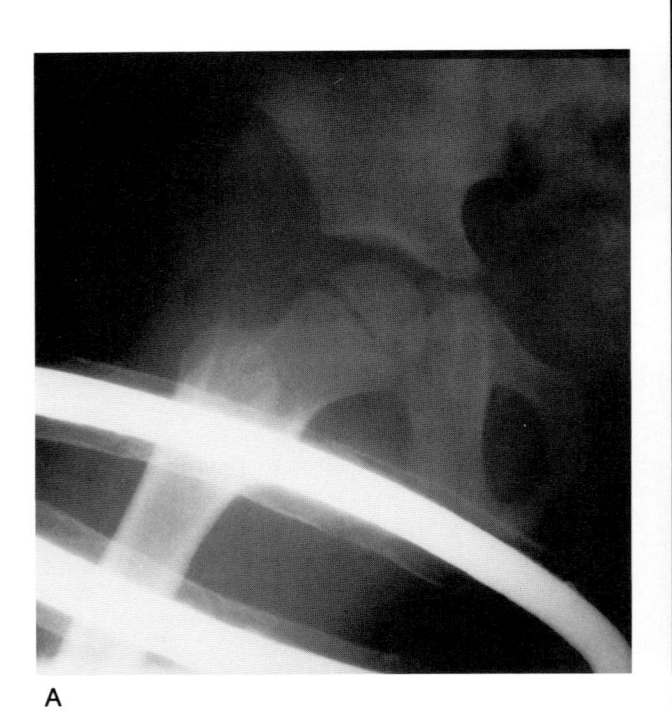

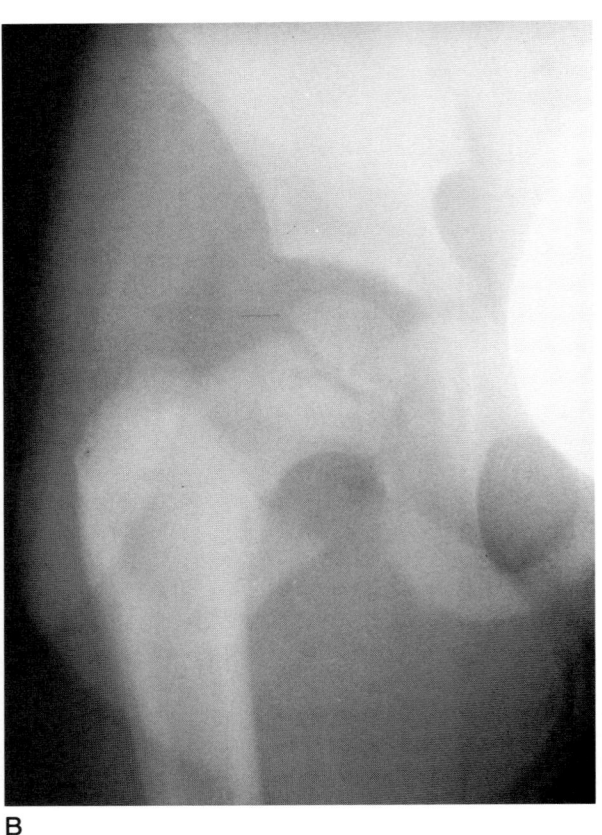

Fig. 26-16. (A) A 7-year-old boy sustained a cervicotrochanteric fracture of the neck of the femur from a fall out of a tree. (B) He was treated in traction but the position could not be maintained and the fracture drifted into a varus position as frequently occurs with this type of management for this fracture. (Courtesy of Dr. Ron Monson, Winnipeg Children's Hospital.)

collapsed at the inferior and posterior fracture surfaces as in adult osteoporotic bone. Therefore the flexed, abducted, internally rotated position of the distal fragment needed to give broader contact between fragments and to compress the fracture to a stable valgus abduction fracture with the head in slight anteversion[43] is usually not necessary in children. However, the distal fragment may be gently manipulated for reduction by moving the foot and limb secured to the fracture table apparatus.

Knowles pins or cannulated hip screws can then be drilled across the fracture site using x-ray or image-intensifier guidance. The pins should not be driven across the femoral capital growth plate unless necessary, as in type I fractures (pins smooth at the tip are shown in Figure 26-11 and are best employed for this fracture). If a cannulated screw is used, the head must be stabilized by one or two additional guidewires or K-wires prior to tapping the drill hole and inserting the screw to prevent the unstable femoral head from spinning. The wound is closed routinely. A spica cast, which is removed in 6 weeks, is recommended to prevent early weightbearing by the child.

COMPLICATIONS

Avascular Necrosis of the Femoral Head

Avascular necrosis is the most serious complication following a fractured hip in a child. Osteonecrosis may occur in up to 42 percent of children with hip fractures

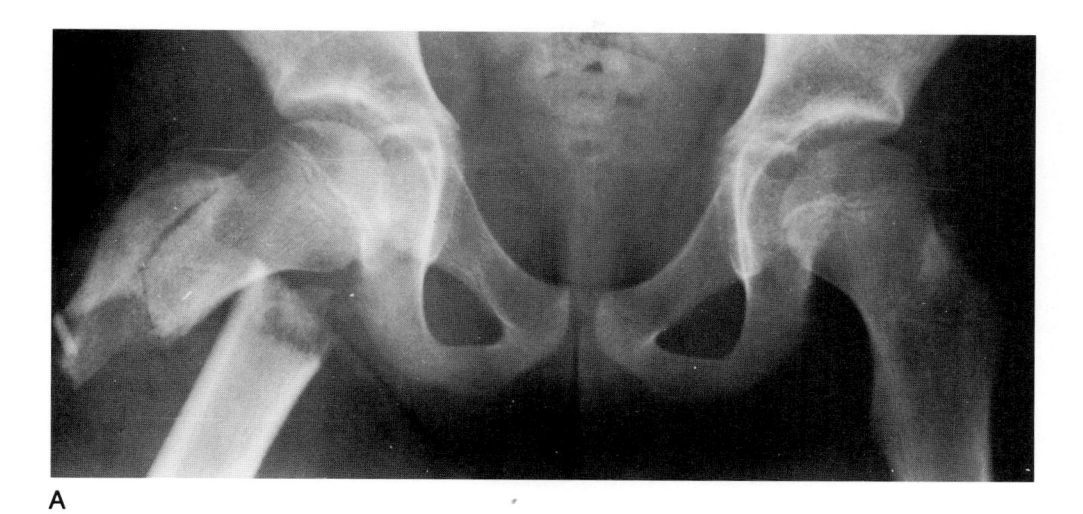

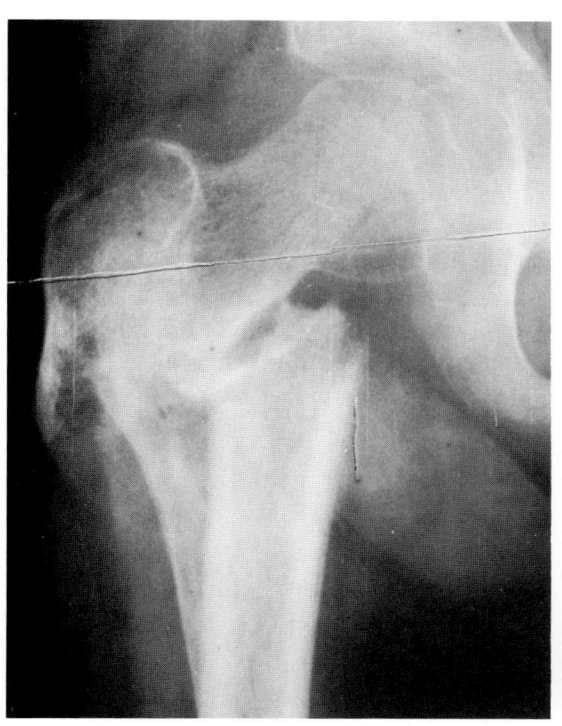

Fig. 26-17. (A) Intertrochanteric type IV fracture in a 13-year old girl. Treated with manipulation and application of an immediate spica. (B) 8 weeks after injury. Fracture is healed. *(Figure continues.)*

C

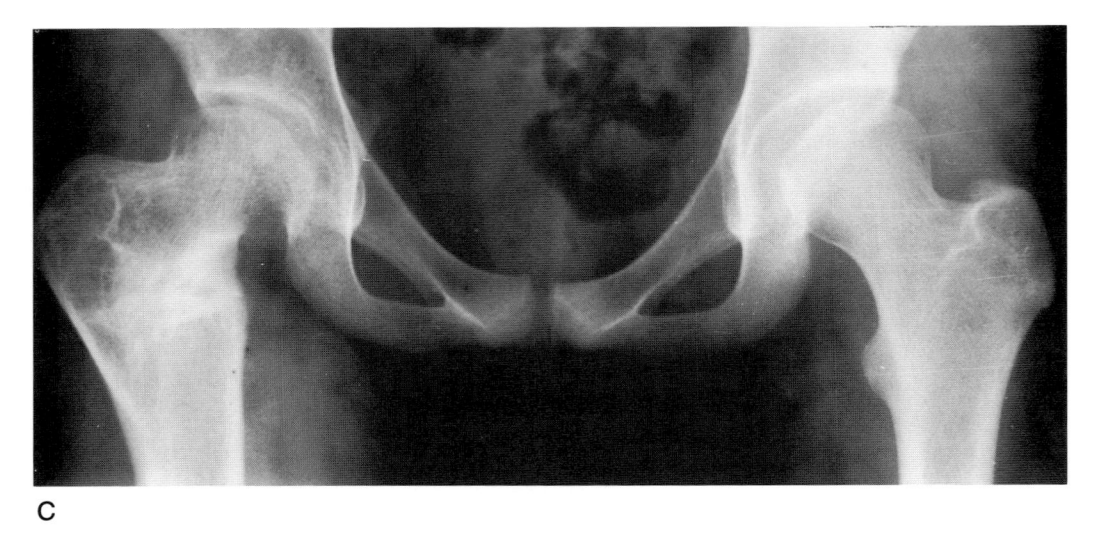

Fig. 26-17 *(Continued.).* **(C)** 6 months later, function is normal.

and is usually apparent within 1 year after injury, but occasionally later (range: 1.5 months to 2 years; average: 9.3 months).[31] The reported incidence of this complication is as follows: type I almost 100 percent; type II, 52 percent; type III, 27 percent; type IV, 14 percent.[31,42] Base of neck fractures (type III) are similar anatomically to those occurring in adults; however, adult fractures rarely result in osteonecrosis, whereas in children, between 20 and 30 percent[38] suffer avascular necrosis. Even intertrochanteric fractures[44] and undisplaced fracture of the cervical neck may develop an ischemic femoral head.

Patterns

There are several patterns of avascular necrosis that may occur in the femoral head and neck[1,41] (Fig. 26-18), which can be explained by injury to the blood vessels shown in Figures 26-1 to 26-4. The types of necrosis that affect the femoral head are as follows:

1. Total head collapse with severe radiodensity of head and neck. [In some cases, although the entire femoral capital epiphysis may be relatively dense on radiographs and have no uptake on radioactive scan, there

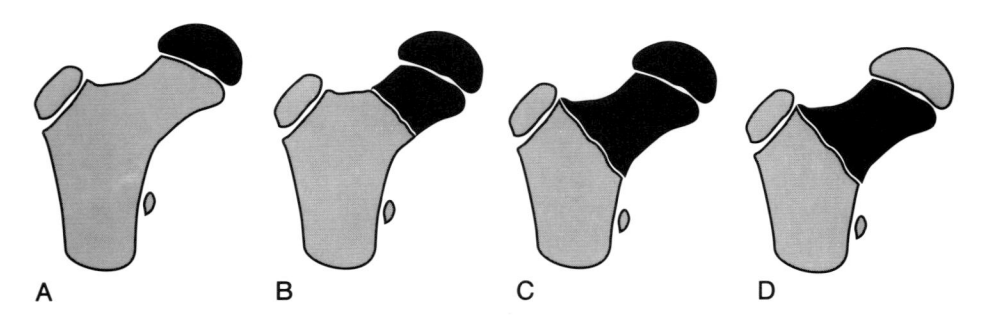

Fig. 26-18. Types of avascular necrosis. **(A)** involvement of the capital epiphysis only; **(B)** capital epiphysis and neck proximal to the transcervical fracture line; **(C)** capital epiphysis and neck proximal to the cervicotrochanteric fracture line; **(D)** necrosis of the femoral neck only.

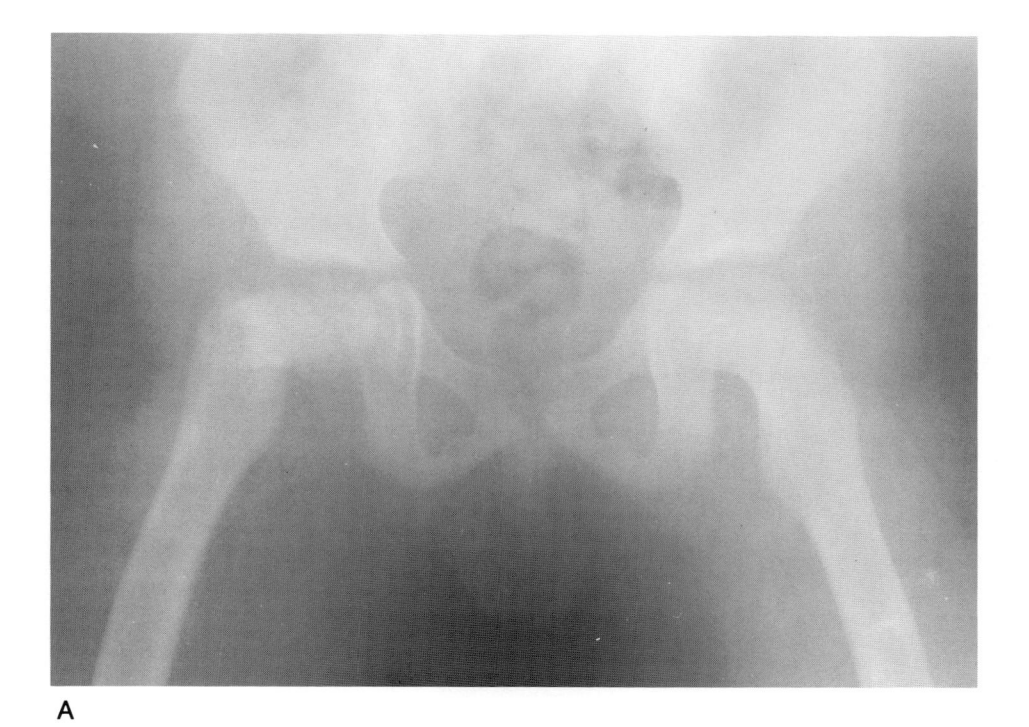

Fig. 26-19. **(A)** This 7-year-old boy sustained a cervicotrochanteric fracture of his right femoral neck in a snowmobile accident. (Courtesy of Dr. Ron Monson, Winnipeg Children's Hospital). **(B&C)** Anatomic reduction was obtained and the fracture internally fixed with three small Knowles pins taking care not to violate the growth plate. *(Figure continues.)*

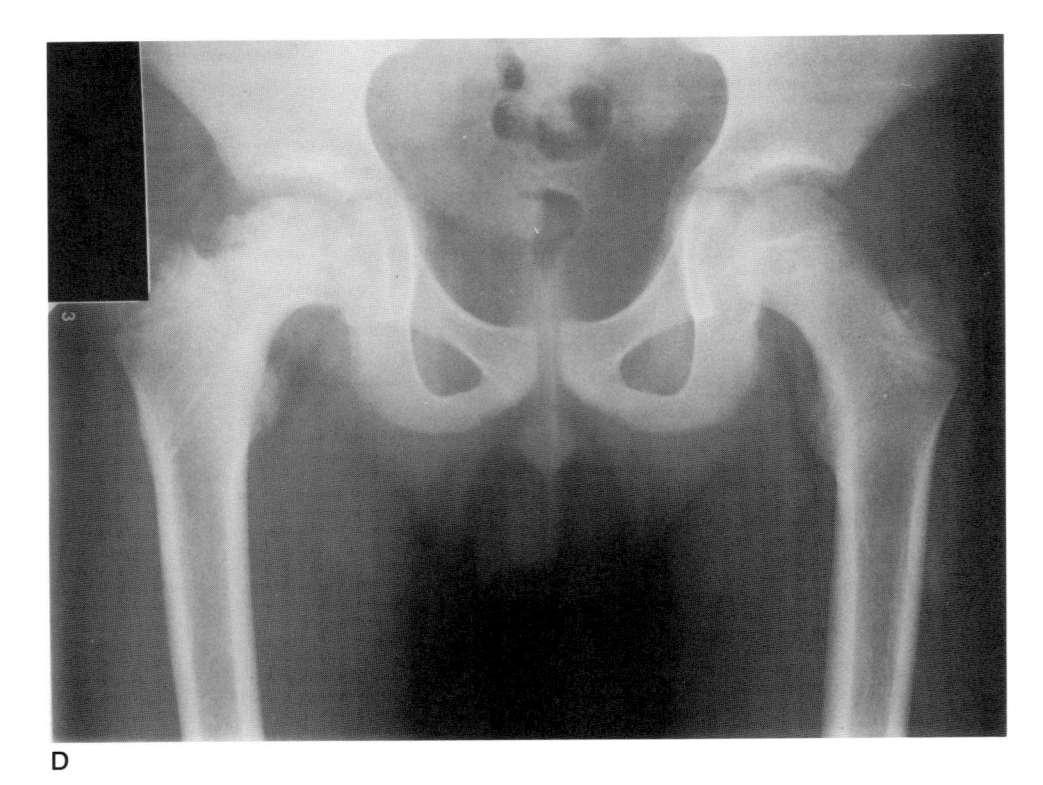

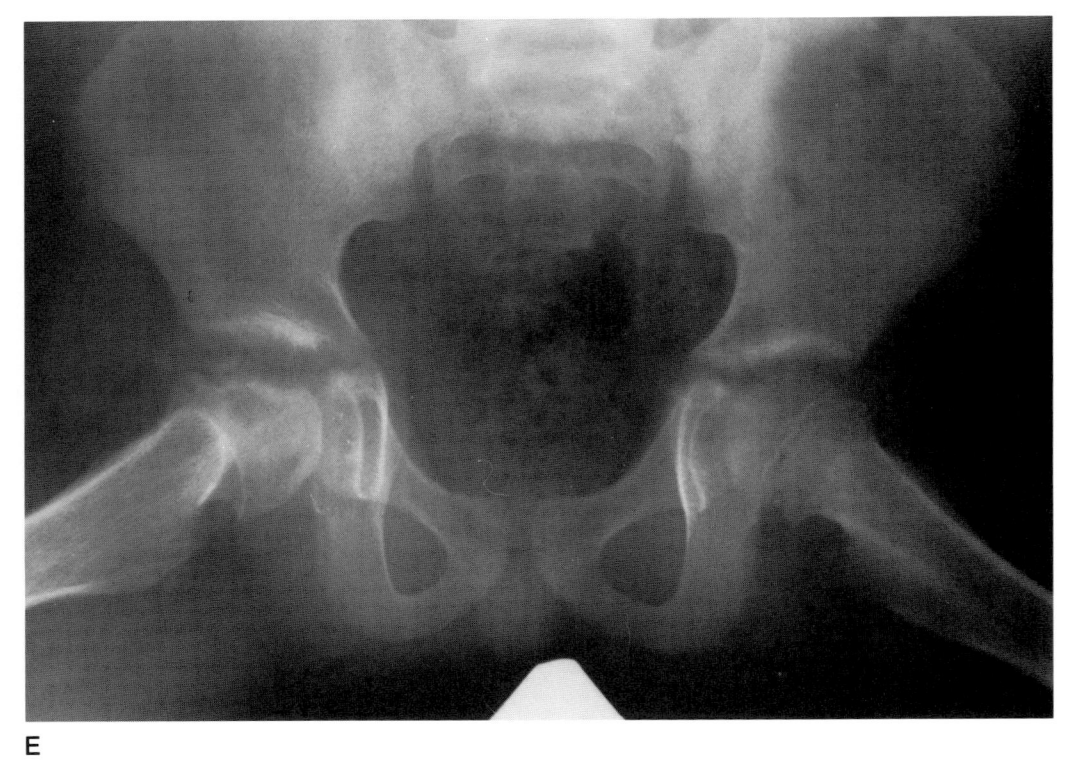

Fig. 26-19. (**D&E**) The pins were removed after 1 year, but the femoral head developed posterolateral segmental collapse with avascular necrosis.

may be minimal or no collapse, or the collapse may be segmental (Fig. 26-19).]
2. In transcervical fractures, necrosis from the fracture line proximal including the femoral head
3. In cervicotrochanteric fractures, necrosis of both the head and neck proximal to the fracture line
4. Necrosis of the neck only proximal to the fracture

If the neck becomes avascular, the bone between the fracture line and epiphyseal plate becomes radiodense shortly after the injury. The capital epiphysis may become radiodense as well, compared to the bone distal to the fracture site and adjacent pelvis. Premature closure of the epiphyseal plate may occur. Avascular necrosis after a hip fracture differs radiographically from typical Legg-Perthes disease. The radiodense and flat femoral head does not fragment and reossify but collapses. Sclerosis, cyst formation, and irregular subchondral bone forms. Femoral neck sclerosis and mild widening or narrowing occur. Coxa vara and articular cartilage loss eventually result.

Contributing Factors

Femoral neck arteriography in adult fractures[46] has demonstrated that avascular necrosis is unlikely when the lateral ascending cervical arteries are intact, providing the fracture line does not cross the nutrient foramina. Femoral head avascular necrosis occurs in most cases when the lateral ascending cervical arteries are interrupted.

Intraosseous venography has shown that arteries and veins run side by side or, at most, 5 mm apart. The lateral descending cervical veins are filled in valgus fractures, but are rarely found intact with varus fractures, indicating an avascular femoral head.[4]

Intraosseous pressures in adult undisplaced valgus fractures, have been shown to be almost identical at both the femoral head and neck, indicating an intact arterial femoral head supply. Absent femoral head pressure in 48 percent of displaced varus fractures was noted by Arnoldi and colleagues,[46] who suggest that the cervical arteries supplying the head have been interrupted. When high femoral head pressures were obtained, the neck readings are lower, indicating that venous drainage from the head is obstructed[46] in the varus position.

Torsion of the femoral head by poor fracture reduction also may impair the blood supply to the femoral head through ligamentum teres vessels. Retrospective review of radiographs of displaced femoral neck fractures developing avascular necrosis or coxa vara have revealed that the head fragment is usually distracted or displaced after percutaneous pin fixation (Figs. 26-12 and 26-15).

Observations at operation in adults whose femoral heads were supplied only by ligamentum teres arteries have also demonstrated that femoral head rotation of more than 115 degrees anteriorly, or 60 degrees posteriorly, or placement in an extreme valgus position, interrupts head fragment bleeding. Ligamentum teres arteries constitute an important femoral head blood supply in 28 percent of children.[2] Malrotation and distraction may occur inadvertently during closed reduction and may both disrupt the blood supply through the ligamentum teres and tear the remaining cervical vessels, so anatomic reposition is essential for femoral head survival for those cases that have some remaining intact vessels. Only when a microsurgical vascular technique is developed to inspect the femoral head vessels, determine patency, and repair lacerations and remove thrombi, will treatment results improve.

Treatment

Prognosis is difficult to establish in avascular necrosis following a hip fracture in children. Treatment should (1) prevent further femoral head collapse, (2) contain the femoral head in the acetabulum, and (3) reduce femoral head forces by nonweightbearing until reossification occurs.

If the child is asymptomatic, treatment may be unnecessary. If the top of the trochanter becomes higher than the top of the femoral head due to physeal arrest of the proximal femoral growth plate, a trochanteric epiphyseodesis may be helpful in children under 10 years of age to prevent a decrease in the resting length of the gluteus medius and minimus. This procedure is usually successful if performed under 10 or 11 years of age as in older children there is not enough growth remaining in the trochanteric physis to render any significant correction.

A Pauwels valgus osteotomy[46] may be performed for coxa vara. If the superior femoral head has collapsed, but the lateral head margin is intact, a varus osteotomy should be considered. Trochanteric arthroplasty may stabilize the hip if the femoral head has been completely resorbed. Another treatment possibility is an abduction brace to contain the femoral head and encourage healing with joint congruity. Treatment results for avascular necrosis reported in the literature are not good especially in older children who have little potential for remodeling.

Bone scintigraphy has been reported not to be useful

in predicting development of femoral head necrosis, subsequent collapse of the femoral head or clinical outcome.[47] Mortensson has suggested that the development of necrosis in the femoral head in spite of a normal presurgical scintigraphy may be due to damage to the blood supply at reposition and osteosynthesis. A normal scintigraphy immediately after surgery does not rule out the risk of future necrosis. Furthermore the strength of dead bone may be preserved for months or years and the child may be asymptomatic. Scintigraphy may be useful for selecting children who require an extended nonweightbearing period to avoid collapse of the femoral head. The test should be done postoperatively in order to include possible ischemic lesions appearing during or after surgery.

Nonunion

Nonunion occurs in 6 to 13 percent of fractures[31,38,41] associated with displaced transcervical fractures may result from distraction by intramedullary pins or traction, from wound infections, interposition of capsule or periosteum in the fracture site or delay in treatment. Nonunion and malunion (usually coxa vara) are more common after closed treatment because the femoral head can more easily fall into a varus position. Nonunion is prevented by accurate reduction and internal fixation.[38]

Delayed or nonunion usually becomes evident 5 to 8 months after fracture fixation. The child complains of pain and has a persistent limp. Radiographs will reveal a persistent radiolucent fracture line and fracture motion may be seen on push-pull films or flouroscopy. Nonunion may be treated with various forms of muscle pedicle grafts or by a valgus osteotomy.

If nonunion occurs, immobilization with a spica cast for more than 3 months should be avoided since the disuse osteoporosis will often result in pathologic fractures and physeal retardation or arrest leading to limb length inequality.[1]

Coxa Vara

Coxa vara can be associated with nonunion, avascular necrosis or premature epiphyseal fusion. This deformity is prevented by accurate reduction and internal fixation.[31] No treatment is necessary for mild deformities. If the capital femoral epiphysis is not damaged, the neck-shaft angle may spontaneously correct especially in younger children.[29,48] If the neck shaft angle is less than 95 to 100 degrees, a Pauwels[48] valgus osteotomy may be required. A persistent coxa vara will result in an abductor lurch, some shortening of the limb, and, later, degenerative changes. A trochanteric epiphiseodesis in children under 10 years of age may help decrease the height of a greater trochanter, which becomes higher than the femoral head.

Premature Closure of the Physis

No definite cause of premature epiphyseal plate closure has been identified, although avascular necrosis, pins crossing the epiphyseal plate, and prolonged immobilization have been associated with this complication. Premature closure of the femoral capital physis will not cause loss of motion or pain unless osteonecrosis is present. Usually minimal leg-length inequality results as the proximal femoral physis contributes only $\frac{1}{8}$ inch per year of growth in the femur or 15 percent of the entire lower extremity length. However, the younger the child at the time of fracture the greater the risk of a significant leg length discrepancy. Reports of up to 5 inches of leg-shortening have occurred within 4 years after the injury.[1,41]

No procedures are available for treatment or prevention of premature epiphyseal fusion, but some children may benefit from a trochanteric epiphyseodesis or greater trochanteric transfer if the trochanter becomes higher than the femoral head. Careful follow-up examinations, including leg length scanograms and bone age determinations must be obtained so leg equalization procedures may be done at the appropriate time if required.

Traumatic Osteochondral Fracture of the Femoral Head

An osteochondral fragment of the femoral head may separate and dislodge into the joint when a hip is dislocated or after indirect trauma applied to the knee (Fig. 26-20). A loose fragment in the hip may be suspected if by radiograph the joint space is abnormally widened between the acetabular teardrop and the femoral head or an unexplained radiolucency is present in the joint space after an injury to the hip. Unexplained pain or loss of hip

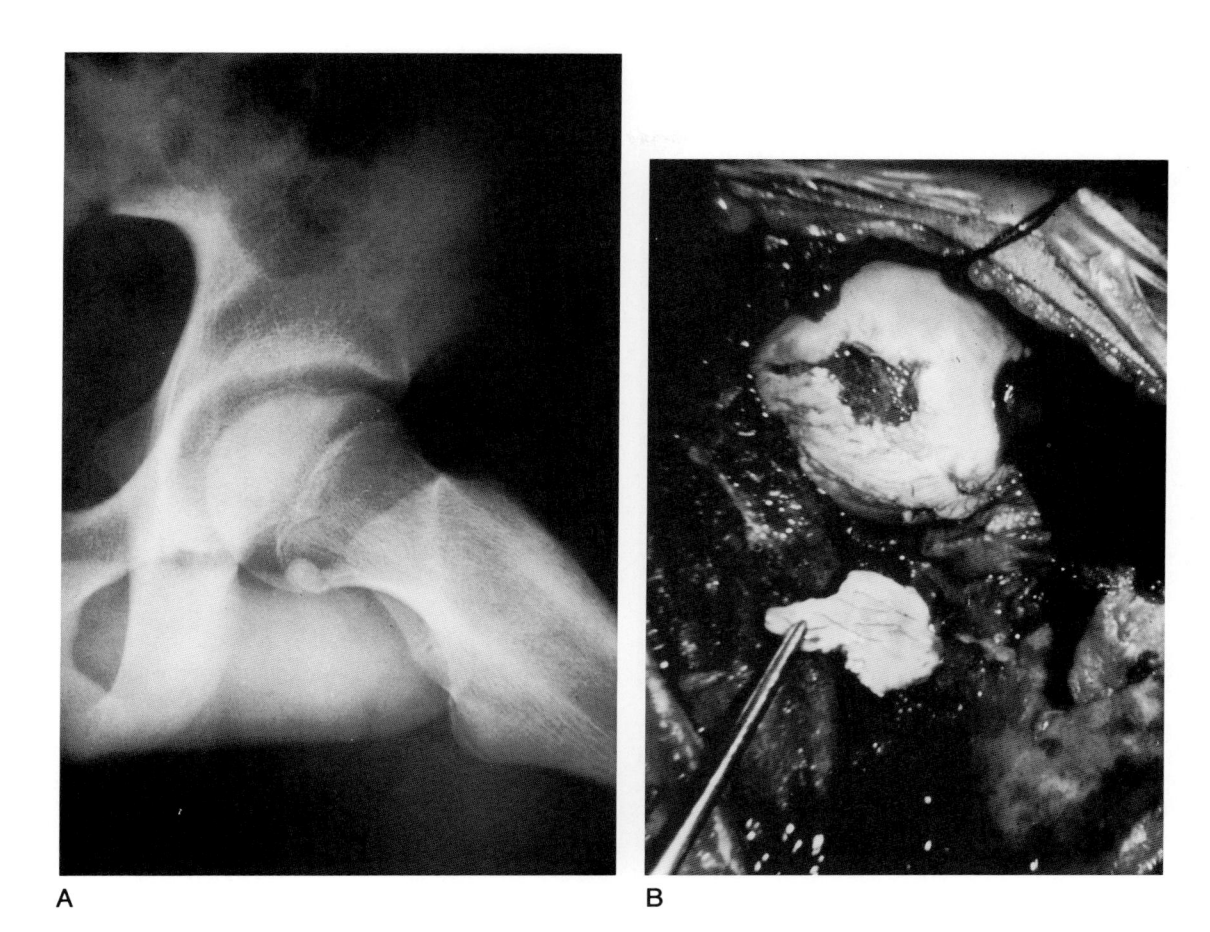

Fig. 26-20. **(A)** A 14-year-old boy whose knee struck the dashboard in an auto accident. The hip did not dislocate, but he developed severe hip pain on motion and a thin flake radiolucency appeared above the superior femoral head. **(B)** At surgery a large articular defect of the superior femoral head was found with several free loose articular cartilage pieces and many cracks in the anterior and lateral articular surface. The posterior surface (to the reader's right) was intact. The free articular pieces were removed. **(C)** A Sugioka rotational osteotomy was done. Two years later he had no pain, had no flexion contracture, but active or passive flexion more than 90 degrees resulted in mild discomfort. (From Chung,[33] with permission.)

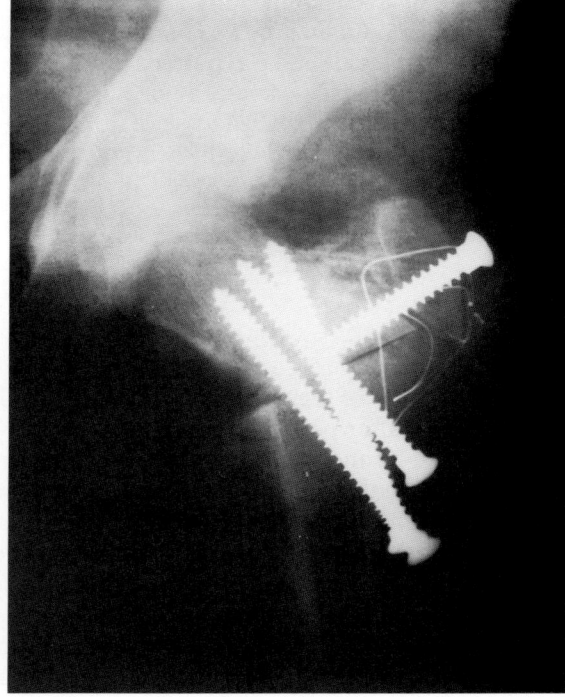

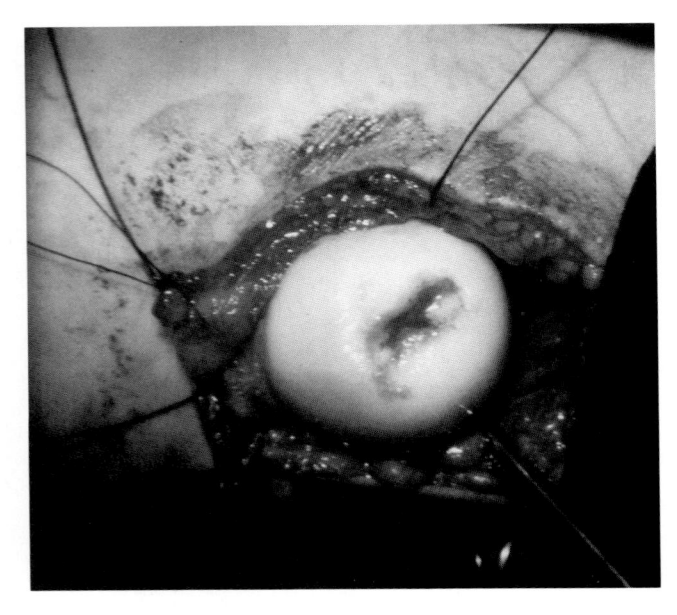

Fig. 26-21. Osteochondral fracture of the femoral head secondary to a posterior dislocation of the hip sustained by an 11-year-old girl in a motor vehicle accident. (Courtesy of Dr. R. Mervyn Letts.)

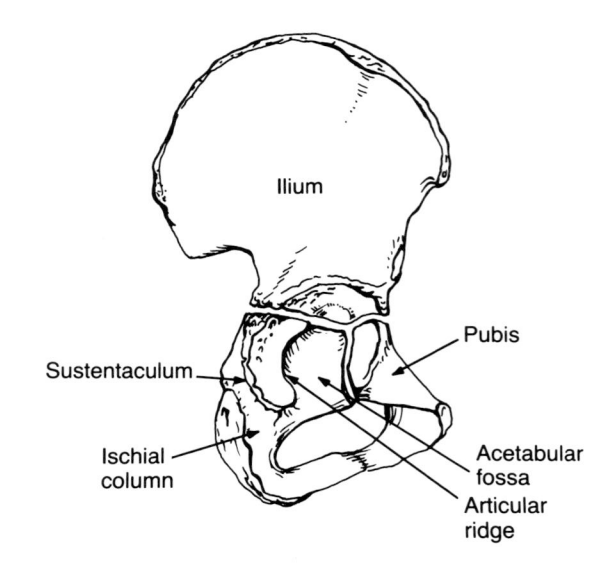

Fig. 26-22. The three components of the acetabulum are: its superior two-fifths composed of ilium, its inferolateral two-fifths of ischium, and its medial one fifth composed of pubis. The triradiate (Y) cartilage is located at the center of the acetabulum where these three bones eventually unite. (From Chung,[33] with permission.)

motion after an apparently successful reduction of a dislocated hip may also be an indication of the presence of a loose osteochondral fragment. If the fragment is small enough, its removal is all that is required (Fig. 26-21). If the defect is large, a varus osteotomy or Sugioka rotational osteotomy may be required to place normal articular cartilage at the superior weight-bearing surface of the femoral head (Fig. 26-20) (also see Ch. 28).

Triradiate Cartilage Injuries

Premature closure of the triradiate cartilage (Fig. 26-22) rarely occurs after pelvic or acetabular injuries in children (Figs. 26-23 and 26-24). This closure produces a wide medial acetabular wall, a "miniacetabulum" and eventual lateral femoral head subluxation, a prominent greater trochanter and lateral acetabular lip compression in children 10 years of age and younger. Older children seldom experience significant growth disturbance. A possible treatment is a combination of Chiari osteotomy and varus osteotomy (Fig. 26-24). Long-term results are not available.[33,49,50]

SUMMARY

Hip fractures are uncommon in children and are serious fractures with a high complication rate of nearly 60 percent. These fractures occur most frequently in the 10 to 12 age group, 60 to 75 percent in boys. Avascular necrosis is the most frequent and serious complication. Age-related differences in mechanical properties of bone may account for the more frequent hip fractures among adults than among children.

Generally these hip fractures do not require immediate emergency treatment, but should be treated promptly within 24 hours. If hip joint aspiration is performed to relieve tamponade as soon as possible after the fracture, osteocyte death may be prevented. Type I fractures with dislocation of the femoral head should be treated preferably within 6 hours, by open reduction and internal fixation. In children less than 3 years of age type I fractures may be treated successfully with gentle closed reduction and immobilization in a spica cast.

Ideally, the types II and III fractures should be reduced to an anatomic position, then percutaneous pins used to transfix the fracture. If an anatomic or near-anatomic reduction cannot be obtained by gentle closed manipulation, an open arthrotomy and reposition of the frag-

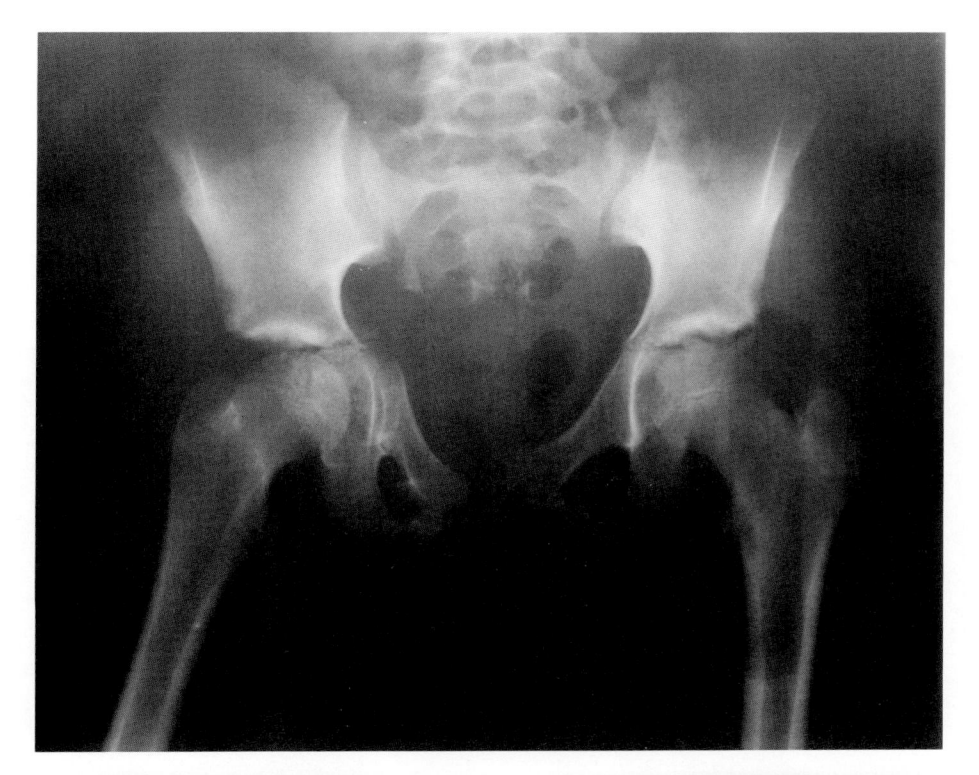

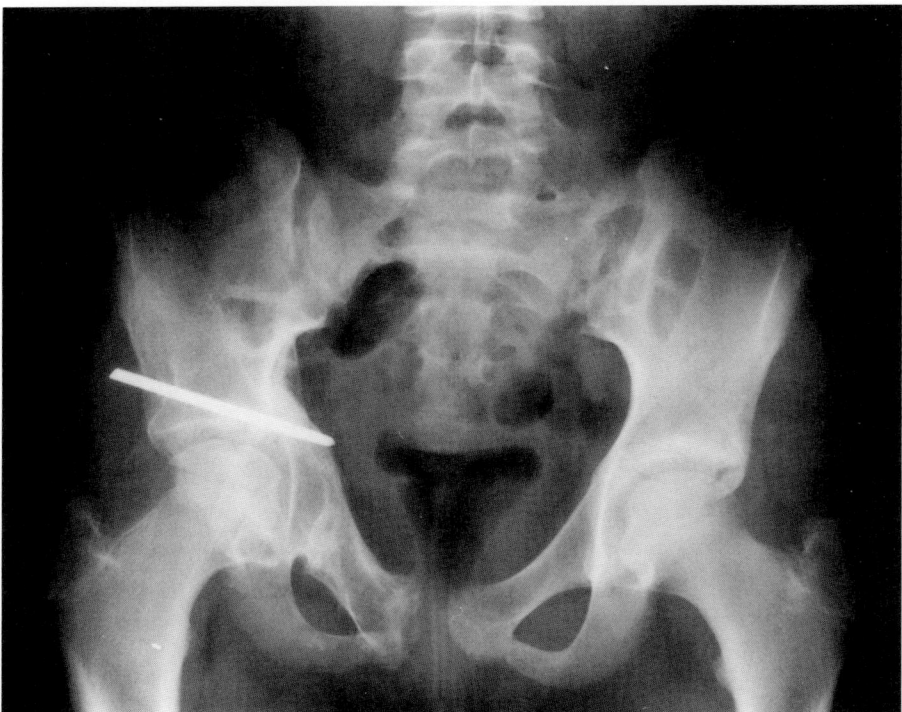

Fig. 26-23. Central dislocation of the hip separating the triradiate cartilage. The separation was surgically reduced and pinned. (Courtesy of Dr. William McIntyre, Children's Hospital of Eastern Ontario, Ottawa, Canada.)

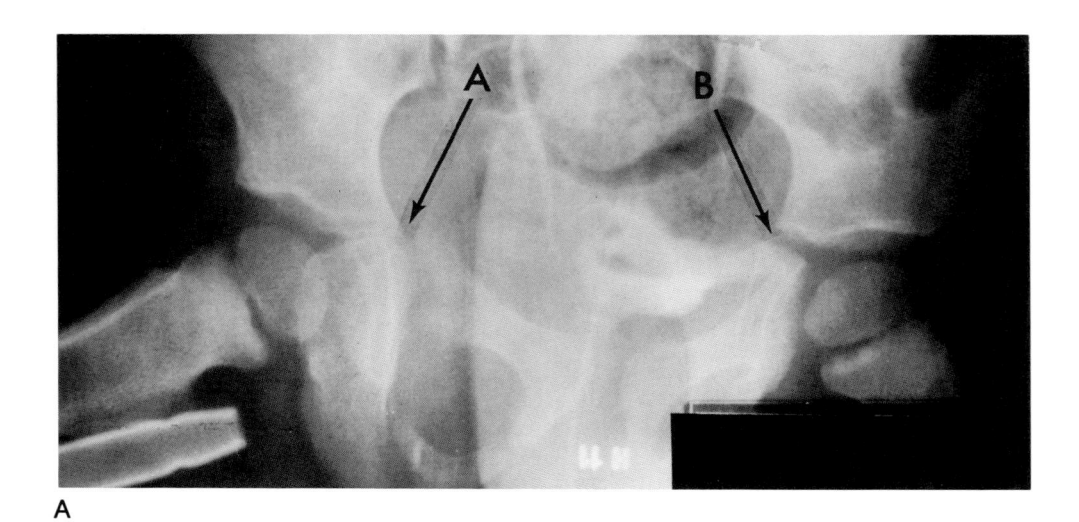

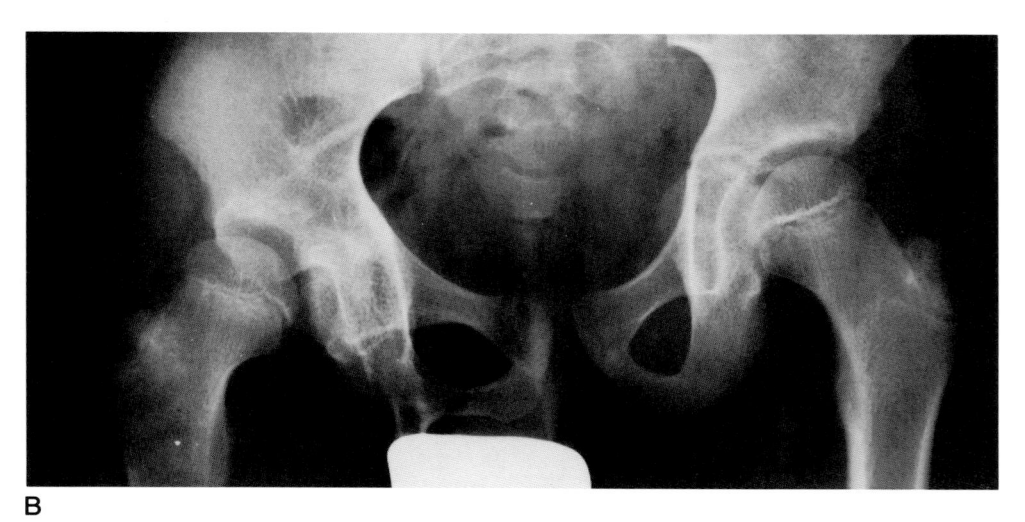

Fig. 26-24. (A) A 5-year-old boy with right femoral shaft and pubic and ischial rami fractures. The triradiate cartilage appears narrow on the right *(A)* compared to the left *(B)*. **(B)** Follow-up at age 11. The radiograph shows the lateral femoral head subluxation with a thick medial acetabulum. The acetabulum appears too small to accommodate the femoral head. The triradiate cartilage has fused prematurely. He has hip discomfort with athletics and an increasingly prominent greater trochanter. *(Figure continues.)*

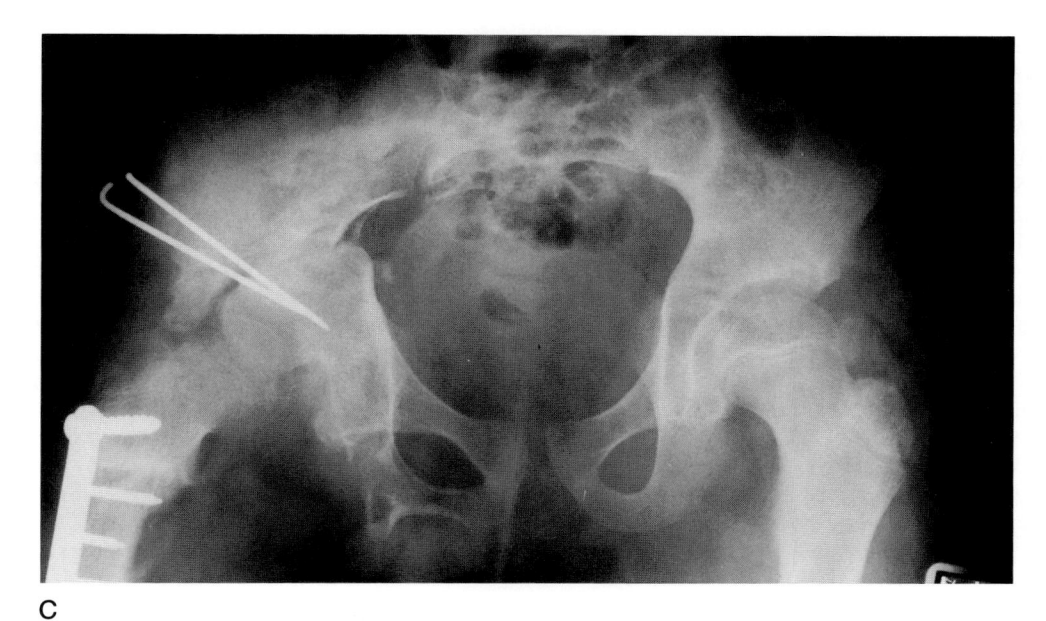

Fig. 26-24 *(Continued).* **(C)** At 3 months after a Chiari osteotomy and varus osteotomy; 5 months after surgery the patient had no pain and had good hip motion. The eventual result has yet to be determined. (From Chung,[33] with permission.)

ments followed by internal fixation probably will result in the least tension on remaining intact vessels.

REFERENCES

1. Ratliff AHC: Fractures of the neck of the femur in children. J Bone Joint Surg [Br] 44:528, 1962
2. Chung SMK: The arterial supply of the developing proximal end of the human femur. J Bone Joint Surg [Am] 58:961:970, 1976
3. Chung SMK: Embryology, growth, and development. p. 3. Steinberg ME (ed): The Hip and Its Disorders. WB Saunders, Philadelphia, 1991
4. Hulth A: Intraosseous phlebography and tracer injection in femoral neck fractures. Angiology 21:413, 1970
5. Shiba T: Study of Perthes disease: radiological examination of circulation, especially venous in the femoral head. (In Japanese). J Jpn Orthop Assoc 39:377, 1965
6. Chung SMK, Batterman SC, Brighton CT: Shear strength of the human femoral capital epiphyseal plate. J Bone Joint Surg [Am] 58:94, 1976
7. Currey JD, Butler G: The mechanical properties of bone tissue in children. J Bone Joint Surg [Am] 57:810, 1975
8. Griffiths WEG, Swanson SAV, Freeman MAR: Experimental fatigue fracture of the human cadaveric femoral neck. J Bone Joint Surg [Br] 53:136, 1971
9. Colonna PC: Fractures of neck of the femur in children. Am J Surg 6:793, 1929
10. Canale ST, Bourland WL: Fracture of the neck and intertrochanteric region of the femur in children. J Bone Joint Surg [Am] 59:431, 1977
11. Lam SF: Fractures of the neck of the femur in children. J Bone Joint Surg [Am] 53:1165, 1971
12. Savage R: Transepiphyseal fracture-dislocation of the femoral neck. Injury 21:187, 1990
13. Mass DP, Spiegel PG, Laros GS: Dislocation of the hip with traumatic separation of the capital femoral epiphysis: report of case with successful outcome. Clin Orthop 146:184, 1980
14. Wolfgang GL: Stress fracture of the femoral neck in a patient with open capital femoral epiphyses. J Bone Joint Surg [Am] 59:680, 1977
15. Coldwell D, Gross GW, Boal DK: Stress fracture of the femoral neck in a child. Pediatr Radiol 14:174, 1984
16. Hoekstra HJ, Binnendijk B: Fractures of neck and shaft of same femur in children. Arch Orthop Trauma Surg 100:197, 1982
17. Baynham GC, Lucie RS, Cummings RJ: Femoral neck fracture secondary to in-situ pinning of slipped capital femoral epiphysis. J Pediatr Orthop 11:187, 1991
18. Fairhurst MJ, McDonald I: Transepiphyseal femoral neck fracture at birth. J Bone Joint Surg [Br] 72:155, 1990
19. Fiddian NJ, Grace DL: Traumatic dislocation of the hip in adolescence with separation of the capital epiphysis. J Bone Joint Surg [Br] 65:148, 1983

20. Greene WB, Torre BA: Femoral neck fracture in a child with autosomal dominant osteopetrosis. J Pediatr Orthop 5:483, 1985
21. Goldman AB, Jacobs B: Femoral neck fractures complicating Gaucher disease in children. Skeletal Radiol 12:162, 1984
22. Devas MB: Stress fractures of the femoral neck. J Bone Joint Surg [Br] 47:728, 1965
23. Johansson C, Ekenhman I, Tornkvist H, Eriksson E: Stress fracture of the femoral neck in athletes: the consequence of a delay in diagnosis. Am J Sports Med 18:524, 1990
24. Volpin G, Hoerer D, Groisman G et al: Stress fractures of the femoral neck following strenuous activity. J Orthop Trauma 4:394, 1990
25. Ammann W, Matzinger J, Lloyd-Smith DR et al: Femoral stress abnormalities; improved scintigraphic detection with frog-leg view. Radiology 169:844, 1988
26. Swiontkowski MF, Winquist RA: Displaced hip fractures in children and adolescents. J Trauma 26:384, 1986
27. Pforringer W, Rosemeyer B: Fractures of the hip in children and adolescents. Acta Orthop Scand 519:91, 1980
28. Harper WM, Barnes MR, Gregg PJ: Femoral head blood flow in femoral neck fractures. J Bone Joint Surg [Br] 73:73, 1991
29. Forlin E, Guille JT, Kumar SJ, Rhee KJ: Transepiphyseal fractures of the neck of the femur in very young children. J Pediatr Orthop 12:164, 1992
30. Heiser JM, Oppenheim WL: Fracture of the hip in children. Clin Orthop 149:177, 1980
31. Canale ST: Fractures of the hip in children and adolescents. Orthop Clin North Am 21:341, 1990
32. Hensinger RN: Operative Management of Lower Extremity Fractures in Children. AAOS Monograph Series, 1992
33. Chung SMK: Hip Disorders in Infants and Children. Lea & Febiger, Philadelphia, 1981
34. Chung SMK, Hirata T: Multiple pin repair of the slipped capital femoral epiphysis. In Black J, Dumbleton JH (eds): Clinical Biomechanics. Churchill Livingstone, New York, 1981
35. Boitzy A: Fractures of the proximal femur. In Weber BG, Brunner CH, Freuler F (eds): Treatment of Fractures in Children and Adolescents. Springer-Verlag, Berlin, 1980
36. Watson-Jones R: Fracture of the neck of the femur. Br J Surg 23:787, 1935–1936
37. Manninger J, Biro T, Zolczer L et al: The diagnostic role of the intraosseous phlebography in the affections of the hip in childhood. Arch Orthop Trauma Surg 96:203, 1980
38. Leung PC, Lam SF: Long-term follow-up of children with femoral neck fractures. J Bone Joint Surg [Br] 68:537, 1986
39. Irani R, Chung SMK, Nicholson JT: Long-term results in the treatment of femoral shaft fractures in young children by immediate spica immobilization. J Bone Joint Surg [Am] 58:945, 1976
40. Hoekstra HJ, Lichtendahl D: Pertrochanteric fractures in children and adolescents. J Pediatr Orthop 3:587, 1983
41. Ratliff AHC: Fractures of the neck of the femur in children. Orthop Clin North Am 7:625, 1976
42. Davison BL, Weinstein SL: Hip fractures in children: long-term follow-up study. J Pediatr Orthop 12:355, 1992
43. Muller ME, Allgower M, Schneider R, Willenegger H: Manual of Internal Fixation: Techniques Recommended by the A-O Group. p. 216. 2nd Ed. New York, Springer-Verlag, 1979
44. Nielsen PT, Thaarup P: An unusual course of femoral head necrosis complicating an intertrochanteric fracture in a child. Clin Orthop 183:79, 1984
45. Brunner S, Christiansen J, Kristensen JK: Arteriographic prediction of femoral head viability in medial femoral neck fractures. Acta Chir Scand 133:449, 1967
46. Arnoldi CC, Lemperg R, Linderholm H: Intraosseous pressure in patients with different types of fractures of the femoral neck. Angiology 21:403, 1970
47. Mortensson W, Rosenborg M, Gretzer H: The role of bone scintigraphy in predicting femoral head collapse following cervical fractures in children. Acta Radiol 31:291, 1990
48. Deluca FN, Keck C: Traumatic coxa vara. Clin Orthop 116:125, 1976
49. Hallel T, Salvati EA: Premature closure of the triradiate cartilage. Clin Orthop Rel Res 124:278, 1977
50. Rodrigues KF: Injury of the acetabular epiphysis. Injury 4:258, 1973

27

Acute Slipped Capital Femoral Epiphysis

Dennis S. Weiner

Examination of the hip is part of the examination of the knee.

DESCRIPTION AND INCIDENCE

An acute slipped capital femoral epiphysis is analogous to a Salter-Harris type I epiphyseal growth plate separation. It is a disorder of puberty resulting in a structurally weakened proximal femoral growth plate. This weakening of the physis renders it susceptible to rather innocuous degrees of stress that otherwise would fail to cause any damage to the physis. Characteristically, the inciting event is no more traumatic than an unguarded slip, twist, fall, stumbling off a curb, or jumping up and down.

Acute slipped capital femoral epiphysis is a very uncommon condition, accounting for roughly 10 percent of all cases of slipped capital femoral epiphysis. Even this figure is likely inflated, inasmuch as many reported cases of acute slipped capital femoral epiphysis have been included on the basis of temporal factors alone (i.e., symptoms occurring within a 2- to 3-week precedent time interval before recognition). Extensive experience with open bone graft epiphysiodesis, directly observing the site of slipping of the head/neck interface, has demonstrated that the femoral head is firmly anchored to the neck (i.e., chronic stable slip), in spite of recent symptomatology. This concept of head/neck mobility versus stability is the most significant differentiating feature between an acute and chronic slip.[1]

ANATOMY

Although the anatomic site of epiphyseal separation is propagated through the same growth plate zone as the fissure plane of an acute epiphyseal traumatic separation (Salter-Harris type I epiphyseal fracture), there is little else in common between the two conditions. Acute traumatic epiphyseal fractures generally occur at a younger age (2 to 12 years), are associated with a very significant traumatic episode, and other areas of traumatic body involvement are present in over two-thirds of the cases. The corrugated undulating separation line primarily extends through the zone of hypertrophy, although some of the fissure lines extend into the zone of proliferation and the zone of provisional ossification (Figs. 27-1 and 27-2). It has been shown on gross histologic and electron microscopy studies of human growth plate from slipped capital femoral epiphysis cases that there is clearly a cellular and matrix disorder at all active metabolic layers of the growth plate.[2,3]

MECHANISM OF INJURY

The exact etiology, whether biochemical or biomechanical or both, is as yet not fully clear but is of sufficient magnitude to render the growth plate deficient in

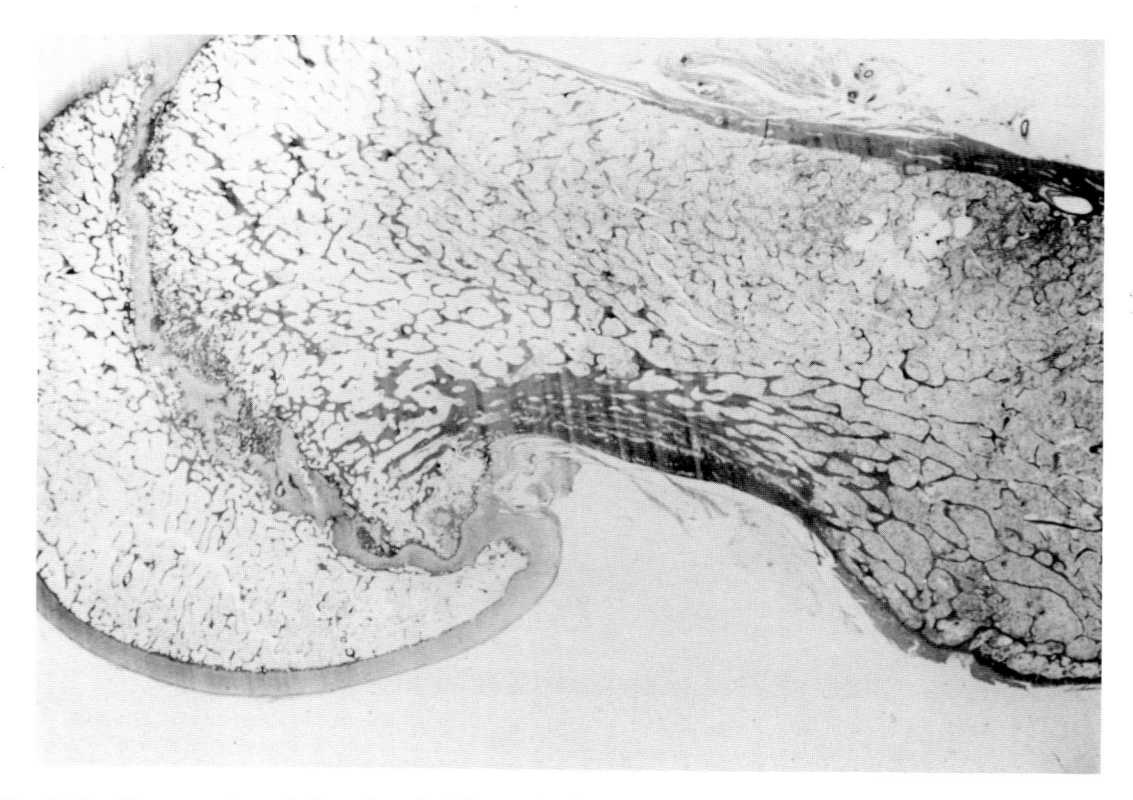

Fig. 27-1. Cross section of slipped capital femoral epiphysis demonstrating femoral head displacement on femoral neck through growth plate.

its ability to resist routine stresses. This similarity of epiphyseal fracture and acute slipped capital femoral epiphysis separation plane is all that the two conditions have in common except for an increased incidence of avascular necrosis. This distinction is also important, inasmuch as in slipped capital femoral epiphysis the opposite hip is involved with the disorder in 25 to 35 percent of the cases. The prognosis of avascular necrosis is substantially higher with an acute traumatic epiphyseal fracture separation.

CLASSIFICATION

The classification of acute slipped capital femoral epiphysis is identical to chronic slipped capital femoral epiphysis and generally consists of the biplanar radiographic assessment of the degree of slipping (Fig. 27-3). Grade I, or minor degrees of slipping, reflect femoral neck on head displacement of up to one-third the diameter of the growth plate. Grade II, or moderate degrees of slipping, are those degrees of slipping in which the head is displaced from the femoral neck between one-third and one-half the diameter of the growth plate. Grade III, or severe slipping, is displacement of the femoral head on the neck above 50 percent.

PHYSICAL EXAMINATION

The clinical picture of acute slipped capital epiphysis is striking. In addition to the usual findings of chronic slipped capital femoral epiphysis (limp, external rotation deformity, shortening, diminished flexion, abduction, and internal rotation, discomfort on internal rotation, and flexion) there is the sudden inability to weight bear, accompanied by marked increase in pain, particularly on attempts at internal rotation and flexion. Most commonly, the femoral head is significantly displaced (moderate to severe degree of slip) but occasionally may be minimal. Documentary evidence of a mobile head/neck interface is necessary to confirm an acute slip and

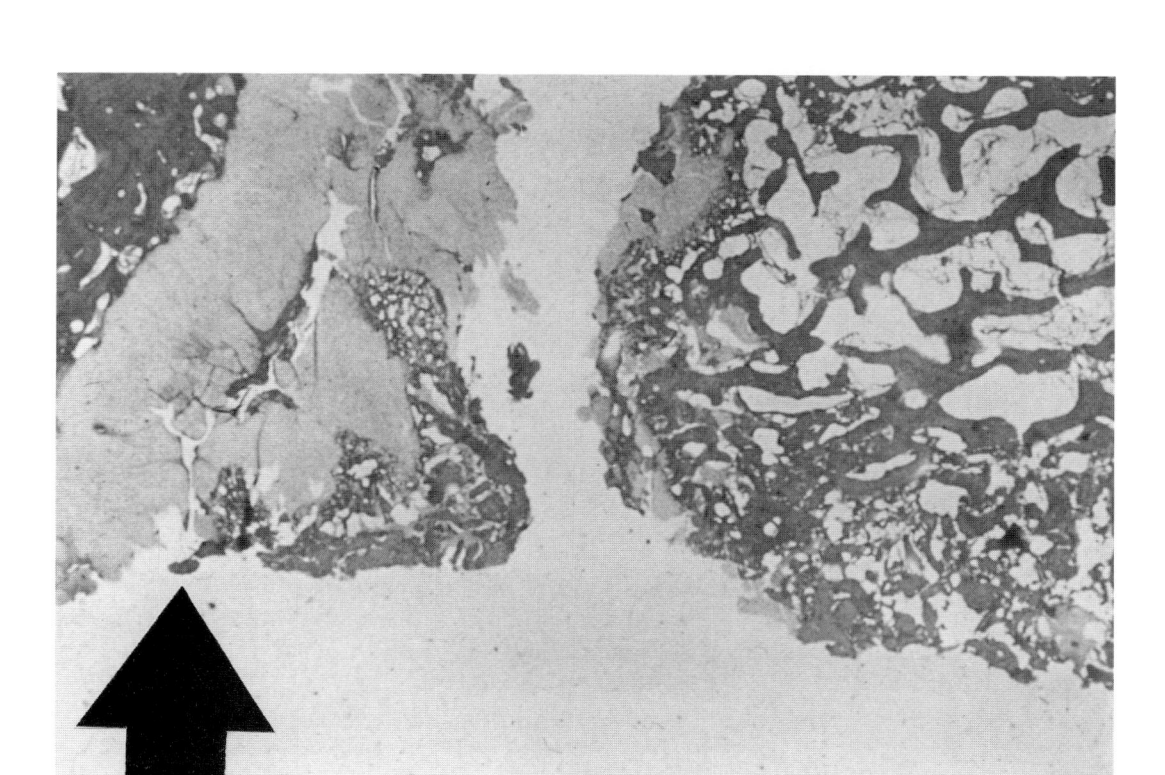

Fig. 27-2. Histologic section of slipped capital femoral epiphysis showing fissure separation primarily through zone of hypertrophy and zone of provisional ossification.

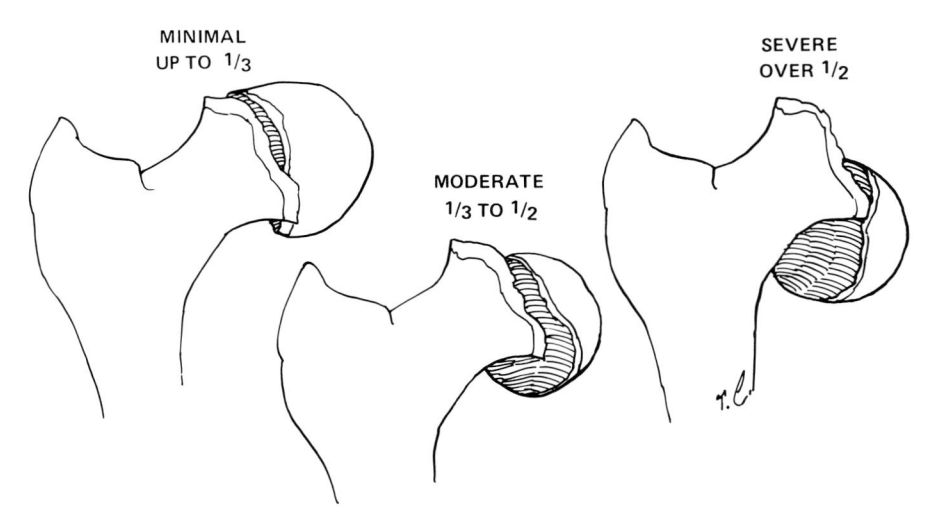

Fig. 27-3. Grading of slipped capital femoral epiphysis.

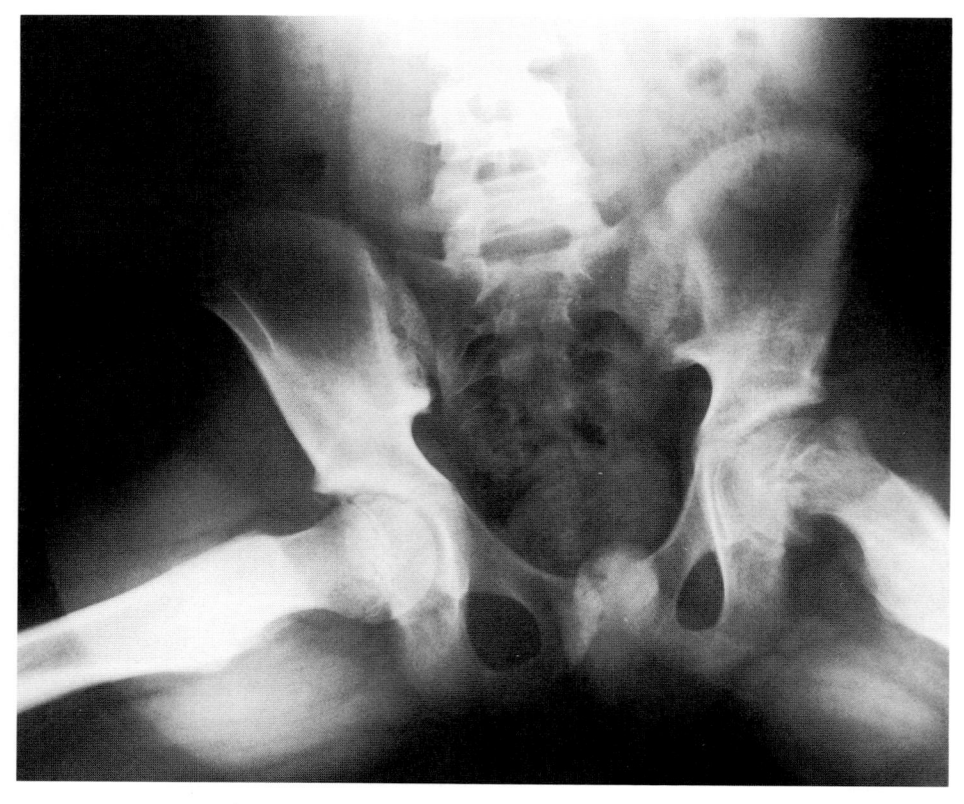

Fig. 27-4. Lateral frog-leg radiograph demonstrating significant acute inferior slipping.

separate it from a chronic stable slip.[1,4] Documentation of a mobile femoral head can be established by radiographically documenting a change in position of the femoral head relative to the neck after closed manipulation, or by directly observing at the time of arthrotomy of the hip that the head is moving on the femoral neck with internal rotation and flexion (Figs. 27-4 to 27-6).

DIFFERENTIAL DIAGNOSIS

Careful separation of acute from chronic slipping is important due to the marked difference in prognosis between an unstable head/neck relationship (acute) and the stable situation (chronic). The incidence of avascular necrosis, further slipping, and eventual osteoarthritis secondary to permanently altered head architectural geometry is substantially higher in an acute unreduced slipped capital femoral epiphysis.

At the present time no firm dogmatic statement on the recommended care of the acute slip can be made. Unfortunately, there is a tremendous deficiency in the number of reported cases of acute slipped capital femoral epiphysis consistently treated in a similar fashion, and statistically reviewed.[4,5]

This is not to imply that the pathophysiology and prognosis of the acute slip is not appreciated. For years it has been common knowledge that the acute slipped capital femoral epiphysis (mobile femoral head) bears a poorer overall prognosis than the chronic, stable head/neck interface, particularly as it relates to avascular necrosis. Acute cartilage necrosis, which occurs in association with treated and untreated slipped capital femoral epiphysiodesis, occurs to a much greater degree in treated cases of acute slipped capital femoral epiphysis. The association of acute cartilage necrosis with pin penetration in the treatment of slipped capital femoral epiphysis has been clearly established.[6-9] Although for many years it was thought that blacks, particularly black females, had a much poorer prognosis in slipped capital

Acute Slipped Capital Femoral Epiphysis / 517

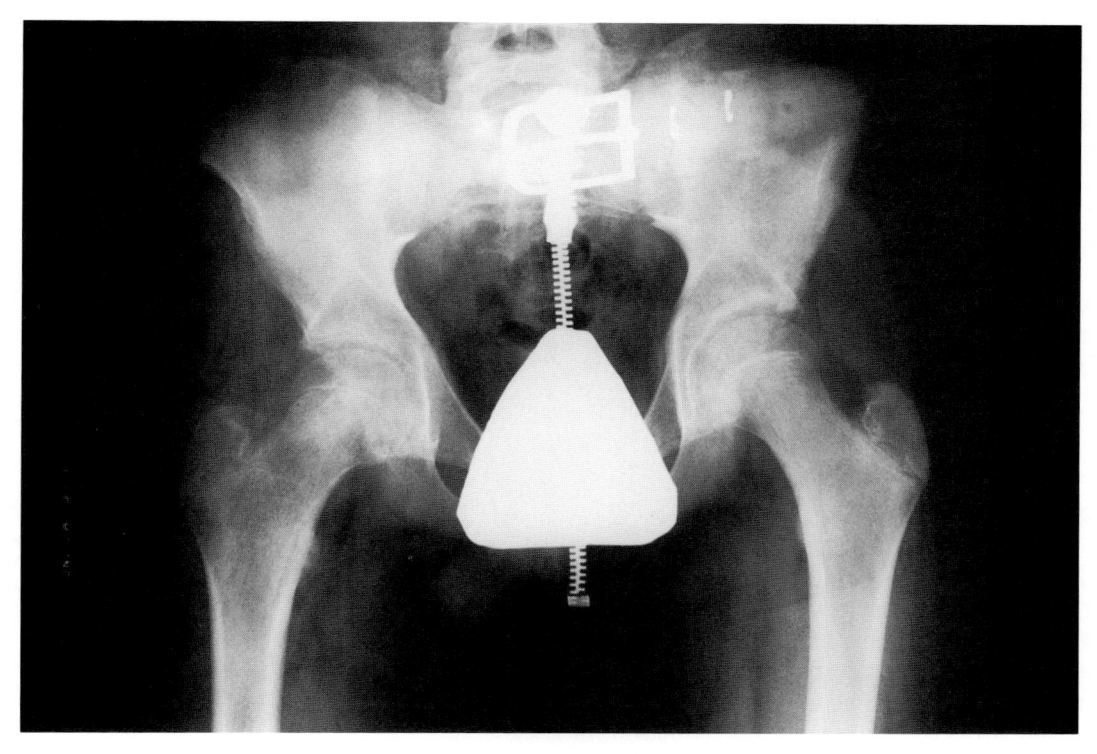

Fig. 27-5. Following reduction of acute slipped capital femoral epiphysis, AP view radiograph shows early growth plate closure.

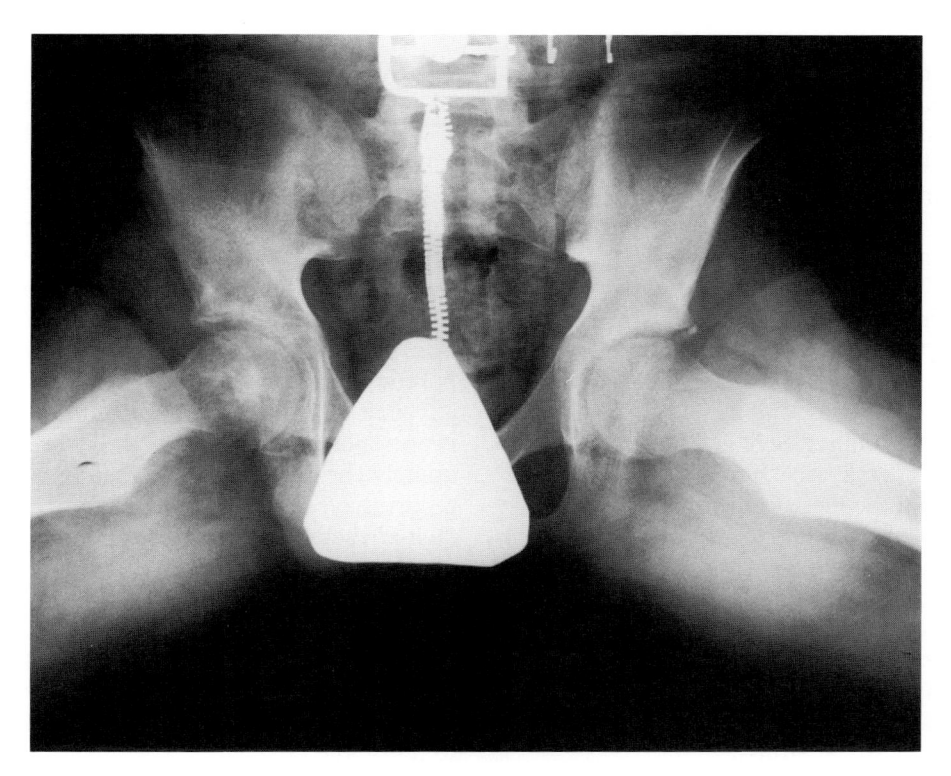

Fig. 27-6. Lateral frog-leg radiograph following reduction and bone graft epiphysiodesis demonstrates advanced growth plate closure.

femoral epiphysis, recent studies have clearly established the inaccuracy of that impression.

The degree of slipping has for many years been linked to prognosis. More advanced degrees of slipping severely distort the architectural geometry of the femoral head and its relationship to the acetabulum. The potential for acetabular remodeling in the age group for slipped epiphysis has been exhausted, commonly resulting in an incongruous relationship with the femoral head, and an implied greater risk of premature osteoarthritis. More severe degrees of acute slipping may also bear a direct relationship to an increased incidence of avascular necrosis.

TREATMENT INDICATIONS

Controversy exists in the literature on nearly every aspect of treatment of the acute slip. These divergent opinions will likely persist until a significant number of similar cases can be carefully analyzed. In spite of a direct relationship between significant head deformity and early-onset osteoarthritis, avoidance of reduction in acute slips has been argued as safer than risking avascular necrosis by replacing the femoral head. This opinion has not in any way been substantiated. In fact, the low incidence of avascular necrosis encountered in many series of reduced slips supports the opposing view. Indeed, in a large series presented, a remarkably low incidence of avascular necrosis was encountered in those hips reduced as a surgical urgency (i.e., within 24 hours).[10]

The peculiar anatomy of the adolescent proximal femur creates a precarious environment for the nutrition to the femoral head, which is provided by the lateral epiphyseal artery. The artery arborizes after piercing the femoral capital epiphysis just above the physeal level and beneath the epiphyseal bone plate. With an acute sudden displacement of the head from the neck, there is a tear in the periosteal sleeve of the neck along its anterior/superior aspect, and the vascular sleeve is stripped from the bony metaphysis and may be "kinked"[1,4] (Fig. 27-7). The displaced edge of the metaphyseal side of the epiphyseal growth plate projects anteriorly. The periosteal sleeve remains intact along the posterior/inferior aspect of the neck. It is likely that some of the retinacular vessels are disrupted at the time of the acute displacement. Others within the periosteal sleeve likely remain attached to the epiphysis, but may be compromised. Theoretically, the circulation may be improved by prompt restoration of the anatomy.

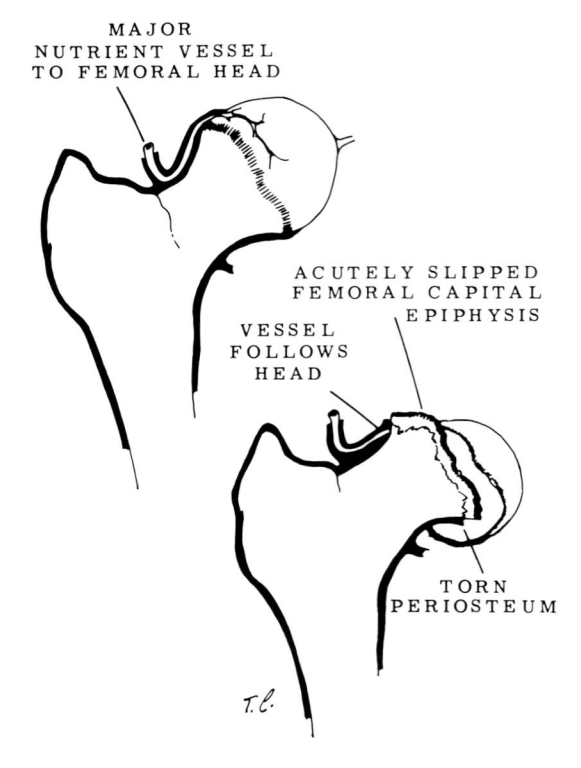

Fig. 27-7. Proposed anatomic disruption of vascular sleeve accompanying an acute slipped capital femoral epiphysis.

COMPLICATIONS

Every treatment technique used to treat chronic slipped capital femoral epiphysis has been applied to the acute form, all with varying degrees of success and all with at least one reported case of avascular necrosis (Figs. 27-8 and 27-9). Casting in situ, casting with reduction, pin or screw fixation with or without reduction, and bone graft epiphysiodesis with or without reduction have all been advocated. Complications secondary to improper placement of pins and screws have been adequately chronicled in the literature, and, most recently, reports have indicated that pin penetration is a causative factor in acute cartilage necrosis and avascular necrosis.[7] Reslipping has occurred in cases treated by both pinning and bone graft epiphysiodesis. The inherent stability imparted by pins or screws is not provided by bone graft epiphysiodesis, and, in fact, bone graft epiphysiodesis in the treatment of acute slips renders the head/neck interface further weakened by the cylindrical tunnel formed to house the bone graft. The hip spica cast, for 6 weeks,

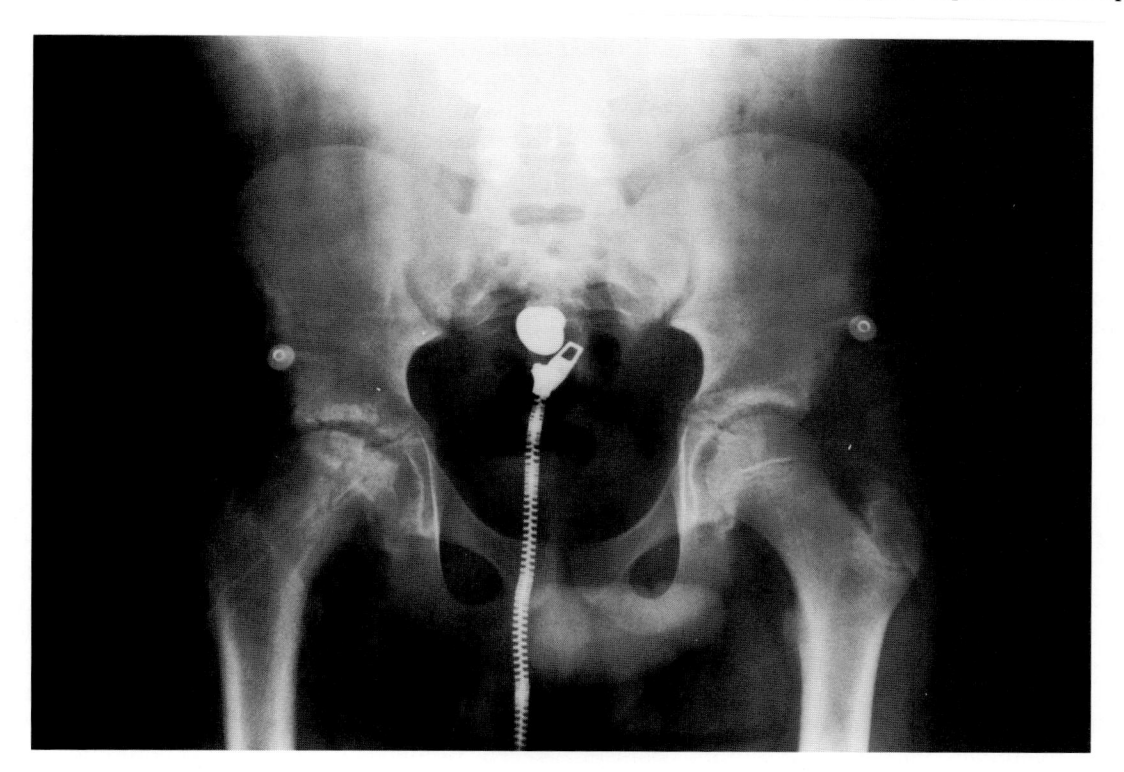

Fig. 27-8. AP view radiograph demonstrating avascular necrosis following pin fixation for acute slipped capital femoral epiphysis.

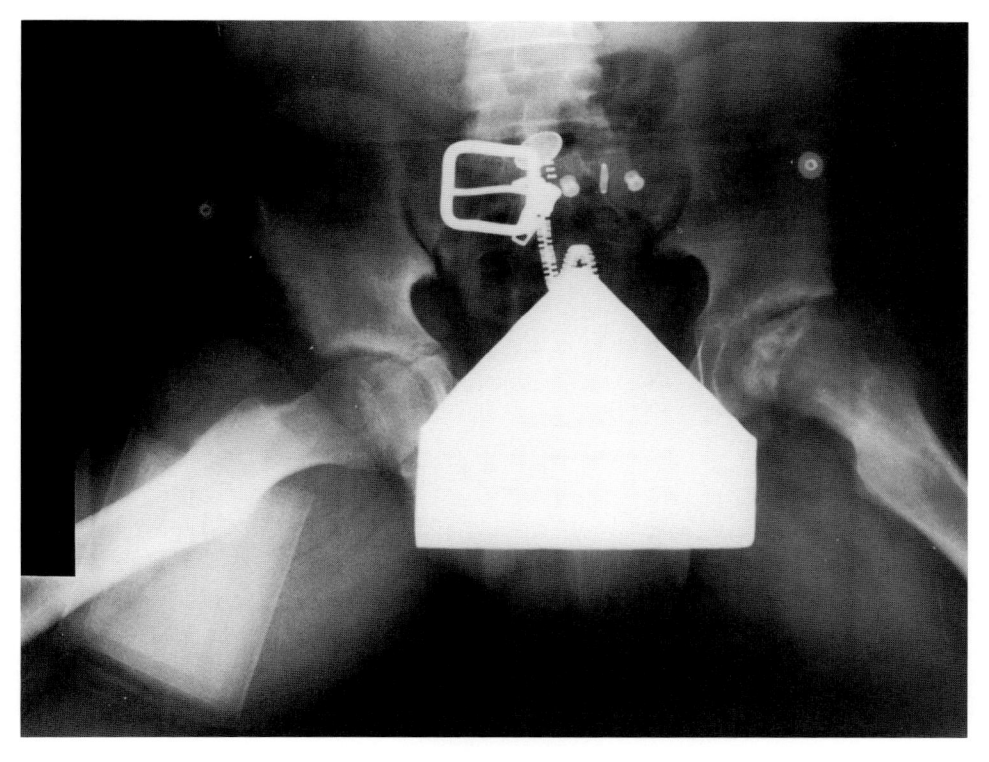

Fig. 27-9. Lateral frog-leg radiograph of avascular necrosis following pin fixation for acute slipped capital femoral epiphysis.

has reduced displacement in cases so treated until the head is firmly anchored to the neck.

Acute cartilage necrosis does not inherently seem to be influenced by the extent of acute displacement or the adequacy of reduction of that displacement. It may be more related to extended periods in a cast with or without reduction of an acute slip. Curiously, it has not been seen as a consequence of cases treated by reduction, bone graft epiphysiodesis, and casting for 6 weeks. In younger children, metallic internal fixation or bone graft epiphysiodesis in the treatment of acute slips may occasionally result in coxa vara, coxa breva, and greater trochanter overgrowth due to premature growth plate closure. These rarely reported complications need to be reviewed in context with the risk of allowing further potential slipping of the femoral head on the femoral neck and the subsequent increased incidence of osteoarthritis.

TREATMENT

Based on the available currently reported literature, the following treatment approaches seem most defensible and least likely to result in later osteoarthritis, and they may reduce the incidence of avascular necrosis. The acute slip is a surgical urgency, and it is essential to proceed with reduction of displacement *within* 24 hours of its recognition. Closed gentle manipulation (traction, internal rotation, slight flexion, and abduction if necessary) (Fig. 27-10), followed by properly placed internal fixation with threaded pins or screws inserted by open technique or percutaneously, is an acceptable option. Limited weightbearing with crutches is generally begun a few days after surgical stabilization. Percutaneous pin or screw fixation is currently in vogue and is certainly an acceptable option providing diligence is exerted in properly placing the devices. Pin placement must be verified by careful radiographic scrutiny and may require recently developed imaging techniques for documentation. A more anteriorly placed pin or screw entry site may be required to avoid the complication of penetration. The use of dye inserted through cannulated screws may be useful in detecting penetration of the head. Clinical data analyzed to date provides support for open bone graft epiphysiodesis and casting as a reliable alternative.[1] Hip spica immobilization for 6 weeks followed by progressive ambulation with crutches is the standard postoperative regimen following bone graft epiphysiodesis.

The rationale for reduction in bone graft epiphysiodesis relates to the theory that the potential of additional vascular communications are opened across the physis,

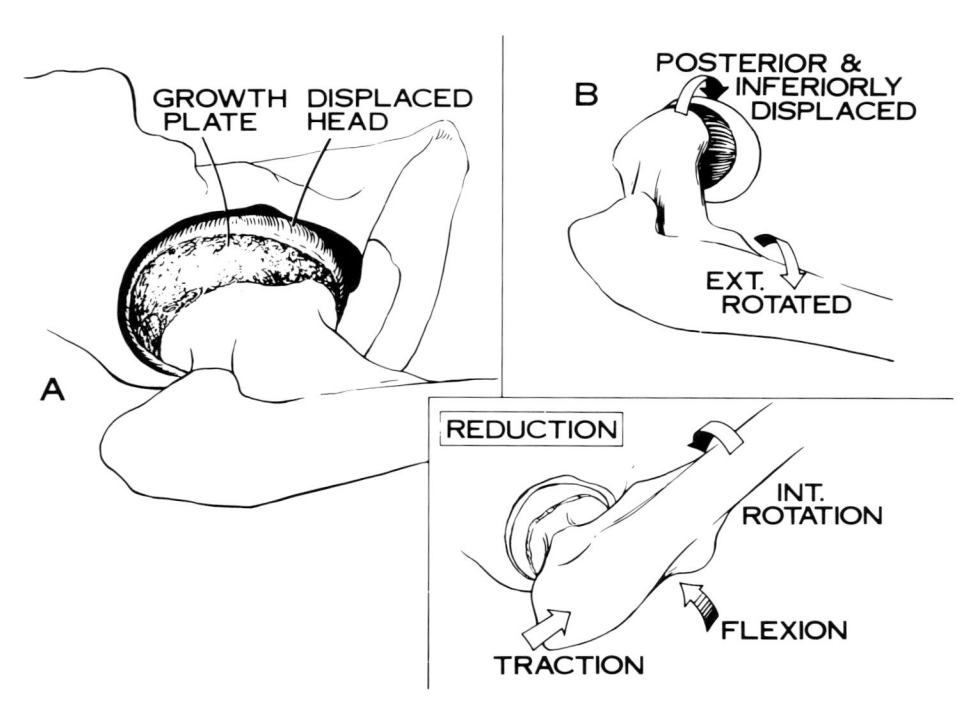

Fig. 27-10. (A&B) Usual mechanism of "gentle" reduction of acute slipped capital femoral epiphysis.

permitting anastomotic channels to be established between the epiphyseal and metaphyseal circulatory beds, and also to hasten growth plate closure. Rapid reliable growth plate closure has been one of the most important contributions in the use of bone graft epiphysiodesis for chronic slipped epiphysis.[1,4]

Reslipping following bone graft epiphysiodesis and casting has not been a problem in spite of the temporary reduction in stability. A very low incidence of avascular necrosis, particularly in those treated within 24 hours lend further support for this treatment. Avascular necrosis may be detected by classic radiographic features or by radionuclide imaging and magnetic resonance imaging if suspicious changes on plain radiography occur. Historically, poor results with reduction and casting alone diminish support for this treatment option.

Regardless of which of the main two options is entertained, there remains an increased risk of avascular necrosis considerably above that seen in chronic slipped capital femoral epiphysis, which has been reported with every treatment technique. Avascular necrosis becomes apparent within 1 year from the time of acute slip, and it is likely related to vascular injury rather than the type of treatment. I believe, on the basis of a personal review of acute slips treated within 24 hours (5 percent avascular necrosis) and compared to those acute slips treated over 24 hours (20 percent avascular necrosis), that the mechanical impairment to the vascularity of the femoral head is relieved by urgent decompression (reduction) and accounts for the very low incidence of avascular necrosis, as compared to those reduced later.[10] Furthermore, it appears that reduction with metallic internal fixation and bone graft epiphysiodesis both yield a high percentage of quality results, although to date bone graft epiphysiodesis has been statistically safer in our hands.

REFERENCES

1. Weiner DS, Weiner S, Melby A et al: A 30-year experience with bone graft epiphysiodesis in the treatment of slipped capital femoral epiphysis. J Pediatr Orthop 4:145, 1984
2. Agamanolis DP, Weiner DS, Lloyd JK: Slipped capital femoral epiphysis: a pathological study. I. A light microscopic and histochemical study of 21 cases. J Pediatr Orthop 5:40, 1985
3. Agamanolis DP, Weiner DS, Lloyd JK: Slipped capital femoral epiphysis: a pathological study. II. An ultrastructural study of 23 cases. J Pediatr Orthop 5:47, 1985
4. Aadalen RJ, Weiner DS, Hoyt W et al: Acute slipped capital femoral epiphysis. J Bone Joint Surg [Am] 56:1473, 1974
5. Weiner DS: Bone graft epiphysiodesis in the treatment of slipped capital femoral epiphysis. Instr Course Lect 38:263, 1989
6. Walters R, Simon S: Joint destruction: a sequel of unrecognized pin penetration in patients with slipped capital femoral epiphysis. Hip 8:145, 1980
7. Riley P, Weiner DS, Weiner S et al: Hazards of internal fixation in slipped capital femoral epiphysis. J Bone Joint Surg [Am] 72:1500, 1990
8. Swiontkowski M: Slipped capital femoral epiphysis: complications related to internal fixation. Orthopaedics 6:705, 1983
9. Greenough CG, Bromage JD, Jackson AM: Pinning of the slipped upper femoral epiphysis: a trouble-free procedure. J Pediatr Orthop 5:657, 1985
10. Peterson M, Weiner DS, Green NE et al: Slipped capital femoral epiphysis: the value of urgent reduction. Presented at the Mid America Orthopaedic Association meeting, 1991. 7-1-93–6-30-94, APA award winning paper.

28

Traumatic Dislocation of the Hip

Morris Duhaime
Marc Isler
Dominique Marton

>An ounce of prevention equals a pound of prosthesis.
>—R.B. Salter

EPIDEMIOLOGY

Acute traumatic dislocation of the hip, although uncommon in children, is nevertheless more common than hip fractures in this age group: 10 percent of all traumatic dislocations of the hip occur in children.[1-3] The hip is one of the most frequent joints to be dislocated. The right side is affected as often as the left, and bilateral cases are rare. The male:female ratio is generally reported to be approximately 3:1.[3,4]

The incidence peaks within two age groups. Between the ages of 2 and 5 years, hip dislocation typically occurs with minimal trauma and few complications.[3,5] The second peak involves children between the ages of 11 and 15 and comprises 50 percent of all cases. These patients characteristically experience greater trauma and the dislocation of their hip is more frequently complicated by associated injuries.[5,6,12,13] Most authors report less favorable prognosis for older children, but there is a significant disparity in the reported significance of the various identified prognostic factors and in the type of traumatic incident. Common causes of traumatic dislocation of the hip in children are falls (50 percent), motor vehicle accidents (30 percent), and sporting activities (20 percent).[1,2,5]

ANATOMY

Certain anatomic features in children are significant in this injury. The capsule inserts proximally along the acetabular junction between bone and cartilage in the area of the anteroinferior iliac spine. Thus the labrum is an intracapsular structure and can be avulsed with the capsule as in a Bankart injury of the shoulder. A significant element reinforcing the capsule anteriorly and medially is the iliofemoral ligament of Bigelow, often referred to as the Y ligament. The stem of the Y represents the proximal origin of the capsule. Distally the two branches insert into the intertrochanteric line, limiting hyperextension and external rotation. Tears commonly occur near the pelvis, that segment being thinner, with or without bone or cartilage avulsion. The ligaments around the hip may undergo midsubstance tears, avulsions, or buttonhole interposition. Anatomic structures, which in the various types of dislocation may be an obstruction to closed reduction include an inverted segment of limbus, osteochondral fragments, buttonholed capsule, and, less frequently, in anterior dislocation, the iliopsoas. The capsule has been noted to tear at any site according to the type of dislocation.[3,6]

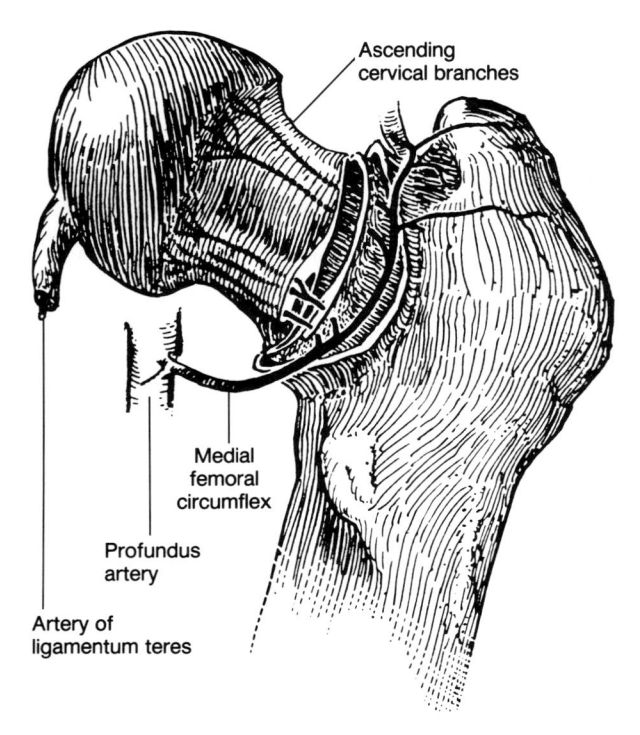

Fig. 28-1. Vascular anatomy of the proximal femur. (Modified from Rockwood and Green.[5])

VASCULAR SUPPLY OF THE HIP

The vascular anatomy of the proximal femur is an important consideration in these injuries, particularly in posterior dislocations (Fig. 28-1). The blood supply to the femoral head is dependent on an extracapsular arterial ring at the base of the femoral neck, ascending cervical branches on the surface of the neck, an intracapsular epiphyseal ring, and the arteries of the ligamentum teres. Although significant variations exist, it is generally believed that the medial femoral circumflex artery gives the predominant blood supply at the level of the extracapsular arterial ring, and of the four ascending cervical arteries, the lateral is the predominant source of vascularization to the femoral head. These critical structures are collectively referred to as the posterior retinacular vessels. They are at risk in a posterior dislocation of the hip, but in younger children the risk of injury is somewhat diminished, probably due to the greater laxity of the investing capsular structures and by the more significant contribution from the ligamentum teres.

CLASSIFICATION

Classification of traumatic dislocation of the hip can be anatomic or related to associated injuries (Table 28-1). The acetabulum can be portrayed as being supported by three ridges sloping away it, the femoral head dislocating into one of the three valleys thus formed. The anteriorly dislocated hip would thus be located between the ilium and the pubis, posterior between ilium and ischium, and, more rarely, obturator dislocation involves the femoral head lodging in the obturator foramen, between the pubis and ischium.[2] Other authors have added to the complexity of this classification by adding variations for vertical displacement, others for associated injuries.[3]

Fracture-dislocations have also been classified by Stewart and Milford according to associated fractures[4] (Table 28-2). Type 1 is a simple dislocation with an acetabular chip of insignificant size equivalent to a moderate to severe capsular tear. Type 2 involves one or more rim fragments of various sizes, the acetabular socket remaining sufficiently stable not to require reconstruction. Type 3 involves an unstable hip due to rim comminution. Type 4 involves associated head or neck fracture.

Perhaps the most severe type of fracture-dislocation of the hip is the central fracture-dislocation. The incidence of the most frequent types in children is reported to be 80 percent for posterior displacement, 16 percent for anterior displacement, and 4 percent for central fracture-dislocations[3,6] (Table 28-3).

TABLE 28-1. Classification of Hip Dislocations

Anterior
   Anteroinferior
   Anterosuperior
Posterior
   Posterosuperior
   Posteroinferior
Obturator

TABLE 28-2. Stewart and Milford Classification of Fracture-Dislocations

1. Stable hip, insignificant acetabular chip
2. Stable hip, significant acetabular fragments
3. Unstable hip, acetabulum requires reconstruction
4. Associated head or neck fracture

TABLE 28-3. Incidence
of the Most Frequent
Types of Hip Dislocation

Type	Incidence (%)
Posterior	80
Anterior	16
Central	4

Differential Diagnosis

Chronic causes of hip dislocation, such as muscular imbalance and dysplastic hips, pose few problems. In children with Down syndrome, however, dislocatable hips may present without obvious dysplasia. The history is usually that of frequent dislocations, and reduction can usually be performed in the emergency department. Finally, a rare pitfall in diagnosis is the obstetrical "hip dislocation," which is in fact a type 1 epiphyseal separation injury of the proximal femur.[3]

Posterior Dislocation

In teenagers the most common type of mechanism is typified by the "dashboard" injury involving an axial blow to the flexed knee on a hip flexed to about 90

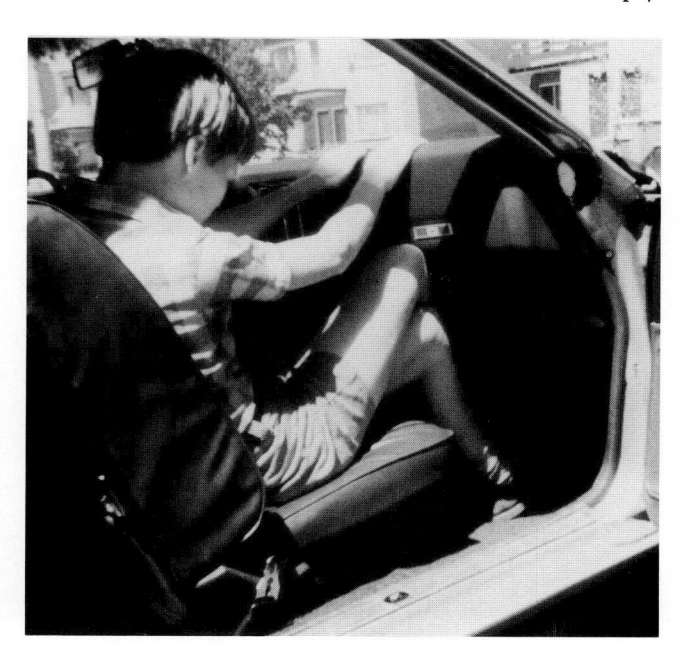

Fig. 28-2. "Dashboard injury" mechanism in posterior dislocation.

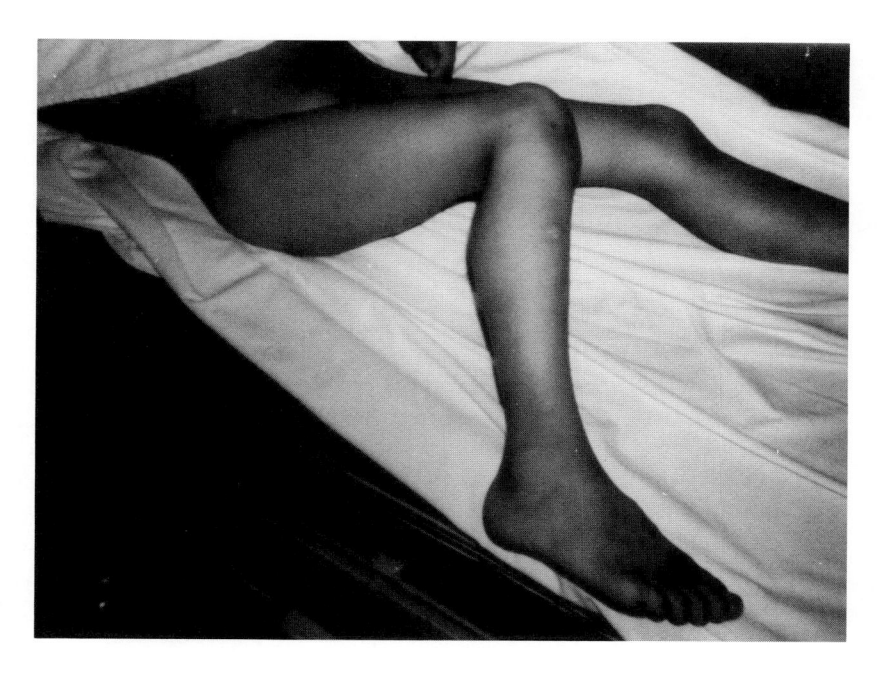

Fig. 28-3. Typical deformity in posterior dislocation. (Courtesy of R. Mervyn Letts.)

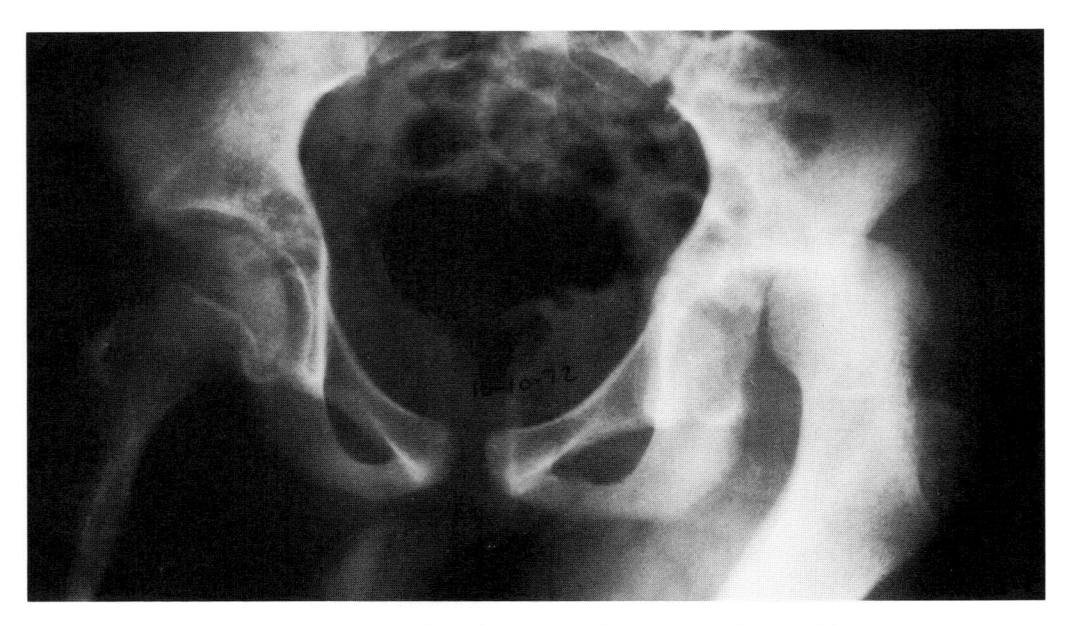

Fig. 28-4. Posterosuperior dislocation of the hip in 13-year-old boy.

degrees[2,4] (Fig. 28-2). In younger children the mechanism of posterior dislocation also involves retropulsion of the femur on a flexed hip in most cases, but this occurs most often in falls. One reported variation of this mechanism is that of a child, crawling on all fours, receiving a blow to the back.[2] As in adults, one of the most common associated injuries is fracture of the posterior lip of the acetabulum. Most hip dislocations are posterior, and can usually be diagnosed with the frequent clinical findings of hip flexion, adduction, and internal rotation with shortening[3,5-7] (Figs. 28-3 and 28-4).

Knee pain may occasionally mislead the unwary clinician to delayed diagnosis of a dislocated hip from which the pain radiates down the medial obturator nerve to the knee. The risk of significant associated injury to the knee region should motivate the clinician to systematic evaluate the knee for any associated ligamentous injury or fracture of the distal femur, proximal tibia, or patella.[3] Sciatic nerve injury may occur from contusion by the posteriorly dislocated head of the femur and often affects the more anterior fibers of the sciatic nerve—the peroneal fibers. Documentation of sciatic nerve function is essential before and after reduction of hip dislocation (Table 28-4).

Femoral shaft fractures are occasionally complicated by ipsilateral hip dislocation in older children. The associated hip injury can be missed, diagnosis being made 4 to 6 weeks later.[3] On the femoral radiographs, adduction of the proximal fragment is pathognomonic[5] of hip dislocation. Radiographs in two planes should be scrutinized for associated bony injury and position of the dislocation. Computed tomography (CT) scanning should be used for further study in a preoperative setting or to further evaluate bony injury discovered on plain radiographs. More often, however, it is used when closed reduction yields a nonconcentric femoroacetabular relationship. A reliable radiographic sign of this is widening of the medial joint space. CT scanning is much more reliable than arthrography in the detection of loose bodies after closed reduction[3,8] (Figs. 28-5 to 28-7).

Treatment of all acute hip dislocations consists of early reduction, detection of associated injury, and, as indicated, further treatment of the concomitant injuries. Closed reduction under general anesthesia is almost always successful when performed within 12 hours of injury.[3,6] Limiting this delay contributes significantly to

TABLE 28-4. Associated Injuries in Traumatic Hip Dislocation

Head trauma
Thoracic contusion
Pelvic fracture
Ipsilateral-contralateral femoral fractures
Fractures and ligamentous injuries about the knee
Sciatic nerve (posterior)

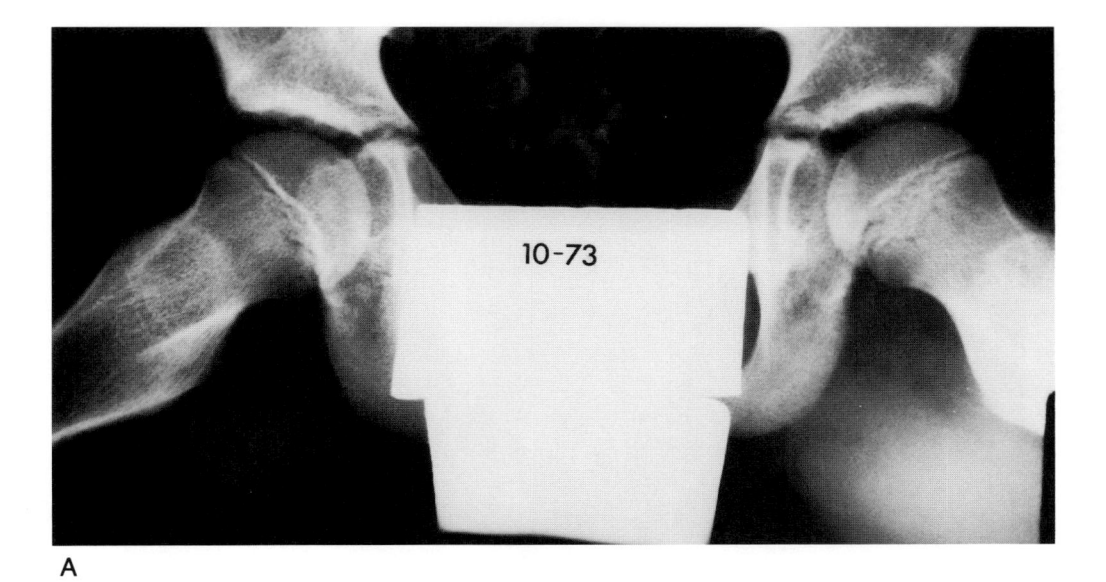

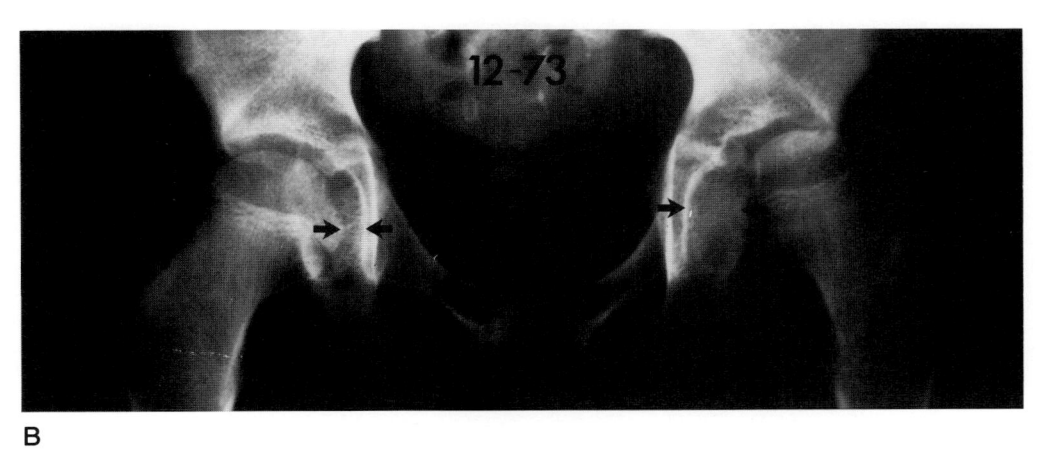

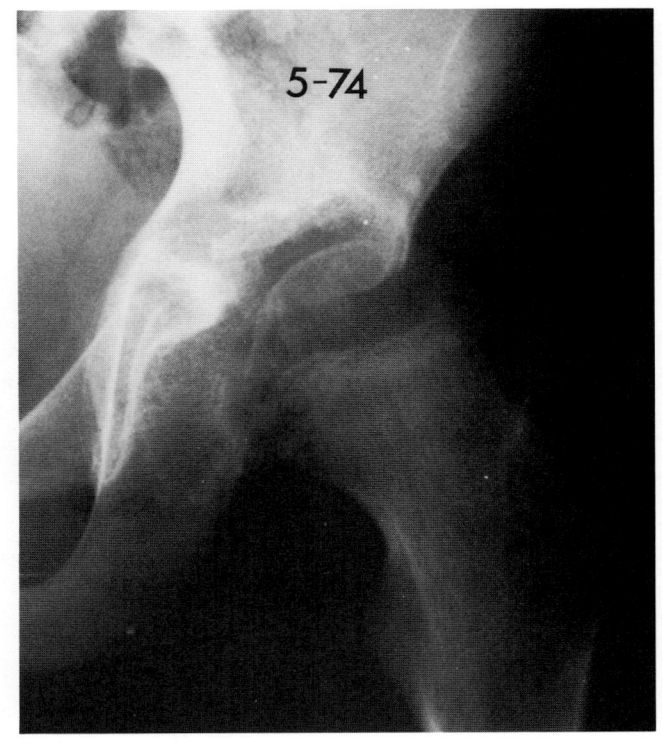

Fig. 28-5. Nonconcentric reduction with widened medial joint space. **(A)** Lateral view immediately postreduction. **(B)** 2 months later AP view shows degenerative changes. **(C)** 7 months postreduction.

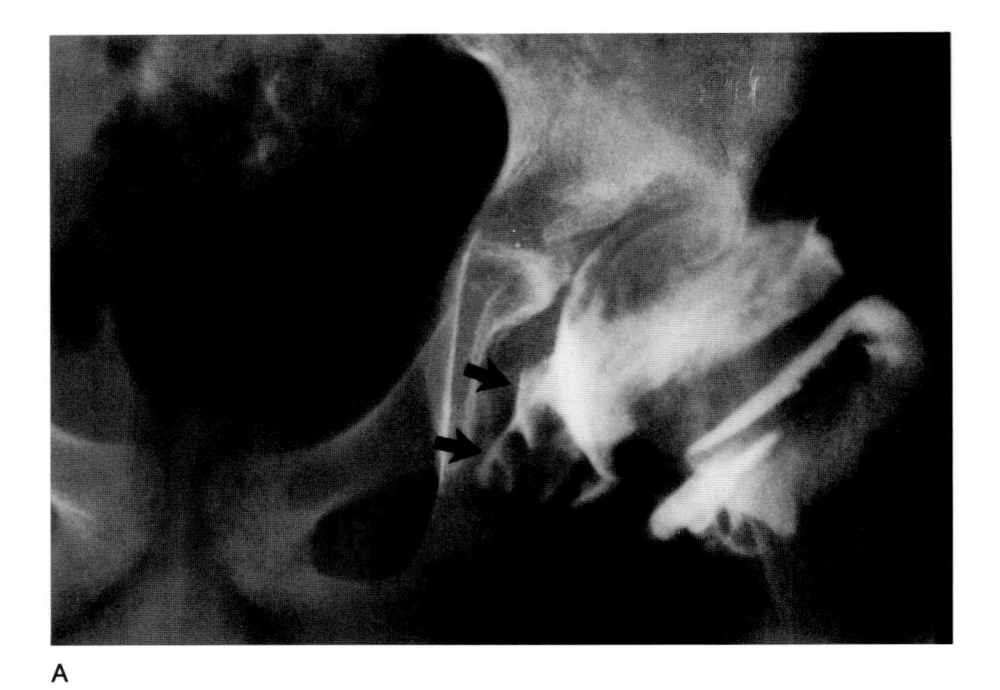

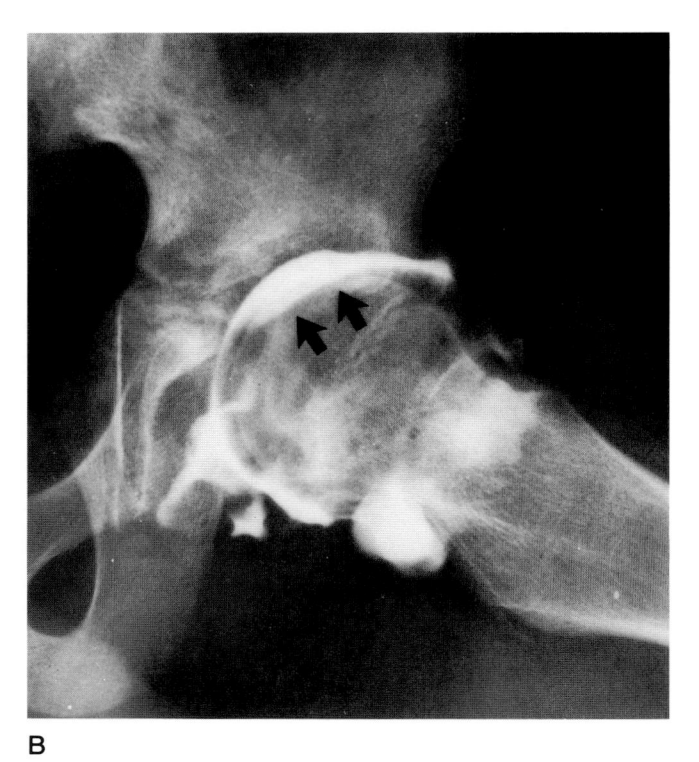

Fig. 28-6. (A) AP and (B) lateral arthrograms of case shown in Figure 28-8 showing femoral head defect.

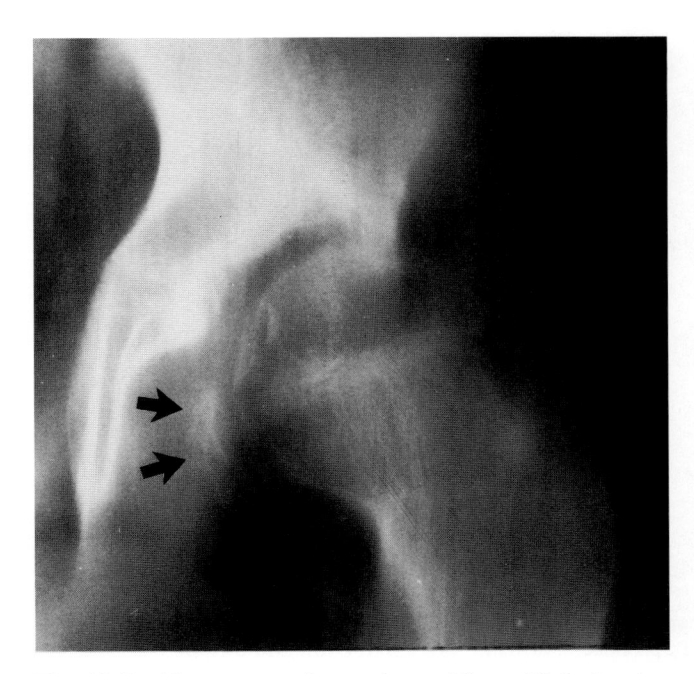

Fig. 28-7. Tomogram of case shown Figure 28-8 showing intra-articular fragment.

decreasing the risk of complications, primarily avascular necrosis, though less so than in the adult.[1,3]

The methods of reduction are chiefly those of Stimson, Allis, and Bigelow.[3,6] Basic to all of these techniques is traction in line with the position of the dislocated limb. The presence of an associated shaft fracture may necessitate the insertion of a trochanteric pin for manipulation of the proximal fragment.[1] In the child the importance of performing a closed reduction in an atraumatic manner is especially pertinent, as epiphyseal separation can result from overly vigorous maneuvers, resulting in the metaphysis being reduced into the acetabular cavity leaving the epiphysis dislocated posteriorly (Fig. 28-8).

Very occasionally, closed reduction will prove impossible. The usual obstacles to reduction include the Y ligament, the piriformis tendon, an inverted ar avulsed limbus, or osteochondral fragments. The latter are, in most cases, of acetabular origin, but occasionally a femoral head fragment is involved[3] (see Fig. 28-6).

Immediately after reduction, one must move the hip through a full range of motion to detect any crepitus or instability. A radiograph should be done immediately postreduction and examined for epiphyseal separation and medial joint space widening, a reliable sign of nonconcentric reduction most often due to a loose body within the joint.[6,7,9] When an intra-articular fragment is suspected on postreduction radiographs, tomograms or a CT scan should be done. This examination is useful to confirm the diagnosis and often indicates the source and position of the loose body. The appropriate surgical approach can then be planned.[4,6] Open reduction is almost always done by a posterolateral approach, with excision of small fragments and repair of large defects, unless the fragment is lying anteriorly[1] (see Figs. 28-6 and 28-7).

Postoperative Management

Following successful reduction, management is controversial.[3] One issue is the duration of nonweightbearing in these children. Even though many authors have recommended a prolonged period of up to 3 months of nonweightbearing, most children will resume full weightbearing as soon as physical constraints are removed, in spite of medical advice.[3] A painful range of motion indicating posttraumatic synovitis is probably the best indicator of the necessary duration of traction.[3] When the patient is pain-free, a gradual return to weightbearing is recommended by most clinicians. It is clear from review of the literature that the duration of nonweightbearing is of no proven prognostic significance.[1,4,7] Some clinicians will immobilize routinely in spica casts, others will reserve this treatment modality for those patients who demonstrate instability at the time of reduction. The hip spica cast, when indicated, should maintain the hip in extension and mild abduction,[4] and is usually maintained for 4 to 6 weeks, depending on the age of the child.[7] Since a torn capsule requires approximately 6 weeks to heal, and since children under the age of 10 are notoriously difficult to limit in activity, we recommend immobilizing such children in a hip spica cast for 6 weeks.

The follow-up regimen we recommend includes a baseline bone scan at around 3 months postdislocation to detect early avascular necrosis.[4,7] By 2 years, the great majority of avascular necrosis will be obvious; therefore, radiographs every 3 months until 2 years of age is recommended.[4] If avascular necrosis does occur it should be managed using treatment criteria established for Legg-Calvé-Perthes disease.[4]

Anterior Dislocation

Anterior hip dislocation represents 16 percent of total acute hip dislocations in children. The usual mechanism is reported to be forced external rotation of the hip, or a blow to the greater trochanter with the hip in external

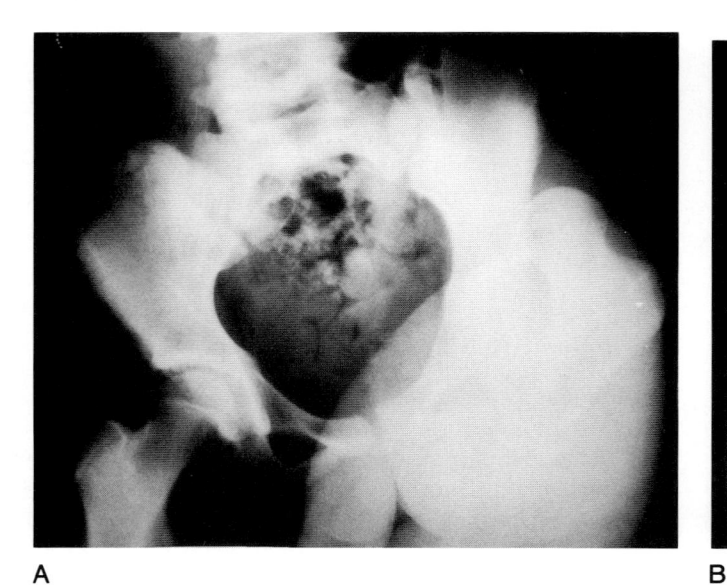

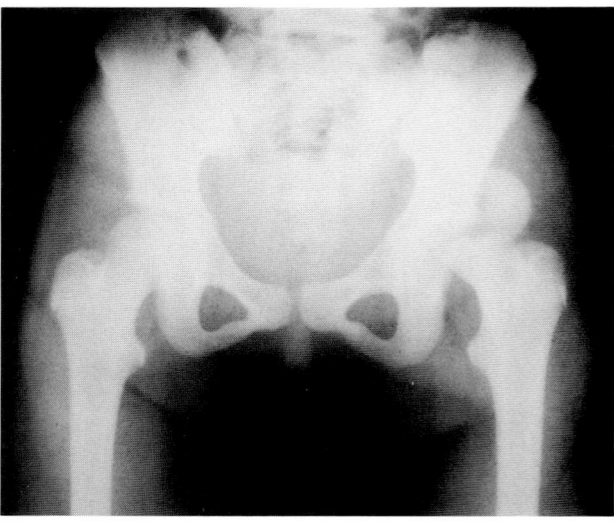

Fig. 28-8. (A) Posterior dislocation of the hip in a 10-year-old girl. (B) Following an attempted closed reduction a type I fracture of the physis was obvious on the radiograph necessitating an open reduction and pinning.

rotation (Fig. 28-9). These are most often found in falls from a height, though motor vehicle accidents may cause them.[2-4] Anatomically, there is a tendency for extrusion of the femoral head through the capsule with occasionally femoral artery damage. Indeed femoral artery thrombosis and acute limb ischemia may complicate the clinical picture. Femoral nerve injury is rare, and occasionally the greater trochanter may present an avulsion-type fracture[3] (Fig. 28-10).

Closed reduction is usually possible in anterior hip dislocation. The knee should be flexed to release the hamstring tension, the hip adducted, and longitudinal traction applied with or without gentle rotational movements. Failure of closed reduction, which is rare, may be due to capsule interposition, buttonholing of the femoral head through the capsule, or psoas tendon interposition. Open reduction in these cases are best achieved by an anterior approach. This exposure requires a minimal amount of surgical trauma and has the theoretical advantage of avoiding compromise of the remaining blood supply to the femoral head. Greater trochanteric avulsion may necessitate open reduction and internal fixation unless anatomy is restored on postreduction radiographs. Management after reduction is essentially the same as that described above for posterior dislocation.[3,4]

Fig. 28-9. Most common mechanism of anterior dislocation, as in a fall from a height.

Obturator Dislocation

The obturator dislocation is a rare form of hip dislocation, caused by a forced abduction of the hip.[2] Reduction may be impossible due to ligament interposition in which case open reduction is reported to yield good results[10] (Fig. 28-11).

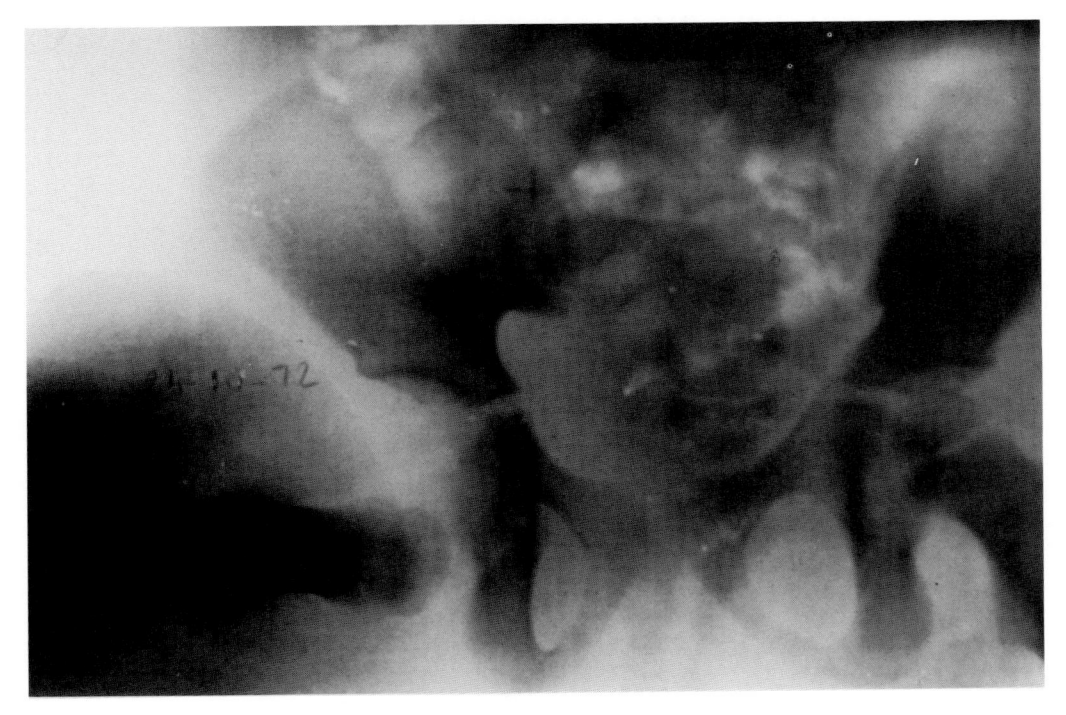

Fig. 28-10. Anteroinferior dislocation in a 3-year-old girl.

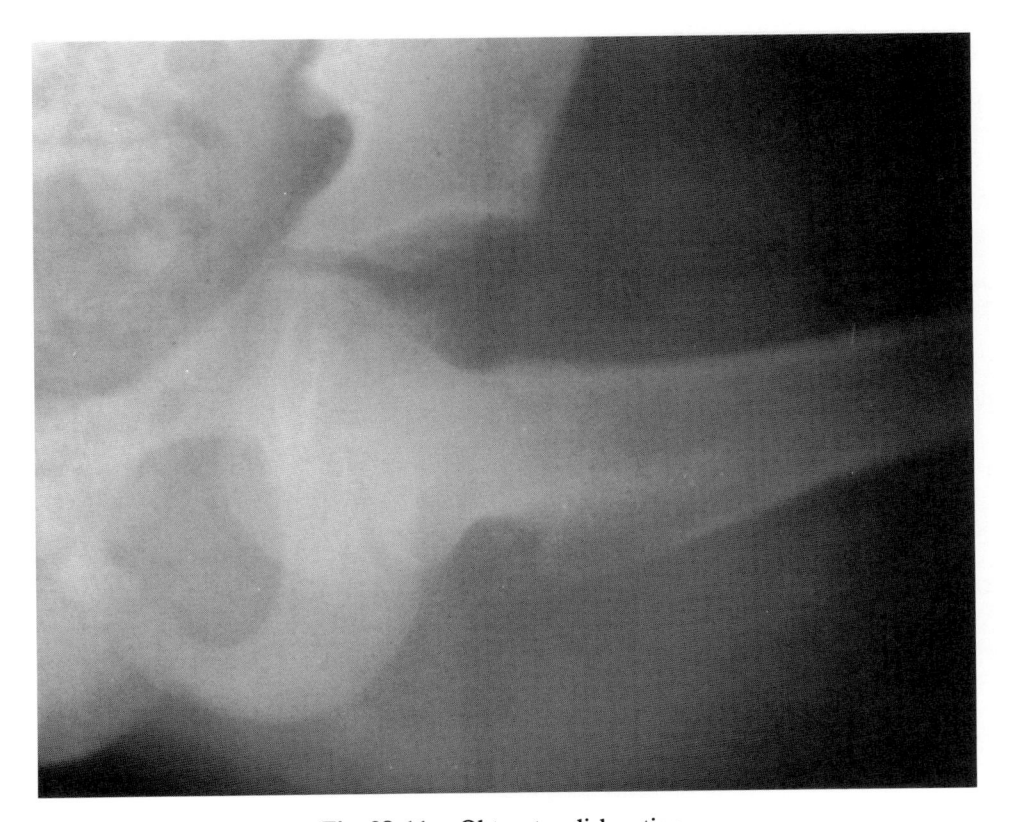

Fig. 28-11. Obturator dislocation.

532 / Management of Pediatric Fractures

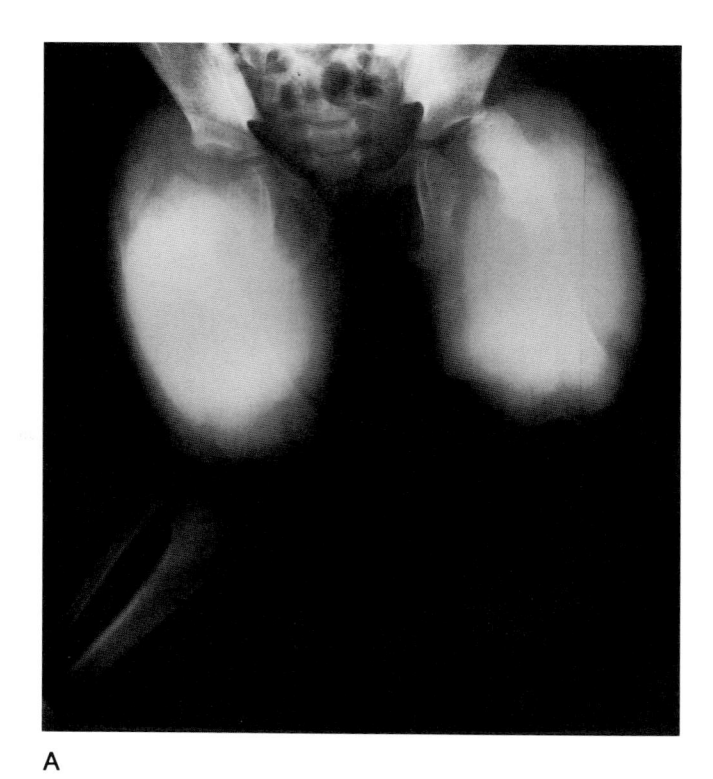

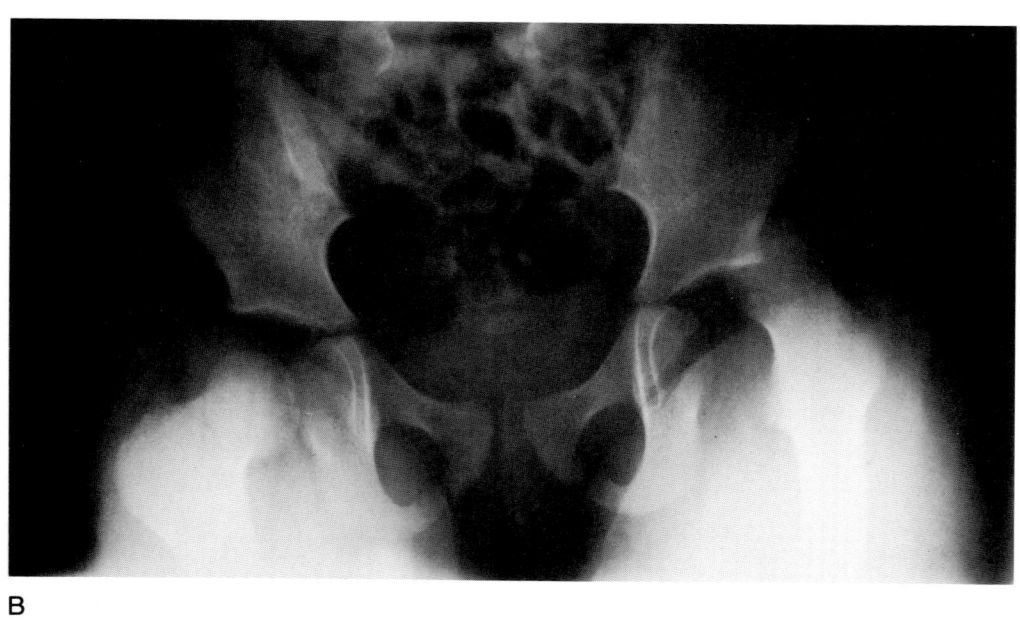

Fig. 28-12. (A) Bilateral dislocations of the hips. (B) Detail view.

Fracture-Dislocation

As noted above, fracture-dislocations can be classified by the Stewart and Milford method. Grades 1 and 2 can be treated as simple dislocations, testing for stability under general anesthesia after simple reduction to evaluate the necessity for immobilization.[2,4] Grades 3 and 4 are rare in children and require open reduction and internal fixation (Fig. 28-12).

Central Fracture-Dislocation

Central fracture-dislocation accounts for 4 percent of the reported cases in children. The cause is usually a fall from a height onto the greater trochanter with adduction and internal rotation of the hip at impact. This severe injury is difficult to treat, and traditionally skeletal traction with addition of lateral trochanteric traction is recommended. Trochanteric traction can be done with a large Schantz screw or equivalent, or alternatively a K-wire passed anteroposteriorly with a tensioning device.[4] This injury is associated in many cases with triradiate cartilage disruption in young children. If traction fails to provide reduction and congruity open reduction and internal fixation may be indicated. The morbidity of such surgery has decreased significantly in the hands of those with appropriate expertise. Furthermore, open reduction and internal fixation can offer not only joint congruity and stability but also can ensure anatomic reduction of the triradiate cartilage.[11] This aggressive approach, though theoretically appealing, remains to be justified in the literature as pertains to a decrease in the incidence of growth related complications for this uncommon injury (see Ch. 25).

Associated Soft Tissue Injuries

Although any soft tissue structure around the hip can conceivably be injured in a hip dislocation, the younger age group sustains few such injuries (Table 28-5). Most frequently, injured structures include the capsule and Y ligament, the ligamentum teres (with or without avulsion of a femoral head fragment), and acetabular labrum avulsion with or without interposition. The sciatic nerve may be contused in posterior dislocations, and the femoral artery may be injured in anterior dislocation. The blood supply to the femoral head may be jeopardized directly by injury to the retinacular vessels or indirectly by an increase in intra-articular pressure secondary to hematoma.[2]

Associated Fractures

The acetabulum, femoral head, and the femoral neck may be fractured in association with a hip dislocation (Table 28-6). Loose bodies accompanying these injuries often present as a widened medial joint space on a postreduction radiograph[2] (Figs. 28-5 to 28-7). Some of these loose bodies may present late, limiting range of motion and causing pain, sometimes associated with degenerative changes in the joint. Even late presentations are improved by excision of the fragments. Chronic labrum injury may lead to acetabular dysplasia, radiographs typically showing a degenerative cyst at the superolateral acetabular margin (Fig. 28-5).

The incidence of neglected hip dislocation is higher when a child presents with a concomitant femoral shaft fracture. Indeed 60 percent of these cases in adults are diagnosed 4 to 6 weeks later.[3] In children, this injury pattern is less common and the dislocation not missed as frequently. However, vigilance must be maintained, and the hip radiographs should always be carefully examined in a child with a fractured femur. A pathognomonic sign seen on radiographs of the femoral shaft fracture is adduction of the proximal fragment.[5] Another sign is absence of the lesser trochanter due to internal rotation of the dislocated fragment. Epiphyseal separations may be associated with overly vigorous reduction maneuvers in posterior dislocations (Fig. 28-8). However, these may be primary and should be looked for on the prereduction

TABLE 28-5. Associated Soft Tissue Injuries in Pediatric Traumatic Hip Dislocation

Capsuloligamentous structures
Acetabular labrum
Sciatic nerve
Posterior retinacular vessels
Femoral artery and nerve

TABLE 28-6. Associated Fractures in Hip Dislocation in Children

Acetabulum
Femoral head
Femoral neck
Pelvis
Femoral shaft

radiographs. Such epiphyseal separations should be treated with open reduction and pin fixation.[3] Pelvic fractures have been reported in conjunction with simple hip dislocations.[2] Finally, an effort should be made to detect fractures around the knee, especially in dashboardlike injuries. These may involve the proximal tibia, the patella, and the distal femur.[2]

COMPLICATIONS

The complications of hip dislocation include nonconcentric reduction, which may present acutely or late, avascular necrosis, recurrent dislocation, heterotopic ossification, chronic or neglected dislocation, coxa magna, neurologic injuries, and early degenerative arthritis.

Nonconcentric Reduction

Nonconcentric reduction occurs with an incidence of approximately 8 percent. It is most often caused by loose bodies, which are osteochondral fragments, usually of acetabular origin[2] (Fig. 28-13). A torn labrum or ligamentum teres may also produce this complication.[12] Open repair or excision should prevent the complication of early degenerative arthritis.[4] Even those cases presenting late, however will benefit from this surgery.[4,8] The less favorable result associated with late diagnosis should motivate the surgeon to always perform a systematic postreduction evaluation by moving the hip through a full range of motion to detect any crepitation indicative of a loose intra-articular fragment. Widening of the medial joint space on radiographs is a reliable sign of nonconcentric reduction. Computed tomography should then be done to further evaluate the source and magnitude of the lesion. Most patients present with an average delay of 2.3 years. Many of these had negative arthrography. A review of postreduction plain radiographs showed a consistently widened medial joint space. Arthrography is unreliable to detect loose bodies after hip dislocation. Prognosis, although always improved, with fragment removal is less favorable if the delay exceeds 1 year, or if signs of avascular necrosis is present at the time of diagnosis[8] (Fig. 28-5).

Avascular Necrosis

Avascular necrosis is the most serious complication of hip dislocation in children. In contrast to the incidence reported for adults, it is rare in children if the delay in reduction is less than 8 hours and unusual even when the delay approaches 24 hours.[2] As a subgroup children less than 5 years of age experience an incidence of avascular necrosis, which approaches 0 percent.[3,4,6] Most adult series report a 15 to 25 percent incidence, whereas children as a group present 10 percent or less. Duration of nonweightbearing is not a significant factor in producing avascular necrosis. Radiographic signs of avascular necrosis usually appear within 15 months of injury, and are more frequent when the dislocations are caused by a severe trauma.[4,6] As noted earlier, treatment for this complication is similar to that recommended for Legg-Calvé-Perthes disease.[4]

Recurrent Dislocation

Traumatic hip dislocation in the child is associated with recurrence in only 1.5 percent. Such cases are usually associated with avascular necrosis.[2,4] Acetabular lip fragments of significant size increase the risk of redislocation and merit fixation. Large posterior capsular tears may heal with a redundant pouch, which can be documented by arthrography. When this lesion is found in a hip presenting with recurrent dislocation, surgical repair followed by spica immobilization is indicated.[2-4]

The risk of recurrence appears to be decreased when hips demonstrating instability after concentric reduction are immobilized for 4 to 6 weeks in a spica cast.[2] Children with marked ligamentous laxity such as Down syndrome or Ehlers Danlos syndrome are particularly prone to recurrent dislocation. Such children may also present with a history of voluntary dislocation of the hip. This is of great concern to the parents, particularly the "clunk" associated with the reduction. It should of course be discouraged and usually becomes more difficult as the child grows older and the hip develops more osseous stability.[13]

Neurologic Injury

The incidence of neurologic injury after hip dislocation approaches 10 percent.[6] The vast majority of these involve the sciatic nerve injury in posterior dislocation. Early reduction decreases the degree and duration of nerve dysfunction. Some authors suggest early exploration if large acetabular segments are present. Although all these cases recover some degree of function, many present significant permanent sequelae.[4,6] When no recuperation is apparent on clinical and electromyogra-

Traumatic Dislocation of the Hip / 535

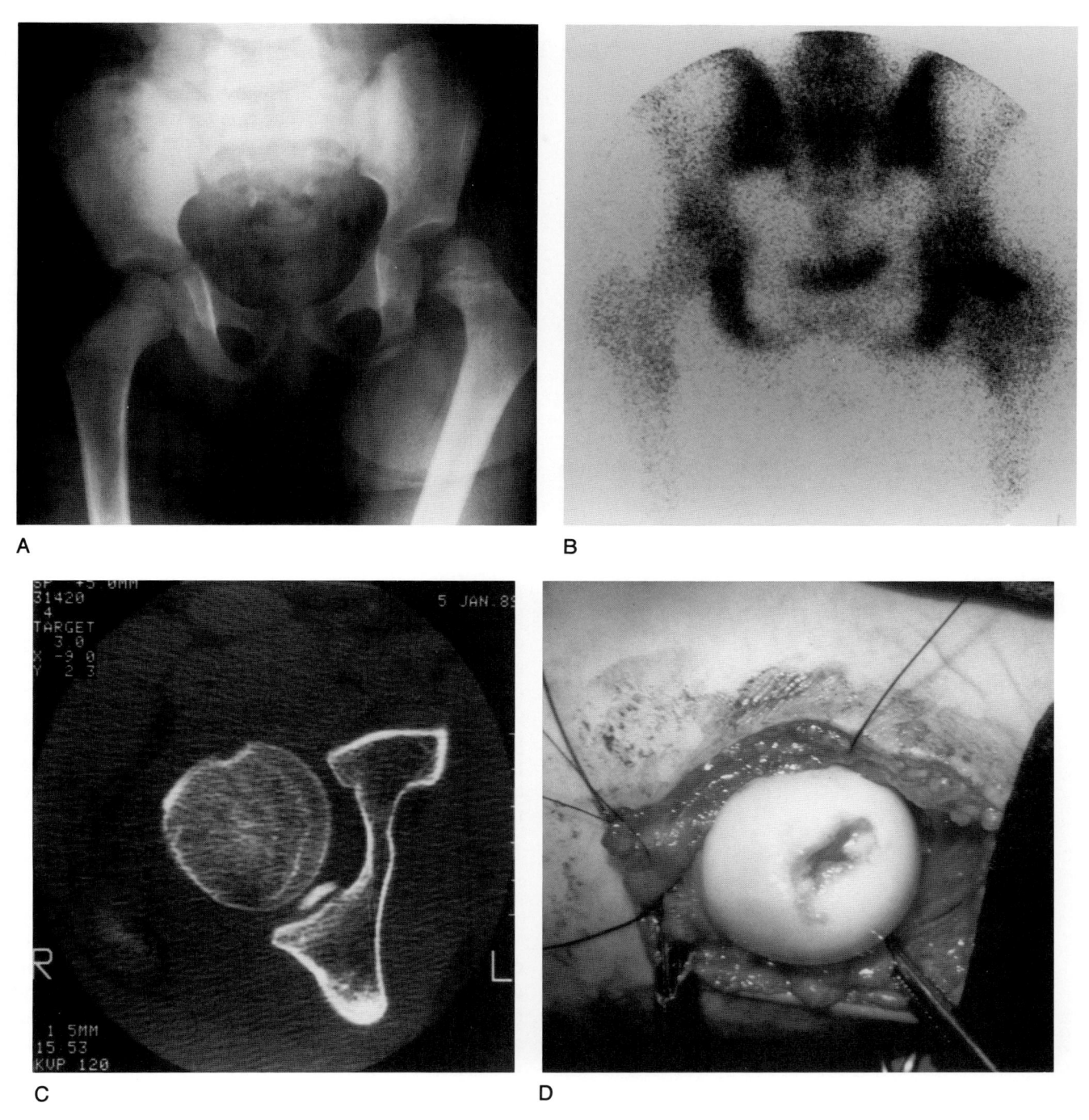

Fig. 28-13. (A) This child's hip could not be properly concentrically reduced — an indication of an intra-articular fragment. (B) A bone scan may assist in diagnosing the presence of an associated obscure fracture indicated by increased uptake at the fracture site but the CT scan (C) is the most useful in detecting the presence and origin of the intra-articular fragment. (D) Femoral head articular fracture, an uncommon source of an intra-articular loose cartilaginous fragment.

phic evaluation after 4 to 8 weeks exploration and neurolysis is indicated.[4]

Heterotopic Ossification

Heterotopic ossification is rare after hip dislocation. Associated head injury is usually present and would appear to be a more significant factor. Treatment should be along standard guidelines, those rare patients showing functional disability being treated by excision once the heterotopic bone has matured.[3]

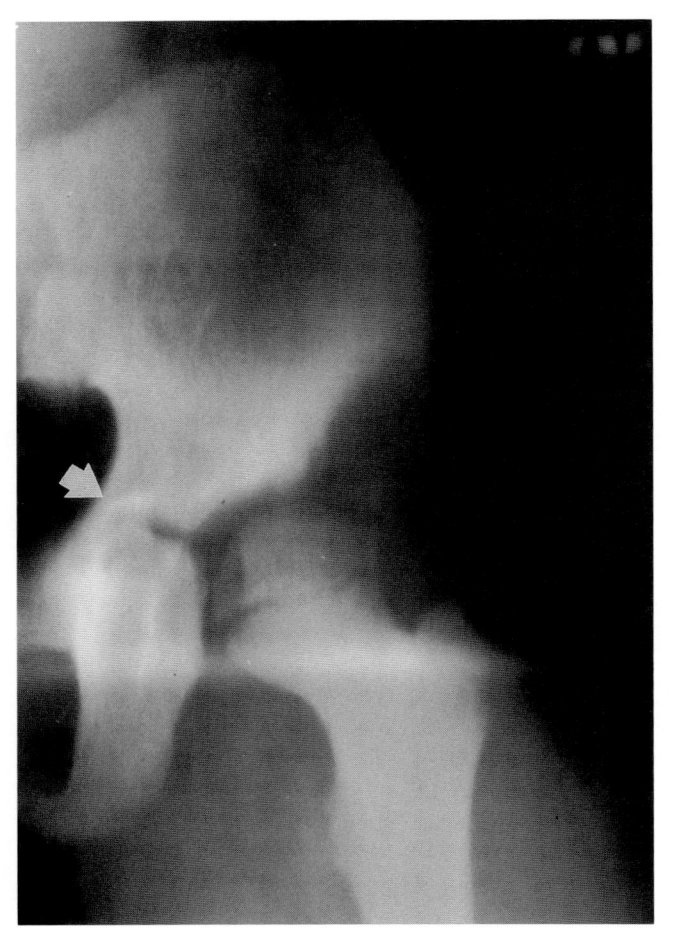

Fig. 28-14. Fusion of triradiate cartilage in a 6-year-old girl subsequent to a traumatic dislocation of her hip sustained in a motor vehicle accident.

Chronic or Neglected Dislocation

Cases of chronic dislocation typically present several years after injury and will usually reduce after prolonged heavy skeletal traction.[4] The cases of reported late open reduction would appear not to give optimal results.[9]

Coxa Magna

Coxa magna is caused by the hyperemia associated with tissue repair following trauma.[7] Alternatively, triradiate cartilage damage may cause premature cessation of growth of the acetabulum with resultant disproportion[3,11] (Fig. 28-14). These both lead to incongruity between the femoral head and the acetabulum. Secondary degenerative arthritis can occasionally be improved or prevented by innominate osteotomy.[7]

Early Osteoarthritis

Early osteoarthritis is related to avascular necrosis or late diagnosis of intra-articular loose bodies. Late reduction is also associated with increased risk of premature degenerative arthritis. Overall children in the lower age groups have a better prognosis.[4] A better understanding of the prognostic factors involved in this entity and their significance may be developed by an analysis of long-term follow-ups of these patients. Even in practice these patients should be followed to skeletal maturity and ideally into adulthood to determine the true evolution of this traditionally benign entity.[3,4]

Prognostic Factors

The most significant factors in the development of complications, particularily avascular necrosis and its degenerative sequelae, are the severity of the trauma and the age at diagnosis.[5,6] It is to be noted that avascular necrosis is particularly unlikely in children of less than 5 years of age, the global incidence in children being under 10 percent. It should also be noted that recurrence is more likely in this age group. Delay in reduction increases the risk of avascular necrosis partly because the success of late closed reduction is less likely. Open reduction is associated with a greater risk of avascular necrosis and early degenerative arthritis. This factor, however, appears to be somewhat less critical in children.[4,6] The duration of nonweightbearing has no correlation with outcome. Nonconcentric reduction, if neglected, predictably leads to early degenerative changes. Finally, late open reduction may give worse results than with prolonged skeletal traction when no surgical indications such as loose bodies exist.[5]

SUMMARY

Treatment of hip dislocation in the child is somewhat less complicationed than in the adult, but similar precautions are necessary to avoid potential complications. An additional consideration in this age group is the presence of an open triradiate cartilage.

Associated injuries must be ruled out. The neurovascular status should be documented and closed reduction, under anesthesia, performed as soon as possible. The delay in reduction should be less than 8 hours and certainly within 12 hours. Only perfect concentric reduction should be accepted. Widening of the medial joint space on postreduction radiographs should prompt CT scanning followed by appropriate open surgical excision or repair. If the hip joint appears unstable at the time of reduction immobilization in a spica cast is advisable. Otherwise, a short period of traction until pain-free range of motion is regained is advisable followed by gradual return to full weight-bearing status. Potential complications, particularily avascular necrosis of the femoral head should be explained to the parents and screened for with radiographs every 3 months until 2 years after the injury. A baseline bone scan at 3 months is recommended. The best prognosis in children occurs with early recognition and treatment of the acute dislocation and its complications.

REFERENCES

1. Canale ST, Beaty JH: Operative pediatric orthopedics. p. 896. Mosby-Year Book, St. Louis, 1991
2. Moseley CF: Fractures and dislocations of the hip. Instr Course Lect 41:397, 1992
3. Ogden J: Skeletal injury in the child. 2nd Ed. p. 661. JB Saunders, Philadelphia, 1990
4. Tachdjian M: Pediatric orthopaedics. Vol. 4. 2nd Ed. JB Saunders, Philadelphia, 1990
5. Rockwood CA, Green DP: Fractures in children. Vol. 3, 3rd Ed. JB Lippincott, Philadelphia, 1992
6. Yang RS, Tsuang YH, Hang YS, Lyu TK: Traumatic dislocation of the hip. Clin Orthop Rel Res 265:218, 1991
7. Rang M: Children's fractures. 2nd Ed. p. 257. JB Lippincott, Philadelphia, 1983
8. Santora SD, Stevens PM, Coleman SS: Intraarticular loose bodies in the adolescent hip: results of treatment of those recognized late. J Pediatr Orthop 10:261, 1990
9. Younge D, Lifeso R: Unreduced anterior dislocation of the hip in a child. J Pediatr Orthop 8:478, 1988
10. Pries P, Gayet LE, Bonnet L, Clarac JP: A case of traumatic obturator luxation of the hip in a 4-year-old child. Rev Chir Orthop Reparat Appareil Mot 77:49, 1991
11. Brooks E, Rosman M: Central fracture-dislocation of the hip in a child. J Trauma 28:1590, 1988
12. Cinats JG, Moreau MJ, Swersky JF: Traumatic dislocation of the hip caused by capsular interposition in a child. J Bone Joint Surg [Am] 78:130, 1988
13. Fowles JV: Skeletal trauma notes. p. 282. Williams & Wilkins, Baltimore, 1985

29

Fractures of the Femoral Shaft

William G. MacKenzie

> In science the most important thing is to modify and change ones ideas as science advances.

DESCRIPTION AND INCIDENCE

Fractures of the shaft of the femur in children are relatively common injuries that, with appropriate management, usually heal with no significant long-term complications.

In Nottingham, England, it was estimated that approximately 1.2 percent of children under 12 years old, suffered a femoral fracture.[1] In a review of 851 femoral shaft fractures in children and adolescents, Hedlund and Lindgren[2] found the maximum incidence occurred between 2 and 5 years of age. In the younger children, less than 3 years of age, falls were the most common cause and in the older children, there was an equal incidence of falls and traffic accidents being the etiologic factor. Many studies have confirmed the high incidence of associated injuries. For example, the combination of head and lower limb injury was seen in 53 percent of children injured in vehicle pedestrian accidents in New Zealand.[3] These children must be carefully examined to rule out injury to the central nervous system, chest, and abdomen.

ANATOMY

The normal femur is gently curved in both the coronal and sagittal planes resulting in an anterolateral convexity. The posterior concavity is buttressed by a strong ridge, the linea aspera, in its middle third. There is a medial inclination of the shaft, which is dependent on the width of the pelvis and the length of the legs. The longer the limb, the more vertical the inclination. The vastus medialis, lateralis, intermedius, and articularis genu surround almost the entire circumference of the shaft, the anterior surface of the lower shaft having no muscular attachment. The femur has a very good blood supply from both endosteal and periosteal sources, an important consideration in healing.

The most common site of fracture of the femoral shaft is in its middle third. Griffin and colleagues[4] reported 70 percent of fractures in the middle third, 22 percent in the proximal third, and 8 percent in the distal third. Most studies report a similar distribution.

The fracture pattern depends on the type of force applied to the femoral shaft. Indirect torsional force usually results in a long spiral or oblique fracture whereas the transverse fracture is usually caused by direct trauma. In young children, low rotational forces can result in a long spiral fracture. When the force is severe, there may be a butterfly pattern, comminution, or a segmental fracture. Torus or buckle fractures usually occur in the distal third of the femur in the metaphyseal region, especially in children with knee stiffness, paralysis, and spasticity.

The displacement and angulation of femoral shaft fractures depends on several factors, including the force and the level of the injury. In fractures of the upper third, the proximal fragment is usually flexed by the iliopsoas muscle, abducted by the gluteus medius and minimus muscles and externally rotated by the external rotators and gluteus maximus muscle. The distal fragment usually lies posteriorly, and is shortened by the pull of the quadriceps and hamstrings and adducted because of the unopposed pull of the adductors. Fractures of the middle third usually result in the proximal fragment being flexed and the distal fragment being posteriorly displaced, but angulation is not consistent. In fractures of the lower third, the gastrocnemius muscle is the primary deforming force. The distal fragment is usually extended and displaced posteriorly.

MECHANISM OF INJURY

Falls and motor vehicle accidents account for the majority of femoral shaft fractures in children. Knowing the mechanism of injury is important as it can help the examining physician look for expected associated injuries. For example, when a child is struck by a car when crossing the street, Waddell has suggested that three injuries should always be looked for, a fractured femur, a thoracic injury, and a head injury.[5]

CLASSIFICATION

Classification of femoral shaft fractures is similar to other long-bone fractures. The fractures can be classified by position; proximal, middle, or distal third, and by the fracture pattern. Open fractures are classified using the Gustilo classification. It must be remembered that, because of the extensive soft tissue envelope, a small open injury indicates extensive underlying soft tissue damage.

There are a group of specific fractures that, in addition to the features that characterize the fracture type, must be considered in the classification of femoral shaft fractures.

Child Abuse

Femoral shaft fractures are a common result of child abuse.[6-10] In two studies, the femur was the third most common fractured bone in battered children.[6,9] Approximately 30 percent of femoral fractures that occur in children under 3 to 4 years of age, are the result of child abuse; 50 percent of these children may present with only a single fracture, and of these the midshaft diaphyseal femoral fracture is the most common pattern.[9] Beals and Tufts[7] reported that child abuse is more common in those under 1 year of age, first-born children, those with preexisting brain damage, the presence of bilateral fractures, no appropriate history of trauma, and when the family delays seeking medical care for the child (see Ch. 51).

Pathologic Fractures

Pathologic fractures occur through weakened bone. This may be the result of generalized osteopenia or a localized area of weakness. The former can occur in myelodsyplasia and children with neuromuscular disease, such as muscular dystrophy, spinal muscular atrophy, cerebral palsy, and paraplegia. Lock and Aronson[11] report that fractures occurring in the lower extremity in children with myelodysplasia were usually distal to the level of neurologic involvement, that is, they occurred predominantly in the femur in children who had thoracic involvement and in the tibia in those with lumbar involvement. These children most commonly have metaphyseal injuries but can present with midshaft fractures. These fractures are often confused with osteomyelitis and cellulitis, as they present with a swollen, warm, erythematous limb. An appropriate history and radiographs usually make the diagnosis. Osteomyelitis[12] and bone tumors may also cause pathologic fractures (see Ch. 56).

Neonatal Fractures

Neonatal fractures are usually due to trauma during vaginal delivery, but there have been several recent reports of femoral fractures occurring at cesarean section.[13] If multiple fractures are present at birth, the diagnosis of osteogenesis imperfecta must be considered. The lack of other fractures or radiologic evidence of metabolic bone disease usually imply a traumatic etiology. Even without evidence of bone disease, which is almost universal in infants born at less than 28 weeks gestation, premature infants are at risk of fracture and appropriate care is essential[14] (see Ch. 57).

Stress Fractures

Femoral stress fractures are more common in the athletic adolescent but have been reported in younger children.[15,16] The most common area of occurrence is in the proximal third, but they can be found in the mid or the distal third. Radiologic characteristics include an uninterrupted layer of periosteal new bone with absence of soft tissue mass and bone destruction. The bone scans usually demonstrate no hyperemia on the vascular phase with a fusiform focus of increased uptake on the delayed images.[16] Computed tomography (CT) scan and magnetic resonance imaging (MRI) are other modalities that can be useful in differentiating the stress fracture from osteomyelitis and bone tumors such as Ewing sarcoma.

PHYSICAL EXAMINATION

The child with a femoral fracture presents with tenderness and swelling in the involved thigh and an inability to move the limb. There often is an obvious deformity with shortening and lateral rotation of the leg. Crepitus may be noted with spasm but should not be actively elicited. The vital signs should be taken and the child carefully examined for any injuries to the head and neck, chest, abdomen, pelvis, genitourinary system, and other extremity injuries. The neurovascular status of the involved limb must be carefully assessed and recorded. Injury to the femoral artery and sciatic nerve can occur. A knee hemoarthrosis may indicate the presence of an intra-articular fracture or possibly injury to the collateral or cruciate ligaments. Associated joint and skeletal injury must also be considered, such as hip dislocation[17] and pelvic fracture, segmental fractures, and ipsilateral tibial fractures.

The fractured femur should be splinted to reduce the discomfort and prevent further injury to the soft tissues and bone. The type of splint used depends on availability and the age of the child. In very young children strapping the legs together about a folded blanket or pillow can be satisfactory preliminary immobilization. Padded boards extending from the axilla to the foot are effective. Ideally, a Thomas splint or one of the newer commercially available splints should be used for immobilization. Whatever the method of immobilization, areas of pressure application should be evaluated for skin breakdown. It is important to institute definitive care of the femoral shaft fracture and not to leave the child in temporary forms of immobilization for long periods.

There can be extensive soft tissue injury to the thigh. Loss of intravascular volume can be secondary to hemorrhage in the thigh as well as edema. Although isolated femoral shaft fracture in adults can be a cause of hypotension, this is rarely seen in children. Barlow and colleagues,[18] in evaluating 50 children with isolated closed femoral fractures, did not observe any hypotension. Only a third of the children had a measurable change in hematocrit, averaging only a 4-point drop. They emphasized that any child with a femoral fracture who develops hypotension should be promptly evaluated for another source of blood loss. Several authors have noted a marked febrile response to injury in 80 percent of children, which lasted an average of 4 days in one study.[18,19]

TREATMENT

A variety of traction and operative techniques are available that are applied, depending on the type of fracture, associated injuries, age and size of the child, availability of the equipment, and experience of the surgeon. Regardless of the method of treatment employed, pain and muscle spasm must be dealt with in the emergency department. Morphine administered either intravenously (0.1 mg/kg) or intramuscularly (0.1–0.2 mg/kg) can be very effective. Femoral nerve block with bupivacaine has been shown to provide effective and prolonged analgesia,[20-22] allowing the transport, radiographic examination, and application of traction in optimal conditions. The side effects are rare. The technique consists of injecting 2 mg/kg of 0.5 percent bupivacane without epinephrine, 1 fingerbreadth lateral to the femoral artery at the level of the inguinal ligament.[22] A femoral sheath catheter can be inserted for continuous analgesia. Once the child is comfortable, temporary below-knee skin traction can be used to reduce the discomfort and allow for appropriate radiographs. The hip and knee joint need to be visualized to rule any other fractures or dislocation.

The simplest, safest, and most effective method of treatment for the fractured femur in a particular age group should be the method of choice. Unfortunately, the choice is not always clear. Some form of skin or skeletal traction and subsequent hip spica is appropriate treatment for most children up to about 10 years of age.[23-27] There is a growing body of evidence that in minimally displaced and shortened fractures, early hip spica is an effective form of treatment in this age group.[28-38] Management of diaphyseal femoral fractures in adolescence is controversial. It is difficult to control alignment and shortening using traction in this age group.[39-45] The remodeling of malunions and growth stimulation is less predictable than in young children.[46-49] Operative stabilization, including some form of intramedullary fixation, plates, or external fixation, seems to be more appropriate and successful in adolescents.

Traction

Many forms of traction have been used in the treatment of femoral shaft fractures in children.[23-27] All consist of either skin or skeletal traction with the leg in various positions. The traction can be continued until the fracture has consolidated to the point that a child can weight bear without producing angulation or shortening. The disadvantage of this method is that it requires a prolonged period of immobilization, from 1 to 3 months, depending on the age of the child. A more common alternative is to place the child into a hip spica cast or cast brace once the fracture is stable enough to prevent shortening. Depending on the age of the child, 1 to 3 weeks of traction is usually satisfactory.

The fracture should be as aligned as anatomically as possible. As to what is acceptable angulation is still controversial. Several studies suggest that angulation of 20 degrees in the coronal plane and 30 degrees in the sagittal plane will result in satisfactory alignment at skeletal maturity.[47,50] Large degrees of angulation do not remodel to a significant degree in adolescent children.[46-48] Most authors accept up to 10 degrees of coronal plane angulation and 15 degrees of an anterior bow and 5 degrees of a posterior bow.[23-27] Rotational malunions are infrequent and not a functional problem.[50-58] In the 2- to 10-year-old group, up to 1.5 cm of shortening can be accepted because of expected overgrowth.[4,49] It can be difficult to measure the amount of shortening in patients who are in skin traction or spica. A tape measure is useful with children in traction. Estimation of shortening by radiography is fraught with difficulty because of magnification problems and the x-ray beam is often not exactly perpendicular to the femoral shaft and at the level of the fracture site. If these problems are taken into consideration, plain radiographs seem to provide an adequate method of assessing the length of the femur where these children are in traction. Once healed, CT leg lengths are the most accurate radiologic measurement technique.

Skak and Jensen[59] found the time required for union of 275 consecutive fractures of the femoral shaft in children followed a log-normal pattern. Newborns healed in about 3½ weeks with the average time to union increasing by 0.7 weeks per year. Multiple injuries increased and operative treatment reduced the mean time for fracture healing.

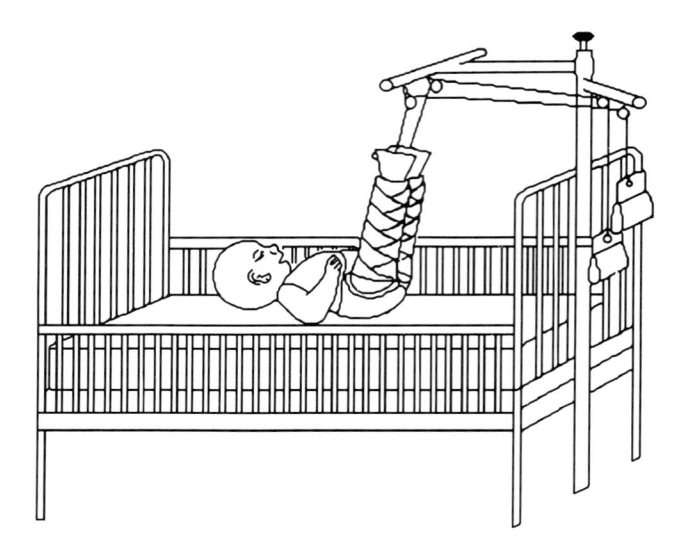

Fig. 29-1. Infant in vertical skin traction.

Bryant's Traction

In young children, up to 2 years of age, some form of skin traction is required, such as overhead (or Bryant's traction) or longitudinal traction (Fig. 29-1). Bryant's traction should not be used in children over age 2 or in those weighing over 25 pounds[25] to avoid vascular injury. Children in Bryant's traction must be closely monitored for neurovascular complications in both lower extremities.[60] The skin traction is always applied to both lower extremities. Padding is placed over the medial and lateral malleoli to prevent pressure sores. Adhesive traction tapes are applied over the medial and lateral aspects of the leg from the malleoli to the greater trochanter. These are then wrapped with an adhesive bandage. This should not be applied tightly. If overhead traction is used, equal weight is applied to either leg such that the infant's buttocks are lifted just off the surface of the mattress. Fixed traction, by tying the legs to an overhead bar, should not be used, as there is a higher incidence of complications with this type of fixed or gallows traction.

Bradford Frame Traction

Another traction method is to place the child on an inclined plane such as a Bradford frame with the foot end elevated 45 degrees. Both legs are placed in longitudinal skin traction. The disadvantage of this technique is the lack of hip flexion with occasional difficulty achieving a satisfactory reduction. By 10 to 14 days, these children usually are quite comfortable with minimum tenderness over the fracture site. There is usually early callus formation on radiograph. They can be placed into a hip spica at this point for 4 to 6 weeks.

In the group of children from 3 to 11 years of age, there have been many successful techniques of management reported. Most involve either skin or skeletal traction.

Early Hip Spica Application

Application of a hip spica immediately or after several days has been gaining popularity, particularly for minimally displaced fractures which are not initially shortened more than 2 cm[28-38] (Fig. 29-2). The chief advantage of closed reduction and application of an immediate hip spica is that it reduces the length of hospital stay. The financial considerations are obvious, but it has also been shown that an early return to the home environment is psychologically beneficial to these children.[32,34,35,37] There have been reports of abnormal renal function occurring in children immobilized in a hip spica for 5 to 9 weeks.[61] This technique of early casting should not be used in children with the following conditions:

1. Older than 10 years of age[31]
2. Greater than 2 cm of shortening at presentation[34]
3. Excessive comminution and subtrochanteric fractures[31]
4. Associated injuries to the central nervous system, chest, or abdomen[37]
5. Unreliable families[37]

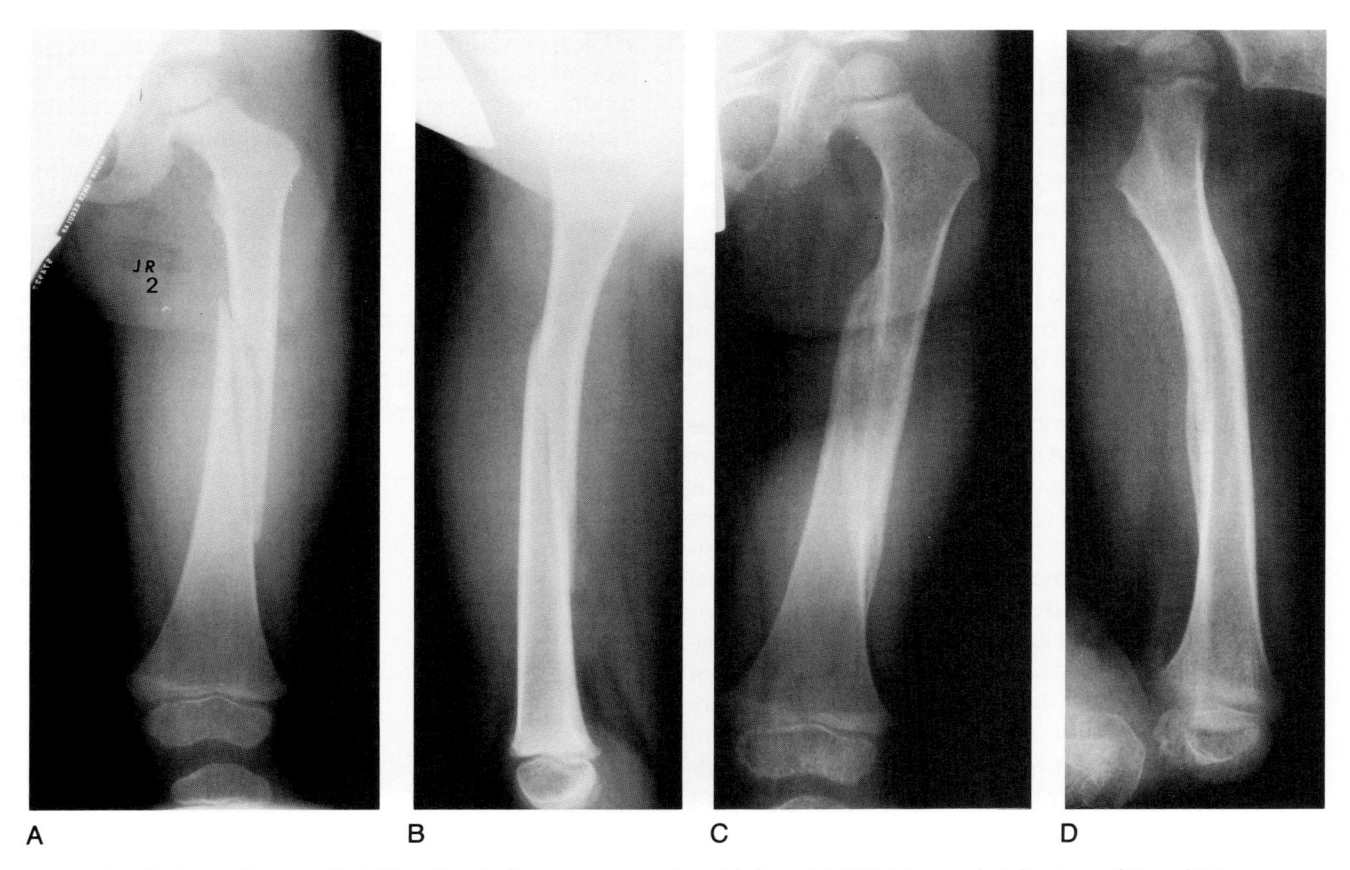

Fig. 29-2. A 2-year-old child suffered a low-energy rotational injury. **(A&B)** A long spiral fracture of the middle third of the femur. Skin traction was used for 10 days and subsequently a hip spica was applied. **(C&D)** Satisfactory early healing. A good result could also have been achieved in this child with immediate application of a hip spica.

Most studies suggest placing the child in skin traction for several days to allow time for full evaluation and then applying a 1½ hip spica (double-hip spica in infants). The hip and knee should be in approximately 45 degrees of flexion. The hip abducted 30 degrees and the leg in 10 to 15 degrees of external rotation. More hip flexion is often required with proximal third fractures. Probably the safest technique is to reduce the fracture, apply an above-knee cast, and then connect this to the body portion of the hip spica. The cast should be snugly applied and well padded about the knee and the upper head of the fibula. The lateral surface of the thigh should be flat, and molding should be done to maintain the natural anterior curve of the femur. Irani and colleagues[32] originally advocated removing the cast over the plantar surface of the foot to avoid telescoping of the fracture when the child actively plantarflexes the foot against the sole of the cast. Other studies have not confirmed the usefulness of this technique. Dameron and Thompson[29] and several more recent papers[31,35,36] report success incorporating a distal femoral K-wire in the spica cast. In most cases, this is not required.

McCarthy[33] described a method for early spica cast application in 1986. He advocated 90-degree flexion of the hip and knee, applying the cast to the torso and unaffected thigh, and applying a below-knee cast, reducing the fracture, and then applying the middle section. Weiss and coworkers[62] recently described four examples of peroneal nerve palsy using this technique. They suggested that, if this technique is to be used, the cast should be extended just above the knee and the lateral aspect of the knee and leg should be well padded to prevent peroneal nerve compression.[62]

If early spica cast immobilization is used, the child has to be closely followed. Angulation is dealt with by either wedging the cast or cast change. There are numerous reports of the results of closed reduction and early spica cast immobilization.[28-38] The results appear to be comparable to those obtained with either skin or skeletal traction. Rotational and angular malunions are uncommon. The main problem appears to be leg length discrepancy. Martinez and coworkers[34] noted that the main factors associated with shortening in this technique, are shortening greater than 2 cm on initial radiograph and shortening greater than 1 cm after the cast has been applied. I prefer to employ traction to maintain alignment until there is adequate callus to prevent shortening and then hip spica immobilization.

There are many different methods of traction that have been described for this age group. Skin traction can be used with a Thomas splint or as one of the variations of Russell traction. Skeletal traction should be applied through the distal femur either in the 90/90 position or on a Thomas splint with a Pearson knee attachment.

Skin Traction

Skin traction can be very useful as long as the traction tapes are carefully applied. It must be emphasized that the skin tapes should be applied while traction is being applied to the leg to avoid skin tension that will occur if the tapes are applied with the fracture overriding and the limb shortened. Inappropriate application or excessive weight (usually over 10 lbs) can cause skin slough. The legs should be carefully cleared of any debris and sprayed with a commercial benzoin compound. Soft synthetic or cotton padding should be applied to the malleolar region and the adhesive traction tape applied to the medial and lateral aspects of the leg, right up to the groin. This should be wrapped from distal to proximal with Elasticized adhesive bandage, being careful not to apply too much circumferential pressure. The leg is then placed on a Thomas splint with firm padding under the thigh to prevent posterior angulation at the fracture site. Depending on the age and weight of the child, up to 12 lb of traction can be safely applied. The amount of hip flexion depends on the level of the fracture with the more proximal fracture requiring more hip flexion. (This technique is inappropriate for most subtrochanteric fractures, which usually require 90 degrees of hip flexion and a femoral traction pin. A more appropriate technique for this fracture would be 90/90 skeletal traction). The Thomas splint can be simply fixed to the bottom of the bed with the foot of the bed elevated to provide countertraction. A more sophisticated form of balanced trac-

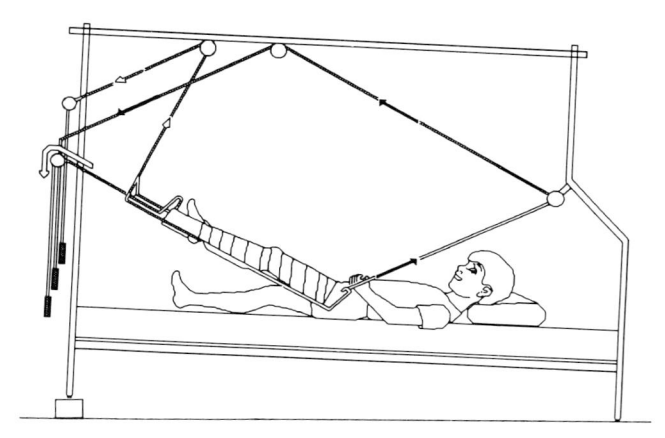

Fig. 29-3. Balanced skin traction using a Thomas splint. Note that the skin traction extends up to the proximal thigh.

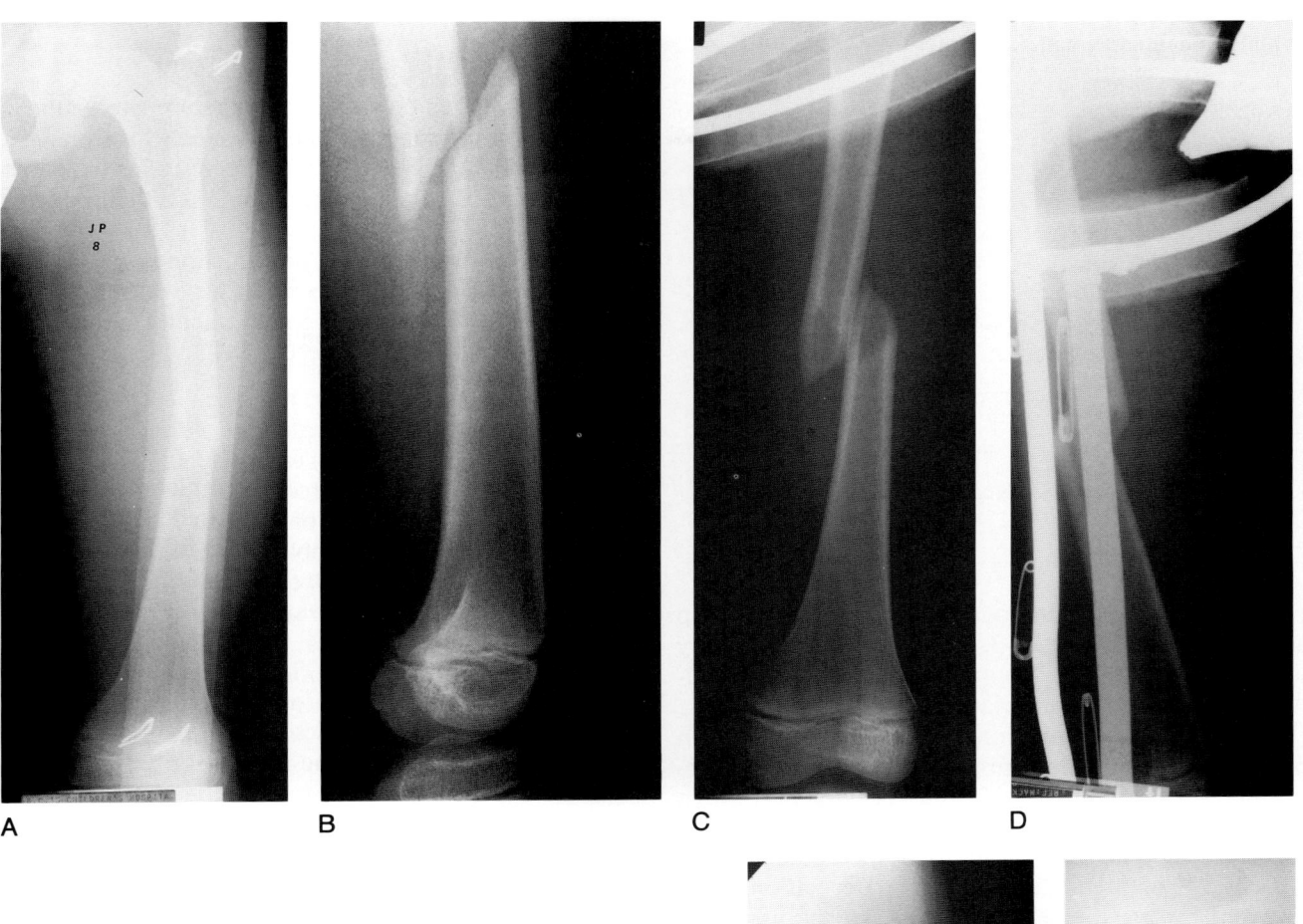

Fig. 29-4. This 8-year-old boy was hit by a car while cycling. **(A&B)** There is an oblique fracture of the middle third of the femur with about 2 cm of shortening. **(C&D)** He was placed in balanced skin traction. There is approximately 1 cm of overlap which is appropriate to allow for expected overgrowth in this age group. **(E&F)** The healed femur undergoing remodeling.

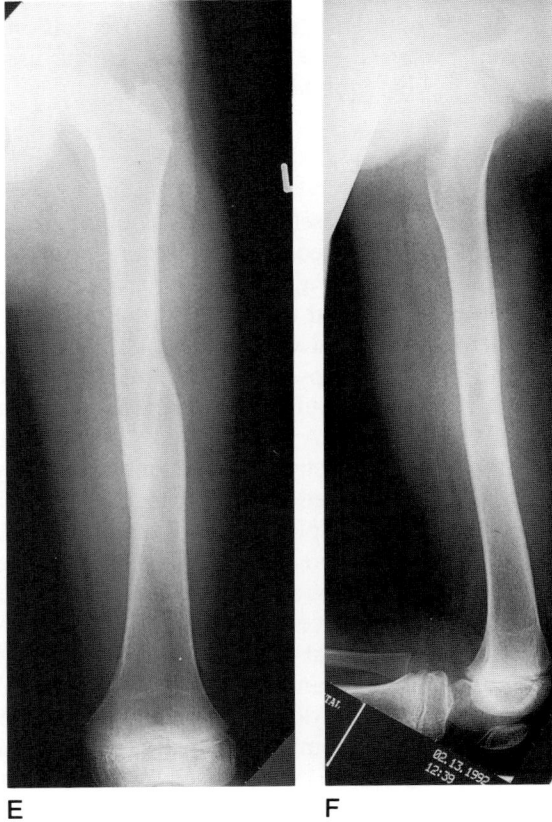

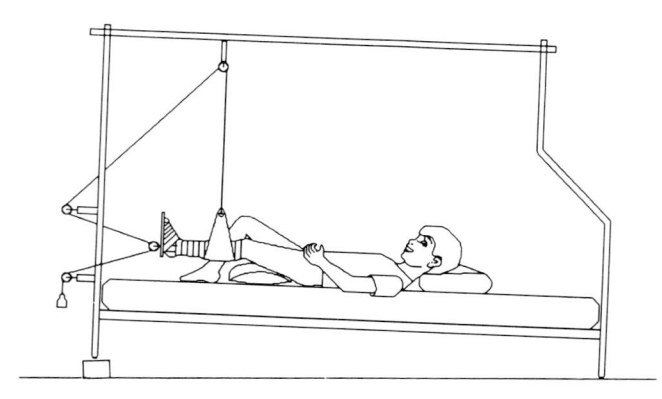

Fig. 29-5. Russell traction.

tion, allowing the patient to move around, can be set up as illustrated in Figure 29-3. This usually requires very little adjustment. The amount of traction can be adjusted to provide appropriate overlap of the fracture (Fig. 29-4). Varus angulation of the distal fragment can be corrected by applying pressure to the apex of the fracture site with padding or with transverse traction with a sling. Valgus angulation is usually corrected by applying skin traction to the opposite leg to the level of the knee.[23] Usually 5 lb of traction is satisfactory. Derotation straps to avoid excessive external rotation can be used, but these are rarely required.

Russell Traction

Russell or split-Russell traction is a popular method of skin traction, but it requires close monitoring and frequent adjustments (Fig. 29-5). The traction is applied below knee in a similar technique to that just described, with medial and lateral adhesive straps and padding over the malleoli. The straps are attached to a footplate, and in Russell traction a pulley is applied to the plantar surface of the footplate. A well-padded sling is placed behind the knee. A traction rope extends vertically to a pulley, which is directed to the bottom of the bed back to the pulley on the footplate and subsequently back over the end of the bed where the weight is attached. The knee is flexed about 30 degrees. The expectation is that the resultant vector of force is along the longitudinal axis of the femur. The vertical traction is approximately equal to the weight applied and the horizontal traction on the limb is approximately double the weight applied because of the double-pull from the footplate to the foot of the bed.[25] The foot of the bed is raised to provide countertraction. A pillow is often required under the thigh to prevent posterior bowing at the fracture site. Staheli[26] notes that if the patient has an extremely heavy leg, the longitudinal force may be excessive, resulting in distraction through the fracture site, which is difficult to control.

An alternative to Russell skin traction is split-Russell traction. This technique provides a little more flexibility in that the vertical and horizontal traction are independent, being attached to different weights.

Skeletal Traction

The 90/90 distal femoral skeletal traction is a useful technique, particularly with proximal third femoral shaft fractures, which require flexion of the distal fragment to maintain alignment (Fig. 29-6). The gastrocnemius, hamstring, and ilipsoas muscles are relaxed reducing some of the deformity forces. The children are usually quite comfortable. The traction wire should be placed in the distal femur proximal to the growth plate. Humberger and Eyring[63] described a method of 90/90 skeletal traction through the proximal tibia. This technique should not be used. The main complication is with proximal tibial growth arrest, but there is also a high incidence of knee pain and occasionally knee subluxation[63,64] and stretching of the collateral ligaments of the knee.

A threaded 7/64th Steinmann pin can be inserted under local or general anesthetic. This should be placed about 2 cm proximal to the adductor tubercle to avoid injury to the distal femoral physis. It is advanced parallel to the knee joint. A traction bow is applied; the type with a broad wing nut allows correction of angular deformity by placing the traction rope at either end of the wing nut as appropriate. The traction rope extends vertically to a pulley. The calf should be supported on a sling with

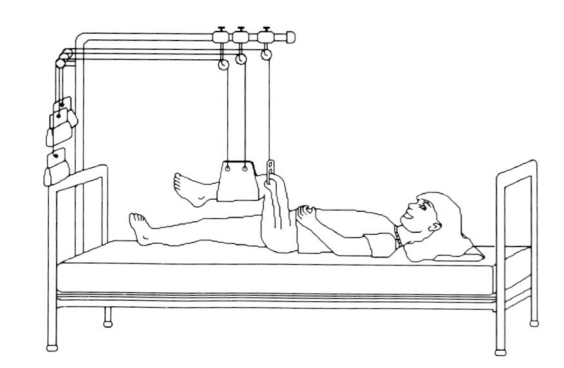

Fig. 29-6. Distal femoral skeletal 90/90 traction.

sheepskin padding. A below-knee cast can be used, but one must be extremely careful to pad this cast and be alert to the possibility of a pressure sore over the heel. The sling under the calf goes vertically to an overhead pulley and enough weight is used to maintain the knee flexed at 90 degrees. As with the other techniques of traction, as soon as the fracture is stable and nontender, a hip spica can be applied. This may take from 2 to 4 weeks, depending on the age of the child.

The 90/90 skeletal traction can be very effective up to early adolescence.[4,42,64] Ryan[65] reported on 59 children between 3 and 13 years of age treated with distal femoral skeletal traction and subsequent immobilization in hip spica. All healed and were back to full activity at 18 months follow-up with no significant rotational or angular deformities. The greatest leg length discrepancy was 1.3 cm. Aronson and colleagues[42] report similar results in children under 11 years of age, but in older children there was a lot of difficulty controlling leg length discrepancy. In 15 of these older children, 8 healed with greater than 1.5 cm of discrepancy.

Cast Bracing

An alternative to traction treatment methods is cast bracing.[40,66-69] The cast brace can be applied early in the management,[40] or after a period of traction as an alternative method of immobilization to the spica cast. It appears that cast bracing in all age groups should be restricted to fractures in the distal third of the shaft because of difficulty controlling varus and anterior angulation in the proximal- and midshaft fractures.[40,67,68] Gross and coworkers[40] had most of their problems with angulation and shortening in older adolescent children. They recommended that this procedure not be used in this age group.

Operative Management

The ideal management of closed isolated diaphyseal femoral fractures in adolescence is not clear. In children up to 12 years of age, 90/90 skeletal traction and subsequent spica cast immobilization can be very effective.[4,42,65] Using this technique, as well as other nonoperative techniques in older children, can result in angular malunions and shortening.[39-44] Despite the remaining growth potential in adolescence, remodeling of a malunion is less predictable than in younger children.[46-48] The overgrowth that is seen in 2- to 10-year-old children is not present to the same extent in adolescents.[49] Their increased muscle mass and strength can make management in traction difficult. Adolescent femoral fractures heal more slowly than in younger children, leading to longer immobilization times.[59] Prolonged immobilization in skeletal traction and subsequent spica casts may have a deleterious psychological effect in this age group.[44]

The alternative of operative stabilization involves risks, the most notable being infection and physeal injury. Recent series comparing the outcomes of operative and nonoperative treatment have noted superior anatomic and functional results with internal fixation (Fig. 29-7). Herndon and colleagues[43] compared the results of traction and spica cast or cast brace immobilization with closed intermedullary nailing in 45 femoral fractures in children aged 11 to 16 years. All fractures healed, but there were malunions in 7 of 24 fractures in the nonoperative group (the malunions were defined as shortening greater than 2 cm, angulation of greater than 10 degrees in the frontal plane and greater than 20 degrees in the sagittal plane). The intramedullary fixation consisted of 12 Kuntschner nails, 4 interlocking nails, 3 Enders rods, and 2 Rush rods. There were no infections, malunions, or growth arrests in the operative group. The economic benefits of a shorter hospital stay in the operative group were significant. Several similar studies reached the same conclusions.[39,44]

Flexible intramedullary nailing using Enders nails[41,70-72] and more flexible rods[73,74] have been reported in adolescent patients (Fig. 29-8). Leg length discrepancies, malunion, and growth disturbances of the proximal femur have not been a problem, but Pankovich[70,71] has found that there are problems when this technique is used for unstable diaphyseal fractures. Sliding of the nails out of the entrance portals, loss of fixation, malrotation, and knee pain can result.

Intramedullary fixation has other complications. One must consider the routine anesthetic complications, which are doubled because of the need for removal of the nail. Although no infections have been reported in this age group, one would expect the infection rates to be similar to those seen in adult series (about 1 percent).[45] Avascular necrosis of the proximal femoral epiphysis can occur, but this is a rare complication.[75] Growth disturbance is a potential complication. Care must be taken not to damage the proximal and distal femoral growth plates. Five cases of trochanteric apophyseal arrest have been reported.[39,75] The clinical results were satisfactory and increase in the articulotrochanteric distance was not symptomatic. In 5 of these arrests, 4 occurred after proximal reaming, and Ziv and colleagues[75] concluded that proximal reaming should be avoided in the young child.

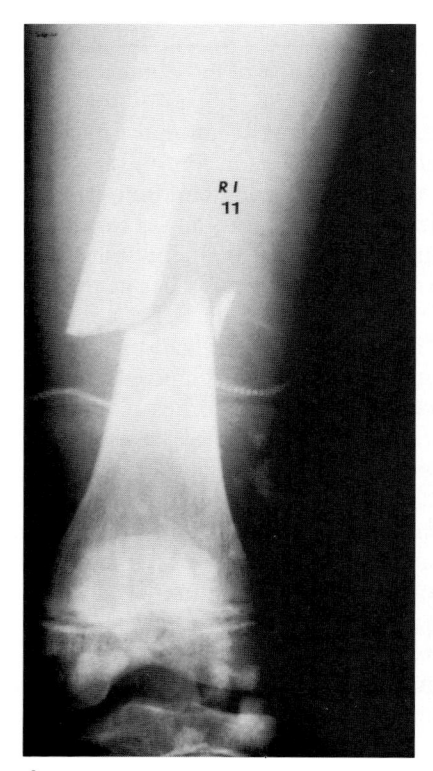

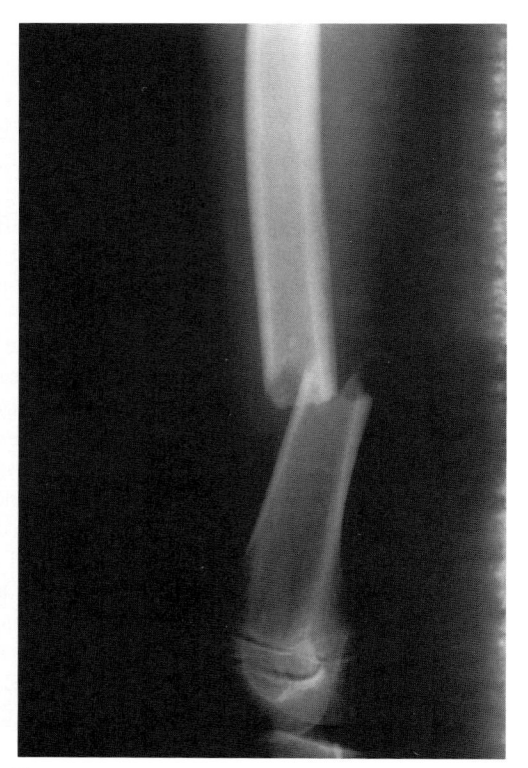

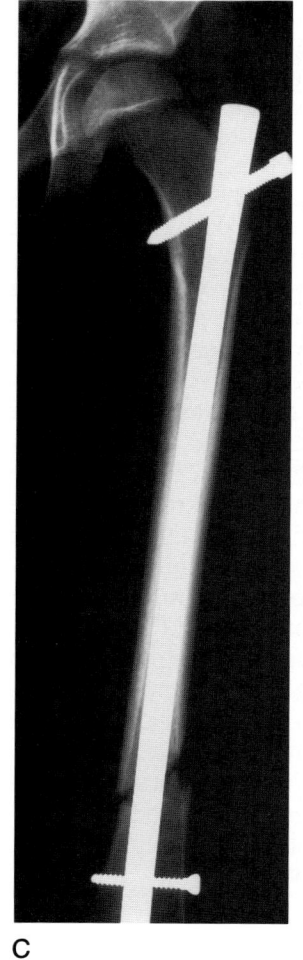

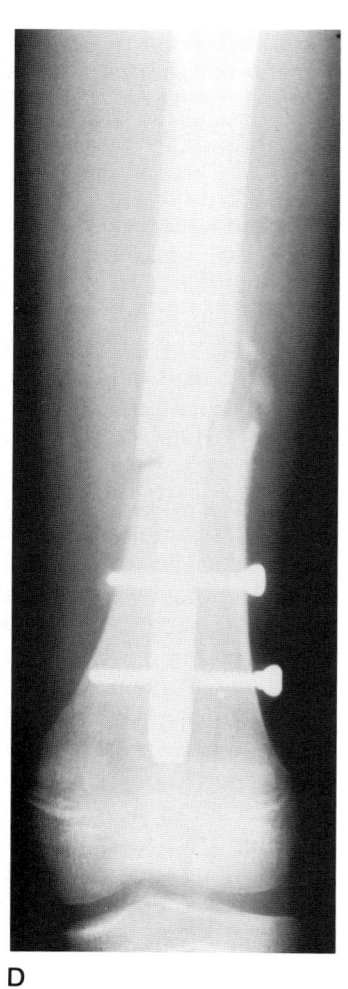

Fig. 29-7. **(A&B)** This 11-year-old child suffered a closed isolated injury to the distal third of the left femur. Note the characteristic extension of the distal fragment due to the unopposed pull of the gastrocnemius muscle. It was elected to treat this child with a closed locked intramedullary nail. **(C&D)** The early results shown.

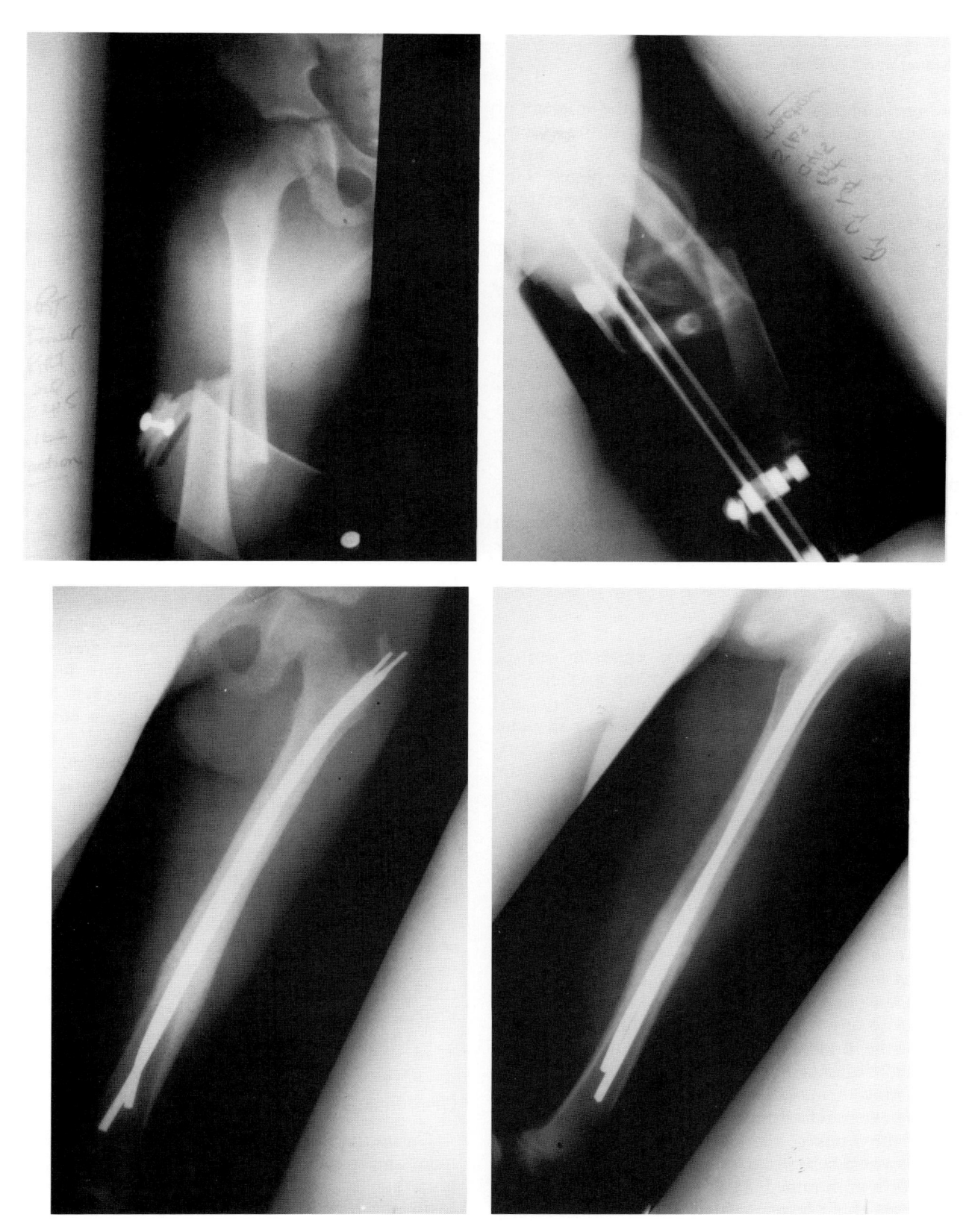

Fig. 29-8. This 8-year-old girl suffered bilateral femoral fractures in a pedestrian/motor vehicle accident. She was treated by closed intramedullary fixation using Enders nails. The nails were inserted through the greater trochanter. An alternate insertion site would be through a window distal to the trochanteric apophysis. (Courtesy of Dr. R. Galpin, London, Ontario, Canada.)

Valdiserri and colleagues[76] reported that the problems of trochanteric arrest and valgus deformity of the femoral neck did not occur in children older than 8 to 9 years of age. A historical concern has been with the potential for overgrowth after operative stabilization of femoral fractures.[4,23,26,51] Viljanto and colleagues[77] reported 35 patients with an average age of 10 who had undergone operative stabilization with various techniques of internal fixation. The mean overgrowth was 9.8 mm, which compared favorably with those treated nonoperatively.

Intramedullary stabilization with careful attention to the site of insertion and avoidance of the proximal and distal growth plates is an effective and safe alternative to nonoperative treatment in adolescent children with femoral shaft fractures.

Indications for Operative Stabilization

Operative stabilization of femoral shaft fractures in younger children is usually unnecessary, but there are certain circumstances where it may be indicated.

HEAD INJURY

Femoral fractures in comatose children can be extremely difficult to treat because of the spasticity, involuntary movement, and agitation.[78-80] Fry and colleagues[78] reported considerable difficulties in management, including malunion, more than 5 cm of shortening, and fracture bone ends eroding through skin. They found proximal tibial skeletal traction and skin traction were ineffective as methods of management. As greater than 90 percent of children in coma for more than 48 hours have an excellent neurologic recovery, a poorly treated fracture may impair future mobility.[78] In those children with severe neurologic injury and elevated intracranial pressure, the head of the bed should ideally be elevated 30 degrees. The head-down position required for countertraction in all methods of traction other than 90/90 skeletal traction is thus contraindicated. Also any manipulation of the fracture tends to increase the intracranial pressure. A 90/90 skeletal traction can be successful if there is no agitation and involuntary movement. The fracture is often best stabilized using an external fixator or intramedullary or plate fixation. In the younger children, an external fixator or plate fixation would be appropriate and, in the older children, some form of intramedullary fixation.

Several centers have reported an increased incidence of heterotopic ossification in head-injured children and adults after intramedullary nailing of femoral shaft fractures.[81,82] This, however, was not confirmed in a recent study by Brumback and colleagues,[83] who noted the degree of heterotopic ossification after intramedullary nailing did not correlate with the presence or absence of a head injury.

External Fixation. External fixators are a safe and effective method of immobilization in head-injured children.[80,84-91] With external fixation, three screws should be used on either side of the fracture and the screws should be 2 cm away from the growth plate to avoid thermal injury and possible contiguous infection[84,85] (Fig. 29-9). These screws should be inserted at the lateral intermuscular septum to avoid muscle transfixion, except in cases where open injuries makes this impossible. In children over age 8, 5- and 6-mm screws can be used, and smaller sizes in younger children. A more rigid frame is needed for fractures with extensive comminution or segmental bone loss. A more flexible frame can be used if there is bone contact in a stable fracture pattern. The frame can be left on until the fracture is fully healed. Tolo[80,86] has reported a 21 percent refracture rate in 5 to 10 months if a rigid frame was used. A more flexible frame should be used in these circumstances, or, if possible, the frame should be dynamized. Aronson and Tursky[91] reported the results of 42 children with 44 femoral shaft fractures treated by external fixation (2-17 years old). Until union, which was usually by 10 to 12 weeks, 50 percent of the children were treated in the external fixator. Pin-tract infection occurred in approximately 11 percent of pins but never resulted in osteomyelitis. Of interest, even though most fractures were reduced anatomically, 6 of 16 patients followed for more than 18 months had only 2 to 10 mm overgrowth, the rest being equal.

If the head injury is minor and expected to improve in several days, the fracture should be treated as it would have been if the head injury had not been present. If traction is used in a child with severe head injury, 90/90 skeletal traction is the most appropriate.

OPEN FEMORAL FRACTURES

The open wound should be treated with early debridement and irrigation and delayed primary closure. Appropriate broad-spectrum antibiotics and tetanus antitoxin are administered as necessary. If the femoral shaft fracture is an isolated injury, 90/90 skeletal traction works well and provides access to the wound. External fixation is often an option, as this also provides good

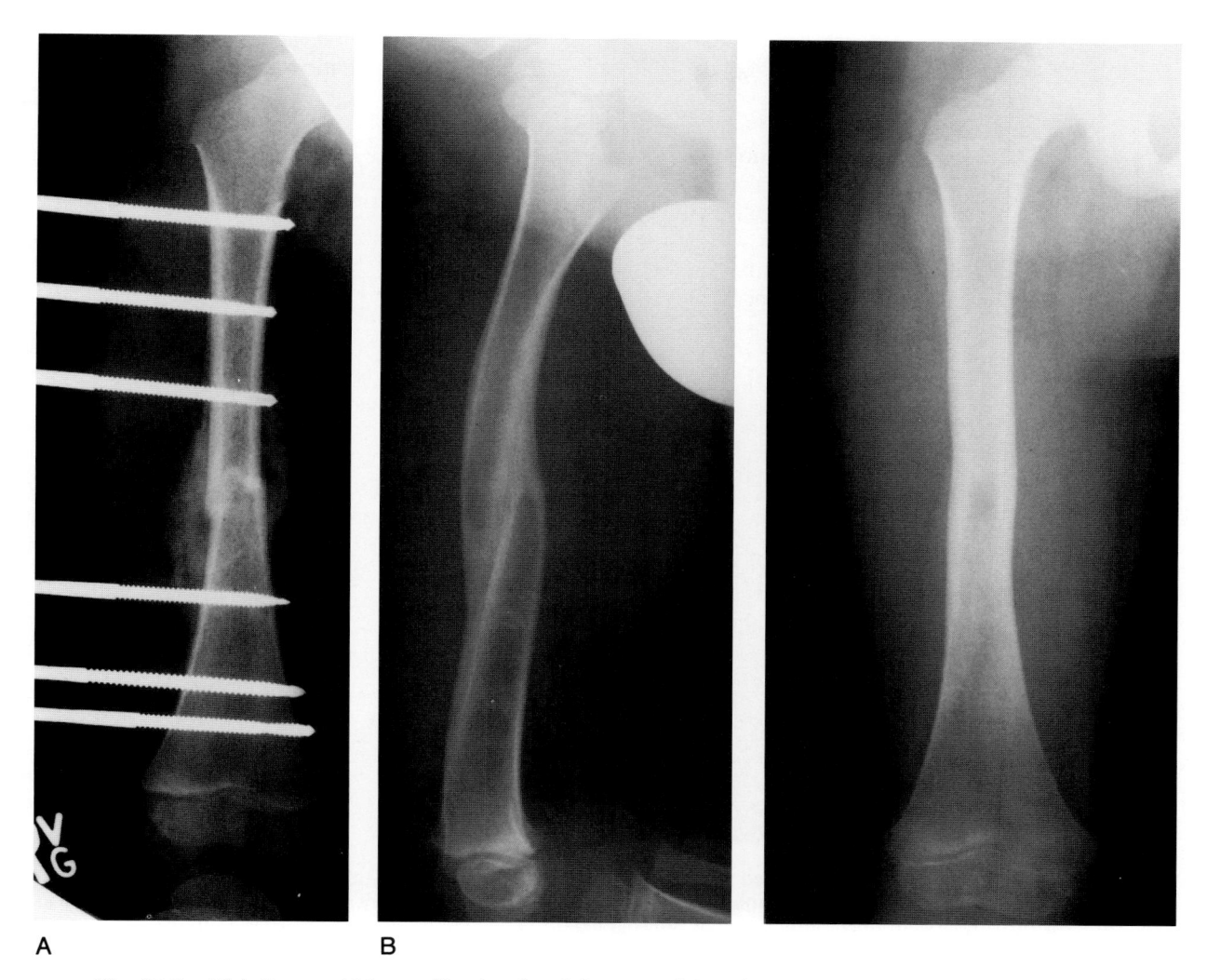

Fig. 29-9. This 3-year-old boy suffered a closed fracture of the middle third of his right femur and liver and spleen lacerations when struck by a car while crossing the road. He required an emergency laparotomy, and the femoral fracture was treated in skin traction. Subsequent laparotomies were needed to manage complications from the liver lacerations. He was in a Trendelenburg position in traction and could not be weaned from the respirator until the external fixator (**A**) was applied. The external fixator was left on until the fracture was fully healed. (**B**) Demonstrates the healed fracture 6 months later.

access to the wound but allows early joint movement and weightbearing.

Multiple Trauma

Early (<24 hours) stabilization of fractures in severely or multiply injured adults has been shown to decrease morbidity and mortality and reduce the cost of care significantly.[92-96] When spine, pelvis, or femoral fractures are not rigidly fixed, the patient must be nursed in a recumbent position. In immobilized patients with unstable fractures, there is increased morbidity due to respiratory complications or sepsis with related multiple organ failure.[92-96]

While there is little information in the literature on early fracture fixation in the multiply traumatized child, similar complications should be expected in the teenaged group. Fat embolism can occur in children after femoral fractures and resembles that which occurs in

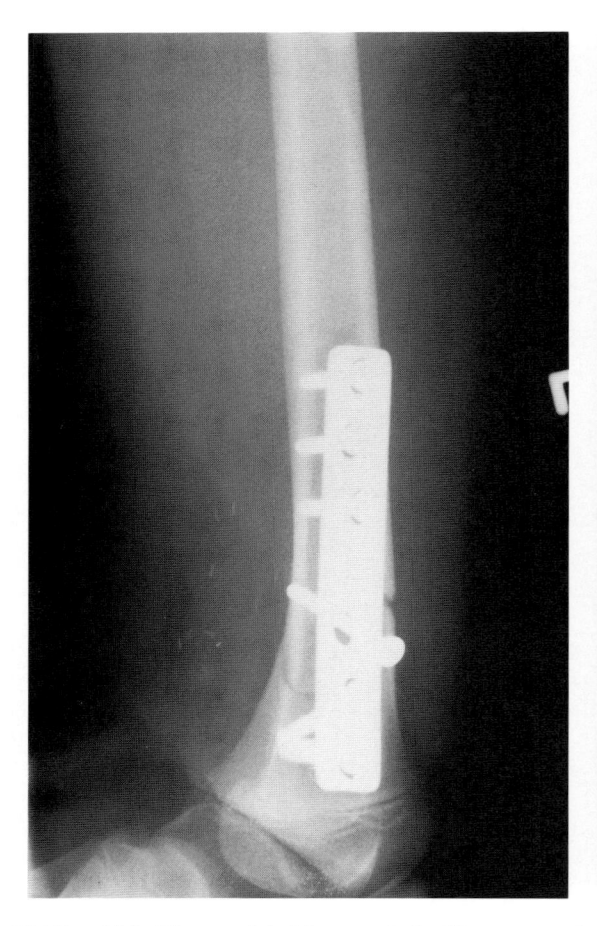

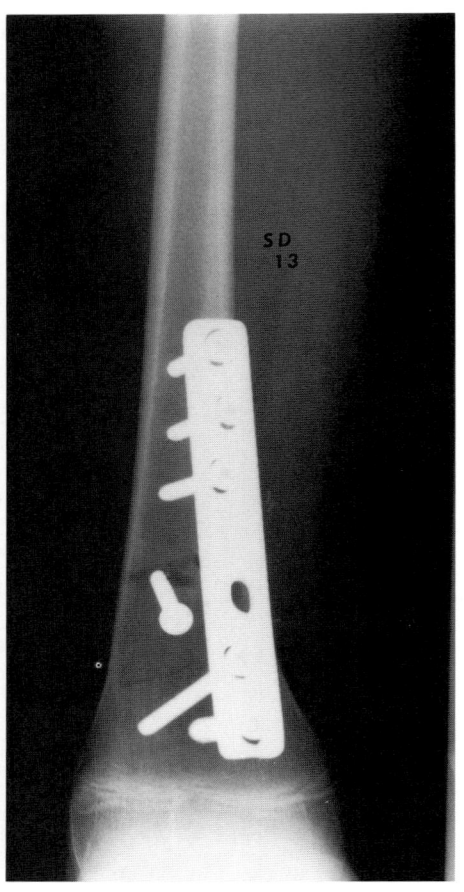

Fig. 29-10. This 13-year-old girl presented with an avascular left lower extremity after suffering a compound fracture of her left distal femur. Arteriography demonstrated a femoral artery injury at the level of the fracture. She subsequently underwent open reduction and internal fixation and vein grafting of the arterial injury.

adults.[97] Rigid fracture fixation in older children should similarly decrease such complications of fracture mobility.

VASCULAR INJURY

Vascular injury is uncommon after a femoral shaft fracture.[98,99] Howard and Makin[98] report 13 vascular injuries after reviewing 1,743 femoral fractures in adults and children. Ideally, the limb should be revascularized within 8 hours. The amputation rate is 50 percent for those who have had more than 8 hours of ischemia.[98] Rigid fixation may protect a vascular repair, but it is essential that the operative stabilization does not delay revascularization (Fig. 29-10). The fracture should be stabilized before the vascular repair only if the delay will not excessively prolong the time of ischemia.

IPSILATERAL FEMORAL AND TIBIAL SHAFT FRACTURES

These injuries are usually secondary to high-energy trauma, usually after a pedestrian or cyclist is struck by a motor vehicle[100-102] (Fig. 29-11). There is a high incidence of associated injuries to the head, chest, and abdomen, and many of these children have other long-bone fractures.[101,102] Ipsilateral knee ligament injuries can occur and Bohn and Durbin[102] describe four children with late problems with the knee secondary to ligamentous injuries. In adults with ipsilateral femoral and tibial fractures, the best results have been in patients who have

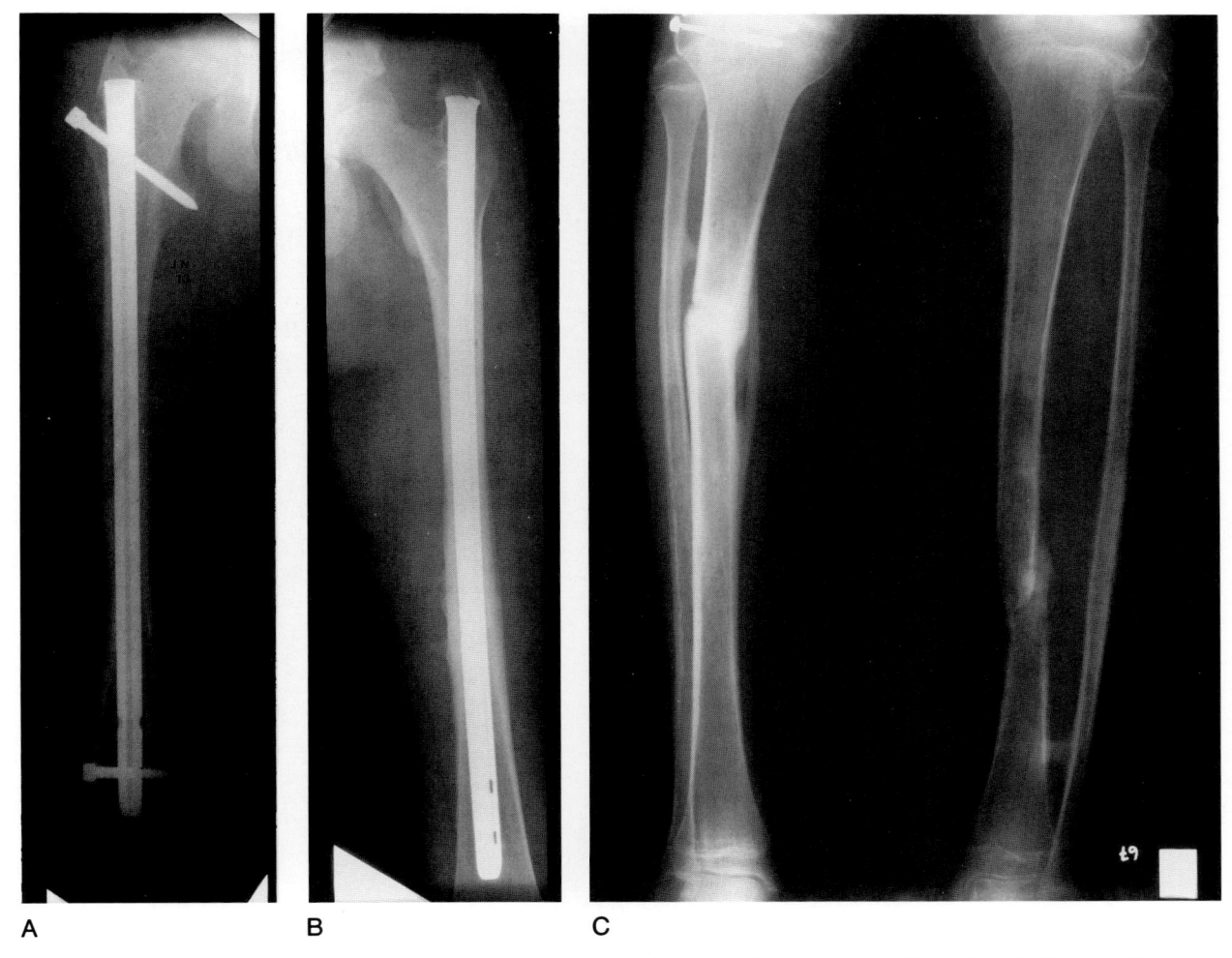

Fig. 29-11. This 13-year-old girl suffered bilateral closed femoral fractures and bilateral grade II open tibial fractures after she was struck by a falling lamppost. **(A)** The femoral fractures were treated with closed intramedullary nails and **(B)** the tibial fractures in external fixators. A local muscle flap was required for coverage of one of the tibial fractures. **(C)** Radiographs of both tibiae taken soon after removal of the external fixators demonstrate a malunion on the right with a delayed union on the left. She was treated in casts and subsequently went on to satisfactory union.

had operative stabilization of both fractures. McBryde and Blake[100] report 20 children who were treated with traction. There were four delayed unions, and six malunions that needed late osteotomy. Letts and colleagues[101] reported the results with 15 children with "floating knee injuries" and recommended that at least one fracture should be rigidly fixed in all cases and that often it was most appropriate for this to be the tibia. They felt that, in older children, intramedullary nailing of the femur would be appropriate.

Bohn and Durbin,[102] in a recent review of 44 ipsilateral, femoral, and tibial fractures in children, concluded that, in children under 10 years of age, the femur should be treated by distal femoral skeletal traction, and the tibia by closed reduction and casting. Operative stabilization would be indicated in instances of head trauma and compound fractures. In children older than 10 years, they recommended internal fixation of the femoral fracture, as there was a high incidence of complications with nonoperative management (see Ch. 35).

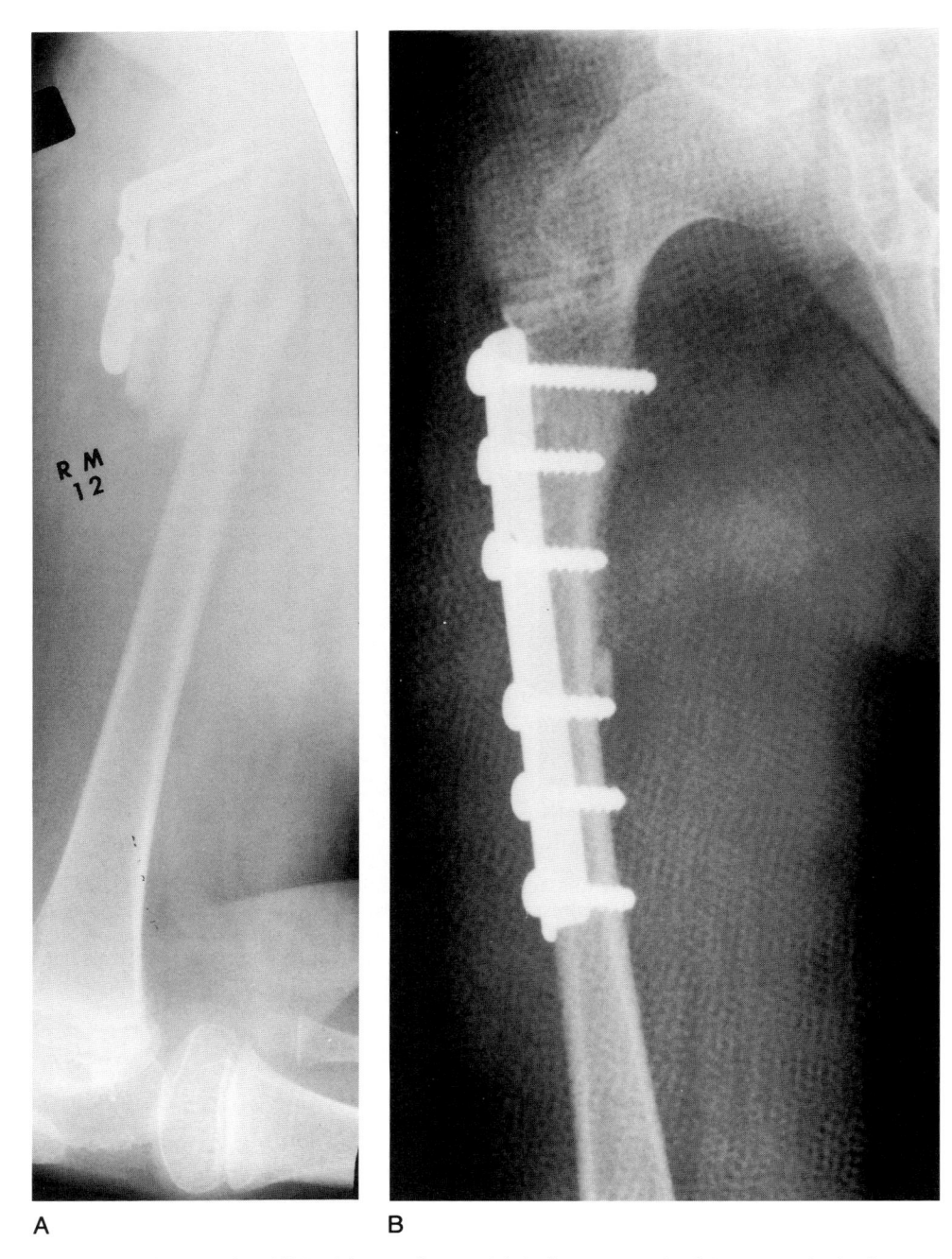

Fig. 29-12. (A) A 12-year-old child with spastic quadriplegia presented with a pathologic fracture after a low-energy injury. (B) The previous internal fixation was removed and the fracture treated with open reduction and internal fixation.

Pathologic Fractures

Occasionally, these fractures require operative stabilization (Fig. 29-12). Flexible intramedullary rods can be useful in children with osteogenesis imperfecta. Children with spastic quadriplegia do not tolerate traction well, and plate fixation can be a good management option.

Excessive Shortening in Cast

If the shortening cannot be managed by osteoclasis and reapplication of traction, external fixation can be successful. The Wagner or Ilizarov fixator can be used to slowly regain the length.

COMPLICATIONS

Malunion

Rotational Malunions

The most commonly observed rotational malunion is increased internal rotation.[26] Verbeek and coworkers[53] estimated that 20 to 40 percent of femoral fractures in children healed with rotational deformity. It is usually considered significant if the difference is in excess of 15 degrees, as Brouwer and coworkers[56] noted the physiologic difference in rotation of a pair of femora ranges from 0 to 15 degrees. The rotational difference can be assessed clinically by measuring hip rotation or radiographically most accurately using the CT scan.

Most authors conclude that rotational malunions are not a major functional problem.[50-52,54-58] There is some debate as to whether rotational deformities remodel; however, several recent animal studies indicate that internal malrotation of femoral fractures remodel about 55 percent.[103,104] Hägglund and colleagues[58] and other studies[51,56,57] indicate that rotational remodeling does occur in children, but it is not clear as to the magnitude or the mechanism of correction.

Angular Malunions

Mild angular malunions are quite common after femoral shaft fractures. The deformity is rarely a cosmetic problem, as the thigh musculature often camouflages the angulation. As mentioned earlier, the acceptable amount of angulation at the time of healing is controversial. This is because there are many factors to consider, including the age of the child and the direction and position of the angulation in the shaft. Up to 10 degrees of coronal plane angulation, 10 degrees of an anterior bow and 5 degrees of a posterior bow have been reported as being acceptable angulation.[25] Using these guidelines, acceptable results will be achieved in most instances. Angular remodeling is generally incomplete, with most of the correction occurring within 5 years after the injury.[48] Coronal plane deformities have been noted by one study to correct to about 50 percent the original angulation (varus, 40 percent; valgus, 60 percent), while sagittal plane angulation corrects up to 70 percent.[48]

Barfod and Christiensen[47] found that 25 degrees of angulation did not affect the final result. A similar conclusion was reached by Malkawi and coworkers[50] who found that coronal plane angulation of 20 degrees and sagittal plane angulation of 30 degrees will result in satisfactory alignment at long-term follow-up. These two studies bring up several important points. The majority of patients in the study of Malkawi and coworkers were 10 years of age or less. These children had between 4 and 6 years of growth remaining, depending on their sex — a tremendous potential for remodeling. Such remodeling would not be seen in the adolescent child with similar degrees of deformity. A 20-degree varus or valgus angulation in the distal femoral diaphysis would result in a significant cosmetic deformity in a child. Many parents would find it difficult to accept this deformity over the many years required for remodeling. There have been no studies that have addressed the effects of residual femoral angulation on the function of the joints of the lower extremities (Fig. 29-13).

If significant angulation occurs after the application of the spica cast, simple wedging of the cast may be all that is required. If the fracture is healed, such that wedging is not possible, remanipulation under an anesthetic, or possibly a drill osteoclasis, can be effective. Late presentation of an angular malunion can be managed in an adolescent by osteotomy and intramedullary fixation if severe and unacceptable (Fig. 29-14).

Leg Length Discrepancy

Leg length discrepancy is probably the most common complication after femoral shaft fractures. After any diaphyseal fracture, longitudinal growth is accelerated, but the exact amount is not always predictable. The final discrepancy is the result of the degree of overlap or distraction of the fracture, the amount of subsequent growth acceleration, any preexisting leg length discrepancy, and subsequent growth arrests in the ipsilateral extremity. The aim of the treating physician is to achieve

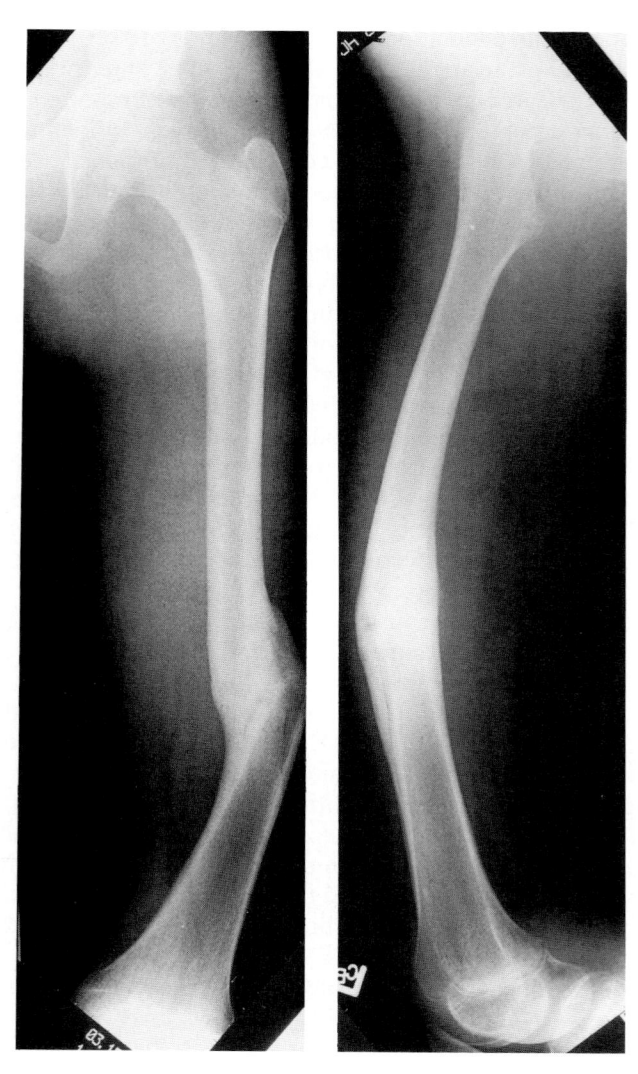

Fig. 29-13. This 11-year-old girl suffered an oblique fracture of her left distal femur and was treated in proximal tibial skeletal traction. She developed an angular and rotational malunion, which was cosmetically unacceptable and had pain over the apex of the deformity. Ideal treatment for this would be an osteotomy and intramedullary locking nail.

limb lengths that are within 1 cm of each other after the period of growth acceleration is complete. Pearson[105] found that 43 percent of schoolchildren evaluated with radiographs of the pelvis, in the standing position, had a discrepancy of 5 mm. Leg length discrepancies over 1.25 cm result in a higher incidence of low-back pain, compared to a control group with no leg length discrepancy.[106,107] There also appears to be a relationship between leg length discrepancy and osteoarthritis of the hip. Gofton and Trueman[108] found osteoarthritis occurred on the long side, possibly due to uncovering of the femoral head from the pelvic obliquity. While leg length discrepancy of more than 1 to 2 cm can result in a limp, there is no evidence that it produces a structural scoliosis.[109-111]

The degree of overgrowth is not predictable. Since Truesdell's original description,[112] many authors have observed that the relative lengthening of the fractured femur averages approximately 1 cm.[4,48-50,113-117] Staheli[49] and Griffin and colleagues[4] have found that children between the ages of 2 and 8 show the most consistent growth acceleration. This generally accepted phenomenon has not been confirmed by others who believe that age is not a factor and that overgrowth is universal.[48,113-118] Although there is much controversy, it does not appear that the site of the fracture, sex, degree of shortening, and soft tissue trauma have much effect on the degree of growth stimulation.

Reynolds[116] has calculated that the normal growth of the femur may increase from the normal rate of 0.13 cm per month to 0.18 cm per month. The increase of growth in the ipsilateral tibia is minor and should not affect the final result.[49,113,114,116] The growth acceleration appears to be maximal about 3 to 6 months postinjury.[116] The majority of the overgrowth occurs in the first 18 months following fracture,[113,114] and by 3½ years after fracture, 85 percent of the children had completed their overgrowth.

In 2- to 10-year-old children, the objective should be to allow the fracture to heal with about 1 to 1.5 cm of overriding to allow for subsequent growth acceleration.

Growth Arrest

Anterior proximal tibial growth arrest with secondary genu recurvatum has been reported after proximal tibial skeletal traction.[64] This method of skeletal traction should not be routinely used. Proximal tibial growth arrest as well as growth arrest of other growth plates in the ipsilateral extremity can occur after femoral diaphyseal fractures with no evidence of trauma to the growth plate.[119-121] In the seven patients described by Hresko and Kasser,[119] the diagnosis was delayed for an average of almost 2 years, indicating these children need to be followed.

SUMMARY

Fractures of the shaft of the femur in children are major injuries that are best managed by skin traction in infants and young children, skeletal traction in juveniles,

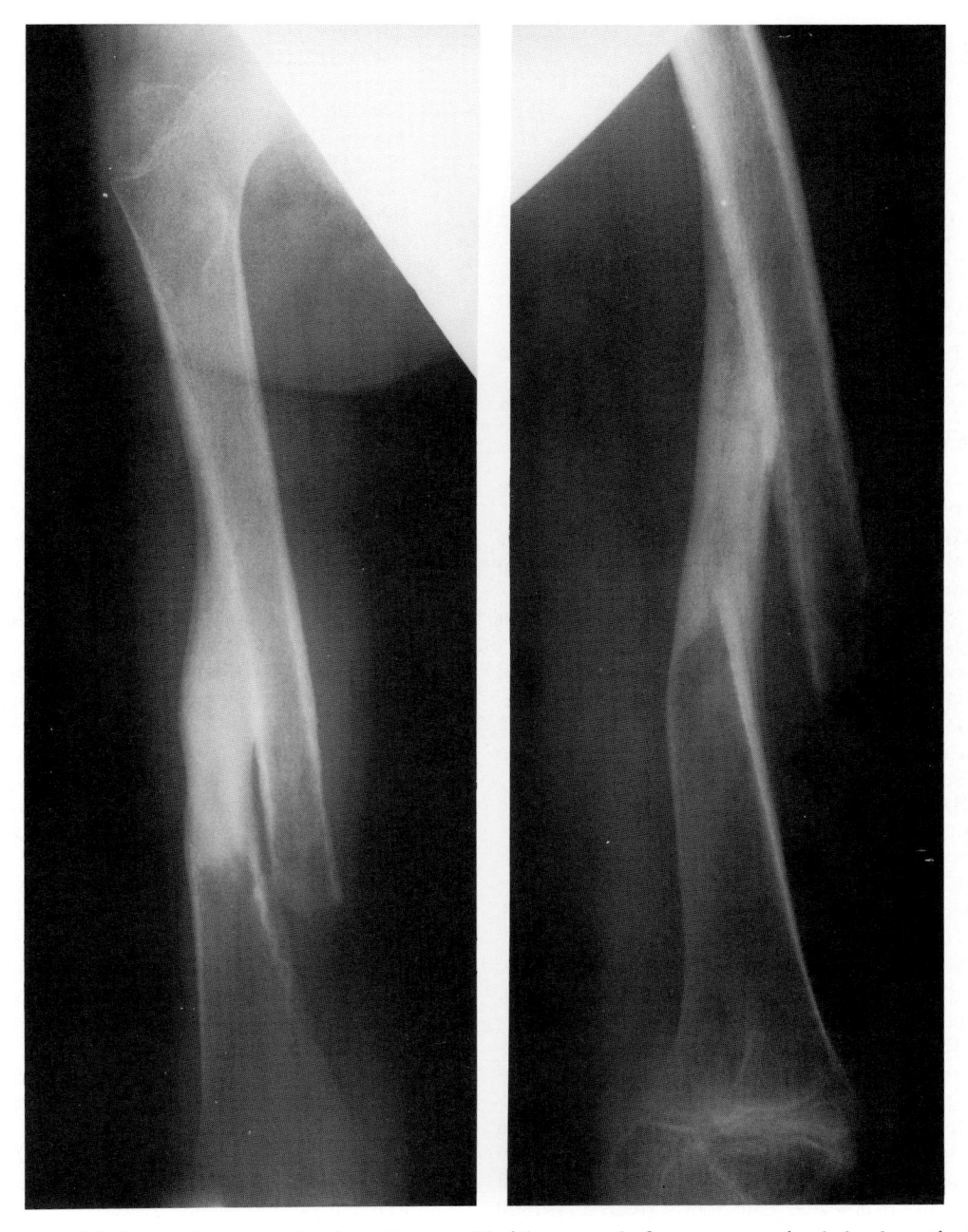

Fig. 29-14. This interesting malunion in a 10-year-old girl occurred after treatment in skeletal traction. Presumably, there was muscle interposition with an intact periosteal sleeve. She has healed her fracture with no angular or rotational deformity. She was ambulatory at the time these films were taken and not having any discomfort.

and intermedullary closed nailing in teenagers. Although potential complications of these fractures are numerous, with careful management and attention to detail most children with fractured femurs will heal satisfactorily with minimal long-term sequelae.

REFERENCES

1. Warlock P, Stower M: Fracture patterns in Nottingham children. J Pediatr Orthop 6:656, 1986
2. Hedlund R, Lindgren U: The incidence of femoral shaft fractures in children and adolescents. J Pediatr Orthop 6:47, 1986
3. Roberts I, Streat S, Judson J et al: Critical injuries in paediatric pedestrians. N Z Med J 104:247, 1991
4. Griffin P, Anderson M, Green W: Fractures of the shaft of the femur in children. Orthop Clin North Am 3:213, 1972
5. Rang M: Children's Fractures. 2nd Ed. p. 271. JB Lippincott, Philadelphia, 1983
6. Arkbarnia B, Torg JS, Kirkpatrick J et al: Manifestations of the battered child syndrome. J Bone Joint Surg [Am] 56:1159, 1974
7. Beals RK, Tufts E: Fractured femur in infancy: the role of child abuse. J Paediatr Orthop 3:583, 1983
8. Wellington P, Bennet GC: Fractures of the femur in childhood. Injury Br J Accident Surg 18:103, 1987
9. King J, Diefendorf D, Apthorp J et al: Analysis of 429 fractures in 189 battered children. J Paediatr Orthop 8:585, 1988
10. Dalton HJ, Slovis T, Helfer RE et al: Undiagnosed abuse in children younger than 3 years with femoral fracture. Am J Dis Child 114:875, 1990
11. Lock TR, Aronson DD: Fractures in patients who have myelomeningocele. J Bone Joint Surg [Am] 71:1153, 1989
12. Park HM, Kernek CB, Robb JA: Early scintigraphic findings of occult femoral and tibial fractures in children. Clin Nucl Med 13:271, 1988
13. Vasa R, Kim MR: Fracture of the femur at cesarian section: case report and review of the literature. Am J Perinatol 7:46, 1990
14. Phillips RR, Lie SH: Fractures of long bones occuring in neonatal intensive therapy units. Br Med J 301:225, 1990
15. Hershman EB, Lombardo J, Bergfeld JA: Femoral shaft stress fractures in atheletes. Clin Sports Med 9:111, 1990
16. Davies AM, Carter SR, Grimer RJ et al: Fatigue fractures of the femoral diaphysis in the skeletally immature simulating malignancy. Br J Radiol 62:893, 1989
17. Casado-Salinas JM, Llamas-Elvira JM, Lorente-Moreno R et al: Traumatic hip luxation associated with ipsilateral and contralateral femoral fracture in a child. Acta Orthop Belg 55:248, 1989
18. Barlow B, Niemirska M, Gandhi R et al: Response to injury in children with closed femur fractures. J Trauma 27:429, 1987
19. Staheli L: Fever following trauma in childhood. JAMA 199:503, 1967
20. Grossbard GD, Love BRT: Femoral nerve block; a simple and safe method of instant analgesia for femoral shaft fractures. Aust NZ J Surg 49:592, 1979
21. Denton JS, Manning MP: Femoral nerve block for femoral shaft fractures in children: brief report. J Bone Joint Surg [Br] 70:84, 1988
22. Ronchi L, Rosenbaum D, Athouel A et al: Femoral nerve blockade using bupivacaine. Anesthesiology 70:622, 1989
23. Blount WP: Fractures in Children. Williams & Wilkins, Baltimore, 1955
24. Rang M: Children's Fractures. 2nd Ed. JB Lippincott, Philadelphia, 1983
25. Ogden JA: Femoral Shaft Fractures. p. 708. In: Skeletal Injury in the Child. 2nd Ed. WB Saunders, Philadelphia, 1990
26. Staheli LT: Femoral Shaft Fractures. p. 1121. In Rockwood CA Jr, Wilkins KE, King RE (ed): Fractures in Children. 3rd Ed. JB Lippincott, Philadelphia, 1991
27. Tachdjian MO: Pediatric Orthopedics. WB Saunders, Philadelphia, 1990
28. Allen BL Jr, Schoch EP, Emery FE: Immediate spica cast system for femoral shaft fractures in infants and children. South Med J 71:18, 1978
29. Dameron TB Jr, Thompson HA: Femoral shaft fractures in children. Treatment by closed reduction and double spica cast immobilization. J Bone Joint Surg [Am] 41:1201, 1959
30. Guttmann GG, Simon R: Three-point fixation walking spica cast: an alternative to early or immediate casting of femoral shaft fractures in children. J Pediatr Orthop 8:699, 1988
31. Henderson OL, Morrissy RT, Gerdes MH et al: Early casting of femoral shaft fractures in children. J Pediatr Orthop 4:16, 1984
32. Irani RN, Nicholson JT, Chung SMK et al: Long term results in the treatment of femoral shaft fractures in young children by immediate spica immobilization. J Bone Joint Surg [Am] 58:945, 1976
33. McCarthy RE: A method for early spica cast application in treatment of pediatric femoral fractures. J Pediatr Orthop 6:89, 1986
34. Martinez AG, Carroll NC, Sarwark JF et al: Femoral shaft fractures in children treated with early spica cast. J Pediatr Orthop 11:712, 1991
35. Miller ME, Bramlett KW, Kissell EU et al: Improved treatment of femoral shaft fractures in children: the "pontoon" 90-90 spica cast. Clin Orthop 219:140, 1987
36. Splain SH, Denno JJ: Immediate double hip spica immobilization as the treatment for femoral shaft fractures in children. J Trauma 25:994, 1985
37. Staheli LT, Sheridan GW: Early spica cast management of femoral shaft fractures in young children: a technique

utilizing bilateral fixed skin traction. Clin Orthop 126:162, 1977
38. Sugi M, Cole WG: Early plaster treatment for fractures of the femoral shaft in childhood. J Bone Joint Surg [Am] 69:743, 1987
39. Kirby RM, Winquist RA, Hansen ST: Femoral shaft fractures in adolescents: a comparison between traction plus cast treatment and closed intramedullary nailing. J Pediatr Orthop 1:193, 1981
40. Gross RH, Davidson R, Sullivan JA et al: Cast brace management of the femoral shaft fracture in children and young adults. J Pediatr Orthop 3:572, 1983
41. Mann DC, Weddington J, Davenport K: Closed ender nailing of femoral shaft fractures in adolescents. J Pediatr Orthop 6:651, 1986
42. Aronson DD, Singer RM, Higgins RF: Skeletal traction for fractures of the femoral shaft in children. J Bone Joint Surg [Am] 69:1435, 1987
43. Herndon WA, Mahnken RF, Yngve DA et al: Management of femoral shaft fractures in the adolescent. J Pediatr Orthop 9:29, 1989
44. Reeves RB, Ballard RI, Hughes JL: Internal fixation versus traction and casting of adolescent femoral shaft fractures. J Pediatr Orthop 10:592, 1990
45. Bucholz RW, Jones A: Fractures of the shaft of the femur: current concepts review. J Bone Joint Surg [Am] 73:1561, 1991
46. Greville N, Ivins J: Fractures of the femur in children: an analysis of the effect on the subsequent length of bones of the lower limb. Am J Surg 93:376, 1957
47. Barfod B, Christensen J: Fracture of the femoral shaft in children with special reference to subsequent overgrowth. Acta Orthop Scand 116:235, 1958
48. Viljanto J, Kiviluto H, Paananen M: Remodeling after femoral shaft fractures in children. Acta Orthop Scand 141:360, 1975
49. Staheli L: Femoral and tibial growth following femoral shaft fracture in childhood. Clin Orthop 55:159, 1967
50. Malkawi H, Shannak A, Hadidi S: Remodelling after femoral fractures in children treated by the modified Blount method. J Pediatr Orthop 6:421, 1986
51. Neer CS, Cadman EF: Treatment of fractures of the femoral shaft in children. JAMA 163:634, 1957
52. Burton V, Fordyce A: Immobilization of femoral shaft fractures in children aged 2–10 years. Injury 4:47, 1972
53. Verbeek H, Bender J, Scavidis K: Rotational deformities after fractures of the femoral shaft in childhood. Injury 8:43, 1976
54. Verbeek H: Does rotation deformity following femoral shaft fractures correct during growth? Reconstr Surg Traumatol 17:75, 1979
55. Benum P, Ertesvag K, Hiseth K: Torsional deformities after traction treatment of femoral fractures children. Acta Orthop Scand 50:87, 1979
56. Brouwer KJ, Molenaar J, Van Linge B: Rotational deformities after femoral shaft fractures in childhood: a retrospective study 27–32 years after the accident. Acta Orthop Scand 52:81, 1981
57. Brouwer KJ: Torsional deformities after fractures of the femoral shaft in childhood: a retrospective study 27–32 years after trauma. Acta Orthop Scand, suppl 52:2, 1981
58. Hägglund G, Hansson LI, Norman O: Correction by growth of rotational deformity after femoral fracture in children. Acta Orthop Scand 54:858, 1983
59. Skak SV, Jensen TT: Femoral shaft fracture in 265 children: log-normal correlation with age of speed of healing. Acta Orthop Scand 59:704, 1988
60. Nicholson JT, Foster RM, Heath RD: Bryant's traction: a provocative cause of circulatory complications. JAMA 157:415, 1955
61. Andrews PI, Rosenberg AR: Renal consequences of immobilization in children with fractured femurs. Acta Paediatr Scand 79:311, 1990
62. Weiss APC, Schennk RC Jr, Sponseller PO, Thompson JD: Peroneal nerve palsy after early cast applications for femoral fractures in children. J Pediatric Orthop 12:25, 1992
63. Humberger FW, Eyring EJ: Proximal tibial 90/90 traction in management of children with femoral shaft fractures. J Bone Joint Surg [Am] 51:499, 1969
64. Van Meter J, Branicke R: Bilateral genu recurvatum after skeletal traction. J Bone Joint Surg [Am] 62:837, 1980
65. Ryan JR: 90/90 Skeletal femoral traction for femoral shaft fractures in children. J Trauma 21:46, 1981
66. Mital MA, Cashman WA: Fresh ambulatory approach to treatment of femoral shaft fractures in children: a comparison with traditional conservative methods. J Bone Joint Surg [Am] 58:285, 1976
67. McCullough N, Vinsant J, Sarmiento A: Functional fracture bracing of long bone fractures of the lower extremity in children. J Bone Joint Surg [Am] 60:314, 1978
68. Scott J, Wardlaw D, McLauchlan J: Cast bracing of femoral shaft fractures in children: a preliminary report. J Pediatr Orthop 1:199, 1981
69. Suman RK: Treatment of fractures of the femoral shaft with early cast bracing. Injury 13:239, 1981
70. Pankovich AM: Flexible intramedullary nailing of femoral shaft fractures. Instr Course Lect 36:324, 1987
71. Fein LH, Pankovich AM, Spero CM et al: Closed flexible intramedullary nailing of adolescent femoral shaft fractures. J Orthop Trauma 3:133, 1989
72. Kissel EU, Miller ME: Closed Ender nailing of femur fractures in older children. J Trauma 29:1585, 1989
73. Ligier JN, Metaizeau JP, Prevot J et al: Elastic stable intramedullary nailing of femoral shaft fractures in children. J Bone Joint Surg [Br] 70:74, 1988
74. Verstreken L, Delronge G, Lamoureux J: Orthopaedic treatment of paediatric multiple trauma patients: a new technique. Int Surg 73:177, 1988
75. Ziv I, Blackburn N, Rang M: Femoral intramedullary nailing in the growing child. J Trauma 24:432, 1984
76. Valdiserri L, Marchiodi L, Rubbini L: Kuntscher nailing in the treatment of femoral fractures in children: is it

77. Viljanto J, Linna M, Kiviluoto H et al: Indications and results of operative treatment of femoral shaft fractures in children. Acta Chir Scand 141:366, 1975
78. Fry K, Hoffer MM, Brink J: Femoral shaft fractures in brain injured children. J Trauma 16:371, 1976
79. Ziv I, Rang M: Treatment of femoral fractures in the child with head injury. J Bone Joint Surg [Br] 65:276, 1983
80. Tolo VT: External fixation in multiply injured children. Orthop Clin NA 21:393, 1990
81. Marks PH, Paley D, Kellam JF: Heterotopic ossification around the hip with intramedullary nailing of the femur. J Trauma 28:1207, 1988
82. Keret D, Harcke HT, Mendez AA et al: Heterotopic ossification in central nervous system-injured patients following closed nailing of femoral fractures. Clin Orthop 256:254, 1990
83. Brumback RJ, Wells JD, Lakatos R et al: Heterotopic ossification about the hip after intramedullary nailing for fractures of the femur. J Bone Joint Surg [Am] 72:1067, 1990
84. Alonso JE, Horowitz M: Use of the AO/ASIF external fixator in children. J Pediatr Orthop 7:594, 1987
85. Alonso JE, Geissler W, Hughes JL: External fixation of femoral fractures: indications and limitations. Clin Orthop 241:83, 1989
86. Tolo VT: External skeletal fixation in childhood fractures. J Pediatr Orthop 3:435, 1983
87. Shih HN, Chen LM, Lee ZL et al: Treatment of femoral shaft fractures with the Hoffman external fixator in prepuberty. J Trauma 29:498, 1989
88. Behrens F: External fixation in children: lower extremity. Instr Course Lect 39:205, 1990
89. Kirschenbaum D, Albert MC, Robertson WW Jr et al: Complex femur fractures in children: Treatment with external fixation. J Pediatr Orthop 10:588, 1990
90. Krettek C, Haas N, Walker J et al: Treatment of femoral shaft fractures in children by external fixation. Injury 22:205, 1991
91. Aronson J, Tursky EA: External fixation of femur fractures in children. J Pediatr Orthop 12:157, 1992
92. Riska EB, Myllynen P: Fat embolism in patients with multiple injuries. J Trauma 22:891, 1982
93. Johnson KD, Cadambi A, Seibert B: Incidence of ARDS in patients with multiple musculoskeletal injuries: effect of early operative stabilization of fractures. J Trauma 25:375, 1985
94. Meek RN, Vivoda EE, Pirani S: Comparison of mortality of patients with multiple injuries, according to the type of fracture treatment: a retrospective age and injury matched series. Injury 17:2, 1986
95. Bone LB, Johnson KD, Weigelt J et al: Early versus delayed stabilization of femoral fractures. J Bone Joint Surg [Am] 71:336, 1989
96. Kotowica Z, Balcewicz L, Jagodzinski Z: Head injuries coexistent with pelvic or lower extremity fractures: early or delayed osteosynthesis. Acta Neurochir 102:19, 1990
97. Weicz GM, Rang M, Salter RB: Post traumatic fat embolism in children. J Trauma 13:529, 1973
98. Howard PW, Makin G: Lower limb fractures with associated vascular injury. J Bone Joint Surg [Br] 72:116, 1990
99. Esposito PW, Crawford AH: Paediatric update: 6. False aneurysm arising from a closed femur fracture in a child. Orthop Rev 18:114, 1989
100. McBryde AM Jr, Blake R: The floating knee: ipsilateral fractures of the femur and tibia. J Bone Joint Surg [Am] 56:1309, 1974
101. Letts M, Vincent N, Gouw G: The "Floating Knee" in children. J Bone Joint Surg [Br] 68:442, 1986
102. Bohn WW, Durbin RA: Ipsilateral fractures of the femur and tibia in children and adolescents. J Bone Joint Surg [Am] 73:429, 1991
103. Schneider M: The effect of growth on femoral torsion: an experimental study in dogs. J Bone Joint Surg [Am] 45:1439, 1963
104. Strong ML, Wong-Chung J, Babikan G et al: Rotational remodelling of malrotated femoral fractures: a model in the rabbit. J Pediatr Orthop 12:173, 1992
105. Pearson WM: A progressive structural study of school children. J Am Osteopathic Assoc 51:155, 1951
106. Giles LGF, Taylor JR: Low back pain associated with leg length inequality. Spine 6:510, 1981
107. Giles LGF, Taylor JR: Lumbar spine structural changes associated with leg length inequality. Spine 7:159, 1982
108. Gofton JP, Trueman GE: Unilateral idiopathic osteoarthritis of the hip. Can Med Assoc J 97:1129, 1967
109. Moe JH, Winter RB, Bradford DS, Lonstein JE: Scoliosis and Other Spinal Deformities. WB Saunders, Philadelphia, 1978
110. Papaioannov T, Stokes I, Kenwright J: Scoliosis associated with limb length discrepancy. J Bone Joint Surg [Am] 64:59, 1982
111. Gibson PH, Papaioannov T, Kenwright J: The influence on the spine of leg length discrepancy after femoral fracture. J Bone Joint Surg [Br] 65:584, 1983
112. Truesdell ED: Inequality of the lower extremities following fracture of the shaft of femur in children. Ann Surg 74:498, 1921
113. Shapiro F: Developmental patterns in lower-extremity length discrepancy. J Bone Joint Surg [Am] 64:639, 1982
114. Shapiro F: Fractures of the femoral shaft in children. Acta Orthop Scand 52:649, 1981
115. Hougaard K: Femoral shaft fractures in children: a prospective study of the overgrowth phenomenon. Injury Br J Accident Surg 20:170, 1989
116. Reynolds DA: Growth changes in fractured long bones. J Bone Joint Surg [Br] 63:83, 1981
117. Clement DA, Colton CL: Growth of the femur after fracture in childhood. J Bone Joint Surg [Br] 68:534, 1986

118. Edvardsen P, Syverson S: Overgrowth of the femur after fracture of the shaft in childhood. J Bone Joint Surg [Br] 58:339, 1976
119. Hresko HT, Kasser JR: Physeal arrest about the knee associated with non-physeal fractures in the lower extremity. J Bone Joint Surg [Am] 71:698, 1989
120. Beals RK: Premature closure of the physis following diaphyseal fractures. J Pediatr Orthop 10:717, 1990
121. Bowler JR, Mubarak SJ, Wenger DR: Tibial physeal closure and genu recurvatum following femoral fracture: occurrence without a tibial traction pin. J Pediatr Orthop 10:653, 1990
122. Hunter LY, Hensinger RN: Premature monomelic growth arrest following the fracture of the femoral shaft: a case report. J Bone Joint Surg [Am] 60:850, 1978

30

Supracondylar (Nonphyseal) Fractures of the Femur

Jacques D'Astous

> A hunch is creativity trying to tell you something.
> —Frank Capra

DESCRIPTION AND INCIDENCE

Supracondylar fractures of the femur occurring proximal to the physis and distal to the diaphysis are uncommon in children, as most occur through the weaker growth plate. These fractures are located in the distal metaphyseal region of the femur just proximal to the origin of the gastrocnemius and are usually secondary to severe direct trauma.[1] However, children with severe osteoporosis or tumors, such as a nonossifying fibroma, may fracture as a result of minor twisting injuries or falls.[2,3]

ANATOMY

Since these fractures occur just proximal to the origin of the gastrocnemius, there is a tendency for the gastrocnemius to pull the distal fragment posteriorly, causing apex posterior angulation at the fracture site, particularly when the knee is in full extension (Fig. 30-1).[3,4] For this reason, once a closed reduction of this fracture has been obtained, it is important to immobilize the fracture with the knee flexed to prevent recurrent apex posterior angulation.

The anatomic proximity of the neurovascular bundle to the distal femoral metaphyseal region, creates a potential for vascular compromise.[1,2] This may occur either in the region of the adductor hiatus through which course the popliteal vein and artery or in the popliteal fossa, especially with apex posterior angulation at the fracture site.

Significant varus or valgus malalignment may occur as it is very difficult to assess the varus/valgus alignment in the metaphyseal region. For this reason, it is important to include as much distal femur and proximal tibia as possible in the postreduction radiographs to accurately assess the varus/valgus alignment at the fracture site.

MECHANISM OF INJURY

The usual mechanism of injury is one of hyperextension of the knee with an anteriorly placed fulcrum just proximal to the knee joint. More frequently, however, in children with open growth plates, the fracture will occur through the physis. Occasionally, supracondylar fractures of the femur may result from a fall from a height

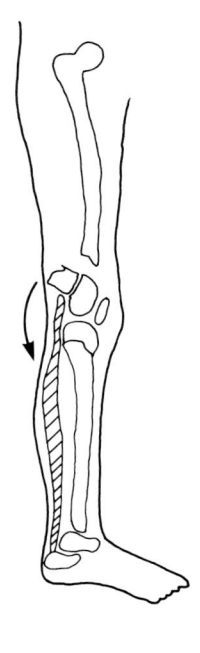

Fig. 30-1. Supracondylar fracture of the femur. Note apex posterior angulation resulting from the pull of the gastrocnemius on the distal fragment.

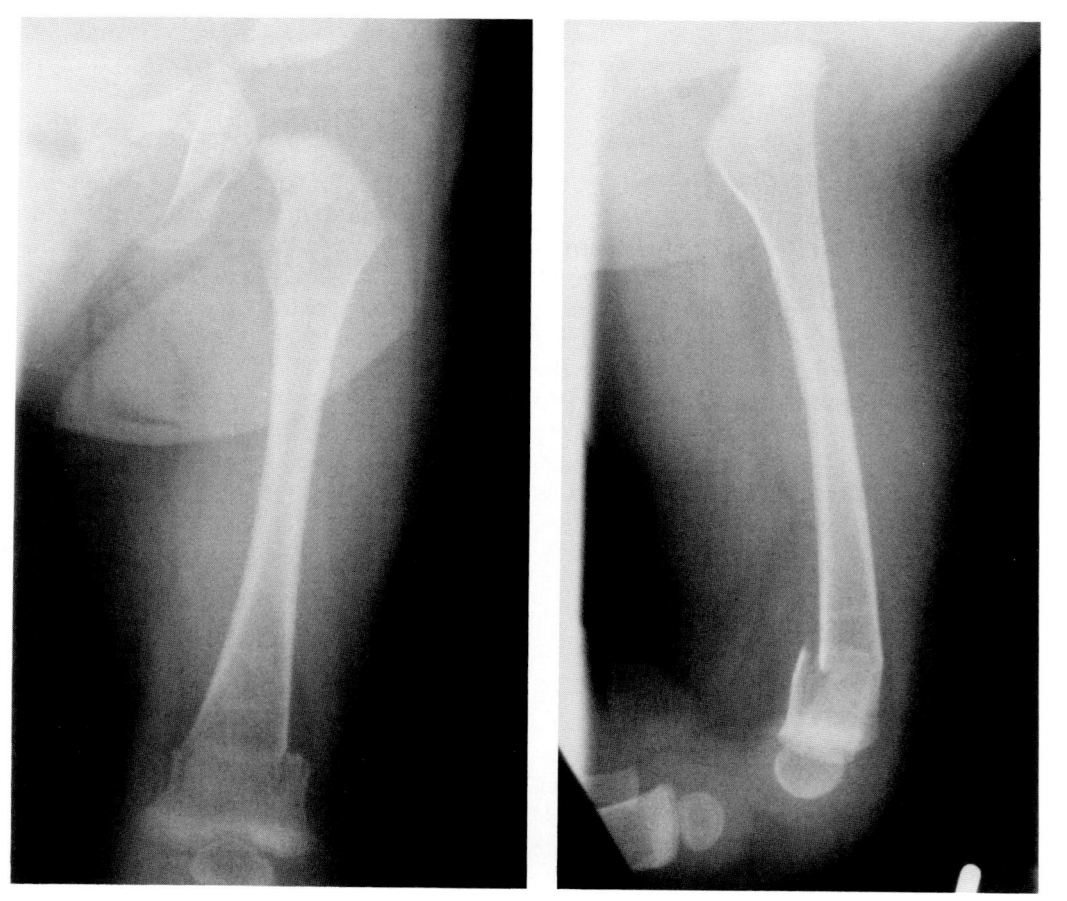

Fig. 30-2. Minimally displaced distal femoral metaphyseal fracture in a 6-month-old child who fell off a changing table, treated by gentle extension of the knee and a single hip spica.

(e.g., changing table, couch) in prewalkers and toddlers (Fig. 30-2).

CLASSIFICATION

1. The fractures may be *open* or *closed.*
2. The fracture may be *undisplaced,* (buckle fracture, stress fracture) *angulated* (apex anterior, posterior, varus, or valgus), or *displaced.*
3. *Pathologic* fractures also occur in the supracondylar region of the femur in conditions that cause osteoporosis: spina bifida, muscular dystrophy, or neoplastic lesions such as a large nonossifying fibroma or fibrous cortical defect[2,3] (Fig. 30-3).

PHYSICAL EXAMINATION

The distal thigh of the involved limb is usually swollen, and, depending on the degree of displacement or angulation, a deformity might be noted. It is important to assess the varus/valgus alignment of the lower extremity and to compare it to the uninjured limb. A detailed neurovascular examination of the limb should be performed because of the close proximity of the neurovascular structures to the fracture. Finally, one should always look for the presence of a knee effusion which might be suggestive of a torn anterior or posterior cruciate ligament or an intra-articular extension of the fracture.

TREATMENT

Simple Plaster Immobilization

If the fracture is undisplaced, a well-molded cylinder or long leg cast with the knee in 20 degrees of flexion is applied for a period of 3 to 6 weeks depending on the age of the child.

Closed Reduction

In the presence of an angulated or displaced fracture, a closed reduction is performed under general anesthesia. In cases of angulated fractures, the angulation is corrected under image intensifier control after which a long leg cast or hip spica cast is applied. Where the fracture is angulated in an apex posterior direction, it is preferable to flex the knee approximately 70 degrees to

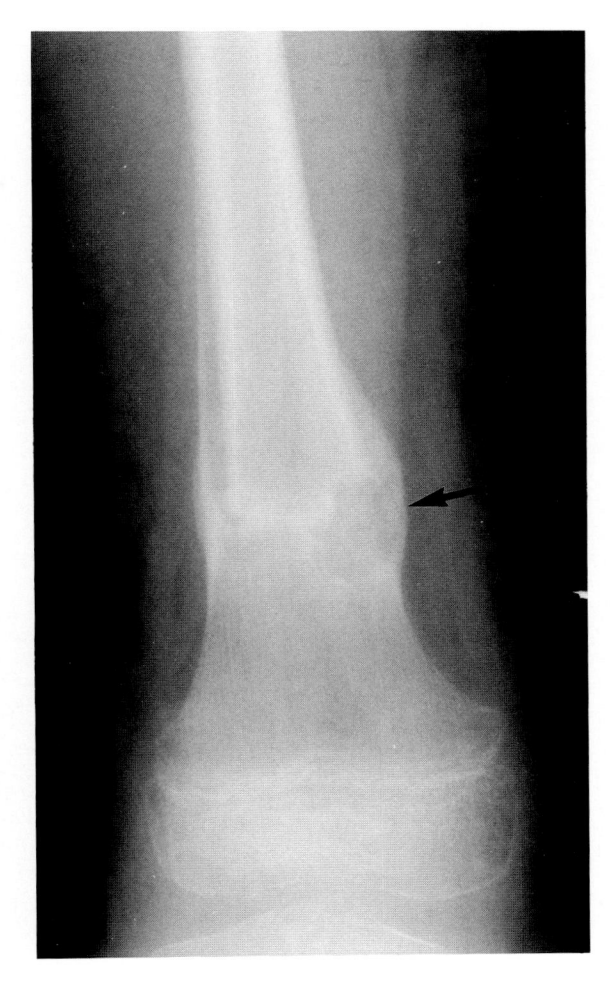

Fig. 30-3. Healed supracondylar fracture of the distal femur through a nonossifying fibroma.

prevent recurrence of the angulation secondary to the pull of the gastrocnemius muscles. In apex anterior angulated fractures, the cast should be applied with the knee in full extension. Care should be taken to obtain an anatomic varus/valgus alignment.

When the fracture is displaced, a closed reduction should be attempted, and, if successful, the fracture may be immobilized in a long-leg cast or spica if the reduction is stable. The unstable fracture may be pinned percutaneously with two appropriately sized crossed smooth pins supplemented by a long-leg cast or spica. Alternatively, reduction and maintenance of reduction may be obtained using skeletal traction with the knee flexed 70 to 90 degrees. Occasionally we have found it useful to use a two-pin technique to obtain better control of the tendency to angulate apex posteriorly[1] (Fig. 30-4). One pin is

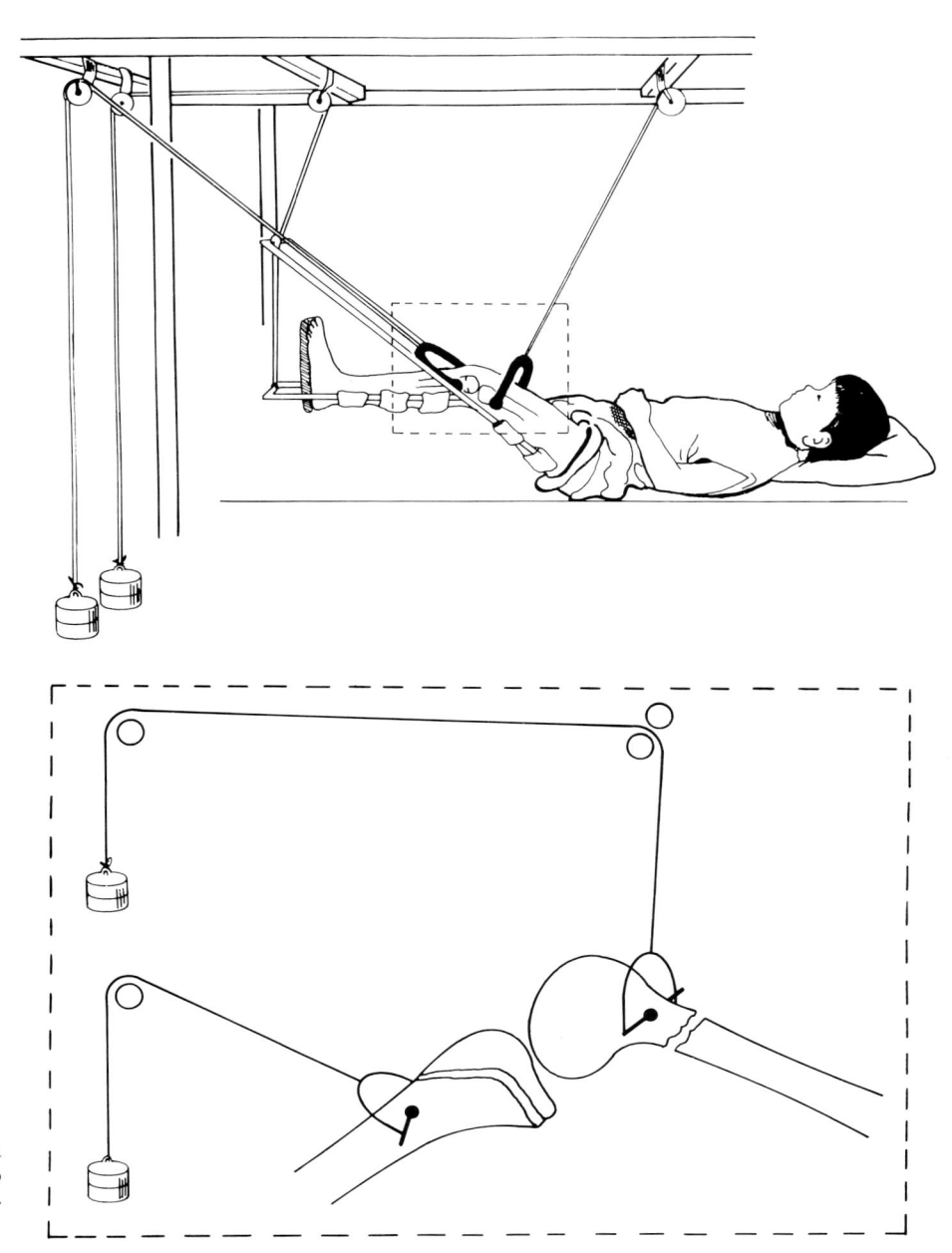

Fig. 30-4. Balanced suspension traction using a two-pin technique to control the tendency for these fractures to angulate apex posterior.

placed transversly in the metaphysis, a second pin in the proximal tibia. Balanced traction is then applied with the knee flexed at 60 to 90 degrees. Another option is the use of an external fixator to stabilize the fracture.

Open Reduction

In cases where a closed reduction cannot be obtained because of soft tissue interposition, an open reduction may be performed using a lateral approach. Once the fracture is reduced, it can be stabilized by using the crossed-pin technique or with a contoured AO direct compression plate and screws (Fig. 30-5). If the growth plate is closed, it is possible to fix these fractures with either a supracondylar type of plate and screws or a blade plate.

In the presence of a vascular injury, the basic principle is to reduce and stabilize the fracture as quickly as possible to permit and protect a good vascular repair. If the arterial injury is in the region of the adductor hiatus, a medial approach to the supracondylar region of the

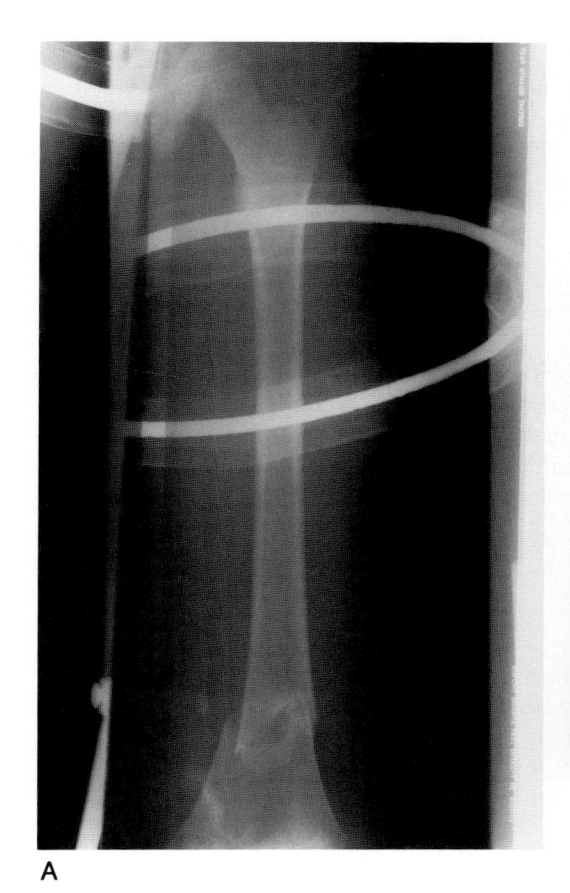

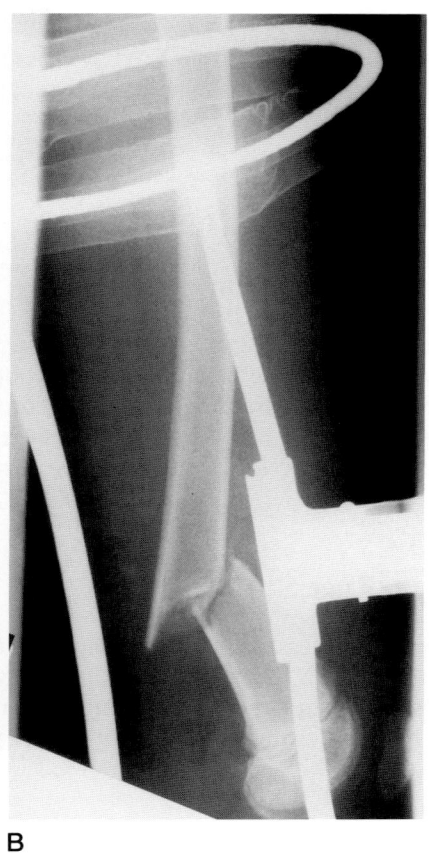

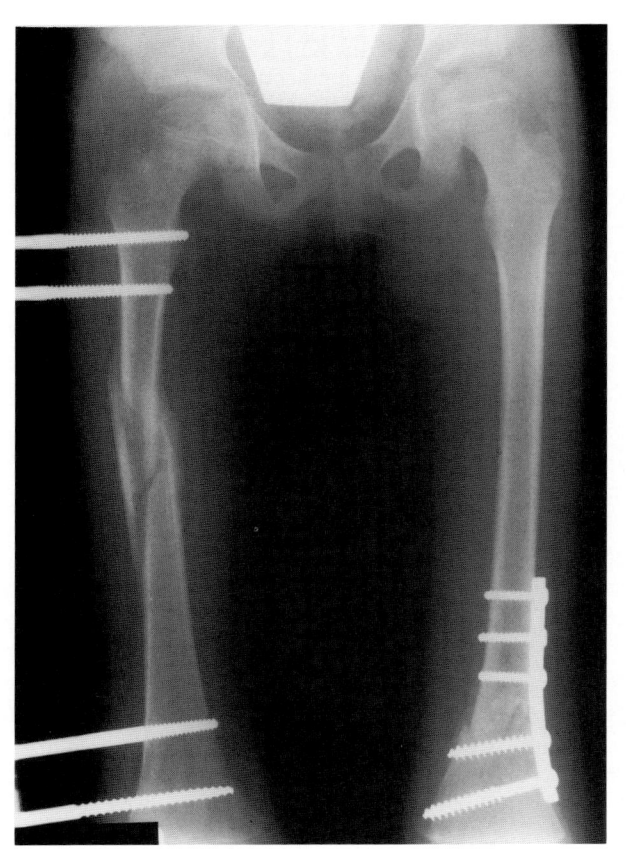

Fig. 30-5. (A&B) Displaced and apex posterior angulated supracondylar fracture of the femur in a patient with bilateral femoral fractures and a head injury. (C) AP view of both femora following open reduction and fixation with a contoured AO plate of the supracondylar fracture of the left femur. Note the external fixator used to stabilize the diaphyseal fracture of the right femur.

femur is performed, the fracture stabilized by cross-pinning or an AO plate, after which the arterial repair is performed.

COMPLICATIONS

Malunion

Failure to correct the apex posterior angulation will result in a genu recurvatum deformity. Failure to obtain anatomic alignment of the fracture site in the coronal plane may result in varus or valgus malalignment.[4] These deformities, when present, may require a corrective osteotomy.

Knee Stiffness

In general, knee stiffness is not frequently seen in a young child. However, in the adolescent, there may be some adhesions in the suprapatellar pouch, which may lead to knee stiffness.[2] For this reason, once the fracture exhibits good callus, a hinged cast may be used in the adolescent patient.

Neurovascular Complications

Vascular injuries, such as intimal tears and lacerations, ideally are treated by a vascular surgeon after first reducing and stabilizing the fracture. In some delayed cases, fixation of the fracture may further delay the vascular repair, and temporary stabilization may be obtained using skeletal traction or cross-pinning; definitive fixation of the fracture may be performed following the vascular repair.

SUMMARY

Supracondylar fractures of the femur not involving the physis are less common than physeal injuries of the distal femur and are usually secondary to severe direct trauma. The major complications encountered are secondary to vascular injury of the associated femoral artery and malunion due to the tendency of the distal fragment to be pulled into flexion due to the unopposed action of the gastrocnemius. Reduction can usually be achieved by closed means with the knee flexed to reduce the pull on the gastrocnemius floating distal fragment.

REFERENCES

1. Crawford AH: Fractures about the knee in children. Orthop Clin North Am 7:639, 1976
2. Rang M: Femoral shaft: supracondylar fractures. p. 277. In: Children's Fractures. 2nd Ed. JB Lippincott, Philadelphia, 1983
3. Staheli L: Fractures of the shaft of the femur. p. 1147. In Rockwood CA, Wilkins KE, King RF (eds): Fractures in Children. 3rd Ed. JB Lippincott, Philadelphia, 1991
4. Ogden JA: Distal femoral metaphyseal injuries. p. 721. In: Skeletal Injury in the Child. 2nd Ed. WB Saunders, Philadelphia, 1990

31

Supracondylar (Physeal) Fractures of the Femur

Jacques D'Astous

Avoid procedures that are a triumph of technique over reason.

DESCRIPTION AND INCIDENCE

Distal femoral epiphyseal injuries account for 1 to 6 percent of all epiphyseal injuries[1-4] and 9 to 16 percent of epiphyseal separations in the lower extremities.[2,5] Two-thirds of the children suffering distal femoral physeal fractures are adolescents. Most injuries occur as a result of an injury suffered in a sports-related activity. The most frequent fracture patterns observed are Salter-Harris types I and II, although Salter-Harris types III, IV, and V are not infrequently seen.[6,7] The type V injury frequently occurs in association with a type II injury and is responsible for growth plate arrest in as high as 40 to 50 percent of physeal fractures of the distal femur.[1,3,7]

Historically, these fractures were most frequently associated with "cartwheel" injuries.[1,4,7,8] Young boys, attempting to jump on a wagon, caught their lower limb in the spokes of the wheel and would sustain a hyperextension injury to the distal femur. In modern times, sports account for 49 percent of distal femoral physeal injuries, pedestrians hit by automobiles, 25 percent, and falls, 12 percent.[3] Among the other less common mechanisms of injury are obstetrical injury to the distal femoral physis occurring at birth.[3,7]

ANATOMY

The distal femoral physis is the largest and most rapidly growing of all the physes in the child and adolescent, accounting for 70 percent of the longitudinal growth of the femur and 37 percent of the longitudinal growth of the lower extremity.[3] The physis itself is extra-articular. The capsule inserts on the epiphysis distal to the growth plate and varus/valgus injuries to the knee may thus transmit considerable forces across the growth plate. These forces, combined with a deep intercondylar notch separating the condyles, imparting a relative weakness of the central epiphysis, may facilitate Salter-Harris types III and IV fractures of the distal femoral epiphysis. The epiphyseal component of the fracture most often begins in the intercondylar notch.

The distal femoral physeal plate is horizontal but undulates from medial to lateral as well as from anterior to posterior.[3,7] Consequently, shearing forces across the growth plate may damage the germinal cells, causing growth arrest even in simple Salter-Harris type I and type II injuries, which are usually associated with a good prognosis in other physes. As well, the high-energy force required to cause this fracture plus impingement of the metaphysis into the germinal layer of the physis results in the highest incidence of growth arrest of any physeal injury in the child (Fig. 31-1).

The distal femoral epiphysis is also in very close proximity to the popliteal artery, which lies directly on the posterior surface of the distal femur and is subject to injury in the extension type of distal femoral epiphyseal fracture with apex posterior angulation[3] (Fig. 31-2). Similarly, the common peroneal nerve can be stretched with varus or medial rotation forces or it may be injured by a direct blow to the posterolateral aspect of the knee as in a blow from a football helmet.[3]

MECHANISM OF INJURY

Direct

A direct anterior blow to the extended knee, such as occurs in a football tackle, causes a hyperextension or valgus type of injury with corresponding angulation and displacement at the fracture site (Fig. 31-3).[1,3,7,9] Similarly, hockey players sliding into the boards on a flexed knee may suffer a fracture of the distal femoral physis with posterior displacement of the epiphysis.

Indirect

Forced bending of the distal femur when the foot is fixed or firmly planted or alternatively, wrenching the lower leg against a fixed thigh, lead to extension or valgus types of injuries to the distal femoral physis.[7,10] As in other joints in children, the medial and lateral collateral ligaments of the knee are extremely strong and well anchored into bone by Sharpey's fibers. They seldom rupture and are much stronger than the adjacent, thick growth plate of the distal femur.

Valgus Force

Valgus injury usually produces a type II physeal fracture in which the periosteum is ruptured on the medial side, the distal femoral epiphysis is displaced laterally,

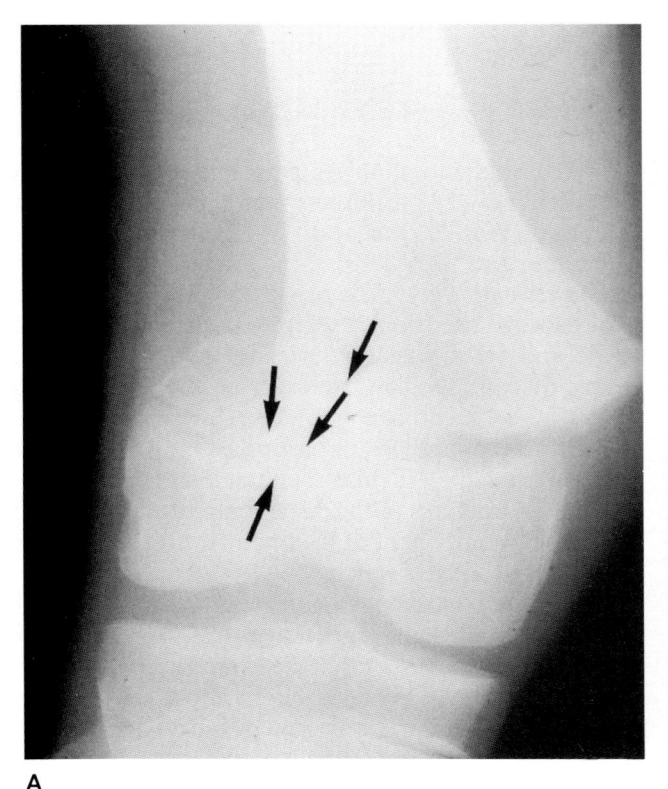

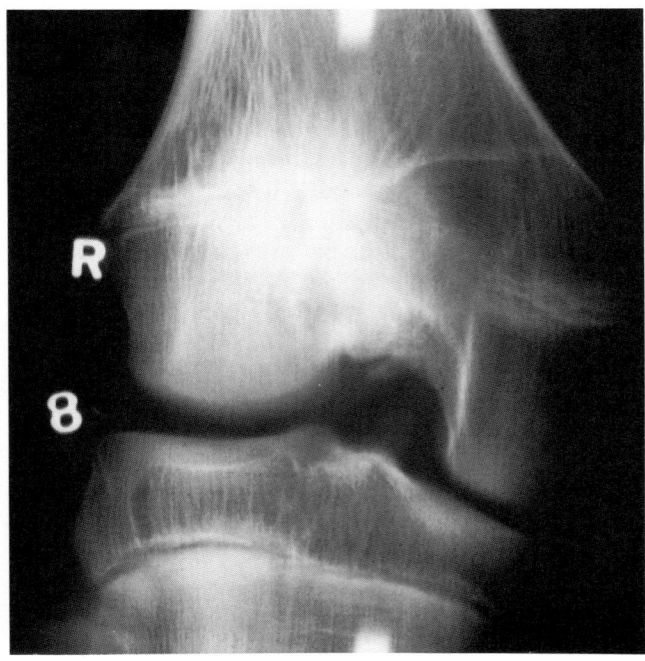

Fig. 31-1. (A) Type II fracture of the distal femur with impingement of the metaphysis into the germinal layer of the physis resulting in a central growth arrest. (B) Two years later.

Supracondylar (Physeal) Fractures of the Femur / 571

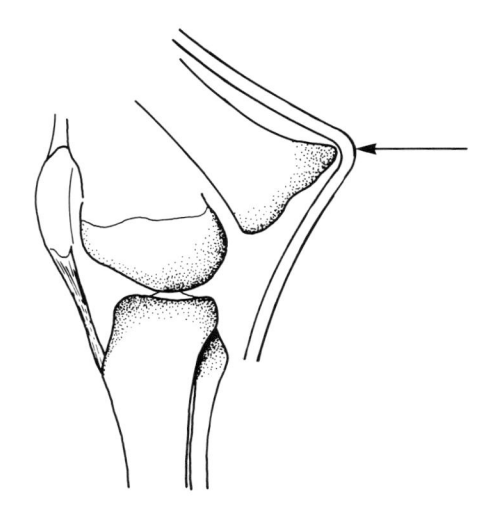

Fig. 31-2. Extension type of supracondylar fracture with apex posterior angulation causing potential injury to the neurovascular structures.

and the metaphyseal fragment is lateral. This same mechanism may also cause a Salter-Harris type III or IV injury of the medial femoral condyle.

Varus Force

Varus injury results in a Salter-Harris type I or type II fracture with medial displacement of the distal femoral epiphysis and the triangular metaphyseal fragment is medial. As with the valgus type of injury, a Salter-Harris type III or IV injury of the lateral femoral condyle may occur.

Hyperextension Force

A hyperextension force to the knee usually results in an anterior displacement of the epiphysis and posterior displacement of the distal femoral metaphysis and may cause direct injury to the popliteal artery.

Hyperflexion Forces

Hyperflexion of the knee or an anterior blow on a flexed knee leads to posterior displacement of the distal femoral epiphysis. This displacement may also cause injury to the posterior popliteal vessels.

CLASSIFICATION

Distal femoral physeal fractures may be classified according to the Salter-Harris classification or according to the direction of displacement.[3]

Salter-Harris

Type I

Type I fractures may be seen in obstetrical injuries of the newborn or they may mimic a sprain of the medial collateral ligament of the knee if undisplaced. This type of physeal injury, although more common in younger children, may also be encountered in teenagers, though less commonly than type II injuries (Figs. 31-4 and 31-5).

Type II

Type II fractures are the most common distal femoral physeal fractures.[3,6,7] The most frequently seen pattern is one of valgus angulation, with lateral displacement of the epiphysis and a lateral triangular metaphyseal fragment, producing the so called Thurston-Holland sign seen radiographically (Figs. 31-6 and 31-7).

Type III

Type III fractures may be unicondylar (Figs. 31-8A and 31-9) or bicondylar. The unicondylar fractures may be medial or lateral and are frequently displaced, al-

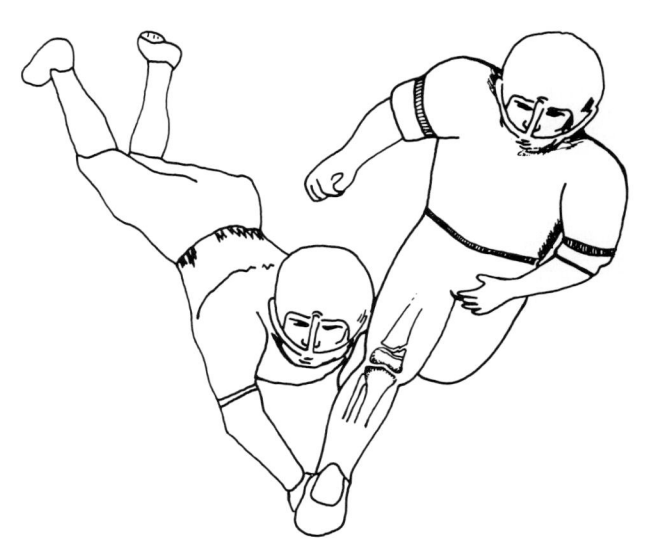

Fig. 31-3. Direct blow to extended knee causing a type II valgus fracture of the distal femur.

Fig. 31-4. Type I fracture distal femoral physis.

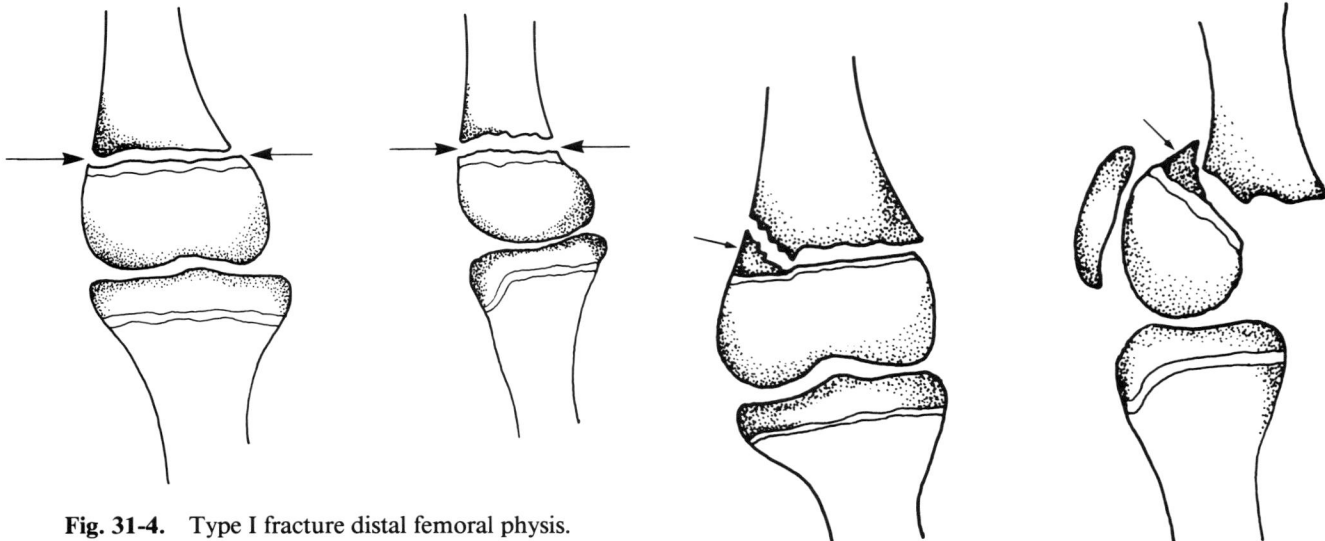

Fig. 31-6. Type II fracture distal femoral physis. The *arrows* point out the triangular metaphysial fragment sometimes referred to as the "Thurston-Holland sign" on the radiograph.

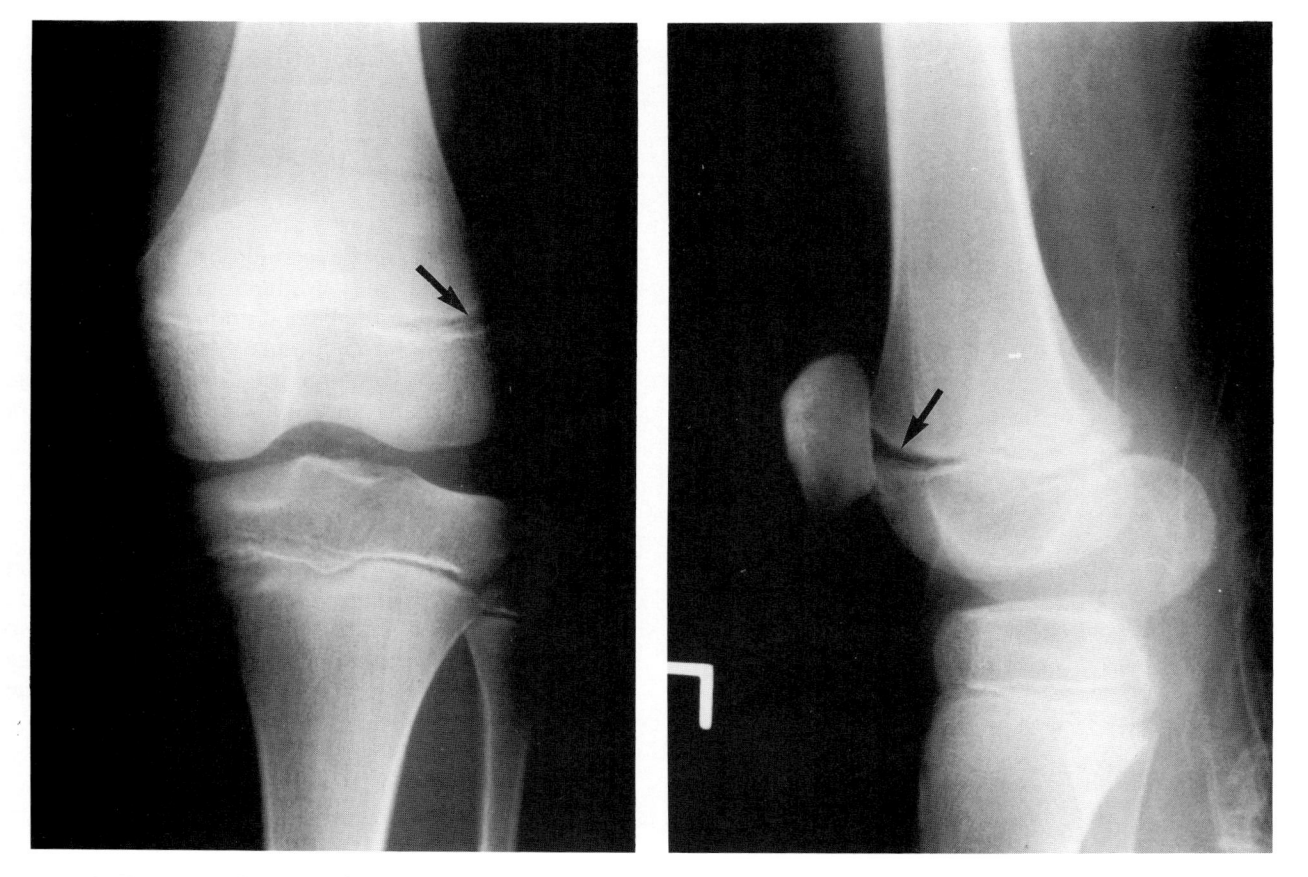

Fig. 31-5. **(Left)** Type I fracture in a 12-year-old boy. **(Right)** Note anterior opening of the physis seen on the lateral view.

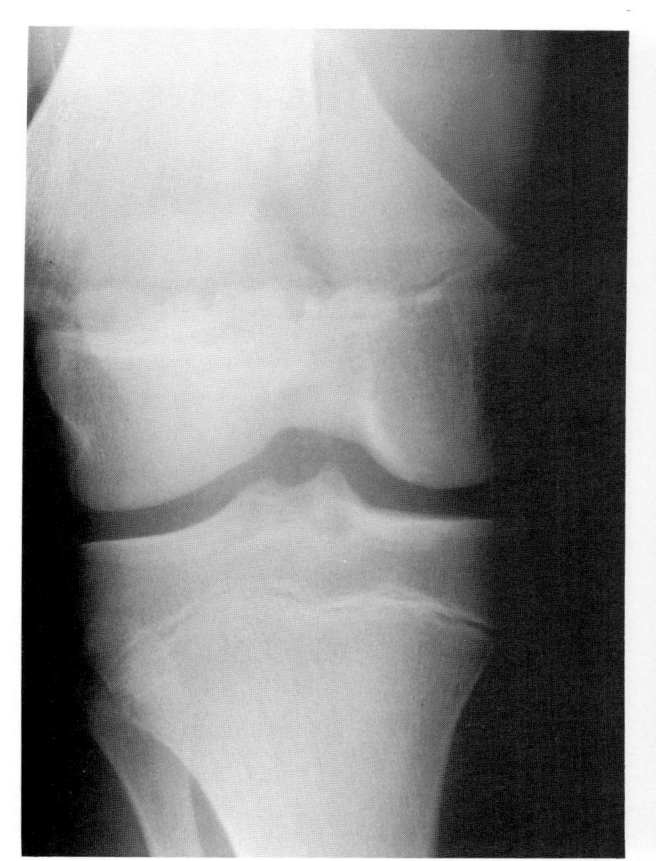

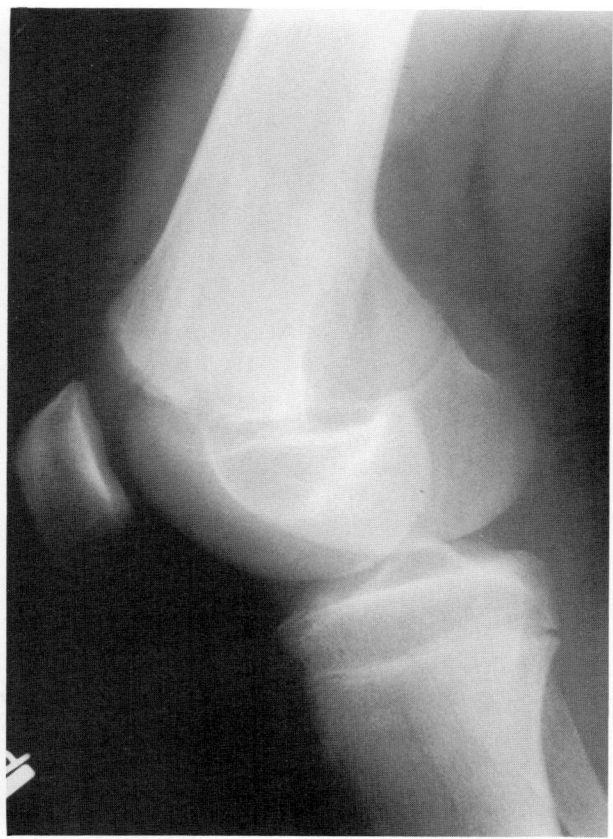

Fig. 31-7. Type II fracture distal femoral physis in a 12-year-old boy secondary to a varus strain of the knee joint, the triangular metaphyseal fragment being located on the medial side.

though wide displacement is usually prevented by the attachment of the anterior cruciate ligament on the medial femoral condyle and the posterior cruciate ligament on the medial femoral condyle. One type of displacement often not appreciated is the open-book deformity in which the epiphyseal fracture gaps open 2 or 3 cm, usually at the front, hinging on the posterior periosteum. The only clue to this displacement on a plain radiograph, anteroposterior (AP) view, will be a widening of the distal femoral growth plate. Rarely, the fracture line through the epiphysis is in the coronal plane (Fig. 31-8B) and usually involves the posterior part of the medial or lateral femoral condyle.

Type IV

Type IV fractures, similar to the type III fractures may be unicondylar (medial, lateral) or bicondylar (T-condylar, Y-condylar). The fragment is usually displaced proximally resulting in a malalignment of both

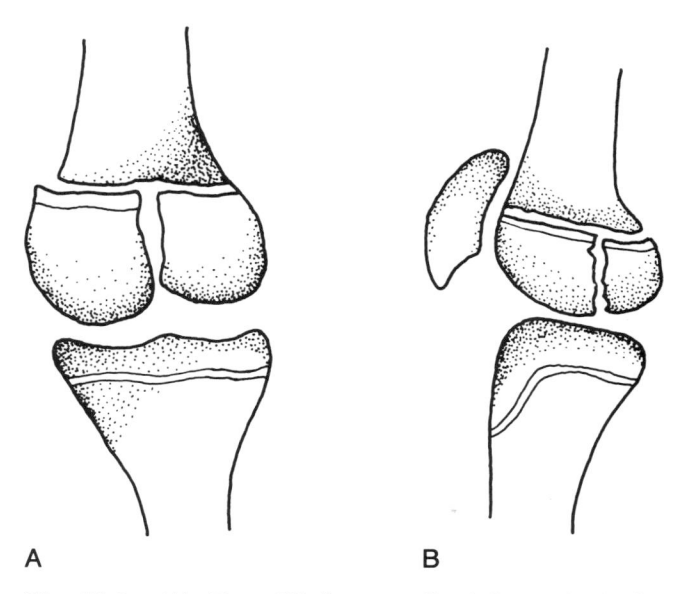

Fig. 31-8. (A) Type III fracture distal femoral physis. (B) Type III fracture occurring in the coronal plane.

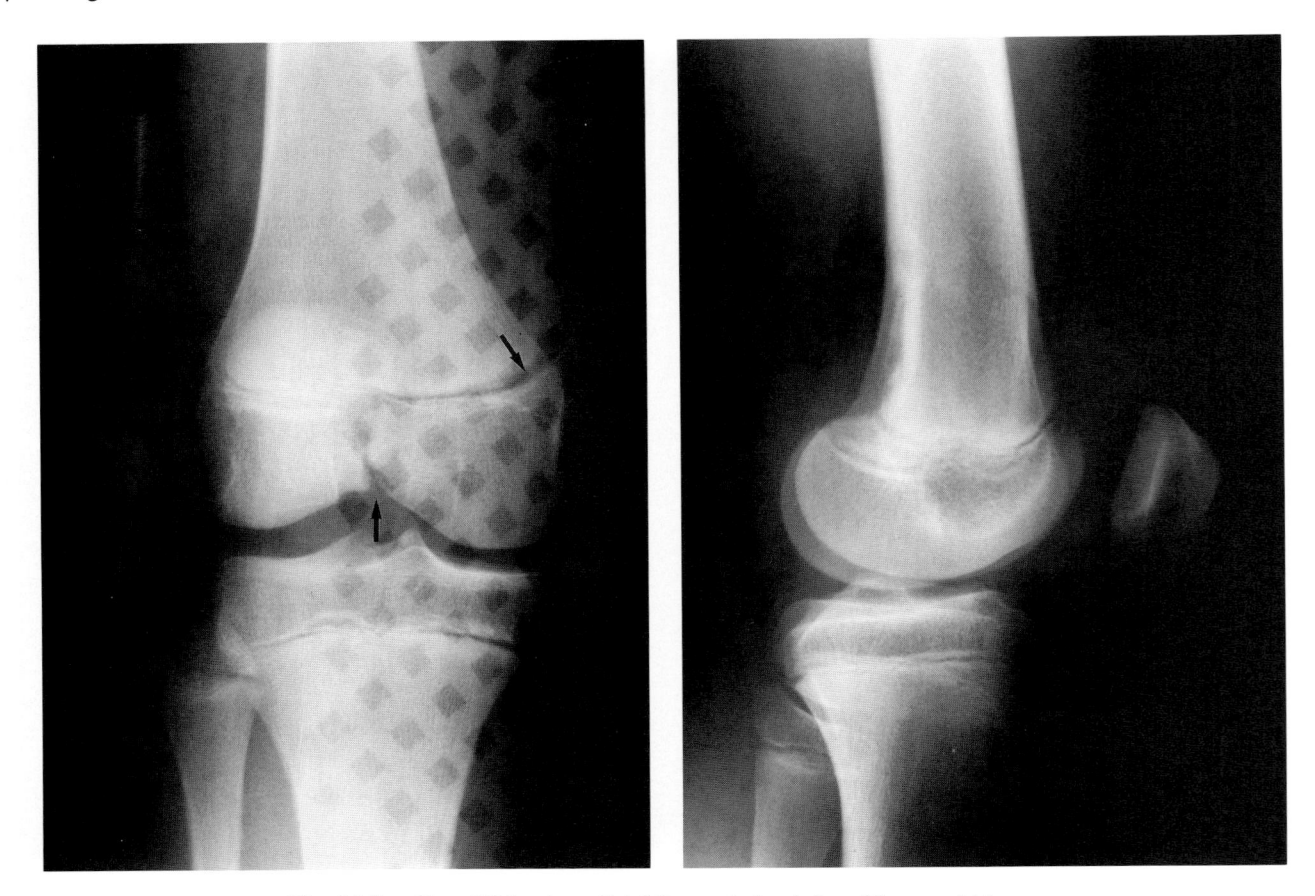

Fig. 31-9. Type III fracture distal femoral physis in a 12-year-old boy.

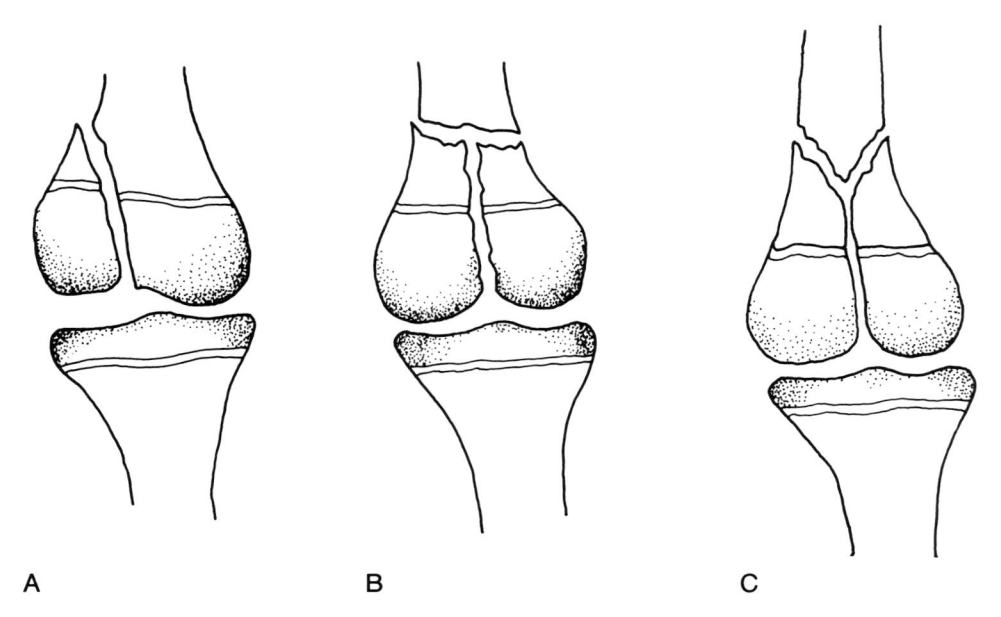

Fig. 31-10. Type IV fractures of the distal femoral physis. **(A)** Unicondylar. **(B)** Bicondylar, T-type **(C)** Bicondylar, Y-type.

the growth plate and articular surface of the joint (Figs. 31-10 and 31-11).

Type V

Type V fractures usually are diagnosed in retrospect and manifest themselves as a growth arrest. It must be emphasized that a type V injury may occur in association with other types of physeal fractures and is seldom encountered as a purely isolated lesion (Fig. 31-12).

Ogden

Type VI

Ogden type VI fractures are difficult to diagnose radiologically as they represent an avulsion of the periphery of the growth plate in which the perichondrium and a sliver of underlying bone are avulsed and may lead to a peripheral bony bridge at the level of the growth plate. These are usually open fractures secondary to a penetrating wound such as a lawnmover blade, which shears off a portion of periosteum and perichondrial ring (Fig. 31-13).

Type VII

Ogden type VII fractures are osteochondral fractures of the femoral condyles, usually caused by a direct blow to the flexed knee, such as bicycle handlebars or the corner of a wall (Fig. 31-13).

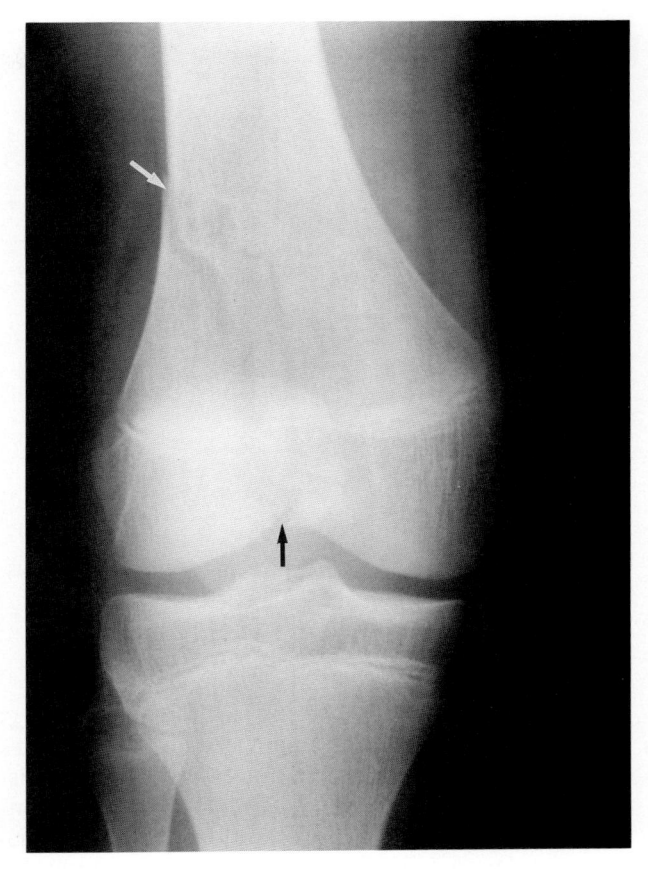

Fig. 31-11. Type IV fracture lateral femoral condyle in a 15-year-old boy.

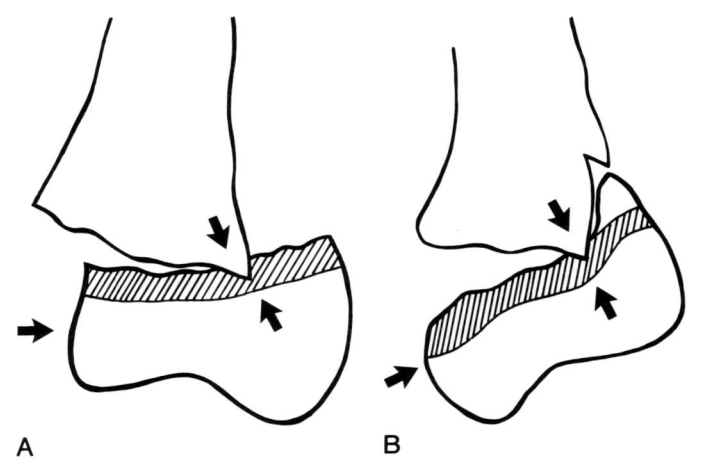

Fig. 31-12. (A) Type I and (B) Type II shear and compression associated with Type V fracture distal femoral physis.

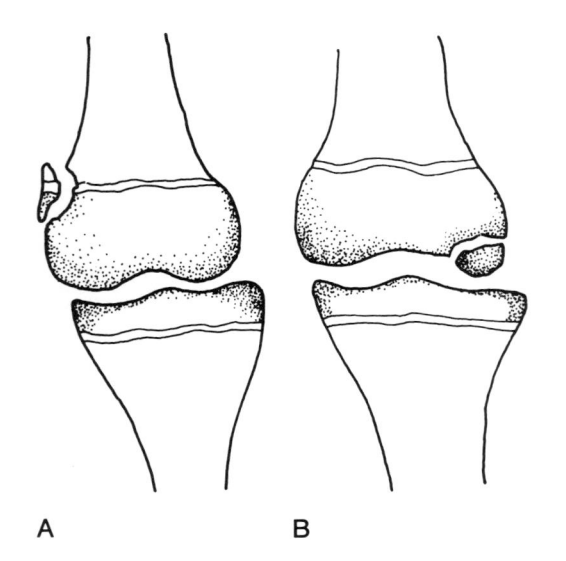

Fig. 31-13. (A) Type VI fracture distal femoral physis. (B) Type VII fracture distal femoral physis.

Direction of Displacement

The direction of displacement classification applies mostly to Salter-Harris types I and II fractures. The displacement of the epiphysis may be *anterior* (hyperextension injuries), *posterior* (birth injuries or direct blow), *medial* or *lateral* (Fig. 31-14). The medial or lateral displacement is the most common displacement and results from varus or valgus stresses applied to the distal femoral physis.

PHYSICAL EXAMINATION

Usually there is a history of major trauma to the knee accompanied by severe pain and inability to weight bear immediately after the accident. In infants with obstetrical injuries to the distal femoral physis, the usual history is one of pseudoparalysis of the injured leg following delivery.

The actual physical findings may vary somewhat, depending on the direction and degree of displacement of the fracture. The child usually keeps the knee flexed, secondary to hamstring spasm, and a knee effusion may be present, especially in the intra-articular Salter-Harris types III and IV injuries. There is soft tissue swelling just proximal to the patella, and the overlying skin may be abraded or lacerated, depending on the mechanism of injury. In the undisplaced fracture, there may be no significant deformity noted, but careful palpation will reveal tenderness at the level of the physis, remembering that the growth plate is located at the upper pole of the patella. The undisplaced fracture can easily mimic an injury to the medial collateral, lateral collateral, or even anterior cruciate ligament; however, such ligamentous injuries are rare in children with open physes. If there is significant doubt between a ligamentous or physeal injury on physical examination, a valgus or varus stress test under anesthesia using the image intensifier can be diagnostic.

In the displaced fracture, there is frequently a deformity noted in the coronal plane resulting in a varus or valgus appearance of the knee. The metaphysis may be

Medial   Lateral   Anterior   Posterior

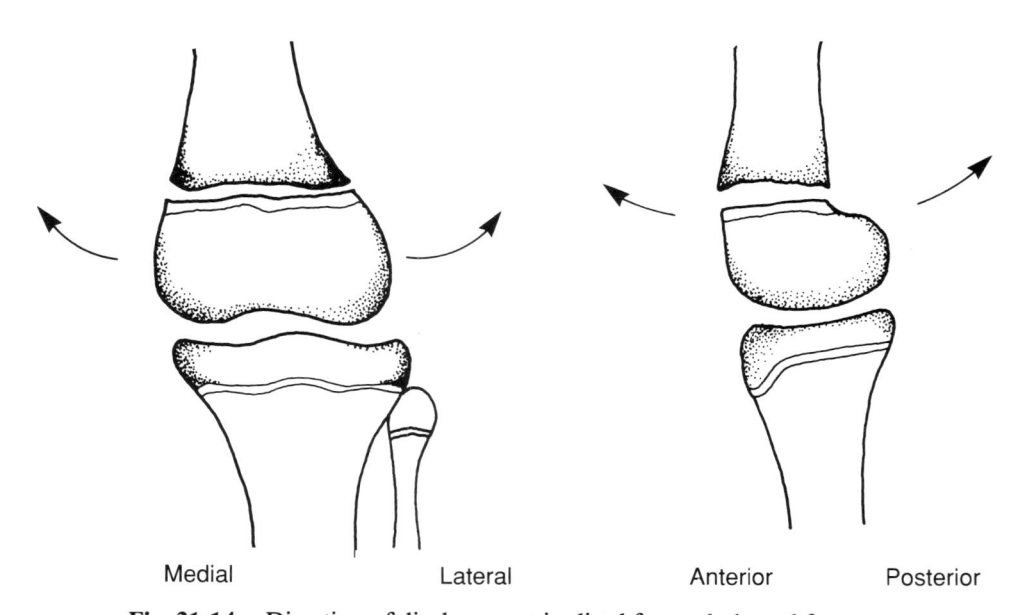

Fig. 31-14. Direction of displacement in distal femoral physeal fractures.

seen protruding medially or laterally beneath the muscle and skin and crepitus may be felt. In rare instances, a puncture wound from within may be produced by the sharp metaphyseal edge, converting the injury to an open fracture. When the epiphysis is displaced anteriorly, the patella looks abnormally prominent, whereas in posterior displacement of the epiphysis, the metaphysis may be prominent just proximal to the patella and a fullness is felt in the popliteal fossa.

Because of the close proximity of the distal femoral physis to the popliteal fossa, it is essential to perform a very careful neurovascular examination of the lower extremities and to document the presence or absence of the posterior tibial and dorsalis pedis pulse. Any evidence of cyanosis (venous compression) or pallor should be noted. Also, it is important to document the status of the common peroneal nerve and posterior tibial nerve with a careful motor and sensory examination. We must always remind ourselves that the fracture position as visualized on the radiograph is only the final resting position of the fragments and that, at the moment of impact, they may have been displaced three or four times this amount!

The signs and symptoms of vascular injury to the popliteal vessels are subtle due to the excellent collateral blood supply about the knee, which is usually sufficient to provide good perfusion of the skin in the entire lower limb. One may be lulled into a false sense of security regarding an intact blood supply if reliance is placed only on the appearance of the limb and good capillary filling. Pulses must be present; if not, an arteriogram should be performed.

As these fractures are high-energy injuries, often the result of a motor vehicle accident or a high-speed collision, it is imperative to look for other associated injuries, in particular, fractures of the patella and hip as well as compartment syndromes secondary to a crush injury to the limb.

RADIOLOGIC CHARACTERISTICS

In the presence of an undisplaced physeal injury, the only finding may be that of soft tissue swelling adjacent to the growth plate. Oblique views may be helpful to visualize a small Thurston-Holland sign, suggestive of a Salter-Harris type II fracture, or an undisplaced intercondylar fracture as seen with a Salter-Harris type III/IV fracture of the distal femur. Stress radiographs to assess the ligamentous stability of the knee may confirm the diagnosis of a Salter-Harris type III/IV fracture of the femoral condyle as evidenced by opening of the growth plate (Fig. 31-15). Repeat radiographs done at 14 to 21 days postinjury may show some periosteal reaction, which would confirm a clinical diagnosis of an undisplaced distal femoral physeal injury (Fig. 31-16).

Radiographic evidence of premature closure of the physis usually becomes evident within 6 months from the time of injury and is best seen by looking for presence of Harris growth arrest lines converging at the site of the physeal bridge.[1,11] Growth plate arrest of the distal physis is frequently central and is best mapped out in extent using tomography (Fig. 31-17) (see Ch. 62).

In the presence of obvious arterial injury, arteriography may not always be necessary, since the general region of the arterial trauma is known, but it may provide some information with respect to the exact location and type of arterial injury as well as the extent of the collateral circulation present.

DIFFERENTIAL DIAGNOSIS

Distal femoral epiphyseal injuries can mimic ligamentous injuries of the knee, such as tears of the medial collateral, lateral collateral, or anterior cruciate ligaments. The key to making the diagnosis is a careful diligent clinical examination. In distal femoral physeal injuries, the area of maximum tenderness is at the growth plate, which is usually at the level of the superior pole of the patella. In medial or lateral ligament injuries, the tenderness often occurs at the distal insertion of the ligaments or along their midsubstance. Occasionally, if stress radiographs are required for a suspected tear of the medial collateral ligament, gapping at the level of the distal femoral physis confirms the diagnosis of a distal femoral physeal injury.

TREATMENT OF PHYSEAL INJURY OF THE DISTAL FEMUR

General Principles

The goal of treatment for distal femoral physeal injuries is to obtain and maintain a near-anatomic reduction. An accurate anatomic reduction is essential if the fracture is intra-articular or if the fracture is in the coronal plane, producing varus or valgus deformity at the fracture site. In the sagittal plane, it is possible to accept 15 to 20 degrees of apex anterior or posterior angulation,

578 / Management of Pediatric Fractures

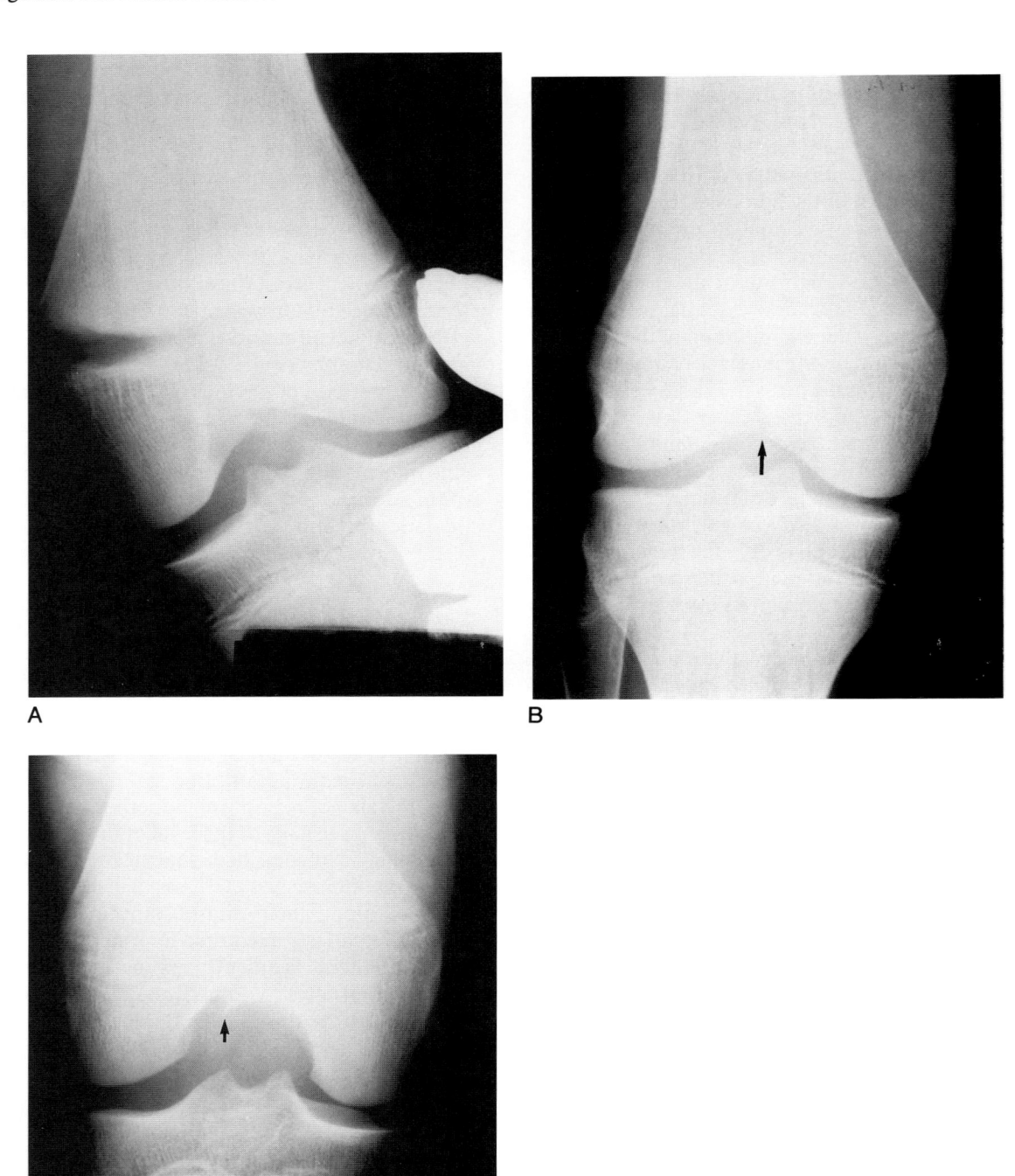

Fig. 31-15. A 15-year-old boy suspected of having a tear of the medial collateral ligament. Valgus stress radiographs revealed the type III fracture of the medial femoral condyle **(A),** which could be seen retrospectively on the AP **(B)** and notch views **(C).**

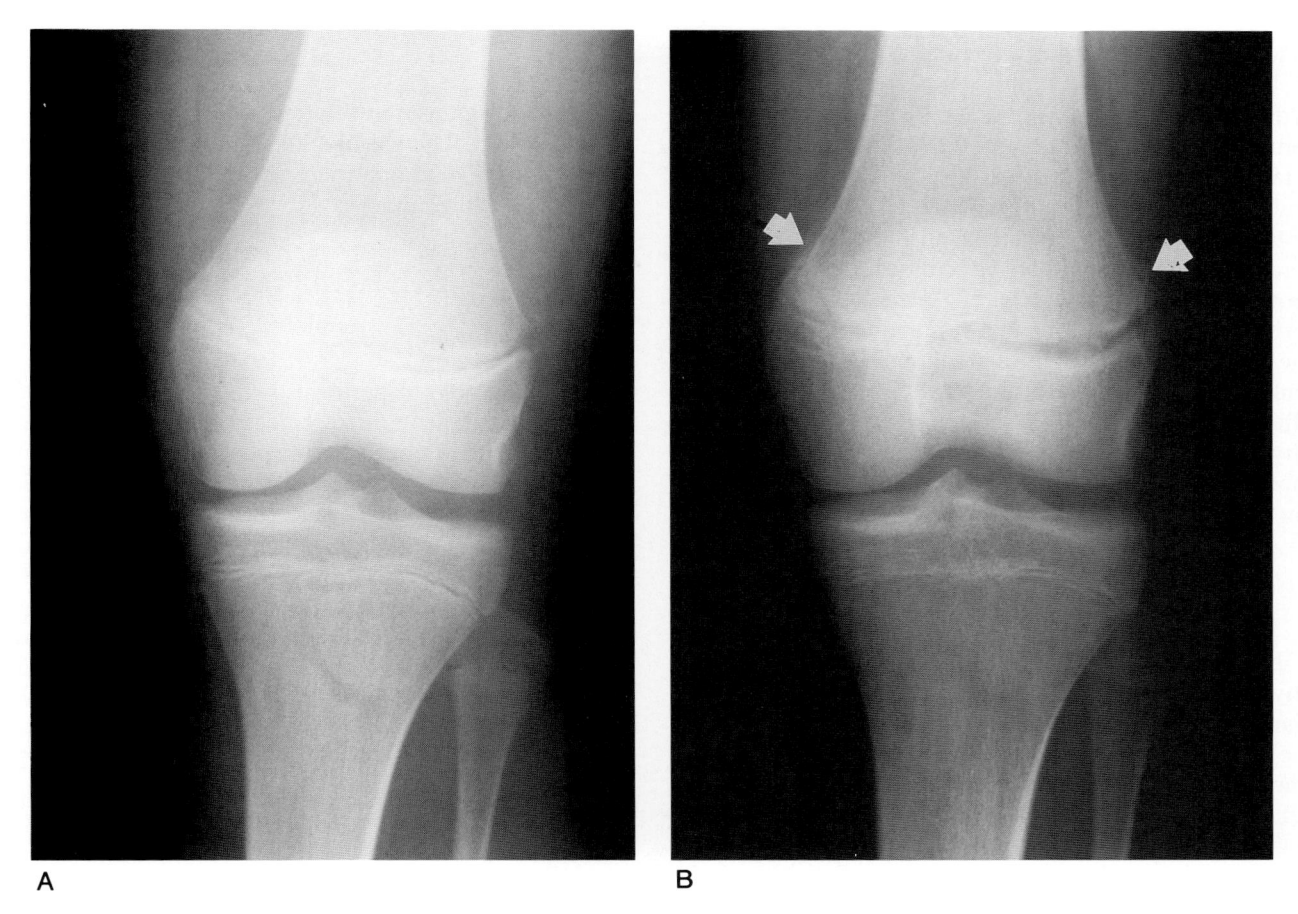

Fig. 31-16. Suspected distal femoral physeal fracture. **(A)** Initial radiographs inconclusive but **(B)** radiograph taken 4 weeks later shows medial and lateral periosteal reaction confirming the distal femoral physeal fracture.

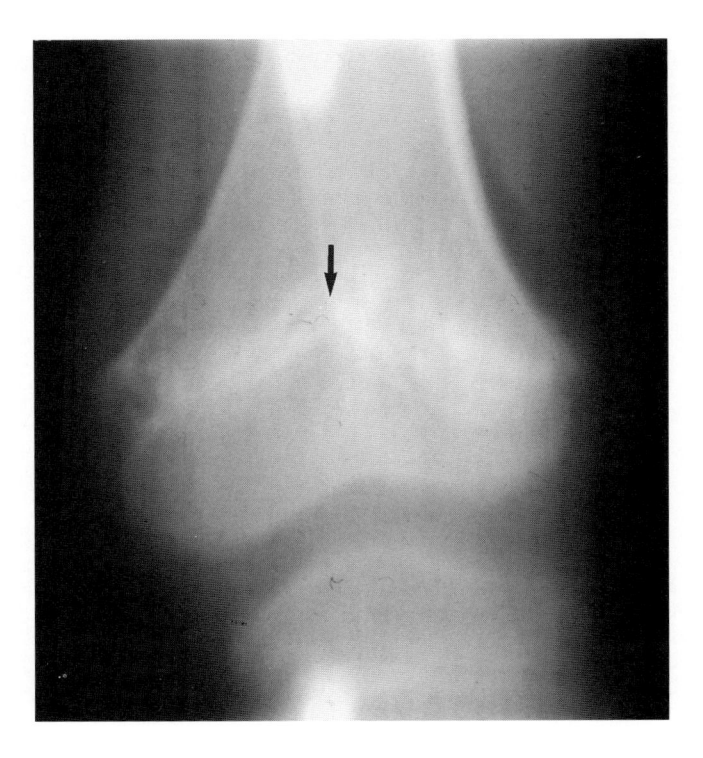

Fig. 31-17. Central growth arrest resulting from a Type II distal femoral physeal fracture treated by closed reduction.

providing that there are at least 3 to 4 years of growth remaining. It is useful to remember that the lower leg is attached to the distal femoral epiphysis by strong collateral ligaments and that the leg may be used as a lever to obtain closed reduction, although it is best to avoid a forceful reduction in order to decrease the possibility of a growth plate injury. The Salter-Harris types I and II injuries are very analogous to a supracondylar fracture of the humerus in children. In small children, placing the child prone and using the same principles of reduction is often helpful[8] (Fig. 31-18). In the case of distal femoral physeal injury in infants, most can be treated by splinting the leg in extension as long as the varus or valgus alignment is satisfactory.

Undisplaced Fractures

The goal of treatment for undisplaced distal femoral physeal fractures is to relieve pain and to prevent displacement. If there is a tense hemarthrosis, aspiration of the knee will make the child more comfortable. The fracture needs to be immobilized in a well-molded cylinder or long-leg cast with the knee in approximately 20 degrees of flexion.

The child should then be seen at approximately 1, 2, 4, and 6 weeks postinjury and radiographs should be performed to ensure that there has been no displacement of the fracture and that healing is progressing satisfactorily. After 4 to 6 weeks, the cast is removed and gentle active-assisted range of motion exercises as well as isometric quadriceps exercises are started and partial weightbearing is allowed. The use of a knee immobilizer is recommended until good quadriceps power and control of the knee has been regained.

Displaced Fractures

Closed Reduction

It is preferable to perform a closed reduction under general anesthesia in order to decrease the muscle spasm and possibility of trauma to the physis and also to ensure maximum comfort for the child. If there is a tense hemarthrosis, it should be aspirated to facilitate the reduction and relieve discomfort. To perform the reduction, gentle longitudinal traction is applied after which the deformity is increased and the edge of the epiphysis and metaphysis are realigned, followed by realignment of the lower leg with respect to the thigh to complete the reduction. It is important to be as gentle as possible to avoid grinding the growth plate against the metaphyseal corner, which could further damage the physis. Anterior displacement of the distal fragment can be reduced with the patient supine or prone. I prefer the supine position. With the hip and knee flexed to approximately 60 degrees, to decrease the muscle tension, longitudinal traction is applied and the anterior displacement is corrected by direct anterior pressure on the epiphysis. Once the reduction is obtained, the knee is flexed to 90 degrees (Fig. 31-19). The neurovascular status must be verified after reduction and the adequacy of the reduction must be confirmed by fluoroscopy. If the fracture feels stable, a long-leg cast with the knee flexed to 90 degrees is applied. Some authors have recommended the use of a hip spica for potentially unstable fractures, but cross-pinning with smooth pins plus a long-leg cast will provide adequate fracture stability (Figs. 31-20 and 31-21).[3,7,12,13,15–17] At approximately 3 weeks, the long-leg cast is changed and the knee is brought out to 45 degrees of flexion and the percutaneous pins removed. By 6 weeks the fracture is usually sufficiently healed to allow knee mobilization. The same therapy program that was outlined for the undisplaced fracture is started at 6 weeks.

In posteriorly displaced fractures, the child is placed in the supine position, longitudinal traction is applied with the knee slightly flexed while an assistant pulls gently upward under the distal femoral epiphysis and pushes downward on the distal femoral metaphysis. Once the reduction is obtained, the knee is immobilized in full extension to tighten the medial head of the gastrocnemius and posterior periosteum thus stabilizing the reduction.

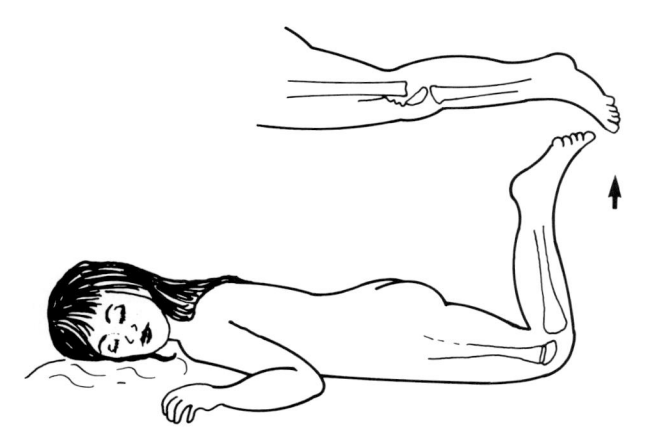

Fig. 31-18. Closed reduction of a distal femoral physeal fracture with the child in the prone position. Longitudinal traction is applied followed by flexion of the knee and an upwardly directed pull similar to reducing an extension type of supracondylar fracture of the humerus. (Adapted from Rang,[8] with permission.)

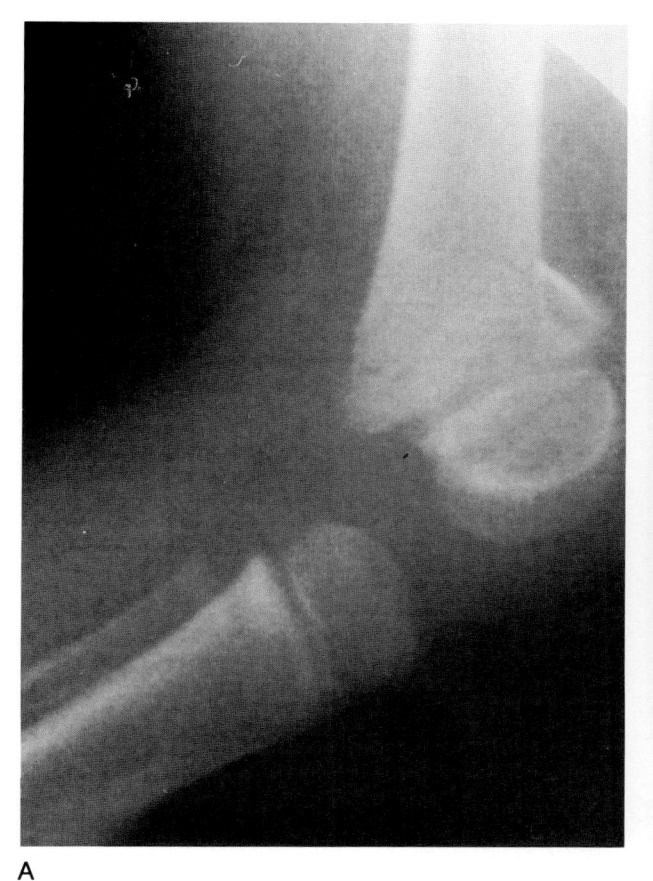

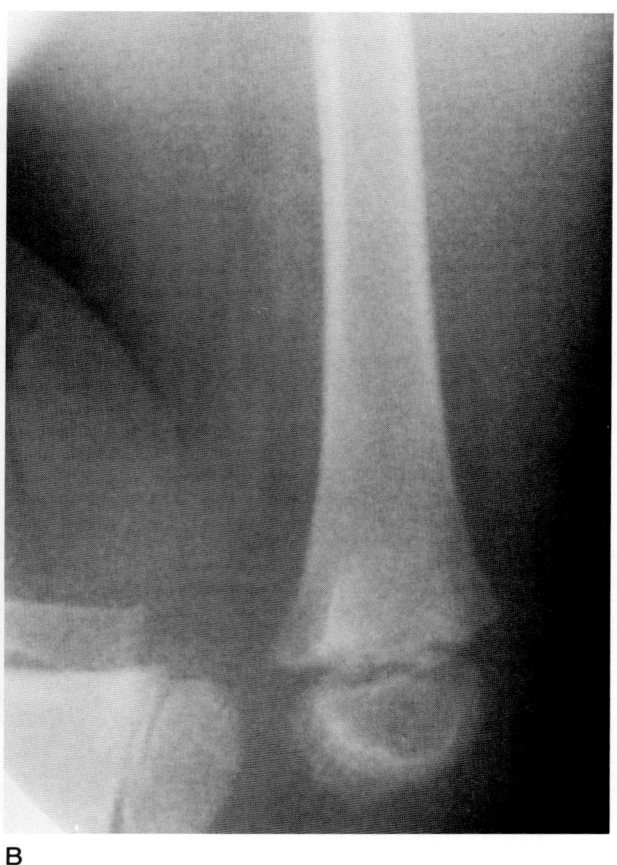

Fig. 31-19. Type II fracture of the distal femur (**A**) treated by closed reduction and a long-leg cast with the knee flexed to 90 degrees in a 3-year-old boy (**B**).

When closed reduction is obtained but is felt to be unstable, the use of crossed smooth pins, inserted from distal to proximal starting just proximal to the articular cartilage of the femoral condyles, is the preferred method of stabilization.[3,7,12,13,15-17] The pins are left protruding through the skin and the ends are bent at 90 degrees to prevent migration of the pins. If there is a large metaphyseal fragment, fixation may also be obtained by using a cannulated cancellous lag screw inserted parallel to the growth plate to fix the metaphyseal fragment to the distal metaphysis and thereby stabilize the fracture (Figs. 31-22 and 31-23). If percutaneous pins have been used, these can be safely removed at 3 weeks as growth plate fractures heal rapidly and are usually stable by 3 weeks postinjury.

Open Reductions

Open reduction should be performed when a stable anatomic reduction cannot be achieved or closed reduction is impossible because of interposed soft tissue. The incision should be centered over the palpable end of the distal femoral metaphysis and after incising the skin, subcutaneous tissue and deep fascia, the muscle fibers are spread, using blunt dissection, and the interposed muscle and periosteum are removed from the fracture

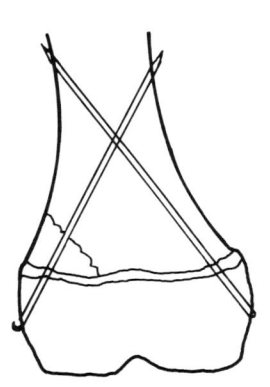

Fig. 31-20. Cross K-wire technique to stabilize unstable Type II fractures of the distal femur.

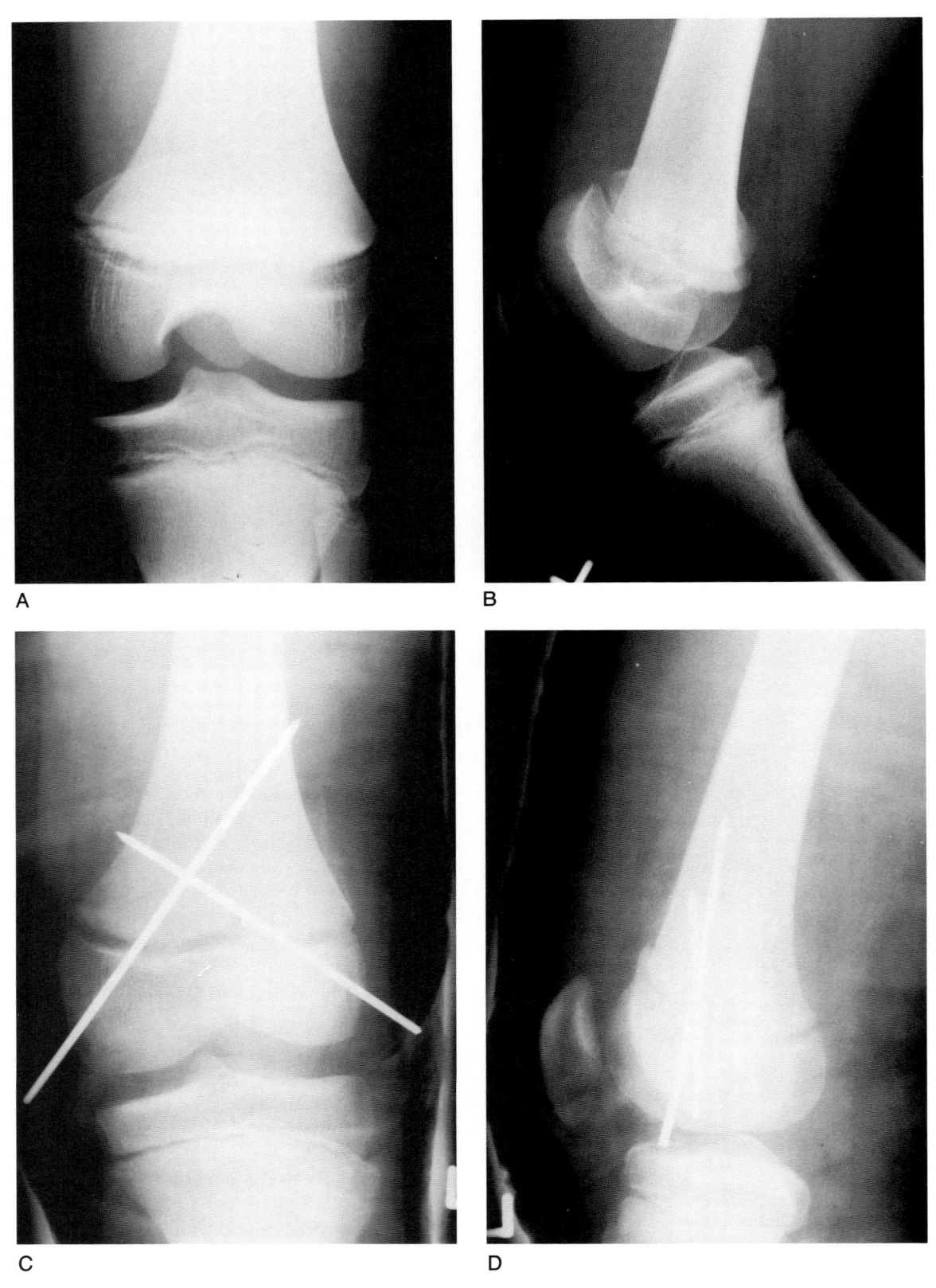

Fig. 31-21. Type II fracture of the distal femur **(A&B)** treated by closed reduction and cross-pinning with smooth K-wires to provide stability **(C&D)**.

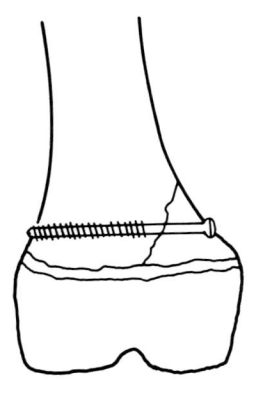

Fig. 31-22. Lag compression screw to internally fix an unstable Type II distal femoral fracture.

site. A gentle reduction is obtained under direct visualization, and it is preferable not to use skids or any type of levering instruments to prevent further trauma to the physis. Following the open reduction, the fracture can be internally fixed by cross-pinning or by using a cancellous lag screw placed parallel to the growth plate fixing the metaphyseal fragment to the main part of the distal femoral metaphysis.[11] Even when the fracture is deemed to be stable at the time of open reduction, internal fixation should still be used, since it is such a simple and safe technique, if only to prevent having to repeat the open reduction.

In the Salter-Harris III/IV fractures of the distal femoral physis, it is imperative to obtain an anatomic reduction at the level of the articular surface of the knee joint as well as at the physis. For this reason an arthrotomy (medial arthrotomy for medial femoral condyle, lateral arthrotomy for lateral femoral condyle) is performed and the fracture is reduced under direct vision and transfixed with smooth K-wires.[3,7,11] Following this, fixation is secured, using a 6.5-mm AO cannulated cancellous lag screw (Figs. 31-24 and 31-25). The T- or Y-supracondylar fracture is somewhat more difficult to stabilize. Initially, the distal femoral joint surface is reduced anatomically and stabilized with one or two large fragment cannulated lag screws. Following this, the femoral con-

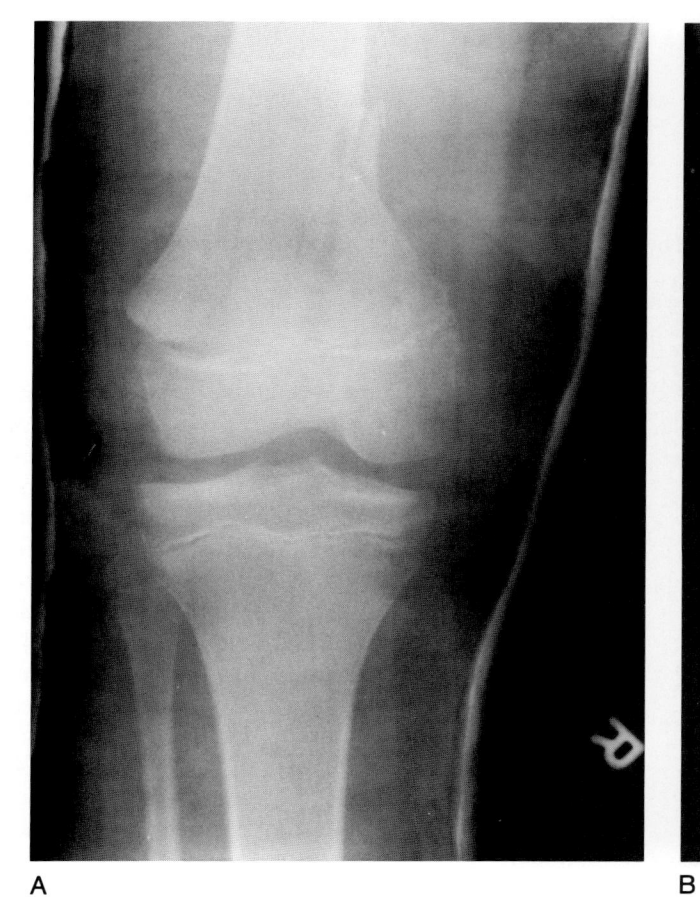

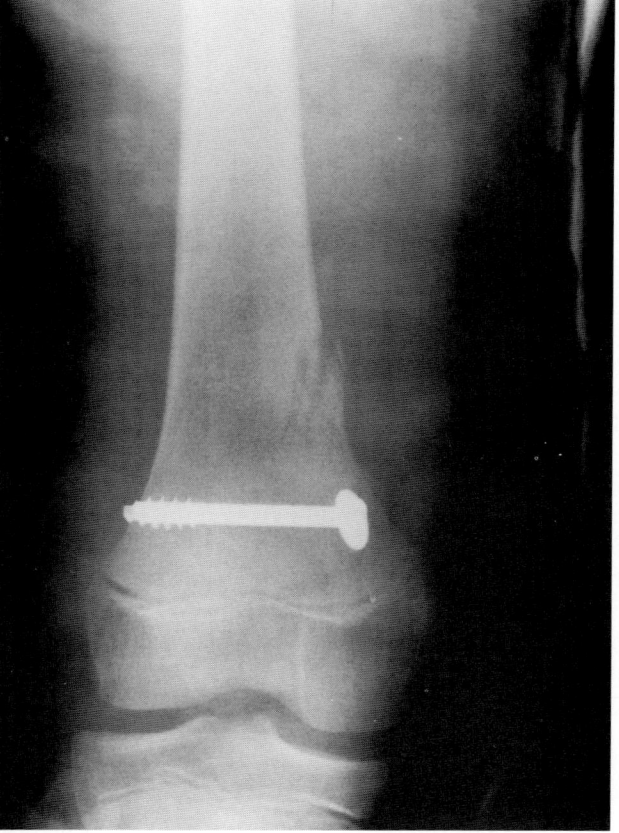

Fig. 31-23. Type II distal femoral fracture (**A**) treated by closed reduction and percutaneous fixation with a 6.5 mm cannulated AO lag compression screw (**B**).

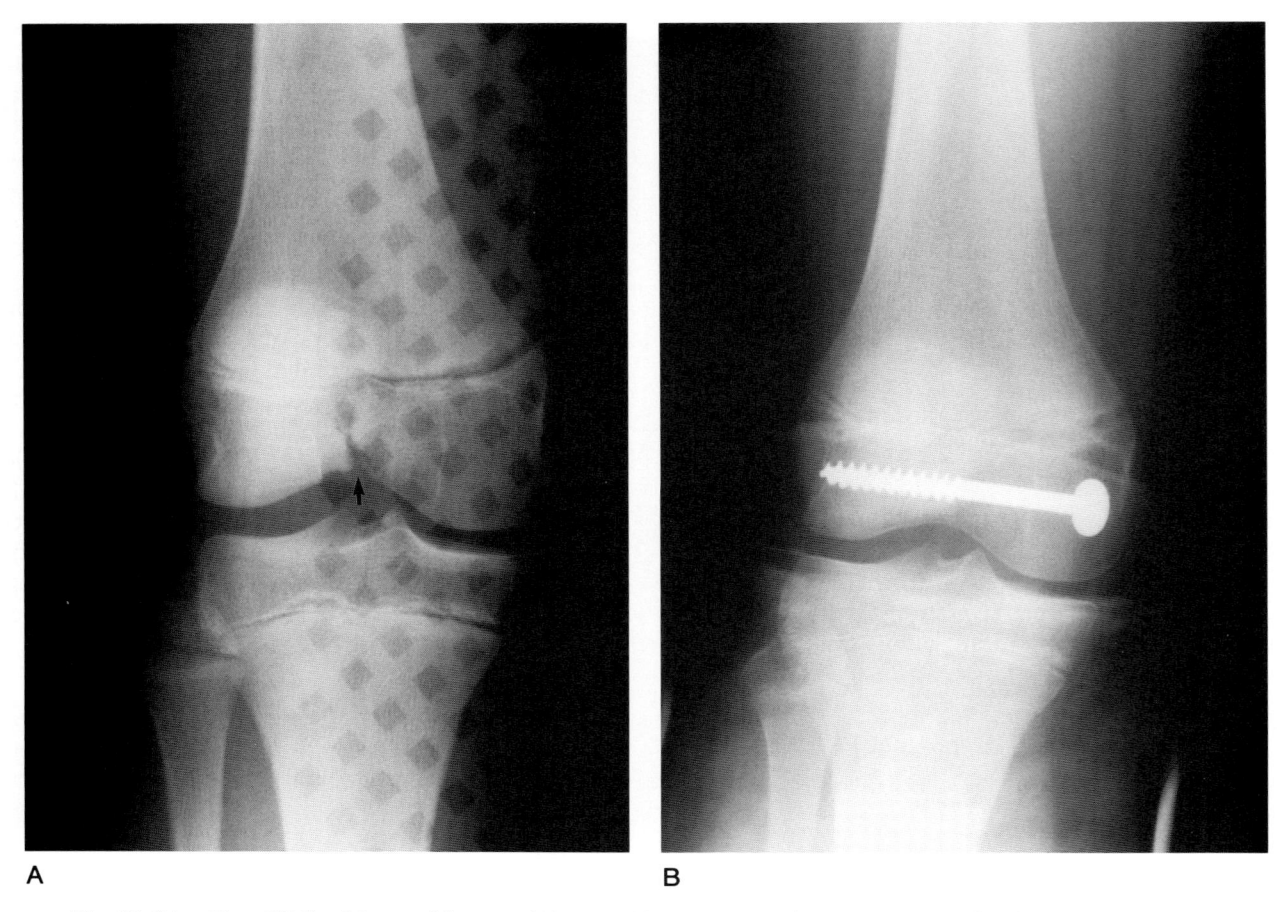

Fig. 31-24. Type III distal femoral fracture (**A**) treated by open reduction and lag screw fixation in a 12-year-old girl who had an ipsilateral fracture of the tibia (**B**).

dyles are reduced onto the metaphysis and fixation is obtained using large smooth crossed K-wires (Figs. 31-26 and 31-27). When the fracture through the physis is in the coronal plane, the reduction is performed under visual and fluoroscopic control, and the fracture may be stabilized by a screw with threads on both ends such as the Herbert screw. Postoperatively, the child should be immobilized in a long-leg cast, which may be changed to a hinged knee cast at 3 weeks if the fixation is stable enough to permit early motion. The lag screws are usually removed 3 to 6 months postoperatively.

Open Fractures

Usually, open fractures of the distal femoral physis are of a hyperextension type, with the distal femoral metaphysis protruding through the skin in the region of the popliteal fossa. The patient should be placed in the prone position, the wound irrigated with copious amounts of saline, after which the limb is prepped and draped in the usual fashion. The skin edges should be excised, any gross contamination removed, and the wound thoroughly irrigated. Any devascularized tissue should be debrided. The distal metaphyseal end of the femur should be inspected and debrided, after which a gentle open reduction should be performed, taking care not to injure the neurovascular bundle. The fracture may then be stabilized with crossed pins and the wound packed open if there was gross contamination or an undue delay in getting the patient to the operating room; otherwise the skin may be loosely approximated. In cases that require vascular repair, it is preferable to perform the open reduction and cross K-wire stabilization prior to the vascular repair, providing that this brief delay does not jeopardize the viability of the limb.

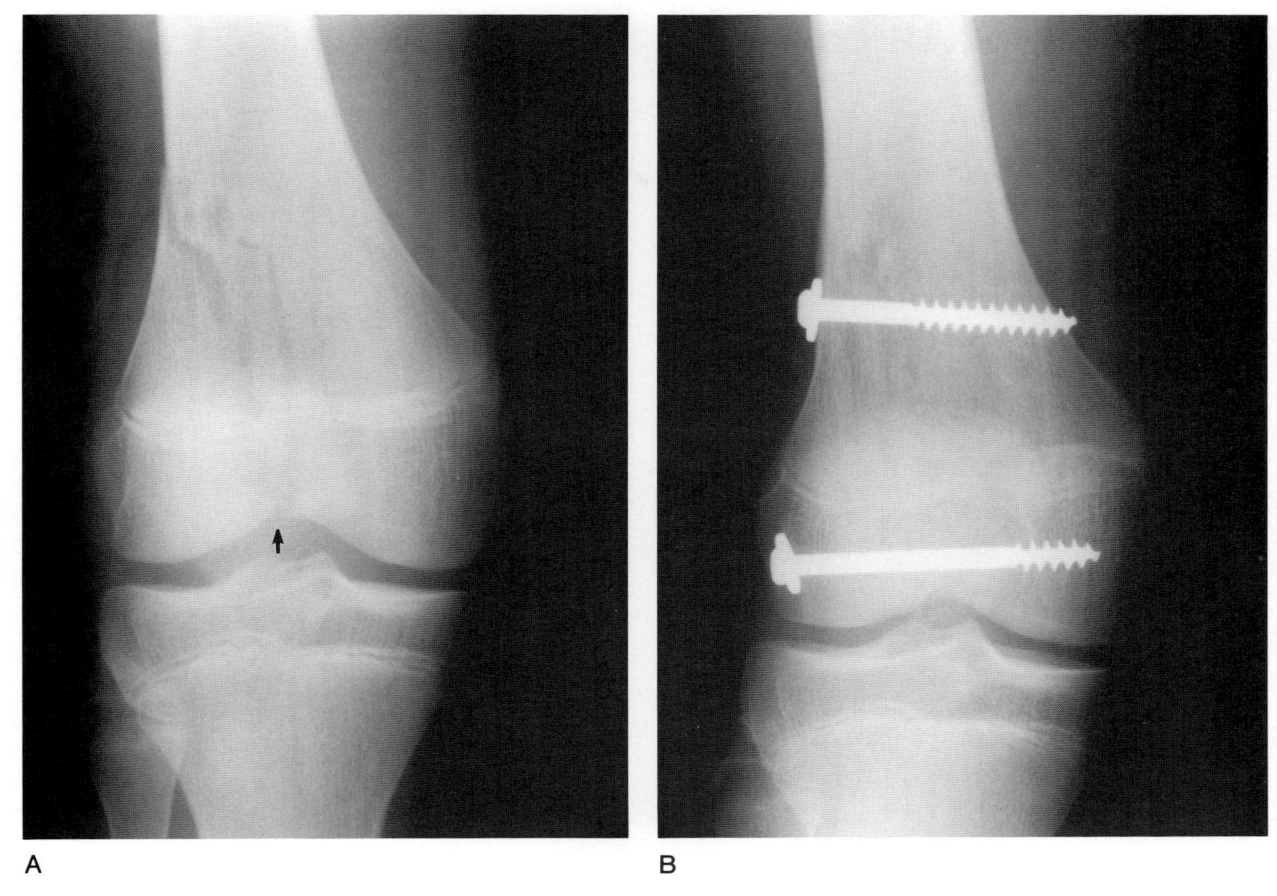

Fig. 31-25. Type IV distal femoral fracture **(A)**, treated by open reduction and fixation with two lag screws, one in the metaphysis and one in the epiphysis, taking care not to cross the growth plate **(B)**.

Fractures with Associated Arterial Injury

In the presence of an arterial injury, the fracture should be reduced and stabilized as quickly as possible to facilitate and protect a good vascular repair. Most commonly, the arterial injury is proximal to the knee joint and therefore a medial approach to the supracondylar region of the femur allows access to the fracture and to the popliteal artery (Fig. 31-28).

COMPLICATIONS

Because of the close proximity of the neurovascular structures to the distal femoral physis, injuries to the *popliteal artery* and *common peroneal nerve* may occur.[3,7,15] The main complications seen in these fractures are late, and include *malunion, progressive angulation, leg length discrepancy* and *knee stiffness.*[1,3,4,6,7,10,13,15-20] These complications are usually related directly or indirectly to physeal arrest. Occasionally, *late ligamentous laxity* may lead to symptoms of knee instability.[3,9,10,14,17]

Approximately 40 percent of children with distal femoral physeal fractures suffer permanent damage to the growth plate at the time of injury,[1,3,7] but fortunately most are close enough to skeletal maturity to make shortening or progressive angulation insignificant. As previously discussed, the distal femoral physis is the largest and fastest growing growth plate in the body, and its shape is more undulating than many other physes.[3,7] Consequently, Salter-Harris type II fractures of the distal femur have a worse prognosis than in other areas of the body, and the prognostic value of the Salter-Harris classification is not as reliable for distal femoral physeal fractures. The probability of physeal injury varies with the degree of displacement, the type of physeal injury,

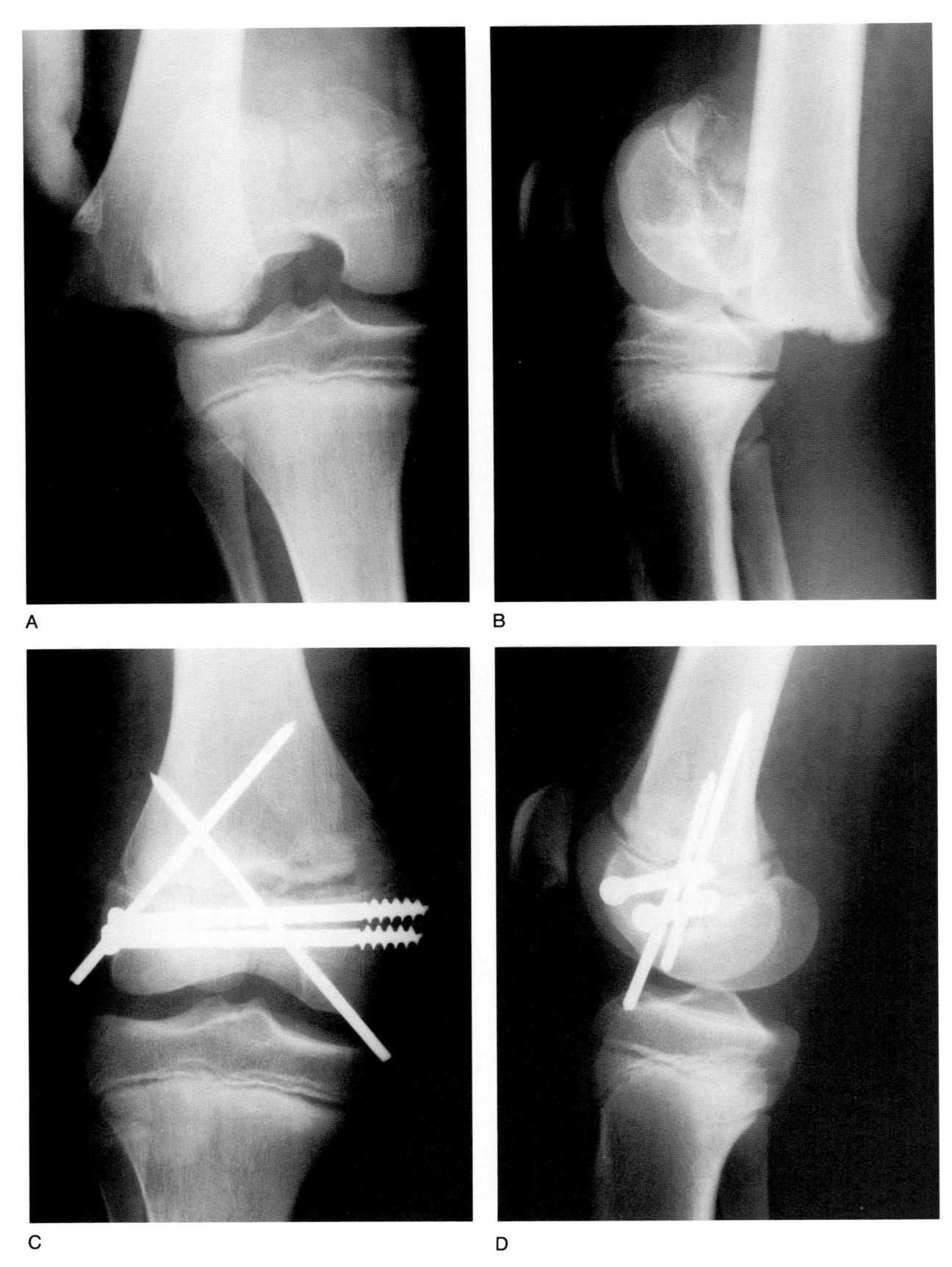

Fig. 31-26. Type IV T-supracondylar distal femoral **(A&B)** fracture treated by open reduction, fixation of the condyles with lag screws, and the supracondylar part of the fracture stabilized with two additional smooth K-wires **(C&D).**

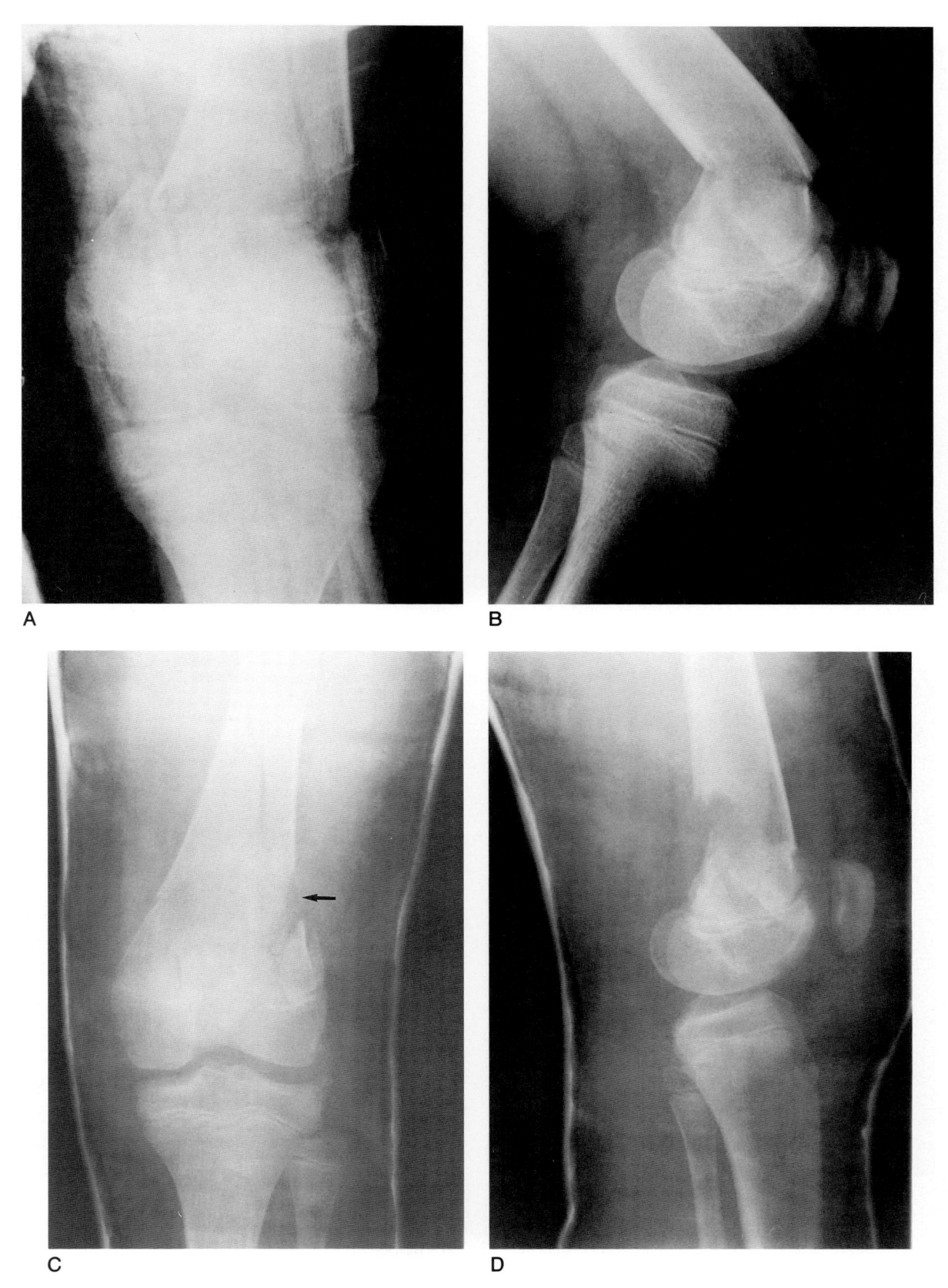

Fig. 31-27. (A&B) Type IV modified Y-supracondylar fracture treated initially by closed reduction. **(C&D)** Immediate postreduction films confirmed an acceptable reduction but the absent posterolateral metaphysis was noted. *(Figure continues.)*

588 / Management of Pediatric Fractures

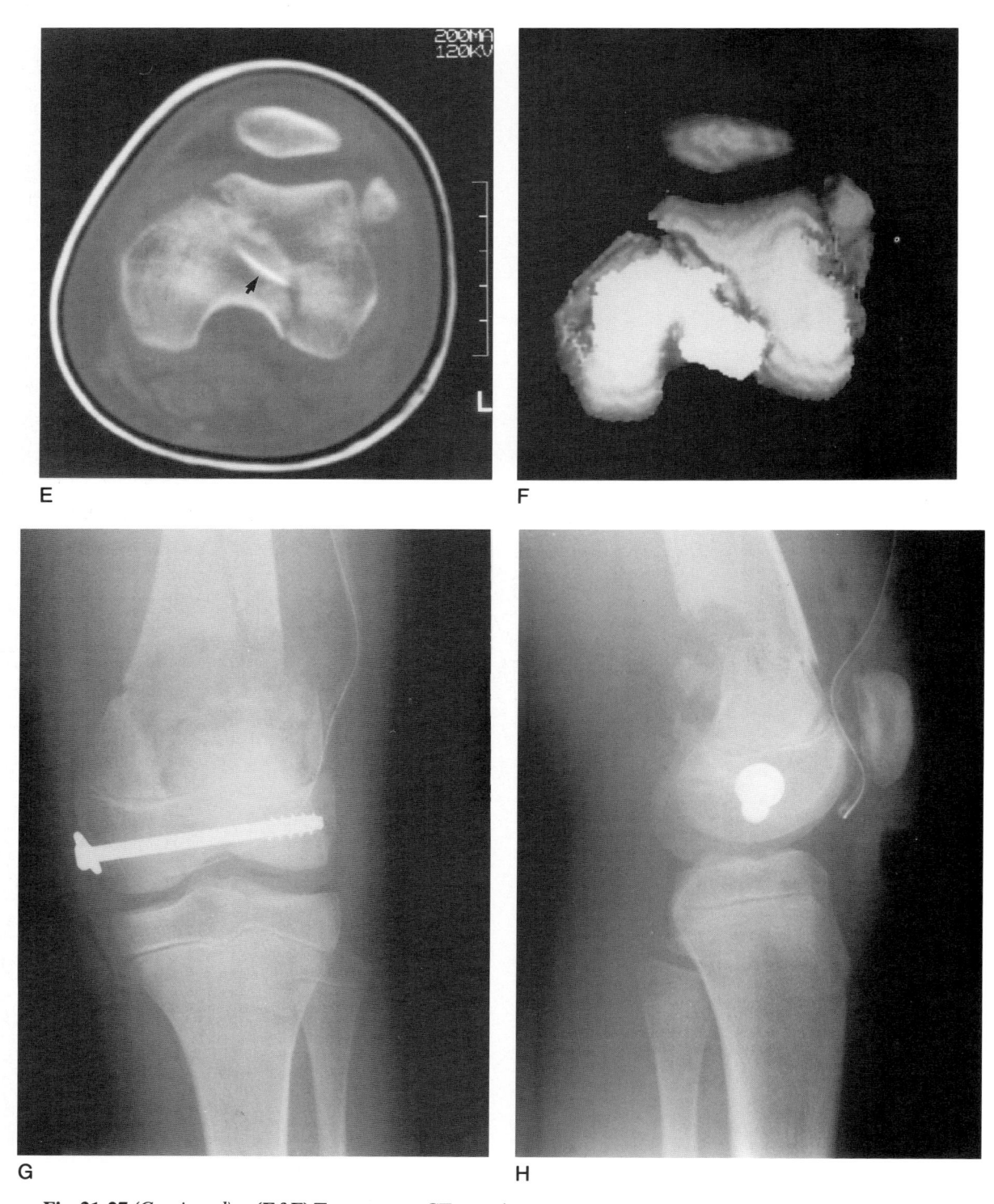

Fig. 31-27 *(Continued).* **(E&F)** Tomograms, CT scan, including three-dimensional reconstructions showed the missing metaphyseal fragment to be trapped between the two condyles and crossing the growth plate. **(G&H)** The fracture required an open reduction and internal fixation of the femoral condyles after removal of the large metaphyseal fragment.

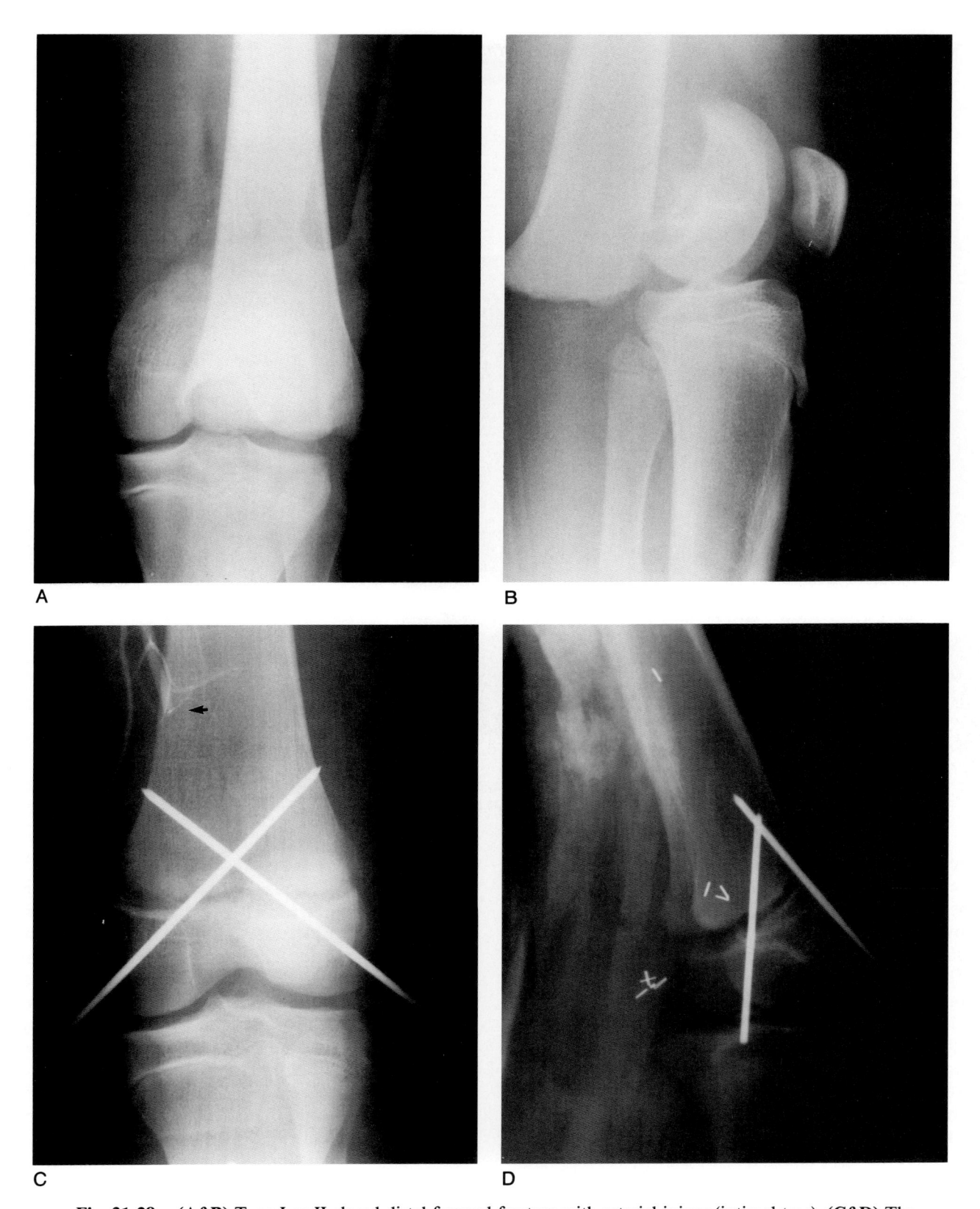

Fig. 31-28. **(A&B)** Type I or II closed distal femoral fracture with arterial injury (intimal tear). **(C&D)** The fracture was close-reduced and stabilized with cross K-wires, after which a saphenous bypass graft was performed by the vascular surgeon.

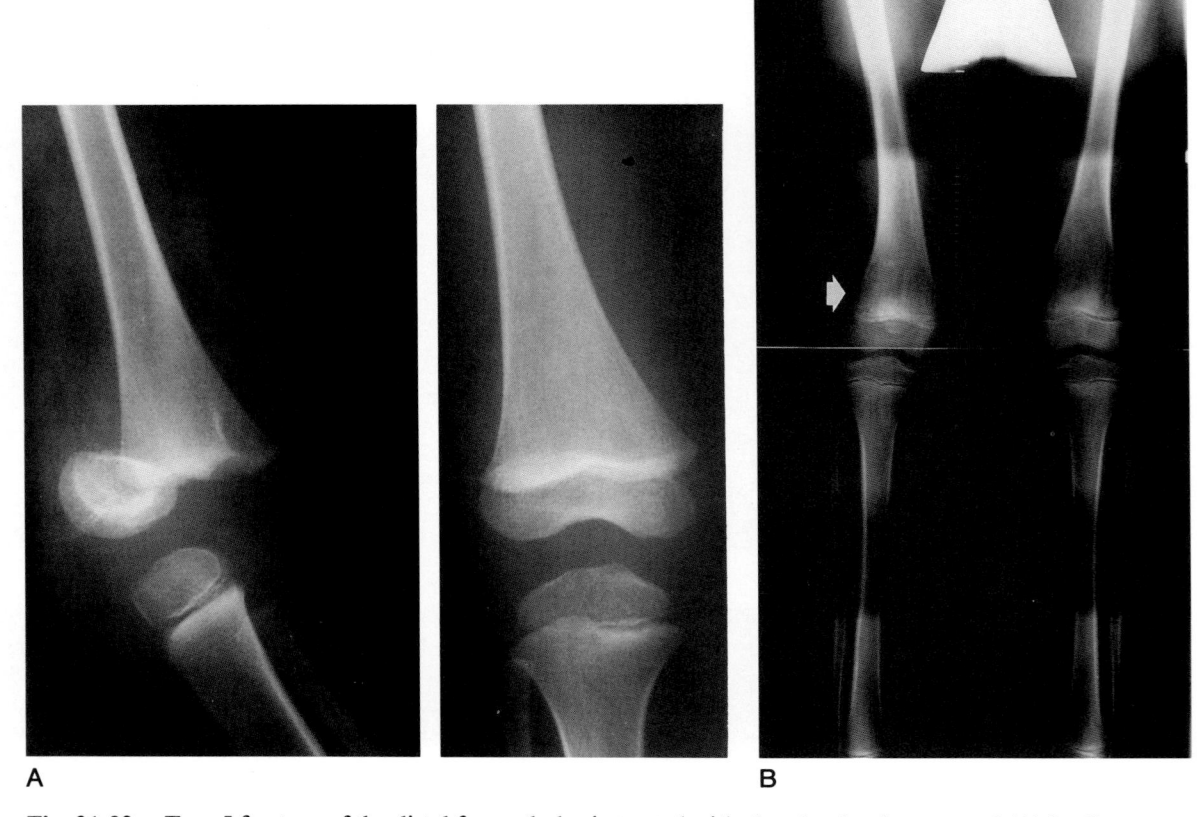

Fig. 31-29. Type I fracture of the distal femoral physis treated with closed reduction at age 5 (**A**) leading to a significant valgus deformity of the distal right femur but no leg length discrepancy at age 8 (**B**).

the exactness of the reduction, the age of the patient at the time of injury, and the magnitude of force producing the injury. Generally, the prognosis for distal femoral physeal fractures in newborns is good because these are usually low-energy fractures, with less propensity to damage the physis, aided by the remarkable remodeling potential of the distal femoral physis in young children.

Malunions are usually secondary to inadequate or unstable reductions with redisplacement. This can usually be prevented by close follow-up in the initial postoperative period or by simply stabilizing the fracture at the time of reduction by percutaneous crossed K-wire fixation.

If there has been damage to the growth plate, progressive angulation may occur in the distal femur, especially if there are 2 years or more of physeal growth remaining (Fig. 31-29). The direction of the angulation is directly related to the location of the physeal bridge; for example, a medial bridge leads to varus deformity. Treatment options for a physeal bridge include bridge resection, epiphysiolysis or epiphysiodesis of the physis in the opposite condyle. These procedures may have to be combined with a supracondylar femoral osteotomy to correct any existing deformity. Leg length discrepancies may occur even in the absence of an obvious physeal bridge secondary to premature closure of the growth plate, especially if there were 2 years or more of growth remaining (Fig. 31-30).

For these reasons, it is very important to follow these children for a minimum of 2 years postinjury and preferably until skeletal maturity. Clinical assessment of limb length, alignment, and knee stability should be performed at each visit to detect early evidence of physeal arrest. Radiographs should be obtained at 6, 12, and 24 months postfracture to ensure normal physeal growth.

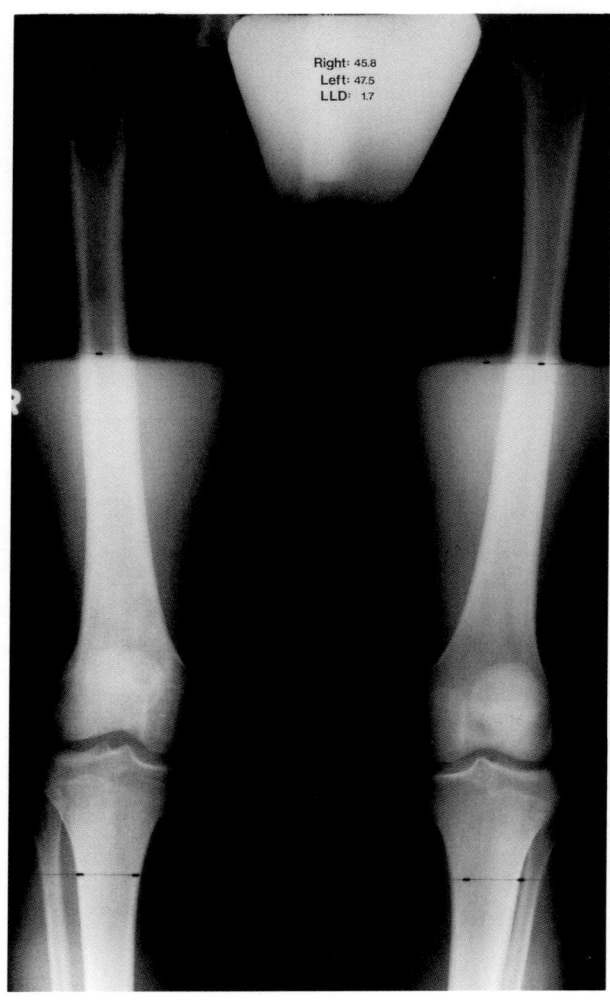

Fig. 31-30. Type IV T-supracondylar fracture (same patient as in Fig. 31-26) showing a 1.7-cm leg length discrepancy at age 18, three years postinjury.

SUMMARY

In summary, fractures of the distal femoral physis are high-energy fractures and carry a significant risk of damage to the growth plate, which may lead to progressive angulation or leg length discrepancy. For this reason, as near an anatomic reduction as possible should be obtained and maintained, and these children should be followed for a minimum of 2 years or until growth is completed.

REFERENCES

1. Neer CS II: Separation of the lower femoral epiphysis. Am J Surg 99:756, 1960
2. Peterson CA, Peterson HA: Analysis of the incidence of injuries to the epiphyseal growth plate. J Trauma 12:275, 1972
3. Roberts J: Fractures and separations of the knee. p. 1165. In Rockwood CA, Wilkins KE, King RF (eds): Fractures in Children. 3rd Ed. JB Lippincott, Philadelphia, 1991
4. Czitrom AA, Salter RB, Willis RB: Fractures involving the distal epiphyseal plate of the femur. Int Orthop 4:269, 1981
5. Mann DC, Rajmaira S: Distribution of physeal and nonphyseal fractures in 2,650 long bone fractures in children age 0–10 years. J Pediatr Orthop 10:713, 1990
6. Crawford AH: Fractures about the knee in children. Orthop Clin North Am 7:639, 1976
7. Ogden JA: Distal femoral epiphyseal injuries. p. 722. In Skeletal Injury in the Child. 2nd Ed. WB Saunders, Philadelphia, 1990
8. Rang M: Femoral shaft: supracondylar fractures. p. 277. In Children's Fractures. 2nd Ed. JB Lippincott, Philadelphia, 1983
9. Torg JS, Pavlov H, Morris VB: Salter-Harris type III fractures of the medial femoral condyle occurring in the adolescent athlete. J Bone Joint Surg [Am] 63:586, 1981
10. Grogan DP, Bobechko WP: Pathogenesis of a fracture of the distal femoral epiphysis. J Bone Joint Surg [Am] 66:621, 1984
11. Brunner C: Fractures in and around the knee joint. p. 294. In Weber BG, Brunner C, Freuler F (eds): Treatment of Fractures in Children and Adolescents. Springer-Verlag, New York, 1980
12. Criswell AR, Hand WL, Butler J: Abduction injuries to the distal femoral epiphysis. Clin Orthop 115:189, 1976
13. Lascombes P, Prévot J, Bardoux J: The prognosis of fracture of the lower end of the femur in children and adolescents: a review of 96 cases. Rev Chir Orthop, suppl 74:438, 1988
14. Lombardo SJ, Harvey JP: Fractures of the distal femoral epiphysis: factors influencing prognosis: a review of 34 cases. J Bone Joint Surg [Am] 59:742, 1977
15. Riseborough EJ, Barett IR, Shapiro F: Growth disturbances following distal femoral physeal fractures-separations. J Bone Joint Surg [Am] 65:885, 1983
16. Roberts JM: Operative treatment of fractures about the knee. Orthop Clin North Am 21:365, 1990
17. Robert M, Moulies D, Longis B et al: Décollements épiphysaires traumatiques de l'extrémité inférieure du fémur. Rev Chir Orthop 74:69, 1988
18. Salter RB, Czitrom AA, Willis RB: Fractures involving the distal femoral epiphyseal plate, abstracted. J Bone Joint Surg [Br] 61:248, 1978
19. Stephens DC, Louis E, Louis DS: Traumatic separation of the distal femoral epiphyseal cartilage plate. J Bone Joint Surg [Am] 56:1383, 1974
20. Telfer C, D'Astous J: Fractures of the distal femoral epiphysis. p. 161. In Uhthoff HK, Wiley JJ (eds): Behaviors of the Growth Plate. Raven Press, New York, 1988

32

Intra-articular Fractures of the Knee

Roger Gallien

> Everything has been thought of before. The problem is to think of it again.

Intra-articular fractures of the knee can be classified as (1) Salter-Harris types III and IV of the distal femoral epiphysis, (2) Salter-Harris types III and IV of the proximal tibial epiphysis, (3) fracture of the intercondylar eminence of the tibia, and (4) osteochondral fractures.

Salter-Harris types III and IV fractures of the distal femoral or proximal tibial epiphysis represent rare injuries and are always serious.[1] They may cause an unacceptable defect in the articular surface and produce serious growth disturbances. Of 1,629 patients reported by Mizuta and colleagues,[2] there were only 10 fractures of the lower femoral epiphysis and 18 of the proximal tibial epiphysis, none of these being of the Salter-Harris types III and IV. Associated lesions emphasize the importance of the initial trauma and may aggravate the prognosis if on the homolateral limb.

INTRA-ARTICULAR FRACTURE OF THE DISTAL FEMORAL EPIPHYSIS (SALTER-HARRIS TYPES III AND IV)

Incidence

Riseborough and colleagues[3] reported 66 fractures of the distal femoral epiphysis, of which 7 were type III and 6 were type IV. In this study the mean age was 12 years for type III and $8\frac{11}{12}$ years for type IV fracture. Lombardo and colleagues[4] reported 34 fractures, of which 5 were type III and 3 were type IV. Lascombes and colleagues[5] reviewed 96 fractures, 5 of them being type III and 5 type IV. These types of intra-articular fractures are thus uncommon but potentially very disabling to both the integrity of the physis and the congruity of the articular surfaces of the knee.

Anatomy

The distal femoral growth plate contributes 70 percent of the growth of the femur and 37 percent of the growth of the lower extremity. The rate of growth is approximately 0.9 cm per year at the distal femur. At 13 years of age (bone age), there is 1 cm growth left in the distal femur of girls and 3.5 cm in boys. At 15 years (bone age), there is no growth left in the distal femur of girls and under 1 cm left in the femur of a boy.

The distal femoral growth plate is completely extra-articular. The strength of the knee joint is derived from the ligaments that surround it. An excessive force applied to the knee joint will put tension on the ligaments, and with sufficient strain the epiphysis will separate from the diaphysis. The popliteal artery is adjacent to the posterior surface of the distal femur. It is vulnerable to injury from a backward thrusting of the distal femoral metaphysis at the time of hyperextension injury.[6] The sciatic nerve divides just above the popliteal space into the peroneal and posterior tibial nerves. The peroneal nerve is subject to stretch if the distal femoral epiphysis is tilted into varus or medially rotated.[6] It is also vulnerable to direct contusion from a blow on the posterolateral aspect of the knee.

Mechanism of Injury

In general, fractures in juvenile patients are associated with severe trauma usually secondary to automobile accidents.[3] In adolescents most of the injuries are sports related. Other common causes are motorcycle accidents or a fall from a height. Special consideration must be given to the recognition of the Salter-Harris type III fracture of the medial femoral condyle. It involves a valgus force applied to the distal part of the femur and the knee caused by a clipping injury (football) or an automobile accident (Fig. 32-1A). Because of the restraining effect of the anterior cruciate and lateral capsular ligaments, spontaneous reduction can occur, making identification difficult.[7]

Classification

The Salter-Harris type III fracture is intra-articular and crosses the epiphysis from the joint surface to the plate and then passes along the plate to its periphery. If not perfectly reduced, it may cause incongruity of the articular surface and later degenerative arthritis. The prognosis is good, provided the blood supply remains intact and the reduction perfect. The Salter-Harris type IV fracture is also intra-articular. A vertical line extends from the metaphysis across the growth plate through the intra-articular surface of the epiphysis. If it heals in a displaced position, a bony bridge forms and angular deformity results. The prognosis is guarded.

In type III fracture, the medial or lateral condyle is involved. The medial condyle fracture is often undisplaced and can be unrecognized. Bicondylar T or Y Salter-Harris type III or IV fractures represent complex problems. Tangential fractures (osteochondral fractures) of the articular surface are the subject of Chapter 55.

Physical Examination

In the majority of these fractures, there is a history of violent injury to the lower limb and severe pain. The child is unable to bear weight on the affected limb. The knee is swollen and a large hematoma may often be felt in the popliteal region. There may be an obvious deformity, and one must be aware of the possibility of associated injuries. One must particularly have a very high index of suspicion of neurovascular problems. A careful examination of the dorsalis pedis and posterior tibial pulses is mandatory. The foot may be cool and pale and the tibial compartments must be examined for increased pressure. It is essential that a motor and sensory examination is done, and special attention must be given to the sensation on the dorsum and plantar aspect of the foot in order to rule out a vascular or neurologic injury. Doppler examination of the pedal pulses may be useful.

Differential Diagnosis

Salter-Harris type III fracture of the medial femoral condyle is the most frequently occurring undisplaced fracture that involves the distal epiphysis.[7] It may be mistaken for disruption of the medial collateral ligament. Torg and coworkers[7] recommend a cross-table lateral radiograph in an attempt to detect fat within the joint fluid and confirm the existence of an intra-articular fracture. An oblique radiograph, a tunnel view, computed tomography, a radiograph with valgus stress applied to the knee (under general anesthesia) can all be very useful in confirming the diagnosis.

Treatment Indications

Type III and type IV fractures of the distal femoral or proximal tibial epiphysis must be reduced perfectly and internally fixed if unstable. Open reduction is the rule rather than the exception in displaced fractures (Figs. 32-1 and 32-2).

Malunion of these articular fractures can produce later joint degeneration. Transverse Kirschner wire fixation of the epiphyseal and metaphyseal fragment is usually sufficient. Alternatively interfragmentary screws parallel to the growth plate can be used. The physeal plate can be crossed if necessary with small smooth pins but never with interfragmentary screws. Repeated closed reduction causes damage to the already endangered growth plate. In open reduction, great care must be given to minimize trauma to the periosteum, perichondrium, and surrounding tissues. Operative intervention may be necessary for wound care in open injury.

Excellent reduction can be achieved by closed methods if the fracture is minimally displaced. This is particularly true with Salter-Harris type III fracture of the femoral condyle, which is the most frequently occurring

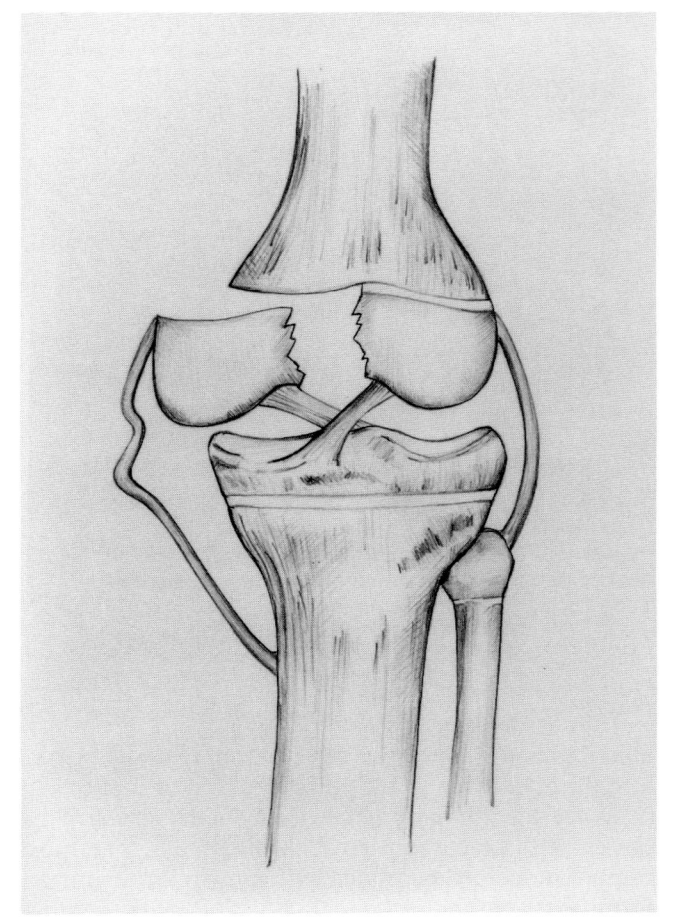

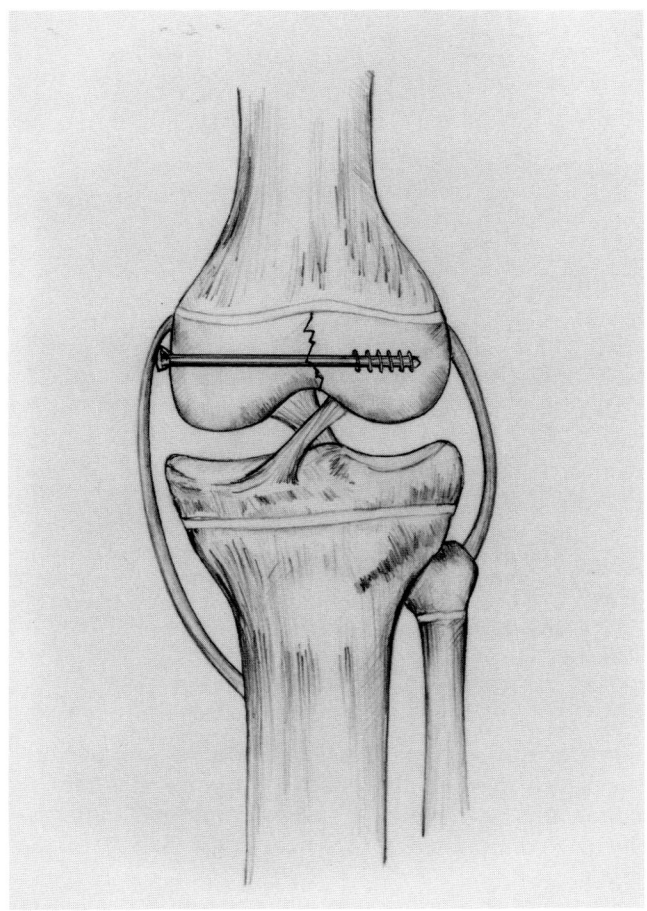

Fig. 32-1. **(A&B)** Salter-Harris type III fracture of distal femoral epiphysis. The displaced condyle is approached through either an anteromedial or anterolateral incision, depending on which condyle is involved. A cancellous screw (a smooth pin) is inserted transversely into the intact opposite condyle without crossing the physis. A cannulated screw lessens the risk of trauma to the growth plate. Arthrotomy is necessary to ensure an anatomic reduction. (Fig. A modified from Torg et al.,[7] with permission.)

undisplaced fracture that involves the distal femoral epiphysis. In these the reduction is maintained in a non-weight-bearing cylinder cast for 4 to 6 weeks. In some displaced types III and IV fractures, the displaced fragment can be controlled with a Steinmann pin introduced percutaneously. Under fluoroscopic control, this is used as a handle to guide the fragment into a reduced position.[8,9] After reduction, one or two pins are inserted horizontally across the epiphysis, taking care not to cross the growth plate. Reduction should be maintained in a long-leg cast for 6 weeks. Open reduction (Figs. 32-1 to 32-3) is reserved for cases in which closed reduction fails. Postoperative reduction can be maintained in a long-leg or hip spica cast. Bicondylar T or Y fractures and triplane fracture-separation present with both the problems of types III and IV injuries (Fig. 32-3) and occur in adolescents close to the end of growth. They represent serious problems. Angled blade plates should be used only near the end of growth.

Complications

Intra-articular types III and IV femoral fractures are always very serious and often associated with complications, particularly in young children where trauma is usually severe. A high index of suspicion must be maintained for the possibility of growth plate arrest with close

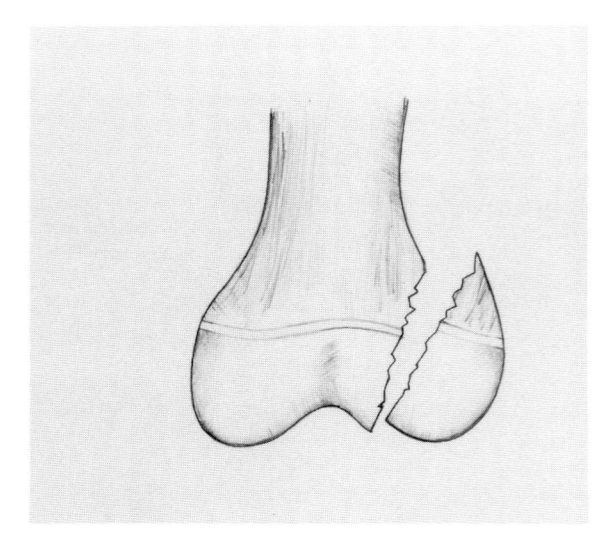

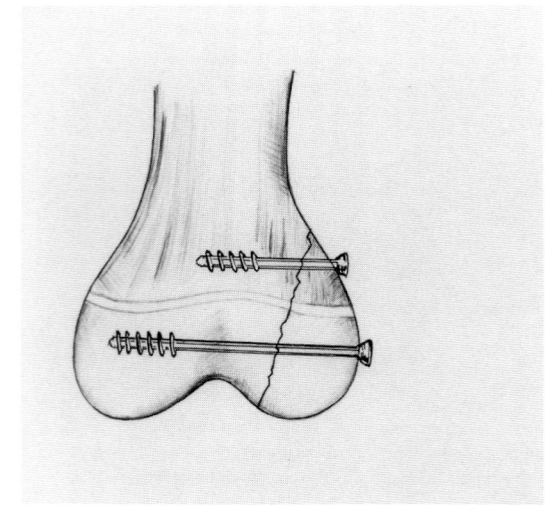

Fig. 32-2. Salter-Harris type IV fracture of distal femoral epiphysis. The same principles apply as for type III fracture. If the metaphyseal spike is not large, a smooth pin can be inserted through the physis. Accurate reduction and fixation is especially important to avoid formation of a bony bridge between a proximally displaced epiphyseal fragment and the adjacent metaphysis.

follow-up during the year following trauma. Serial clinical examination of the patient with investigation by scanograms, tomography, and/or computed tomography are recommended to detect early closure of the physis.

Stretch of the peroneal nerve occurs in 3 percent of separation of distal femoral epiphysis.[6] It rarely requires treatment other than reduction of the separation and is usually a neuropraxia.

The most devastating complication is arterial damage. Injury to the popliteal artery occurs rarely in type IV fracture-separation of the lower femoral epiphysis in juvenile patients.[3]

Unique Characteristics of Fracture

Progressive Angulation

Progressive angulation following separation of the distal femoral epiphysis is usually due to asymmetrical growth inhibition. Riseborough and colleagues[3] studied growth disturbances following these fractures and found clinically and significant angular deformity occurring in 26 percent of patients. Type IV fracture had an especially poor outcome in terms of both length inequality and angular deformity. Damage to the physis is frequently extensive regardless of the pattern of fracture. Permanent damage of the physis can occur in two ways: (1) as a result of damage to the epiphyseal blood supply and (2) as a result of transverse and horizontal fissuring of the physis, with or without gross displacement. The most important factors associated with growth arrest and deformity are not the pathoanatomic types of the injuries but the patient's young age at the time of injury and the severity of injury.

Shortening

Riseborough and colleagues[3] noted significant shortening of the injured femur in 56 percent of the patients with distal femoral separation. This shortening is often combined with angular deviation. This can be a very serious complication depending on the years left before cessation of growth. His study documented the central-arrest phenomenon in 20 percent of the patients. Bone continuity was seen across the middle of the growth plate, with the radiolucency that persisted medially and laterally representing apparently normal growth cartilage. The central growth-arrest phenomenon was ominous, however, in that following its appearance in all children either complete radiographic fusion occurred in a matter of months or the central arrest persisted with little or no further contribution of the physis to femoral length.[3]

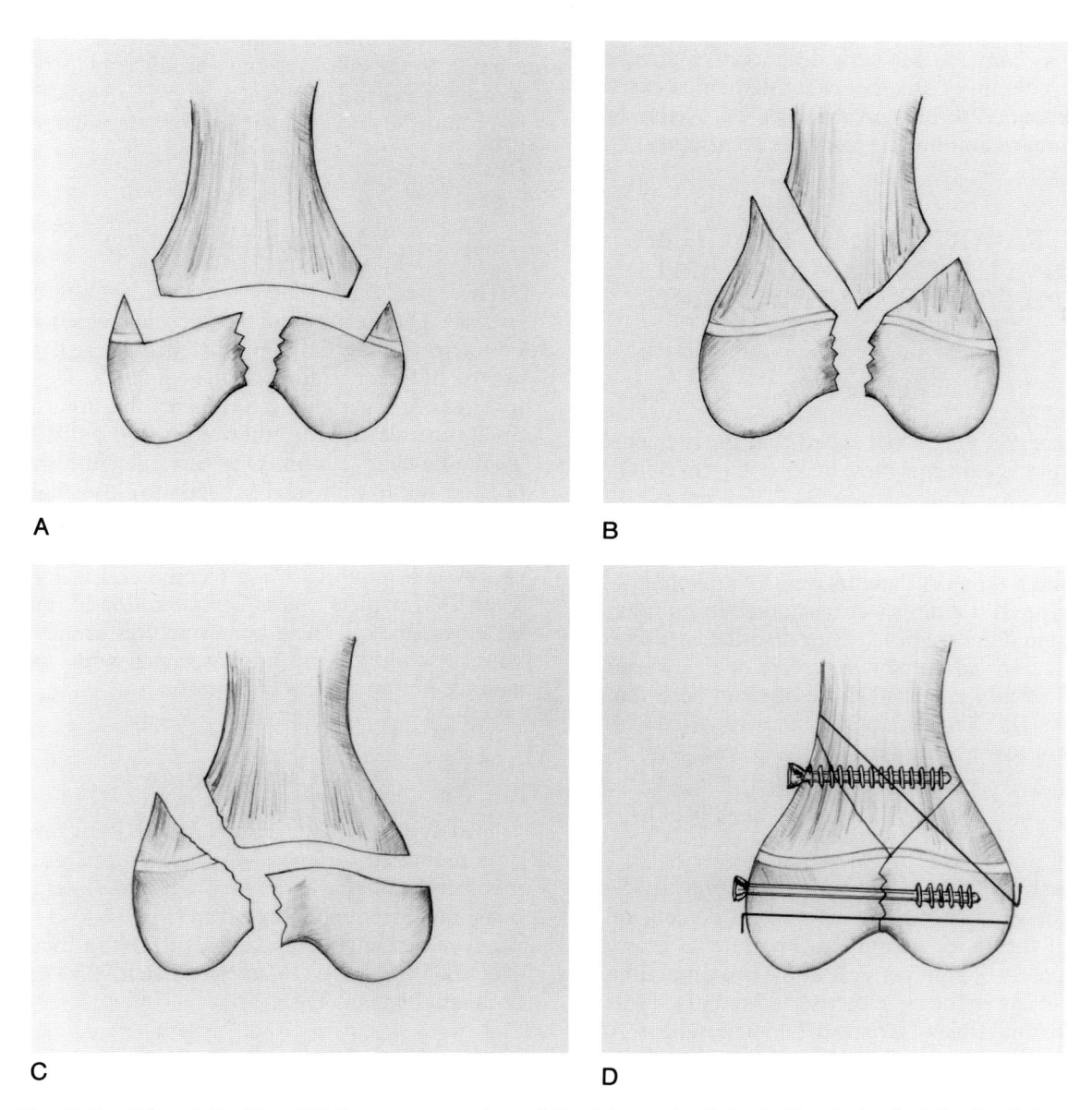

Fig. 32-3. Bicondylar T and Y fracture-separation of distal femoral epiphysis. Surgical principles for Salter-Harris types III and IV apply. Temporary fixation by pins or wires is recommended before final fixation with screws. **(A)** T fracture. **(B)** Y fracture, type IV. **(C)** Combination of type III and IV. **(D)** Y fracture after open reduction and internal fixation. (Fig. D modified from Bonnard and Peres,[10] with permission.)

Stiffness

Types III and IV more severe injuries usually result in slightly greater limitation of motion of the knee and would appear to benefit from internal fixation and the early restitution of knee motion.[3] An irregular cartilage surface may contribute to early degenerative changes. A vigorous program of quadriceps strengthening exercises is recommended to prevent extensor lag. Active hamstring exercises and bicycle exercises are useful.

INTRA-ARTICULAR FRACTURE OF THE PROXIMAL TIBIAL EPIPHYSIS (SALTER-HARRIS TYPES III AND IV)

Incidence

Burkhart and Peterson[11] stated that the incidence of this fracture is extremely low accounting for about 0.5 percent of all epiphyseal injuries. They reviewed 914 cases of epiphyseal fractures and found only 28 that involved the proximal tibial epiphysis, of which 6 were type III and 8 type IV. Patients were 14 and older. Most of their type III fractures were sustained in jumping activities around the age of 15. They described a group of 5 children (2 to 6 years old) with type IV open lawnmower accidents. Injury occurred more often in boys than in girls (23 vs 4).[11] Shelton and Canale[12] reported 39 fractures, 10 of them being type III and 3 type IV.

Anatomy

The proximal tibial epiphysis contributes to 55 percent of the growth of the tibia and 28 percent of the growth of the lower extremity. The rate of growth is approximately 0.6 cm per year at the proximal tibia. At 13 years of age (bone age), there is 0.5 cm of growth left in the proximal tibia of girls and 2 cm left in boys. At 15 years of age (bone age), there is no growth left in the proximal tibia of girls and only 0.5 cm left in boys. Growth of the fibula is proportional to that of the tibia. This must be taken into consideration if growth is altered in the proximal tibia.

The tibial collateral ligaments mostly insert in the metaphysis and *not* the epiphysis. The varus or valgus stresses to the knee are transmitted to the metaphysis and not the epiphysis. Another important consideration is the special tongue-shaped configuration of the epiphysis of the tibial tubercle. The anterior portion of the proximal tibial epiphysis includes the epiphysis of the tibial tubercle into which the patellar tendon inserts. The forces transmitted through that tendon are an important cause of a Salter-Harris type III fracture.[11]

The popliteal artery is often at risk if the proximal part of the tibia is injured. Displacement of the tibial shaft in relation to the epiphysis may produce a laceration or a thrombosis of the popliteal artery. The vessels may also be occluded by internal swelling or external immobilization.

Mechanism of Injury

These fractures usually occur in older children or adolescents. They result from motorcycle accidents, twisting injury in the sagittal plane as encountered in contact sports, and direct trauma to the epiphysis. Type III fracture can occur with jumping and involves avulsion of the tibial tubercle and the anterior portion of the epiphysis by the patellar tendon. One can infer that the central portion of the epiphysis has begun to close, thus anchoring the epiphysis centrally and that a sudden violent contraction of the quadriceps avulses a portion of the epiphysis through its weaker peripheral attachments.[11] Type IV fractures caused by lawnmower injury have been described.[11] These open fractures usually occur in younger children and are associated with open, dirty wounds and some loss of bone.

Classification

Two types of Salter-Harris type III fractures of the proximal tibial epiphysis may be encountered. The first involves the medial or lateral plateau, the lateral condyle being more frequently involved (Fig. 32-4). The second is a displaced intra-articular fracture of the tibial tubercle (Fig. 32-5). The type IV fracture can involve the medial or lateral plateau (Fig. 32-6).

Physical Examination

Physical examination previously described for the distal femur apply here. Vascular occlusion is a serious potential complication of this fracture. The vessels may be lacerated directly or occluded by internal swelling or external immobilization. A high index of suspicion is needed. Nerve injury is relatively uncommon, and in most cases no surgery is needed, as a good recovery can be expected. In tibial tubercle avulsion extending into

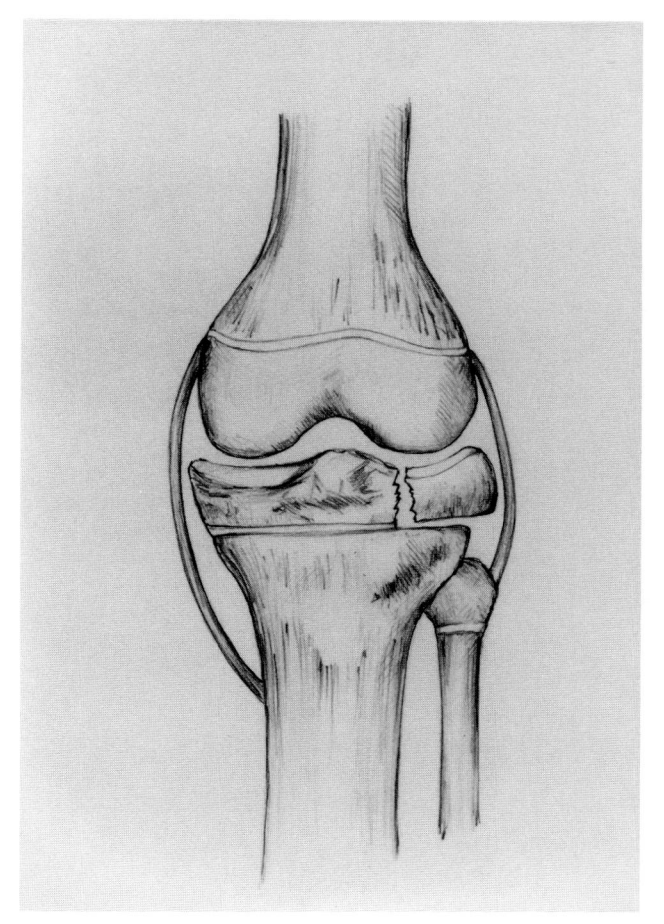

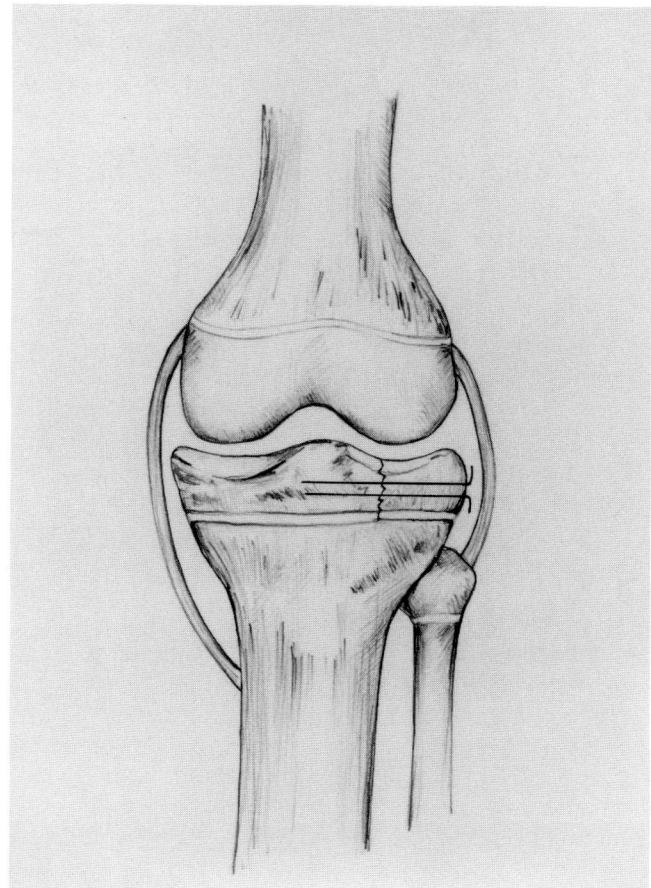

Fig. 32-4. Salter-Harris type III fracture of the proximal tibial epiphysis. Smooth pins are preferred to screws because of the small height of the physis and the danger to injure it and the joint. Insert pins transversely and parallel to the physis. Stress radiograph can show a rupture of the medial collateral ligament. Do not hesitate to bivalve the cast to prevent a compartment syndrome!

the joint (type III fracture), the patient presents with pain and swelling over the tibial tuberosity. There is usually a tense hemarthrosis, loss of knee extension, and proximal displacement of the patella.

Differential Diagnosis

In Salter-Harris type III and IV fractures of the lateral plateau, stress radiographs can diagnose an associated rupture of the medial collateral ligament. As for type III fracture involving the tibial tubercle, a history of significant violence immediately preceding the onset of symptoms suggests that the lesion has been a traumatic one quite different from the chronic Osgood Schlatter lesion.[13]

Treatment Indications

Type III Intra-articular Fractures

Excellent results can be obtained with closed or open methods. In a nondisplaced separation, a long-leg cast with 30 degrees of flexion at the knee is used. The cast and underlying padding must be split and open from top to bottom. The cast is kept for 5 to 6 weeks. If there is displacement, closed reduction and fixation by percutaneous pins may be possible. One must not hesitate to

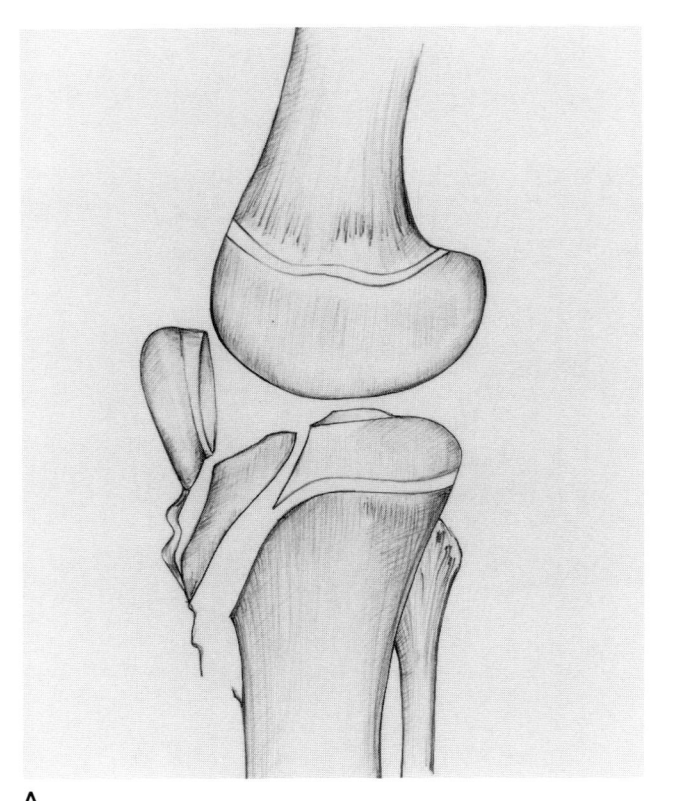

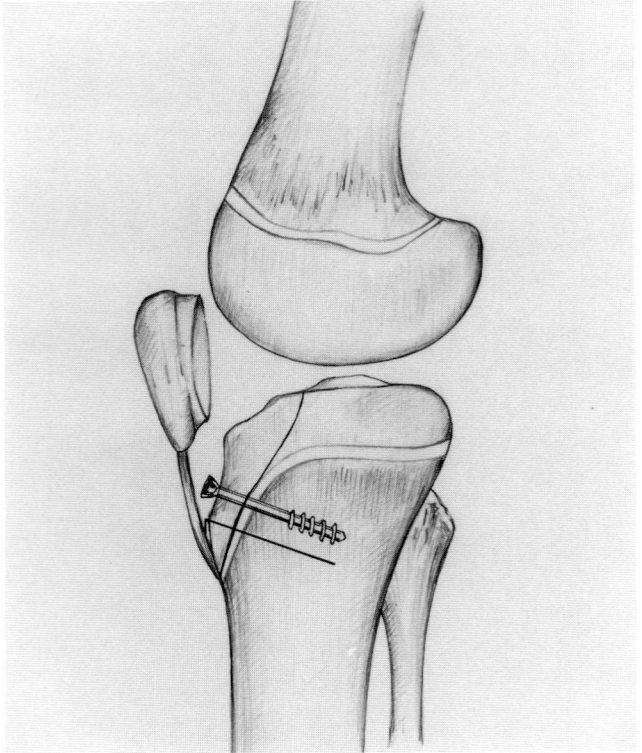

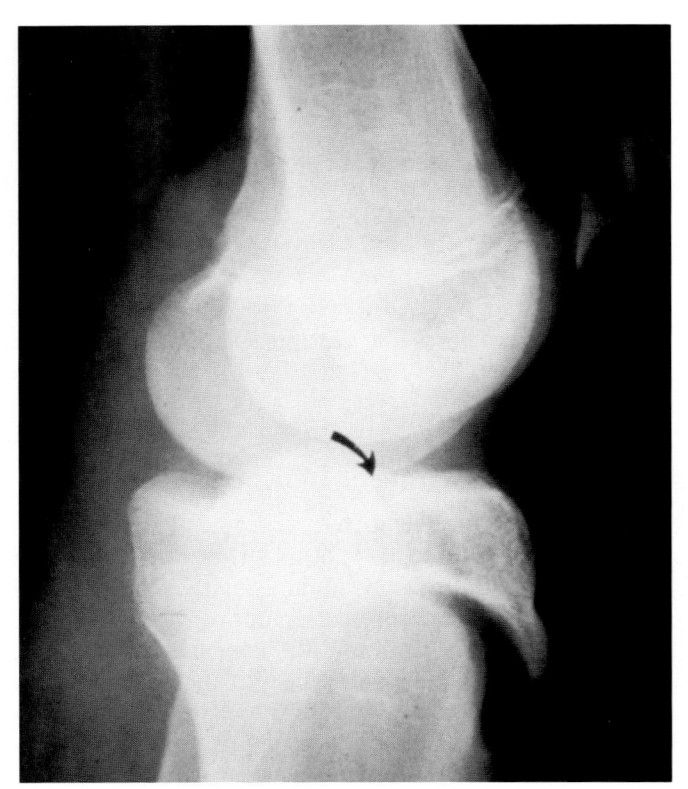

Fig. 32-5. Salter-Harris type III fracture of the proximal tibial epiphysis. Open reduction and internal fixation with one or more screws is indicated if the patient is very closed to the end of growth. Internal fixation by tension band wiring is an alternative. In a young patient, smooth pins or tension band wiring avoiding the physis are preferred. An anterior longitudinal incision is used centered over the tibial tubercle along either its medial or lateral border. The avulsed periosteal flap attached to the fragment distally is sutured for stability. **(A)** Fracture avulsion of tibial tubercle and anterior portion of epiphysis by the patellar tendon. **(B)** After open reduction and internal fixation. **(C)** Radiographic appearance of avulsion of the tibial tubercle extending intra-articularly.

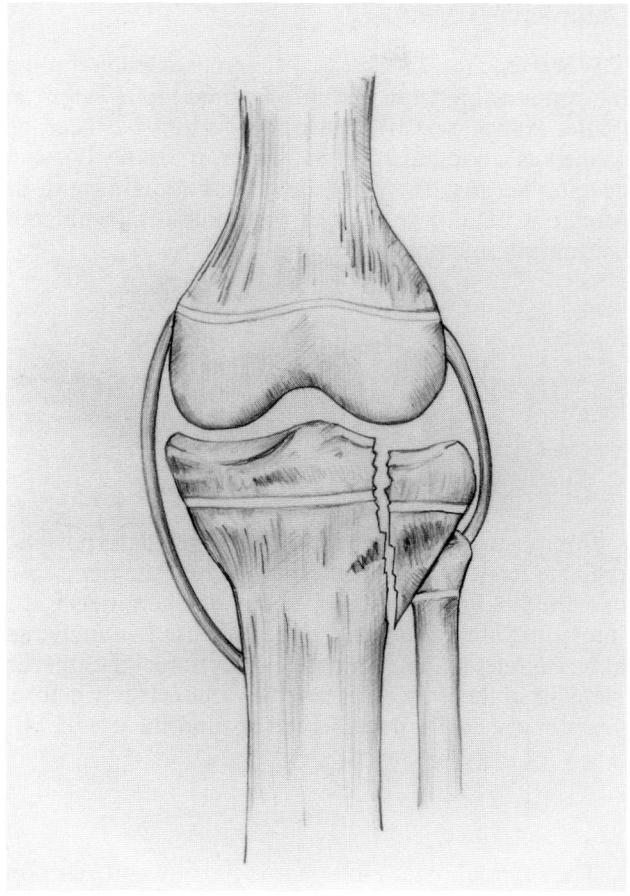

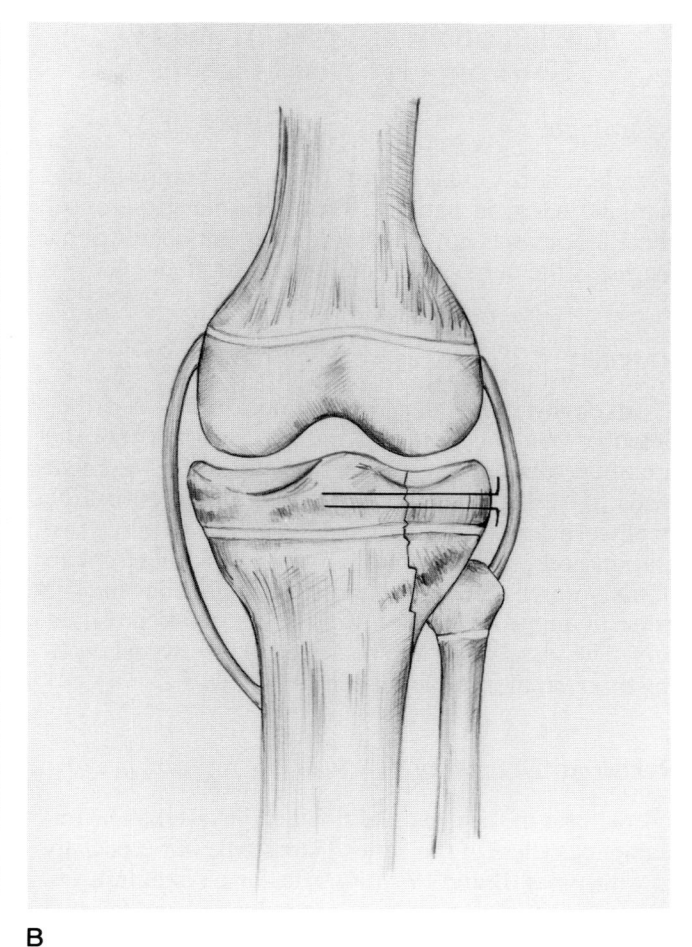

Fig. 32-6. (A) Salter-Harris type IV fracture of the proximal tibial epiphysis. (B) A screw parallel to the growth plate is used if the metaphyseal fragment is big enough.

open the fracture and reduce under direct vision if necessary (Fig. 32-4). Special attention must be given to the type III fracture involving the tibial tubercle and extending into the knee joint. A closed reduction under general anesthesia should be attempted but, failing anatomic reduction, open reduction and internal fixation of the fracture should be undertaken followed by immobilization with the knee in extension in a cylinder cast for 6 weeks (Fig. 32-5). This fracture often occurs when the epiphyseal plate is near closing.[14]

Type IV Intra-articular Fractures

The majority of growth disturbances occur in type IV fractures. Most require open reduction (Fig. 32-6), although closed reduction in a minimally displaced fracture may be possible. Burkhart and Peterson[11] described type IV fractures associated with lawnmower accidents. They were always associated with open dirty wounds that required careful debridement of devitalized tissue, removal of foreign bodies, prolonged and thorough irrigation, and antibiotic therapy.[11]

In fresh fractures associated with arterial injury that is unrelieved by reduction of the fracture, open reduction with internal fixation is required. When acute arterial involvement is evident, the popliteal artery is explored whatever the type of fracture. One must always observe the limb for signs of a developing compartment syndrome. Fasciotomy may also be necessary, either concomitant with surgery to the artery or when anterior compartment syndrome is evident.[12]

Complications of Types III and IV Tibial Intra-articular Fractures

Neurologic

Shelton and Canale[12] found that exploration of the peroneal nerve in patients who had isolated peroneal nerve lesions was not necessary, unless an open wound suggested the nerve had been directly severed.

Vascular

Aitken has shown that vascular occlusion is a serious potential complication of a fracture separation of the proximal tibial epiphysis because the distal fragment tends to be displaced posterolaterally and press on the popliteal artery.[31] Burkhart and Peterson[11] reported two amputations, one in a type III fracture resulting from an initially unrecognized compartment syndrome and the other in a type IV fracture with an associated crush injury. The vessels may also be occluded by internal swelling or external immobilization.

Recurrent Deformity

Fractures of the proximal tibial epiphysis may be unstable regardless of the Salter-Harris type but especially so with types III and IV intra-articular physeal injuries. One must not hesitate to use open reduction and internal fixation to achieve anatomic reduction, as these fractures usually displace after closed reduction and cast immobilization.

Angular Deformity and Shortening

Burkhart and Peterson[11] reported that the most common complication was angular (varus-valgus) deformity due to premature partial closure of the physis often combined with limb-length discrepancy. The majority of these growth disturbances occurred in type IV injuries, mostly in younger children. Corrective surgery for the complications of growth disturbance was required in 9 of 27 patients, and the majority of these surgical procedures were performed on patients with type IV injuries. They did not describe growth disturbance associated with type III fractures, probably because these patients were older, with little or no growth remaining.[11] Shelton and Canale[12] made the same observations, finding no significant growth disturbances with types III or IV fractures. This has also been our experience.

Genu Recurvatum

When fracture of the tibial tubercle extends through the anterior portion of the proximal tibial epiphysis (Salter-Harris type III), genu recurvatum has been described as a complication. However, it usually does not develop because there is little growth remaining in the proximal tibial epiphysis in the adolescent who most commonly sustains this injury.

FRACTURE OF THE INTERCONDYLAR EMINENCE OF THE TIBIA

Description and Incidence

Injuries that cause rupture of the anterior or posterior cruciate ligament in an adult will avulse the tibial spine of a child.[15] The terms tibial spine, tibial eminence, and intercondylar eminence have been used interchangeably. All refer to the interarticular portion of the adjacent plateaus of the tibia. This fracture occurs rarely before 7 years of age and is usually seen around the age of 14.

Anatomy

The intercondylar eminence is the nonarticular bony prominence between the articular surfaces of the medial and lateral plateaus of the knee to which the anterior cruciate ligament is attached anteriorly (Fig. 32-7) and the posterior cruciate posteriorly. The anterior eminence consists of two bony tuberosities: a medial one which receives the attachment of the anterior cruciate ligament and a lateral spine. No structure attaches to the apex of the lateral spine.[25] The avulsion fracture occurs through the cancellous bone beneath the subchondral plate. Its extent can involve the weight-bearing portion of the articular surface of the tibia in the region of the medial plateau. The reduction of this fracture can be impeded by the medial meniscus and/or the anterior horn of the lateral meniscus. Roberts[17] examined fresh amputation specimens in which fractures of the anterior intercondylar eminence had been simulated. In each specimen, the displaced fragment could be reduced into its bed by extension of the knee joint. The anterior portion of the femoral condyles pushed the hinged fragment down and overrode the increasing tightness of the anterior cruciate ligament.[17] The posterior cruciate ligament attaches to a shallow depression immediately behind the region of the

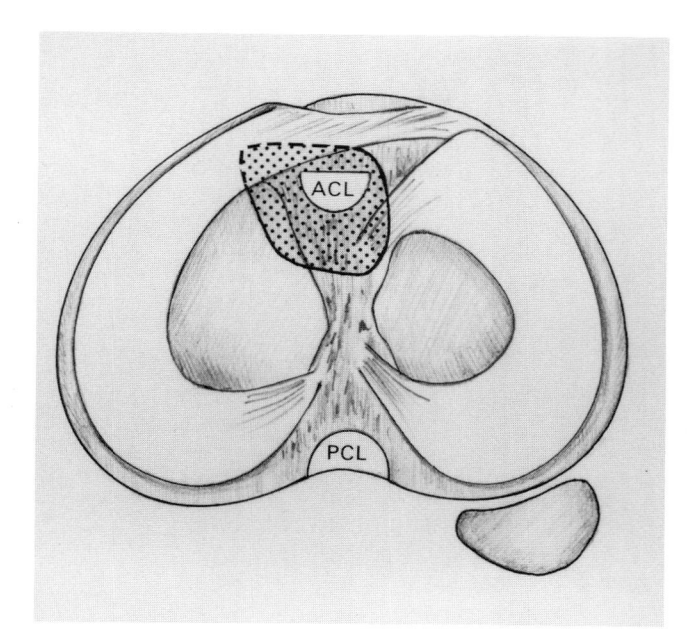

Fig. 32-7. Superior surface of the tibia. The detached bone fragment corresponds to the hatched area. It is larger than the attachment of the anterior cruciate ligament *(ACL)*. *PCL,* posterior cruciate ligament.

intercondylar eminence, at the posterior part of tibia and is much less commonly avulsed.

Mechanism of Injury

The trauma is often violent and the mechanism complex. Most of the fractures are caused by bicycle or car accidents and sports injuries. It can be speculated that traction is exerted on the anterior cruciate ligament in one of two ways: (1) a direct blow to the front of a flexed knee will drive the femur posteriorly on the fixed tibia; another example is a forced hyperextension of the knee, the tibia being projected forward, and (2) less frequently an indirect blow on a flexed knee will bring the tibia in valgus-external rotation or varus-internal rotation.

Classification of Anterior Tibial Spine Avulsions

Plain radiograph investigation is usually diagnostic. If standard anteroposterior or lateral views are not satisfactory, a tunnel (notch) view is added. Tomography and computed tomography will assist in the assessment of the characteristics of the fragment itself, its possible fragmentation, its size, and displacement. The Meyers and McKeever[18] classification is practical and recommended (Fig. 32-8).

Physical Examination

There are no specific signs of fractures of the tibial spines. The child presents with a painful, slightly flexed swollen knee and is reluctant to bear weight. Sometimes the diagnosis is delayed, the child being able to walk with a slight extension deficit. Extension of the knee is limited by hemarthrosis and hamstring spasm. On palpation, the local tenderness is on the central region of the anterior aspect of the joint line and not on the medial or lateral side.[19] The physical examination may reveal a positive drawer sign or an associated medial collateral ligament lesion. A stable knee without an anterior drawer sign may often be found with an undisplaced fracture on radiograph. However, it is frequently difficult or impossible to assess the knee joint for concomitant ligament injury because of pain and apprehension. An examination under general anesthesia may be necessary if ligament injury is suspected. After needle aspiration of the hematoma, one can examine the knee for a drawer sign or an associated tear of the medial collateral ligament with valgus stress.

Posterior Tibial Spine Avulsions

If seen late, the fractures of the tibial spines can be misdiagnosed as a foreign body (Fig. 32-9). Avulsion of the anterior tibial spine occurs both in young adults and children as opposed to avulsion of the posterior intercondylar eminence, which is a rare injury in children. In 1977, Torisu[20] reported 21 patients with an isolated fracture of the tibial attachment of the posterior cruciate ligament. It is considered an adult injury; the youngest patient in their series was 15. Isolated fracture of the tibial attachment of the posterior cruciate ligament is caused by a direct force that strikes the proximal part of the flexed tibia and drives it posteriorly. Sometimes it results from an hyperextension injury to the knee joint.[19] Occasionally the fragment may be avulsed from the femoral attachment of the cruciate.[16] Motorcycles accidents are the commonest cause of this injury, followed by automobile accidents in which the knee hits the dashboard. The fracture is usually seen on a lateral radiographic view of the knee at the back of the intercondylar

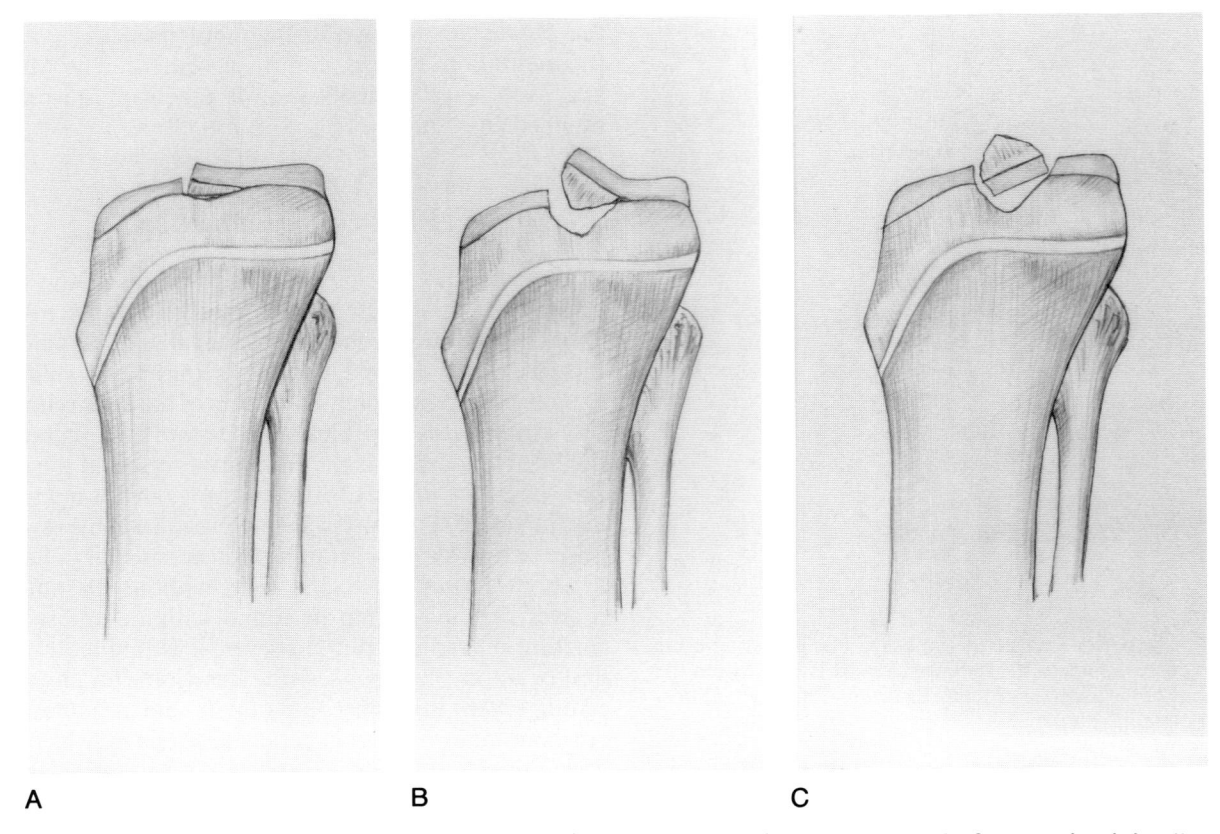

Fig. 32-8. Fractures of intercondylar eminence of the tibia. Lateral view. **(A)** Type I: The fragment is minimally displaced. **(B)** Type II: The anterior third to half of the avulsed fragment is elevated from its bone bed. **(C)** Type III: The avulsed fragment is completely lifted from its osseous bed, and there is no bone apposition. Rotation can be so marked that the cartilaginous surface of the avulsed fragment faces the bare bone of the eminence. (Modified from Meyers and McKeever,[18] with permission.)

space. The fragment may be single or comminuted, minimally displaced or pulled upward, often much larger than it appears on radiograph due to the cartilagenous component. In fresh fractures, conservative treatment gives good result if the fragment is small and minimally displaced.[21-23] Torisu[20] recommends a plaster cast for 6 weeks holding the knee in 20 degrees of flexion and the tibia pulled forward to relax the tension on the posterior cruciate ligament. Open reduction is recommended for a large single or comminuted fragment that is displaced upward and/or rotated. The adolescent is placed in a prone position and the lesion is approached through a posterior incision. The attachments of the posterior horns of the menisci to the fragment are checked. Any free fragment not attached to the posterior cruciate ligament is removed. The fragment is fixed to its bed by a small screw or a staple.[20] If one is afraid of splitting the fragment, insertion through a drill hole is recommended. In a delayed repair, the fragment is freshened and the tibial bed cleared of granulation tissue. The fracture is internally fixed. A cast is applied for 4 to 6 weeks with 20 degrees of flexion.[20]

Treatment of Tibial Spine Fractures

It has been previously thought that tibial spine avulsions seldom cause any long-term disability. Recently several authors have reported variable amounts of ligamentous laxity after this fracture, residual symptoms, and instabilities regardless of the methods of treatment.[24,25]

An attempt should be made to reduce the fracture by closed methods whatever the type of injury. With type I injury (Fig. 32-8), there is little or no displacement. All this fracture requires is a long-leg cast applied without anesthesia with the knee in extension. Hyperextension is

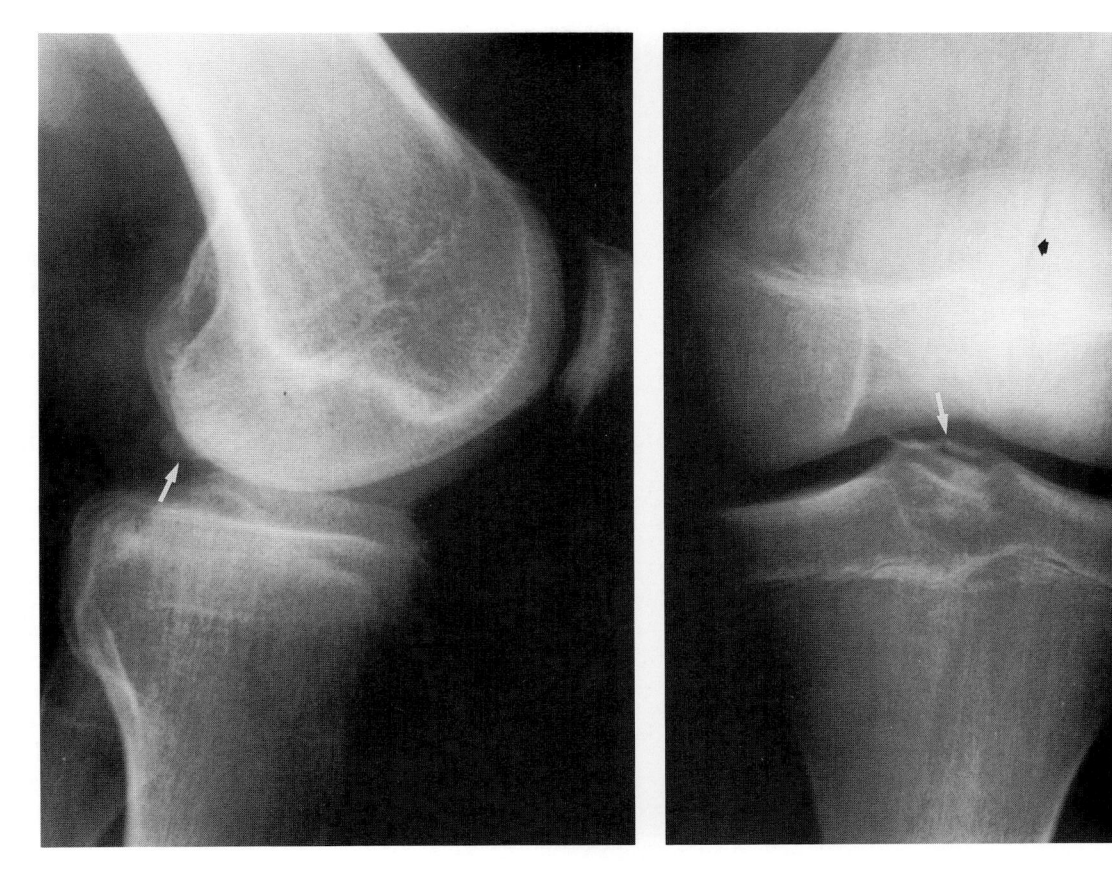

Fig. 32-9. Posterior cruciate avulsion secondary to a blow on the knee with knee flexed and foot fixed. Note the associated fracture of the patella.

avoided not only because of patient discomfort but also because of increased tension on the anterior cruciate that can cause displacement of the fragment. Placement of the knee in full extension will reduce the fragment in type I and usually type II fractures (Fig. 32-8). Aspiration of the hemarthrosis can be beneficial to relieve pain and facilitate extension and reduction. Hyperextension must be avoided, as it can detach and displace the fragment.

Rigault and colleagues[26] have stressed the importance of the initial clinical examination under general anesthesia if necessary. It is important to test stability and evaluate injuries to other ligaments around the knee. The hematoma is aspirated and gentle extension of the knee brings the anterior portion of the femoral condyles into contact with the avulsed fragment pushing it back down into its bed. A good criteria of a successful reduction is a degree of knee extension symetrical with the opposite knee. After the reduction is obtained, it is maintained in a non-weight-bearing long-leg cast for 6 weeks with the knee in 20 to 30 degrees of flexion or until union of the bone fragment to its bed on the tibia is demonstrated on the radiograph.

Closed reduction may not be possible in type III fractures (Fig. 32-8). Sometimes the lateral edge of the fragment is displaced above the anterior horn of the lateral meniscus. Simultaneous ligament tears can coexist and open repair is necessary. Open reduction is performed through a longitudinal anteromedial incision or can also be accomplished with the aid of arthroscopy. Sometimes the extension of the knee and the opposed distal femur will maintain reduction. If unstable, it should be internally fixed. Meyers and McKeever[18] reported excellent results by a simple absorbable catgut suture between the reduced avulsed fragment and the adjacent anterior pole of the lateral meniscus. The reduction is maintained in an above-knee cylinder cast in partially flexed position. The use of a small pin or screw through the fragment into the adjacent epiphysis is an alternative method of fixation. Rigault and colleagues[26] recommend, and I prefer, the following technique: mandatory internal fixation for

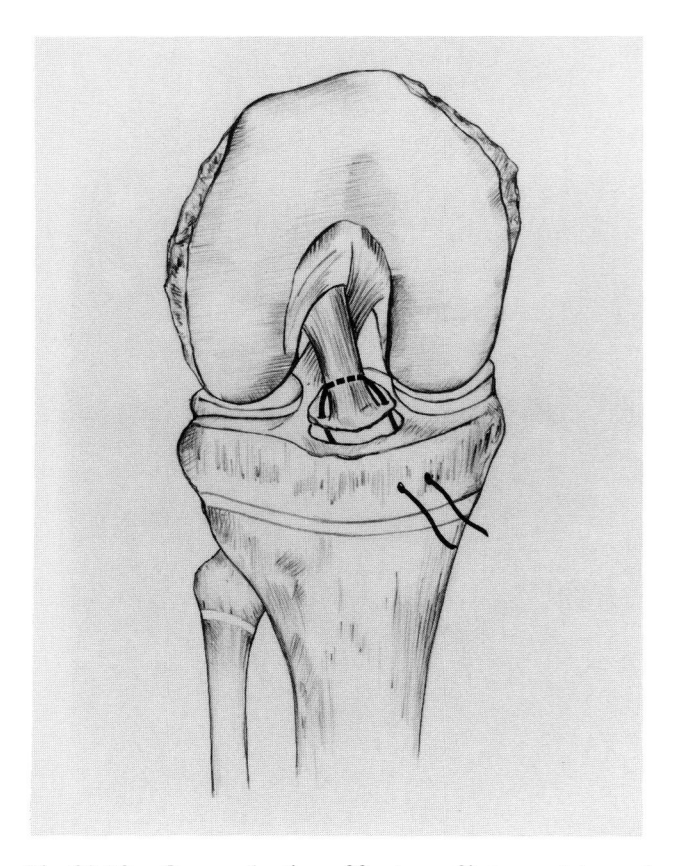

Fig. 32-10. Open reduction of fracture of intercondylar eminence. Internal fixation by nonabsorbable suture through the distal portion of the anterior cruciate ligament just proximal to the fractured fragment. Ends of suture are passed through the drill holes proximal to the physis and tied on themselves after the reduction is satisfactory. (Modified from Seriat-Gauthier et al.,[27] with permission.)

type III fractures and a lacing suture through the distal anterior cruciate ligament before reduction, bringing the fragment down into its bed (Fig. 32-9). Ischemic effects have been attributed to tight figure-of-8 lacing of the tendon. When the bone fragment is large and solitary, a loop (nonabsorbable suture) is passed over the superior surface of the fragment behind the distal part of the ligament (Fig. 32-10). A figure-of-8 lacing suture is used with multiple small fragments.[27] Through short stab incisions over the anterior aspect of the proximal tibia drill two holes from distal to proximal through the tibial epiphysis. The holes should enter the joint (1) just medial and lateral to the fractured fragment(s) or (2) into the defect and into the fragment itself if it is large enough.[28] Reduction is maintained in a non-weight-bearing long-leg cast with the knee in slight flexion. If internal fixation is indicated, it should be solid and perfect (Fig. 32-11).

Late Unrecognized Displaced Fractures of the Anterior Tibial Spine

The natural history of these untreated fractures is to heal in an elevated position or to present as pseudarthrosis (Fig. 32-12). If the drawer sign is not marked and stability relatively good, active exercises are recommended. If symptomatic, open reduction with curetting the bed of the lesion and the corresponding side of the fragment followed by reduction and internal fixation can be offered with a guarded prognosis.[27]

Complications

Malunion of a displaced fracture will limit extension of the knee joint. In this fracture the anterior cruciate ligament is not torn, but this does increase its length. Wiley and Baxter[25] reported a measurable degree of cruciate ligament laxity after tibial spine fractures. However, the children were generally asymptomatic. An anatomic reduction of the fracture does not prevent the cruciate laxity or the loss of full extension. Recent reports in the literature have documented residual knee symptoms, mainly giving-way episodes and catching sensations. Symptoms can be of such magnitude as to cause reduction of physical activities.[28] This should not be confused with retropatellar pain most likely secondary to patellofemoral disorders common in adolescents and usually present in the uninjured knee as well.

As for the undetected old anterior tibial spine avulsion, some patients may do relatively well except for some catching sensations or giving-way episodes in athletic activities. Others present as having chronic "sprains" with chronic swelling of the knee, anterior draws sign and laxity in valgus. These patients may need surgical repositioning of the fragment and their prognosis is uncertain.[26]

OSTEOCHONDRAL FRACTURES

Osteochondral fractures occur on the patella and the cartilaginous portion of the medial or lateral femoral condyle. A medial tangential osteochondral fracture of the patella is not infrequently associated with the trauma of recurrent dislocation of the patella or with the trau-

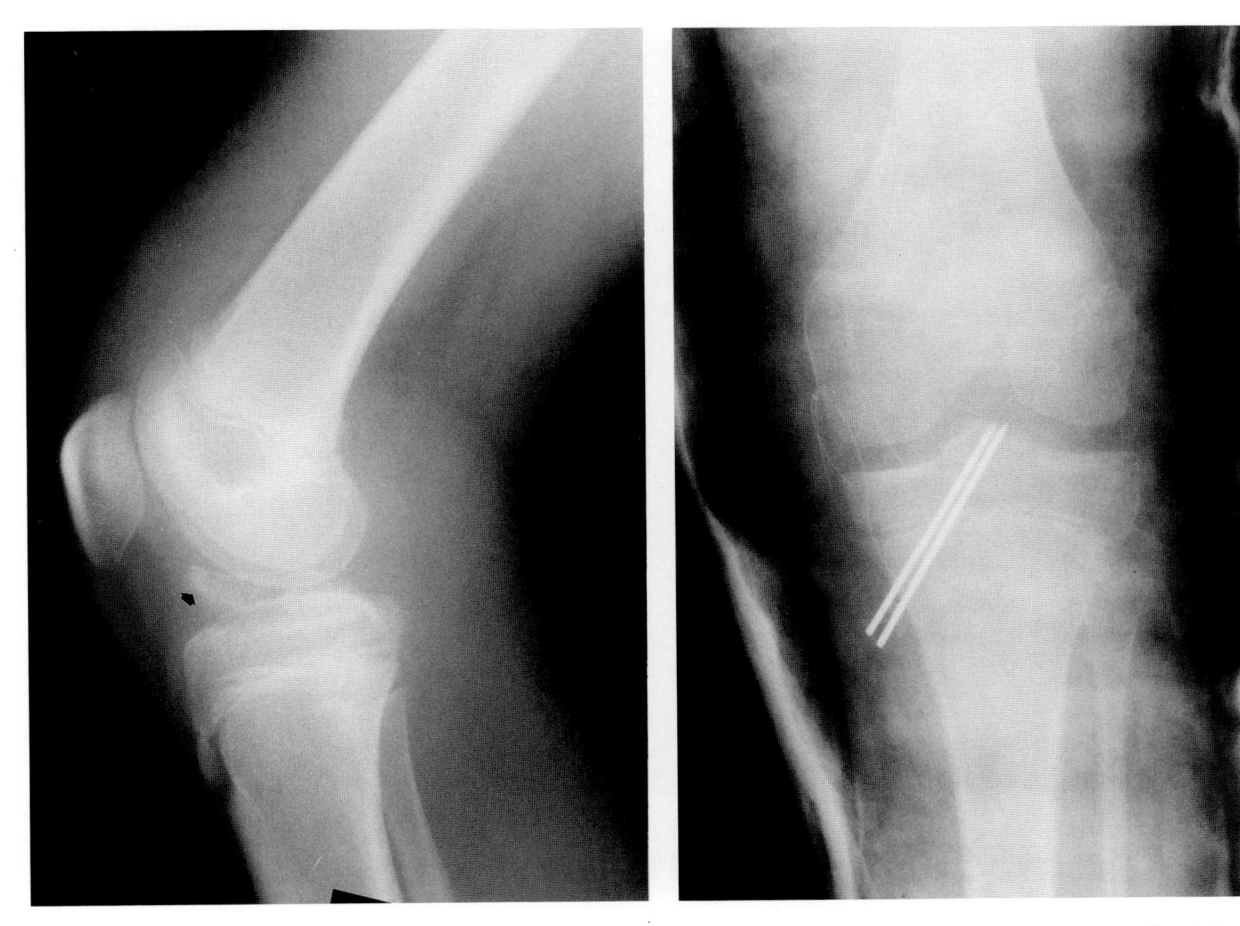

Fig. 32-11. A type III anterior tibial spine avulsion reduced and internally fixed with two smooth K-wires left subcutaneous for easy removal.

matic dislocation of the patella. Flexion of the knee combined with a direct blow during sporting activities may chip a small piece of bone and cartilage from the femoral condyle or from the patella.[13] Pain and swelling of the knee with hemarthrosis is characteristic. Ligament strength is normal. Diagnosis can be very difficult and the fragment impossible to see on regular radiographs or the tunnel anteroposterior view, especially if largely cartilaginous. Arthroscopic examination is useful to identify and locate the lesion and to remove the loose body. Only large fragments should be replaced. The lesion can usually be differentiated from osteochondritis dissecans of the knee due to the direct association with trauma. The site of osteochondritis is usually in the lateral aspect of the medial femoral condyle.

Replacement of the fragment, if large, should be undertaken using bone pegs, K-wires, small interfragmentary screws, or a Herbert screw. This may be accomplished arthroscopically, but if the fragment is difficult to accurately reduce, a formal arthrotomy is usually required. If K-wires are used, they can be extended through the adjacent cortex and left subcutaneously for easy removal in 4 to 6 weeks. Recent techniques using synthetic polyglycolic acid pegs or bonding with Tisseal are attractive, but await further critical assessment of their efficacy.[29,30]

SUMMARY

Intra-articular fractures of the knee in children are serious injuries, often difficult to diagnose and frequently requiring open reduction and internal fixation to ensure an anatomic restoration with an optimum re-

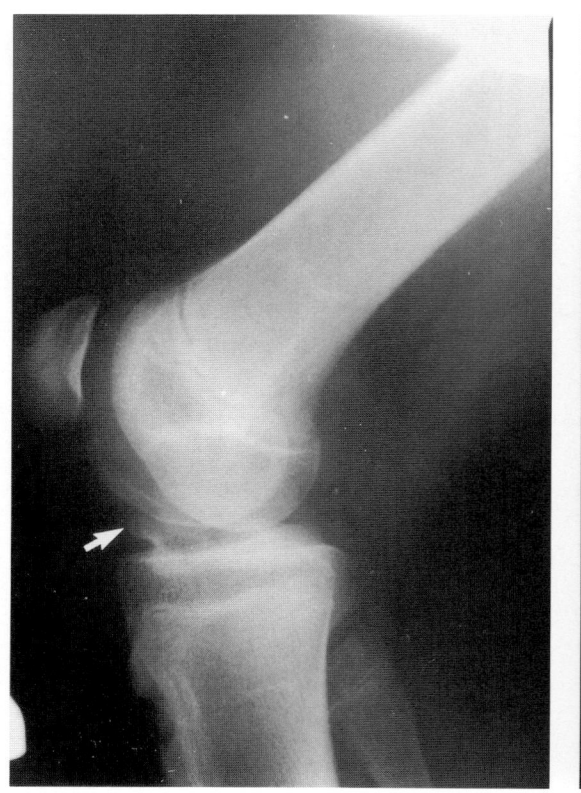

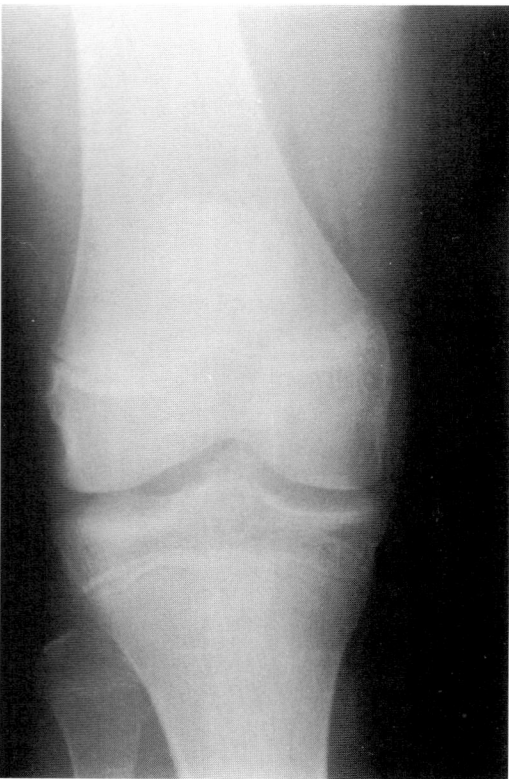

Fig. 32-12. Unreduced type III anterior tibial spine in a 15-year-old boy has healed in an elevated position and resulted in increased anterior tibial glide with a slight limitation of full extension of the knee.

sult. The maintenance of the integrity of the articular surface as well as the accurate alignment of the epiphyseal plate is essential. The rapid and significant physeal growth about the knee makes it susceptible to intra-articular epiphyseal fractures as well as having significant potential for functional disability secondary to physeal arrest, degenerative arthritis, or knee instability especially if these fractures are not treated promptly, accurately, and diligently.

REFERENCES

1. Salter RB, Harris WR: Injuries involving the epiphyseal plate. J Bone Joint Surg [Am] 45:587, 1963
2. Mizuta T, Benson WH, Foster BK: Statistical analysis of the incidence of physeal injuries. J Pediatr Orthop 7:518, 1987
3. Riseborough EJ, Barrett LR, Shapiro F: Growth disturbances following distal femoral physeal fracture-separation. J Bone Joint Surg [Am] 65:885, 1983
4. Lombardo SJ, Harvey P: Fractures of the distal femoral epiphysis. J Bone Joint Surg [Am] 59:742, 1977
5. Lascombes P, Prévot J, Bardoux J: The prognosis of fracture of the lower end of the femur in children and adolescents: a review of 96 cases. Rev Chir Orthop, suppl 74:438, 1988
6. Roberts JM: Fractures and dislocations of the knee. p. 891. In Rockwood CA, Wilkins KE, King RE (eds): Fractures in Children. Vol. 3. JB Lippincott, Philadelphia, 1984
7. Torg JS, Pavlov H, Morris VB: Salter-Harris type III fracture of the medial femoral condyle occurring in the adolescent athlete. J Bone Joint Surg [Am] 63:586, 1981
8. Padovani JP, Rigault P, Raux P, Lignac F, Guyonvarch G: Décollements épiphysaires traumatiques de l'extrémité inférieure du fémur. Rev Chir Orthop 62:211, 1976
9. Roberts JM: Operative fractures about the knee. Orthop Clin North Am 21:365, 1990
10. Bonnard C, Peres E: Fracture du genou de l'enfant. p. 331.

In Clavert JM, Metaizeau JP (eds): Les fractures des membres chez l'enfant. Sauramps Médical, Montpellier, 1990
11. Burkhart SS, Peterson HA: Fractures through the proximal tibia epiphysis. J Bone Joint Surg [Am] 61:996, 1979
12. Shelton WR, Canale T: Fractures of the tibia through the proximal tibial epiphyseal cartilage. J Bone Joint Surg [Am] 61:167, 1979
13. Sharrad WJW: Paediatric Orthopaedics and Fractures. 2nd Ed. Vol. 2. Blackwell, London, 1979
14. Christie MJ, Dvonch V: Tibial tuberosity avulsion fracture in adolescents. J Pediatr Orthop 1:391, 1981
15. Rang M: Children's Fractures. 2nd Ed. JB Lippincott, Philadelphia, 1983
16. Itokazu M, Yamane T, Shoen S: Incomplete avulsion of the femoral attachment of the posterior cruciate ligament in a twelve year old boy. Arch Orthop Trauma Surg 110:55, 1990
17. Roberts JM: Fractures and dislocations of the knee. p. 940. In Rockwood CA, Wilkins KE, King RE (eds): Fractures in Children. Vol. 3. JB Lippincott, Philadelphia, 1984
18. Meyers MH, McKeever FM: Fracture of the intercondylar eminence of the tibia. J Bone Joint Surg [Am] 52:1677, 1970
19. Tachdjian MO: Pediatric Orthopaedics. 2nd Ed. Vol. 4. WB Saunders, Philadelphia, 1990
20. Torisu T: Isolated avulsion fracture of the tibial attachment of the posterior cruciate ligament. J Bone Joint Surg [Am] 59:68, 1977
21. Kennedy J, Grainger RW: The posterior cruciate ligament. J Trauma 7:367, 1976
22. McMaster WH: Isolated posterior ligament injury: literature review. J Trauma 15:1025, 1975
23. Sanders WE, Wilkens KE, Neidre A: Acute insufficiencey of the posterior ligament in children. J Bone Joint Surg [Am] 62:129, 1980
24. Smith JB: Knee instability after fractures of the intercondylar eminence of the tibia. J Pediatr Orthop 4:462, 1984
25. Wiley JJ, Baxter MP: Tibial spine fractures in children. Clin Orthop 255:54, 1990
26. Rigault P, Moulies D, Padovani JP, Lesaux D: Les fractures des épines tibiales chez l'enfant: étude de 26 cas. Ann Chir Inf 17:237, 1976
27. Seriat-Gauthier B, Frick M, Pieracci M: Fractures des epines tibiales chez l'enfant. Rev Chir Orthop 69:221, 1983
28. Canale ST, Beaty JH: Operative Pediatric Orthopaedics. Mosby-Year Book, St. Louis, 1991
29. Plaga BR, Royster RM, Donigian AM et al: Fixation of osteochondral fractures in rabbit knees. J Bone Joint Surg [Br] 74:292, 1992
30. Scapinelli R: Treatment of fractures of the humeral capitellum using fibrin sealant. Acta Orthop Trauma Surg 109:235, 1990
31. Aitken AP: Fractures of the proximal tibial epiphyseal cartilage. Clin Orthop 41:92, 1965

33

Fractures and Dislocations of the Proximal Tibia and Fibula

James A. Harder

> The least questioned assumptions are often the most questionable.
> —PAUL BROCA

FRACTURES OF THE PROXIMAL TIBIA SHAFT

Incidence

Fractures of the tibia and fibula are the most common fractures in the lower limb in childhood.[1] Fractures located in the proximal tibial region and dislocation of the knee are, on the other hand, the least common injuries of this group but have the highest complication rate.[2-6]

Anatomy

Tibia and Fibula

It is important to understand the biomechanics and the anatomic characteristics of these fractures in order to understand the mechanism of injury, and institute a logical approach to the management and rehabilitation of the injured extremity. The tibia articulates with the femoral condyles proximally, and the tibia and fibula join to form the tibiofibular syndesmosis distally. They terminate at the ankle joint, forming the tibial plafonde. The two bones are joined together proximally by the tibiofibular synovial joint, and along their length by the interosseous membrane, which travels downward and laterally from the tibia to the fibulae.

Vessels and Nerves

The popliteal artery and veins pass behind the knee joint and are firmly held against the femur, tibia, and joint capsule[7] deep to the gastrocnemius heads (Fig. 33-1). Significant translation of the tibia will therefore result in injury or disruption of the vessels. The popliteal nerve, in contrast, is more superficial and therefore less likely to suffer damage during tibial translation-type injuries (Fig. 33-1). The anterior tibial artery branches from the popliteal artery and passes through a hiatus in the proximal interosseous membrane to supply the anterior compartment muscles. The anterior tibial artery is anchored in the interosseous hiatus, and significant translation of the proximal tibia will result in arterial disruption (Fig. 33-2). The gastrosoleus sling posteriorly and distally, under which the vascular bundle travels, also limits the movement of the vessels. The vascular bundle is at significant risk during high-energy translational injuries about the knee (Fig. 33-3).

The peroneal nerve passes around the proximal fibula to divide into the deep and superficial branches to serve

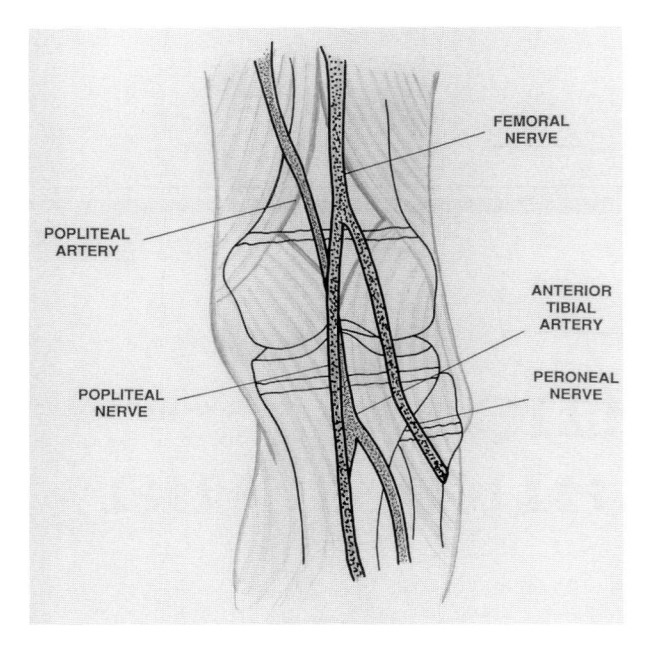

Fig. 33-1. Anatomy of popliteal fossa. The arteries lie next to the joint capsule. The nerves are immediately superficial to the arteries.

the anterior and lateral compartment muscles, respectively. The nerves are the most superficial layer and are the least constrained behind the popliteal fossa. Damage to the nervous structures is less frequent than damage to the vascular structures (Fig. 33-1).

Muscles

The muscles are rigidly contained in four compartments, which offer very little expandibility when they become filled with extravasated fluid from the injured bone and soft tissue. Compartment syndrome is therefore a serious concern, particularly when soft tissue damage has failed to disrupt the fascial compartments, or when soft tissue damage is associated with vascular compromise. When the fascial compartments are completely disrupted, blood will extravasate out of the compartment and into the subcutaneous tissues. The muscles and neurovascular structures are no longer confined, and pressure will be less likely to increase within the compartment. The period that the distal limb is avascular will determine the amount of cell death and

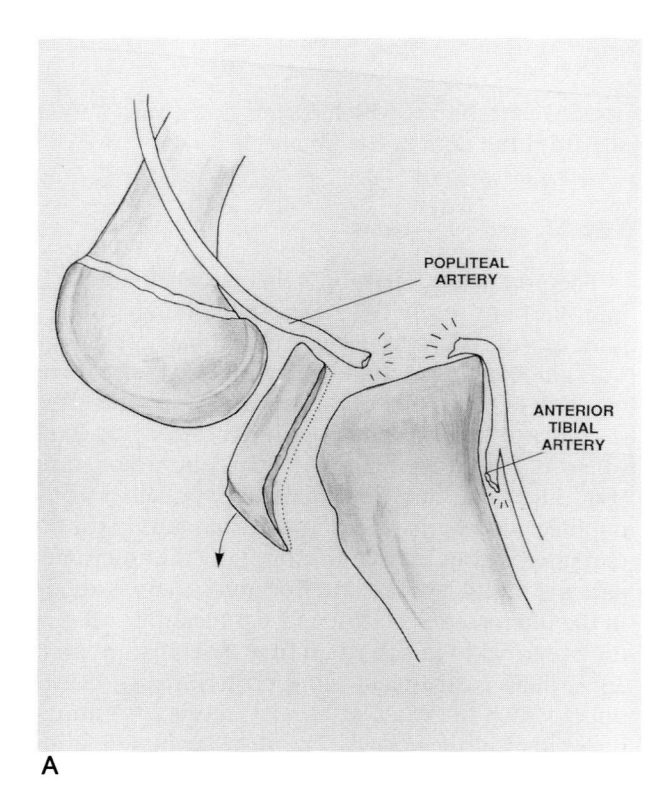

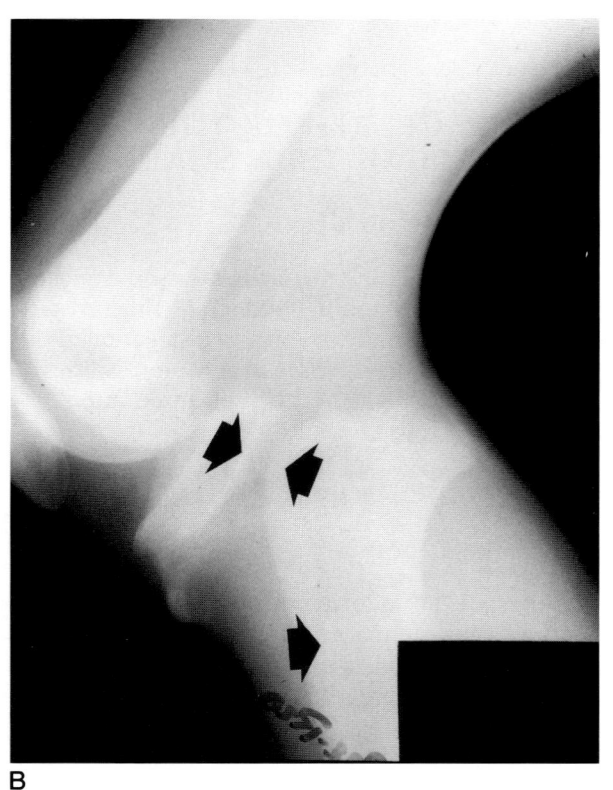

Fig. 33-2. (A) Salter-Harris type I epiphyseal plate fracture of the proximal tibia with popliteal artery disruption. (B) Compression of the plate may cause an associated type V injury to the posterior physis (arrows indicate direction of forces.).

Fractures and Dislocations of the Proximal Tibia and Fibula / 613

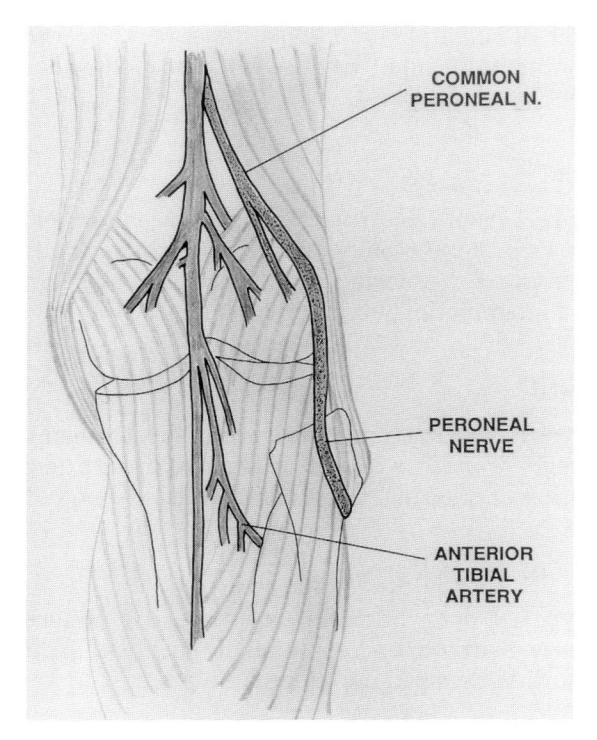

Fig. 33-3. The medial and lateral gastrocnemius muscles hold the posterior tibial artery, anterior tibial artery, and posterior tibial nerve closely to the proximal tibia.

the degree of cell membrane breakdown. After 6 hours of vascular compromise the likelihood of infection or failure to reestablish blood flow is high.[8] Immediately following revascularization there is significant exudation of edematous fluid into the compartments from the damaged tissues. Compartments that have maintained their integrity will experience significant rise in pressure, and the soft tissues are at significant risk to compromise by compartment syndrome.

Tibial Physis

The growth plate at the proximal end of the tibia is extracapsular but surrounded by the knee ligaments and is protected from direct valgus and varus strain (Fig. 33-4). The patellar tendon inserts into the tibial tubercle apophysis, which may be part of or separate from the proximal tibial epiphysis. Growth of the tibia and fibula is distributed such that approximately 60 percent of the total length of the bone is contributed by the proximal tibial growth plate, and 40 percent is contributed by the distal tibial physis. This becomes important when growth arrest occurs due to physeal damage and estimation in leg length discrepancy is required.[9,10]

The proximal tibial physis is more stable than most other epiphyseal plates. Considerable force is required to disrupt the physis. This stability is due both to the protection of the medial and lateral collateral ligaments as well as many mammillary processes protruding from the tibial metaphysis into the physis.

Mechanism of Injury

Injury to the proximal tibia and fibula occur when forces are exerted on the proximal aspect of the lower leg either independently or associated with a rotational and angular component. High velocity and contact are the key ingredients to an obvious fracture, whereas more subtle stress fractures will occur after repeated microstress. Some examples are the pedestrian automobile accident in the teenage patient where the proximal tibia is high enough to be contacted by the car bumper, or the vehicular passenger who moves forward against the dashboard or seat ahead, striking the knee and lower leg area. Sporting activities such as soccer, basketball, hockey, tobogganing, skating, skiing, snowboarding, and track and field are other examples of activities where a fracture may occur suddenly, or after prolonged repeated fatigue injury to the bone or soft tissues.[11]

The toddler, when properly restrained in a moving vehicle is still subject to lower limb injury. Uphold and

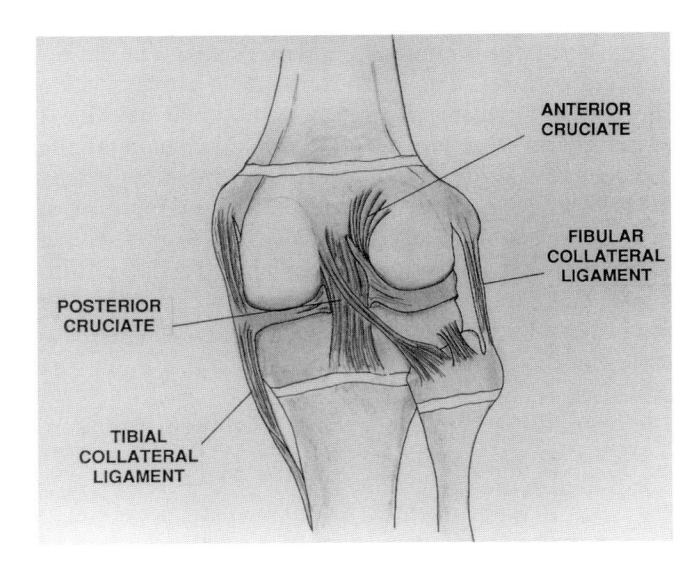

Fig. 33-4. The capsule of the knee joint attaches from the distal femoral epiphysis to the proximal tibial epiphysis. The medial collateral ligament runs from the proximal femoral epiphysis and attaches proximal and distal to the proximal tibial growth plate, thus offering some protection from proximal tibial physeal disruption.

colleagues,[12] in a study of 10 properly restrained toddlers, reported fractures of the tibia and fibula, with minimal displacement. Diagnosis was made on radiograph and not by observing the soft tissue swelling or obvious angulation.

Classification of Proximal Tibial Fractures and Dislocation

The classification of proximal tibial fractures and dislocation is as follows:

I. Closed or open fractures of the proximal tibia
II. Fractures involving the tibial physis or apophysis
III. Fractures of the proximal tibial metaphysis
IV. Dislocation of the knee joint
V. Dislocation of the tibiofibular joint

Management

Closed Fractures

Closed fractures of the proximal tibia and fibula are treated by manipulation and external splinting. The complexity of the splint will depend upon the stability of the fracture, and the severity of damage to the soft tissues. Methods may be as simple as a removable splint or plaster slab if the fracture is inherently stable. The plaster or fiberglass cast is used for more unstable patterns where shortening, angular deformity, or rotational stability is required. The knee joint and the foot are included in the cast to give rotational stability. The external fixator may be considered, particularly when soft tissue injury is of prime concern, and significant swelling, or soft tissue viability are a major concern. The stability of the fixation device becomes more important the more unstable the fracture, and must meet a number of management principles:

1. Maintain acceptable fracture alignment (rotation, angulation, length)
2. Stabilize the soft tissues
3. Help to relieve pain
4. Allow adequate clinical observation of the injured limb

Open Fractures: Gustilo Classification

Open fractures[13] are treated according to the size of the open injury, the degree of soft tissue damage, and the degree of contamination. Open fractures are classified according to Gustilo,[14] as discussed in the following sections.

TYPE I

Type I open fractures have a skin laceration of less than 1 cm long, usually caused by a bone spike from within or a low-velocity bullet. The soft tissue damage and contamination are minimal.

TYPE II

Type II open fractures have a wound greater than 1 cm in length or width, with little devitalized tissue extensive avulsion or crushing. Contamination is moderate.

TYPE III

Type III open fractures have extensive soft tissue damage, avulsion, and contamination. These fractures are further classified into three subtypes.

Type IIIa. In type IIIa fractures, soft tissue coverage of the fractured bone is adequate, despite heavy contamination of the fracture and extensive soft tissue damage, with or without segmental bone loss.

Type IIIb. Type IIIb fractures demonstrate extensive injury to soft tissue and bone, with massive contamination. After debridement and irrigation is complete, there remains an area of soft tissue loss exposing a segment of bone.

Type IIIc. Type IIIc injuries are associated with an arterial injury, which requires repair, regardless of the soft tissue injury.[13]

GENERAL PRINCIPLES

Management of the open wound is based on well-established principles of debridement, irrigation, intravenous antibiotics, and gaining stability of the bone, and soft tissues.[8] The fracture is managed according to its pattern, location, and inherent stability and will include splinting, casting, external fixation, internal fixation, or amputation. A type I fracture requires a first-generation cephalosporin administered intravenously for 48 to 72 h. Intramedullary nailing and reaming is not recommended for early stabilization of open tibial fractures due to the increased incidence of infection.[14,15] Types II and III fractures require a cephalosporin plus an aminoglycoside to cover both gram-positive and gram-negative organisms. Penicillin is added if the patient sustained the injury in a farmyard or there is other reason to suspect clostridial contamination. All antibiotics for the type III fractures are administered intravenously, at doses prescribed for severe infection for no longer than 3 days at a time. Antibiotics may be restarted after reculturing, if there is evidence of infection, or if a surgical procedure is performed.

FRACTURES OF THE PROXIMAL TIBIAL PHYSIS

Isolated fractures of the proximal tibia are a relatively uncommon injury[2] due to the protection offered the physis by the collateral ligaments of the knee (Fig. 33-4). Forces required to disrupt the physis are therefore significant, and there is a high probability of fracture instability after reduction. The fracture is usually of the Salter-Harris type I or type II and the tibial tubercle may stay with the epiphysis or form a separately avulsed fragment (Fig. 33-5).

Physical Examination

On physical examination the knee joint area will be significantly swollen, with the primary areas of tenderness related to the proximal tibia. With complete disruption of the ligamentous structures on the medial or lateral side of the knee, there will be no knee effusion, as the blood will have extravasated into the soft tissues. As movement of the tibial plateau can easily damage the posterior neurovascular structures, assessment and documentation of the neurovascular status of the lower leg is of great importance. Because of a fairly good collateral cutaneous blood supply, the skin of the distal leg and foot often appears well vascularized in spite of complete disruption of the popliteal artery. Unless one maintains a high degree of suspicion of arterial injury, one may be lulled into a false sense of security. The history of the injury is very important, to ascertain the magnitude and duration of the forces involved. Should the limb distal to the fracture be cool and pulseless, further investigation of the vascularity is indicated. Angiograms should not delay the operative intervention significantly, and therefore it is suggested that they be done in the surgical suite during the exploration and debridement phase of treatment. Delaying revascularization of the distal limb by more than 6 hours significantly increases the incidence of muscle necrosis and amputation.[8]

Radiologic Assessment

Radiologic examination of the knee should include anteroposterior, lateral, and oblique views of the joint, including the distal femur and the proximal tibia. Usually the fracture is clearly evident on the radiograph. Sometimes the radiograph may be normal in appearance except for soft tissue swelling and a widened physeal line. Careful physical examination will help to confirm the diagnosis of a type I growth plate fracture. The proximal tibial physis is very superficial and can be easily palpated. Pain on pressure directly over the growth plate assist in the differentiation between a type I growth plate injury and a ligamentous injury. If there is still doubt about the extent of the injury, stress views under anesthesia may be necessary (Fig. 33-5A&B).

Management of Physeal Injury

With the child supine on a stretcher or the operating table under general anesthesia, the knee is examined. If there is a large hemarthrosis, the knee joint is aspirated under sterile conditions. Aspiration of the knee is best accomplished with a large 18-gauge needle introduced under the lateral aspect of the patella. Hemarthrosis is evidence that the soft tissues in continuity with the joint have been disrupted, and a ligamentous injury to the knee is likely. If the fluid is bloody with fatty globules floating on the top, then an associated intra-articular fracture is likely. *Fracture and ligamentous tears of the knee may coexist, but this is uncommon in children.*

After the knee is aspirated, it should be stressed in all directions for instability. The examination is observed with the image intensifier and the origin of the instability identified, that is, ligamentous, physeal separation, or both.

Closed Reduction

Gentle closed reduction is the preferred method of treatment for physeal injuries of the tibia. The patient may be positioned supine if there is no suspicion of a vascular injury. If a vascular injury is suspected, however, it is best to position the patient prone on the operating table, and perform the closed reduction by grasping the proximal tibia, in much the same way a supracondylar fracture of the humerus might be manipulated (Fig. 33-6). If vascular compromise is confirmed post-closed reduction, exploration of the vascular structures in the popliteal fossa is facilitated in the prone position. With the fracture reduced under the image intensifier, stability of the fracture is assessed. If the fracture is stable, the leg

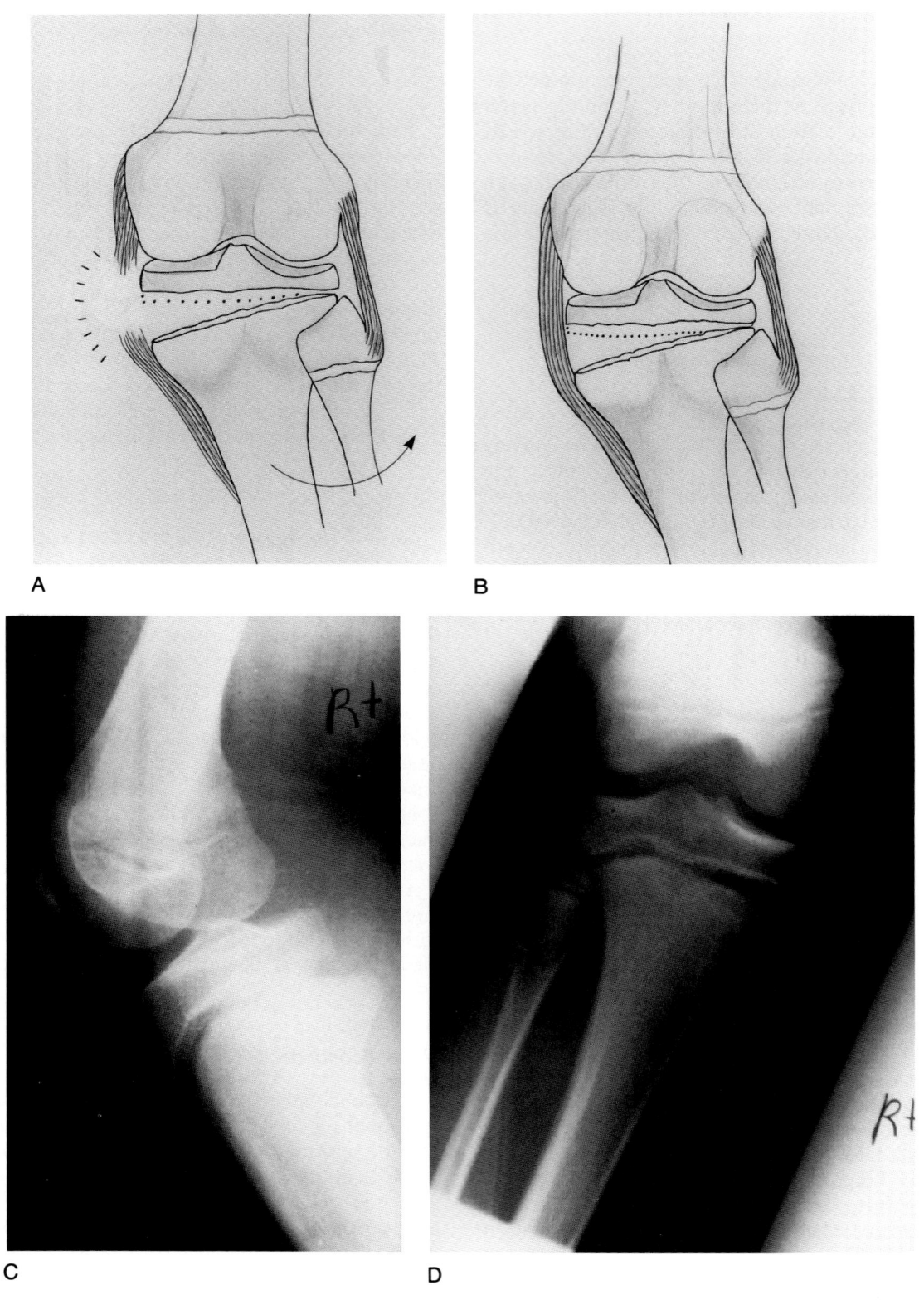

Fig. 33-5. (A & B) Salter-Harris type I fracture of the proximal tibial physis, with a valgus strain being applied under general anesthesia. (A) The disruption of the medial collateral ligament inferiorly. (B) The medial collateral ligament may also be intact. (C & D) Valgus injury to the knee with a minimally displaced Salter-Harris type I fracture of the proximal tibia and a metaphyseal fracture of the proximal fibula. (D) The "notch view" of the femur indicates the knee is in flexion, and therefore valgus angulation cannot be accurately assessed on this AP radiographic view. In spite of minimal displacement of the tibial epiphysis, a physeal arrest of the anterior plate occurred which resulted in genu recurvatum over several years. *(Figure continues.)*

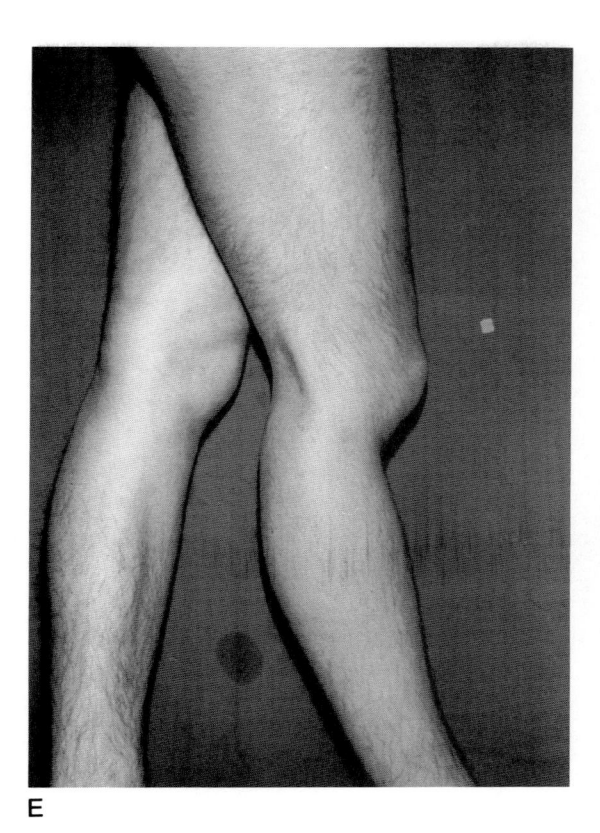

Fig. 33-5 *(Continued).* **(E)** In spite of minimal displacement of the tibial epiphysis, a physeal arrest of the anterior plate occurred which resulted in the development of genu recurvatum over several years of growth.

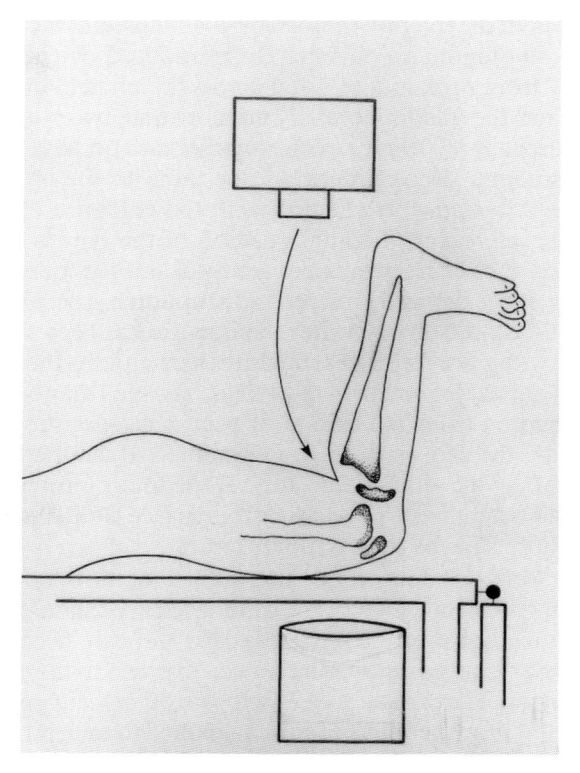

Fig. 33-6. A method of reduction of a displaced proximal tibial epiphysis in younger children that is often helpful is to place the child prone on the operating table and deal with the fracture like a supracondylar fracture of the humerus. Percutaneous pinning is recommended postreduction using the image intensifier.

is immobilized in a posterior plaster slab. This allows for inspection of the knee when at rest, and the application of ice packs. If a vascular repair was necessary, the leg should be placed in a cylinder cast to stabilize the fracture and protect the vascular repair. Cylinder casts are notorious for sliding down and chafing the medial and lateral maleolei. This can be prevented to some extent by using tincture of benzoin on the skin, by molding the cast in the area above the femoral condyles and by extending the cast only to the mid-calf area. *Whether a splint or a cast is used, the knee should be in full extension,* as this is the only way to adequately assess the presence of angulation at the fracture site. If the vascular repair will not allow full extension, the fracture should be securely stabilized with two percutaneus Steinmann pins, before the vascular repair takes place. A stabilized fracture may be placed in some flexion at the knee to protect the vascular repair, without the danger of malunion. Radiographic assessment for varus or valgus drift at the fracture site is difficult, with the knee in any amount of flexion. *The cylinder cast will not stabilize rotation.* If there is any evidence of rotational instability, the cast should be extended to include the foot. Knee extension will be difficult to obtain if there is a large hemarthrosis present. The effusion should be aspirated under sterile conditions, to allow ease of extension without undue tension on the posterior soft tissues. The patient should ambulate with crutches—partial weightbearing. Total immobilization of the knee should be continued for 3 to 4 weeks as epiphyseal fractures stabilize more rapidly than osseous fractures. Gentle range of motion is then encouraged, under the guidance of a physiotherapist, and splinting is continued for another week while up with crutches. The splint is then discontinued, and the limb is rehabilitated with gradual increasing range of motion and muscle strengthening. Swimming is an excellent exercise to rehabilitate the injured limb and to maintain cardiopulmonary fitness during the early stages of rehabilitation. Contact sports are permitted again after the patient is able to run without a limp.

Should the fracture be unstable after closed reduction, smooth Steinmann pins may be introduced percutaneously from proximal to distal across the physeal line to stabilize the fracture. Usually no more than two pins are required, at 45 degrees to one another and because they are smooth, little damage will be done to the growth plate. After pin introduction with the guidance of the image intensifier, the final position of the pins is confirmed and the fracture again gently examined for instability. If coexisting ligamentous disruption has occurred, it will become obvious after the fracture has been stabilized with pins. As physeal fractures heal rapidly, the pins need only be left in for 14 to 21 days. The pins may be left protruding from the skin, and bent at 90 degrees just outside the skin to prevent migration and facilitate removal in the outpatient clinic. Betadine ointment is placed around the pin and skin interface under sterile conditions at the time of pin insertion.

As long as the sterile dressing applied in the operating room is left intact, pin care is unnecessary. Should the dressing, however, be replaced, daily pin care becomes necessary, as the pin sites have been exposed to the environment. The pin site is cleansed with 50 percent peroxide, and more betadine ointment applied to each pin site on a daily basis. This can be done after a shower or wash with soap and water, if the fracture was stable enough to have been immobilized in a posterior slab or knee immobilizer. Soaking the leg and pin sites in the bath is not recommended.

Open Reduction

Open reduction is reserved for irreducible fractures secondary to soft tissue interposition of the ligamentous structures into the fracture site or the Salter-Harris types III and IV fractures where the articular surface and the physis must be accurately aligned. Soft tissue interposition into the physis is evident by appreciating a persistently widened epiphyseal line after closed reduction. A medial or lateral approach to the growth plate is performed and the offending interposed soft tissues removed. Stability postreduction is tested intraoperatively, and percutaneous pins introduced across the fracture site if indicated by existing instability.

After stability has been achieved, the leg is treated as a closed fracture as described above. If the fracture involves the joint space as in the Salter-Harris type III or IV, an anteromedial or anterolateral approach to the joint is indicated, to expose the joint as well as the fracture site. The fracture site is inspected and washed clean of all clot, as well as small loose pieces of bone. Comminution at the fracture site may result in some loss of

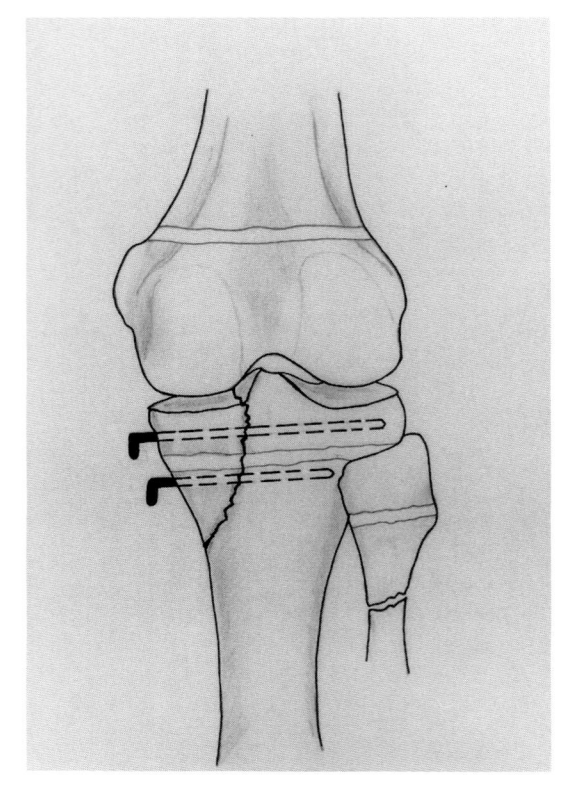

Fig. 33-7. Parallel percutaneous pinning of a Salter-Harris type IV fracture of the proximal tibia. The articular surface is aligned preferentially in the presence of comminution. Small comminuted fragments of bone near the epiphysis should be irrigated free and discarded. The gaps near the physis are best left open or filled with fat if large enough.

epiphyseal integrity. The articular surface is aligned preferentially and the larger fragments held with threaded Steinmann pins or a single screw passed parallel to the growth plate (Fig. 33-7). Threaded Steinmann pins or screws must not be passed across the physis. The gap is not packed with the removed comminuted pieces of bone, as this will likely encourage the formation of an epiphyseal bar and lead to growth disturbance. The gap is simply left open, to fill in spontaneously, and the patient kept nonweightbearing until evidence of radiologic healing is present. Fat from the adjacent subcutaneous tissue may be placed into the defect at the level of the physis if it is large enough. The fat may help prevent epiphyseal bar formation.[16] As the pins do not go across the growth plate, there is no hurry to remove them. The likelihood of Salter-Harris type V physeal damage with subsequent epiphyseal bar formation, is much greater if there is evidence of comminution at the time of open reduction.[17]

Complications

As the forces necessary to produce this injury are significant, growth plate arrest and ligamentous instability of the knee may occur. After the fracture has been stabilized by percutaneous pin fixation, the knee should be examined clinically with the image intensifier to assess any associated ligamentous damage.[18]

An associated Salter-Harris type V physeal injury or an Ogden type 6 injury to the perichondral ring[19] will become obvious on follow-up radiographs of the proximal tibia at 6 to 12 months postinjury (Fig. 33-8). An epiphyseal bar will be seen and depending on its size and position, may result in angular deformity of the tibia. The bar should be evaluated by three-dimensional CT scan to determine its exact location and extent. If three-dimensional CT is not available, tomography should be used. Surgical excision of the bar may then be indicated.[18] Vascular damage to the popliteal artery may be confirmed at the time of the injury by arteriography and the appropriate steps taken to repair and restore the arterial flow to the lower leg. Reduction of the fracture, must not be unduly delayed in order to perform arteriography. The likely site of neurovascular disruption is in the popliteal fossa. If adequate circulation is not restored to the distal portion of the leg after closed reduction and pinning of the fracture, exploration of the popliteal fossa and repair of the arterial injury is indicated with or without an arteriogram. Reduction and possible exploration of the popliteal fossa can sometimes be facilitated by reducing this fracture with the patient in the prone position. The fracture is then manipulated much like a supracondylar fracture of the humerus (Fig. 33-6). Compartment fasciotomy is indicated in the case of major vascular disruption at the time of vessel repair as the likelihood of developing compartment syndrome is high.

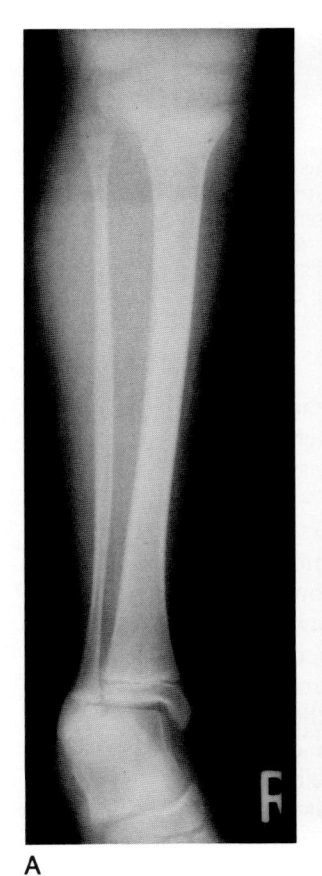

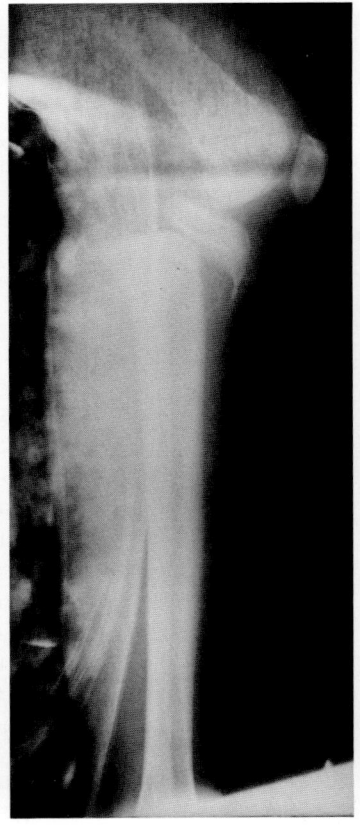

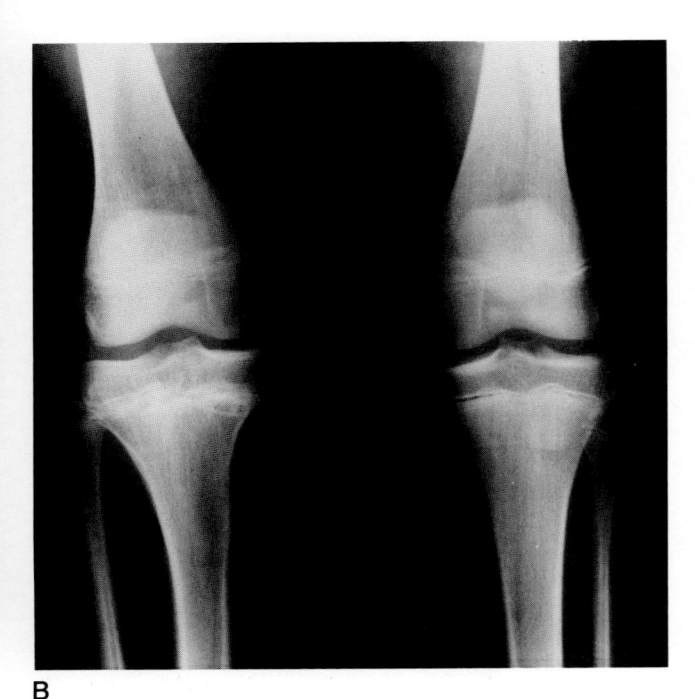

Fig. 33-8. (A) Salter-Harris type I fracture of the proximal tibia with significant posterior displacement of the distal tibia in a 10-year-old boy who struck a tree branch while on a snowmobile driving the tibia posteriorly. (B) One year later a physeal arrest of the proximal growth plate was obvious.

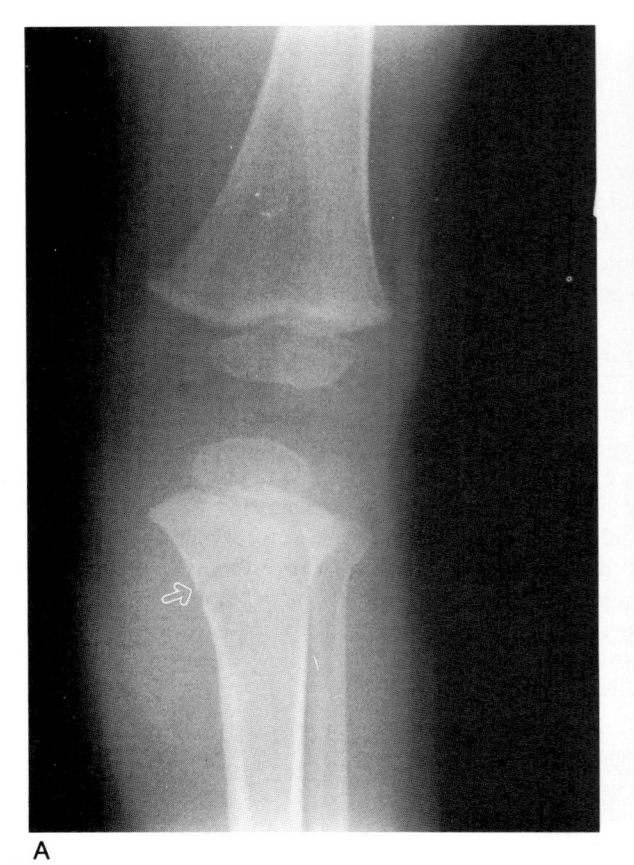

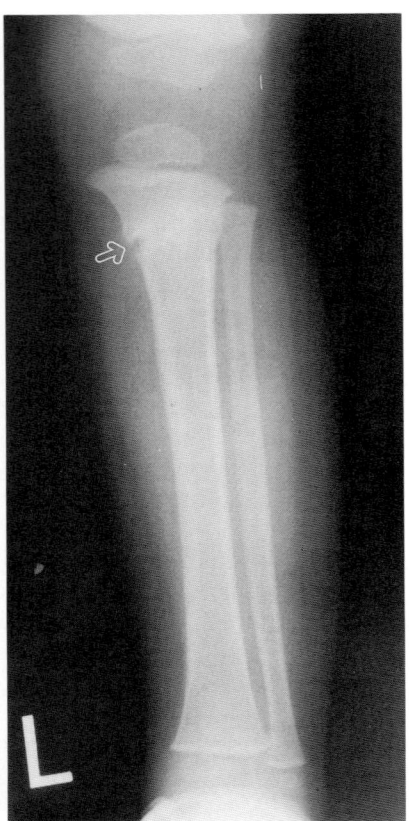

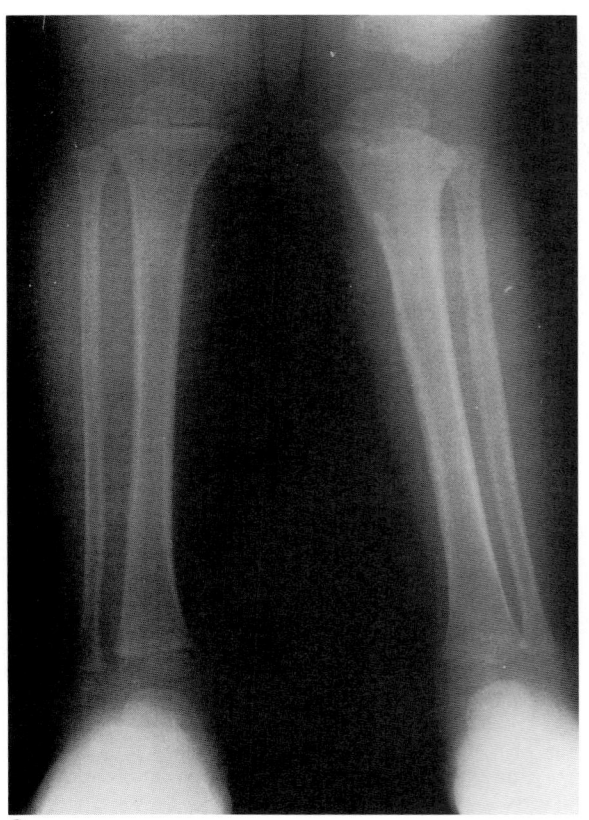

Fig. 33-9. A valgus injury to the left knee with an oblique fracture of the proximal tibia and an intact fibula, which may cause a valgus deformity if not well casted. **(A)** The fracture is hardly visible and appears innocuous *(arrow)*, whereas **(B)** 2 months later it has opened medially and a valgus deformity is beginning *(arrow)*, but **(C)** 1 year later is quite marked.

Isolated Fractures of the Proximal Tibia with Intact Fibula

Fracture of the proximal tibia in the area of the pes anserinus is a relatively common fracture in the pediatric age group and is usually caused by a direct valgus force to the tibia during a high-velocity activity[1-6] (Fig. 33-9).

The child will complain of significant pain along the medial aspect of the knee, and there will be accompanying swelling about 1.5 cm distal to the joint space. There may be some valgus angulation of the tibia evident on examination. The differential diagnosis lies between separation of the physis (Salter-Harris type I) a medial tibial metaphyseal fracture, or disruption of the medial soft tissue structures of the knee.

Radiologic examination of the knee joint by anteroposterior lateral and oblique views will show a transverse fracture line along the medial tibial metaphysis passing into the metaphysis laterally anywhere from 5 mm in length to involving the entire extent of the metaphysis. Angulation is usually in the valgus plane and seldom is there any rotational malalignment in the common variety of injury. Soft tissue disruption is confined to the pes anserinus, and the periosteum at the fracture site on the medial side of the tibia.

Management

Closed Reduction

Management of this fracture appears simple, but beware that this fracture is fraught with a significant incidence of residual persistent valgus malalignment. Theories as to the etiology of the valgus deformity are numerous, and all include reference to the complex growth relationship of the proximal tibial physis, the pes anserinus, the tibial tubercle apophysis, and the proximal fibula.[20] The proposed etiologies that are still popular include the following[3-6]:

1. Inadequate fracture reduction
2. Weightbearing too early
3. Soft tissue imbalance
4. Soft tissue interposition in the fracture site
5. Tethering by the fibula
6. Salter-Harris type V fracture of the lateral tibial physis
7. Asymmetric overgrowth secondary to an increased vascular response.

There are factors that have been identified, which can be easily remedied by following three recognized principles of fracture management:

1. There must be no residual valgus deformity at the fracture site after the reduction. This can only be assessed with the knee in full extension.
2. Valgus deformity must not be allowed to develop during the healing process. Complete reduction can only be accomplished and maintained by holding the knee in a cast in complete extension.
3. The pes anserinus and the periosteum must not be entrapped in the fracture site. This will be seen by persistence of the fracture line on the anteroposterior radiographic view.

A closed reduction is accomplished under general anesthesia, by correcting the valgus deformity. *As the knee must be in extension to reduce the fracture, so must it be held in extension to maintain the reduction.* Observation of the reduction with the image intensifier or standard anteroposterior and lateral radiographic views postreduction, will demonstrate the quality of the reduction. If valgus angulation has been completely corrected and the fracture line has closed, the fracture is held reduced in a well-molded cast with the knee in *full extension.* Varus force is applied to the knee while the cast is setting, and an assistant should mold the cast above the femoral condyles to help prevent the cast from slipping downward. If the fracture line remains open on the postreduction radiograph, the pes anserinus and periosteum are likely entrapped in the fracture. Persistent soft tissue interposition may result in prolonged hyperemia and prolonged healing at the fracture site[3] with the development of a valgus deformity of the tibia immediately distal to the fracture site. *Open reduction is therefore indicated if the fracture line is widened after closed reduction.*[6]

Open Reduction

Open reduction is accomplished by making a short oblique incision over the pes anserinus of the proximal medial tibia. The pes anserinus area is exposed and will be found to be enfolded into the fracture site with the periosteum.[6] The soft tissues are elevated out of the fracture site, and the fracture reduced. It will be necessary to hold the knee in extension to reduce the fracture, and therefore it is also important to keep the knee extended in the cast to maintain the reduction. No internal fixation is required. The leg should be immobilized in a cyclinder cast as described in the section on closed treatment.

Complications

The complications of fracture of the proximal tibia are the following:

1. Failure to reduce the valgus angulation at the time of closed reduction
2. Failure to maintain the reduction by allowing the knee to be flexed in the cast
3. Failure to recognize the presence of soft tissue in the persistently opened fracture site postreduction
4. The development of valgus deformity unrelated to any of the above factors

Management of Valgus Deformity

The development of valgus deformity of the proximal tibia after a proximal tibial fracture, is a frequent complication.[5,21,22] The valgus angulation will develop during the first 12 months postfracture, and will then usually remain stable. The development of valgus deformity is predictable if there is persistent valgus after closed reduction, or if the fracture remains wide due to soft tissue interposition after closed reduction. The degree of valgus that occurs is, however, not predictable. Braces and shoe lifts have been used to control or correct the valgus deformity, but the efficacy of these treatments is not known.[22] The valgus deformity does not cause functional impairment, but is cosmetically unsightly. Angulation beyond 15 degrees is thought to be significant enough to correct by osteotomy.[22] Slow correction of the valgus deformity by remodeling of the distal tibia creating an s-shaped or serpentine tibia is possible in the infant or juvenile.

Correction of the deformity can be accomplished surgically by osteotomy of the tibia and fibula. If a dome or wedge osteotomy is selected, the osteotomy must be performed well below the tibial tubercle so as not to endanger further growth in this area. This results in a dog leg deformity of the tibia, which will be evident on radiograph for some time (Fig. 33-9C).

My own preferred method of correction is an oblique osteotomy, which is made along the coronal plane pass-

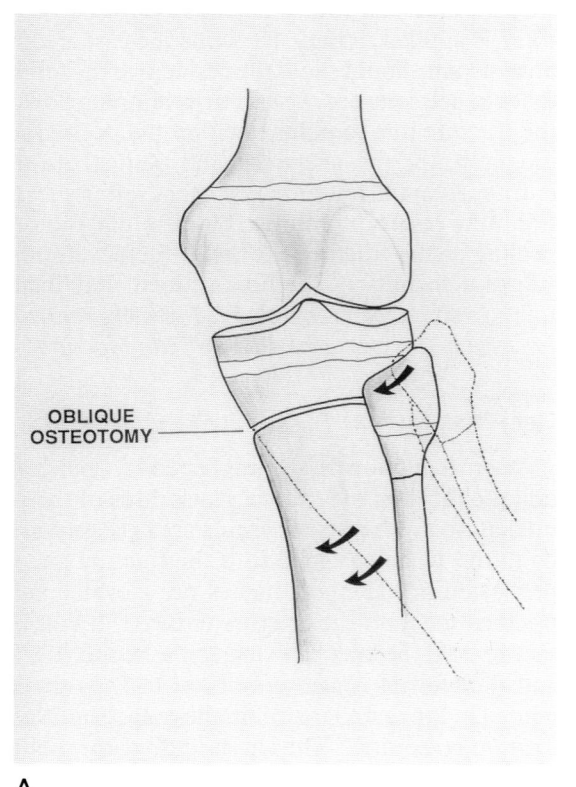

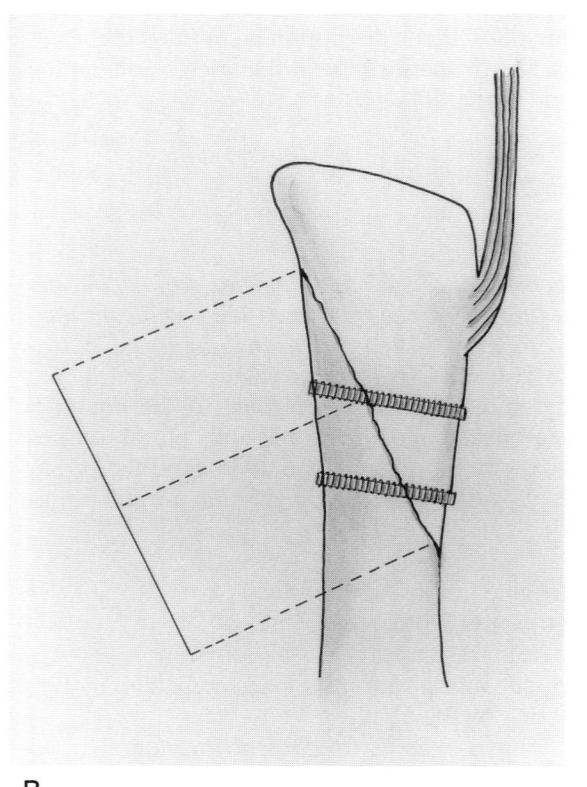

Fig. 33-10. An **(A)** AP and **(B)** lateral view of the proximal tibia is shown. The osteotomy is indicated by the oblique line in Fig. B and is cut so that a central threaded Steinmann pin can be placed across the osteotomy from anterior to posterior, and used as a pivot point. The more distal Steinmann pin secures the osteotomy after the angular correction is made. The tibial osteotomy must be inferior and completely clear of the physis posteriorly. The fibular osteotomy should be near the same level as the tibial osteotomy to allow ease of rotation.

ing from the posterior and proximal tibia, under the tibial tubercle, to exit anteriorly and distal to the tibial tubercle. After the osteotomy of the tibia and fibula are complete,[23] as illustrated in Fig. 33-10, a threaded Steinmann pin must be inserted from the anterior tibia, through the midpoint of the osteotomy, so that rotational correction of the valgus can be facilitated. The central Steinmann pin stabilizes the osteotomy and allows controlled rotation of the osteotomy without displacement. The midpoint of the osteotomy must therefore fall just distal to the tibial tubercle, so that the central pin does not interfere with the tibial tubercle. Another

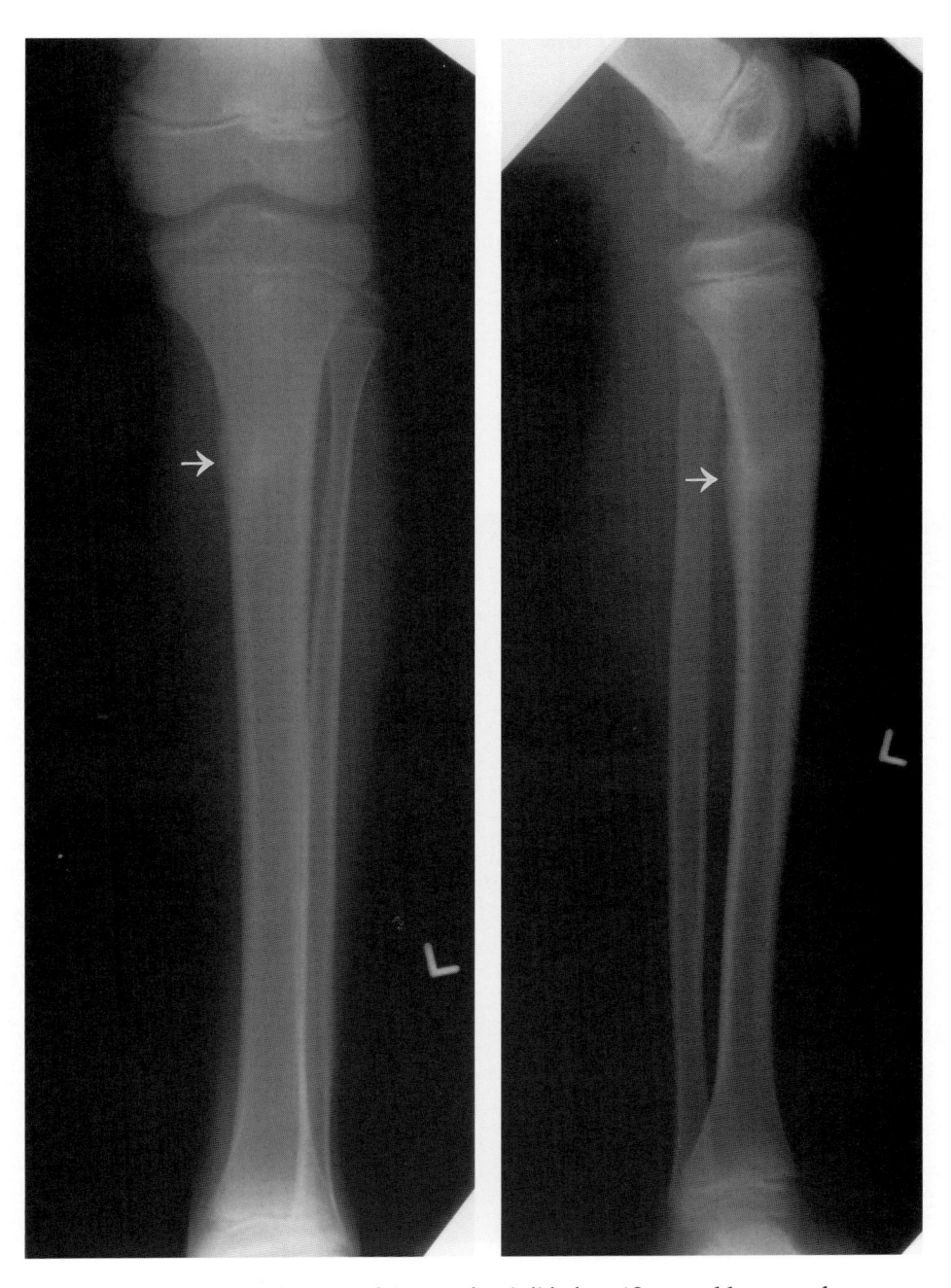

Fig. 33-11. A stress fracture of the proximal tibia in a 12-year-old soccer player.

Steinmann pin is then used distally to fix the osteotomy after correction of the valgus deformity. The leg is then placed in a long-leg cast. The pins are left in place for approximately 3 weeks or until there is radiologic evidence of stability. The pins are then removed, and a further cast applied, until the osteotomy is clinically healed.

Stress Fractures of the Proximal Tibia

Stress fractures of the proximal tibia are commonly encountered in teenage athletes, usually in association with a particularly rigorous game or training schedule. The adolescent complains of pain and aching in the upper tibia although the complaint may be of "knee pain." Initial radiographs of the proximal tibia often show no fracture, although a bone scan is usually positive at this early stage. Radiographs taken 5 to 7 days later will usually reveal periosteal elevation and a faint line across the tibial metaphysis (Fig. 33-11).

Treatment with 3 weeks of a cylinder cast, primarily to prevent participation in athletics as much as to rest and immobilize the fracture, is usually successful in healing the injury. Nonunion is rare.

Pathologic Fractures of the Proximal Tibia

The upper tibia is a common site for cyst, tumors, and infection, all of which predispose to pathologic fractures in this area. Usually the diagnosis is self-evident with the cyst or tumor being obvious, as in the unicameral bone cyst in Fig. 33-12, which first presented in a 12-year-old girl with a pathologic fracture. Occasionally, however, it may be more subtle, as in the 16-year-old girl shown in Fig. 33-13, with a metaphyseal fracture through a small nonossifying fibroma that may have been a combination of a pathologic and a stress fracture in this very athletic teenager. Treatment consists of immobilization in a cylinder cast for 4 to 6 weeks until the fracture has consolidated followed by a treatment plan for the underlying pathologic lesion. If a malignant lesion has been suspected, an immediate biopsy is of course indicated.

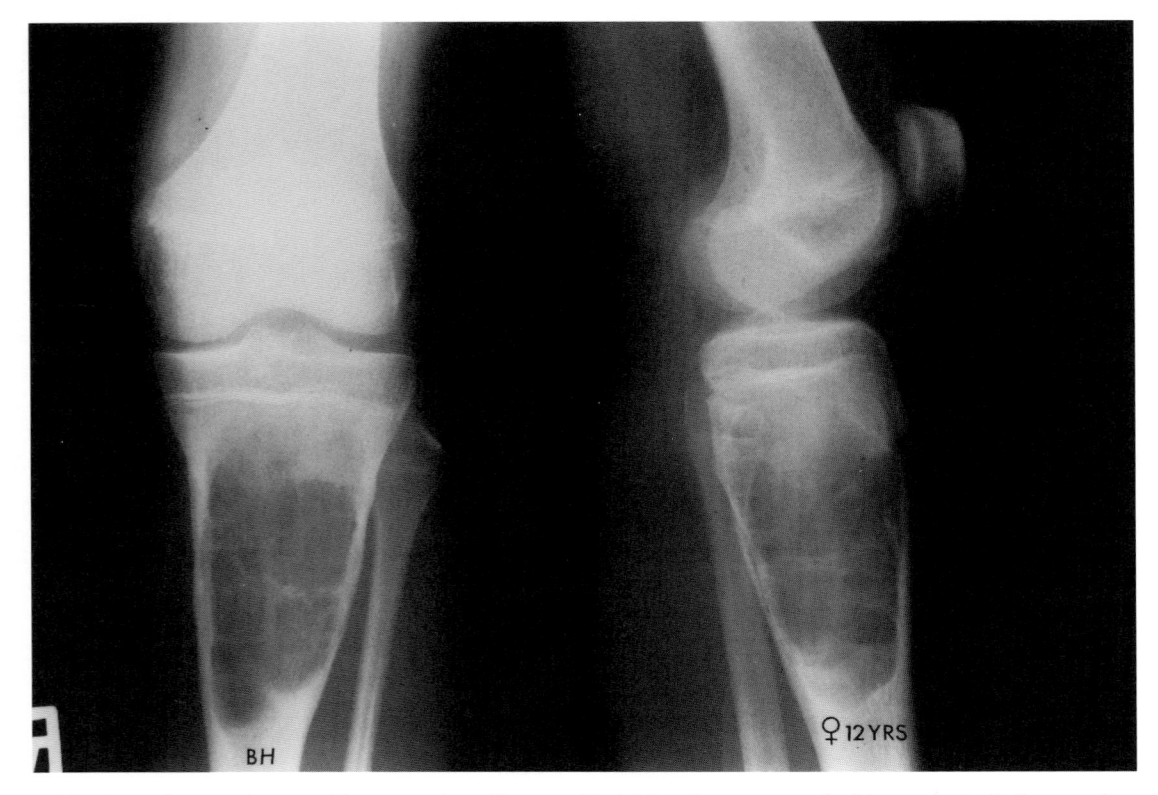

Fig. 33-12. A large unicameral bone cyst in a 12-year-old girl that first presented with a pathologic fracture from a minor fall.

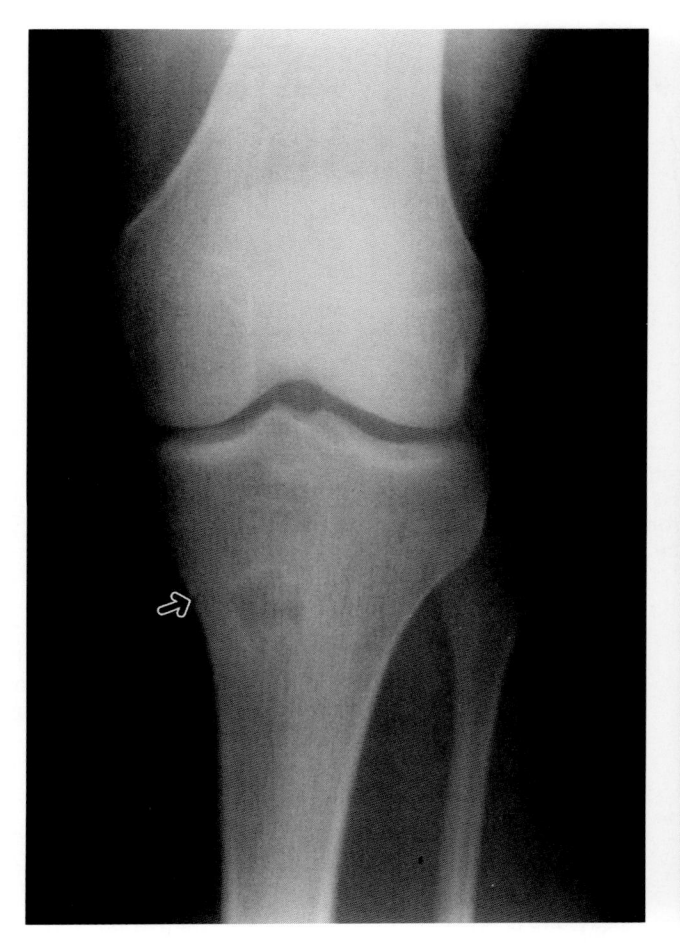

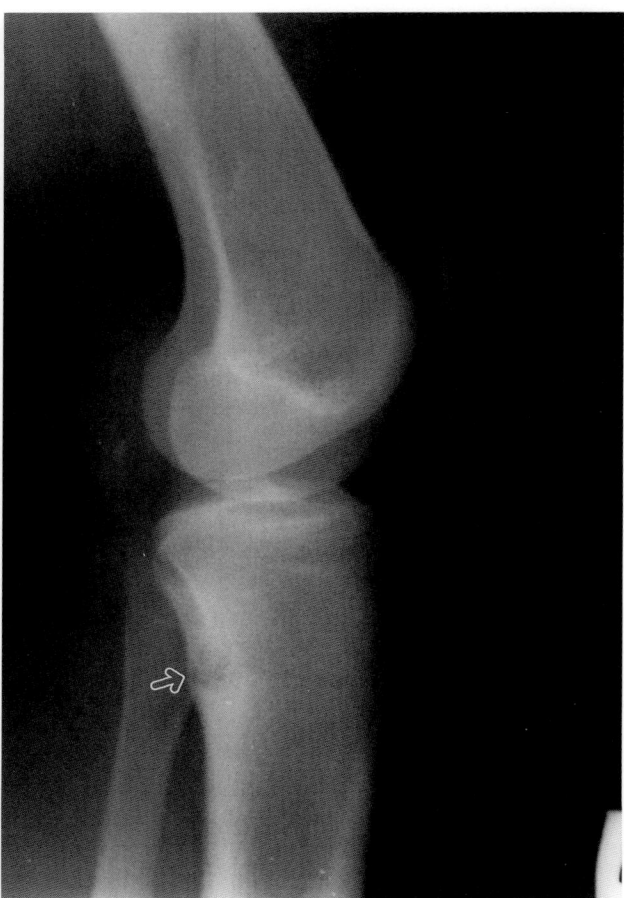

Fig. 33-13. A pathologic plus stress fracture in a 16-year-old basketball player. A small nonossifying fibroma can just be visualized.

Avulsion of the Tibial Apophysis

The tibial apophysis is at risk for avulsion in the adolescent age group when the physeal plate of the proximal tibia becomes partially fused. The tonguelike extension of the tibial apophysis is slower to fuse, and this remains the weakest portion of the proximal tibial epiphyseal plate.

In younger children, the apophysis may be affected by microscopic avulsion of Sharpy's fiber attachments to the subcondral bone, and this is reflected in pain and some swelling known as tibial apophysitis or so-called Osgood-Schlatter syndrome (Fig. 33-14). This is an aggravating problem, but one that usually does not leave any long-term disability for the child. It is often seen in very active child athletes, especially those who train in running sports such as soccer or football. The syndrome disappears once the tibial apophysis becomes ossified.

Occasionally, a small nonossified ossicle will cause persistent problems into the late teens and may require removal to relieve symptoms. Seldom is surgery necessary to cause early fusion of the tibial apophysis, and the syndrome usually responds to rest and occasional immobilization with an orthosis or a cast to allow the chronic avulsion to heal and to protect the adolescents from their own overactivity. Rare premature fusion of the tibial apophysis leading to genu recurbation has been reported.[24,25]

Complete avulsion of the tibial apophysis is uncommon and may be partial or complete. Partial avulsions that are minimally displaced need only treatment with cast immobilization; however, those that are completely avulsed, usually secondary to a sudden impediment of forward motion of the tibia with the quadriceps contracting maximally, will require open reduction (Fig. 33-15).

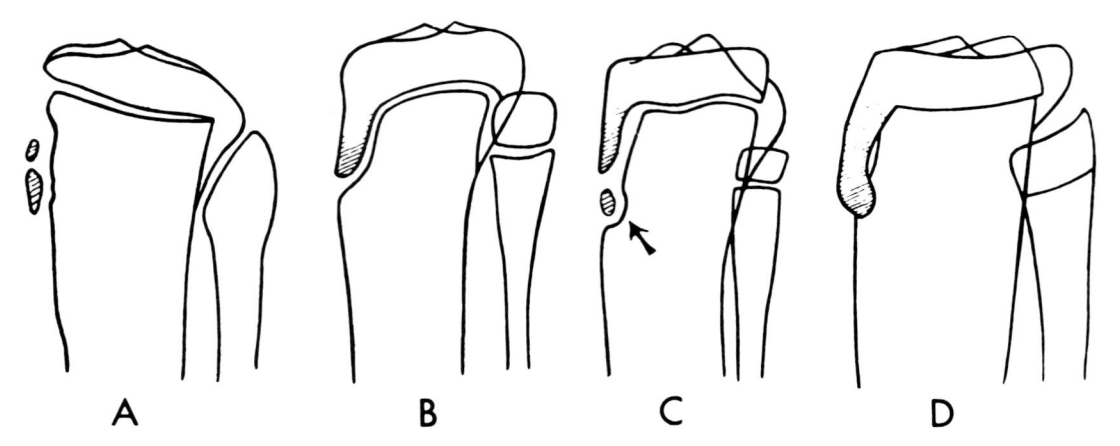

Fig. 33-14. (A–D) Normal variations in the size and configuration of the anterior tibial process. Avulsion of the attachment of the patellar tendon to the tibial apophysis is a commonly seen overuse syndrome in active children, the so-called Osgood-Schlatter syndrome. (Modified from Caffey, J: Pediatric X-ray Diagnosis. Section 8: The Extremities. p. 935. Year Book Medical Publishers, Chicago, 1972.)

DISLOCATION OF THE KNEE JOINT

Pathogenesis in Children

Acute dislocation of the knee joint in children is rare. It may be predisposed to by ligamentous laxity or a neuropathic joint as in myelomeningocele children (Fig. 33-16). The dislocation is brought about by high-velocity sporting activities, such as water- or snow-skiing, farm injuries involving power equipment, or motor vehicle accidents.[26] Physical examination will reveal a patient who has multiple severe injuries of multisystems. The knee joint will be swollen and grossly unstable in all directions indicating disruption of all intra- and extra-articular ligamentous structures. A tense effusion is uncommon, as the blood has usually escaped into the soft tissues. The knee joint will probably have reduced spontaneously subsequent to the accident except in the case of the posterolateral dislocation. A posterolateral dislocation may prove irreducible, due to invagination of medial soft tissues into the knee joint, or due to buttonholing of the medial femoral condyle through the medial retinaculum. A medial skin dimple is present and accentuated with attempts at reduction; the femoral condyle can be palpated just beneath the skin. Failure to achieve an adequate reduction is reported to result in significant soft tissue necrosis along the medial aspect of the knee.[27] Roman and colleagues[27] state that the incidence of vascular injury is as high as 32 percent overall and results primarily from disruption of the popliteal artery posteriorly. Observation of a cool or pulseless lower extremity requires urgent exploration and saphenous repair of the popliteal artery. Eger and Huler[28] reported a 90 percent likelihood of amputation with knee dislocation and vascular injury in the 1970s.

Management of the Dislocated Knee in Children

If there is no evidence of vascular impairment, following closed reduction, splinting the limb to protect from further injury to the soft tissues is all that is necessary in the short-term resuscitative period. If the vascularity of the distal limb is intact and the knee joint dislocation is reduced on radiographs continued nonoperative treatment of the knee can result in a functional knee.[28] The knee is immobilized in a cylinder cast or removable knee splint, slightly flexed, for a period not exceeding 6 weeks.

The knee is then mobilized and strengthened. Immobilization beyond the 6 weeks results in prolonged stiffness. Taylor obtained a stable painless knee with 90 degrees of flexion in 18 of 26 adult patients by conservative management.

Many authors, however, support operative repair of the soft tissues about the knee[26] to improve stability and function. The repair should ideally take place within 5 days of the injury. When vascularity of the knee is intact the knee must be approached from both the medial and lateral sides to expose the intra- and extra-articular structures. An external fixator should be applied in approximately 30 degrees of flexion after complete congruous reduction is accomplished, and the ligaments

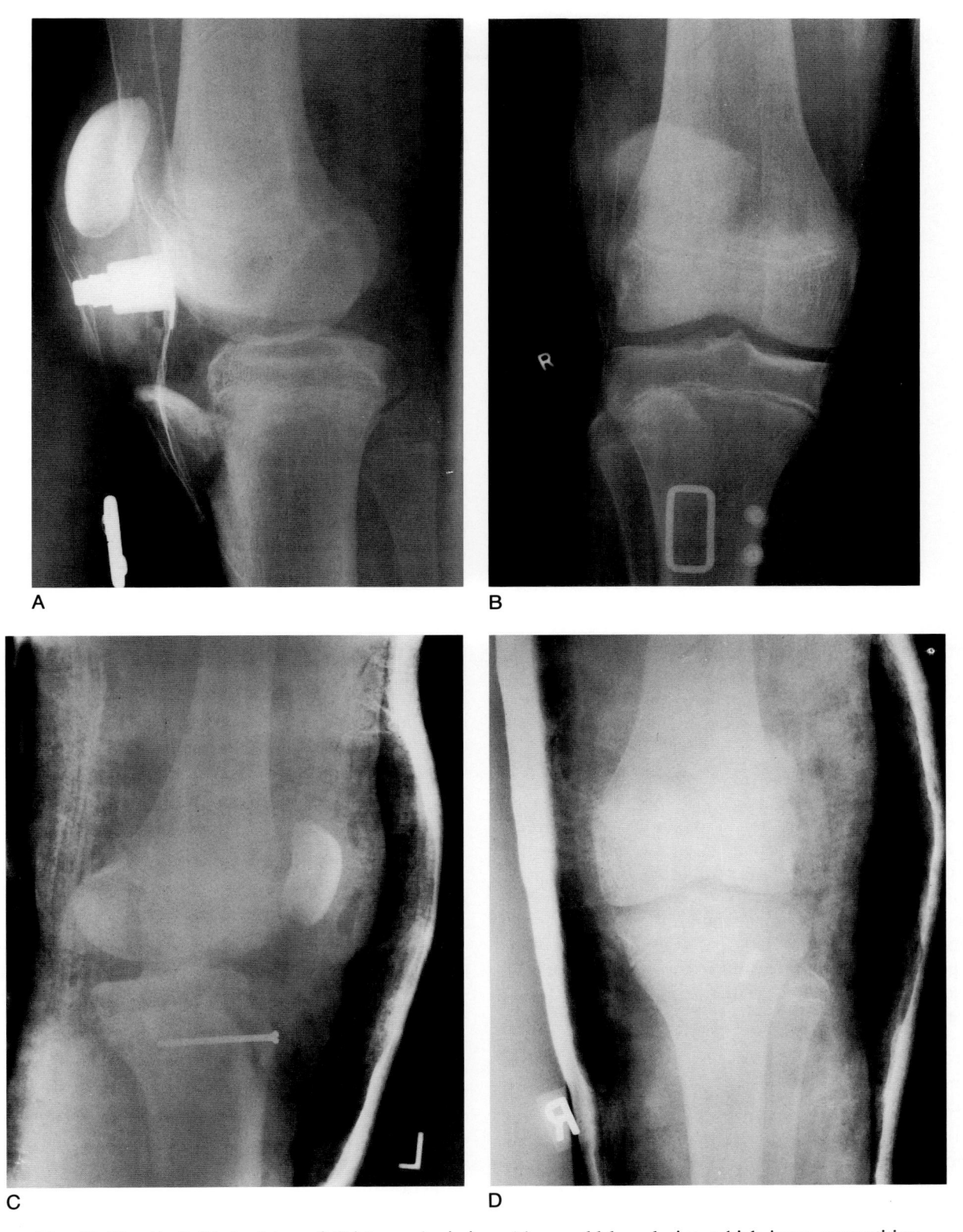

Fig. 33-15. **(A & B)** Avulsion of tibial apophysis in a 14-year-old boy during a high jump competition. **(C & D)** Post-open reduction and internal fixation of the avulsed fragment, which went on to uneventful union.

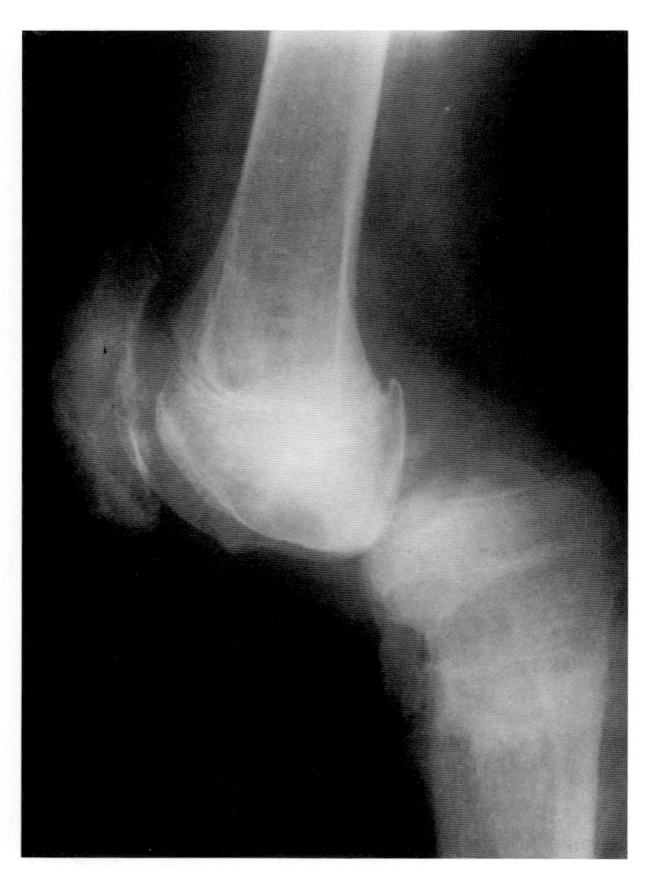

Fig. 33-16. Posterior dislocation of the tibia in a 12-year-old boy with a neuropathic joint secondary to an L3 level myelomeningocele.

then sutured or stapled as required giving consideration to protection of the growth centers. Immobilization with the external fixator is necessary for 4 to 6 weeks depending on age. This is followed by range of motion and muscle strengthening exercises, guarding the knee joint against accidental varus, valgus, or rotational strain with the appropriate bracing. Results in the literature are retrospective and indicate 50 percent excellent and 50 percent good results in adults.[26]

Complications

The knee joint dislocation that has an associated vascular injury and will require prompt exploration and vascular reconstruction. In order to protect the vascular repair, an external fixator should be applied across the knee joint, and the subsequent repair of the ligamentous structures accomplished. Fasciotomy of the lower leg compartments may become necessary, depending upon the degree of soft tissue damage, and the length of time the limb was dysvascular. Knee instability due to cruciate rupture may be a late complication necessitating cruciate reconstruction procedures.

ACUTE DISLOCATION OF THE PROXIMAL TIBIOFIBULAR JOINT

Acute dislocation of the proximal tibiofibular joint is a rare injury in children[29] but is predisposed to associated ligamentous laxity. The joint may dislocate anteriorly or posteriorly, anterior dislocations being twice as common as posterior. The peroneal nerve, as it winds around the proximal fibula anteriorly, is most vulnerable to injury with the posterior dislocation. The anterior dislocation occurs during sporting events, or falls during the landing, while parachute jumping or hang gliding, where the foot is in supination and some plantar flexion, while the knee is flexed with some varus strain. The peroneal muscles contract strongly, pulling the proximal fibula forward unapposed by the lateral hamstring forces, with the knee in flexion. The posterior dislocation occurs by a direct blow to the proximal fibula, with the knee in some flexion. Damage to the peroneal nerve and subsequent foot drop is more frequently associated with the posterior dislocation.

Management of the Acute Dislocation

Closed Reduction

Treatment of the acute anterior or posterior tibiofibular joint dislocation is by direct manipulation of the proximal fibula back into its anatomic position. General anesthesia is required, and the knee is flexed to relax the hamstrings during the manipulation. The fibula pops back into position and feels stable. Radiographs are taken to assure a congruous reduction. Immobilization in a cast is unnecessary, but a period of non- or partial weightbearing is advised as one-sixth of the weight borne at the ankle joint is distributed through the fibula. Post-reduction instability or a widened joint space are signs of irreducibility likely secondary to soft tissue interposition.

Open Reduction

Open reduction is then indicated. Exposure is through an anterolateral oblique incision over the tibiofibular joint taking care not to damage the peroneal nerve laterally or the anterior tibial artery as it passes through the interosseous hiatus just beneath the joint. After reduction is accomplished, the anterior ligament may be repaired with sutures, and the fibula held in position with one or two parallel threaded Steinmann pins. Care must be taken not to damage the proximal fibular or tibial growth plates. Weightbearing with the pin in place is contraindicated. The pin should remain in place for approximately 4 weeks, and thereafter partial weightbearing with range of motion and muscle strengthening is carried out. Occasionally there is a communication of the synovial tibiofibular joint with the knee joint. The pin should be placed under the skin at the time of open reduction to reduce the likelihood of knee joint infection.

Complications

Peroneal Nerve Injury

Damage to the peroneal nerve with sensory changes and foot drop is most common with the posterior dislocation, and is treated conservatively for about 3 months to await recovery before further investigations are undertaken. The foot should be splinted at 90 degrees with an articulated polypropylene ankle foot orthosis, with a 90-degree plantar flexion stop, to prevent posterior soft tissue contracture. Exploration of the nerve acutely is not indicated.

Recurrent Dislocation of the Tibiofibular Joint

Recurrent dislocation will occur in only 5 percent of acute dislocations.[29] It may result from failure to achieve an adequate closed reduction of the acute dislocation,

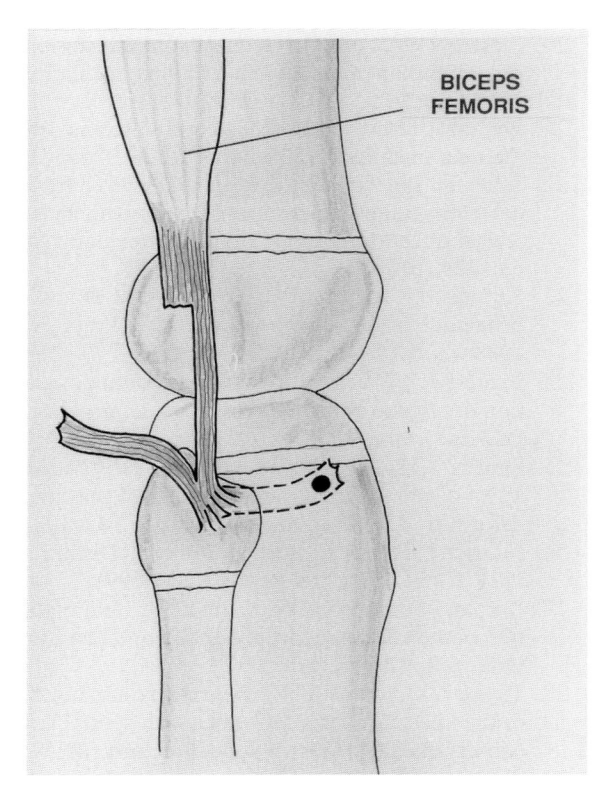

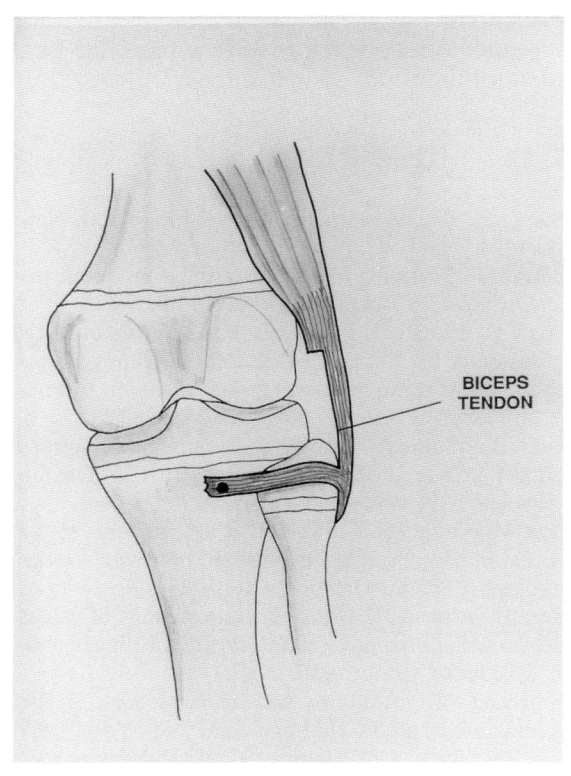

Fig. 33-17. Technique for repairing a tibiofibular subluxation. **(A)** A strip of biceps tendon attached to the fibular head is removed and routed posteriorly. **(B)** The strip of tendon, when routed posteriorly, may be tunneled anteriorly through the proximal tibia if the growth plates are closed or anchored posteriorly with a screw inferior and clear of the growth plate in the younger patient.

inherent anatomic joint instability, and ligamentous laxity may occur spontaneously.[30,31] The dislocation is usually present in athletically active adolescents, and limits their activities. The recurrent dislocation is usually anterior.

Treatment consists of proximal fibular resection in the later teens if severe, or tethering of the proximal fibula with a strip of biceps tendon as described by Weinert (Fig. 33-17). In the presence of open physeal lines it would be advisable to tunnel the tendon through the periosteum distal to the growth plate. The biceps tendon could also be anchored with a screw inferior to the tibial physeal line. Fusion of the tibiofibular joint is not advised, as it alters ankle joint mechanics distally.

SUMMARY

Injuries about the knee and the proximal tibia are common and complex. They require thoughtful analysis of the magnitude of force and mechanism of injury in order to anticipate the damage to the soft tissue, bone, and physis. Carefully well-established principles of fracture management must be followed to achieve the best result with a minimum of complications.

REFERENCES

1. Wilkins KE: Fractures in children. JB Lippincott, New York, 1984
2. Roberts JM: Operative treatment of fractures about the knee. Orthop Clin North Am 21:365, 1990
3. Zionts LE, Harcke HT, Brooks KM, MacEwen GD: Posttraumatic tibia valga: a case demonstrating asymmetric activity at the proximal growth plate on technetium bone scan. J Pediatr Orthop 7:458, 1987
4. Wood KB, Bradley JP, Ward WT: Pes anserinus interposition in a proximal tibia physeal fracture. Clin Orthop Rel Res 264:239, 1991
5. Robert M, Khouri N, Carlioz H, et al: Fractures of the proximal tibia metaphysis in children: review of a series of 25 cases. J Pediatr Orthop 7:444, 1987
6. Jordan SE, Alonso JE, Cook FF: The etiology of valgus angulation after metaphyseal fractures of the tibia in children. J Pediatr Orthop 7:450, 1987
7. Hollinshead WH: Anatomy for Surgeons. Vol. 3: The back and limbs. 2nd Ed. Harper Collins, New York, 1969
8. Lange RH, Bach AW, Hansen ST, Jr. Johansen KH: Open tibial fractures with associated vascular injuries: prognosis for limb salvage. J Trauma 25:203, 1985
9. Anderson M, Green WT, Messner MB: Growth and prediction of growth in the lower extremities. J Bone Joint Surg [Am] 45:1, 1963
10. Green WT, Anderson M: Skeletal age and the control of bone growth. Instr Course Lect 17:199, 1960
11. Schneider RC, Kennedy JC, Plant ML: Sports injuries. Williams & Wilkins, Baltimore, 1985
12. Uphold R, Harvey R, Misselbeck W, Hill S: Bilateral tibial fractures in properly restrained toddlers involved in motor vehicle collisions: case reports. J Trauma 31:1411, 1991
13. Gustilo RB, Merkow RL, Templeman D: Current concepts review: the management of open fractures. J Bone Joint Surg [Am] 72:299, 1990
14. Gustilo RB, Anderson JT: Prevention of infection in the treatment of one thousand and twenty five open fractures of long bones: retrospective and prospective analysis. J Bone Joint Surg [Am] 58:453, 1976
15. Klemm KW, Borner M: Interlocking nailing of complex fractures of the femur and tibia. Clin Orthop 212:89, 1986
16. Langenskiold A: An operation for partial closure of an epiphyseal plate in children and its experimental basis. J Bone Joint Surg [Br] 57:325, 1975
17. Salter RB, Harris WR: Injuries involving the epiphyseal plate. J Bone Joint Surg [Am] 45:587, 1963
18. Eger M, Huler T, Hirsch M: Popliteal artery occlusion associated with dislocation of the knee joint. Br J Surg 57:315, 1970
19. Ogden JA: Injury to the growth mechanism of the immature skeleton. Skelet Radiol 6:237, 1981
20. Jackson DW, Cozen L: Genu valgum as a complication of proximal tibial metaphyseal fractures in children. J Bone Joint Surg [Am] 53:1571, 1971
21. Balthazar DA, Pappas AM: Acquired valgus deformity of the tibia in children. J Pediatr Orthop 14:538, 1984
22. Salter R, Best T: Pathogenesis and prevention of valgus deformity following fractures of the proximal metaphyseal region of the tibia in children. J Bone Joint Surg [Am] 55:1324, 1973
23. Kumar SJ, Pizzutillo PD: Treatment of Blount's disease: behaviour of the growth plate. Raven Press, New York, 1988
24. Lynch MC, Walsh HPJ: Tibia recurvatum as a complication of Osgood Schlatter's disease: a report of two cases. J Pediatr Orthop 11:543, 1991
25. Pappas AM, Anus P, Toczylowski HM: Asymmetrical arrest of the proximal tibial physis and genu recurvatum deformity. J Bone Joint Surg [Am] 66:575, 1984
26. Frassica FJ, Sim FH, Staeheli JW et al: Dislocation of the knee. Clin Orthop Rel Res 263:200, 1991
27. Roman PD, Hopson CN, Zenni EJ, Jr: Traumatic dislocation of the knee: a report of 30 cases and literature review. Orthop Rev 16:33, 1987
28. Taylor AR, Arden GP, Rainey HA: Traumatic dislocation of the knee: a report of 43 cases with special reference to conservative treatment. J Bone Joint Surg [Br] 54:96, 1972
29. Rockwood CA, Green D: Fractures and dislocations of the knee: fractures. 2:1214, 1975
30. Weinert CR, Raczka R: Recurrent dislocation of the superior tibiofibular joint. J Bone Joint Surg [Am] 68:126, 1986
31. Halbrecht JL, Jackson DW: Recurrent dislocation of the proximal tibiofibular joint. Orthop Rev 20:957, 1991

34

Degloving Injuries in Tibial Shaft Fractures

R. Mervyn Letts
Eric Robinson

I dressed him and healed him.
— AMBROÍSE PARÉ

DESCRIPTION AND INCIDENCE

Fractures of the tibia and fibula are very common, being the most frequently encountered injuries of the lower extremity in the pediatric age group.[1,2] As is true of any fracture, the nature and severity of the injury will vary according to the age of the patient, the mechanism of injury, and the anatomic location.

They may occur from either an indirect force or a direct blow. In infants and young children the most common injury patterns include spiral fracture (Fig. 34-1) and torus or "buckle" fracture (Fig. 34-2) of the tibia with the fibula often intact. In older children, including toddlers, the patterns are more variable and can range from toddler's fracture (Fig. 34-3) to greenstick fractures of the metaphysis or diaphysis with or without associated fracture of the fibula (Fig. 34-4). Spiral fractures are also frequently encountered in this age group. In the preadolescent children, direct trauma will often produce a transverse fracture with or without displacement. Finally, the adolescent will frequently experience fractures that are reminiscent of the adult type, that is, frequently comminuted, associated butterfly fragment, and displacement[3] (Fig. 34-5).

ANATOMY

Neurovascular injury is a well-known entity in lower limb trauma. Certain anatomic characteristics of the proximal tibial region predisposes the lower leg to potential vascular insufficiency following trauma.

The popliteal artery courses through the popliteal fossa to the lower border of the popliteus muscle where it then divides into anterior and posterior tibial arteries. The anterior tibial artery angles anteriorly between the two heads of the tibialis posterior muscle and then through an aperture above the upper border of the interosseous membrane. Here it lies close to the medial aspect of the head of the fibula and courses distally on the interosseous membrane where it comes to lie on the anterior aspect of the distal tibia and ankle joint, at which time it is called the dorsal pedal artery. The posterior tibial artery, which is larger than its anterior counterpart, descends distally in the deep posterior compartment between the superficial and deep muscle layers. Distal to the medial malleolus it divides into the medial and lateral plantar arteries.[4]

Although direct neurovascular injuries are uncommon in closed fractures, they unfortunately occur and

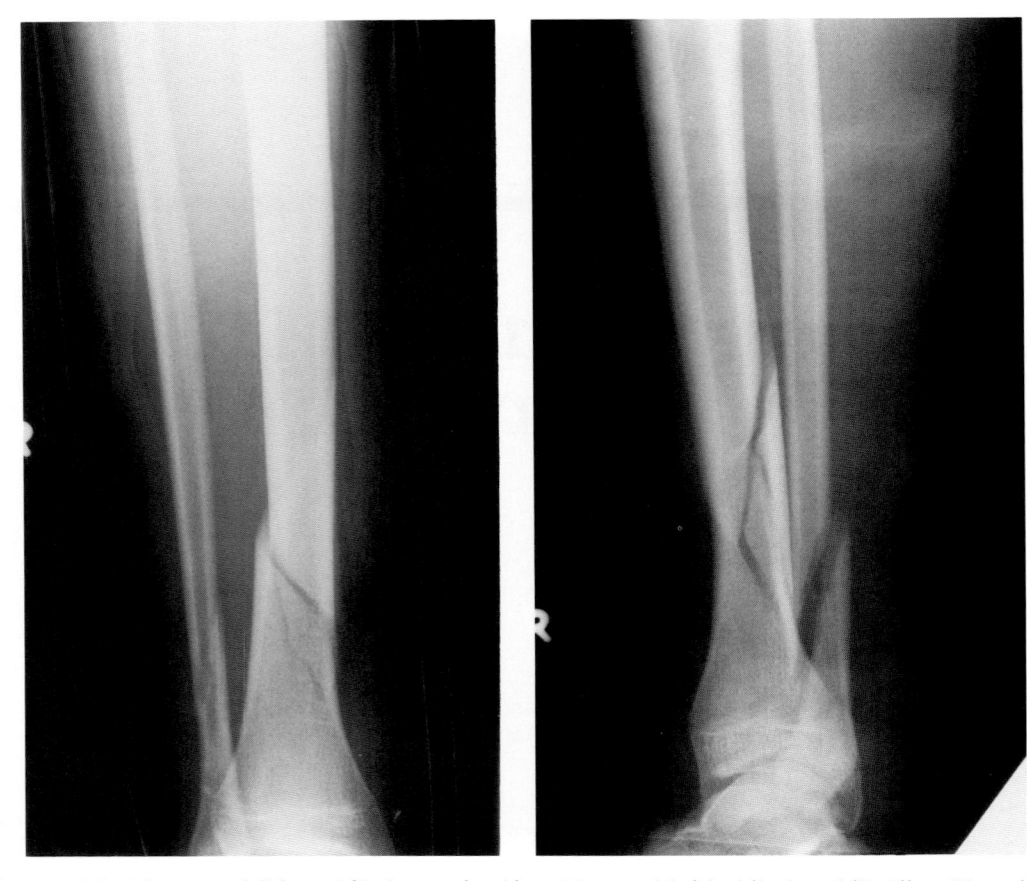

Fig. 34-1. Spiral fracture of tibia and fibula sustained in a 14-year-old girl while downhill skiing. The spiral has started at the top of the rigid boot, which usually protects the ankle but facilitates spiral fractures of the tibial shaft.

the complications can be disabling. The most common area of vascular injury is the proximal metaphysis of the tibia just distal to the bifurcation of the popliteal artery where the anterior tibial artery penetrates the interosseous membrane (Fig. 34-6).

The paucity of soft tissue on the anterior border of the tibia predisposes to open fractures of the tibial diaphysis, especially in the adolescent.

MECHANISMS OF INJURY

The mechanisms of injury of nonphyseal fractures of the tibia and fibula are multiple and vary according to age. Direct trauma is usually associated with the older child and often results in transverse or comminuted types of fractures. In younger children, indirect rotational forces from simple falls, resulting in spiral fractures, appear more common.

In 102 fractures of the tibia reported by Hansen and his associates,[5] approximately 30 percent were the result of severe trauma such as motor vehicle accidents or falls from heights.

Sporting injuries are another common source of tibial fractures in children (Fig. 34-7). In a recent review by Beitzer and associates,[6] the incidence of tibial shaft fractures associated with skiing varied significantly with age. In children less than 11 years of age, fractures of the tibia accounted for 13.3 percent of the injuries associated with skiing. In children of 11 years and older, and in adults, this proportion decreased to 3.3 percent.

In 1986, Bayer and his colleagues[7] reported their experience with seven proximal tibial fractures caused by trampoline jumping. Izant and associates[8] reviewed 60 cases of bicycle-spoke injuries (Fig. 34-8). Severe injuries to the extremities may also result from "propeller" boating injuries, lawnmower trauma, or farm machinery accidents.[9]

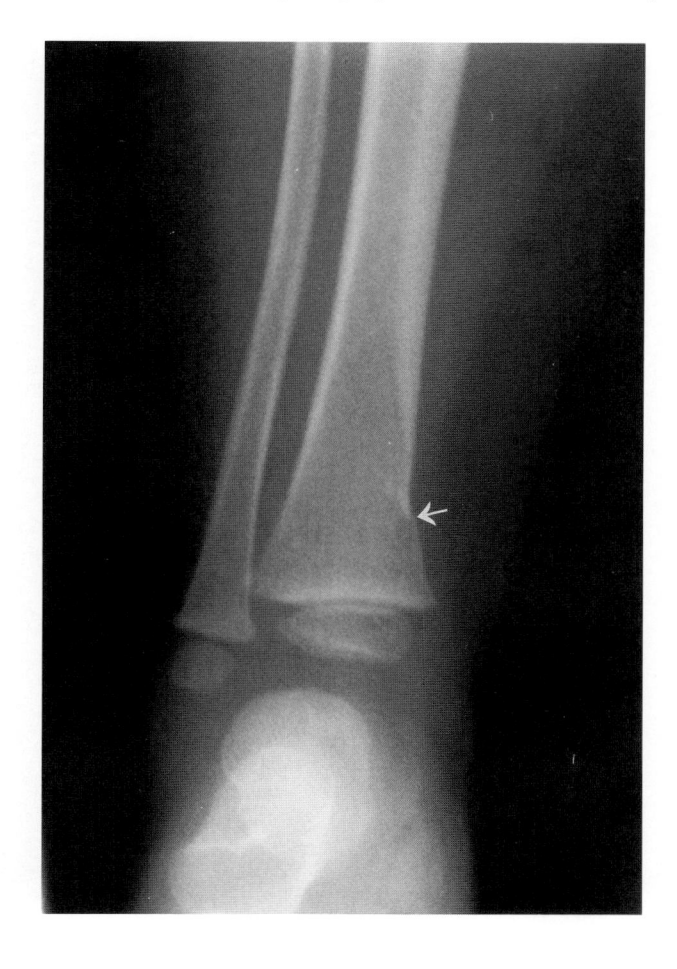

Fig. 34-2. The buckle or "torus" fracture of the tibia is a very subtle compression failure of the cortex that occurs only in the metaphyseal region of the tibia.

Unfortunately, physical abuse is another etiologic factor that should not be overlooked. These children may present with diaphyseal fractures, sometimes associated with exuberant callus, because of delay in seeking medical attention. Multiple lesions of various stages of healing is another important diagnostic clue.

Metaphyseal fractures may also be seen and include impaction fractures, buckle fractures, and the classic corner fractures (see Ch. 51).

In an extensive review of 489 fractures in battered children, King and associates[10] found the tibia to be the second most commonly fractured bone after the humerus.

CLASSIFICATION

Fractures of the tibia and fibula can be divided into various regional categories as proposed by Dias[2] (Table 34-1). This section of the chapter will deal specifically with fractures of the tibial and fibular diaphysis.

PHYSICAL EXAMINATION

The findings on physical examination will vary according to the age of the patient and the severity of the injury.

Pain is the major symptom in tibial and fibular shaft fractures. A young child will often rub the area of maximal tenderness. In toddlers, refusal to weight bear or a characteristic antalgic gait may be present. In this young age group, palpating or percussing the tibial shaft gently will elicit a constant painful response when compared to the contralateral limb.

In older children and adolescents, apprehension is often present, and the patient must be reassured. Deformity, which is common in the adult, may not be present in the younger patient, as fractures are frequently undisplaced. When deformity is present, the limb should be splinted prior to movement for physical examination or radiographs.

Local swelling will occur quickly after the injury secondary to bleeding. Soft tissue must be carefully in-

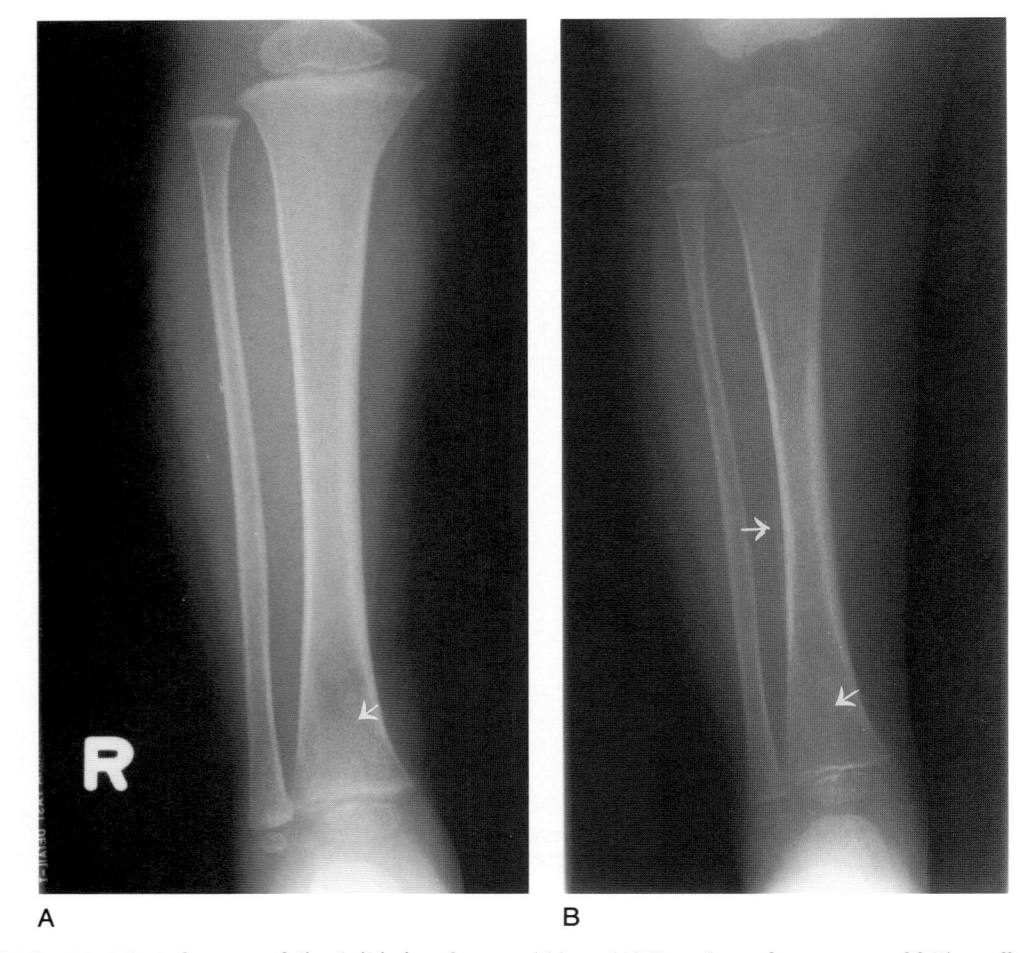

Fig. 34-3. Toddler's fracture of distal tibia in a 2-year-old boy. **(A)** Two days after trauma of falling off a coffee table with refusal to weight bear. Radiograph shows very fine subtle oblique crack in distal metaphysis. **(B)** Three weeks later with increased sclerosis of fracture site and periosteal elevation of the lateral cortex of the tibia.

spected for any evidence of crush injury or a puncture wound that indicates an open fracture. Puncture wounds must be opened for a thorough debridement.

Although neurologic and arterial damage are infrequent in shaft fractures, they may occur in severely displaced fracture patterns and with proximal metaphyseal fractures, hence the vascular integrity must always be carefully evaluated. It should also be remembered that the radiograph indicates only the final resting site of the fracture fragments. The clinician must speculate the trajectory of the fragments at the moment of impact in accordance with the force exerted on the limb.

Any child who has sustained significant trauma should undergo a full musculoskeletal examination to rule out any other fractures. Often the most important fracture is the one that's missed!

RADIOGRAPHIC EVALUATION

When injuries to the tibia or fibula are suspected clinically, good quality anteroposterior and lateral radiographs must be obtained. In keeping with basic orthopaedic principles, the joint above and the joint below should be included. Comparison views may occasionally be necessary to assess an undisplaced greenstick or torus fracture in the young child. The fracture pattern, displacement, angulation, and shortening should be assessed and recorded.

The presence of an associated fracture of the fibular shaft may have some implication for the treatment with regard to the deforming forces acting on the fracture site. In contradistinction to adults, the pediatric patient may often present with an intact fibula. This prevents short-

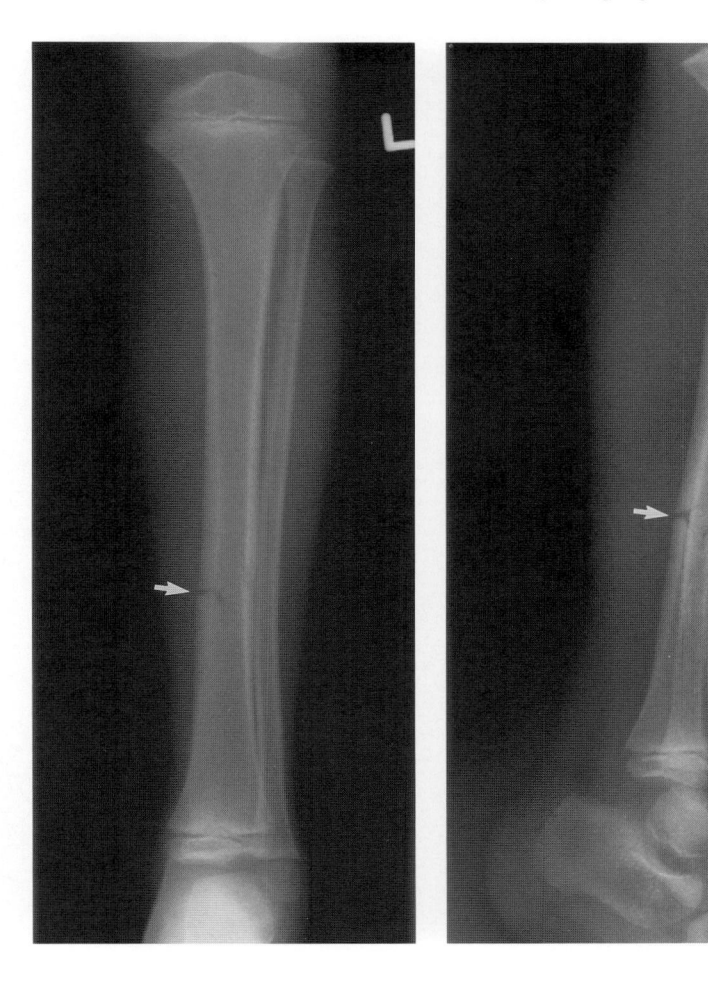

Fig. 34-4. Greenstick fractures of the tibia are uncommon but are occasionally encountered, being best treated by a well-molded cast. If significant angulation is encountered, controlled fracturing of the intact cortex under general anesthesia will be necessary.

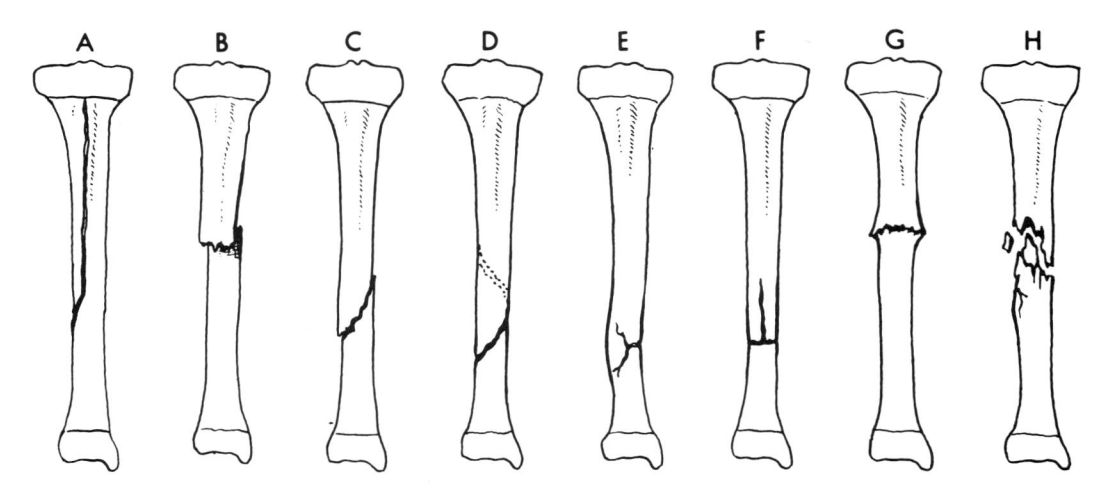

Fig. 34-5. Classification of diaphyseal fractures of the tibia according to the course and nature of the fracture line. **(A)** Longitudinal. **(B)** Transverse. **(C)** Oblique. **(D)** Spiral. **(E)** Greenstick or torus. **(F)** Longitudinal transverse. **(G)** Transverse impacted. **(H)** Comminuted. (From Caffey J: Pediatric X-ray Diagnosis. Section 8: The Extremities. p. 1084. Yearbook Medical Publishers, Chicago, 1972, with permission.)

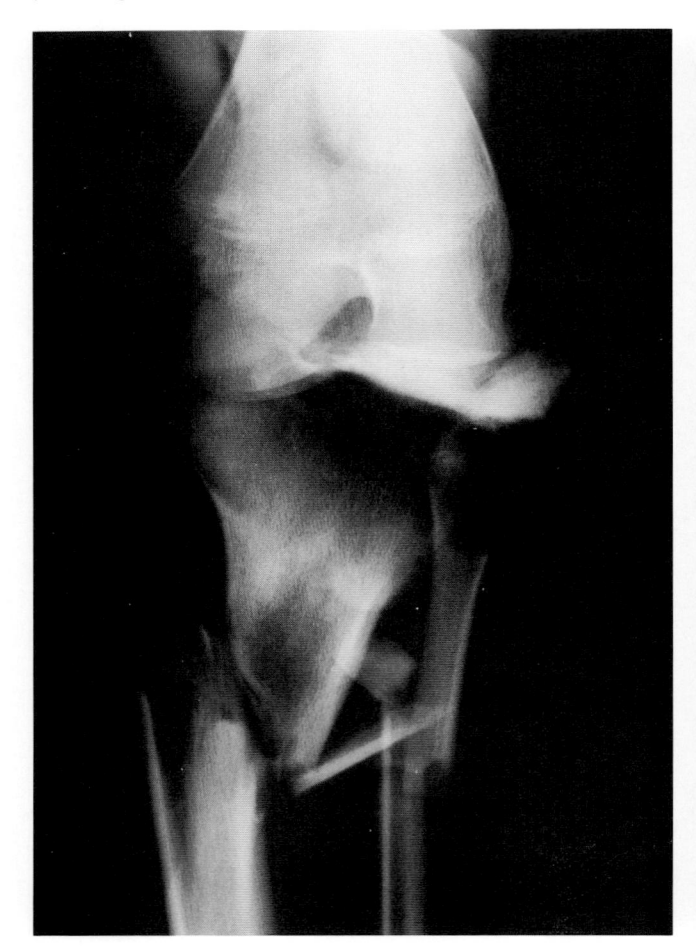

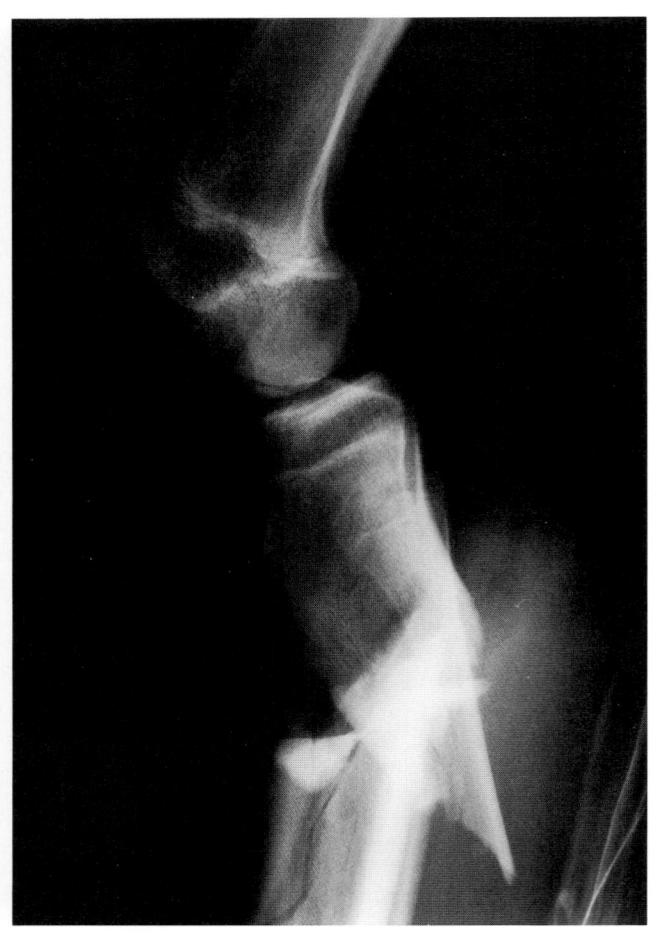

Fig. 34-6. A 16-year-old boy involved in a boating (propellor) accident while riding a jet ski. The patient sustained an open grade III fracture of the proximal tibia and fibula. The AP view **(left)** reveals the comminution of the fracture, and, on the lateral view **(right)**, one can see that the anterior 25 percent of the tibial plateau is missing. This type of fracture has a high incidence of vascular injury, as this is the region where the popliteal artery divides into the anterior and posterior tibial arteries and the vessel are relatively fixed.

ening but may also result in mild varus alignment due to the deforming forces of the flexor tendons in the posterior compartment of the leg. This is especially true when the fracture is oblique. Although this is rarely significant, it should be kept in mind when applying and molding a long-leg cast.

When the tibial fracture is associated with a fibular fracture, both shortening and angulation may result. In this instance, the angulation is often valgus secondary to the deforming forces of the muscle in the anterior and lateral compartments.

Isolated fractures of the proximal fibula, although uncommon, may occur from direct blows to the lower limb. These are rarely complicated and treatment is symptomatic. They must, however, be differentiated from the more ominous distal tibial physeal injury associated with a proximal fibular fracture, the so-called "Maisonneuve" type of ankle fracture. The differentiation is usually easily accomplished by careful examination of the ankle and radiographic evaluation of the entire tibia and fibula.

Tomography, computed tomography, and radionuclide imaging are rarely indicated in the evaluation of simple uncomplicated tibial and fibular diaphyseal fractures. They can, however, be of value in the diagnosis of stress fractures. These more commonly occur in training athletes and young army recruits and are usually located on the medial aspect of the proximal tibial metaphyseal-diaphyseal junction (Fig. 34-7).

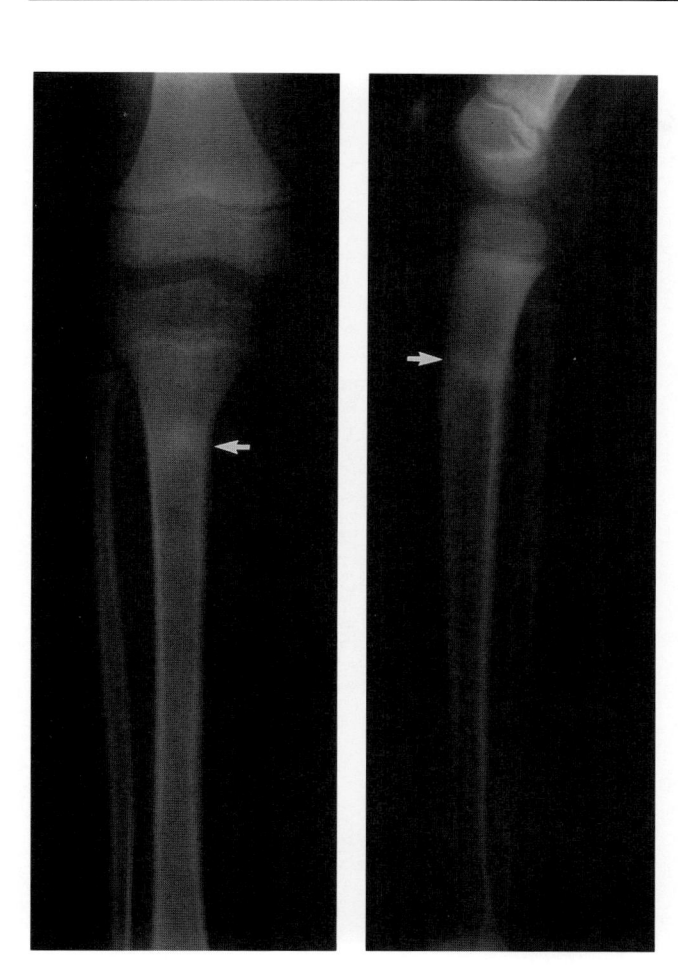

Fig. 34-7. Typical stress fracture of the tibia in a 13-year-old boy who started playing soccer daily after a sedentary winter.

TREATMENT INDICATIONS

Closed Methods

Diaphyseal fractures in children can usually be treated with simple manipulation and immobilization in a long-leg cast.[2,3,11-13] Uncomplicated fractures unite rapidly. In a study of tibial fractures in 117 children, all shaft fractures united in an average period of 30 days.[11] In this age group, incorporating the knee in a long-leg cast rarely leads to knee stiffness.

If the fracture required manipulation, it is recommended that the child be observed closely for 12 to 24 hours postoperatively. During that time the neurovascular status of the limb should be monitored at frequent intervals to detect the early signs and symptoms of compartment syndrome.

The cast may be applied with the child supine and the affected leg hanging over the side of the table or the limb held by an assistant. If manipulation is required, intramuscular analgesics or intravenous sedation may be used. Monitoring of the child's blood pressure and respiratory status are essential with the use of intravenous sedation (see Ch. 5). For marked displacement of fragments, general anesthesia will be required.

A well-padded cast is then applied initially extending to the knee and subsequently extended above knee to the thigh area. To provide rotational stability, 90 degrees of knee flexion is recommended. It is preferable to immobilize the ankle in neutral position, but this will occasionally lead to posterior angulation, especially in fractures of the distal third of the tibia. If this occurs, some ankle equinus is permitted to achieve correct alignment. Flexing the knee to 90 degrees will also prevent weight-bearing in young uncooperative children. Proper rotatory alignment of the fracture fragments is critical, and the tibial rotation of the contralateral limb should be assessed.

As described previously, isolated fractures of the tibial shaft tend to drift into varus because of the force exerted by the extrinsic toe flexors and ankle plantar flexors. When both the fibula and tibia are fractured, shortening frequently ensues. Valgus drift may occur because of the deforming forces of the muscles in the anterior and lateral compartments. These potentially deforming forces should be considered in the molding of the cast for these fractures.

When manipulating and applying a long-leg cast, one should not accept more than 5 degrees of midshift varus or valgus angulation, while anteroposterior deformity should be kept below 10 degrees angulation.[2,12] Residual deformity may be amenable to wedging at the time of the initial reduction or after a few days, but since cast wedging is often a frightening and painful procedure for the child, care should be taken to "get it right the first time!"

In infants and toddlers, the fracture will usually unite within 3 weeks. In adolescents, union will usually require 10 to 12 weeks. A patellar tendon-bearing cast can be used after 6 weeks. Limb rehabilitation after fracture healing is usually not a problem, and children are their own best physiotherapists. A limp following removal of the cast is always encountered and is secondary to mild calf atrophy and weakness as well as a habit cast walk with the leg externally rotated. The natural history of the limp must always be shared with the parents to avoid undue concern regarding the occurrence of an abnormal gait, which may persist for several weeks.

Isolated fractures of the fibula shaft are best managed with a "protective cast" that protects the child from both

638 / Management of Pediatric Fractures

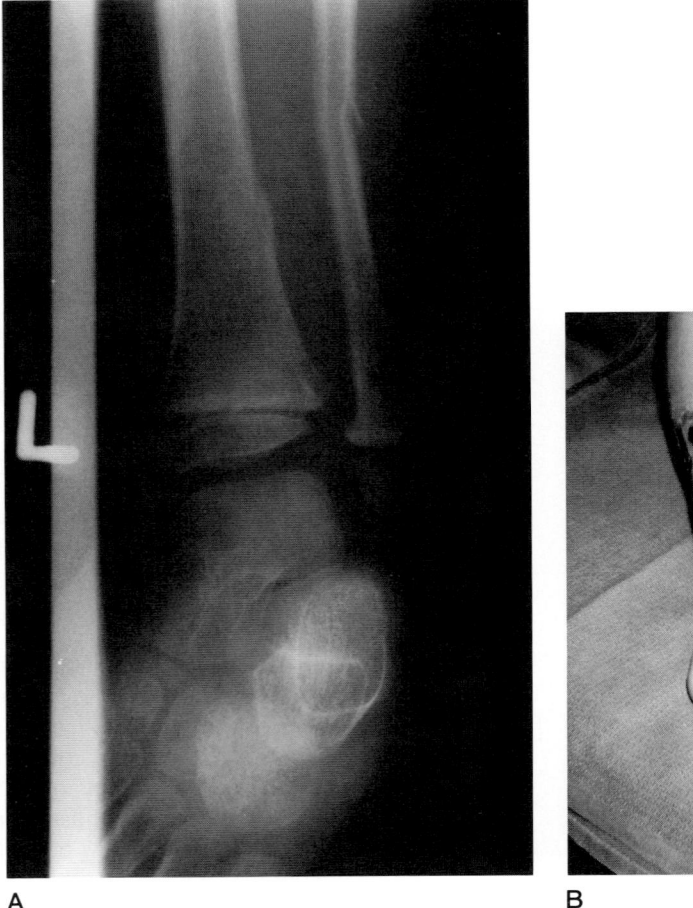

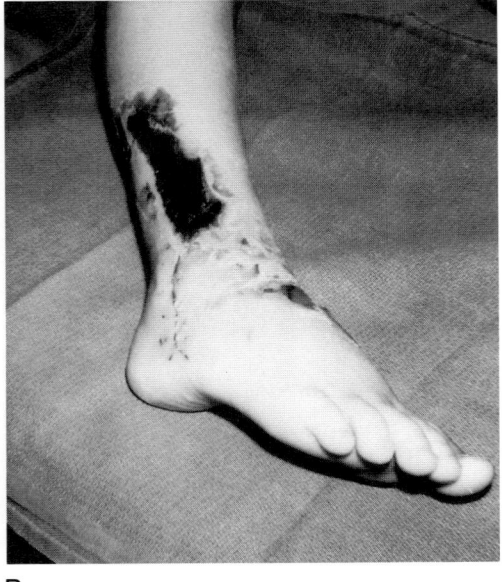

Fig. 34-8. (A) Greenstick fracture of the tibia and fibula in a 7-year-old boy injured when his leg became entangled in the spokes of a bicycle while riding double sitting on the seat with legs dangling unsupported. (B) Skin loss is frequently encountered in bicycle-spoke injuries.

TABLE 34-1. Classification of Tibial Fractures in Children

A. Fractures of the proximal tibia and fibular physes
B. Fractures of the proximal tibial metaphysis
C. Fractures of the tibial and fibular diaphysis
   1. Isolated fractures of tibial shaft
   2. Fractures of both tibial and fibular shafts
   3. Isolated fractures of fibular shaft
D. Fractures of the distal tibial metaphysis
E. Fractures of the distal tibial and fibular physis

Each of these fracture patterns generates different forms of treatment and associated complications

local trauma, and their own exuberant activity and is aimed at ambulatory comfort. Children under 5 years can seldom manage crutches. About 50 percent of those between 5 and 6 will be effective on crutches and most over 6 years will be successful in their use. Hence the walking cast for the young child often avoids constant carrying of the child by the parents and contributes to a happier family!

Operative Indications

Although the majority of tibial diaphyseal fractures can be managed by closed techniques, surgical stabilization is warranted in some circumstances.

An open fracture is the prime example of an injury requiring operative management. Other indications include polytrauma and in the severely head-injured child where multiple long-bone fractures may require surgical stabilization[14] to avoid prolonged recumbency. This treatment will facilitate nursing care[15] and enhance the mobilization of the child. Direct vascular injury, although uncommon, will also require operative osseous stabilization and repair of vascular insult.[16] In 1986 Letts and Vincent[17] reported on their experience with fractured tibia and ipsilateral femurs and recommended that at least one fracture should be rigidly fixed. McBryde and Blake[18] reported a 20 percent rate of delayed union and an incidence of 30 percent of malunion in children with floating knees treated by nonoperative management. In the very young—under 7 years—an argument can be made for closed management of such injuries in traction followed by hip spica cast (see Ch. 35).

Open Fractures

In children with compartment syndrome requiring fasciotomies or severely comminuted fractures, fixation of the tibial fracture should be strongly entertained.[14] In treating open fractures of the tibia in the pediatric population, decision-making is frequently based on soft tissue injuries and the age of the patient. The most commonly accepted grading system has been proposed by Gustilo and Anderson[19,20] and is outlined in Table 34-2.

When treating open injuries, basic orthopaedic principles apply. The wound should be inspected in the emergency department and debridement planned for the operating room. The tetanus status should be verified and intravenous antibiotics started. Generally, for a minimally contaminated wound, a first-generation cephalosporin with gram-positive and gram-negative coverage is used. For more contaminated wounds an aminoglycoside for specific gram-negative coverage is added. In severe contamination, such as a farm injury, penicillin should be added to reduce the risk of clostridial infection. Prior to operative debridement, the wound should be cultured and dressed, and the limb splinted.

Most children's open fractures, will fall into the grade I open fracture category. These fractures are usually stable and can be immobilized in plaster after adequate debridement. If the fracture pattern is unstable, minimal internal fixation, such as a Kirschner wire or a single Steinmann pin, introduced at the fracture site in conjunction with casting, may provide enough stability. Alternatively, an external fixator can be used.

TABLE 34-2. Classification of Soft Tissue Trauma

Type	Description
Type I	Wound less than 1 cm, relatively clean, and no crush component
Type II	Wound more than 1 cm, no extensive soft tissue damage, flaps and minimal to moderate crush component
Type III	Extensive damage to soft tissues; high velocity or severe crushing component; type III open fractures include 1. Segmental fractures irrespective of size of wound 2. Gunshot wounds 3. Farm or soil contamination irrespective of size of wound 4. Neurovascular injuries irrespective of size of wound 5. Traumatic amputations 6. Open fractures over 8 hours old 7. Mass casualties
Subtype IIIA	Adequate soft tissue coverage despite extensive location and flaps
Subtype IIIB	As above but associated with periosteal stripping and bony exposure
Subtype IIIC	Associated with arterial injury requiring repair, irrespective of soft tissue damage

(From Gustillo and Anderson,[19] with permission.)

External Fixation

Grade II open injuries usually require external fixation for rigid stabilization. The same is true for grade III-A, III-B, and III-C injuries to the tibial diaphysis.

External fixators in children's tibial fractures have unique capabilities that assist in the management of multitissue injury:

1. Skeletal stabilization at a distance from the site of injury
2. Free access to an injury site for primary and secondary procedures
3. Great versatility in accommodating a wide variety of bone and soft tissue lesions, including
   a. Ability to stabilize injuries across two adjacent limb segments
   b. Adjustability of alignment, length, and mechanical properties of the device after its application
   c. Ability to use simultaneous or sequential internal fixation
   d. Minimal interference with adjacent joints
   e. Mobilization of the limb and child
   f. On occasion, full weightbearing

Many reports have suggested that external fixators are well tolerated in children[22-25] (Fig. 34-9). The most se-

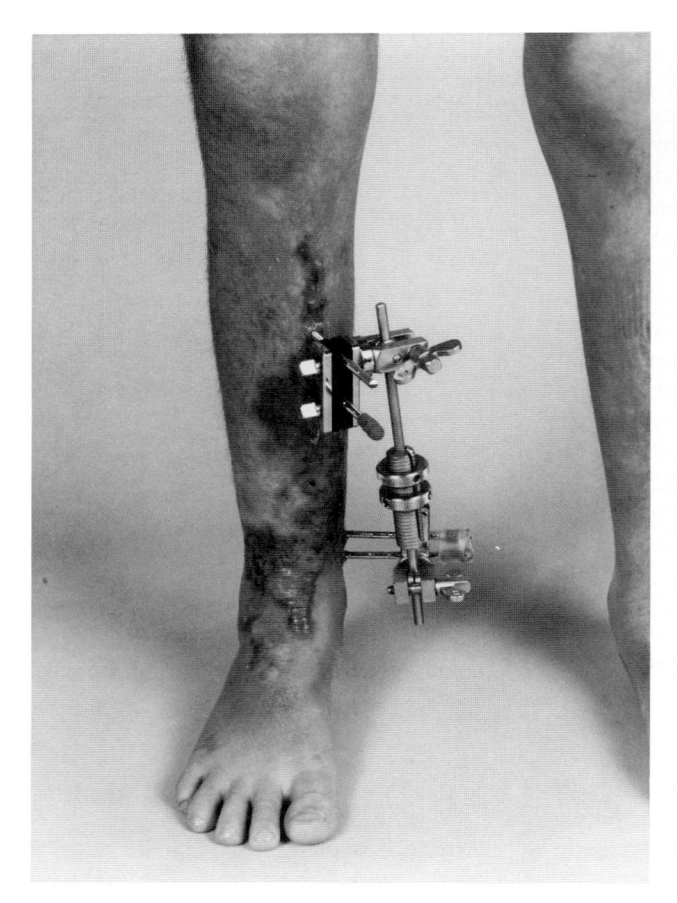

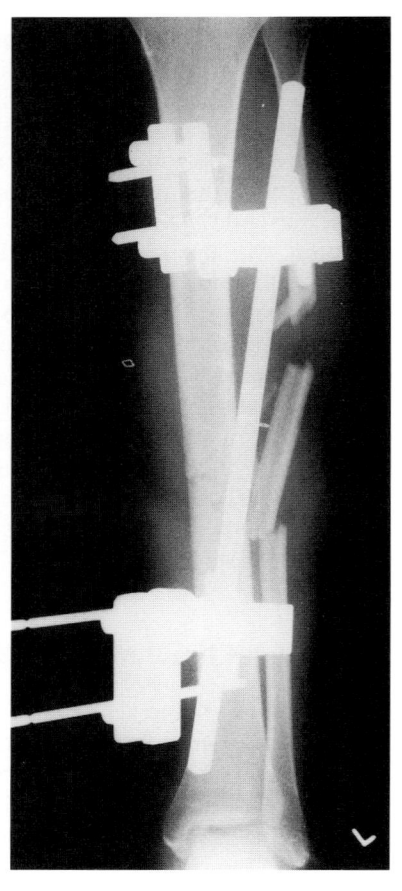

Fig. 34-9. External fixation is amazingly well tolerated by children and adolescents. It has now become a useful alternative to traction or internal fixation in this age group.

vere complications are related to the improper insertion of pins and wires and includes injuries to nerve, vessels, and musculotendinous units[22] (Fig. 34-10). Most of these injuries are preventable by relevant knowledge of limb anatomy and a basic understanding of application techniques, mechanical demands, and adaptation of frame to particular injuries.

Behrens[22,26] has emphasized the concept of "safe corridors" during application of the pins. "Safe corridors" contain no musculotendinous units nor important neurovascular structures. They occur in eccentric limb segments and are usually subcutaneous.[22] In such areas, pin-tract infection and loosening are reduced by 50 percent.[27] "Hazardous corridors" contain musculotendinous units but no significant neurovascular structures. Compartment syndrome and joint stiffness from tendon tethering may result[22] as well as increased pin-tract infection.[27] Finally, the "unsafe corridor" contains both musculotendinous units as well as important neurovascular structures and the resulting complications are obvious. Pins in this area should be inserted under direct vision.[22]

Frame configuration for lower limb injuries are multiple but can be grouped into[1] unilateral frames and bilateral frames. Unilateral frames are safe and provide excellent wound access, but are not always rigid enough for very unstable fractures or to permit early weightbearing.[26,28] Unilateral frames can be constructed in one plane or two planes.[26,30] Bilateral frames, although stronger, require the use of transfixing pins. They are therefore more prone to pin-tract infection and complications such as impalement of musculotendinous units or neurovascular structures.[25,26,29] Bilateral frames can also be constructed in one plane or two planes.[26,30] In children unilateral frames are usually sufficient (Fig. 34-11).

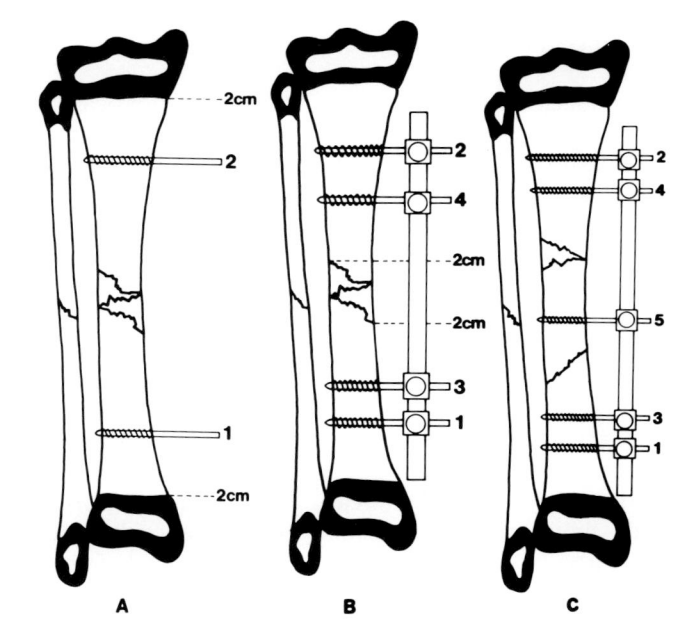

Fig. 34-10. Application of external fixators in children. **(A)** Insertion of fixation pins 2 cm away from the growth plate. **(B)** Bar attached and other pins inserted 2 cm from fracture site. **(C)** With a segmental fracture a fifth pin can be inserted into the fragment to prevent displacement. (From Alonzo JE, Horowitz M: Use of AO/ASIF external fixator in children. J Pediatr Orthop 7:596, 1987, with permission.)

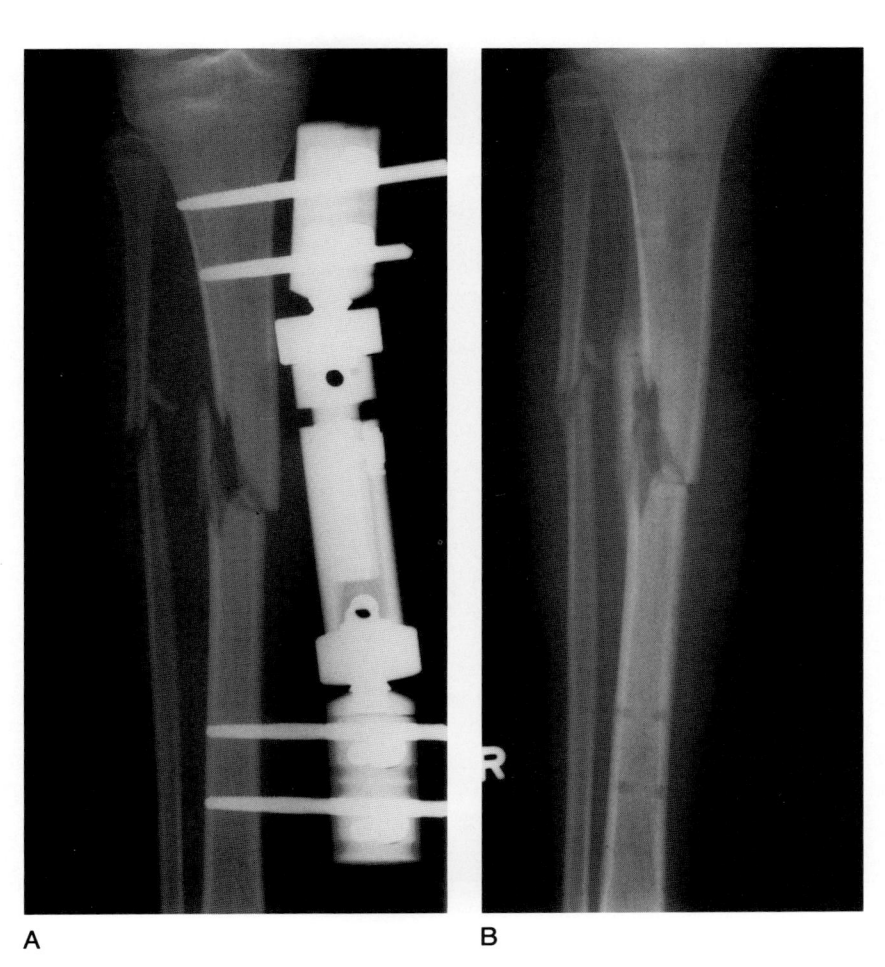

Fig. 34-11. **(A)** The Orthofix external fixator effectively immobilizing the tibia in a 10-year-old boy until **(B)** callus has stabilized the fracture and soft tissue damage has healed.

Biomechanical properties of external fixators can be altered at the level of the components, frame geometry, or the site of injury.[22,31] Increasing the number of pins per cluster is not necessarily mechanically more effective and may result in increased complications.[32] Increasing its dimension, however, will increase the bending stiffness and resistance to torsion.[33] Behrens and colleagues[33] also describe advancing the wider pin shaft into the cortex, which will double the stiffness, reduce stress at the pin-bone interface, and decrease soft tissue irritation. This is important as the pin-bone interface is probably the weak link in the system. Other methods of increasing construct stiffness include double-stacked unilateral frames,[22,31] increasing the spread of pins in each main fragment, reducing the distance between bone and longitudinal rod,[26] and keeping the length of the construct to a minimum (Fig. 34-12).

Experience has shown that simple one-plane unilateral frames in children are usually adequate.[23,25] Full early weightbearing is often possible if there is no bone loss.[23] Fractures in the adolescent are often comparable to those in adults, and the external fixation is therefore taxed with increased mechanical demands. The above-described methods of increasing construct stiffness are routinely used. As in adults, transfixing pins and bilateral frame constructs are rarely indicated for routine fracture care.[23]

The consequences of physeal injuries by inappropriate pin placement are self-explanatory and should be avoided at all cost. Due to the undulating nature of plate growth an unsafe zone of 1–2 cm exists adjacent to the physis. With the use of fluoroscopy, the pins can be safely introduced into the epiphysis itself if necessary.

The postoperative and long-term management must

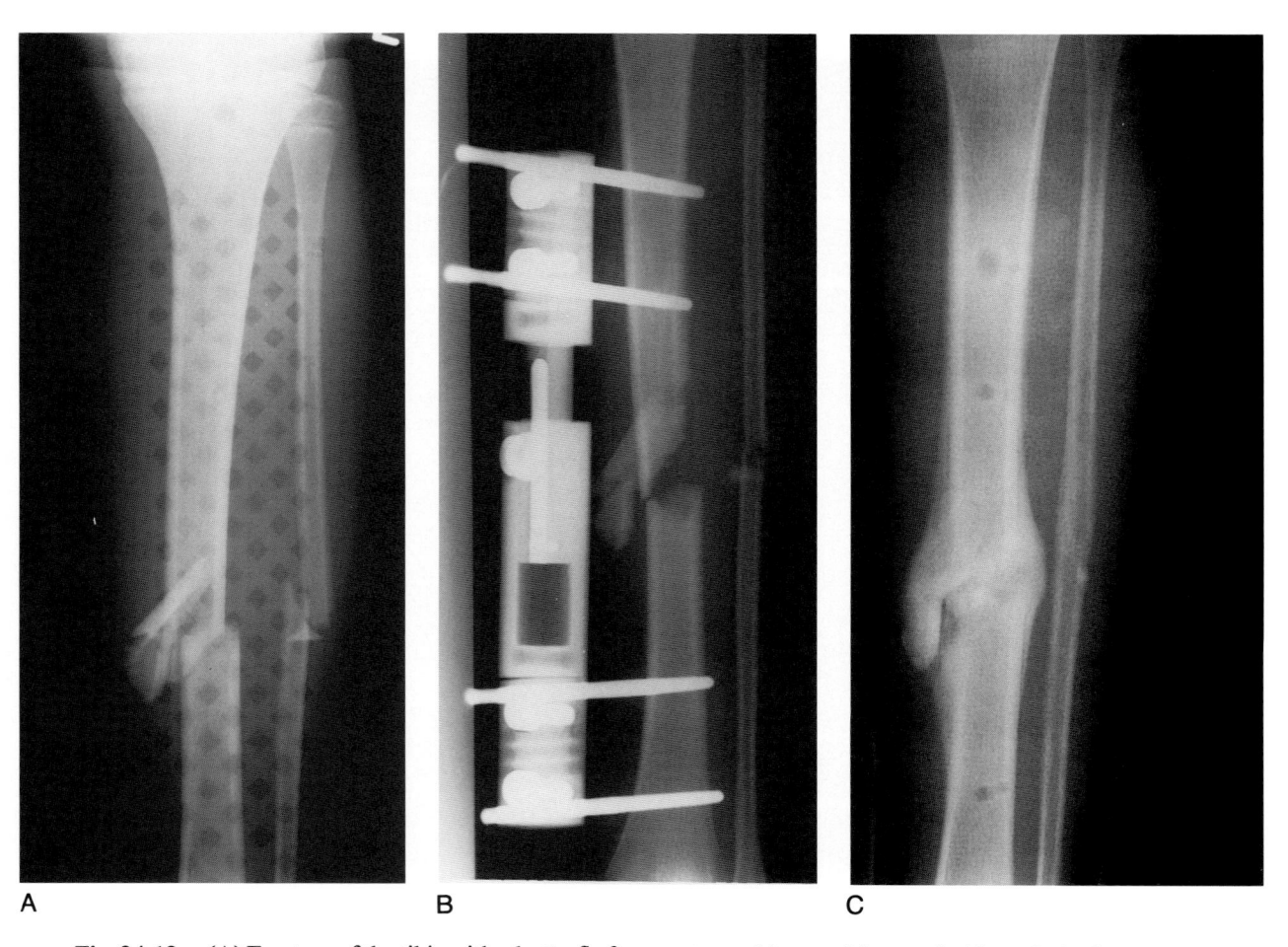

Fig. 34-12. (**A**) Fracture of the tibia with a butterfly fragment on a 14-year-old treated with an Orthofix external fixator. (**B&C**) With resultant healing in 8 weeks. Care must be taken not to distract the fragments, and early weightbearing should be encouraged with the fixator dynamized.

be clearly delineated and often individualized. In stable fractures, unilateral frames in "safe corridors" may be the only treatment necessary until fracture union. Alternatively, the frame can be removed and substituted by plaster immobilization when union of the fracture has been initiated.

Intramedullary Nailing of the Tibia

Intramedullary nailing has enjoyed wide acceptance in the management of open injuries of the tibia, especially since the introduction of the unreamed nail, which is said to preserve the endosteal blood supply. These are now routinely used in type II and even type IIIA and IIIB in adults. The presence of open growth plates in children precludes their use, but they may be a reasonable alternative in the older adolescent. Occasionally, intramedullary Kirschner wires or small Steinmann pins will provide alignment for tibial fractures associated with severe soft tissue injury in young children.

Fractures Associated with Extensive Soft Tissue Injury

The timing of soft tissue reconstruction in open injuries is of crucial importance. In the past, the standard treatment of such injuries included debridement and irrigation, antibiotics, stabilization of the fracture, and delayed closure of the wound. It has been shown, however, that the healing of fractures that have an ischemic soft tissue envelope does not begin until after neovascularization of the muscle layer.[34] Additionally, an intact viable muscle layer helps to avoid infection. Mathes and colleagues[35] demonstrated that muscle flaps could clear a larger inoculum of bacteria than those with poor muscle coverage. Fisher and Gustilo[36] recently reviewed their cases of type IIIB fracture of tibial shaft with special attention to timing of flap coverage and secondary bone grafting. Their data supported other studies[37] reporting the highest rate of complications for muscle flap coverage occurred when the procedure was done at 2 to 6 weeks. Their final recommendations were early flap coverage within 10 days after aggressive debridement. Osseous reconstruction, if necessary, should then be carried out after soft tissue healing[36] (Fig. 34-13).

A recent study by Cramer and colleagues[38] in 1992 reviewed 35 children with open diaphyseal fractures of the lower extremity. They concluded that immediate and repeated debridement, adequate stabilization, early wound coverage, and bone graft, when necessary, produced few problems of growth arrest, limb length discrepancy, or angular deformity. However, 50 percent of their type IIIC fractures of the tibia eventually required amputation. The severity of these injuries must not be underestimated. At the 1992 Combined Meeting of the Orthopedic Associations of the English Speaking World, Obrien[39] stated that he prefers to perform primary amputation in type IIIC in older patients, although salvage procedures may be indicated in children.

DEGLOVING INJURIES ASSOCIATED WITH FRACTURES OF THE TIBIA

Degloving injuries of the extremities in children, although fortunately infrequent, are nevertheless being more commonly encountered due to increasing exposure of children to motorized all-terrain vehicles, motor scooters, snowmobiles, sea-doos and other recreational high-energy motorized vehicles (Fig. 34-14). The lesion most commonly results from a severe shearing force to the limb, most commonly the result of the extremity being run over by a wheeled or tracked vehicle or the part being caught in a piece of moving machinery.[40] Since it is frequently the orthopaedic surgeon who first encounters the degloved extremity in association with fractures of the long bones, it is paramount that the lesion be recognized and treated appropriately in order to avoid the prolonged morbidity that may result from massive skin loss. The lower extremity is the most frequently involved body part, although it may occur at virtually any body site that is exposed to a shearing force. We have encountered the lesion on the buttocks and back of children being dragged by vehicles on the road.

The Degloving Lesion

Degloving injuries occur secondary to a severe shearing strain, such as the limb experiences in being run over by a tire or tracked vehicle, somewhat analogous to an electric cord being run over by a car (Fig. 34-15). Most degloving injuries are fairly obvious with a natural anatomic peeling-off of the skin sometimes appearing like a long stocking that has fallen down (Fig. 34-16). However, it may also be "concealed" with no actual break in the skin but complete disruption of all connections between the skin and the underlying fascia (Fig. 34-17A). Suspicion of concealed degloving should be aroused in a child with multiple abrasions over the skin and a history

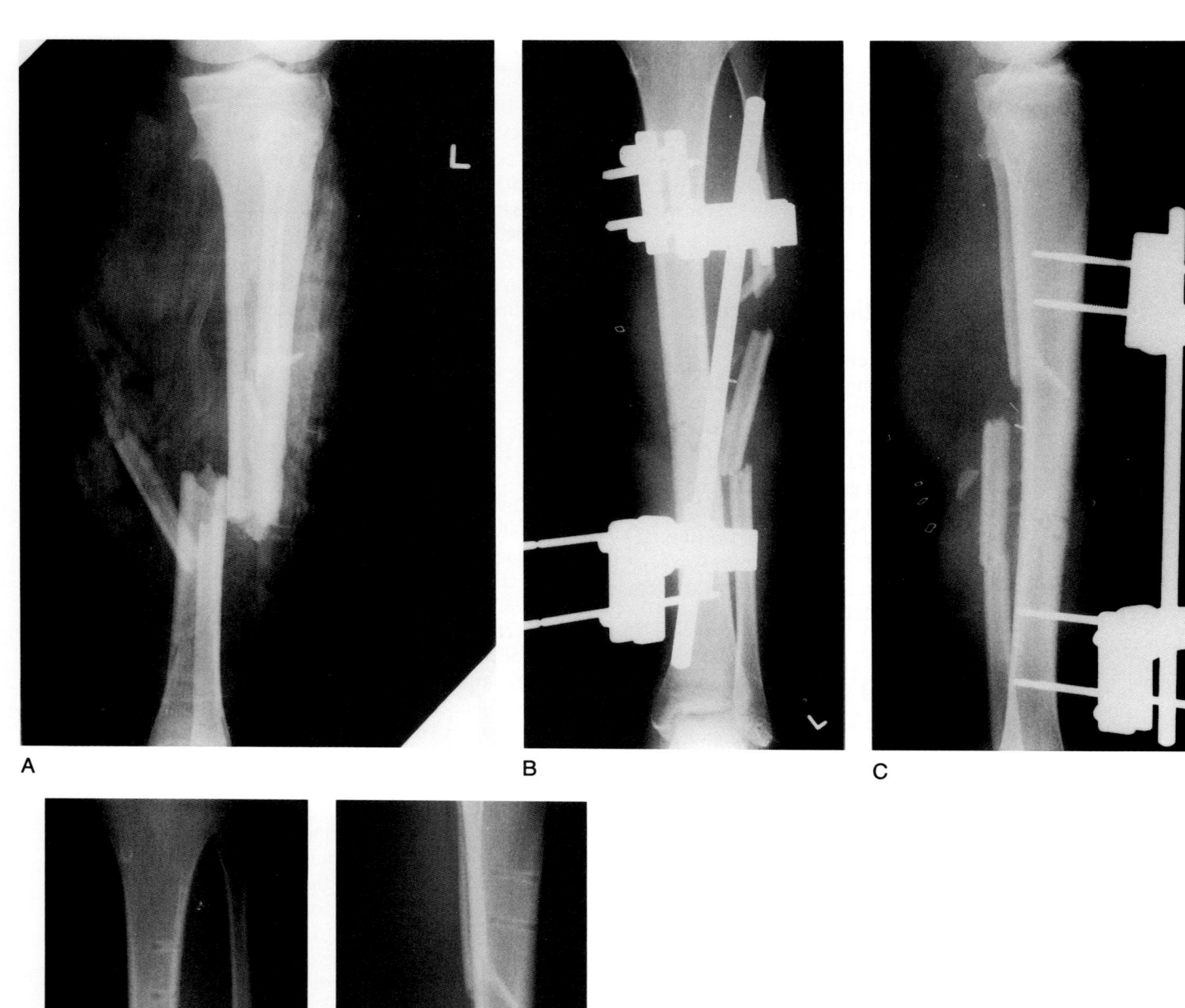

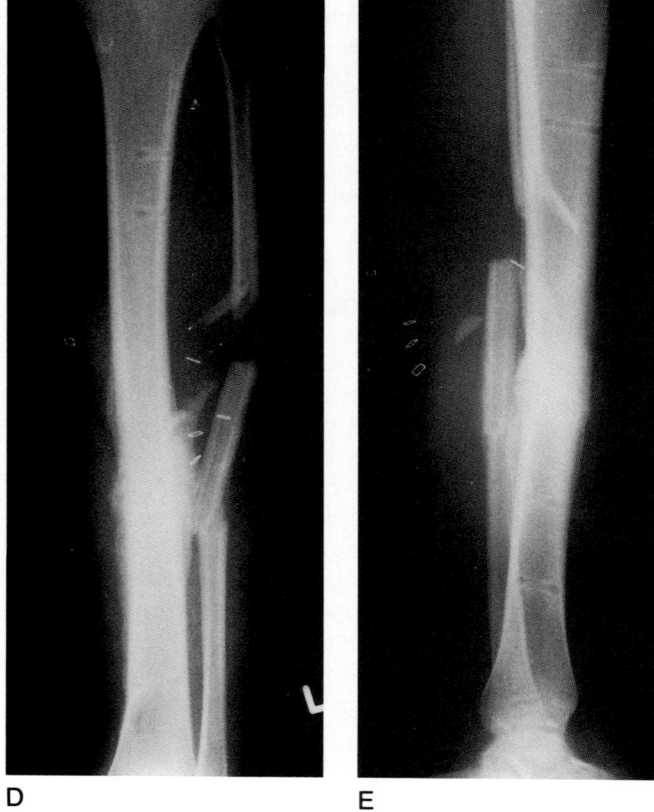

Fig. 34-13. (A–E) A 15-year-old girl involved in an all-terrain vehicle accident sustained a grade III open fracture of the midshaft tibia and fibula with marked soft tissues distruction. An osteochondroma on the medial and proximal aspect of the tibia is also present. The fractures were debrided and rigid stabilization was achieved with a unilateral uniplanor external fixator. The soft tissue defects were managed using local muscle flaps and split thickness skin grafts, the external fixator facilitating dressing changes. The external frame was maintained until union was solid. At the latest follow-up the patient is fully weightbearing on a sensate foot. She does, however, experience problems with the venous return of the lower leg, resulting in significant edema.

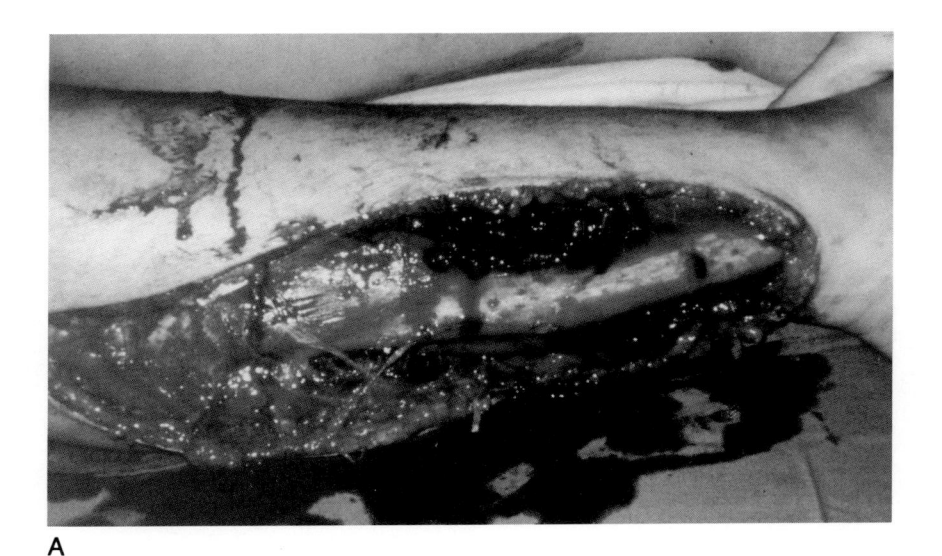

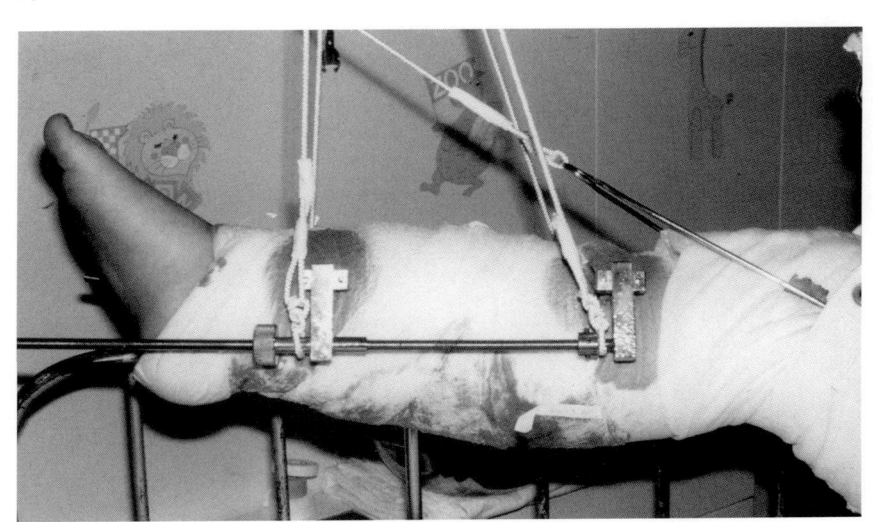

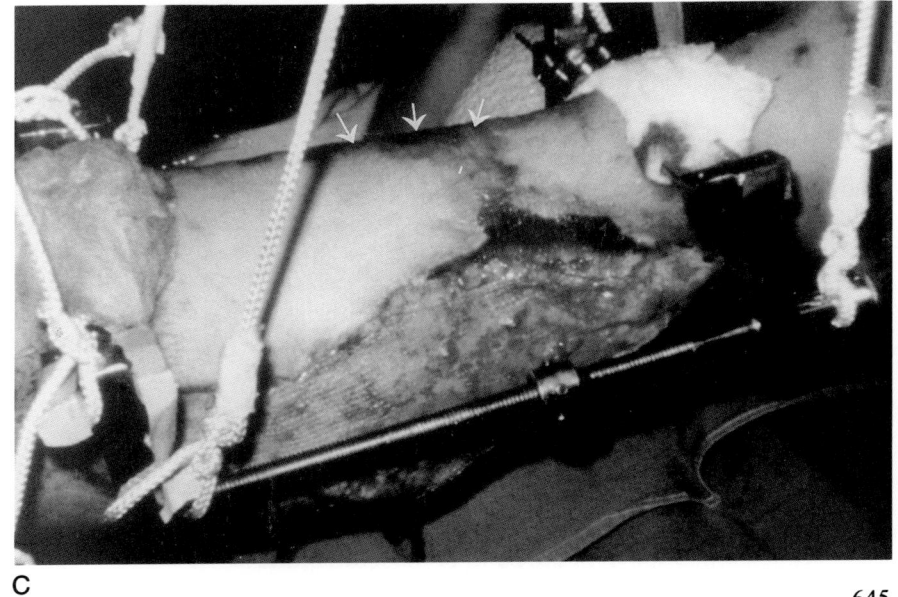

Fig. 34-14. (A) A 14-year-old boy on a motorbike was struck by a Mack truck sustaining a fractured tibia and a degloving injury. This was debrided and covered with a splint thickness skin graft and the tibia stabilized with an external fixator. (B) Unfortunately, the leg was elevated using only the ropes on the fixator with no sling. (C) The weight of the edematous calf resulted in skin ischemia over the anterior tibia, resulting in further skin loss. In such cases always use a sling to support the calf and avoid tension on the anterior tibial skin.

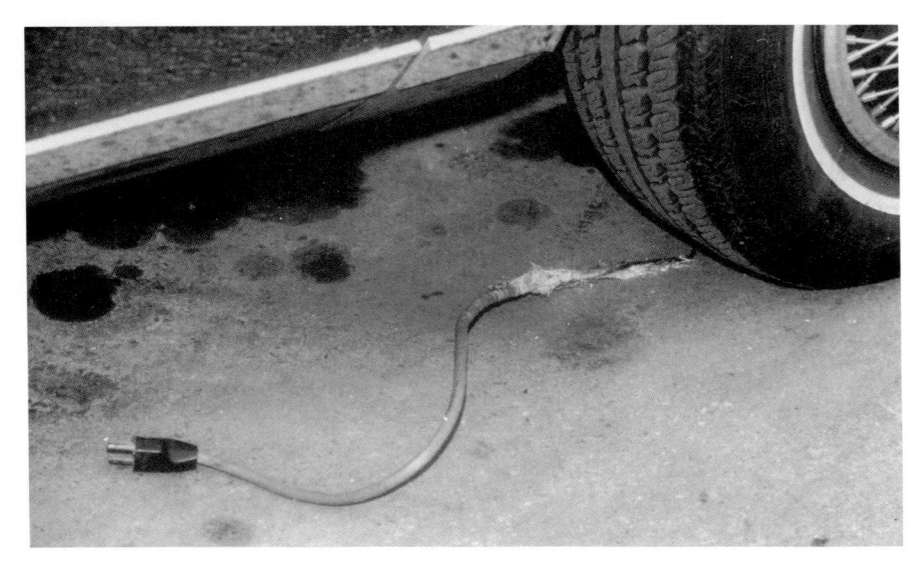

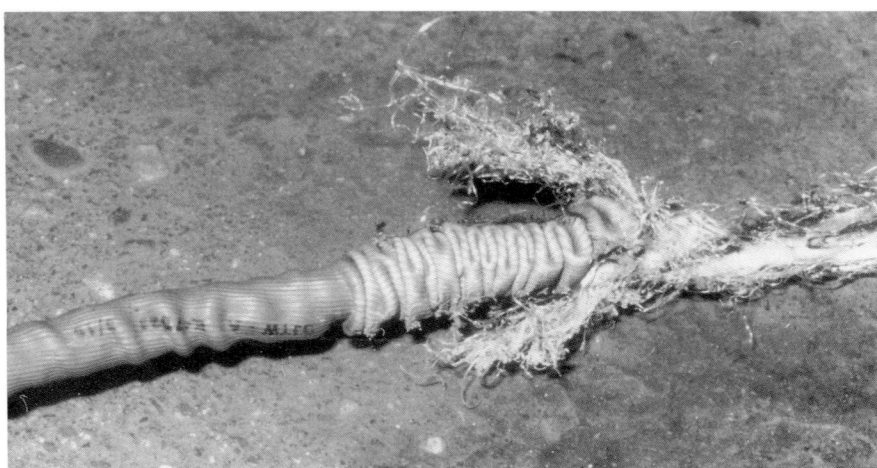

Fig. 34-15. An electrical cord when run over by a car is analogous to the degloving injury sustained by a child's limb.

of the extremity being run over. The diagnosis can be made by placing a hand over the skin and producing a mild shearing force. If the skin has been degloved it will be extremely loose with obvious detachment from the underlying fascia. Skin necrosis will inevitably occur in the degloved portion, since the blood supply to the skin has been disrupted (Fig. 34-17B). The skin is supplied primarily by large vessels that come up into the dermis. The dermal vascular pattern of capillaries, however, remains intact and thus allows the skin to be replaced as a full-thickness graft.[41-45] The plane of cleavage in the degloving injury lies between the skin and superficial fascia, except where the skin is densely attached to the underlying fascia, such as in the palm of the hand or the sole of the foot. Here the skin and fascia may be both involved as a degloved portion, the plane then being between the fascia and the layers of tenosynovium. Most degloving injuries are attached distally and disrupted proximally, hence the appearance of the skin being rolled down the extremity like a stocking or glove.

It is important to emphasize that degloving and crushing injuries often coexist with major underlying soft tissue damage as well as limb instability from underlying fractures. In some instances, the underlying soft tissue may be so traumatized as to be incapable of accepting a full-thickness skin graft. The skin itself may also be so damaged that it will not be amenable for use as a skin graft.

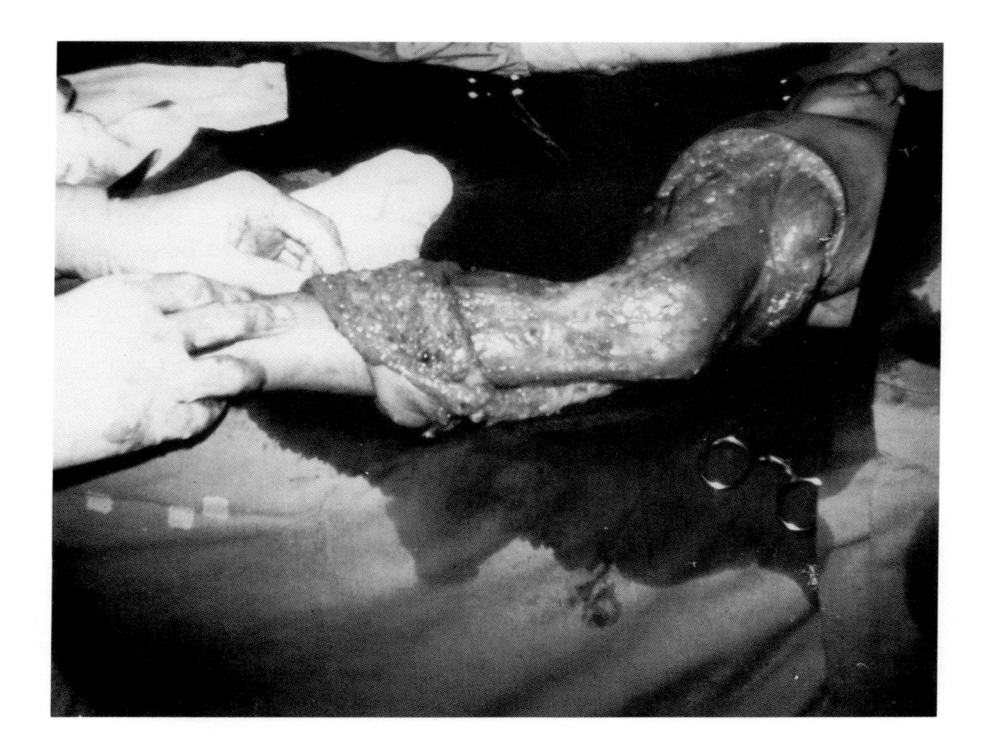

Fig. 34-16. The degloving injury illustrating the skin rolled down the leg like a stocking. (From Letts,[40] with permission.)

Fig. 34-17. **(A)** Mechanism of concealed degloving, which may occur without actual laceration of the skin. **(B)** Degloved skin that was simply sutured back in place without being defatted and reapplied as a full-thickness graft illustrating the inevitable development of skin gangrene. (From Letts,[40] with permission.)

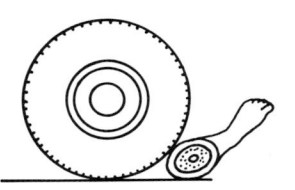

FRICTIONAL FORCE APPLIED

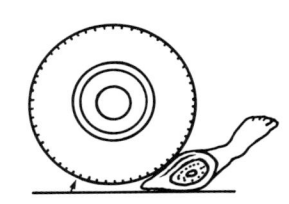

WHEEL MOUNTS LIMB
SKIN DRAWN ROUND

A

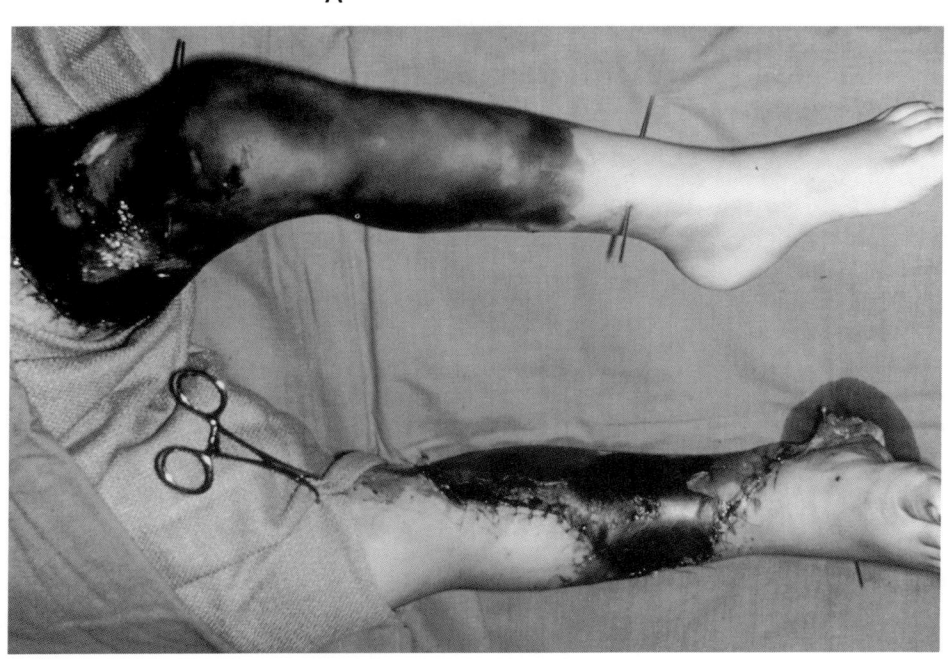

B

Management of the Fractured Tibia in the Presence of Degloving

The initial recognition and management of the degloved limb is critical. In the absence of obvious anatomic degloving, the presence of tire tracks over the clothes, increased mobility of the skin or the presence of a large subcutaneous hematoma should alert the surgeon to the possibility of a concealed degloving. The integrity of the degloved skin must be carefully assessed as to whether it can be utilized as a full-thickness skin graft, and, as well, the underlying soft tissues must be capable of accepting such a graft.

One of the pitfalls in the assessment of degloved skin is the excellent appearance and the impression that the skin is viable and well vascularized. The confirmation of skin devascularization is very difficult at the time of the initial debridement and care of a severely injured extremity in a child. Such clinical signs as failure of the skin to blanch when pressed, with no return of color when the pressure is released or the absence of dermal bleeding from a skin edge is suggestive of the vascular disruption to the skin.[42,43] A tourniquet test has been used with success by Grabb and Smith[44] to assess skin viability. This test is performed by elevating the limb for a minute and inflating a thigh cuff. The limb is then lowered and the cuff deflated, and if the skin is viable there should be return of color to the flap accentuated by the vasodilatation induced by a short period of ischemia. All of these tests, however, may be equivocal and, in some instances, depending upon the site of the lesion, may be impractical. Farmer[45] first advocated the replacement of degloved skin as a full-thickness graft in 1943. However, in spite of this early recognition of a successful method of treatment for this serious problem, many surgeons do not appreciate the importance of this concept. As a result, many surgeons learn by bitter experience as they watch degloved skin they meticulously resutured the previous night gradually turn dusky and black over the next several days, requiring replacement with split-thickness skin grafts and all the morbidity that such grafting entails (Fig. 34-17).

It must be emphasized that the degloved extremity is a very contaminated wound and demands meticulous wound toilet. The general principles of wound debridement apply, and devitalized tissues and debris must be removed. Frequently, the magnitude of the wound is often underestimated in the emergency department, and it is only in the operating theatre that the true extent of the massiveness of the degloving is truly appreciated. Skin that has been severely crushed at the point of impact usually requires resection. The entire noncrushed degloved area of the skin should be excised and carefully defatted. This can be achieved by pinning the skin on a skin board and using a large scalpel to scrape off the subcutaneous fat (Fig. 34-18). The defatted skin can then be applied to the degloved area, sutured in place with several apertures made in the graft with a scalpel to allow drainage of any hematoma (Table 34-3). A moderate pressure dressing should then be applied to the limb using Kerlex bandaging rather than a tensor bandage, which has the potential of producing too much pressure and the danger of ischemia. Most full-thickness grafts will have a very successful take in the pediatric age group and thus avoid the need for future split-thickness grafting.

If the underlying soft tissue has been severely traumatized or contaminated and is not capable of accepting a full-thickness skin graft, the skin can be simply defatted and stored in glycerol in the refrigerator and reapplied several days later when granulation tissue has formed and graft acceptance is more likely.

Fractures are frequently associated with the degloved extremity. These should be treated with an external fixator or skeletal pin traction so that the extremity can be completely accessible and the soft tissues and skin monitored (Fig. 34-19). In younger children, a K-wire or small Steinmann pin can be inserted into the tibia to maintain alignment. Portions of the tibia that have been denuded of soft tissue as well as skin should be covered with muscle flaps.[46,47] Depending on the amount of soft tissue

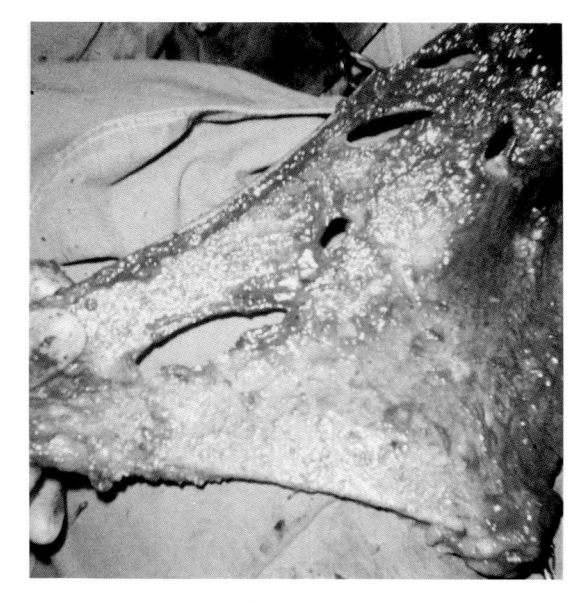

Fig. 34-18. Degloved skin can be defatted and replaced as a full-thickness skin graft.

damage and skin loss, split-thickness skin grafting may still be required, but using the degloved skin as a full-thickness graft will greatly reduce the amount required.

In the unfortunate event of a full-thickness skin graft necrosis, the graft should be removed in 2 to 3 days and replaced with split-thickness graft.

Another pitfall to be avoided in the management of the degloved extremity is to avoid hanging the limb from the attached external fixator (Fig. 34-13). As the calf becomes edematous and heavy, considerable traction will be exerted over the pretibial skin, with the result that a previously precarious blood supply may be obliterated by the downward traction and further skin loss accentuated.

In summary, recognition of a degloving lesion affords an opportunity to considerably decrease the child's morbidity by defatting the degloved skin, reapplying it as a full-thickness skin graft, and treating the fractured tibia with either external fixation or skeletal pin traction.

TABLE 34-3. The Skin Flap

1. Excise the flap
2. Meticulous defatting of flap
3. Debridement of wound bed
4. Apply as full thickness graft

The Degloved Heel

Heel degloving, unfortunately, is often associated with degloving of the lower leg and fractures of the tibia, particularly secondary to motorcycle accidents among teenagers. The driver is often thrown across the road, resulting in degloving of the dependent leg. The management of heel degloving is even more difficult than the associated proximal degloving.[48] Because the skin is attached to the heel with a thick fibrous septa, even a full-thickness skin graft is seldom effective. Split-thick-

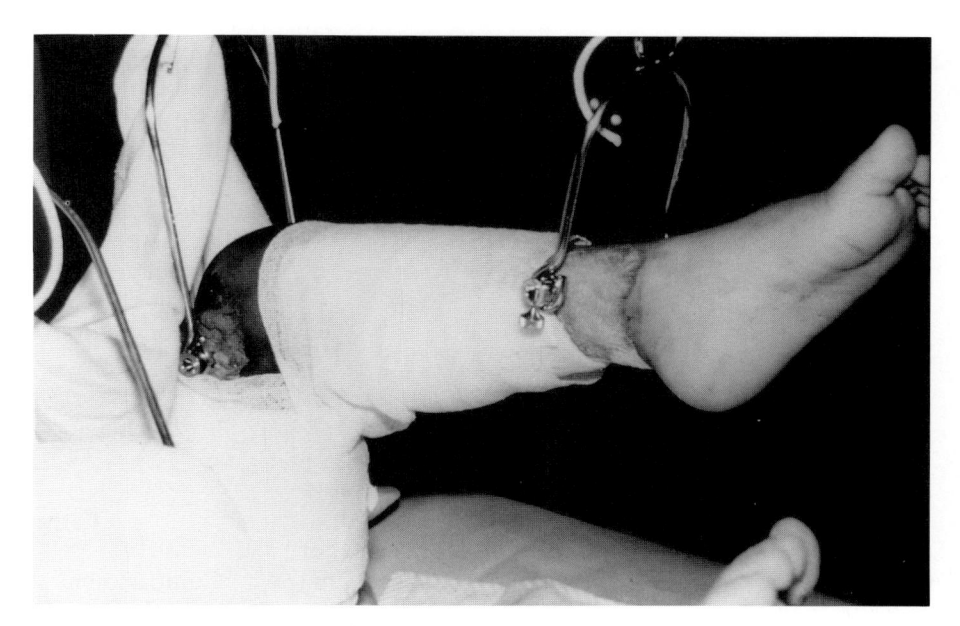

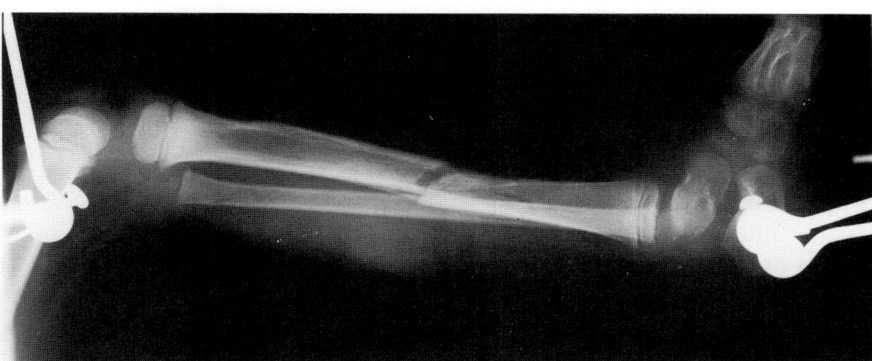

Fig. 34-19. Skeletal traction allows treatment of both the fractured tibia and the associated soft tissue injury.

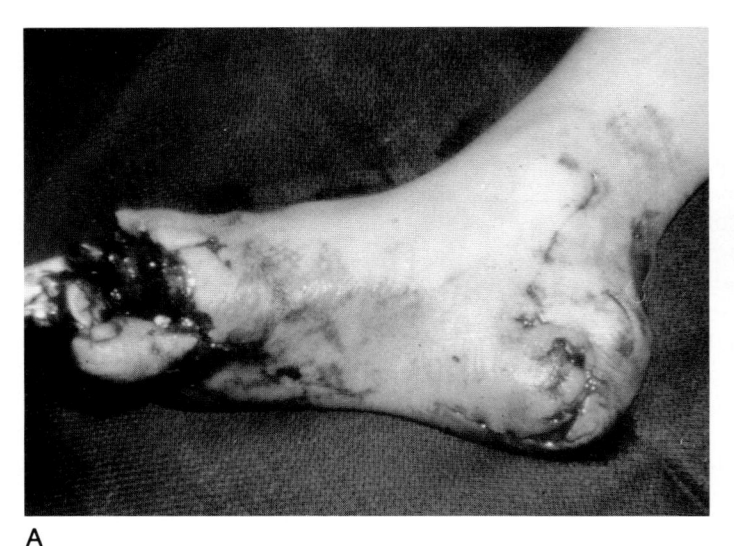

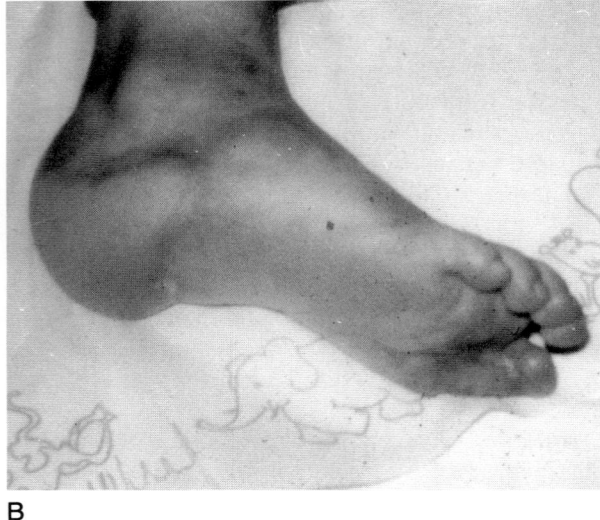

Fig. 34-20. (A) Degloved heel. (B) Heel coverage utilizing a deltoid myocutaneous transplant. (Courtesy of Dr. Ken Murray, Winnipeg, Manitoba, Canada.)

ness skin grafts almost always break down, hence more substantial coverage is usually required. The recent techniques of microvascular flap coverage have answered this need very effectively. Various flaps can be utilized with a deltoid myocutaneous transplant illustrated in Figure 34-20.

THE MANGLED EXTREMITY

Unfortunately, children are prone to become entangled in machinery for which they have a fascination rather than a fear. On farms this includes the various forms of farm machinery, but augers, in particular, as well as snowmobiles and motorbikes, are the major dangers. In the city the lawnmower and traffic trauma result in many severely traumatized lower extremities. Fortunately, with the advances in microsurgical techniques combined with the tremendous resiliency and healing powers of young children, limb salvage in the pediatric age group is a more rewarding and successful venture than in adults.

Indeed, providing the child with a mangled extremity can reach the operating room in less than 6 hours, the vascular integrity can usually be reconstituted, and, if there is not major nerve loss, the limb can usually be reconstructed. The mangled extremity severity score (MESS), which has been developed by Helfet and co-workers[49] for decision-making regarding limb salvage or amputation in the adult population, must be modified for young children (Table 34-4).

In adults, MESS scores for injuries that resulted in a viable limb range from 3 to 6 points. Those requiring amputation usually have scores from 7 to 12 points. The MESS score is a reliable quantitative criteria that has the potential to assist surgeons in decision-making regarding limb salvageability. It still needs to be fine-tuned a little more for children, but the concept is a good one.

COMPLICATIONS

Compartment Syndrome

Compartment syndrome may occur after relatively uncomplicated tibial fractures, particularly when the interosseous membrane remains intact, thus maintaining a confined compartment, facilitating a rise in intracompartmental pressure with persistent bleeding. Fractures located in any area of the tibia can develop compartment syndrome, but classically the metaphyseal tibial fracture is most vulnerable for this complication. In more severe injuries, compartment syndrome can occur even if the interosseous membrane has been disrupted. It is important to remember that open fractures are not immune to this problem, and a 5 percent incidence of compartment syndrome has been reported with such open injuries.[14]

TABLE 34-4. Mangled Extremity Severity Score

Type	Characteristics	Injuries	Points
Skeletal/soft-tissue Group			
1	Low energy	Stab wounds, simple closed fractures, small-caliber gunshot wounds	1
2	Medium energy	Open or multiple-level fractures, dislocations, moderate crush injuries	2
3	High energy	Shotgun blast (close range) high-velocity gunshot wounds	3
4	Massive crush	Logging, railroad, oil rig accidents	4
Shock Group			
1	Normotensive hemodynamics	BP stable in field and in OR	0
2	Transiently hypotensive	BP unstable in field bu responsive to intravenous fluids	1
3	Prolonged hypotension	Systolic BP less than 90 mmHg in field and responsive to intravenous fluid only in OR	2
Ischemia Group			
1	None	A pulsatile limb without signs of ischemia	0^a
2	Mild	Diminished pulses without signs of ischemia	1^a
3	Moderate	No pulse by Doppler, sluggish capillary refill paresthesia, diminished motor activity	2^a
4	Advanced	Pulseless, cool, paralyzed and numb without capillary refill	3^a
Age Group			
1	<30 years		0
2	>30 <50 years		1
3	>50 years		2

OR, operating room; BP, blood pressure.
^{a} Points × 2 if ischemic time exceeds 6 hours.
(From Helfet et al.,[49] with permission.)

In a cooperative child, the symptom of increasing pain (out of proportion to what is expected) and the later signs of paresthesia, paralysis, and tense swelling should alert the examiner to impending problems of increasing pressure. Capillary refill and pulses are not accurate signs of vascular sufficiency. Passive stretching of the toes will consistently exacerbate the pain due to the stretch of ischemic deep muscles and nerves of the leg.

In the case of an unconscious child or uncooperative child, one may use compartment pressure measurements if compartment syndrome is suspected. All four compartments (anterior, lateral, superficial, and deep posterior) should be recorded. Decompression by fasciotomy is indicated if the compartment pressure rises to within 20 to 30 mmHg of the diastolic pressure or if the absolute value is greater than 35 mmHg.

Decompression should be performed without delay after the diagnosis is made, as muscle and nerve damage are time-related. All four compartment should be decompressed either by a single lateral incision or more commonly by an anterolateral incision for the anterior and lateral compartments and a medial incision for the superficial and deep compartments.

Fasciotomy is also considered an indication for surgical stabilization of the fracture (see Ch. 64).

Vascular Injuries

Although rare in children, vascular complications are disastrous. As previously stated Cramer and coworkers[38] have reported a 50 percent amputation rate with type IIIC wounds.

The most frequently involved area for vascular injury is the proximal tibial metaphysis where the anterior tibial artery enters the anterior compartment at the proximal end of the interosseous membrane.[2,50] The anterior tibial artery may also be damaged when there is major displacement in the distal third of the tibia. Injuries to the posterior tibial artery are uncommon.[2]

The most critical aspect for a satisfactory outcome is a high index of suspicion, prompt diagnosis, and immediate repair. Surgical stabilization and fasciotomies are recommended in combination with the vascular repair.

Angular Deformities

As previously discussed, the final residual deformity should not exceed 5 degrees of varus or valgus angulation or 10 degrees of anteroposterior angulation to avoid cosmetic and functional malalignment.

Due to their remaining growth, children have the ability to remodel many fractures, especially in the metaphyseal regions. The same does not apply for diaphyseal fracture of the tibia. Infants and young children (up to age 8) can remodel a greater degree of deformity. In children between the ages of 9 to 12 years, only 50 percent of the angulation magnitude can be expected to correct. In children over 13, 25 percent or less of the angulation will be achieved.[2,14] Hansen and his colleagues[5] have estimated an overall correction of diaphyseal tibial angulation to be only 13.5 percent. Shannack[11] obtained similar results and also reported that deformity in two planes has an even poorer prognosis for correction. The least amount of correction was found to occur in posterior angulation, followed by valgus angulation.[2,14]

The best management is undoubtedly prevention of these deformities by good initial reduction and close follow-up. If a tibial angular deformity has developed, a closed wedge osteotomy at the fracture site is the best option.[2] If this is unsuccessful, a formal remanipulation under a general anesthesia is recommended. Failure of manipulation may necessitate open reduction or application of an external fixator.

Malrotation

Healing in malrotation is a permanent deformity and should be avoided.[14] Excessive rotation will change the biomechanics of the limb, resulting in an increased load on the medial aspect of the foot in external rotation and forced pronation of the foot in internal rotation. Compensatory rotation at the knee joint may also occur.[2] In children, the cosmetic appearance of malrotation will engender considerable parental concern. At the time of reduction, the rotation of the normal limb and tibia should be used as the template for the reduction of the tibial fracture.

Leg Length Discrepancy

Accelerated growth is a well-known phenomenon after fractures in children and has been best documented in femoral fractures. The mechanism of growth stimulation includes the effects of the periosteal stripping and callus formation, resulting in an increased blood flow to the limb. This includes an increased epiphyseal blood flow resulting in enhanced physeal activity. Although also documented in the tibia, the increased growth is not as significant in the tibia as in the femur following fracture. In his series of tibial fractures in children, Shannack[11] reported an average tibial overgrowth of only 1.3 mm. Young age and comminution of the fracture appear to be important factors.[2] In the child, shortening is a much more frequent potential problem than overgrowth.

Delayed Union and Nonunion

Delayed union and nonunion are not common in children,[2] but occasionally occur. Predisposing factors include open injury, bone loss, severe comminution, infection, excess motion of fracture site, external fixation distraction. The definition of nonunion as proposed by a U.S. Food and Drug Administration panel states that a nonunion is "established when a minimum of nine months has elapsed since the injury and the fracture shows no visible progressive signs of healing for a minimum of three months."[51] Practically, most orthopaedic surgeons will consider a tibial fracture ununited in the skeletally mature if after 6 months or more there is no progression toward union as evidenced by physical testing and radiographic evidence such as callus bridging the gap. The decision to treat nonunion is often individualized according to factors such as age, fracture pattern, and soft tissue injuries. In a child, failure to unite after 3 months is forboding. In infants and children with excessive anterior bowing of the tibia, congenital pseudarthrosis of the tibia should be kept in mind.

The differential diagnosis in a fracture that fails to unite includes delayed union, nonunion, synovial pseudarthrosis, infection, and unrecognized pathologic fractures. Diagnostic studies should include plain radiographs in multiple planes, including stress views and radionuclide scanning.

Technetium scintigraphy is useful for the detection of synovial pseudarthrosis. A nonunion is often characterized by an intense uniform uptake, whereas pseudarthrosis will often present as a photodeficient area between two intense areas of uptake.[51] The diagnosis of pseudarthrosis is significant because, if electrical stimulation is chosen as the method of treatment, it will not succeed in the presence of a synovial fluid gap.

A nonunion may be predicted by radionuclide scanning with a sensitivity of 70 percent and 90 percent.[52] Radionuclides may also be used in the investigation of a suspected infected nonunion. Although evaluation with sequential technetium and gallium scintigraphy is usually used, recent studies report an accuracy of only 50 to

60 percent.[53,54] Leukocyte labeling with indium[III] appears promising and has been found to be 100 percent sensitive in acute osteomyelitis but only 60 percent sensitive in the chronic form.[51] Biopsy remains the gold standard for evaluation of a suspicious nonunion. Osteomedulloangiography is another technique occasionally used to evaluate the medullary circulation at the fracture site.[53]

The treatment of nonunion of the tibia can be problematic, but with the evolution of new technology more options are becoming available for the treating surgeon (Fig. 34-21).

Delayed union of the tibia may respond to increasing weightbearing on the fractured limb. The intermittent cyclic loading is often sufficient to induce healing. Most children with a fractured tibia can weight bear by 3 to 4 weeks postfracture. Osteogenesis is induced by biomechanical factors that influence the undifferentiated stem cells to develop into osteoblasts.[55] The stress potential thus generated also promotes remodeling.

Treatment of tibial nonunion with fibular osteotomy remains popular, although controversial. The rationale for such treatment includes the concept that in fractures of both the tibia and fibula, the latter often unites first and thus becomes load-sharing, thereby decreasing axial loads across the tibia. The same phenomenon probably occurs with fracture of the tibia where the fibula remains intact.

Larger defects often require more extensive procedures. The time-honored bone grafting (autogenous) such as onlay and dual onlay grafts are not commonly used today. They are well described in *Campbell's Operative Orthopaedics.*[56] The posterolateral approach to bone grafting has a definite clinical indication in the treatment of nonunion with poor soft tissue coverage and in infected nonunions.[57] Surgical fixation of the fracture is used to augment stability and bone graft to promote osteosynthesis when indicated. These include compression plating, compressive external fixation, and intramedullary nailing in the older adolescent. More recently, procedures such as the Ilizarov technique for bone transport and vascularized graft for massive defects are becoming widely accepted (see Ch. 37).

Electrical Stimulation in Tibial Nonunions

Electrical stimulation remains an area of controversy in the treatment of nonunion. Three types of endogenous electrical signals have been described. Piezoelectric potentials, which are believed to originate from the collagenous portion of bone arising from stress-induced orientation of electrical dipoles in the organic material. Streaming potential results from the streaming of fluid through the solid matrix when bone is deformed and may be the electrical basis of Woff's law, that is, that bone is laid down in areas of stress and resorbed in areas of no stress. Finally, there are endogenous bioelectrical currents generated by electric pumps associated with living cells.[49,50,59] The response of bone to external current are numerous and fall outside the scope of this chapter.[51,58] Three modalities of treatment exist and include (1) totally invasive methods, (2) semiinvasive methods, and (3) noninvasive methods (indirective coupling and capacitive coupling).[51,59] The results of treatment are difficult to interpret, as many of the studies have been poorly controlled. In a recent double-blind study by Sharrard,[60] union was obtained in 45 percent compared to 12 percent in the control group. In children external or implantable electrical devices are preferable to percutaneous wire insertion.

SPECIAL TIBIAL SHAFT FRACTURES

Toddler's Fracture

A common injury pattern in infants and young children is torsion of the leg causing a spiral fracture of the tibia. The fibula remains intact. The child is usually seen in the emergency department because of refusal to weight bear on the affected leg. Careful physical examination consistently reproduces pain in the affected area. Examination should always be initiated on the contralateral limb to gain the child's confidence. There may be a slight increase in skin temperature.[61]

Radiographs will usually reveal an undisplaced spiral fracture of the tibial shaft. Additional views may be required to fully visualize the fracture. Occasionally, the fracture line may not be defined initially, only to become visible after a few days to 2 weeks post injury. A periosteal reaction is usually obvious at that time. The treatment consists of a long-leg cast for 3 to 4 weeks (Fig. 34-3).

Stress Fractures

Stress fractures, although relatively uncommon, may occasionally pose a diagnostic dilemma. This injury is usually activity-related and is more common in males.[2] It is most frequently located at the metaphyseal-diaphy-

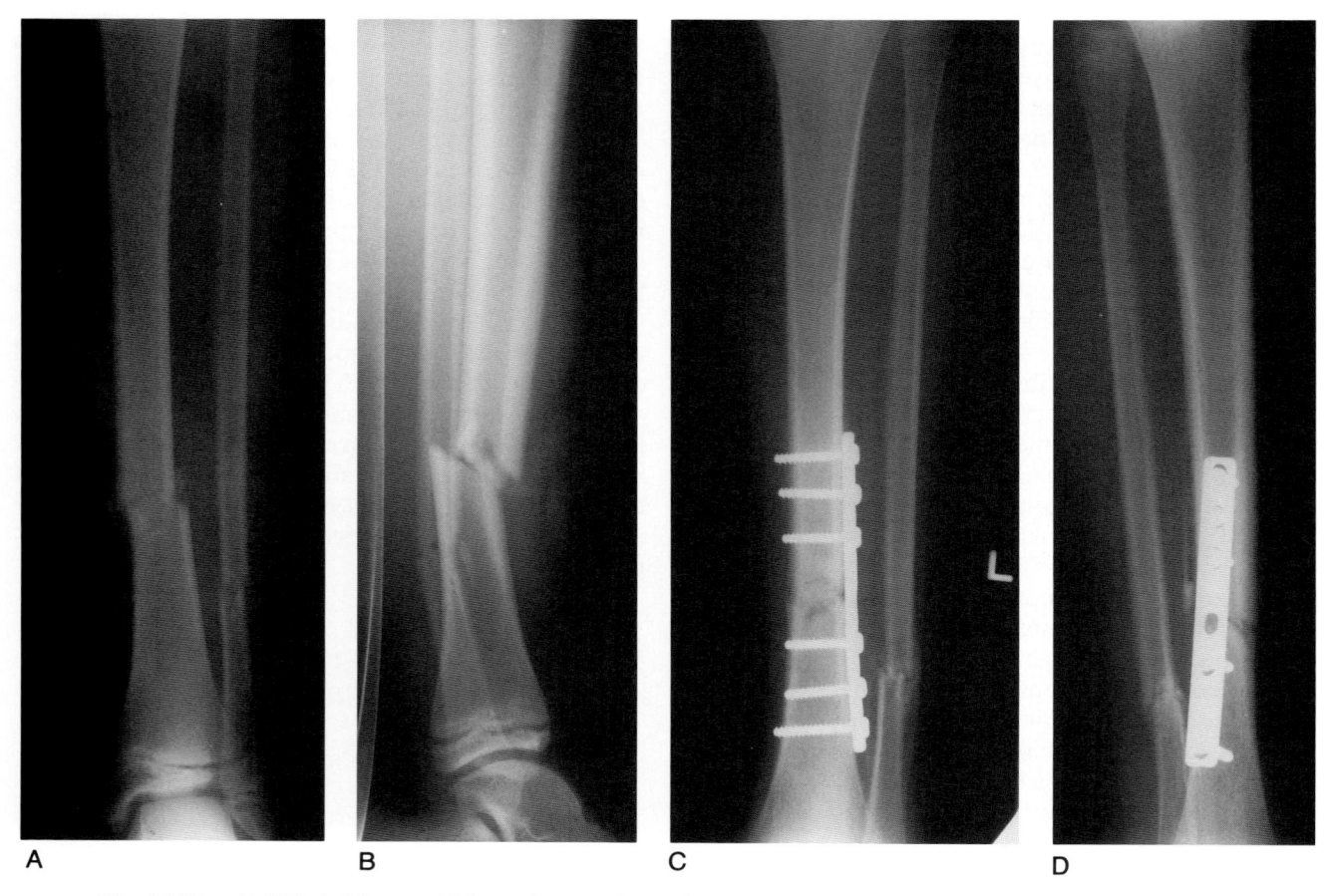

Fig. 34-21. (A&B) A 14-year-old boy who sustained bilateral fractures of the tibia and fibula and proximal femur. The injuries occurred when the patient was hit by a snowmobile after landing from a ski jump. All the injuries were closed fractures. (C&D) These multiple injuries were treated by open reduction internal fixation of the tibia using compression plate. The femur was stabilized using a reamed locked intramedullary nail. *(Figure continues.)*

seal junction. There is no history of specific trauma, and the child presents with a painful limp. Swelling is occasionally present, and local tenderness is constant (Fig. 34-7).

The diagnosis may be difficult as the radiographs are often initially negative. This may be followed by a small radiolucent zone with increased metaphyseal bone density and periosteal reaction in subsequent radiographs. A fracture line rarely becomes visible as this is a compression injury.[2] Radionuclide scanning is an effective and sensitive modality to investigate such an injury.[62] The treatment consists of rest and long-leg cast for 4 to 6 weeks. Nonunions have been described.[63]

Stress fracture may also occur in the fibula and may cause a problem in diagnosis as described in the tibia. Again treatment consists of rest and immobilization (see Ch. 53).

Tibial Fractures Associated with Paralysis

With the increasing life expectancy of patients afflicted with myelomeningocoele, fractures in this pediatric group are more commonly encountered. Because of lack of sensation, fractures are not always appreciated

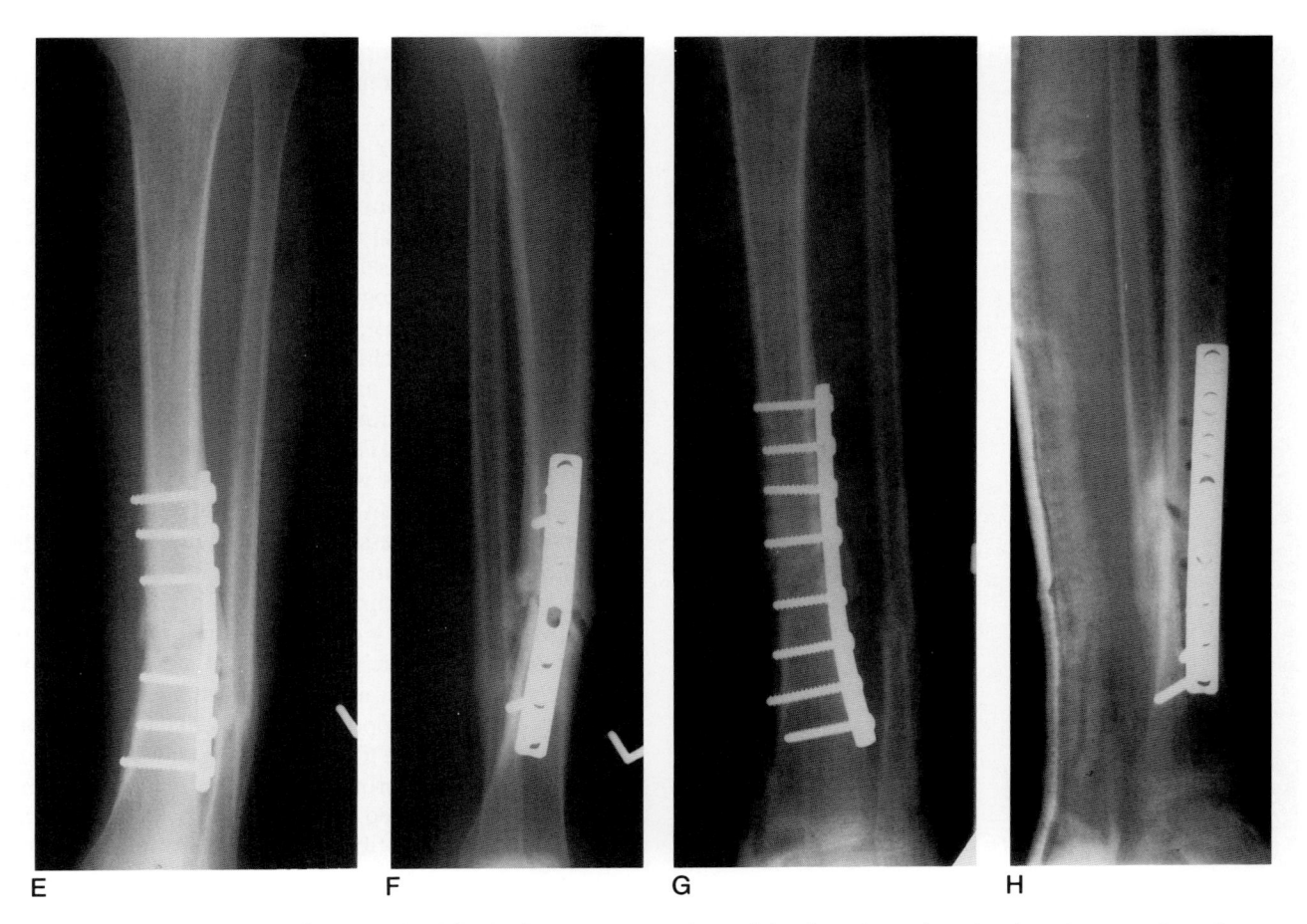

Fig. 34-21 *(Continued).* **(E&F)** While the femur progressed to solid union, the patient developed a nonunion of the tibia. Breakage of the compression plate is seen at 3 months in these radiographs especially on the lateral view at the level of one screw hole spanning the fracture site. **(G&H)** The nonunion was debrided and bone grafted and a new compression plate was applied. The patient progressed to solid union in the next 12 weeks. (Courtesy of Dr. Timothy Carey, Children's Hospital of Eastern Ontario, Ottawa, Canada.)

acutely. Fractures more commonly affect the knee region and are more frequent in the totally flaccid limb than in spastic paralysis or in patients with some quadriceps function. Occasionally, however, the tibial diaphysis is also affected. Radiographs will often show definite periosteal new bone and occasional widening of the growth plate, as these injuries are usually juxta-acticular.[64] The treatment consists of immobilization rest followed by protected ambulation. Complications are rare and are usually related to pressure by casts or orthoses. These fractures are especially common after the child has been immobilized in hip spica for unrelated reasons. In poliomyelitis, sensation is normal, and the injuries are therefore painful (see Ch. 60).

Pathologic Fractures

Stress risers in the tibial shaft may be generated from cortical defects resulting from an array of malignant or benign neoplasms. More commonly encountered lesions include nonossifying fibroma, unicameral bone cysts, aneurysmal bone cysts, and eosinoplilic granuloma. Trauma is usually minor and the fractures frequently undisplaced. Biopsy may be required for diagnosis of the underlying lesion (Fig. 34-22).

Pathologic fracture may also be encountered postbiopsy, postradiation, and in a variety of metabolic bone disease. Most respond to immobilization in a walking cast.

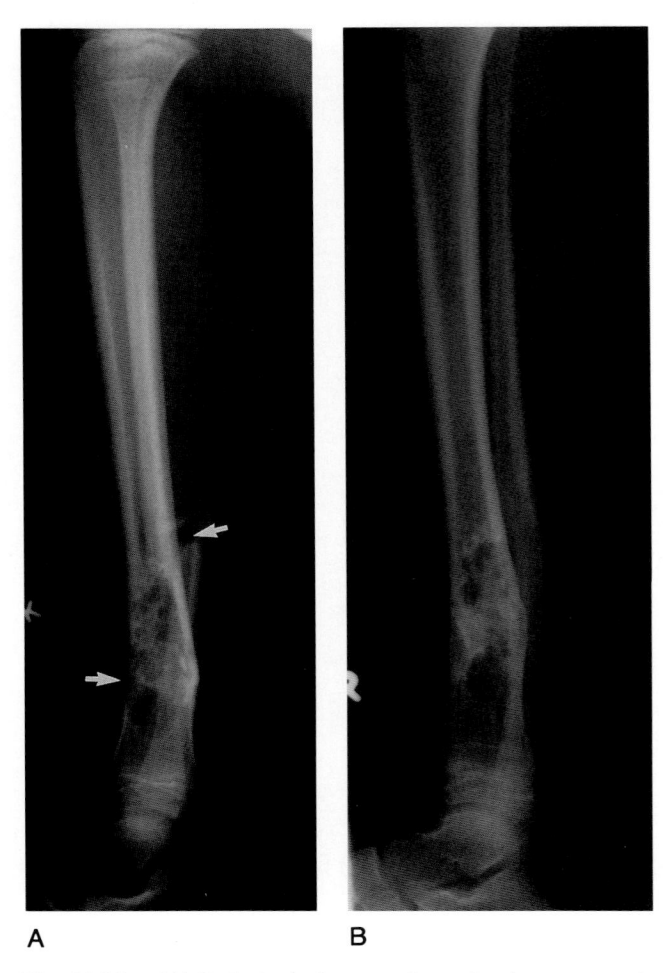

Fig. 34-22. (A) Pathologic fracture through a large nonossifying fibroma. (B) Such fractures usually heal uneventfully, sometimes with obliteration of a portion of the pathologic cyst.

CONGENITAL PSEUDARTHROSIS OF THE TIBIA

Congenital pseudarthrosis of the tibia is the most difficult nonunion of the tibia to ultimately achieve bony healing (Fig. 34-23). Over the years many techniques have been tried to achieve union, and many children's limbs have required amputation because of the complications from this very difficult entity.[65]

Several classifications of congenital pseudarthrosis of the tibia are in existence, but we find the most practical to be the classification illustrated in Table 34-5.[66]

About 50 percent of congenital pseudarthrosis of the tibia are secondary to neurofibromatosis, which may not be evident initially in a young child, although there is usually a family history. Cafe-au-lait spots are uncommon in young children and usually appear during the teens.

The type III variety, including anterior angulation of the tibia, must always be kept in mind in fractures of the tibia that go on to nonunion. The major problems associated with congenital pseudarthrosis of the tibia, aside from the nonunion itself, is the marked angulation of the tibia that develops together with a major limb length inequality. In the past, because of the multiple operations most of these children required, many clinicians recommended early amputation of the limb using a Symes or Boyd technique.[67] Function with a below-knee prosthesis in the child is usually excellent, and morbidity from many surgeries was thus avoided. Although this approach is always an option, recent techniques have met with more success. These have included vascularized fibular grafts, bone grafting and intramedullary fixation, the Ilizarov technique, and the addition of electrical stimulation to any of these procedures.[68,69] It is not sufficient to merely achieve union of the tibia, the limb has to be kept functional with minimal limb length inequality. The best opportunity to achieve a functional limb and union of the tibia is in young children who have not undergone numerous other procedures. Although in the infant vascularized grafting is not practical, it is important to keep the tibia from angulating, shortening, and deforming. Intramedullary fixation utilizing the Charnley technique with bone grafting, may result in union but, almost as important, will keep the tibia in an anatomic position, allow weightbearing, and maintain biomechanical function of the growth plates until such time as a more definitive procedure, such as the more recent Ilizarov technique, can be applied (Fig. 34-23). Even though union may be achieved, vigilance can never be relaxed, since refracture is not uncommon. It is recommended that intramedullary fixation be maintained no matter what technique is used to provide extra strength to the tibia. These children are also advised to use a high-laced boot or polypropylene total contact below knee orthosis until skeletal maturity to minimize the chance of recurrent pseudarthrosis.

TABLE 34-5. Classification of Congenital Pseudoarthrosis of the Tibia

Type 1	Fracture present at birth
Type 2	Develops following a fracture through congenital cyst
Type 3	Develops following a fracture through congenital bowed tibia
Type 4	Develops after a fracture through an area of tibial insufficiency, e.g., narrowed canal, sclerosis

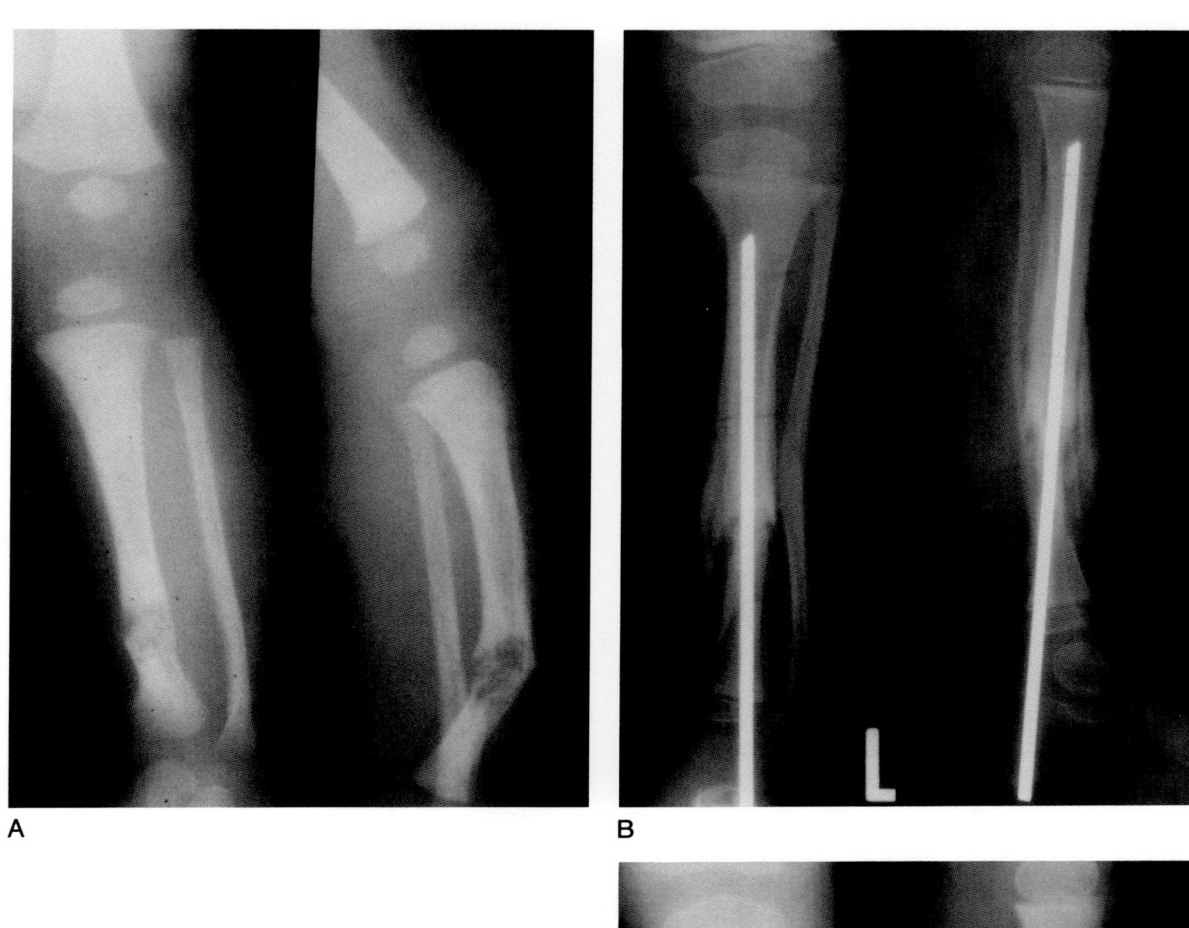

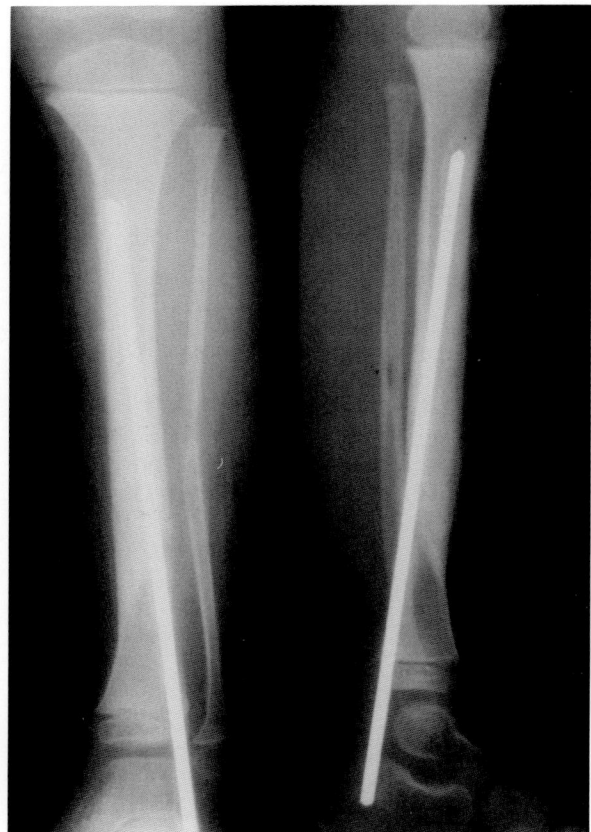

Fig. 34-23. Congenital pseudarthrosis of the tibia. **(A)** At 6 months of age. **(B)** At 2 years of age following bone grafting and intramedullary fixation through the calcaneus (Charnley technique). **(C)** At 6 years of age illustrating complete healing of the tibia, a straight limb and minimal limb length inequality.

SUMMARY

Fractures of the tibia and fibular shafts in the pediatric age group are the most common major fracture involving the lower extremity. The mechanisms of injury are numerous ranging from seemingly benign falls to severe trauma. Accordingly, the fracture patterns are various and include undisplaced low-energy injuries to severe crush injuries and occasional traumatic amputations. Most fractures can be treated by simple manipulation and casting techniques but occasionally requiring the full spectrum of operative management, including debridement, stabilization, and reconstruction of bone and soft tissues. Complications in simple fractures are uncommon but are increased as the complexity of the injury increases. These include malunion, nonunion, compartment syndrome, leg length discrepancy, infection, and vascular injuries.

REFERENCES

1. Blount WP: Fractures in Children. p. 183. Williams & Wilkins, Baltimore, 1955
2. Rockwood CA, Jr, Wilkins FrE, King EK: Fractures in Children. 3rd Ed. p. 1217. JP Lippincott, Philadelphia, 1991
3. Tachdjian MO: Pediatric Orthopedics. 2nd Ed. p. 3295. WB Saunders, Philadelphia, 1990
4. Clemente CD: Gray's Anatomy. 36th Ed. p. 773. Lea & Febiger, Philadelphia, 1985
5. Hansen BA, Grieff J, Bergmann F: Fractures of the tibia in children. Acta Orthop Scand 47:448, 1976
6. Beitzer CM, Johnson RH, Ettlinger CF, Aggeboin K: Downhill skiing injuries in children. Am J Sports Med 12:142, 1984
7. Boyer BS, Jaffe RB, Nixon GN, Condon UR: Trampolin fractures of the proximal tibia in children. AJR 146:83, 1986
8. Izant RJ, Jr, Rothmann BF, Franke VH: Bicycle spoke injuries of the foot and ankle in children: an underestimated minor injury. J Pediatr Surg 4:654, 1969
9. Morrisy RT: Lovell and Winter's Pediatric Orthopedics. 3rd Ed. Vol. 1. p. 370. 1990
10. King J, Diefendarf D, Apthorp J et al: Analysis of 429 fractures in 189 battered children. J Pediatr Orthop 8:583, 1988
11. Shannack AO: Tibial fractures in children: follow-up study. J Pediatr Orthop 8:306, 1988
12. Rang M: Children's Fractures. 2nd Ed. 297. JB Lippincott, 1987
13. Halderman WD: Results following conservative treatment of fractures of the tibial shaft. Am J Surg 99:593, 1959
14. Hensinger R: Operative management of lower extremity fractures in children. Am Acad Orthop Surg Monogr Ser 51, 1992
15. Verstreken L, Defrange G, Lamoureux J: Orthopedic treatment of pediatric multiple trauma patients: a new technique. Int Surg 73:177, 1988
16. Hansen ST: Internal fixation of children's fractures in the lower extremity. Orthop Clin North Am 21:353, 1990
17. Letts M, Vincent M: The floating knee in children. J Bone Joint Surg [Br] 68:442, 1986
18. McBryde AM, Jr, Blake R: The floating knee: ipsilateral fractures of the femur and tibia. J Bone Joint Surg [Am] 56:1309, 1974
19. Gustilo RB, Anderson JT: Prevention of infection in the treatment of one thousand and twenty-five open fractures of long bones: retrospective and prospective analysis. J Bone Joint Surg [Am] 58:453, 1976
20. Gustilo RB: Orthopaedic Infection, Diagnosis and Treatment. p. 87. WB Saunders, Philadelphia, 1989
21. Behrens F: General theory and principles of external fixation. Clin Orthop Rel Res 241:15, 1989
22. Behrens F: External fixation in children. Instr Courses Lect 39:205, 1990
23. Porat S, Milgron C, Nyska M et al: Femoral fracture treatment in head injured children: use of external fixation. J Trauma 26:81, 1986
24. Quintin J, Eurard H, Govat P et al: External fixation in child traumatology. Orthopaedics 1987:463, 1984
25. Tola VT: External fixation in children's fractures. J Pediatr Orthop 3:435, 1983
26. Behrens F, Seaels K: External fixation of the tibia: basic concepts and prospective evaluation. J Bone Joint Surg [Br] 68:246, 1986
27. Burny F: The pin as a percutaneous implant: general and related research. Orthopaedics 7:610, 1984
28. Schmidt A, Rorabeck GA: Fractures of the tibia treated by flexible external fixation. Clin Orthop Rel Res 193:162, 1978
29. Kimmel RB: Results of treatment using the Hoffman external fixator for fractures of the tibial diaphysis. J Trauma 22:960, 1982
30. Behrens F: A primer of fixator devices and configurations. Clin Orthop Rel Res 241:5, 1989
31. Behrens F, Johnson WD: Unilateral external fixation: methods to increase and reduce frame stiffness. Clin Orthop Rel Res 241:48, 1989
32. Briggs BT, Chao EYS: The mechanical performance of the standard Hoffman-Vidal external fixation apparatus. J Bone Joint Surg [Am] 64:566, 1982
33. Behrens F, Johnson WD, Kouk TN, Kovacevic N: The bending stiffness of unilateral and bilateral external fixator frames. Clin Orthop Rel Res 178:103, 1983
34. Holden GEA: The role of blood supply to the soft tissue in the healing of diaphyseal fractures: an experimental study. J Bone Joint Surg [Am] 54:993, 1972
35. Mathes SJ, Alpert BS, Chang Ning: Use of muscle flaps in

chronic osteomyelitis: experimental and clinical correlation. Plast Reconstr Surg 69:815, 1982
36. Fisher MD, Gustilo RB, Uorecka TF: The timing of flap coverage, bone grafting, and intramedullary nailing in patients who have fractures of the tibial shaft with extensive soft tissue injury. J Bone Joint Surg [Am] 73:1316, 1991
37. Byrd HS, Spices TE, Cierny G: Management of open tibial fractures. Plast Reconstr Surg 76:719, 1985
38. Cramer KE, Limbird TJ, Green NE: Open fractures of the diaphysis of the lower extremity in children: treatment results and complications. J Bone Joint Surg [Am] 74:218, 1992
39. OBrien P: Personal communication presented at the Combined Meeting of the Orthopaedic Associations of the English Speaking World, Toronto, Canada, June 1992
40. Letts RM: Degloving injuries in children. J Pediatr Orthop 6:193, 1986
41. Saact MN: The problems of traumatic skin loss of the lower limbs, especially when associated with skeletal injury. Br J Surg 57:601, 1970
42. Corps BV, Littlewood M: Full thickness skin replacement after traumatic avulsion. Br J Plast Surg 12:229, 1966
43. Coryllos E, Dabbert O, Tracey E et al: Treatment of an avulsed skin flap involving the circumferences of the entire lower leg. Ann Surg 151:437, 1960
44. Grabb W, Smith J: Plastic surgery, a concise guide to clinical practice. Little, Brown, Boston, 1973
45. Farmer AW: Whole skin removal and replacement. Surg Clin North Am 23:1440, 1943
46. Shapiro J, Akbarnia BA, Hanel DP: Free tissue transfer in children. J Pediatr Orthop 9:590, 1989
47. Louton RB, Harley RA, Hagerty RC: A fasciocutaneous transposition flap for coverage of defects of the lower extremity. J Bone Joint Surg [Am] 71:988, 1989
48. Rooks MD: Coverage problems of the foot and ankle. Orthop Clin North Am 20:723, 1989
49. Helfet D, Howey T, Sanders R, Johansen K: Limb salvage versus amputation: preliminary results of the mangled extremity severity score. Clin Orthop 256:80, 1990
50. Hoover NW: Injuries of the popliteal artery associated with fractures and dislocations. Surg Clin North Am 41:1099, 1961
51. Orthopaedic Advisory Panel: Guidance on the Investigational Device Exemptions on Premarket Approval Applications for Bone Growth Stimulation Devices. p. 5. Food and Drug Administration, Washington, DC, 1986
52. Smith MA, Jones EA, Strachan RK et al: Prediction of fractures healing in the tibia by quantitative radionuclide imaging. J Bone Joint Surg [Br] 69:441, 1987
53. Puramen J, Punto L: Osteomedulloangiography: a method of estimating the consolidation prognosis of tibial shaft fractures. Clin Orthop Rel Res 161:8, 1981
54. Merkel KD, Brown ML, Dewangee MK et al: Comparison of indium-labeled leucocyte imaging with sequential technitium-gallium scanning in the diagnosis of low grade musculoskeletal sepsis: a prospective study. J Bone Joint Surg [Am] 67:465, 1985
55. Reddi AH, Wientroub S, Mutlukumaran N: Biologic principles of bone induction. Orthop Clin North Am 18:207, 1987
56. Campbell's Operative Orthopaedics. 8th Ed. p. 1287. CV Mosby, St. Louis, 1991
57. Maurer RG, Dillan L: Multistaged surgical management of posttraumatic segmental tibial bone loss. Clin Orthop Rel Res 216:162, 1987
58. Albright JA, Brand RA: The Scientific Basis of Orthopaedics. 2nd Ed. Appleton & Lange, E. Norwalk, CT, 1987
59. Lavine LS, Godzinsky AJ: Current concept review: electrical stimulation of repair of bone. J Bone Joint Surg [Am] 69:626, 1987
60. Sharrard WJW: A double blind trial of pulsed electromagnetic fields for delayed union of tibial fractures. J Bone Joint Surg [Br] 72:347, 1990
61. Dunbar JJ, Owen HF, Norgrady MB, McLesse R: Obscure tibial fracture of infants: the toddler's fracture. J Can Assoc Radiol 25:136, 1964
62. Roub LW, Gumaman LW, Hawley EN et al: A radionuclide imaging perspective. Radiology 132:431, 1979
63. Gruen NE, Rogers RA, Lipscomp AB: Nonunions of stress fractures of the tibia. Am J Sports Med 13:171, 1985
64. Gyepes MT, Newbern DH, Newhower EBD: Metaphyseal and physeal injuries in children with spina bifida and myelomeningocoele AJR 95:168, 1965
65. Staheli LT: The lower limb. In Morrissy RT (ed): Pediatric Orthopaedics. 3rd Ed. p. 755. JP Lippincott, Philadelphia 1990
66. Sage FP: Congenital anomalies. p. 1812. In Edmonson AS, Crenshaw AH (eds): Campbell's Operative Orthopaedics. 8th Ed. CV Mosby, St. Louis, 1991
67. Umber JS, Moss SW, Coleman SS: Surgical treatment of congenital pseudoarthrosis of the tibia. Clin Orthop 166:28, 1982
68. Fabry G, Lammens J, Mekebeek J et al: Treatment of congenital pseudoarthrosis with the Ilizarov technique. J Pediatr Orthop 8:67, 1988
69. Paterson DC, Simonis RB: Electrical stimulation in the treatment of congenital pseudoarthrosis of the tibia. J Bone Joint Surg [Br] 67:454, 1985

35

The Floating Knee

R. Mervyn Letts
Guy Moreau

Always examine the joint above and the joint below a fracture.

DESCRIPTION AND INCIDENCE

Ipsilateral fractures of the femur and tibia in children, "the floating knee" have received little attention in the literature until relatively recently (Fig. 35-1). The problem in management of two major bone fractures in the same limb has long been recognized in adults as being fraught with complications.[1-6] Over the past decade there has been much more interest in this fracture pattern in children undoubtedly due to the increasing incidence of this complex fracture pattern secondary to a more motorized pediatric population. As well, several reviews have pointed out the difficulty in managing ipsilateral fractures of the femur and tibia in children, particularly in the adolescent age group.[7,8] Most trauma resulting in this injury pattern is of a severe nature, with many children sustaining injury to other areas of the body. In children, the fracture pattern may involve the growth plate resulting in further long-term sequelae secondary to physeal arrest and subsequent limb deformity or shortening.

Reviews of this fracture pattern in children have consistently reported a male:female ratio of 4:1, with an average age of 8 to 10 years.[7,8] In the majority of instances, the trauma is secondary to either a car-pedestrian collision or a car-bicycle encounter. Injury severity scores averaging 14 were noted in Bohn and Durbin's[8] review of 44 children sustaining this injury. In the adult population incurring this injury, 12 percent are complicated by the fat embolism syndrome. Associated injuries must be carefully looked for, since the energy required to produce a fracture of the femur and tibia almost invariably causes other serious injuries. In particular, the ipsilateral knee must be carefully examined for ligamentous rupture.

The exact incidence of the floating knee is difficult to determine, but in a 3-year study of children admitted to the Winnipeg Children's Hospital, only 4 of 154 fractured femurs had floating knees, an incidence of 2.6 percent.

ANATOMY

Fractures of the femur are common in children, especially in the 6- to 12-year age group. In these children the midshaft of the femur is approximately at the level of a car bumper and most sustain a transverse fracture of the femur when struck by a car. The high incidence of the floating knee in association with bicycle accidents is probably due to the tibia and femur being directly struck, the femur by the hood of the car and the tibia by the bumper, resulting in a floating segment, including the knee. Because children at this age have open physes and

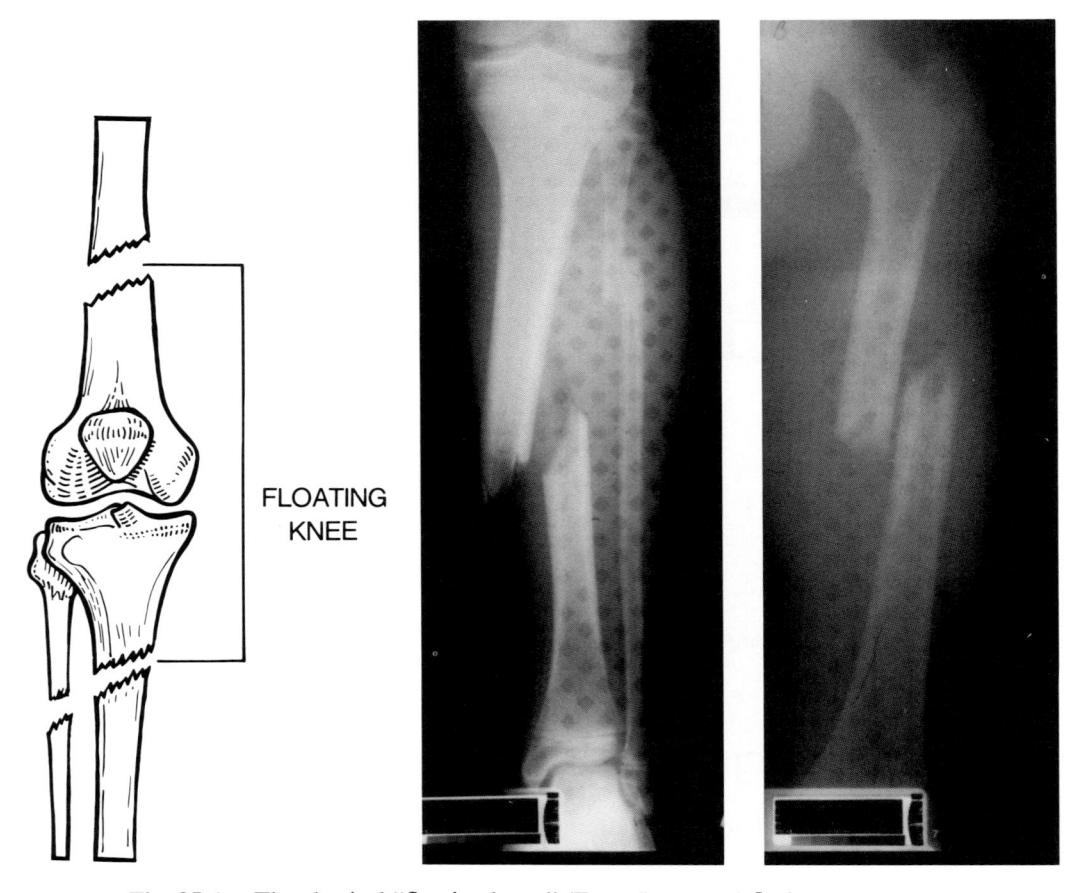

Fig. 35-1. The classical "floating knee." (From Letts et al.,[7] with permission.)

since the growth plate is relatively weaker than the surrounding bone, fractures through the distal femoral physis and less commonly the proximal tibial physis add a further dimension to the treatment of this complex injury. Unfortunately, due to the massive transfer of energy, fractures involving the growth plate have a high incidence of physeal arrest—in the neighborhood of 40 to 50 percent. This is primarily due to marked compression of the physis that occurs in association with the translation of the epiphysis on the metaphysis. Although in children between 3 and 12 years of age some overgrowth can be expected as a result of a fractured femur, shortening due to excessive overlap and angulation usually occurs in floating knee fractures treated nonoperatively.

To emphasize this difference and to draw attention to the involvement of the growth plate, a classification of the floating knee in children was devised by Letts and colleagues[7] (Fig. 35-2).

MECHANISM OF INJURY

The type of trauma required to inflict a fracture of the tibia and femur is of a violent nature. In two major reviews[7,8] the commonest mechanism of injury occurred when the child was either hit as a pedestrian or riding a bicycle. As illustrated in Figure 35-3, a child on a bicycle is usually struck by the bumper of the car in the lower leg, thus sustaining the fractured tibia and in the thigh by the hood of the car resulting in the fractured femur, with other injuries being sustained as the child rolls off the hood striking the head or sustaining an abdominal injury. A similar mechanism has been pointed out by Waddell to explain the characteristic injuries of fractured femur, abdominal trauma, and head injury often seen in younger children struck by a car[9] (Fig. 35-4). The added insult of a wheel passing over an extremity adds further to the trauma sustained by these unfortunate children.

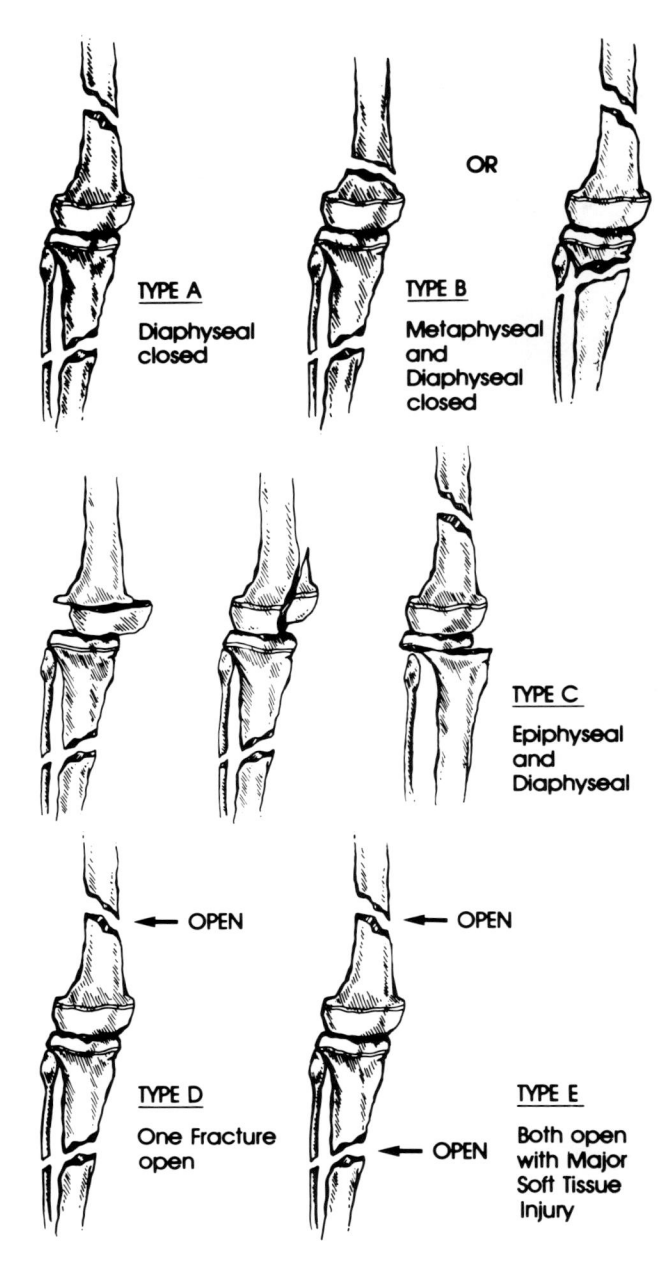

Fig. 35-2. Classification of the floating knee in children showing the variations induced by associated physeal injury. (From Letts et al.,[7] with permission.)

PHYSICAL EXAMINATION

Children sustaining this magnitude of trauma obviously need a meticulous physical examination to rule out other associated injuries. The fractures of the femur and tibia are usually the most self-evident injuries. A complete search for evidence of other fractures and possible intra-abdominal injury must be performed. The ABC's of trauma evaluation must be instituted immediately in the emergency department on the child's arrival. The limb will demand splinting in a Thomas splint with a tibial aluminum splint or plaster slab. Once respiratory function has been ensured, the limb must be carefully examined for neurovascular integrity. If either of the fractures are open, a clean sterile dressing should be applied while waiting to take the child to the operating theater. It will be difficult, if not impossible, to adequately examine the integrity of the ipsilateral knee; however, the presence of a hemarthrosis is highly suggestive of an associated ligamentous disruption or cruciate avulsion of the knee. A careful limb examination is mandatory under general anesthesia at the time the fractures are treated.[10-13] Occasionally an associated fracture of the femoral neck will be encountered, emphasizing the importance of examining the joint above and below each fracture (Fig. 35-5).

Adequate radiographs of all suspected osseous trauma must be obtained. If a head injury has been incurred, good films of the cervical spine should be taken at the time of the skull films to rule out cervical spine fracture.

TREATMENT

Treatment of the floating knee in children by traction and nonoperative methods is fraught with difficulty due to the requirements of maintaining a balancing act in a limb with 4 degrees of freedom of motion, that is, the hip, the fractured midshaft femur, the knee, and the fractured midshaft tibia. The result with this method of treatment is usually that one or other of the fracture ends up with a malunion and a less than adequate result with an associated limb length inequality due to shortening (Fig. 35-6). Some fracture patterns will absolutely demand an open reduction. This includes physeal injuries that are displaced and those fractures that are open and require debridement and wound care. It has been our experience[7] and recently that of others[8,14,15] that in most children over 7 years of age at least one fracture should be reduced and maintained with fixation. In older teenagers both fractures would probably benefit from external and/or internal fixation[16] (Fig. 35-7). All physeal injuries should be internally stabilized following an accurate open or closed reduction with K-wires or screw fixation, providing the latter do not cross the physis. Smooth K-wires may cross the growth plate without danger of causing a growth plate arrest.

In the classic type A floating knee in a teenager, closed

664 / Management of Pediatric Fractures

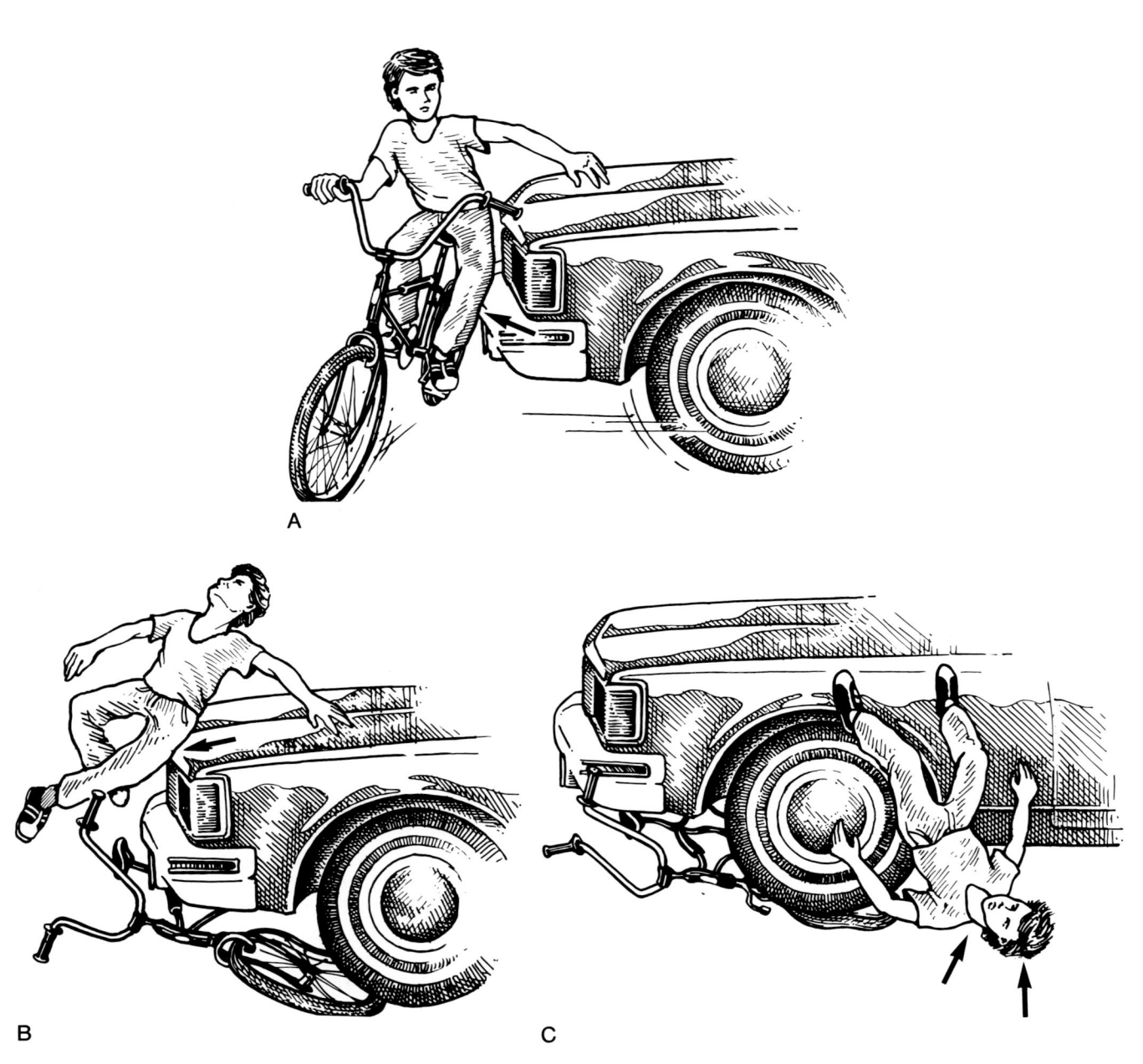

Fig. 35-3. A common mechanism of injury resulting in a floating knee in children. **(A)** The bumper of the car strikes the tibia of the cyclists extended leg, fracturing the tibia and fibula. **(B)** The cyclist is then struck on the thigh by the hood of the car sustaining a fracture of the femur. **(C)** The cyclist is thrown over the hood and onto the road, sustaining head, chest, or abdominal injuries and possible skin trauma from the wheels. (From Letts et al.,[7] with permission.)

Fig. 35-4. Young children involved in car-pedestrian accidents frequently sustain fractures of their femur or tibia from the bumper impact, chest or abdominal injury from the hood impact, and a head injury when thrown from the hood—Waddell's triad. (From Rang M.,[9] with permission.)

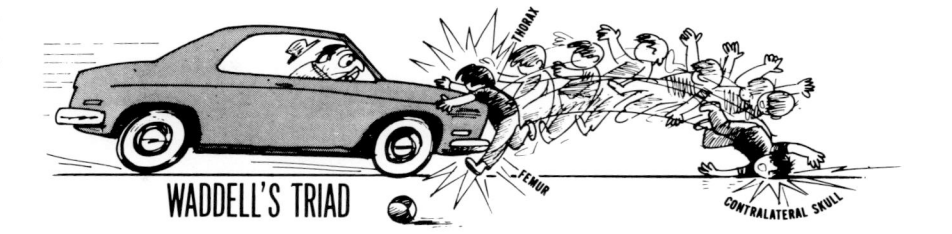

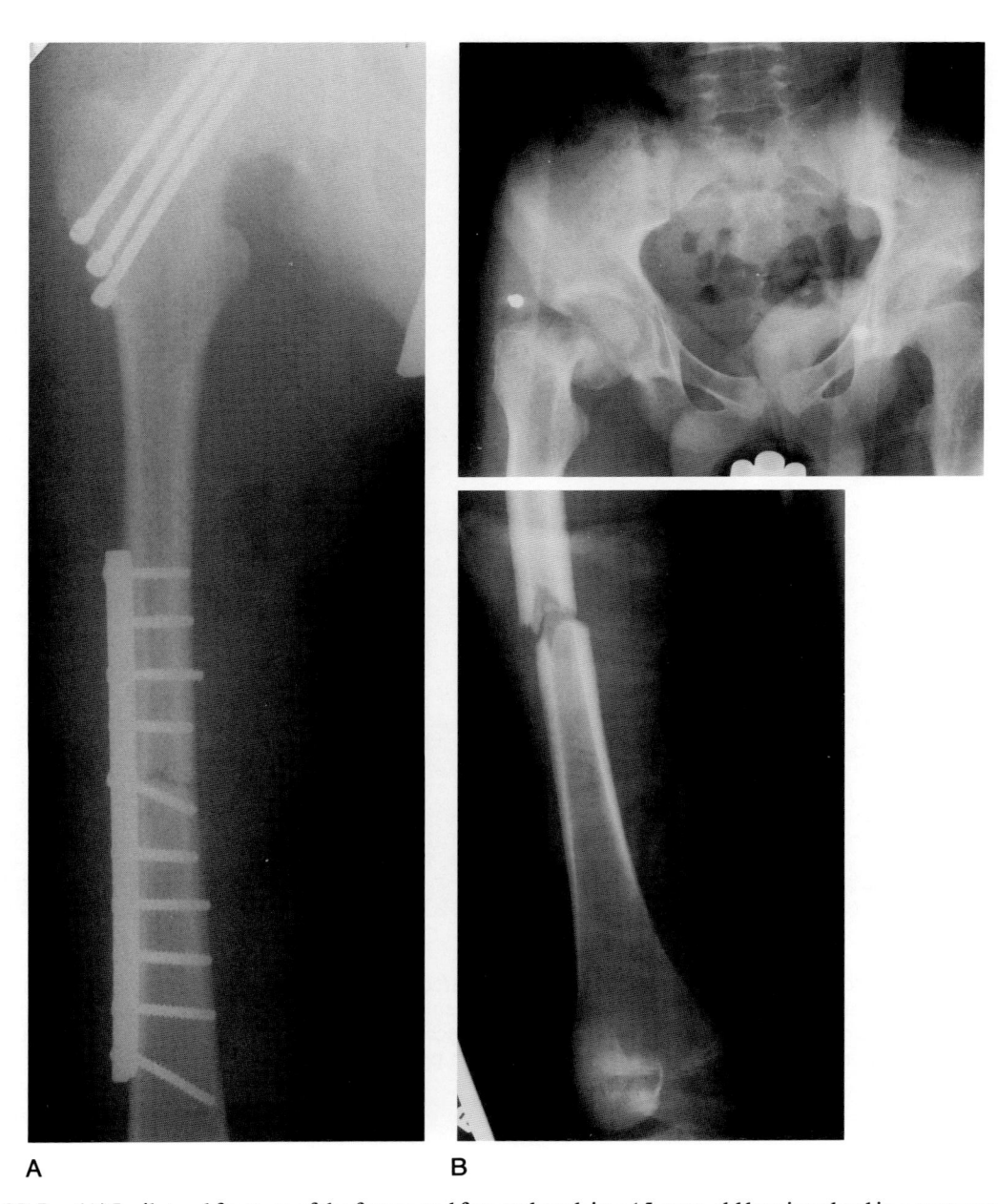

Fig. 35-5. (A) Ipsilateral fracture of the femur and femoral neck in a 15-year-old boy involved in a motor vehicle accident. (B) Treated by cannulated screws and a femoral plate. (Courtesy of Dr. Jay Jarvis, Children's Hospital of Eastern, Ontario, Ottawa, Canada.)

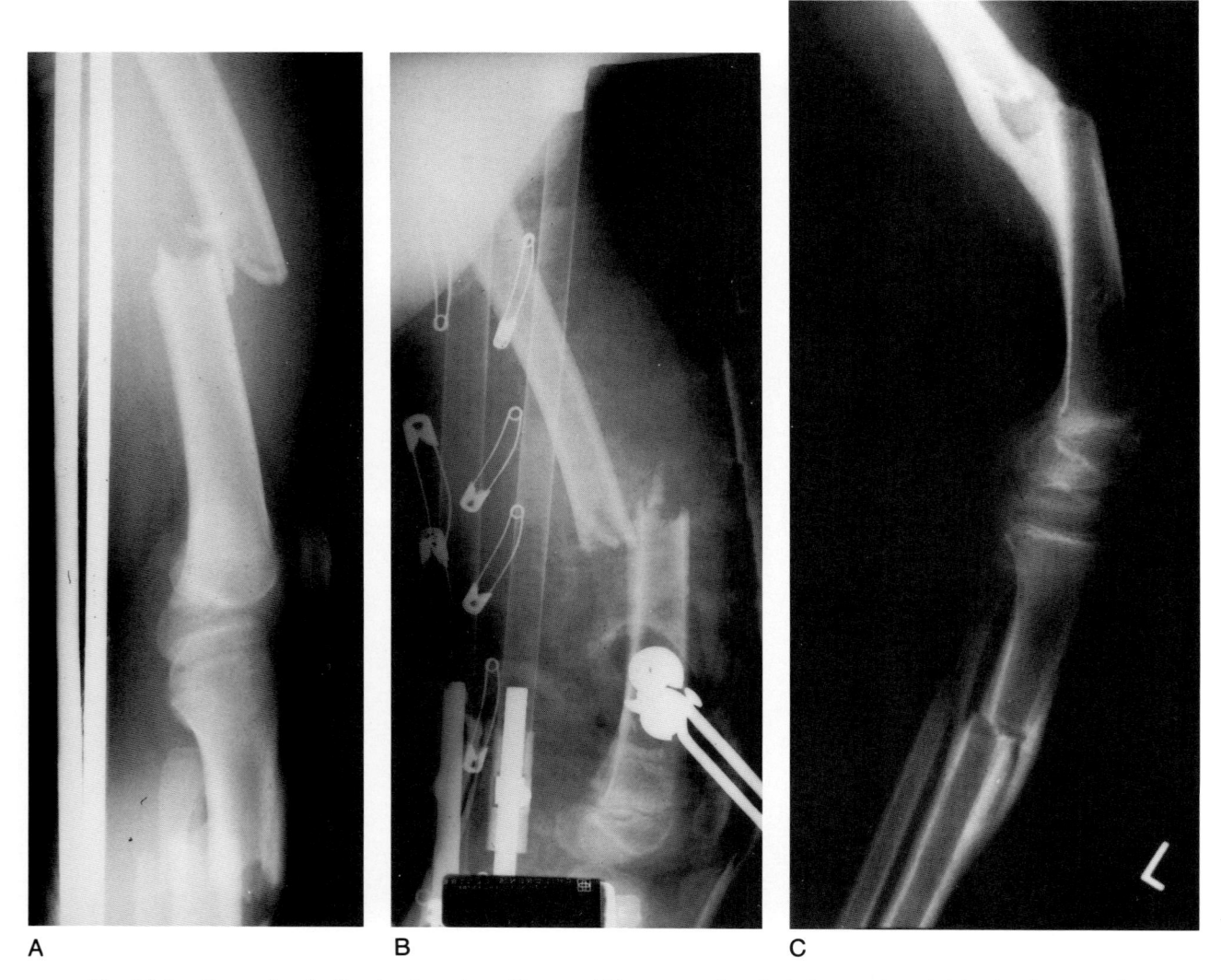

Fig. 35-6. Example of a floating knee in a 12-year-old boy treated entirely by traction. **(A)** Reduction unsatisfactorily with skin traction. **(B)** Traction with a femoral pin, resulting in angulation of the distal femoral fragment. **(C)** The tibia treated by manipulation and casting has an acceptable result, but the femur has healed or an acceptable marked anterior bowing. (From Letts et al.,[7] with permission.)

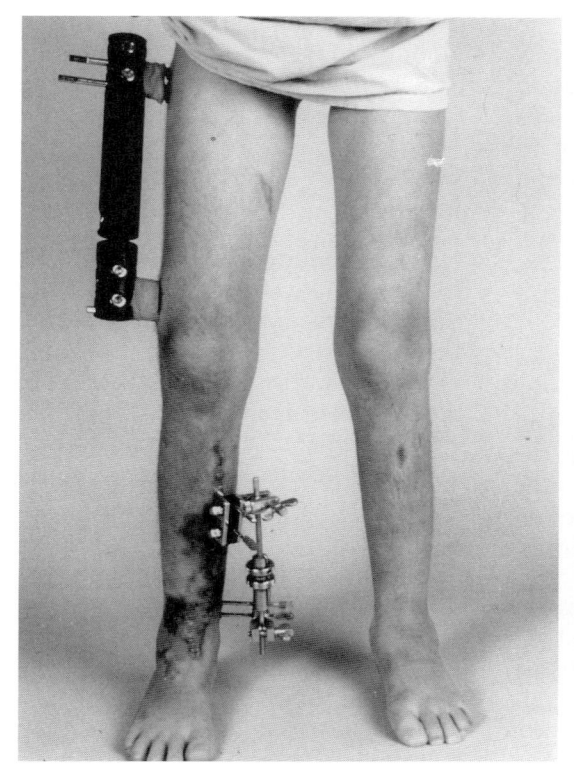

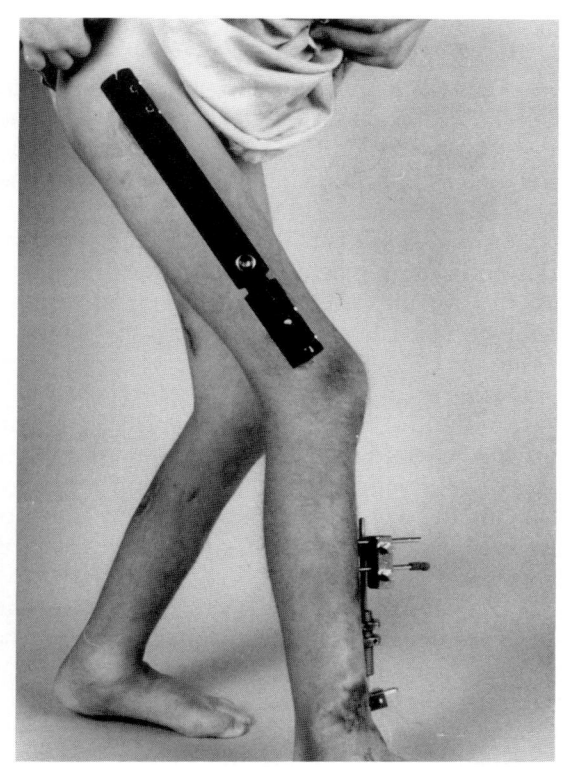

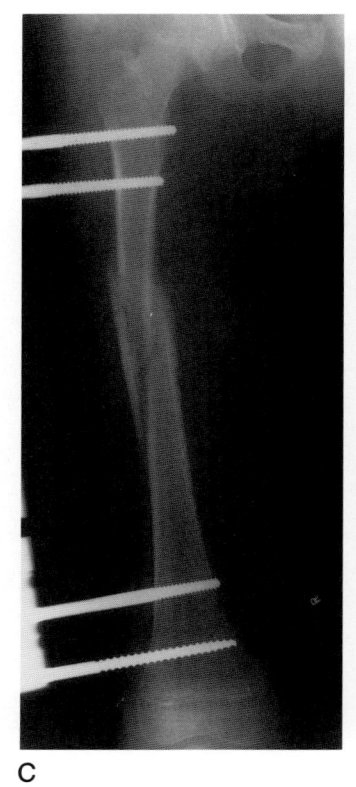

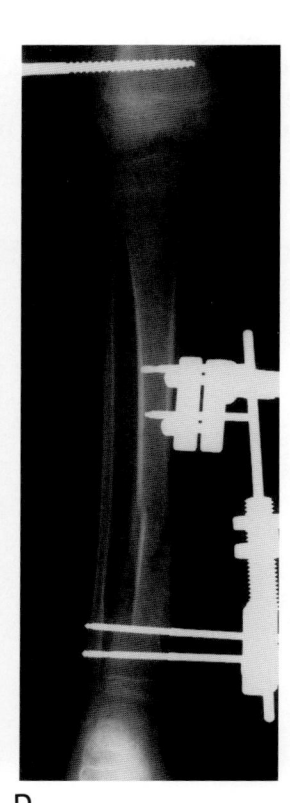

Fig. 35-7. **(A&B)** Floating knee in a 14-year-old boy struck by a car in whom both fractures of the tibia and femur were treated with external fixation. (Courtesy of Dr. Tim Carey, Children's Hospital of Eastern Ontario, Ottawa, Canada.) **(C&D)** Radiographs of child treated with external fixator of both the tibia and femur, using an Orthofix for the femur and a Hoffman external fixator for the tibia.

intramedullary nailing of the femur and plating of the tibia transforms an extremely unstable situation into a very manageable limb. An alternative is the application of an external fixator to either the femur or the tibia. This should be the method of choice in the presence of an open fracture to allow monitoring of the wound and surrounding skin.

In the type B injury with a high metaphyseal fracture, the diaphyseal fragment should be stabilized either internally or with an external fixator; the metaphyseal fragments being managed by casting or traction.

The type C injury in which there is both a physeal and diaphyseal lesion, the physeal fracture must be accurately reduced and pinned. The diaphyseal fracture can be treated by open reduction, external fixation, or, in the case of the tibia, casting, depending on the age of the child and the type of fracture. Traction is not an option in this type of floating knee, since it may place undue stress on the injured physis.

The type D and E floating knees with open injuries can be effectively stabilized with external fixators, so that full attention can be given to dealing with the soft tissue trauma. The presence of other injuries may well influence the type of treatment options for the floating knee.

A child with severe head trauma and irritability will be better managed with both fractures internally or externally fixed. Fractures in teenagers near skeletal maturity where reduction and maintenance of traction may be extremely difficult, especially in association with other injuries, fixation of both fractures will be advantageous.

If the ipsilateral knee has also been disrupted early knee motion will then be facilitated after the ligamentous repair. In this instance fixation of the femoral and tibial fracture fragments is recommended.

Closed Management

Young children under the age of 7 years can usually be managed quite effectively with 90/90 femoral pin traction. The fractured tibia can be reduced and held in a below-knee cast, which can rest comfortably in a sling. Usually 4 weeks of traction is sufficient to allow the application of a hip spica cast, and the results of this type of management for the floating knee in young children is usually quite successful (Fig. 35-8).

COMPLICATIONS

Malunion

Malunion has been the major complication of this fracture pattern in older children in whom the fractures were both treated by closed methods (Fig. 35-6). Usually one fracture was successfully treated but at the expense of angulation and malunion in the other. With most of these children with floating knees now being treated by internal or external fixation this complication is becoming less frequent.

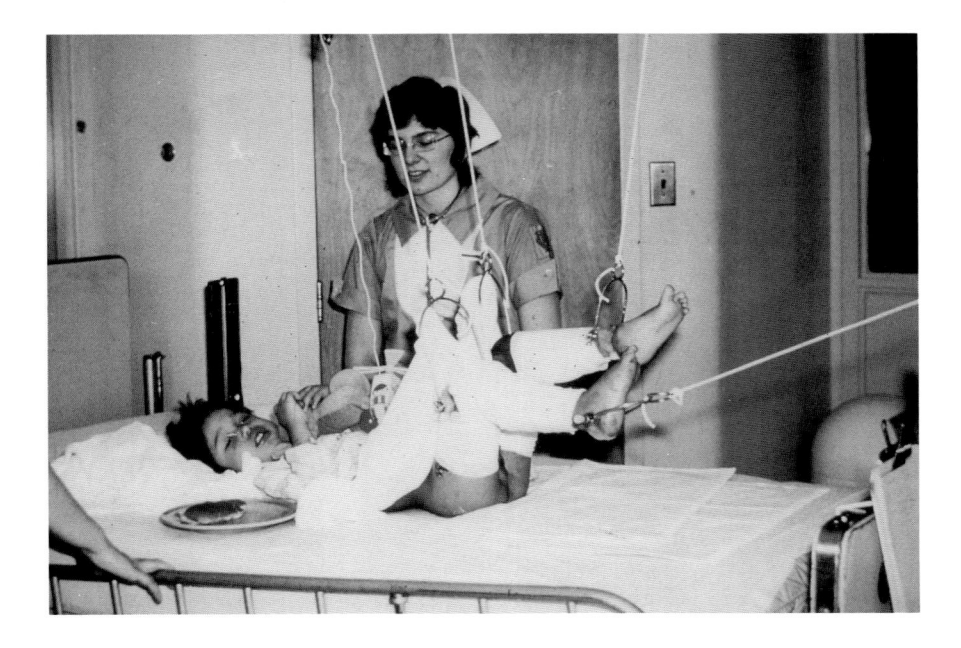

Fig. 35-8. Management of the floating knee by traction techniques in children under 7 years can be successful with careful monitoring of the fractures and traction set up as shown in this 4-year-old boy with bilateral floating knees following a jump out of a second-story window to escape a fire. (From Letts RM: J Ped Orthop 6:193, 1986, with permission.)

Compartment Syndrome

Because of the combination of fracturing plus limb crushing, compartment syndrome must be carefully searched for over the initial 48 to 72 hours. In Bohn and Durbin's series,[8] compartment syndrome was felt to be the most common cause of peroneal nerve dysfunction with three patients developing increased compartmental pressures. This complication lends further support for open reduction and fixation of the tibial fracture, since compartmental decompression can be performed at the same time (see Ch. 64).

Ligamentous Injury to the Ipsilateral Knee

Ligamentous injury to the ipsilateral knee is frequently missed. It is difficult to examine the knee adequately, especially if the fractures above and below have not been stabilized. The incidence of associated ligamentous injury to the knee in most series is 20 percent. The incidence is the same in children as in adults.[7,8,10,12] Examination of the knee for associated ligamentous disruption is mandatory in all children with ipsilateral fractures of the tibia and femur.

Physeal Growth Arrest

Complete or partial growth arrest occurs in 40 to 50 percent of children sustaining displacement of the distal femoral growth plate or proximal tibial growth plate. Obviously the younger the child at the time of this injury the more serious is the physeal arrest, and the more interference with limb growth that will be encountered. This may necessitate other procedures being recommended to ensure equal limb lengths, including contralateral epiphyseodesis, osteotomies to correct varus or valgus deformity and limb lengthening or shortening (see Ch. 62).

Femoral and Tibial Overgrowth

If both the femur and tibia are fixed out to length, some overgrowth of the limb may be encountered between the ages of 6 to 12.[17] The overgrowth is seldom more than 2 cm and usually is not associated with any major limb length discrepancy. If such should occur, an epiphyseodesis of the affected limb could be offered the parents at an appropriate time in accordance with the Mosely or Green Anderson growth charts. Occasionally these fractures may be associated with premature physeal closure even in the absence of obvious physeal injury[18] (see Ch. 61).

SUMMARY

Floating knee in children is a serious injury, often associated with other serious injuries, particularly the head, ipsilateral knee, abdomen, and soft tissue trauma to the limb. In children over 7 years of age it is recommended that at least one fracture, usually the tibia be stabilized with internal fixation or an external fixator with the femoral fracture treated in 90/90 traction. In teenagers, consideration should be given to stabilizing both the femoral and tibial fractures with either internal fixation or an external fixator. Fracture fixation is also indicated in severe head injured children and those in whom ligamentous injury to the knee has occurred. All physeal injuries require accurate open reduction and internal fixation with smooth K-wires. This fracture pattern has had a very high incidence of complications, primarily malunion when treated by traction techniques alone.

REFERENCES

1. Winquest RA: Segmental fractures of the lower extremity and the floating knee. p. 218. In Myers MH (ed): The Multiple Injured Patient with Complex Fractures. Lea & Febiger, Philadelphia, 1984
2. Veith RG, Winquest RA, Hansen ST, Jr: Ipsilateral fractures of the femur and tibia: a report of 57 consecutive cases. J Bone Joint Surg [Am] 66:991, 1984
3. Winston ME: The results of conservative treatment of fracture of the femur and tibia in the same limb. Surg Gynecol Obstet 134:985, 1972
4. Fraser RD, Hunter GA, Waddell JP: Ipsilateral fracture of the femur and tibia. J Bone Joint Surg [Br] 60:510, 1978
5. McAndrew MP, Pontarelli W: The long-term follow-up of ipsilateral tibial and femoral diaphyseal fractures. Clin Orthop 232:190, 1988
6. Omer GE, Moll J, Hand Bacon WL: Combined fractures of the femur and tibia in a single extremity. J Trauma 6:1026, 1966
7. Letts M, Vincent N, Gouw G: The floating knee in children. J Bone Joint Surg [Br] 68:442, 1986
8. Bohn WW, Durbin RA: Epiphyseal lateral fractures of the tibia in children and adolescents. J Bone Joint Surg [Am] 73:429, 1991
9. Rang M: Children's Fractures. 2nd Ed. JP Lippincott, Philadelphia, 1983

10. Paul GR, Sawka MW, Whitlaw GP: Fractures of the ipsilateral femur and tibia: emphasis on intra-articular and soft tissue injury. J Orthop Trauma 4:309, 1990
11. Shelton ML, Heer CS II, Granthan SA: Occult knee ligament ruptures associated with fractures. J Trauma 11:853, 1971
12. Szalay MJ, Hosking OR, Annear P: Injury of knee ligament associated with ipsilateral femoral shaft fractures and with ipsilateral femoral and tibial shaft fracture. Injury 21:398, 1990
13. Van Raay JJAM, Raaymakers ELFB, Dupree HW: Knee ligament injuries combined with ipsilateral tibial and femoral diaphyseal fractures: the "floating knee." Arch Orthop Trauma 110:75, 1991
14. Ogden JA: Skeletal Injury in the Child. p. 578. Lea & Febiger, Philadelphia, 1982
15. Kasser JR: Femur fractures in children. Instr Course Lect 41:403, 1992
16. Rooser E, Hanson P: External fixation of ipsilateral fractures of the femur and tibia. Injury 16:371, 1985
17. Staheli LT: Femoral and tibial growth following femoral shaft fracture in childhood. Clin Orthop 55:159, 1967
18. Beals RK: Premature closure of the physis following diaphyseal fractures. J Pediatr Orthop 10:717, 1990

36

Fractures and Dislocations of the Patella

Walter B. Greene

> Tell me and I will forget.
> Show me and I will remember.
> Involve me and I will understand.

DESCRIPTION AND INCIDENCE

The patella is the largest and most injured sesamoid bone. Fractures of the patella occur in all ages but are uncommon in children. In large reviews, children comprise only 1 to 3 percent of all patella fractures.[1,2] Relative to other pediatric knee injuries, fractures of the patella are also uncommon. In a review of 48 children with fractures about the knee joint, Benz and colleagues[3] observed only four avulsion fractures of the patella.

The reasons for the decreased incidence of patella fractures in children is partly sociological and partly physiologic. The most common cause for patella fractures in young adults is motor vehicle accidents, and in older adults, falling.[2] Young adults are more likely to be involved in a motorcycle or high-speed car accident, which causes the patella to be slammed against the ground or an unyielding dashboard.[4] Children are less likely to be involved in traffic accidents and are less likely to be front-seat passengers whose patella is propelled into an unyielding dashboard. Older adults frequently sustain patella fractures after falls on a bone weakened by osteoporosis. Children fall frequently, but, compared to older adults, their bone demonstrates greater force absorption before breaking.[5]

ANATOMY

Greater plasticity of pediatric bone,[5-7] coupled with a relatively large mass of surrounding cartilage, is another major factor for the low incidence of pediatric patella fractures. Ossification of the patella does not commence until 20 to 40 months of age in girls and 32 to 76 months in boys.[8] Initially, ossification is a multifocal process, but these foci rapidly coalesce into a single center.[9] Ossification of the patella proceeds in a centrifugal fashion, but even at 9 to 10 years of age approximately one-third of the patella remains unossified, that is, cartilaginous.

Greater elasticity of surrounding soft tissues is also a factor reducing injury to the patella in children. In Blount's classic textbook,[6] the only child with a displaced transverse fracture of the patella was a 6-year-old boy who had previously sustained an extensive laceration of the quadriceps mechanism that caused limited knee flexion. The stiffness in his quadriceps muscle concentrated forces at the patella so that a transverse fracture occurred when the knee was suddenly and forcefully flexed.

MECHANISMS OF INJURY

Fractures of the patella may be uncommon in children, but certain patterns of injury do occur in this age group that are strikingly different from those seen in adults. Indeed, "sleeve" fractures of the patella are unique even among pediatric fractures.

The patella is also subject to repetitive stresses of weight-bearing forces, rapid knee movements, and quadriceps contractions. The bone-cartilage and cartilage-tendon junction is susceptible to failure, particularly during the preadolescent and adolescent years when the child combines increased activity, rapid growth, and enough size and coordination to contract the quadriceps muscle with considerable force. The result from acute trauma is either a sleeve or avulsion fracture, whereas chronic repetitive stress injuries cause a traction tendonitis. Although other terms, such as juvenile osteochondritis and traction epiphysitis, have been used to describe chronic stress injuries of the patella in children, I prefer traction tendonitis. Repeated minor or microscopic tears of the tendon at its insertion and the resultant inflammation with possible heterotopic ossification seem to provide the best explanation for these chronic injuries.

Traumatic lateral dislocation of the patella is considerably more common in children than fractures. This is an injury of adolescents and young adults with the reported mean age of the initial dislocation ranging from 14 to 21 years of age.[10-14] Indeed, it is very unusual, although not impossible, for a child younger than 8 or an adult older than 40 to sustain a traumatic dislocation of the patella.

Patterns of patella fractures and dislocations occurring in children are listed in Table 36-1. These injuries will be the focus of this chapter. Other disorders, such as congenital dislocation of the patella or lateral marginal fractures, will be briefly described to clarify and differentiate them from acute traumatic injuries of childhood.

FRACTURES OF THE BODY OF THE PATELLA

Transverse Fractures

Transverse fractures of the patella are typically located in the midportion of the bone. Direct trauma is the usual mechanism of injury in children.[15] An indirect force such as a sudden contraction of the quadriceps muscle with the knee flexed can cause this fracture when the quadriceps muscle has less elasticity.[6]

Pain is noted after the fall, but the degree of pain, swelling, and tenderness may be considerably less than that seen in adults. Belman and Neviaser[15] reported an 11-year-old boy who did not present until 2 days after injury despite having a palpable defect in the patella and apparent separation of the fracture fragments (Fig. 36-1). The reason for the relative paucity of symptoms was discovered at surgery. Even though the bony portion of the patella was completely disrupted and the quadriceps retinaculum was torn, this child's thick and relatively elastic posterior cartilage remained intact. The intact posterior hinge explained the greater anterior displacement of the fracture (Fig. 36-1) and also explained why this child had less separation of his fracture fragments than an adult with a transverse patella fracture and disrupted quadriceps retinaculum.

Diagnosis

Diagnosing a transverse patella fracture is relatively easy. The exception would be the child whose patella has not begun to ossify. This unusual situation was described

TABLE 36-1. Injury Patterns of the Patella in Children

Fractures of the body of the patella
  Transverse
  Comminuted

Inferior pole fractures
  Displaced sleeve fractures
  Minimally displaced avulsion fractures
  Traction tendonitis
    (Sinding-Larsen-Johansson disease)

Superior pole fractures
  Displaced sleeve fractures
  Minimally displaced avulsion fractures
  Traction tendonitis

Traumatic separation bipartite patella

Medial margin fractures
  Medial margin avulsion injuries
  Osteochondral fractures

Lateral margin fractures

Dislocation
  Congenital
  Habitual
  Lateral
  Central

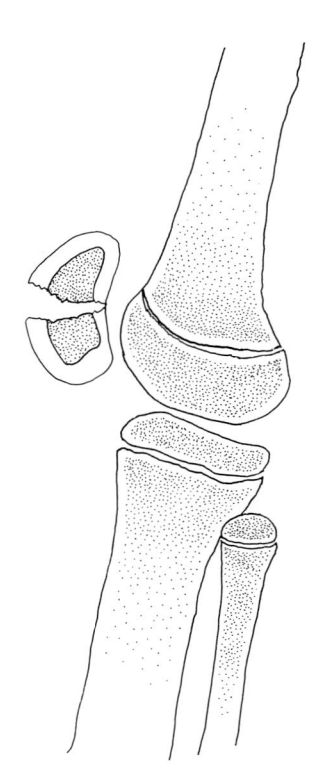

Fig. 36-1. Schematic drawing of a lateral view apparently showing a complete and displaced transverse fracture of the patella. (Adapted from Vainionpää et al.,[14] with permission.)

in a 1918 report[16] of a 2-year-old child whose physical examination suggested a significant knee injury but whose radiographs were nondiagnostic. Exploratory surgery was necessary to diagnose a completely displaced patella fracture. Ultrasonography could now confirm this injury in a child whose patella had not commenced ossification.

Treatment

Due to the rarity of transverse patella fractures in children, guidelines for closed versus open treatment are based on experience in adults with similar injuries. In a remarkable series of 40 patients followed for an average of 30 years, Edwards and coworkers[17] found that patella fractures that healed with more than 2 mm diastasis or greater than 1 mm articular surface incongruity had a significantly greater incidence of pain, reduced quadriceps strength, and narrowing of the patellofemoral joint. Restoring anatomic congruity of the articular surface is important in children if disabling osteoarthritis is to be avoided in later years when their employment and/or avocation demand an effective and efficient patellofemoral joint.

Closed Reduction

Closed treatment is indicated for transverse patella fractures that have 1 mm or less stepoff at the joint surface or 2 mm or less diastasis of the articular surface. The hemarthrosis should be aspirated to make the child more comfortable and to minimize the inflammatory effect of blood breakdown products on the synovium. Immobilization of the knee in full extension for 4 to 6 weeks is usually satisfactory. A loss or reduction is unlikely but possible. Repeat anteroposterior (AP) and lateral radiographic views of the knee, made 7 to 10 days after injury, should rule out that possibility.

Transverse fractures of the patella with disruption of the quadriceps retinaculum are characteristically displaced more than 1 cm. For fractures that have borderline or slight displacement, repeat radiographs should be done after the joint is aspirated and the knee immobilized in extension. That procedure will minimize tension in the quadriceps and may provide acceptable alignment of the fracture.

Open Reduction and Internal Fixation

Techniques of internally fixing transverse patella fractures in children range from interrupted catgut sutures to tension band wiring with supplemental Kirschner-wire fixation. I prefer fixation of displaced patella fractures in children by the intraosseous tension band loop technique described by Lotke and Ecker.[18] Cerclage wiring of the patella is *not* recommended, since the strength of fixation is inferior to other techniques[19] and a circumferential wire around the patella may compromise blood supply to the bone.[20] Compared to the intraosseous tension band loop, the AO technique of tension band wiring with Kirschner-wire fixation has only slightly greater strength of fixation for patella fractures.[19] This minimal increase in fixation strength is *not* necessary in children. Kirschner wires also have a tendency to migrate in this technique of patella fracture fixation.

Open reduction of patella fractures may be performed through either a longitudinal or transverse incision. Location of abrasions may dictate the choice of incision, but, if possible, I prefer a transverse incision in children. This incision is more cosmetic and, in most cases, may be closed with a running subcuticular suture. The knee joint is thoroughly irrigated to remove blood and small osteochondral fragments. The joint is then inspected for damage to the articular surface, the status of the knee ligaments and menisci, and for any remaining loose osteochondral fragments. Polyglactin sutures are placed in the torn retinaculum but are not tied until the intraosseous wire has been secured. This sequence allows accurate placement of the retinacular sutures without compromising insertion of the intraosseous wires and permits inspection of the articular surface of the patella after tightening the wires.

Insertion of the intraosseous wire loop (Fig. 36-2) is started by drilling two small Kirschner wires retrograde into the proximal fragment. Holding the patella fracture reduced, the pins are then drilled through the distal patella fragment, exiting on either side of the patella tendon. The two ends of a No. 22 stainless-steel wire are inserted into the drill holes of the distal patella fragment as the pins are backed out. The fracture fragments are displaced and the ends of the wire are then passed through the drill holes in the proximal fragment. A midportion loop of wire is brought to the anterior surface of the patella. One end of the wire is passed through this loop, and the two ends of the wire are then twisted or tied together. Before tying the sutures in the quadriceps retinaculum, the articular surface of the patella is inspected and palpated to ensure that anatomic congruity has been restored.

The intraosseous loop technique allows secure fixation without disruption of blood supply or bone growth, permits early weightbearing in a cylinder cast, and allows early institution of knee motion at 2 to 3 weeks after operation. As the knee is flexed, the wire is tightened and the fracture surfaces are compressed. Although unlikely, if the posterior fracture surface gaps open with flexion, then the surgeon can change to tension band and Kirschner-wire fixation.

Comminuted Fractures

Comminuted fractures of the patella result from a direct blow. Given the strength and plasticity of the patella in children, this injury requires a significant impact. Comminuted patella fractures in children, therefore, are very uncommon and are usually open injuries. Spills from motorbikes and all-terrain vehicles are common causes of this fracture.

No series or even case reports of comminuted patella fractures in children have, to my knowledge, been reported. In a symposium on pediatric fractures, Crawford[21] recommended patellectomy for fractures containing more than three fragments. Based on present knowledge of patella biomechanics, immediate patellectomy in a child would, in my opinion, be indicated only for a fracture that cannot be reassembled. If symptomatic patellofemoral osteoarthritis develops, patellectomy can always be done at a later date.

A 45 degree "trauma" oblique view radiograph[22] may help delineate the fracture pattern and aid in preoperative planning (Fig. 36-3). Operative treatment starts with meticulous debridement of the open injury. Intraosseous wiring, as previously described, may adequately secure a three-part comminuted fracture. As previously noted, cerclage wiring of the patella is avoided if possible. Sometimes this technique and/or supplemental Kirschner wires must be combined with intraosseous tension band wiring to provide adequate fixation of a multiple fragment fracture. Since the patella receives its blood supply from the two superior and two inferior geniculate arteries,[23] avascular necrosis does not necessarily develop. Meticulous and gentle technique will minimize the risk of surgical trauma to the blood supply.

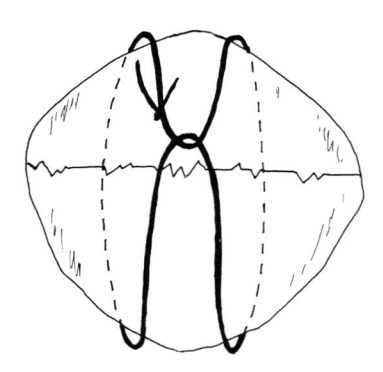

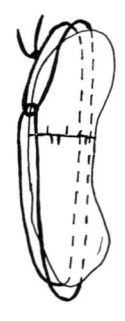

Fig. 36-2. Intraosseous wire loop technique. (Adapted from Lotke and Ecker,[18] with permission.)

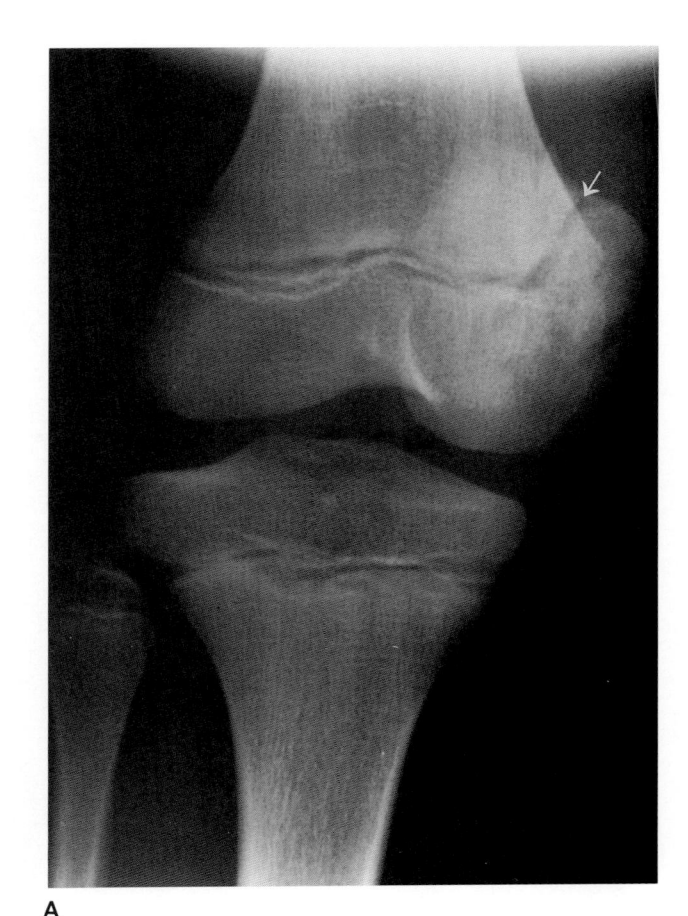

Fig. 36-3. (A) 30-degree oblique and (B) lateral views of the knee in a 12-year-old boy who sustained a comminuted patella fracture and other injuries after a high-speed fall from a dirt bike. The fracture was treated by irrigation and debridement. Alignment was considered acceptable. *(Figure continues.)*

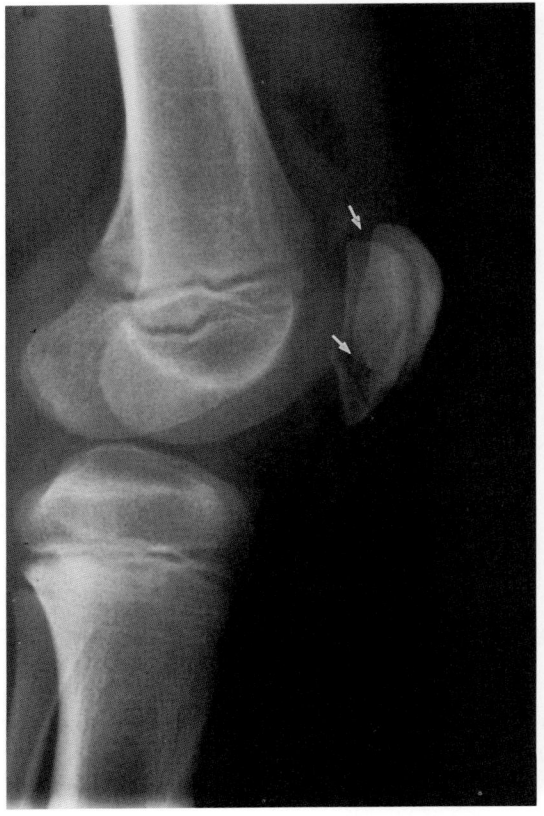

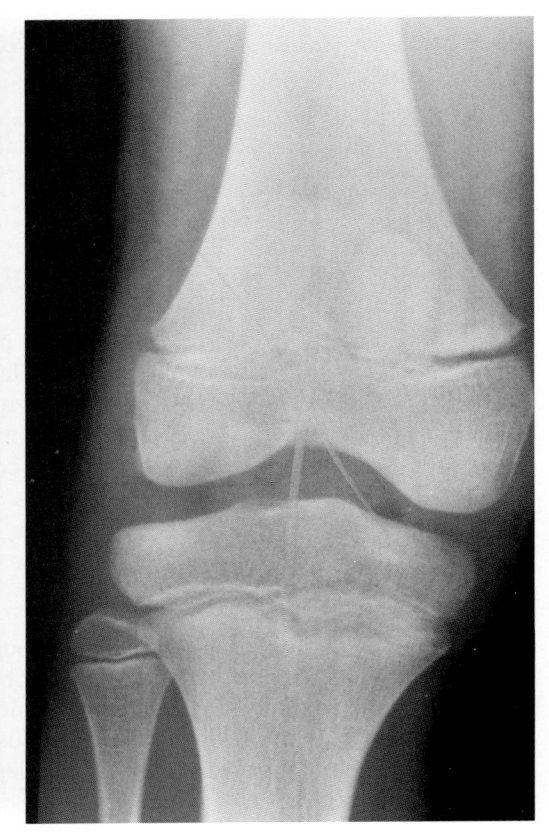

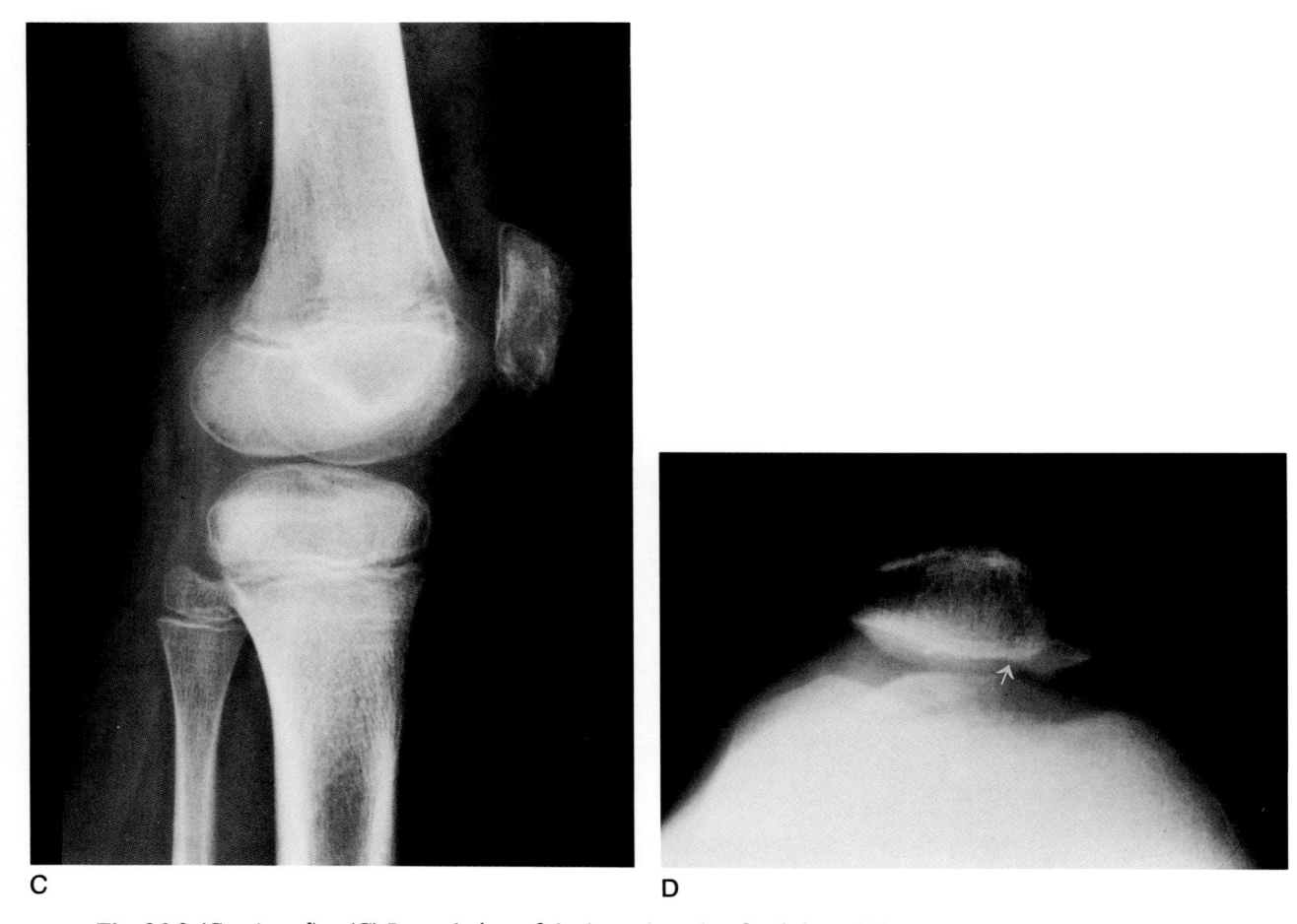

Fig. 36-3 *(Continued).* **(C)** Lateral view of the knee 4 weeks after injury. **(D)** Tangential view of the patella 3 years after injury. Articular surface demonstrates 3-mm step-off. Patient is likely to develop patellofemoral osteoarthritis.

INFERIOR POLE FRACTURES

Injuries to either the superior or inferior pole of the patella range from traction tendonitis to displaced sleeve fractures. Inferior pole injuries are more frequent, perhaps due to the smaller width of the inferior pole and the resultant concentration of quadriceps contraction forces.

Sleeve Fractures

The term *sleeve fracture* was coined by Houghton and Ackroyd[24] to describe the large covering, or sleeve, of cartilage that is pulled off the main body of the bony patella (Fig. 36-4). A small bony fragment usually, but not always, accompanies the sleeve of cartilage.

Sleeve fractures at the inferior pole of the patella typically occur in the preadolescent years, a time when the patella still has a large unossified portion. The cartilage-bone interface is a weak link, much like the physis in long bones at this age. The preadolescent has also developed enough muscular coordination and body weight to provide forceful contraction of the quadriceps. Children with this injury are typically jumping or pushing off the injured leg.[24,25] The sleeve fracture results from an indirect force when sudden flexion of the knee is opposed by a forceful quadriceps contraction. The broad expanse of the quadriceps tendon diffuses the force at the proximal pole and therefore, the inferior pole of the patella sustains the injury.

A displaced sleeve fracture effectively disrupts the quadriceps mechanism. The sudden and severe pain associated with this injury results in prompt referral for

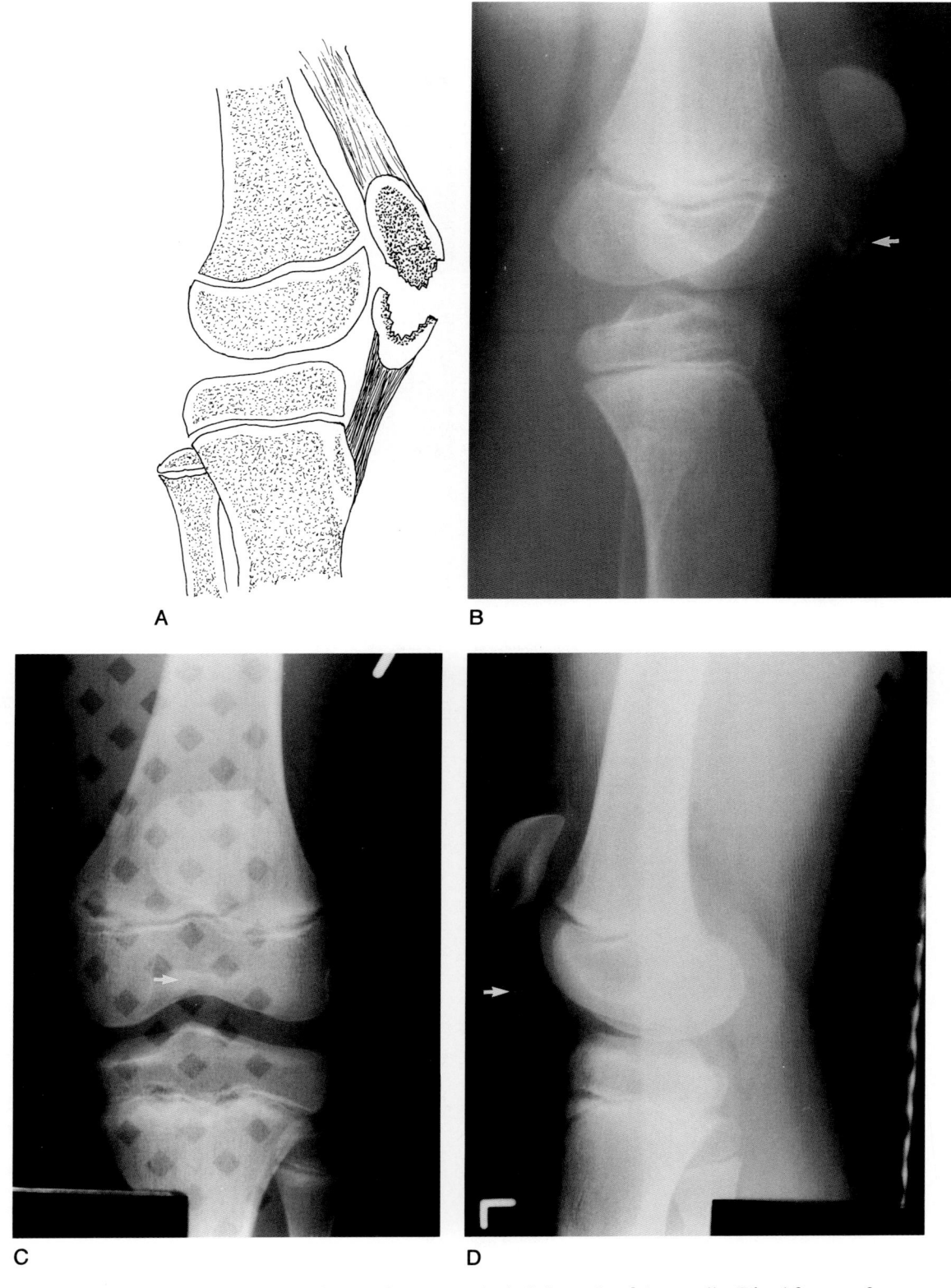

Fig. 36-4. **(A)** Schematic diagram of sleeve fracture at the inferior pole of the patella. Distal fracture fragment has large component of cartilage. **(B)** Radiograph of a sleeve avulsion in a 12-year-old soccer player who tripped and fell over another player. **(C&D)** AP and lateral radiograph at knee showing inferior avulsion at patellar tendon attachment in a 12-year-old girl sustained while high jumping. At operation this was found to be a sleeve fracture, and it was repaired with 0 chromic suture followed by immobilization of the knee in a cylinder case for 6 weeks. (Fig. A from Bishay,[32] with permission. Fig. B courtesy of Dr. Carl L. Stanitski, Detroit, MI. Fig. D courtesy of Dr. R. Mervyn Letts, Ottawa, Canada.)

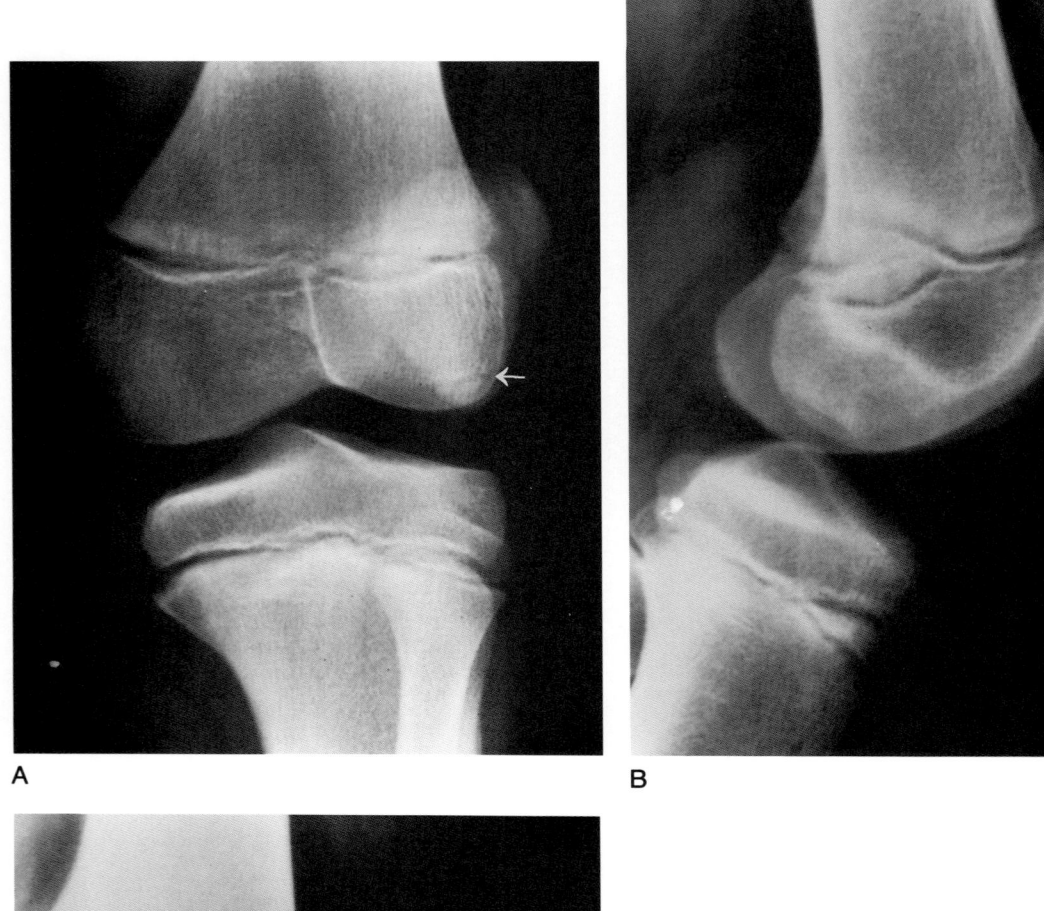

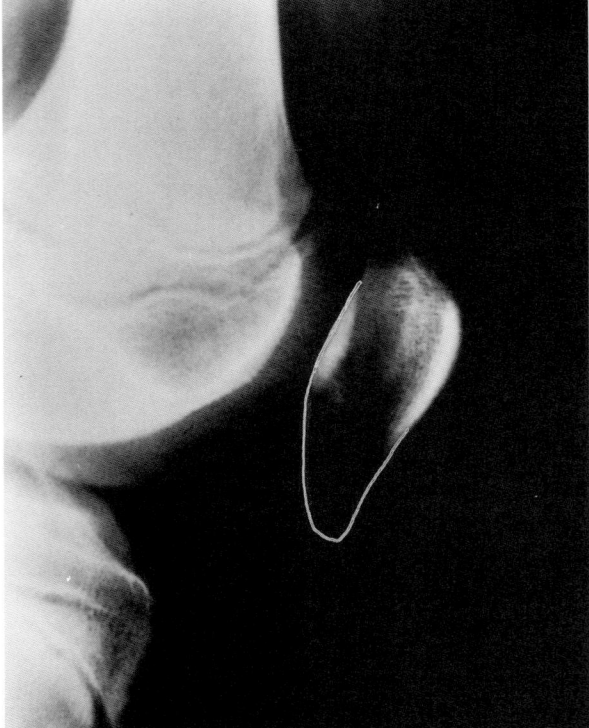

Fig. 36-5. (A) 30-degree oblique and (B) lateral views of the knee in a 10-year-old boy who fell while playing softball. Arthrocentesis of the knee obtained 60 cc of bloody fluid. Radiographs showed a minimally displaced avulsion fracture of the inferior pole. The patella is in a normal position, i.e., not high riding. This provides evidence that the quadriceps mechanism is intact. (C) Lateral view of the knee 2 years after injury. Mild overgrowth of the inferior pole of the patella has occurred, but this does not involve the articular surface and should not affect patellofemoral joint mechanics.

medical evaluation. Despite marked swelling of the knee, a gap may be palpated at the disrupted end of the patella. Radiographs reveal a high-riding patella with a small avulsed bony fragment remaining with the patella tendon. In a variant of the typical sleeve fracture, Peterson and Stener[26] described displaced medial and lateral avulsion fractures of the patella and disinsertion of the patella tendon at the tibial tuberosity.

With less severe injuries, the avulsed fragment is only displaced a few millimeters. Enough of the quadriceps mechanism remains in continuity that knee extension is maintained.[27] The initial injury is often dismissed as a trivial fall, but with persistent pain during running and jumping activities the child is brought for evaluation. Physical examination will reveal tenderness over the avulsed fragment. Full extension of the knee will be possible, but knee extension against resistance may reproduce the pain. Radiographs will demonstrate a small avulsion fragment at the inferior pole of the patella (Fig. 36-5).

Displaced sleeve fractures need operative intervention. If untreated, these injuries will cause a persistent deficit in knee extension and quadricep strength.[26] Even though the fracture defect will reossify without treatment, the result is an enlarged patella, persistent quadriceps insufficiency, persistent limitation of knee extension and unknown long-term consequences on the patellofemoral joint.[26,27]

Displaced sleeve fractures and the associated tears of the quadriceps retinaculum can be satisfactorily repaired in children with large-caliber polyglactin sutures. Suture fixation is supplemented with 6 weeks of cylinder cast immobilization. Moving the knee earlier is not necessary with this injury. The sleeve fracture has limited, if any, involvement of the articulating surface and children regain joint motion easier than adults.

Minimally Displaced Avulsion Fractures

If the avulsed pole of the inferior patella is separated by only a few millimeters, one must decide whether the injury is a stable or unstable fracture. Lateral radiographs of the knee taken in extension and flexion may be helpful.[27] Cast immobilization is all that is necessary for the child who demonstrates full, active extension of the knee and no widening of the fracture gap on radiographs taken with the knee in flexion. With an extension lag and radiographic evidence of increased fracture separation on stress radiographs (Fig. 36-6), operative repair should be considered, especially if the avulsed fragment remains separated from the patella with the knee held in extension.

Traction Tendonitis

Traction tendonitis at the inferior pole of the patella in growing children is called Sinding-Larsen-Johansson disease.[28] The typical child with Sinding-Larsen-Johansson disease is an athletic youngster of 10 to 12 years of age who presents with pain in the anterior aspect of the knee that is accentuated by sports activities and stair climbing.[27,28] Findings on physical examination are typically limited to tenderness at the inferior pole of the patella. Radiographs in the early stage of the disease will be normal, but subsequent views may demonstrate heterotopic ossification that eventually coalesces with the inferior pole of the patella.

Sinding-Larsen-Johansson disease will consistently resolve with time and symptomatic treatment.[27,28] Restriction of activities, with or without a short period of immobilization, is usually the only treatment that is necessary. I do not favor the routine use of nonsteroidal anti-inflammatory drugs (NSAIDs) for these patients, since their symptoms are usually not severe enough to warrant possible adverse reactions from the medication.

Differentiating a traction tendonitis from a minimally displaced avulsion fracture may be difficult. If a child presents with a definite history of a recent fall and radiographs demonstrate a well-demarcated linear bony fragment adjacent to the inferior pole of the patella, then that child should be classified as having an avulsion fracture. Likewise, if the patient presents with chronic pain at the inferior pole of the patella, no history of a traumatic injury, and radiographs that initially are normal but subsequently develop heterotopic ossification at the inferior pole of the patella, then that child's problem can be easily classified as Sinding-Larsen-Johansson disease. The history and radiographs, however, may not permit differentiation of these conditions. A chronic problem may have been preceded by a fall of questionable significance, and radiographs of an acute avulsion injury will not show any abnormality if only the cartilage portion of the patella is torn. The physical examination also overlaps, since both conditions are characterized by point tenderness at the inferior pole of the patella, minimal restriction of knee motion, and minimal swelling. Fortunately, the treatment for the two

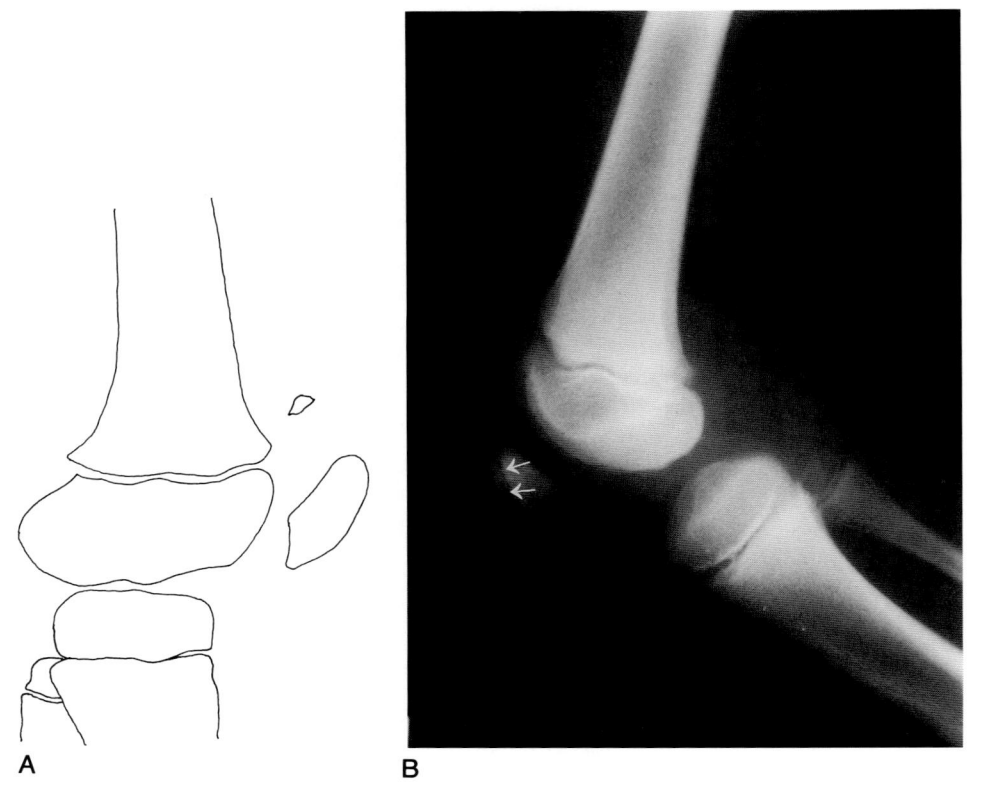

Fig. 36-6. (A) Schematic diagram of the lateral view of a radiograph of the knee in a 9-year-old girl who fell directly on her knee. Displaced sleeve fracture of the superior pole was indicated by high-riding small bony fragment. At operation, a large chondral fragment was repaired by figure-of-8 sutures. (B) Lateral radiograph of the knee showing sleeve fracture of the proximal patella with minimal displacement. (Fig. A from Bishay,[32] with permission. Fig. B courtesy of Dr. R. Mervyn Letts, Ottawa, Canada.)

conditions is similar, although short-term cast immobilization is more frequently utilized for an avulsion fracture.

Children with cerebral palsy may have symptomatic fragmentation of the inferior pole of the patella.[29,30] The typical patient tends to be an older adolescent with moderately severe diplegia who has patella alta and walks with the hips and knees flexed. Fragmentation of the patella probably develops from a crouched posture requiring constant quadriceps activity during standing and walking. The pain may be difficult or recalcitrant to treatment. Modalities, such as short-term immobilization, NSAIDs, patella tendon debridement and repair, and even lengthening of the hamstring tendons as suggested by Rosenthal and Levine[29] are not always successful.

SUPERIOR POLE FRACTURES

The spectrum of injuries at the superior pole of the patella in children is similar to those at the inferior pole. As previously noted, superior pole injuries are less frequent. Indeed, fragmention at the proximal pole of the patella may be a variation of normal development, as many of these children have been recorded as having no symptoms or signs.[31]

Sleeve fractures at the superior pole of the patella have a different mechanism of injury compared to their counterparts at the inferior pole of the patella. These injuries result from a direct blow to the upper pole of the patella[32] (Fig. 36-6). Continued force will cause a central dislocation of the patella.

Treatment for traction tendonitis, avulsion fractures,

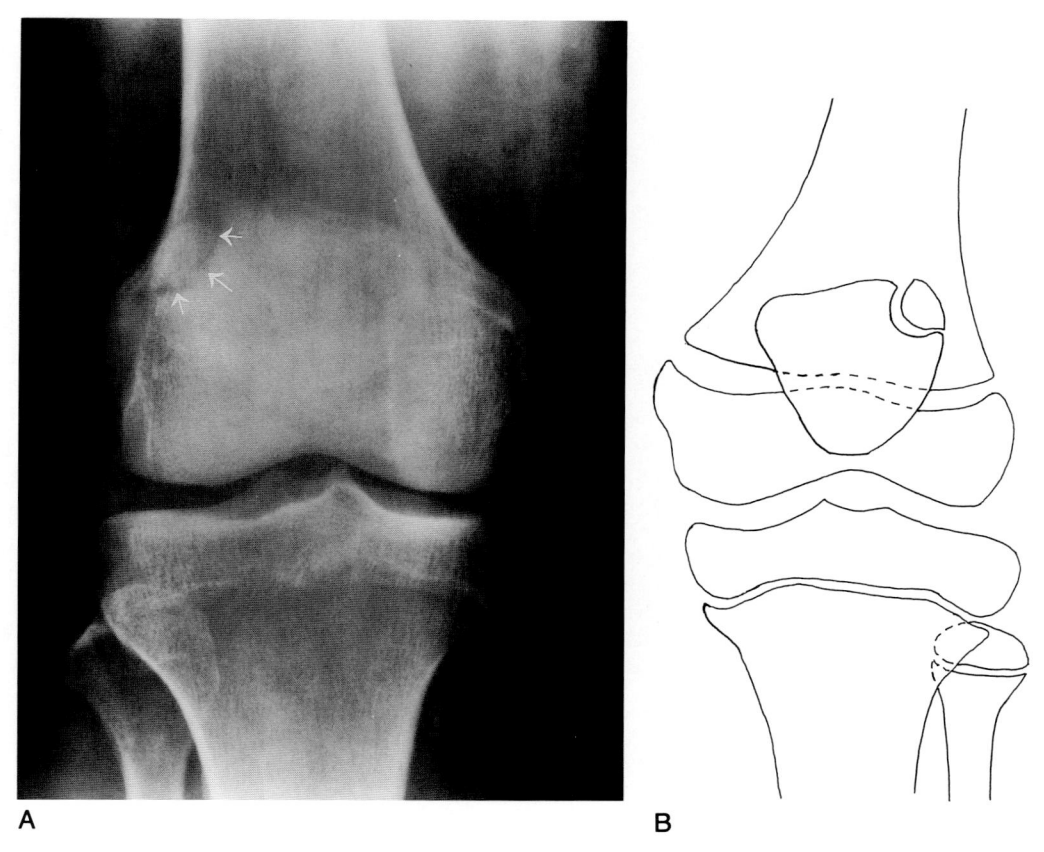

Fig. 36-7. (A) AP view and (B) schematic diagram of the knee demonstrate typical appearance of an asymptomatic bipartite patella in an adolescent boy.

and sleeve fractures at the superior pole of the patella are based on the same principles utilized in managing similar injuries at the inferior pole of the patella.

TRAUMATIC SEPARATION OF BIPARTITE PATELLA

The bipartite patella has an accessory ossification center in the superior, lateral portion of the patella that fails to fuse. This developmental anomaly persists into adult life and is usually an incidental radiographic finding of no clinical significance[9] (Fig. 36-7). The actual incidence of bipartite patella is variously reported but is probably around 1 percent.[33,34] The lesion usually appears during the adolescent years, is more frequent in males, and is unilateral in a slight majority of cases. The radiolucent zone connecting the two bony portions of the patella is comprised of fibrocartilaginous tissue.[9]

Although uncommon, adolescents may present with a painful bipartite patella that frequently commences after a traumatic episode. The teenager usually presents several days to several months after the onset of symptoms. The typical history is one of pain over the superiolateral portion of the patella that is aggravated by sports activities and stair climbing.[27,33-35]

Radiographs show a bipartite patella. If previous radiograph of the knee are available, then increased separation is seen at the superolateral corner of the patella (Fig. 36-8). The amount of separation, however, may not be increased and is usually only a few millimeters. Technetium bone scans show increased uptake in the superolateral corner of the patella with a symptomatic

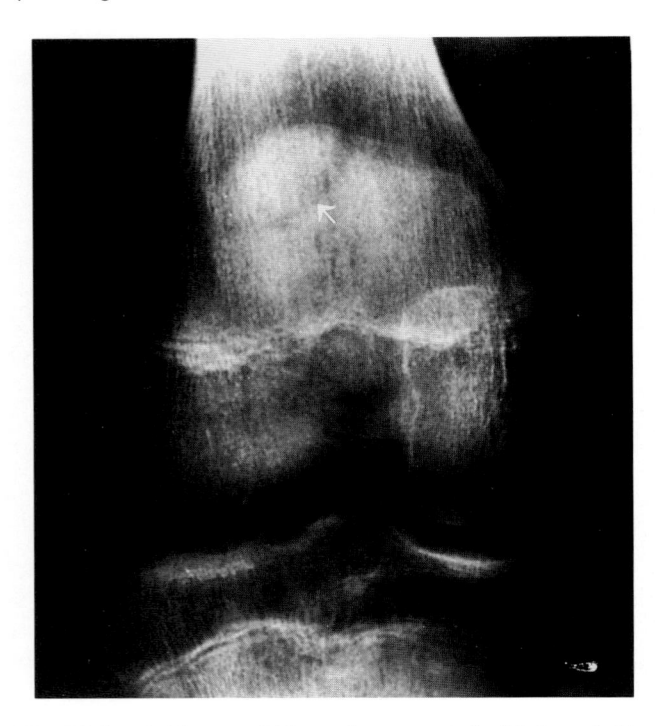

Fig. 36-8. A 15-year-old boy who presented with 1-week history of pain at the superolateral corner of the patella following a forceful flexion injury. Fibrocartilaginous interval of bipartite patella increased by 1 mm, compared to a radiograph made 1 year previously for unrelated problems. Four weeks of cylinder cast immobilization resolved the patient's symptoms.

bipartite patella.[34] This study, however, is not necessary, as the diagnosis can be made with a typical history, physical examination, and routine radiographs that demonstrate a bipartite patella but no other lesion.

Treatment options include restriction of activities, short-term immobilization of the knee in extension, or excision of the bipartite patella if recalcitrant to conservative management. In my experience, restriction of activities without prior cylinder cast immobilization has not been efficiently effective. Even with discontinuation of sports and running activities, normal daily activities have enough repetitive flexion of the knee to preclude effective healing. By comparison, 3 weeks of cast immobilization seems to enhance fibrous repair of the partially disrupted fibrocartilaginous tissue.

Even the adolescent who presents with chronic symptoms (≥ 1 month) should have a 3- to 4-week period of immobilization in a cylinder cast. Carter[36] reported successful resolution of symptoms with 4 weeks of cast immobilization in a 62-year-old man whose treatment began 9 weeks after a hyperflexion injury. Ogden and colleagues[34] also observed good results in a 12-year-old boy who had symptoms for 3 months and who was casted for 3 weeks.

Surgical excision of the superolateral portion of the patella is utilized for patients who do not respond to nonoperative therapy. The bipartite fragment is identified by probing with a Keith needle or by visualizing the white line of fibrocartilaginous tissue at the superolateral corner of the patella. The fragment is excised and the involved quadriceps tendon is reattached to the patella. The length of postoperative immobilization varies depending on the size of the excised fragment but typically ranges from 1 to 4 weeks.[34,35]

Results following surgical excision are usually good. In the largest reported series, Bourne and Bianco[35] noted that 13 adolescents had complete relief of symptoms and total recovery to full activities, two were markedly improved with only occasional discomfort, and only one child had no relief of symptoms. No difference in final outcome was observed for patients who recalled a precipitating traumatic event versus those who presented with an insidious onset of knee pain.

MEDIAL MARGIN FRACTURES

Avulsion fractures of the medial margin of the patella and osteochondral fractures that involve the medial facet of the patella are primarily and perhaps exclusively associated with lateral dislocation of the patella. In the study of Grogan and coworkers,[27] all 22 medial margin fractures were associated with dislocation of the patella.

It is important to differentiate a medial margin avulsion fracture from an osteochondral fracture of the medial portion of the patella.[13] Unfortunately, most studies on patella dislocations do not distinguish these lesions and use the terms interchangeably. The avulsion fracture is contained within the medial capsule (Fig. 36-9) and, by itself, is not an indication for surgery. The osteochondral fracture extends into the articular surface of the medial facet (Fig. 36-10). Osteochondral fractures will become loose bodies within the joint and should be excised or repaired.

In Runow's[13] study of 140 dislocated patella, 46 had associated fractures, 30 knees had an avulsion fracture of the medial margin of the patella, 12 knees had an osteochondral fracture of the medial patella, and 12 knees had an osteochondral fracture of the lateral femoral condyle. Some patients had simultaneous fracture of the lateral

Fractures and Dislocations of the Patella / 683

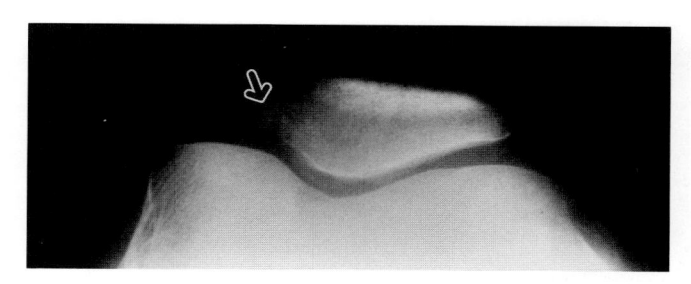

Fig. 36-9. An old avulsion fracture of the medial margin of the patella in a patient seen for follow-up evaluation of a previous patella dislocation.

femoral condyle combined with either an avulsion fracture or osteochondral fracture of the medial patella.

Although both fractures are caused by dislocation of the patella, the mechanism of injury is different for avulsion fractures versus osteochondral fractures. An osteochondral fracture of the patella is caused by shearing of the medial facet of the patella as it slides over the lateral femoral condyle with the knee in a flexed position.[37] By contrast, an avulsion fracture is caused by rupture of the vastus medialis as the patella is laterally dislocated.

Recognition of these fractures requires tangential views of the patella in addition to routine AP and lateral views of the knee. These radiographs, usually obtained after the patella has been relocated, will routinely identify the osteochondral fracture. Avulsion fractures, however, may not be apparent at the time of injury even with special radiographic studies. In one representative series,[27] 32 percent of the medial margin avulsion fractures were diagnosed when ossification developed at the periphery of the patella several weeks after the acute dislocation. The original avulsion fracture may have been missed, but it is more likely that in most cases only peripheral cartilage was detached from the patella. This avulsed cartilage was eventually recognized when it underwent osseous transformation and bony healing.

Osteochondral fractures are typically small and can be treated by excision rather than repair.[27,37] Occasionally, the osteochondral fragment may involve a large portion of the articular surface of the medial facet. Recent case reports support the use of a Herbert screw as an effective technique in internally fixing these injuries.[38] The differential pitch in the two threaded portions of the Herbert screw allow interfragmentary compression of the fracture. This screw can also be entirely buried beneath the articular surface of the patella.

It may be difficult to differentiate an avulsion fracture that is contained within the medial capsule versus an osteochondral fragment of the medial margin of the patella. If this be the case, then arthroscopy or arthrotomy of the knee should be performed.

LATERAL MARGINAL FRACTURES

Lateral marginal fractures are vertical cleavage fractures extending along the full extent of the lateral margin of the patella. These injuries should be differentiated from traumatic separation of a bipartite patella. Although stress fractures of the lateral margin of the patella have been described,[39] a direct blow to the periphery of the patella is the mechanism of injury in most of these fractures.[4] Although these fractures are minimally displaced, they often do not heal because of the nature of the soft tissue attachments and frequently require excision of the fragment[4] (Fig. 36-11).

I question whether lateral marginal fractures of the patella occur in children. The review by Grogan and colleagues[27] of 47 children with avulsion fractures of the patella did not describe any patients with this injury. The other case reports of this injury in children that I reviewed either appeared to be a symptomatic bipartite patella or provided insufficient information to rule out that possibility. If this injury does occur in a child, particularly an older teenager, then it would be reasonable to treat this person by the same guidelines used for adults, that is, excision of a persistently symptomatic fragment followed by early mobilization.[4]

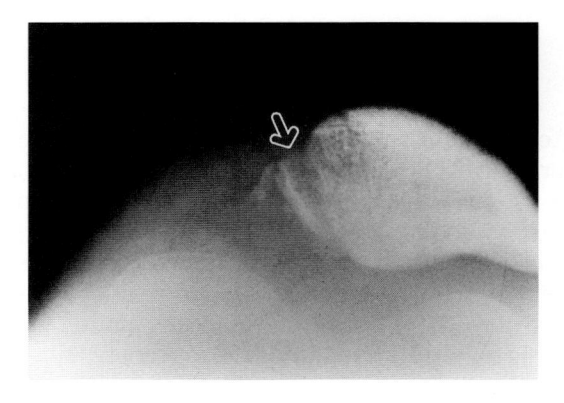

Fig. 36-10. Tangential view of the patella in a 15-year-old boy who sustained a traumatic dislocation of the patella after a "twisting" injury to his knee. An osteochondral fracture of the medial facet was shown on radiographs. The fragment was excised and the tear in the medial quadriceps retinaculum was repaired.

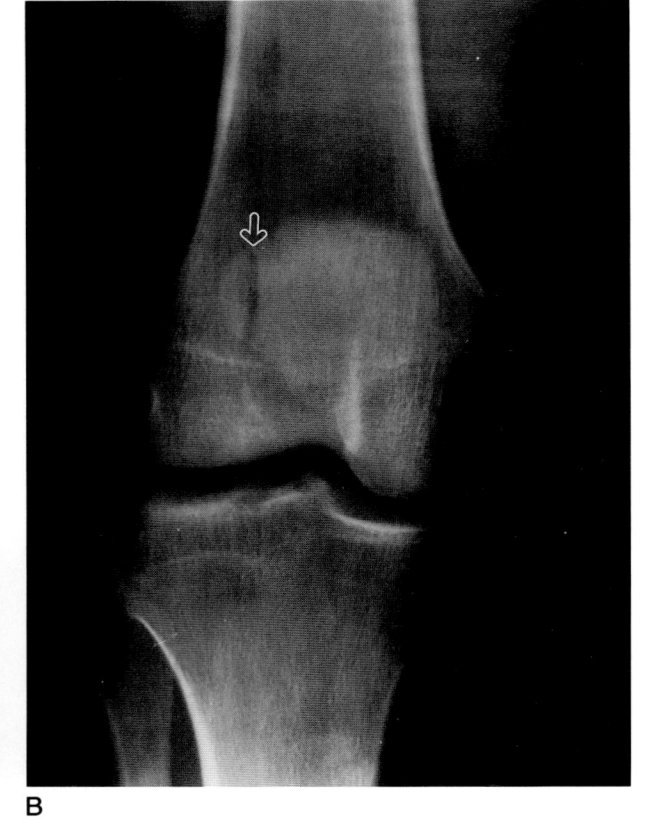

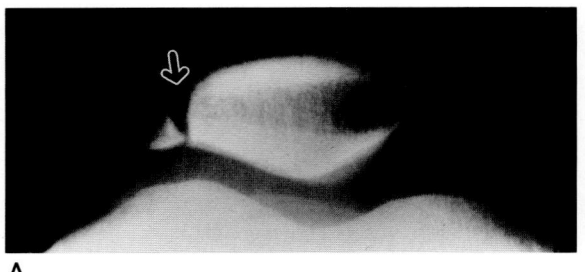

Fig. 36-11. (A) Tangential view of the patella and (B) AP view of the knee in a 24-year-old man who, 3 months previously, sustained a direct blow to the lateral aspect of his knee. Radiographs show persistent nonunion of lateral margin patella fracture. Note that fracture occupies full lateral margin of the patella. Excision of the fragment eliminated patient's symptoms.

DISLOCATIONS OF THE PATELLA

Dislocations of the patella in children can be classified as congenital, habitual, lateral, or central. The latter two are secondary to traumatic injuries and will be discussed in greater detail.

Congenital dislocation of the patella is present at birth, associated with a knee flexion deformity, and not reducible by closed means.[40] Habitual dislocation typically presents during the first decade. The patella dislocates laterally every time the knee is flexed.[40]

Habitual dislocation of the patella typically occurs in children who have had repeated intramuscular injections or in conditions such as Down syndrome that have marked ligamentous laxity.

Lateral Dislocation

Acute traumatic lateral dislocation of the patellae is an injury that occurs during the adolescent and young adult years. A direct blow may cause the dislocation, but the most common mechanism of injury is a rotational stress to the knee. This rotational stress frequently occurs during sports activities such as ball games and gymnastics, but it may also occur during routine running or even walking on level ground. In Runow's series,[13] the initial dislocation occurred during athletics or dancing in 55 percent of the patients, while the remaining 45 percent sustained their initial dislocation during minor trauma described as a slip or giving way of the knee during a trivial fall or walking.

The patella typically dislocates with the knee stressed

in a valgus, external rotation direction and flexed 20 to 30 degrees. To paraphrase Hughston's[41] classic description, the athlete is running full speed and suddenly "cuts back," pivoting on a moderately flexed knee, with the foot fixed on the ground. The sudden change in direction imposes a lateral displacing force on the patella. Dislocation of the patella does not occur with the knee in full extension because the quadriceps mechanism is fully lax in that position. Dislocation also does not occur with the knee flexed greater than 30 to 40 degrees, since the patella is now seated in the deeper portion of the intercondylar notch. In addition, more knee flexion puts increasing tension on the quadriceps muscle, a factor which by itself can centralize the patella.

Amateur softball players have been noted to dislocate their patella when they take a full, uncontrolled swing at the ball and miss, similar to the saga of "Mighty Casey in Mudville."[42] In this situation, a massive contraction of the quadriceps muscle occurs with the knee in the predisposing posture of slight flexion while the femur is internally rotated relative to the fixed tibia.

Predisposing Factors to Dislocation

Predisposing factors to patella dislocation include female gender, ligamentous laxity, patella alta, and genu valgum.[10,12,13,43-45] Genu valgum places a lateral stress on the patella. Ligamentous laxity affects the stabilizing constraint of the medial capsule. The increased association of females is probably related to greater genu valgum and ligamentous laxity in this sex. Patella alta causes the patella to be positioned in a very shallow portion of the intercondylar notch at the typical posture of dislocation. These anatomic characteristics are more likely to be present in patients whose primary dislocation is secondary to minor trauma.[13]

Traumatic dislocation of the patella primarily spans the age group from adolescence to young adults. Indeed, all but one study on patella dislocation include children and adults. The report by McManus and colleagues[46] was reportedly on children but did not specify the mean or upper age of their patients. Since another study on osteochondral patella fractures from the same institution[37] had some patients as old as 18, it is likely that even this often-quoted study included several "adult" patients who had completed growth at the knee when they sustained the initial patella dislocation.

On the other hand, it is now becoming apparent that age is an important factor in traumatic dislocation of the patella. Larsen and Lauridsen[12] found that the risk of redislocation was significantly greater in their teenage patients compared to patients who were 20 or older. These results were confirmed and amplified in another large series reported by Cash and Hughston,[11] who observed a 60 percent incidence of recurrent dislocation in the 11- to 14-year-old age group compared to 33 percent in the 15- to 18-year-old group.

Diagnosis of Dislocation

Acute dislocation of the patella may be easy or difficult to diagnose. The problem is obvious in the child who comes to the emergency room with the patella sitting on the lateral aspect of the knee. Many patients, however, have patella dislocations that either spontaneously reduce or that are reduced by the patients themselves. The latter group may provide an adequate history of the patella being laterally dislocated, but the former group can only describe their injury in terms of the knee "giving out" or "slipping."

With spontaneous reduction of the patella, the diagnosis can be established by corroborating a suggestive history with a physical examination demonstrating the following three signs: (1) tenderness along the medial border of the patella, (2) a hemarthrosis, and (3) a positive apprehension sign. The tenderness and the hemarthrosis result from tearing or stretching of the medial capsular structures. The apprehension sign is elicited by stretching these torn structures. With the knee extended and the quadriceps muscle relaxed, the examiner uses the thumb to push the patella laterally. The knee is then flexed. A positive apprehension sign is noted by an increase in the patient's anxiety and pain as the patella starts to subluxate and the examiner's arm may be grabbed by the patient.

Physical examination should also include assessment of surrounding soft tissue and bony structures. The medial quadriceps retinaculum is either torn or attenuated.[14] Either circumstance will cause tenderness at the superomedial margin of the patella and a hemarthrosis. Other structures are uncommonly injured with dislocation of the patella; however, since many teenagers give only a history of the knee giving way, a physical examination should also exclude other injuries that can cause a knee hemarthrosis. Collateral and cruciate ligament injuries are particularly important to rule out, especially if the injury occurred in a sports activity.

Generalized ligamentous laxity is also assessed as this characteristic makes a patient prone to recurrent dislocation. Hyperextension of the elbow greater than 10 degrees, hyperextension of the contralateral knee joint greater than 10 degrees, and passive apposition of the thumb to within 0.5 cm of the volar aspect of the forearm are three easy tests to perform. In a study by Runow,[13] these three tests were positive in 57 percent of the males and 69 percent of the females with recurrent dislocation of the patella. By comparison, only 11 percent of the age and sex match controls had all three signs of ligamentous laxity present.

Treatment of Traumatic Dislocation

Radiographs obtained with the patella dislocated provide dramatic pictures but limited information about osteochondral fractures or patella alignment (Fig. 36-12). Assuming that the examination does not suggest any other injuries, I prefer to relocate the patella before obtaining radiographs. This is usually successful without parenteral analgesics or local anesthesia, but if quadriceps spasm and pain are too intense, then one or both of these modalities may be prescribed. The patella is relocated by flexing the hip to relax the rectus femoris and then applying pressure to the lateral aspect of the patella while extending the knee.

After the patella is relocated, the joint is aspirated. The hemarthrosis is often quite large, being greater than 50 ml in about half of the patients.[14] Evacuating the hemarthrosis will make the patient more comfortable and may improve apposition of the torn quadriceps retinaculum. Through the same needle used for the arthrocentesis, the physician may also inject a long-acting local anesthetic. After completing the arthrocentesis, the physician should reexamine the knee with particular emphasis on assessing cruciate and collateral ligament stability. The aspirated blood should also be examined for fat globules as their presence makes an osteochondral fracture more likely.

Radiographic Assessment

Radiographs are the next step in the evaluation. For an acute dislocation, the radiographs are specifically scru-

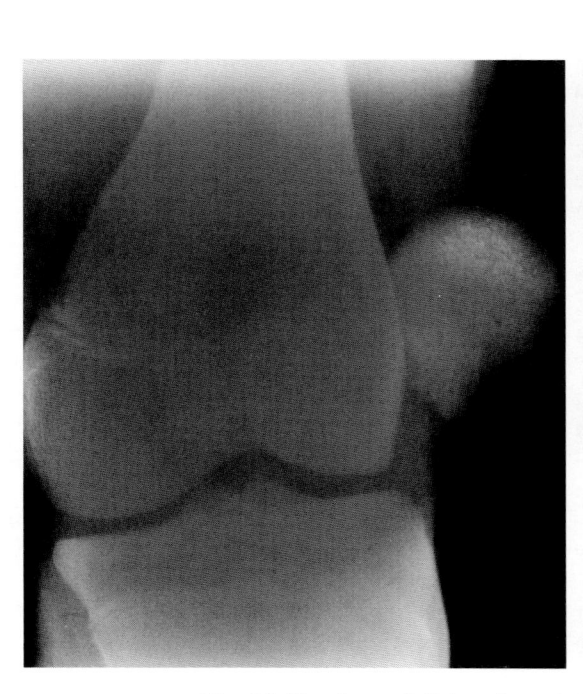

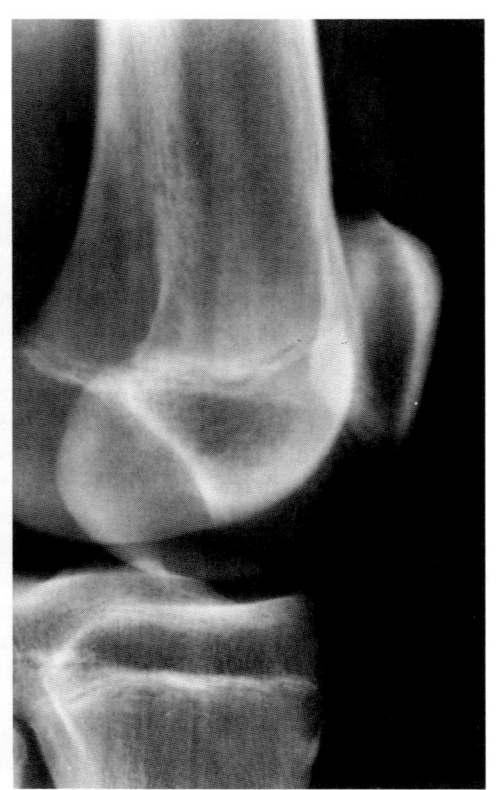

Fig. 36-12. Lateral dislocation of the patella in a 15-year-old boy.

tinized to rule out osteochondral and avulsion fractures as well as other injuries. For a patient with recurrent dislocation of the patella, radiographic studies are primarily utilized to evaluate patella alta, patella tilt, and lateral subluxation of the patella. For each situation, the three basic views are an AP and lateral radiographic view of the knee and a tangential view of the patella.

The lateral view of the knee defines the relative position of the patella, that is, whether patella alta is present. On a lateral view made with the knee flexed 30 degrees, the lower pole of the patella is normally transsected by a line drawn along the intercondylar notch, the so-called Blumenstat line. Insall and colleagues[44,47] and other subsequent authors[13,48,49] have shown that the ratio of the length of the patella to the length of the patella tendon is a more reproducible and accurate assessment of patella alta (Fig. 36-13). In patients with recurrent dislocation, the ratio averages approximately 0.8 compared to an average ratio of 1.0 in control populations.[44] Patella alta is also more frequent in patients who have sustained a primary, acute dislocation. In this group, the incidence of patella alta ranges from 23 to 43 percent compared to a 5 percent incidence of patella alta in the general population.[14,47,50] Measurement of patella alta is less precise in a child who has a larger proportion of cartilage comprising the patella,[47] but in an adolescent the difference is probably insignificant.

The tangential view of the patella profiles the patellofemoral joint as well as the medial and lateral margins of the patella. Some options for this radiograph include the Settegast or "sunrise" view and other techniques described by Hughston,[41] Merchant and colleagues[51] and Laurin and colleagues.[52] Any of the tangential views may be used to inspect for avulsion or osteochondral fractures. Each radiographic technique has relative advantages and disadvantages. The routine "sunrise" view and the technique described by Hughston[41] are relatively easy to obtain, but have the disadvantage of flexing the knee to a degree that tightens the quadriceps muscle and centralizes the patella. Therefore, accurate evaluation of patella tilt and patella subluxation is precluded.

Merchant and colleagues[51] described a radiographic technique that exposes the patellofemoral joint with the knee flexed 45 degrees. To obtain this radiograph, the patient lies supine on the table with the hips extended and the legs allowed to flex at a 45-degree angle over the end of the table. With the quadriceps muscle relaxed, a tangential view of the patellofemoral joint is obtained. Merchant and colleagues[51] also described a congruence angle to assess lateral subluxation of the patella and a sulcus angle to measure the depth of the intercondylar notch (Fig. 36-14). Normal values in their study were -6 ± 11 degrees for the congruence angle and 138 ± 6 degrees for the sulcus angle.

Noting that 45 degrees of knee flexion could still tighten the quadriceps muscle enough to preclude demonstration of patella subluxation, Laurin and colleagues[52] described a tangential view of the patella with the knee flexed 20 degrees. In addition to measuring the congruence angle as described by Merchant and colleagues,[51] these authors also devised a measurement that assessed lateral tilt of the patella (Figs. 36-15 and 36-16).

In recent years, the concepts espoused by Laurin and colleagues[52] have been generally accepted for the radiographic evaluation of recurrent patella dislocation or patella femoral pain. The disadvantage of the Laurin technique is the difficulty in obtaining these radiographs. With the knee flexed only 20 degrees, it is consistently difficult to profile the patellofemoral joint. For that reason, other authors have advocated computed tomogra-

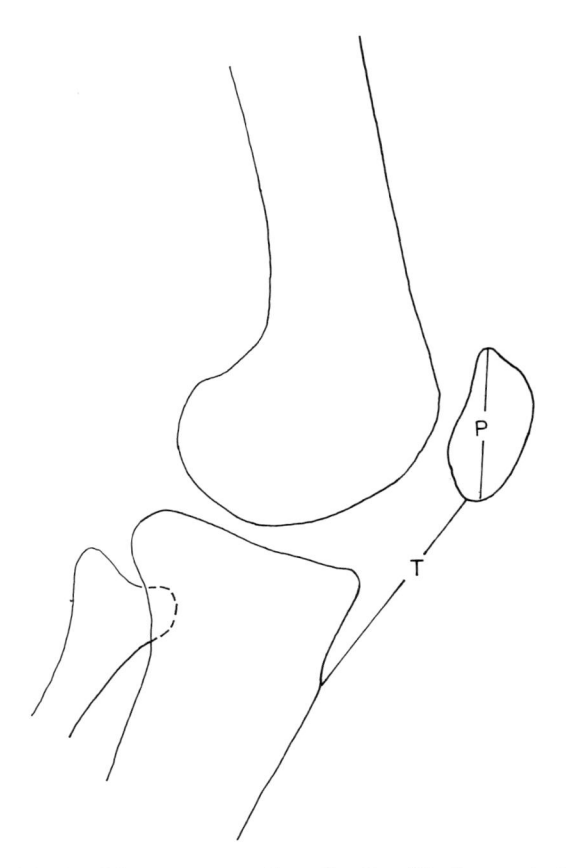

Fig. 36-13. Measurement of patella alta. P is the greatest diagonal length of the patella. T is the length of patella tendon measured from the inferior pole of the patella to the tibial tuberosity. The ratio of P/T averages 1.0 in normals compared to 0.8 in patients with recurrent dislocation of the patella. (Adapted from Insall and Salvati,[47] with permission.)

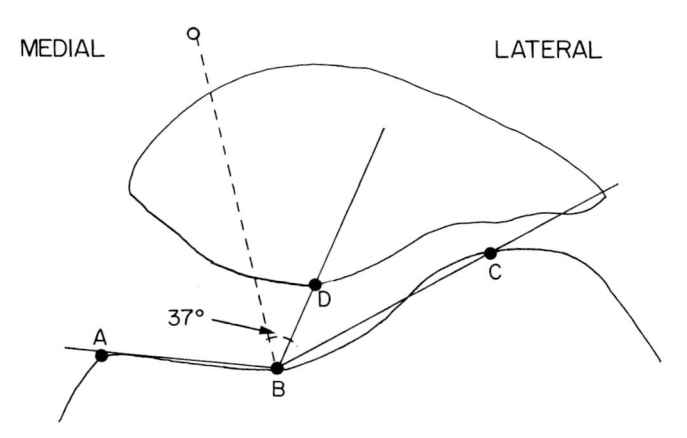

Fig. 36-14. Measurement of congruence and sulcus angle. *A* is the highest point on the medial femoral condyle, *B* is the lowest point of the intercondylar sulcus, *C* is the highest point on the lateral femoral condyle, and *D* is the lowest point on the articular surface of the patella. The sulcus angle is *ABC*. The congruence angle is measured by line *BD* and the bisector line of the sulcus angle. (Adapted from Merchant et al.,[51] with permission.)

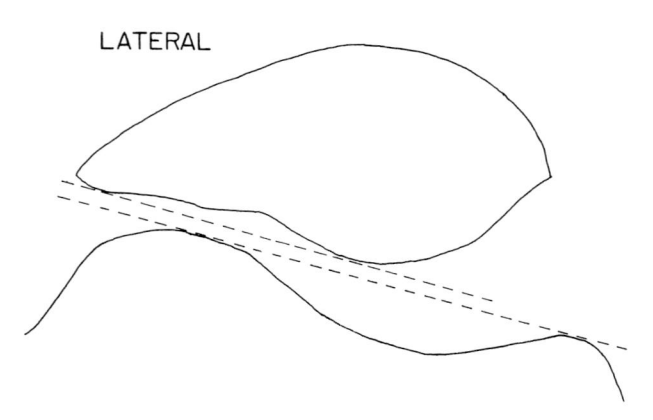

Fig. 36-16. Schematic diagram of Laurin view from a patient with chronic patellofemoral instability. With a tight lateral retinaculum, the tilt angle is decreased. (Adapted from Laurin et al.,[52] with permission.)

phy (CT)[53–56] or magnetic resonance imaging.[57] With these special studies, the patellofemoral joint can be consistently seen with the knee extended or in slight flexion. Indeed, my own routine preoperative evaluation of a patient with either recurrent patella dislocation or patella tracking problems is a transverse CT scan of the midpatella with the knee extended and flexed 15 degrees. Patella tilt and the congruence angle are measured as described by Schutzer and coworkers[55,56] to determine lateral retinacular tightness and patella subluxation. (Normal values for tilt angle are greater than 8 degrees and normal values for congruence angle are greater than 0 degrees.)

Limited information is available on using either the Laurin or Merchant view in the evaluation of an acute, primary dislocation. Vainionpää and coworkers[14] obtained Laurin views in 64 consecutive acute dislocations of the patella and noted that reproducible radiographs were difficult to obtain. This study, unfortunately, did not report absolute values for the sulcus angle, congruence angle, or tilt angle. The tilt angle was described as abnormal in 19 patients, but, otherwise, the radiographic measurements on the injured leg were compared to the contralateral side. Since the contralateral side may have had a predisposing anatomic factor, this information is of limited value. Indeed, the study by Vainionpää and colleagues[14] found many patients who had abnormal radiographic measurements on the contralateral limb.

The Merchant view is the radiographic technique I use in the evaluation of an acute dislocation. This view is relatively easy to obtain, even with a tender knee. The sulcus angle is not affected by the acute situation. The congruence angle is measured as a standard of comparison, but whether this angle provides meaningful information in the acute situation is presently unknown.

Treatment of Acute Traumatic Dislocation

The only absolute indication for surgery in a primary patella dislocation is an osteochondral fracture, an associated injury that occurs approximately 10 to 15 percent of the time.[13,46] Avulsion fractures of the medial margin of the patella do not require surgery. If an operation is required to remove an osteochondral fragment, then repair of the quadriceps retinaculum, and, if necessary, realignment of the quadriceps mechanism should also be

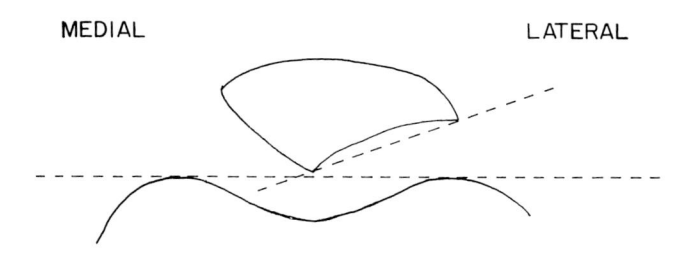

Fig. 36-15. Measurement of patella tilt. Schematic diagram was made from a patient with a normal patella. (Adapted from Laurin et al.,[52] with permission.)

performed. Rorabeck and Bobechko[37] observed redislocation in 2 of 5 patients treated only by excision of the osteochondral fragment but no recurrent dislocation in 10 patients who had excision of the fragment plus realignment of the quadriceps.

For the remaining patients, indications for nonoperative versus operative therapy of the time of the initial dislocation are not precisely established at this time. For that reason, I believe that nonoperative therapy should be presented as an alternative to every patient.

Nonoperative therapy starts with aspiration of the hemarthrosis and immobilization of the knee in extension by medial and lateral plaster splints. A compressive dressing and a foam pad placed laterally will enhance reapproximation of the torn medial structures. The patient is instructed in isometric quadriceps strengthening exercises and crutch-assisted ambulation. Weightbearing is permitted as tolerated. The maximum time of immobilization is 6 weeks. The patient, however, is examined at 2-week intervals and if there is no tenderness or hypermobility of the patella, then the immobilization can be discontinued. Physical therapy should be continued until knee motion and quadriceps strength has been regained. Using this protocol, Cash and Hughston[11] did not observe differences in the rate of redislocation or subsequent realignment procedures for patients immobilized 2, 4, or 6 weeks.

Operative treatment for all patients at the time of the initial dislocation has been advocated or tried by some authors.[14,50,58,59] The theory of immediate operative repair is that pathologic changes in the quadriceps mechanism can be prevented. With disruption or attenuation of the medial quadriceps retinaculum, contraction of the surrounding muscles may result in the vastus medialis healing in a lengthened or lax position. Concomitant shortening of the vastus lateralis may also occur. The subsequent loss of the medial stabilizing forces and tightness of the lateral retinaculum will cause recurrent dislocation of the patella and/or patellofemoral instability. The knee "giving way" probably represents transient episodes of patella subluxation. Repeated episodes of patella subluxation and/or dislocation cause shearing forces across the articular surface and will ultimately produce patellofemoral osteoarthritis.[10,53] This is supported by Bowker and Thompson's[10] study of patients undergoing quadriceps realignment for recurrent patellar instability. Patients who had a longer duration of symptoms had more extensive erosion of the articular cartilage.

Limited data are presently available on the results of immediate operative repair of an acute patella dislocation.[14,50,59] The incidence of redislocation is certainly less after immediate operative repair,[11,59] but the incidence of subsequent patellofemoral instability and anterior knee pain is not affected as much. In fact, in a small series reported by Hawkins and coworkers,[59] the proportion of patients with patellofemoral instability and anterior knee pain was similar in the operative and nonoperative group.

Since some patients do quite well with nonoperative treatment, I favor a selective approach to treating an adolescent who has sustained an initial dislocation of the patella. Operative therapy is considered more seriously for patients who are at greater risk for recurrent dislocation.

Redislocation Following Acute Traumatic Dislocation

Recurrent instability following patella dislocation is more likely in younger teenagers, in patients with ligamentous laxity, and in patients who have predisposing anatomic factors. Cash and Hughston[11] found a redislocation rate of 60 percent in the 11- to 14-year-old age group, whereas the 15- to 18- and 19- to 27-year-old age groups had a redislocation rate of 33 and 28 percent, respectively. No redislocations occurred in a patient over the age of 28. Therefore, nonoperative therapy is preferred for "older" adults.

The presence of ligamentous laxity and other anatomic factors affects the results of therapy.[11-13,59] Cash and Hughston[11] retrospectively grouped their patients into those with and those without predisposing factors (Table 36-2). The predisposing factors they evaluated included lateral hypermobility of the patella, a dysplastic vastus medialis obliquus, a high and/or lateral position of the patella, and a history of previous patella instability in the unaffected knee. Those with predisposing factors had a much higher rate of recurrent dislocation, recurrent symptoms of patellofemoral instability, and the need for subsequent reconstruction operations. However, if predisposing factors were absent, then the results of nonsurgical treatment was similar to an acute repair with the exception of a slightly lower rate of recurrent dislocation (Table 36-2).

The high incidence of redislocation in younger teenagers may be primarily related to a greater proportion of these patients having anatomic predisposing factors. Data proving that concept, however, are not currently available. In any circumstance, predisposing anatomic factors do affect the results of nonoperative treatment, and, in my opinion, most patients, no matter what their age, should have some of these anatomic factors present

TABLE 36-2. Results in Acute Dislocation of the Patella

	N	Recurrence (%)	Poor Result[a] (%)	Subsequent Reconstruction (%)
Predisposing factors present				
Closed treatment[b]	58	43	41	26
Acute repair	11	0	9	0
No predisposing factors				
Closed treatment[b]	29	17	21	3
Acute repair	5	0	20	0

[a] Poor result defined as more than one redislocation or frequent episodes of moderate or severe knee pain with limitation of activity.
[b] Includes patients who underwent diagnostic arthroscopy with removal of osteochondral fragment but no repair/realignment of the extensor mechanism.
(Adapted from Cash and Hughston,[11] with permission.)

before operative therapy is recommended for the initial dislocation. The exception to this requirement is the patient who has a large defect in the vastus medialis or an ostrochondrial fracture.

Operative Repair of Dislocation

The predisposing factors that I assess before recommending operative repair of an acute dislocation are listed in Table 36-3. Patella alta and a decreased sulcus angle are radiographic signs that can be determined with reasonable accuracy in the acute situation. Ligamentous laxity is defined by the three tests previously described. A defect in the vastus medialis obliquus should be ascertained after aspiration of the hemarthrosis. Persistent swelling in the knee may make this sign difficult to quantify.

Current knowledge does not allow numerical rating of these predisposing factors, but obviously a decision to recommend operative therapy is based on the number and severity of the positive predisposing factors. In addition, operative therapy is considered more seriously for patients who not only have predisposing factors but who are also active in sports activities. The parents and the patient should understand that operative therapy may not prevent subsequent problems but that the incidence of these problems, particularly that of recurrent dislocation, is reduced in patients who have predisposing factors. Even when the orthopaedic surgeon thinks that operative repair is a better alternative, the possibility of nonoperative therapy should also be discussed.

The technique of operative repair for an acute primary patellar dislocation is usually not as elaborate as the surgery required for a patient with recurrent dislocation. An acute primary repair always includes inspection of the joint for any osteochondral fragments and repair of the torn medial retinaculum. Release of the lateral retinaculum and advancement of the vastus medialis, two common components of reconstructive surgery for chronic patella instability, are usually not necessary and, indeed, may cause complications, since medial subluxation of the patella has been reported after lateral retinacular release.[60] Jensen and Roosen[50] also noted that a lateral capsulotomy did not decrease the incidence of chondromalacia following an acute repair. Therefore, a lateral retinacular release is only done in patients who conclusively demonstrate abnormal lateral tracking of the patella following repair of the torn vastus medialis. I have not used advancement of the vastus medialis in a patient undergoing an acute primary repair. Transfer of the tibial tubercle has never been considered in an acute repair, as that procedure has a significant incidence of chondromalacia, even in patients with chronic patellofemoral instability.[61]

Nonoperative therapy is used initially for all patients with a history of previous patella dislocations. These patients most likely have already developed secondary changes, such as patella tilt and lateral subluxation of the patella, that should be corrected when the patella is realigned. Therefore, after the acute situation resolves, a CT scan or other special imaging studies can be obtained to

TABLE 36-3. Predisposing Factors Assessed in Determining Acute Repair of Patella Dislocation

Patella alta
Decreased sulcus angle
Ligamentous laxity
Genu valgum > 15°
Previous history of patella instability in the unaffected knee
Age < 15 years
Large defect in vastus medialis

identify these problems. Not all these patients, however, require these special studies. The decision to obtain additional tests depends on the presence of predisposing factors and on the frequency of previous dislocations. Frequent dislocators typically have more than two dislocations per year and, more importantly, usually have a perception of knee instability between the episodes of frank dislocation.[13] As one would expect, frequent dislocators also have a high incidence of ligamentous laxity and other anatomic factors. Infrequent dislocators typically average one dislocation every other year, only have symptoms of instability for 2 to 3 weeks following the episode of frank dislocation and are less likely to have predisposing factors. Therefore, continued nonoperative therapy may be a better choice for the infrequent dislocator who is otherwise functioning quite well.

Summary

Unless an osteochondral fracture fragment is present, acute traumatic dislocation of the patella may be treated by nonoperative or operative means. The decision to operate should be made after assessing predisposing factors to recurrent patella instability. Future studies, no doubt, will provide more precise guidelines for treatment of an acute traumatic patella dislocation.

CENTRAL DISLOCATION

Central or intra-articular dislocation of the patella is an injury that typically occurs in the preadolescent knee and is another example of the greater elasticity of soft tissues in children.[62-65] The mechanism of injury is direct trauma to the upper portion of the patella. The patella becomes lodged in the joint with the articular surface facing distally (Fig. 36-17). The quadriceps tendon is typically stripped from the upper pole of the patella, but the medial and lateral retinaculum remain intact.

Physical examination frequently reveals an abrasion over the anterior aspect of the knee at the site of the direct trauma. The inferior pole of the patella is quite prominent. The knee is typically held in slight flexion.

In two case reports[63,64] closed reduction under general anesthesia was successful. Two other cases[62,65] required an open reduction through a limited incision. Closed reduction should be attempted under general anesthesia. Pushing on the inferior pole may lever the patella back into position. If there is a large defect in the quadriceps tendon or if postreduction radiographs show a displaced sleeve fracture, then the quadriceps mechanism should be repaired. The knee is immobilized in extension for 4 to 6 weeks. No long-term abnormalities or disability have been reported.

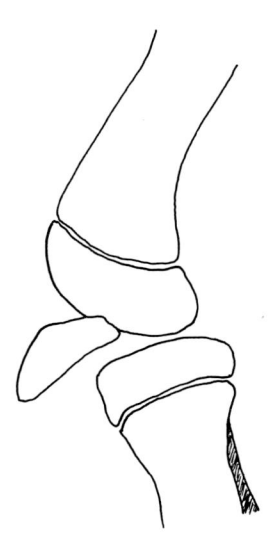

Fig. 36-17. Schematic diagram of radiograph demonstrates central dislocation of the patella in a 12-year-old boy. (Adapted from Donelson and Tomaiuouli,[62] with permission.)

ACKNOWLEDGMENT

The author gratefully acknowledges the technical assistance of Terry Murphy in preparing this chapter.

REFERENCES

1. Bostrom AKE: Fracture of the patella: a study of 422 patellar fractures. Acta Orthop Scand, suppl 143:10, 1972
2. Nummi J: Fracture of the patella: a clinical study of 707 patellar fractures. Ann Chir Gynaecol Fenn [Suppl] 179:1, 1971
3. Benz G, Roth H, Zachariou Z: Frakturen und Knorpelverletzungen des kindlichen Kniegelenkes. Z Kinderchir 41:219, 1986
4. Smillie IS: Injuries of the Knee Joint. 5th Ed. Churchill Livingstone, Edinburgh, 1978
5. Currey JD, Butler G: The mechanical properties of bone tissue in children. J Bone Joint Surg [Am] 57:810, 1975
6. Blount WP: Fractures about the knee. p. 171. In: Fractures in Children. Williams & Wilkins, Baltimore, 1955
7. Borden S: Traumatic bowing of the forearm in children. J Bone Joint Surg [Am] 56:611, 1974

8. Girdany BR, Golden R: Centers of ossification of the skeleton. AJR 68:922, 1952
9. Ogden JA: Radiology of postnatal skeletal development: patella and tibial tuberosity. Skelet Radiol 11:246, 1984
10. Bowker JH, Thompson EB: Surgical treatment of recurrent dislocation of the patella: a study of forty-eight cases. J Bone Joint Surg [Am] 46:1451, 1964
11. Cash JD, Hughston JC: Treatment of acute patellar dislocation. Am J Sports Med 16:244, 1988
12. Larsen E, Lauridsen F: Conservative treatment of patellar dislocations: influence of evident factors on the tendency to redislocation and the therapeutic result. Clin Orthop 171:131, 1982
13. Runow A: The dislocating patella: etiology and prognosis in relation to generalized joint laxity and anatomy of the patellar articulation. Acta Orthop Scand, suppl 201:1, 1983
14. Vainionpää S, Laasonen E, Pätiälä A et al: Acute dislocation of the patella: clinical, radiographic and operative findings in 64 consecutive cases. Acta Orthop Scand 57:331, 1986
15. Belman DAJ, Neviaser RJ: Transverse fracture of the patella in a child. J Trauma 13:917, 1973
16. Spalding CB: Fracture of patella in child two years old. Int Clin 4:245, 1918
17. Edwards B, Johnell O, Redlund-Johnell I: Patella fractures: a 30-year follow-up. Acta Orthop Scand 60:712, 1989
18. Lotke PA, Ecker ML: Transverse fractures of the patella. Clin Orthop 158:181, 1981
19. Weber MJ, Janecki CJ, McLeod P et al: Efficacy of various forms of fixation of transverse fractures of the patella. J Bone Joint Surg [Am] 62:215, 1980
20. Scapinelli R: Blood supply of the human patella: its relation to ischaemic necrosis after fracture. J Bone Joint Surg [Br] 49:563, 1967
21. Crawford AH: Fractures about the knee in children. Orthop Clin North Am 7:639, 1976
22. Daffner RH, Tabas JH: Trauma oblique radiographs of the knee. J Bone JOint Surg [Am] 69:568, 1987
23. Shim SS, Leung G: Blood supply of the knee joint: a microangiographic study in children and adults. Clin Orthop 208:119, 1986
24. Houghton GR, Ackroyd CE: Sleeve fractures of the patella in children: a report of three cases. J Bone Joint Surg [Br] 61:165, 1979
25. Gardiner JS, McInerney VC, Avella DG, Valdez NA: Injuries to the inferior pole of the patella in children. Orthop Rev 19:643, 1990
26. Peterson L, Stener B: Distal disinertion of the patellar ligament combined with avulsion fractures at the medial and lateral margins of the patella. Acta Orthop Scand 47:680, 1976
27. Grogan DP, Carey TP, Leffers D, Ogden JA: Avulsion fractures of the patella. J Pediatr Orthop 10:721, 1990
28. Medlar RC, Lyne ED: Sinding-Larsen-Johansson disease: its etiology and natural history. J Bone Joint Surg [Am] 60:1113, 1978
29. Rosenthal RK, Levine DB: Fragmentation of the distal pole of the patella in spastic cerebral palsy. J Bone Joint Surg [Am] 59:934, 1977
30. Lloyd-Roberts GC, Jackson AM, Albert JS: Avulsion of the distal pole of the patella in cerebral palsy: a cause of deteriorating gait. J Bone Joint Surg [Br] 67:252, 1985
31. Batten J, Menelaus MB: Fragmentation of the proximal pole of the patella. J Bone Joint Surg [Br] 67:249, 1985
32. Bishay M: Sleeve fracture of upper pole of patella. J Bone Joint Surg [Br] 73:339, 1991
33. Green WT: Painful bipartite patellae: a report of three cases. Clin Orthop 110:197, 1975
34. Ogden JA, McCarthy SM, Jokl P: The painful bipartite patella. J Pediatr Orthop 2:263, 1982
35. Bourne MH, Bianco AJ: Bipartite patella in the adolescent: results of surgical excision. J Pediatr Orthop 10:69, 1990
36. Carter SR: Traumatic separation of a bipartite patella. Injury 20:244, 1989
37. Rorabeck CH, Bobechko WP: Acute dislocation of the patella with osteochondral fracture: a review of eighteen cases. J Bone Joint Surg [Br] 58:237, 1976
38. Rae PS, Khasawneh ZM: Herbert screw fixation of osteochondral fractures of the patella. Injury 19:16, 1988
39. Devas MB: Stress fractures of the patella. J Bone Joint Surg [Br] 42:71, 1960
40. Gao GX, Lee EH, Bose K: Surgical management of congenital and habitual dislocation of the patella. J Pediatric Orthop 10:255, 1990
41. Hughston JC: Subluxation of the patella. J Bone Joint Surg [Am] 50:1003, 1968
42. Gross RM: Acute dislocation of the patella: the Mudville mystery—report of five cases. J Bone Joint Surg [Am] 68:780, 1986
43. Gartland JJ, Benner JH: Traumatic dislocations in the lower extremity in children. Orthop Clin North Am 7:687, 1976
44. Insall J, Goldberg V, Salvati E: Recurrent dislocation and the high-riding patella. Clin Orthop 88:67, 1972
45. Reider B, Marshall JL, Warren RF: Clinical characteristics of patellar disorders in young athletes. Am J Sports Med 9:270, 1981
46. McManus F, Rang M, Heslin DJ: Acute dislocation of the patella in children: the natural history. Clin Orthop 139:88, 1979
47. Insall J, Salvati E: Patella position in the normal knee joint. Radiology 101:101, 1971
48. Dowd GSE, Bentley G: Radiographic assessment in patellar instability and chondromalacia patellae. J Bone Joint Surg [Br] 68:297, 1986
49. Lancourt JE, Cristini JA: Patella alta and patella infera: their etiological role in patellar dislocation, chondromalacia, and apophysitis of the tibial tubercle. J Bone Joint Surg [Am] 57:1112, 1975

50. Jensen CM, Roosen JU: Acute traumatic dislocations of the patella. J Trauma 25:160, 1985
51. Merchant AC, Mercer RL, Jacobsen RH, Cool CR: Roentgenographic analysis of patellofemoral congruence. J Bone Joint Surg [Am] 56:1391, 1974
52. Laurin CA, Dussault R, Levesque HP: The tangential x-ray investigation of the patellofemoral joint: x-ray technique, diagnostic criteria and their interpretation. Clin Orthop 144:16, 1979
53. Fulkerson JP, Shea KP: Disorders of patellofemoral alignment. J Bone Joint Surg [Am] 72:1424, 1990
54. Inoue M, Shino K, Hirose H et al: Subluxation of the patella: computed tomography analysis of patellofemoral congruence. J Bone Joint Surg [Am] 70:1331, 1988
55. Schutzer SF, Ramsby GR, Fulkerson JP: The evaluation of patellofemoral pain using computerized tomography: a preliminary study. Clin Orthop 204:286, 1986
56. Schutzer SF, Ramsby GR, Fulkerson JP: Computed tomographic classification of patellofemoral pain patients. Orthop Clin North Am 17:235, 1986
57. Kujala UM, Osterman K, Kormano M et al: Patellofemoral relationships in recurrent patellar dislocation. J Bone Joint Surg [Br] 71:788, 1989
58. Bassett FH: Acute dislocation of the patella, osteochondral fractures, and injuries to the extensor mechanism of the knee. Instr Course Lect 25:40, 1976
59. Hawkins RJ, Bell RH, Anisette G: Acute patellar dislocations: the natural history. Am J Sports Med 14:117, 1986
60. Hughston JC, Deese M: Medial subluxation of the patella as a complication of lateral retinacular release. Am J Sports Med 16:383, 1988
61. Crosby EB, Insall J: Recurrent dislocation of the patella: relation of treatment to osteoarthritis. J Bone Joint Surg [Am] 58:9, 1976
62. Donelson RG, Tomaiuouli M: Intra-articular dislocation of the patella. J Bone Joint Surg [Am] 61:615, 1979
63. Murakami Y: Intra-articular dislocation of the patella: a case report. Clin Orthop 171:137, 1982
64. Nsouli AZ, Nahabedian AM: Intra-articular dislocation of the patella. J Trauma 28:256, 1988
65. Sarkar SD: Central dislocations of the patella. J Trauma 21:409, 1981

37

Treatment of Posttraumatic Sequelae by the Ilizarov Technique

Deborah F. Bell

> A surgeon should have the eyes of a hawk, the heart of a lion, and the hands of a woman.
> —Christina Hill

Trauma to the extremities in children may have sequelae that lead to difficulties in orthopaedic management. Malunion and nonunion, with or without infection, can occur irrespective of patient age. Injury to the immature skeleton has the additional potential, due to the location and importance of the physes, of producing potential limb length inequality with or without accompanying angular deformity.

Conventional osteotomy techniques usually enable the surgeon to eliminate most angular deformity. Although closing wedge osteotomy may produce some mild shortening, judiciously executed opening wedge corrections can eliminate this problem. Unfortunately, however, standard techniques are ill-equipped to manage the problem of deformity with significant limb shortening due to partial or complete physeal arrest. Similarly, confounding problems of translational and/or rotational malunion make conventional solutions often impossible.

THE ILIZAROV TECHNIQUE

The Ilizarov technique, initiated in Russia in the 1950s, provides the ability to correct deformity and restore limb length simultaneously through distraction osteogenesis.[1-4] In more complex situations, it can also be used to restore bony continuity in the case of significant bone loss caused either by trauma or by the need to debride the necrotic or infected tissue. Additionally, posttraumatic soft tissue contractures such as those related to fracture care, compartment syndrome, or burn can be gradually eliminated using this technique.[5]

The technique employs bony fixation through transosseous small-caliber wires to rings under tension allowing circumferential or nearly circumferential fixation of most limb segments.[6] Gradual distraction, with or without accompanying osteotomy, at no more than 1 mm daily in at least four increments allows correction of bone or soft tissue deformity through distraction histogenesis.[7-10] Bone formation is largely by a direct intramembranous process, rather than through the sequence of endochondral ossification.[7] Once correction is achieved, a fixation period ensues. The length of this period depends on the extent of deformity or lengthening, that is, the length of the regenerate bone segment.

ADVANTAGES OF THE ILIZAROV TECHNIQUE

There are several advantages of the Ilizarov technique, in the treatment of complex problems. The system affords a multiplanar "grip" on the limb segment. This allows the surgeon to correct angulation, rotation, or translation simultaneously or sequentially. The Ilizarov apparatus, properly applied, is stable to full weightbearing. Biomechanical studies have shown this fixator in various configurations to be at least as stable as other uniplanar and delta configuration fixators to torsion and shear, known to be deleterious to bone formation.[11] On the other hand, it is the least stable of conventionally applied external fixators to axial loading due to the use of small-caliber wires rather than large-diameter half-pins. This allows cyclic axial micromotion, known to promote bone healing.[12] Thus, the patient is encouraged to be as functional as possible in the fixator. Additionally, the use of pools for recreation or therapy and showering are recommended during treatment, usually aiding in the local pin site care.

Due to the great modularity of the system and multiple ring sizes, the Ilizarov apparatus is applicable to virtually any limb segment in nearly any size patient. In my own experience, patients have been treated as early as 2 years of age and as large as 150 kg! Finally, the system can be applied to treat or control joints adjacent to the limb segment in question. For example, knee instability in the presence of a posttraumatic femoral deformity with shortening is no longer a contraindication to limb lengthening. One can extend the fixator across the joint in question to the adjacent limb segment with the use of hinges to allow motion during treatment and to prevent potential joint subluxation or dislocation.

DISADVANTAGES OF ILIZAROV EXTERNAL FIXATION

No discussion of the merits of a given treatment scheme is complete without mentioning the actual or potential disadvantages. External fixation, in general, is commonly less well-tolerated in the pediatric patients than internal fixation or, in fact, than a short period of cast-immobilization. All such devices require daily pin care and prevent truly normal activities. Circular external fixation carries the additional problem of being more bulky than many cantilever type half pin systems. Finally, the treatment time may often be measured in months rather than weeks. Thus, this type of treatment should not be used for problems in which more simple solutions are readily available and should not replace standard procedures which have stood the test of time. Rather, this technique is another weapon in the orthopaedic surgical armamentarium for difficult problems.

Detailed specific instructions on the application of this fixator system to each limb segment is beyond the scope of this chapter. In general, for a given limb segment, stable bone fixation must be achieved both proximal and distal to the site of correction of deformity or the site of lengthening.[6] It is possible to produce bony correction at more than one site in a given limb segment if necessary. Stable fixation, by the traditional Ilizarov techniques, is achieved with four transosseous wires under tension proximal and distal to the planned osteotomy or existing nonunion site. Two wire sizes are currently available, 1.5 and 1.8 mm. The former are used in smaller tibiae and in the upper extremity. The larger wires are used in femoral and large tibial applications. Additionally, these wires are available with "stoppers" to prevent bone translation along the wire and to act as a fulcrum for angular correction when necessary.

MANAGEMENT OF POSTTRAUMATIC DEFORMITY

Angular deformity is common as a part of trauma sequelae. Not infrequently partial physeal arrest will lead to incomplete growth arrest with subsequent deformity and shortening. When indicated, that is, if physeal mapping demonstrates a reasonable quantity if viable physis and there is an adequate period of skeletal growth remaining, bar resection should be performed as a first procedure. In the event, however, that there is inadequate growth remaining, extensive physeal involvement or residual deformity and shortening despite bar resection and resumed growth, one may consider the Ilizarov technique.[2] Limb fixation is achieved as described below. The general principle of deformity correction, however, is restoration of limb segment anatomic axes, and overall limb mechanical axis. In general, one attempts to correct the deformity where it exists[13] This is

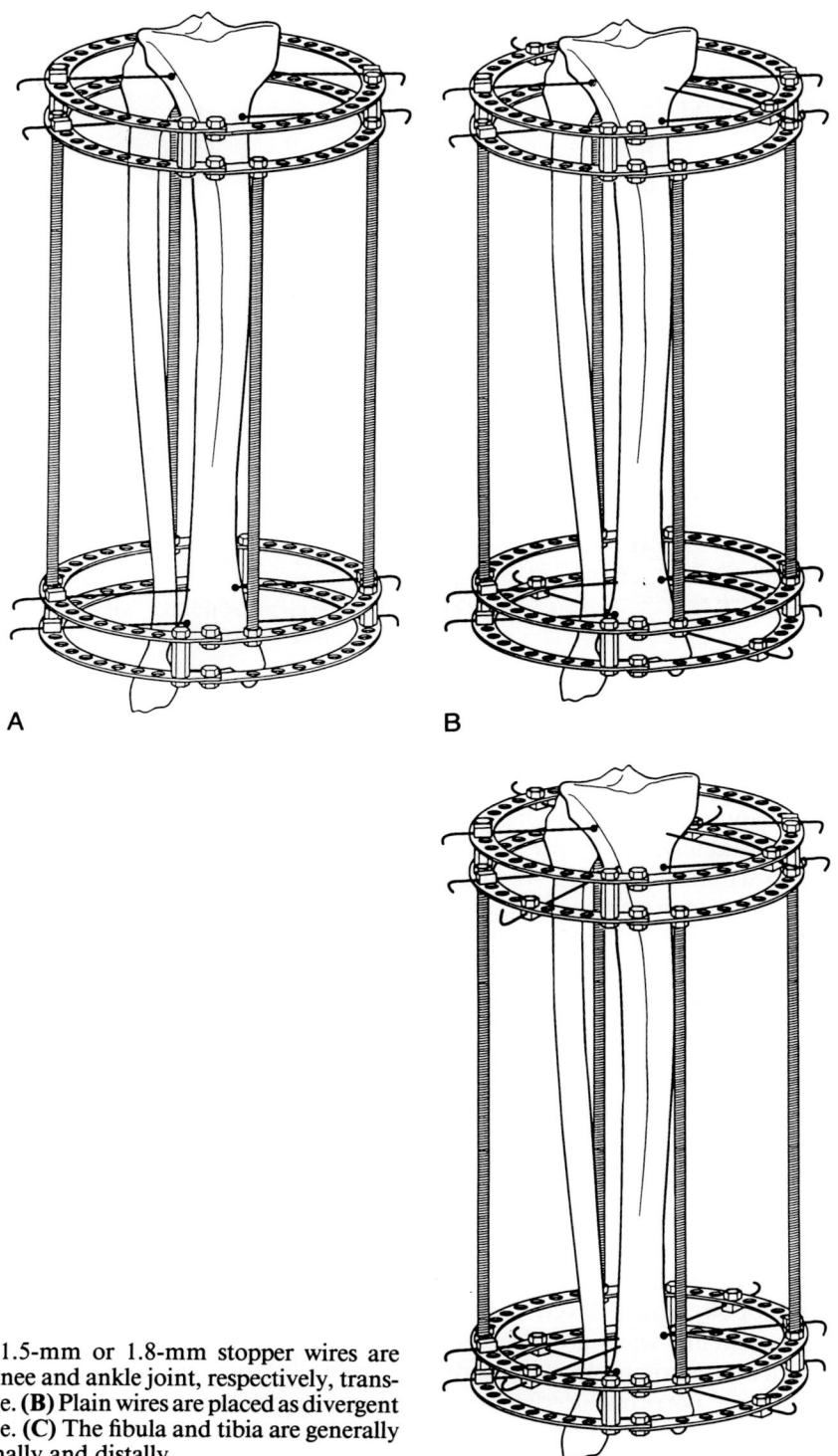

Fig. 37-1. **(A)** Two 1.5-mm or 1.8-mm stopper wires are placed parallel to the knee and ankle joint, respectively, transverse in the cornal plane. **(B)** Plain wires are placed as divergent as anatomically feasible. **(C)** The fibula and tibia are generally transfixed both proximally and distally.

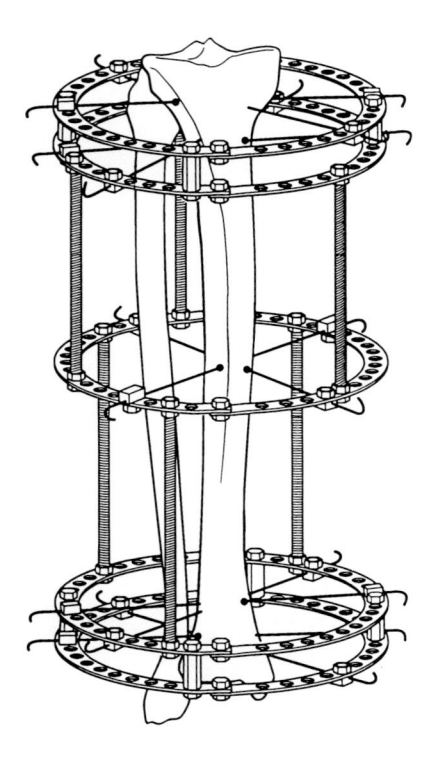

Fig. 37-2. Two-level correction or bone transport requires an additional "middle" ring, generally with two-wire fixation.

relatively straightforward in, for example, a diaphyseal malunion. Unfortunately, many pediatric deformities have their origin within the physis. As such, an osteotomy must be performed at a site somewhat distant from the true deformity. Even so, limb alignment may be restored as long as the axis of rotation (or hinge) for the correction is actually located at the level of the deformity.

Correction by the Ilizarov Technique

The Tibia

The most straightforward limb segment for treatment is the tibia. Four wires are placed proximally essentially parallel to the knee joint, and four distally, parallel to the ankle joint for monofocal (one-level) treatment. In skeletally immature patents, wires are placed distal to the proximal growth plate and proximal to the distal growth plate in order to avoid potential interference with growth or physeal arrest. The wire formula is as outlined in Figure 37-1A–C with two plain and two stopper wires proximally and distally. The stopper wires are generally placed transversely in the coronal or frontal plane (Fig. 37-1A). The plain wires are as divergent from these as are anatomically feasible and transfix both the fibula and tibia (Fig. 37-1B) proximally and distally. Finally, the last two wires are again plain wires, which are placed parallel to the medial face of the tibia (Fig. 37-1C). In the event that two-level bony correction is desired, a middle ring with two additional wires can be added (Fig. 37-2). The wires should fix an adequate bone "sandwich." That is, they cannot all be located at exactly the same level in the bone. The greater the proximal-distal spread between the wires the more stable the "block" of fixation.

Variations in fixation can be achieved by the substitution of certain wires by half-pins (either 4 or 5 mm) depending on the patient's size, if desired.[14] The advantage of wires is one of small scars and dynamic axial micromotion. The disadvantage is that of potential muscle transfixion, which may cause restricted joint motion or pain with muscle excursion. The "medial face" wire (those plain wires parallel to the medial face of the tibia) can quite easily be replaced with a half-pin directed from anterior to posterior in the tibial crest with little soft tissue transfixion. The technique is also applicable to the treatment of nonunions of the tibia—even congenital pseudarthrosis of the tibia.[15]

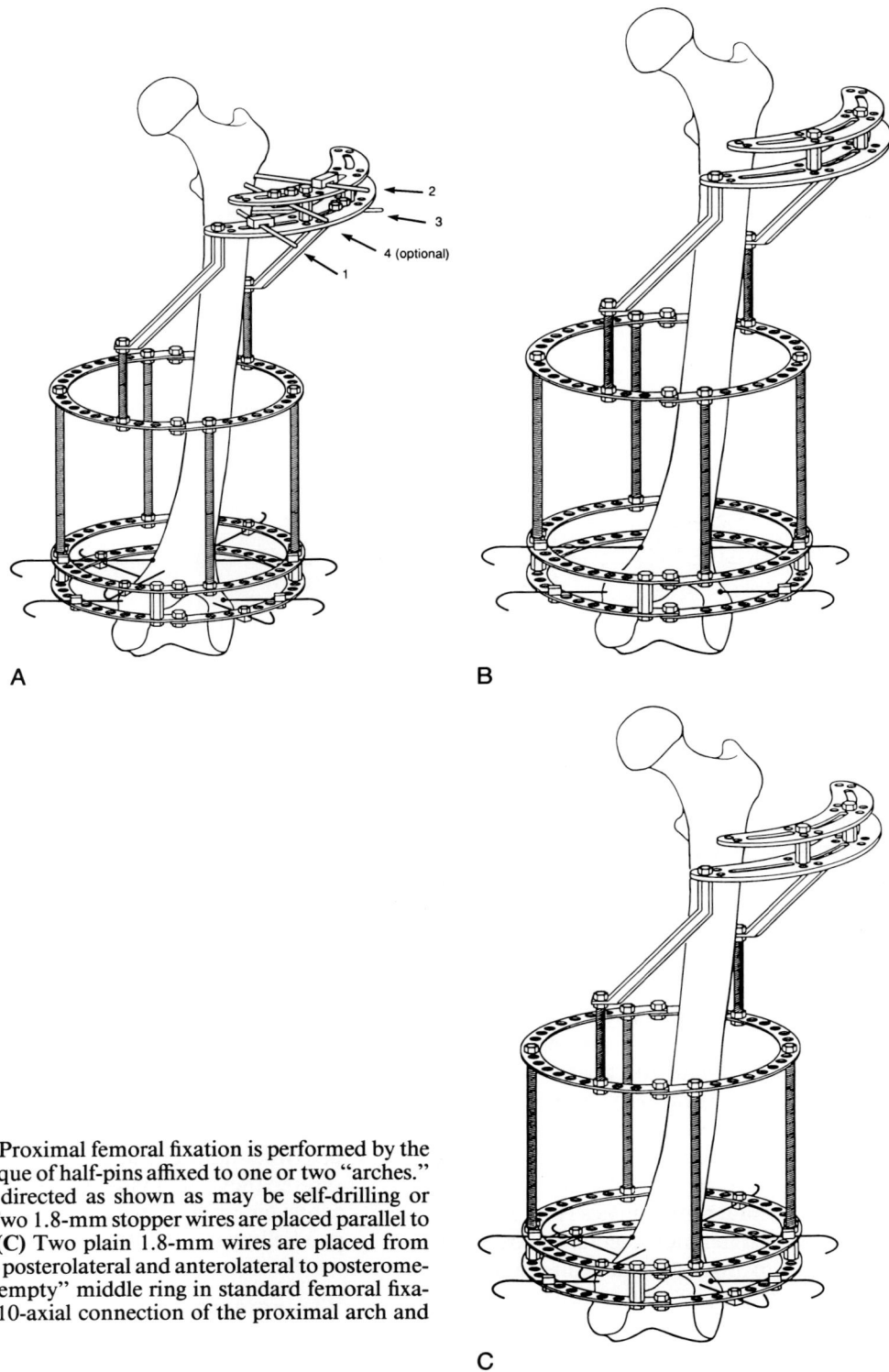

Fig. 37-3. (A) Proximal femoral fixation is performed by the "Italian" technique of half-pins affixed to one or two "arches." These pins are directed as shown as may be self-drilling or predrilled. (B) Two 1.8-mm stopper wires are placed parallel to the knee joint. (C) Two plain 1.8-mm wires are placed from anteromedial to posterolateral and anterolateral to posteromedial. Note the "empty" middle ring in standard femoral fixation ficilitating 10-axial connection of the proximal arch and distal rings.

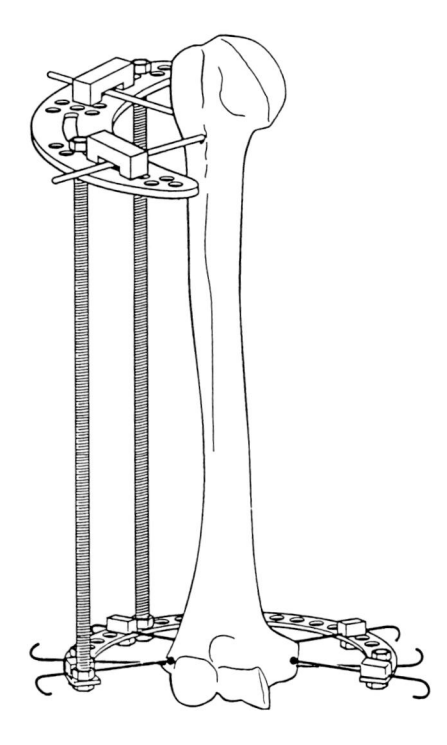

Fig. 37-4. "Standard" humeral fixation construct with 2 proximal half-pins affixed to an arch and 3 wires distally.

The Femur

Historically, the Russian technique of Ilizarov femoral fixation was achieved both proximally and distally with transfixing wires. Circumferential proximal thigh fixation, however, proved to be extremely cumbersome, requiring special mattress cutouts, and so on, due to a large posterior thigh ring. Modification of this technique by the Italian surgeons Catagni, Cattaneo, and Villa led to the fabrication of a special arch to which one could attach half-pins in the proximal thigh. These half-pins are generally 5 or 6 mm in diameter and can be self-drilling or predrilled, depending on the surgeon's preference. An arc of fixation of about 100 to 120 degrees can be achieved by placement of these pins perpendicular to the mechanical axis (not to the anatomic axis) in an anterolateral, lateral, and posterolateral direction (Fig. 37-3A). Distal fixation is in the traditional manner with transosseous 1.8-mm wires. Two stopper wires are placed parallel to the knee joint or distal femoral transcondylar axis, proximal to the physis (Fig. 37-3B). Two plain wires are placed in anteromedial to posterolateral, and anterolateral to posteromedial directions, respectively. Generally an "empty" ring is used in the middle of the femur (Fig. 37-3A–C) to facilitate connection between the proximal arches and distal ring. Half-pins may be attached to this if bifocal femoral treatment is indicated.

The Humerus

Fixation in the upper extremity requires less stability due to the fact that this is not a weightbearing limb.[16-18] Humeral fixation can be achieved with proximal and distal 1.5-mm wires or, more commonly, proximal half-pins (usually 4 mm) and distal wires, similar to the femoral construct (Fig. 37-4). Arches can be applied proximally and a ⅝ ring distally with the opening anteriorly, to allow elbow flexion during treatment. If one chooses half-pin fixation proximally and distally, it may be advisable to introduce the distal half-pins through open incisions to avoid potential radial nerve injury. Humeral osteotomy for the purpose of lengthening is performed through an anterolateral incision distal to the deltoid insertion to avoid excessive shoulder abduction during lengthening. Figure 37-5A demonstrates humeral shortening secondary to a Salter-Harris type IV fracture of the proximal humerus at the age of 8, resulting in a 10-cm discrepancy at maturity (Fig. 37-5B). The patient achieved approximately 8.5 cm of lengthening with good clinical function (Fig. 37-5C–G).

The Forearm

As in the humerus, forearm fixation requires less stability than in the lower extremity.[18] Depending on the treatment indicated, fixation of both or one bone may be

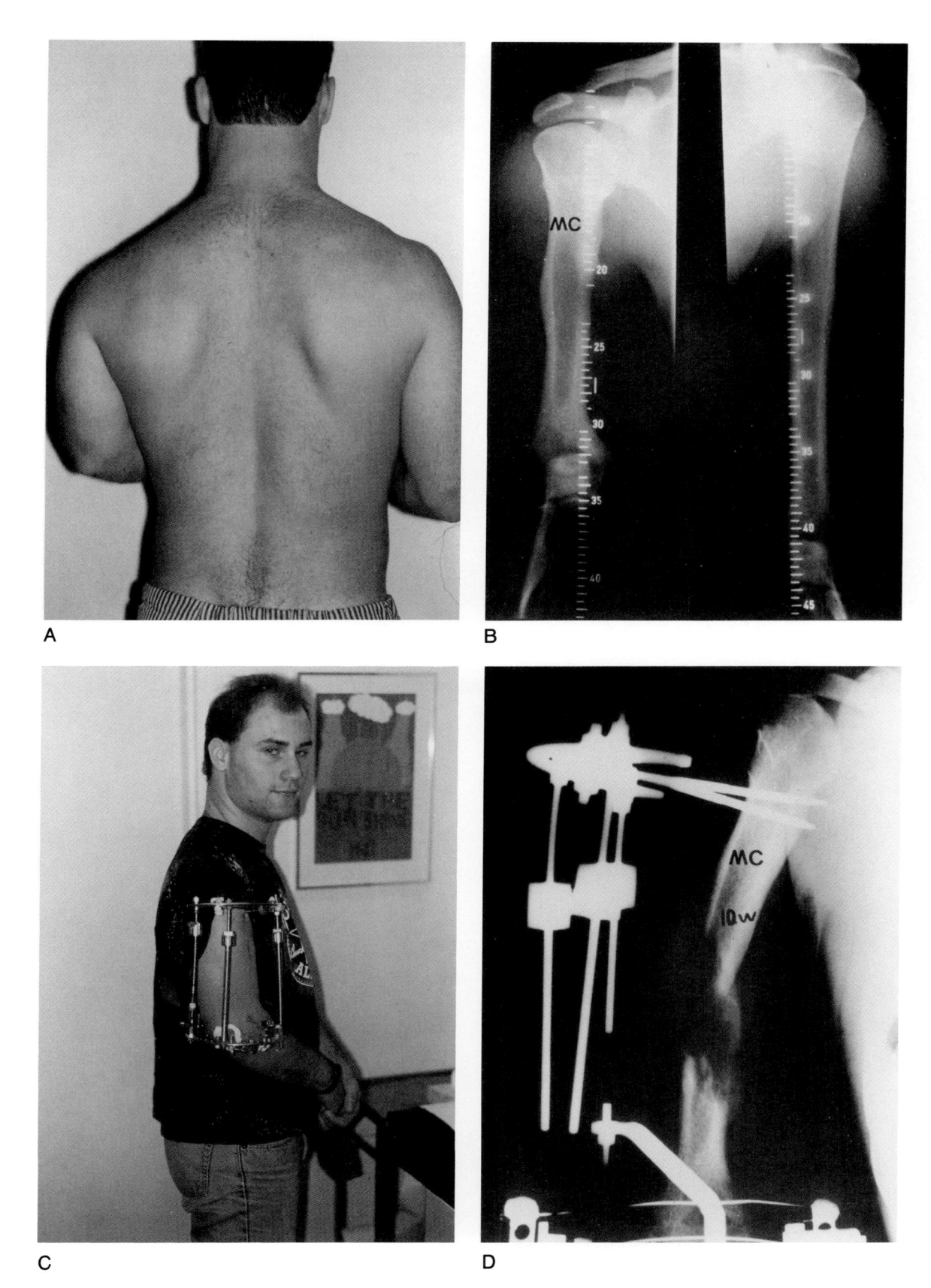

Fig. 37-5. (A) Clinical photograph and (B) scanogram of 17-year-old teenager nine years after type IV proximal humeral fracture. (C) Clinical photograph and (D) radiograph during humeral lengthening. *(Figure continues.)*

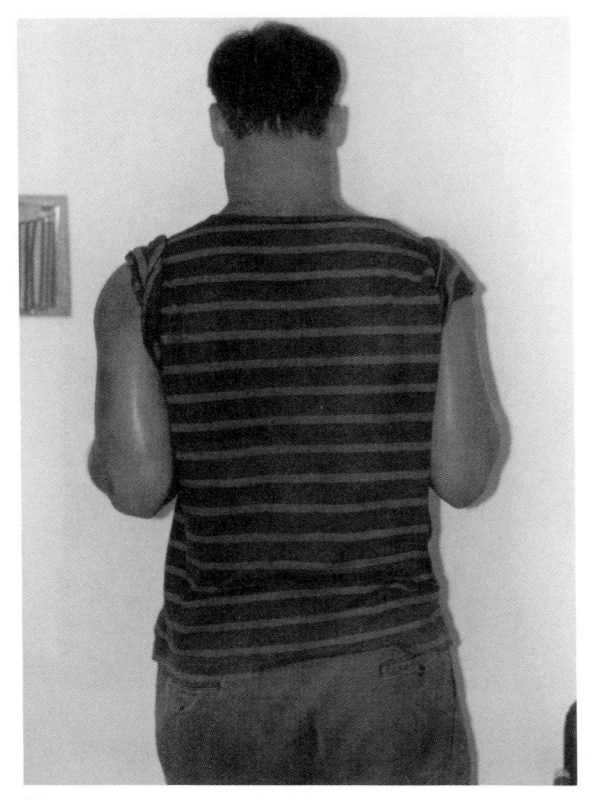

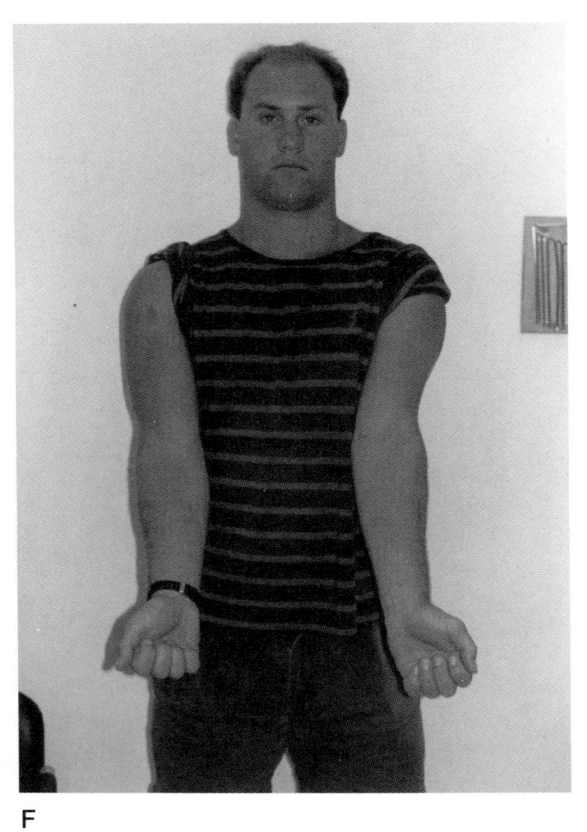

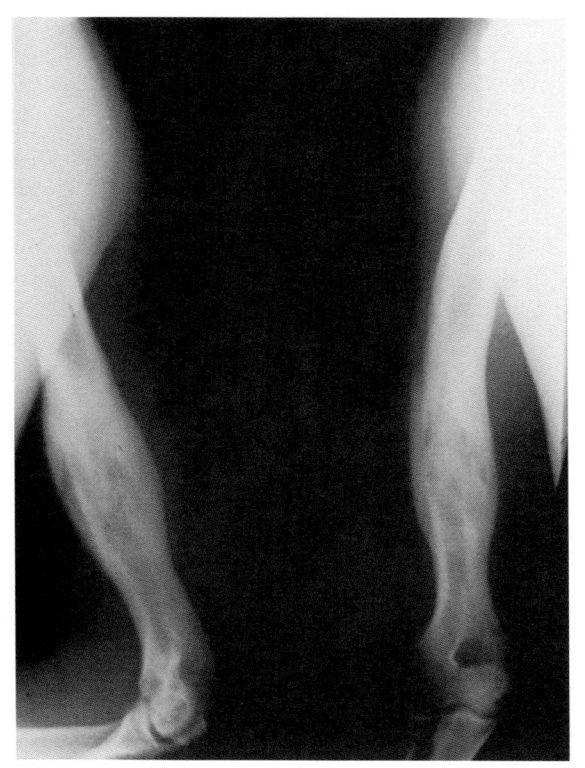

Fig. 37-5 *(Continued).* **(E&F)** Clinical and **(G)** radiographic results at the conclusion of treatment.

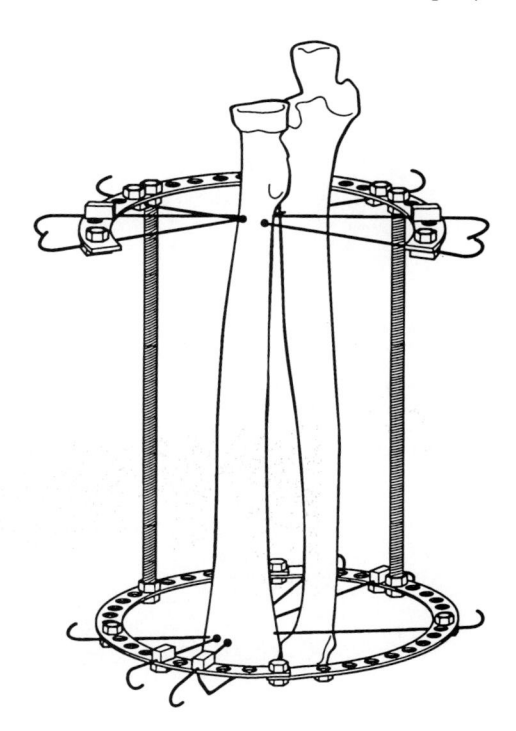

Fig. 37-6. Standard construct for Ilizarov forearm application.

achieved by three-wire proximal and three-wire distal fixation. If feasible, the most proximal "ring" can be a ⅝ ring with the opening oriented anteriorly to allow full elbow extension (Fig. 37-6). A single metacarpal wire is often used through the second and third metacarpals to stabilize the wrist and to avoid a palmar flexion contracture during correction. Certain portions of the radius (particularly distal) and ulna are uniquely subcutaneous and afford convenient fixation with 4-mm half-pins if desired. Figure 37-7 demonstrates treatment of a radial malunion by the Ilizarov technique with hinge application for angular correction.

THE ILIZAROV HINGE CONCEPT FOR CORRECTION OF ANGULAR DEFORMITY

Two basic types of hinge placement are possible for angular correction: (1) opening wedge and (2) distraction hinges. The former creates a simple opening wedge by the hinge placement directly over the cortex on the convex side of the deformity without additional lengthening. The distraction hinge is placed away from the cortex on the convex side of the deformity, thus providing lengthening as well as simultaneous angular correction resulting in a trapezoidal rather than triangular section of new bone formation.[19] The further the hinge is displaced relative to the cortex, the greater the resultant lengthening achieved. Once deformity has been eliminated, the hinge and "distractor" rods may be replaced and lengthening continued as needed. Figures 37-8 to 37-10 demonstrated further extensions of the hinge concept in posttraumatic deformity. Figure 37-8 shows severe recurvatum in a 13-year-old secondary to an unrecognized tibial tubercle injury when the patient sustained a femoral fracture at the age of 8 and was treated by distal femoral skeletal traction. Correction of the deformity was achieved through application of a standard tibial apparatus, proximal tibial osteotomy, and gradual anterior distraction.

The patient in Figure 37-9 sustained a left distal femoral Salter-Harris type II fracture with lateral growth arrest. Bar resection resulted in resumption of growth, but a residual valgus deformity with 3.5 cm of shortening. Application of the Ilizarov technique to the femur achieved correction of residual deformity and shortening. Simultaneous application to the tibia and femur is possible as demonstrated in Fig. 37-10 where angular correction and lengthening was required in both limb segments due to posttraumatic incomplete growth arrest of both the distal femoral and proximal tibial physes.

Soft tissue corrections without osteotomy are an ex-

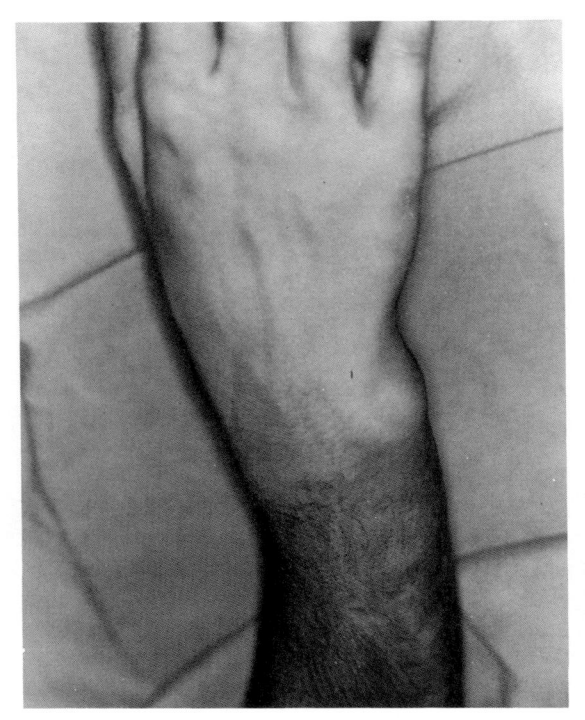

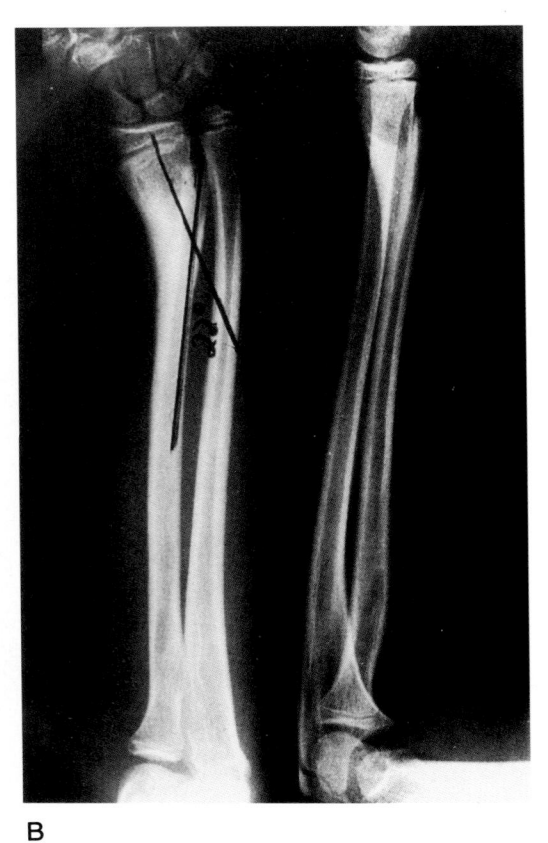

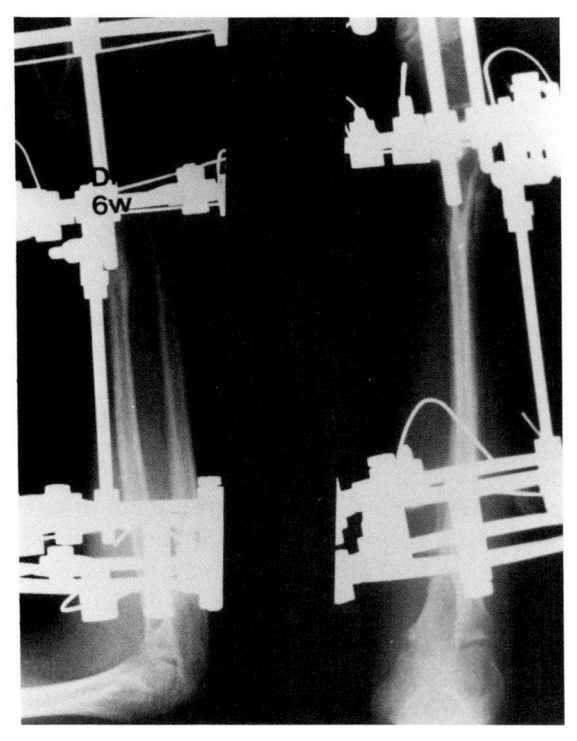

Fig. 37-7. (A) Clinical and (B) radiographic appearance of a 12-year-old girl with a 22-degree distal radius malunion with shortening. (C) Radiographs at the conclusion of angular correction. *(Figure continues.)*

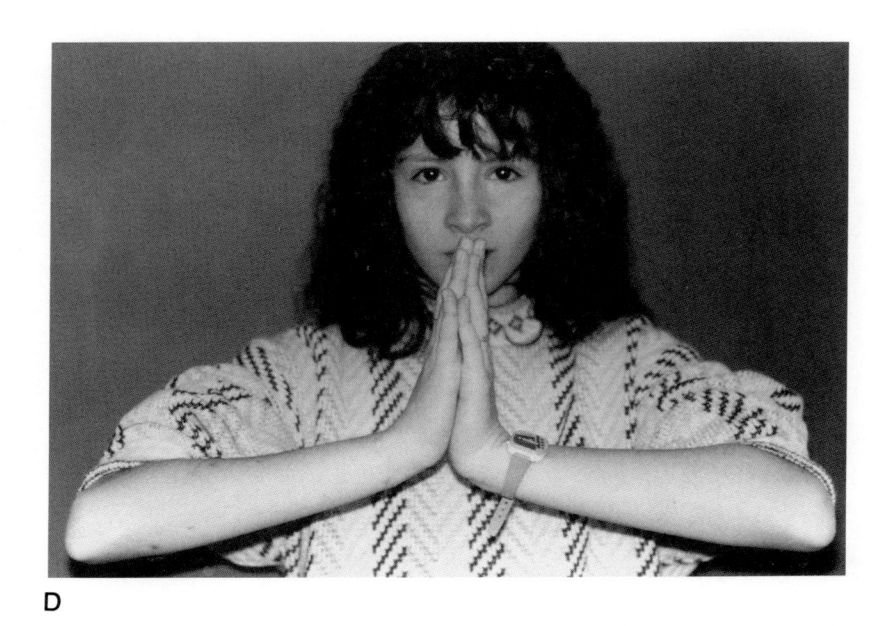

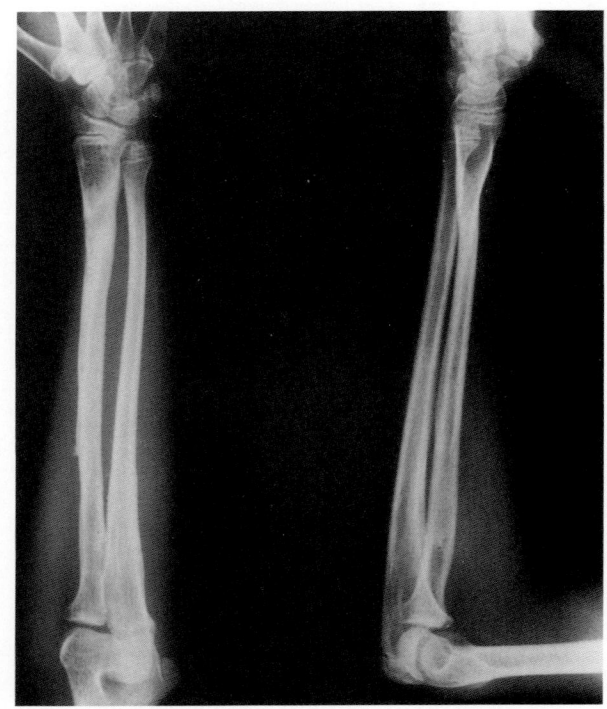

Fig. 37-7 *(Continued).* **(D)** Clinical and **(E)** radiographic appearance after removal of the Ilizarov apparatus.

706 / Management of Pediatric Fractures

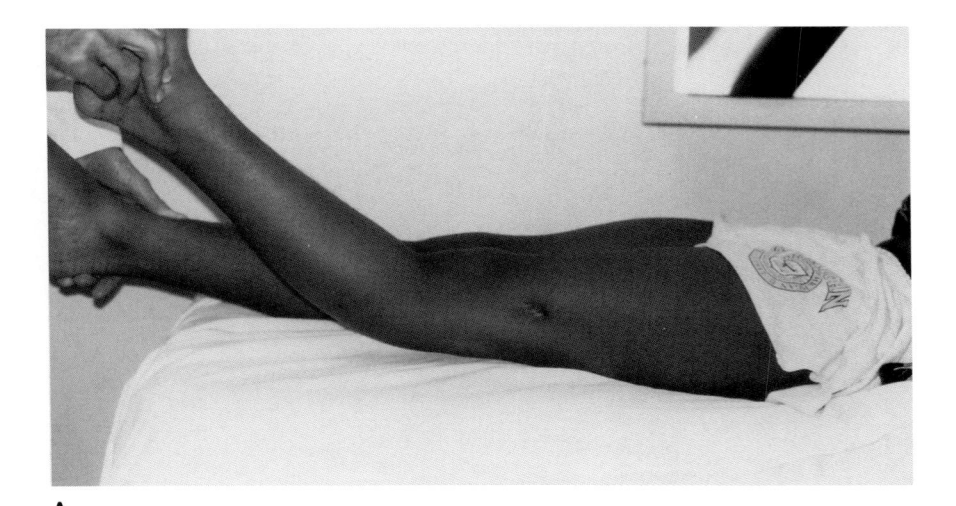

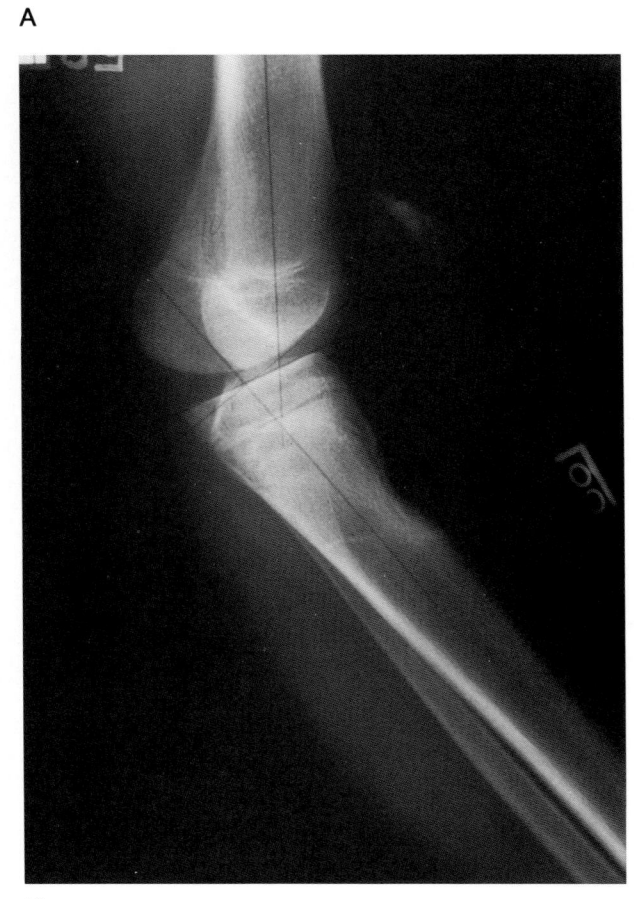

Fig. 37-8. (A) Clinical and (B) radiographic appearance of proximal tibial recurvature deformity following unrecognized tibial tubercle injury at the age of 8. *(Figure continues.)*

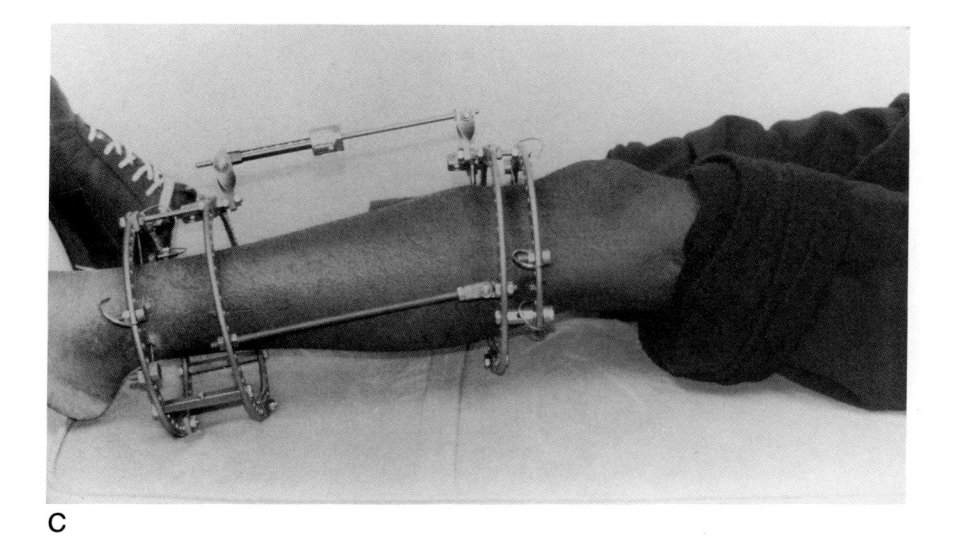

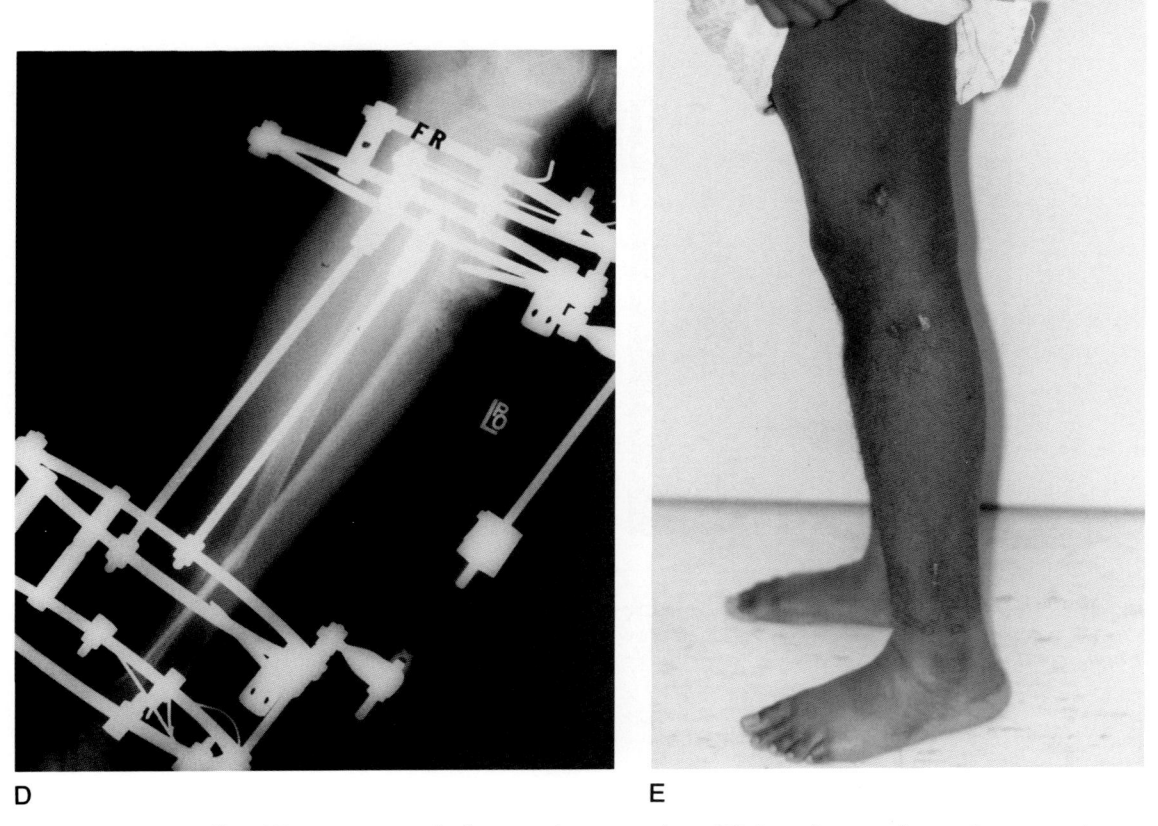

Fig. 37-8 *(Continued).* **(C)** Appearance during angular correction. **(D)** Anterior opening wedge correction to restore normal sagittal alignment. **(E)** Clinical appearance at the conclusion of treatment.

708 / Management of Pediatric Fractures

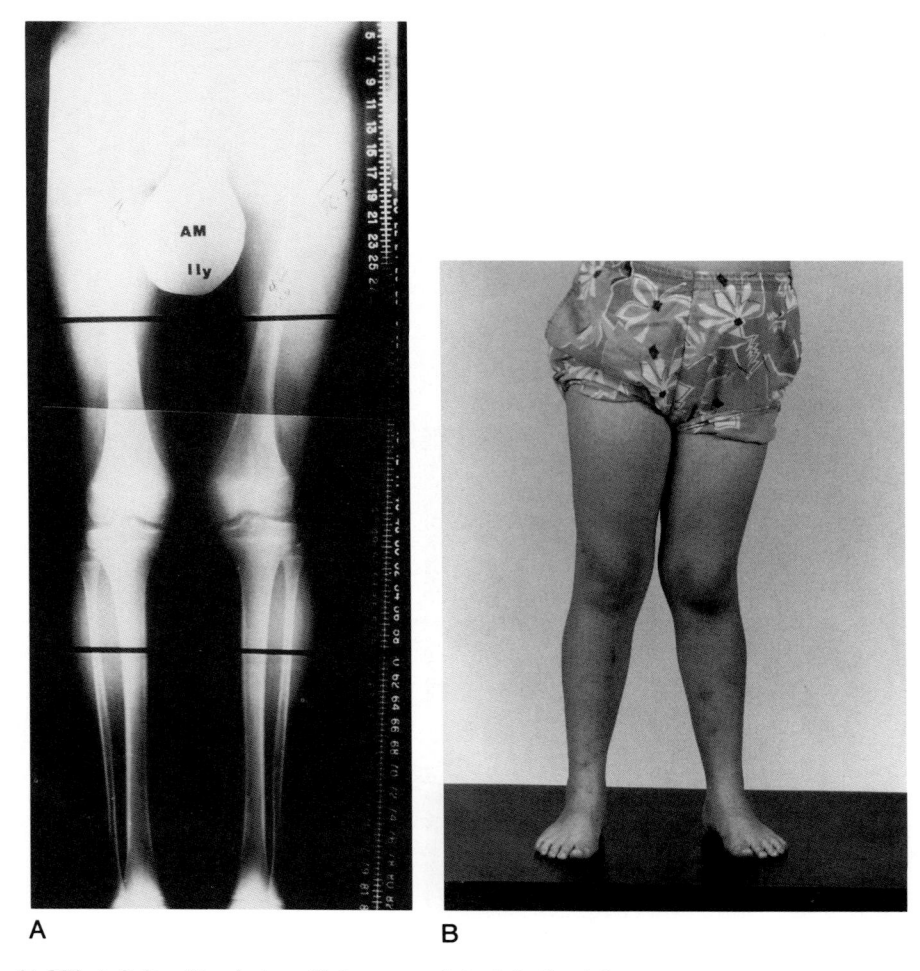

Fig. 37-9. **(A&B)** A Salter-Harris type II fracture of the left distal femur resulted in a partial lateral physeal arrest. Successful bar resection led to resumed growth but residual valgus deformity with 3.5 cm of shortening. *(Figure continues.)*

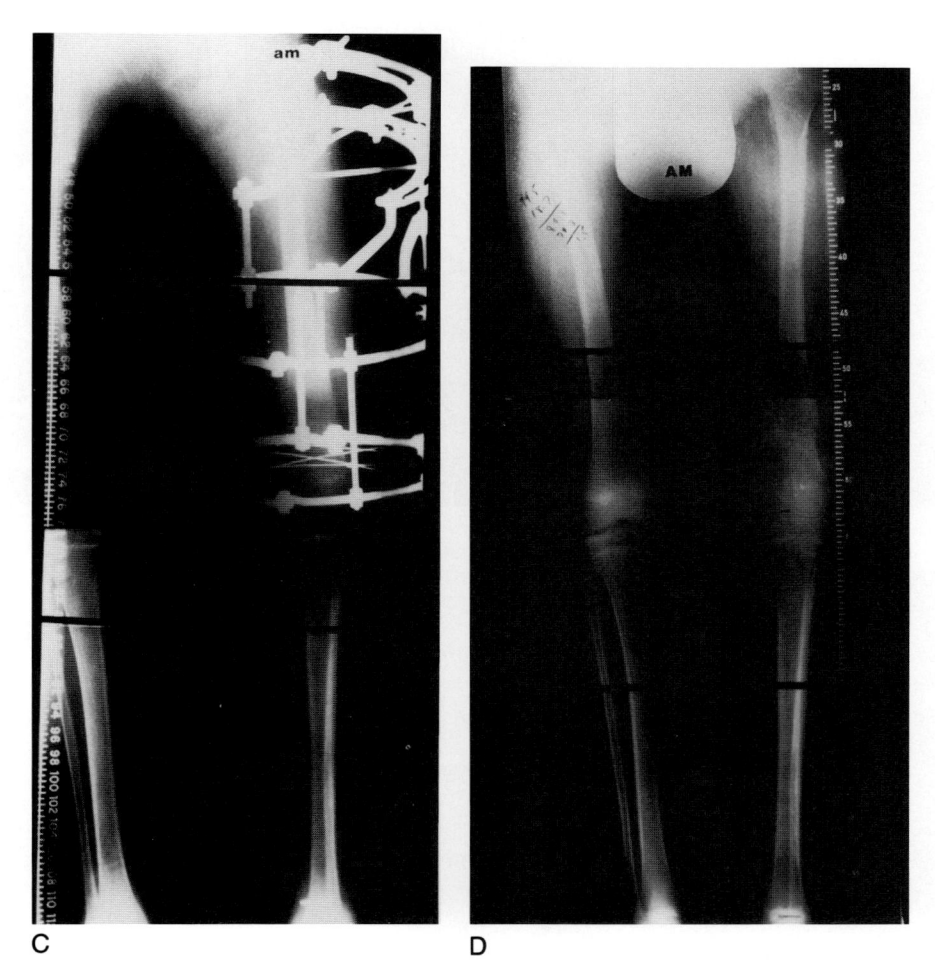

Fig. 37-9 *(Continued).* **(C&D)** Angular correction and lengthening restored limb length equality and axial alignment.

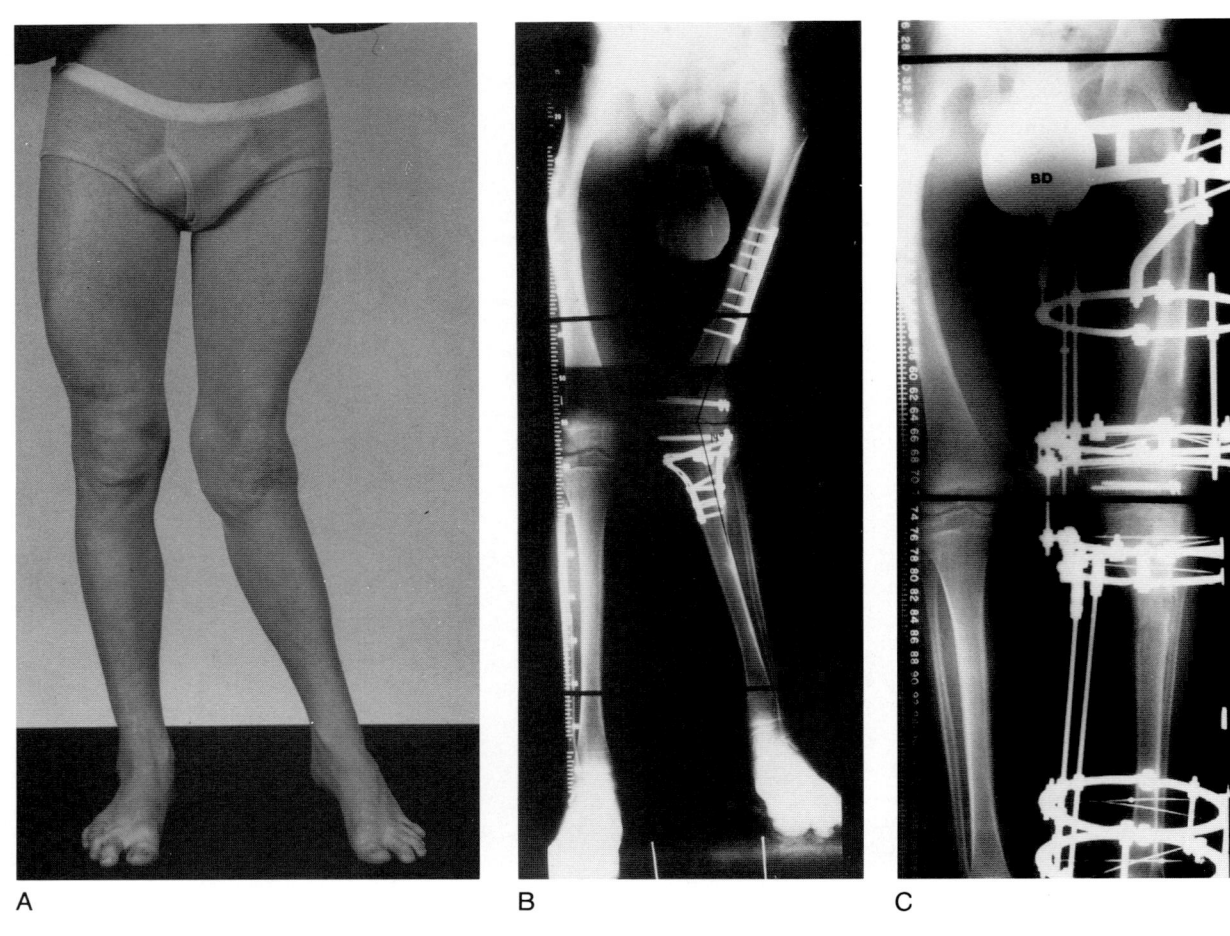

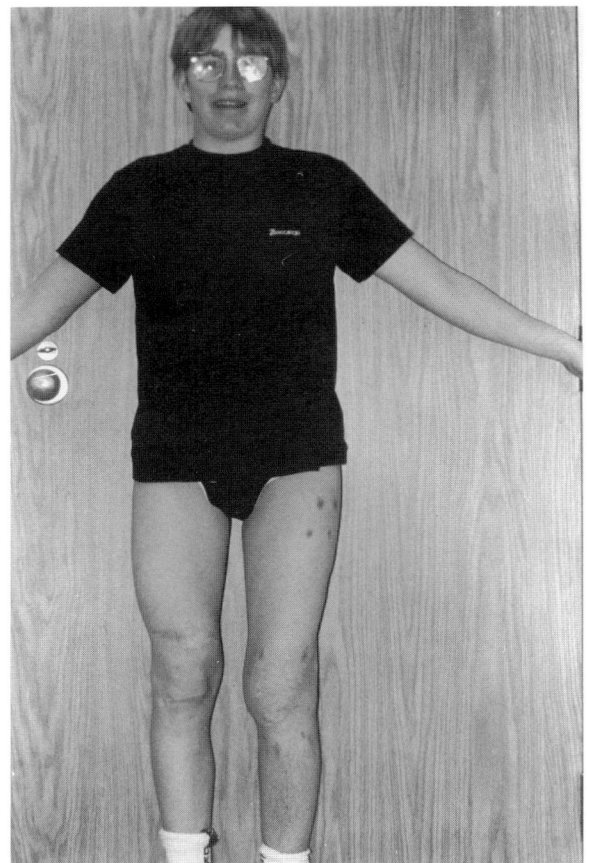

Fig. 37-10. **(A&B)** Posttraumatic lateral growth arrest of proximal tibia and distal femur resulted in severe valgus deformity and shortening in this 15-year-old boy. **(C&D)** Removal of hardware, femoral and tibial osteotomy, and correction of deformity plus lengthening restored limb alignment.

tension of the hinge concept. Adjacent limb segments must be first fixed in the usual manner with the exception that the number of wires or pins can generally be reduced by half. The limb segment should be spanned so as to provide the greatest lever arm for the correction. For example, in a knee flexion contracture, the apparatus should span the femur from below the lesser trochanter to the distal metaphysis as one would do for a standard lengthening. Similarly, the leg is fixed from the proximal to the distal metaphysis. The intervening hinges, both medial and lateral, must be coaxial and must approximate the center of rotation of the knee joint in order to be functional. Care must be taken to place the hinges in such a manner that correction of the deformity does not result in articular surface compression or in fact in joint subluxation. During correction of, for example, knee flexion or ankle equinus contracture, lateral radiographs of the joint in question are useful to assess potential translation resulting in subluxation or compression of the articular surface. Posterior distraction or anterior compression rods can then be used to achieve deformity correction. The rate of deformity correction is then directly related to the tolerance of the soft tissue, neurovascular structures, and patient discomfort.

SUMMARY

In summary, the Ilizarov technique of circular transsosseous skeletal fixation provides the ability to address the multiple problems often encountered in posttraumatic deformities in children. Limb shortening with deformity can be addressed in one operative intervention. The presence of joint contractures and/or instability does not preclude treatment. Finally, it is even possible to address the problems of nonunion or frank bone loss and to thus restore limb integrity.

REFERENCES

1. Frankel VH, Gold S, Golyakhovsky V: The Ilizarov technique. Bull Hosp Joint Dis 48:17, 1988
2. Grill F: Correction of complicated extremity deformities by external fixation. Clin Orthop 241:166, 1989
3. Ilizarov GA: The tension-stress effect on the genesis and growth of tissues: Part I. Clin Orthop 238:249, 1989
4. Ilizarov GA: The tension-stress effect on the genesis and growth of tissues: Part II. Clin Orthop 239:264, 1989
5. Leong JCY, Ma RYP, Clark JA et al: Viscoelastic behavior of tissue in leg lengthening by distraction. Clin Orthop 139:102, 1979
6. Green SA: Ilizarov external fixation: technical and anatomic considerations. Bull Hosp Joint Dis 48:28, 1988
7. Aronson J, Harison BH, Stewart CL, Harp JH: The histology of distraction osteogenesis using different external fixators. Clin Orthop 241:106, 1988
8. Aronson J, Harrison B, Boyd CM et al: Mechanical induction of osteogenesis: the importance of pin rigidity. J Pediatr Orthop 8:396, 1988
9. Kojimoto H, Yasui N, Goto T et al: Bone lengthening by callus distraction. J Bone Joint Surg [Br] 70:543, 1988
10. White SH, Kenwright J: The timing of distraction of an osteotomy. J Bone Joint Surg [Br] 72:356, 1990
11. Fleming B, Paley D, Kristiansen T, Pope M: A biomechanical analysis of the Ilizarov external fixator. Clin Orthop 241:95, 1989
12. Goodship AE, Kenwright J: The influence of induced micromovement upon the healing of experimental tibial fractures. J Bone Joint Surg [Br] 67:650, 1985
13. Tetsworth K, Krome J, Paley D: Lengthening and deformity and correction of the upper extremity by the Ilizarov technique. Orthop Clin North Am 22:689, 1991
14. Green SA: The Ilizarov method: Rancho technique. Orthop Clin North Am 22:677, 1991
15. Catagni M, Paley D, Argnani F et al: Treatment of congenital pseudarthrosis by the Ilizarov methods. Presented at the annual meeting of the American Academy of Orthopaedic Surgeons, New Orleans, Feb. 9, 1990
16. Cattaneo R, Villa A, Catagni M, Bell D: Lengthening of the humerus using the Ilizarov technique. Clin Orthop Rel Res 250:117, 1990
17. Paley D: The principle of deformity correction by the Ilizarov technique: technical aspects. Tech Orthop 4:15, 1989
18. Villa A, Paley D, Catagni M, Bell D: Lengthening of the forearm by the Ilizarov technique. Clin Orthop Rel Res 250:125, 1990
19. Ilizarov GA, Deviatov AA: Operative elongation of the leg with simultaneous correction of the deformities. Ortop Travmatol Protez 30:32, 1969

38

Fractures of the Ankle

Anthony Ashworth
Douglas Hedden

> More mistakes are made from want of a proper diagnosis than from any other reason.
> —F. G. St. Clair Strange

DESCRIPTION AND INCIDENCE

Injuries about the ankle occur while the child's foot is in contact with the ground, the relationship between the foot below and the leg and torso above determining the pattern of injury that will occur. The translation of force through the foot depends upon the structure and mobility of the foot. The cavovarus foot, for example, is more predisposed to inversion-type injuries than is the pronated foot. Likewise, the foot with limited hindfoot motion will transmit forces proximally, especially those of inversion and eversion, to a greater degree than will the flexible foot.

In the study by Mizuta and colleagues[1] of almost 2,000 fractures in children, 7 percent occurred about the ankle. Of these, 34 percent involved either the distal tibial or distal fibular physis. Furthermore, of the 353 physeal injuries included in their study, only injuries at the distal end of the radius (28.3 percent) or involving the phalanges of the fingers (25.8 percent) were more common than those involving the distal tibial physis (9.4 percent).

Not surprisingly, a significant proportion of injuries about the ankle occur during participation in athletics. Jumping sports such as basketball frequently cause inversion-type injuries as the athlete plants the plantar-flexed foot. Goldberg and Aadalen,[2] in their study of 53 fractures of the distal tibial physis, reported that almost two-thirds of the injuries they studied occurred while their patients were participating in athletics.

ANATOMY

The ankle joint is essentially a hinge. The following anatomic features are important when considering injuries in this area:

1. The dome of the talus is wider anteriorly. More rotatory and translational motion may occur within the joint when the foot is plantar-flexed, hence injury to the ankle is more common in this position (Fig. 38-1).
2. The level of the distal fibular physis is the same as is the tibiotalar joint and is thus exposed to stress with inversion and eversion of this joint (Fig. 38-2A).
3. The lateral malleolus extends more distally than does the medial. Thus, the medial malleolus is more likely to function as a pivot point when the foot is inverted, whereas the lateral malleolus functions as a solid barrier to eversion. Angular forces applied in eversion, with the distal tibiofibular ligament as a hinge, may cause fracturing in the distal fibular diaphysis (Fig. 38-2C).
4. The anteroinferior tibiofibular ligament serves as a firm attachment between the anteromedial epiphysis of the tibia and the fibula. This is an important structure contributing to the fracture of Tillaux (Fig. 38-3).
5. The distal tibial physis closes first centrally, then medially and finally anterolaterally. This phenomenon thus predisposes the lateral physis to epiphyseal plate injuries well into the teens (Fig. 38-4).

Posterior

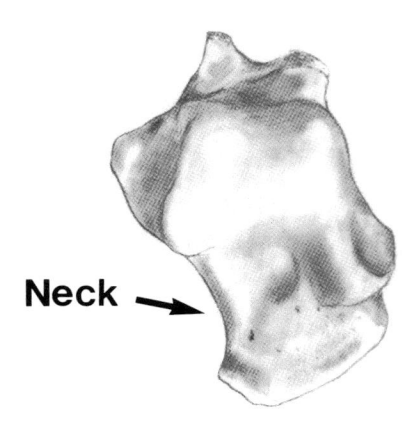

Neck →

Fig. 38-1. The dome of the talus from above. Note that the articular surface is wider anteriorly. The ability to dorsiflex will be limited if the mortise is narrowed. The ankle joint is more unstable in plantar flexion.

6. The anterior talofibular and calcaneofibular ligaments provide resistance to excessive inversion or pivoting under the tip of the medial malleolus. When stressed, these structures generate a distracting force on the lateral aspect of the distal fibular physis.
7. The deltoid ligament, with its deep and superficial fibers, applies a distraction force to the medial malleolus on eversion.
8. Accessory ossification centers, which may be confused with fractures, are often present in the distal tibia and fibula, most commonly at the tip of the medial malleolus (Fig. 38-5). Ogden and Lee[3] surveyed a large number of radiographs, obtained for various reasons. They identified 61 cases of accessory ossification involving the medial malleolus and 19 cases involving the lateral. In addition, 23 children had accessory ossification centers present in both malleoli. They pointed out that a "smooth appearance on both sides of the radiolucency" usually differentiates this growth variant from an acute fracture.

MECHANISM OF INJURY

The mechanism of an individual injury can usually be postulated from the radiologic picture. In describing the mechanism causing an injury about the ankle, one usually refers to the position of the foot relative to the mortise.

As the foot is invariably in contact with the ground at the moment of impact, some degree of axial force is always present. Angular, and often rotational forces, occur concomitantly in most injuries. Severe axial compression may damage the resting and dividing cells of the physis with resulting future growth disturbance—the Salter-Harris type V injury.

Inversion is the most common injuring force. It may cause injuries with the relatively mild severity of a "sprain" of the lateral ligamentous complex of the ankle to the more serious oblique fracture of the medial malleolus that disrupts both the physis and the articular surface. In children, however, the ligamentous attachment to bone via Sharpey's fibers is usually much stronger than the epiphyseal plate, hence growth plate injuries are more common than ligamentous strains (Fig. 38-6).

Eversion injuries are less common. As the deltoid ligaments are stronger in the child than is the physis, the usual injury occurs through the physis, often with a fracture of the fibula occurring proximal to the physis. Occasionally the medial malleolus may be avulsed through the epiphysis.

Force applied in dorsiflexion is not common. When it does occur, it is most likely to cause a fracture of the tibial metaphysis or talus.

The plantar-flexed foot stressed translationally in the anteroposterior direction may result in a fracture through the distal tibial physis, almost always with a large posterior metaphyseal fragment attached. The fibula may or may not fracture, and in the younger child may undergo plastic deformation. Such deformation can cause difficulties in reduction.

Rotatory forces are seen typically in the triplane fracture and in the fracture of Tillaux. Both of these injuries tend to occur in teenaged children who have undergone the early stages of distal tibial physeal closure.

CLASSIFICATION

Injuries about the ankle may be classified in several ways. An anatomic approach, with reference to the site of major involvement, is simple and practical:

1. Metaphyseal fractures
2. Physeal injuries
3. Epiphyseal fractures
4. Ligamentous injuries
   a. Sprains
   b. Disruptions

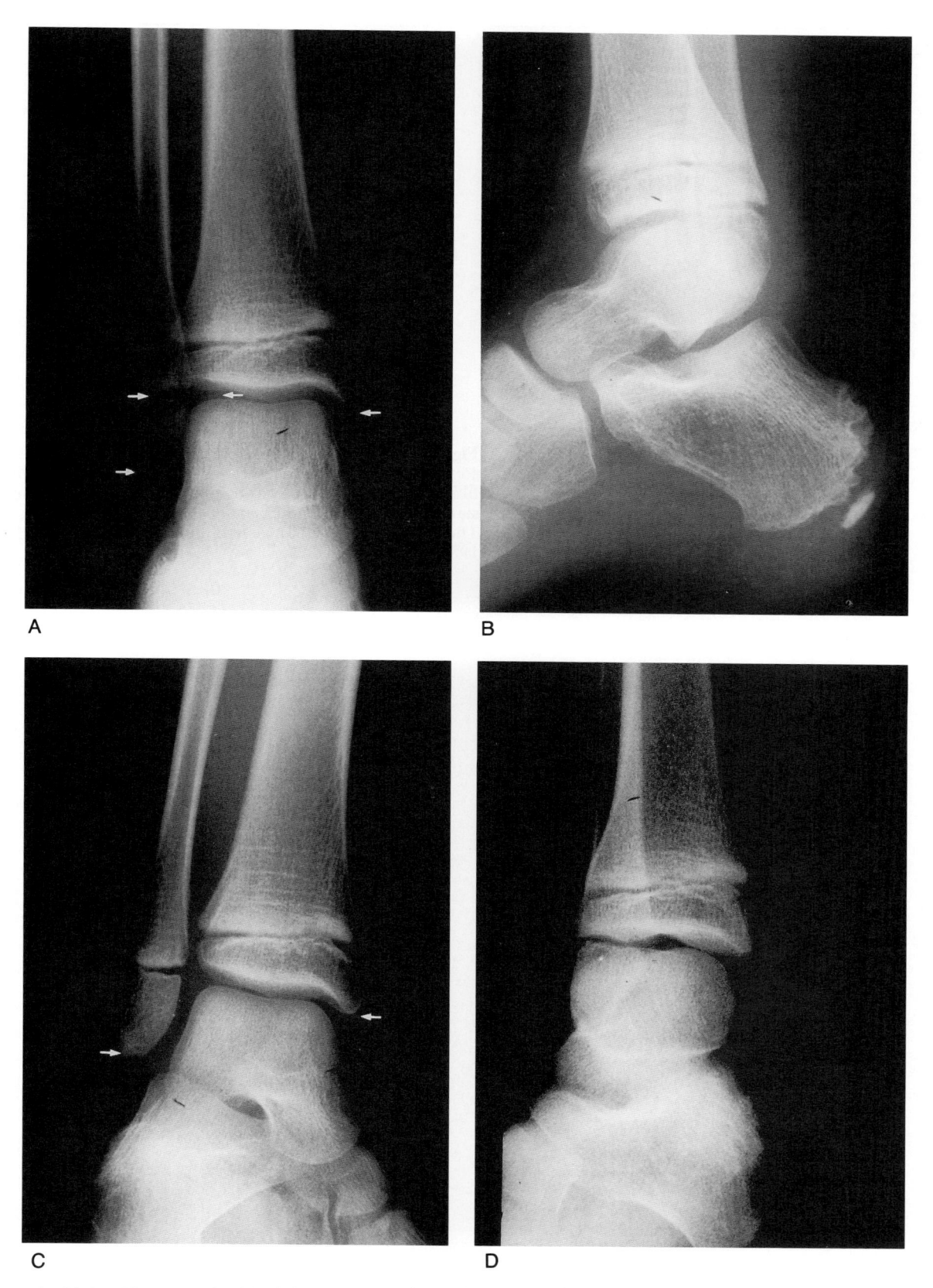

Fig. 38-2. The normal ankle. **(A)** Anteroposterior, **(B)** lateral, **(C)** internal oblique (mortise), and **(D)** external oblique views provide complete visualization of the various surfaces.

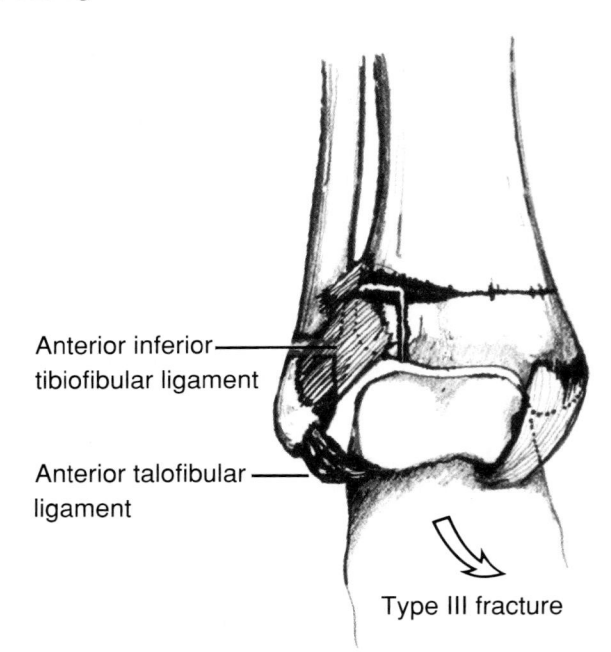

Fig. 38-3. The anterior inferior tibiofibular ligament. Everson and external rotation forces will be transmitted to the distal tibial epiphysis. The latter is of special importance in understanding the Tillaux and triplane fractures. (From Letts M: The hidden adolescent ankle fracture. J Pediatr Orthop 2:161, 1982, with permission.)

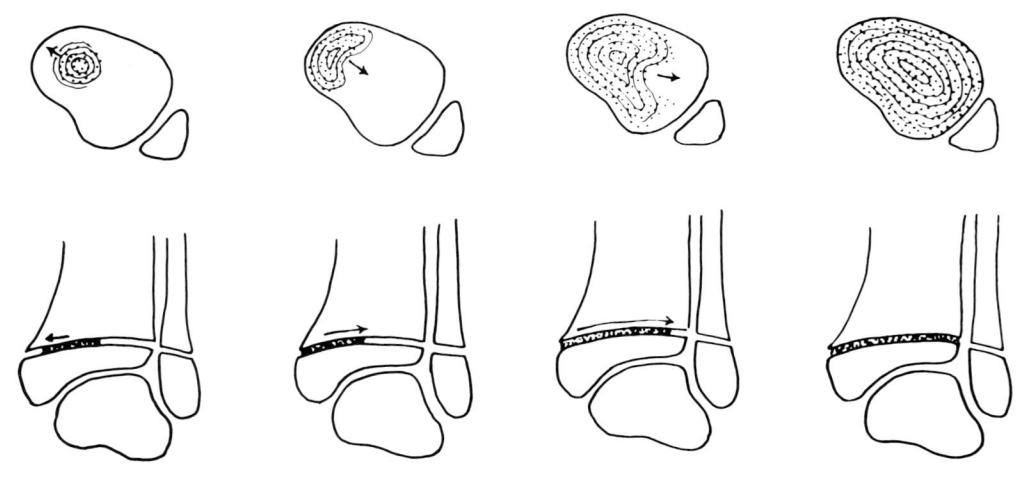

Fig. 38-4. The distal tibial physis begins to fuse centrally, proceeds medially, and finally laterally. The lateral physis therefore remains open and vulnerable to physeal fracture into late adolescence. (From Feldman F et al: Distal tibial triplane fractures: diagnosis with CT. Radiology 164:429, 1987, with permission.)

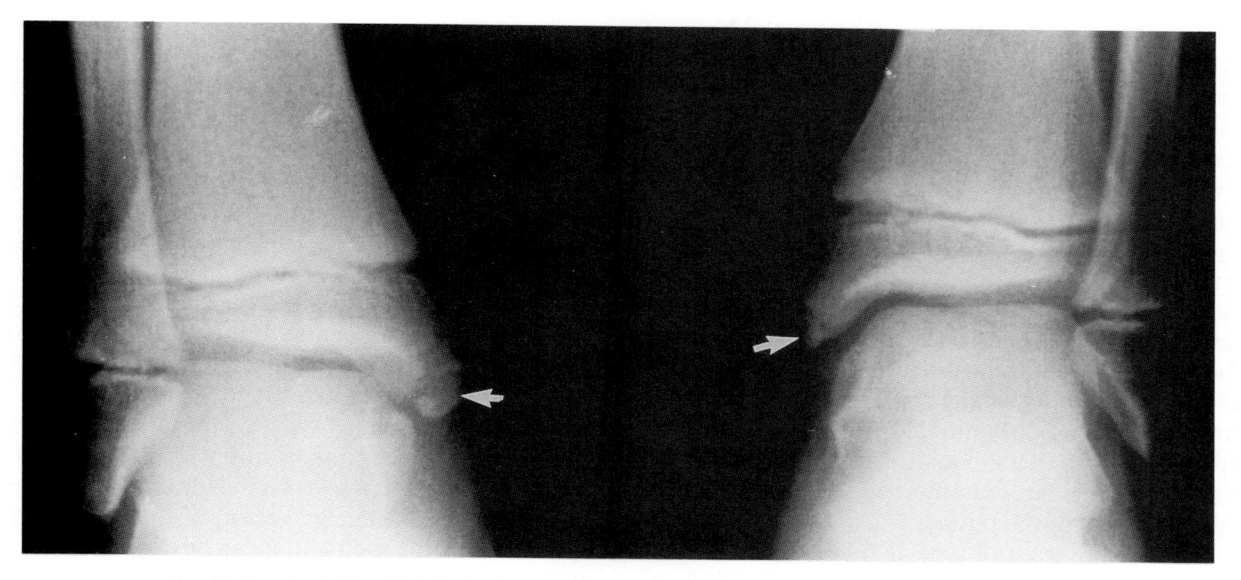

Fig. 38-5. A child with bilateral accessory ossification centers of the medial malleolus.

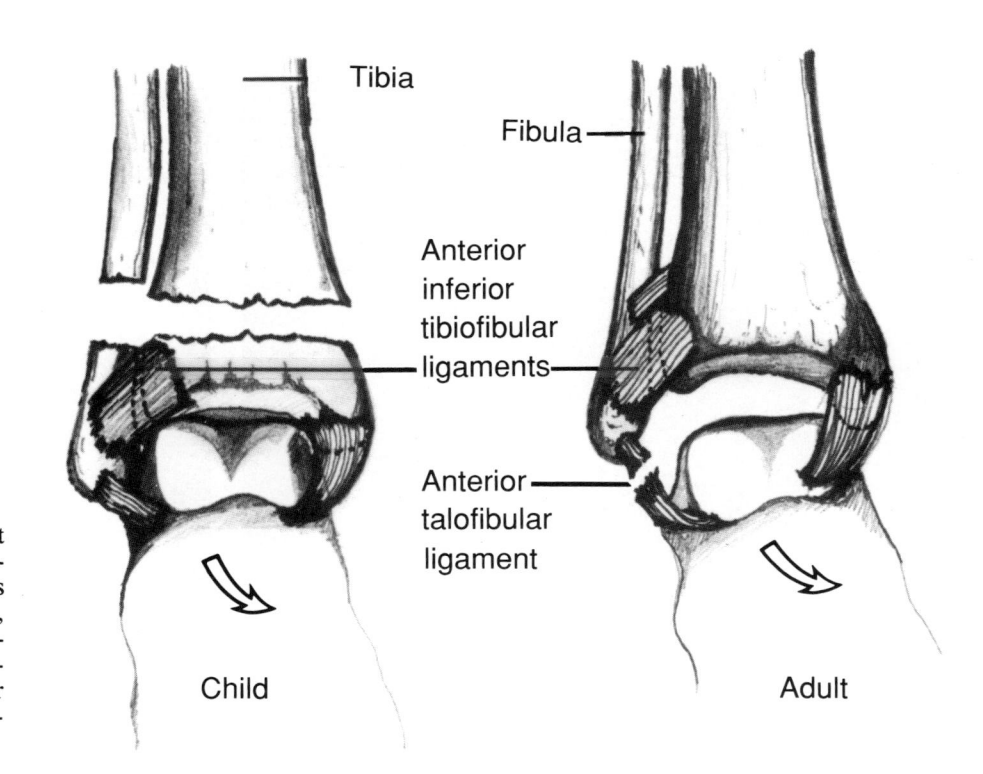

Fig. 38-6. In children the adjacent physis is weaker than the ankle ligaments, hence sprains or partial tears of ankle ligaments are uncommon, whereas physeal injuries are common. (From Letts M: The hidden adolescent ankle fracture. J Pediatr Orthop 2:161, 1982, with permission.)

The injuries may also be classified on the basis of deforming forces. Most authors have used this approach to classify adult fractures of the ankle, with varying degrees of complexity, such as Johnson and Fahl[4] or Lauge-Hansen.[5] Dias and Tachdjian[6] have devised a pediatric classification. Though angular forces tend to predominate, rotation often plays a significant role.

The most important classification of growth plate injury about the ankle is that of Salter and Harris.[7] The importance of their classification is its implications for management and prognosis.

Their type I physeal injury is most commonly seen as an avulsion-type injury of the distal fibula, but may also occur as the result of rotational force (Fig. 38-7). It is commonly seen in metabolic disorders such as rickets, where the physis is structurally weak because of the increased thickness of the physis.

As in most physes, the type II fracture is the most common (Fig. 38-8). About the ankle it results from many patterns of injury. Fortunately, with appropriate reduction, growth disturbance and angular deformity seldom occur unless associated with high velocity forces producing a concomitant type V injury.

Type III fractures are uncommon except in teenagers. A classic type III fracture is that of Tillaux, occurring in teenagers, who are close to skeletal maturity with partial fusion of the tibial growth plate leaving the lateral physis open and vulnerable to the type III injury. Type III fractures other than that of Tillaux can occur, though uncommonly (Fig. 38-9).

The type IV fracture about the ankle is often seen as a part of the triplane fracture. It may also occur as a result of a shearing force on the medial malleolus with inversion of the ankle (Fig. 38-10).

Fortunately, isolated type V injuries, which may not be identified at the time of initial evaluation, are rare. They are the result of severe axial force that has not been dissipated by an angular vector. If the plafond is not comminuted, the radiograph can be expected to be normal. It is assumed that these injuries occur when the traumatic force is sufficient to devitalize the resting and dividing cells of the physis. These injuries may lead to

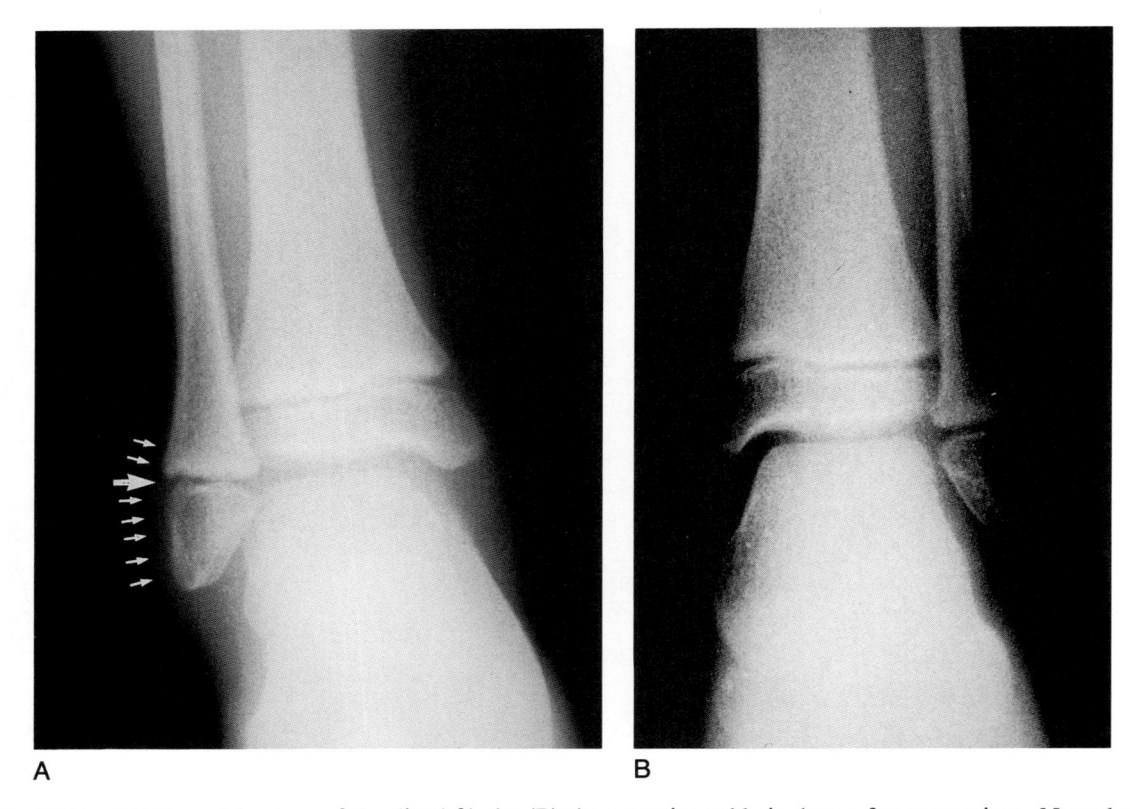

Fig. 38-7. **(A)** Type I fracture of the distal fibula; **(B)** the opposite ankle is shown for comparison. Note the localized swelling that coincided with the site of maximum tenderness (arrows). Often a small fragment of metaphysis is visible, indicating a type II fracture. Though a stress view in inversion would prove the injury, it is unnecessary for management and probably meddlesome.

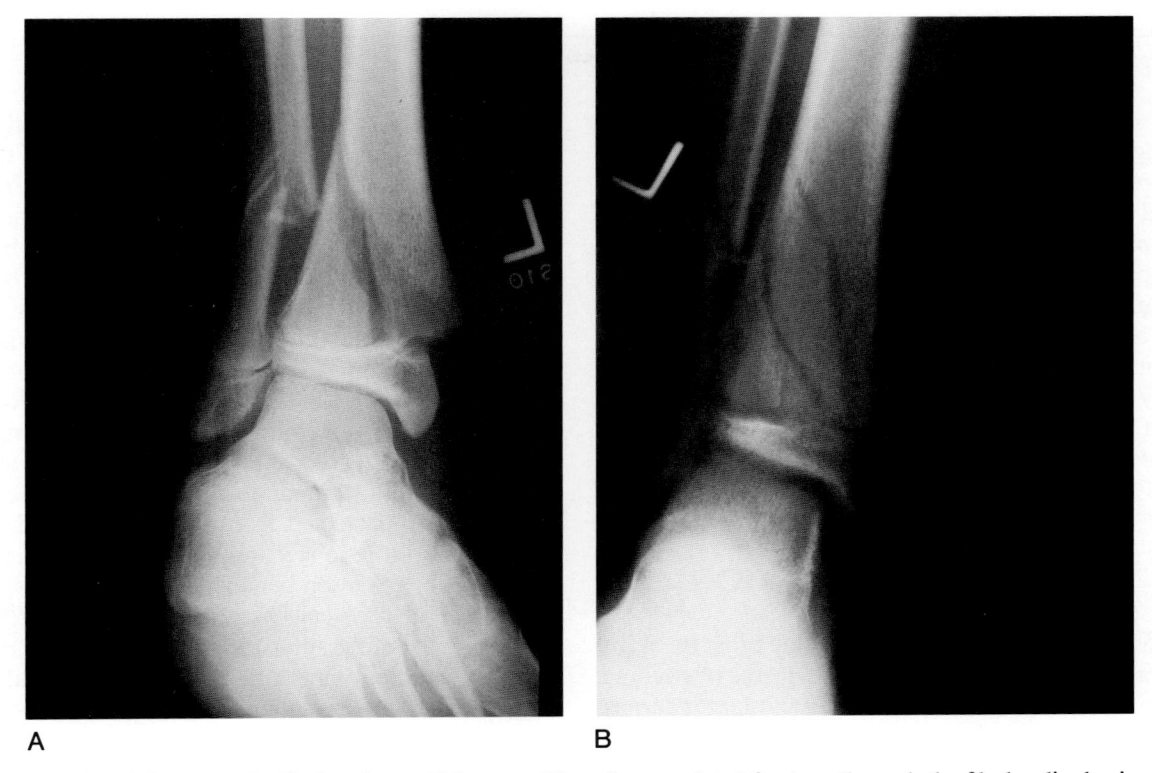

Fig. 38-8. (A) A severely displaced type II fracture. Note the associated fracture through the fibular diaphysis. (B) As is usually the case, the injury was managed successfully by closed reduction.

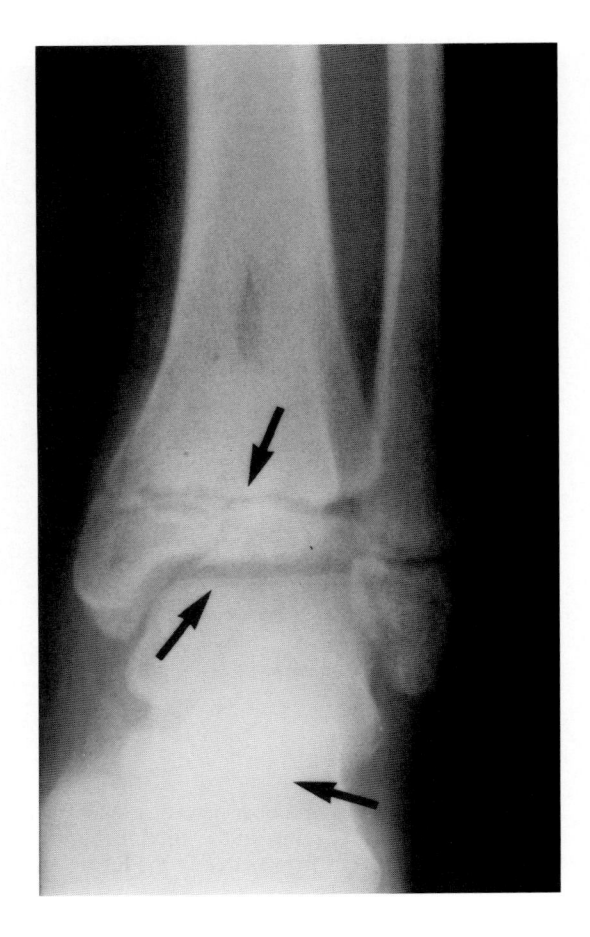

Fig. 38-9. Type III fracture in a 10-year-old boy. Note the widening of the physis laterally. The *arrows* depict the lines of force that produced this physeal injury.

partial or complete cessation of growth. Longitudinal and angular deformities may result. If only the central cells are destroyed, as growth continues peripherally, physeal "tenting" and incongruity of the joint surface develop.

A type VI fracture has been described associated with degloving of the perichondrium (Fig. 38-11). This removes a source of growth plate cells and also can lead to a bony bridge that can subsequently produce angular deformity with growth. This injury may be caused by any trauma that can deglove the skin and perichondrium such as a lawnmower or a bicycle-spoke injury (Fig. 38-12).

PHYSICAL EXAMINATION

As in the case of all injuries, the ankle must be examined with care in the acute state. The degree of swelling, its specific location, and the site of maximal tenderness are important factors in decision-making. As in all situations, it is best to gain the confidence of the child by commencing one's examination at a distance from the area of primary pain and tenderness. A careful physical examination, as well as an understanding of the likely forces applied at the time of injury, is essential in making a primary decision as to the level of intervention that is appropriate. The grossly swollen ankle, even in the absence of radiologic evidence of bony injury, is best managed by immobilization. Not only does this provide maximum comfort for the child, but it also will help to limit swelling. As children are not prone to joint stiffness, except about the elbow, immobilization is seldom contraindicated. Upon coming out of a cast, the child can be expected to return to full activity and thus be at risk for further trauma immediately. Children, therefore, often have to be "protected from themselves" and, as such, erring on a little longer immobilization to ensure complete healing is often beneficial.

A careful physical examination should precede the ordering of radiographs. It is only through the identification of the sites of swelling and tenderness that one can appreciate the area of maximal injury and thus order the appropriate films. Emergency care may appear to be speeded by the ordering of radiographs by a triage person. However, if this is done without an adequate physi-

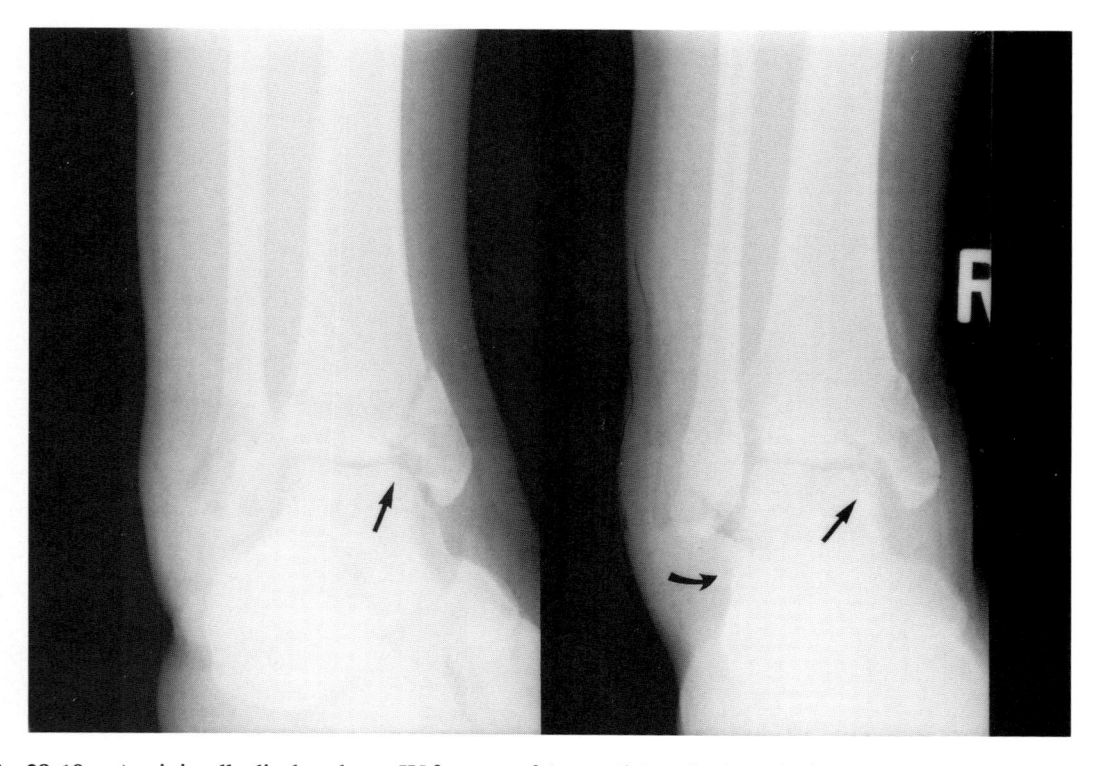

Fig. 38-10. A minimally displaced type IV fracture of the medial malleolus. The internal oblique (mortise) view allows better visualization of the fracture. Note the soft tissue swelling adjacent to the fibular physis suggestive of a type I fracture. The *arrows* depict the forces producing these injuries.

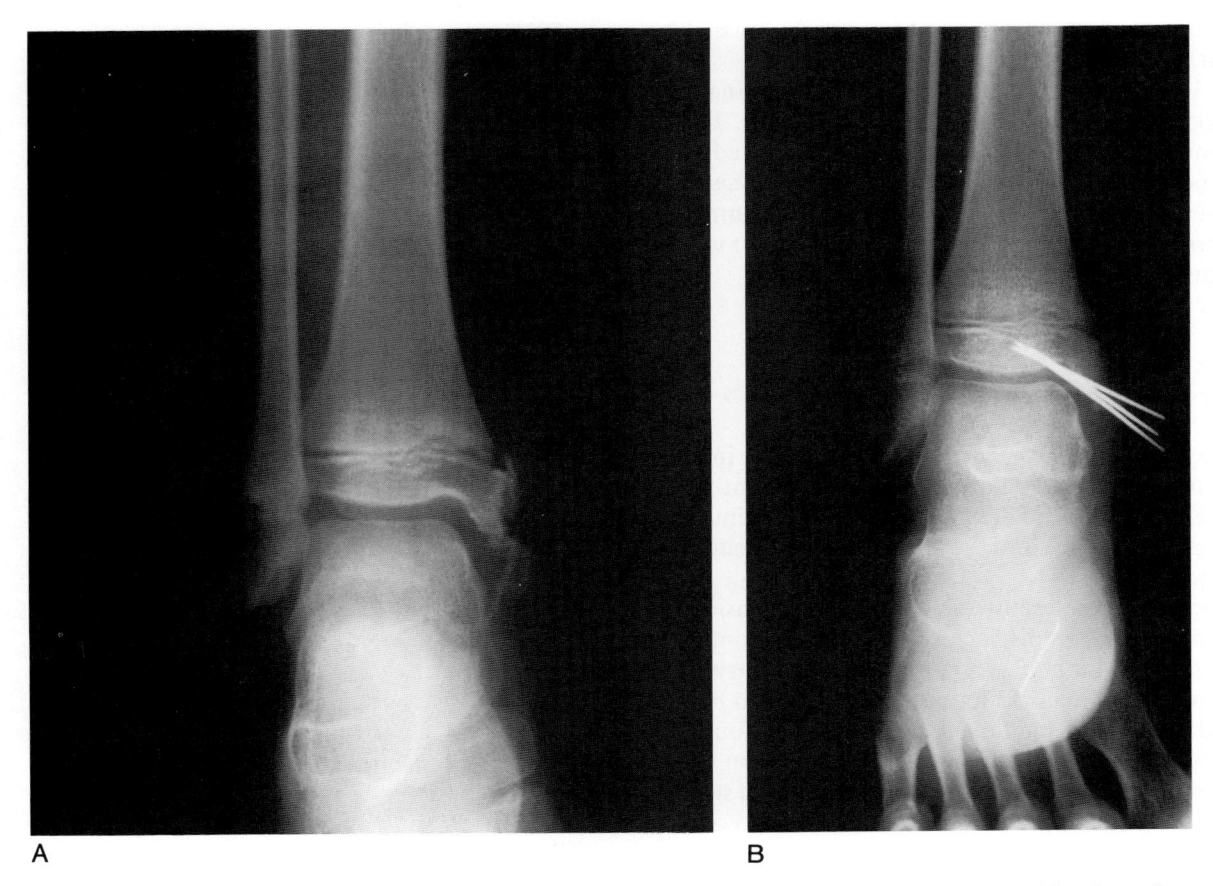

Fig. 38-11. (A) A shearing type VI periosteal avulsion with some subchondral bone secondary to a bicycle-spoke injury. (B) The periosteal fragment was replaced and held with three Kirschner wires avoiding an almost certain medial tethering bar.

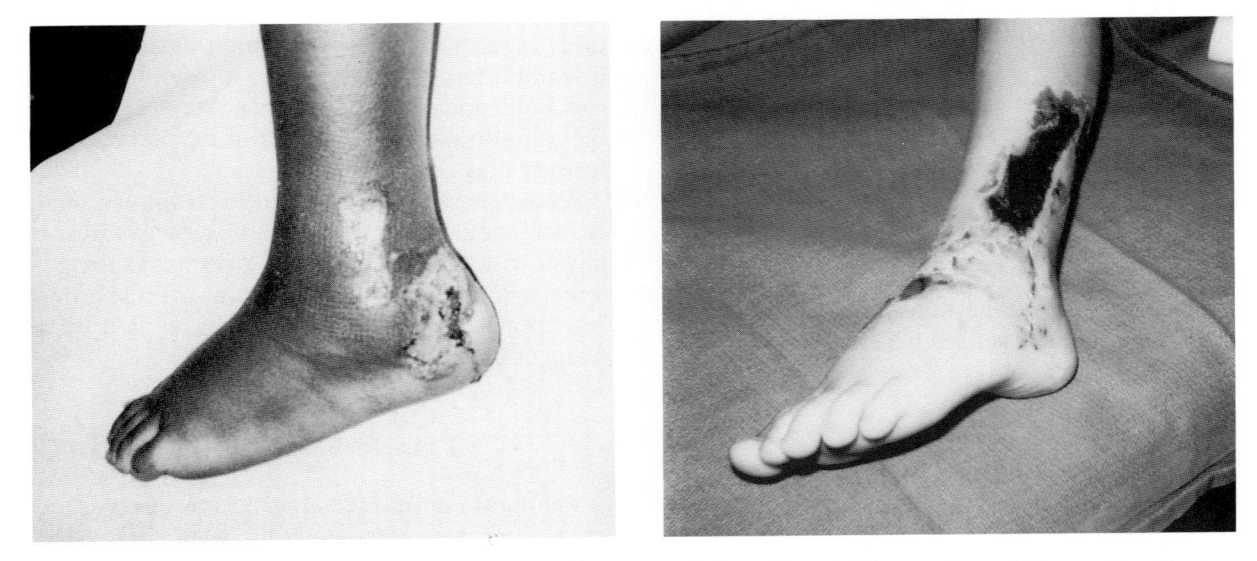

Fig. 38-12. Bicycle-spoke injury of foot and ankle may result in periosteal injury to the periphery of the distal fibular or tibial growth plate—the so-called type VI epiphyseal injury described by Mercer Rang.

cal examination, not only will injuries be missed but repeat films will be often required.

An important adjunct to the physical examination is the appreciation of swelling on the radiograph. Though the physis may not appear to be disrupted, radiologic evidence of swelling at the location of the physis, coincident with the clinical appreciation of maximum point tenderness at that site, will avoid the failure to identify and treat a type I fracture of the distal fibula.

DIFFERENTIAL DIAGNOSIS

The radiograph is the most important factor in differentiating injuries. Fractures with displacement should be easily recognized. Those without displacement can be suspected on the basis of the location of soft tissue swelling and tenderness.

If no displaced fracture exists one must consider the possibility of an undisplaced fracture, as is commonly seen in the distal fibula, or a ligamentous injury. If the swelling is minimal it is unlikely that the child has sustained a major ligamentous injury. When in doubt, immobilize the limb in a walking cast with review in 1 week; children are not prone to permanent ankle joint stiffness.

If the patient returns for follow-up of what was diagnosed as a sprain of the lateral ligaments and there is ecchymosis extending to the toes, assume that there has been total disruption of the anterior talofibular ligament. Ecchymosis does not extend to the toes unless the short extensor compartment is violated. There must be significant tearing of the lateral ligamentous attachments at the site of their insertion to cause extension of the ecchymosis.

TREATMENT OF SPECIFIC ANKLE INJURIES

Though multiple configurations and combinations of injuries may occur about the ankle joint, the most common patterns seen are discussed here in relation to their major deforming force.

Dorsiflexion Injuries

The most common injury pattern that results from this type of force is a metaphyseal fracture with a greenstick fracture of the posterior cortex (Fig. 38-13).

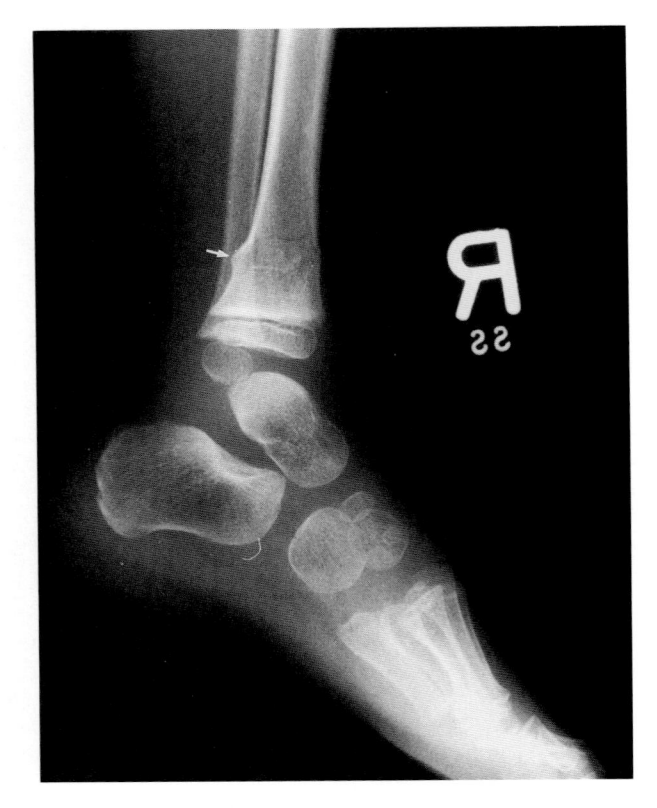

Fig. 38-13. A greenstick metaphyseal fracture. This particular injury did not require reduction.

This fracture, except in the rare case of complete displacement, is usually managed by closed reduction. The deformity, having a tendency to recur, is best immobilized in a cast with the foot in plantar-flexion. In addition, it is important to mould the cast carefully beneath the calf and tendoachilles. If this is not done, as the inevitable calf atrophy occurs, posterior sag and recurrent deformity may develop.

As the physis is not involved in this injury, abnormal growth should not occur due to growth arrest of the physis. If a small degree (5–15 degrees) of angulation remains in the actively growing child, future growth can be expected to correct the angulation, as it lies in the plane of the ankle joint.

Plantar-Flexion Injuries

The most common plantar-flexion injury is a type II physeal fracture that tends to have a large posterior metaphyseal fragment attached to the intact physeo-epiphyseal segment (Fig. 38-14). Often there is a small

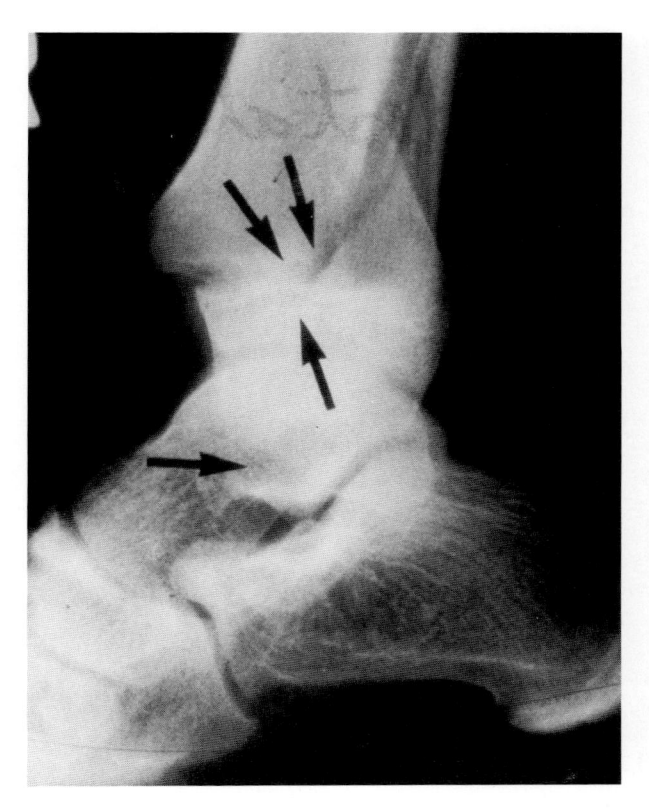

Fig. 38-14. A type II fracture. Downward force of the body weight is countered by upward and posterior forces on the planted foot (arrows). This is a common fracture encountered in skateboarders.

amount of rotation, usually internal, of the distal fragment. Less commonly a metaphyseal fracture, similar to that which was described in the previous section, may occur (Fig. 38-13). This injury is best immobilized with the ankle joint in neutral or slight dorsiflexion, tightening the flexor hallucis longus over the posterior fragment.

A particular problem in reduction occurs when plastic deformation of the fibula occurs at the time of tibial fracturing. This can be very difficult to reduce. The extreme force that may be required to accomplish reduction in this instance can place the physis at risk. In these extreme situations an osteotomy of the fibula may be necessary in order to accomplish an adequate reduction. Once the fracture is reduced, as in most type II physeal injuries, the reduction is usually quite stable. Overreduction is almost impossible due to the presence of the posterior metaphyseal fragment and the periosteum that is usually intact posteriorly as well. The ankle should be immobilized in neutral or slight dorsiflexion. The flexor hallucis will assist in preventing posterior displacement in this position.

With these injuries it is rare for subsequent growth disturbance to occur.

Eversion Injuries

Severe eversion places a lateralizing force on the distal fibula. In the child, the most common injury pattern is that of a Salter-Harris type II fracture of the tibia that usually includes a posterolateral metaphyseal fragment. The fibula, being firmly attached distally to the tibial epiphysis through the anterior tibiofibular ligament, tends to fracture about the distal diaphyseometaphyseal junction. A rotatory force that is insufficient to disrupt the tibia may be sufficient to produce a spiral fracture of the fibula alone (Fig. 38-15).

A variant of this injury occurs when the deltoid ligaments avulse the medial malleolus. The fracture line is usually transverse. This injury should not be mistaken for an accessory ossification center, as these are usually round and bear little resemblance to the sharp outline seen in an acute fracture (Fig. 38-16).

Inversion Injuries

The most common group of injuries about the ankle are those that occur when the dominant force is that of inversion. A variety of patterns are seen, from the mild ligamentous sprain of the talo- and calcaneofibular ligaments to the type IV fracture of the medial malleolus.

As the normal subtalar joint allows for a greater degree of inversion than eversion, a greater degree of medial displacement of the foot below the mortise can occur as axial force is applied. This may lead to complete tearing of the anterolateral ligaments of the ankle, a distraction (type I) injury to the distal fibular physis, or the rare transverse fracture through the distal fibular epiphysis itself (Fig. 38-17). A type II fracture of the distal tibial physis is usually accompanied either by a distraction injury to the fibular physis or a shearing injury to the medial malleolus. This latter injury tends to have a Salter-Harris type IV pattern and usually requires open reduction.

Both eversion and inversion injuries are usually managed by closed reduction, unless the joint surface is violated.

When a Salter-Harris type III or IV pattern is a component of the injury, displacement is almost always present. If the position of the fracture fragment in rela-

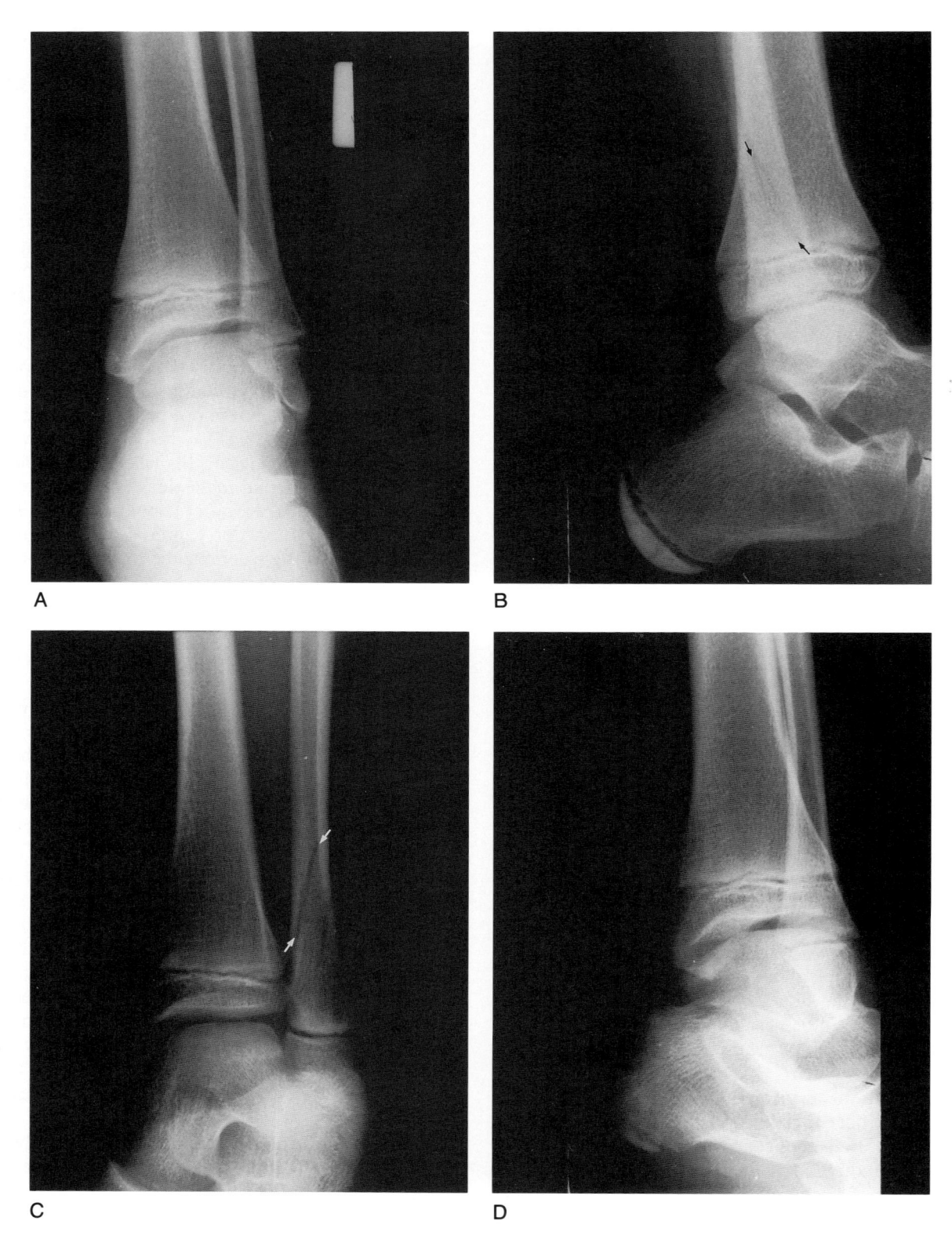

Fig. 38-15. A spiral fracture of the distal fibula. **(A)** Anteroposterior, **(B)** lateral, **(C)** internal oblique, and **(D)** external oblique views. Note that the fracture is clearly visible in Fig. C, barely in Fig. B, and not at all in Figs. A and D, emphasizing the need for oblique views in ankle trauma in children.

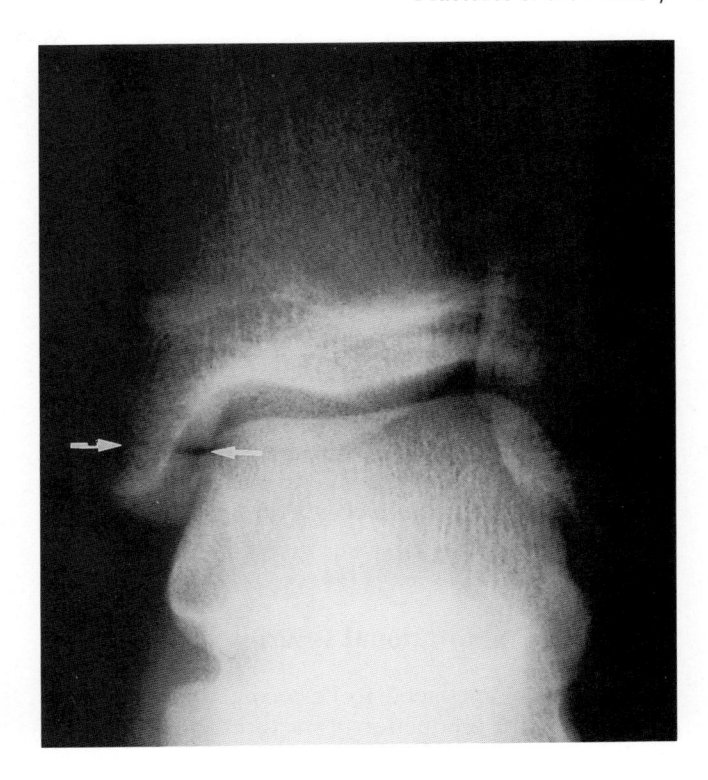

Fig. 38-16. A transverse fracture across the medial malleolus. This injury with its sharp outline, should not be confused with an accessory ossification center.

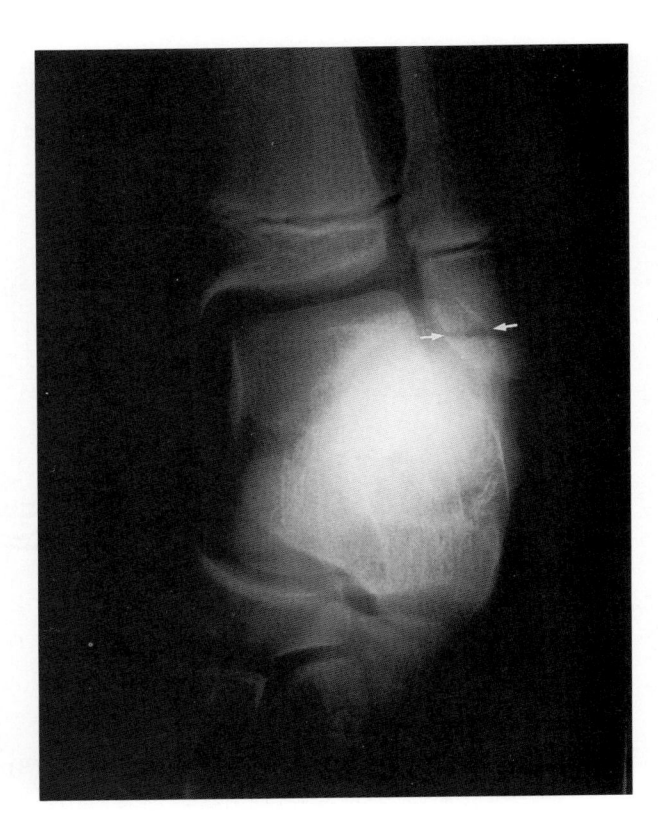

Fig. 38-17. A transverse fracture across the lateral malleolus. This uncommon fracture, being intra-articular, is one of the few lateral malleolar fractures that may require open reduction.

tion to the physis and the articular surface is not anatomic, open reduction is recommended. Although a type III fracture fragment may be stable following a closed reduction, a type IV fragment is not. In this circumstance, the reduction may be maintained using a single screw through the metaphyseal fragment into the body of the metaphysis itself (Fig. 38-18) or across the epiphysis. In instances where the metaphyseal fragment is small, or in type III injuries, it may be appropriate to place a small screw or two Kirschner wires transversely across the fracture line in the epiphysis (Fig. 38-19). If the child's growth is almost complete, fixation across the physis is not contraindicated (Fig. 38-20). Fractures through the distal fibula rarely require open reduction in children. An exception to this is the uncommon instance when a transverse fracture occurs through the distal fibular epiphysis.

Rotational Injuries

Rotational forces tend to be secondary rather than dominant in the production of fractures about the ankle in children. Two particular injuries, however, have an important rotational element in their occurrence. These are the fracture of Tillaux and the triplane fracture.

The Fracture of Tillaux

The Tillaux fracture almost always occurs in the adolescent within a year of complete closure of the distal tibial physis. As it is the lateral aspect of this structure that fuses last, a distraction force translated to the anterolateral aspect of the tibial physis through the anterior tibiofibular ligament may cause a Salter-Harris type III injury. Central closure of the tibial physis maintains the integrity of the major part of the epiphyseometaphyseal relationship. As the fibula rotates externally in relation to the tibia, a rectangular or pie-shaped defect, which is wider anteriorly, results (Fig. 38-21). A mortise view is essential with this fracture as the fibula may obstruct its visualization (Fig. 38-22). This fracture may reduce with internal rotation of the foot but if good reduction is not obtained, open reduction should be performed. This is an anterior fracture and can easily be dealt with through an anterolateral approach.

This adolescent version of the Tillaux fracture was well described by Kleiger and Mankin.[8] It is of interest that, on careful scrutiny of their illustrations, one of their cases appears to have been a triplane fracture as later described by Marmor.[9]

The need for a thorough radiographic examination of the ankle area, including a mortise view, cannot be over-

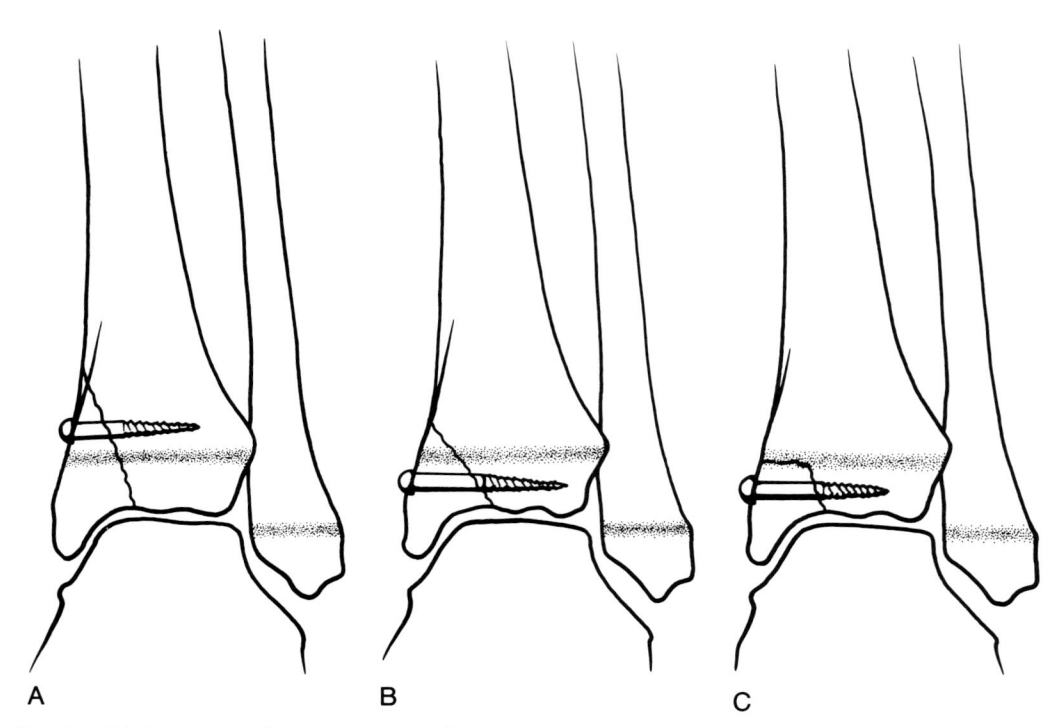

Fig. 38-18. (A) Transmetaphyseal screw fixation. (B) Trans-epiphyseal screw fixation (Type IV). (C) Transepiphyseal screw fixation (Type III).

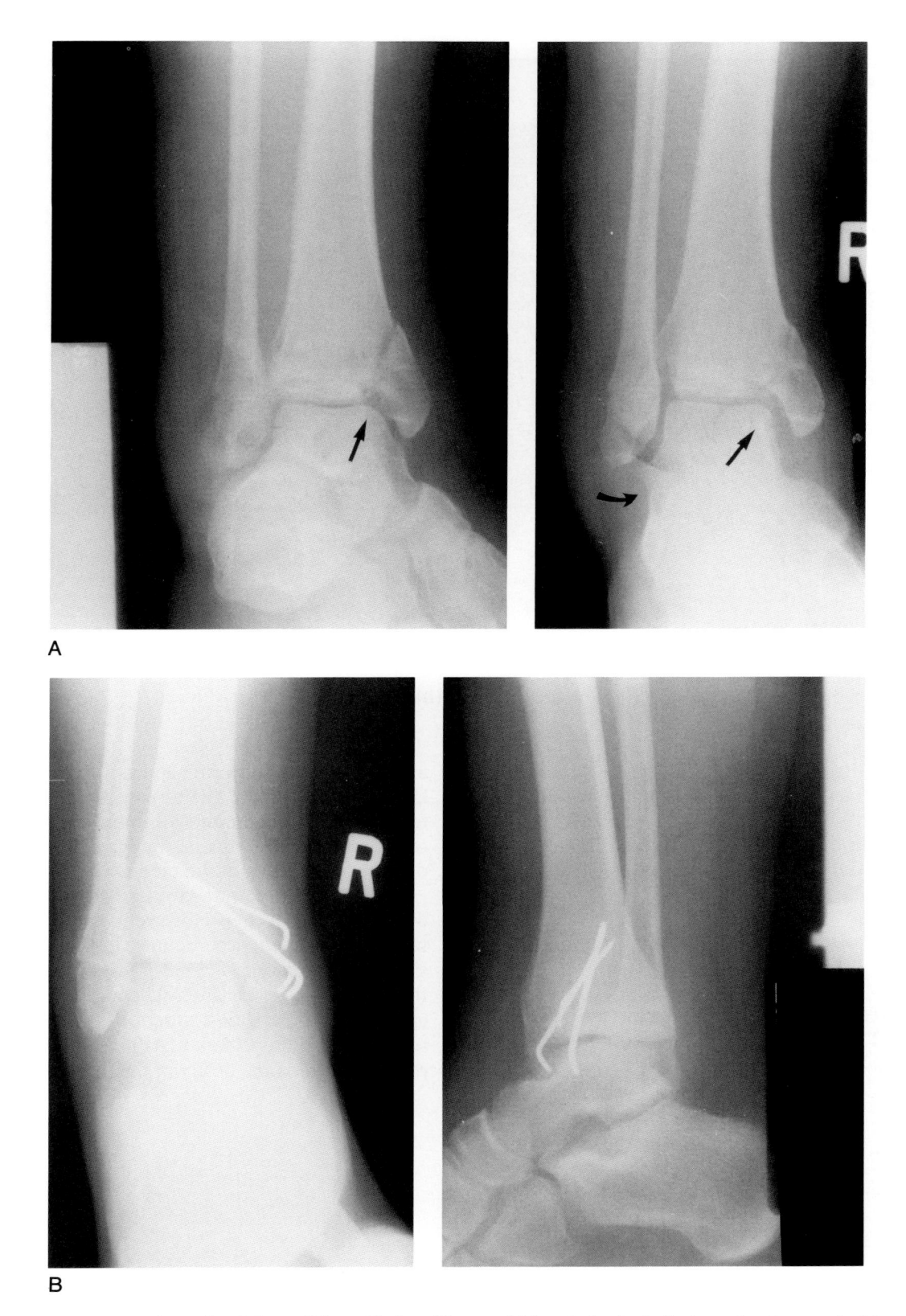

Fig. 38-19. (A) An inversion injury of the ankle in a 13-year-old female basketball player that has resulted in a type IV shear fracture of the medial malleolus and a type I fracture of the fibula. (B) An open reduction with smooth Kirschner wire fixation. *Arrows* show direction of force.

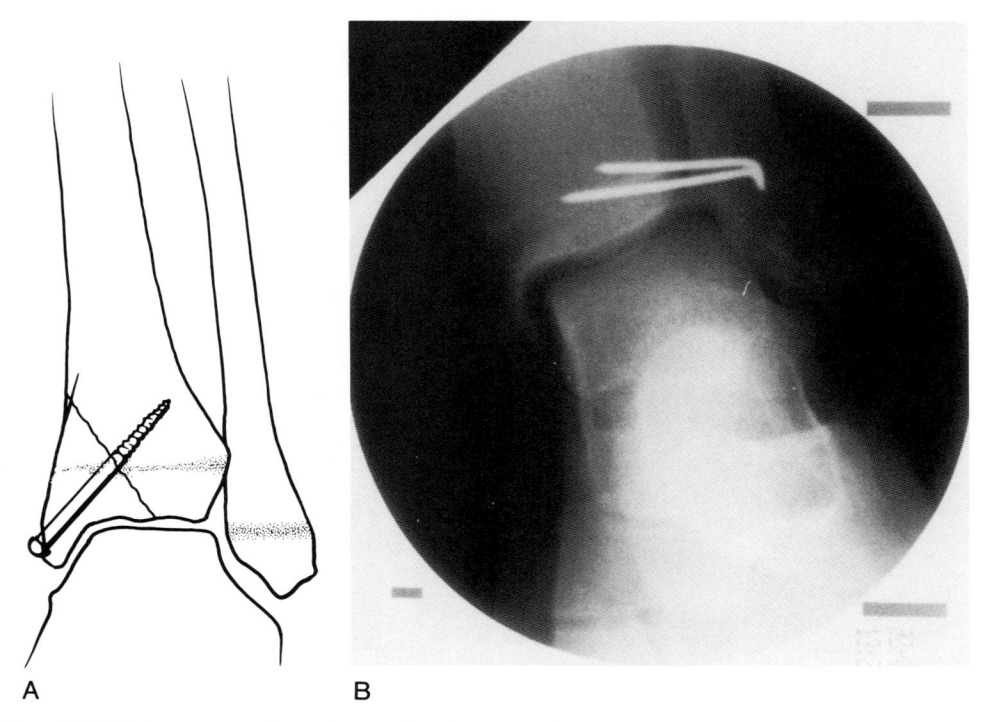

Fig. 38-20. (A) Epiphyseometaphyseal screw fixation. (B) Tillaux fracture fixed with two Kirschner wires.

emphasized. Beaty and Russell,[10] in their description of an unusual fracture of the medial malleolus, were only able to identify the inverted intra-articular fragment of bone on the mortise projection. A shear fracture of the lateral malleolus may also be visible only in this view (Fig. 38-23).

The Triplane Fracture

Two, three, and four-part triplane fractures have been described. The most common is the two-part form. Classically, this fracture appears as a type III injury in the anteroposterior radiograph and as a type II injury on the lateral view. It is the lateral part of the epiphysis that tends to be involved more commonly, as in the fracture of Tillaux. Medial triplane fractures can occur in children prior to fusion of the medial physis.

In the most common two-part form, a Tillaux-like defect usually occurs. However, a posterolateral metaphyseal fragment accompanies the portion of epiphysis that is displaced (Fig. 38-24). Again, in this injury there tends to be an anterolateral defect in the tibial epiphysis that is widest anteriorly. The displacement seen in the anteroposterior (AP) radiographic view represents the maximal defect of the "crust" of the pie.

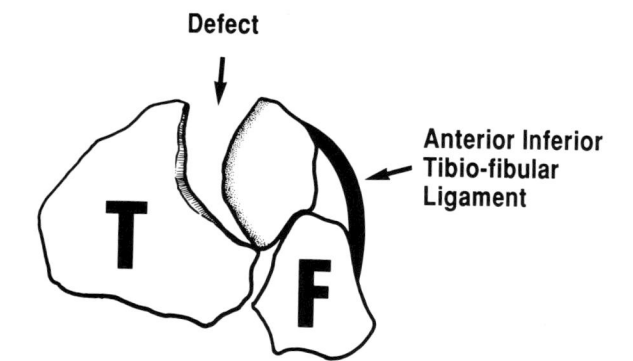

Fig. 38-21. The Tillaux fracture from below. The fragment is avulsed by the anterior tibiofibular ligament.

Fractures of the Ankle / 729

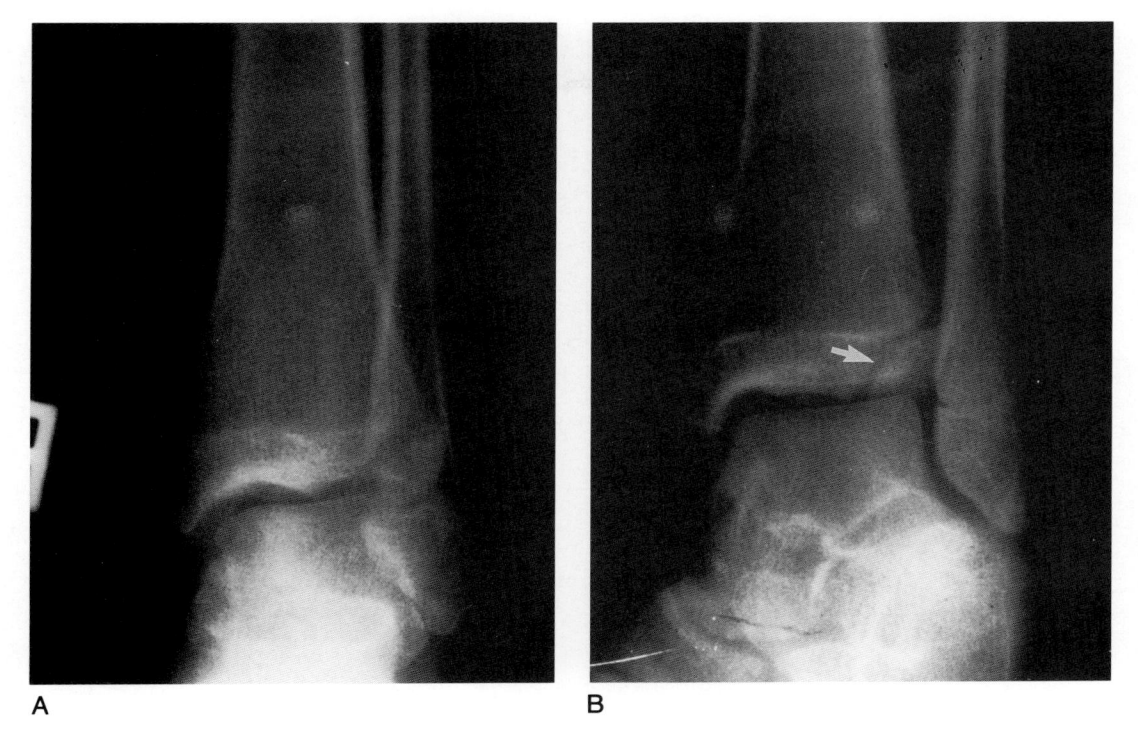

Fig. 38-22. The Tillaux fracture—importance of the mortise view. **(A)** Fracture of lateral plafond of tibia partially hidden by the fibula. **(B)** Oblique (mortise) view uncovers the tibia and reveals the underlying fracture clearly.

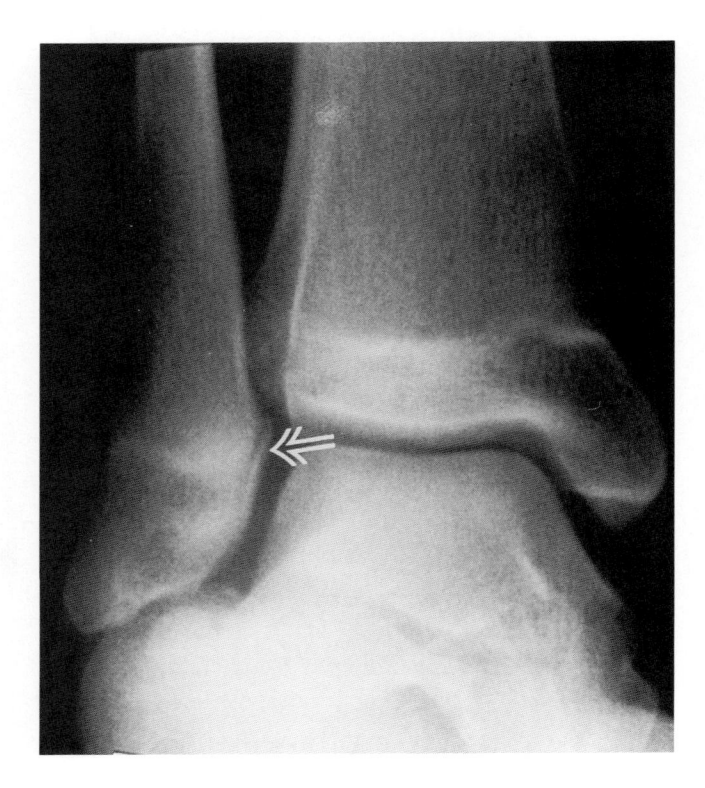

Fig. 38-23. A shear fracture of the lateral malleolus, visible only on the mortise view.

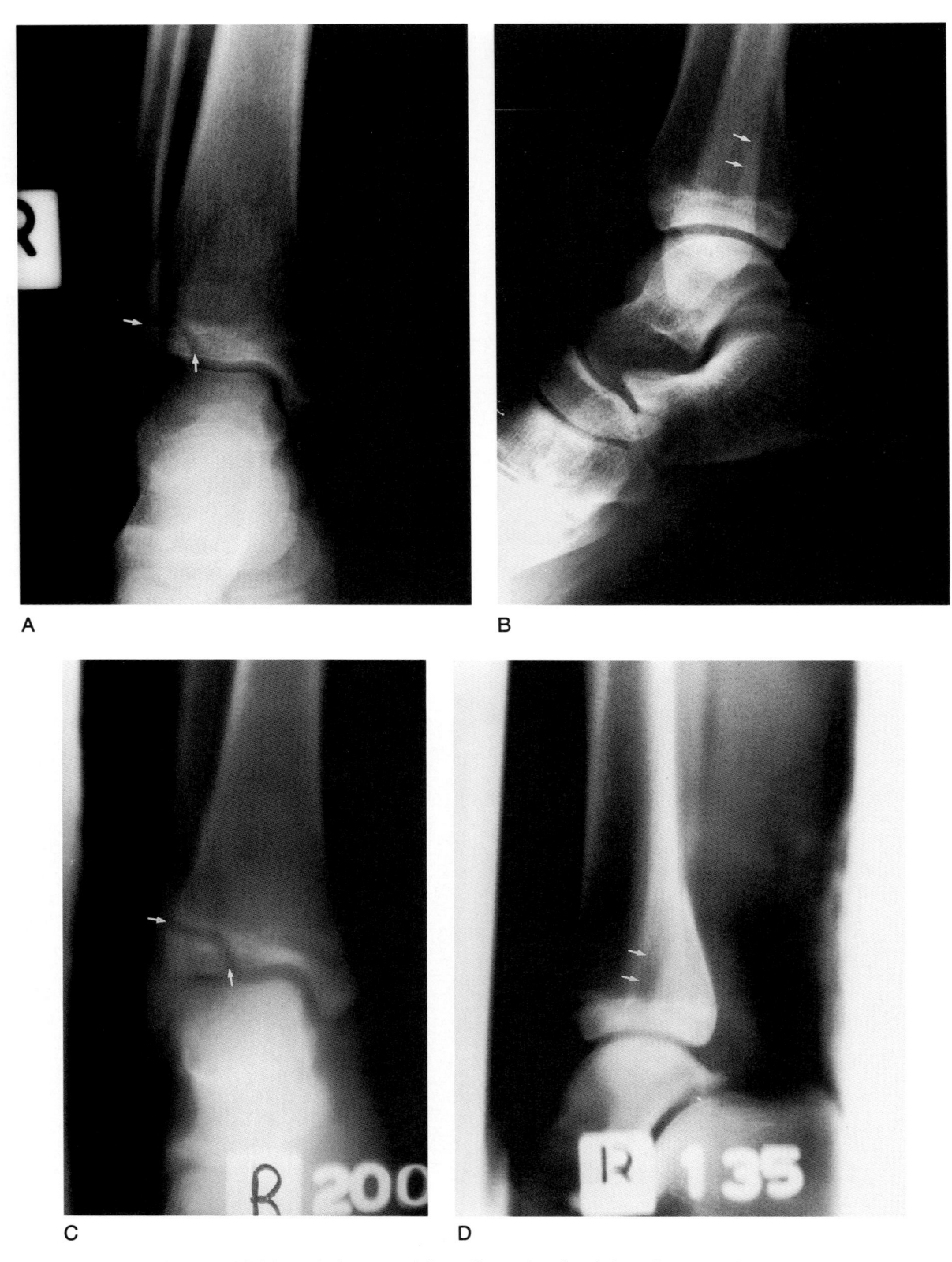

Fig. 38-24. **(A)** AP and **(B)** lateral views on plain radiographs of a triplane fracture. **(C&D)** Tomographs better delineate fracture lines.

Though it is conventional practice to recommend open reduction and internal fixation of these V-shaped defects that enter the joint, some are reduced by internally rotating the foot within the mortise. Should open reduction and internal fixation be performed, the reduction may be fixed either by a metaphyseal screw, Kirschner wires, a screw placed transversely through the epiphysis, or even by internal fixation that crosses the physis itself. Though not recommended in the younger patient, transphyseal fixation is appropriate in the almost-mature individual or when other means are difficult. If significant future growth is expected, smooth wires are recommended. As noted earlier, these particular fractures, especially that of Tillaux, tend to occur in the individual who has essentially no growth remaining in the distal tibial physis.

The most controversial question is whether all of these fractures require anatomic reduction. Remembering that it is the "crust" of the pie that is visualized and that there is some magnification present in the radiograph of the AP position, it has been our practice to accept a 1-mm defect but not one of 2 mm. Individual judgment must prevail. This complex set of fractures is discussed more thoroughly in Chapter 39.

Direct Axial Compression

These forces are potentially the most destructive to both the ankle joint and the distal tibial physis. Classically, the Salter-Harris type V injury is not recognizable at the time of initial radiographic examination. It is assumed that the forces are sufficient to disrupt the vascular supply of the resting and dividing cells throughout a portion of the physis. Partial or complete growth arrest result in shortening, deformity, and incongruity (Fig. 38-25).

In the most severe of these injuries the tibial plafond is comminuted. Not only will abnormalities of growth follow in this instance but even the short term prognosis for the joint is ominous. Type V injuries may occur in association with other types of physeal fractures.

Special Treatment Considerations

In the face of proven damage to the distal tibial physis, a decision must be made as to the best long-term management that is appropriate to each case. Because the anatomy of the ankle joint involves not only the tibia but

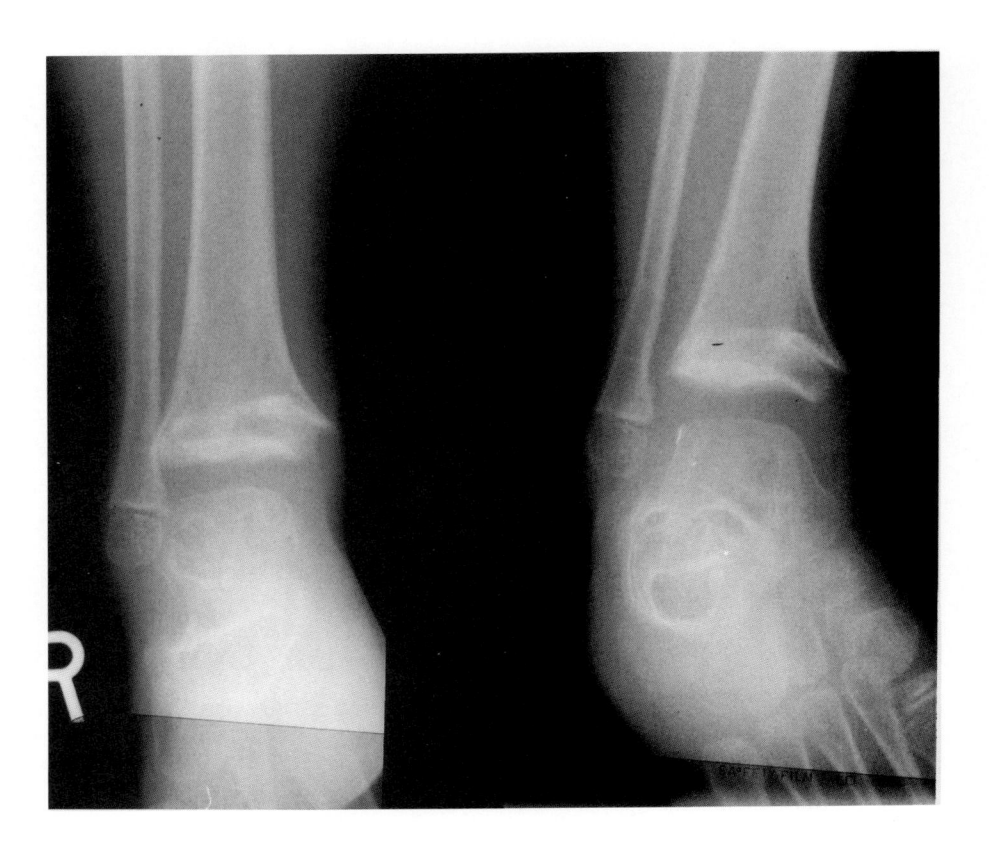

Fig. 38-25. Growth plate arrest of distal tibia in a 5-year-old girl who had been involved in a high-speed motor vehicle accident at age 3 years, in which her parents were killed. She sustained a crushing type V injury of the distal tibia, resulting in almost complete fusion of the physis.

732 / Management of Pediatric Fractures

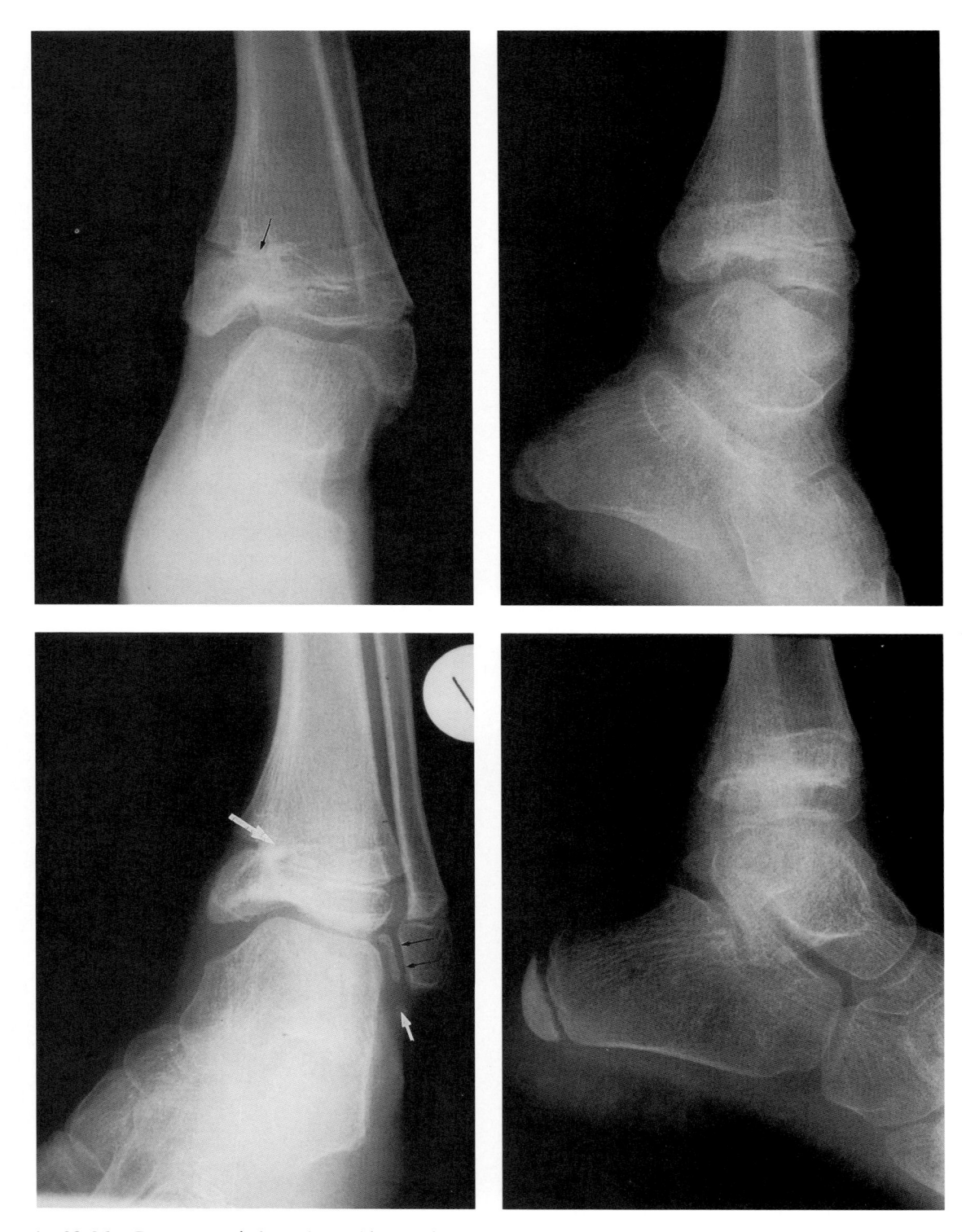

Fig. 38-26. Posttraumatic bony bar. This "tenting" deformity followed an unrecognized type IV injury in an 8-year-old boy who sustained multiple injuries in a motor vehicle accident. Note fibular cartilage avulsion and shear fractures that have now ossified.

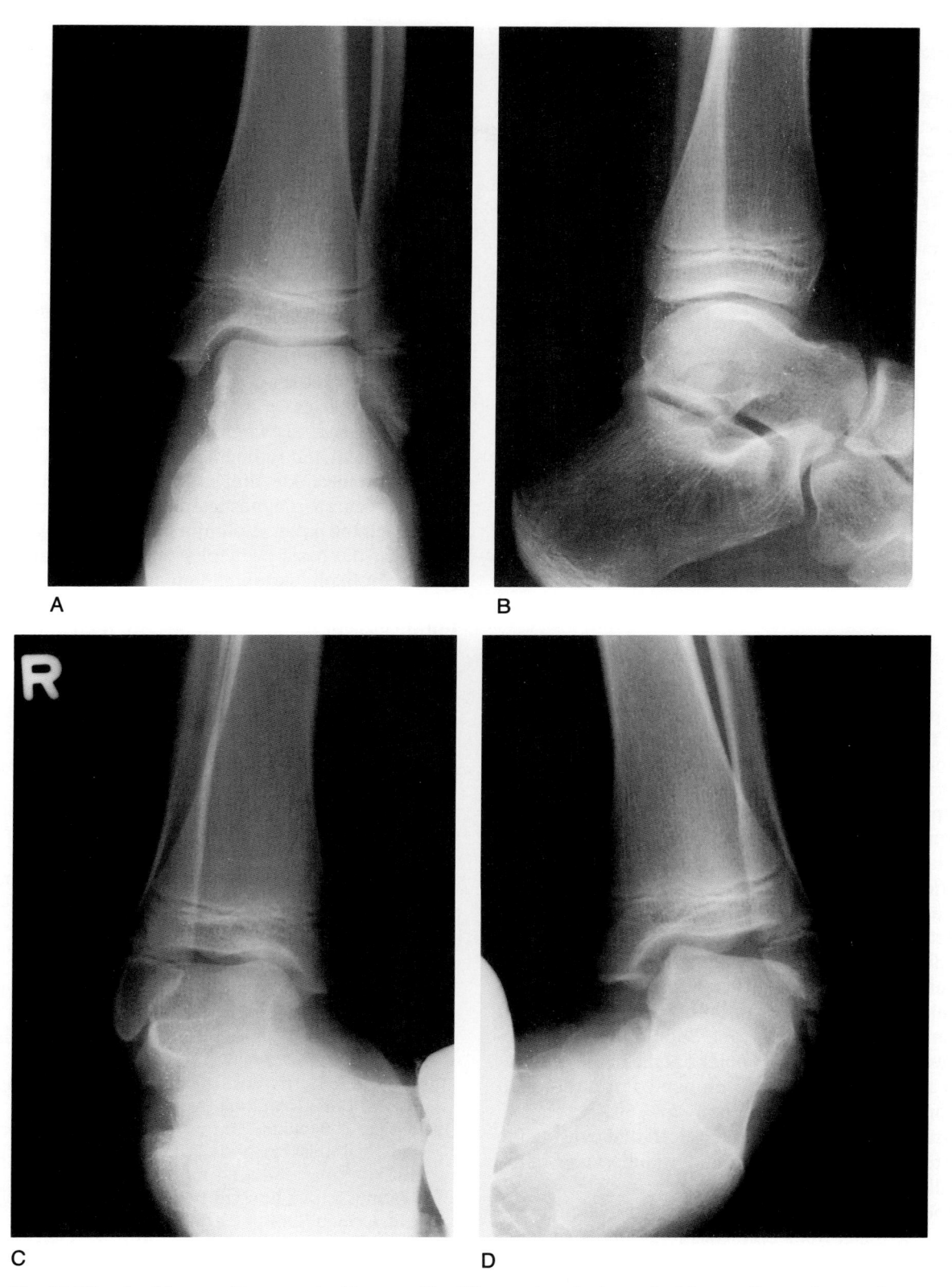

Fig. 38-27. An 11-year-old gymnast with generalized ligamentous laxity and a history of several severe inversion injuries to her left ankle continued to experience ankle instability. **(A&B)** An old avulsion fragment of the distal fibula is indicative of the previous trauma. **(C&D)** Stress views of the ankle revealed a marked talar tilt as compared to the normal right ankle, suggesting both a previous osseous injury and a ligamentous tearing and stretching.

also the fibula, the implications of continuing relative overgrowth of the other member (usually the fibula) must be considered. If one is fortunate enough to recognize that serious damage has occurred before significant deformity results in the older child, completion of the growth arrest of both distal tibia and fibula may be the most appropriate treatment. Even if one deems it necessary to perform a contralateral epiphyseodesis, this approach may be superior in the end to one that requires multiple osteotomies and accepts gradually increasing incongruity either from "tenting" of the tibial physis, fibular overgrowth, or both (Fig. 38-26).

In the younger child, excision of the bony bar and grafting of the physeal defect may allow growth to continue at a normal or almost normal rate. Should this fail, multiple osteotomies and/or epiphyseodesis, followed by lengthening, may be the most appropriate form of management. In this situation it may also be appropriate that contralateral epiphyseodesis be carried out toward the latter stages of longitudinal growth.

COMPLICATIONS

Complications involving fractures about the ankle are similar to those secondary to injuries at other sites. The management of open injuries must include debridement with or without secondary closure and/or skin grafting. The appropriate use of antibiotics, giving consideration to the environment in which the injury occurred, is fundamental.

Injuries about the ankle are rarely associated with neurovascular damage in children. Usually reduction of the fracture is sufficient to restore circulation. If a sensory deficit is present, it is usually due to an injury in continuity that will recover. Occasionally, severe trauma to the ankle and hindfoot will result in a compartment syndrome in the sole of the foot. Should this occur, decompression of the neurovascular bundle in the posteromedial ankle area must be accompanied by a thorough fasciotomy of the sole of the foot.

If a fracture is significantly displaced and causing the skin to tent, rapid reduction should be undertaken as the skin will necrose if left under stretch.

Kennedy and Weiner[11] have reported avascular necrosis of the distal tibial epiphysis following a Type IV distal tibial fracture. Total growth plate closure allowed revascularization of the epiphysis and no deformity developed.[11]

Occasionally ligamentous tearing will occur and if untreated with rest and immobilization, the ligaments may heal with lengthening, resulting in ankle instability (Fig. 38-27).

SUMMARY

Other than the hand and wrist, the area about the ankle joint is the most frequently fractured site in the child. The particular anatomic features, the weight of the body above and the subtalar joint and ground below provide a unique set of factors that contribute to a wide variety of injuries.

As in other areas where skeletal injury occurs, thorough physical and radiographic examination are essential. About the ankle, the "mortise view" is often the key to both accurate diagnostic and therapeutic evaluation.

Though the patterns of injury about the ankle may be complex, the basic principles of fracture management prevail. Both physeal and articular disruptions should be accurately reduced, by open surgical means if necessary. Future growth potential can be both used and abused.

REFERENCES

1. Mizuta T et al: Statistical analysis of the incidence of physeal injuries. Pediatr Orthop 7:518, 1987
2. Goldberg VM, Aadalen R: Distal tibial epiphyseal injuries: the role of athletics in 53 cases. Am J Sports Med 6:263, 1978
3. Ogden JA, Lee J: Accessory ossification patterns and injuries of the malleoli. J Pediatr Orthop 10:306, 1990
4. Johnson EW, Jr, Fahl JC: Fractures involving the distal epiphysis of the tibia and fibula in children. Am J Surg 93:778, 1957
5. Lauge-Hansen N: Fractures of the ankle. Arch Surg 60:957, 1950
6. Dias LS, Tachdjian MO: Physeal injuries of the ankle in children. Clin Orthop Rel Res 136:230, 1978
7. Salter RB, Harris WR: Injuries involving the epiphyseal plate. J Bone Joint Surg [Am] 45:587, 1963
8. Kleiger B, Mankin HJ: Fracture of the lateral portion of the distal tibial epiphysis. J Bone Joint Surg [Am] 46:25, 1964
9. Marmor L: An unusual fracture of the tibial epiphysis. Clin Orthop Rel Res 73:132, 1970
10. Beaty JH, Linton RC: Medial malleolar fracture in a child. J Bone Joint Surg [Am] 70:1254, 1988
11. Kennedy JP, Weiner DS: Case report: avascular necrosis complicating fracture of the distal tibial epiphysis. J Pediatr Orthop 11:234, 1991

39

Tibial Triplane Fractures

James G. Jarvis

> Triplane fractures strain the spatial imagination of the surgeon.
> —L. Von Laer

Tibial triplane fractures are complex fractures involving the distal tibial growth plate, which, according to Von Laer,[1] "strain the spatial imagination of the surgeon." In 1978 Cooperman and colleagues[2] defined the tibial triplane fracture as one in which the fracture plane has sagittal, transverse, and coronal components, and courses in part along and in part through the epiphyseal plate and enters the ankle joint. In 1985 Von Laer[1] introduced the term transitional fracture to the English literature. This referred to the age-dependent fractures and tibial triplane fractures were included in this group. It is estimated that tibial triplane fractures account for 6 to 10 percent of epiphyseal injuries.[3]

In 1957 Johnson and Fahl,[4] in describing fractures involving the distal epiphysis of the tibia and fibula in children, described a fracture with plantar flexion type of epiphyseal displacement and this probably represented one of the earliest descriptions of the triplane fracture. In 1964 Kleiger and Mankin[5] reported a series of lateral epiphyseal fractures, some of which had posterior metaphyseal fragments, and which most likely represented triplane fractures. In 1970, Marmor[6] published a diagram of an unusual tibial epiphyseal fracture, depicting three fragments (Fig. 39-1) and this was repeated by Lynn,[7] Rang,[8] and Torg.[9] Cooperman and colleagues[2] first used computed tomography (CT) to clarify the definition of the two-part triplane fracture (Fig. 39-2). Peiro and colleagues,[10] MacNealy and colleagues[11] and Dias and Giegerich[12] subsequently described three-part triplane fractures based on radiographic studies only, while numerous subsequent authors[1,3,13-18] reported cases, which had been studied using computed tomography. As pointed out by Von Laer,[1] these fractures of the distal aspect of the tibia, with their complicated course of fracture lines in different planes, challenge the imagination of the surgeon. Therefore, it is not surprising that discussions of these fractures in the literature have frequently been contradictory.

ANATOMY

The triplane fracture occurs as a result of the special anatomic circumstances surrounding the nature of closure of the distal tibial growth plate. The features of this phenomenon have been documented by several authors.[3,5,11] Closure proceeds in two directions from an initial site in the near central area (Fig. 39-3). This is followed by fusion of the posteromedial and finally the anterolateral segments of the growth plate. Mineralization and closure of the growth plate progresses in a proximal (metaphyseal) to distal (epiphyseal) direction until the physis is ossified. Prior to this, the weakest part of the open physis is the zone of provisional calcification. At a transitional age, that is, during the stage of epiphyseal closure—fracture represents an incomplete epiphysiolysis with deviation of the fracture from the mineralized area into the joint space.[1]

Kump[21] noted that the initial fusion site occurred at a central tibial "bump" overlying the medial edge of the

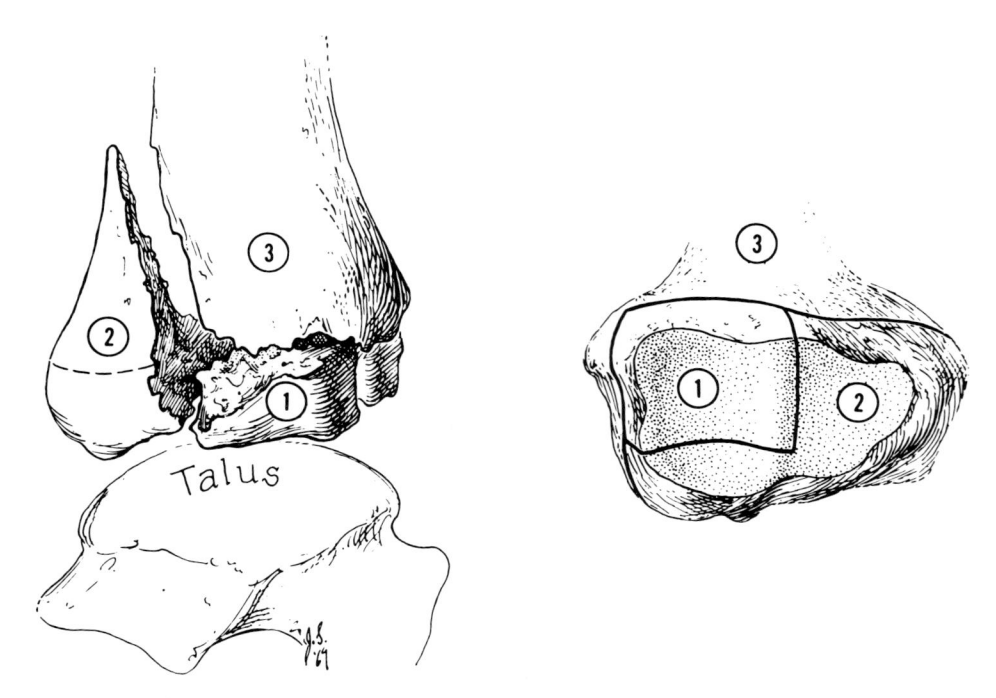

Fig. 39-1. Three-fragment fracture as depicted by Marmor. (From Marmor et al.,[6] with permission.)

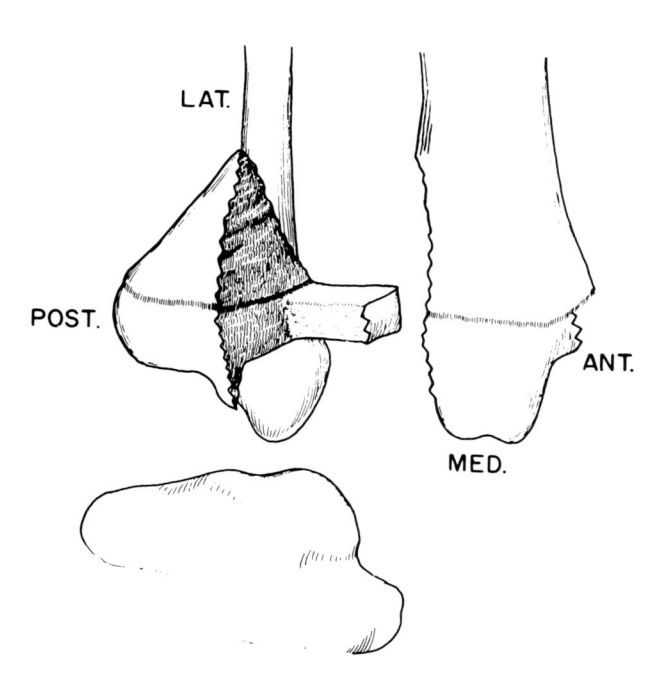

Fig. 39-2. Typical two-part triplane fracture as depicted by Cooperman. (From Cooperman et al.,[2] with permission.)

talus (Fig. 39-3). This medial-central "bump" is felt to represent a strong area with a relatively weaker area in the anterolateral physis.[5]

Many authors[1,3,5,10–13,20] feel that the pattern of fracture is dependent on the timing of growth plate closure and the resulting strong and weak zones. Clement and Worlock[13] noted that triplane fractures can also occur in younger children because the undulation or "bump" is found even before that part of the physis is fused.

MECHANISM OF INJURY

It is nearly universally agreed that most triplane fractures are the result of an external rotation of the foot on the leg (Fig. 39-4).[22] Karrholm and coworkers,[22] in an exhaustive review of supination-eversion injuries, felt that there was a continuum depending on the degree of trauma involved. This commenced with the juvenile Tillaux fracture progressing to the triplane fracture and finally the triplane fracture with associated fibular fracture. Dias and Giegerich[12] and others[10] felt that the position of the foot at the time of injury influenced the type of fracture. Some authors[22] have implicated the severity of trauma as the determinant of the type of fracture, while others[1] feel that the type of fracture depends solely

EPIPHYSEAL PLATE

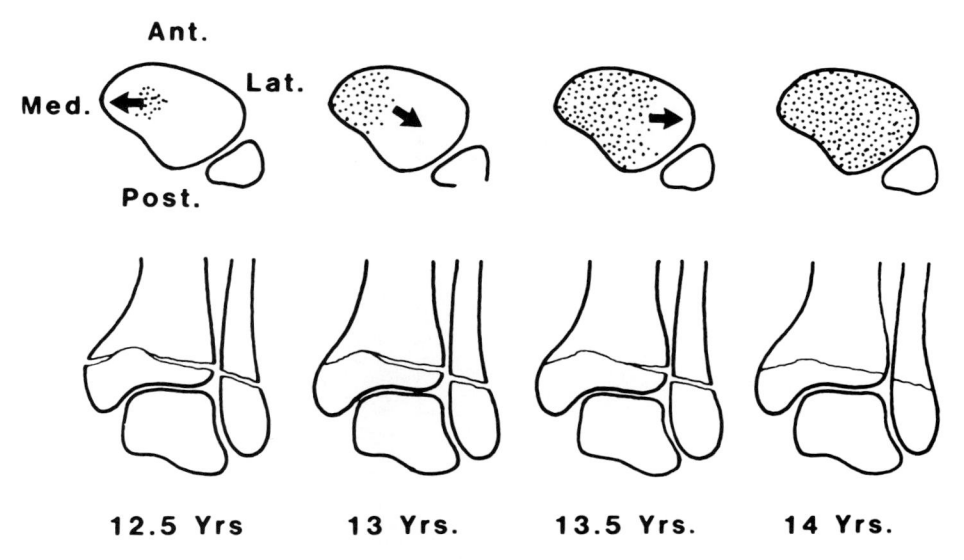

Fig. 39-3. The average age of onset and normal fusion pattern of the distal tibial growth plate. (From MacNealey et al.,[11] with permission.)

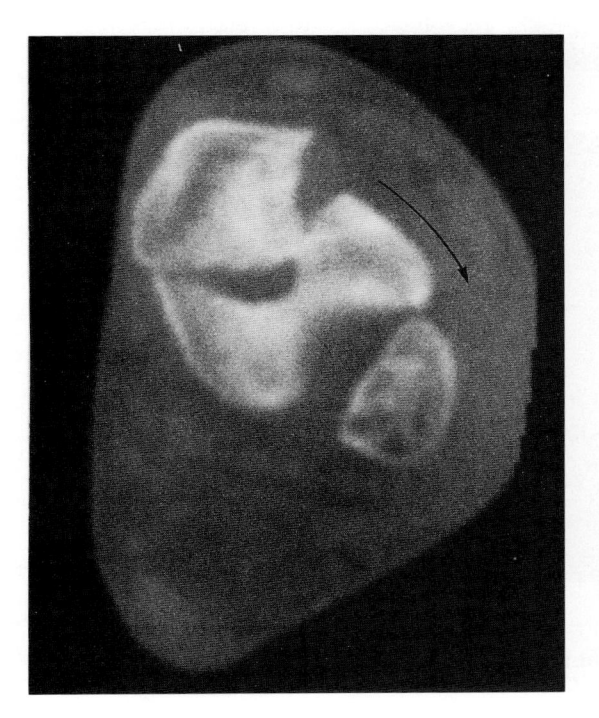

Fig. 39-4. Lateral triplane fracture: CT scan at the level of the epiphysis showing typical external rotation deformity (prior to reduction). (Modified from Jarvis et al.,[16] with permission.)

on the stage of growth plate closure and not on the magnitude of trauma.

There are several reports of medial triplane fractures.[19,23,24] These authors agree that this fracture occurs as a result of an internal rather than an external rotation force. This is a much rarer occurrence.

CLASSIFICATION

There has been much confusion in the literature as to the exact nature of the triplane fracture. Although the early descriptions depicted lateral triplane fractures in either two or three fragments, in general the fracture was felt to be intra-articular. Karrholm and colleagues[22] first described an extra-articular variant, while Denton and Fischer[23] first differentiated a medial variety.

Perhaps the most significant tool in classifying these fractures has been CT scanning, which has been used in many of the later reports,[1-3,13-18,20] adding greatly to our knowledge of this enigmatic fracture. In general, most classification systems are based on three factors: (1) medial or lateral, (2) number of parts, and (3) intra- or extra-articular. It is well recognized that plain radiographs alone are not sufficient to determine whether a fracture is in two or three parts. This requires use of CT scans. Fractures of the fibula may be seen with any type of triplane fracture.

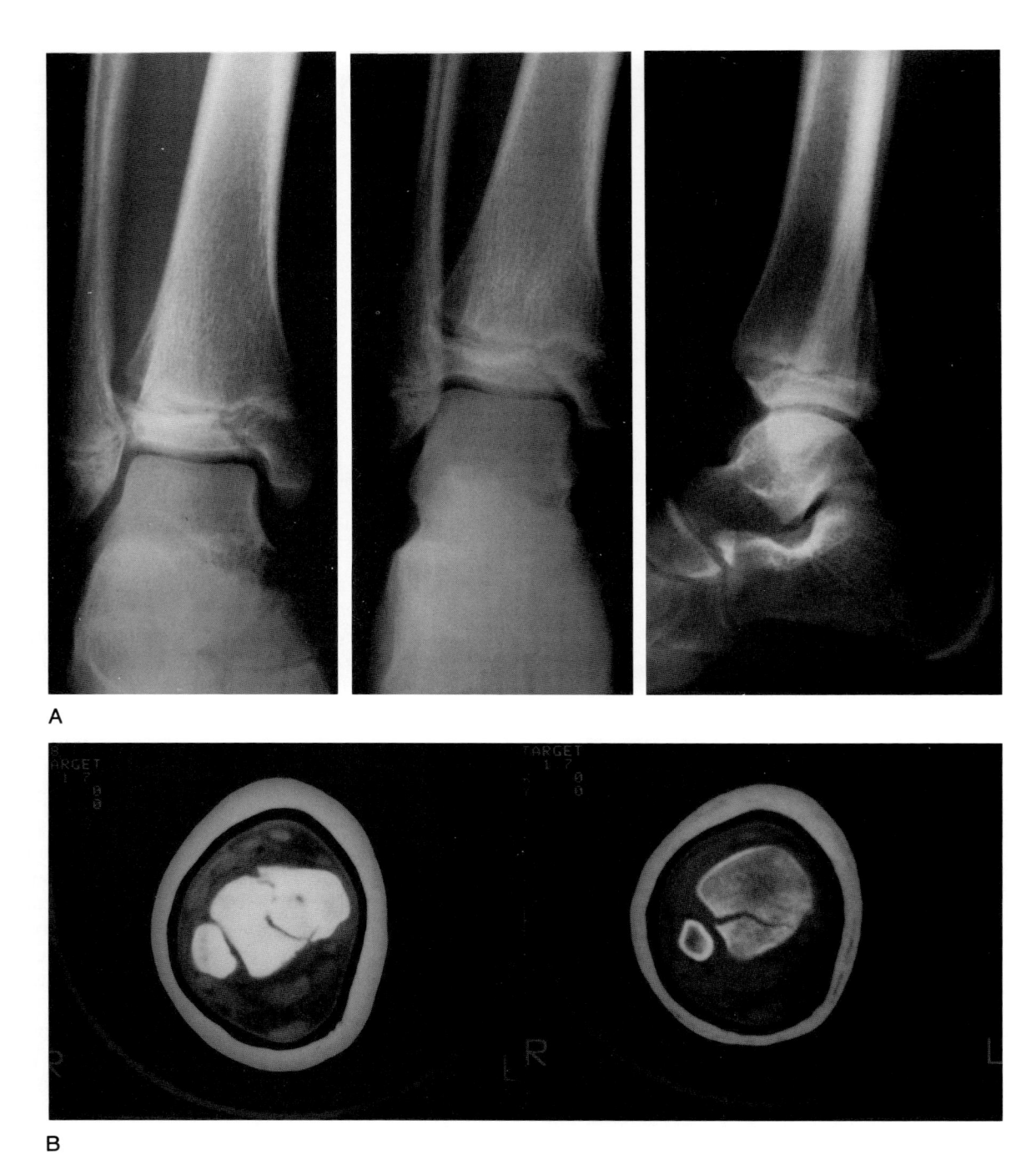

Fig. 39-5. (A) Intra-articular two-part lateral triplane fracture. (B) CT scan at the level of the epiphysis (**left**) and the metaphysis (**right**). (From Jarvis et al.,[16] with permission.)

The most common triplane fractures are discussed in the following sections.

Two-Part Lateral Fractures

Intra-articular

The intra-articular two-part lateral fracture (Fig. 39-5) appears as a Salter-Harris[25] type III fracture on AP radiographic views, but as a type II or IV on the lateral view (Fig. 39-5A). At the epiphyseal level, two discrete fragments are seen on CT scans, namely, an anterolateral and posterior segment tethered to the fibula, and a smaller anteromedial fragment constituting most of the medial malleolus (Fig. 39-5B). At the metaphyseal level the coronal fracture separates a posterior metaphyseal fragment (attached to the posterior and lateral epiphyseal segment), whereas the remainder of the tibial shaft remains as an intact medial pillar that includes the anteromedial quadrant of epiphysis (Figs. 39-2 and 39-6).

Extra-articular

In the extra-articular two-part lateral fracture, the sagittal fracture line is seen on the AP or mortise view radiographs coursing through the medial malleolus (Fig. 39-7A). CT sections through the epiphysis reveal this fracture to be outside the weight-bearing zone (Fig. 39-7B).

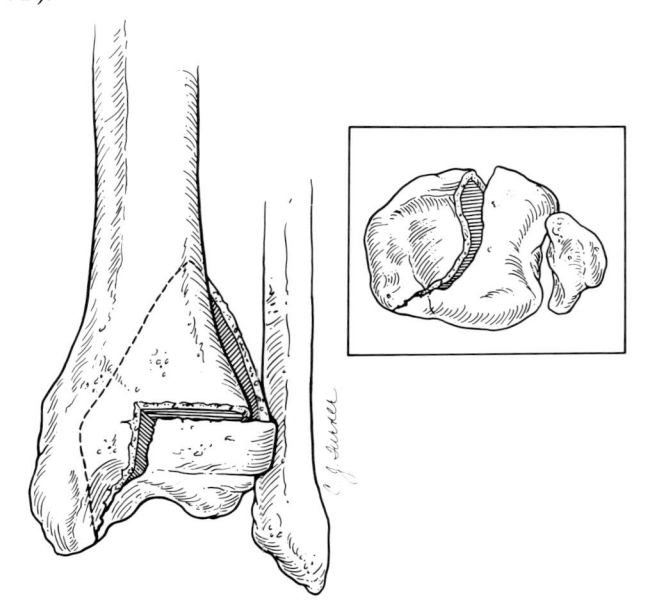

Fig. 39-6. Intra-articular two-part lateral triplane fracture. **Inset** shows articular surface. (Courtesy of Cynthia J. Turner, Dallas, Texas.)

Three-Part Lateral Fractures

Three-part fractures cannot be readily distinguished on plain radiographs (Fig. 39-8A). With CT scanning, the fracture pattern proximal to the physis is identical to that seen in two part fractures. At the epiphyseal level, however, a coronal fracture separates the anterolateral beak as a free third fragment (Figs. 39-8B and 39-9).

Medial Fractures

On the AP radiographic view both the sagittal epiphyseal fracture and the posterior metaphyseal spike are more medially oriented (Fig. 39-10A). CT scans at the level of the epiphysis reveal a distinctive large posterior and medial fragment whereas the anterolateral portion of the epiphysis constitutes the smaller fragment (Fig. 39-10B). The metaphyseal sections are unique in that the fracture line is in a sagittal (instead of coronal) plane and more medially situated on the shaft. Medial fractures may also be in two or three parts.

Four-Part Fractures

Four-part fractures are comminuted fractures representing combinations of the above types.

DIFFERENTIAL DIAGNOSIS

The differential diagnosis includes the juvenile Tillaux fracture or the "hidden adolescent fracture" of Letts.[26] These fractures do not have a metaphyseal component. The Salter-Harris type II distal tibial fracture includes a metaphyseal component but does not extend distal to the physis. In uncertain situations, a single-cut CT scan at the epiphyseal and at the metaphyseal level will clarify the diagnosis (Fig. 39-11).

EXAMINATION

Patients with distal triplane fractures, typically present with a swollen foot and ankle. Neurovascular compromise is rare. In the typical displaced external rotation fracture there often is a clinically discernible increase in external tibial torsion, compared to the normal side. Occasionally, in widely displaced fractures, anterior tenting of the skin over fracture fragments may lead to skin necrosis if reduction is not carried out expediently.

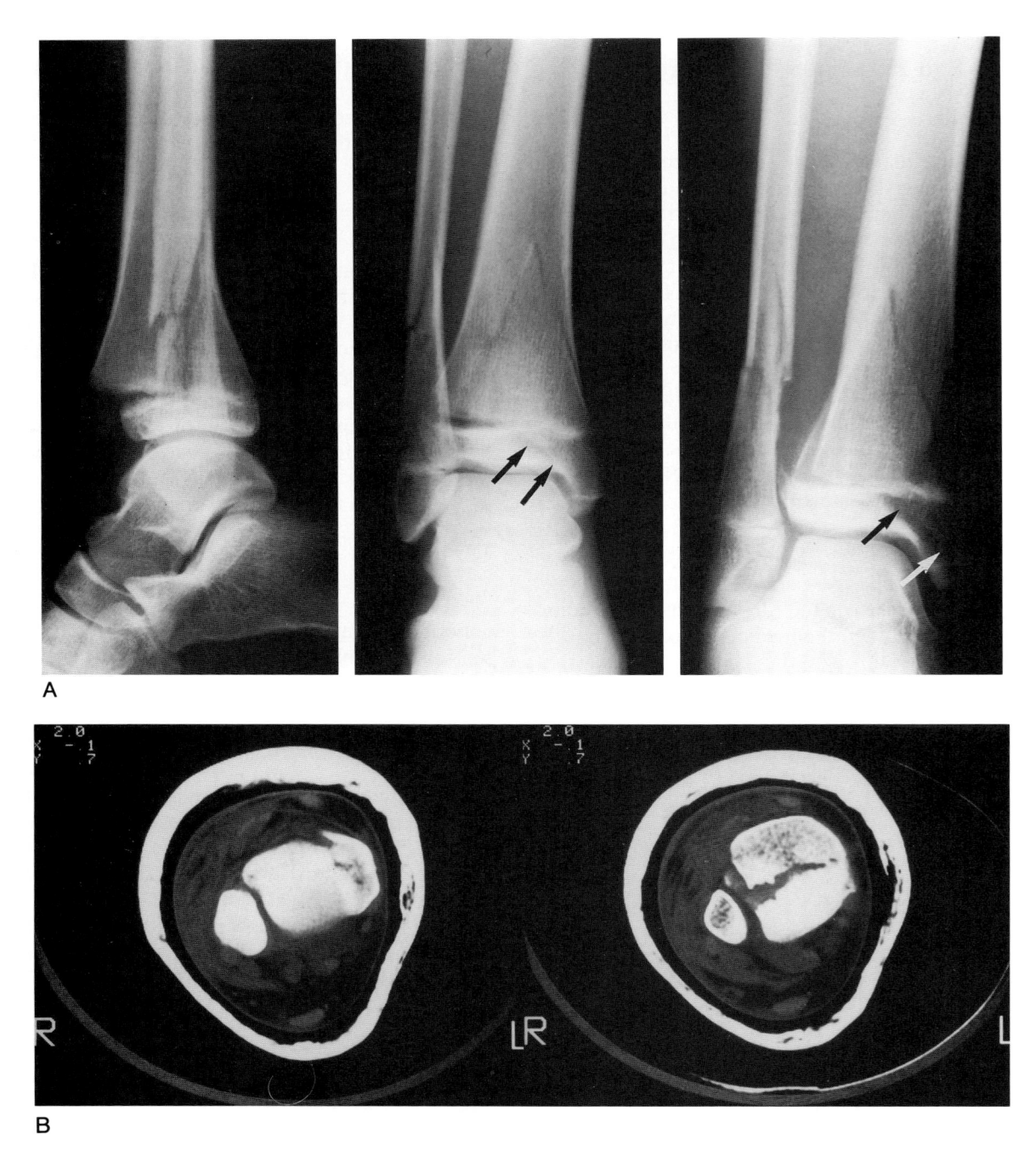

Fig. 39-7. **(A)** Extra-articular two part lateral triplane fracture showing fracture coursing through medial malleolus *(arrows)*. **(B)** CT scan at the level of the epiphysis **(left)** and the metaphysis **(right)**. (Modified from Jarvis et al.,[16] with permission.)

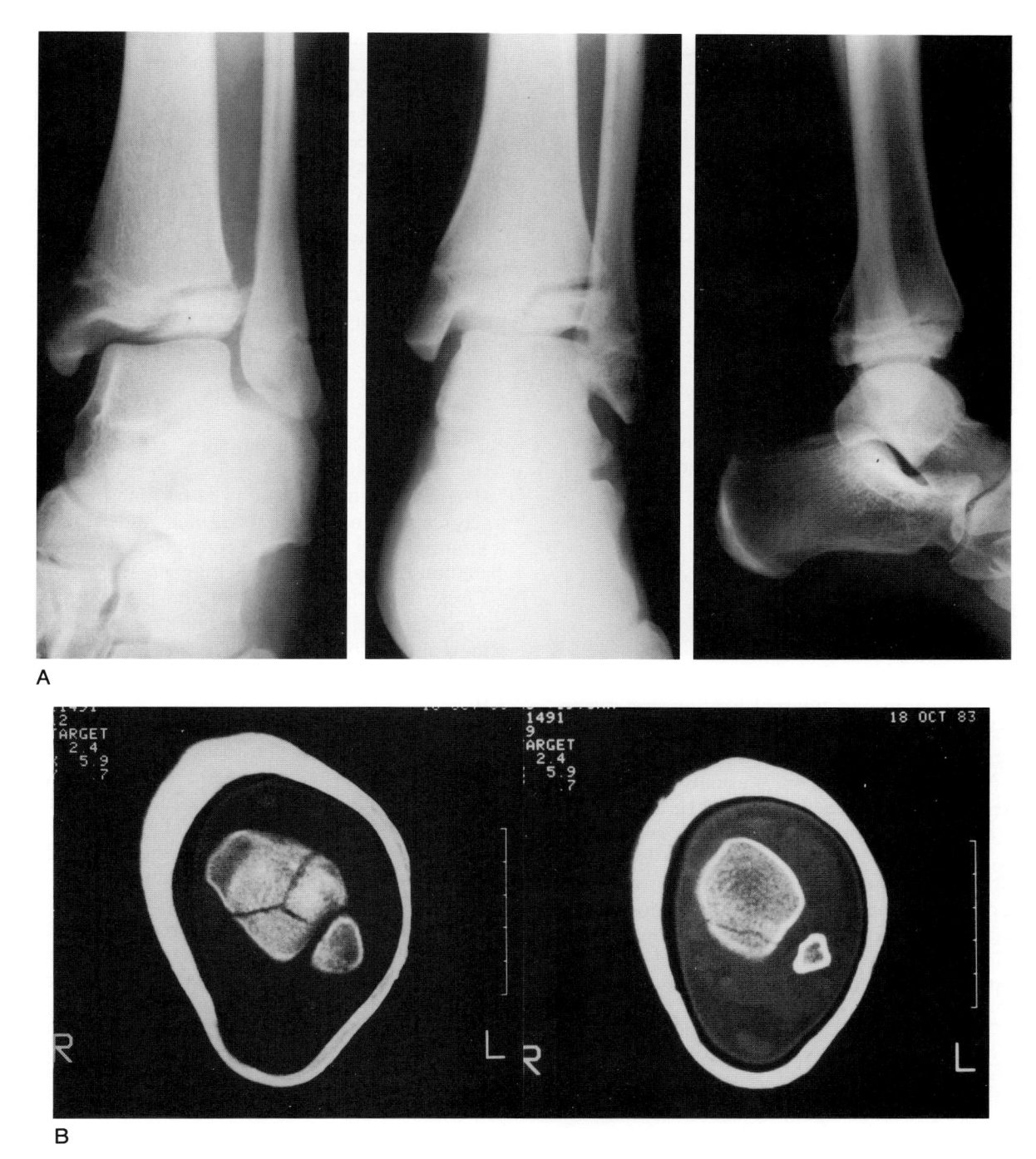

Fig. 39-8. (A) Three-part lateral triplane fracture. (B) CT scan at the level of the epiphysis **(left)** and the metaphysis **(right)**.

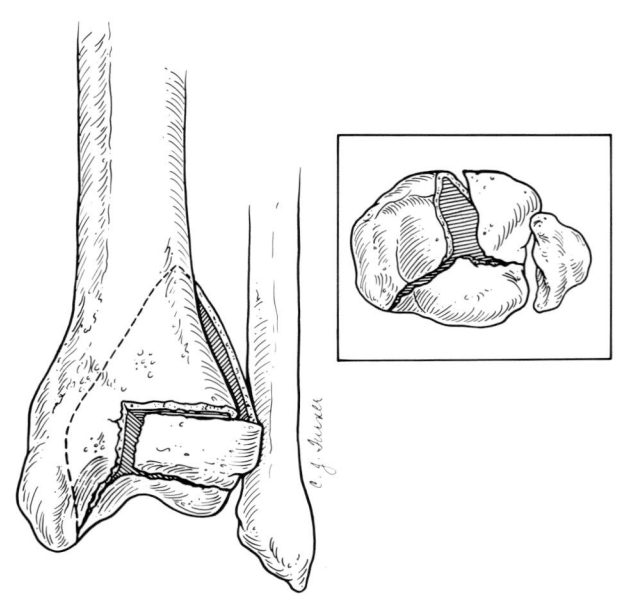

Fig. 39-9. Three-part lateral triplane fracture. **Inset** shows articular surface. (Courtesy of Cynthia J. Turner, Dallas, Texas.)

TREATMENT

Closed Methods

Although in the initial description of the triplane fracture open reduction and internal fixation was recommended,[3,6,9] it is now widely accepted that accurate closed reduction is the usual mainstay of treatment.[1,2,20,27] General anesthesia is usually necessary for adequate relaxation. Reduction should be achieved by traction and internal rotation of the foot, usually with the foot in plantar flexion. The exception is the rare medial fracture which may require external rotation. A long-leg cast is then applied maintaining the foot in medial rotation (not varus). Weightbearing should be restricted for about 3 weeks followed by 2 to 4 weeks immobilization in a patellar tendon weight-bearing cast.

Open Methods

There is general agreement in the literature that the maximum acceptable residual displacement is 2 mm in the weight-bearing area. Open reduction should be reserved for these fractures. For the extra-articular variant, where the fracture line is outside the weight-bearing area, less stringent requirements may apply.[15,22] In our experience, open reduction is more frequently necessary for medial fractures and some three-part fractures. Fixation proceeds from metaphyseal to epiphyseal or vice versa depending on the fracture circumstances.[20] In two fragment fractures, metaphyseal fixation may be sufficient for anatomic reduction. Typically, the lateral triplane fracture has been approached using an anterolateral incision for the free third part (made up of the anterolateral quadrant of the epiphysis). A second posterior incision may be medial or lateral depending on the fracture configuration. CT scans are invaluable in planning operative intervention. In general, interfragmentary screws have been used for fixation with occasional plating of displaced fibular fractures (Fig. 39-12). Smooth pins are less desirable for maintenance of an anatomic reduction as they do not compress the fracture fragments adequately.[20]

Pitfalls

The most significant pitfall in treating tibial triplane fractures is in not recognizing and understanding the fracture pattern. Three part fractures cannot be appreciated on the basis of plain roentgenograms alone. The CT scan is an invaluable tool and is the best way to differentiate two part from three part fractures.[15] The CT scan is also the optimum way to accurately assess residual rotatory displacement at the joint surface (Fig. 39-13).

Three-part fractures are recognized for their propensity to cause intra-articular incongruity. The three-part fracture may leave a posterior metaphyseal-epiphyseal fragment which behaves like a Salter-Harris type IV fracture. This may migrate proximally leaving a residual step in the joint surface. This type of incongruity can best be appreciated with lateral tomograms or CT reconstructions (Fig. 39-14).

Overzealous attempts at closed reduction can be detrimental. It is possible to convert a two-part fracture into a three-part fracture by overly aggressive internal rotation and forceful dorsiflexion before the distal fragment is reduced (Fig. 39-15). This maneuver can fracture the anterolateral beak of epiphysis which then becomes a free third fragment.

Finally, we have seen several triplane fractures in conjunction with ipsilateral tibial shaft fractures (Fig. 39-16). Although we have been successful in reducing these fractures using closed methods, this particularly rare and challenging combination may represent an indication for open reduction.

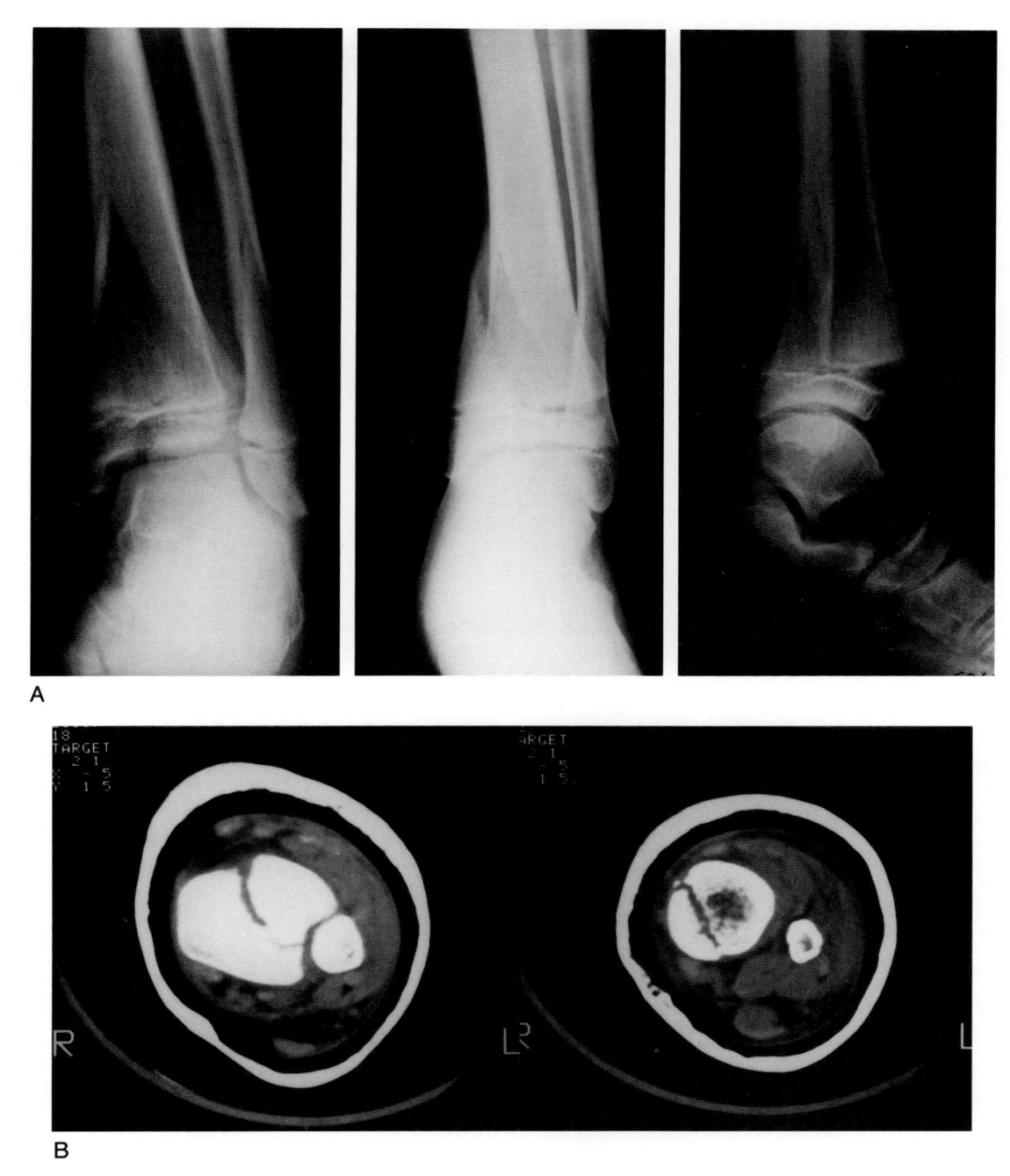

Fig. 39-10. (A) Medial triplane fracture. (B) CT scan at the level of the epiphysis **(left)** and the metaphysis **(right)**. (From Jarvis et al.,[16] with permission.)

744 / Management of Pediatric Fractures

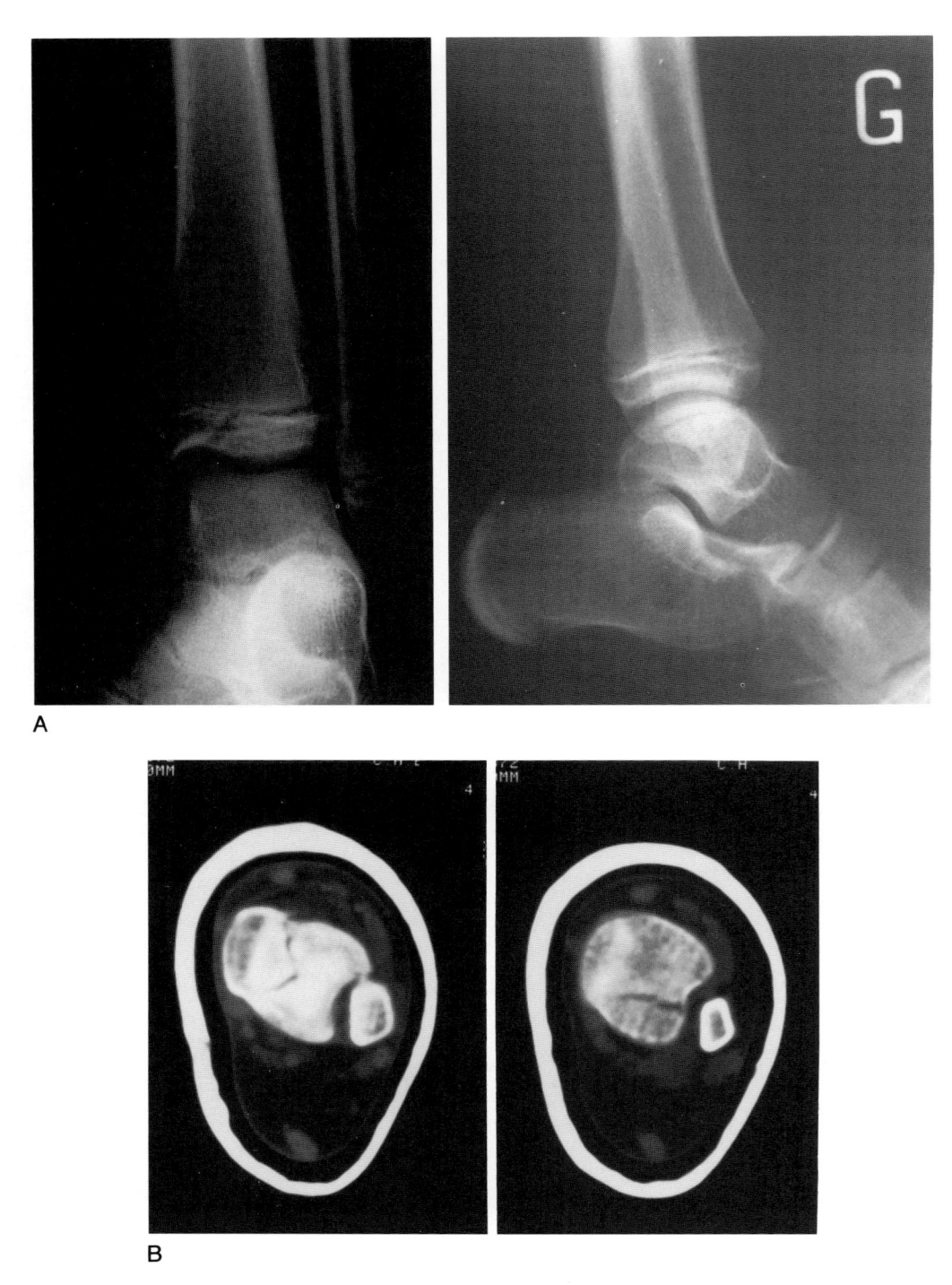

Fig. 39-11. (A) AP and lateral radiographic views show presumed juvenile Tillaux fracture. (B) CT scan at the level of the metaphysis **(right)** confirms triplane fracture.

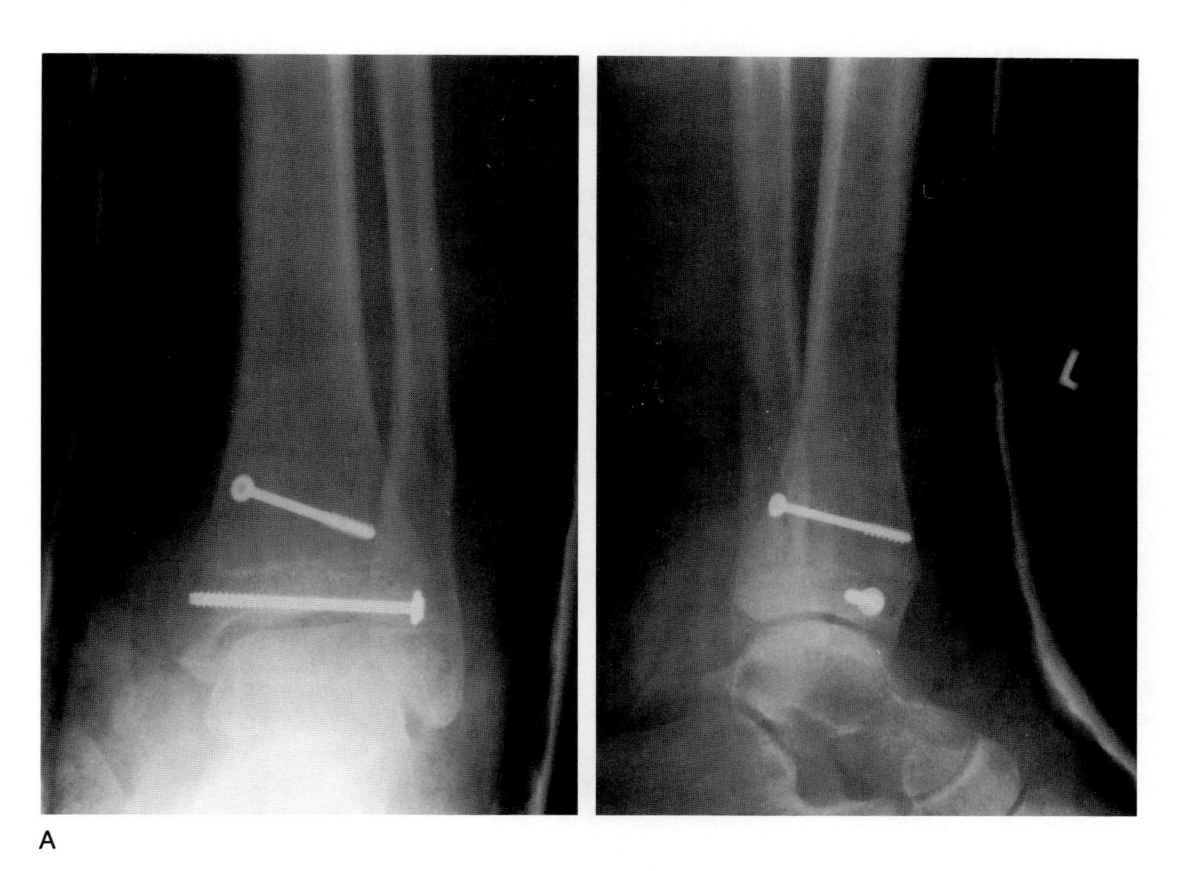

Fig. 39-12. (A) Three-part lateral triplane fracture following open reduction and internal fixation. *(Figure continues.)*

746 / Management of Pediatric Fractures

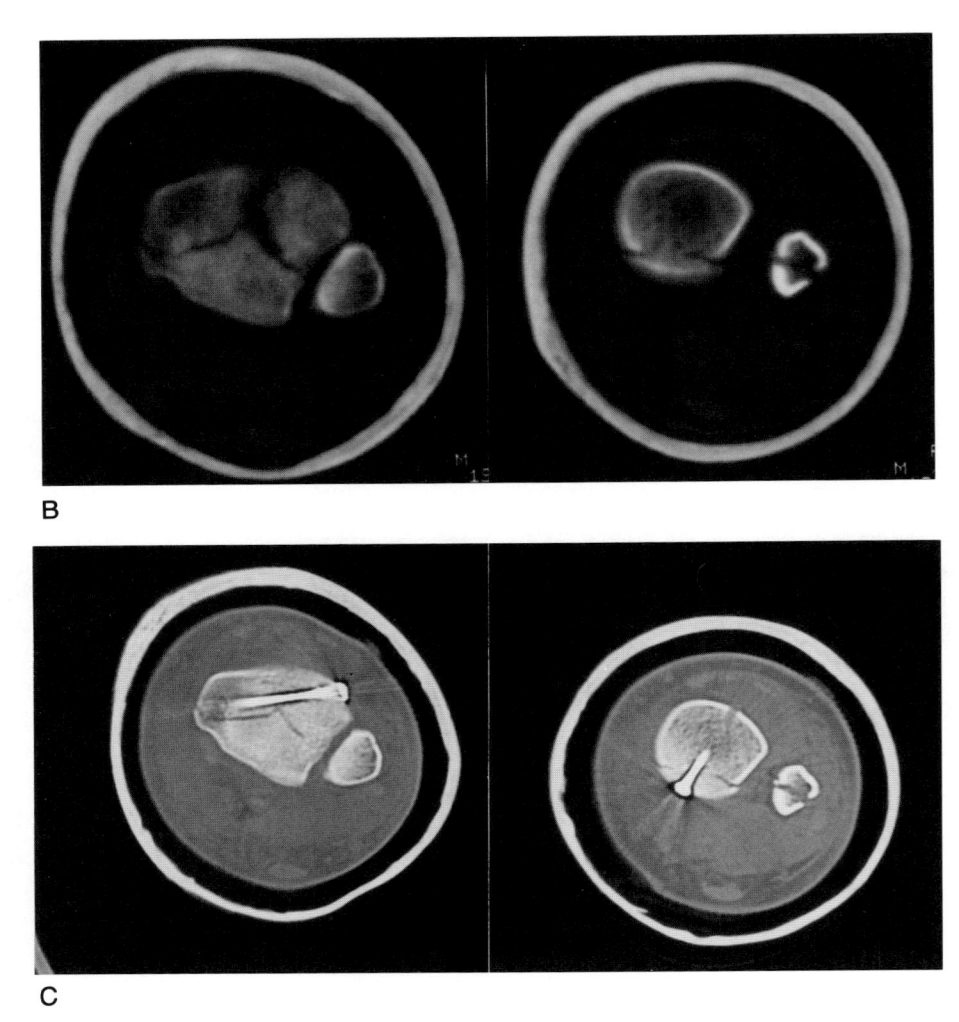

Fig. 39-12 *(Continued).* **(B)** CT scan prereduction at level of epiphysis **(left)** and metaphysis **(right)**. **(C)** CT scan following open reduction and interfragmentary fixation.

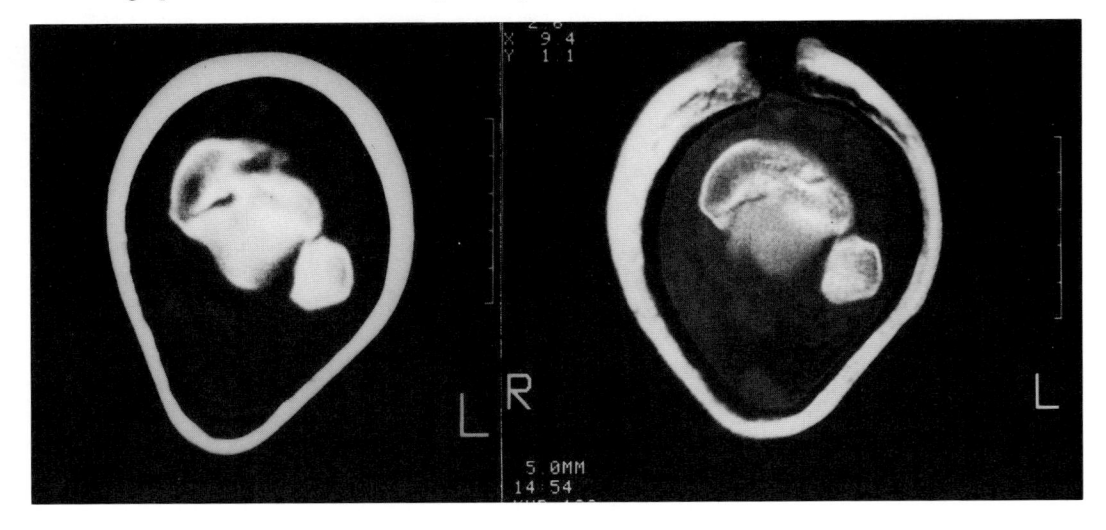

Fig. 39-13. Two-part intra-articular lateral triplane fracture: initial reduction with residual deformity **(left)** and final reduction **(right)**. (From Jarvis et al.,[16] with permission.)

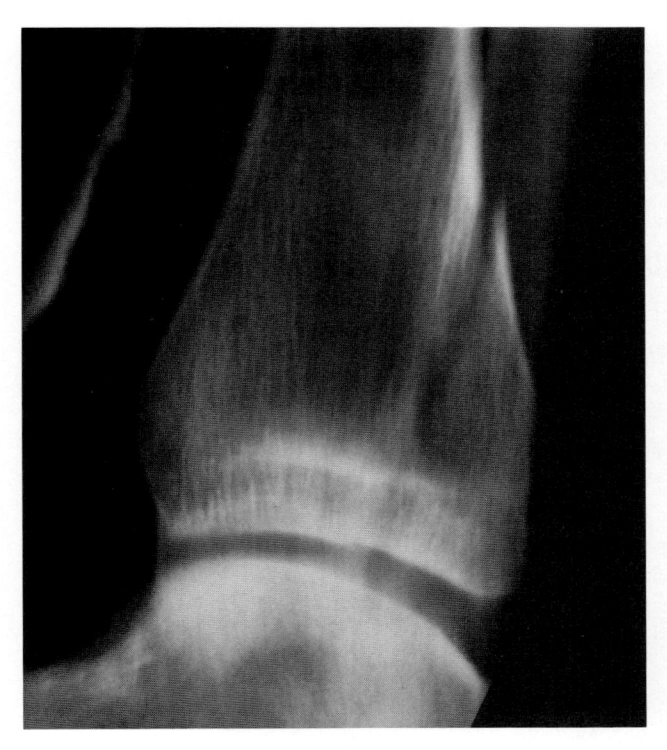

Fig. 39-14. Posterior type 4 fragment with intra-articular step (lateral view tomogram). (From Jarvis et al.,[16] with permission.)

COMPLICATIONS

In general, the tibial triplane fracture seems to have a good prognosis with few complications, but there are very few long-term studies reviewing the outcome of treatment. Ertl and coworkers[15] found that those fractures healing with greater than 2 mm of displacement were often associated with pain on activity. Conversely, Dias and Giegerich[12] reported similar pain in two patients who had undergone open reduction. Cooperman and colleagues[2] noted a residual external rotation deformity of 5 to 10 degrees in 3 of his 12 cases. As the distal tibial articular surface is hemicylindrical in shape, it is likely that rotatory displacement would produce more incongruity than pure parallel gap displacement.

The tibial triplane fracture occurs during the transitional period of partial growth plate closure. As the remaining longitudinal growth is limited, angular growth changes are typically not found.[1,10,20,28] The only exception was noted by Karrholm and colleagues[29] in his stages 3 and 4b injuries, which occurred in younger age groups where growth remaining exceeded 1 cm.

SUMMARY

The tibial triplane fracture is a unique fracture involving the distal tibial growth plate—usually in adolescents—and occurs during the transitional time of

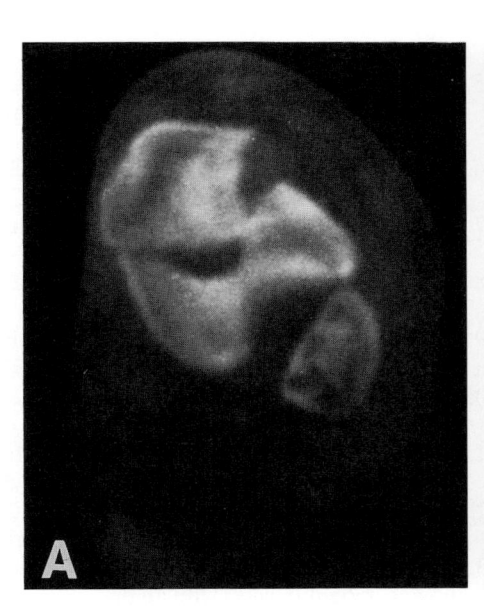

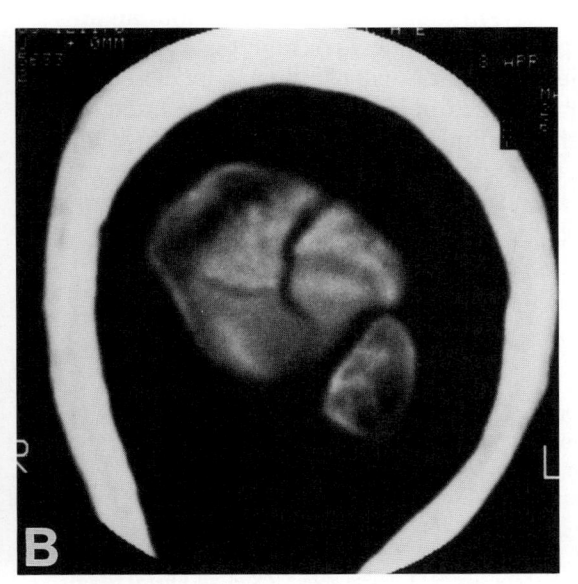

Fig. 39-15. (A) Two-part lateral triplane fracture before reduction (CT scan at level of epiphysis). (B) Postreduction CT scan shows conversion to three-part fracture following manipulation by internal rotation.

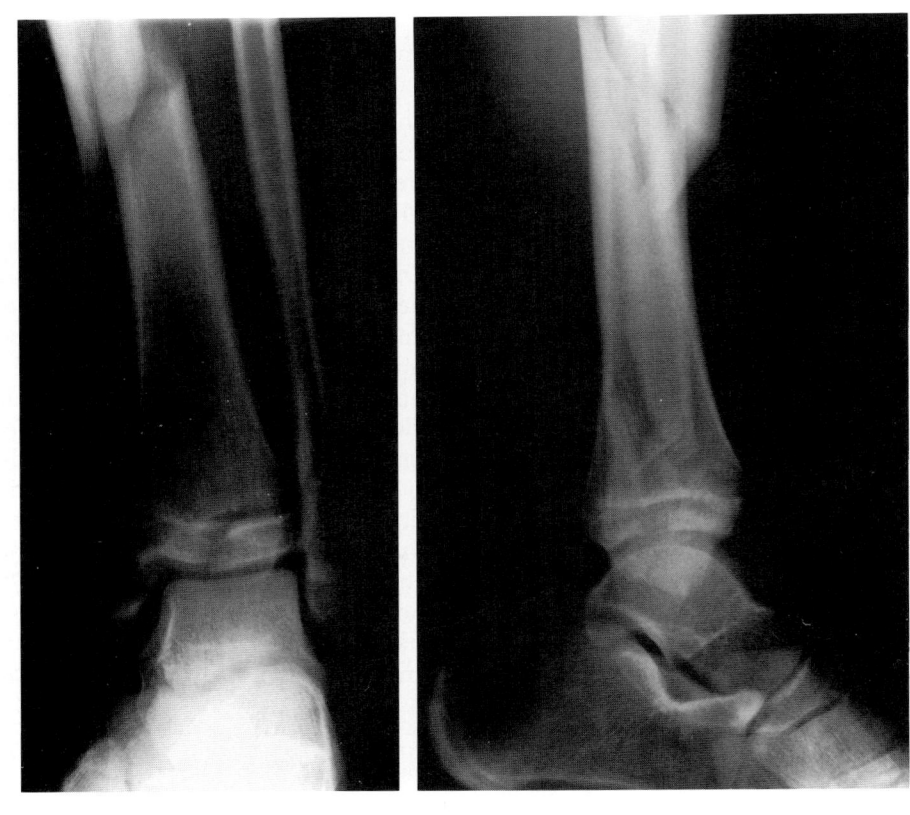

Fig. 39-16. Triplane fracture with ipsilateral tibial shaft fracture.

growth plate closure. It is usually in two, sometimes in three, and, rarely, in four parts with or without an accompanying fibular fracture. Typically it is an external rotation injury and can usually be treated by closed reduction. Open reduction is reserved for those fractures with more than 2 mm displacement at the weight-bearing surface. CT scans are frequently necessary to assess the deformity and the adequacy of reduction. In general, the prognosis for this complex fracture is good.

REFERENCES

1. Von Laer L: Classification, diagnosis, and treatment of transitional fractures of the distal part of the tibia. J Bone Joint Surg [Am] 67:687, 1985
2. Cooperman DR, Spiegel PG, Laros GJ: Tibial fractures involving the ankle in children. J Bone Joint Surg [Am] 60:1040, 1978
3. Feldman F, Singson RD, Rosenberg ZS et al: Distal tibial triplane fractures: diagnosis with CT. Radiology 164:429, 1987
4. Johnson EW, Fahl JC: Fractures involving the distal epiphysis of the tibia and fibula in children. Am J Surg 93:778, 1957
5. Kleiger B, Mankin HJ: Fracture of the lateral portion of the distal tibial epiphysis. J Bone Joint Surg [Am] 46:25, 1964
6. Marmor L: An unusual fracture of the tibial epiphysis. Clin Orthop 73:132, 1970
7. Lynn MD: The triplane distal tibial epiphyseal fracture. Clin Orthop 86:187, 1972
8. Rang M: Ankle fractures. In: Children's Fractures. JB Lippincott, Philadelphia, 1974
9. Torg JS, Ruggiero FA: Comminuted epiphyseal fracture of the distal tibia. Clin Orthop 110:215, 1975
10. Peiro A, Aracil J, Martos F, Mut T: Triplane distal epiphyseal fracture. Clin Orthop 160:196, 1981
11. MacNealy GA, Rogers LF, Hernandez R, Poznanski AK: Injuries of distal tibial epiphysis. AJR 138:683, 1982
12. Dias LS, Giegerich CR: Fractures of the distal tibial epiphysis in adolescence. J Bone Joint Surg [Am] 65:438, 1983
13. Clement DA, Worlock PH: Triplane fracture of the distal tibia: a variant in cases with an open growth plate. J Bone Joint Surg [Br] 69:412, 1987
14. Cone RO, Nguyen V, Flournoy JG, Guerra J: Triplane

fracture of the distal tibial epiphysis: radiographic and CT studies. Radiology 153:763, 1984
15. Ertl JP, Barrack RL, Alexander AH, VanBuecken K: Triplane fractures of the distal tibial epiphysis: long-term follow-up. J Bone Joint Surg [Am] 70:967, 1988
16. Jarvis J, McIntyre W, England R: Computerized tomography and the triplane fracture. p. 165. In Uhthoff HK, Wiley JJ (eds): Behaviour of the Growth Plate. Raven Press, New York, 1988
17. Karrholm J, Hansson LI, Laurin S: Computed tomography of intra-articular supination-eversion fractures of the ankle in adolescents. J Pediatr Orthop 1:181, 1981
18. Marcus NW: Comminuted triplane fractures of the distal tibial epiphysis. Orthop Trans 7:448, 1983
19. Seitz WH, LaPorte J: Medial triplane fracture delineated by computerized axial tomography. J Pediatr Orthop 8:65, 1988
20. Spiegel P, Mast J, Cooperman D, Laros GS: Triplane fractures of the distal tibial epiphysis. Clin Orthop 188:74, 1984
21. Kump WL: Vertical fractures of the distal tibial epiphysis. Am J Radiol 97:676, 1966
22. Karrholm J, Hansson LI, Laurin S: Supination-eversion injuries of the ankle in children: a retrospective study of radiologic classification and treatment. J Pediatr Orthop 2:147, 1982
23. Denton JR, Fischer SJ: The medial triplane fracture: report of an unusual injury. J Trauma 21:991, 1981
24. Ogden JA: Skeletal injury in the child. Lea & Febiger, Philadelphia, 596, 1982
25. Salter RB, Harris WR: Injuries involving the epiphyseal plate. J Bone Joint Surg [Am] 45:587, 1963
26. Letts RM: The hidden adolescent ankle fracture. J Pediatr Orthop 2:161, 1982
27. Tinnemans JG, Severijnen RS: The triplane fracture of the distal tibial epiphysis in children. Injury 12:393, 1981
28. Cass JR, Peterson HA: Salter-Harris type-IV injuries of the distal tibial epiphyseal growth plate, with emphasis on those involving the medial malleolus. J Bone Joint Surg [Am] 65:1059, 1983
29. Karrholm J, Hansson LI, Selvik G: Roentgen stereophotogrammetric analysis of growth pattern after supination-eversion injuries in children. J Pediatr Orthop 2:25, 1982

40

Fractures and Dislocations of the Tarsal Bones

Norris Carroll

> There is nothing so captivating as new knowledge.
> —PETER LATHAM

Fractures and dislocations of the tarsal bones in children are relatively uncommon injuries. When I canvased my colleagues at The Children's Memorial Hospital for examples they only came up with half a dozen names. Gross[1] found that at his hospital, over a 5-year period, 150 children were admitted with fractures of the femoral shaft, but there were only 2 talar fractures and 1 fracture of the calcaneus in skeletally immature children. In his book, *Children's Fractures,* Rang[2] states "Injuries to children's feet, despite all the little bones and joints, are remarkably uninteresting. Very few fractures will be encountered that display any subtleties or tricks; few are even displaced."

When examining the radiographs of an injured foot in a child it is important not to confuse ossification centers and accessory bones with fractures (Figs. 40-1 and 40-2).

If the symptoms and signs are much worse than one would anticipate, given the history of injury, suspect a pathologic fracture (Fig. 40-3).

The pliable child's foot dissipates energy and avoids fractures with "routine" trauma but major severe injuries can occur in lawnmower, automobile, all-terrain vehicle, motorbike, and snowmobile accidents[3,4,5] (Fig. 40-4).

ANATOMY

The medial border of the foot, from the heel to the tip of the great toe, is longer than the lateral border of the foot, from the heel to the tip of the fifth toe. Therefore a line joining the midpoints of the medial and lateral borders of the foot is oblique. In front of this line are the metatarsals, and behind this line are the bones of the tarsus osseous.[6] The tarsus osseous is divided into the midfoot and the hindfoot. The midfoot consists of the navicular, cuboid, and three cuneiforms. These bones have a cubical shape. The navicular has a medial tuberosity where the tibialis posterior tendon inserts. This tuberosity can remain as an "accessory" navicular and be confused with a fracture. The cuboid which forms the blunt apex of the wedge-shaped midfoot has a groove for the tendon of the peroneus longus. The forefoot is "keyed" to the midfoot by the second metatarsal, which is slotted between the middle and lateral cuneiforms. This mortising locks the second metatarsal and prevents side to side shifting of the forefoot in relation to the midfoot.

The hindfoot comprises the two largest tarsal bones;

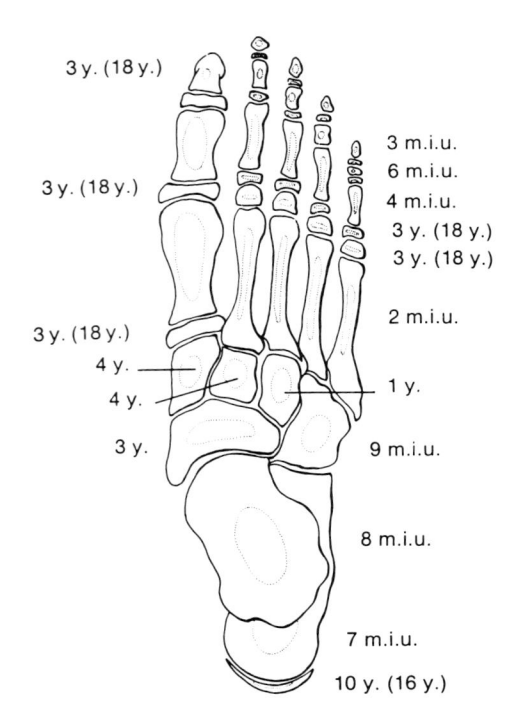

Fig. 40-1. Ossification centers of the tarsal bones in children. Numbers in parentheses indicate the time of fusion of primary and secondary ossification centers. y, years; miu, months in utero. (Redrawn from Aitken JT, Joseph J, Causey G, Young J: A Manual of Human Anatomy. 2nd Ed. Vol. IV. p. 80. E & S Livingstone, London, 1966, with permission.)

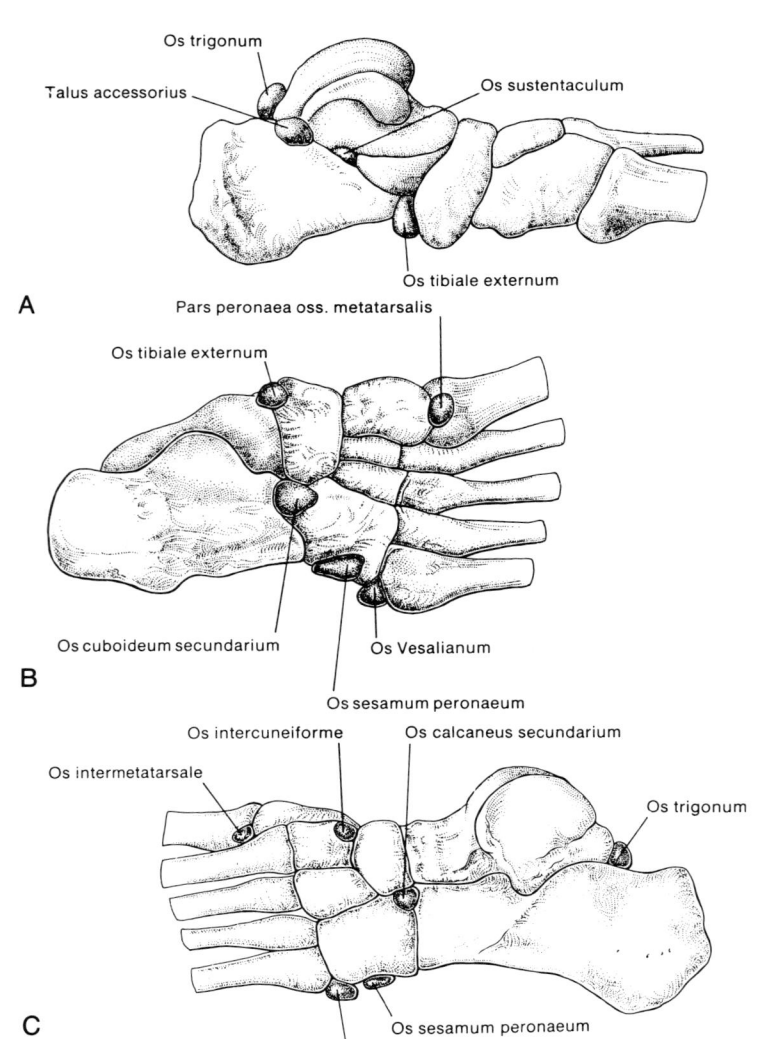

Fig. 40-2. Diagrammatic representation of the supernumerary tarsal bones. **(A)** Medial view. **(B)** Plantar view. **(C)** Lateral view. (Redrawn from Schaeffer JP: Morris' Human Anatomy. 11th Ed., p. 279. McGraw-Hill, New York, 1953, with permission.)

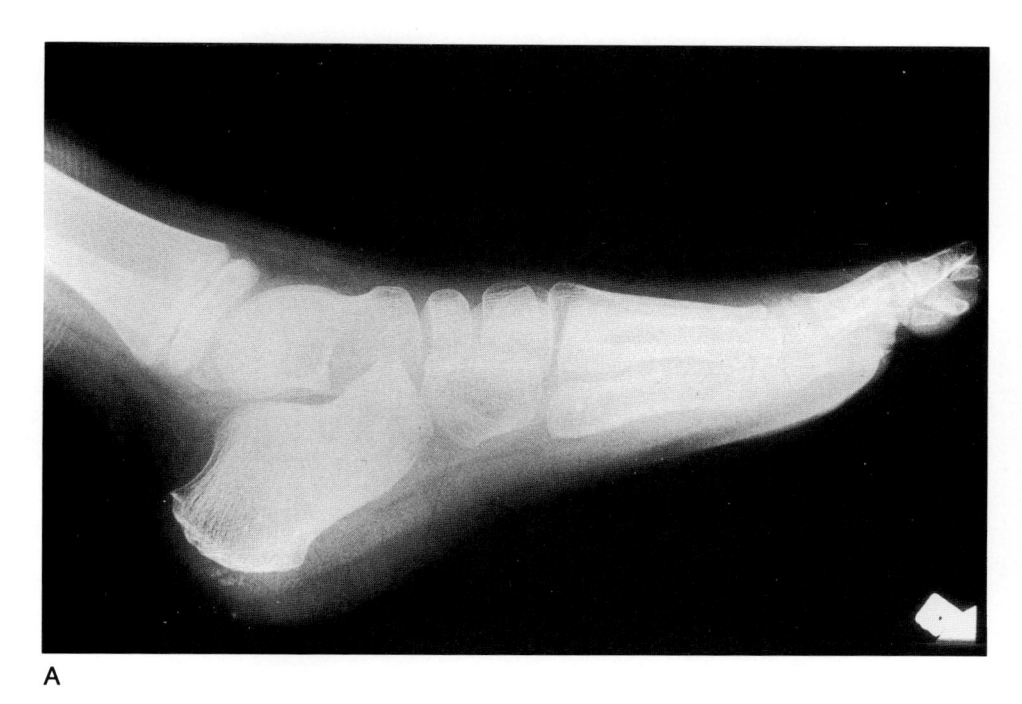

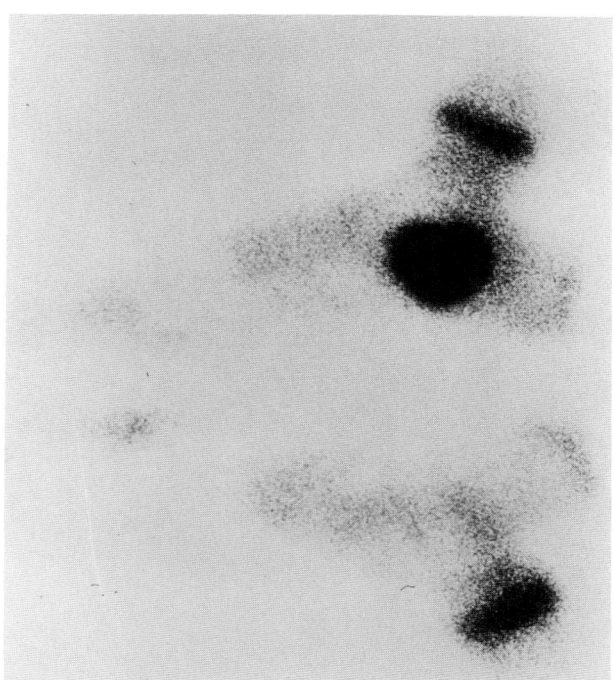

Fig. 40-3. (A) A 10-year-old boy complained of heel pain following a trivial injury. A lateral radiograph was read as negative. (B) The bone scan was very hot. *(Figure continues.)*

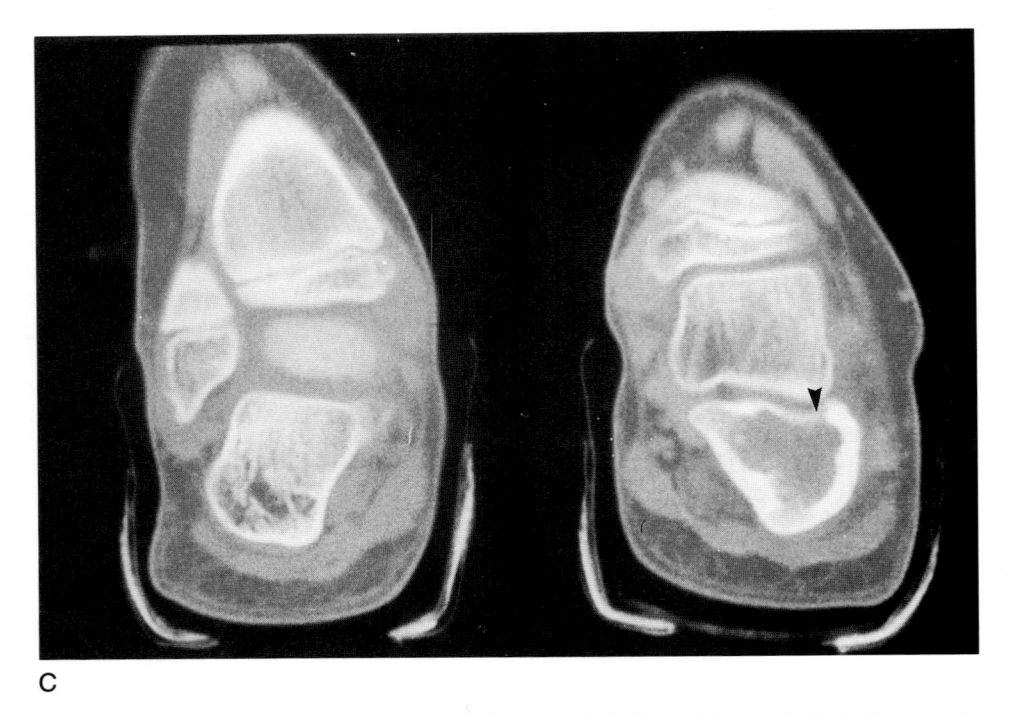

Fig. 40-3 *(Continued).* **(C)** CT scans demonstrate a large cystic lesion with a pathologic fracture through the posterior facet *(arrowhead).*

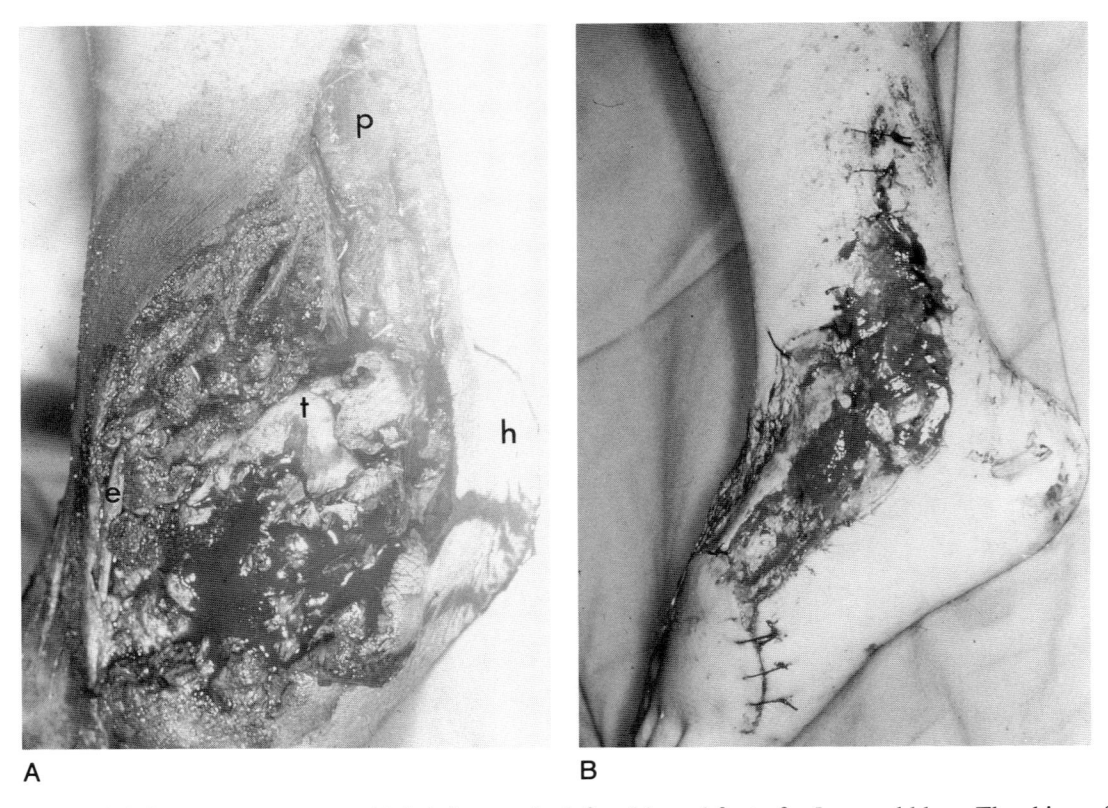

Fig. 40-4. **(A)** Severe open motor vehicle injury to the left ankle and foot of a 5-year-old boy. The skin, soft tissue, lateral malleolus, part of the calcaneus, and part of the talus have been sheared away. (e, extensor tendon; h, heel; p, peroneus brevis muscle; t, talus. **(B)** Five days later, prior to skin grafting (the peroneus brevis was used to cover the bony architecture).

the talus and calcaneus. The talus articulates with the tibia and fibula.

ANKLE JOINT

The ankle joint is a hinged joint. The axis of this hinge motion passes from a point slightly below the lowest point of the anterior part of the middle malleolus to a point under the tip of the fibula. As the fibular malleolus is lower and more posterior than the medial malleolus the axis of the hinge motion of the ankle is inclined downward and backward in the medial lateral direction.[7]

EVERSION AND INVERSION

Inversion of the foot is defined as a movement in which the lateral margin of the sole is depressed, while the medial border of the foot is elevated. Conversely, eversion is defined as a movement in which the medial margin of the sole is depressed and the lateral border of the foot is elevated.[7] To permit inversion and eversion it is apparent that a joint or joints in which convex surfaces are in articulation with concave surfaces are a requisite.[6] This condition is found where the head of the talus, which is globular, fits into the posterior surface of the navicular, which is cup shaped, and where the anterior surface of the calcaneus, which is cut away inferior medially, articulates with the posterior surface of the cuboid, which has a backwardly projecting process called the calcaneal process. It is at the talonavicular and calcaneocuboid joints (known as the transverse tarsal joint), in combination with the subtalar joint, that the movements of inversion and eversion take place.

TALUS

The talus rests on the anterior two-thirds of the calcaneus and projects slightly in front of it. It has a body, neck, and head. The upper surface of the body supports the tibia; it is entirely articular and is saddle shaped. The sides of the body are grasped by the malleoli and the facets that result correspond in length and shape with those of the malleoli. The lateral facet tapers from front to back and medially. The lateral border of its superior articular surface is correspondingly curved and is longer than the medial border. There are two tubercles on the posterior surface of the body of talus; a medial and a lateral, separated by a groove for the flexor hallucis longus tendon and therefore running downward and medially. The upper surface of the nonarticular neck is rough, while the head is rounded to articulate with the navicular. The part of the talus that projects laterally and downward toward the horizontal platform of the os calcis is called the lateral process. On the undersurface of the talus between the lateral process and the tubercles is the concave articulation for the posterior facet of the calcaneus. Medially there is a convex facet that articulates with the sustentaculum.

Fracture of the Talus

Signs and Symptoms

Signs and symptoms of a fracture of the talus are as follows:

1. History of forced dorsiflexion of the foot
2. Swelling
3. Pain and tenderness in the region of the talus
4. Painful dorsiflexion

All of the above should make one suspicious that there is a fracture of the talus.

With trauma to a child's foot the soft tissue injury may be more significant than the fracture and initial treatment must be directed toward managing the swelling and the damage to the skin (abrasions, fracture blisters), muscles, and the neural and vascular structures.[9] The foot must be carefully examined for evidence of circulatory or neurologic complications. One must be on the lookout for compartment syndrome. Septa from the plantar aponeurosis attach to the first and fifth metatarsals, dividing the plantar surface of the foot into three compartments.[10] The medial plantar compartment encloses the abductor hallucis and the flexor hallucis brevis and the tendon of the flexor hallucis longus. The midplantar compartment encloses the adductor hallucis, the tendon of the flexor digitorum longus, the quadratus plantae, and the flexor digitorum brevis. The lateral plantar compartment encloses the flexor digiti minimi brevis and the abductor digiti minimi. The dorsal compartment encloses the lateral four metatarsals, the extensor tendons of the toes, and the interossei. Most foot injuries must be treated initially with a bulky dressing and elevation. Definitive treatment of the fracture will have to be delayed until it is safe to manipulate the foot and apply a plaster or make incisions for open reduction and internal fixation.

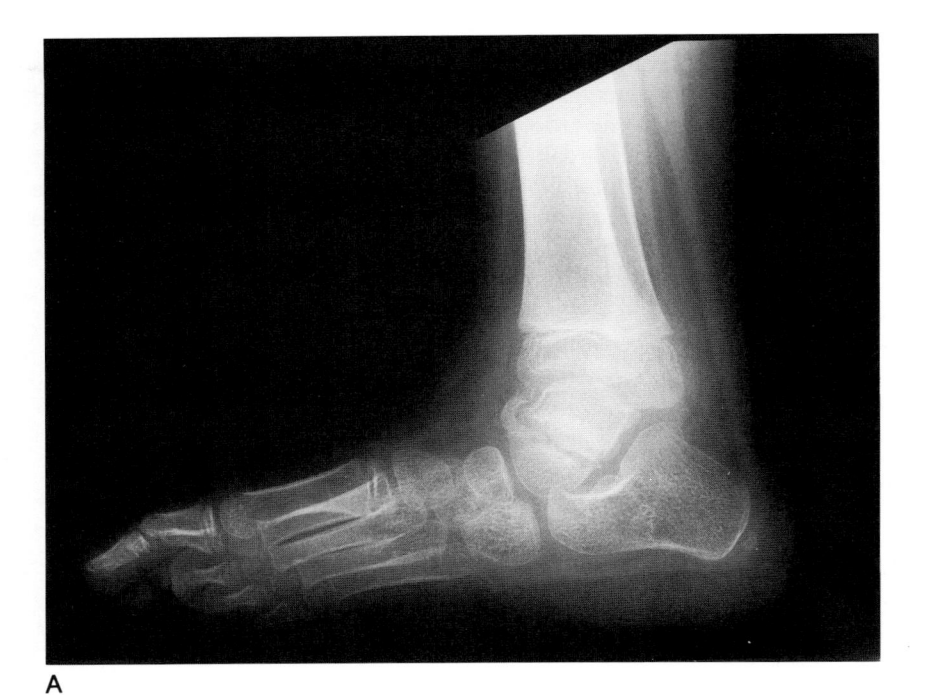

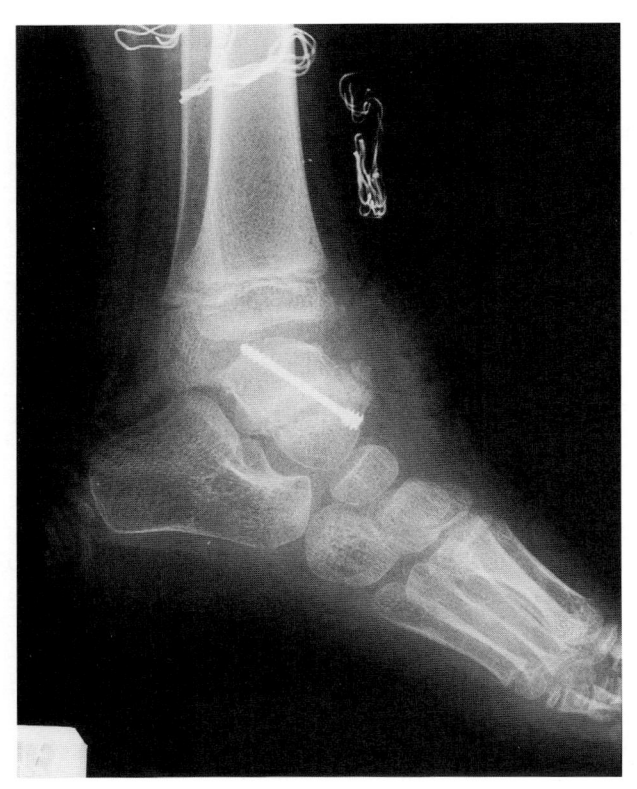

Fig. 40-5. (A) A 16-year-old girl with a sacral level myelomeningocele is an independent ambulator with bilateral AFOs. She injured her right ankle while playing without her braces. Her initial radiographs were interpreted as being negative, but subsequent films demonstrated a talar neck fracture. (B) As the fracture did not heal with 6 months of immobilization she was treated with a compression screw and bone graft.

The most common injury is a vertical fracture through the talar neck and the most common mechanism of injury is forced dorsiflexion[11] (Fig. 40-5).

Classification

The fracture pattern and displacement will depend not only on the direction and magnitude of the force but also with the age of the child, that is, how much of the talus is still cartilaginous.

Because so much of the talus is articular, it has a precarious blood supply. Vessels enter the bone on the dorsum of the talar neck in the sinus tarsi and medially deep to the deltoid ligament.[12] The key to the successful treatment of talus fractures is a knowledge of the anatomy of the talus and its blood supply. Classifications should aid in management strategies and predict prognosis therefore Szyszkowitz and colleagues[13] proposed the Classification in Table 40-1.

Crush fractures of the lateral process and medial and lateral tubercles, fractures through the head, avulsion fractures of the lateral process, and fractures through the distal neck are not associated with avascular necrosis of the body. Nondisplaced fractures through the proximal neck and through the body have a rare incidence of avascular necrosis. Displaced fractures through the neck and through the body have frequently had avascular necrosis and a fracture through the neck with dislocation of the body is always associated with avascular necrosis.[14]

AP, lateral, and oblique radiographic views should be taken of the hindfoot and ankle.[11,15,16] In any instance, when it is difficult to define the nature and extent of a talus injury, a CT scan or magnetic resonance image (MRI) is recommended. Nondisplaced fractures can be treated in a non-weight-bearing cast (Fig. 40-6). The easiest way to keep a child non-weight-bearing is to apply a long-leg cast with the knee flexed. Displaced fractures will require manipulative or open reduction (Fig. 40-5). If a fracture of the talar neck requires open reduction, it can be approached dorsally between the tendons of the extensor hallucis longus and the tibialis anterior. Minimal stripping of the soft tissues from the bone will lessen the chance of an avascular necrosis (Fig. 40-7). Displaced fractures of the dome of the body of the talus that cannot be adequately reduced can be approached by doing an osteotomy of the medial malleolus. The osteotomy should be fixed with smooth pins and the patient should be kept non-weight-bearing until there is radiographic evidence of healing. I have never had to use this approach in a child nor have I seen a subtalar dislocation in a child.

It is difficult to differentiate a dome fracture from an osteochondritis dissecans.[17] The osteochondral fracture demonstrated in Figure 40-8 was treated by arthroscopic debridement.

CALCANEUS

The calcaneus is large, oblong, and is divided into three parts. The anterior two-thirds supports the talus, while the posterior third forms the prominence that rests

TABLE 40-1. Classification of Talus Fractures

Type	Circulation	Necrosis

Type I
Peripheral fractures
  Lateral processe
  Medial & lateral tubercles
  Distal neck
  Head
	Intact	None

Type II
Central fractures without displacement
  Proximal neck
  Body
	Mainly intact	Seldom

Type III
Central fractures with displacement
  Proximal neck
  Body
	Interrupted, intraosseous; intact auxiliary	Often

Type IV
Dislocation fractures
  Proximal neck
  Body dislocated in the ankle and/or subtalar joint
	Interrupted interosseous and auxiliary	Nearly always

(Modified from Szyszkowitz et al.,[13] with permission.)

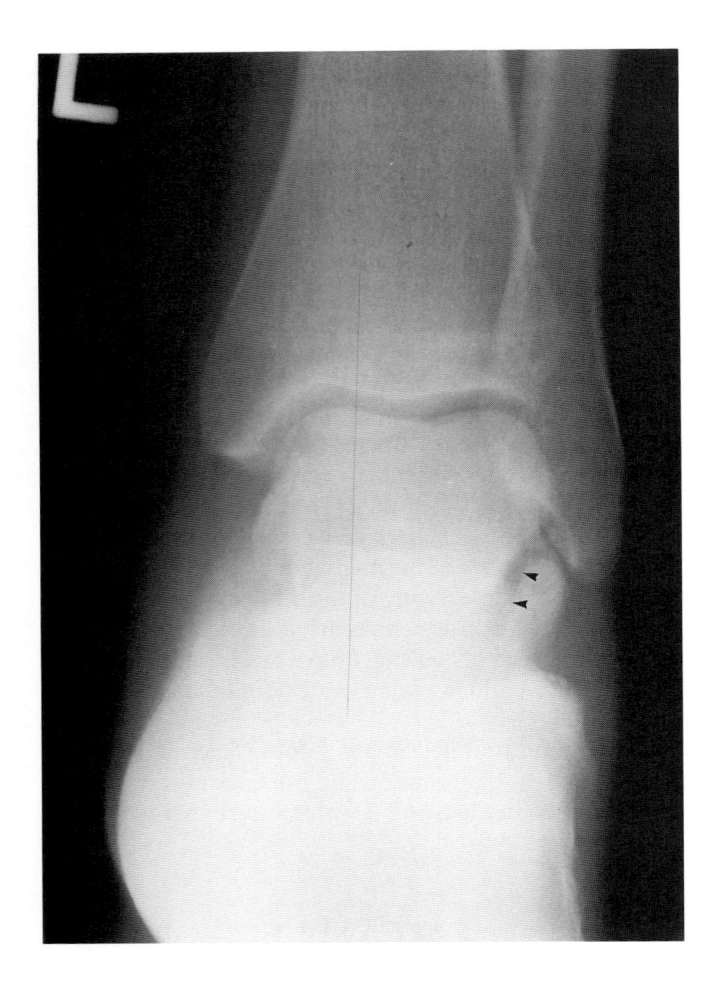

Fig. 40-6. AP view of the ankle of a 15-year-old boy who was injured in a gymnastic accident. There is an avulsion fracture of the lateral process of his talus *(arrows)*.

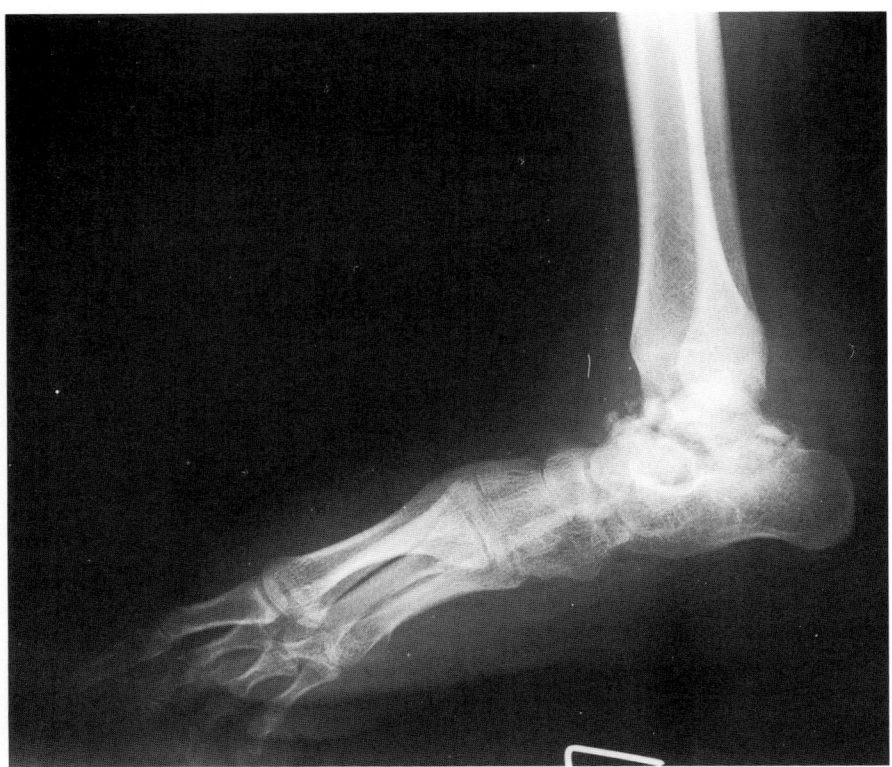

Fig. 40-7. This 18-year-old female has a lumbar myelomeningocele, an Arnold Chiari malformation, and an L-P shunt. She injured her right ankle in a motor vehicle accident. Her radiographs demonstrated a comminuted fracture of the talus. She was treated in a cast. The main fragments united and the loose pieces were debrided at a later date. (There was no avascular necrosis.)

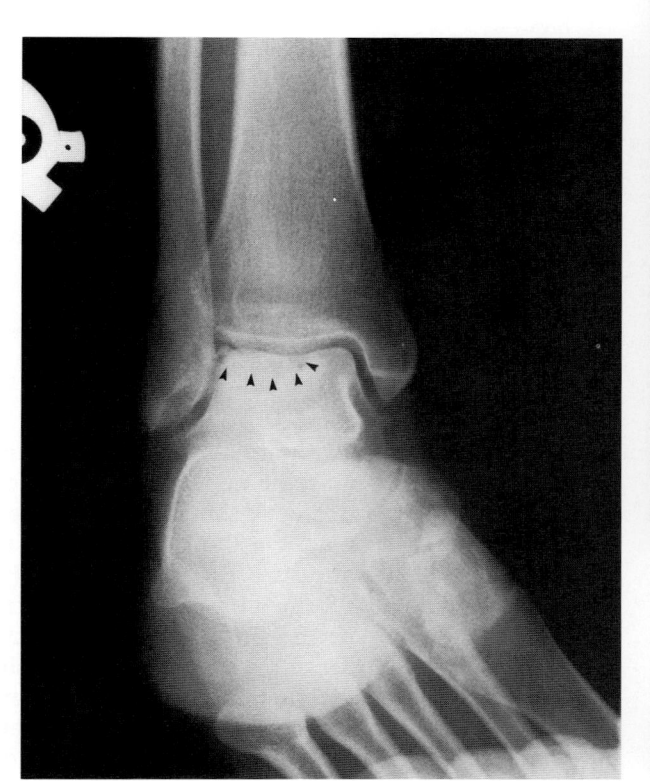

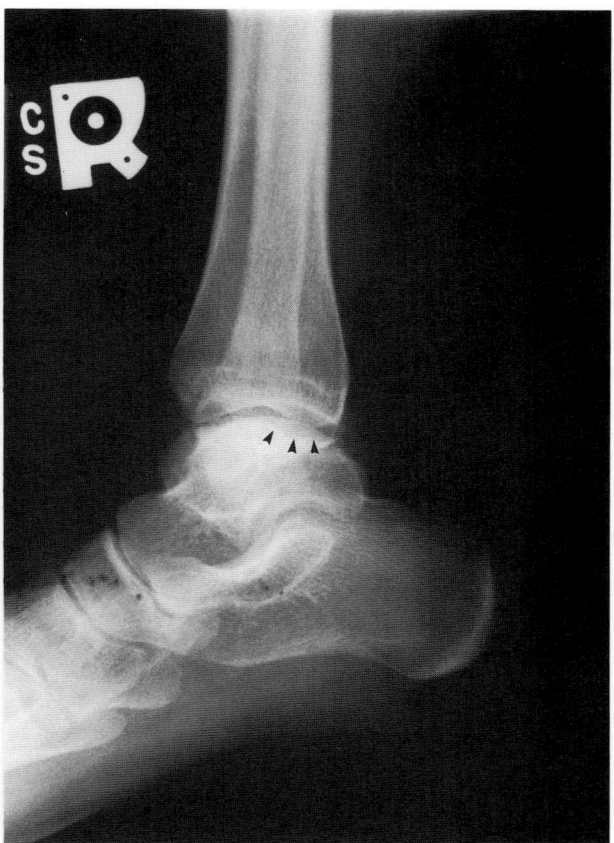

Fig. 40-8. This 17-year-old girl presented with pain and locking in her right ankle. Three years prior to presentation she developed acute lymphocytic leukemia, which was treated with vincristine and prednisone. Her radiographs demonstrate a large osteochondritic fragment on the dome of her talus *(arrowheads)*. This was treated by arthroscopic debridement.

on the ground during stance. The entire anterior surface articulates with the cuboid. The posterior third of the superior surface is free. The intermediate third of the superior surface comprises the posterior facet of the subtalar joint, while the anterior third forms a nonarticular horizontal platform laterally and a small facet medially for the head of the talus. This facet may or may not be continuous with the middle facet on a medially projecting shelf called the sustentaculum tali. A deep groove, separating the posterior facet from the middle facet, is called the sinus tarsi. The lateral surface of the calcaneus is almost flat and vertical. It has the peroneal tubercle placed below the lateral malleolus and a fullness behind this where the calcaneofibular ligament attaches. The medial surface is hollowed out between the sustentaculum and the posterior surface. The posterior surface (tuberosity) is nonarticular and is wider below than above. The plantar surface has a large medial tubercle and a smaller lateral tubercle.

The foot is described as having two longitudinal arches. These arches are more apparent in a child over the age of 4. The three medial digits, their metatarsals and cuneiforms, the navicular and talus are collectively known as the medial longitudinal arch of the foot, while the lateral two digits, their metatarsals, the cuboid and the calcaneus collectively form the lateral longitudinal arch. The foot is also arched transversely; the dorsum being convex both anteroposteriorly and from side to side. The plantar aspect is concave in both directions. The foot with its complex bony architecture, supporting ligaments and intrinsic and extrinsic motors is a remarkable structure that is both flexible and rigid during the gait cycle. During the third interval of the stance phase (foot flat to toe-off) the foot is converted from the flexible structure that was present during the first interval (heel strike to foot flat) and the partially stabilized foot that was present in the second interval (period of foot flat) into a rigid arch.[8]

Fractures of the Calcaneus

Mechanism of Injury

Calcaneal fractures are rare in children. Most are sustained as a result of a fall from a height. The inferiorly protruding lateral process of the talus is jammed into the superior surface of the calcaneus on impact.

Classification

A classification of calcaneal fractures is shown in Table 40-2.[18]

Signs and Symptoms

Calcaneal injuries usually present with the following signs and symptoms, confirmed on radiologic examination.

1. History of a fall from a height
2. Local swelling (broad heel flat arch)
3. Pain and tenderness over the heel
4. Radiographic examination
   A. Anteroposterior
   B. Lateral
   C. Axial
   D. Oblique

TABLE 40-2. Os Calcis Fracture Classification

I. Tuberosity Fractures
II. Involving subtalar joint with displacement
   A. Tongue type
      Primary fracture line
      a. Medial to posterior facet
      b. Central to posterior facet
      c. Lateral to posterior facet
   B. Joint depression
      Primary fracture line
      a. Medial to posterior facet
      b. Central to posterior facet
III. Avulsion fractures
   A. Extra-articular
   B. Intra-articular

(Adapted from Ross and Sowerby,[18] with permission.)

Schmidt and Weiner[19] reported the presence of compression fractures of the spine in association with calcaneal fractures so these children should also have lateral radiographs of their spine. On the lateral view of the hindfoot one should measure Bohler's[20] angle (Fig. 40-9). Bohler's angle is formed by a line parallel to the articular surfaces of the calcaneus with a line drawn along the superior border of the tuberosity. Depression of the subtalar joint decreases this angle. Most fractures of the calcaneus in children involve the tuberosity and heal uneventfully (Fig. 40-10) immobilization and non-

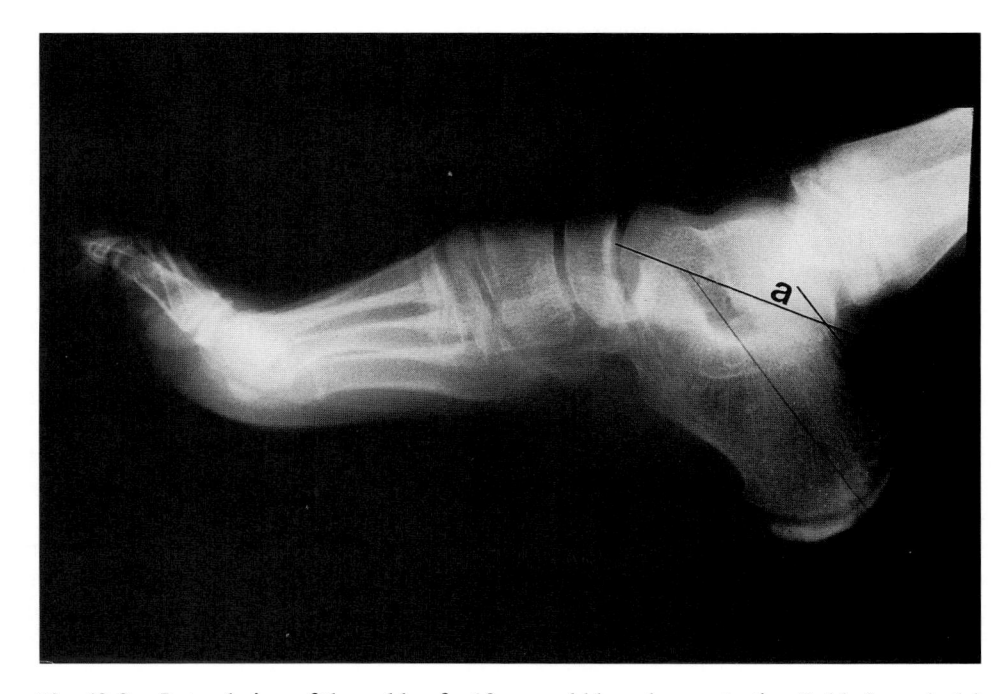

Fig. 40-9. Lateral view of the ankle of a 13-year-old boy demonstrating Bohler's angle *(a)*.

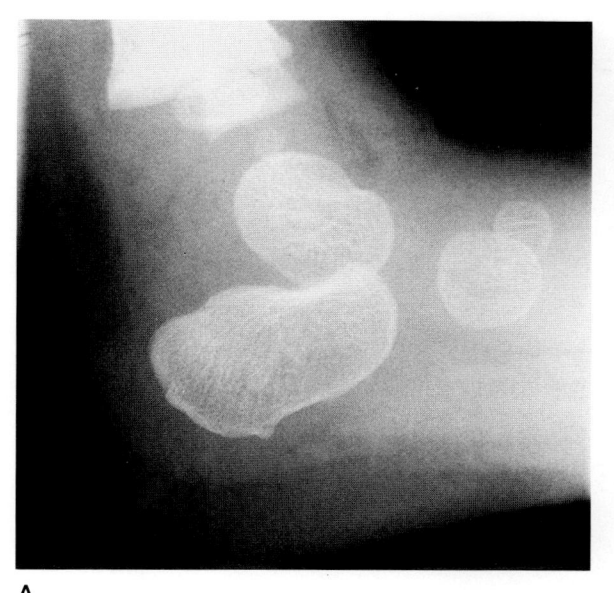

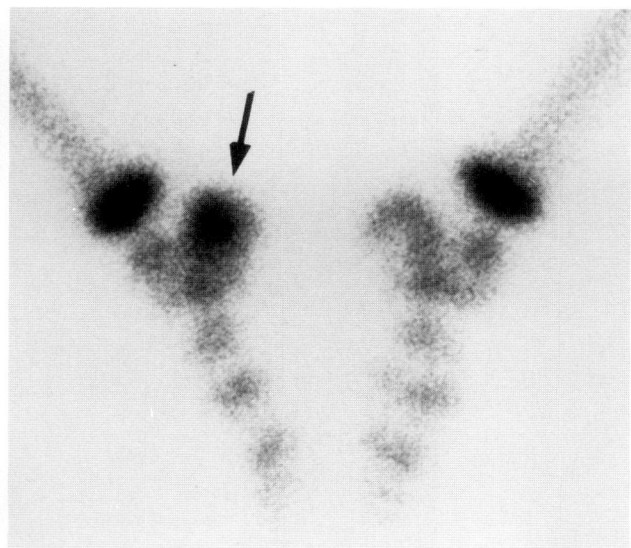

Fig. 40-10. (A) This 13-month-old boy developed a limp after jumping off a step. He walked with his left knee stiff and kept the limb externally rotated. Physical examination and initial radiographs were negative. (B) A bone scan demonstrates a hot left heel (black arrow). (C) Five weeks later one can see the sclerotic line in the os calcis *(arrowheads)*.

weight-bearing until union is achieved is all that is necessary.[21] Thomas[22] demonstrated five fracture patterns in his five patients. He reported good results even when Bohler's angle was flattened. He observed that the inferior articular facet of the talus appeared to overgrow to such a degree as to precisely accommodate the joint depression of the calcaneus. He concluded that the remodeling potential of the talus minimized the affect of the depression of the calcaneal facet. Very satisfactory clinical results were reported in these five patients.

In an older child with a calcaneal fracture if the anterior, posterior, lateral, oblique, and axial views indicate that there is a comminuted interarticular fracture I think that computed tomography (CT) should be used to better define the fracture pattern. We have reported on the use of CT in the evaluation of five calcaneal fractures in three patients. Three of the fractures were comminuted and the CT gave graphic additional information to the plane radiographs. Three fractures were undisplaced and were managed conservatively. In the other two there was displacement of bony fragments and these were treated operatively.

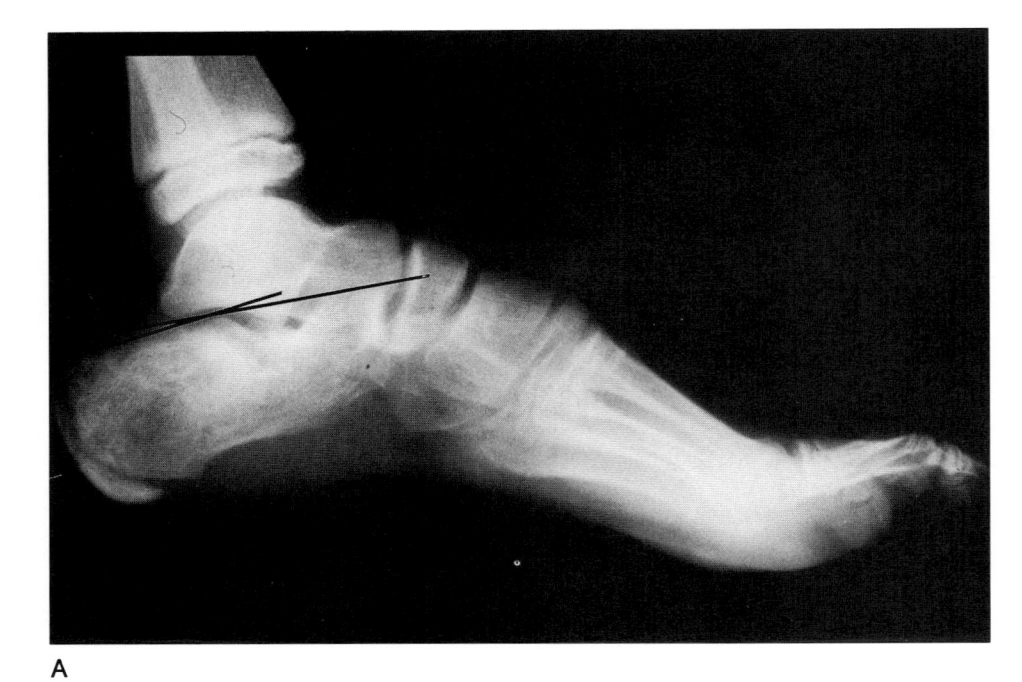

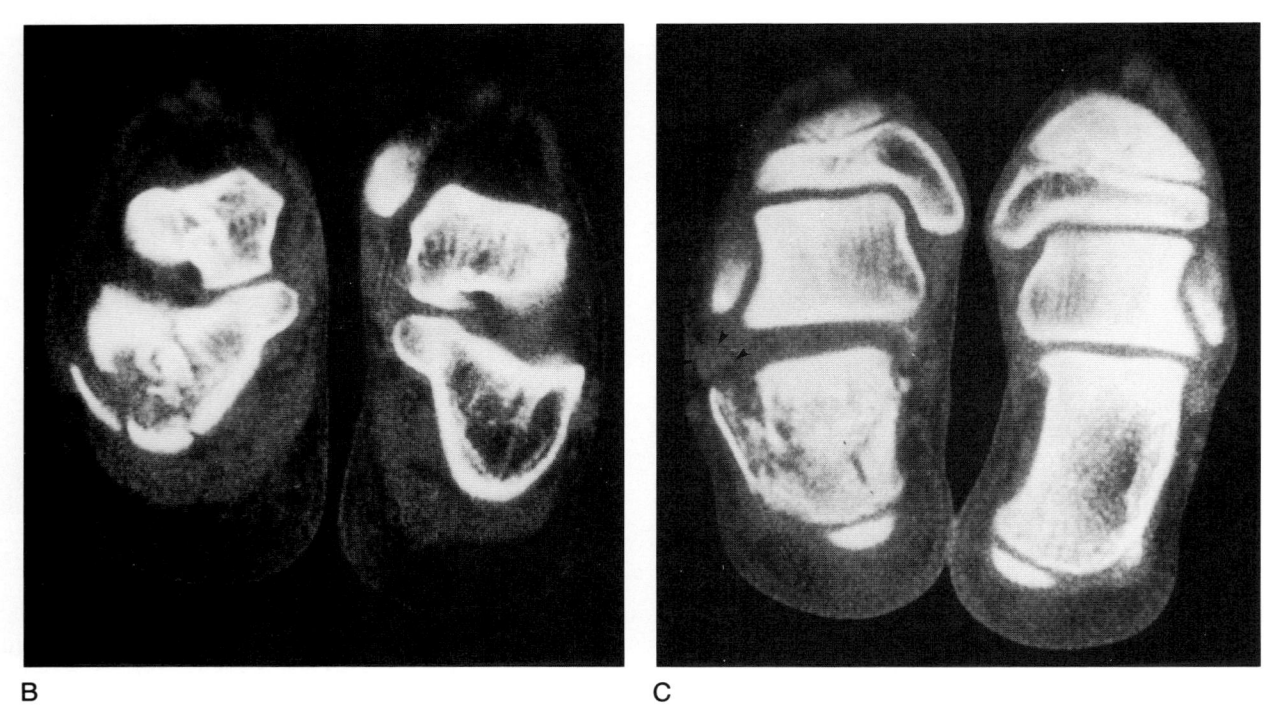

Fig. 40-11. **(A)** A 13-year-old boy jumped 15 ft, landing on his right foot. Plane radiographs showed a joint compression fracture with a poorly seen fragment on the lateral aspect of the calcaneus, loss of Bohler's angle, and disruption of the lateral margin of the calcaneus. **(B–D)** CT scan demonstrated a comminuted fracture with multiple fragments in the body, posterior and lateral aspects of the calcaneus, marked AP compression of the calcaneus and widening and disruption of the posterior talocalcaneal joint. The middle and anterior talocalcaneal joints and the calcaneocuboid joint were intact. The peroneal tendons appeared closely related to the displaced fragments along the lateral margin *(arrows). (Figure continues.)*

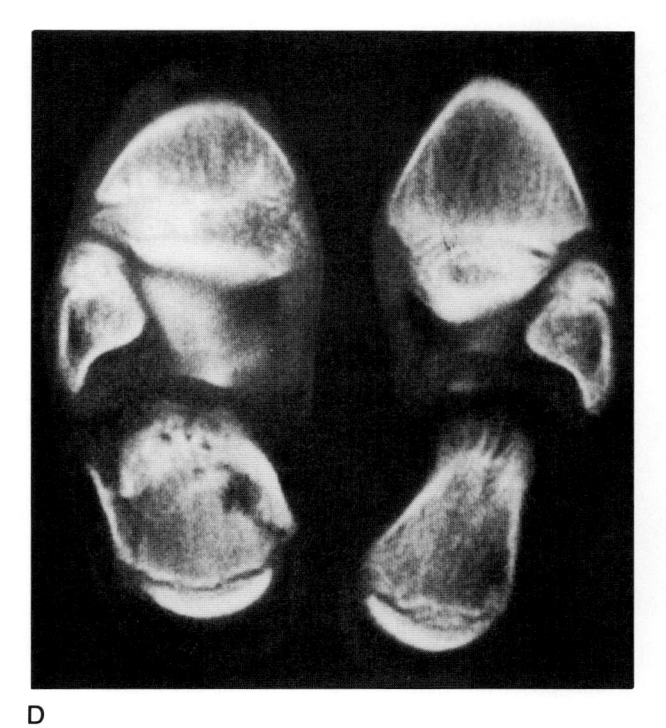

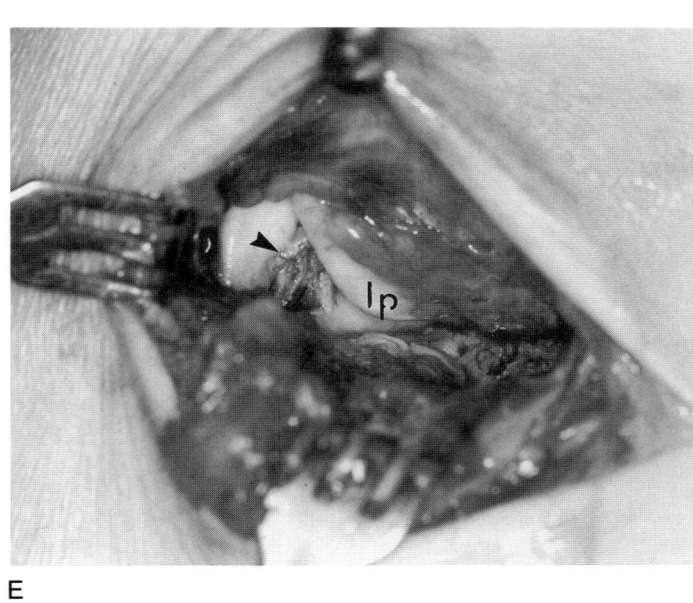

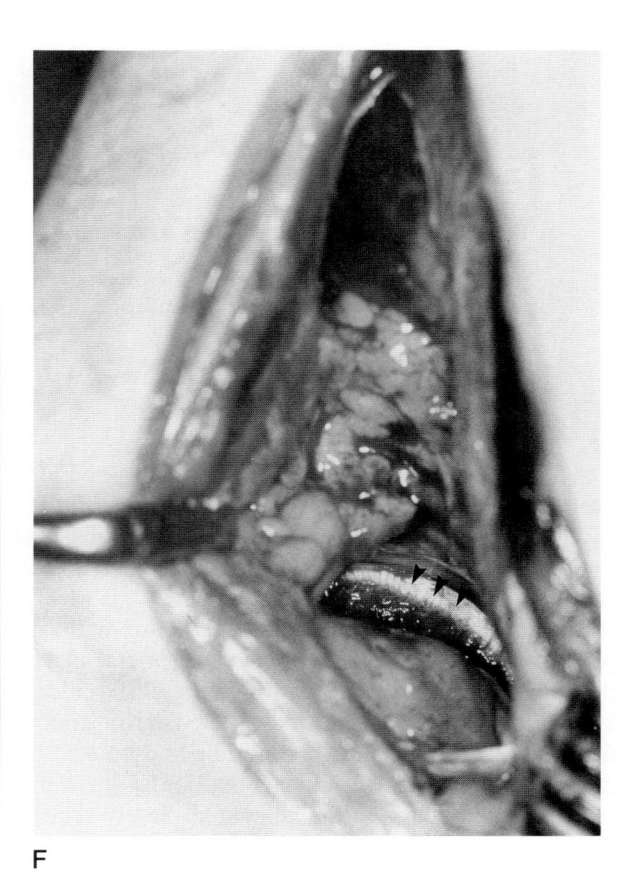

Fig. 40-11 *(Continued).* **(E)** Lateral exposure of subtalar joint demonstrating lateral process (*lp*) of talus and comminuted fracture of the posterior facet of the subtalar joint *(arrowhead)*. **(F)** Posterior exposure demonstrating fracture of the posterior facet of the subtalar joint *(arrowheads)*. *(Figure continues.)*

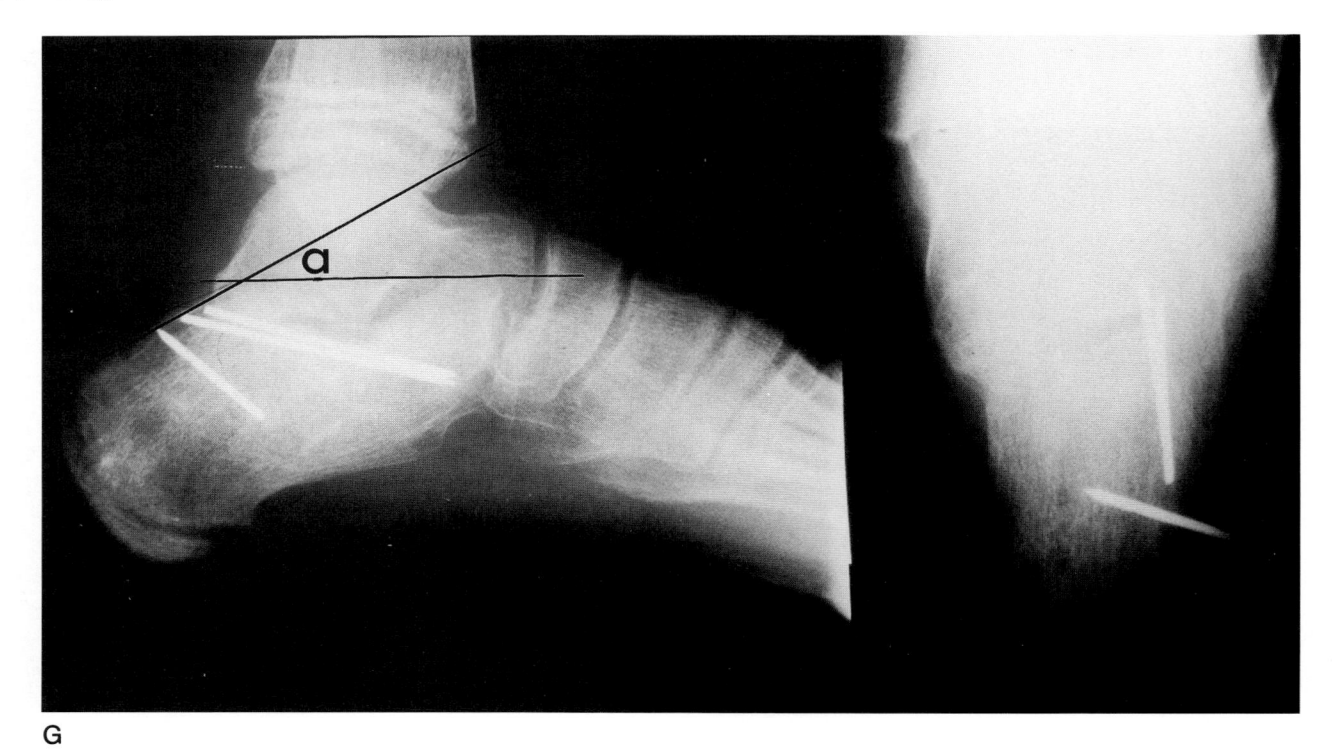

Fig. 40-11 *(Continued).* **(G)** At operation, through lateral and posterior incisions, the posterior depressed fractures were elevated and disimpacted. The lateral cortex of the calcaneus was reduced anatomically. Bone graft was used to fill the defect left in the subarticular portion of the bone and the bone fragments were held in position with multiple K-wires. [Note improvement in Bohler's angle *(a)*.]

Case Example

A 13-year-old boy jumped 15 feet landing on his right foot. Plain radiographs showed a joint compression fracture with a poorly seen fragment on the lateral aspect of the calcaneus, loss of Bohler's angle, and disruption of the lateral margin of the calcaneus (Fig. 40-11A). CT scans demonstrated a comminuted fracture with multiple fragments in the body, posterior and lateral aspects of the calcaneus, marked AP compression of the calcaneus and widening and disruption of the posterior talocalcaneal joint (Fig. 40B–D). The middle and anterior talocalcaneal joints and the calcaneocuboid joint were intact. The peroneal tendons appeared closely related to the displaced fragments along the lateral margin. At operation, through lateral and posterior incisions (Fig. 40-11E&F), the posterior depressed fracture was elevated and disimpacted. The lateral cortex of the calcaneus was reduced anatomically. A bone graft was used to fill the defect left in the subarticular portion of the bone, and the bony fragments were held in position with multiple K-wires (Fig. 40-11G). The patient had a good result. He has lost some subtalar motion but has no pain and participates in all athletic activities.

PRINCIPLES OF TREATMENT: CALCANEUS FRACTURES

The principles in treating these complex injuries are as follows:

1. Define nature and extent of the injury preoperatively.
2. Use an operative approach that will permit an accurate reduction of all the bony fragments.
3. Reduce the fragments of the posterior facet of the subtalar joint (support with bone graft if necessary).
4. Reduce the sustentaculum tali fragment.
5. Restore Bohler's angle and heel height.
6. Reduce the heel width to normal.
7. Adequate internal fixation.
8. Early motion.

FRACTURES OF THE LESSER TARSAL BONES

Fractures of the navicular, cuneiforms, and cuboid are rare in children, but they can occur when the foot is subjected to direct trauma such as being struck by a falling object. However, Sangeorzan and colleagues[23] reported on 21 patients who had a displaced fracture of the body of the tarsal navicular treated with open reduction and internal fixation. One of these patients was a 12-year-old boy. These authors devised a classification system based on the direction of the fracture line, the pattern of disruption of the surrounding joints and the direction of displacement of the foot.

Type I: The fracture line is in the coronal plane and there is no angulation of the forepart of the foot.

Type II: The primary fracture line is dorsolateral to plantar medial, and the major fragment and forepart of the foot are displaced medially.

Type III: There is a comminuted fracture in the sagittal plane of the body of the tarsal navicular and the forepart of the foot is laterally displaced; the lateral displacement of the forepart of the foot is associated with injuries to the cuboid or the anterior process of the calcaneus.

These fractures were treated by open reduction and internal fixation using a medial approach between the tendons of the tibialis anterior and tibialis posterior.

Blumberg and Patterson[24] have reported on two proven and two presumed cases of cuboid fractures in toddlers. These children were seen because of their inability to weight bear on the affected foot following a fall. The initial radiographs were normal; however, early scintigraphy revealed focal uptake in the cuboid. Follow-up radiographs demonstrated characteristic sclerosis of the base of the cuboid.

Dr. James Conway, Chief of Nuclear Medicine at The Children's Memorial Hospital in Chicago, has collected a series of occult bony injuries in children. He calls these

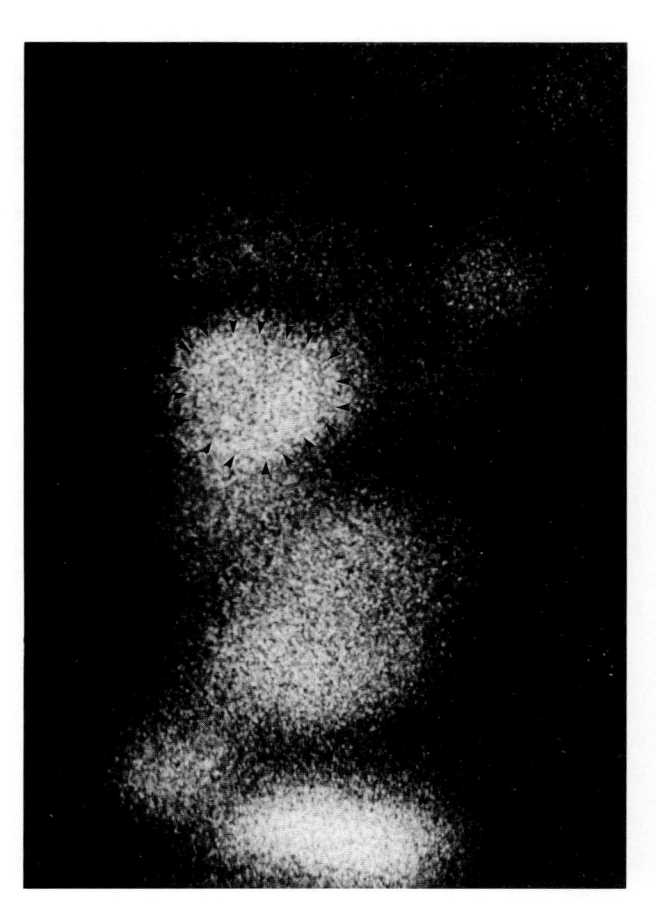

Fig. 40-12. This 2½-year-old boy presented with an unexplained limp of 2 months duration. His initial radiographs were negative. His bone scan demonstrated intense localization of radionuclide in the third cuneiform and cuboid of the left foot *(arrowheads)*. This most likely represents a compression injury.

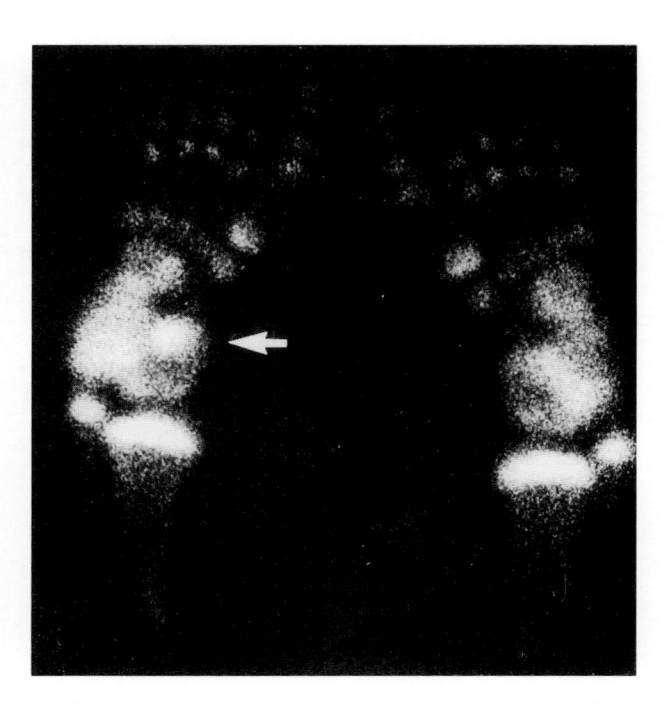

Fig. 40-13. This 1 year, 10-month-old boy had a persistant limp after falling from a couch. His radiographs were negative. His bone scan demonstrated increased localization of radionuclide in the anterior aspect of the left talus *(arrow)*. This likely represents a compression injury.

trabecular fractures or elastic injuries. They are undetected on routine initial radiographic examination (Fig. 40-7). The evidence for such an injury may only be documented by delayed evidence such as radiographic changes seen 3 weeks after the injury (a zone of sclerosis at the trabecular fracture site). Bone scintigraphy has been shown to be sensitive for detecting this type of injury. Most of the patients in Dr. Conway's study were toddlers who had an injury and then refused to weight bear. The patients were tender over the affected bone, but their initial radiographs were all normal. The diagnosis was made with scintigraphy and then substantiated with computed tomography or magnetic resonance imaging of the affected bone. Dr. Conway has documented occult injuries to the cuboid (Fig. 40-12), head of the talus (Fig. 40-13), calcaneus (Fig. 40-10), and navicular. He has noted that these injuries are commonest in cube-shaped bones that have a high trabecular to compact bone ratio. Treatment consists of immobilization until symptoms subside.

REFERENCES

1. Gross RH: Fractures and dislocations of the foot. p. 1043. In Rockwood CA Jr (ed): Fractures in Children. Vol. 3. JB Lippincott, Philadelphia, 1984
2. Rang M: Foot. p. 323. In: Children's Fractures. 2nd Ed. JB Lippincott, Philadelphia, 1974
3. Letts RM, Cleary J: The child and the snowmobile. Can Med Assoc J 113:1061, 1975
4. Peterson HA, FitzGibbons TC, Arata MA: Snowmobile injuries in children. Minn Med 62:193, 1979
5. Ross PM, Schwentker EP, Bryan H: Mutilating lawn mower injuries in children. JAMA 236:480, 1976
6. Grant JCB: A Method of Anatomy. 5th Ed. p. 442. Williams & Wilkins, Baltimore, 1952
7. Kelikian H, Kelikian AS: Physiological and forced movements. p. 40. In: Disorders of the Ankle. WB Saunders, Philadelphia, 1985
8. Mann RA: Biomechanics of the foot and ankle. p. 1. In Mann RA (ed): Surgery of the Foot. 5th Ed. CV Mosby, St. Louis, 1986
9. Ogden JA: Foot. p. 621. In: Skeletal Injury in the Child. Lea & Febiger, Philadelphia, 1982
10. Hollinshead WH: Anatomy for Surgeons. 2nd Ed. Vol. 3. p. 857. Hoeber Harper, New York, 1968
11. Letts RM, Gibeault D: Fractures of the neck of the talus in children. Foot Ankle 1:74, 1980
12. Mulfinger GL, Trueta J: The blood supply of the talus. J Bone Joint Surg [Br] 52:161, 1970
13. Szyszkowitz R, Reschauer R, Seggl W: Eighty-five talus fractures treated by ORIF with five to eight years of follow-up study of 69 patients. Clin Orthop Rel Res 199:98, 1985
14. Weber BG, Brunner C, Freuler F: Treatment of Fractures in Children and Adolescents. p. 365. Springer-Verlag, New York, 1980
15. Canale ST, Kelly FB Jr: Fractures of the neck of the talus: long term evaluation of 71 cases. J Bone Joint Surg [Am] 60:143, 1978
16. Smith GR, Winquist RA, Allan TNK, Northrop CH: Subtle transchondral fractures of the talar dome: radiological perspective. Radiology 14:667, 1977
17. Berndt AL, Harty M: Transchondral fractures (osteochondritis dissecans) of the talus. J Bone Joint Surg [Am] 41:988, 1959
18. Ross SDK, Sowerby MRR: The operative treatment of fractures of the os calcis. Clin Orthop Rel Res 199:135, 1985
19. Schmidt TL, Weiner DS: Calcaneal fractures in children: an evaluation of the nature of the injury in 56 children. Clin Orthop 171:150, 1982
20. Harty M: Anatomic considerations in injuries of the calcaneus. Orthop Clin North Am 4:179, 1973
21. Trott A: Fracture of the foot in children. Orthop Clin North Am 7:677, 1976
22. Thomas HM: Calcaneal fractures in childhood. Br J Surg 56:664, 1969
23. Sangeorzan BJ et al: Displaced intra-articular fractures of the tarsal navicular. J Bone Joint Surg [Am] 71:1504, 1989
24. Blumberg K, Patterson RJ: The toddler's cuboid fracture. Radiology 179:93, 1991

41

Fractures and Dislocations of the Metatarsals and Phalanges of the Foot

Maureen P. Baxter

> For most diagnoses all that is needed is an ounce of knowledge, an ounce of intelligence, and a pound of thoroughness.

FRACTURES AND DISLOCATIONS OF THE METATARSALS

Description and Incidence

Fractures of the metatarsals in children are a common injury. In a review of fractures seen at the Children's Hospital of Eastern Ontario, these injuries represented 1.25 percent of all fractures. Metatarsal fractures accounted for 56 percent of the foot fractures. 62 percent occurred in males, and the mean age at the time of injury was 11 years. The classification of metatarsal fractures in children is shown in Table 41-1.

Anatomy

Bones

The five metatarsals form the most proximal portion of the part of the foot referred to as the forefoot (Fig. 41-1). Each metatarsal bone tapers from a broad base to a thin neck, then enlarges into a round head that articulates with the proximal phalanx. The secondary ossification centers of the second through fifth metatarsals are curvilinear structures located distally at the level of the necks. They appear between the ages of 3 and 4 years and fuse with the diaphyses between the ages of 16 and 18 years. The secondary ossification center of the first metatarsal is located proximally at the base of the bone. It appears and fuses at the same time as the other metatarsals. The base of the first metatarsal is expanded on its plantar-medial aspect to form a tuberosity for the insertion of peroneus longus. The plantar-lateral surface of the fifth metatarsal has a similar tuberosity for the insertion of peroneus brevis. This tuberosity may form a seprate ossification center known as os vesalianum. If ununited, it can be confused with a fracture. The blood supply to the metatarsals pierces the bone dorsally at the junction of the proximal and middle thirds.

Metatarsal Joints

The base of the first metatarsal forms a proximal convex articulation with the medial cuneiform. (Fig. 41-2) The base of the second metatarsal has a flatter articular surface with the middle cuneiform proximally and the

TABLE 41-1. Classification of Metatarsal Fractures in Children

Neck, Shaft
  Undisplaced
  Displaced
Base of fifth metatarsal
First metatarsal
Associated with tarsometatarsal injury
Compound
Stress
Sesamoid

medial cuneiform medially. The base of the third metatarsal articulates with the lateral cuneiform slightly distally to the second. The fourth metatarsal articulates with the cuboid at the same level as the third. The fifth metatarsal articulates with the lateral half of the cuboid. The second, third, and fourth metatarsals have medial and lateral articulations with each other. The fifth has a medial articulation with the fourth, and the first, a lateral articulation with the second. These surfaces of the metatarsals form gliding joints, hence apposed or corresponding facets are not exact counterparts of each other, one being more extensive than the other. The extent of forward projection of the first, second, and third metatarsal bones varies. The heads of the metatarsals are all joined to each other by the transverse capitular liga-

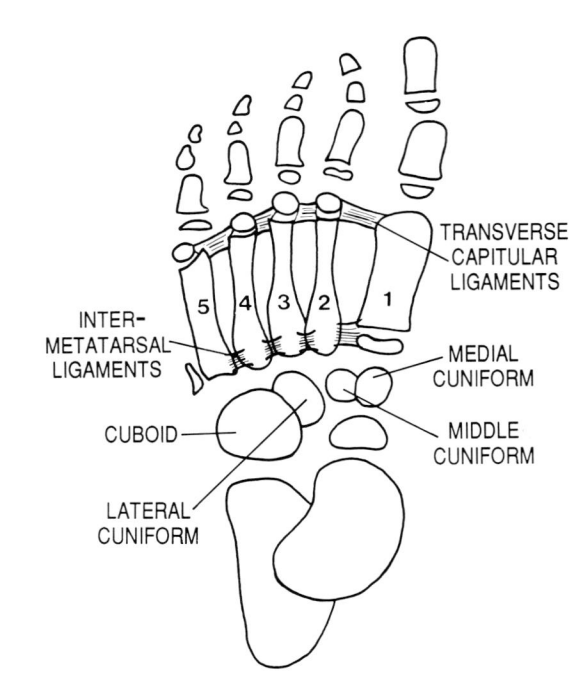

Fig. 41-2. Metatarsal bones and joints of the child's foot.

ments at the level of the capsule of the metatarsophalangeal joints. Proximally, the metatarsals are joined to the tarsals by the dorsal and plantar tarsometatarsal ligaments and to each other by the interosseous metatarsal ligaments.

Muscles

The muscular attachments to the metatarsals are as follows:

First: Insertions of tibialis anteromedial base, peroneus longus-lateral base.
Second, third, fourth: Plantar origins of adductor muscles. Insertions of small parts of tibialis posterior on plantar bases of second and fourth. Dorsally, small expansion of peroneus tertius at base of fourth.
Fifth: Plantarly, origin of flexor digiti V. Dorsally, peroneus tertius insertion along medial shaft and peroneus brevis at tuberosity of base.

Surface Anatomy

The metatarsal heads are beneath the fat pads proximal to the distal foot crease. The first metatarsal cuneiform joint is at the medial midfoot crease. The tuberosity of the fifth is easily palpable subcutaneously (Fig. 41-1).

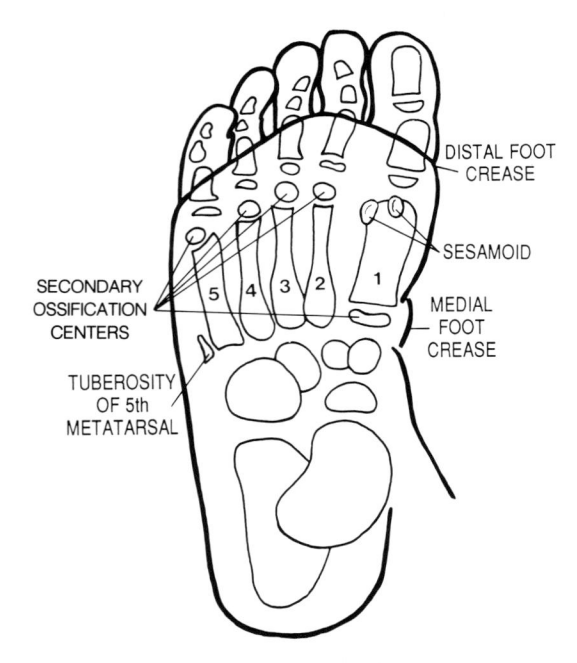

Fig. 41-1. Surface anatomy of the child's foot.

Mechanism of Injury

The metatarsal bones can be injured either directly or indirectly. A direct injury due to a falling object results in a variable fracture pattern depending on the nature of the object and the height from which it fell. Frequently, the fracture itself appears innocuous and the soft tissue damage is the more significant component of the injury. The indirect injuries occur with violent abduction and/or plantar flexion of the forefoot. Torsional forces applied to the forefoot produce fractures of the metatarasal necks. Chronic repetitive loading can produce stress fractures.

Physical Examination

The history will elicit a mechanism of direct or indirect trauma to the foot. The signs will vary according to severity of the impact. Fractures with minimal displacement may have slight swelling and no ecchymosis. The presence of localized tenderness is the real clue to the diagnosis. The more severely injured foot will be associated with greater swelling, ecchymosis, and, possibly, clinical deformity.

Since children do not know anatomy, a complaint of 'sore foot' must be carefully assessed. A child's verbal description of the location of the pain is invariably inaccurate. A child may point to a very general region as the source of the pain. However, a careful, gentle physical examination will usually delineate the exact anatomic site of the child's symptoms.

Differential Diagnosis

Plain radiographs are usually sufficient to confirm the diagnosis. Standard anteroposterior, oblique, and lateral views should be performed. However, undisplaced Salter-Harris type 1 fractures remain a clinical diagnosis. If there is concern with respect to a secondary ossification center, comparison views with the opposite foot may be necessary.

Treatment Indications

Rang[1] best summarized the treatment of metatarsal fractures when he wrote: "Injuries to children's feet, despite all the little bones and joints, are remarkably uninteresting. Very few fractures will be encountered that display any subtleties or tricks; few are even displaced."

The most serious and frequently neglected aspect of treatment of foot fractures is the soft tissue injury. A circular cast should never be applied in cases with moderate to severe swelling secondary to a crush injury. These children require hospital admission, elevation of the foot, application of ice, and observation for development of a compartment syndrome. The interossei and short plantar muscles are enclosed in fascial compartments. Fasciotomy is indicated in the presence of taut skin, marked swelling, venous congestion of the toes, and increasing pain in the foot. In the multiple trauma victim, this pathology is frequently overlooked, resulting in progressive muscle fibrosis with an intrinsic minus foot with claw toes (Fig. 41-3).

Treatment of Fractures of The Metatarsal Neck and Shaft

Closed Methods

It is generally accepted that minimally displaced fractures of the metatarsal shaft and neck occur frequently and present no particular difficulty in management. These injuries heal rapidly in the pediatric population. I prefer to offer the patient and the parents the option of casting versus bandaging and the use of crutches. Casting

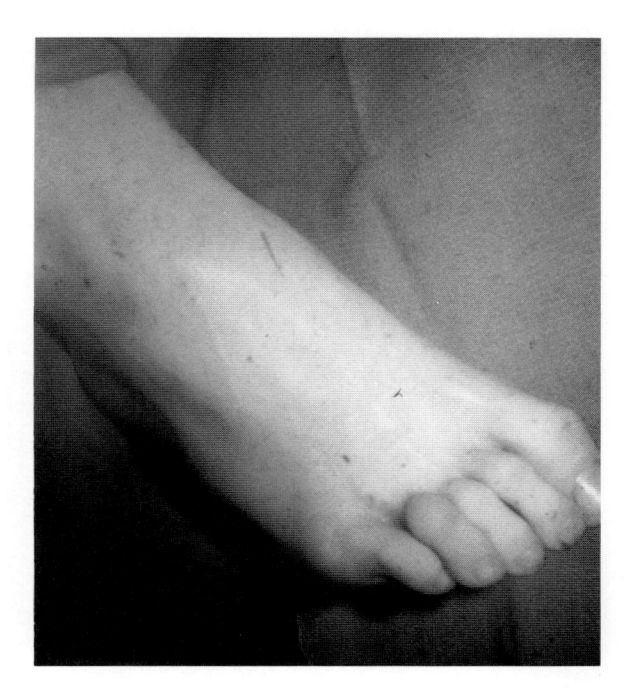

Fig. 41-3. Claw toes in an 18-year-old patient resulting from fractures of the second, third, and fourth metatarsals sustained 2 years earlier after dropping a 20-kg drum on his foot.

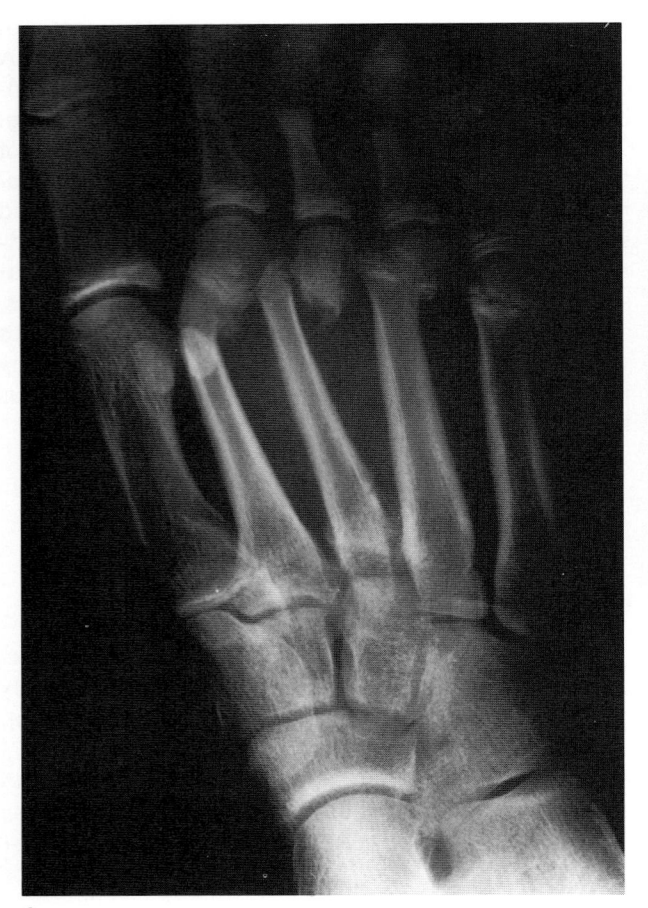

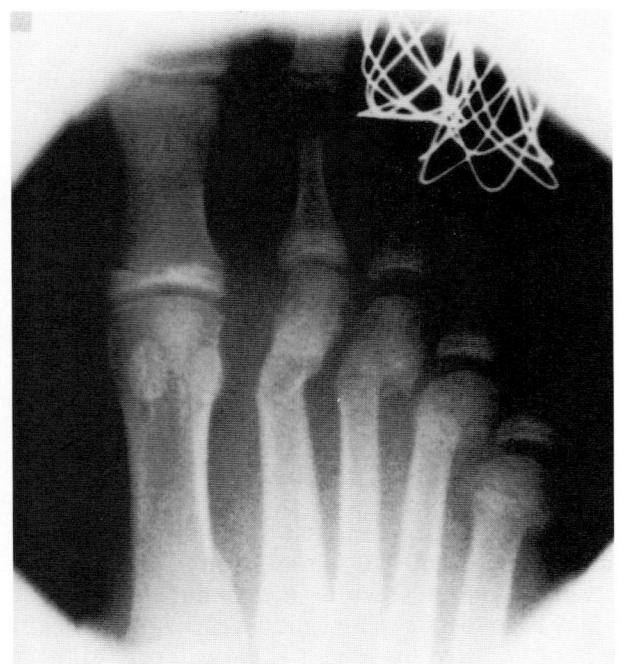

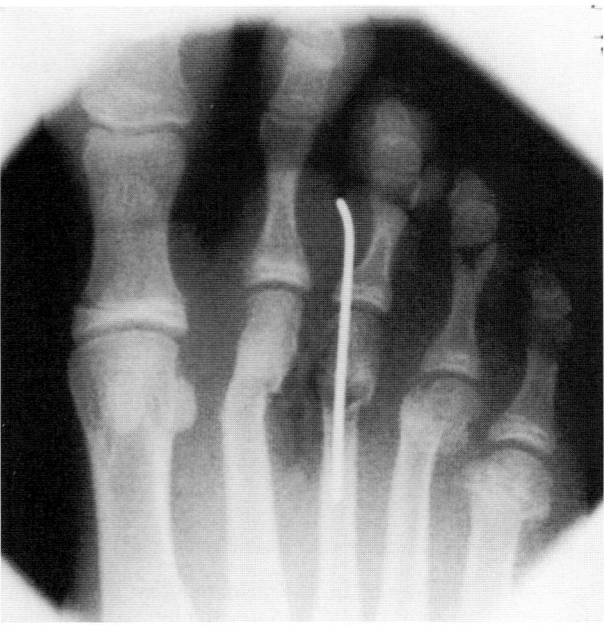

Fig. 41-4. (A) Fractures of the second through fifth metatarsals in a 12-year-old boy whose foot became entangled in the spokes of a bicycle wheel. (B) Closed reduction with Chinese finger traps could not achieve a stable reduction of the third metatarsal. (C) Percutaneous pinning of the unstable third metatarsal was performed. *(Figure continues.)*

Metatarsals and Phalanges of the Foot / 771

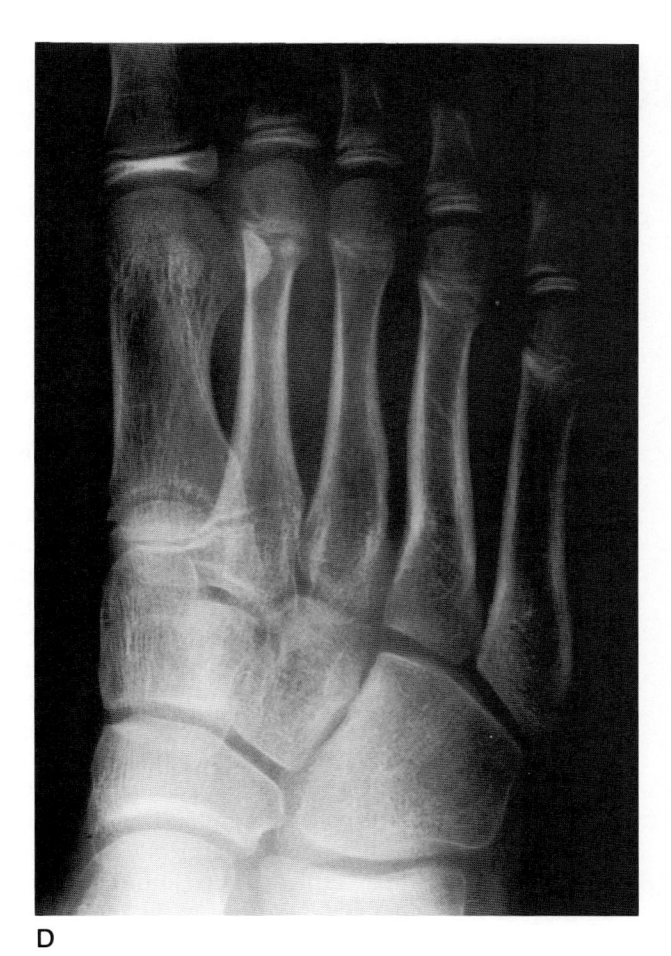

Fig. 41-4 *(Continued).* **(D)** A radiograph taken 2 years post-injury shows the fracture remodeling.

is valuable in the active preschooler who cannot manage crutches safely. A below-knee walking cast for a maximum of 10 days to 2 weeks is sufficient. These children usually return with their casts destroyed. Compression bandaging to relieve swelling and early partial weight-bearing with crutches is particularly valuable for some adolescents. In the warm months, it permits aquatic activity, and makes bathing and showering at any time of the year easier. It will not delay healing. Displaced fractures of the second, third, and fourth metatarsals require reduction (Fig. 41-4A–C). Closed manipulation is usually successful. This can best be accomplished with the use of Chinese finger traps applied to the corresponding toes of the fractured metatarsals. Countertraction is applied to the distal tibia. If the first and fifth metatarsals are not fractured as well, I still favor short casting periods, 2 weeks or less, followed by protected weightbearing and joint mobilization in physiotherapy. The displaced fractures are associated with greater soft tissue injury are slower to become pain-free.

If the first and/or fifth metatarsal are fractured and displaced as well, these fractures of the first or fifth can be reduced by closed traction and held by percutaneous K-wire fixation into the midfoot. This maintains metatarsal length and assists in preserving reduction of the other metatarsals by casting when the swelling subsides. I have found K-wire fixation of any individual metatarsal shaft necessary only if the reduction is unstable. A considerable degree of lateral displacement of the middle metatarsals is acceptable, as is angulation of the metatarsal necks in the range of 45 degrees, since this will remodel in the growing child (Fig. 41-4D). In the child nearing maturity, much less angulation may be accepted, since abnormal weight-bearing pressure will result if there remains inadequate remodeling potential. Casting for 3 weeks is generally necessary for sufficient healing prior to protected weightbearing and physiotherapy. Weightbearing is not recommended while K-wires are still in place to minimize migration of the pins or breakage.

Open Methods

An open reduction is rarely necessary and should be reserved for the unreducible fracture. It can be performed through a dorsal longitudinal exposure, K-wire placement through the fracture site exiting distally through the plantar skin, fracture reduction, then retrograde intramedullary fixation through the proximal fragment and into the midfoot if necessary.

Fractures of the Base of the Fifth Metatarsal

Injuries to the base of the fifth metatarsal are common in children. The ossification process at the proximal end of the fifth metatarsal merits further description. The secondary center of ossification appears as a small, shell-shaped fleck of bone oriented slightly obliquely to the metatarsal shaft. The apophysis was present in 198 out of 200 children studied by serial radiographs.[2] It is not often visible on the anteroposterior or lateral radiographic views; however, it is almost always visible on the oblique view.[3] The apophysis appears in girls at about 9.7 years and in boys at 12.1 years, and fuses with the shaft of the fifth metatarsal by 11.6 years in girls and 14.1 years in boys.[3]

Differentiation of a fracture of the tuberosity from the apophysis of the fifth metatarsal is difficult (Fig. 41-5). The apophyseal line traverses the tubercle almost parallel to the long axis of the shaft, whereas a fracture line through the tuberosity is more transverse. The apophyseal line also does not extend proximally into the metatarsal joint or medially into the joint between the fourth and fifth metatarsal.[3] (Fig. 41-6A). This apophysis can be confused with the os vesalianum, a rare sesamoid found in the peroneus brevis tendon. This sesamoid was present in only 1 of 1,000 feet examined radiographically by Dameron[4] and in none of the 2,249 feet studied by Gruber.[5] The sesamoid presents a smooth, sclerotic border on both opposing surfaces with a wider gap than usually seen with a fracture (Fig. 41-6B).

Anatomic studies by Dameron[4] showed that the center of ossification of the tuberosity of the fifth metatarsal was located within the cartilaginous flare onto which the peroneus brevis inserted. The injury is therefore traditionally described as an avulsion of the site of insertion of the peroneus brevis on the metatarsal. However, Giachino[6] refutes this theory. He describes the minimal displacement, and the direction of the fracture line perpendicular to the longitudinal axis of the shaft being more consistent with the insertions of the tendinous portion of the abductor digiti minimi and the lateral cord of the plantar aponeurosis.

This fracture is suspected clinically by point tenderness at the base of the fifth metatarsal and minimal to mild swelling. Healing is generally rapid. Cast immobilization is not absolutely necessary but can be used in active or noncompliant teenagers to avoid prolonged symptoms. If used, it should be discontinued as soon as the local tenderness disappears. This will occur well before evidence of radiographic union.

This avulsion fracture must be differentiated from the Jones fracture, which takes place 1.5 cm distal to the tuberosity (Fig. 41-7A&B). Kavanaugh and coworkers[7] have emphasized that the Jones fracture occurs in the proximal part of the diaphysis of the fifth metatarsal. It occurs in late adolescence (15–20 years) and bears a high rate of delayed or nonunion (67 percent in their series) and refracture. More aggressive treatment with 6 weeks of cast immobilization is therefore warranted. Open reduction and internal fixation with a cancellous screw is recommended in cases of nonunion. These authors stress that the diagnosis can be a clinically important decision, especially in an athlete where some consideration may be given to a primary open reduction.

The avulsion fracture also must be differentiated from traction apophysitis, referred to as Iselin's disease. This disorder was first described in 1912 in the German literature by Iselin. Canale and Williams' 1992 review[3] suggests this apophysitis is rare but perhaps more common than generally appreciated. Over a 3-year period, the diagnosis was found in four of their patients. These patients differ from those with an avulsion injury in that a history of significant trauma is usually absent, although symptoms may begin after an inversion injury. Children who participate in sports that cause inversion stress on the forefoot appear to be especially prone to development of the condition. Clinically, the tuberosity of the affected foot is larger than that of the uninvolved side. Local soft tissue edema and erythema may be present. The site of insertion of peroneus brevis is tender. Pain can be elicited by maximum plantar flexion or dorsiflexion and resisted eversion. Oblique radiographs show enlargement of the apophysis and often fragmentation of the ossication center. The chondro-osseous junction may be widened. If the radiographs are normal, ^{99}Tc bone scanning is indicated to confirm the diagnosis.[8]

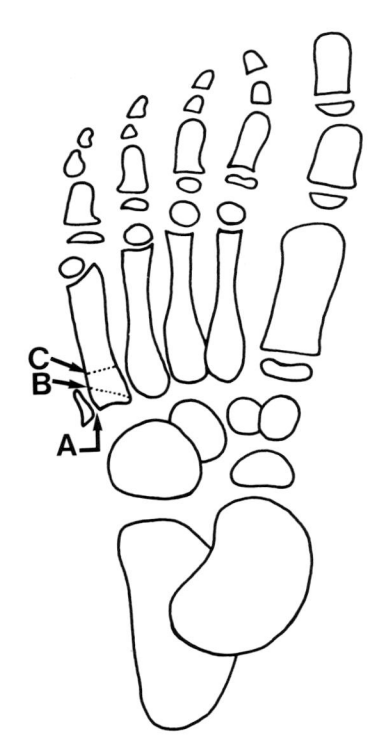

Fig. 41-5. (A) Physis between the apophysis and the base of the fifth metatarsal. (B) Fracture of the base of the fifth metatarsal. (C) Joint fracture.

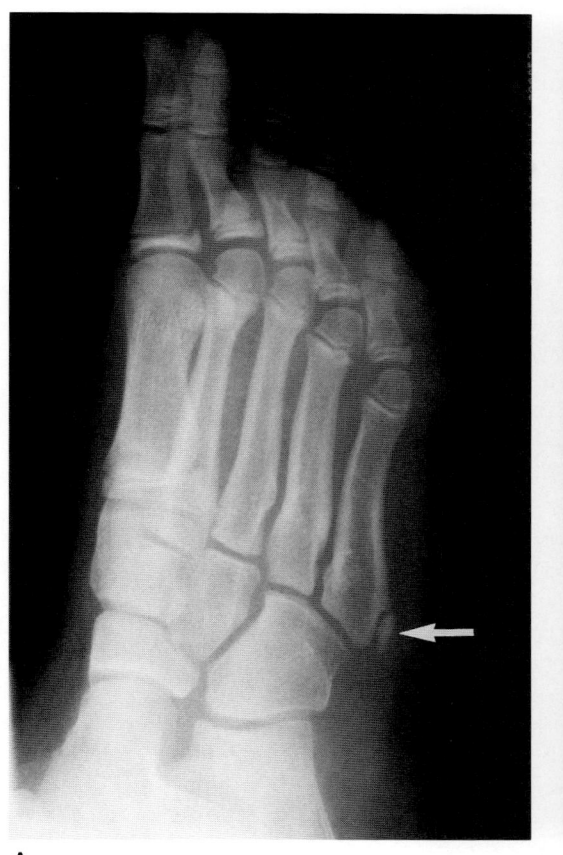

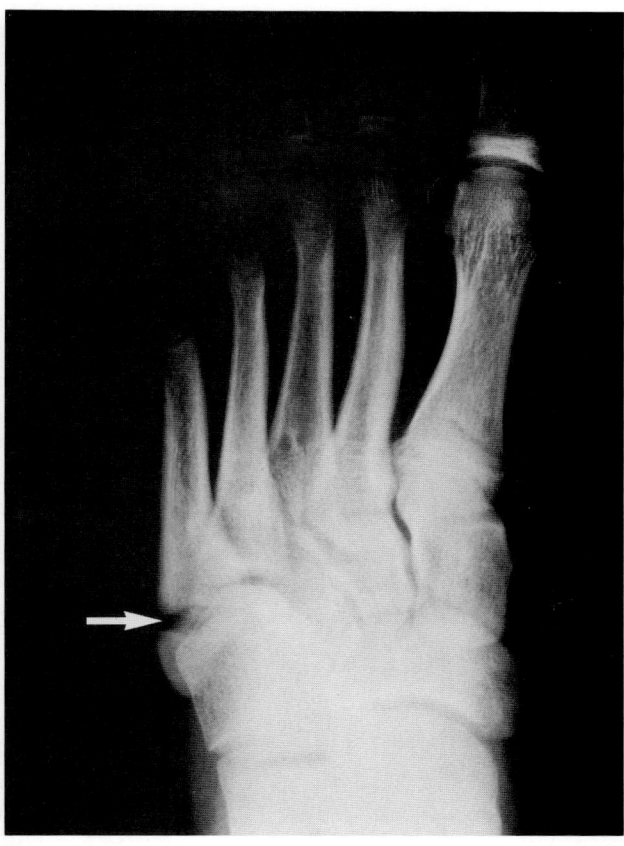

Fig. 41-6. (A) Normal apophysis. (B) Fracture of the base of the fifth metatarsal.

Fractures of The First Metatarsal

Fractures of the first metatarsal proximally may damage the physis resulting in shortening of the medial side of the foot. Johnson[9] described a variation of the Lisfranc injury occurring in children under the age of 10 years and affecting the first metatarsal. A jump from a height, notably a bunk bed, may cause a fracture of the lateral (or occasionally medial) side of the proximal first metatarsal with concomitant damage to the first cuneiform. The fracture may involve the proximal physis (Fig. 41-8). The diagnosis is frequently retrospective after sclerotic healing becomes radiographically evident.

Crush injuries of the first metatarsal require restoration and maintenance of the normal length of the bone during healing. Closed reduction with percutaneous pinning of the distal portion of the metatarsal to adjacent metatarsals for 3 to 4 weeks will suffice. If the distal portion of the metatarsal is severely damaged, the pinning to the proximal phalanx of the great to the lateral toes will maintain metatarsal length.

Undisplaced fractures of the shaft may be treated with simple cast immobilization and protected weight-bearing.

Fractures Associated with Tarsometatarsal Dislocations

This is an easily overlooked injury of the older child. The anatomy and mechanism of injury were described by Wiley[10] as an acute, forced, plantar flexion of the forefoot, usually combined with a rotational force. The foot posture at the time of injury occurs in at least three situations: striking an object while in the tiptoe position, heel-to-toe compression where the victim is in a kneel-

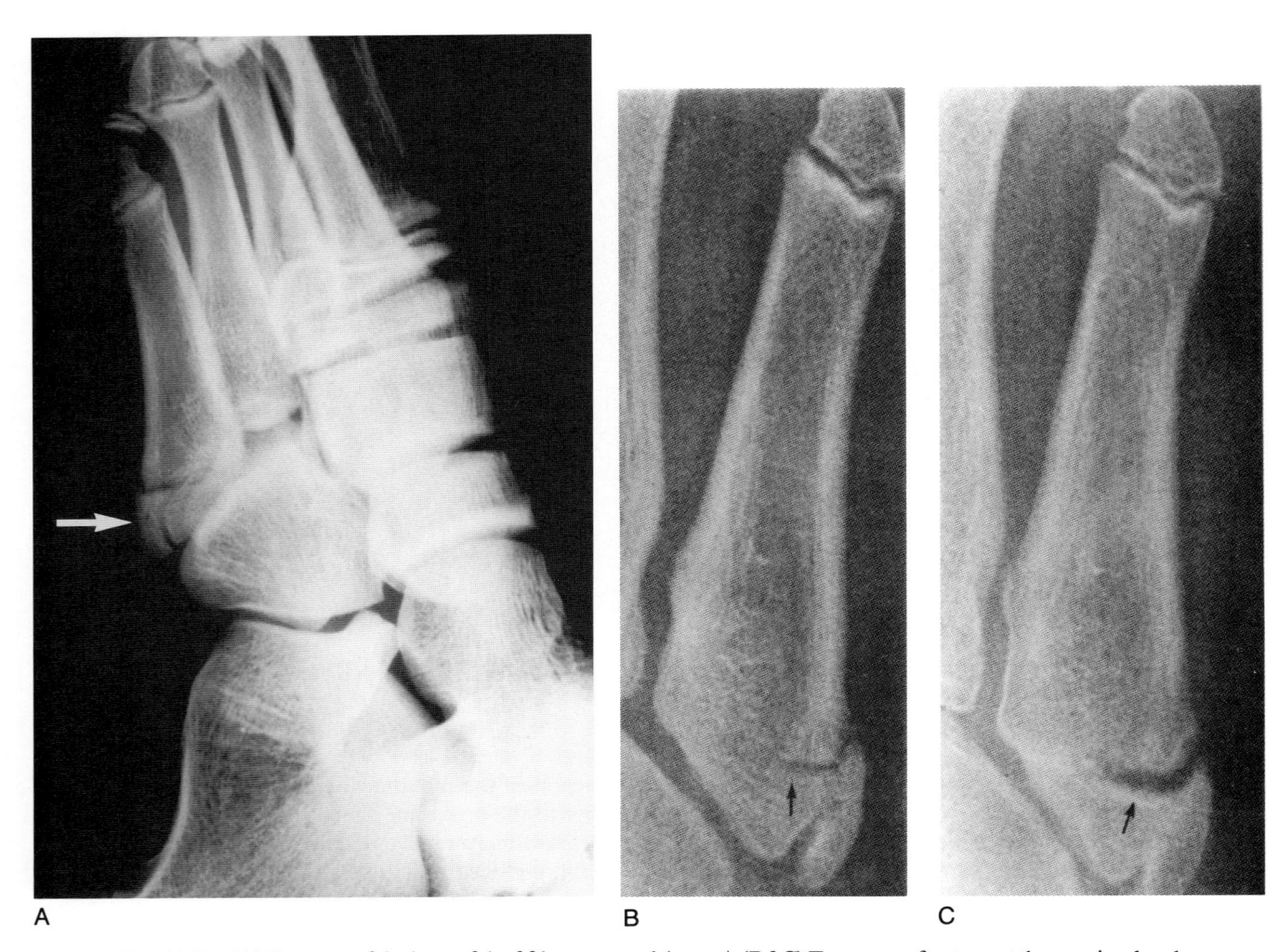

Fig. 41-7. **(A)** Fracture of the base of the fifth metatarsal *(arrow)*. **(B&C)** Transverse fracture at the proximal end of the fifth metatarsal of a girl 10 years of age. **(B)** Immediately after a twisting injury the *arrow* is directed at the incomplete transverse fracture. The independent small mass of bone lateral to the end of the shaft is the normal apophyseal center. **(C)** 34 days later, the fracture line is widened *(arrow)* and the apophyseal center is more completely fused. Fusion has probably been accelerated by the local chronic hyperemia induced by the fracture. This is known as a Jones' dancing fracture. (Figs. B&C from Caffey J: Pediatric X-ray Diagnosis. Section 8: The Extremities. p. 1109. Year- Book Medical Publishers, Chicago, 1972, with permission.)

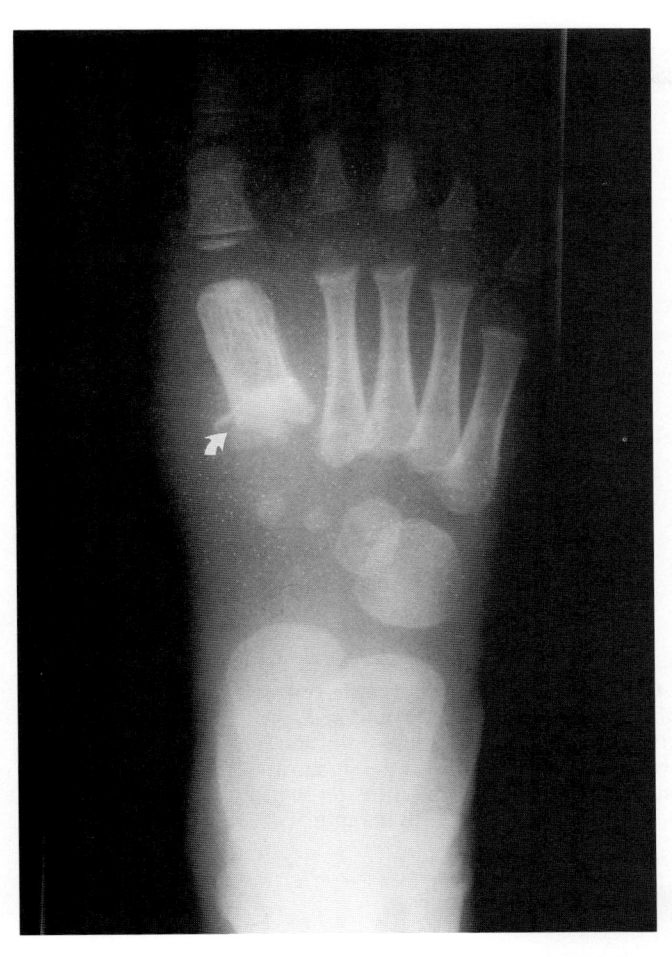

Fig. 41-8. Displaced fracture of the base of the first metatarsal in a 5-year-old who jumped off the top of a bunk bed.

ing position when the impact load strikes the heel, and the fixed forefoot while the patient falls backward (Fig. 41-9). A considerable amount of force is required to produce the injury. The metatarsals generally displace in a plantar and lateral direction, rupturing the plantar ligaments. The second metatarsal most often fractures because of the more proximal fixed position of its base.

Clinical examination usually shows no obvious deformity because spontaneous reduction most often occurs (Fig. 41-9A–D). Marked local pain, swelling, and tenderness, accompanied by an inability to bear any weight, should suggest this diagnosis.

Radiographic examination should include anteroposterior, lateral, and oblique views (Fig. 41-9E&F). Since spontaneous reduction is the rule, the associated fractures may be the only clues to the diagnosis. The physician must carefully look for fractures of the base of the second metatarsal, the cuboid or the cuneiforms (Fig. 41-9D). Initial management is directed toward the severe soft tissue injury. Ice, compression, and elevation are required to minimize the swelling. Admission to hospital is warranted to observe for vascular compromise. Fasciotomy could be required in severe cases.

Specific treatment for the fractured metatarsal associated with the tarsometatarsal injury is not required if it is undisplaced. In the case of a displaced injury, closed reduction is usually successful. In Wiley's series[10], 7 of 18 cases required operative reduction, which was accomplished through a dorsal incision. Internal fixation, if necessary, includes Kirschner wires left protruding through the skin and bent at a right angle to prevent migration. The wires can be removed at 2 weeks. When the initial swelling subsides, the foot should be placed in a short-leg cast for 3 to 4 weeks. Weightbearing may be permitted when the patient can tolerate it and the wires have been removed.

Complications were minimal in Wiley's series[11] despite the extensive joint disruption. Only two patients had minimal residual abduction of the forefoot that did not interfere with shoewear or function. In his series, there were no neurovascular complications.

Open Fractures

The most devastating injury to a child's foot results from the crushing of a car tire or the laceration of a power lawnmower. Compound fractures of the metatarsals can be caused by sharp penetrating objects or crushing and tearing of skin. The initial management includes wound debridement down to the bone, copious irrigation, tetanus, and antibiotic prophylaxis and secondary closure when all nonviable tissue has been excised. In severe cases, this may involve multiple debridement procedures. After appropriate wound management, any fractures can be treated as discussed earlier with K-wire fixation if necessary.

Stress Fractures

Stress fractures of the metatarsals in children are unusual.[12] They most frequently involve the second or third metatarsal.[13] In a series of 368 stress fractures in athletes, 32 fractures (8.7 percent) occurred in children under 16, and 117 (31.8 percent) occurred in the 16 to 19-year age group. Stress fractures of the metatarsals accounted for 73 of the cases (19.8 percent).[14] However, the diagnosis should not be overlooked in the differential diagnosis of the limping toddler.

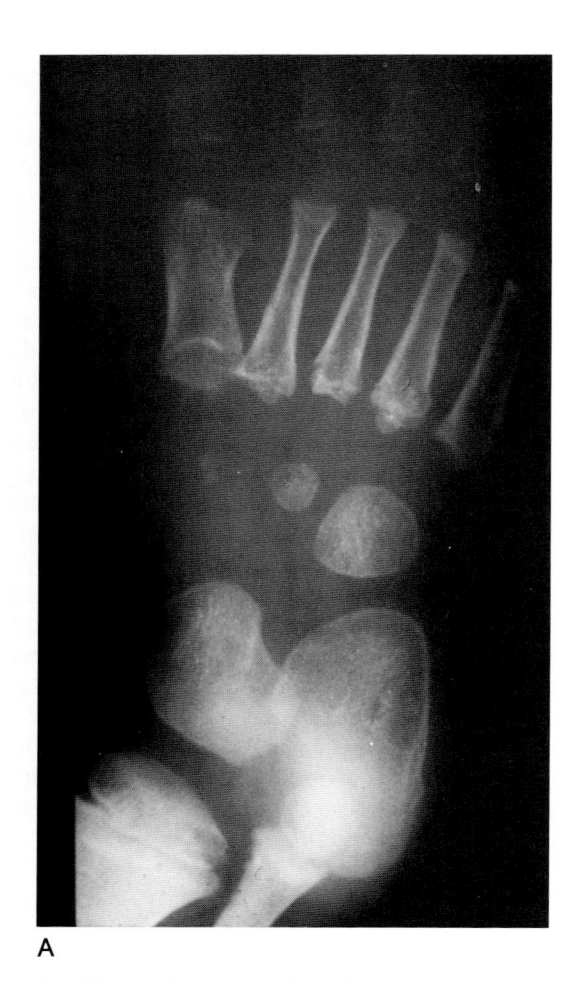

Fig. 41-9. **(A)** This 7-year-old girl fell backward with her foot caught under a fallen drawer and sustained this innocuous looking foot injury. **(B)** A close-up of the metatarsals on the anteroposterior view confirms the fractures of the shaft of the second and the bases of the third through fifth metatarsals. This is a typical pediatric Lisfranc injury. *(Figure continues.)*

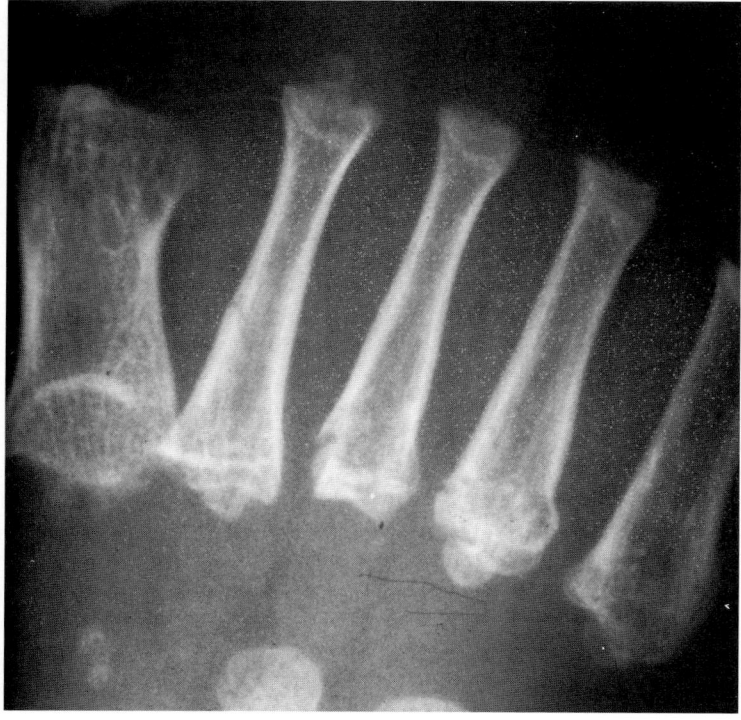

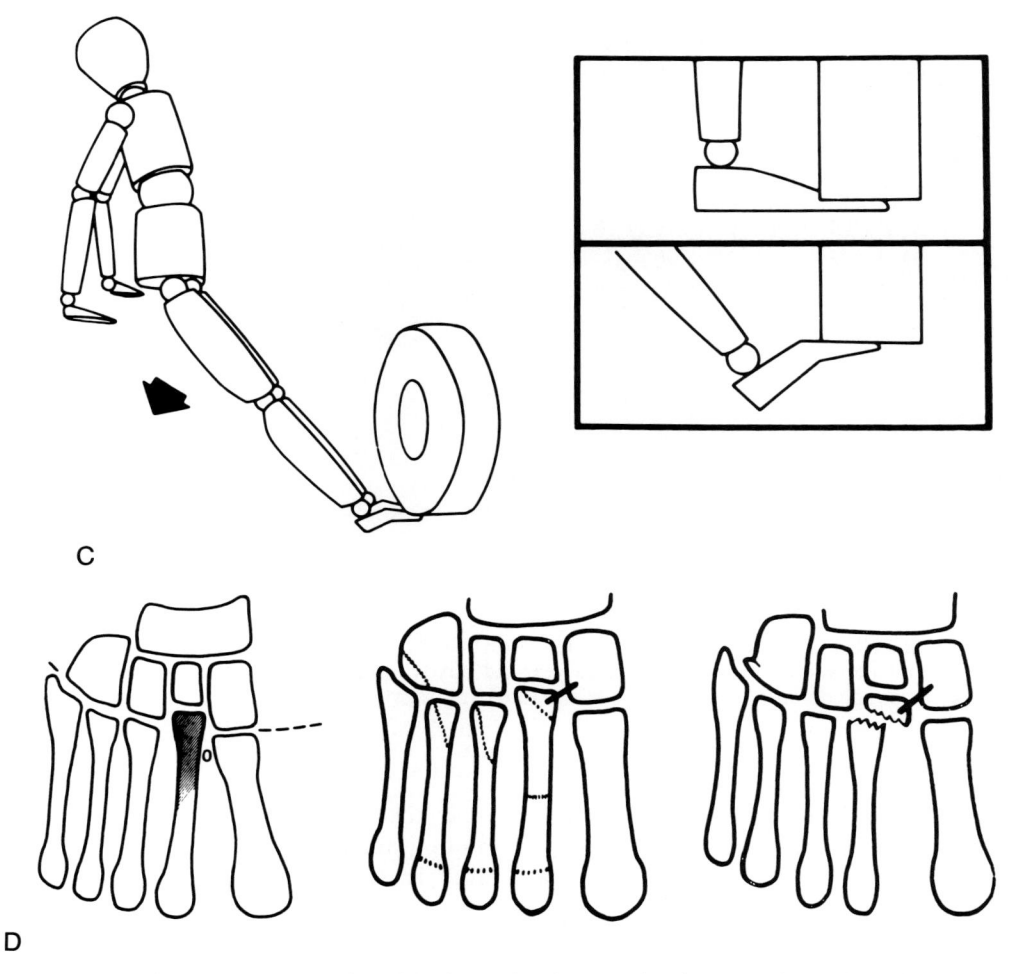

Fig. 41-9 *(Continued).* **(C)** Backward fall with pinned forefoot causing fracture dislocation of the tarsometatarsal joint. **(D)** Second metatarsal bone represents the keystone of the locking mechanism. The fractures of the cuboid and second metatarsal bones are the pathognomonic signs of disruption of the tarsometatarsal joints. Fractures of the first and fifth metatarsals are uncommon. *(Figure continues.)*

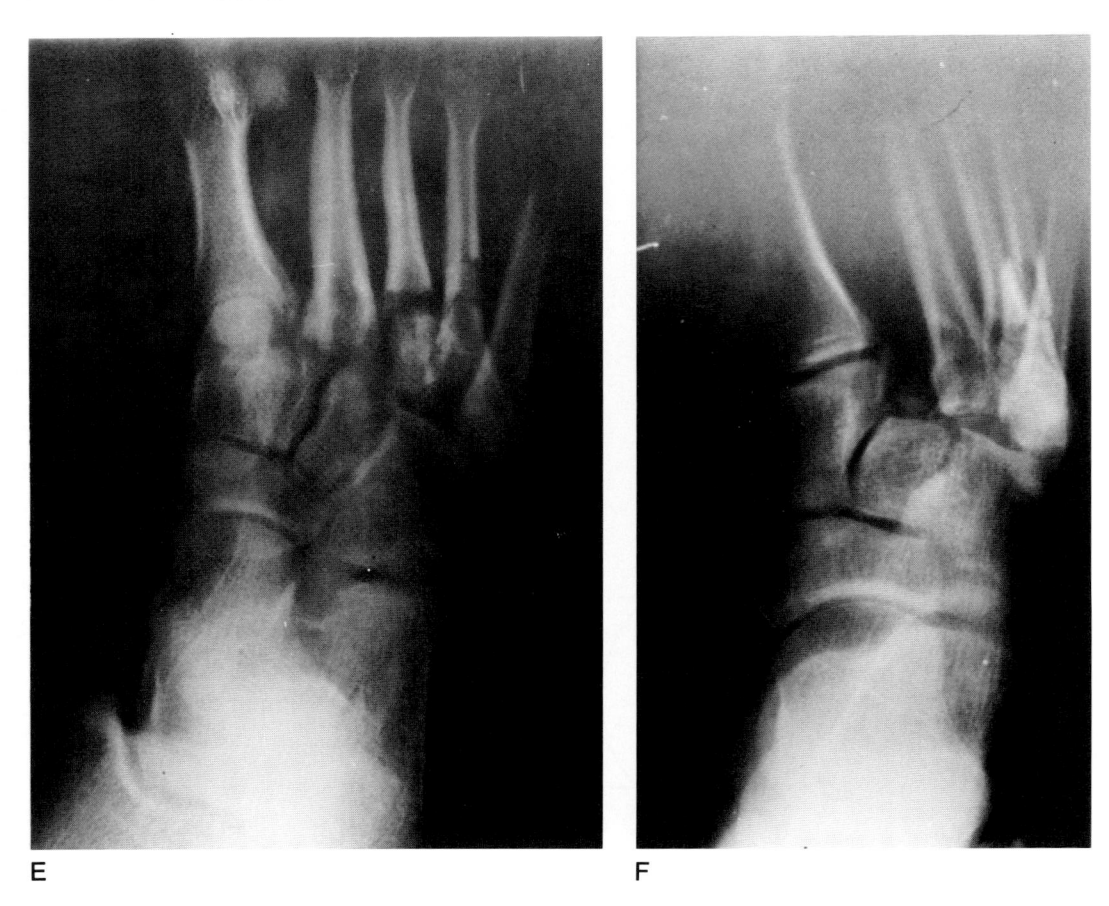

Fig. 41-9 *(Continued).* **(E)** An anteroposterior view shows the disruption of the Lisfranc joint, especially at the base of the second metatarsal, sustained by a 15-year-old boy who jumped 15 ft from a train bridge. **(F)** The oblique view shows the detail of the fractures of the third and fourth metatarsals. *(Figure continues.)*

The etiology is thought to be repetitive microfractures of the involved area. The force is applied on the bone in a normal physiologic manner, but the frequency and magnitude of the force are increased. The physiologic response of the bone is increased osteoclastic activity with an increase in osteoblastic activity. When small microinfractions occur and the bone does not have time to heal, a stress fracture across the entire shaft results. Drez and coworkers[15] disproved the belief that a short first metatarsal was a contributing factor.

The onset of symptoms is usually insidious. There is no associated swelling or ecchymosis. The pain is persistent and progressive. The gait is altered such that the patient avoids weightbearing on the tender area. The physical examination may show some diffuse swelling over the affected area. There is always localized tenderness over the involved bone. If the process has been prolonged, there may be some palpable callus formation.

In the first 2 weeks after the symptoms appear, the radiographs are normal. During the third week, a fine line in the metatarsal shaft representing bone resorption along the fracture becomes evident. This is followed by slight periosteal thickening representing early callus formation (Fig. 41-10A). Gross callus is noted 4 weeks after the onset of symptoms (Fig. 41-10B).

Immobilization in plaster is very effective in relieving acute symptoms. It also serves to limit the patient's activity to permit healing to take place. The cast can be removed within 2 to 3 weeks. This can be followed by the use of a metatarsal pad applied to the plantar aspect of the foot just behind the metatarsal heads, thus altering weightbearing and permitting further healing to continue. This is particularly valuable in athletes participating in running and jumping sports. This fracture heals without any complications.

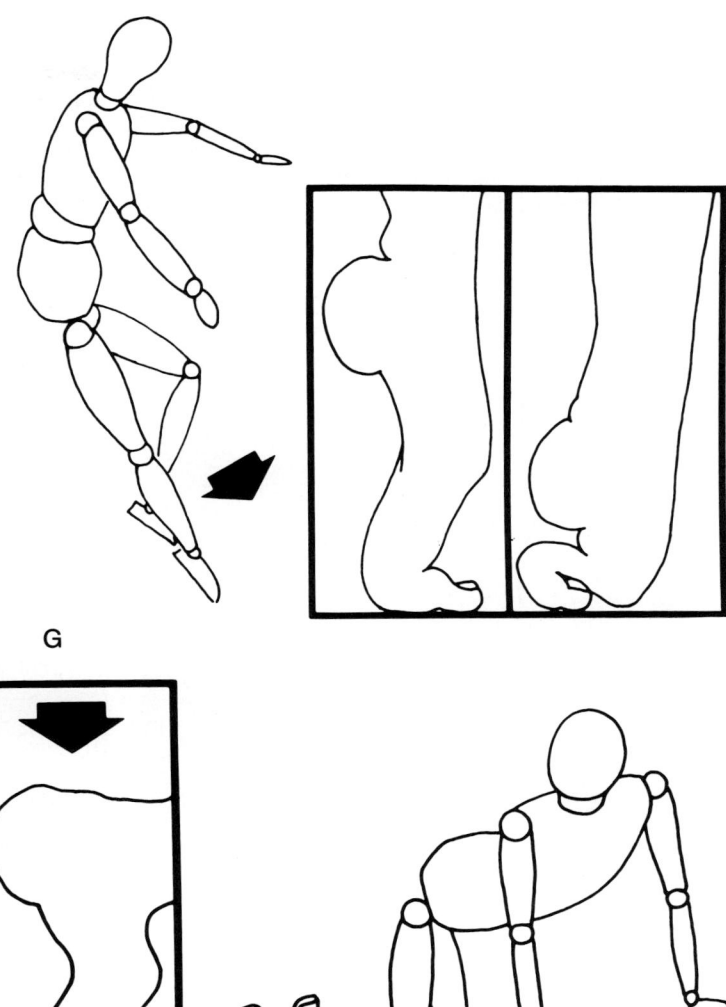

Fig. 41-9 *(Continued).* **(G)** Tiptoe landing from a height produces forced plantar flexion of the forefoot causing fracture dislocation of the tarsometatarsal joint. **(H)** The third mechanism of injury resulting in a Lisfranc fracture dislocation is a heel to toe compression injury of foot resulting in complete collapse of the tarsometatarsal joint. (Figs. C, G, & H from Wiley,[11] with permission. Fig. D from Wiley,[10] with permission.)

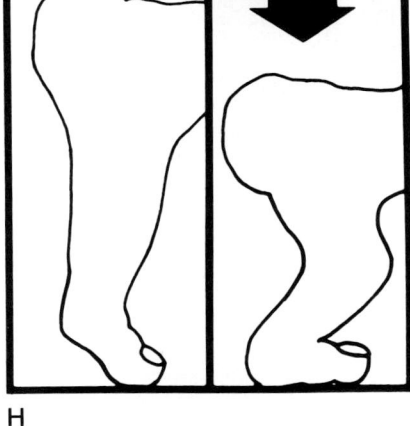

Fracture of Sesamoid

The ossification of the medial and lateral sesamoids of the great toe usually takes place between 12 and 14 years of age, but may occur as early as 8 years. They are located on the plantar aspect of the first metatarsal at the level of the neck and are contained within the tendons of flexor hallucis brevis. They are present in 100 percent of feet. Sesamoids may exist at the same level for the remaining metatarsals, but their presence is much less frequent. A medial sesamoid of the second metatarsal is seen in 5.4 percent; a lateral sesamoid of the fifth metatarsal, 13.3 percent; and the remaining sesamoids, less than 2 percent.[16] The sesamoids may have two ossification centers, making them bipartite and difficult to differentiate from fracture (Fig. 41-11A). Bone scanning is helpful.[17]

Fractures of this bone are a rare occurrence in children. They are caused by a fall onto the forefoot with the great toe dorsiflexed at the metatarsophalangeal joint (Fig. 41-11B). Stress fractures at this level can occur and are usually produced by prolonged standing or running. In Hulkko and Orava's series,[14] sesamoid stress fractures accounted for 4.1 percent of all stress fractures.

Treatment is conservative. Weight-bearing relief is

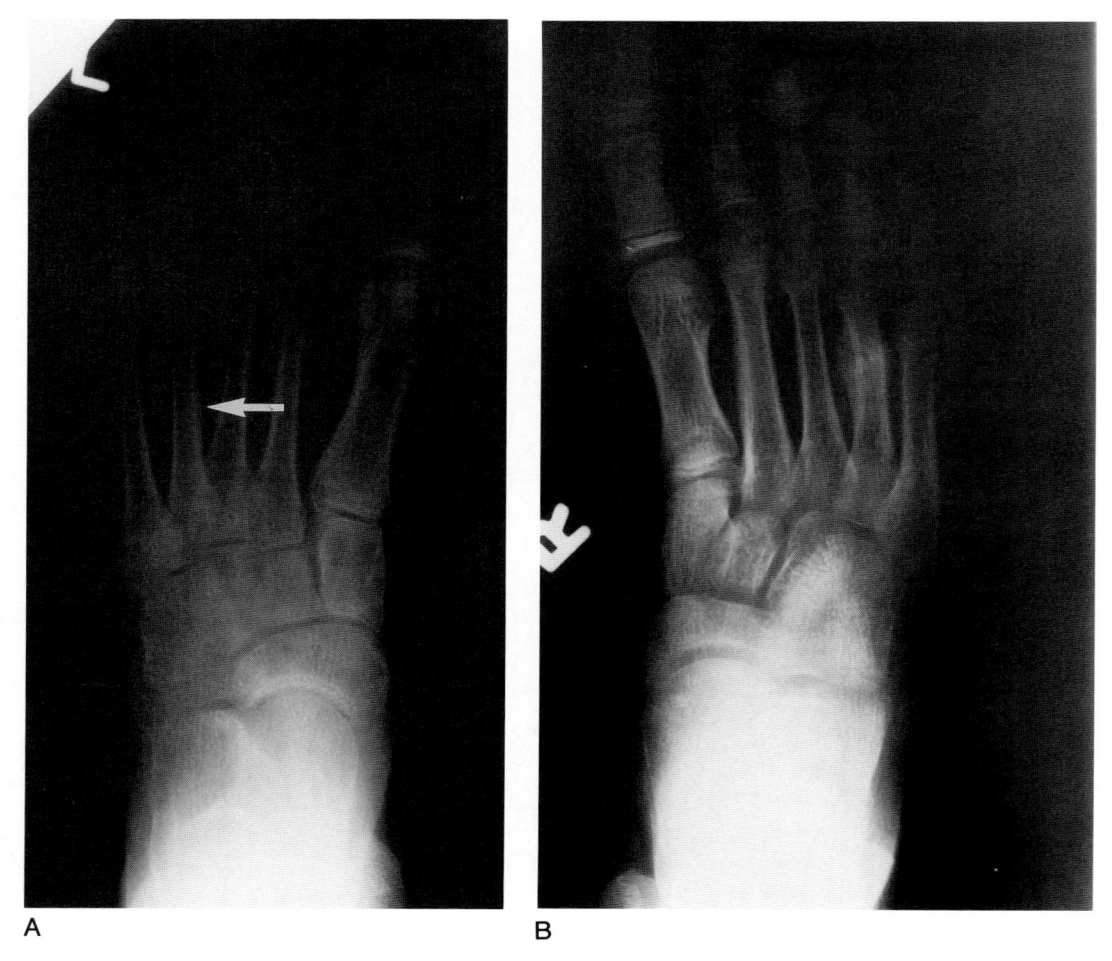

Fig. 41-10. (A) Subtle stress fracture of the fourth metatarsal in a 16-year-old female rhythmic gymnast with a 2-week history of foot pain. Note small periosteal elevation. (B) Stress fracture of the fourth metatarsal in a 12-year-old springboard diver with a 4-week history of foot pain-periosteal callus formation more obvious.

provided by orthotics. These are useful for altering weightbearing by moving it more proximally. The use of modalities in physiotherapy to decrease pain and to mobilize the great toe are beneficial. Immobilization is not necessary. Cortisone injection is done in adults. I have not performed it in children. Avoidance of the offending activity assists in healing. This is sometimes difficult in athletes such as gymnasts and ballet dancers. Healing can be expected within 2 to 3 months. Nonunion should be considered in cases with persistent pain (Fig. 41-11C).

Osteochondritis of the first metatarsal sesamoids is a rare entity. This condition may not be associated with a history of trauma, although Irwin and colleagues[18] describe three cases of fibular sesamoid fracture they believe progressed secondarily to osteochondritis. Patients show localized tenderness of the first metatarsal sesamoid, and radiographic finding of fragmentation, irregularity, and mottling of the sesamoid. An axial view of the sesamoids can be obtained by maximum dorsiflexion of the great toe and best demonstrates the radiographic changes. Ilfeld and Rosen[19] described three cases that were refractory to conservative management, including shoe modifications, nonsteroidal anti-inflammatory medications, and local injection of cortisone. All three patients required excision of the painful sesamoid with good relief of their complaints. His patients were all women between 17 and 24 years old. Histologic examination of the excised tissue confirmed the diagnosis of osteochondritis.

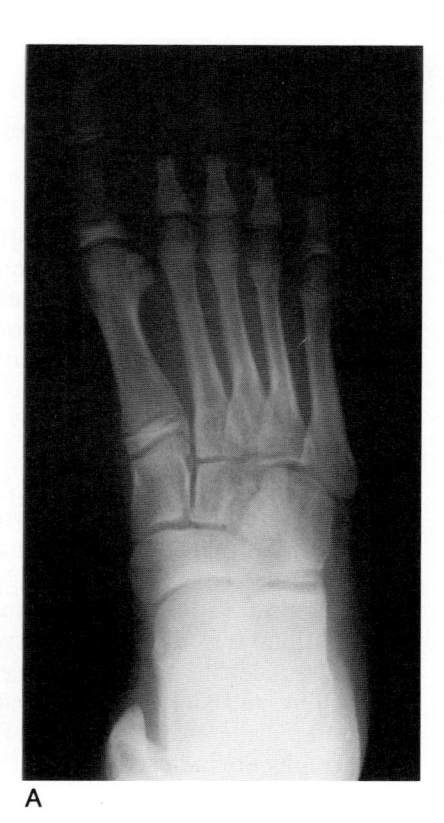

Fig. 41-11. **(A)** Bipartite sesamoid. **(B)** Fracture of the sesamoid in a 17 year old tower diver who hit his foot on the edge of the concrete platform after takeoff. **(C)** The athlete complained of persistent pain and was unable to return to this sport. This radiograph taken 6 months postinjury showed a nonunion of the fracture had developed. An excision of the offending sesamoid was performed.

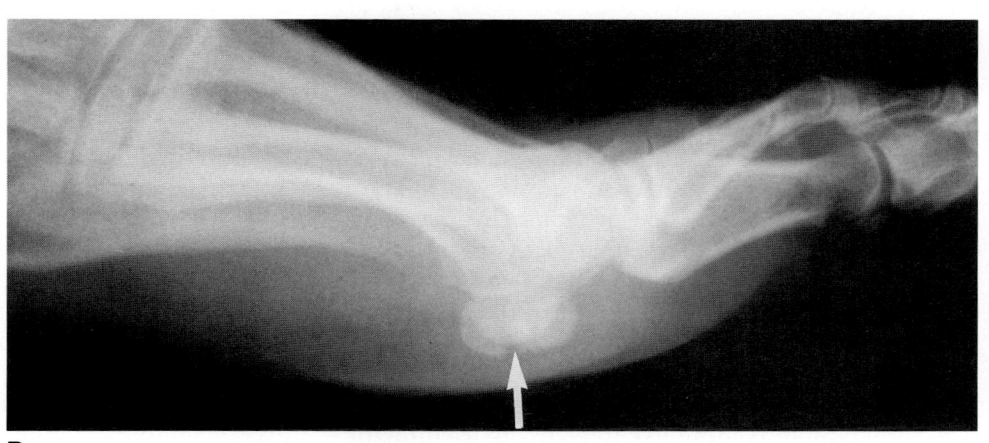

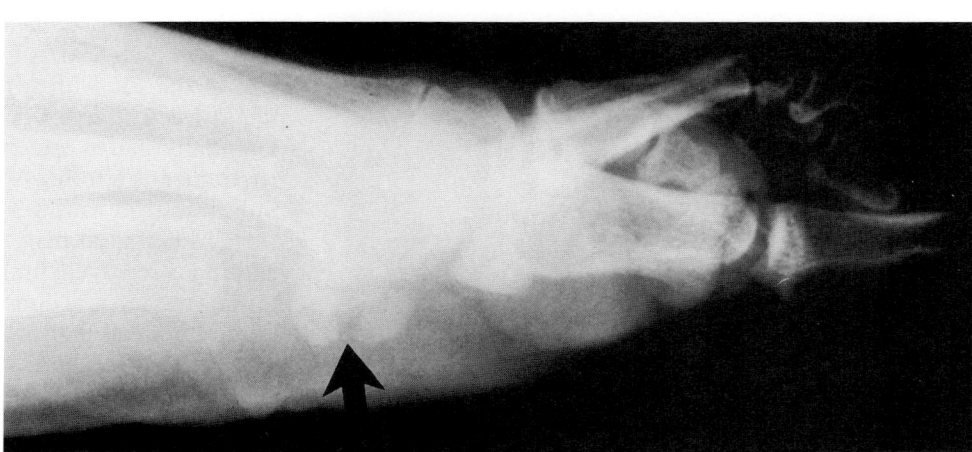

Complications

Neurologic

Volkman's ischemia can be prevented by recognition of the warning signs of vascular compromise and performing early fasciotomy. Avoidance of circular casting in very swollen feet allows better monitoring of the neurovascular status and prevents circulatory compromise due to the cast itself.

Vascular

Penetrating and crushing injuries to the dorsum of the foot could injure the dorsalis pedis artery. If a vascular injury is suspected clinically, debridement of the penetrating wound without a tourniquet should be performed initially. In the massively swollen foot, a pulse will not be palpable. In the presence of increasing pain and swelling, and cool, blue toes, a vascular injury can be suspected. Further investigation via Doppler studies and arteriography are indicated. Whether the vessel requires repair remains a subject of some controversy.

Premature Physeal Closure

Premature physeal closure appears to be a very rare complication of metatarsal fractures. It may occur in a completely displaced fracture of the metatarsal neck. As in physeal injury, this could lead to growth arrest and a progressive shortening of the metatarsal with gradual recession of the toe. Lengthening methods similar to those used in congenital shortening of the metatarsal may be indicated. Premature closure of the base of first metatarsal presents a more difficult problem, since it will significantly affect the shape of the foot. I have never seen complete displacement of a fracture in this region. The early closure is more likely related to asymmetric crushing of the physis.

FRACTURES OF THE FOOT PHALANGES

Incidence and Description

Fractures of the phalanges of the toes in children are not common. They represent about 2 percent of all fractures of the foot seen at the Children's Hospital of Eastern Ontario. The injuries are usually due to a crush from a dropped object or a stub of the toe against another object, which may result in an avulsion fracture (Fig. 41-12).

The child presents with an appropriate history, and a painful, swollen toe. In severe cases with rotation and displacement, the toe may appear deformed.

The diagnosis can usually be confirmed radiographically, although, as in the hand, AP, lateral, and oblique views should be obtained. The degree of rotation and displacement, however, are best evaluated clinically.

Treatment

Treatment is generally nonoperative. Reduction is rarely necessary and immobilization consists of taping to the adjacent toe. Any rotational malalignment must be corrected by aligning the nailbed of the injured toe with the adjacent noninjured ones.

Occasionally, a closed reduction may be required. The proximal phalanx of the great toe will not accommodate much angular deformation and therefore should be reduced as anatomically as possible. Simple taping may not be sufficient. A percutaneous pinning will then maintain the reduction (Fig. 41-13). In fractures of multiple phalanges of multiple toes, position may also be difficult to maintain without percutaneous pinning of some or all of the toes. Salter-Harris type III or IV physeal fractures of the phalanges of the great toe require accurate reduction to prevent symptomatic growth arrest. Therefore, an open reduction may even be necessary (Fig. 41-14).

Healing progresses rapidly in the child. Weightbearing is permitted as soon as tolerated. Taping can be discontinued when the fracture site is nontender. If the toe has been pinned, the Kirschner wire is removed at 10 to 14 days.

These injuries rarely cause any complications. However, symptomatic growth arrest is possible in cases of fracture of the base of the proximal or distal phalanx of the great toe. Also, as with the finger, the child may sustain a Salter-Harris type I fracture of the distal phalanx of the toe with a nailbed injury creating a compound fracture (see Ch. 24). If unrecognized, this can potentially lead to osteomyelitis. Infection related to the percutaneous pinning is very rare, probably because the pin is removed within 3 weeks.

The differential diagnosis of phalangeal fractures in children is relatively limited. Osteoid osteoma, enchondroma, aneurysmal bone cyst, and unicameral bone cyst are rare but can first present following trauma. Subungual exostosis is a bony overgrowth from the dorsal surface of the distal part of the distal phalanx of the great toe

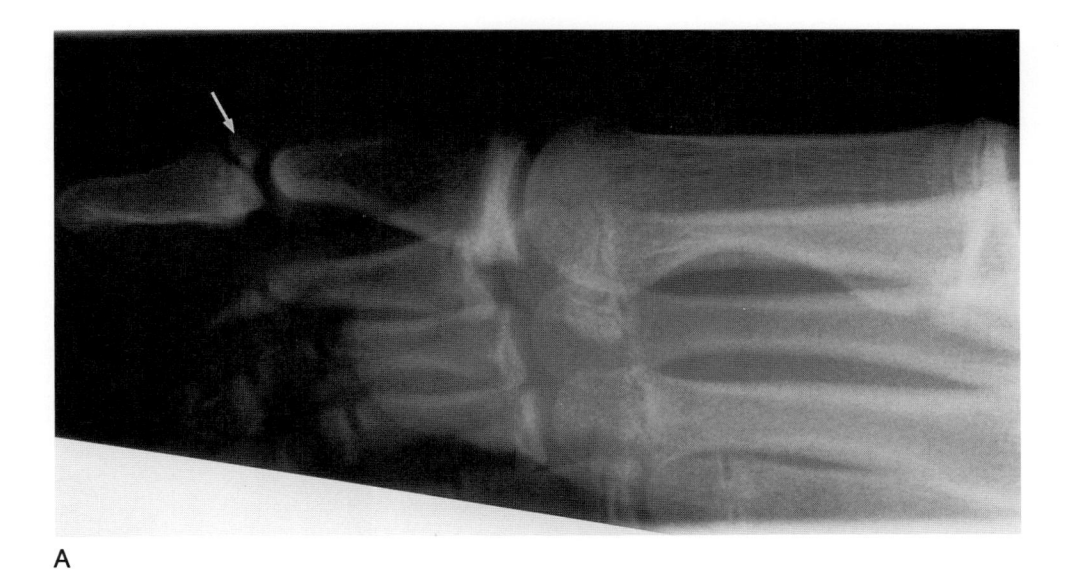

Fig. 41-12. (A) Avulsion of the extensor tendon attachment of the distal toe phalanx. This occurs in a manner similar to the adolescent mallet finger resulting in a type III physeal fracture. (B) The AP view does not demonstrate this fracture, emphasizing the need for several views in children's physeal injuries.

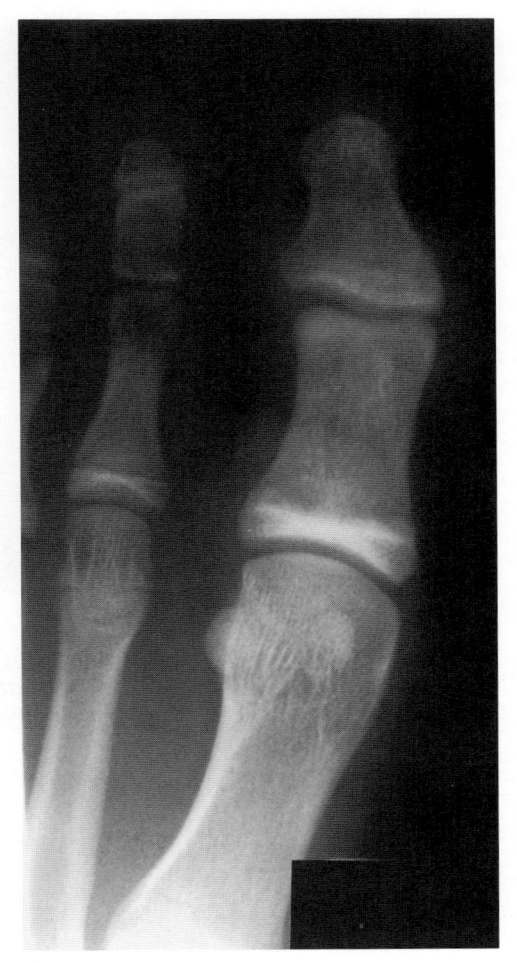

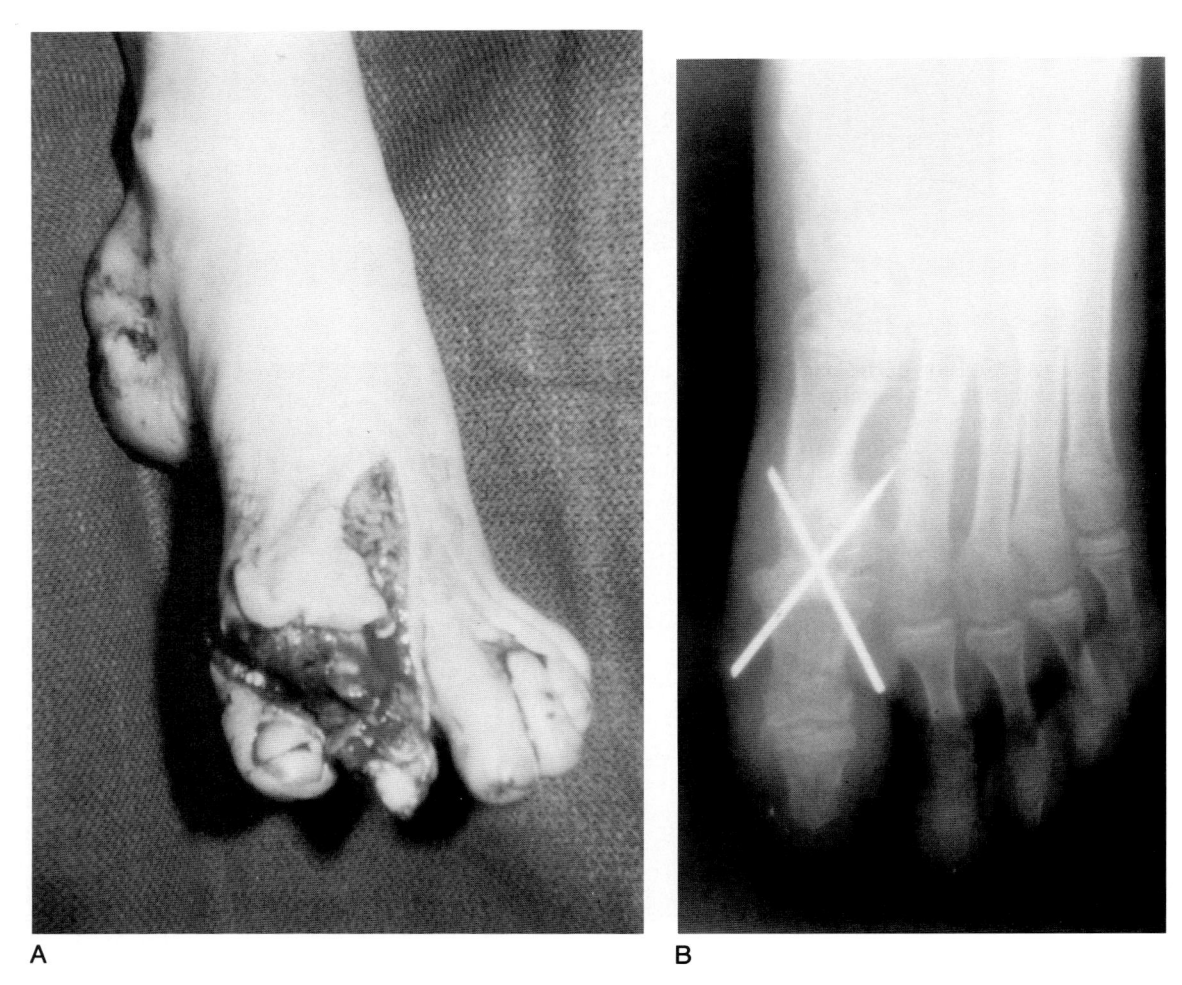

Fig. 41-13. (A) Partial amputation of the great toe through the metatarsophalangeal joint with fracture of the proximal phalanx by a lawnmower. (B) Radiograph 2 months later. The toe was stabilized with crossed K wires. The toe was salvaged and although a fibrous fusion of the metatarsophalangeal joint was produced the foot was functional and pain free.

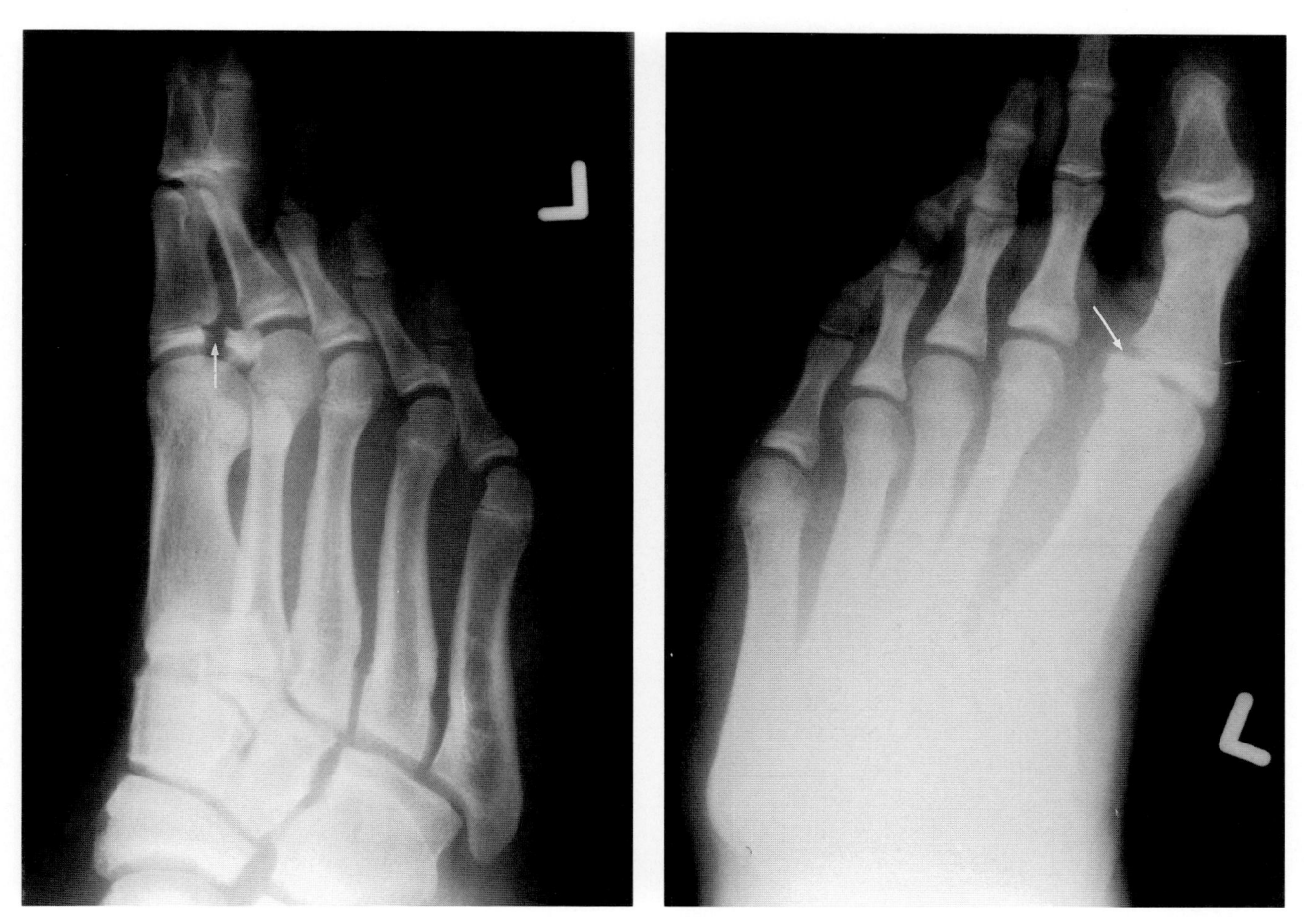

Fig. 41-14. Oblique and AP views of type III fracture of the proximal phalangeal epiphysis of the great toe in a 15-year-old boy sustained when he kicked a wall. This required open reduction and internal fixation with fine K-wires. Separation by more than 3 mm warrants reduction of the fragments.

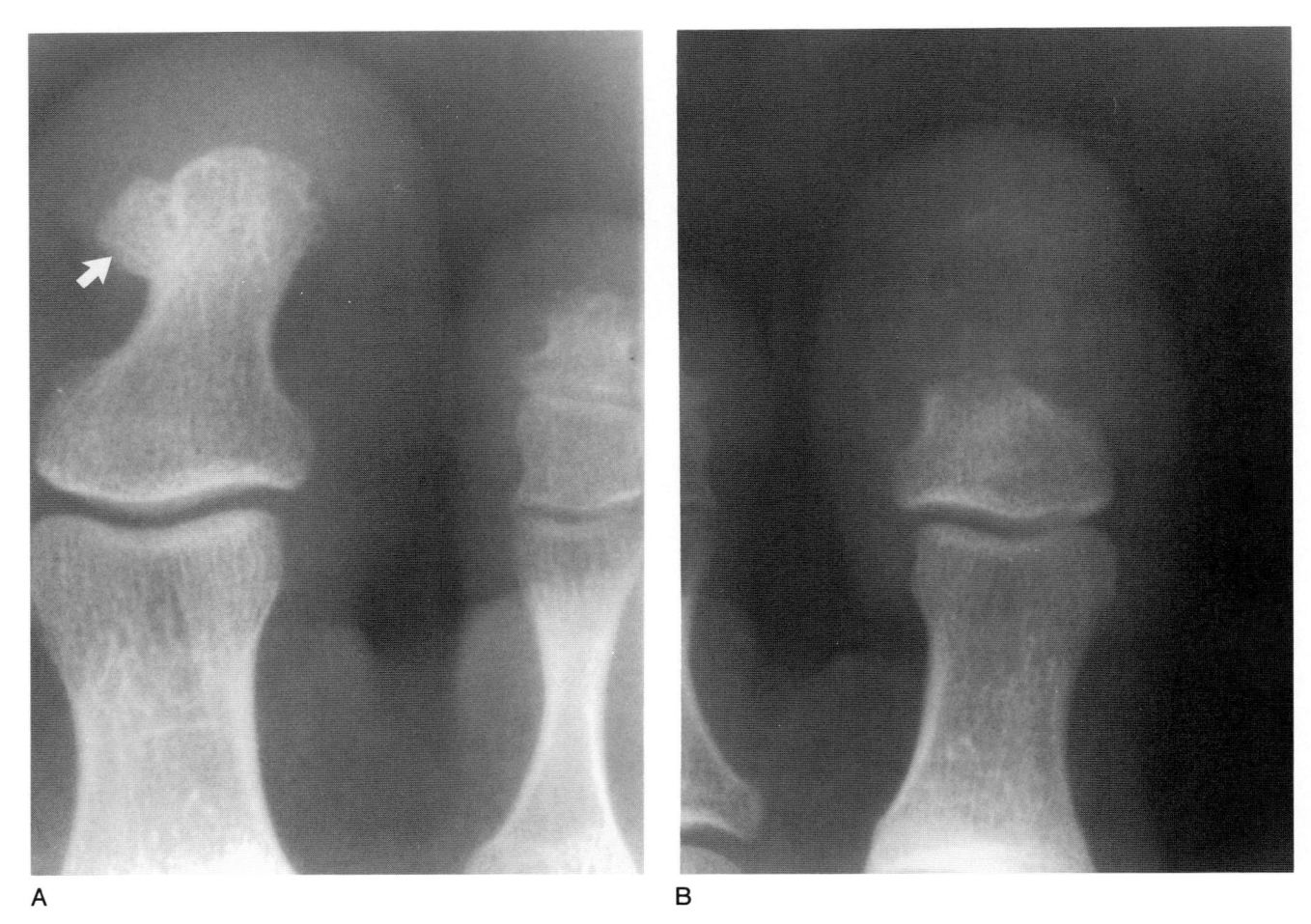

Fig. 41-15. (A) Third recurrence of a subungual exostosis of the great toe in a 15-year-old girl. (B) Appearance after radical resection of the distal portion of the distal phalanx. The patient suffered no further recurrences.

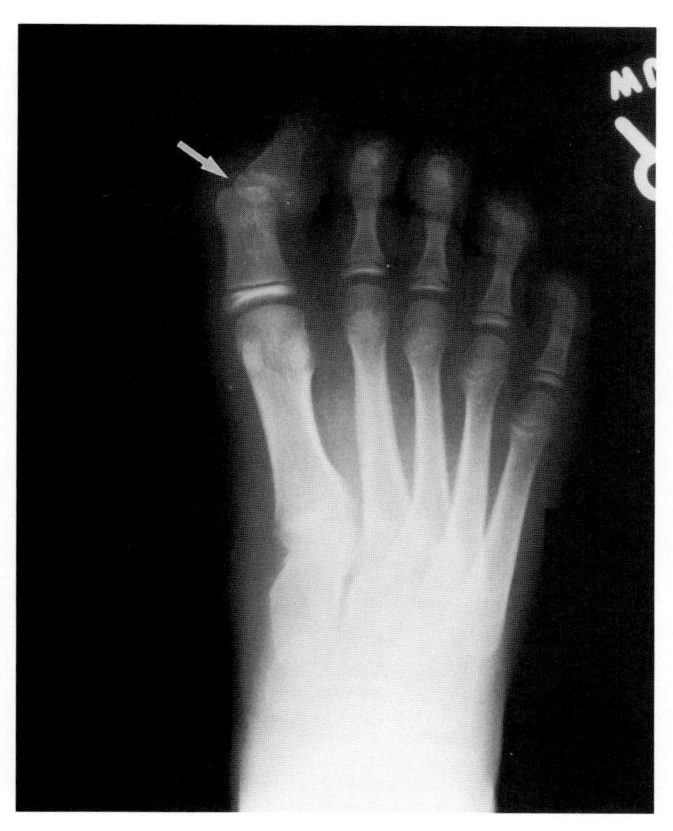

Fig. 41-16. Dislocation of the distal interphalangeal joint of the right great toe *(arrow)* in an 8-year-old boy who stubbed his toe while running barefoot.

that can present in the weeks or months following trauma (Fig. 41-15). Its etiology is unknown. It is more common in adolescent females. The disorder causes severe pain with pressure over the exostosis. The nailbed becomes deformed. Treatment is surgical. The exostosis is excised through a transverse incision at the distal end of the nail. Unfortunately, the recurrence rate is high. Sometimes, a more radical resection of the distal tip of the distal phalanx is required to permanently correct the problem.

Dislocations of the metatarsophalangeal and interphalangeal joints of the toes are also quite rare (Fig. 41-16). They are related to direct trauma to the toe usually by striking another object. They are easily reduced by traction and typically are quite stable after reduction. Immobilization consists of taping to an adjacent toe. Occasionally, the toe may not be reducible. Then an open reduction should be performed with removal of the offending piece of soft tissue from the joint.

SUMMARY

Fractures of the metatarsals are a common foot injury in children. Operative intervention is rarely required, as most heal rapidly with immobilization. Anatomic reduction is not necessary due to the excellent remodeling potential of the metatarsals in children. Fractures of the base of the fifth metatarsal can present some diagnostic difficulty. Stress fractures, although uncommon, should be considered in the teenage athlete. Fractures of the phalanges of the foot are usually secondary to crush injury. Proper alignment of the fractures can usually be achieved by manipulation, but occasionally percutaneous K-wire fixation will be necessary.

REFERENCES

1. Rang M: Children's Fractures. p. 323. JB Lippincott, Philadelphia, 1983
2. Hoerr NL, Pyle SI, Francis CC: Radiographic atlas of skeletal development of the foot and ankle. CC Thomas, Springfield, IL, 1962
3. Canale ST, Williams KD: Iselin's disease. J Pediatr Orthop 12:90, 1992
4. Dameron TB: Fractures and anatomical variations of the proximal portion of the fifth metatarsal. J Bone Joint Surg [Am] 57:788, 1975
5. Gruber W: Virchows Arch 1885. Cited in Ref. 3, p. 92.
6. Giachino A: Personal communication. Rockwood CA, Wilkins KE, King RE (eds): In, Fractures in Children. p. 1088. JB Lippincott, Philadelphia, 1984
7. Kavanaugh JH, Brower TD, Mann RV: The Jones fracture revisited. J Bone Joint Surg [Am] 60:776, 1978
8. Lehman RC, Gregg JR, Torg E: Iselin's disease. Am J Sports Med 14:494, 1986
9. Johnson GF: Pediatric Lisfranc injury: "Bunk bed" fracture. AJR 137:1041, 1981
10. Wiley JJ: The mechanism of tarsometatarsal joint injuries. Jour Bone Joint Surg [Br] 53B:474, 1971
11. Wiley JJ: Tarsometatarsal joint injuries in children. J Pediatr Orthop 1:255, 1981
12. Engh CA, Robinson RA, Milgram J: Stress fractures in children. J Trauma 10:532, 1970
13. Ogden JA: Skeletal Injury in the Child. p. 894. WB Saunders, Philadelphia, 1990
14. Hulkko A, Orava S: Stress fractures in athletes. Int J Sports Med 8:221, 1987
15. Drez D, Young JC, Roy D et al: Metatarsal stress fractures. Am J Sports Med 8:123, 1980

16. Tachdjian MO: The Child's Foot. p. 35. WB Saunders, Philadelphia, 1985
17. Maurice HD, Newman JH, Watt I: Bone scanning of the foot for unexplained pain. J Bone Joint Surg [Br] 69:448, 1987
18. Irvin CM, Witt CS, Zielsdorf LM: Traumatic osteochondritis of the lateral sesamoid in active adolescents. J Foot Surg 24:219, 1985
19. Ilfeld FW, Rosen V: Osteochondritis of the first metatarsal sesamoid. Clin Orthop Rel Res 85:38, 1972

42

Crush Injuries and Compartment Syndrome of the Foot

R. Baxter Willis
Robert D. Galpin

> Experience is a hard teacher because she gives the test first, the lesson afterward.

Compartment syndrome to the upper and lower extremity is now well recognized as a complication of trauma to the upper and lower extremity. Much has been written about the pathophysiology, investigation, and treatment of compartment syndromes of the limb in the past 20 years.[1-9] Only in recent years; however, has attention focused on the foot as a site of this potentially severe complication of trauma.[1,10-14]

DESCRIPTION AND INCIDENCE

Compartment syndrome is defined as a symptom complex caused by elevation of tissue fluid pressure within a closed osseofascial compartment of the limb, which interferes with the circulation to the muscles and nerves of that compartment. Following crush injury to the foot, bleeding occurs into closed spaces resulting in increased compartmental pressure. This will eventually result in obstruction to venous outflow from the compartment leading to further swelling and further increases in tissue pressure. If the pressure within the compartment rises above the arteriolar pressure to muscle and nerve, no further blood will enter the capillary anastomosis, and muscle and nerve ischemia will occur, leading to irreversible damage to the contents of the compartment(s).

Many theories have been proposed to document the exact series of events leading from injury to a full-blown compartment syndrome. Rorabeck and Clarke,[7] using a canine model, demonstrated that the extent of injury to the contents of the compartment are time- and pressure-dependent. If the pressure within the anterior compartment of the leg was maintained at 30 mmHg or more for 8 hours, changes in conduction velocity of the peroneal nerve were noted. If higher pressures were introduced and maintained, conduction velocity changes occurred much sooner.

Local venous hypertension may also play a role in the pathogenesis of compartmental ischemia. Local increases in venous pressure will lower the arterivenous gradient and further reduce capillary blood flow. Compartment syndrome of the foot may also occur after arterial injury in the foot, ankle, or leg. Compartment syndrome usually does not occur in this instance until after restoration of arterial flow. The period of ischemia leads to myoneural hypoxia, allowing a transudation of fluid

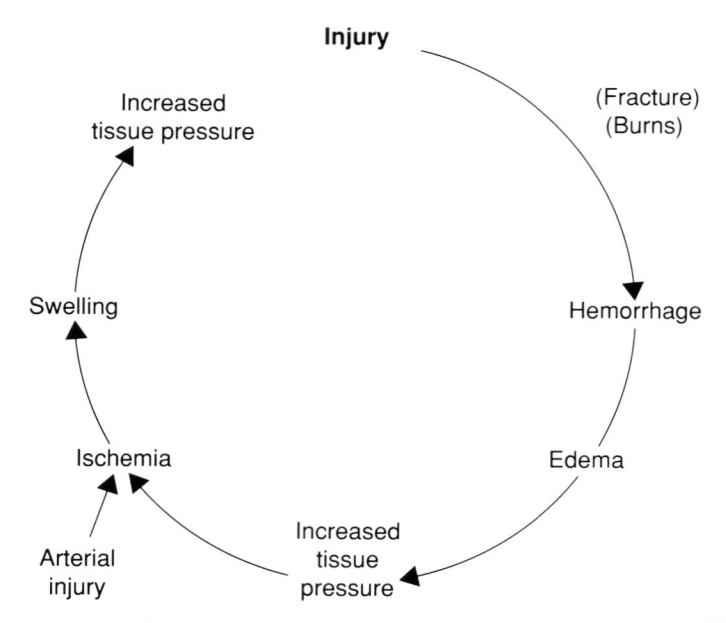

Fig. 42-1. The pathophysiology of compartment syndrome is "a vicious cycle." (From Willis RB: Orthopaedic trauma. p. 206. In Sibbald WJ (ed): Synopsis of Critical Care. 2nd Ed. Williams & Wilkins, Baltimore, 1983, with permission.)

through capillary basement membranes and in muscle, thus increasing the content of the compartment. When vascular repair has been accomplished, fluid will continue to leak across the basement membrane into the interstitial space. The pressure will continue to rise until it exceeds the end-closing pressure of the arterioles to muscle, at which point no further blood will enter the muscle of the compartment involved and shunting will occur (see Fig. 42-1). The pressure within the compartment is not great enough to occlude or obstruct the major arterial vessels, therefore pulses are present in an acute compartment syndrome.

The incidence of compartment syndrome involving the foot is rare but still must be considered. Isolated reports of compartment syndrome of the foot have been associated with crush injuries of the foot, fractures of the metatarsals, Lisfranc fracture-dislocations, and, more recently, with fractures of the calcaneus.[12,14] The true incidence of compartment syndrome of the foot in children is not known, but the treating physician must be aware of the potential for this complication in treating fractures, dislocations, and crush injuries of the foot.

ANATOMY

Classically the anatomy of the foot is considered in layers, but for the purposes of surgical anatomy it should be considered in a coronal section. Traditionally four distinct osseofascial compartments are noted: medial, central, lateral, and the interosseous compartment.[15,16]

The *medial* compartment contains the abductor hallucis and flexor hallucis brevis muscles. It is bounded medially and inferiorly by an extension of the plantar aponeurosis and on its dorsal surface by the first metatarsal.

The *central* compartment is bounded by the plantar aponeurosis inferiorly, the osseofascial tarsometatarsal structures dorsally and the intermuscular septae medially and laterally. It contains the flexor digitorum brevis, lumbricals, quadratus plantae, and abductor hallucis muscles.

The *lateral* compartment contains the flexor, abductor, and opponens muscles of the fifth toe. It is bounded dorsally by the fifth metatarsal, medially by an intermuscular septum, inferiorly by the plantar fascia, and dorsally by the fifth metatarsal.

The *interosseous* compartment is bounded by the metatarsals and interosseous fascia and contains the seven interossei.

Recently, Manoli and Weber[12] introduced the concept of nine compartments in the foot. The medial and lateral exist as previously described. The central compartment consists of superficial and deep portions. The deep portion is called the calcaneal compartment and is the only compartment in the foot to communicate with the leg, namely, the deep posterior compartment of the leg. Manoli and Weber found four separate interossei compartments deep in the forefoot and a separate compartment containing the adductor muscles. The importance of this distinction obviously lies in adequate decompression at the time of fasciotomy.

MECHANISM OF INJURY

Probably the most common cause of a compartment syndrome of the foot is a crush injury. These can occur in children when a large heavy object falls on a child's foot causing severe soft tissue damage and possibly bony injury as well. The condition may also occur with Lisfranc fracture-dislocation, multiple fractures of the metatarsal bones, and fractures of the calcaneus.[12,14]

CLASSIFICATION

Classification of compartment syndromes have been divided into intrinsic and extrinsic causes.[9] *Intrinsic* causes are those that lead to increased compartment content and pressure and include hemorrhage following fracture or severe soft tissue injury. Hereditary bleeding disorders and postischemic swelling following arterial injury are additional intrinsic causes.[10,17] *Extrinsic* causes occur from external pressure affecting compartment pressure and include bandages and casts that are excessively tight.

The type or cause of compartment syndrome is not important. What is vitally important for the child's limb is its prompt recognition and treatment.

PHYSICAL EXAMINATION

The diagnosis of compartment syndrome of the foot is extremely difficult to make on clinical grounds alone. A high index of suspicion based on pain out of proportion to the injury, increased pain with passive stretching of the foot intrinsic muscles and severe swelling is necessary to affect a successful diagnosis.

Gentle passive dorsiflexion of the toes stretches the intrinsic muscles of the foot and should raise alarms about the potential of increased pressure within the compartments of the foot. However, it is not pathognomonic of the condition.[14] Sensory changes in the distal distribution of nerves that pass through the compartment are not reliable in the foot. The presence or absence of dorsalis pedis or posterior tibial pulses should not be used as reliable indicators of a compartment syndrome.

Because of the lack of definitive clinical signs it is recommended to assess compartment pressures with the use of one of the commercially available catheter systems.[6,18-20] This is mandatory if the patient has a severe foot injury with significant swelling and is unconscious or has a spinal cord or peripheral nerve injury. It is highly recommended as an objective measurement in any equivocal situation.

The slit catheter designed by Rorabeck and colleagues[6] employs a polyethylene catheter with five slits cut into its end. The system is calibrated after filling the tubing with saline in conjunction with a pressure transducer and recorder. A large, 16- or 18-gauge needle is introduced obliquely into the compartment and the catheter fed through until appropriate readings are obtained. The system can be checked for accuracy by applying local pressure to the compartment or by having the patient use the muscle(s) in question to produce a deflection in the recording (Figs. 42-2 and 42-3).

The threshold pressure for fasciotomy is 30–35 mmHg but must be considered in conjunction with the patient's clinical findings.

DIFFERENTIAL DIAGNOSIS

A high index of suspicion in a child with a crush injury, multiple fractures, or dislocations is necessary to make the diagnosis. Other conditions that may mimic compartment syndrome include:

1. Musculoskeletal injury alone
2. Vascular (arterial) injury
3. Neurologic injury

Immobilization after appropriate reduction should alleviate much of the child's pain in most musculoskeletal injuries. Careful physical examination after removal of constricting bandages or casts is necessary to adequately examine the child. If the pain fails to subside, objective assessment for compartment syndrome using the slit catheter system is indicated.

Arterial injury without penetrating injury of the foot or ankle is extremely rare. Pain with arterial injury results from tissue ischemia, and true ischemia is unlikely unless both arterial sources are disrupted. True compartment syndrome occurs well below systolic blood pressure so peripheral pulses are usually present and other signs of arterial ischemia absent.

Compartment syndrome may cause neurologic dysfunction in its late stages but the signs are not confined to one neurologic structure and are therefore diffuse not discrete.

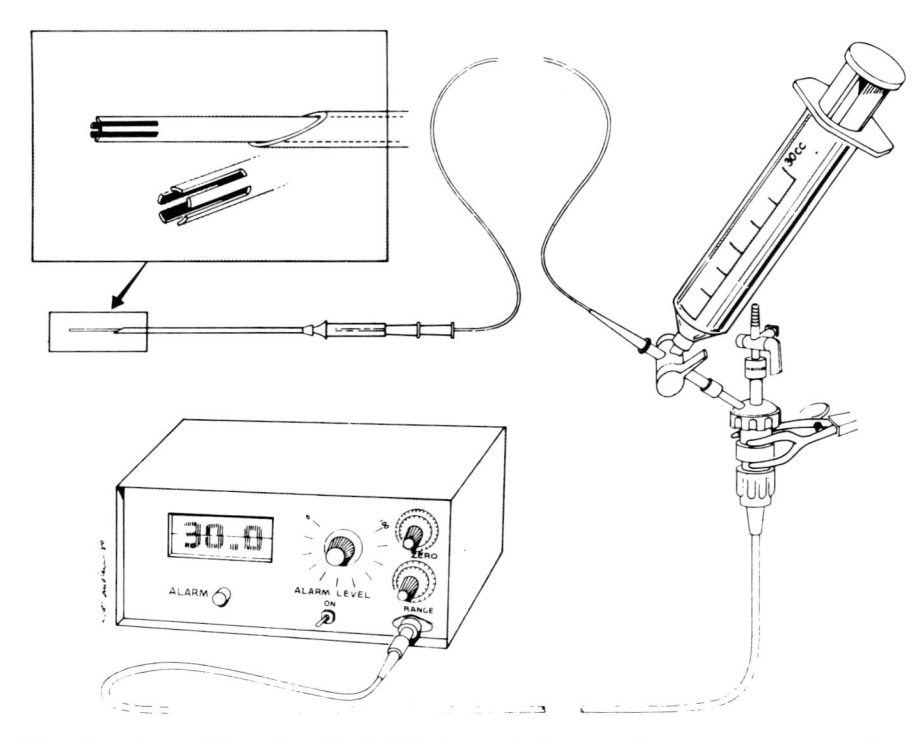

Fig. 42-2. The slit catheter. (From Rorabeck CH: A practical approach to compartment syndromes. Part III. Management. Instr Course Lect 32:88, 1983, with permission.)

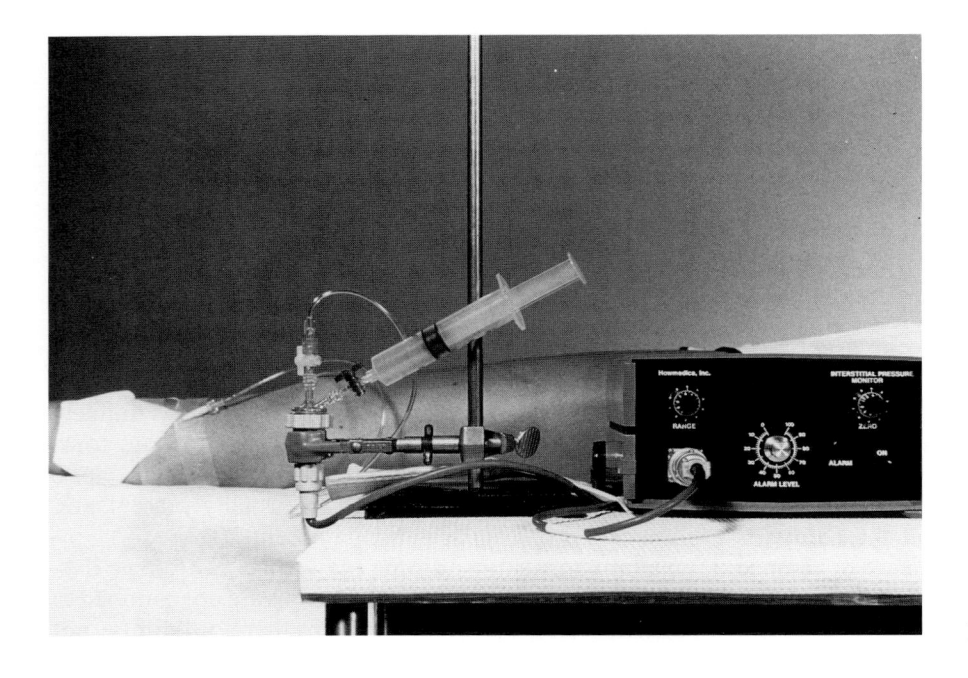

Fig. 42-3. The slit catheter monitoring system. Note the transducer dome is at the same height as the catheter. (From Rorabeck CH: A practical approach to compartment syndromes. Part III. Management. Instr Course Lect 32:88, 1983, with permission.)

```
                SUSPECTED
                COMPARTMENTAL
                SYNDROME
                     │
         ┌───────────┴───────────┐
         ▼                       ▼
  unequivocally positive    patient not alert/unreliable
  clinical findings         polytrauma victim
                            inconclusive clinical findings
         │                       │
         │                       ▼
         │              compartmental pressure
         │                  measurement
         │                       │
         │              ┌────────┴────────┐
         │              ▼                 ▼
         │         >30 mmHg*         <30 mmHg*
         │              │                 │
         │              │                 ▼
         │              │           continuous
         │              │           compartmental
         │              │           pressure monitoring
         │              │           and serial clinical  ◄──┐
         │              │           evaluation              │
         │              │                 │                 │
         │              │                 ├──► <30 mmHg* ───┘
         │              │                 │
         │              │        ┌────────┴────────┐
         │              │        ▼                 ▼
         │              │    clinical          >30 mmHg*
         │              │    diagnosis
         │              │    made
         ▼              ▼        ▼                 ▼
    ████████████████████████████████████████████████████
    ██                  FASCIOTOMY                    ██
    ████████████████████████████████████████████████████
```

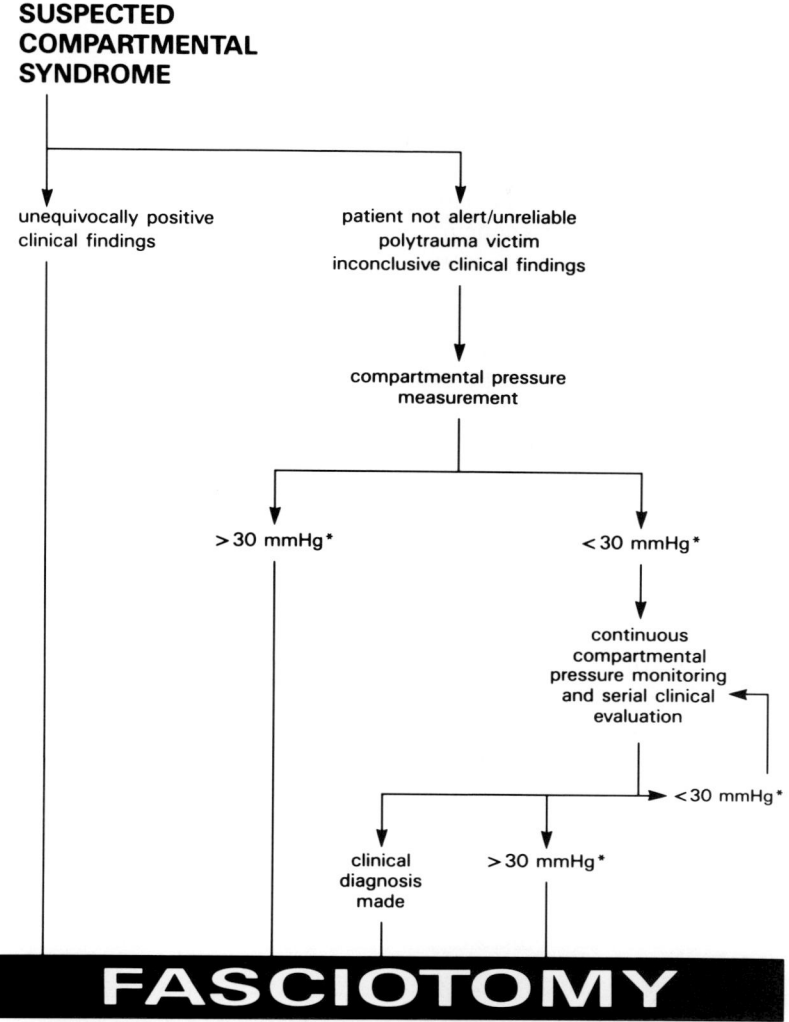

*In patients with hypotension, compartmental syndromes may occur at pressures less than 30 mmHg. Currently we use 25 mmHg as the critical pressure in these patients.

Fig. 42-4. Algorithm used in diagnosing and treating acute compartment syndrome. (From Bourne RB, Rorabeck CH: Compartment syndromes of the lower leg. Clin Orthop Rel Res 240:97, 1989, with permission.)

TREATMENT INDICATIONS

Fasciotomy is indicated in established compartment syndrome. This would include any situation where there are conclusive clinical findings, where objective compartment pressure measurements exceed 30 mmHg or at lower pressures when patients have been hypotensive. In the equivocal patient who is unable to cooperate or where the diagnosis is suspected but not confirmed, continuous pressure measurement is indicated. If the pressures exceed 30mm Hg at any time, fasciotomy is indicated (Fig. 42-4).

Technique of Fasciotomy

Fasciotomy of the compartments of the foot is best accomplished through two dorsal incisions and an additional medial incision.[11,14,16] The two dorsal incisions are in line with the second and fourth metatarsals. The incision is carried down to bone without subcutaneous dissection to avoid further tissue trauma, especially to the narrow skin bridge between the two dorsal incisions. Once the bone is identified, the fascia overlying the interosseous compartments is incised. The first dorsal and plantar interossei are stripped from the shaft of the second metatarsal. The fascia of the adductor compartment is located deep within the interspace after the interossei are retracted medially.

The medial incision follows the inferior surface of the first metatarsal extending about 6 cm proximally to end 4 cm from the posterior portion of the heel. The incision is developed to the fascia of the medial compartment and subcutaneous dissection exposes the plantar aponeurosis. Fasciotomy of the medial compartment is accomplished about 1 cm from its inferior border. The lateral fascial wall of the medial compartment is exposed by retracting the abductor hallucis muscles superiorly and releasing its attachment to the lateral fascial wall. The lateral fascial wall is incised very carefully to avoid the lateral plantar nerve and artery lying just deep to this fascia. The fasciotomy is carried distally to decompress the calcaneal compartment.

A second incision is placed inferior to the original fascial strip remaining to decompress the superficial compartment. In the most proximal portion of this fascial incision fasciotomy of the lateral compartment is accomplished by incising the overlying fascia on the inferomedial aspect extending to the lateral side of the foot (Fig. 42-5). All the wounds are left open and delayed primary closure and/or split thickness skin grafting is carried out at approximately the fifth postoperative day.

Reduction of fractures and dislocations and fixation by small fragment plates and screws or K-wires is advised. Stability of fractures and dislocations enhances the environment for soft tissue healing and allows earlier rehabilitation of the foot.[9,14]

Pitfalls to Avoid

The most common pitfall is the failure to recognize and treat an established compartment syndrome. If any doubt about the diagnosis exists, objective measurement with the slit catheter technique should be performed. If the treating surgeon is unfamiliar with this equipment or it is not available and there are clinical findings of increased compartment pressure, fasciotomy should be performed. A high index of suspicion in crush injuries is critical to the successful management of these rare injuries. A thorough knowledge of the anatomy of the osseofascial compartments of the foot is essential to perform an adequate decompression.

Failure to act may result in permanent damage to the foot. Crush injuries in the growing child may lead to premature growth arrest and subsequent deformity. Parents should be warned of these potential complications at the outset of treatment.

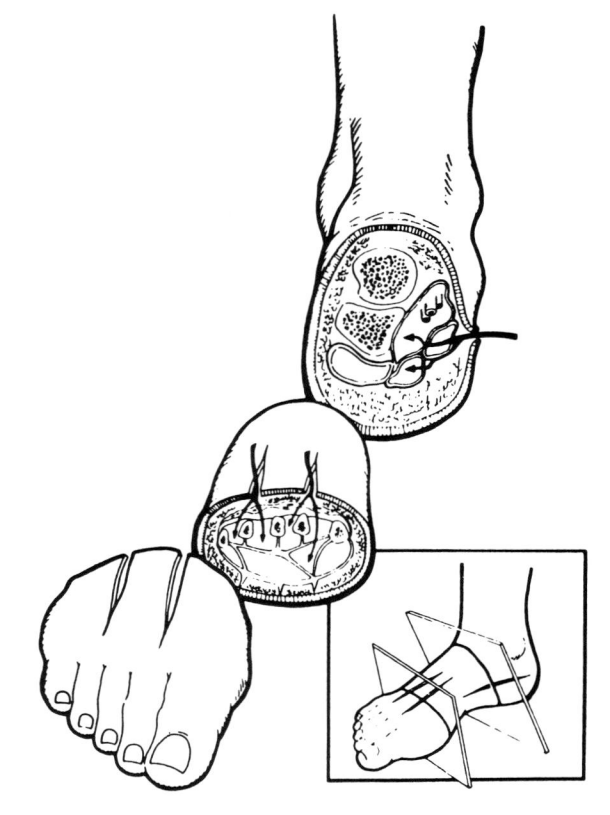

Fig. 42-5. Two dorsal forefoot incisions and one medial hindfoot incision are used to decompress all of the foot compartments. (From Manoli and Weber,[12] with permission.)

SUMMARY

A high index of suspicion in crush injuries is critical to the successful management of these rare injuries. A thorough knowledge of the anatomy of the osseofascial compartments of the foot is essential to perform an adequate decompression. Prevention of compartment syndrome is impossible to attain, but early recognition and prompt surgical decompression will ensure the best possible results.

REFERENCES

1. Bonutti PM, Bell GR: Compartment syndrome of the foot. J Bone Joint Surg [Am] 68:1449, 1986
2. Delee JC, Stiehl JB: Open tibia fracture with compartment syndrome. Clin Orthop Rel Res 160:175, 1981
3. Gelberman RH, Garfin SR, Hergenroeder PT et al: Compartment syndromes of the forearm: diagnosis and treatment. Clin Orthop 161:252, 1981

4. Matsen FA: Compartmental syndrome: a unified concept. Clin Orthop 110:113, 1975
5. Mubarak SJ, Carroll NC: Volkmann's contracture in children: aeteiology and prevention. J Bone Joint Surg [Br] 61:285, 1979
6. Rorabeck CH, Castle GSP, Hardie R et al: The slit catheter: a new device for measuring intracompartmental pressure. Proc Can Orthop Res Soc 1980:12, and Surg Forum 31:513, 1980
7. Rorabeck CH, Clarke KM: The pathophysiology of the anterior tibial compartment syndrome: an experimental investigation. J Trauma 18:299, 1978
8. Willis RB, Fowler PJ: Vascular compartment syndromes. Can J Surg 18:157, 1975
9. Willis RB, Rorabeck CH: Treatment of compartment syndromes in children. Orthop Clin North Am 21:401, 1990
10. Heim M, Martinowitz U, Horoszowski H: The short foot syndrome: an unfortunate consequence of neglected raised intra-compartment pressure in a severe hemophilic child: a case report. Angiology 37:128, 1986
11. Manoli A: Compartment syndromes of the foot: current concepts. Foot Ankle 10:340, 1990
12. Manoli A, Weber TG: Fasciotomy of the foot: an anatomical study with special reference of the calcaneal compartment. Foot Ankle 10:267, 1990
13. Myerson M: Acute compartment syndromes of the foot. Bull Hosp Joint Dis Orthop Inst 47:251, 1987
14. Myerson M: Diagnosis and treatment of compartment syndrome of the foot. Orthopaedics 13:711, 1990
15. Garfin SR: Anatomy of the extremity compartments. p. 44. In Mubarak SJ, Hargens AR (eds): Compartment Syndromes and Volkmann's Contractures. WB Saunders, Philadelphia, 1981
16. Loeffler RD, Ballard A: Plantar fascial spaces of the foot and a proposed surgical approach. Foot Ankle 1:11, 1980
17. Hieb LD, Alexander AH: Bilateral anterior and lateral compartment syndromes in a patient with sickle cell trait: case report and review of the literature. Clin Orthop 228:190, 1988
18. Garfin SR, Mubarak SJ, Evans KL et al: Quantification of intracompartmental pressure and volume under plaster casts. J Bone Joint Surg [Am] 63:449, 1981
19. Matsen FA III, Mayo KA, Sheridan GW et al: Monitoring of intramuscular pressure. Surgery 79:702, 1976
20. Mubarak SJ, Hargens AR, Owen CA et al: The wick catheter technique for measurement of intramuscular pressure: a new research and clinical tool. J Bone Joint Surg [Am] 58:1016, 1976

43

Atlanto-Occipital Fractures and Dislocations

James G. Jarvis

> We are constantly misled by the ease with which our minds fall into the ruts of one or two experiences.
> —Sir William Osler

DESCRIPTION AND INCIDENCE

In general, cervical spine injuries are uncommon in children. Bohlman,[1] in his series of 300 cervical spine injuries, reported only 15 children aged less than 15 years. Henrys and colleagues[3] reported a series of 631 cervical lesions over a 20-year period, which included only 12 patients (1.9 percent) under 15. Rang[4] estimated an incidence of 1.3 cases per year at a busy children's hospital.

Injuries of the craniocervical junction are very rare. They are almost exclusively atlanto-occipital dislocations (AOD) (Fig. 43-1). Although these lesions are usually traumatic, they can also result from inflammatory causes such as rheumatoid arthritis or ankylosing spondylitis.[2]

Although atlanto-occipital dislocation is a rarely reported injury, Bucholz and Burkhead,[5] in an autopsy study of multiple-trauma victims, found 9 of 26 cadavers with cervical spine injuries had suffered atlanto-occipital dislocation—the most common cervical spine injury in this group. He also noted AOD was 2.5 times more common in children than in adults and that in no child was there an associated fracture. It is estimated that AOD accounts for up to one-third of all deaths from traumatic cervical spine injury.[1,6-8]

Traumatic AOD has been estimated to account for only 0.7 to 1 percent of all cervical spine injuries encountered in trauma centers.[3,9] Many physicians, therefore, have little experience with this entity. With the development of specialized trauma centers and improved mechanisms for transporting injured patients, survival of AOD, at times with complete neurologic recovery, has been reported with increasing frequency.[10] Thus, an understanding of the nature of this injury coupled with knowledge of the management of survivors is imperative to reduce the associated morbidity and mortality.

ANATOMY

The occipitoatlantoaxial joints function as a unit during the cervical movements of flexion, extension, lateral flexion, and rotation. The atlas serves as a bearing between the occipital condyles and the superior articular surfaces of the axis. Movement in the craniovertebral region is determined by the occipital condyles and the axis.

Numerous ligaments and synovial joints comprise the occipitoatlantoaxial unit (Fig. 43-2). The only direct

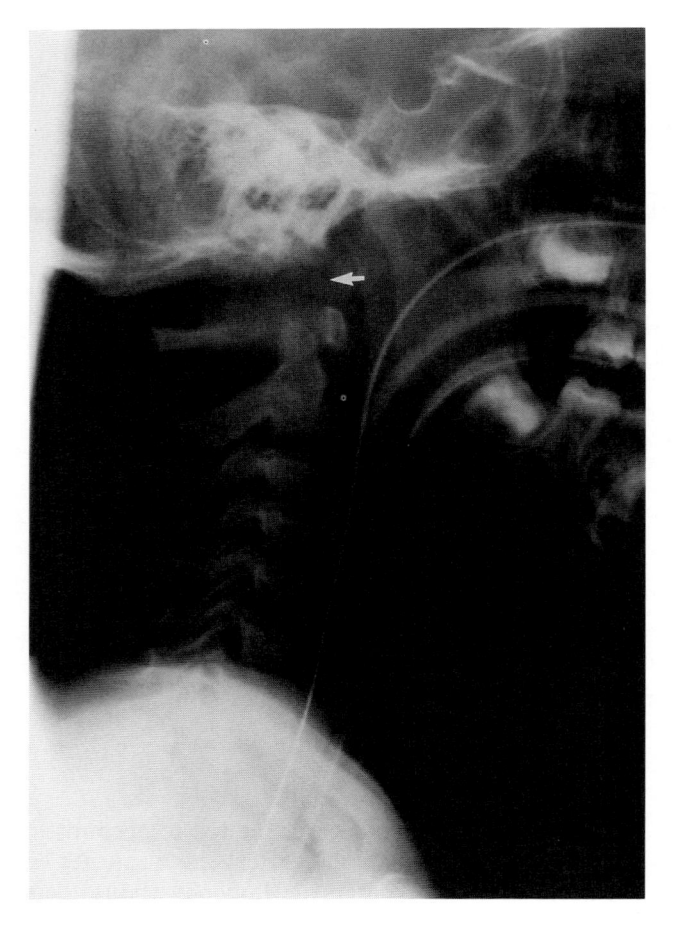

Fig. 43-1. Traumatic atlanto-occipital dislocation in a 4-year-old child.

TABLE 43-1. Range of Motion of the Occipitoatlantoaxial Complex

Unit of Complex	Type of Motion	Degrees of Motion
Occipitoatlantal joint (ocp-C1)	Flexion/extension	13° (Moderate)
	Lateral bending	8° (Moderate)
	Axial rotation	0° (Negligible)
Atlantoaxial joint (C1–C2)	Flexion/extension	10° (Moderate)
	Lateral bending	0° (Negligible)
	Axial rotation	47° (Extensive)

(Modified from White and Panjabi,[12] with permission.)

connections between the occiput and the axis are the tectorial membrane, cruciate ligament, apical dental ligament, and paired alar ligaments. The most important are the tectorial membrane and the alar ligaments. Werne[11] showed that the range of forward occipitoatlantal flexion is limited by skeletal contact between the anterior margin of the foramen magnum and the odontoid apex. Hyperextension is limited by the tectorial membrane and by skull contact between the posterior arch of the atlas and the occiput. Lateral tilting is controlled by the alar ligaments (Fig. 43-2B). The apical dental ligament is a rudimentary structure and does not prevent motion.

The range of motion of the occipitoatlantoaxial complex in adults has been well described by White and Panjabi[12] (Table 43-1). In children, the occipital condyles are small and the plane of the occipitoatlantal joint is almost horizontal. The steep inclination of the occipitoatlantal joints develops with aging. Therefore, dislocation without fracture is possible in children but rare in adults.

MECHANISM OF INJURY

The mechanism of injury in atlanto-occipital dislocation is controversial. Alker and associates[6] thought that it was a hyperflexion injury but provided no data to support that contention. Bucholz and Burkhead[5] noted the high frequency of submental lacerations, mandibular fractures, and lacerations to the posterior pharangeal wall as being more consistent with injury caused by hyperextension with a distraction force applied to the head. An intact posterior atlanto-occipital membrane in one of their cadavers implied a primary hyperextension injury. Gabrielsen and Maxwell[13] felt lateroflexion was responsible in their one case, while Fielding and Hensinger[14] felt that in "short-stop" accidents, the head was inertially carried forward with cranial vertebral dislocation followed by immediate spontaneous reduction. This could account for the normal radiographic findings in some cases.

Autopsy evaluation after atlanto-occipital dislocation has frequently shown direct mechanical injury to the lower brainstem and upper cervical spinal cord. In 1908 Blackwood[15] studied a patient who survived for 34 hours following a shipboard accident. He showed the spinal cord to be compressed between the posterior rim of the foramen magnum and the posterior surface of the dens. More recent reports have described complete transection of the cord at the spinal medullary junction,[1,8,9] partial transection of the cord,[16] and laceration of the pontomedullary junction plus contusion of the brainstem and upper cervical spinal cord.[17] Fruin and Pirotte[18] reported a case of AOD with bilateral sixth cranial nerve palsies, felt to be due to avulsion of the nerve roots resulting from distraction of the skull.

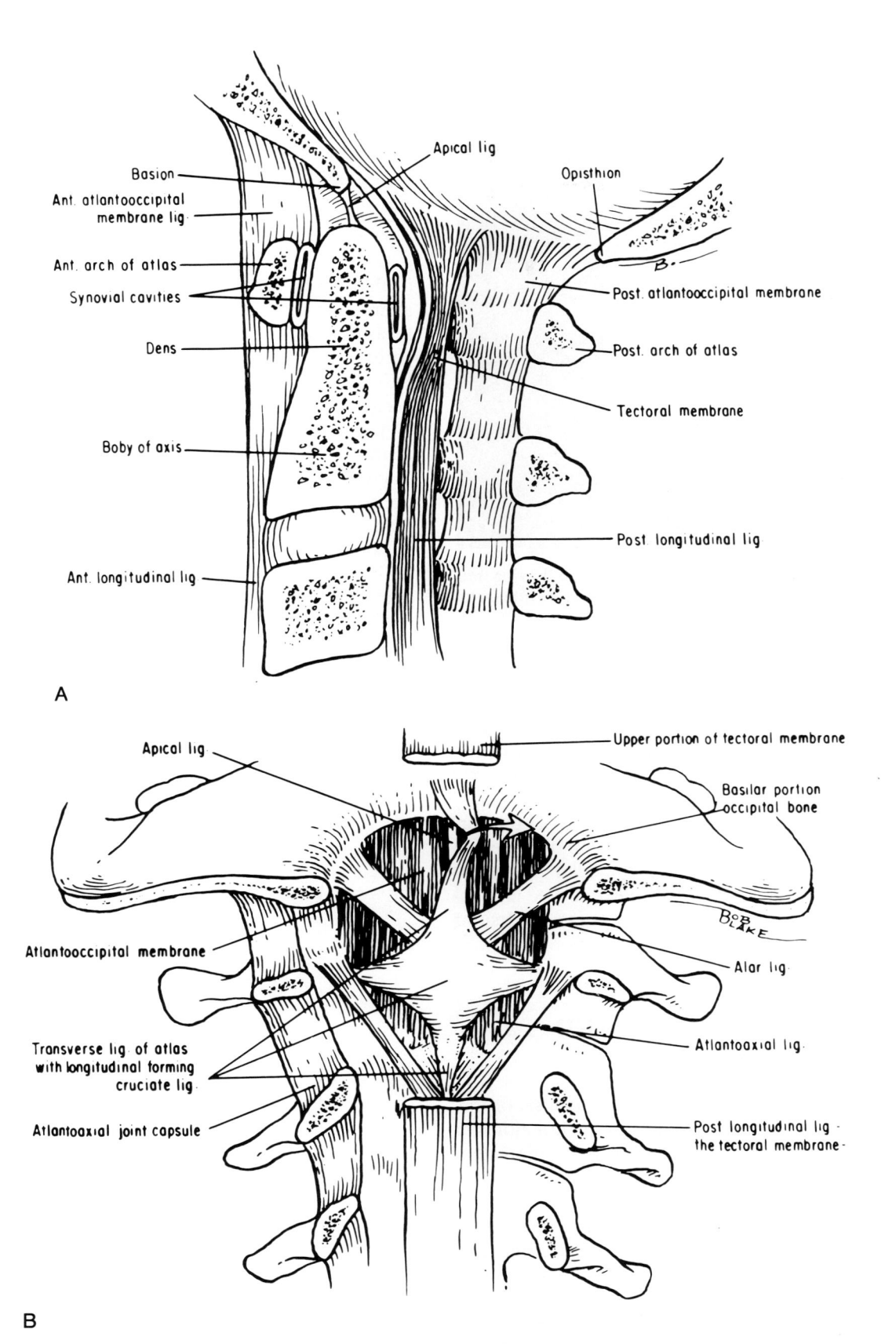

Fig. 43-2. Joints and ligaments of the occipitoatlantoaxial region. **(A)** lateral view. **(B)** Posterior view. Ant, anterior; Post, posterior; lig, ligament. (Modified from Powers et al.,[9] with permission.)

800 / Management of Pediatric Fractures

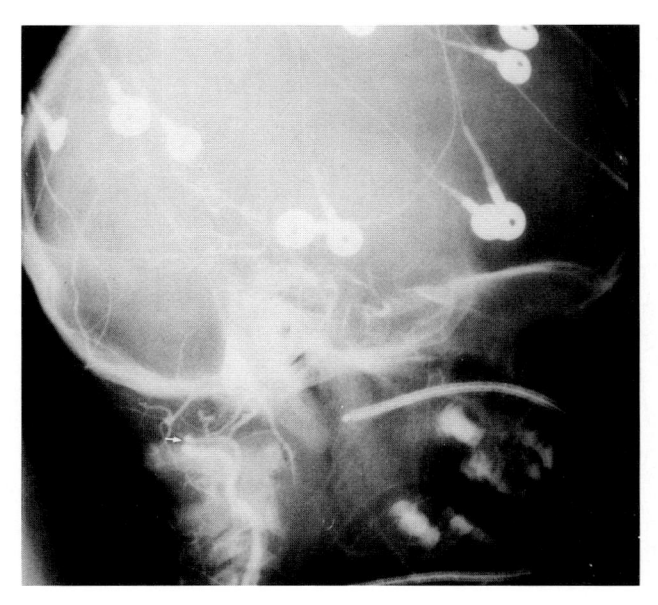

Fig. 43-3. Vertebral artery vascular occlusion following traumatic atlanto-occipital dislocation in a 4-year-old child (same patient as in Fig. 43-1).

More recently, reports of survivors suggest that post-traumatic vascular insufficiency of the brainstem and cord may be clinically significant in causation of the neurologic dysfunction in many patients with atlanto-occipital dislocation[10,19] (Fig. 43-3). Farthing[20] illustrated the clinical syndrome of compression of both vertebral arteries with an immediate cessation of pulse and respiration following extension of the head. These parameters returned to normal with flexion. Lee and coworkers[10] showed that some of these vascular lesions may be completely reversible.

CLASSIFICATION AND RADIOLOGY

Accurate and prompt radiographic diagnosis of this injury is essential so that the craniocervical junction can be stabilized to prevent further damage to the brainstem and spinal cord with resultant permanent paralysis, neurologic deficit, or death.[17] Evaluation of the atlanto-occipital articulation is difficult at best. Gross dislocation may be obvious, but subtle degrees of longitudinal distraction can be difficult to evaluate. Instability can be either anterior, posterior, or longitudinal (distraction).

White and Panjabi and associates[21] have outlined stability criteria for the occipitoatlantal junction in adults

TABLE 43-2. Occiput-C1 Instability

Dens (tip) to basion of occiput	4 to 5 mm
Flexion-extension translation	1 mm
Neurologic signs or symptoms	

(From White and Panjabi,[21] with permission.)

(Table 43-2). Most of the methods for analyzing the atlanto-occipital articulation are based on dens-basion measurements. The method of Powers and coworkers[9] is perhaps the most sensitive (Fig. 43-4). He claims that the BC/AO ratio is a good discriminator of anterior atlanto-occipital dislocation when greater than or equal to 1.0.

Although few methods address the actual longitudinal distraction-dislocation injury, Kaufman and colleagues[17] suggested using the actual distance between the occipital condyle and the condylar facet of C1 rather than using adjacent structures, such as the mandible, basion, or dens as markers. This can be carried out in both the lateral and the anteroposterior (AP) radiographic positions. They found the distance between the cortical margin of the occipital condyle and the ossified condylar facet was between 1.5 and 3.5 mm in most cases (Fig. 43-5). They found no cases where the distance in normal children exceeded 5 mm, regardless of age.

In young children radiographic evaluation is difficult for a number of reasons. The tip of the odontoid process is cartilaginous and difficult to assess radiologically.

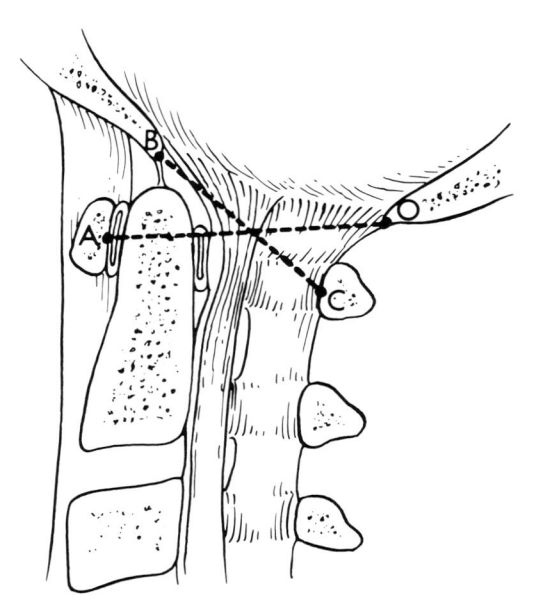

Fig. 43-4. Radiographic criteria for atlanto-occipital dislocation. B, basion of occipital bone; O, opisthion of occipital bone; A, anterior arch of C1; C, posterior arch of C1. (From Powers et al.,[9] with permission.)

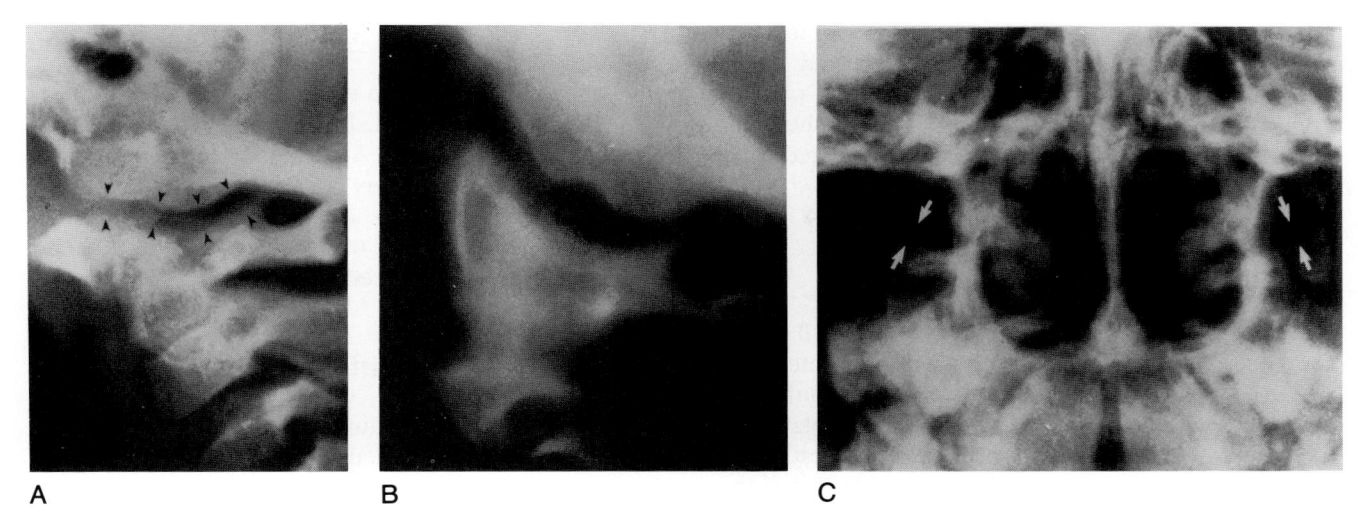

Fig. 43-5. Determination of longitudinal atlanto-occipital dislocation from radiographs. (A) Brow-up lateral view showing normal atlanto-occipital junction in a 3-year-old child. (B) Lateral polytone through normal atlanto-occipital joint in a 9-year-old. (C) Anteroposterior skull film. Normal atlanto-occipital joint. (Modified from Kaufman et al.,[17] with permission.)

There is frequently bony superimposition further compromising assessments. Congenital anomalies of the atlas or foramen magnum can affect the reliability of measurement. No truly reliable measurement between the skull and the atlas has yet been defined.

PHYSICAL EXAMINATION

Survival after traumatic atlanto-occipital dislocation is rare. Pang and Wilberger[22] reviewed the spectrum of clinical manifestations of atlanto-occipital dislocation in those few cases of survival. Although there have been reports of cases of dislocation with a normal neurologic examination on presentation,[20] neurologic compromise is usually significant. Cranial nerve palsy is among the most common findings. Frequently, patients are comatose on presentation or have varying degrees of neurologic deficit. As many of these injuries are the result of motor vehicle accidents, associated visceral and musculoskeletal injuries are also quite common. This may include other fractures in the cervical spine.[9,17]

DIFFERENTIAL DIAGNOSIS

The differential diagnosis of atlanto-occipital instability includes conditions resulting in maldevelopment of bone and ligamentous laxity. This includes various syndromes such as mucopolysaccharidosis, spondyloepiphyseal dysplasia, and Down syndrome, as well as severe rheumatoid disease of the cervical spine.[23-25] Other abnormalities caudal to the atlas, such as spina bifida occulta or congenital malformations can also result in atlanto-occipital instability.

TREATMENT

Closed Methods

The management of all patients surviving traumatic atlanto-occipital dislocation begins with immediate immobilization of the head and neck to prevent further spinal cord injury. Respiratory distress should be treated, taking care not to move the head or neck during intubation. The well-known principles of cardiorespiratory resuscitation should be followed, with maintenance of an adequate airway assuming priority.[26]

The use of traction has been controversial. Earlier reports advocate the use of minimal skeletal traction (2–4 lb).[27,28] More recently, traction has been felt to be contraindicated, especially in longitudinal distraction injuries.[10,17] Immediate immobilization of the head to prevent further injury to the cord and arteries should be employed. A halo vest may be more beneficial than even minimal skeletal traction, since the cord and arteries may be further stretched by traction.

Angiography should be undertaken to assess the vertebral and carotid arterial supply. If an intimal tear is found, anticoagulation has been suggested to prevent thrombosis formation.[10] Vasospasm has been shown to be potentially reversible and should be treated with maintenance of blood pressure and volume.[10]

Halo Fixation in Children

In 1986 Garfin and colleagues[29] studied skull osteology using computed tomography scans to determine optimal sites for placement of halo pins. They confirmed that halo fixation pins should be placed anterolaterally and posterolaterally where the bones are thickest. They also felt that, because of the thinness of the skull and the risk of pin penetration, alternative methods of immobilization should be utilized in children under the age of 2 years. Subsequently, Letts and colleagues[30] in a biomechanical analysis and later Mubarak and colleagues[31] in a clinical follow-up, showed that halos can be utilized in infants and children under the age of 2. CT scanning of the skull prior to application of the halo is recommended to determine the safest pin sites. Multiple pins or the "ring of thorns" technique can be utilized with low torques, in the range of 2 in. lb (Fig. 43-6). Custom bivalved polypropylene vests can be made from a plaster mold of the trunk.

Open Methods

About half the children reported as long-term survivors of atlanto-occipital dislocation have undergone occipitocervical arthrodesis. A safe and effective method of fusing this area in children has been reported by Letts and Slutsky[24] (Fig. 43-7). Adequate postoperative immobilization of the skull using the halo is essential to achieving successful arthrodesis.

Pitfalls

The main pitfall in dealing with atlanto-occipital dislocation involves initial identification and recognition of the injury. As survival from this injury is rare, few centers have experience in dealing with this dislocation. Interpretation of radiographs of the craniovertebral junction is notoriously difficult. The difficulty is compounded in young children where there are no reliable measurements.

Failure to immobilize the spine can lead to aggravation of vascular and neurologic injury.[10] Application of traction, particularly in longitudinal distraction injuries, can further potentiate neurovascular complications.

Numerous complications can ensue during attempts to fuse the upper cervical spine.[32] Of these, iatrogenic neurologic deterioration is the most feared. Occipitocer-

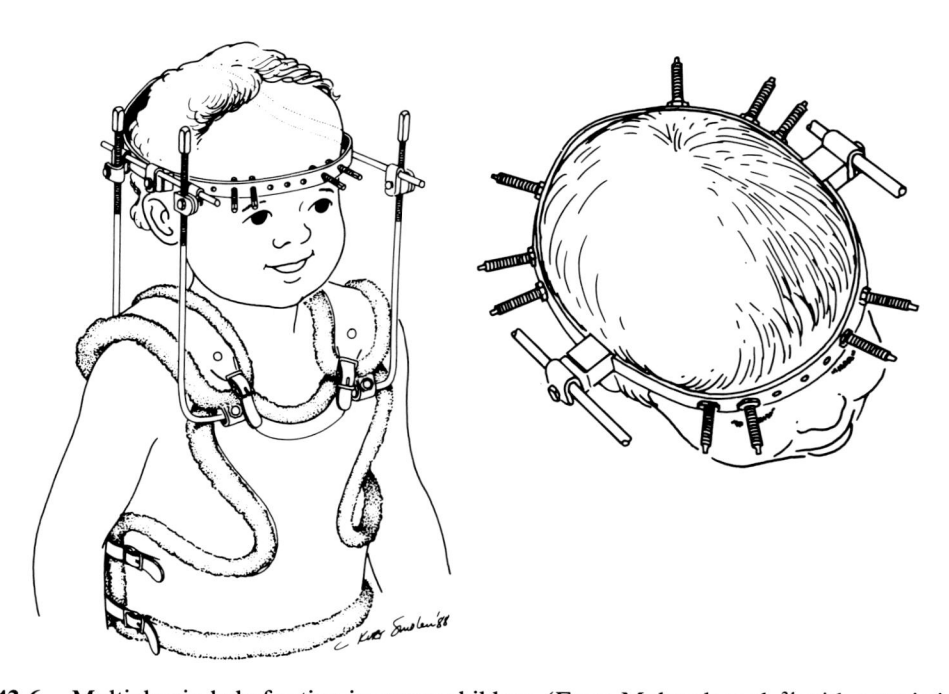

Fig. 43-6. Multiple-pin halo fixation in young children. (From Mubarak et al.,[31] with permission.)

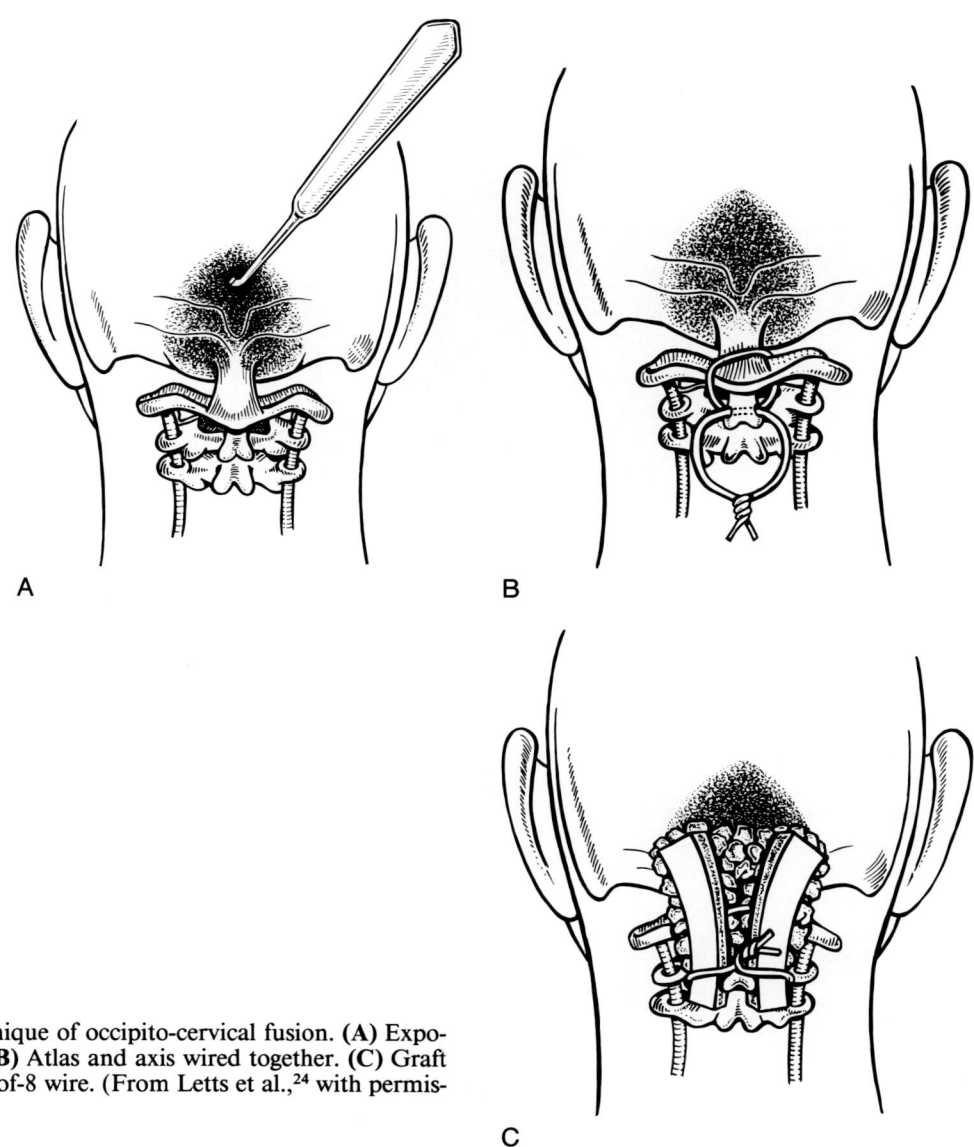

Fig. 43-7. Technique of occipito-cervical fusion. **(A)** Exposure of occiput. **(B)** Atlas and axis wired together. **(C)** Graft secured by figure-of-8 wire. (From Letts et al.,[24] with permission.)

vical arthrodesis is not commonly performed in children but can be safe and effective with careful attention to detail[24] (Figs. 43-8 and 43-9).

COMPLICATIONS

Due to the rarity of atlanto-occipital dislocations and fractures, recognized complications are few. Most patients have a neurologic deficit on presentation. Although cranial nerve lesions are reported to be most common,[22] deficits range from partial lesions to complete quadriplegia. It is now recognized that the initial neurologic deficits may be secondary to vascular injury rather than mechanical transection. With appropriate immobilization as well as attention to the vascular injury, the potential complication of conversion to a permanent deficit can be avoided. However, a few of the early survivors of this injury have died after several months, reportedly secondary to cardiorespiratory causes.[10,17,33]

Complications associated with the use of halo fixation devices are well known.[34] These include pin-loosening, pin-site infection, pressure sores under the plastic vest or cast, nerve injury, dural penetration, dysphasia, cosmetically disfiguring scars, and severe pin discomfort. The

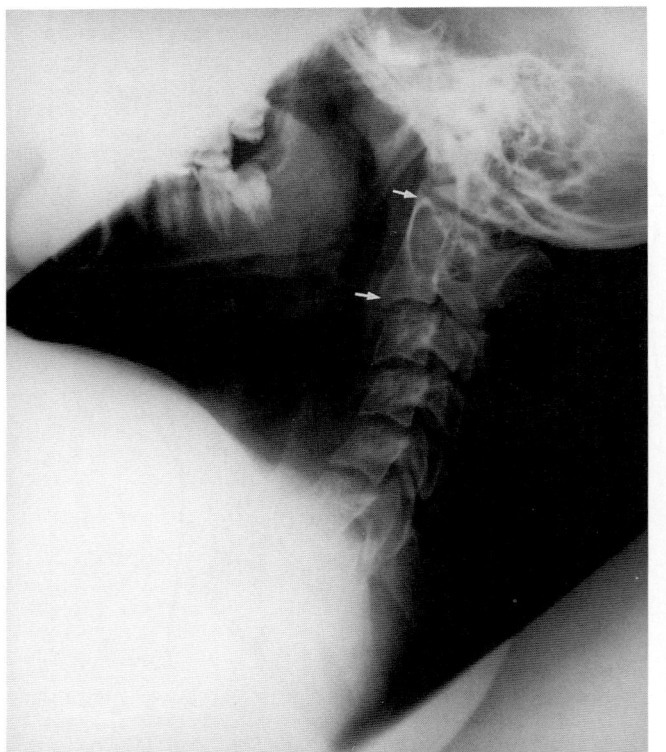

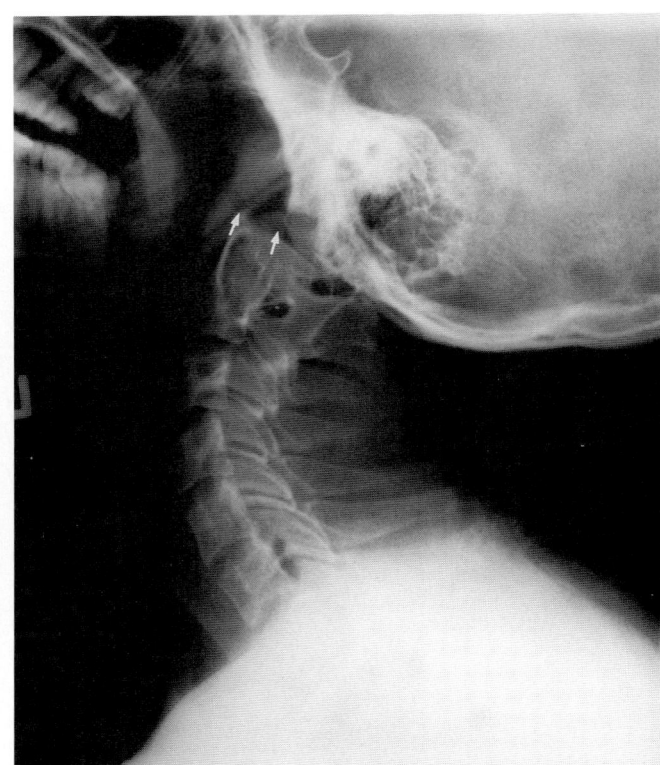

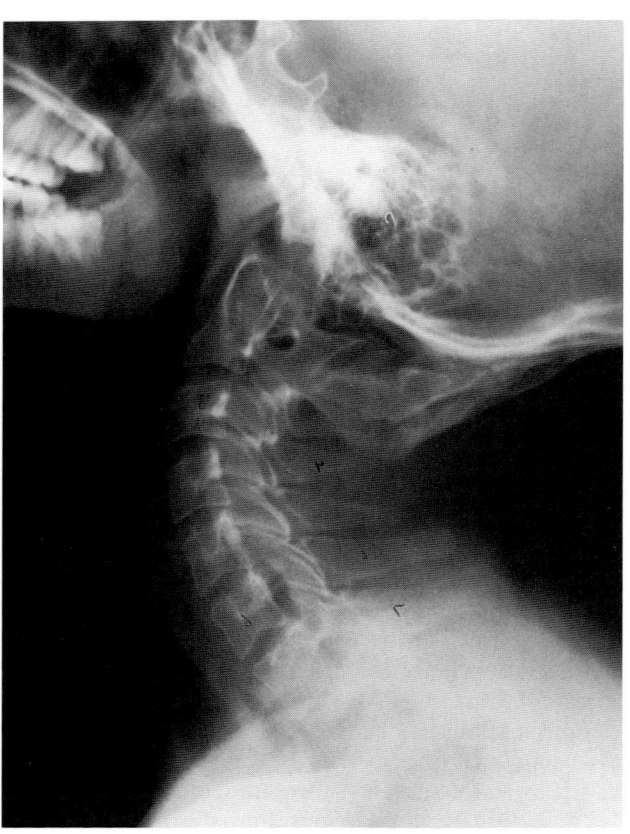

Fig. 43-8. (A) Congenital malformation of upper cervical spine segments including the cervico-occipital articulation. Note C1-C2 block vertebrae. (B) In extension, occiput slides posteriorly on the block vertebrae. This 13-year-old girl was experiencing increasing cervical and occipital pain. (C) Following an occipital-cervical fusion her symptoms disappeared.

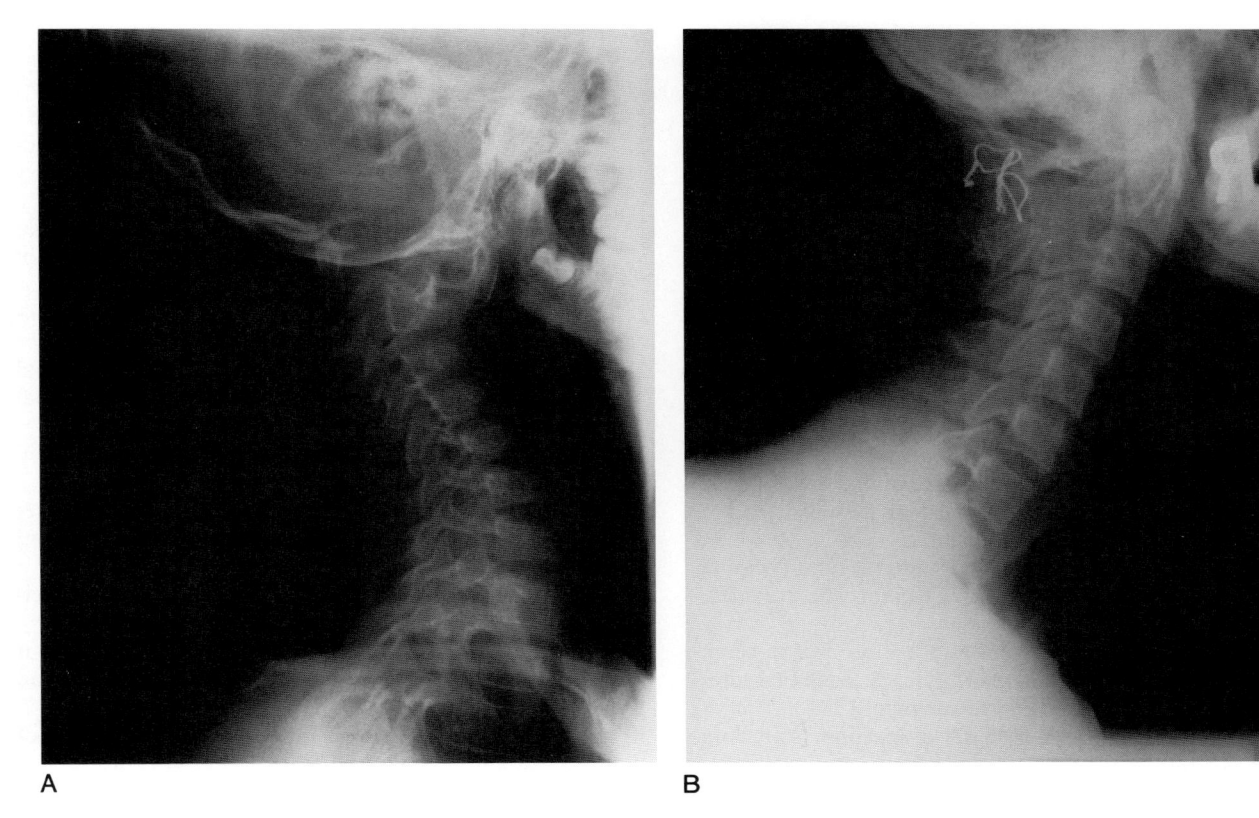

Fig. 43-9. **(A)** Congenital C1-occipital fusion with later fracture of odontoid and occipital-C1 forward instability. **(B)** Following occipital-C2 fusion with restoration of normal cervical alignment and odontoid healing.

use of halos in infants carries further risks, including that of pin-site penetration.[30,31] These can be minimized through the use of CT scanning prior to halo application as well as by special techniques, including multiple pin fixation.

Finally, occipitocervical arthrodesis in young children can be difficult, complicated by loss of reduction and nonunion.[24,32] These problems can be minimized with careful attention to technique, coupled with the use of secure postoperative immobilization.

SUMMARY

Atlanto-occipital dislocation is a rare and devastating injury. Although most cases have been fatal in the past, recent reports show an increasing frequency of survival. Previously thought to be simply a mechanical disruption of the spinal cord, it is now known that vascular injury plays a major part in the pathology of this lesion and may be reversible. Treatment involves immediate immobilization of the neck, without traction. This is followed by occipitocervical fusion when the patient is stabilized. Although residual neurologic deficit is the rule, complete recovery has been reported in children.

REFERENCES

1. Bohlman HH: Acute fractures and dislocations of the cervical spine. J Bone Joint Surg [Am] 61:1119, 1979
2. Martel W: The occipito-atlanto-axial joints in rheumatoid arthritis and ankylosing spondylitis. AJR 86:223, 1961
3. Henrys P, Lyne D, Lifton C, Salciccioli G: Clinical review of cervical spine injuries in children. Clin Orthop Rel Res 129:172, 1977
4. Rang M: Children's Fractures. 2nd Ed. JB Lippincott, Philadelphia, 1983
5. Bucholz RW, Burkhead WZ: The pathological anatomy of fatal atlanto-occipital dislocations. J Bone Joint Surg [Am] 61:248, 1979
6. Alker GJ, Young SO, Leslie EV: High cervical spinal and

craniocervical junction injuries in fatal traffic accidents: a radiological study. Orthop Clin North Am 9:1003, 1978
7. Bucholz RW, Burkhead WZ, Graham W et al; Occult cervical spine injuries in fatal traffic accidents. J Trauma 19:768, 1979
8. Davis D, Bohlman H, Walker AE et al: The pathological findings in fatal craniospinal injuries. J Neurosurg 34:603, 1971
9. Powers B, Miller MD, Kramer RS et al: Traumatic anterior atlanto-occipital dislocation. Neurosurgery 4:12, 1979
10. Lee C, Woodring J, Walsh J: Carotid and vertebral artery injury in survivors of atlanto-occipital dislocation: case reports and literature review. J Trauma 31:401, 1991
11. Werne S: Studies in spontaneous atlas dislocation. Acta Orthop Scand [Suppl] 23:1, 1957
12. White A, Panjabi M: The clinical biomechanics of the occipitoatlantoaxial complex. Orthop Clin North Am 9:867, 1978
13. Gabrielsen TO, Maxwell JA: Traumatic atlanto-occipital dislocation with case report of a patient who survived. Radiology 97:624, 1966
14. Fielding J, Hensinger R: Injuries of the cervical spine. p. 683. In Rockwood C, Wilkins K, King R (eds): Fractures in Children. JB Lippincott, Philadelphia, 1984
15. Blackwood NJ: Atlanto-occipital dislocation. Ann Surg 47:654, 1908
16. Dublin AB, Marks WM, Weinstock D et al: Traumatic dislocation of the atlanto-occipital articulation (AOA) with short-term survival. J Neurosurg 52:541, 1980
17. Kaufman RA, Dunbar JS, Botsford JA et al: Traumatic longitudinal atlanto-occipital distraction injuries in children. AJNR 3:415, 1982
18. Fruin AH, Pirotte TP: Traumatic atlanto-occipital dislocation: case report. J Neurosurg 39:394, 1973
19. Schneider RC, Schemm GW: Vertebral artery insufficiency in acute and chronic spinal trauma. Neurology 9:643, 1959
20. Farthing JW: Atlanto-cranial dislocation with survival. NC Med J 9:34, 1948
21. White AA, Panjabi MM, Posner I et al: Spinal stability: evaluation and treatment. Instr Course Lect 30:457, 1981
22. Pang D, Wilberger JE: Traumatic atlanto-occipital dislocation with survival: case report and review. Neurosurgery 7:503, 1980
23. Georgopoulos G, Pizzutillo P, Lee M: Atlanto-occipital instability in children: a report of five cases and review of the literature. J Bone Joint Surg [Am] 69:429, 1987
24. Letts M, Slutsky D: Occipitocervical arthrodesis in children. J Bone Joint Surg [Am] 72:1166, 1990
25. Shapiro R, Youngberg A, Rothman S: The differential diagnosis of traumatic lesions of the occipito-atlanto-axial segment. Radiol Clin North Am 11:505, 1973
26. Stauffer S, Mazur J: Cervical spine injuries in children. Pediatr Ann 11:502, 1982
27. Evarts CM: Traumatic occipital-atlantal dislocation: report of a case with survival. J Bone Joint Surg [Am] 52:1653, 1970
28. Woodring JH, Selke AC, Duff DE: Traumatic atlantooccipital dislocation with survival. AJR 137:21, 1981
29. Garfin SR, Roux R, Botte MJ et al: Skull osteology as it affects halo pin placement in children. J Pediatr Orthop 6:434, 1986
30. Letts M, Kaylor D, Gouw G: A biomechanical analysis of halo fixation in children. J Bone Joint Surg [Br] 70:277, 1988
31. Mubarak S, Camp J, Vuletich W et al: Halo application in the infant. J Pediatr Orthop 9:612, 1989
32. Smith M, Philips W, Hensinger R: Complications of fusion to the upper cervical spine. Spine 16:702, 1991
33. Evans D, Bethem D: Cervical spine injuries in children. J Pediatr Orthop 9:563, 1989
34. Garfin S, Botte M, Waters R, Nickel V: Complications in the use of the halo fixation device. J Bone Joint Surg [Am] 68:320, 1986

44

C1-C2 Fractures and Dislocations

Francois Fassier

> Anatomy is to physiology as geography to history: it describes the theatre of events.

DESCRIPTION AND INCIDENCE

Cervical spine fractures and dislocations in skeletally immature children are rare, but present unique characteristics quite different from adult cervical fractures. Pediatric spinal injuries, although uncommonly reported,[1] are increasing in frequency with the childhood use of powered recreational vehicles, such as motor scooters, all-terrain vehicles, snowmobiles, and water scooters.

At the Pediatric Orthopaedic Society of North America Meeting in 1990, Benoit and Jarvis[2] reported on 72 children with cervical spine trauma, 29 percent of them sustaining upper cervical segment fractures.

During the period 1980 to 1990, in Ste-Justine Hospital in Montreal, 7,961 children were admitted with the diagnosis of a fracture or dislocation. During the same 10 years, 68 children were admitted for the treatment of a fracture of the cervical spine, an incidence of 0.8 percent (Table 44-1). This is greater than the 0.2 and 0.34 percent incidences of spine fractures reported by Becker[3] in 1963 and Hubbard[4] in 1974. The greater incidence of upper cervical injuries in children reported by Hubbard,[4] 46 percent, Hasue and colleagues,[5] 70 percent, Birney and Hanley,[6] 56 percent, and Benoit and Jarvis,[2] 29 percent, was confirmed in the Ste-Justine review with 47 percent involving C1-C3 vertebrae. This is in contradistinction to adult series where fractures of the lower cervical spine predominate.

Radiologic abnormalities of the pediatric cervical spine vary from benign (physiologic) C2-C3 subluxation to the almost always lethal atlanto-occipital dislocation. Fractures of the dens in children present particular diagnostic problems due to the presence of the apical apophysis and base of odontoid growth plate (Fig. 44-1). Fortunately, these heal quite well and do not have the same rate of complication as in adults. The incidence of neurologic deficit in pediatric cervical spine fractures has been reported to be as high as 50 percent of cases by Birney and Hanley,[6] the pure ligamentous injuries exhibiting the highest risk. In 1987 Denis and coworkers,[7] at the Scoliosis Research Society annual meeting, reported a series of 186 consecutive spinal injuries in children, 22 having had a cervical spine fracture. In this group 16 children died, with 50 percent of deaths being related to injuries of the occipitoatlantoaxial complex.

ANATOMY

Ligamentous laxity allows a much greater mobility of the cervical spine in children compared to the adult. The more horizontal alignment of the articular facets in young children further contributes to the hypermobility in the sagittal plane in flexion. This results in the "pseudosubluxation" appearance at C2-C3 and C3-C4 level

TABLE 44-1. 68 Fractures and Dislocations of the Cervical Spine

Upper Cervical Spine		32 (47%)
Atlanto-occipital dislocation	3	
C1 fractures	8	
C2 fractures	8	
Hangman's	4	
Odontoid	4	
C1–C2 rotatory dislocation	4	
C2–C3 pseudosubluxation	7	
C1 + C2 fracture	2	
Lower cervical spine		36 (53%)
		68

Study from Ste-Justine Hospital, Montréal, 1980–1990.

that can engender serious concern in the emergency department assessment of children who have sustained cervical trauma, especially by clinicians not familiar with assessing children's cervical spines (Fig. 44-2). This increased laxity also preserves motion in the pediatric cervical spine following cervical fusion of one or two segments and in association with congenital malformations of the cervical spine.

Incomplete ossification, epiphyseal variations, and secondary ossification centers may cause confusion when interpreting cervical radiographs. By the age of 8 to 10 years, most children have achieved an adult cervical spine configuration radiographically, but significant cervical ligamentous laxity and associated mobility may persist until skeletal maturity.

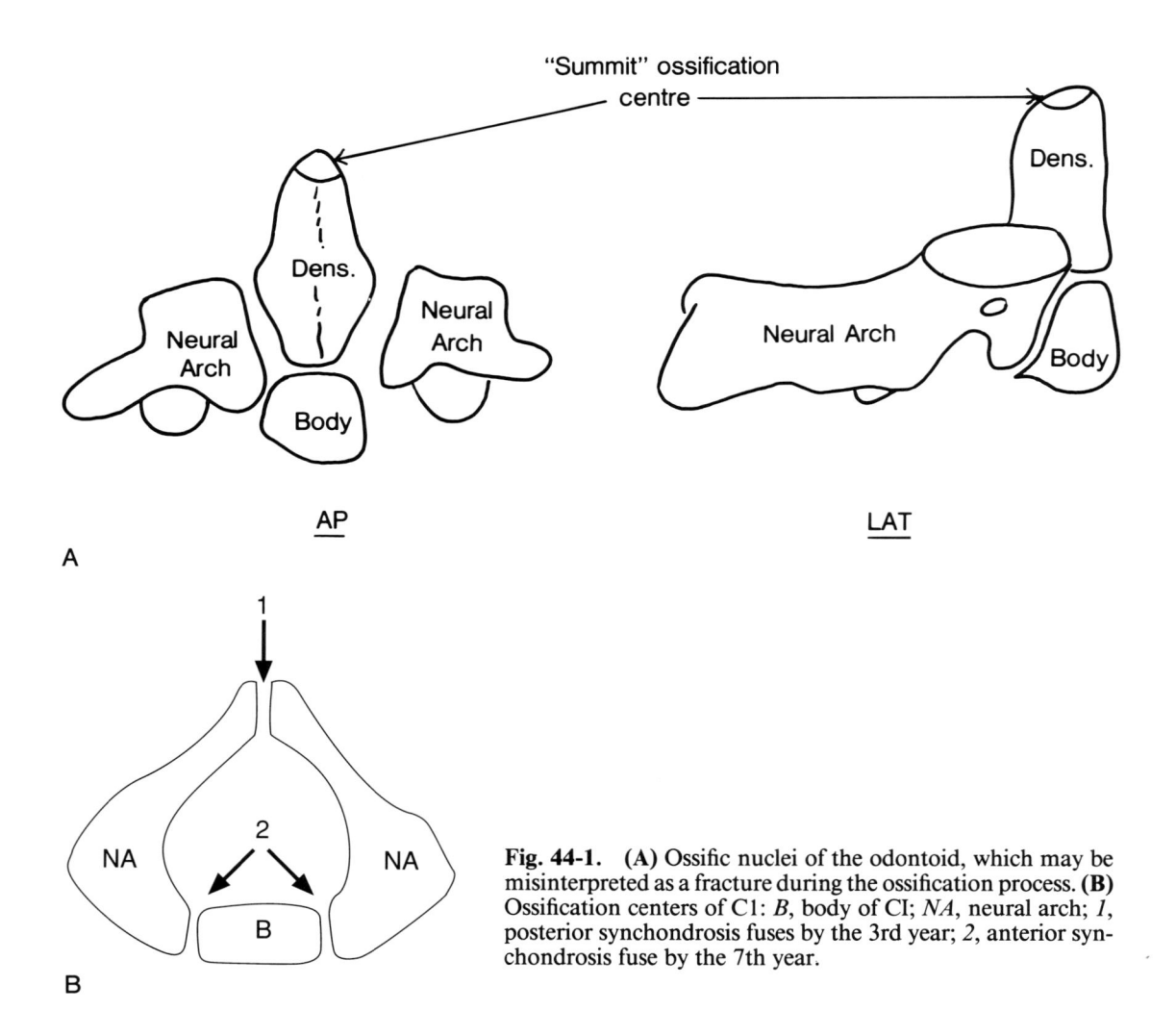

Fig. 44-1. (A) Ossific nuclei of the odontoid, which may be misinterpreted as a fracture during the ossification process. (B) Ossification centers of C1: *B*, body of CI; *NA*, neural arch; *1*, posterior synchondrosis fuses by the 3rd year; *2*, anterior synchondrosis fuse by the 7th year.

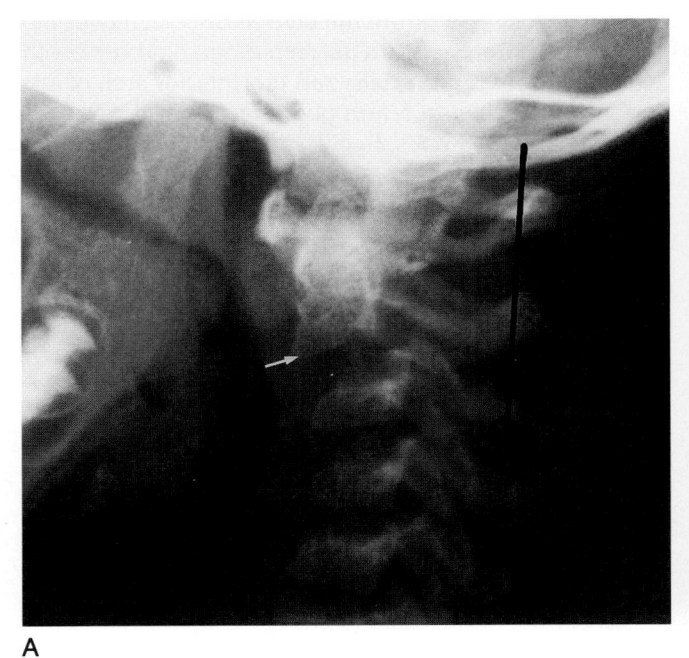

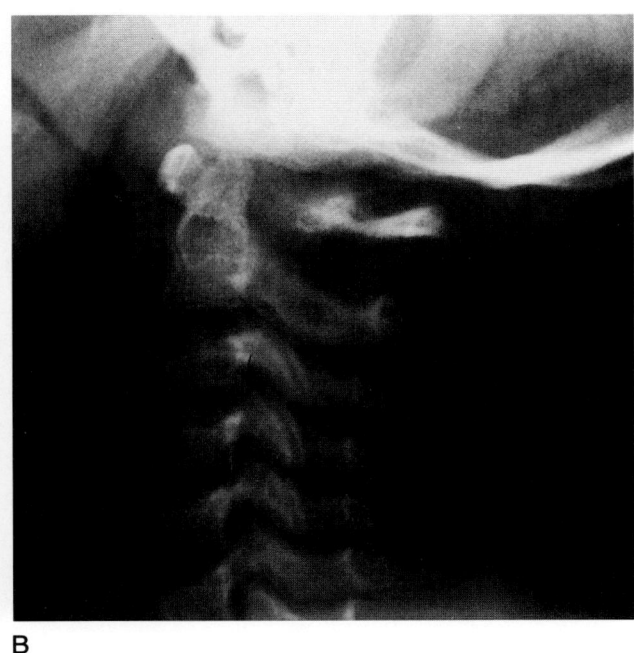

Fig. 44-2. Physiologic pseudosubluxation of C2 on C3 in a 2-year-old boy. **(A)** Aspect of pseudosubluxation of C2 on C3. The posterior cervical line (Swischuk) touches the anterior aspect of the posterior arch of C2 indicative of physiologic pseudosubluxation. **(B)** Same patient, radiograph taken in hyperextension of the cervical spine. Pseudosubluxation is reduced.

Proportional increased size and weight of the head in a child relative to the body is the major biomechanical reason for the increased incidence of upper cervical spine fracture in children. The head size also contributes to difficulties in immobilization of neck-injured children requiring specially designed cervical spine boards.

Development and Normal Ossification

Atlas

The atlas (C1) is composed of three ossification centers, one for the body (which appears during the first year of life) and one for each of the two neural arches (which unite posteriorly by the 3rd year, and fuse with the body by the 7th year)[8] (Fig. 44-1).

Axis

The axis (C2) is composed of four ossification centers: (Fig. 44-1) one for the body, one for the odontoid process (dens), and one for each of the two neural arches. The synchondrosis between the neural arches fuses posteriorly by the 2nd or 3rd year, while the anterior synchondrosis between the body and neural arches is united by the 7th year. The basilar odontoid synchondrosis fuses by age 7, but may be still radiologically visible up to age 10.

Apical Center

The apical or "summit" ossification center of the dens appears between 3 and 6 years and is not fused before 12 years.

Ligamentous Stability of the Occipitoatlantoaxial Complex

The stability of the occipitoatlantoaxial complex is provided mainly by the following:

1. Occipitoatlantal joint (cup-shaped) and anterior and posterior atlanto-occipital membrane
2. Connections between the occiput and the dens (alar and occipital ligaments, tectorial membrane)
3. Transverse portion of the cruciate ligament, prevent-

ing forward displacement of C1 over C2; the most important structure

Atlantoaxial Motion

There is little rotary movement at the occipitoatlantal level, but the atlantoaxial joint provides axial rotation of 45 degrees, flexion of 5 degrees, and extension of 10 degrees. During flexion, the sagittal displacement of C1 on C2 is appreciated on a lateral radiographic view by the distance between the dens and the anterior arch of atlas (Fig. 44-3A). Up to 5 mm of displacement is normal in children under 8 years. In older children, the ligamentous laxity decreases and the atlantodens interval is characteristically 3 to 4 mm. It must be emphasized, however, that in some children with a more generalized laxity, such as Down syndrome, cutis laxita, and syndromic hypotonia,

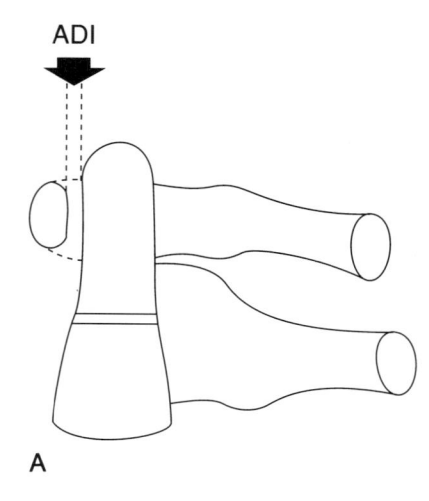

Fig. 44-3. (A) Atlantodens internal *(ADI)* as it appears on a lateral radiograph of the upper cervical spine. (B&C) Atlantoaxial instability in a 2-year-old boy with Down syndrome and extreme hyperflexibility. The atlantodens interval is 9 mm—excessive even for a child with increased laxity.

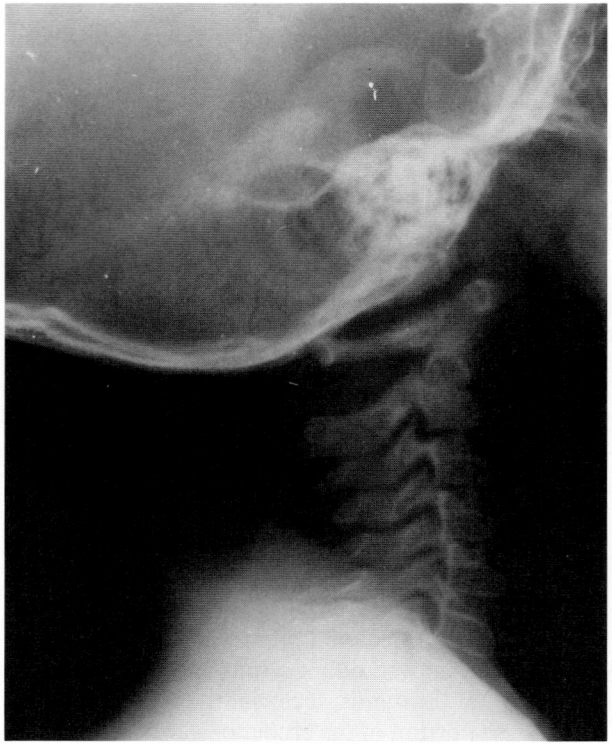

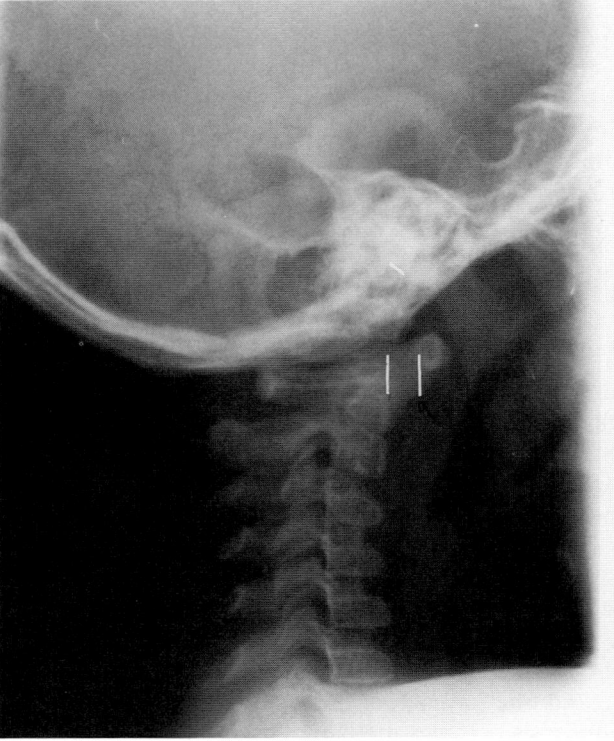

this interval may be normally as high as 5 to 7 mm. Cattell and Filtzer[9] mention a "distance of 3 mm or more" in 20 percent of the children between 1 and 7 years, and Locke and colleagues,[10] in their series, found that the greatest atlantodens interval was 3.5 mm (Fig. 44-3).

Therefore, most normal children with an interval of 4 mm or greater should be suspected of having an injury at that level[11] if the clinical signs and symptoms of a neck injury are also present.

In extension, hyperlaxity often allows the anterior arch of the atlas to override the dens so that two-thirds of the visible anterior arch of atlas may lie above the superior margin of the odontoid process (Fig. 44-4).

Normal Variations of the Pediatric Cervical Spine

Variations in ossification centers are numerous and may lead clinicians not familiar with the immature cervical spine to arrive at a misdiagnosis when interpreting radiographs. Common normal anatomic configurations seen in the pediatric cervical spine that often engender confusion are as follows:

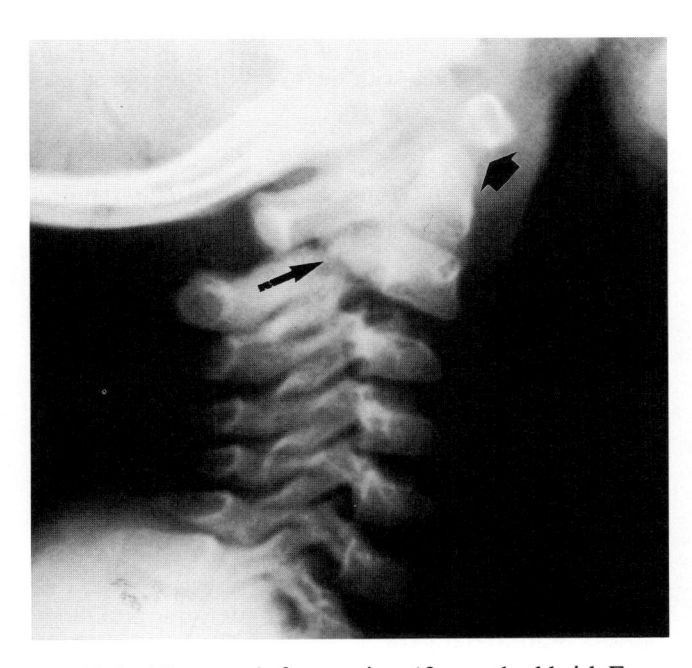

Fig. 44-4. Hangman's fracture in a 12-month-old girl. Fracture through the pedicles is obvious *(thin arrow)*. There is apparent superior subluxation of the anterior arch of C1 over the dens *(wide arrow)*. In extension, hyperlaxity often allows the anterior arch of the atlas to override the dens so that over two-thirds of the arch may lie above the superior margin of the odontoid process.

1. The center of ossification of the body of C1 may be bifid, sometimes absent.[8]
2. Neural arches may not fuse posteriorly.
3. Angulation of the odontoid process can be seen in 4 percent of normal children.[12]
4. The tip of the dens may show a V-shaped aspect.
5. Anterior wedging of the immature vertebral body is frequent.
6. Secondary ossification centers of the spinous and transverse processes may simulate avulsion fractures.

Variations in mobility due to hyperlaxity are common. The physiologic pseudosubluxation of C2 on C3 in flexion has been reported to be present in 40 percent of children under 8 years.[9] This also can be seen in some children at the C3-C4 level (Fig. 44-2).

Loss of the normal cervical lordotic curve occurs in 14 percent of children between 8 and 16.[9,13] The presence of a straight cervical spine in a child is therefore not necessarily indicative of cervical muscle spasm secondary to trauma.

Absence of uniform angulation between adjacent vertebrae, and sometimes kyphotic angulation at a single interspace can be suggestive of ligamentous injury, but usually reflect the hypermobility of the pediatric cervical spine secondary to ligamentous laxity (see Ch. 4).

MECHANISM OF INJURY

Very few reviews are available in the literature concerning cervical spine fractures in children,[4,6,7,14,15] and even fewer addressing C1-C2 injuries only!

Traffic accidents (motor vehicle accidents, pedestrian/car collision, bicycles, three-wheels, all-terrain vehicles) are the most common causes of cervical spine fractures in children under 8 years of age, whereas sports-related injuries, particularly diving accidents, are most frequent in the older child.[2] In 1988, however, Birney and Hanley[6] reported 84 cervical spine injuries in which 38 percent were secondary to a fall from a height, while motor vehicle accidents accounted for only 17 percent. When looking at the Ste-Justine series of C1-C2 injuries (Table 44-2), we note the high incidence of minor trauma in very young children (e.g., a fall from a chair or from his own height). The second most frequent etiology was traffic accidents. Most sporting accidents involving the cervical spine in children are flexion-compression fractures seen after diving in shallow water. These usually occur below C2, hence the small number of C1-C2 injuries secondary to sports-related causes seen in this review.

TABLE 44-2. Anatomic Classification of Fractures of the Upper Cervical Spine in Children

1. Fractures of C1-atlas
2. Fractures of C2-axis
   Fractures of the odontoid process (dens)
   Fractures of the ring
3. Atlantoaxial dislocation (without fracture of dens)
   Rotatory subluxation
   Traumatic ligament disruption
4. C2-C3 subluxation
5. Injuries of the abnormal cervical spine

Birth trauma has also been reported as a cause of fracture of the odontoid process after rotational stresses induced by forceps delivery in difficult cephalic presentations.[16]

Battered children may also present with trauma to the cervical spine, often secondary to whiplash (in the shaken infant syndrome).[17,18] At the 1986 Pediatric Orthopaedic Society of North America meeting, King and colleagues[19] reported an incidence of 3 percent of spine fractures among 189 abused babies with a mean age of 7 months.

Gunshot wounds to the spine are now being reported as a major cause of all pediatric spinal cord injuries.[20] In Macielak's report of 34 gunshot-wounded children, 10 were shot in the neck, sustaining vertebral injury. Cord lesions were complete in 59 percent of these children.

CONGENITAL MALFORMATIONS OF THE CERVICAL SPINE

Congenital anomalies may occur in the upper cervical spine that can either predispose to injury or cause confusion with traumatic lesions (Fig. 44-5). Congenital fusion of C1 to the occiput results in increased biomechanical forces being exerted at the C1-C2 interval, predisposing to injury at this site. Children with congenital fusions of the cervical spine should be discouraged from participating in contact sports, such as football, where cervical spine contact is common, or sophisticated gymnastics, where the cervical spine may be exposed to considerable impact forces. Congenital absence of the odontoid, the so-called *os odontoideum*, predisposes to C1-C2 instability. Controversy exists as to whether this entity is a true congenital lesion or a nonunion of the odontoid secondary to a previous unrecognized odontoid fracture, but the end result is the same: a predisposition to C1-C2 instability that usually requires a C1-C2 fusion if only to protect the child from a catastrophic cord injury.

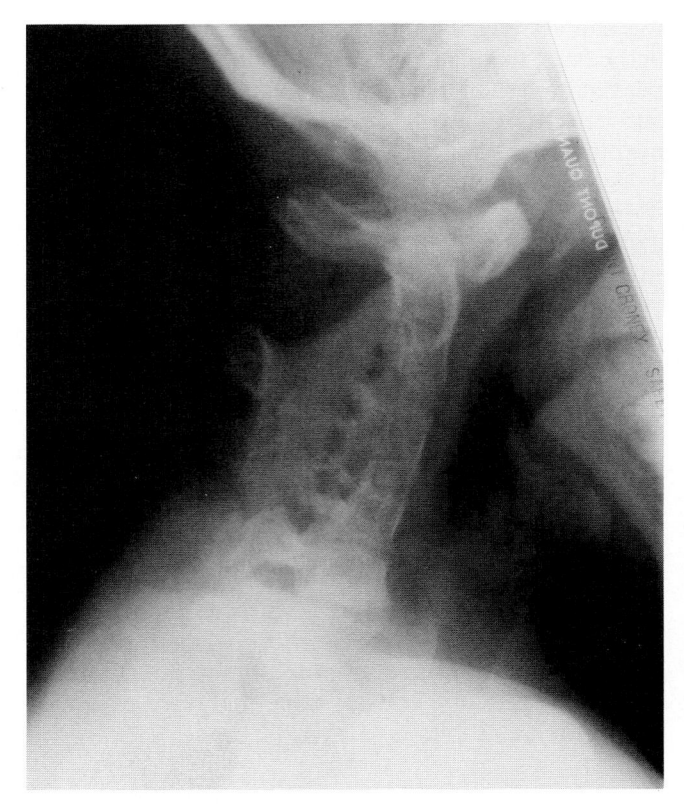

Fig. 44-5. Congenital fusion of the cervical spine typically encountered in children with the so-called Klippel-Feil syndrome.

PHYSICAL EXAMINATION

Neck pain is the most prevalent symptom associated with cervical spine fractures or dislocations in children.[21] If absent, one should seriously question the presence of an acute neck injury in a child. Occasionally, a child will splint the neck in an unusual position to eliminate pain and discomfort. The neck, however, will appear distorted as in a torticollis, indicating underlying pathology in spite of minimal pain.

Torticollis or the "cock robin position," a cervical rotation and tilt directed toward opposite side, is observed in many neck-injured children due either to a rotatory displacement of C1 or cervical muscle spasm. Careful palpation of the paracervical musculature will reveal the side of the muscle spasm. Spasmodic sternocleidomastoid muscular torticollis occurs on the side of the head tilt, while in rotary subluxation of C1, the muscle spasm is on the *opposite* side of the deformity, as the muscle attempts correction of the osseous deformity.

Two different clinical situations may be encountered in children:

1. There may be a definitive history of trauma either cervical or cranial.
2. There may be no observed trauma history and the neck pain has been present for several days. Other etiologies of muscle spasm include tumors of the posterior fossa, tumors of the cord, syringomyelia, bulbar palsies, and dysfunctions of either the ocular or the vestibular systems.

Movement of the child's injured neck should be performed with great care, as any forced maneuver can elongate the neurologic structures or narrow the spinal canal and create further damage. Most often, active range of motion is limited by pain, and attempts at passive movement is useless in very young children who cry and show fear, whether or not the motion elicits pain.

Diagnosis of cervical spine injury is particularly difficult in the comatose child where no local signs may indicate traumatic injury to the cervical spine. Thus, it is mandatory to obtain plain anteroposterior and lateral radiographic views of the cervical spine in all unconscious patients following polytrauma.

Injuries known to occur concomitantly with high frequency in association with cervical fractures are head and facial trauma.[23] A simple cut under the chin of an unconscious patient may be a sign of forced hyperextension with possible associated cervical spine injury.

Cervical fractures frequently occur in association with head and facial trauma. A pediatric neurologic assessment sheet is helpful to facilitate such recordings. It must also be emphasized that, in upper cervical spine trauma, the brainstem may also be damaged, resulting in respiratory depression or cardiac arrest as the initial clinical presentation. Children with occiput, C1, and C2 fracture dislocations are now being resuscitated at the accident scene and maintained in pediatric intensive care wards with upper cervical spine injuries and high spinal paralysis that will require later orthopaedic management.

The upper cervical nerves and the lower cranial nerves may also be stretched in severe trauma. Occiput to C2 ligamentous injuries have been reported with as high as 50 percent rate of neurologic deficit, usually permanent.[6]

RADIOLOGIC EVALUATION

After prior adequate immobilization of the cervical spine, routine anteroposterior (AP) and lateral radiographic views still remain the best initial screening examination. The "open-mouth" AP view of the odontoid process, though important, is technically difficult to obtain in a noncooperative crying child.

Plain tomograms are helpful to assess the position of the lateral masses of C1 in relation to the odontoid process as well as detecting odontoid fractures (Fig. 44-6). Computed tomography (CT) is very helpful in the diagnosis of rotatory displacements, in differentiating fractures from the normal synchondrosis, and in detecting subtle laminar fractures at the C1 level. Cineradiographs are less helpful in emergency cases, but during the course of treatment, they can provide important information

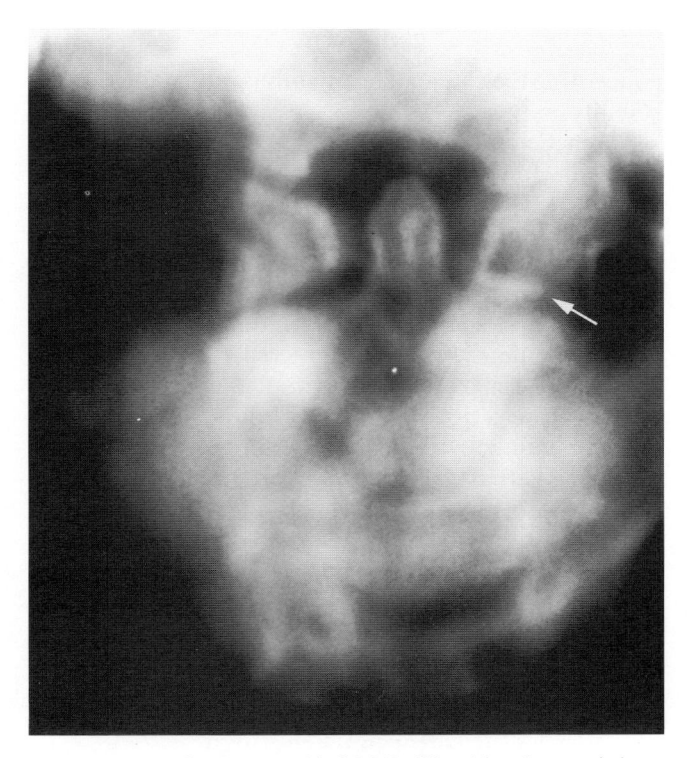

Fig. 44-6. This 12-year-old girl fell off her bicycle sustaining a fractured clavicle and acute torticollis. Her fractured clavicle healed uneventfully, but the torticollis persisted for 6 months. When seen at the Children's Hospital of Eastern Ontario, a fixed rotatory subluxation on C1 was present with marked anterior displacement of C1 on C2 and long-tract signs of clonus and hyperreflexia. An AP tomogram showed only mild asymmetry of the lateral masses but obliteration of the left C1-C2 facet secondary to the dislocation of the C1 facet anteriorly. (Courtesy of Dr. Mervyn Letts, Children's Hospital of Eastern Ontario, Ottawa, Canada.)

TABLE 44-3. Possible Causes for Confusion in the Assessment of the Radiograph of the Pediatric Cervical Spine

Variations due to ossification
  Absence or incomplete ossification of C1
  Apical ossification of the odontoid process
  Transverse and spinous processes ossification centers
  Persistence of the synchondrosis at the base of the dens
  Angulation of the dens
  Articular facets horizontally oriented
  Congenital anomalies (spina bifida, Klippel-Feil syndrome, etc.)

Variations due to hyperlaxity
  Increase in atlantodens interval up to 5 mm
  Subluxation at the C2-C3 level
  Apparent posterior displacement of C1 or apparent superior subluxation of the anterior arch of C1 over the dens in extension

Other causes of confusion
  Absence of cervical lordosis
  Prevertebral soft tissue swelling, which may be due to deep inspiration (child crying); take a new film with mouth closed if any doubt
  Overlying anatomy (ears, teeth, braids)

concerning the extent of ligamentous injury and cervical stability.

Magnetic resonance imaging (MRI) can assist in classifying the injuries and correlating them with spinal cord lesions. A correlation between the MRI pattern and prognosis for spinal cord recovery has been demonstrated in the adult population.[24] Such studies are not yet available for children.

Many physiologic normal variations of the pediatric cervical spine may be encountered (Table 44-3) and create concern that the radiographic appearance indicates a more serious underlying injury. It is only with experience and reviewing many "normal" pediatric cervical spines that these normal variations can be diagnosed with confidence.

TYPES OF INJURIES TO THE UPPER CERVICAL SPINE

Fractures of the Atlas (Jefferson Fracture)

Fractures of the first cervical vertebra are extremely rare in children,[25,26] probably because of the flexibility due to the synchondrosis.

Mechanism of Injury

Axial transmission of forces through the skull and occipital condyles concentrates stress on the lateral masses of C1. Sherk[27] stated that "if the head is in slight extension, the occiput can produce a fracture through the narrow part of the atlantal ring where the vertebral arteries pass behind the lateral masses." Most often, a fall on the vertex of the head causes such fractures.

Physical Examination

Immediate neck pain is usually associated with a diminished range of motion of the cervical spine due to muscle spasm. Head tilt and the child's support of the head with the hands may be observed when attempts are made to flex or extend the neck.

Neurologic injury is rare in children with this fracture, whereas Jefferson,[28] in his initial description in 1920, reported a 41 percent incidence of spinal cord injury. In children, "Steel's Rule of Thirds" is most applicable, that is, $\frac{1}{3}$ space, $\frac{1}{3}$ cord, and $\frac{1}{3}$ odontoid.[29] In fact, in a child under 10 years, the space is closer to $\frac{1}{2}$, hence the low incidence of spinal cord impingement with fractures of the atlas.

Radiologic Evaluation

Plain radiographs of the atlas can be confusing in very young children when the synchondrosis of C1 have not yet ossified. Widening of the atlas on a frontal view, that is, unilateral or bilateral offsetting of the lateral masses (Fig. 44-7) may be difficult to detect and pseudospread of the atlas is a normal variation in 30 percent of young children. A true AP view is difficult to obtain if the child has an associated painful torticollis and the bone ring of the atlas may be fractured at only one site. Lateral and oblique views can be helpful but tomograms (Fig. 44-8) can more precisely delineate the lesion; however, the CT scan (Fig. 44-9) provides the best recognition of this fracture. The scan also reveals the margins of synchondrosis more accurately. Differentiation of congenital defects from true traumatic disruption of the atlas ring can also be difficult. Both the location and appearance of the defect are helpful clues.[30] Fractures are most often located adjacent to the lateral masses, while congenital defects are in the midportion of the arch and a smooth regular appearance versus the irregular, jagged appearance of a fracture. Nevertheless, it is important to emphasize that disruption may also occur through a synchondrosis.[31] This may go undetected on plain films due to the cartilaginous site of the fracture and will require computed tomography or MRI to accurately delineate the site of the fracture.

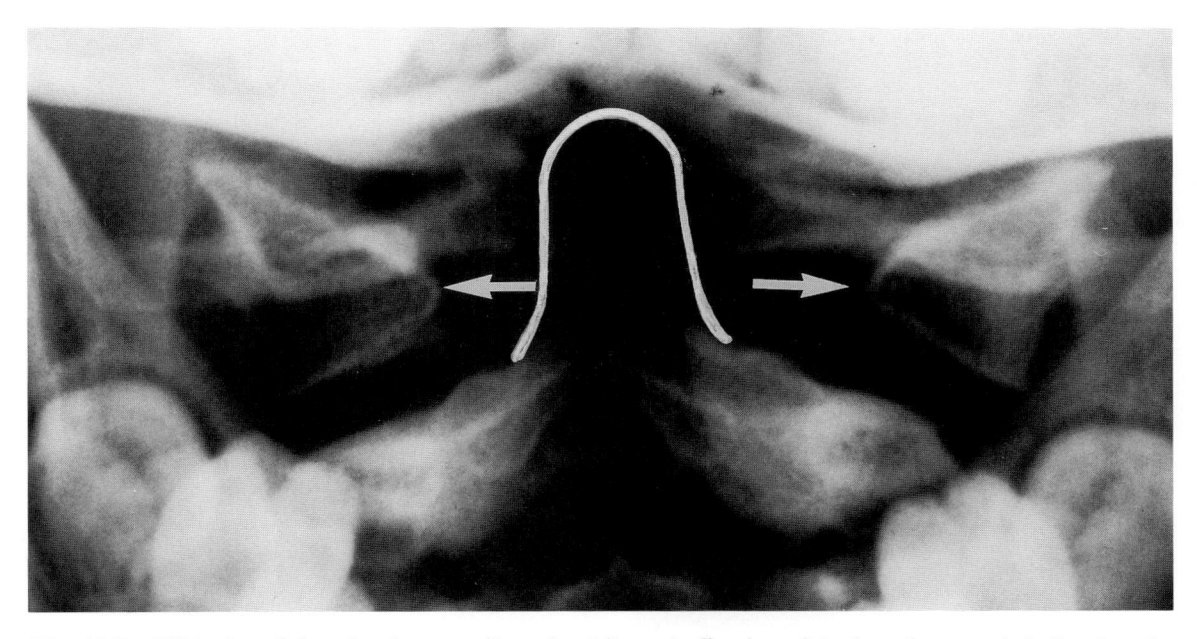

Fig. 44-7. Widening of the atlas due to unilateral or bilateral offsetting of the lateral masses is indicative of a Jefferson fracture of C1. This 6-year-old-boy fell from a height onto his head and the AP view illustrated bilateral offsetting lateral masses.

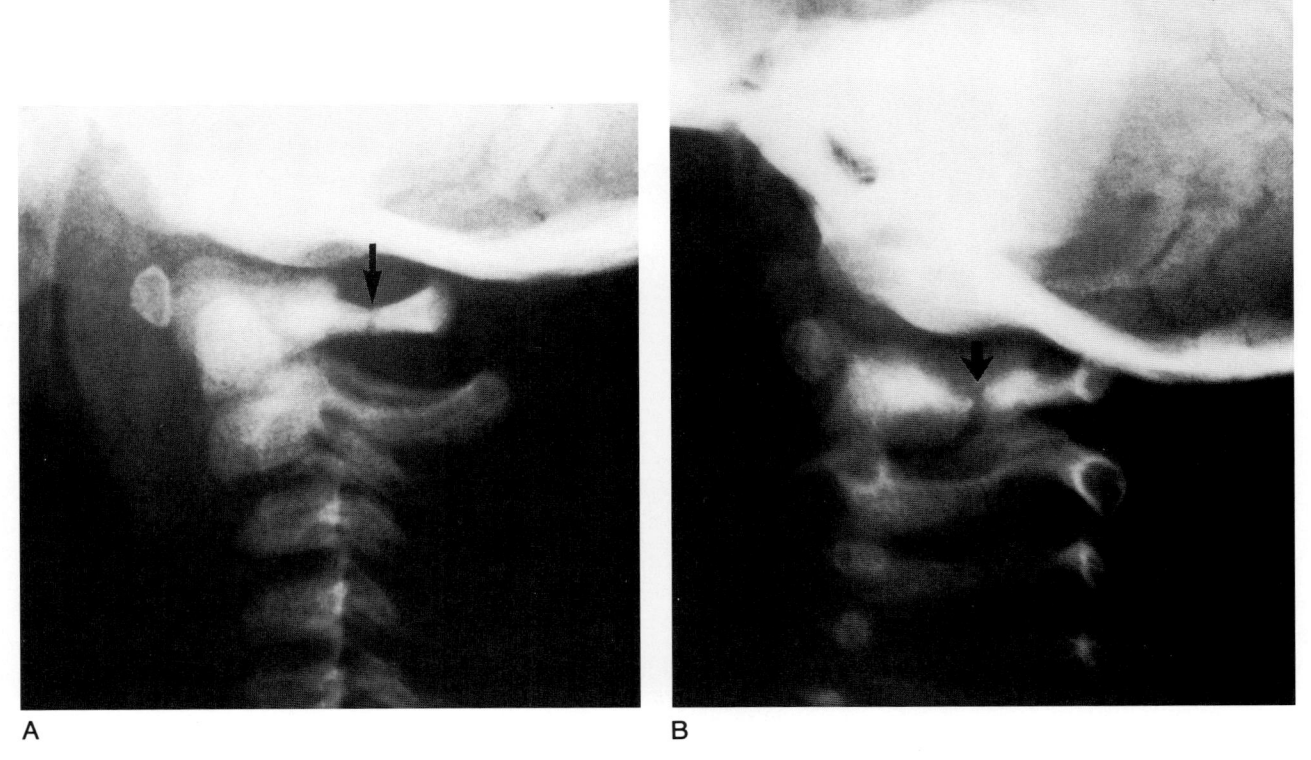

Fig. 44-8. (A) A lateral tomogram illustrating a fracture of the arch of the atlas. (B) An oblique view of the same fracture illustrating the fracture a little more clearly.

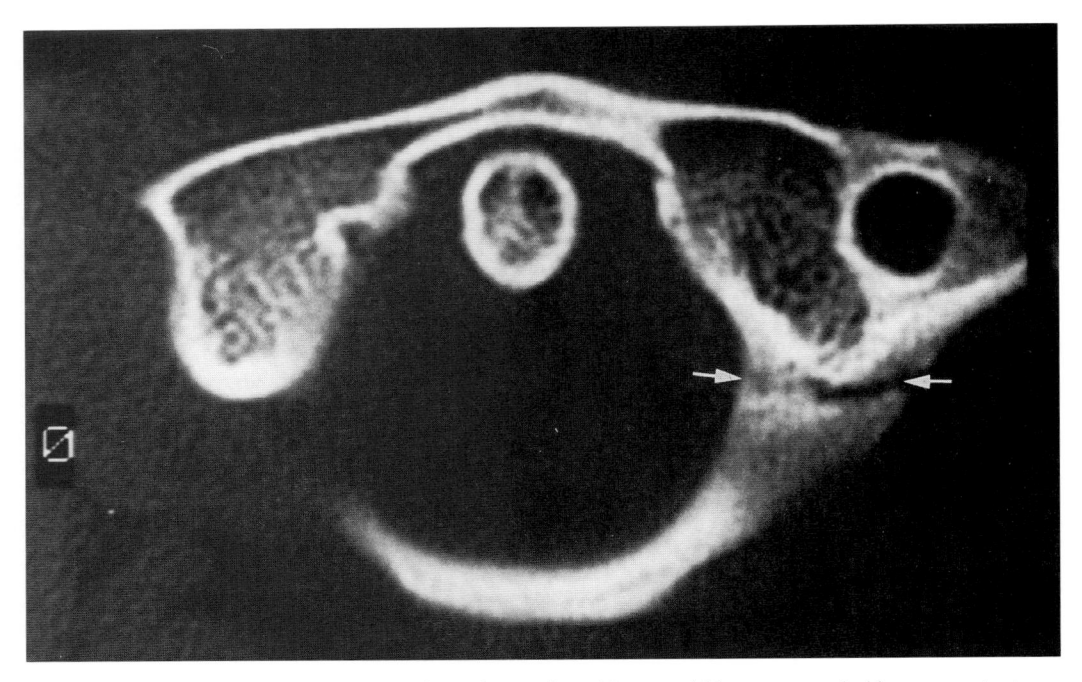

Fig. 44-9. Fracture of atlas, adjacent to the lateral mass in a 14-year-old boy as revealed by computer tomography. Note the irregular aspect of the fracture line.

A   B

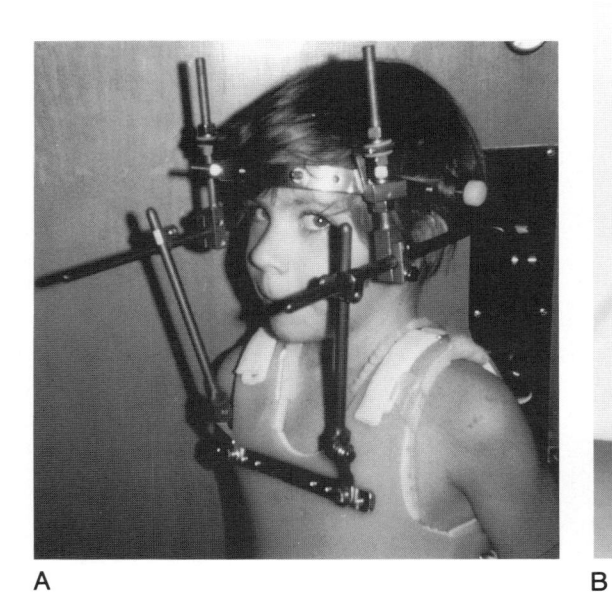

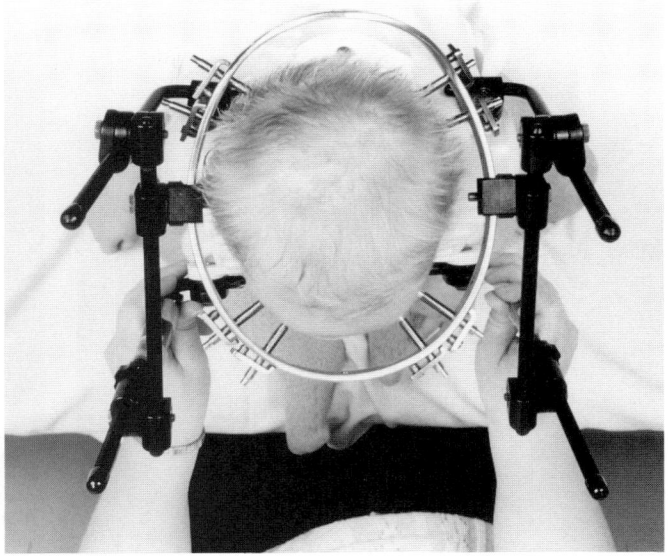

Fig. 44-10. **(A)** Halo fixation provides the most rigid immobilization of the cervical spine for children with unstable cervical spine injury. As they are very active even in halos, pin complications such as loosening, infection, and penetration are more frequent than with adults. These may be minimized by the use of 6 to 8 multiple pins with less penetration. **(B)** In infants and young children double pins are recommended at each pin site to minimize loosening. (Courtesy of Dr. Jacques D'Astous, Children's Hospital of Eastern Ontario, Ottawa, Canada.)

Treatment

Simple undisplaced and stable fractures of C1 can be treated in the child with a rigid collar. For unstable fractures of the atlas involving both arches, good immobilization is mandatory. Such can be obtained with either a Minerva cast, a custom-made plastic orthosis[29] or the halo apparatus, which is more popular and can be used in young children with safety (Fig. 44-10). Healing time varies from 2 months in younger children to 3 to 4 months[32] in teenagers. Surgical fusion is unnecessary, and this fracture usually heals quite satisfactorily in children when properly immobilized.

Complications

Neurologic complications are rarely reported in children with an isolated Jefferson fracture, but with an associated fracture of C2, the incidence of neurologic deficit increases significantly.[33-35] Quadriparesis and Brown-Séquard syndrome are the most frequently reported spinal cord injury.

Fractures of the Axis

Fractures of the Odontoid Process (Dens)

Fractures of the dens are reported to represent as high as 75 percent of cervical spine injuries in children under 7 years.[16] The cartilaginous plate separating the odontoid process from the body of the axis is the weakest area of the C2 vertebra. Most fractures of the odontoid in children under 7 years occur through this synchondrosis and are referred to as epiphysiolysis of the dens.[36] The average age of children reported in the literature with this type of synchondral odontoid fracture is less than 5 years.

MECHANISM OF INJURY

There is still controversy about the pathomechanics of fracture of the odontoid process. Flexion injuries seem to be the most prone to cause dens fractures in children.[37] This also explains the consistent anterior displacement of the dens. Traffic accidents and falls from heights are the most common causes of such fractures in children[27,38] (Table 44-4). An unusual but well-documented cause of the odontoid fracture in infants is the occasional birth trauma,[16] where the mechanism of injury is believed to be the rotational stress of forceps when changing the presentation of the head. The transverse odontoid ligament, as with all ligaments in children, is much stronger than the adjacent odontoid growth plate and undoubtedly contributes to the flexion moment during forced hyperflexion of the neck.

TABLE 44-4. Mechanisms of Injury and Mean Age at the Time of Trauma: 32 Fractures and Dislocations of C1-C2 in Children

	No. of Patients	Age (yr)
Traffic accident	10 (31%)	3.3
Minor trauma	11 (34%)	7.9
Fall from a height	5 (15%)	7
Sports	3 (9%)	14.6
Inflammatory Related	2	3
Unknown Etiology	1	1.5
Total	32	6.2

Study from Ste-Justine Hospital, University of Montréal, 1991

CLASSIFICATION

Prior to age 7, epiphysiolysis of the odontoid is the only type of dens fracture that has been reported.[35] After closure of the synchondrosis at the base of the odontoid process, which usually occurs around 7 to 8 years of age, the classification of Anderson and D'Alonzo[39] is applicable to children (Table 44-5).

PHYSICAL EXAMINATION

Although "there is no diagnostic clinical syndrome for a dens fracture" as stated by Ogden,[32] it has been reported that pain from a fractured odontoid is most often occipital, and Seimon[40] noticed that the children were most comfortable when either lying supine or standing. Movement of the neck is painful and the children often hold their heads with their hands.

In the Griffiths series,[38] all 4 children had delayed diagnosis (1 to 3 days), all were involved in traffic acci-

TABLE 44-5. Fractures of the Odontoid in Children

Type I
Fracture of the tip of the dens without vascular compromise
Type II
Fracture through the base of the dens with potential instability
Type III
Fracture through the upper part of the body of C2 within cancellous bone
Type IV
Fracture through odontoid synchondrosis in children under 7 years

dents, and 3 of the 4 presented with associated head injuries. This frequent association—head trauma/odontoid fracture—has also been reported by Nachemson.[41]

RADIOLOGIC EVALUATION

Plain lateral films of the upper cervical spine (Fig. 44-11), as well as tomograms, are the most helpful diagnostic radiographs. The open-mouth view is of little value in young children, being difficult technically to obtain, as well as to interpret.

Anterior displacement of the odontoid can be calculated in millimeters or in terms of the width of the odontoid process.[16] Angulation of the dens is not a reliable sign of odontoid fracture, as it can be observed in 4 percent of normal children. When observed in association with neck injury and symptoms, however, it should be an indication for tomograms or a CT scan of the odontoid.

Widening of the prevertebral space can be helpful for the diagnosis if the film has been taken in appropriate circumstances (mouth closed, child not crying) to eliminate physiologic soft tissue widening, which may occur during inspiration or when the child cries (Fig. 44-12).

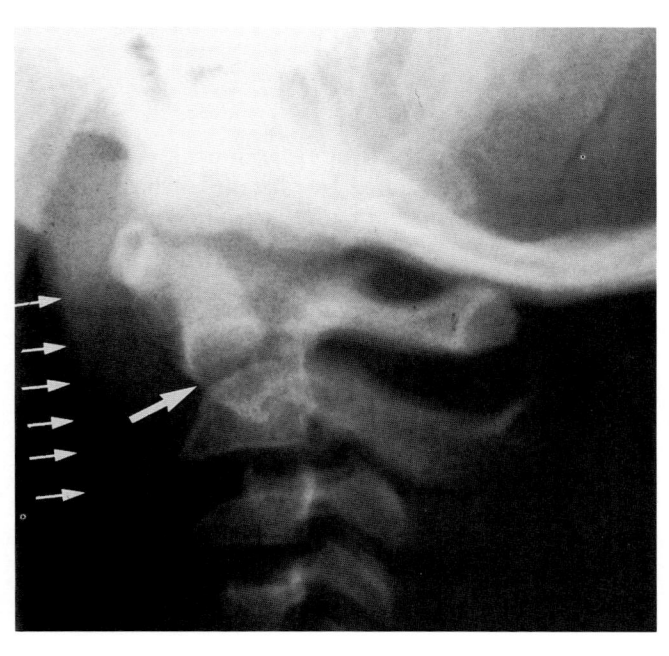

Fig. 44-11. Fracture of the odontoid in a 3-year-old child seen on the lateral view on a plain radiograph. Slight anterior displacement as well as angulation of the odontoid is evident. Prevertebral swelling secondary to edema and hemorrhage is also present.

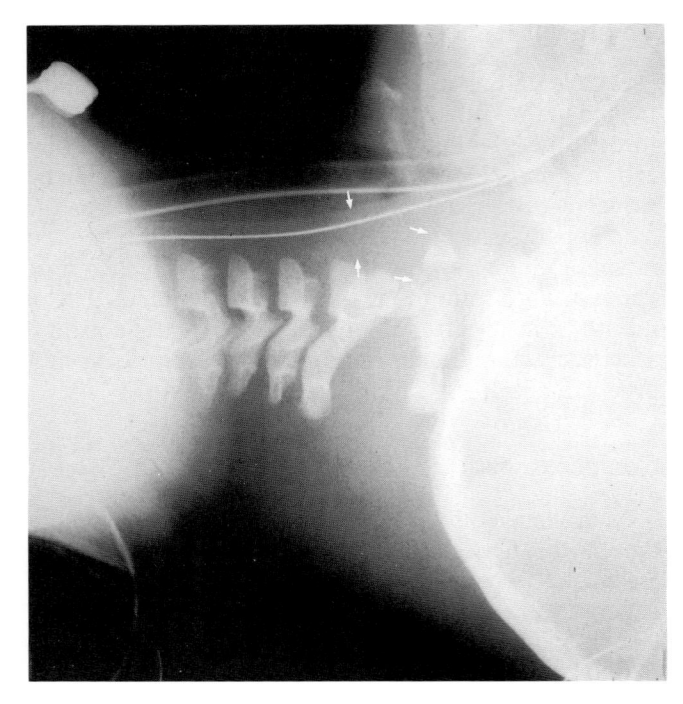

Fig. 44-12. This acutely traumatized 2-year-old boy had no obvious fracture seen on plain films but presented following a motor vehicle accident with C1 dislocation and complete quadriplegia below C3. Halo traction was instituted with only 3 lb when this film was taken. Note the distraction at C1-C2 with only this small amount of traction emphasizing the need to be cautious with cervical traction in young children. Note also the widened paravertebral soft tissue space often indicative of an underlying cervical spine injury.

TREATMENT

The management of undisplaced fractures of the odontoid in children is usually nonoperative. Reduction of anterior displacement of the dens may be achieved by hyperextension of the neck over the edge of a mattress with halter cervical traction in older children or halo traction. No more than 5 percent of the body weight should be initially applied (Fig. 44-12). Daily neurologic evaluation is mandatory, as further cord or root damage can be done if there is associated ligamentous lesions. Sherk and colleagues[16] reported good reduction with gentle manipulation under sedation or general anesthesia in 4 of 11 children. This technique should be reserved for those children who do not respond to traction. Immobilization can be achieved by Minerva jackets or Minerva-like neck braces or four-poster cervical orthosis in most cases. A halo cast is less frequently used in children under 7 years, but is an option for noncompliant children and families.

Fielding and Hensinger[8] have recommended that immobilization should be kept in place for 12 weeks and stress films done following the removal of the brace. In children under 8 years, undisplaced odontoid fractures are usually healed by 2 months. Sherk and colleagues[16] in reviewing 24 children with fracture of the odontoid in the literature, found only 1 child who was treated with a primary fusion of C1-C2.

In adolescents, indications for treatment are similar to adults. In this age group, halo immobilization is the most effective method of immobilization restricting motion by 75 percent at the atlantoaxial complex, whereas a neck orthosis only restricts cervical motion by 45 percent.[42]

COMPLICATIONS

Neurologic. As with fractures of the atlas, odontoid fractures are rarely accompanied by spinal cord injury in children. Birney and Hanley[6] noted none in 4 children, Griffiths,[38] only 2 with transient arm weakness. Sherk,[27] in his 11 cases, noticed that "the only neural deficits occurred in patients who had associated cranial lesions."

Damage to the cord is unlikely to occur because of the space available for the cord when there is simultaneous forward shift of atlas and the odontoid process. This is quite different from odontoid fractures in adult patients where mortality is reported to be as high as 5 to 10 percent. Lesion of the greater occipital nerve causes referred occipital pain, commonly encountered in children with odontoid fractures.

Nonunion. Nonunion of the odontoid is very rare in children, and most heal very satisfactorily. Only one case of nonunion has been reported by Sherk[27] in his review of odontoid fractures in children reported in the literature. In that instance, the fracture had been recognized, but not treated.

Growth Disturbances. As the cartilaginous plate at the base of the odontoid is much more a synchondrosis rather than an epiphyseal plate, no reports of growth arrest have been reported. In contradistinction to other physeal areas of the growing skeleton, growth arrest is not a problem in odontoid epiphyseal plate fractures.

Os Odontoideum. Several reports[43,44] strongly suggest that this lesion is an acquired one, following an unrecognized fracture through the base of the dens in early infancy. Nonunion of the fracture may compromise the blood supply to the proximal segment resulting in bony resorption or failure of development. This is an attractive theory, but has not yet been substantiated.

Fractures of the Ring of C2

Fracture of the pedicles of the axis results in a traumatic spondylolisthesis of C2 and is historically known as the *hangman's fracture* (Fig. 44-13). Birney and Hanley[6] reported 6 children with this fracture in 1989, Pizzutillo and coworkers,[45] 5 cases, and we found 4 such fractures in Ste-Justine's review of upper cervical fractures in children.

MECHANISM OF INJURY

While hanging, hyperextension and distraction cause pedicle fractures, motor vehicle accidents cause different pathomechanisms, resulting in similar fractures. Axial loading, associated with either flexion, or more often hyperextension of the cervical spine, separates the "cervicocranium," (skull, atlas, odontoid process, and body of C2), from the remainder of the cervical spine,[46] resulting in fracturing of the C2 pedicles and a forward displacement of C1 and the body of C2 on C3.

Associated lesions of C3, anterosuperior avulsion fracture in hyperextension, or C3 compression fracture with C2-C3 subluxation in flexion, as well as associated ligamentous disruptions, have been described.[46]

PHYSICAL EXAMINATION

No specific physical findings related to traumatic spondylolisthesis of C2 have been reported, but the high incidence of associated facial fractures and scalp injuries should draw attention to a possible C2 injury. Davidson and Birdsell[23] noted that in patients with facial fractures in cervical spine fractures, one-third of these occurred at the C2 level.

RADIOLOGIC EVALUATION

Most pedicle fractures of C2 can be readily seen on a standard lateral radiographic view of the spine. AP views are of little value, and oblique views may better demonstrate the fracture line. Tomograms or CT scans are less useful than in fractures of the atlas.

Cineradiography or flexion-extension films may assess the stability of the fracture. Nevertheless, such investigations are difficult in young children where muscle spasm "splints" the injury.

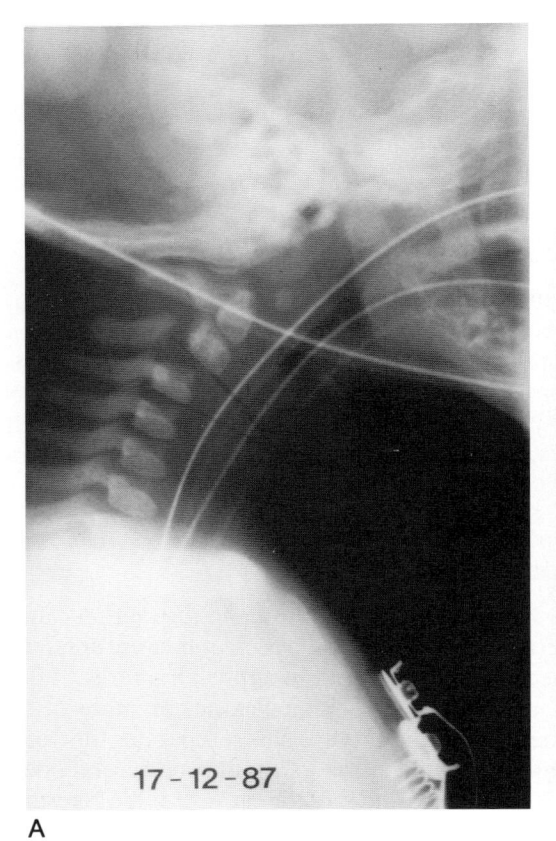

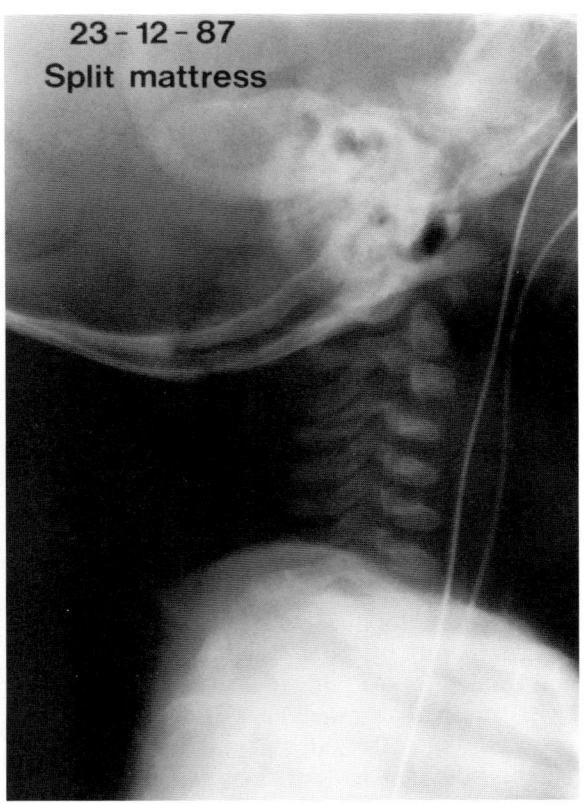

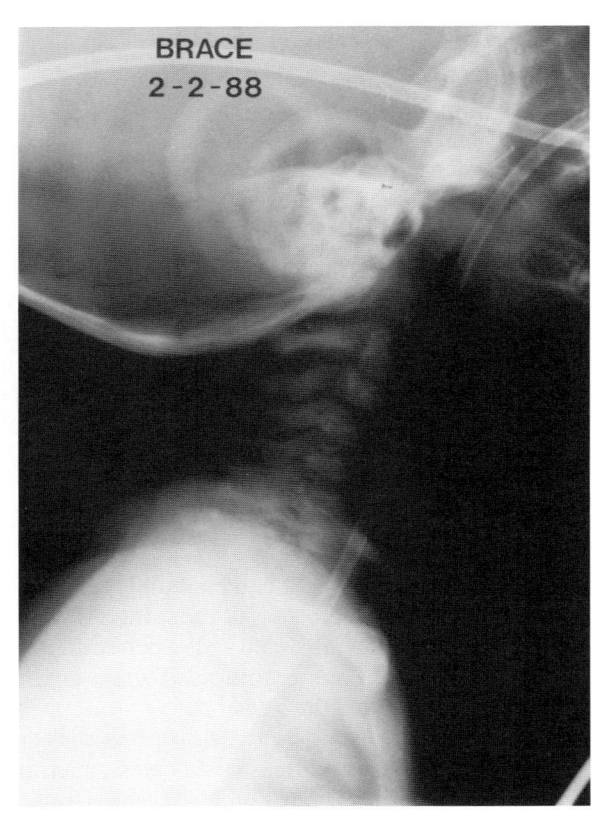

Fig. 44-13. (A) Hangman's fracture of C2 with instability in a 5-month-old boy whose father caught him by the head and neck as he was falling. (B) Reduction with a split mattress and the head in slight extension. (C) Maintenance of reduction 3 months later. *(Figure continues.)*

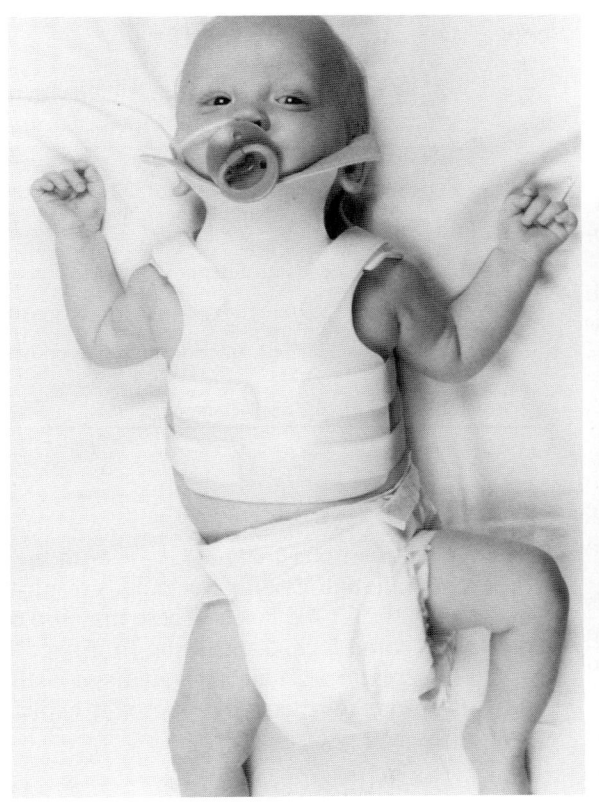

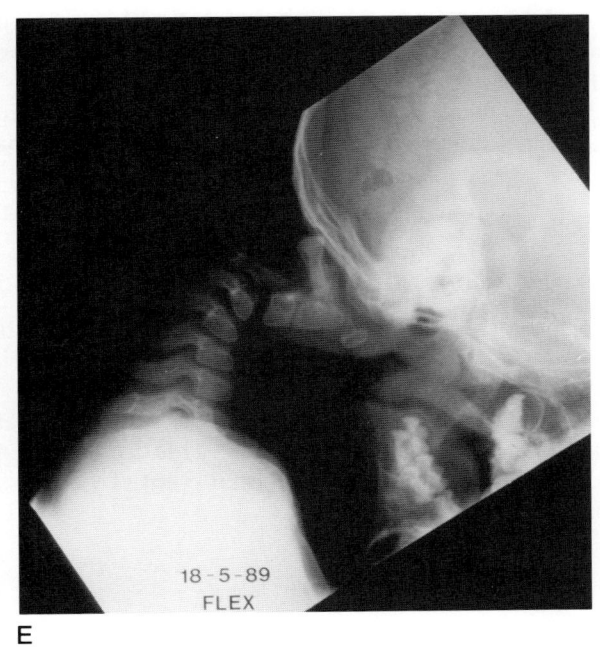

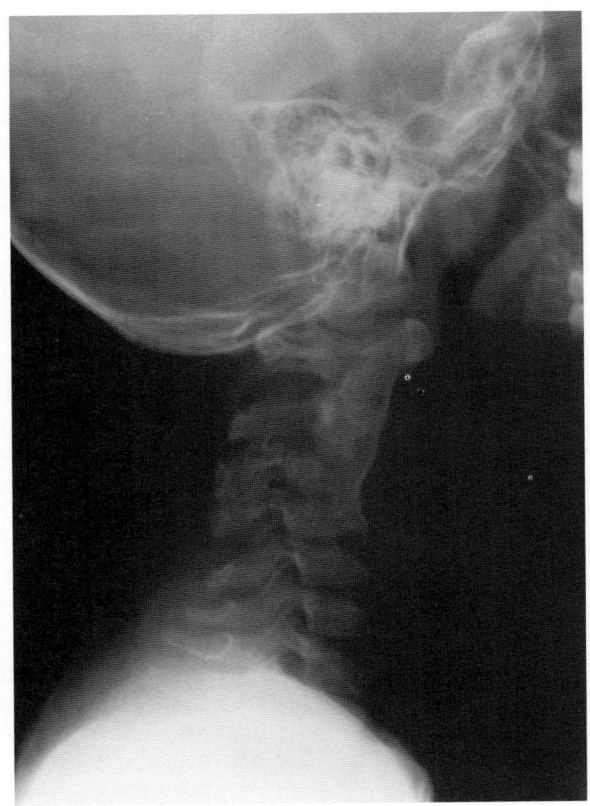

Fig. 44-13 *(Continued).* **(D)** The child in a customized polypropylene thoracic orthosis. In spite of good compliance and immobilization for over 1 year, there was persistent instability at C2-C3. **(E)** An anterior spinal fusion was performed, **(F)** which fused and stabilized C2-C4. (Courtesy Dr. Jacques D'Astous, Children's Hospital of Eastern Ontario, Ottawa, Canada.)

Treatment

Immobilization with a cervicothoracic brace and early ambulation are recommended in non- or minimally displaced fractures. Healing time is usually 12 weeks. Unstable fractures may necessitate more rigid halo immobilization after a few days of recumbency.

Surgical fusion is recommended only for children with an unstable delayed union, or for noncooperative patients.

Complications

Neurologic involvement is rarely seen in traumatic subluxation of C2 in children. Nonunion is rare, even in adult series.

Malunion can be observed, as this fracture often heals with anterior displacement of C2.[46] This does not seem to be detrimental from a functional point of view or to predispose to future instability.

Atlantoaxial Displacements

Atlantoaxial Rotatory Displacement

The most significant movement at the C1-C2 level is rotation with almost 50 percent of all rotatory cervical motion occurring at this level. During childhood, the occurrence of *torticollis* is frequent, and most children with so-called "wry neck" recover spontaneously or with minimal treatment. If the deformity persists, it may be secondary atlantoaxial rotary subluxation. This is probably the most common cervical spine injury in childhood.[6,47]

A wide spectrum of lesions may be hidden behind such terminology, varying from a simple rotatory displacement of one facet to complete C1-C2 dislocation, which can be associated with anterior displacement of C1 and C2 with neurologic compromise and even vertebral artery damage (Fig. 44-14).

Mechanism of Injury

Often, secondary to a twist of the neck beyond normal range, rotatory displacement of the atlas on the axis may occur after trivial trauma. It may also follow regional cervical or throat infection or inflammation (Grisel-Bourgeois syndrome) (Fig. 44-15). The infection predisposes to ligamentous laxity at C1-C2 with the ligaments becoming edematous and weakened, resulting in subluxation of the C1-C2 facets. These may slip completely off and become locked, resulting in a fixed torticollis. Local hyperemia with capsular and synovial interposition are among the theories proposed to explain the fixation of the rotary displacement.

TABLE 44-6. Classification of Atlantoaxial Rotatory Subluxation

Type I
Rotatory displacement without anterior shift of C1; the axis of rotation is the dens (most common type in the series)
Type II
Rotatory displacement with anterior shift of 3 to 5 mm (the pivot is one lateral mass)
Type III
Rotatory displacement with anterior shift of more than 5 mm
Type IV
Rotatory and posterior displacement

After Fielding.[8]

Classification

Fielding and colleagues[48] have classified atlantoaxial rotatory subluxation as shown in Table 44-6. Types III and IV are rare and potentially dangerous for neurologic structures (Fig. 44-16).

Clinical Findings

The child with a rotatory atlantoaxial subluxation usually presents with a painful torticollis. The head is tilted to one side and rotated to the opposite side. Slight flexion of the neck is usual. Palpation of the paracervical muscles will demonstrate associated muscle spasm on the side *opposite* the anterior displacement of C1 as an attempt to correct the deformity.

The range of cervical motion is severely restricted by pain in the acute stage, but in long-standing cases, the child is often able to increase rotation and tilt, but cannot correct and hold the head in a neutral position. With persistent atlantoaxial subluxation that is not recognized or treated for weeks or months, there is a tendency for C1 to slide anteriorly on C2, thus changing an initial type I or II lesion to type III.

As seen with congenital muscular torticollis, flattening on one side of the face may be seen in young children with long-standing fixed rotatory subluxation.

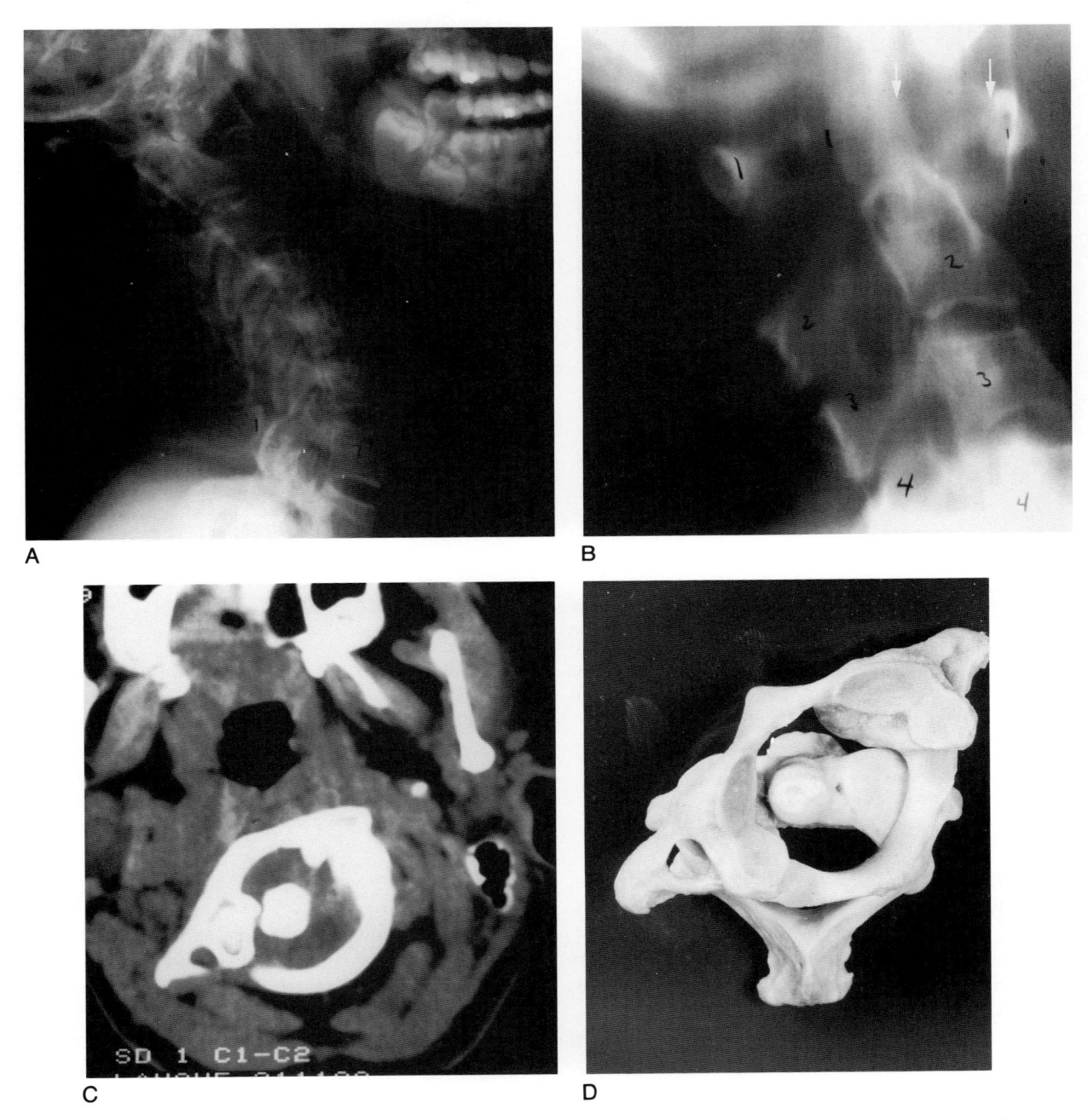

Fig. 44-14. Fixed rotatory subluxation of C1 with anterior subluxation shown in the (**A**) plain film lateral view and (**B**) more clearly with a tomogram. The atlantodens interval *(between the arrows)* is in excess of 1 cm. (**C**) CT scan at C1 level illustrating the rotatory subluxation of C1 on C2, (**D**) with the facets locked as demonstrated in the specimen.

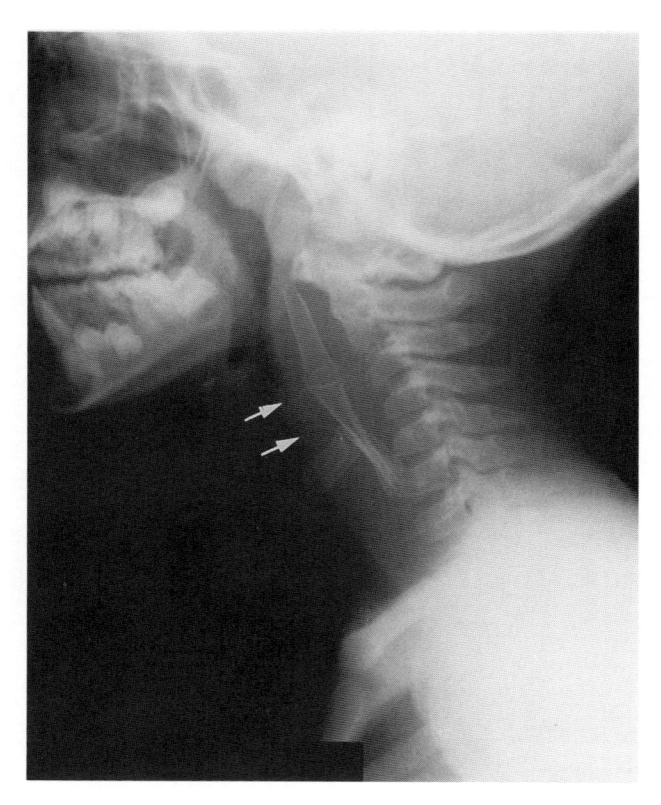

Fig. 44-15. A 4-year-old child presented with a rotatory subluxation of C1 on C2 secondary to a severe tonsillar infection that progressed to involve the paravertebral space—so-called "quinsy." Note the Penrose drain and gross swelling of the prevertebral space in excess of 1 cm. This symptom complex is sometimes referred to as the "Grisel syndrome."

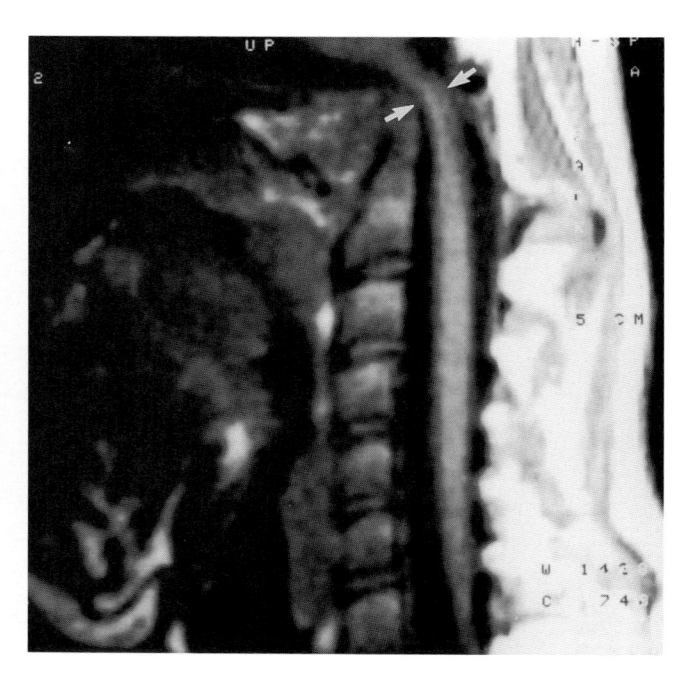

Fig. 44-16. MRI demonstrating canal narrowing at C1 secondary to the rotatory subluxation with anterior displacement of C1. This 12-year-old girl had increased clonus and hyperreflexia indicative of cord compression.

RADIOLOGIC EVALUATION

On the standard AP open-mouth view, the following may be observed (Fig. 44-17):

1. The lateral mass, which is displaced forward, appears wider and closer to the dens than the lateral mass, which is displaced backward.
2. There is a narrowing of the joint between the lateral mass (displaced forward) and axis.
3. The spinous process of the axis and the chin are on the same side of the midline.

On the lateral projection, the most important measure is the interval between the dens and the anterior part of C1 (atlantodens interval). Because of the rotation, this measurement can be difficult and lateral view tomograms are then helpful (Fig. 44-14).

CT techniques are also very helpful to confirm the type of atlantoaxial rotatory injury (Fig. 44-14). Cineradiography may be helpful when the pain has subsided to demonstrate that the atlas and axis move as a unit in fixed rotatory subluxation, whereas in the normal cervical spine, the atlas rotates independently on the axis.

TREATMENT

Most mild episodes of rotary subluxation of the atlas or the axis reduce spontaneously and resolve with minimal treatment using a soft collar, analgesics, and muscle relaxants. In more severe cases of type I injury, cervical traction with muscle relaxants and physiotherapy can be used to reduce the subluxation over several days and is usually successful.

After reduction of these minor short episodes of atlantoaxial subluxation, a soft collar should be worn for 2 to 3 weeks and contact sports avoided for 3 months. Reduction of persistent rotatory displacements can also be attempted by gentle manipulation under sedation.[32] Manipulation under general anesthesia is not recommended.[48]

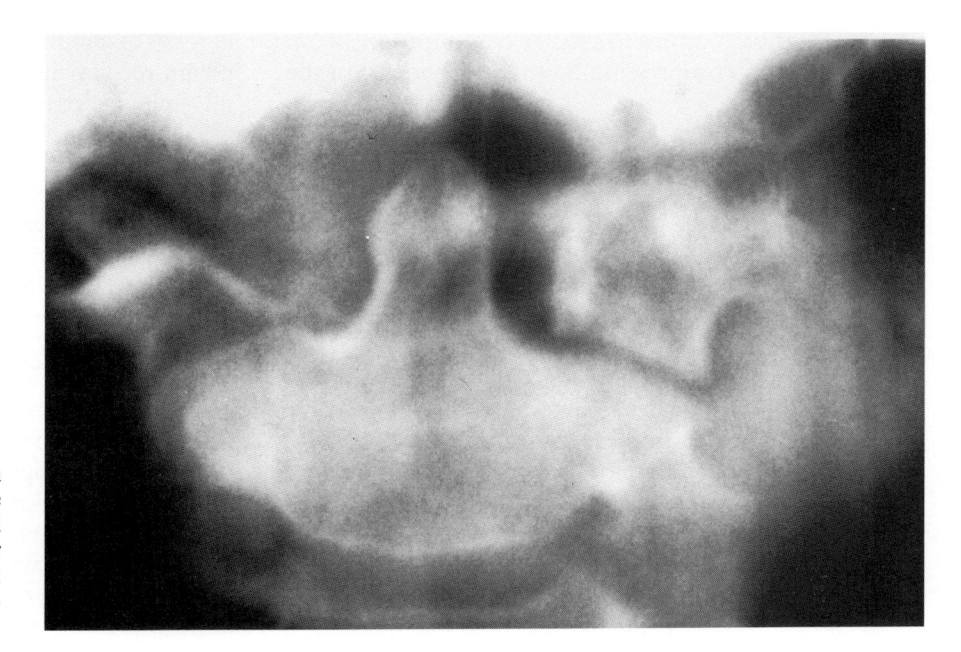

Fig. 44-17. A 15-year-old girl with fixed rotatory subluxation of C1. The lateral mass on the left is displaced forward and appears wider and closer to the dens than the lateral mass on the right, which is displaced backward.

According to Fielding and Hensinger,[8] the indications for C1-C2 fusion are as follows:

1. Neurologic involvement
2. Anterior displacement
3. Failure to achieve and maintain correction of the deformity that has been present for longer than 3 months
4. Recurrence of the deformity following an adequate trial of conservative management, consisting of at least 6 weeks of immobilization

Preoperative traction is recommended for 2 to 3 weeks to achieve as much reduction as possible in the longstanding fixed rotational deformities (Fig. 44-18).

Postoperatively, halo-vest immobilization should permit early ambulation. If this is not available, skull traction should continue for 6 weeks to ensure correction while the fusion is becoming solid. This should be followed by immobilization of the neck with a Minerva-type orthosis or four-poster cervicothoracic orthosis.

Complications

As most children sustain the type I atlantoaxial rotary subluxation, neurologic complications are fortunately rare. Cord compression can be encountered in the other types of rotatory luxations where there is associated anteroposterior displacement. Often, the first indication of cord impingement is clonus and mild sensory deficits

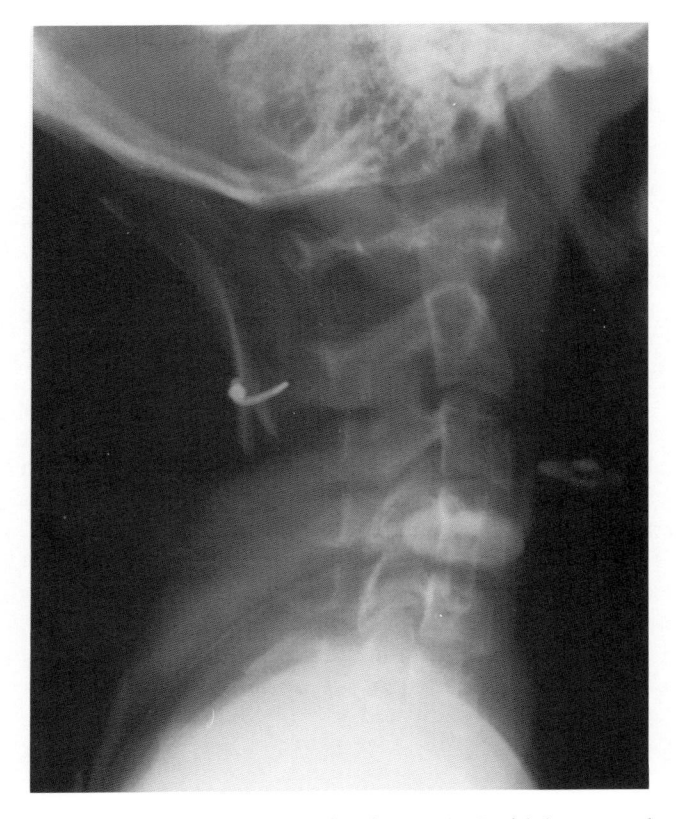

Fig. 44-18. Same patient as in Figure 44-17 with long-standing fixed rotatory subluxation. Following halo traction, the forward displacement of C1 on C2 was corrected and the head centered cosmetically over the torso. Although the rotatory dislocation could not be reduced, a C2-occiput fusion was performed to ensure maintenance of reduction.

in the upper extremities. Vascular complications from vertebral artery compression have been reported in the adult literature.

The most frequent problem associated with C1-C2 rotatory injuries is the inability to correct the subluxation and, thus, the torticollis. Recurrence of the displacement after adequate immobilization may also occur. Surgical fusion of the atlantoaxial complex may be required in these instances. Usually, the longer the subluxation has been present, the more difficult it is to reduce.

Posttraumatic instability seems to be rare, but can occur in long-standing rotatory subluxations. C1-C2 fusion is also indicated in these children.[49,50] After C1-C2 fusion, lower segments may show increased mobility[32] and thus compensate to a much greater extent for loss of motion at the fused segments than it does in adults.

Traumatic Atlantoaxial Ligamentous Disruption

In children, the ligaments are very strong and more resistant to trauma than adjacent growth plates. This probably explains why C1-C2 dislocations are so rare. The mechanism will more likely produce a fracture of the base of the dens (epiphysiolysis) before rupture of the C1-C2 ligaments or transverse odontoid ligament.

Birney and Hanley[6] reported only 2 children with dislocation of C1 on C2 among 26 cases of C1-C2 ligamentous injuries. Henrys and colleagues[51] described 1 dislocation of C1 on C2 of 12 patients with cervical spine injuries. Such dislocations are more frequent after the end of growth.

The atlantodens interval measured on the lateral view of the cervical spine in flexion is the best indicator for ligamentous instability. Displacement of C1 on C2 with an atlantodens interval over 5 mm indicates ligamentous compromise[8] and potential instability of C1 on C2.

The treatment consists of reduction of C1 on C2 in extension and stabilization by either a Minerva or halo cast for 8 to 12 weeks. After the immobilization period, stress films must be done to assess the stability. If the anterior displacement of C1 on C2 persists, posterior C1-C2 fusion is indicated.

C2-C3 Displacement: Pseudo- or Pathologic Subluxation?

Normal variations giving an appearance of subluxation between C2 and C3 are reported in as many as 33 percent of children's radiographs.[52] But how can the clinician recognize true traumatic subluxation from such physiologic "pseudosubluxations"?

Papavasiliou[53] reported three children with traumatic C2-C3 subluxation and stated that because of confusion with the known physiologic subluxation that commonly occurs at this level, considerable delay before the true diagnosis was confirmed was common, even though the children were under medical observation! He noted also the persistence of the subluxation of C2 on C3, even if radiographs were taken in the neutral position or hyperextension of the cervical spine. This appears to be an important differentiating feature and should be used if the C2 subluxation is felt to be posttraumatic rather than physiologic in origin.

Another method to differentiate "pathologic" from "physiologic" subluxation of C2 on C3 was described by Swischuk,[54] who defined the "posterior cervical line." This line is drawn from the cortex of the posterior arch of C1 to the cortex of the posterior arch of C3. This line may pass either through the cortex of the posterior arch of C2, touch the anterior aspect of the posterior arch of C2, or come within 1 mm of this anterior cortex (Fig. 44-2). Pathologic disclocations of C2 on C3 should be assumed when the posterior cervical line misses the posterior arch of C2 by 2 mm or more.

Injuries of the Abnormal Cervical Spine

Congenital deformities of the occipitocervical junction as well as aggravated hyperlaxity (as seen in Down syndrome, for example) may lead to upper cervical spine instability. The marked laxity and/or facet abnormalities create a hypermobile upper cervical spine with less resistance to trauma. Serious neurologic damage can therefore occur secondary to extremes of hyperflexion or hyperextension with minor trauma.

In 1984, the American Academy of Pediatrics recommended that children with Down syndrome participating in high-risk sports should be screened with a dynamic series of lateral views of the cervical spine in neutral position, flexion, and extension. Children with abnormal odontoid or an atlantodens interval exceeding 4.5 mm were advised not to be allowed to participate in stressful sports[55] (Fig. 44-19).

Patients with a diagnosis that indicates marked decrease in cervical motion or increased hyperlaxity are also at risk for cervical trauma (Table 44-7).

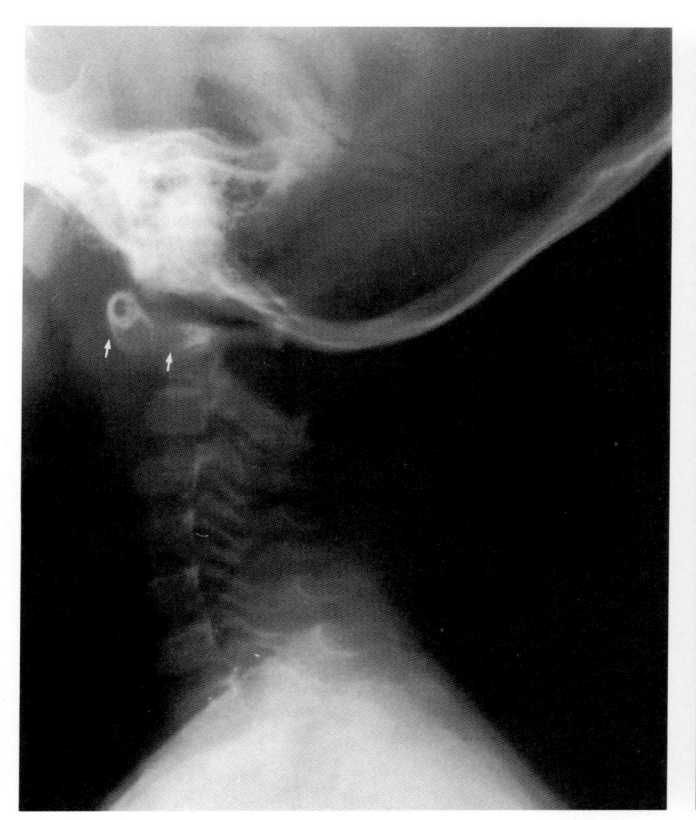

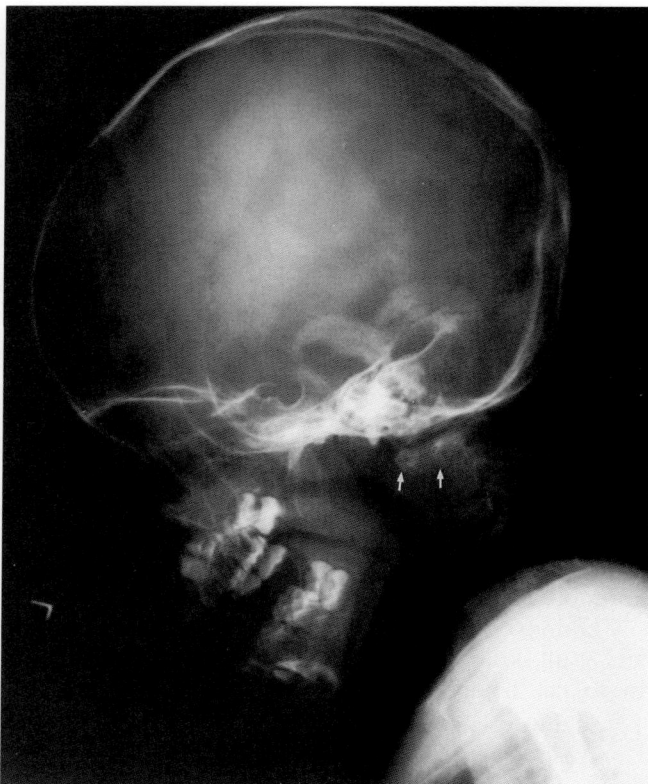

Fig. 44-19. C1-C2 asymptomatic instability in a 3-year-old child with Down syndrome who was screened prior to enrolling in a nursery school program.

TABLE 44-7. Children "at Risk" for Cervical Injury

Spondyloepiphyseal dysplasia
Morquio disease
Chondrodysplasia punctata (Conradi syndrome)
Diastrophic dwarfism
Juvenile rheumatoid arthritis
Klippel-Feil syndrome
Congenital anomalies of the odontoid
Os odontoideum
Occipitocervical synostosis
Larsen's syndrome
Cervical laminectomy
Cervical fusions

TREATMENT GUIDELINES

Transport of Neck-Injured Children

Children with cervical injury must be immobilized as soon as possible to prevent neurologic complications or to minimize further damage if already present. Transport of such young patients on a standard spine board leads to problems in the positioning of the head. As noted by Hensinger and colleagues,[56] because of the relatively large head of the child in comparison with the rest of the body, the neck is usually in hyperflexion on such spine boards, whereas most cervical displacements are reduced in extension. All ambulance attendants and emergency physicians should follow their suggestion to use either a special board with a recess cut out for the back of the head or, more simply, to place a roll under the shoulders of young subjects with cervical trauma during transport.

No traction should be instituted, the stabilization of the head being obtained by either sandbags, taping, or other device.

Immobilization of the Neck

As demonstrated by Johnson and coworkers,[42] conventional orthoses are able to restrict only 45 percent of normal flexion/extension at the C1-C2 level, whereas with a halo, 75 percent of the same motion is reduced. Such cervical braces also do not control lateral bending or axial rotation (Table 44-8).

It has been said that "if the patient can talk and chew, there is some motion between C1 and C2."[57] The Minerva cast can be used in very young patients (less than 2 years old) where halo fixation is more difficult (Fig. 44-20). But the technique of applying the Minerva cast must be meticulous or it will slip down and be worse than no immobilization at all!

Children over 6 years old may be considered as having an "adult skull" and standard halo fixation[58] (4 pins at 8 in.-lb) can be used safely. It is different for younger patients where the skull osteology has some peculiar aspects.[59] It is recommended to use multiple pins (6 or 8) at 4 to 6 in.-lb for children 2 to 5 years old[55] primarily because of their hyperactivity at this age and their tendency to loosen the halo pins.

In children less than 2 years old, alternative methods of immobilization should be considered. Nevertheless, if the halo is to be used, 10 pins at 2 in.-lb, as mentioned by Mubarak and coworkers[60] can be used.

TABLE 44-8. Cervical Orthoses

Type	Effect
Soft collar (variable firmness)	Does not provide any immobilization; slightly reduces cervical flexion
Philadelphia collar	Cervical flexion and extension are reduced, but little effect on lateral flexion and rotation
SOMI (sterno-occipital mandibular immobilizer)	
Four-poster cervical collar	
Custom molded (Minerva jacket)	Lateral flexion is better restrained
Halo (cast or vest)	Provides the greatest control

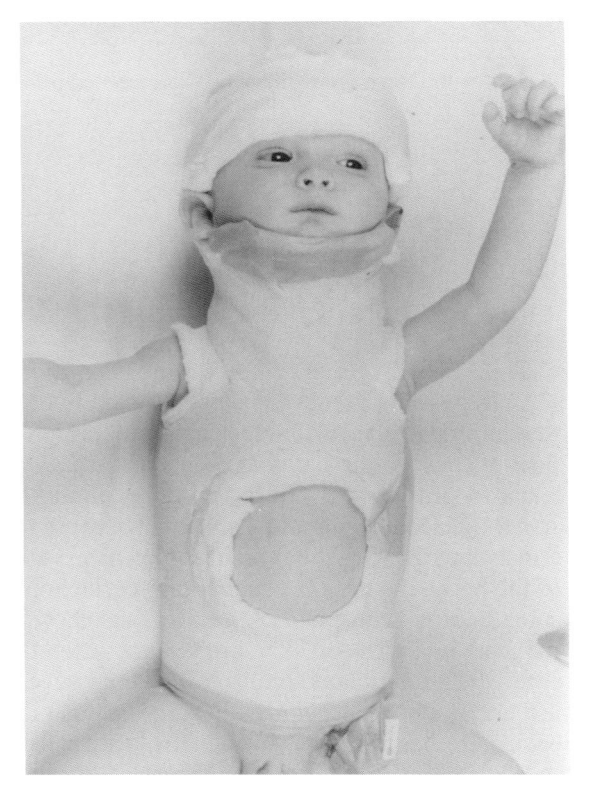

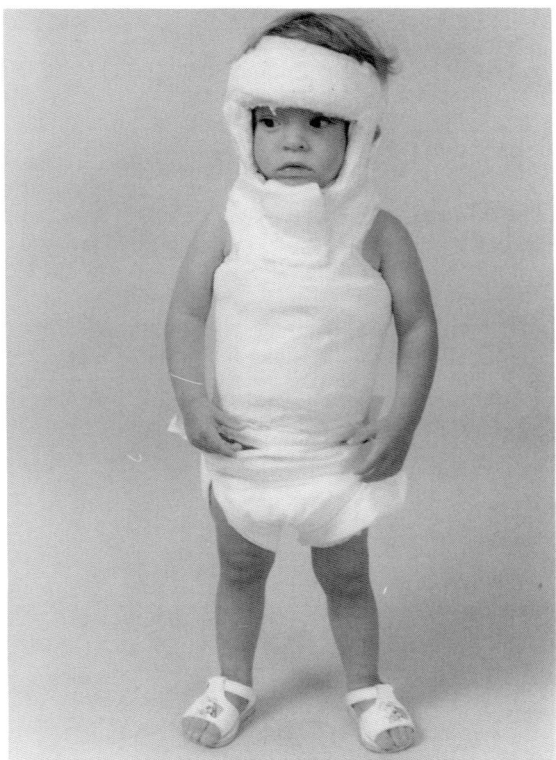

Fig. 44-20. A well-molded Minerva cast can be employed to provide cervical immobility if a halo is contraindicated.

Whatever the age of the child, the frontal sinus area and temporal fossae should not be chosen as pin placement sites because of the limited bone thickness in these regions. Halo pins should rather be placed anterolaterally and posterolaterally where the skull is thicker. CT scanning of the skull in young children before elective halo application is recommended.[61]

Fusion of C1-C2

C1-C2 fusion is usually performed according to the Rogers technique,[62,63] but the following principles must be followed in children to reduce postoperative complications:

1. The patient must be safely positioned and the reduction assessed radiologically.
2. Avoid exposing more than C1-C2, due to "creeping fusion."
3. Use internal fixation (sublaminar wiring) to secure the reduction and decrease the length of postoperative immobilization (in patients with either congenital anomalies, preoperative neurologic deficit, or unreducible C1-C2 dislocation, it may be safer to perform an in situ fusion without wiring or a decompressive laminectomy with occipitocervical fusion)[64] to avoid neurologic complications. Two types of wiring are used:
   Sublaminar wiring of C1 and C2.
   Sublaminar wiring of C1 with distal fixation under the spinous process of C2.
4. Use preferentially autograft bone (from iliac crest). A corticocancellous graft of either H or M shape is fixed between the posterior elements of C1 and C2.
5. Provide adequate postoperative immobilization (depending upon the stability of the internal fixation). With internal fixation, the duration of halo-cast or halo-vest immobilization is reduced by 50 percent.[64]

SUMMARY

Most cervical spine injuries in children can be diagnosed by plain radiographs and physical examination. Do not use skull radiographs to evaluate the upper cervical spine! Ask for specific views of the C1-C2 region.

Fractures of the atlas, as well as odontoid fractures, heal well in children with proper immobilization. Neurologic complications are less often observed than in adult fractures.[65]

Facial injuries have a high incidence of associated fracture of the cervical spine, particularly traumatic spondylolisthesis of the axis, and are often related to motor vehicle accidents.

True ligamentous disruptions are rare in the pediatric age group, but hyperlaxity may explain the frequency of subluxations. Lasting torticollis should arouse suspicion of fixed rotatory displacements of C1 on C2.

REFERENCES

1. Rang M: Children's Fractures. JB Lippincott, Philadelphia, 1974
2. Benoit M, Jarvis JG: Stability of the injured cervical spine in children. p. 71. Proceedings of the 1990 annual meeting, Pediatric Orthopaedic Society, San Francisco, California, May 6–9, 1990
3. Becker F: Luxationfraktur zwischen Atlas und Epistropheus im Kleinkindesaiter. Arch Orthop Unfall-Chir 55:682, 1963
4. Hubbard DD: Injuries of the spine in children and adolescents. Clin Orthop 100:56, 1974
5. Hasue M, Hoshino R, Omata S et al: Cervical spine injuries in children. Fukushima J Med Sci 20:114, 1974
6. Birney TJ, Hanley EN Jr: Traumatic cervical spine injuries in childhood and adolescence. Spine 14:1277, 1989
7. Denis F, Winter RB, Lonstein JE: Pediatric spinal injuries. p. 74. Proceedings of the 22nd annual meeting of Scoliosis Research Society, Vancouver, BC, Canada, Sept. 15–19, 1987
8. Fielding JW, Hensinger RN: Fractures of the spine. p. 683. In Rockwood CA, Wilkins KE, King RE (eds): Fractures in Children. JB Lippincott Philadelphia, 1984
9. Cattell HS, Filtzer DL: Pseudosubluxation and other normal variations in the cervical spine in children: a study of one hundred and sixty children. J Bone Joint Surg [Am] 47:1295, 1965
10. Locke GR, Gardner JI, Van Epps EF: Atlas-dens internal (ADI) in children: a survey based on 200 normal cervical spines. Am J Radiol 97:135, 1966
11. Mann DC: Spine fractures in children and adolescents: Spine 4:25, 1990
12. Vigouroux RP, Baurance C, Choux M et al: Injuries of the cervical spine in children. Neurochirurgia 14:689, 1968
13. Weir DC: Roentgenographic signs of cervical injury. Clin Orthop 109:9, 1975
14. Sherk HH, Schut L, Lane JM: Fractures and dislocations of the cervical spine in children. Orthop Clin North Am 7:593, 1976
15. Aufdermaur M: Spinal injuries in juveniles: necropsy findings in twelve cases. J Bone Joint Surg [Br] 56:513, 1974
16. Sherk HH, Nicholson JT, Chung SMK: Fractures of the

odontoid process in young children. J Bone Joint Surg [Am] 60:921, 1978
17. Caffey J: The whiplash shaken infant syndrome. Pediatrics 54:396, 1974
18. Swischuk LE: Spine and spinal cord trauma in the battered child syndrome. Radiology 92:733, 1969
19. King J, Diefendorf D, Apthorp J: Computer analysis of 429 fractures in 189 battered children. p. 57. Proceedings of the 1986 annual meeting of the Pediatric Orthopaedic society, May 4–7, Boston, 1986
20. Macielak JR, Swank S, Brown J, Barras D: Gunshot wounds to the spine in children. p. 75. Proceedings of the 22nd annual meeting Scoliosis Research Society, Vancouver, BC, Sept. 15–19, 1987
21. Benoit M, Jarvis JG: Cervical spine injuries in children. p. 65. Proceedings of the Pediatric Orthopaedic Society of North America. Annual Meeting, Hilton Head, South Carolina, May 17–20, 1989
22. Stauffer ES, Mazur JM: Cervical spine injuries in children. Pediatr Ann 11:502, 1982
23. Davidson JS, Birdsell DC: Cervical spine injury in patients with facial skeletal trauma. J Trauma 29:1276, 1989
24. Kulkarni MV, Bondurant FJ, Rose SL, Narayana FA: 1.5 Tesla magnetic resonance imaging of acute spinal trauma. Radiographics 18:1059, 1988
25. Marlin AE, Wiliams GR, Lee JF: Jefferson fractures in children case report. J Neurosurg 58:277, 1983
26. Routt ML Jr, Green NE: Case report: Jefferson fracture in a 2-year-old child. J Trauma 29:1710, 1989
27. Sherk HH: Fractures of the atlas and odontoid process. Orthop Clin North Am 9:973, 1978
28. Jefferson G: Fracture of the atlas vertebra: report of four cases and a review of those previously recorded. Br J Surg 7:407, 1920
29. Steel HH: Anatomical and mechanical consideration of the atlanto-axial articulation. J Bone Joint Surg [Am] 50:1481, 1986
30. Swischuk LE: The cervical spine in childhood. Curr Probl Diagn Radiol 13:1, 1986
31. Mikawa Y, Watanabe R, Yamano Y, Ishii K: Fracture through a synchondrosis of the anterior arch of the atlas. J Bone Joint Surg [Br] 69:483, 1987
32. Ogden JA: Skeletal injury in the child. 2nd Ed. Ch. 14. WB Saunders, Philadelphia, 1990
33. Richards PG: Stable fractures of the atlas and axis in children. J Neurol Neurosurg Psychiatry 47:781, 1984
34. Shacked I, Rappaport ZH, Barzilay Z, Ohri A: Two-level fracture of the cervical spine in a young child. J Bone Joint Surg [Am] 65:119, 1983
35. Dickman CA, Hadley MN, Browner C, Sonntag VKH: Neurosurgical management of acute atlas-axis combination fractures: a review of 25 cases. J Neurosurg 70:45, 1989
36. Blockey NJ, Purser DW: Fractures of the odontoid process of the axis. J Bone Joint Surg [Br] 38:794, 1956
37. Alker GI Jr, Oh YS, Leslie EV: High cervical spine and cranio-cervical junction injuries in fatal traffic accidents. Orthop Clin North Am 9:1003, 1978
38. Griffiths SC: Fracture of odontoid process in children. J Pediatr Surg 7:680, 1972
39. Anderson LD, D'Alonzo RT: Fractures of the odontoid process of the axis. J Bone Joint Surg [Am] 56:1663, 1974
40. Seimon LP: Fracture of the odontoid process in young children. J Bone Joint Surg [Am] 59:943, 1977
41. Nachemson A: Fracture of the odontoid process of the axis (26 cases). Acta Orthop Scand 29:185, 1960
42. Johnson RM, Hart DL, Simmons EF et al: Cervical orthoses: a study comparing their effectiveness in restricting cervical motion in normal subjects. J Bone Joint Surg [Am] 59:332, 1977
43. Fielding JW, Griffin PP: Os odontoideum: an acquired lesion. J Bone Joint Surg [Am] 56:187, 1974
44. Schuler TC, Kurz L, Thompson DE et al: Case report: natural history of os odontoideum. J Pediatr Orthop 11:222, 1991
45. Pizzutillo PD, Rocha EF, D'Astous J et al: Bilateral fracture of the pedicle of the second cervical vertebra in the young child. J Bone Surg [Am] 68:892, 1986
46. Francis WR, Fielding JW: Traumatic spondylolisthesis of the axis. Orthop Clin North Am 9:1011, 1978
47. Fielding JW, Hawkins RJ: Atlanto-axial rotary fixation. J Bone Joint Surg [Am] 59:37, 1977
48. Fielding JW, Hawkins RJ, Hensinger RN, Francis WR: Atlanto-axial rotary deformities. Orthop Clin North Am 9:955, 1978
49. Filipe G, Berges O, Lebard JP, Carlioz H: Instabilités post-traumatiques entre l'atlas et l'axis chez l'enfant: a propos de cinq observations. Rev Chir Orthop 68:461, 1982
50. Arlet V, Rigault P, Padovani JP et al: Instabilités et luxations méconnues ou négligées du rachis cervical supérieur de l'enfant: a propos de 20 observations. Rev Chir Orthop 78:300, 1992
51. Henrys P, Lyne ED, Lifton C, Salciccioli G: Clinical review of cervical spine injuries in children. Clin Orthop 129:172, 1977
52. Sullivan CR, Bruwer AJ, Harris LE: Hypermobility of the cervical spine in children: a pitfall in the diagnosis of cervical dislocation. Am J Surg 95:636, 1958
53. Papavasiliou V: Traumatic subluxation of the cervical spine during childhood. Orthop Clin North Am 9:945, 1978
54. Swischuk LE: Anterior displacement of C2 in children: physiologic or pathologic?—a helpful differentiating line. Radiology 122:759, 1977
55. Reider B: Sports Medicine: The School-Age Athlete. WB Saunders, Philadelphia, 1991
56. Hensinger RN, Herzenberg JE, Dedrick DK, Phillips WA: Emergency transport and positioning of the young child with a cervical spine injury: the standard backboard may be hazardous. p. 73. Proceedings of the Scoliosis Research Society 22nd annual meeting, Vancouver, BC, Canada, Sept. 15–19, 1987

57. White AA, Panjabi MM: The clinical biomechanics of the occipito atlanto axial complex. Orthop Clin North Am 9:867, 1978
58. Nickel VL, Perry J, Garret A, Heppenstall M: The halo. J Bone Joint Surg [Am] 50:1400, 1968
59. Garfin SR, Roux R, Botte MJ et al: Skull osteology as it affects halo pin placement in children. J Pediatr Orthop 6:434, 1986
60. Mubarak SJ, Camp JF, Vuletich W, Wenger DR: Halo immobilization for cervical spine instability in the infant. p. 60. Proceedings of the Pediatric Society of North America annual meeting, Colorado Springs, Colorado, May 5–8, 1988
61. Letts M, Kaylor D, Gouw G: A biomechanical analysis of halo fixation in children. J Bone Joint Surg [Br] 70:277, 1988
62. Canale ST, Beaty JH: Spine fractures and dislocations. p. 934. In: Operative Pediatric Orthopaedics. Mosby-Year Book, St. Louis, 1991
63. Holmes JC, Hall JE: Fusion for instability and potential instability of the cervical spine in children and adolescents. Orthop Clin North Am 9:923, 1978
64. Smith MD, Phillips WA, Hensinger RN: Fusion of the upper cervical spine in children and adolescents: an analysis of 17 patients. Spine 16:695, 1991
65. McGrory BS, Klassen RA, Chao EYS et al: Acute fractures of the cervical spine in children and adolescents. J Bone Joint Surg [Am]75:988, 1993

45

C3-C7 Fractures and Dislocations

Stephen J. Tredwell

> It is that which we do know which is the great hinderence to our learning that which we don't know.
> —Claude Bernard

DESCRIPTION AND INCIDENCE

This chapter discusses trauma to the middle and lower cervical segments in the child and the younger adolescent. The discussion addresses the maturing cervical spine, its anatomy, the radiographic description of the cervical spine in the child, the initial assessment of the patient with a cervical injury, and operative and nonoperative management.

Spinal injury in childhood is rare and comprises less than 2 percent of all spine injuries.[1] However, injuries to the cervical spine form a larger percentage of pediatric spine trauma than do injuries to the cervical spine in the adult. In a series of pediatric injuries reported in 1974 by Burke[2] 9 of 24 complete spinal cord lesions occurring after the neonatal period were in the cervical spine. Within the cervical spine itself, injuries to the upper cervical segment (C1-C2) constitute the majority of injuries in the first 7 to 8 years of life. Following age 8, the distribution of cervical spine injuries begins to approximate that of the adult, and injuries to the middle (C3-C4) and lower (C5-C7) become more common.[1-3] Mid- and lower-segment injuries in the child are associated with more severe injuries.[3] In the child, cord injuries are more likely to be complete, as in Burke's review, with 80 percent of cord injuries being complete.[2]

ANATOMY

The unique and changing anatomy of the neck in children places the neck at higher risk in the younger child than in the adult.[1,3,4] In the child, the head is relatively larger than it is in the adult, and the effect of violent flexion-extension injuries is magnified by the large load that the head places upon the cervical spine. In the child, there is also a relative ligamentous laxity, and the facet joints of the cervical spine are more horizontal. The joints of Lushka, which in the adult protect against hyperflexion injury, are not well developed in the child until 8 or 9 years of age, hence this protection is absent. The immature cervical vertebrae have an anterior wedge configuration as growth centers are located anteriorly in the vertebral body. These growth centers are cartilaginous and do not provide the same support as the more squared-off bony contour in the adult (Fig. 45-1). The lack of cervical supporting musculature leaves the child's neck a rather slender column. The cervical muscles strengthen in late childhood and early adolescence and add secondary support and protection (Fig. 45-2). As the child matures, therefore, the neck becomes relatively less at risk.

From ages 1 to 8 years, cervical spine injuries are caused by distraction forces with rupture of the osseous

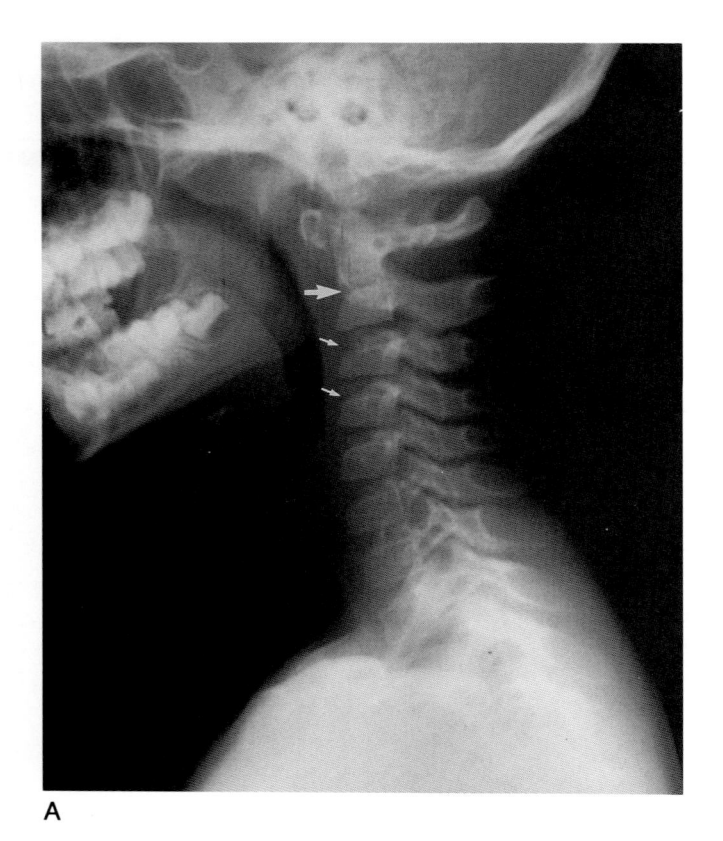

Fig. 45-1. A normal 5-year-old child without neck pain. **(A)** Note the remnant of the growth center at the base of the dens, the angulation between C2 and C3, the anterior wedging of the vertebral bodies especially C3 and C4. **(B)** On the AP through the mouth view, note the apical ossification center of the dens (ossicle terminale) and the superimposed incisor, which can occasionally be mistaken for a fracture of the odontoid.

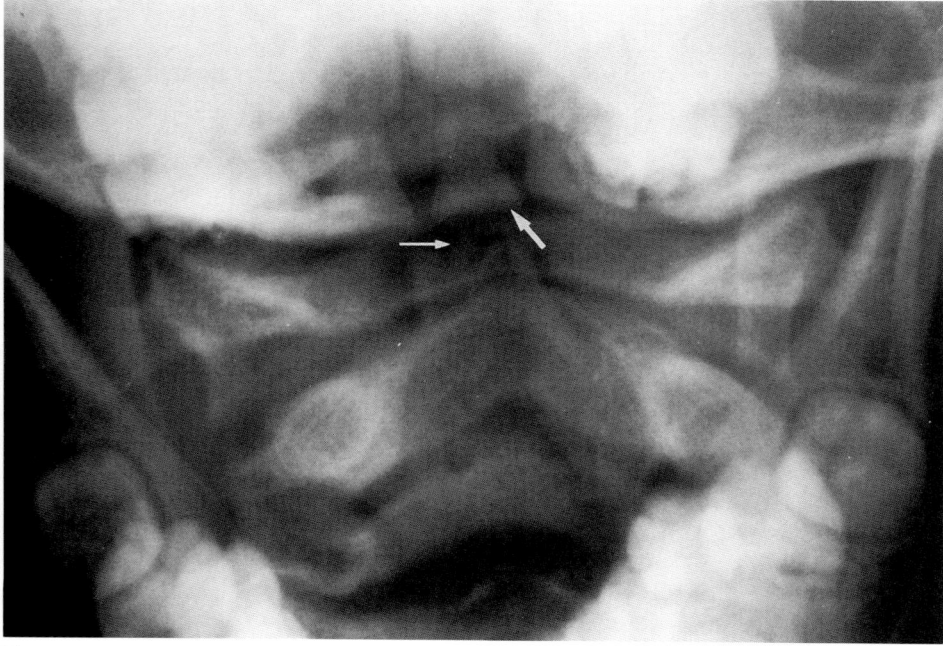

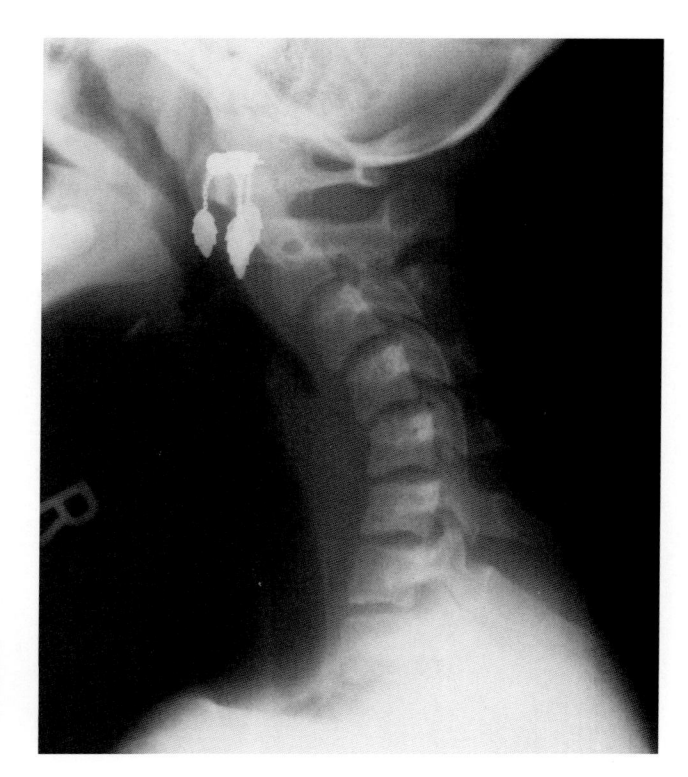

Fig. 45-2. Cervical kyphosis secondary to a cervical spine injury in a 15-year-old gymnast with a long slender neck. This girl had been treated in a cervical collar for a long period of time, which resulted in weakening of the cervical paraspinal musculature.

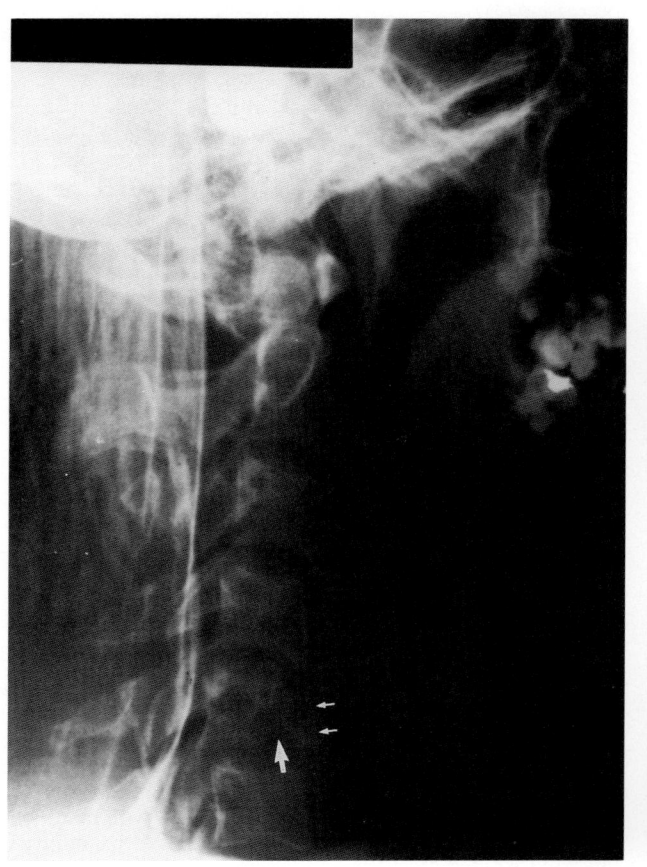

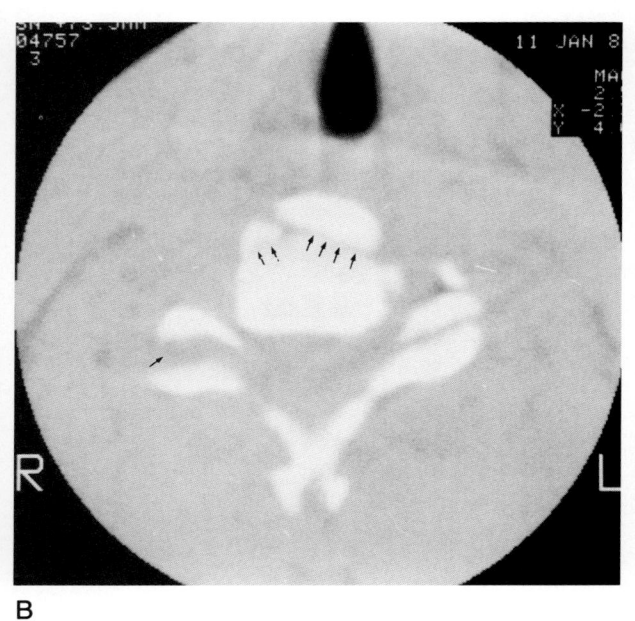

Fig. 45-3. (**A&B**) Teardrop fracture of C5 secondary to a distraction force similar to the lumbar Chance fracture also resulting in a laminar fracture seen best on CT (**B**).

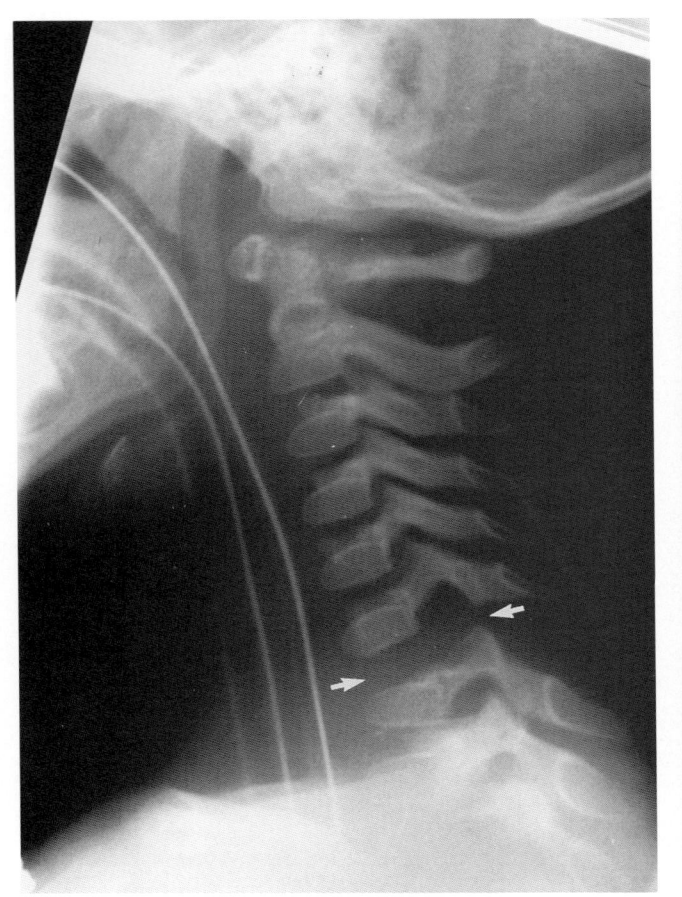

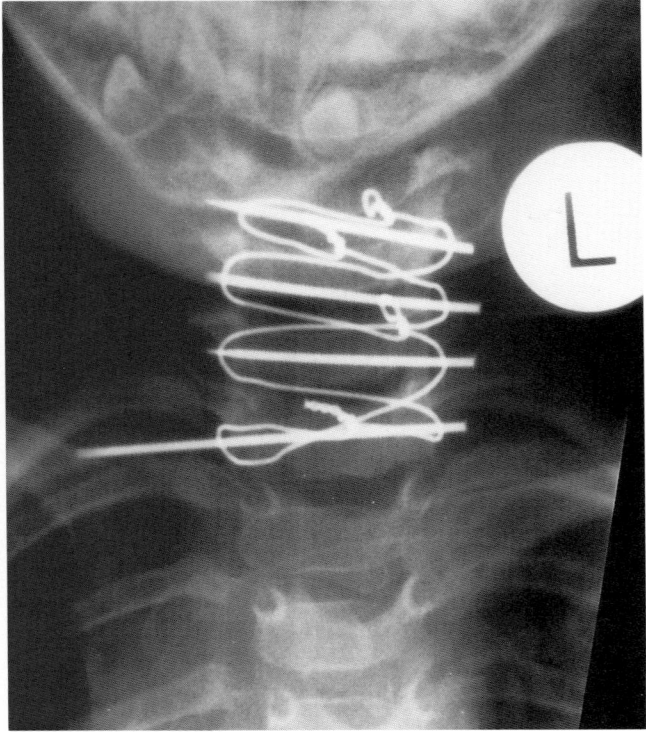

Fig. 45-4. This 3-year-old child was involved in a violent flexion injury as a seat-belted passenger wearing only a lap belt. **(A)** The disproportionately large head when thrown violently forward produces excessive traction on the cervical spine and the resultant injury was one of flexion distraction at C6-C7. **(B&C)** This was a complete spinal cord injury with no function below the level of trauma. The gross clinical instability demanded immediate fusion to allow for appropriate nursing care. With this mechanism of injury, one must also suspect a distraction injury of the lumbar spine (chance fracture). *(Figure continues.)*

D E

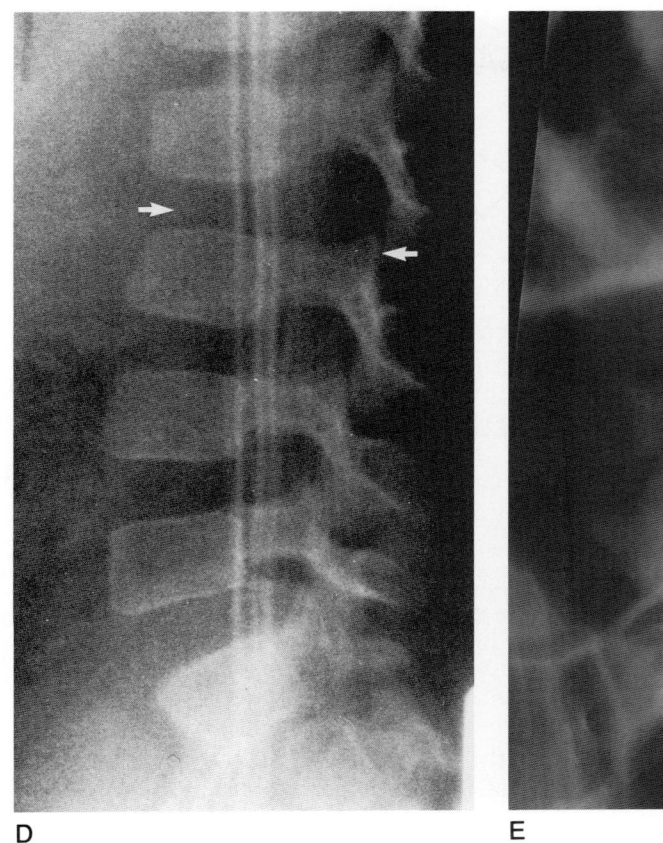

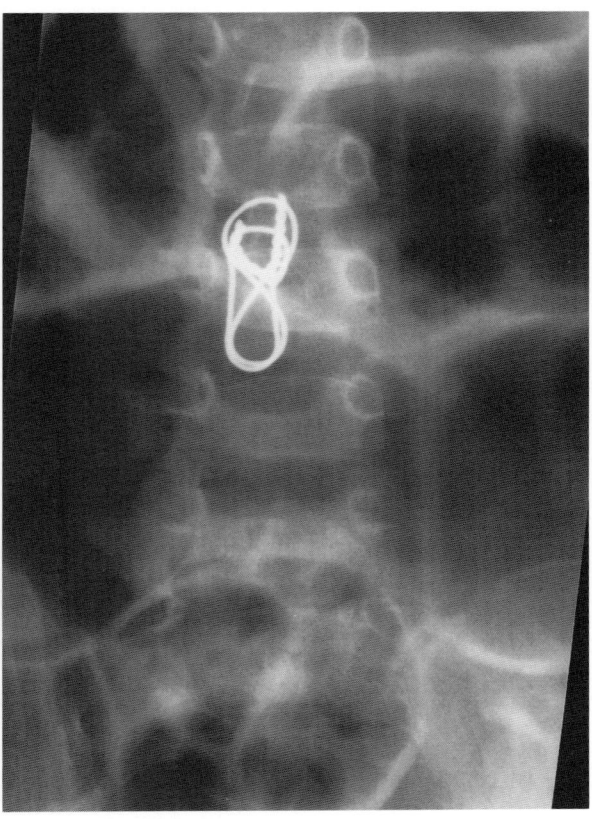

Fig. 45-4 *(Continued).* **(D&E)** Radiographs of the lumbar spine in this child were done on history alone as all clinical findings were masked by the complete cord lesion. A flexion distraction fracture was found at L2 which was also fused to facilitate nursing care.

ring (Fig. 45-3) or rupture of the cartilaginous elements[4] (Fig. 45-4). This contrasts with the compression and/or comminution patterns commonly seen in the adolescent and in the adult (Figs. 45-5 and 45-6). In children, compression and burst fractures are rare in the middle and lower segment presumably because of the higher axis of flexion-extension, skeletal geometry, and weaknesses in the bone and growth plate junctions.

The synchondroses are most vulnerable in the upper cervical segment (dens fracture and Jefferson fracture) but they are also vulnerable in the mid- and lower segments at the neurocentral-posterior elements synchondroses. From age 8 to adulthood, the injury pattern in the cervical spine begins to mirror that of the adult. Facet joint injury and compression fracture do not start appearing as clinical entities in the child until early- to mid-adolescence (Fig. 45-7). The youngest facet injury has been reported in a 14-year-old child by Ehara and coworkers.[4]

MECHANISM OF INJURY

The causes of cervical injury in the child mirror that of adults with a few exceptions. Birth trauma has been reported to cause spinal injury as has the excessive whiplash effect of the shaken child in the child abuse cases.[2] In Burke's series, 16 of the 29 complete lesions were secondary to motor vehicle accidents, the child being either a passenger or pedestrian. Dietrich and colleagues,[5] reporting in 1991, reviewed 50 injuries to the cervical spine in children and found the average age to be 11 years.

In their group, motor vehicle related accidents accounted for 54 percent of the cases, sports injuries were 18 percent and falls were 12 percent. Of this group, 58 percent had an associated head injury. Also within the motor vehicle group, poorly fitting car seats, which allow the child to hyperflex, have been implicated as a cause of cervical spinal injury. In this group, it is postulated that the brachial plexus acts as a distal tether when the head is

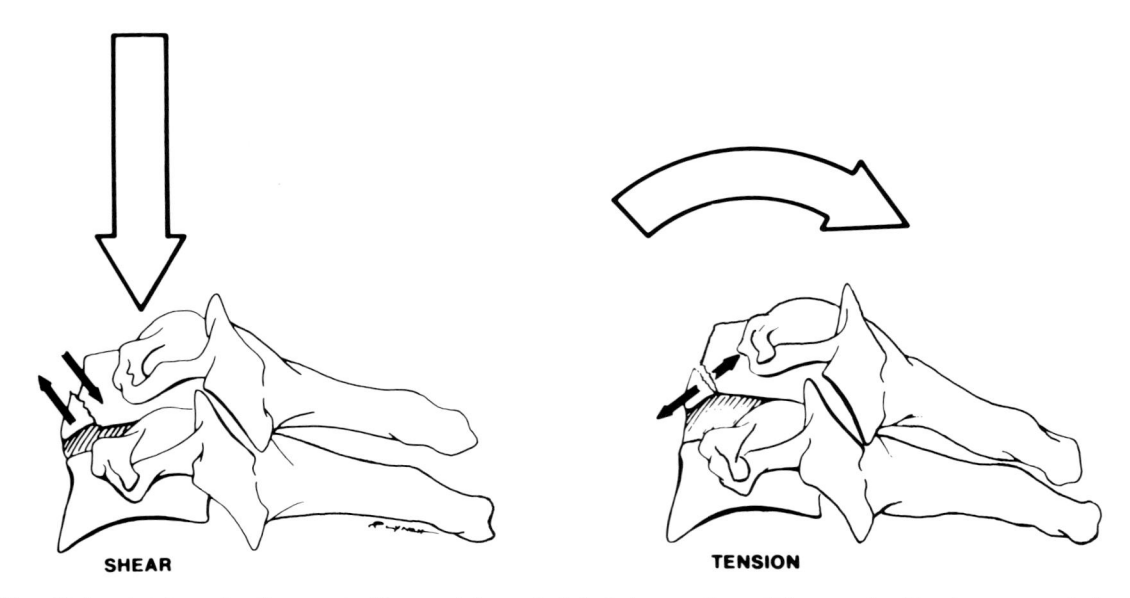

Fig. 45-5. A triangular fragment of bone at the anteroinferior portion of the vertebral body may result from either shear or tensile failure. In compressive loading there are shear stresses along a line about 45 degrees to the force vector. In extension loading, the same region of bone is subjected to tensile stresses. (From White and Panjabi,[7] with permission.)

thrown forward, thus applying a traction injury to the upper cord. Fuchs and colleagues[6] reported on five children less than age 2 years who were injured in forward-facing car seats (Fig. 45-4).

The changing relationships between the size of the head, the supporting cervical musculature and the relative ligamentous laxity produces a fulcrum of flexion extension at C3-C4 in the child (Fig. 45-8), whereas in the adult the change in size increase in strength and decrease in ligamentous laxity produces a center of rotation as C5-C6. As the center of rotation moves distally, the forces focused on the spine likewise move distally and the injury pattern changes. An adult osseous configuration is present in the child at approximately age 8 and adult supporting musculature present by approximately age 14 to 15 years. Under 8 years of age the greater cartilaginous component of the vertebrae plus the ligamentous resiliency of the cervical spine protects the middle and lower segments from major trauma. After this age the conditions conducive to causing fractures in these cervical spinal segments depend on the impact magnitude, direction, point of application and the rate of application of the force applied. Thus a child falling out of a tree onto the head or from a bicycle or motorcycle may strike the ground with the neck flexed, the resultant force then being directly borne by the nonlordosis cervical vertebrae[7] (Fig. 45-9). Such an injury will result in mechanical buckling or compression fractures of the bodies (Fig. 45-10). If the neck has a component of axial rotation at impact, shear forces may cause avulsion injuries in children due to the strong ligamentous attachments.

CLINICAL ASSESSMENT

The emergency department assessment of cervical spine injury in children ranges from the examination of the child with the isolated neck injury and pain, to the polytraumatized patient. All children who present with a history of neck injury and pain must have the cervical spine supported until an investigation has been completed. The more severely traumatized children should be treated according to the routines outlined in the advanced trauma life-support system protocols. Children are significantly different from adolescents and adults with regard to their head size.[8] Given their relatively larger head size, positioning the injured child supine on the standard fracture board will result in a relative forward flexion of the head on the neck. To align the head and neck correctly on the child, they must be positioned with the ear in line with the shoulder. A simple modification of the standard fracture board can be made by creating a small hole for the head, which allows the relative extension needed to align the child's head more correctly. Failing this, a small mattress can be placed on

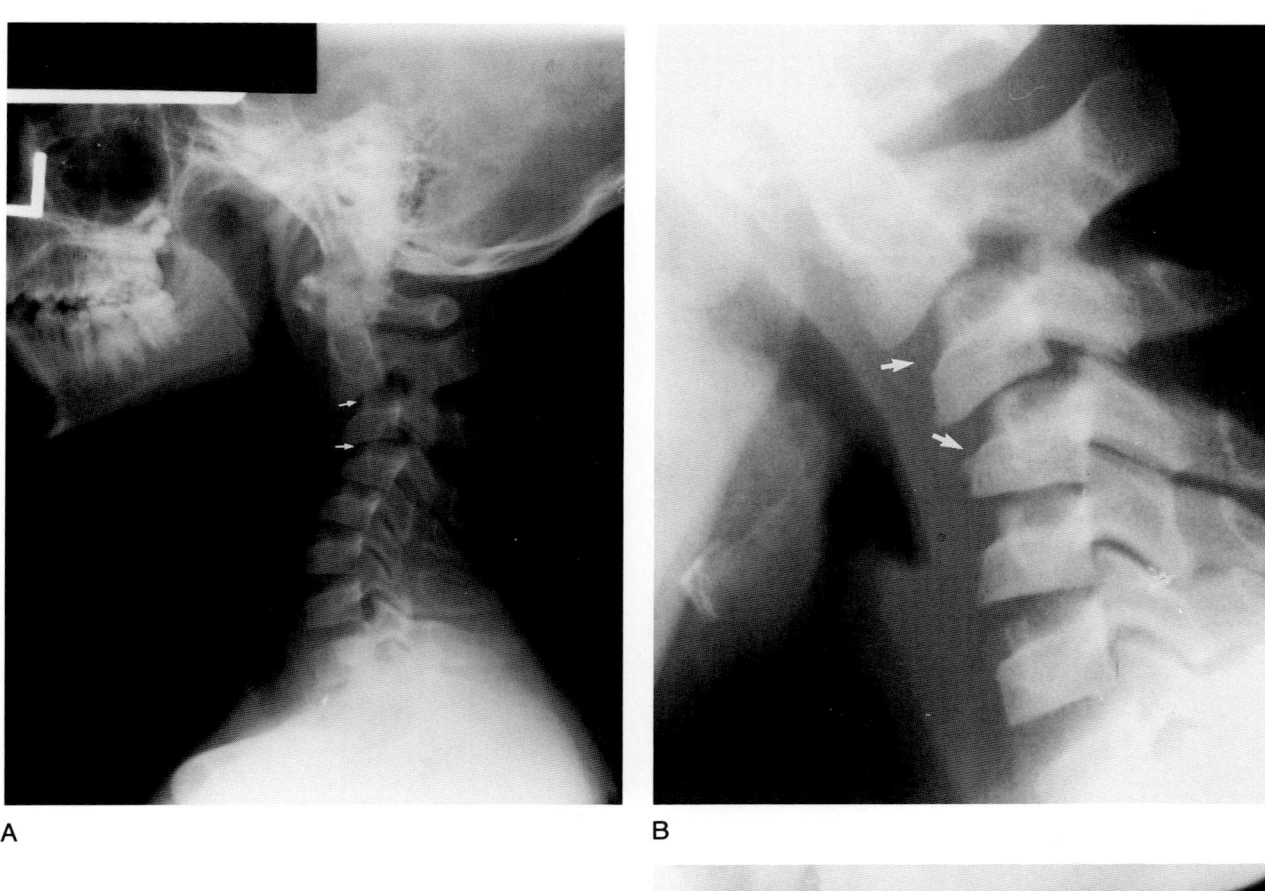

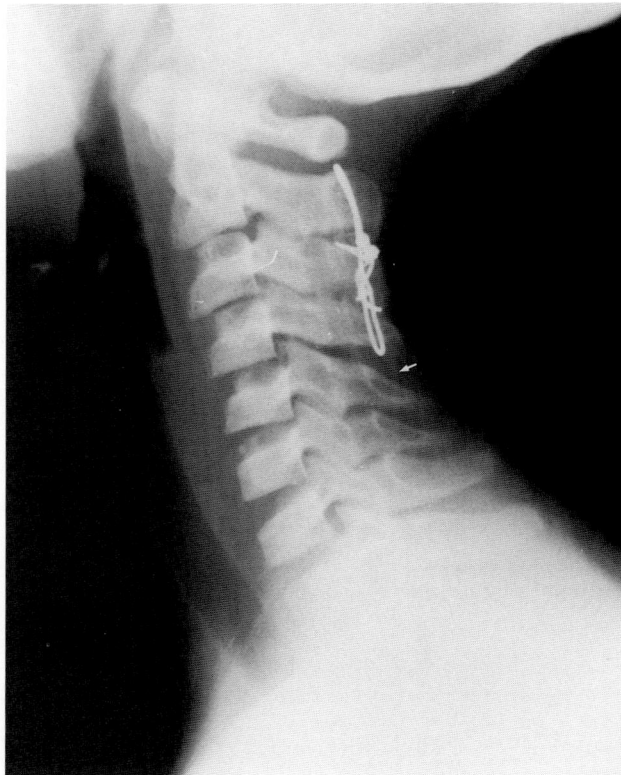

Fig. 45-6. (A&B) C2-C3 and C3-C4 instability with compression fracture of C4 in a 14-year-old boy due to a hyperflexion injury due to a dive into shallow water. **(C)** Postfusion C2-C4. Note slight creep of fusion mass to C5.

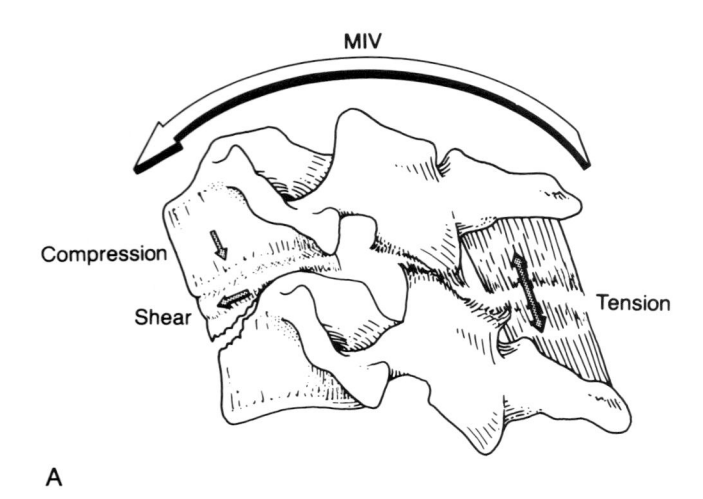

Fig. 41-7. **(A)** Diagrammatic representation of major injuring vector *(MIV)* mechanism of injury and the specific structures involved. **(B&C)** Fracture of superior ring of C7 secondary to hyperflexion injury of spinal cord in a 16-year-old boy sustained in a shallow dive. Note the importance of visualization of C7 by pulling down shoulders with arm traction in muscular teens. (Fig. A from White and Punjabi,[7] with permission.)

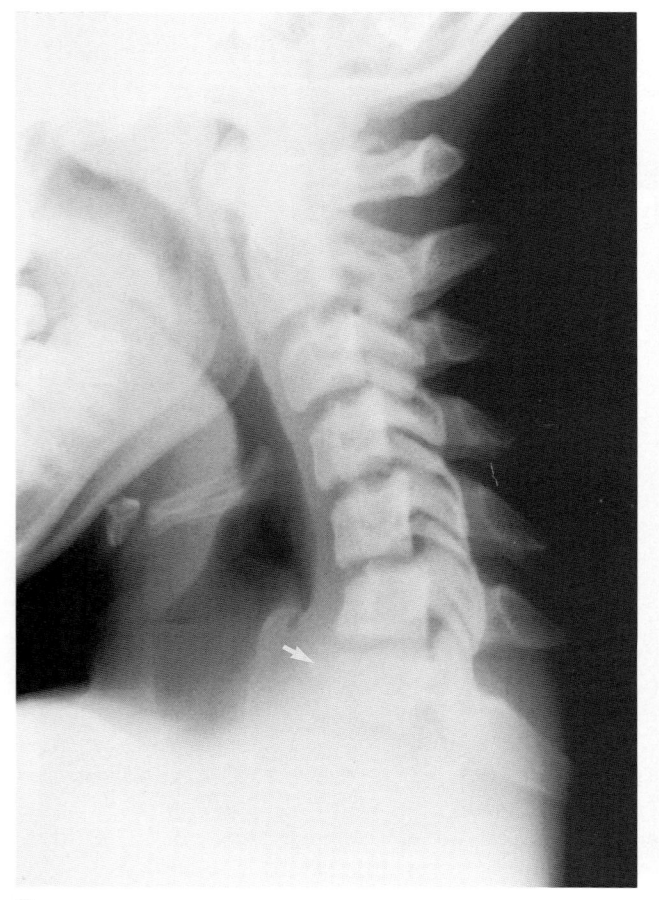

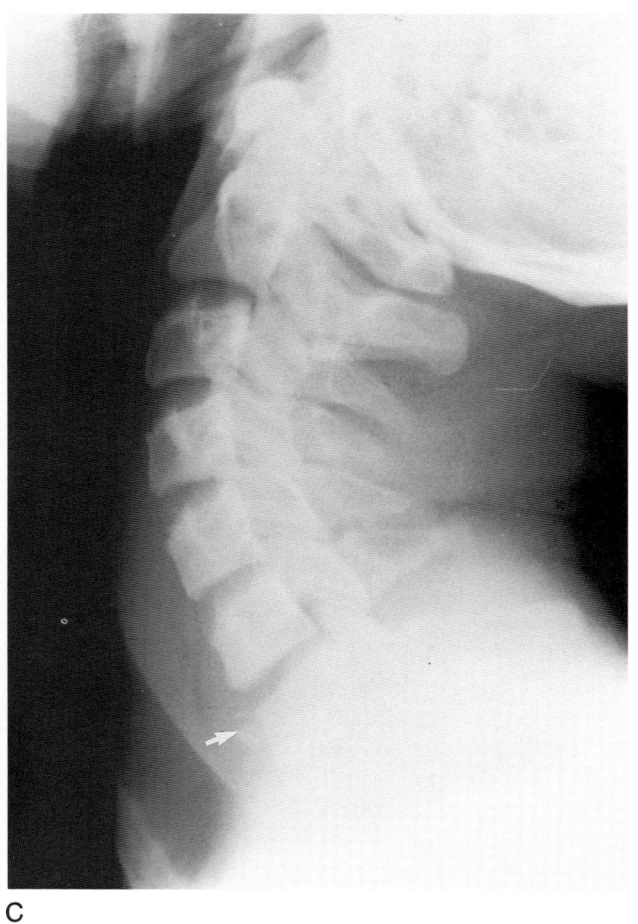

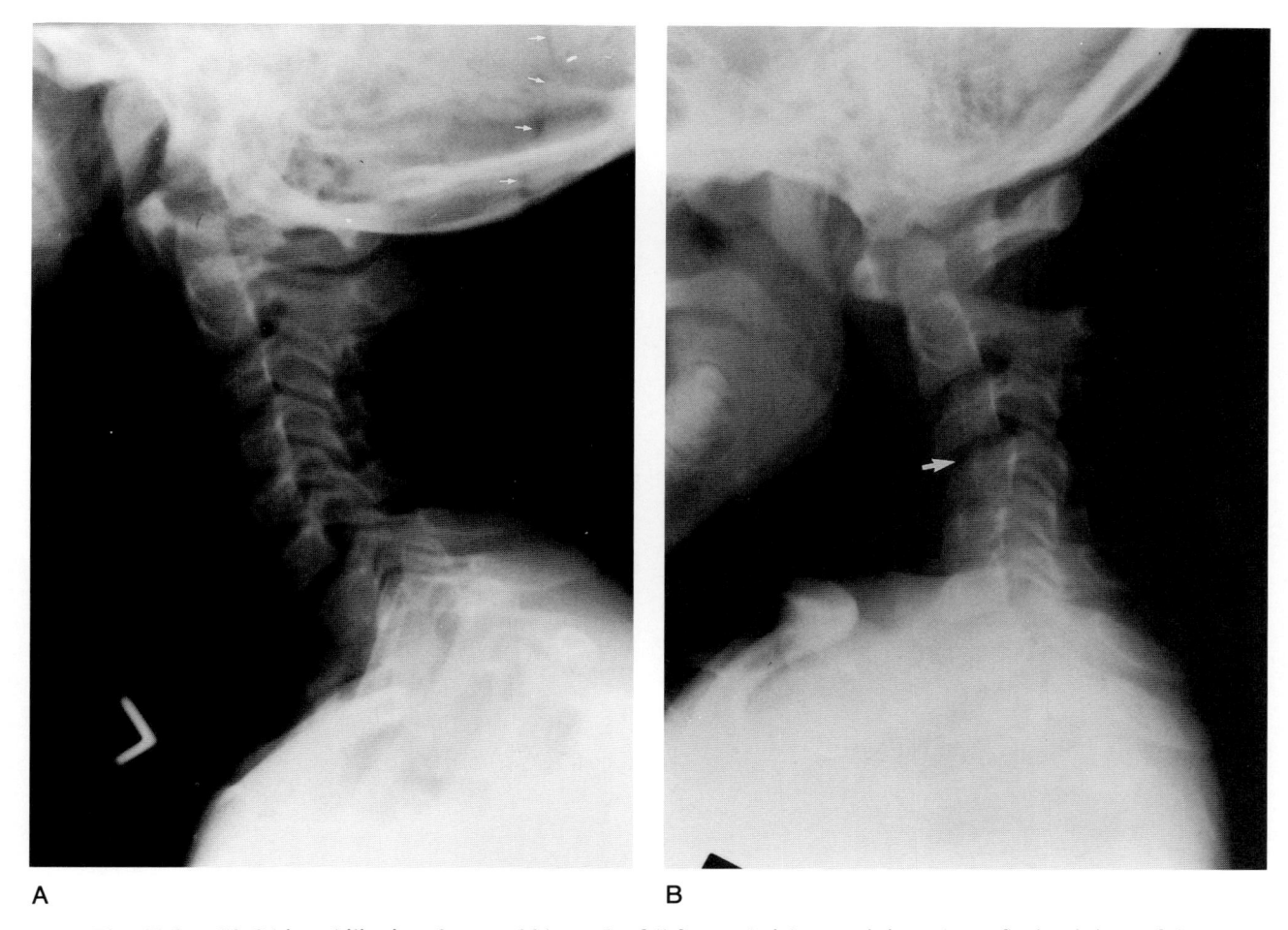

Fig. 45-8. C3-C4 instability in a 9-year-old boy who fell from a height sustaining a hyperflexion injury of the cervical spine. Note the fracture of the occiput which was associated with a laceration of the scalp. **(A)** Extension. **(B)** Flexion.

the standard fracture board, which will again allow the head to extend slightly. Failure to appreciate this anatomic difference between children and adults will stress the neck in flexion.

The extreme flexibility of the child makes attempts at undressing the child in the emergency department more hazardous than the same attempts in the adult. Restricting clothing should be cut away to allow appropriate examination. Examinations of the child in pain can be difficult. A neurologic examination must be attempted. Observation of movement is exceedingly important as is gentle testing of sensation. If the neck is to be stabilized, we prefer sandbags or similar bolsters on either side. If a halter must be used, extreme care must be taken not to overdistract the neck in the young child. If paraplegia or paraparesis is present, one must determine if it is complete or incomplete. Cord concussion can result in temporary paralysis. These lesions are rarely complete and therefore compulsive examination is required. Commonly spared functions are toe movement and sphincter tone. If a history is given of transient paralysis or paraparesis and the patient is now normal, one must identify the area of instability with appropriate imaging studies.

With the child stabilized from other injuries, and with the neck supported in line, and with as detailed a neurologic examination as possible having been completed and recorded, radiographic examination of the cervical spine can then proceed. In the adult, much controversy has arisen as to the number of radiographs required. In the child, visualization of C7 on the lateral film is usually not as difficult as in the adult. Routine antroposterior lateral and through the mouth views of the odontoid, are

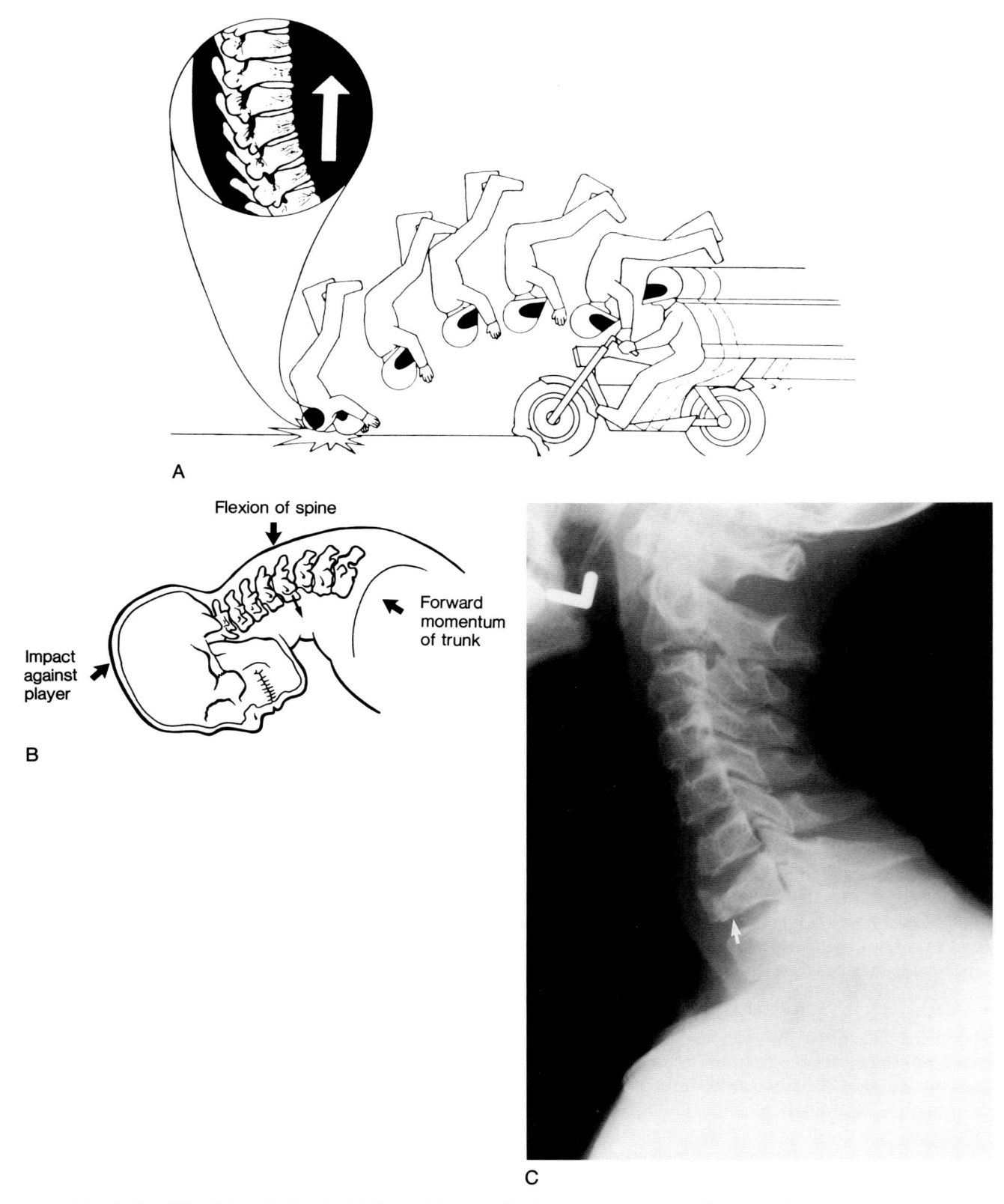

Fig. 45-9. (A) A fall on the head with the neck in some flexion tends to straighten the normal lordotic posture of the cervical spine predisposing the vertebrae to more direct compressive forces. (B) With the neck flexed, the normal lordosis is lost and compression injury to the middle and lower cervical vertebrae is facilitated as in a football "spearing" maneuver. (C) Compression fracture of C7 in a 14-year-old high-school lineman sustained during a high velocity impact tackle.

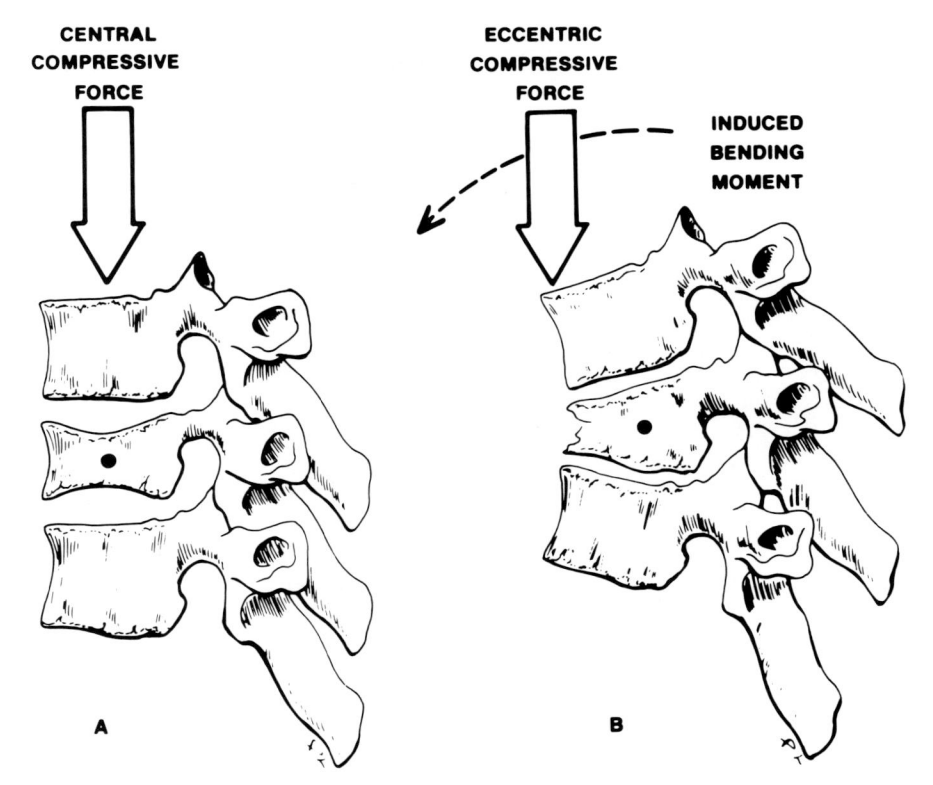

Fig. 45-10. Different configurations of fractures produced by compression. **(A)** A centrally located axial compressive force close the neutral axis (represented by the *black dot*) produces biconcave deformities of the endplate. **(B)** An eccentrically located force away from the neutral axis results in a greater bending moment and produces a compressive fracture of the body, with characteristic wedging. (From White and Panjabi,[7] with permission.)

usually sufficient. Of these radiographic views, the lateral is the most important. If the neck has a superimposed torticollis, then lateral views of the upper cervical spine are sometimes difficult to obtain. If the technician is instructed to take a lateral view of the base of the skull, this will assure a lateral view of C1 and possibly C2. This, plus a routine lateral view of the neck, should allow adequate visualization of all cervical levels.

RADIOGRAPHIC INTERPRETATION OF THE CERVICAL SPINE

When interpreting the cervical radiographs in the emergency department, one must be able to differentiate between normal variation, congenital anomaly, and true pathology. Unlike injuries in the extremities, contralateral views are not available (Fig. 45-11).

In normal development, the vertebrae from C3 to C7 have three ossification centers; one in the centrum, and a left and right neuroarch, which includes the posterior elements pedicle and the posterior corner of the body. Secondary ossification centers can stimulate injury, especially those at the tip of the spinous process, which may stimulate avulsion. In the seventh cervical vertebrae, occasionally a separate ossification center appears for each of the costal processes. This usually fuses with the rest of the transverse process by age 6, but it may remain separate and when large may become a cervical rib.[3] The secondary center at the tips of the spinous process does not usually fuse to the remainder of the process until age 16.

One of the most extensive reviews of normal cervical spine variations was carried out in 1965 by Cattell and colleagues.[9] The authors addressed two major areas, the first were changes in the alignment of the vertebrae due to displacement that simulated subluxation and were actually normal, and the second, were changes in the normal curvatures of the spine that simulated ligamentous injury and muscle spasm.

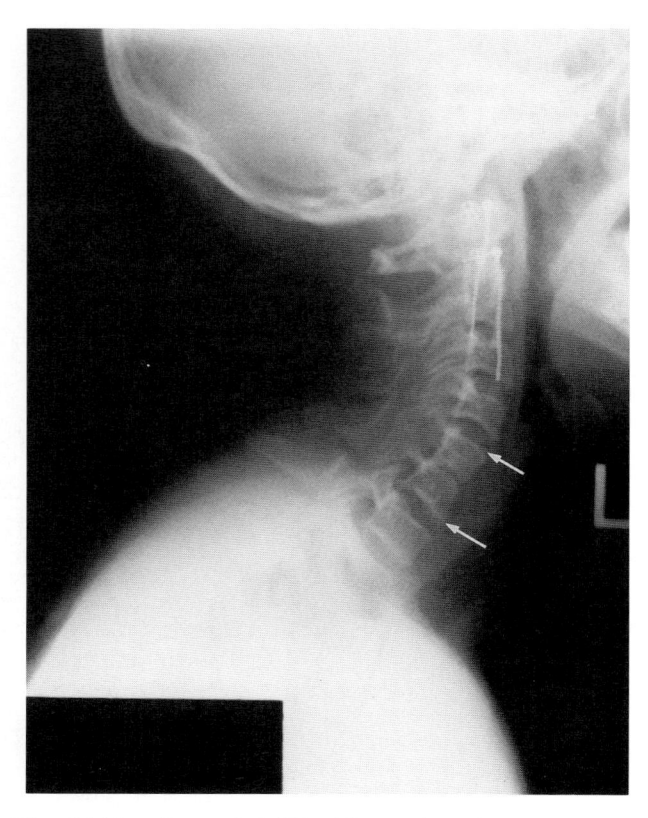

Fig. 45-11. Congenital "block" vertebrae in a 12-year-old gymnast who injured her neck in a tumbling accident. This partial fusion creates increased stress above and below the fused area.

The authors studied 160 normal children from ages 1 to 16. Of this group, 19 percent of the children ages 1 to 7 showed marked inferior displacement of C2 on C3, a further 21 percent showed moderate displacement for a total of 40 percent of children between the ages of 1 and 7 showing some pseudosubluxation of C2-C3 in flexion. In the total group aged 1 to 16 years, a marked displacement was seen in 9 percent and moderate in 15 percent for a total of 24 percent. When the authors measured all antroposterior movement of 3 mm and above, the finding were 44 percent of the entire group had displacement. Anterior displacement was also noted at C3-C4 in 14 percent of the entire group, and 20 percent of the subgroup ages 1 through 7. Of this group, over 90 percent had associated C2-C3 pseudosubluxation.

Absence of uniform angulation between adjacent vertebral segments in flexion and extension is often taken to be a sign of underlying soft tissue injury (see Fig. 44-2). In Cattell's group, angulation at a single level was seen in 16 percent of normal children. The absence of lordosis in the neutral position is also taken to be a sign of soft tissue injury, but is also present in 14 percent of normal children. A group of 16 percent of the normal children also showed straightening of the neck contour in flexion, which simulated splinting. Cattell and coworkers[9] attributed these findings to the above-mentioned combination of ligamentous laxity, relative horizontal inclination of facet joints, immature joints of Lushka, and the anterior wedge configuration of the developing vertebral body.

To further compound matters, although the uninjured spine can simulate injury in the child, absence of bony pathology is very common in the significant neck injury showing neurologic involvement. This is termed *Spinal Cord Injury without Radiographic Abnormality* (SCIWORA) (see Ch. 50).

In Burke's 1974 series,[2] reported in *Paraplegia,* 12 of 29 cord injuries showed no radiographic abnormality and a further 7 showed minimal bony injury. Aufdermaur[10] reported on the autopsies of 12 children with spinal cord injury who subsequently died. In only one case was there radiographic evidence of bony injury.

Postmortem examination of the cervical spine by the same author showed a split in the cartilaginous zone between the endplate and the vertebral body. O'Brien and coworkers[11] reporting on adult cervical spine following a fatal motor vehicle accident, showed separation of the cartilage endplates from the osseous endplate in those patients less than 23 years of age. In these 22 patients, the cause of death was cranial cerebral injury, and no apparent cervical injury was suspected.

The pathology of the injuries sustained without radiographic anomaly would suggest that these are distraction injuries (Figs. 45-12 and 45-13). Pathology is over several segments in the cord and is not focused in one area as might be seen with sudden angulation (Figs. 45-14 and 45-15). To return to the interpretation of the investigation, if the clinical symptoms persist, then more sophisticated imaging techniques may be needed, such as contrast-enhanced CT or magnetic resonance imaging.

Young children in motor vehicle accidents restrained by seat belts may also sustain flexion/distraction injuries of the cervical as well as the lumbar spine[12] (Fig. 45-4).

PITFALLS IN DIAGNOSIS

In 1982 Stauffer and Mazur[3] listed the most frequent pitfalls in the interpretation of the cervical injury in the child (Table 45-1). The difficulty in examining the child in pain, coupled with somewhat ambiguous radiographic findings, often leads to a management problem.

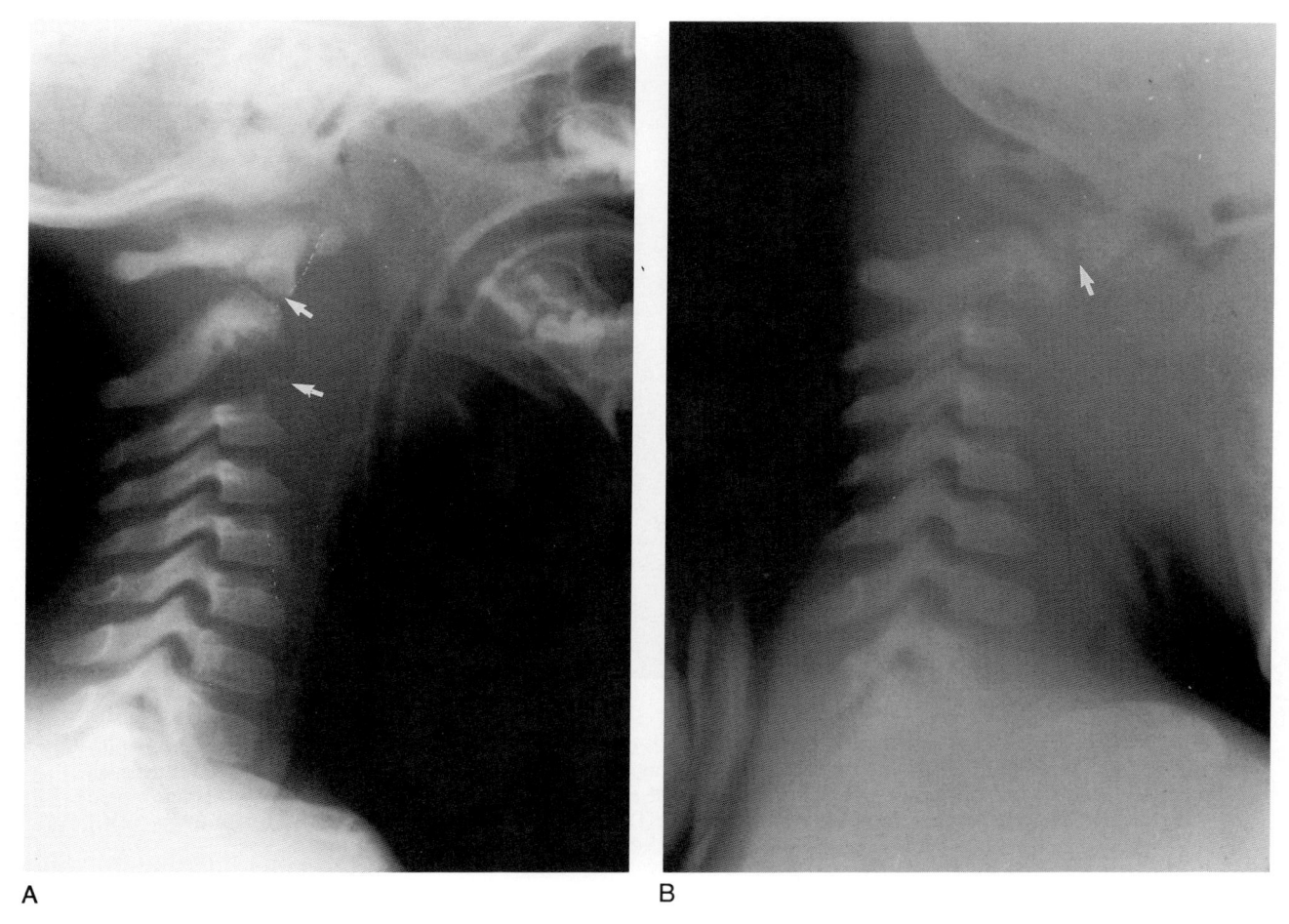

Fig. 45-12. **(A)** Postmortem extension and **(B)** flexion views of the cervical spine in a 1-year-old child with a fractured odontoid and C2-C3 fracture dislocation which resulted in a severed cord at C1. Note the marked separation between C2 and C3 in extension plus the avulsed realignment of C3 lying superiorly suggesting a primary extension distraction force.

Some diagnosis may have to be made in retrospect. The child with minimal findings and rapid resolution of the pain is obviously one in whom the presumed abnormal findings are probably radiographic variants of normal, whereas the child who has persistent pain, especially the child with a torticollis or decreased range of motion, must be vigorously investigated, even if the initial radiographic examination appeared normal.[5,13]

TABLE 45-1. Pitfalls in the Interpretation of Cervical Radiographs in Children

1. Children with neck pain believed to have traumatic subluxation of C2 on C3 vertebrae, which is later proven to be a normal range of motion.
2. Children thought to have fractures of the odontoid process which were later proven to have a vestigial basal or growth plate.
3. Children thought to have fractures of the atlas which failed to heal were found to be a failure of fusion of the ossification center.

TREATMENT

In the younger child under age 8 years, fractures of the middle and lower cervical segments will often show spontaneous fusion. Consequently, reduction and immobilization in traction followed by brace or halo cast is often all that is needed. These children should be followed to skeletal maturity both to assure stability and to document any growth disturbances. If follow-up radiographic examination shows instability, posterior fusion

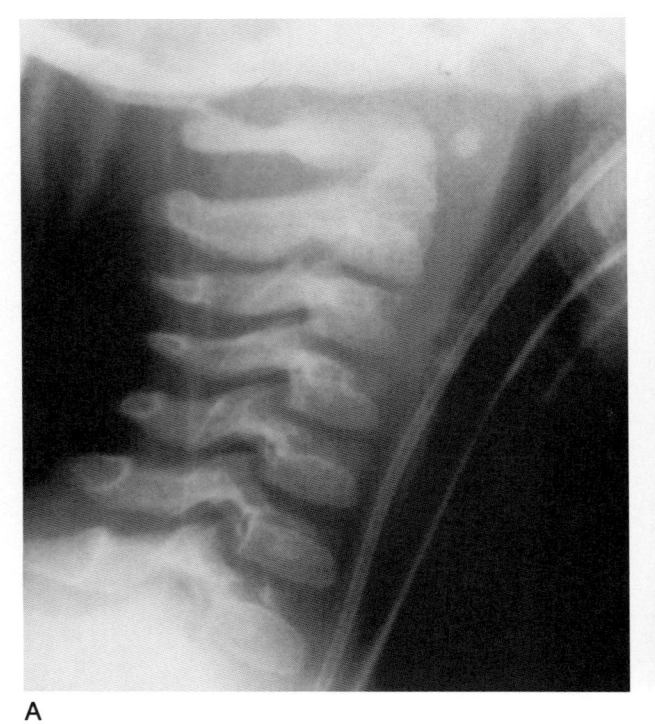

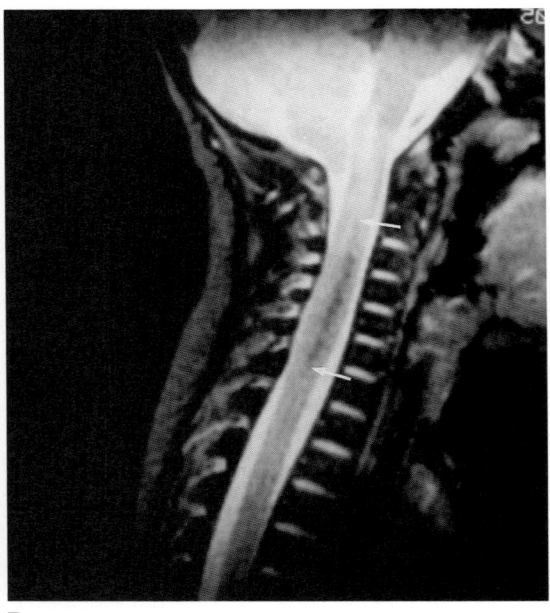

Fig. 45-13. This 17-month-old infant presented with quadraparesis secondary to violent shaking and child abuse. **(A)** The plain films of the cervical spine as well as cineradiography were normal. **(B)** The MRI illustrates cord substance injury extending over several cervical segments. There has been no recovery of neurologic function at 6 months postinjury. (Courtesy of Dr. Eric T. Jones, West Virginia University, Morgantown, WV.)

is indicated. Wire and graft fusion after the method of Dewar is usually appropriate.[14-16]

Posterior fusion alone is usually adequate (Fig. 45-4). In the younger child, where bone graft is difficult to obtain, subperiosteal dissection of the posterior 4 to 5 cm of one of the ribs will usually provide sufficient bone graft. In the older child, iliac crest graft is preferred.

In the adolescent, spontaneous fusion is uncommon, and in this group, instability following nonoperative treatment is probably more common than in the adult. Our practice is primary surgical stabilization in those adolescents who show significant instability (Fig. 45-16 and 45-17). In minor degrees of instability, conservative treatment with bracing followed by fusion if the neck still shows instability on flexion-extension radiographs at 12 weeks, is the management of choice (Fig. 45-16).

In the younger child with significant disruption of the cervical spine such as the child shown in Figure 45-4, instability compromises adequate nursing care. In these children, in the presence of a complete or partial cord lesion, immediate surgical stabilization will allow appropriate care in the intensive care unit and early mobilization. Early fusion will also protect the last functioning cervical nerve root.[1]

There is no demonstrable role for laminectomy in cervical spine injuries in the child. When performed in the young child, a postlaminectomy swan neck deformity can occur.

OBSTETRICAL CERVICAL SPINE INJURY

In Burke's series[2] of complete injuries, 5 of the 29 were birth injuries, and of these, 3 were injuries in the cervical spine, 1 in the midsegment and 2 in the lower segment. Again, tethering of the cord by the brachial plexus is thought to contribute to distraction injury in these children.

Cervical injury to children during delivery can occur in two situations, the first is traction during a breach delivery. The second is associated with intrauterine hyperextension of the head or, "the star-gazing fetus." If

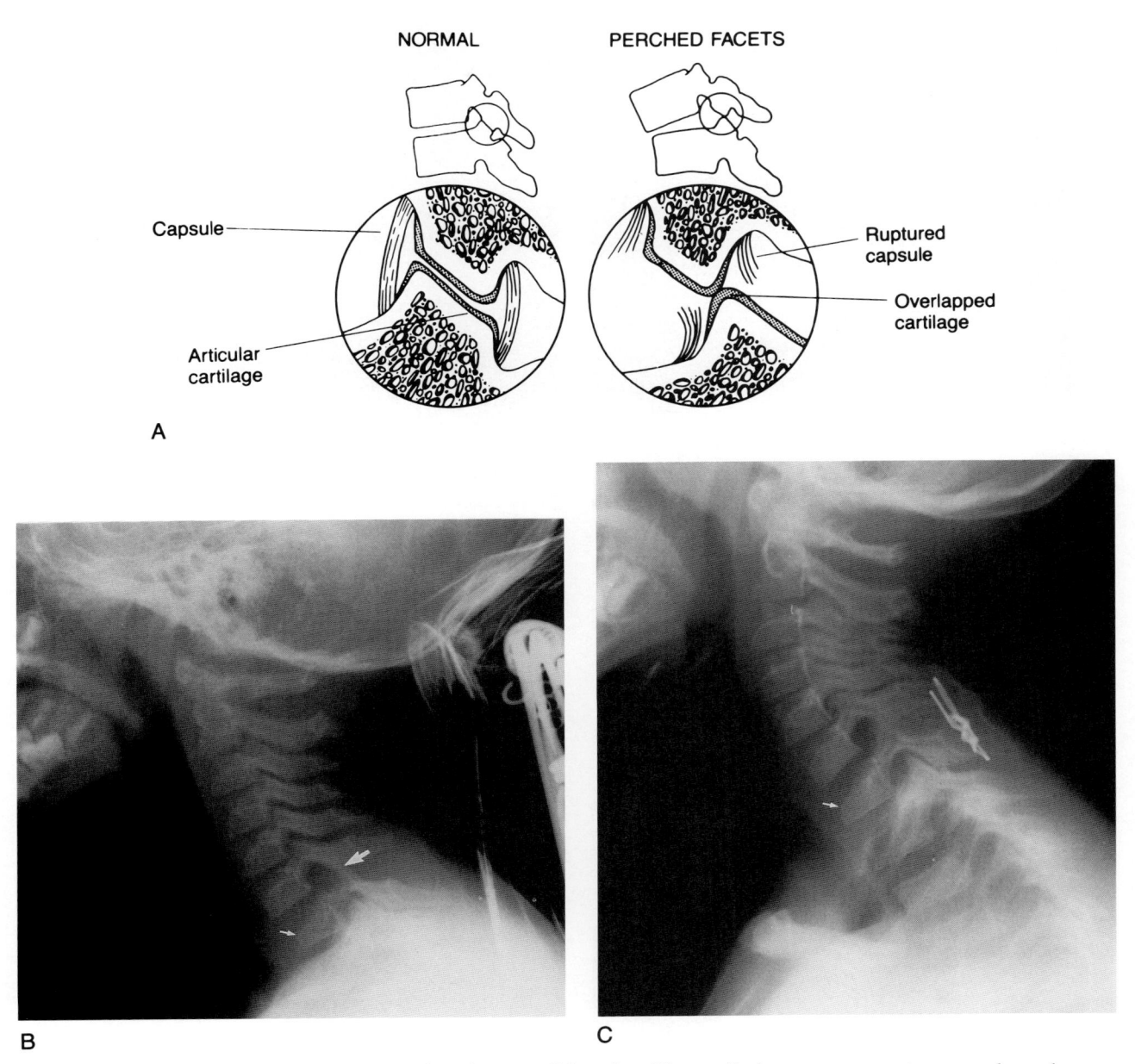

Fig. 45-14. **(A)** The so-called perched facet is a true dislocation. The cartilaginous components are overlapped and locked, as shown here. It appears on the radiograph as "perched" because the overlapped cartilage cannot be seen. **(B&C)** This 5-year-old girl fell from a snowmobile at high speed sustaining a hyperflexion injury of her cervical spine with a compression fracture of C7; disruption of the posterior ligamentous complex at C6-C7 resulting in persistent instability and perched facets but no cord damage. **(C)** A C6-C7 fusion provided permanent realignment and stability even though the facet remained perched. (Fig. A from White and Panjabi,[7] with permission.)

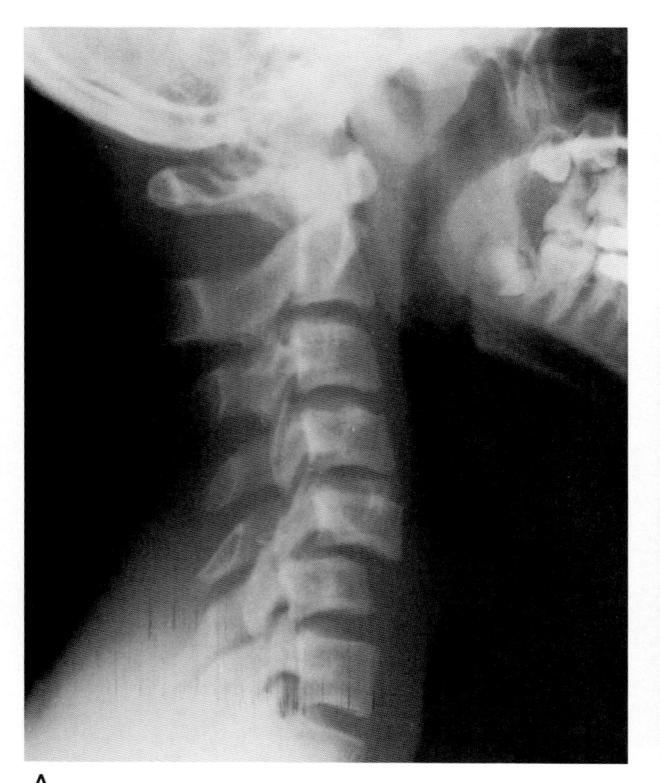

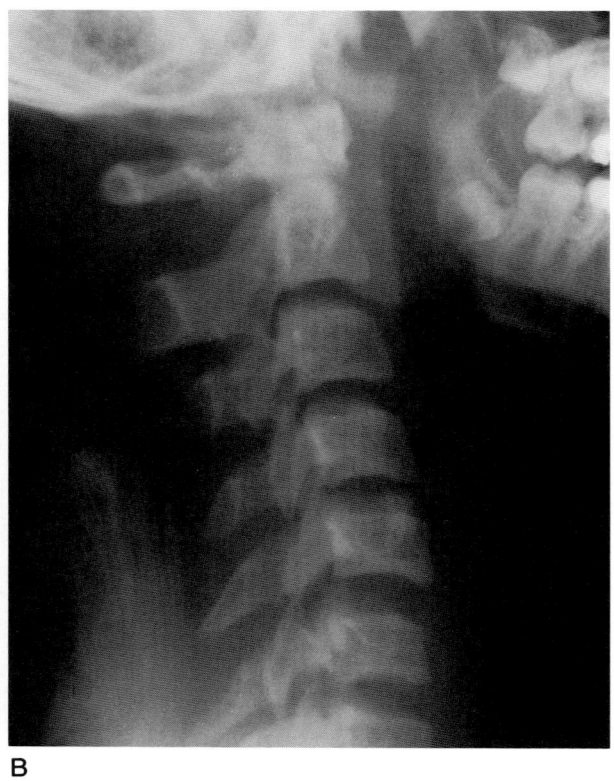

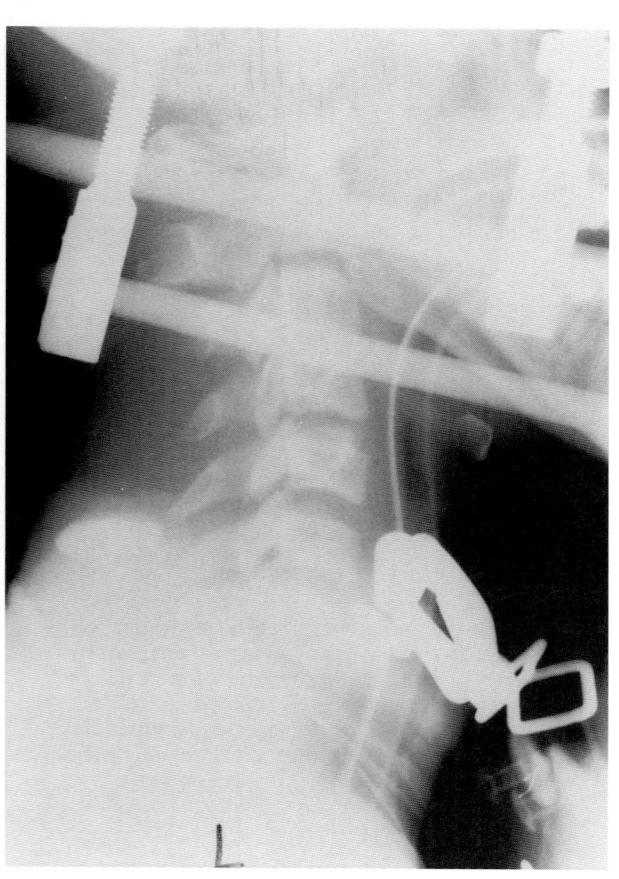

Fig. 45-15. (A) Hyperflexion injury in a 14-year-old boy which resulted in locked facets at C5-C6. (B) Halo traction improved this to perched facets. (C) Extension of the neck and application of a halo-vest reduced the facet dislocation.

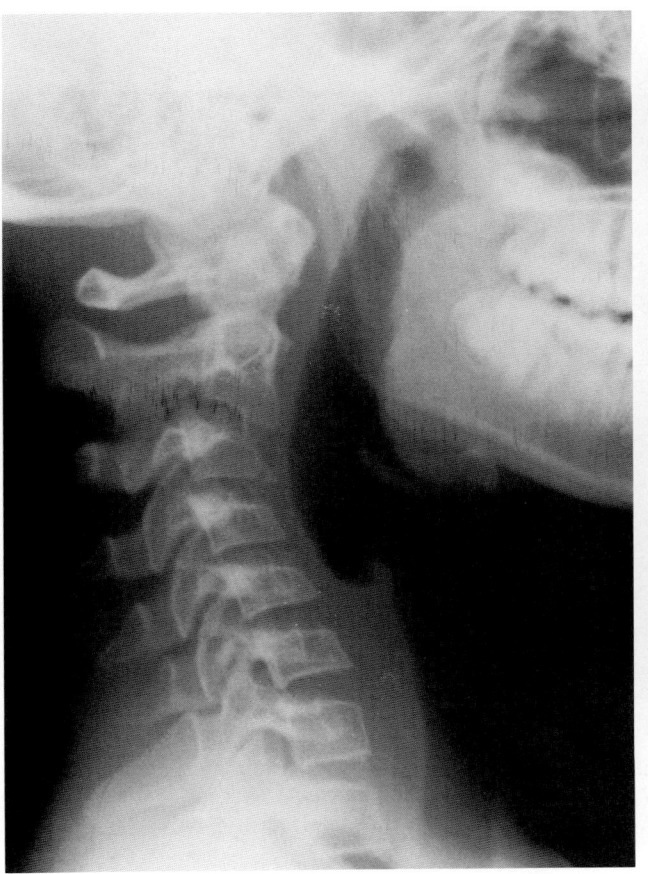

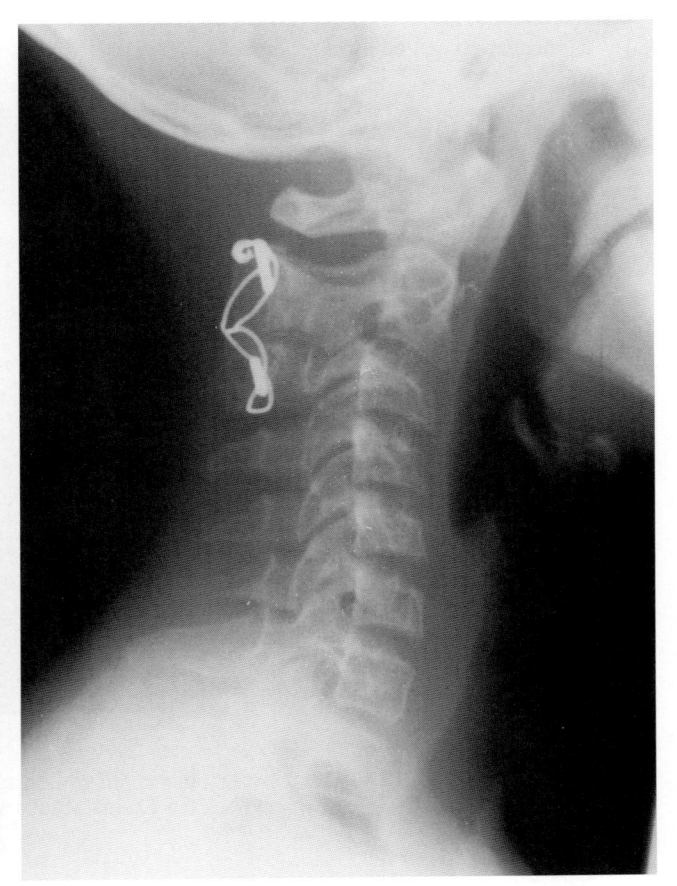

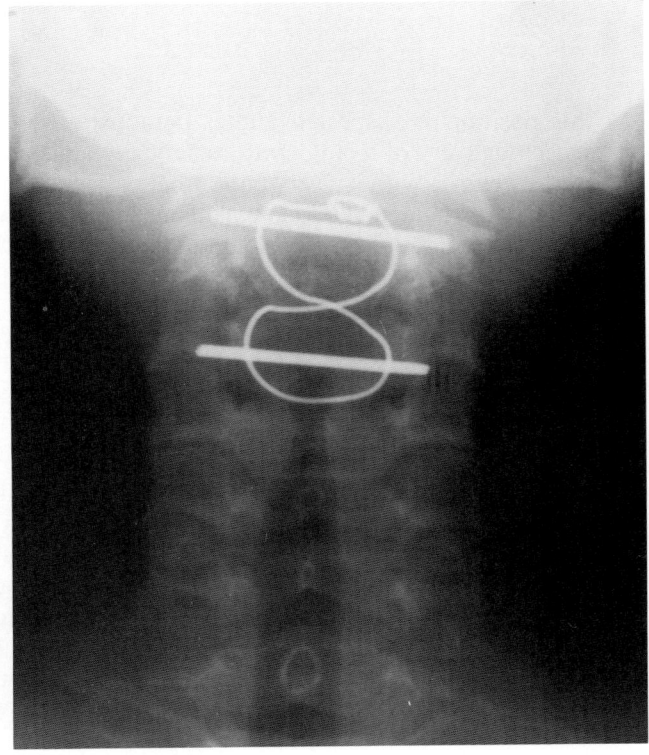

Fig. 45-16. (A) Flexion injury of the cervical spine in a 15-year-old boy which resulted in a rupture of the posterior ligamentous complex, compression of C3 vertebral body and a tear drop fracture of C3. (B&C) Poststabilization of C2-C3 using figure-of-8 wiring around K-wires inserted through the spinous process.

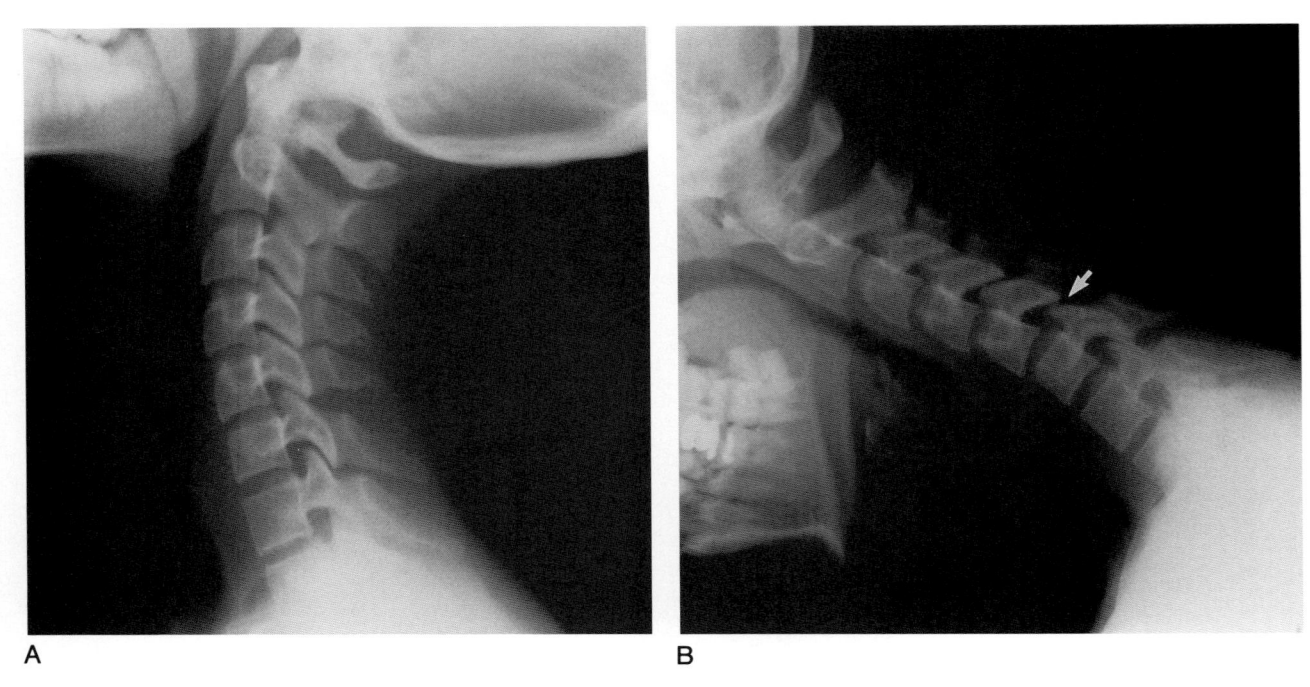

Fig. 45-17. (A) This 14-year-old girl fell while vaulting at a gymnastic competition sustaining acute hyperflexion of her cervical spine. (B) A C5-C6 instability was evident on flexion. *(Figure continues.)*

this position is suspected and is demonstrated, then breach delivery of a child with this hyperextension deformity carries with it a very poor prognosis with almost 25 percent incidence of significant neurologic injury.[3] Such patients should be considered for cesarian section.

PREEXISTING MALFORMATION OF THE CERVICAL SPINE

Congenital malformations of the cervical spine are not uncommon in children (Fig. 45-11). Not only may their presence cause confusion in the interpretation of a radiograph taken to ascertain injury in the traumatized cervical spine, but they also may predispose and facilitate such an injury. Children with decreased motion in some cervical segments due to congenital fusion, such as in the Klippel-Feil syndrome may be hypermobile in adjacent segments. Hyperflexion or hyperextension will focus stress at these more mobile areas creating an increased risk for injury.

SUMMARY

Fractures of the middle and lower segments of the cervical spine in children are more common in children over age 8 as the cervical spine becomes more mature. Prior to that age C1-C2 injuries are the most common. There are many anatomic pitfalls that suggest injury to the cervical spine in the lower segments, such as the wedged appearance of the vertebrae, pseudosubluxation at C2-C3, C3-C4, and the ossifying endplates. Because of the marked ligamentous laxity of the pediatric cervical spine, locked facets may be encountered. As the spine becomes more mature, compression fractures of the lower cervical vertebrae are more frequently encountered in injuries in which the cervical spine is slightly

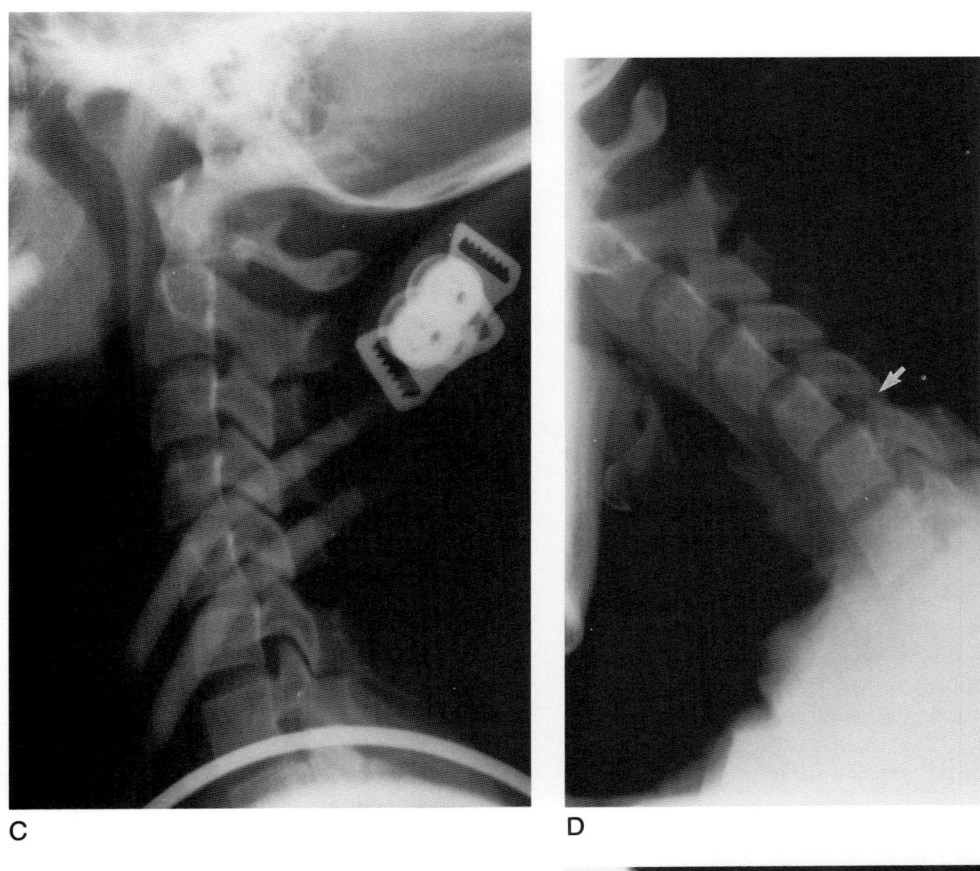

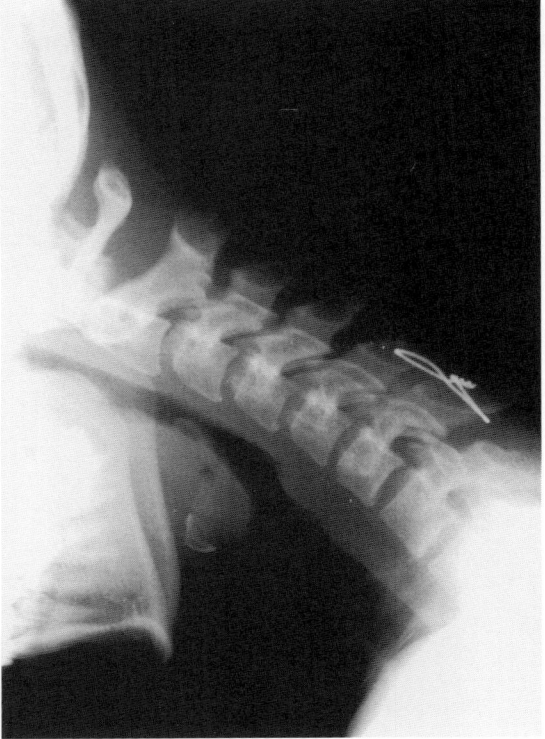

Fig. 45-17 *(Continued).* **(C)** She was treated for 3 months in a four-poster cervical orthosis, **(D)** but the instability persisted. **(E)** A C5-C6 fusion provided permanent alignment and stability. (Courtesy of Dr. Jay Jarvis, Children's Hospital of Eastern Ontario, Ottawa, Canada.)

flexed. This allows the cervical vertebrae to be lined up in a straight column, which transmits force to the vertebral bodies more efficiently and effectively, often resulting in burst fractures. Ligamentous instability of the posterior ligamentous complex is also seen in teenagers and necessitates stabilization by posterior spinal fusion of the unstable cervical components. Cervical spine injuries in children are uncommon but are potentially devastating when they occur. A good knowledge of the developing cervical spine is necessary to assist in the accurate diagnosis of cervical spine trauma in the pediatric age group. Surgical stabilization to ensure stability of the cervical spine is equally as important in children as in the skeletally mature.

REFERENCES

1. Crawford AH: Operative treatment of spine fractures in children. Orthop Clin North Am 21:326, 1990
2. Burke DC: Traumatic spinal paralysis in children. Paraplegia 11:268, 1974
3. Stauffer ES, Mazur JM: Cervical spine injuries in children. Pediatr Ann 11:502, 1982
4. Ehara S, El-Khoury GY, Satoy Y: Cervical spine injury in children: radiographic manifestations. AJR 151:1175, 1988
5. Dietrich AN, Ginn-Pease ME, Bartkowski HM, King DR: Paediatric cervical spine fractures: predominantly subtle presentation. J Paediatr Surg 26:995, 1991
6. Fuchs S, Bartel MJ, Flannery AM, Christoffel KK: Cervical spine fractures sustained by young children in forward facing car seats. J Paediatr 84:348, 1989
7. White AA, Punjabi MM: Practical biomechanics of spine trauma. p. 169. In: Clinical Biomechanics of the Spine. 2nd Ed. JB Lippincott, Philadelphia, 1990
8. Herzenberg JE, Hensinger RN, Dedrick DK, Philipps WA: Emergency transport and positioning of young children who have an injury of the cervical spine. J Bone Joint Surg [Am] 71:15, 1989
9. Cattell HS, Filtzer DL: Pseudo subluxation and other normal variations of the cervical spine in children. J Bone Joint Surg [Am] 47:1295, 1965
10. Aufdermaur M: Spinal injuries in juveniles, neuropsy findings in twelve cases. J Bone Joint Surg [Br] 56:513, 1974
11. O'Brien JP, Jonson H, Rauchning W: Whiplash injury of the cervical spine. Presented at the annual meeting of the British Orthopaedic Association, Sept. 1991
12. Conry BG, Hall CM: Cervical spine fracture and rear car seat restraints. Arch Dis Child 62:1267, 1987
13. Fesmire FM, Luten RC: The paediatric cervical spine. J Emerg Med 11:133, 1989
14. Simmons EH, Bernstein AJ, Capicotto WN, Simmons ED: The Dewar posterior cervical fusion. Presented at the ninth combined meeting of the Orthopaedic Association of the English Speaking World, June 21, 1992
15. Sherk HH, Schut L, Lane JN: Fractures and dislocations of the cervical spine in children. Orthop Clin North Am 7:593, 1976
16. Holmes JC, Hall JE: Fusion for instability and potential instability of the cervical spine in children and adolescents. Orthop Clin North Am 9:923, 1978

46

Fractures and Dislocations of the Thoracolumbar Spine

Rudolph A. Klassen

> Facts do not cease to exist because they are ignored.
> —ALDOUS HUXLEY

DESCRIPTION AND INCIDENCE

North America probably has the highest rate of vertebral column and spinal cord injuries in all age groups. The precise incidence of these injuries in children has not been assessed. Most series of patients relate to those who were hospitalized and actively treated.[1-12] It is estimated that approximately 50 percent of the children with these severe injuries die at the scene of the accident or shortly thereafter and, therefore, are not well tabulated.[13-15] It is also estimated that between 0.65 and 9.25 percent of all spinal injuries occur in children. About 40 to 60 percent are in the cervical area. Children under the age of 10 are most frequently injured secondary to falls from height or motor vehicle accidents. Older children's injuries are the results of sports and recreational activities and motor vehicle accidents. In the age group 2 to 12 the highest incidence of injuries is between ages 7 and 9. The incidence then rises very rapidly after the age of 13 to 16. In the thoracic and lumbar spine the upper thoracic vertebrae T4 to T10 are more frequently injured than the lower thoracic. The thoracolumbar junction, T12 to L2, is the next most frequently injured.[16-18] One series, however, reported that the area between T7 and T10 was most frequently injured.[19]

Multiple level vertebral fractures are common and in the series of Hegenbarth and Ebel[19] 80 percent had multiple lesions (Fig. 46-1). The incidence of a neurologic deficit is reported higher in children than in adults in some series and equal in others.[20-22]

FRACTURE CHARACTERISTICS AND VERTEBRAL MATURATION

The effect of maturation of the skeleton and the cord and their relationships as to the outcome of trauma is unknown. However, a temporal relationship does exist between the radiologic evidence of maturation and clinical manifestations.[20,23] It is noted that the younger child has more upper cervical ligamentous lesions, and this diminishes with maturation. The adult spine morphology is usually seen at about age 11. In the series of Dickman and coworkers,[21] of 38 patients with thoracolumbar spine injuries ages 0 to 8, 35 had complete neurologic deficit, and 3 were incomplete. The 5 that were in the lumbar region 1 was complete and 4 were incomplete. In the group ages 9 to 16, there were 12 thoracic injuries, 6 had complete neurologic deficit and 6 were incomplete.

There were three lumbar lesions, one was complete and two incomplete.[21]

Fracture characteristics change with vertebral maturation.[23] Young children may sustain apophyseal separation, growth plate fractures, and spinal cord injuries without evidence of fractures. Adolescents more frequently have adult pattern injuries with burst fractures, fracture dislocations, and limbus fractures[24-30] (Fig. 46-1). In the Mayo Clinic registry from 1976 to 1990, 156 children were treated with spine injuries of the thoracic and lumbar spine: 99 (64 percent) were compression fractures, primarily thoracic, 41 (26 percent) were fracture dislocations, and 16 (10 percent) were burst fractures. The age ranges were from 3 to 16, the majority being from age 14 to 16. There was almost an equal ratio of male to female patients in the compression and fracture dislocations, whereas in the burst fractures the male to female ratio was 2:1. All of the burst fractures occurred in children ages 14 to 16 and the majority of fracture dislocations also occurred in this age range (R.A. Klassen, unpublished observations).

ANATOMY

The spinal lesion that occurs is dependent on the mechanism of injury and the stage of maturation of the child.[31-34] The ligaments in young children are initially more elastic than the adults. The supporting musculature is smaller and immature. The bone is well mineralized. Intervertebral discs are healthy, well hydrated, and have strong annular fibers. Bone growth is both enchondral and appositional so initially there is a greater cartilage to bone ratio. Vertebral morphology changes with maturation. The facets are initially more horizontal and incompletely ossified and gradually achieving mature configuration by about age 8. Full adult morphologic patterns are not manifested until about age 15. Each vertebra has two ossification centers for the neural arch and one for the centrum. The neural arches fuse at ages 2 to 6 and radiographically may have an appearance of a spina bifida occulta or could also be confused as a vertical linear fracture. The spinal canal achieves a mature diameter size before longitudinal growth is complete. This is probably the reason for a fracture with spinal cord sparing despite significant encroachment of the canal in some burst fractures or dislocations. The vertebral bodies, particularly in the thoracic area, initially appear somewhat wedge shaped because of complete enchondral ossification. The ring apophyses appear as separate ossification centers about age 8 to 12 and mature and close at about age 21 to 25. They do not contribute to vertebral growth as such. The disk, annular fibers, and anterior and posterior ligamentous fibers, however, attach to the ring apophyses and avulsion of this structure or its mature limbus can occur.[35]

Vertebral morphology growth and development depends, as do all skeletal structures, partially on physical stresses applied to them.[36] Therefore, in a child with a paralyzed trunk we will note that the vertebrae are longer and narrower as compared to the normal spine. The developing spine has a significant capacity to remodel and this is best noted in the vertebral body which has undergone a compression fracture and may regain it's height, particularly in the young person. This capacity is, however, limited, and if the wedge is greater than about 20 to 30 degrees it may well not fully reconstitute itself. Vascular channels can be noted in the young child anteriorly and posteriorly and may be present for some time and should not be confused with fractures in this area. Severe vertebral injury may also result in avascular necrosis of the vertebral body preventing reconstitution of the spine. The disk is a very firm structure with dense annular fibers and is much more resistant to injury than the vertebral body. With compression or bursting injury of the vertebral body the disk will compress itself into the vertebral body. The vertebral body with its very vascular and cancellous centrum will also act as a shock absorber and absorb some of the shock before compressing or bursting.[37]

MECHANISM OF INJURY

The most common vertebral injury is compression fracture due to hyperflexion. Burst fractures and subluxations, dislocations, and avulsions are much less common. The disc is more resistent to injury than the vertebral body. Roaf demonstrated that with axial loading the spine and the vertebrae will initially bulge, while the disk will demonstrate little change. With more pressure the endplates will fracture with implosion of the disk into the vertebral body giving a radiographic appearance of thinning of the disk space.[37] Following trauma the narrowed disc space radiographically may also represent an extrusion of the disc into the canal and must be considered if there is a neurologic deficit or a progressive one. The force can be transmitted to several disk spaces. When shear forces occur the separation is again not through the disc but usually through the endplate, ligament, or osseous structures.

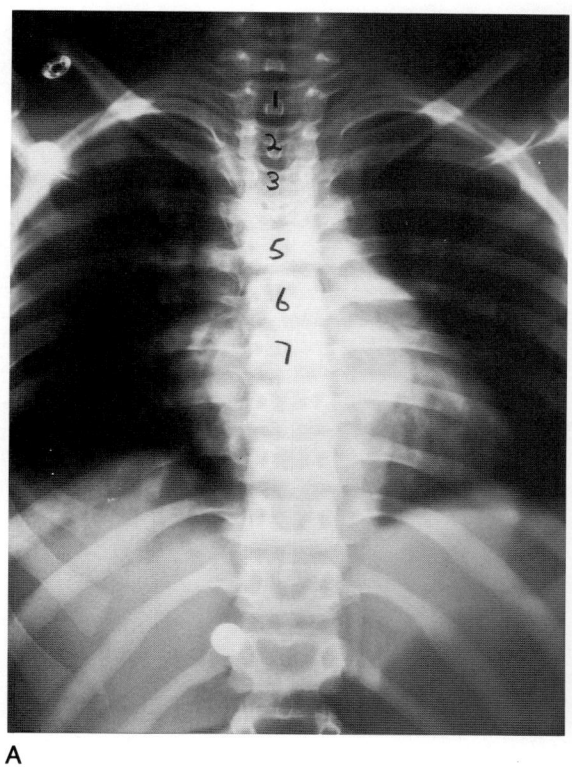

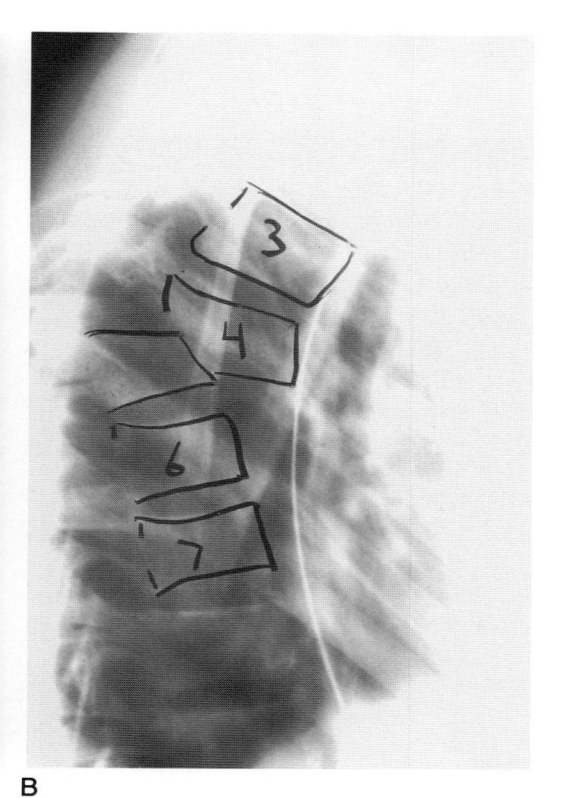

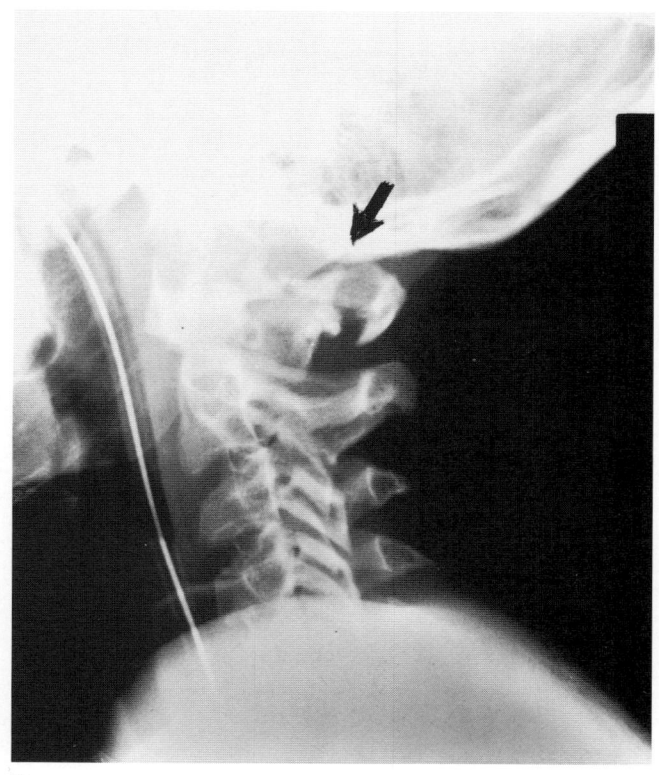

Fig. 46-1. (A) This 13-year-old boy was a passenger in a motor vehicle accident. He had a T4-T5 fracture dislocation with spinal cord transection and also a C2 hangman's fracture. (B) Fracture dislocation of T4-T5. T4 rib was locked and T5 reduction was achieved with distraction and unlocking of the rib followed by reduction. Most of these patients die at the scene of the accident. (C) Associated hangman's fracture C2, treated with halo brace. *(Figure continues.)*

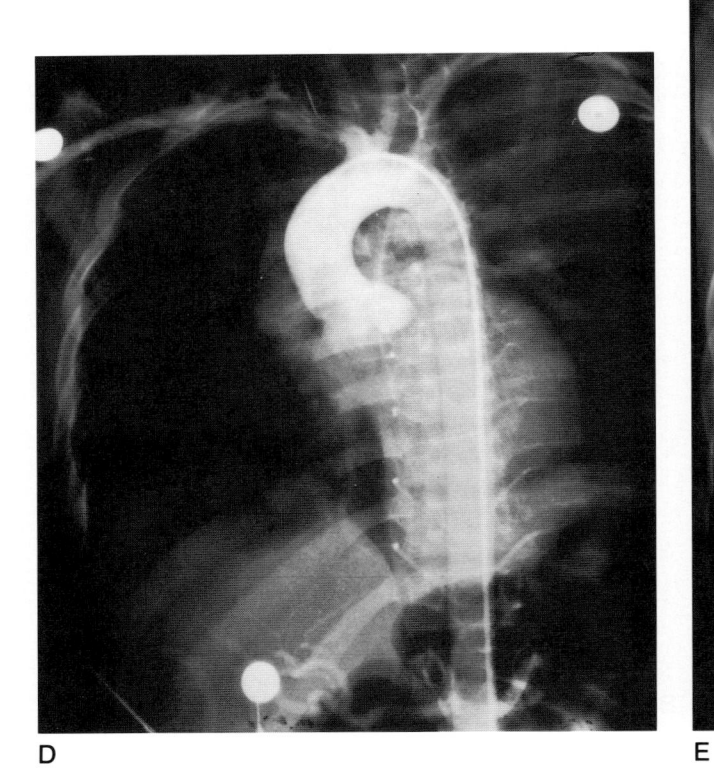

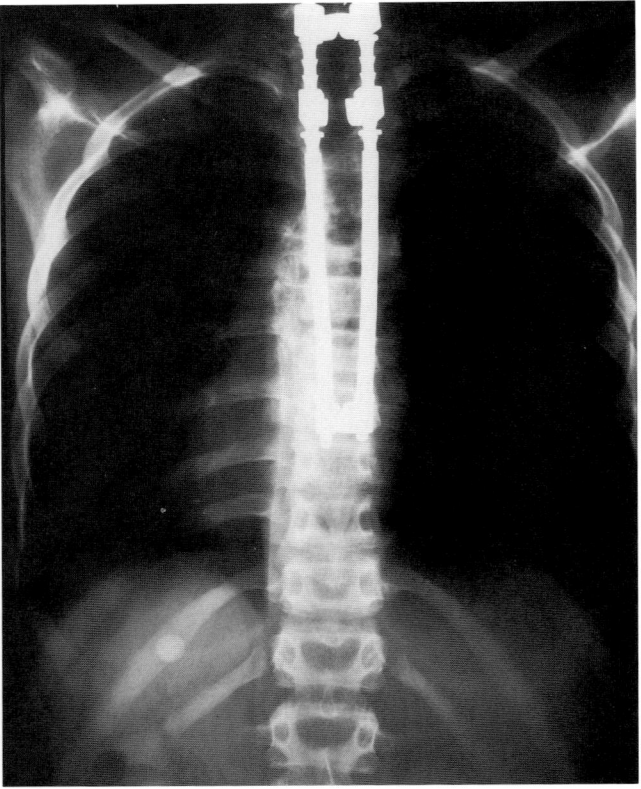

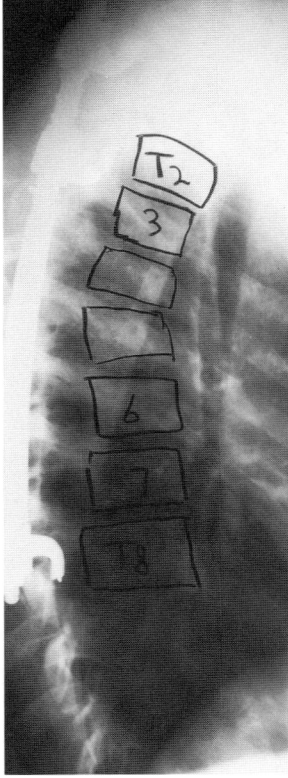

Fig. 46-1 *(Continued).* **(D)** The aorta was evaluated because of the widened mediastinum. **(E)** Open reduction and fixation with Harrington rods. The C2 fracture was stabilized with a halo cast. **(F)** Open reduction of T4-T5 fracture-dislocation. A 30-degree thoracolumbar scoliosis developed but did not require any additional fusion. *(Figure continues.)*

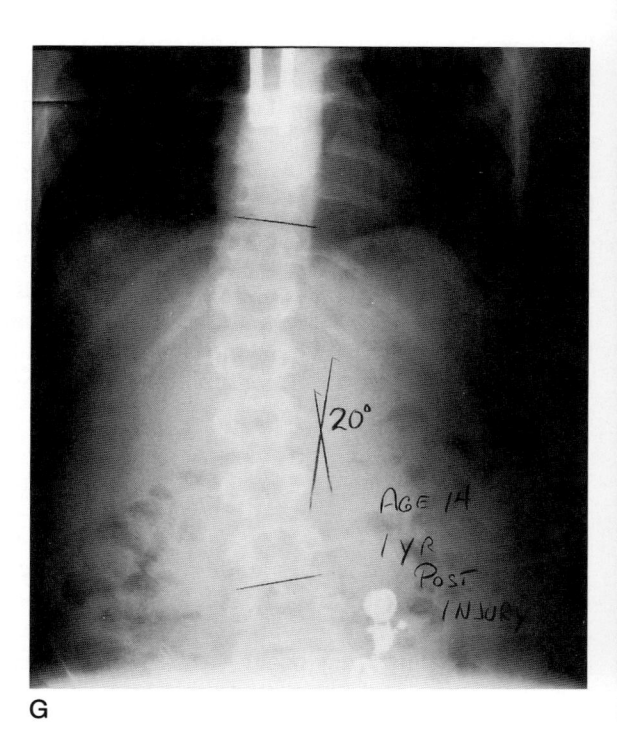

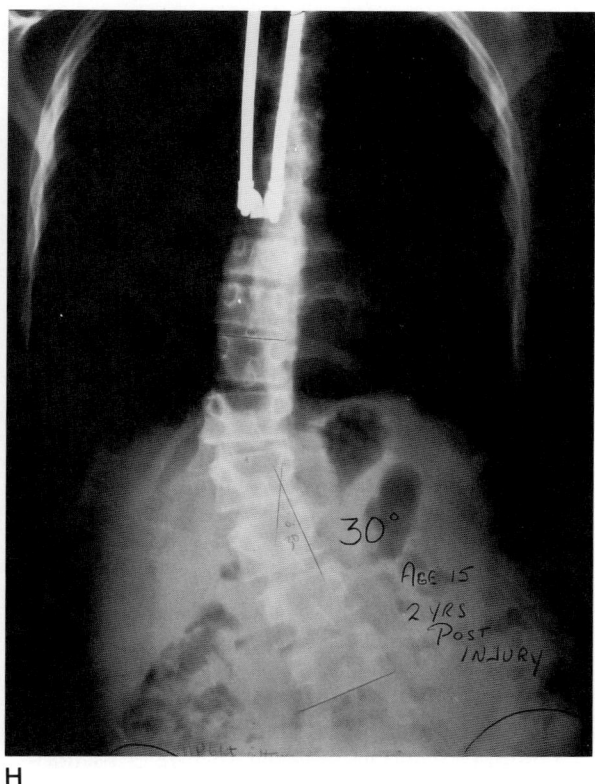

Fig. 46-1 *(Continued).* **(G)** Spinal deformity secondary to T4 paraplegia. **(H)** Progressive scoliosis, 2 years postinjury; 30-degree deformity.

CLASSIFICATION

Denis[38] has noted that burst fractures occur with compression through the anterior and middle columns, whereas fracture dislocations occur through compression, rotation, and shear of the anterior column, and distraction and rotation shear of the middle column, and distraction and rotation shear through the posterior column. A burst fracture can occur with pure axial loading, axial load and flexion, axial load and rotation, or axial load and lateral flexion or combinations of the above (Fig. 46-2). Denis classified these fractures as types A, B, C, D, and E. Types A, B, and C are best evaluated with a lateral view and D and E with an AP view.[38]

Fracture dislocations usually occur with flexion and rotation or shearing. Shearing may occur in either the AP, lateral, or oblique directions or through flexion and distraction. The endplates may still be quite cartilaginous, and when these forces are applied the fractures and separations occur through the cartilaginous endplates or ligamentous and osseous structures. Denis' evaluation[38] was made on the analysis of adult fractures; however, the mechanisms probably apply to children and adolescents as well (Figs. 46-3 to 46-7).

Fractures of the limbus of the vertebral body may be due to trauma or inherent weakness of the limbus (Figs. 46-8 to 46-10). They may occur traumatically or atraumatically. This may be due to the fragmentation of the limbus, which becomes avulsed by chronic pressure or by actual trauma, such as hyperextension or hyperflexion, with impingement of the disk against the endplate.[24-25,28-30,39]

PHYSICAL EXAMINATION

Physical findings are dependent on the age of the patient, the degree of trauma, and associated injuries. Birth trauma with fractures of the upper thoracic spine and fracture dislocations of the upper thoracic spine have been reported. In this instance, it may be difficult to note any physical findings except for neurologic deficits

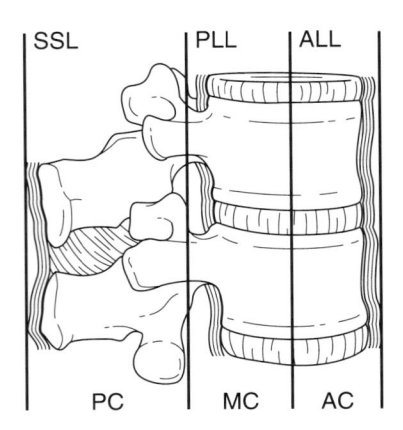

Fig. 46-2. Anterior, middle, and posterior column complexes. *AC*, anterior column: *ALL*, anterior longitudinal ligament; anterior annulus fibrosis and anterior vertebral body. *MC*, middle column: *PLL*, posterior longitudinal ligament; posterior annulus fibrosis and posterior vertebral body. *PC*, posterior column: *SSL*, supraspinous ligament; supraspinous to interspinous ligaments, ligamentum flavum, joint capsule, and posterior bony arch. (Adapted from Denis,[38] with permission.)

if they are present. If the infant has pain, it may not wish to move voluntarily and assume the posture of pseudoparalysis. It may be possible to elicit some localized tenderness. The history of the delivery is important. The diagnosis of the injury may be elicited with the use of magnetic resonance imaging and somatosensory evoked potentials. Most of the severe spinal injuries, however, occur in the older child with multiple injuries who often cannot provide a good history. It has been estimated that about 50 percent of children with severe spinal trauma die at the scene of the accident and there is about 20 percent mortality following acute phase because of associated injuries. Therefore, it must be assumed that a child with multiple injury may have a spinal injury until proven otherwise. Care must be taken in resuscitation efforts to protect the spine with appropriate transport systems.

The comatose or obtunded and neurologically deficited patient presents difficult diagnostic problems.[26] Head, chest, and abdominal injuries must be quickly assessed and localizing neurologic findings noted. Bruising such as from a seat or shoulder belt or the back of a seat, localized tenderness over the spine, defects in the interspinous ligaments or an interspinous process step off on palpation are indicative of a structural spine injury. If there are no neurologic deficits, one must still assume that there could be a spinal injury until full radiographic assessment has been made. This may be technically difficult with severe injuries. A critical evaluation of a good AP radiographic view will demonstrate asymmetry of the spinal structures indicating an injury. Narrowing of the vertebral body, widened interpediculate space, and malalignment of the spinous process are all indicative of skeletal injury. Major rotational changes are readily seen (Fig. 46-3). If direct axial loading, hyperextension, or extension has been the major force the injuries are best seen on a lateral radiographic view[34] (Fig. 46-1).

In the otherwise physically intact patient, complete history of the injury noting mechanism of the injury, whether motor vehicle accident, a fall, or an athletic injury such as football or wrestling should be obtained. Symptoms, progression of symptoms, localization of pain or loss of sensory or motor function should be accurately documented.

DIFFERENTIAL DIAGNOSIS

Error in diagnosis is often underdiagnosis of the neurologic deficit which can be masked in the very young, comatose, or multiple-injured child. Mass reflex withdrawal movements may occur with stimulation and be mistaken for normal response to the stimulation. Crying with stimulation may be mistaken for sensory perception when in fact it is actually a response to the mass motion or simply to the situation the child is in following injury. In a very young child, it may be necessary to use electrodiagnostic techniques such as somatosensory or motor evoked potentials to determine the continuity of the spinal cord.[40] All lesions of bone that can cause weakness and collapse may mimic a spinal fracture. Benign tumors or diseases such as eosinophilic granuloma, lipoidoses, chondrodystrophy, Gaucher's, metabolic bone diseases such as idiopathic osteoporosis, osteogenesis imperfecta, osteomalacia, or osteopenia may all present as a vertebral fracture. Bone malignancies, metastatic bone disease, Ewing's sarcoma, leukemia may have an initial presentation as spine pain and vertebral fractures. Most of the above lesions usually, however, present as compression fractures and do not resemble the burst or fracture dislocation injuries. The history of minimal or inappropriate degree of trauma relevant to the degree of the lesion is frequently a good clue as to the nature of the process.

The appropriate imaging techniques, plain radiographs, tomograms, CT scans, or MRIs, will help to distinguish these lesions. The infant and very young child can present a significant problem in diagnosis due to the hypermobility of the spine and incomplete ossification.[41]

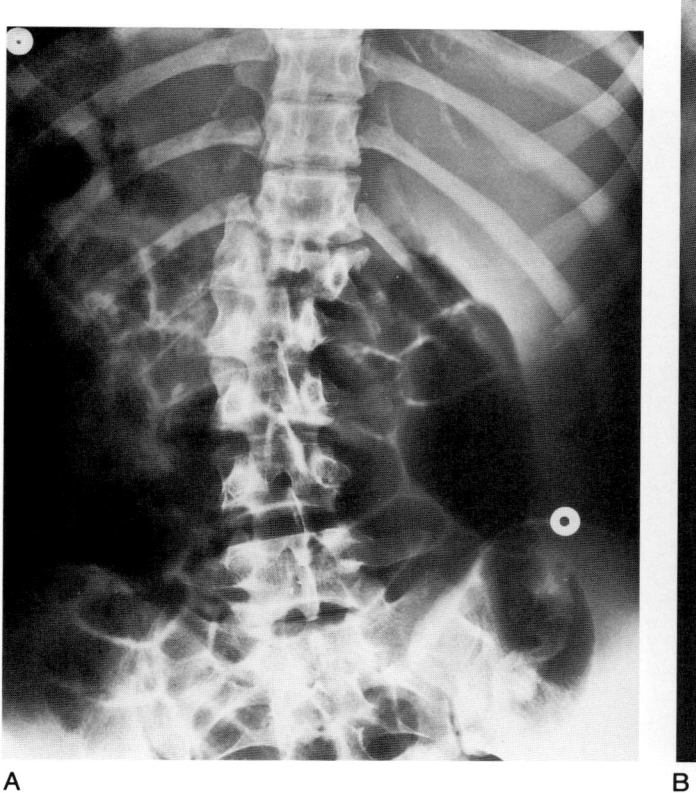

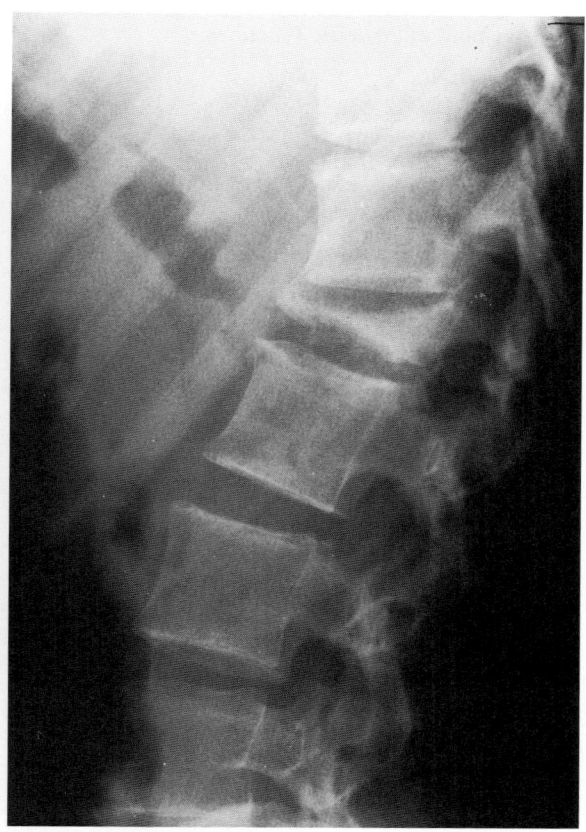

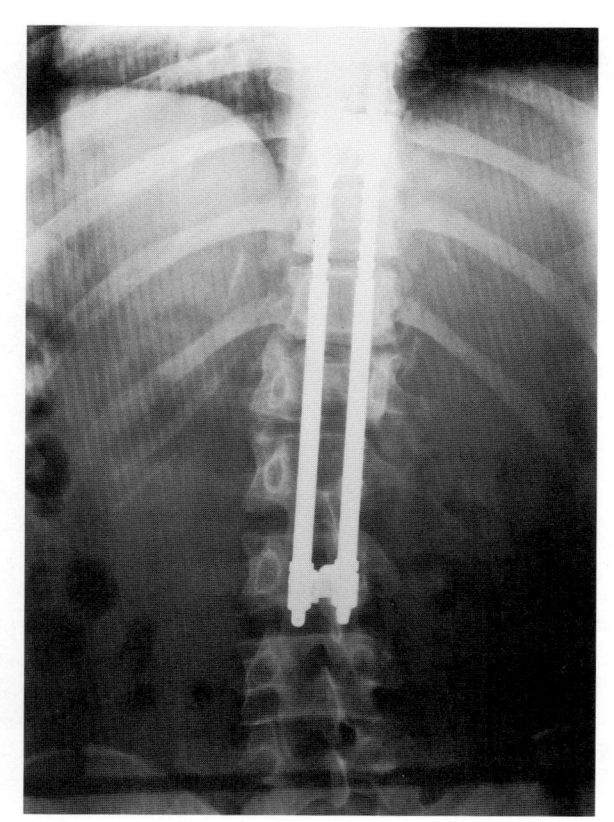

Fig. 46-3. (A) A 16-year-old girl was an unrestrained passenger in a motor vehicle accident. Motor function was intact, but there was thoracolumbar pain, sensory deficit of lower extremities, and fractures of T12, L1, and L2 facets and L1 vertebral body. (B) Fracture-dislocation L1-L2 with neurologic sparing. (C) Fracture-dislocation L1-L2. Open reduction with laminectomy L1-L2 and Harrington rod instrumentation and fusion.

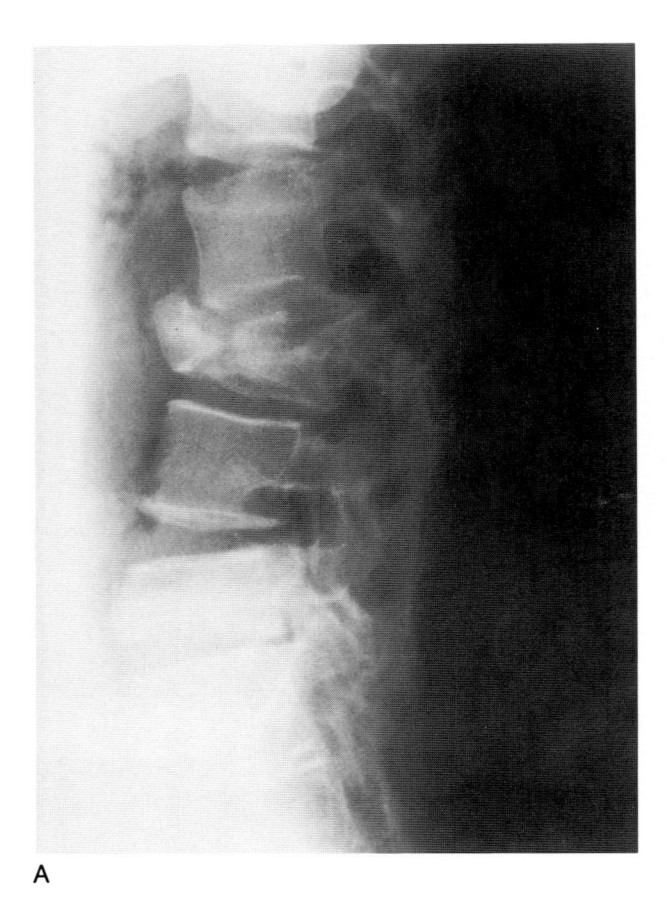

Fig. 46-4. **(A)** A 12-year-old boy who fell from a fourth story window. L3 and L5 burst fractures. Neurologically intact. **(B)** CT scan of L3 shows 33 percent compromise of his spinal canal. **(C)** CT scan of L5 shows a fragment retropulsed into the canal. He was neurologically intact and fused in situ.

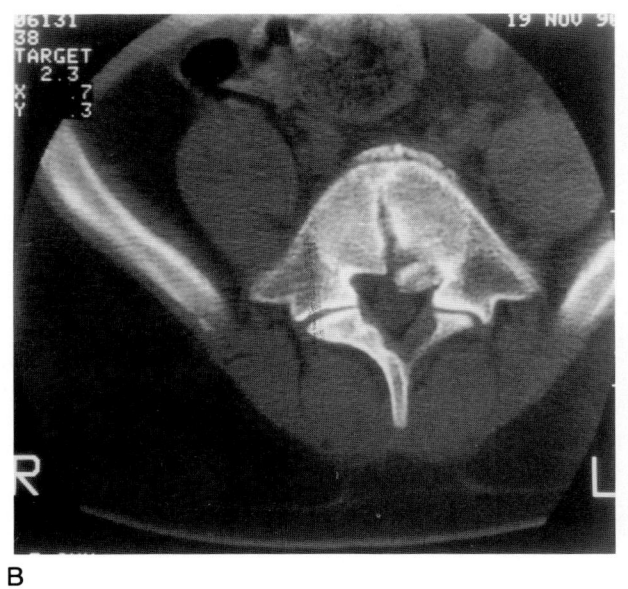

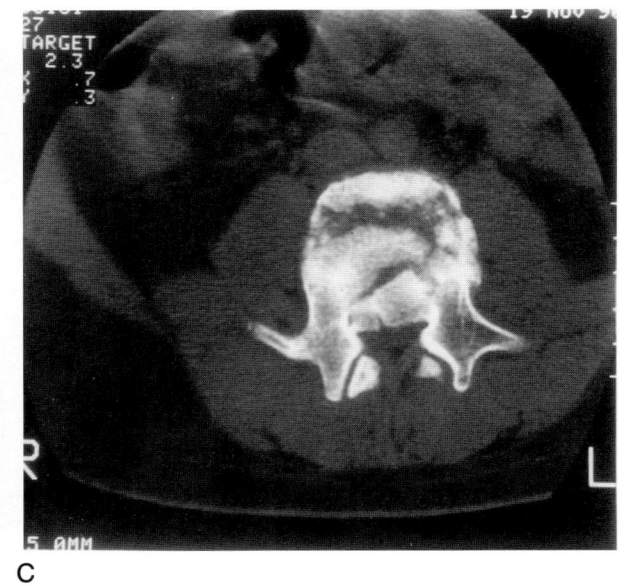

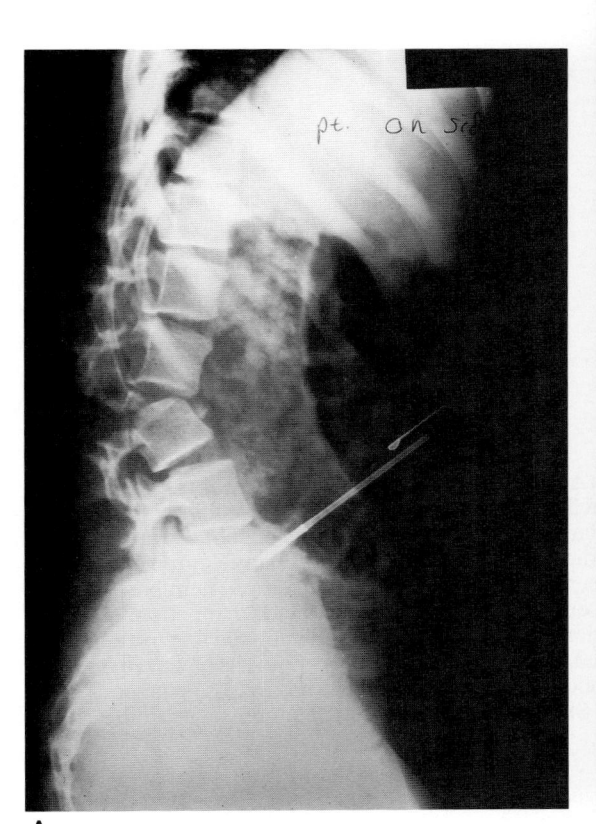

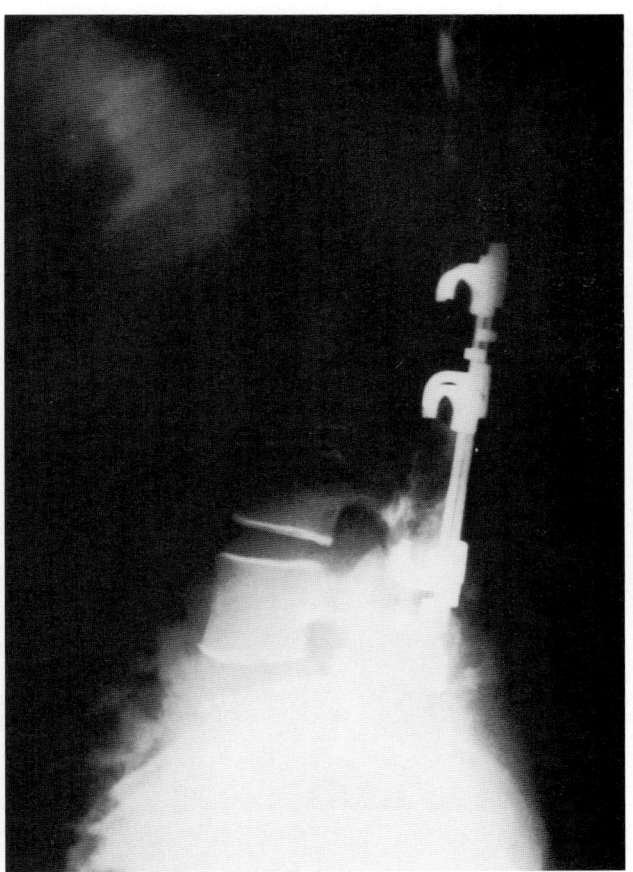

Fig. 46-5. (A) A 12-year-old girl was a restrained passenger in a motor vehicle accident. Fracture L3 facets, transverse process superior anterior rim L3. Neurologically intact. (B) Open reduction compression rod fixation and fusion L1-L4. (C) AP view illustrating bilateral compression fixation.

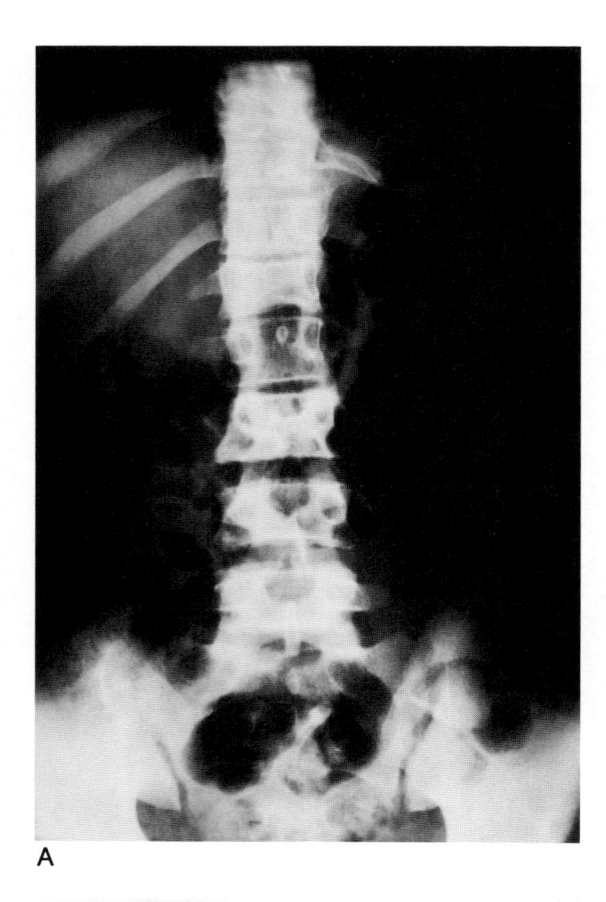

Fig. 46-6. **(A)** 6-year, 11-month-old girl. She was riding on a tractor and fell off and was driven over. Three-column injury, fractures of laminas, pedicles, and global ligament disruption. Note L1 pedicle widening and vertebral body compression. **(B)** 75 percent anterior T12-L1 subluxation hemiparesis. Motor and sensory sparing but absent bladder function. **(C)** Open reduction with Harrington compression rod fixation and fusion T10-L3 and body cast immobilization. **(D)** Open reduction with good alignment. Rods were removed 1 year postoperatively. She had significant but incomplete neurologic recovery.

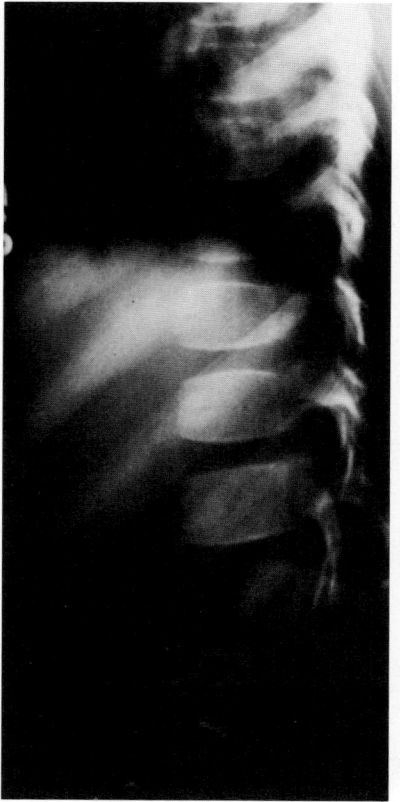

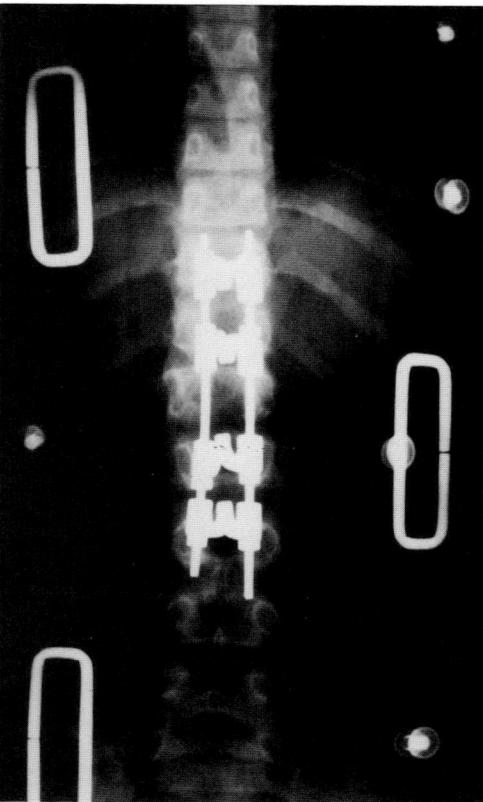

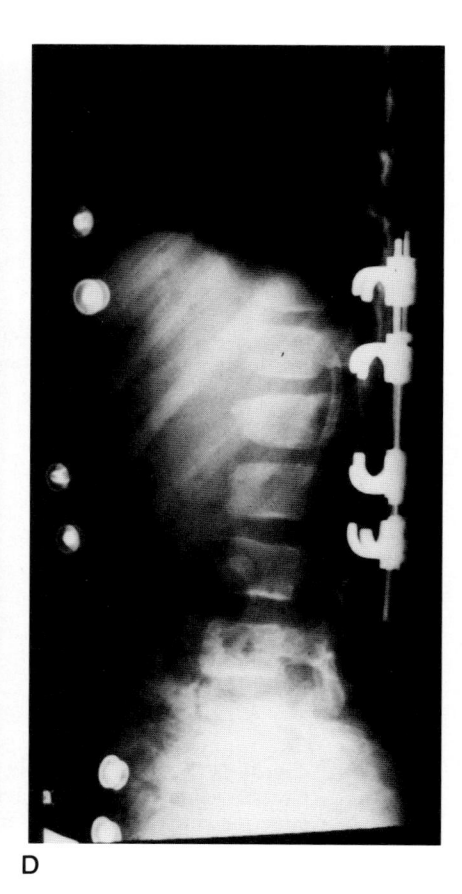

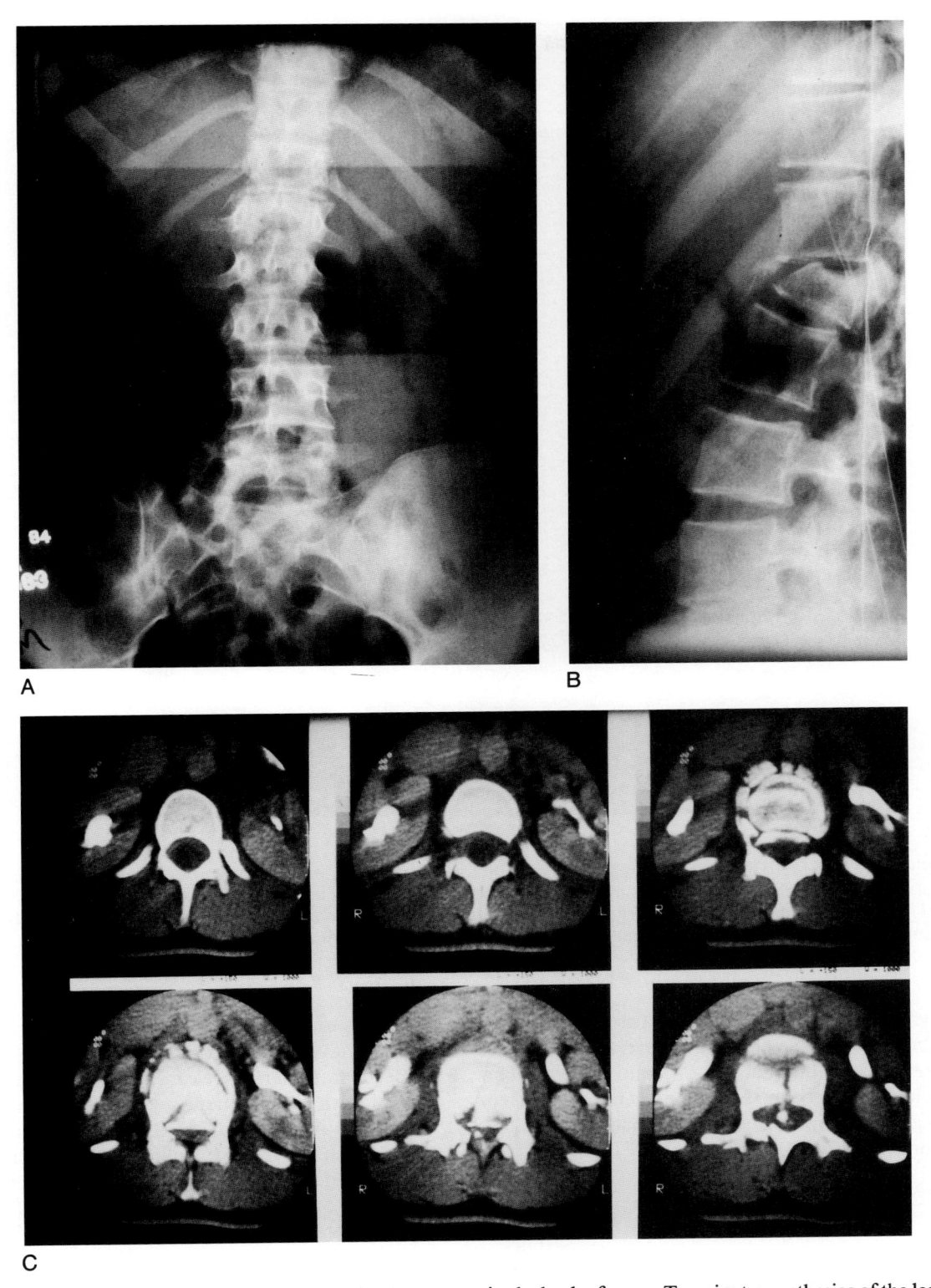

Fig. 46-7. **(A)** A 15-year-old girl, unrestrained passenger in the back of a van. Transient paresthesias of the legs and neurologically intact. Burst fracture dislocation T12-L1. Note pedicle widening. Transverse process fracture L1-L2. **(B)** Burst fracture subluxation T12-L1, 50 percent displaced. Note anterior fragment. **(C)** CT scan of burst fracture of L1. Note the fragmentation of the vertebral body, 50 percent obstruction of the spinal canal and laminar fracture. *(Figure continues.)*

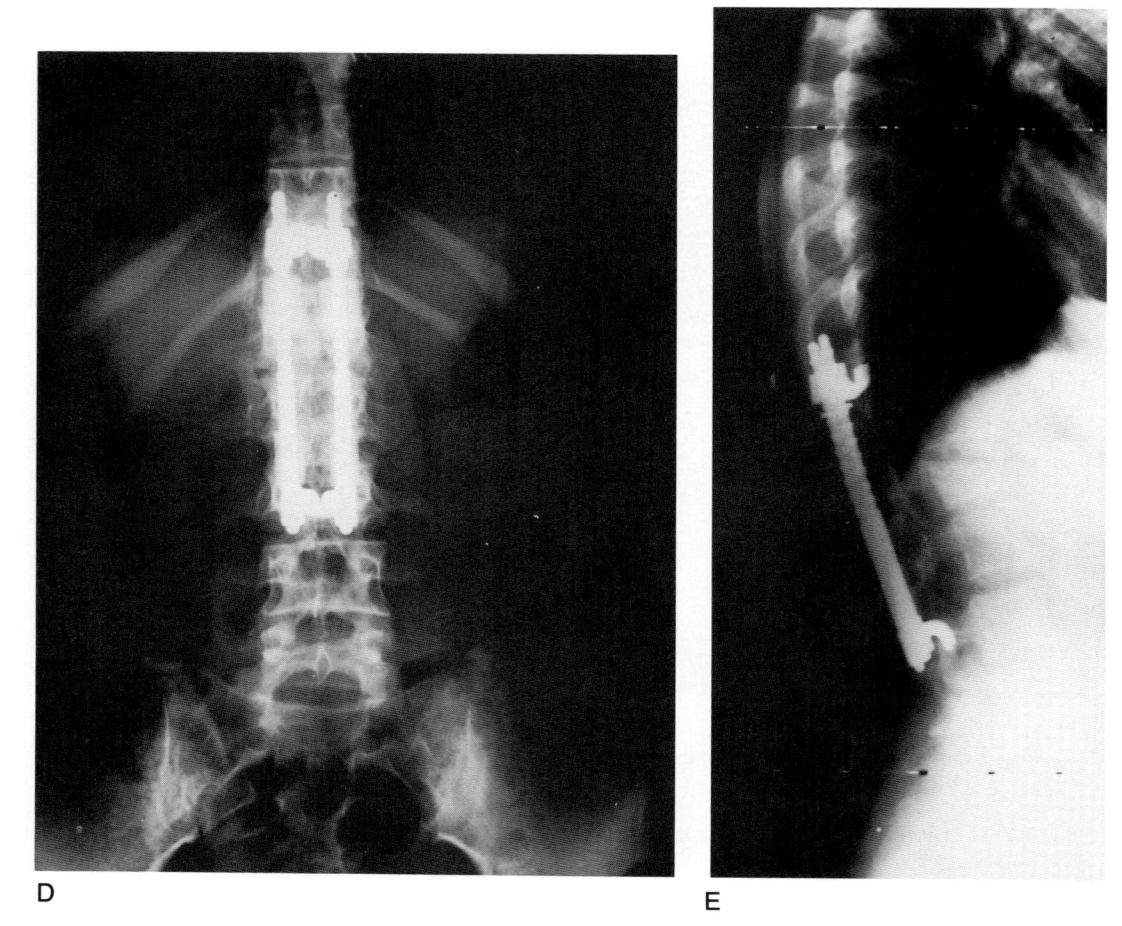

Fig. 46-7 *(Continued).* **(D)** Open reduction of the fracture with a right L1 laminectomy and anterior reduction of the fragment in the canal. Fixation with Harrington distraction rods and Edwards sleeves and fusion T11-L3. **(E)** Open reduction and decompression T12-L1 with Harrington rod stabilization. Note the reduction of the large anterior fragment. Immobilized by a body brace for 3 months.

Another problem in diagnosis may arise when a vertebral limbus fracture occurs that is purely cartilaginous and therefore is not visualized on routine films. This patient's lesion may be mistaken for a herniated nucleus pulposus giving symptoms similar to that seen in a disc protrusion[42] (Fig. 46-10).

TREATMENT

Burst Fractures

Burst fractures and fracture dislocations of the spine are uncommon in young children, and when they occur the child usually has multiple other associated injuries. Nonoperative treatment of the child is indicated in the survivors until appropriate resuscitation of other organ systems have been achieved, as there is a high incidence of death in the first week from these injuries. Thoracic spine injuries are frequently stable as they are supported by the ribs and sternum. Nonoperative treatment is indicated when the relative height of this vertebral body is maintained because the burst fracture affects primarily the upper or lower endplate of the vertebra, with minimal displacement posteriorly into the canal. If the relative height of the vertebra is maintained, due to asymmetrical burst fracture of the vertebral body and one lateral wall is maintained, then the fracture is relatively stable and requires no operative intervention. The child can be maintained in a bed and nursed by log rolling and can be fitted with a molded body jacket as soon as he is able. Fractures of the upper thoracic spine, T1 to T5, are

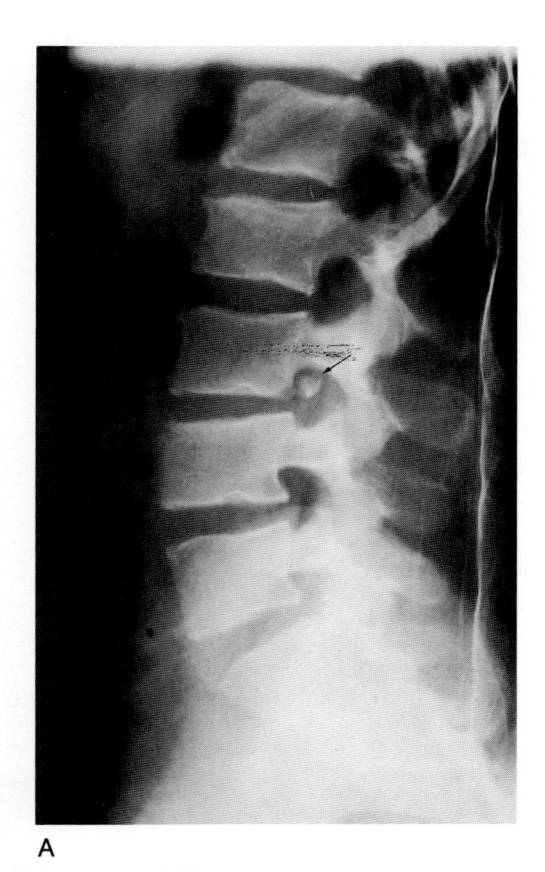

Fig. 46-8. (A) A 15-year-old boy in a motor vehicle accident, unrestrained passenger. Head struck the windshield. Pain mid-lumbar area. Neurologically intact. Treatment: lumbar corset. Healed asymptomatically. (B) 15-year-old type II traumatic apophyseal separation. Treatment: lumbar corset.

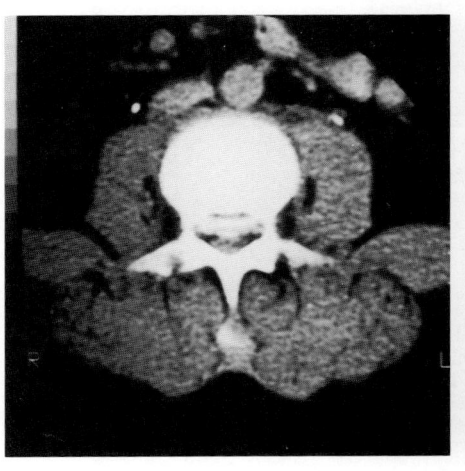

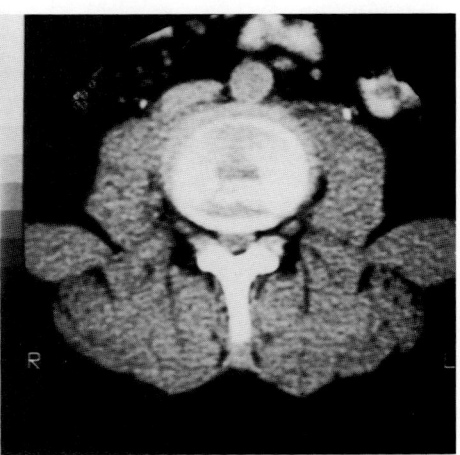

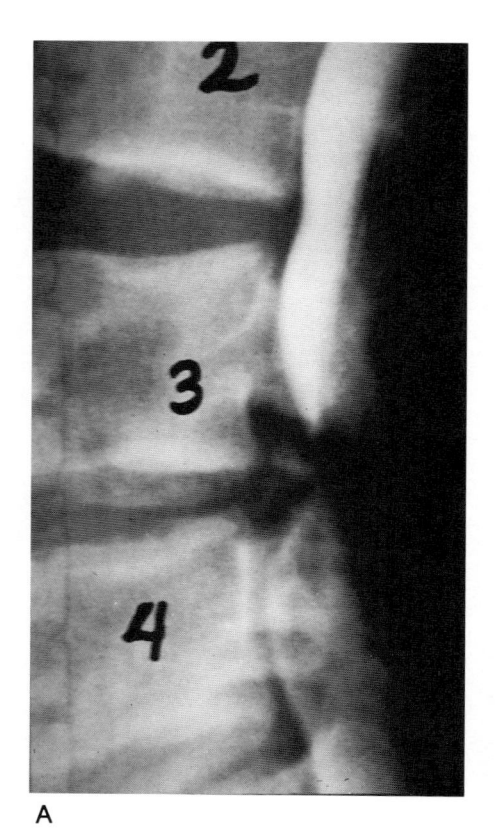

Fig. 46-9. **(A)** A 16-year-old boy, weight lifter, became unbalanced and acute back and leg pain developed. **(B)** A 16-year-old with acute type II fracture of inferior apophyseal rim requiring resection. (Fig. B courtesy of Dr. T. Lowe, Denver, CO.)

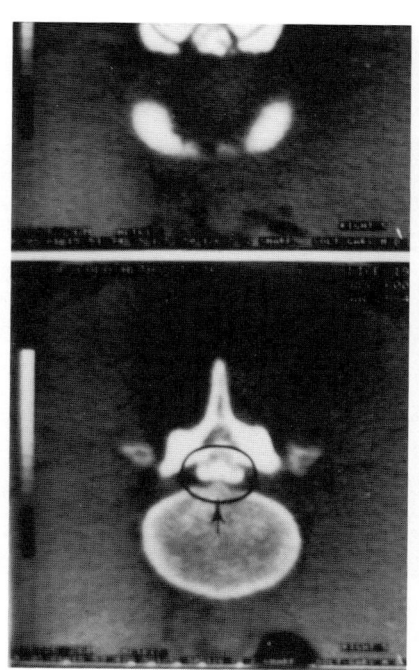

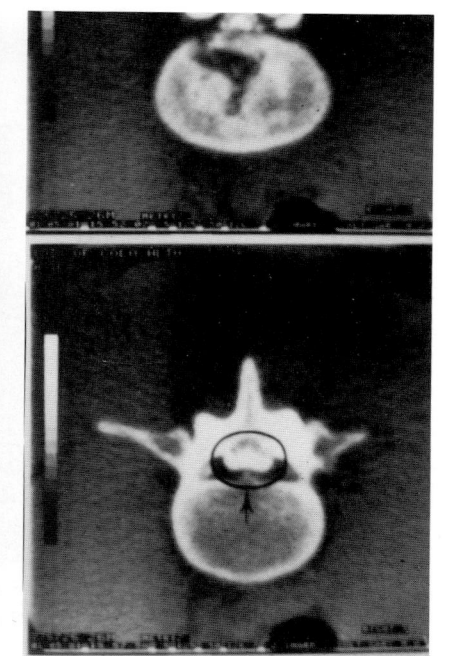

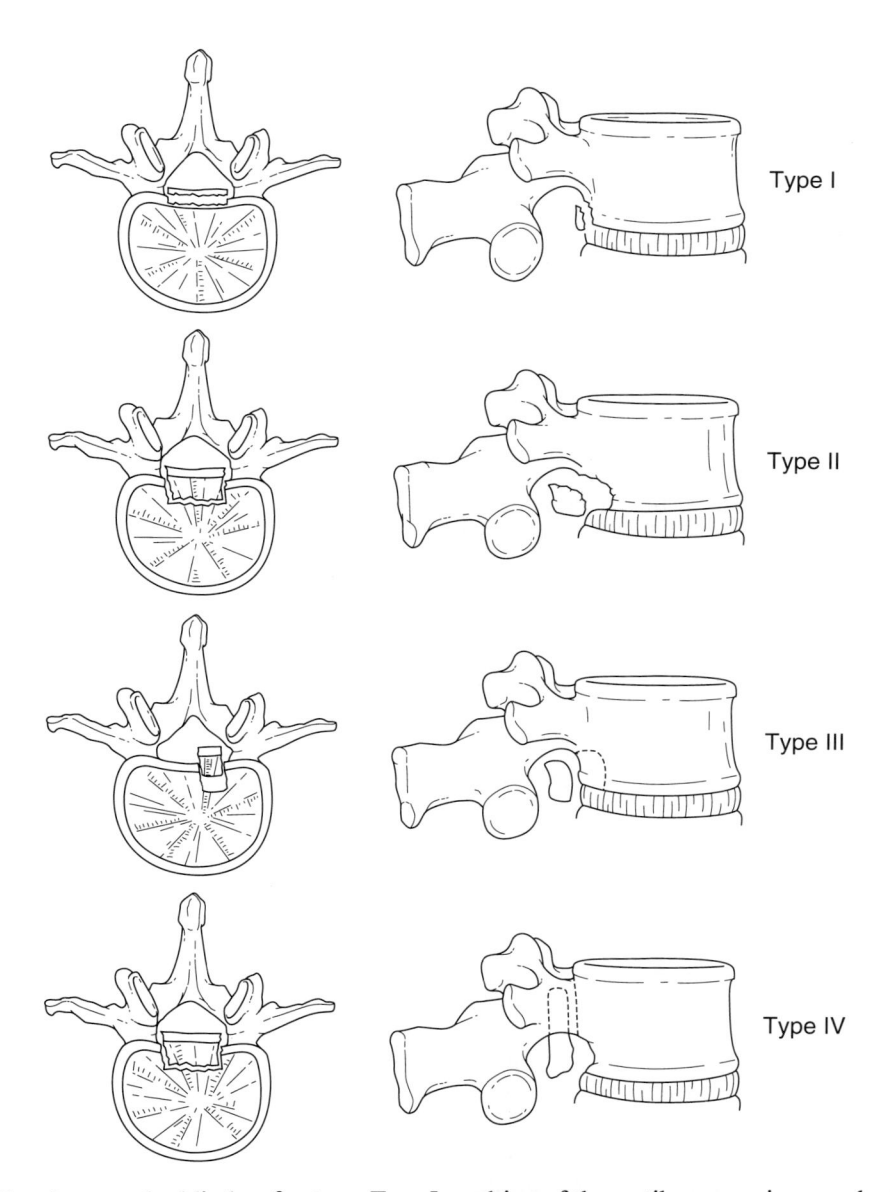

Fig. 46-10. Lumbar vertebral limbus fracture. *Type I:* avulsion of the cartilagenous ring apophysis posterior rim. May not be visualized on routine radiographs. *Type II:* fracture consisting of the apophyseal cartilage plus a rim of cortical bone. *Type III:* a chip fracture of cartilage and cortical bone usually more laterally placed. *Type IV:* a large fragment of cartilage plus cortical cancellous bone of the entire posterior face of the vertebral body. (Adapted from Epstein and Epstein,[24] with permission.)

difficult to immobilize with a body jacket and may require a halo jacket to immobilize and stabilize that spinal level. Commercially produced body jackets are usually not satisfactory for children and a custom-molded jacket needs to be manufactured. Full-time use of the brace may be necessary for 6 to 8 weeks and the patient needs to be closely monitored to note if there is any progression in his deformity or symptoms.

Surgical Treatment

Children present some unique problems in the surgical management of their fractures. In the younger child the small and immature posterior spinal elements require internal stabilization devices of the appropriate size. The most common sites for grossly unstable injuries are the lower thoracic and thoracolumbar spine.

The indications for surgical management are (1) open fractures, (2) neural deficits static or progressive due to compressive lesions, and (3) unstable fractures that will result in significant spinal malalignment or neural deficit or both. If there is more than a 20 percent collapse of vertebral height and/or 50 percent encroachment of the spinal canal resulting in less than 100 mm^2 of space in a mature spinal canal open reduction should be considered.

The object of surgical management is threefold: (1) decompress neural elements, (2) restore anatomic alignment, and (3) maintain alignment with minimal involvement of the unaffected spine.[43-45]

Preoperative Planning

1. Rule out all other organ injuries, i.e., aortic, cardiac, pulmonary, renal, splenic.

2. Imaging should include routine AP and lateral films of the entire spine to note the extent of and nature of other spine injuries (Fig. 46-1). Appropriate tomography, CT, or CT myelography or MRI to note the details of the fracture and neural elements. A split in the spinous process may indicate entrapment of neural elements. A narrowed disc space may indicate a retropulsed fragment of disc. The disk may be transected with a traumatic spondylolisthesis.

3. Decide what type of instrumentation should be used. There are currently over 20 types being utilized. Small children require the appropriate size. The instrumentation should involve as little of the uninjured spine as possible—ideally only one level proximal and distal to the injury should be immobilized and fused; however, mechanical stability can frequently only be achieved with fixation of two vertebrae proximal and distal to the lesion.

4. Decide what surgical approach fits the pathology best. If there is a fracture dislocation with jumped facets, a posterior approach is necessary. If there is marked destruction of the vertebral body with a large fragment into the canal an anterior retroperitoneal or retropleural surgical approach might be most appropriate. The ideal fixation is that which restores and maintains the spinal alignment with the least disturbance of the normal spine.

Posterior spinal distraction techniques with internal fixation such as use of the Harrington rod or one of the other numerous internal fixation devices have been very effective in reducing an acute burst fracture. The longitudinal spinal ligaments are frequently intact and with distraction will reduce the fragments. Multiple level fixation may be achieved with the use of multiple hooks, spinous process wires using Drummond's techniques, or sublaminar wires. It is usually necessary to involve at least two vertebral levels above and below the lesion in the construct to achieve stability (Fig. 46-11). Combinations of distraction and compression rods, as well as transverse stabilizers may be used. It might be noted that the spinal canal achieves its adult size at an early age and so the above instrumentations can be utilized. If there is a retropulsed fragment in the canal and a posterior surgical approach is used, this can frequently be reduced by costal transversectomy, wide laminectomy, or transpedicular route on the appropriate side by applying a traction device to reestablish vertebral height and pushing the fragment back into the body of the vertebra with special impactors or removing the fragments. Depending on the degree of injury, an anterior retroperitoneal or retropleural approach can be used as well if it is necessary to reconstitute the entire vertebral body with a strut graft. Reduction of a retropulsed fragment in the canal can be viewed intraoperatively with the use of ultrasound. If there is any question of a free-floating fragment that tends to retropulse following reduction this is an excellent way of monitoring it. Fracture dislocations require restoration of alignment. If the fractures are massive and the spine is totally unstable, reduction can sometimes be achieved with recumbancy; however, internal fixation will usually be necessary to maintain it.

When rod instrumentation with segmental fixation is used in treating a burst fracture or fracture dislocation the fixation should extend at least two levels above and below the level of fracture and these levels should be grafted. Homologous bone can usually be used for graft-

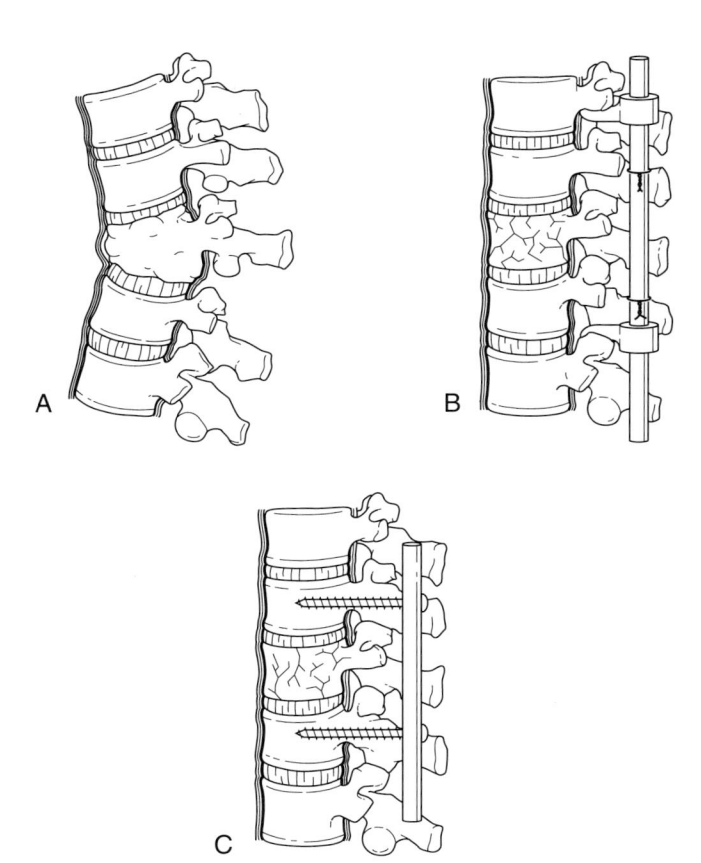

Fig. 46-11. (A) Burst fracture requiring decompression and reduction. Note that the ALL (anterior longitudinal ligament) is intact and the retropulsion of the body into the canal. (B) Burst fracture treated with distraction, reduction, hooks and rods plus segmental spinous process wiring (Drummond). Various configurations can be used, hooks above or below to form a claw, or distraction and compression rods and hooks. This is particularly applicable in the thoracic spine. Laminectomy should be performed to observe the dura during reduction. (C) In the lumbar spine plates and pedicular screws may be used. It may be necessary to use anterior strut grafting to gain stability.

ing purposes, although I have two instances of pseudarthrosis in the adolescents with the use of this product. In the older adolescent, plates and pedicle screws may also be used for fixation in the lumbar spine. Although it is tempting to fix just one level above and below the fracture with the pedicle screws and plates there is significant risk of fracture of the screws if the deficit in the body of the vertebra is not strut grafted. If one elects not to strut graft the body of the vertebra, then two levels above and below the fracture is preferable. When distraction systems are used it is important to monitor radiographically the degree of distraction that is achieved. Excessive stretching can occur and if the cord or cauda equina are intact this can lead to iatrogenic injury. Reduction of the vertebral body may also result in decompression of a torn segmental artery and massive bleeding may occur. It may be necessary to reduce the distraction force and permit collapse of the vertebra to control the bleeding. Radiographically controlled blood vessel embolization techniques may be necessary to control this problem. If root lesions had been noted in the preoperative evaluation, it is important that these be decompressed at the time of surgery. Spinal cord monitoring with the use of SSEP and SMEP is a standard treatment that I have employed when instrumentation is used and neurologic deficits are only partial or if there are no deficits. Autotransfusion systems should also be used, although coagulation problems have been associated with their use when massive trauma and bleeding has occurred.

Limbus Fractures

Limbus fractures may be chronic atraumatic or traumatic. They may mimic a disc protrusion or present with massive canal compromise. It is important to establish radiographically, with an MRI or CT myelogram, the site of the protrusion so that the appropriate surgical approach may be made and one is not confused by the notion that this is a simple disc protrusion.[24-25] The fragment is best treated with simple removal if they are causing symptoms (Fig. 46-10).

Pitfalls

The usual pitfall in the management of a child is an incomplete examination and failure to note other serious injuries to major organs.[26] It is important that good imaging be obtained so that the appropriate surgical exposure and treatment can be made. Accepting poor visualization of the entire spine may well result in missing other lesions of the spine that are as critical as the one that is about to be operated on. If there is retropulsion of fragments into the canal, one should determine which side these are best approached from so that they can be reduced. This is important both in the management of burst fracture, as well as the limbus fractures. Depending on the surgical technique used, the first rule of course is not to compromise the cord with the fixation and, therefore, placement of the instrumentation at the fracture site may well be inappropriate. Using interspinous process wiring is probably the least invasive but perhaps not the sturdiest. Using the pediatric size hooks in claw formation may be quite safe. Excessive distraction may apply added traction on the cord and this should be monitored intraoperatively and avoided. This problem can occur when the burst fracture is being distracted to reconstitute its height. This maneuver may release the compressive effect of the crushed vertebral body on the vertebral arteries and excessive arterial bleeding may occur in a rather dramatic manner. This may be resolved with reduction of distraction. One author had suggested arterial embolization prior to attempting surgical vertebral distraction on a routine basis; however, I found that this problem occurs rather infrequently and doubt the efficacy of embolization prereduction as a routine method of avoiding this problem. Distraction may also cause the increased neurologic deficit if the retropulsed bony or disc fragment is not reduced as distraction is being achieved. The cord is then drawn tightly over the fragment causing further constriction of the cord. If the injury is over a week old, it also may be very difficult to push the fragment back into the defect in the vertebral body and the fragment must be extracted. This may require an anterior approach or very wide total laminectomies in order to tease the fragment out of the canal. Special slim-bladed impactors are helpful in impacting the fragments into the vertebral defect.

COMPLICATIONS

Neurologic

The worst neurologic complication, of course, is paraplegia. It is important to quickly assess whether the neurologic deficit is due to a compressive lesion such as in a burst fracture, a transection of the cord as with a fracture dislocation, or is due to cord injury without any apparent skeletal damage. Steroid therapy should have begun in the field promptly on recognition of the injury following the protocol of the National Acute Spinal Cord Injury study in which methylprednisolone was given at 30 mg per kg body weight as a bolus followed by an effusion of 5.4 mg per kg per hour for the next 23 hours following injury.[46] If there is reason to believe that the paraplegia is secondary to compressive lesion, very prompt decompression of the cord with laminectomy and reduction of the compressive fragment should be performed as this is perhaps the only opportunity of restoring partial cord function. The spine should be stabilized and fused at the same time. Although rare, there have been occasions in which cord function has returned following a neurologic evaluation which would indicated complete cessation of cord function. Lesions of the cauda equina should always be decompressed as these are peripheral nerves and may have the ability to recover significantly although a total lesion may be present. If there is a partial neurologic deficit, this should routinely be decompressed. Care and familiarity with neural decompression, spinal reduction, and instrumentation techniques is prerequisite for the appropriate management of these injuries.

Vascular Injuries

Major vascular injuries may be sustained at the time of the accident in which a rupture or contusion of the aorta or heart may occur. With severe comminution or dislocation of the vertebral body segmental vertebral arteries are frequently torn and massive bleeding can occur if vascular spasm and clotting of these vessels does not occur. This is uncommon; however, at the time of manipulation of the fracture, severe bleeding may ensue. Injury to the vertebral body may be severe enough to cause avascular necrosis. This may result in postreduction increasing collapse of the vertebral body or failure of healing if the area has not been adequately instrumented and grafted.

UNIQUE CHARACTERISTICS OF PEDIATRIC SPINAL FRACTURE

Burst fractures may occur to a varying degree with either just the upper or lower vertebral endplates being involved, both endplates being involved, a varying degree of retropulsion of the fragment into the canal. Comminution may be more on one side than the other resulting in scoliosis as healing proceeds (Figs. 46-12 and 46-13). It also may be a protective mechanism so that if one lateral wall is maintained the fracture is relatively stable from preventing further compression and may not require any instrumentation or fusion and heal in situ. Bridging may or may not occur to the adjacent vertebra, depending on the degree of fracture, but it cannot be relied upon to stabilize the fracture with healing. In a fracture dislocation, the degree of fracture is highly variable, as is the degree of subluxation and dislocation. In some instances the facets are fractured and the level of fracture is highly unstable and readily reduced with instrumentation. In other instances, the facets may be intact and dislocated, which may result in varying degree of locking anteriorly. Reduction can often be achieved surgically by distraction and manipulation or osteotomy

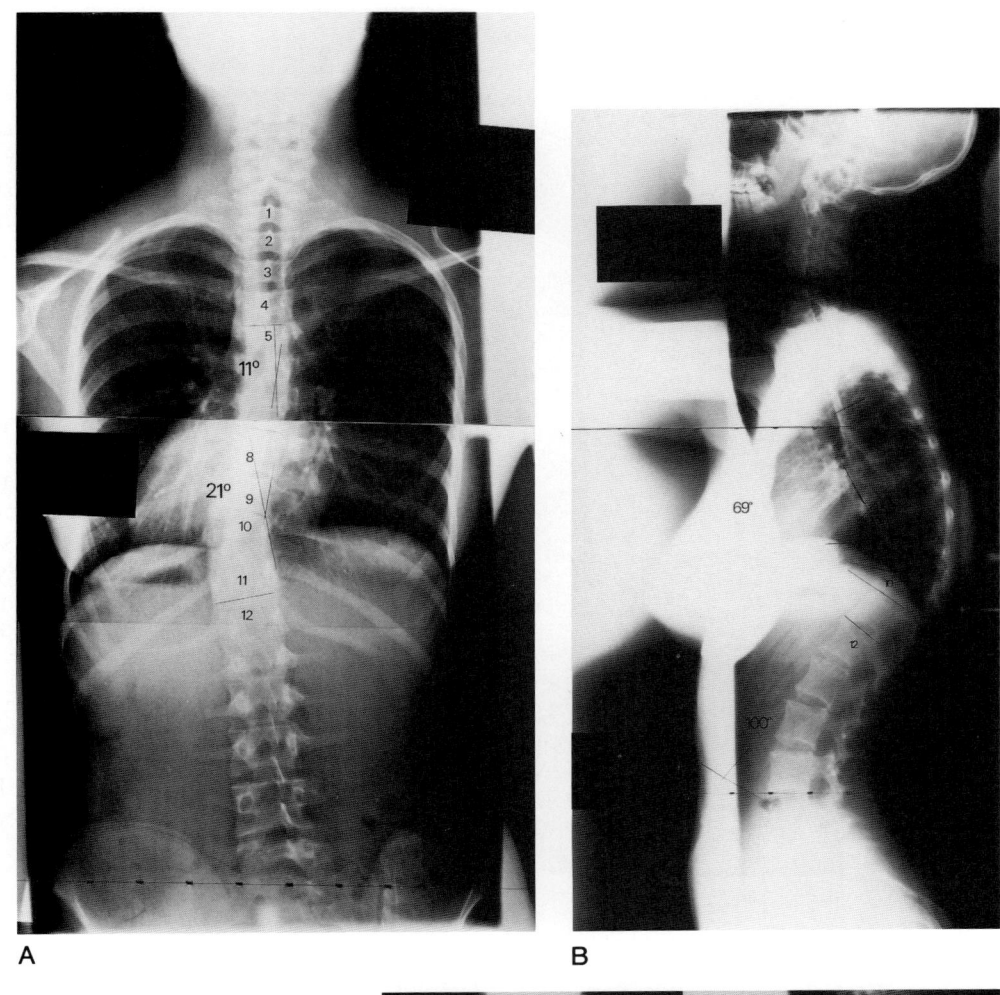

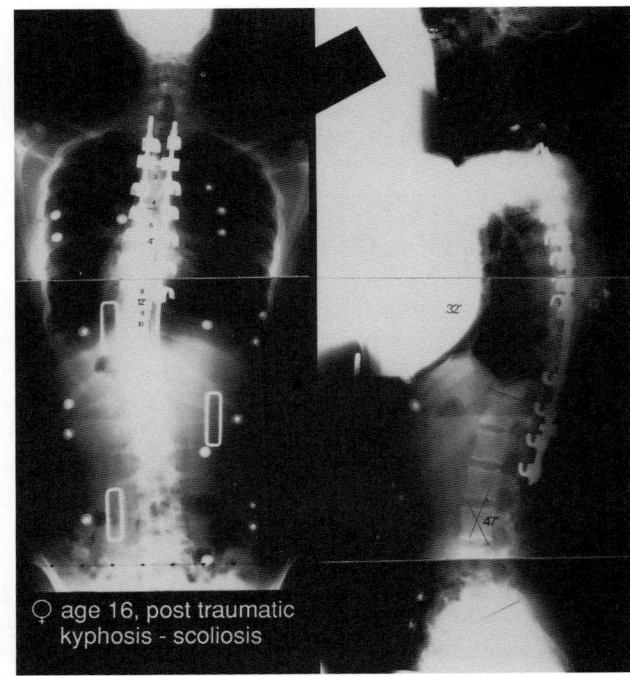

Fig. 46-12. **(A)** A 16-year-old female, 2 years post–burst fracture T10 treated with a corset. She now has progressive deformity. **(B)** Lateral view showing progressive kyphosis. **(C)** Treatment with Harrington compression rods.

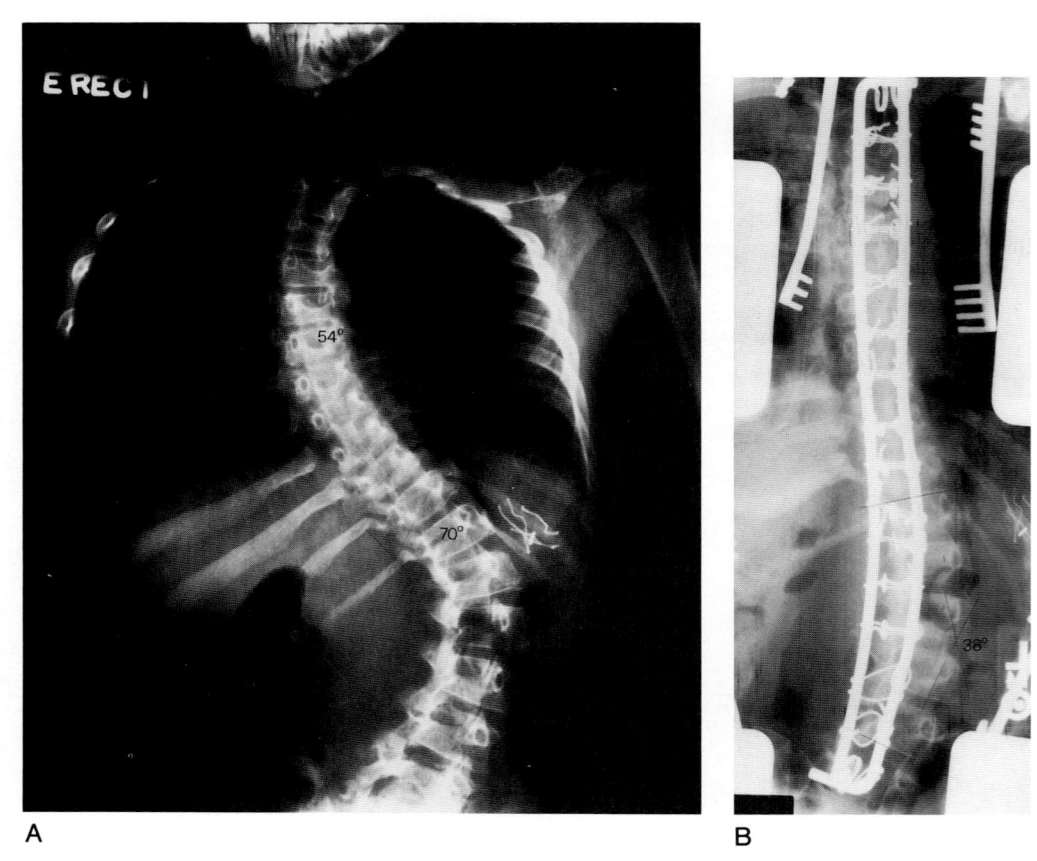

Fig. 46-13. (A) A 10-year-old girl. Spinal trauma at age 1. She has a severe progressive deformity. (B) Initial treatment was posterior fusion, Luque instrumentation and Drummond wire. *(Figure continues.)*

of the facets with care being taken not to injure the cord. Limbus fractures may be unique in that the fragment is totally cartilaginous and cannot be visualized.

LATE COMPLICATIONS

Late complications of spinal fractures are common if neurologic deficits occur. Spinal cord cysts may develop with progressive deficits.[47] The higher the level of paraplegia and the younger the child the greater likelihood for severe late deformity[48-56] (Figs. 46-11 to 46-13). These children may require early bracing and later fusion. The older adolescent can be managed similar to that in which adult fractures are managed (Fig. 46-1).

The Denis classifications of these fractures seem to apply to children as well as they do to the adults. Long-term studies of treatment of these fractures in children are not available, hence the outcome of conservative versus operative management as compared to the adults is not known. Whether children treated operatively will develop pain problems late degenerative changes needs to be assessed.[57] However, if the information that is known regarding child and adolescent fusions for scoliosis may be applied to fracture management then these young patients should do well in the future.

SUMMARY

Thoracolumbar fractures in children are always serious injuries and demand an appreciation of the unique anatomical characteristics of the pediatric spine to facilitate both diagnosis and treatment. An appreciation of the natural history of the fracture's influence on further spinal growth is essential for good treatment planning. An awareness of associated complications both early and late will assist in avoiding functional impairment to further normal growth and development of the traumatized spine in childhood.

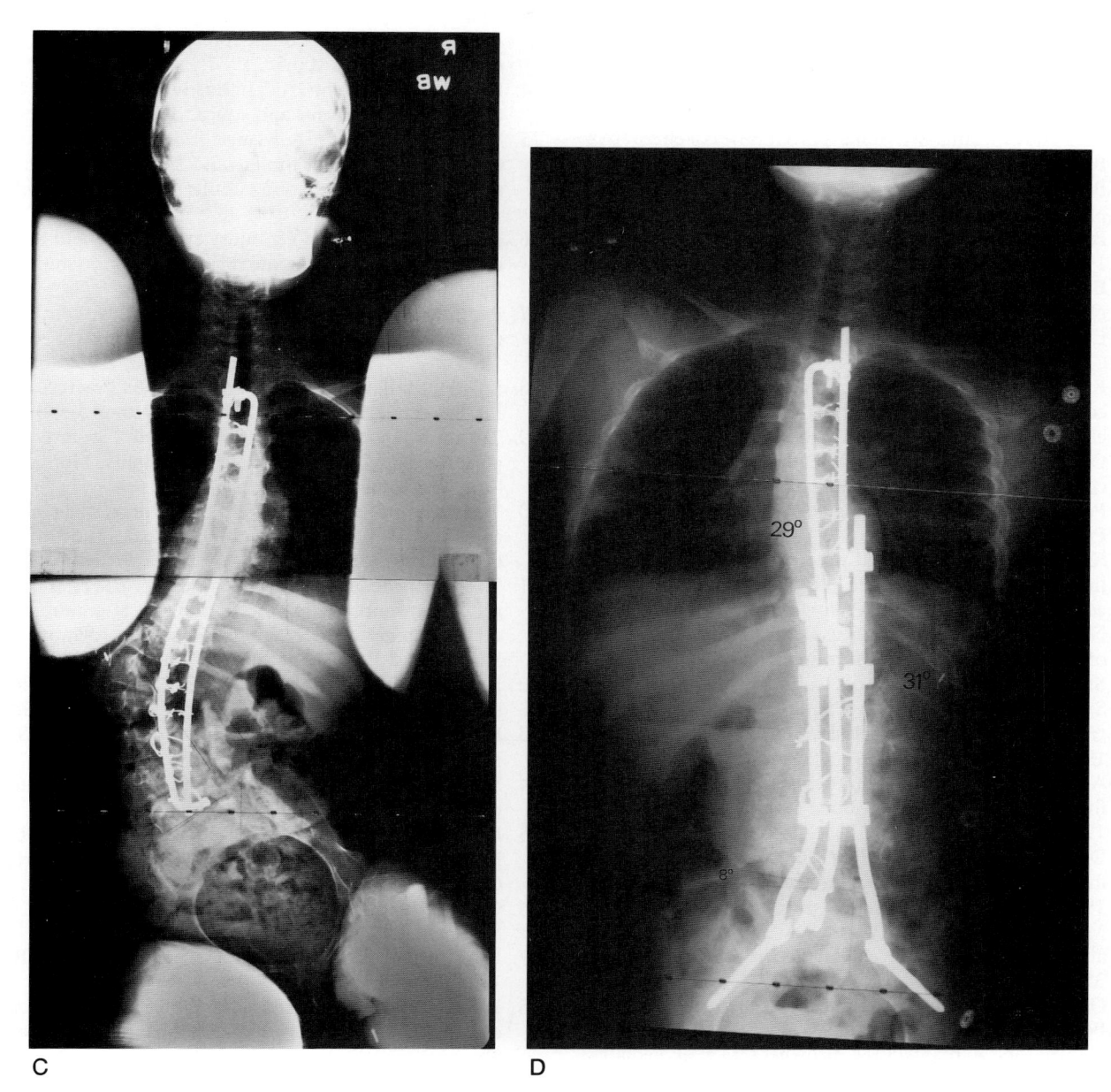

Fig. 46-13 *(Continued).* **(C)** Initial treatment failed due to lumbar pseudoarthrosis. **(D)** Anterior lumbar fusion with posterior fusion.

REFERENCES

1. Bracken MB, Freeman DH Jr, Hellenbrand K: Incidence of acute traumatic hospitalized spinal cord injury in the United States, 1970–1977. Am J Epidemiol 113:615, 1981
2. Anderson JM, Schutt AH: Spinal injury in children: a review of 156 cases seen from 1950 through 1978. Mayo Clin Proc 55:499, 1980
3. Andrews LG, Jung SK: Spinal cord injuries in children in British Columbia. Paraplegia 17:442, 1979
4. Babcock JL: Spinal injuries in children. Pediatr Clin North Am 22:487, 1975
5. Burke DC: Spinal cord trauma in children. Paraplegia 9:1, 1971
6. Burke DC: Traumatic spinal paralysis in children. Paraplegia 11:268, 1974
7. Campbell J, Bonnett C: Spinal cord injury in children. Clin Orthop Rel Res 112:114, 1975
8. Kewalramani LS, Kraus JF, Sterling HM: Acute spinal-cord lesions in a pediatric population: epidemiological and clinical features. Paraplegia 18:206, 1980
9. Ohry A, Rozin R, Brooks ME: Pediatric traumatic spinal cord injuries in Israel. Isr J Med Sci 21:526, 1985
10. Paulson JA: The epidemiology of injuries in adolescents. Pediatr Ann 17:84, 1988
11. Kraus JF: Epidemiological aspects of acute spinal cord injury: a review of incidence, prevalence, causes, and outcome. p. 313. In Becker DP, Povlishock JT (eds): Central Nervous System Trauma Status Report. National Institute of Neurological and Communicative Disorders and Stroke. National Institutes of Health, Bethesda, MD, 1985
12. Sneed RC, Stover SL, Fine PR: Spinal cord injury associated with all-terrain vehicle accidents. Pediatrics 77:271, 1986
13. Aufdermaur M: Spinal injuries in juveniles: necropsy findings in twelve cases. J Bone Joint Surg [Br] 56:513, 1974
14. Davis D, Bohlman H, Walker AE et al: The pathological findings in fatal craniospinal injuries. J Neurosurg 34:603, 1971
15. Mesard L, Carmody A, Mannarino E, Ruge D: Survival after spinal cord trauma: a life table analysis. Arch Neurol 35:78, 1978
16. Garrick JG, Requa RK: Injuries in high school sports. Pediatrics 61:465, 1978
17. Hadley MN, Zabramski JM, Browner CM et al: Pediatric spinal trauma: review of 122 cases of spinal cord and vertebral column injuries. J Neurosurg 68:18, 1988
18. McPhee IB: Spinal fractures and dislocations in children and adolescents. Spine 6:533, 1981
19. Hegenbarth R, Ebel K-D: Roentgen findings in fractures of the vertebral column in childhood: examination of 35 patients and its results. Pediatr Radiol 5:34, 1976
20. LeBlanc HJ, Nadell J: Spinal cord injuries in children. Surg Neurol 2:411, 1974
21. Dickman CA, Rekate HL, Sonntag VKH et al: Pediatric spinal trauma: vertebral column and spinal cord injuries in children. Pediatr Neurosci 15:237, 1989
22. Kewalramani LS, Tori JA: Spinal cord trauma in children: neurologic patterns, radiologic features, and pathomechanics of injury. Spine 5:11, 1980
23. Hubbard DD: Injuries of the spine in children and adolescents. Clin Orthop 100:56, 1974
24. Epstein NE, Epstein JA: Limbus lumbar vertebral fractures in 27 adolescents and adults. Spine 16:962, 1991
25. Epstein NE, Epstein JA, Maurit T: Treatment of the fractures of the vertebral limbus and spinal stenosis in five adolescents and five young adults. J Neurosurg 24:595, 1989
26. Hachen HJ: Spinal cord injury in children and adolescents: diagnostic pitfalls and therapeutic considerations in the acute stage. Paraplegia 15:55, 1977
27. Pang D, Wilberger JE: Spinal cord injury without radiographic abnormalities in children. J Neurosurg 57:114, 1992
28. Sovio OM, Bell HM, Beachamp RD et al: Fracture of the lumbar vertebral apophysis. J Pediatr Orthop 5:550, 1985
29. Takata K, Inque S-I, Takahashi K et al: Fracture of the posterior margin of a lumbar vertebral body. J Bone Joint Surg [Am] 70:589, 1988
30. Techahapuch S: Rupture of lumbar cartilage plate into the spinal canal in an adolescent. J Bone Joint Surg [Am] 63:481, 1981
31. Heizenberg JE, Hensinger RN, Dedrick EK et al: Emergency transport and positioning of young children with cervical spine injuries: standard back board movement hazardous. J Bone Joint Surg [Br] 71B:347, 1989
32. Ruge JR, Sinson GP, McLone DG, Cerullo LJ: Pediatric spinal injury: the very young. J Neurosurg 68:25, 1988
33. Scher AT: Trauma of the spinal cord in children. S Afr Med J 50:2023, 1976
34. Swischuk LE: Spine and spinal cord trauma in the battered child syndrome. Radiology 92:733, 1969
35. Hensinger R: Fractures of the thoracic spine. p. 706. In Rockwood CA, Wilkins KE, King RE (eds): Fractures in Children. JB Lippincott, Philadelphia, 1984
36. Ogdon JA: Skeletal Injury in the Child. 2nd Ed. WB Saunders, Philadelphia, 1990
37. Roaf R: Studies of the mechanics of spinal injuries. J Bone Joint Surg [Br] 42:810, 1960
38. Denis F: The three column spine and its significance in the classification of acute thoracolumbar spinal injuries. Spine 8:817, 1983
39. Handel SF, Twiford TW, Reigel DH, Kaufman HH: Posterior lumbar apophyseal fracture. Radiology 130:629, 1979
40. Bell HJ, Dykstra DD: Somatosensory evoked potentials as an adjunct to diagnosis of neonatal spinal cord injury. J Pediatr 106:298, 1985
41. Burke DC, Murray DD: The management of thoracic and thoracolumbar injuries of the spine with neurological involvement. J Bone Joint Surg [Br] 58:72, 1986

42. DeOrio J, Bianco AJ: Lumbar disk excision in children and adolescents. J Bone Joint Surg [Am] 64:991, 1982
43. Benner B, Moiel R, Dickson J et al: Instrumentation of the spine for fracture dislocations in children. Child Brain 3:249, 1977
44. Crawford AH: Operative treatment of spine fractures in children. Orthop Clin North Am 21:325, 1990
45. Godersky JC, Menezes AH: Optimal management for children with spinal cord injury. Contemp Neurosurg 11:1, 1989
46. Bracken MB, Shepard MJ, Collins WF et al: A randomized, controlled trial of methylprednisolone or naloxone in the treatment of acute spinal-cord injury: results of the Seconde National Acute Spinal Cord Injury Study. N Engl J Med 322:1405, 1990
47. Gabriel KR, Crawford AH: Identification of acute post-traumatic spinal cord cyst by magnetic resonance imaging: a case report and review of the literature. J Pediatr Orthop 8:710, 1988
48. Audic B, Maury M: Secondary vertebral deformities in childhood and adolescence, abstracted. Paraplegia 8:105, 1969
49. Banta JV: Rehabilitation of pediatric spinal cord injury: the Newington Children's Hospital experience. Conn Med 48:14, 1984
50. Bradford DS: Neuromuscular spinal deformity. p. 271. In Bradford DS, Lonstein JE, Moe JH, Ogilvie JW, Winter RB (eds): Moe's Textbook of Scoliosis and Other Spinal Deformities. 2nd Ed. WB Saunders, Philadelphia, 1987
51. Brown H, Bonnett C: Spine deformity subsequent to spinal cord injury. Presented at the American Academy of Orthopedic Surgeons, 1973
52. Lonstein JE: Post-laminectomy spine deformity. p. 513. In Bradford DS, Lonstein JE, Moe JH, Ogilvie JW, Winter RB (eds): Moe's Textbook of Scoliosis and Other Spinal Deformities. 2nd Ed. WB Saunders, Philadelphia, 1987
53. Yasuoka S, Peterson HA, MacCarty CS: Incidence of spinal column deformity after multilevel laminectomy in children and adults. J Neurosurg 57:441, 1982
54. Kilfoyl RM et al: Spine and pelvic deformity in childhood and adolescent paraplegia. J Bone Joint Surg [Am] 47:659, 1965
55. Lancourt JE, Dickson JH, Carter RE: Paralytic spinal deformity following traumatic spinal-cord injury in children and adolescents. J Bone Joint Surg [Am] 63:47, 1981
56. Mayfield JK, Erkkila JC, Winter RB: Spine deformity subsequent to acquired childhood spinal cord injury. Am Acad Orthop Surgeons 3:281, 1979
57. An HS, Simpson JM, Ebraheim NA et al: Low lumbar burst fractures: comparison between conservative and surgical treatments. Orthopedics 15:367, 1992

47

Seat Belt Fractures

James G. Jarvis

> The most important fracture is the one you missed.
> —ROBERT TUCKER

DESCRIPTION AND INCIDENCE

Traffic accidents represent a leading cause of pediatric death and disability.[1] Seat belts significantly reduce the risk of injury or death in a collision by preventing ejection from the car, decreasing the rate of deceleration, and modifying the impact pattern with the vehicle interior.[2-4] Seat belts also change the distribution of forces in a collision. Although accident data indicate a reduction of serious injury or death in seat-belted children, recent evidence suggests an increased frequency of seat belt injuries.[5-10]

In 1948, Chance[11] first reported three cases of "an unusual flexion fracture of the spine." There have been numerous subsequent reports of these injuries in adolescents and adults.[12-15] Although seat belt fractures in young children are uncommonly reported (only 30 reported cases in the literature[8,12,16-21]) their incidence is increasing—with most pediatric trauma centers noting an increase in frequency.

Seat belt fractures of the spine represent a failure in tension of the middle and posterior columns (Fig. 47-1). They are caused by hyperflexion or flexion-distraction of the trunk over a seat belt. Typically these injuries result from high-speed motor vehicle accidents, often head-on collisions. They are usually associated with the use of lap-only seat belts. However, the injury pattern can be seen without seat belts[22,23] or, more commonly, with the incorrect use of shoulder belts.[24-27] These fractures are often associated with abdominal injuries.[28-29] Other associated injuries, including long-bone fractures and paraplegia, are also seen, but their incidence and overall injury severity score (ISS[30]) are lower in restrained occupants of motor vehicles.[4] The lumbar spine is most often involved, although other areas of the spine may be injured, especially the cervical spine.[31-36]

ANATOMY

Several characteristics of the child's spine modify the response to this injury. The child's thoracic and lumbar spine is known to be more flexible than that of its adolescent and adult counterpart. This mobility may account for the higher incidence of paraplegia seen in young children sustaining this injury.[21,37] The healthy intravertebral disc of the child tends to transmit forces to the vertebral bodies,[38] making disc space narrowing and spontaneous interbody fusion following injury, as is seen in adults, an uncommon occurrence. This, coupled with the presence of apophyseal growth centers, both in the body and the spinous process, can result in dissipation of forces and injury over several levels[21] (Fig. 47-2).

One of the unique characteristics of this injury is the association of significant abdominal injuries related to the seat belt. Rutledge and colleagues[5] showed that, although the incidence of abdominal injury was similar in belted and unbelted accident victims, there was a different spectrum of organs injured, with the belted victims

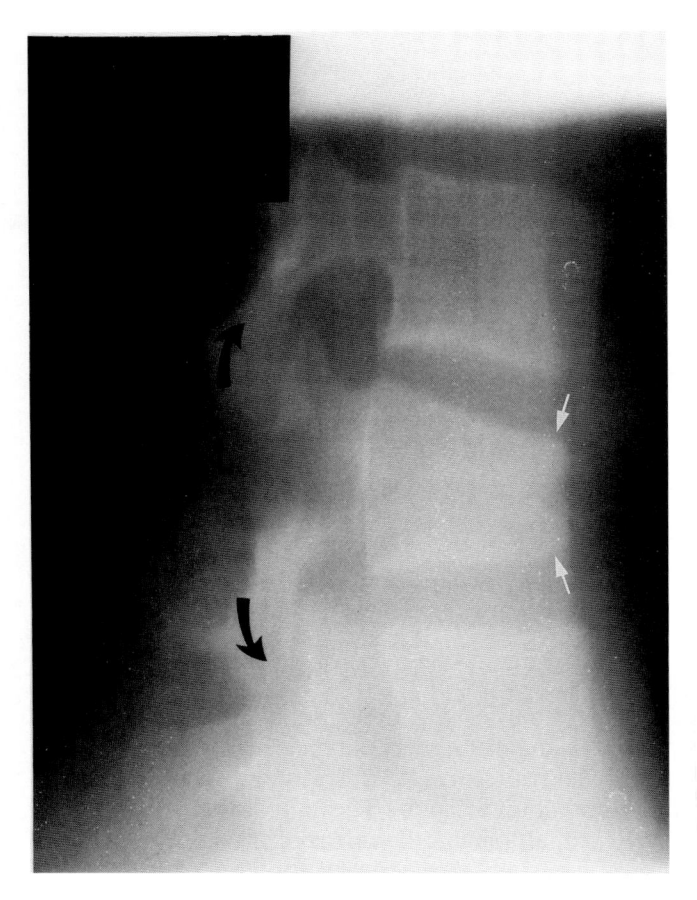

Fig. 47-1. Lateral tomogram of typical seat belt fracture showing tension failure of the posterior and middle columns *(black arrows)*. Note also anterior compression of vertebral body *(white arrows)*.

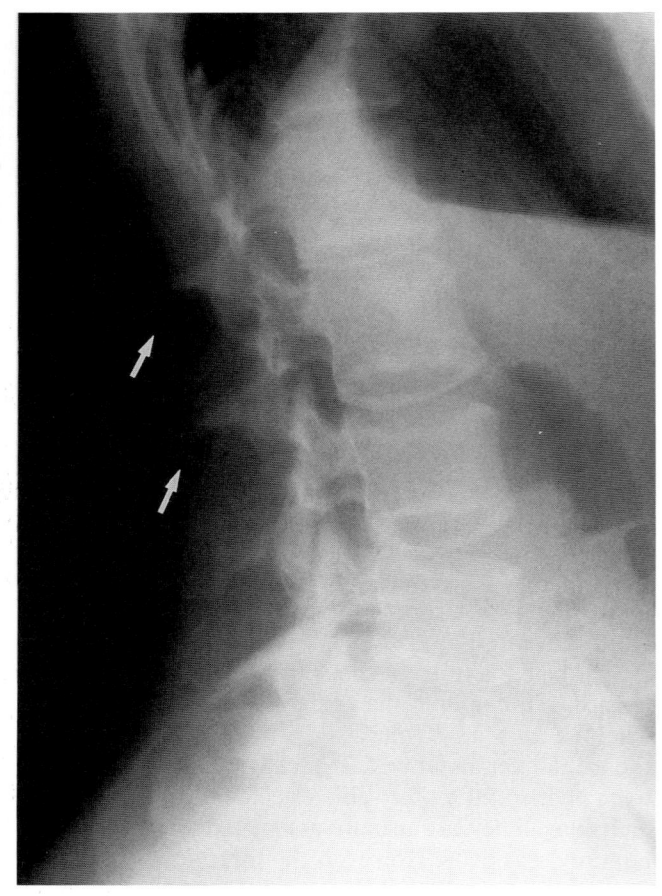

Fig. 47-2. Healed spinous process avulsions *(arrows)* indicates injury extent over several levels.

umn.[14,40] This may be another refection of the healthy intervertebral disc in the child.[21]

The child's center of gravity is higher than that of the adult.[41] This results in an increased moment arm and probably greater distraction. This may contribute to the occurrence of paraplegia in children.

Ideal placement of a lap belt across the hip joint is difficult in young children because of the lack of development of the iliac crest. This leaves the intra-abdominal organs unprotected and susceptible to injury. The child's difficulty in maintaining an upright posture tends to allow the lap belt to locate over the abdomen.[7] Reports of seat belt marks on the upper abdomen indicate that some children "submarine" or actually slide under the belt[13,42] (Fig. 47-4). This can occur because of loosely or incorrectly applied restraints[42] or incorrect use of shoulder belts under the arm.[24,27] We have seen several young children with lap-only belts correctly applied low across the iliac crests — as documented by "seat belts signs" — tending to sustain hollow viscus injuries. Pedersen and Jansen[39] described the four most common types of abdominal injuries seen with this complex (Table 47-1).[8] The intra-abdominal structures that are fixed in the retroperitoneum at the midlumbar region are most vulnerable to injury[20] (Fig. 47-3).

MECHANISM OF INJURY

A seat belt fracture results from hyperflexion over a lap belt during rapid deceleration. It is still widely held that the axis of flexion of the spine is the point of contact between the seat belt and the anterior abdominal wall.[12] In the younger child, however, the presence of anterior compression fractures[19,21] (Fig. 47-1) suggests a more posterior axis, somewhere within the anterior col-

TABLE 47-1. Mechanisms of Intra-abdominal Injury Secondary to Seat Belt Compression

1. Avulsion of fixed retroperitoneal structures
2. Compression of intra-abdominal organs against the vertebral column
3. Closed loop burst of antimesenteric hollow viscus from local increased pressure
4. Shock wave burst of hollow and solid viscus from generalized increased intra-abdominal pressure

(From Reid et al.,[8] with permission.)

who in fact sustain fractures of the iliac wings without concomitant spinal injuries (Fig. 47-5).

CLASSIFICATION

Several classifications of the seat belt injury have been presented in the literature. Smith and Kaufer[12] presented 20 cases and coined the term "Chance fracture." They felt the mechanism was purely tension. Gumley and colleagues[13] further subdivided the Chance fracture into three types, noting particularly the occurrence of unipedicular fractures with fractures through the facets on the opposite side. Denis[14] described the flexion-distraction mechanism while Gertzbein and Court-Brown[15] further expanded the classification based on the type of injury to bone or soft tissue and the state of the vertebral body. They noted the possible bursting component with the potential for retropulsion of fragments into the canal, although this is not common in children.

Review of the literature involving purely skeletally immature patients shows two primary injury patterns. These include posterior ligamentous failure with facet joint disruption and horizontal fracture of the spinous process and neural arch. Our experience with 11 such injuries in skeletally immature children showed four distinct patterns of injury[21] (Fig. 47-6).

PHYSICAL EXAMINATION

The "seat belt sign" is the harbinger of this injury[8,20,43] (Fig. 47-7). This transverse abdominal wall contusion is frequently seen in association with seat belt fractures. Vandersluis and O'Connor[28] reported its association with intra-abdominal injuries is as high as 78 percent in the pediatric population.

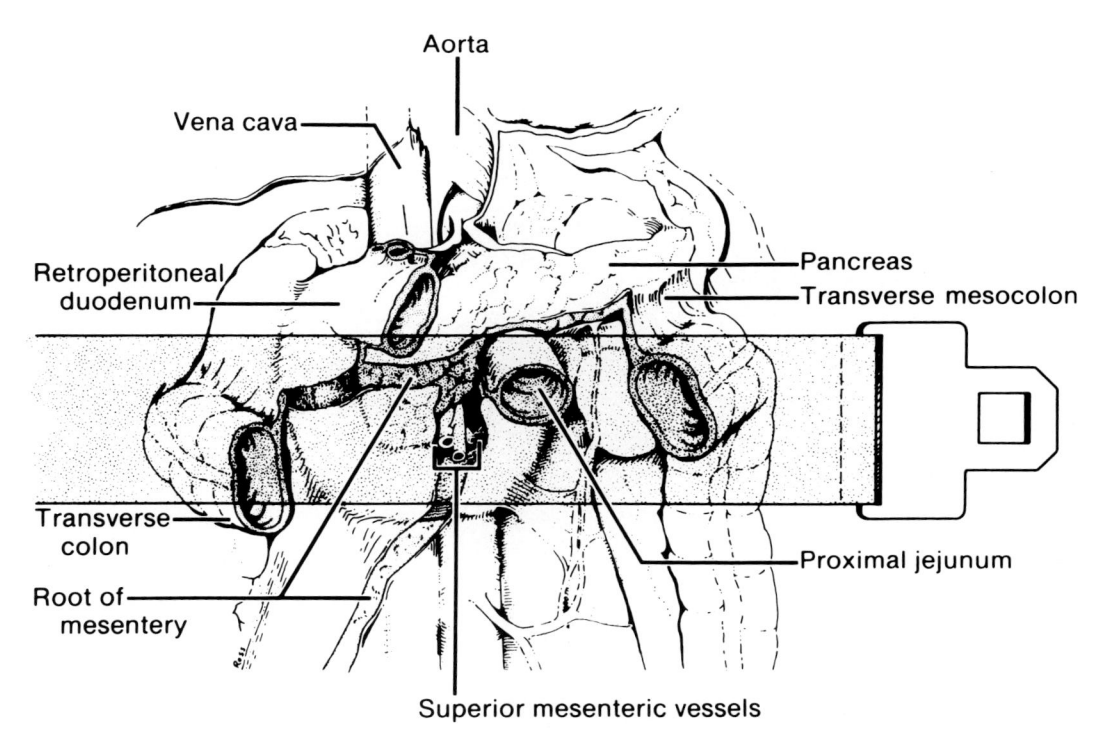

Fig. 47-3. Intra-abdominal structures that are fixed in the retroperitoneum at the midlumbar region are vulnerable to injury. (From Johnson and Falci,[20] with permission.)

880 / Management of Pediatric Fractures

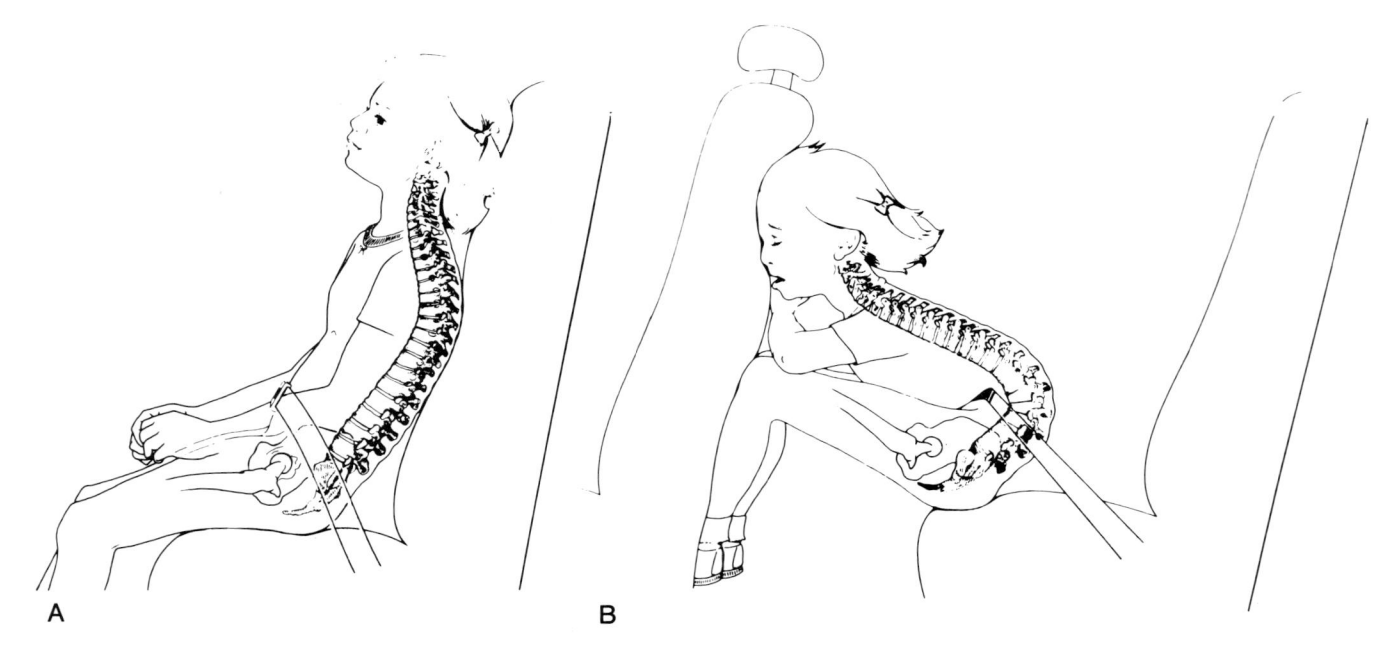

Fig. 47-4. (A) Child with typical "slouch" posture. (B) In frontal collision lap belt slips over iliac crest to focus bending force in midlumbar region. (Modified from Johnson and Falci,[20] with permission.)

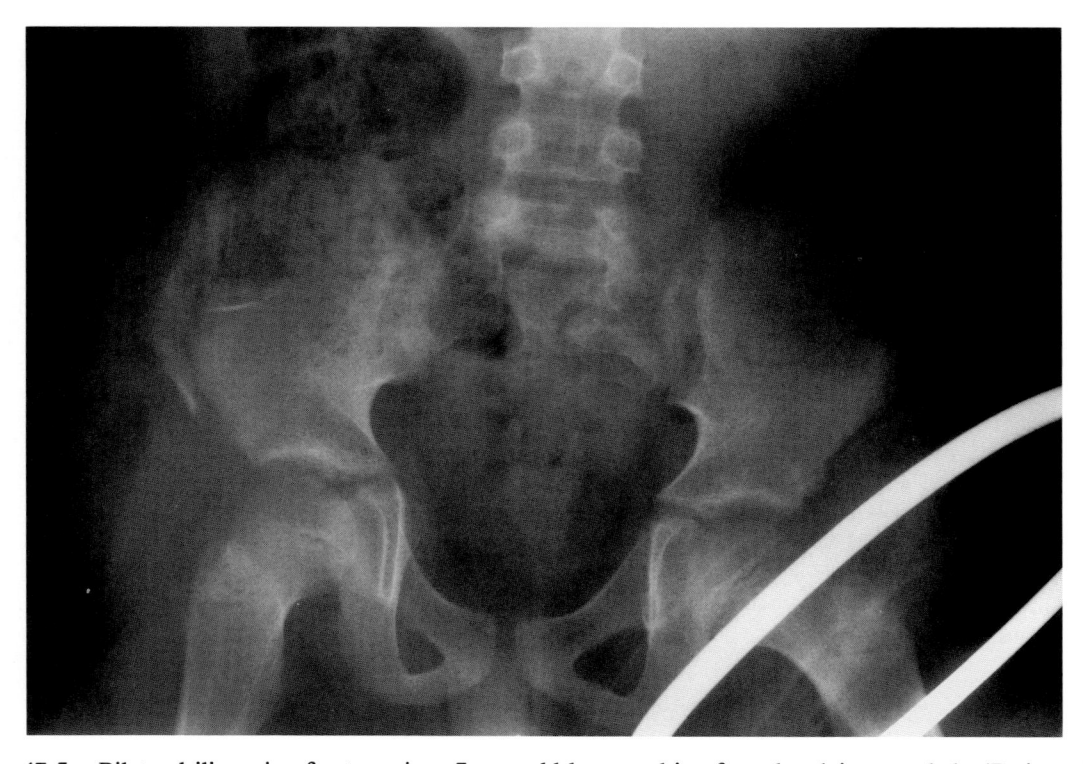

Fig. 47-5. Bilateral iliac wing fractures in a 7-year-old boy resulting from low-lying seat belt. (Patient also sustained a fracture of the left femur.)

TYPE A **TYPE B**

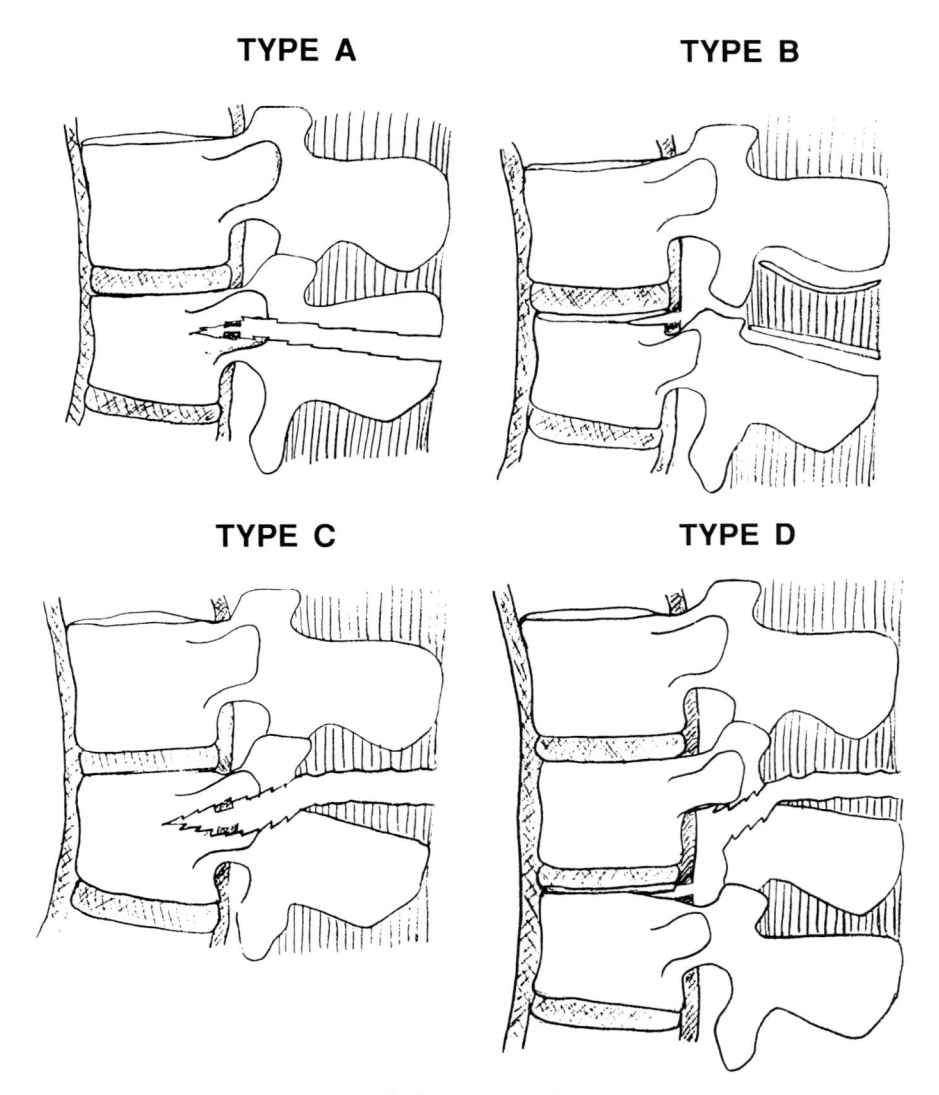

TYPE C **TYPE D**

Fig. 47-6. Seat belt fracture patterns in skeletally immature children. *Type A:* Bony disruption of the posterior column extending just into the middle column. *Type B.* Avulsion of the posterior elements with facet joint disruption or fracture and extension into the apophysis of the vertebral body. *Type C.* Posterior ligamentous disruption with a fracture line entering the vertebra close to the pars interarticularis and extending into the middle column. *Type D.* Posterior ligamentous disruption, with a fracture line traversing the lamina and extending into the apophysis of the adjacent vertebral body. (From Rumball and Jarvis,[21] with permission.)

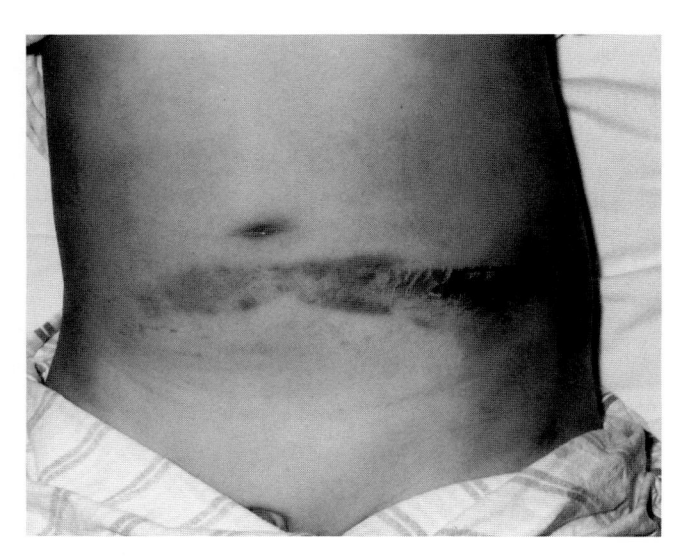

Fig. 47-7. Abdominal contusion or "seat belt sign."

In a child with a fractured spine and a badly bruised abdomen it is often difficult to assess abdominal signs. This can be further aggravated by the occurrence of paraplegia or significant head injuries. Mild tenderness may be attributed to a bruised abdominal wall or the ileus resulting from the fracture. Swelling with local tenderness is usually seen posteriorly over the fractured spinal segments.

IMAGING

Although the vertebral injury can usually be detected on standard anteroposterior and lateral radiographs, the full extent of vertebral injury may not be appreciated. Lateral tomograms are the best additional investigation to assess the vertebral column injury (Figs. 47-1 and 47-8). In a review by Hudson and Kavanagh,[9] decubitus radiographs showed free air in only 3 of 47 cases with ruptured retroperitoneal viscus. Computed tomography (CT) scans may be valuable for assessing the abdominal injury; however, they can fail to detect the transverse fracture, as it is in the same plane as the image.[31,43] Recently, magnetic resonance imaging (MRI) scans have been shown to be the best additional investigation when there is spinal injury with neurologic deficit[19,44] (Fig. 47-9).

TREATMENT

Closed Methods

Many of these injuries in young children are stable in extension, and accordingly the initial treatment should be focused on the abdominal injury. Peritoneal lavage has been shown to be unreliable and early laparotomy is necessary for diagnosis and treatment of ruptured viscus injuries. This approach becomes essential if the patient is unconscious or there is paralysis. Spinal cord injuries are treated following the standard protocols for acute management.[45] The patient must be kept recumbent with frequent log rolling until medically stable. At that point, a hyperextension body cast can be applied. This should be extended down one leg, in pantaloon fashion, for low lumbar fractures (Fig. 47-10).

Open Methods

Although the majority of young children can be treated conservatively with hyperextension casting, open reduction and internal fixation using Harrington compression rods is appropriate for those injuries with wide separation following attempted closed reduction[13,46] (Fig. 47-11). Distraction should be avoided in these injuries. LeGay and colleagues[47] found that in mature patients assessment of initial kyphosis was important, with those measuring in excess of 17 degrees having a poor prognosis.

PITFALLS

The consequences of seat belt injuries are often missed as emphasized in the literature.[8,48] This may result in increased morbidity and even mortality.[2] Delays in diagnosis of both the spinal and the bowel injury are common.[8,47] A high index of suspicion, coupled with appropriate physical examination and adequate radiographic studies, can decrease the incidence of this pitfall. It is also important to be aware that associated injuries are common and that other areas of the spine may be involved. The cervical spine is most frequently fractured when shoulder restraints are utilized.[32,33,49]

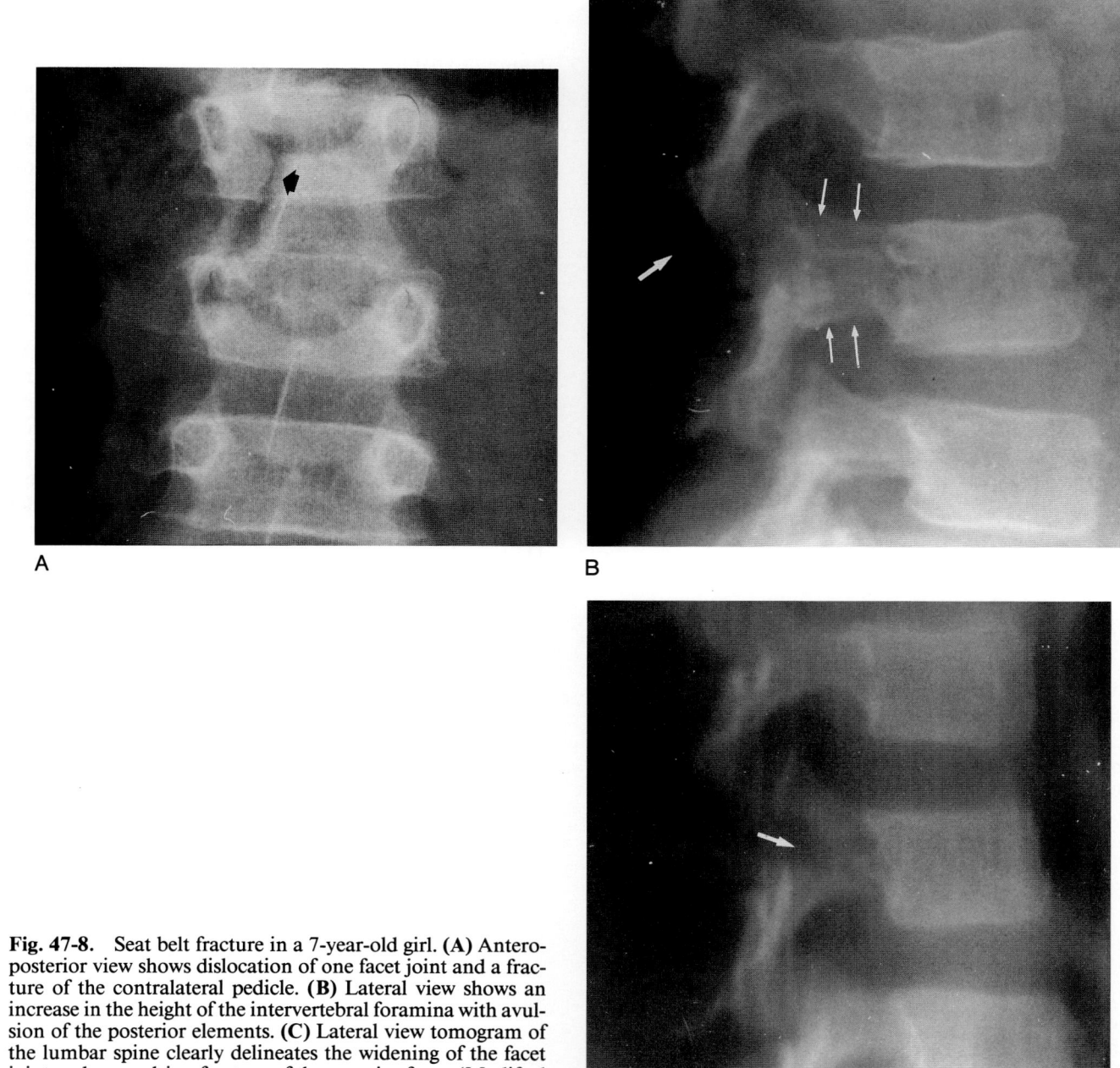

Fig. 47-8. Seat belt fracture in a 7-year-old girl. **(A)** Anteroposterior view shows dislocation of one facet joint and a fracture of the contralateral pedicle. **(B)** Lateral view shows an increase in the height of the intervertebral foramina with avulsion of the posterior elements. **(C)** Lateral view tomogram of the lumbar spine clearly delineates the widening of the facet joint and an avulsion fracture of the superior facet. (Modified from Rumball and Jarvis,[21] with permission.)

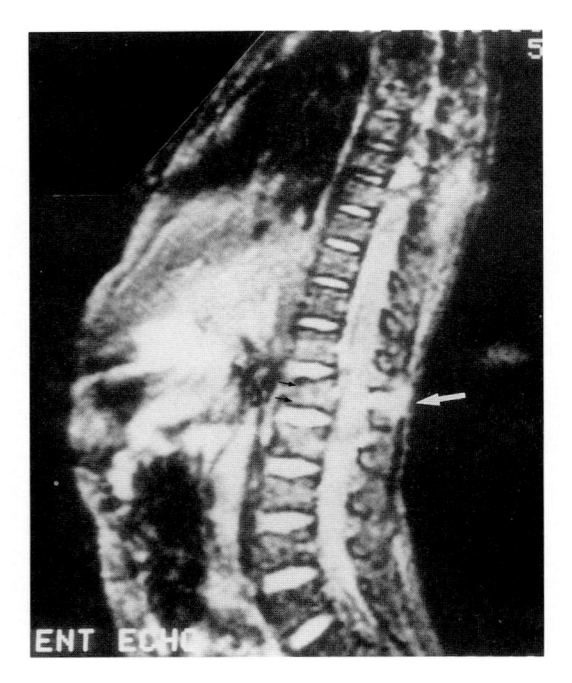

Fig. 47-9. Magnetic resonance image showing anterior compression of the vertebral body and hematoma in the soft tissue posterior to L1. (From Gallagher and Heinrich,[19] with permission.)

COMPLICATIONS

Neurologic

In the adolescent and adult, neurologic injury is uncommon and paraplegia has not been reported. In the skeletally immature, however, paraplegia has been reported as high as 30 percent.[21] In the young child, paraparesis may have a delayed onset and is probably vascular in origin.[50]

Osseous

Residual kyphosis has not been problematic in the young child, although it may develop in the adolescent and adult.[47] Gumley and coworkers[13] felt that it resulted from initial inadequate reduction. Scoliosis, requiring surgical fusion, is a well-recognized complication of traumatic paraplegia in the young child (Fig. 47-12). In those over 10 years of age scoliosis may result from structural wedging associated with the fracture. This may be due to unequal compression of endplates[38] and is most commonly seen with anterolateral compression fractures resulting from the use of three-point restraints.[26]

PREVENTION

Concerns have been raised regarding the suitability of lap belts as a means of restraining children.[51] Several authors have pointed out that seat belt injuries may result from improper use of restraints.[24,25,52] Prevention requires optimal use of restraints.[53,54] The use of special restraints for children under the age of 10 has been recommended,[7,55] while there has been a call for shoulder restraints in the rear seats of North American cars.[8] However, despite these changes, if extreme collision forces are involved, significant injuries will likely still occur.[34,35,54]

SUMMARY

The pediatric seat belt fracture is a unique and potentially devastating injury, frequently associated with the incorrect use of seat belts. Delays in diagnosis of both the

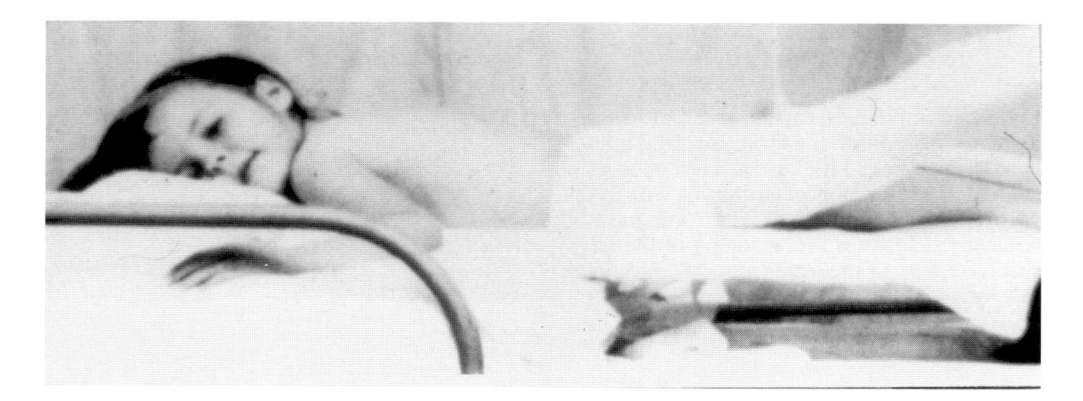

Fig. 47-10. Application of hyperextension body cast extended down legs in pantaloon fashion.

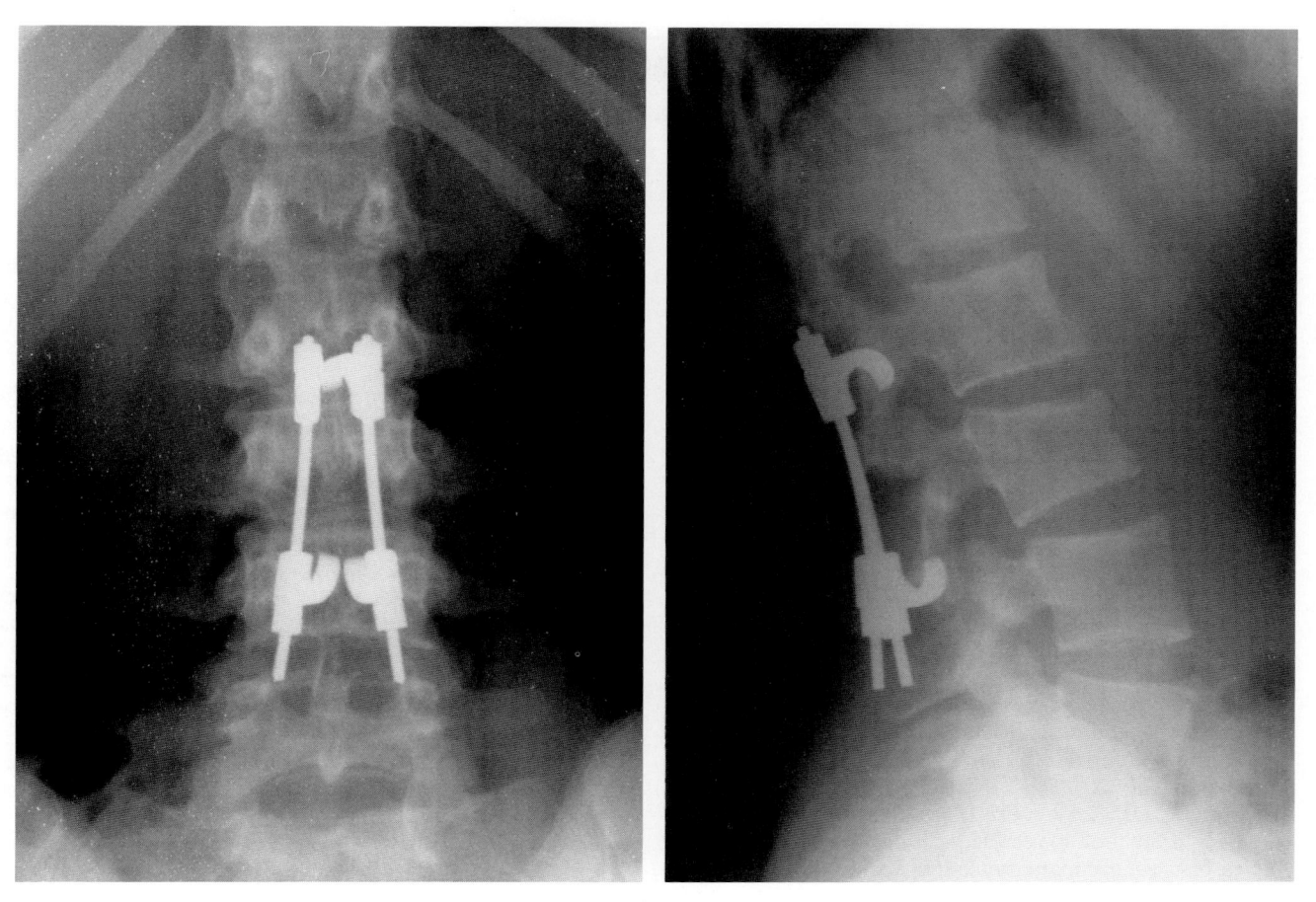

Fig. 47-11. Open reduction and internal fixation using Harrington compression instrumentation.

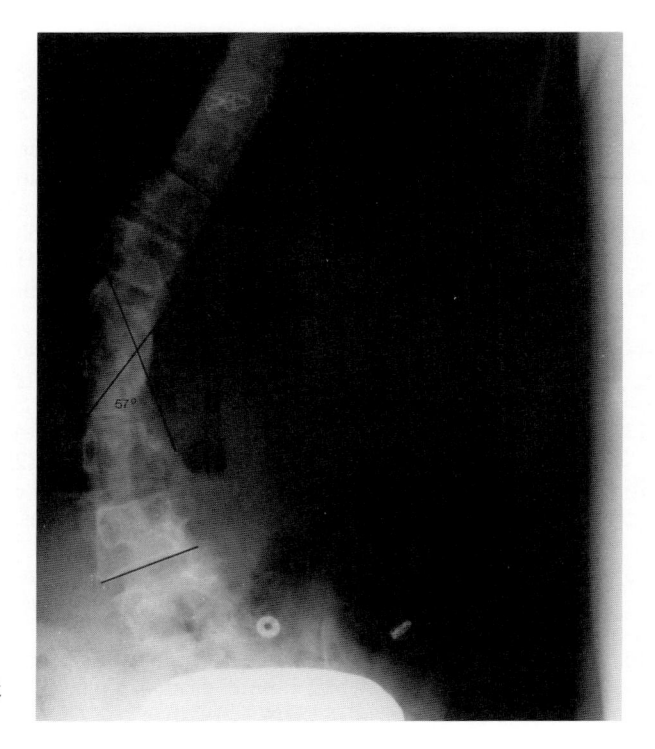

Fig. 47-12. Scoliosis in a 15-year-old girl who sustained a seat belt fracture with paraplegia at age 10.

spinal column and abdominal injuries are common. A high index of suspicion is necessary when a "seat belt sign" is found. Closed treatment usually results in a good outcome in the younger child, with open reduction and internal fixation reserved for the older child and adolescent when reduction cannot be obtained by closed means.

REFERENCES

1. Baker SP: Injuries: The neglected epidemic. J Trauma 27:343, 1987
2. Williams JS, Kirkpatrick JR: The nature of seat belt injuries. J Trauma 11:207, 1971
3. Dooley B: Medical significance of occupant restraint on road-crash victims and the role of the medical profession. Can J Surg 30:400, 1987
4. Christian MS, Bullimore DW: Reduction in accident injury severity in rear seat passengers using restraints. Injury Br J Accident Surg 20:262, 1989
5. Rutledge R, Thomason M, Oller D et al: The spectrum of abdominal injuries associated with the use of seat belts. J Trauma 31:820, 1991
6. Dalmotas DJ, Krzyzewski J: Restraint system effectiveness as a function of seating position: restraint technologies: rear seat occupant protection. Society of Automotive Engineers, Warrendale, PA, 1987
7. Agran PF, Dunkle DE, Winn DG: Injuries to a sample of seatbelted children evaluated and treated in a hospital emergency room. J Trauma 27:58, 1987
8. Reid A, Letts RM, Black GB: Pediatric chance fractures: association with intra-abdominal injuries and seatbelt use. J Trauma 30:384, 1990
9. Hudson I, Kavanagh TG: Duodenal transection and vertebral injury occurring in combination in a patient wearing a seat belt. Injury 15:6, 1983
10. Anderson P, Rivara F, Maier R, Drake C: The epidemiology of seatbelt-associated injuries. J Trauma 31:60, 1991
11. Chance GQ: Note on a flexion fracture of the spine. Br J Radiol 21:452, 1948
12. Smith WS, Kaufer H: Patterns and mechanisms of lumbar injuries associated with lap seat belts. J Bone Joint Surg [Am] 51:239, 1969
13. Gumley G, Taylor TKF, Ryan MD: Distraction fractures of the lumbar spine. J Bone Joint Surg [Br] 64:520, 1982
14. Denis F: The three column spine and its significance in the classification of acute thoracolumbar spinal injuries. Spine 8:817, 1983
15. Gertzbein SD, Court-Brown CM: Flexion distraction injuries of the lumbar spine: mechanisms of injury and classification. Clin Orthop Rel Res 227:52, 1988
16. Ritchie WP, Ersek RA, Bunch WL, Simmons RL: Combined visceral and vertebral injuries from lap-type seat belts. Surg Gynecol Obstet 131:431, 1970
17. Rogers LF: The roentgenographic appearance of transverse or chance fractures of the spine: the seat belt fracture. Am J Roentgenol Radium Ther Nucl Med 3:844, 1971
18. Blasier RD, Lamont RL: Chance fracture in a child: case report with nonoperative treatment. J Paediatr Orthop 5:92, 1985
19. Gallagher DJ, Heinrich SD: Pediatric chance fracture. J Orthop Trauma 4:183, 1990
20. Johnson DL, Falci S: The diagnosis and treatment of pediatric lumbar spine injuries caused by rear seat lap belts. Neurosurgery 26:434, 1990
21. Rumball K, Jarvis J: Seat-belt injuries of the spine in young children. J Bone Joint Surg [Br] 74:571, 1992
22. Appleby JP, Nagy AG: Abdominal injuries associated with the use of seatbelts. Am J Surg 157:457, 1989
23. Hall H, Robertson W: Another chance: a non-seatbelt related fracture of the lumbar spine. J Trauma 25:1163, 1985
24. States J, Huelke D, Dance M, Green R: Fatal injuries caused by underarm use of shoulder belts. J Trauma 27:740, 1987
25. Hope PG, Houghton GR: Spinal and abdominal injury in an infant due to the incorrect use of a car seat belt. Injury 17:368, 1986
26. Miniaci A, McLaren AC: Anterolateral compression fracture of the thoracolumbar spine. Clin Orthop Rel Res 240:153, 1989
27. Green D, Green NE, Spengler DM, Davito D: Flexion distraction injuries of the lumbar spine associated with ruptured abdominal viscus abstracted. J Orthop Trauma 4:214, 1990
28. Vandersluis R, O'Connor HMC: The seat belt syndrome. Can Med Assoc J 137:1023, 1987
29. Denis R, Allard M, Atlas H, Farkouh E: Changing trends with abdominal injury in seatbelt wearers. J Trauma 23:1007, 1983
30. Committee on Injury Scaling, American Association for Automobile Medicine: The abbreviated injury scale. Society of Automotive Engineers, Morton Grove, IL, 1985
31. Taylor GA, Dunne Eggli K: Lap belt injuries of the lumbar spine in children: a pitfall in C.T. diagnosis. AJR 150:1355, 1988
32. Keller J, Mosdal C: Traumatic odontoid epiphysiolysis in an infant fixed in a child's car seat. Injury 21:191, 1990
33. Tolonen J, Santavirta S, Kivilvote O, Lindquist C: Fatal cervical spinal injuries in road traffic accidents. Injury 17:154, 1986
34. Golger H, Anthanasiadis S, Adomeit D: Fatal cervical dislocation related to wearing a seat belt: a case report. Injury 10:196, 1979
35. Sköld G, Voigt GE: Spinal injuries in seat belt wearing car occupants killed by head-on collisions. Injury 9:151, 1977
36. Fletcher BD, Brogden BG: Seatbelt fractures of the spine and sternum. JAMA 200:167, 1967
37. Rockwood CA, Wilkins KE, King RE: Fractures in Children. JB Lippincott, Philadelphia, 1984
38. Hubbard DD: Fractures of the dorsal and lumbar spine. Orthop Clin North Am 7:605, 1976

39. Pedersen S, Jansen U: Intestinal lesions caused by incorrectly placed seat belts. Acta Chir Scand 145:15, 1979
40. White A, Panjabi M: Clinical biomechanics of the spine. JB Lippincott, Philadelphia, 1978
41. Palmer CE: Studies of the center of gravity in the human body. Child Dev 15:99, 1944
42. Dance M, German A, Nowak ES, Green RN: An in-depth analysis of multiple fatal head-on motor vehicle collisions. p. 69. Proceedings of American Association for Automotive Medicine, San Francisco, 1981
43. Newman KD, Bowman LM, Eichelberger MR et al: Lap belt complex: intestinal and lumbar spine injury in children. J Trauma 30:1133, 1990
44. Kerslake RW, Jaspan T, Worthington BS: Magnetic resonance imaging of spinal trauma. Br J Radiol 64:386, 1991
45. Tator C: Spinal cord injuries: acute management. Medicine [North Am] p. 3, 1990
46. Moskowitz A: Lumbar seatbelt injury in a child: case report. J Trauma 29:1279, 1989
47. LeGay DA, Petrie DP, Alexander DI: Flexion-distraction injuries of the lumbar spine and associated abdominal trauma. J Trauma 30:436, 1990
48. Asbun HJ, Irani H, Roe EJ, Block JH: Intra-abdominal seatbelt injury. J Trauma 30:189, 1990
49. Taylor TFK, Nade S, Bennisten JH: Seat belt fractures of the cervical spine. J Bone Joint Surg [Br] 58:328, 1976
50. Laing JHE, Sptiz L: Chylothorax and delayed paraparesis in an infant following improper use of a front seat belt. Br J Surg 76:129, 1989
51. National Transportation Safety Board: Safety Study: Performance of Lap Belts in 26 Frontal crashes. NTSB/SS-86/03 Washington, DC, 1986
52. Hoffman M, Spence L, Wesson D et al: The pediatric passenger: trends in seatbelt use and injury patterns. J Trauma 27:974, 1987
53. ISBN-O-7743 Ministry of Transportation and Communications: What You Should Know About Seat Belts. Ontario, 1990
54. Dooley B: The role of seat-belts in reducing road toll. J Bone Joint Surg [Br] 64:518, 1982
55. Dalmotas DJ, Dance DM, Gardner WT et al: Current activities in Canada relating to the protection of children in automobile accidents. In: Advances in Seatbelt Restraints: Design, Performance and Usage. Society of Automotive Engineers, Warrendale, PA, 1985

48

Fractures of the Sacrum and Coccyx

Guillermo R. Viviani

> Nothing is more fatal to health, than an over-care of it.
> —BENJAMIN FRANKLIN

DESCRIPTION AND INCIDENCE

In children, sacral fractures are uncommon, probably related to the rather flexible nature of the sacroiliac joints and as well the persistence of articulating fibrocartilage segments. As in adults, sacral fractures are usually part of a major pelvic injury with serious visceral lesions.

A recent review of sacral trauma by Denis and colleagues[1] entitled "Sacral Fractures, an Important Problem, Though Frequently Undiagnosed and Untreated," summarizes the present status of sacral fractures in both the skeletally mature and immature. The true incidence of sacral fractures in children is not well known, as the fractures are difficult to see in plain radiographs and are frequently missed. In large reviews of children's pelvic fractures, the incidence of sacral fractures varied between 1.5 and 12 percent.[2,3]

In 1939, a special radiologic study was performed in adults to ascertain the true incidence of fractures of the sacrum, which were diagnosed in 44 percent of 50 pelvic fractures.[4] This high incidence was related to the very careful scrutiny of the radiographs but emphasizes that the sacrum is frequently injured in association with pelvic fractures and are often underdiagnosed!

In adolescents, as in adults, severe sacral fractures are frequently associated with neurologic lesions, but this does not occur in younger children, as no reports of significant neurologic deficits have been found.

There are no specific references of the incidence of coccygeal fractures in children. A series of nine pediatric cases with a mean age of 13.5 years has been reported.[3]

Coccydynia, or coccygodynia, is a term used for a syndrome defined as pain in and around the coccyx and is not a specific diagnosis. Usually the word is reserved for the "idiopathic" condition in which no specific cause for the pain has been found, and this is by far the most common type. Coccydynia is about five times more frequent in women than in men. The most common age affected by this condition is the midthirties, but it does occur as well in the early teens.[5,6] It appears that, in early adolescence, there is usually a history of a traumatic incident that initiated the pain.[3] The true incidence of traumatic coccydynia in adolescence is unknown, but it appears to be increasing in frequency, possibly related to increased participation in vigorous sports and physical training programs. As in adults, it seems to be more common in adolescent girls.

ANATOMY

At 5 weeks the human embryo has a free-moving tail containing 7 to 11 coccygeal vertebrae. However, this becomes concealed by the buttocks and regresses to 4 or 5 rudimentary vertebrae, which are fused together in the

2 yrs.   **8 yrs.**   **10 yrs.**   **13 yrs.**   **16 yrs.**

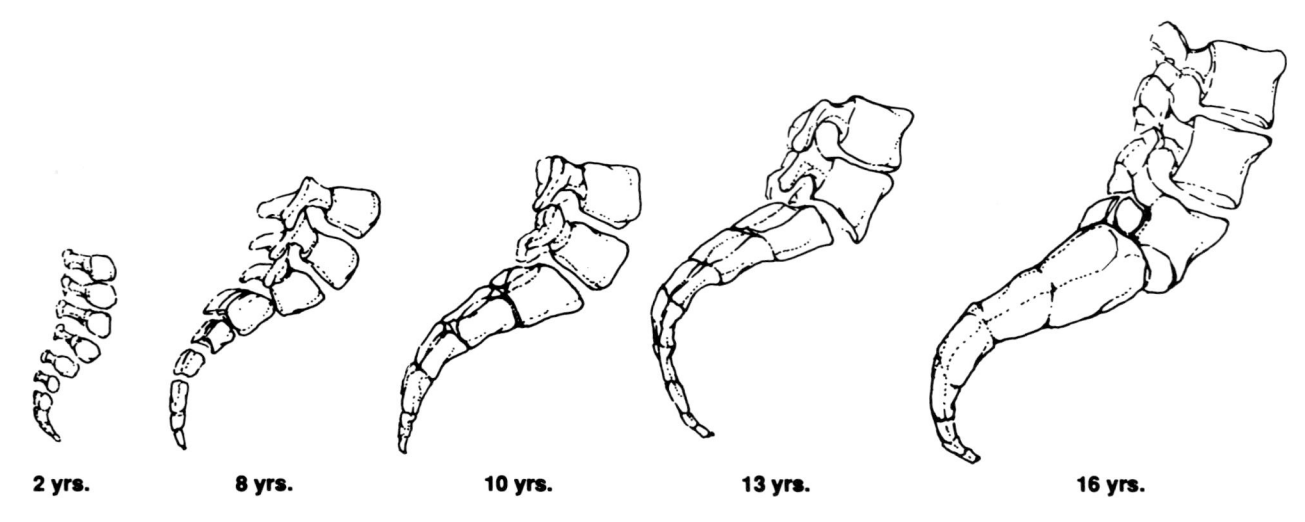

Fig. 48-1. Female sacral development based on radiographs from age 2 to 16.

coccyx. The costal processes become the ribs in the thoracic spine, the transverse processes become incorporated in the lumbar spine and the lateral portion of the vertebrae of the sacrum. The ossification of the five sacral segments is slow and may not be completed until the age of 25 fusing from distal to proximal[7] (Fig. 48-1). In adolescence, this occasionally results in misinterpretation of the unfused segment as a fracture line. Incomplete fusion of the first and second sacral vertebrae produces "lumbarization" of the segment. Also, the fifth lumbar vertebra may be fused on one or both sides to the sacrum, becoming "sacralized." There are also several other sacral developmental anomalies often associated with spina bifida, spondylolisthesis, or other congenital anomalies of the spine. Variations in the shape of the coccyx are common, and may result in a predisposition to traumatic coccydynia.

The sacrum and coccyx have a triangular shape with the base proximally (Fig. 48-2). The base of the sacrum is angulated posteriorly about 30 degrees in relation to L5. The body of the sacrum is oval where it articulates with the disc. The anterior part forms the "promontory." Posteriorly, there is the triangular, flattened, and somewhat wide sacral canal covered in this part by the ligamentum flavum. Lateral to it, is the projection of the superior articular facets of the sacrum with the articular surface somewhat like a concave vertical cylinder to articulate with L5. There are common variations in the orientation and shape of this joint. Distal to the facet is a wide, short, S1 pedicle that continues laterally with the fan-shaped *ala.* The S1 pedicle is separated from the next pedicle by the first sacral foramina. The ala and *lateral mass* of the fused three proximal sacral vertebrae ends laterally into the *auricular facet* (ear-shaped) that articulates with the ilium. The lateral aspect of the sacrum becomes thinner distal to the auricular facet and forms the medial aspect of the *greater sciatic notch,* giving attachments to the sacrospinous and sacrotuberous ligaments. At the apex it articulates with the base of the coccyx with a thin disc and two tiny synovial joints at the level of the *cornu.*

In the front of the sacrum (Fig. 48-3) the promontory and the ala are part of the pelvic brim that is the landmark between the greater and lesser pelvis. The medial part of the ala is crossed by the sympathetic trunk and in sequence lateral to this by the lumbosacral trunk, iliolumbar vessels, psoas, and obturator nerve. The fifth lumbar ventral ramus is so taut that it grooves the anterior border of the ala, with the fourth lumbar root also very close, as well as the iliac veins. Due to this anatomic relationship, this area is considered an "unsafe zone" for fixation with surgical screws.[8,9] The remaining anterior or pelvic surface of the sacrum is concave and crossed horizontally by four rudimentary ridges at the sites where the segments fused together. On each side there are four large anterior or pelvic sacral foramina. The mass of bone lateral to them is called the *pars lateralis* that is grooved by the close four ventral rami of the sacral plexus.

The posterior wall is more irregular. It has a *medial sacral crest* or ridge formed by the spinous processes, decreasing in size from S1 to the distal end, where a variable-sized hiatus or opening is present. Lateral to this and following a line projected from the articular proc-

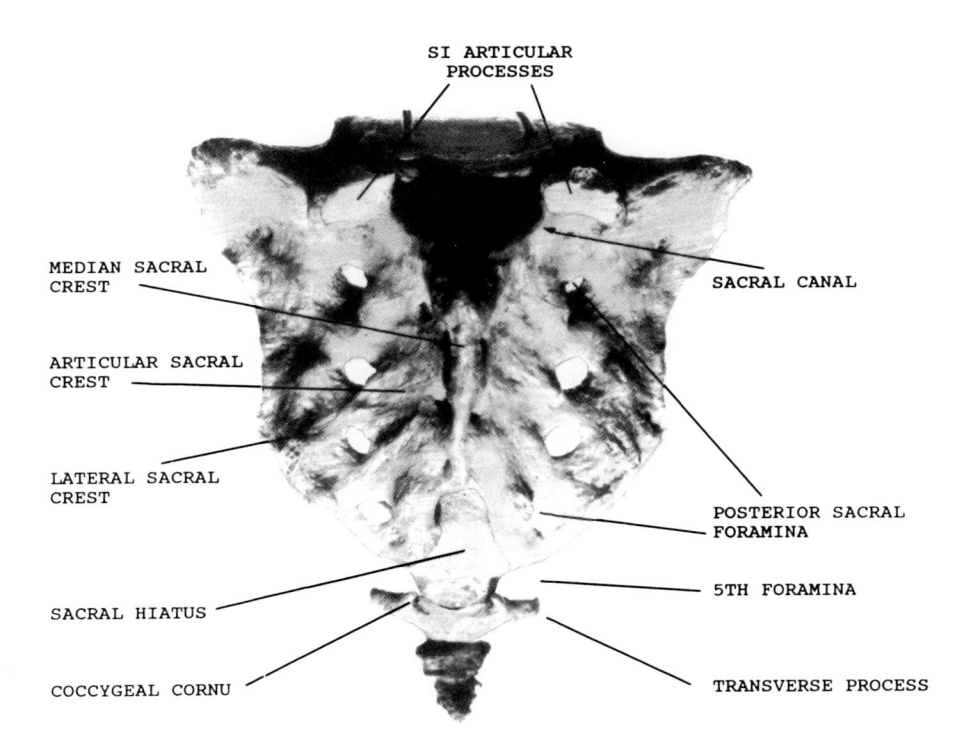

Fig. 48-2. Posterior view of the sacrum. Denis fracture zones are marked.

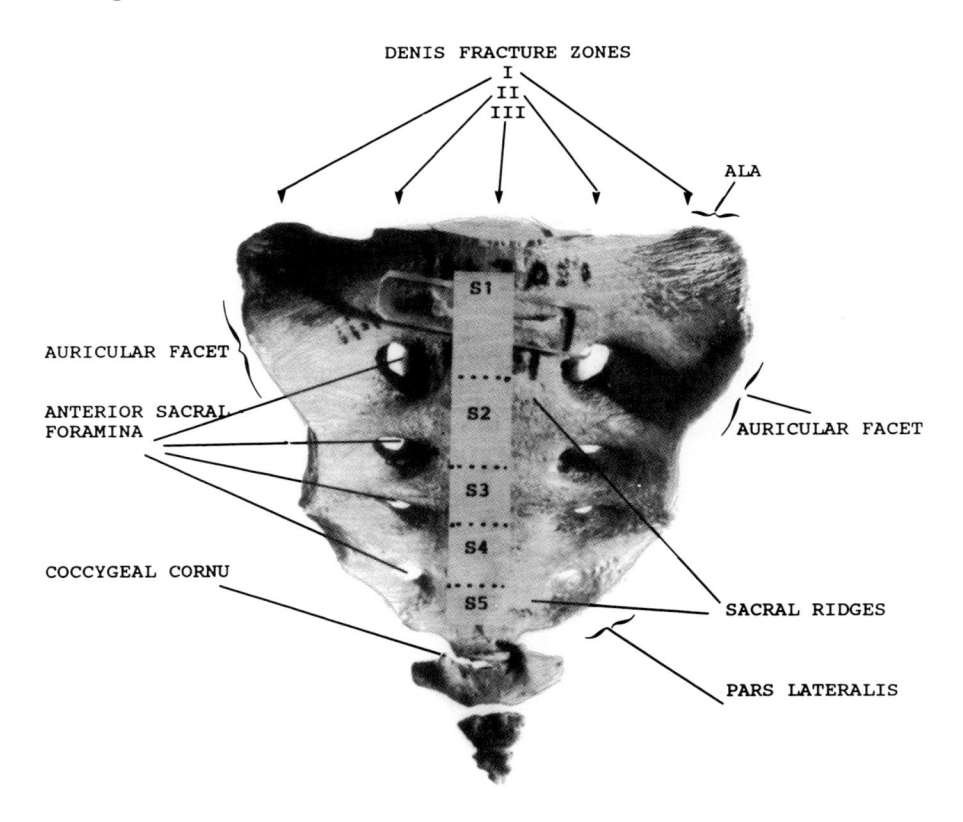

Fig. 48-3. Anterior view of the sacrum.

esses is a ridge formed by small tubercles called the *articular crest*. This ends in the *sacral cornu* that articulates with the corresponding pieces in the base of the coccyx. This articular ridge forms the medial border of the four posterior sacral foramina. The fifth foramen is between the sacrum and coccyx lateral to the cornua. The dorsal foramina are large, and they can admit a lead pencil to communicate directly to the ventral foramina, as well as medially to the sacral canal. Lateral to the foramina is a third ridge called the *lateral sacral crest,* which is a remnant of the transverse processes fusion. The erector spinae muscles are attached between the median and lateral crest. Lateral to this are the attachments of the strong weight-bearing posterior sacral iliac ligaments.

In the sacral canal the dura mater usually ends around S2, thus permitting injection through the hiatus of S2, S3, S4 roots and coccygeal plexus, after their exit through the dura mater, with caudal anesthesia technique.

The coccyx is a small triangular bone usually formed by four segments fused together. It provides attachment to a mass of ligaments and muscles. These include the sacrospinous ligaments, coccygeous muscles, anococcygeal raphe, and external anal sphincter. Anteriorly it is separated from the rectum by a fibrous and muscle tissue mass called the anococcygeous body. The rectum begins at the level of the third sacral vertebrae and ends slightly below the tip of the coccyx, about 3 cm in front of this.

MECHANISM OF INJURY

Sacral fractures in children are usually associated with major pelvic injury. The injury is frequently secondary to motor vehicle accidents or a running child being hit by a vehicle or some unusual crushing injury. Isolated fractures can occur after a hard fall onto the sacral area. The fractures are mainly vertical or oblique, related to compression or shearing forces acting in the sacrum or SI joints. A more uncommon type is a transverse fracture related to a direct force onto the sacrum. Also, combinations of these fractures associated with comminution can occur.[10] The kinematics of the sacroiliac joint suggests that this joint may constitute primarily a shock-absorbing function, but even this strong ligamentous joint will disrupt with extremes of energy.[11]

Stress fractures have been reported in the sacrum, but they are unusual. In our literature review, the youngest case reported was a 20-year-old runner performing 80 km per week.[12] These types of fractures may represent a rather puzzling cause of pain that is difficult to diagnose, without awareness of its existence and the use of CT imaging and/or bone scans.

CLASSIFICATION

Frequently, a sacral fracture in childhood is part of an SI joint disruption. The weakest portion of the bone is along the foramina where often vertical lines of fractures occur. To explain the specific incidence of neurologic lesions, Denis and associates[1] have proposed a classification in three zones. In zone 1 or ala, occasionally the fifth lumbar root may be damaged. Zone 2 is the foramina and can be associated with sciatica. Zone 3 or central sacral canal is associated with saddle anesthesia and a sphincter dysfunction (Fig. 48-3). CT imaging and/or tomograms permit the precise localization of these zones where the fractures are located.

PHYSICAL EXAMINATION

A precondition to arrive at the proper diagnosis of a sacral fracture is awareness of the high incidence of this lesion in any major pelvic injury. Apart from the usual assessment of the pelvic lesions, attention should be directed to the sacrum with proper manual examination. It has been stated that clinical examination of the sacrum is more accurate than radiographs.[3] Palpation and visualization of the area may reveal some swelling and pain. If present, this examination should be gently combined with a rectal bimanual palpation. Plain routine films are almost useless, due to the imprecise direction of the radiographs and the superimposition of bowel images over this poorly visible bone structure.[13] Special pelvic and sacral views, and particularly the use of CT and/or tomograms, will usually identify the fractures.

Proper neurologic examination is absolutely necessary to rule out commonly associated neurologic lesions. This most frequently affects L5, obturator nerve or other lumbosacral roots, with the corresponding variable degree of weakness and sensory deficit in the lower limbs and/or saddle anesthesia and loss of sphincter control. Often, the neurologic lesions are not detected in the early assessment of these patients with multiple trauma, and only when the patient has been stabilized and is conscious can this be properly reassessed. It is worthwhile to remember that transverse fractures are more commonly associated with severe neurologic lesions.

DIFFERENTIAL DIAGNOSIS

The most common problem is lack of diagnosis due to poor examination and imaging. In children and adolescents, anatomic variations that are related to the development of the sacrum, could present further difficulties for the diagnosis. Persistence of segmental disc lines could be interpreted as a fracture (Fig. 48-4). Also, variations in the transitional lumbosacral zone may add difficulties to diagnosis in this particular area. Other pathologic conditions of the sacrum such as cysts or tumors can also be associated with pathologic fractures.

TREATMENT

In young children, most undisplaced pelvic and sacral fractures require only bed rest for 2 to 6 weeks, followed by ambulation with or without crutches according to pain tolerance. Significant remodeling occurs and persistent serious sequelae are uncommon (Fig. 48-5). In adolescents, due to the different nature of the injury and healing process, treatment considerations are similar to adults. Unstable pelvic injuries affecting the SI joints, may require more prolonged bed rest and leg traction and/or the need for external or internal fixation procedures (Fig. 48-6A&B). Major neurologic lesions may benefit from surgical decompression and stabilization of the fracture (Fig. 48-7A&B).

COMPLICATIONS

In children under the age of 10, sacral lesions are treated usually with bed rest and are unlikely to have complications related to instability or neurologic problems. Complications are common in association with major pelvic injuries in which the sacral fracture is part of the pelvic ring disruption. They are related to hemorrhage and associated visceral lesions.

In adolescents, as shown in the two examples, complications can occur in relation to the sacral lesion even without associated major pelvic injuries. Figure 48-6A&B shows radiographs of a 16-year-old female in which an unstable lesion of the right SI joint was identified in the early assessment, and treated with surgical internal fixation, with screws through the joint, that permitted early mobilization and adequate healing of the joint lesion. Figure 48-7A&B is a 16-year-old boy who woke up 2 days after a motor vehicle accident with bilateral leg weakness, urinary retention, and saddle anesthesia. After CT myelogram demonstrated compression of the sacral canal, a laminectomy and root decompression was performed that may have helped the significant recovery that followed. Lack of early diagnosis of sacral fractures with associated instability or neurologic injuries, may contribute to poor final results, and should be avoided with awareness for adequate clinical assessment and proper imaging.

TRAUMATIC COCCYDYNIA

Etiology and Classification

The term *coccydynia* appears to be the preferred term in a 1991 review of this topic in the *British Journal of Bone and Joint Surgery*,[6] but the word "coccygodynia" also appears frequently in the literature.

The exact etiology of this condition remains unknown, but frequently a history of a direct trauma to this region or repetitive mechanical irritation with specific exercises is a precursor of the syndrome.[3,5,6] Numerous possible etiologies have been postulated for truly idio-

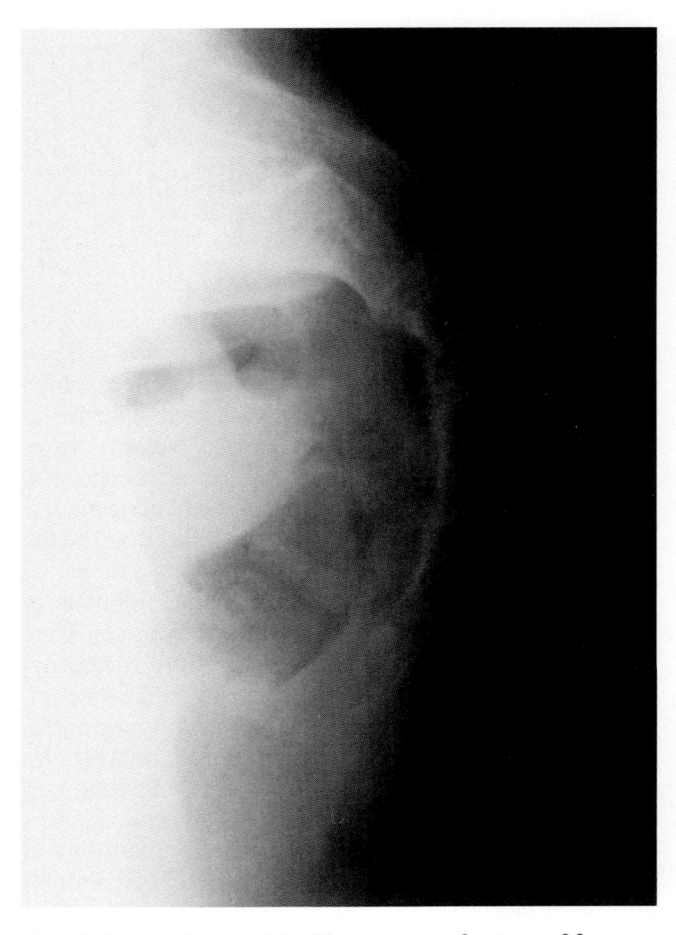

Fig. 48-4. A 13-year-old with transverse fracture of fracture of S3 and clearly visible lines of partially fused sacral segments.

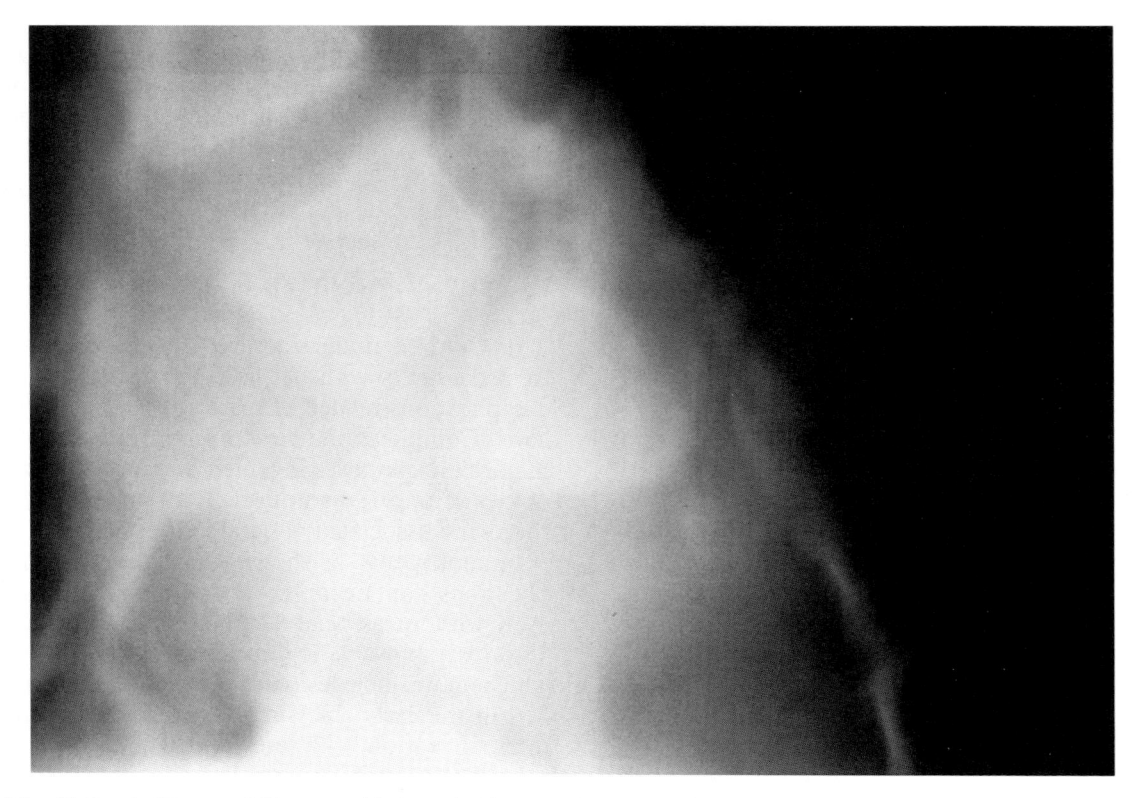

Fig. 48-5. A 10-year-old boy was hit from behind by a front-end loader. A fracture dislocation of S1 on S2 was sustained. Clinically, he suffered no neurologic sequelae; he was treated with bed rest and body cast and healed uneventfully with a local prominence but no progression of the traumatic spondylolisthesis. (Courtesy of Dr. M. Letts.)

pathic cases of coccydynia, as mentioned by Postacchini and Massobrio.[5] These include functional neurosis, a spasm of the muscles of the pelvic floor, anomalies of the soft tissues in the midsacral region, chronic inflammations, lesions of the lumbar discs, arachnoiditis of the lower sacral nerve roots, posttraumatic osteoarthritis of the sacral coccygeal joints, ununited fractures, and subluxations and sprains of the coccyx. Also, some rare but well-defined pathologies have been reported.[6] These include chordoma, giant cell tumor, intradural schwannoma, perineural cyst and intraosseous lipoma.

To our knowledge, no published review of coccygeal injury have been reported in children, but teenagers are being seen complaining of posttraumatic coccygeal pain with increasing frequency. Usually, there is a history of some form of traumatic injury that initiates the pain. In my opinion, the most likely pathogenesis is the mechanism described by Postacchini and Massobrio.[5] They postulate that coccygodynia is related to a developmental instability of the first sacral coccygeal joint at which level the coccyx is angulated or subluxated. This instability may remain asymptomatic or may become symptomatic even at a very young age, usually after coccygeal trauma. The stretching of the articular and periarticular structures of these abnormally mobile joints, may be the cause of the pain.

These authors also examined the radiographic variations of the anatomy of the coccyx in 120 subjects. They found significant variations in the fusion of the coccygeal segments and/or fusion of segments to the sacrum, as well as in the position and angulation of the segments. Four types of configurations of the coccyx were described with variable degree of forward angulation or curvature (Fig. 48-8). They noticed that types 2, 3, and 4 have a more significant forward angulation pattern and are more prone to become painful. Types 2 and 3 might also predispose to injury during childbirth and development of coccygeal symptoms in the postnatal period.

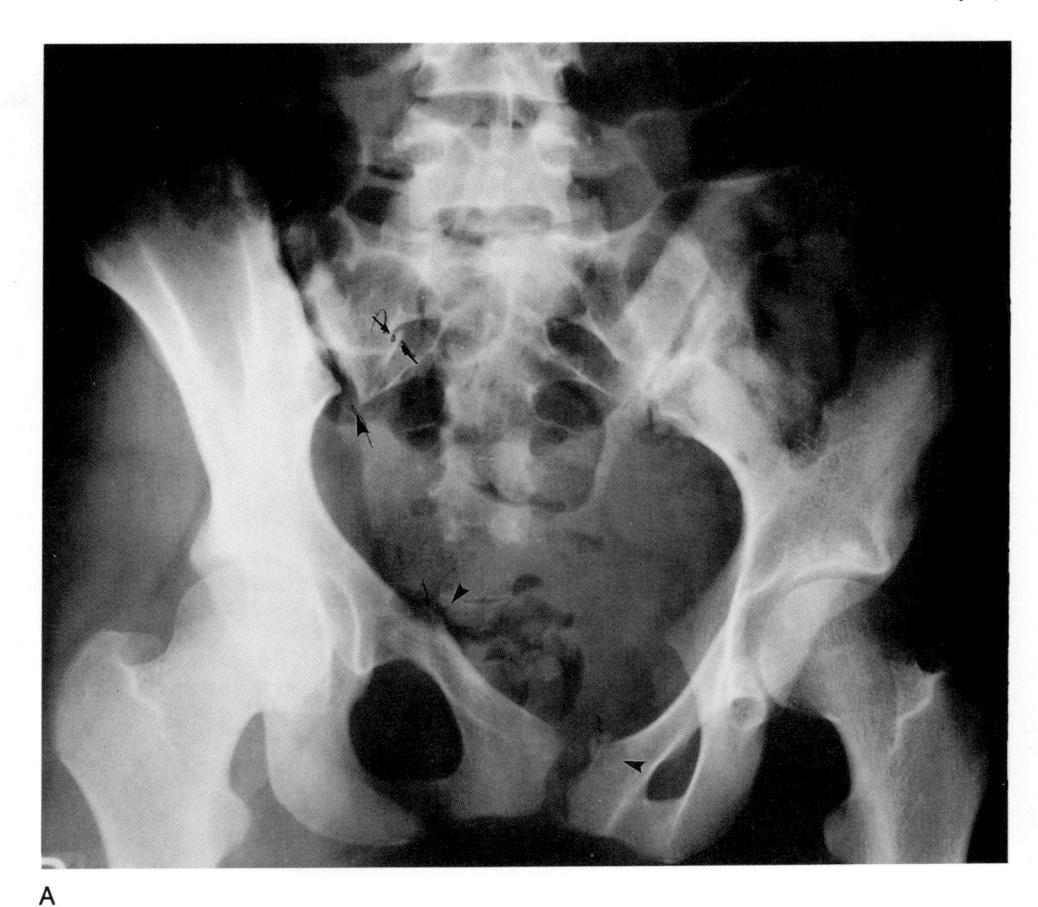

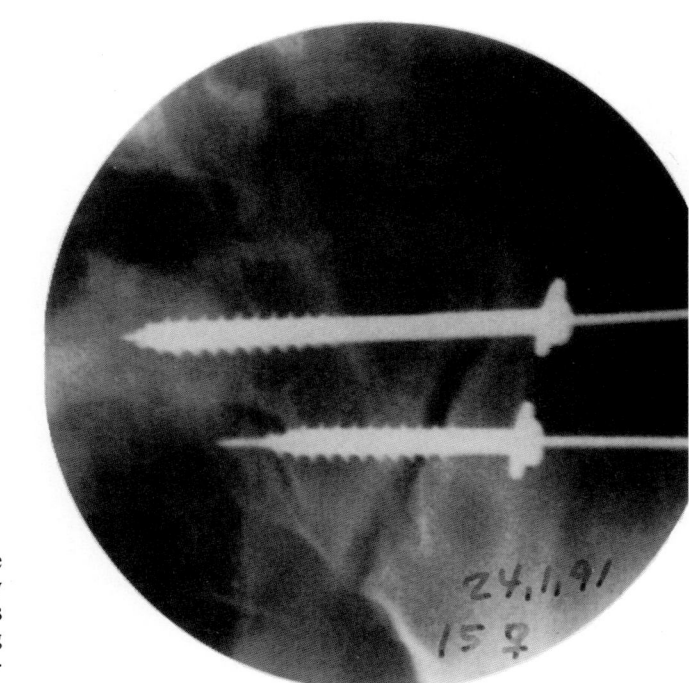

Fig. 48-6. (A) A 15-year-old girl with an undisplaced fracture of sacrum and disruption of the right sacroiliac joint secondary to a motor vehicle accident. (B) The sacroiliac disruption was reduced and held with two percutaneous screws inserted using biplane radiograph control allowing early ambulation and uneventful healing. (Courtesy of Dr. D. Punthakee.)

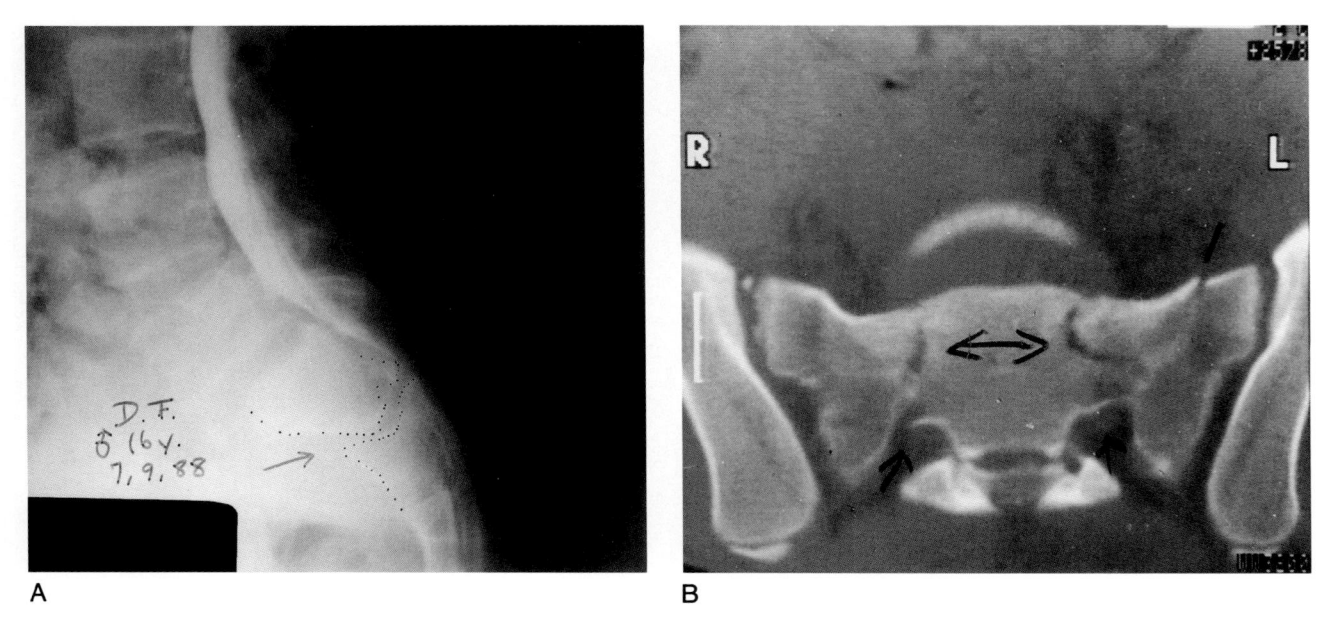

Fig. 48-7. (A) A 16-year-old boy involved in a motor vehicle accident, awoke from a head injury with no sphincter control and bilateral leg weakness. Radiographs illustrate tilting of S1 on S2 with disruption of anterior cortical margin of S2 and a myelogram block at the S1-S2 angulation. A traumatic spondylolysis bilaterally was noted at L5. This progressed and required fusion 2 years later. (B) CT scan shows a comminuted fracture of S1 primarily involving the lateral segments and foramina. Surgical decompression with laminectomy was performed followed by almost complete recovery of the neurologic deficit.

Physical Examination

In a child with a history of pain in or around the coccyx that is increased with sitting or with specific physical activities, the examination of the area becomes essential for the diagnosis of coccydynia. The coccyx can be examined in teenagers with the child lying on one side with external pressure and gentle manipulation of the coccygeal tip. This will reproduce the typical coccygeal pain in a well-localized area. Furthermore, injection of a local anesthetic in the mobile region between the sacrum and the coccygeal segments will usually relieve the pain at least temporarily. If felt necessary, a rectal examination can then be performed and a bimanual examination

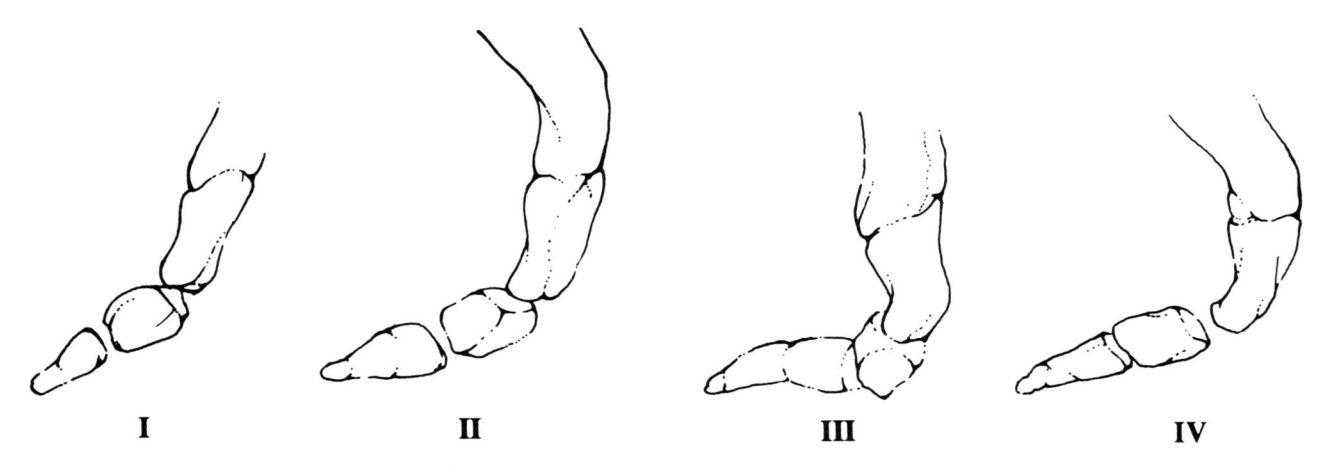

Fig. 48-8. Types of coccygeal configuration. (After Postacchini and Massobrio.[5])

of the coccyx performed to determine mobility. In younger children, examination of the coccyx with the child prone facilitates access to the coccyx. In the history and examination, other conditions, as previously described, should be ruled out. In the examination, the anatomic type of the coccyx and its angulation can also be assessed.

Differential Diagnosis

The differential diagnosis is made on the basis of the history, physical examination and good quality radiographs of the sacrum, coccyx, and lumbar spine. In more doubtful cases, CT scans of the area, or isotope bone scans and/or psychiatric assessment, should be included.

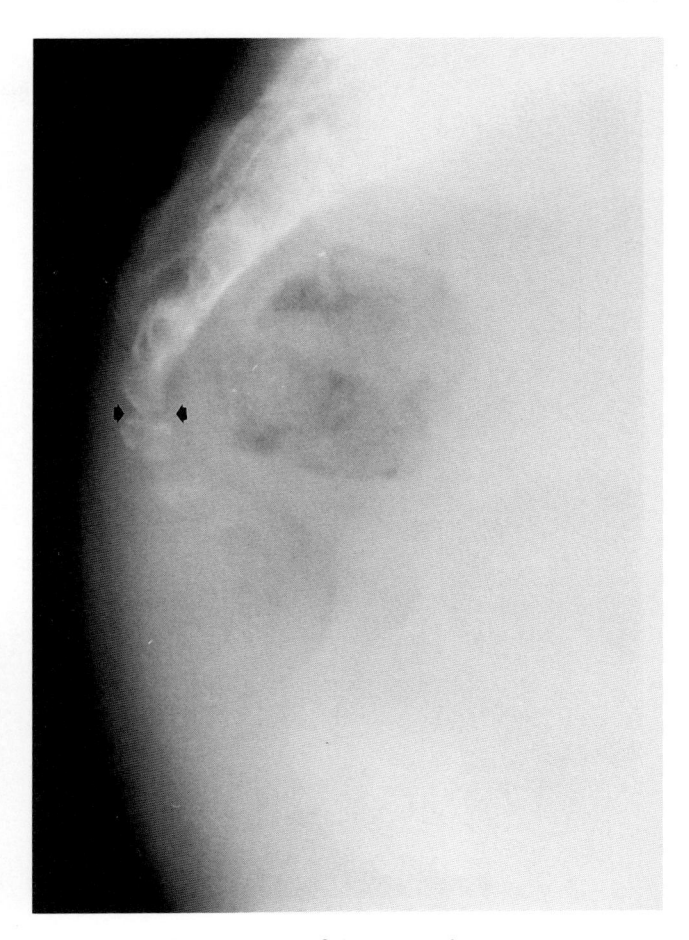

Fig. 48-10. Fracture of the coccyx in a 14-year-old.

In cases of very prolonged pain, like in other chronic pain syndromes, important psychological problems may develop.

Treatment

Most cases of traumatic coccygodynia appear to resolve spontaneously within 3 to 6 months (Fig. 48-9). At the outset, reassurance and explanation of the frequently prolonged course of the condition is extremely important to avoid unnecessary anxiety and mislabeling of the condition. In children with a clear history of a traumatic onset, the pain may last for 6 months or more. The most useful treatment in this stage, is the regular use of a soft cushion that can be carried around by the patient. Teenagers will often accept the football or baseball seat cushions that are made for carrying and attract less attention.

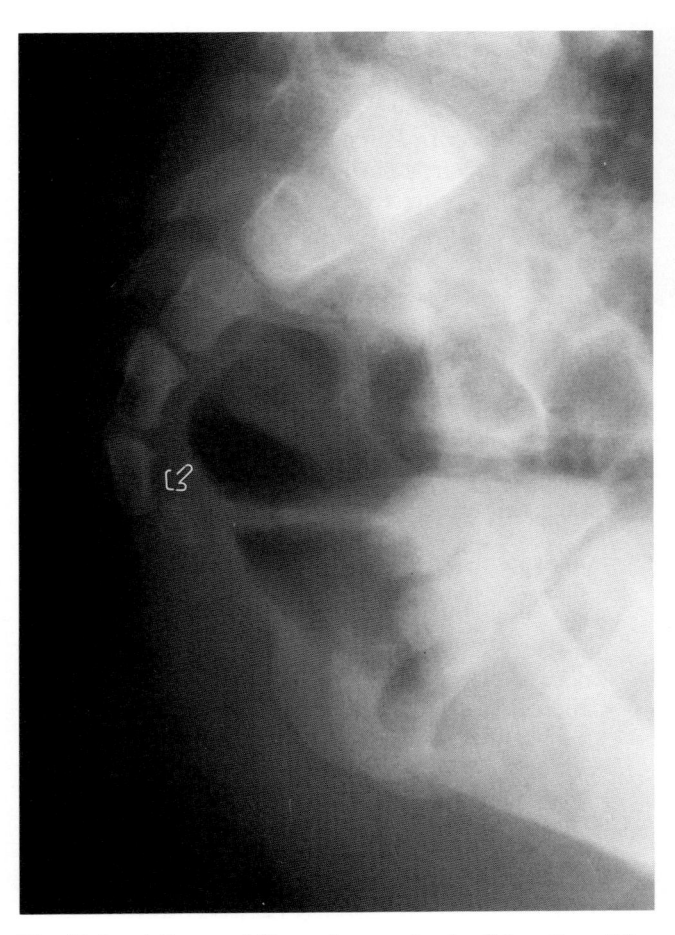

Fig. 48-9. A 7-year-old boy who sustained a dislocation of the last coccygeal vertebrae in a fall downstairs. Treated symptomatically, the symptoms subsided over 6 to 8 weeks. (Courtesy of Dr. R. Mervyn Letts.)

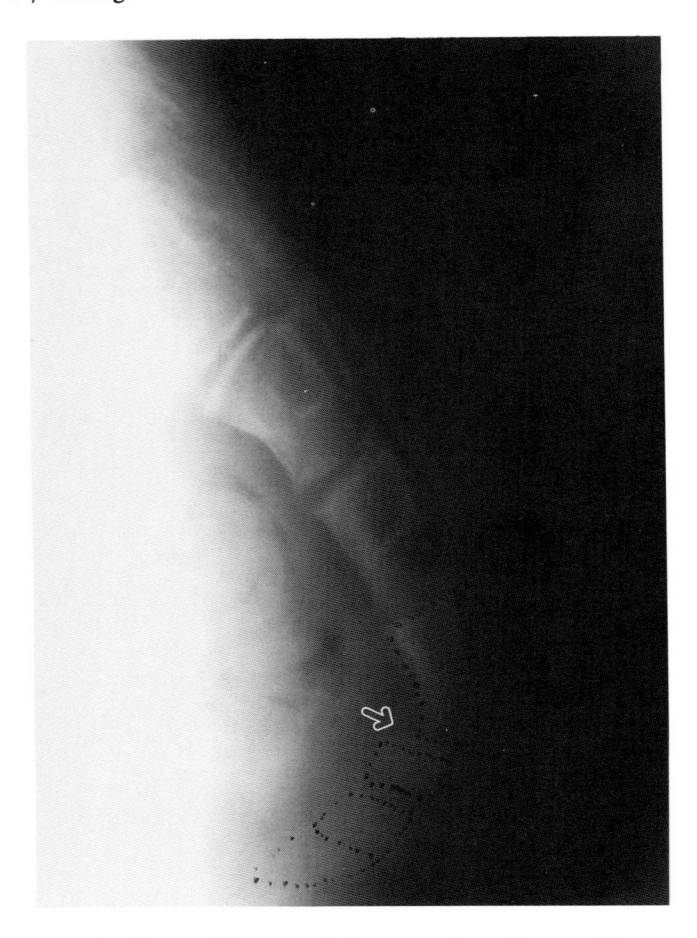

Fig. 48-11. Fracture of the coccyx in a 12-year-old.

Physiotherapy has been used, but there is little information on its efficacy. In one prospective study,[6] in 16 percent of the cases the addition of ultrasound and shortwave diathermy appeared to have helped. When the pain is severe or prolonged, local injection with a mixture of 40 mg Depomedrol in 2 percent xylocaine is often helpful in relieving symptoms. This can be repeated after 1 or 2 months if necessary. In my experience, this has eradicated the symptoms in most teenagers. For pain that persists in spite of local injections, surgery can be considered, although, in my experience, surgery has not been necessary in children and teenagers. However, severe congenital malformation of the coccyx which is predisposed to minor trauma and fracture may necessitate excision in rare instances. Although various kinds of surgical procedures are reported in the literature, including tenotomy of coccygeal ligaments and rhizotomies of the lower sacral roots, the preferred surgical treatment remains removal of the coccyx with smoothing down of bony prominences at the lower end of the sacrum. A vertical incision should be used because transverse incisions do not heal as well in this region.[6,14]

There is a wide divergence of opinions on effectiveness of coccygectomy. Reported results vary from 95 percent satisfactory to significant failures and strong advice against surgery.[6,5,14-16] In children, it is seldom necessary.

Complications

Lack of proper diagnosis and clear explanations regarding the nature of the condition and its natural prolonged course may create unnecessary family anxiety and problems. Fractures are difficult to see on standard radiographs (Figs. 48-10 and 48-11). Not infrequently, the child is labeled as neurotic without proper justification. Noncompliance of the sensitive teen to use a cushion regularly, sometimes prolongs the coccydynia due to constant irritation from the hard desk seats at school.

With surgery, complications can occur including perforation of the rectum, superficial infections, and unsatisfactory scars, particularly with transverse incisions. Persistence of pain may be due to inadequate bone removal or persistence of a rough area at the end of the sacrum.

REFERENCES

1. Denis F, Davis S, Comfort T: Sacral fractures, an important problem, though frequently undiagnosed and untreated (retrospective analysis of 203 consecutive cases): orthopaedic transactions. J Bone Joint Surg [Am] 11:118, 1987
2. Denis F, Winter RB, Lonstein JE: Pediatric spinal injuries: orthopaedic transactions. J Bone Joint Surg [Am] 12:232, 1988
3. Canale ST, King RE: Pelvic and hip fractures. p. 733. In Rockwood CA, Wilkins KE, King RE (eds): Fractures in Children. Vol. 3. JB Lippincott, Philadelphia, 1984
4. Medelman JP: Incidence of associated fractures of the sacrum. AJR 42:100, 1939
5. Postacchini F, Massobrio M: Idiopathic coccygodynia: analysis of fifty-one operative cases and a radiographic study of the normal coccyx. J Bone Joint Surg [Am] 65:1116, 1983
6. Wray CC, Easom S, Hoskinson J: Coccydynia: aetiology and treatment. J Bone Joint Surg [Br] 73:335, 1991
7. McKern TW, Stewart TD: Skeletal age changes in young American males, analysed from the standpoint of age identification. Smithsonian Institution, 1957

8. Esses SI, Botsford DJ, Huler RJ, Rauschning W: Surgical anatomy of the sacrum: a guide for rational screw fixation. Spine 16:S283, 1991
9. Mirkovic S, Abitbol JJ, Steinman J et al: Anatomic consideration for sacral screw placement. Spine 16:S289, 1991
10. Yasuda T, Shikata J, Iida H, Yamamuro T: Upper sacral transverse fracture. Spine 15:589, 1990
11. White III, AA, Panjabi MM: Clinical Biomechanics of the Spine. 2nd Ed. JB Lippincott, Philadelphia, 1991
12. Haller J, Kindynis P, Resnick D et al: Fatigue fracture of the sacrum: a case report. Can Assoc Radiol J 40:277, 1989
13. Rang M: Pelvis. p. 150. In Parks J, Rang M (eds): Children's Fractures. JB Lippincott, Philadelphia, 1974
14. Hellberg S, Strange-Vognsen HH: Coccygodynia treated by resection of the coccyx. Acta Orthop Scand 61:463, 1990
15. Duncan GA: Painful coccyx. Arch Surg 34:1088, 1937
16. Wray AR, Templeton J: Coccygectomy: a review of 37 cases. Ulster Med J 51:121, 1982
17. Nelson DW, Duwelius PJ: CT-guided fixation of sacral fractures and sacroiliac joint disruptions. Radiology 180:527, 1991

49

Acute Spinal Cord Injury

Garth Johnson

> Beware of fake knowledge, it is more dangerous than ignorance.
> —George Bernard Shaw

DEFINITION AND INCIDENCE

Spinal cord injuries occur at the rate of approximately 30 per million population annually, and, of these, fewer than 10 percent occur in children.[1] Differences in the injuries to the spinal cord in the pediatric population exist, such as the increased frequency of spinal cord injury in the absence of vertebral damage,[2] the predilection of the spinal injury to occur in the upper thoracic and upper cervical areas.[3] There may also be an increased proportion of complete neurologic injuries and delayed onset of neurologic signs.

Factors that may account for these differences include disproportionate head size and a higher fulcrum of neck motion. Structural changes, such as the horizontal facet orientation, and wedge-shaped vertebral bodies may also be contributory. Other factors that may account for these observed differences may be maturation of the spinal cord and its blood supply as well as the paraspinal musculature and ligaments.

Structural variations exist in the spine within the pediatric age group. Up to 3 years of age, the vertebra consists of three ossification centers, which unite by 10 or 12 years. After 13 years of age, the spine closely resembles the adult, with the exception of the presence of annular ossification centers.

ANATOMY

The dura is a prolongation of the fibrous layer of the dura mater from the posterior cranial fossa extending through the foramen magnum. It is attached firmly to the membrana tectoria and the posterior longitudinal ligament on the body of the axis. As each spinal nerve root pierces it, the dura is prolonged over the root extending into the intervertebral foramen, further anchoring the dura within the neural canal. Below, the spinal cord is tethered by the lumbar roots, leaving the thoracic spinal cord relatively unsupported and possibly more vulnerable to trauma. The spinal cord is suspended within the dura by thin lateral projections of the pia mater called the dentate ligaments, which attach to the dura as a series of interdigitations between the exiting nerve roots.

There is a centrifugal lamellar arrangement of fibers within each of the ascending and descending tracts, such that fibers arising most distally lie peripherally within their tract. Thus vascular injury to the central part of the cervical spinal cord will result in the preservation of perianal sensation and long toe flexion in the central cord syndrome. The blood supply to the spinal cord consists of the anterior spinal artery and smaller paired posterior spinal arteries arising from branches of the ver-

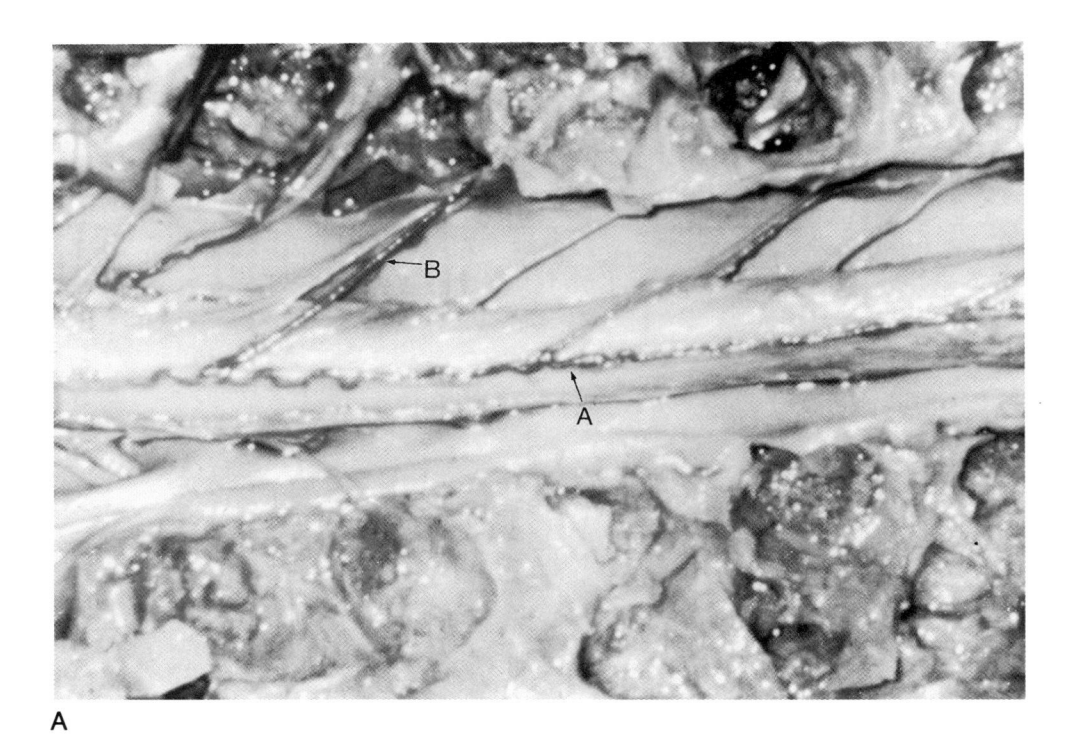

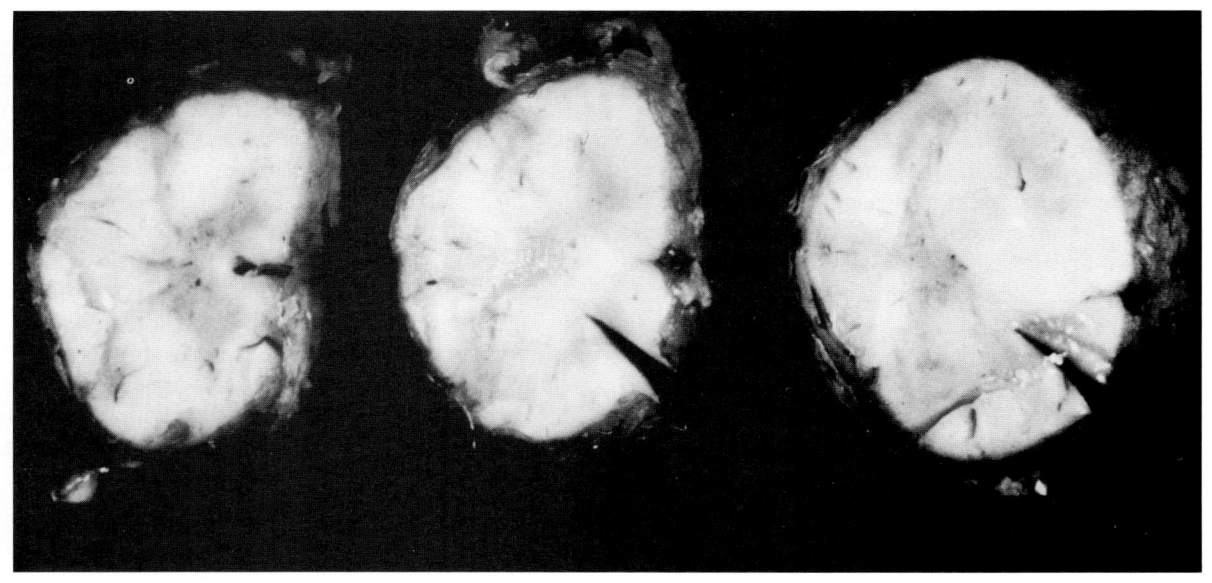

Fig. 49-1. (A) Spinal cord illustrating *(A)* longitudinal vessels; *(B)* feeder vessels associated with nerve roots and supplying the cord independently. (B) Cross-sectional views 1 year after an incomplete spinal cord injury demonstrating the asymmetrical scarring secondary to ischemia. Posterior column function was incompletely preserved.

tebral and posteroinferior cerebellar arteries, respectively. At each vertebral level, the blood supply is enhanced by paired segmental branches of the aorta. There is a relative watershed created in the lower thoracic level as there are fewer segmental vessels; however, there is a rich anastomosis created within the intervertebral foramen providing collateral blood flow to the cord at all levels.

The intrinsic blood supply of the spinal cord is predominantly from central sulcus branches of the anterior spinal artery, which supply the central part of the cord (the medulla) and then branch centrifugally. A small rim of the anterior portion of the cord and a larger portion of the posterior cord are supplied by coronal branches from each of the anterior and posterior spinal arteries (Fig. 49-1A).

MECHANISM OF INJURY

The spinal cord, lying within the protective neural canal, can be subjected to forces of compression or tension. It is, however, extremely rare that in closed injuries there is true physical disruption of the cord[1] (Fig. 49-1).

Primary Injury

Seconds following impact, small hemorrhages occur in the gray matter and pia arachnoid. After several minutes, the hemorrhages extend into the white matter. At the same time, changes in the microcirculation occur. Initially, there is extravasation of blood and fluid and, after several days, significant edema.[5,6]

Within minutes, there is significant increase in the periaxonal space. Hours later, variable degrees of damage are recognized up to an endpoint characterized by shrunken axons and extensive tissue necrosis. The late stage shows focal gliosis (Fig. 49-2), with formation of microcysts, which may coalesce.

Secondary Injury

Multiple factors contribute to the further progression of the injury. Release of lysosomal enzymes from damaged local cells, as well as invading inflammatory cells, promote further tissue breakdown.

Local tissue ischemia following the initial physical injury (as evidenced by increased lactate) results in propagation of the injury. The alterations in the microcirculation have been attributed to many factors. Local release of norepinephrine,[7,8] other vasoactive amines, and endogenous opioids[9] have all been implicated in extending the local area of spinal cord injury. Further injury may also be aggravated by local electrolyte imbalance or oxygen free radicals as part of the reperfusion phenomenon.[10]

CLINICAL PRESENTATION

In addition to the usual patterns of complete or incomplete spinal cord injury seen in adults, spinal cord injuries in the pediatric age group may have a higher incidence of spinal cord concussion, spinal cord injury without vertebral injury, and delayed onset of signs and symptoms.

Spinal Cord Concussion

Spinal cord concussion may be defined as a transitory state of neurologic signs and symptoms following spinal cord injury followed by complete resolution within 48 hours. Initially thought to be rare, it is now becoming more commonly recognized.[11] The neurologic symptoms are usually incomplete—burning dysesthesia, numbness, and weakness. Objective neurologic signs resolve quickly. Many reported cases have preexisting abnormalities of the neural canal. Torg and colleagues[12] has emphasized the significance of a narrow spinal canal

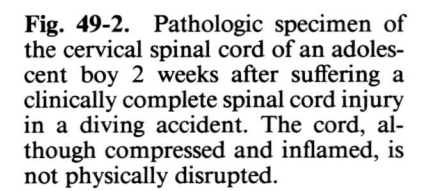

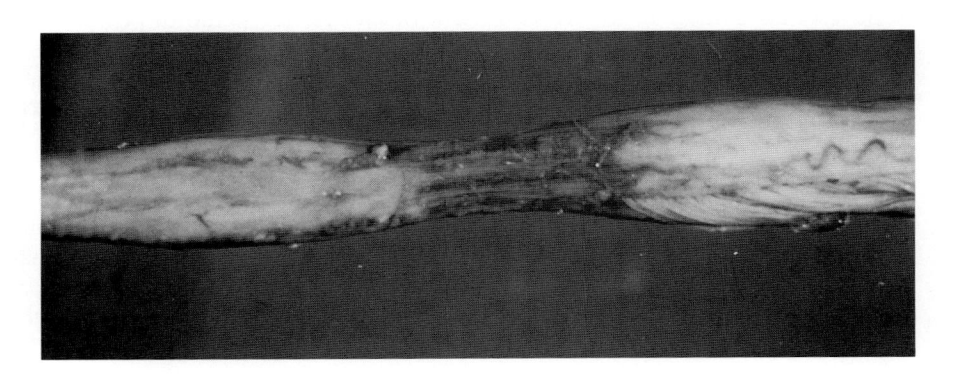

Fig. 49-2. Pathologic specimen of the cervical spinal cord of an adolescent boy 2 weeks after suffering a clinically complete spinal cord injury in a diving accident. The cord, although compressed and inflamed, is not physically disrupted.

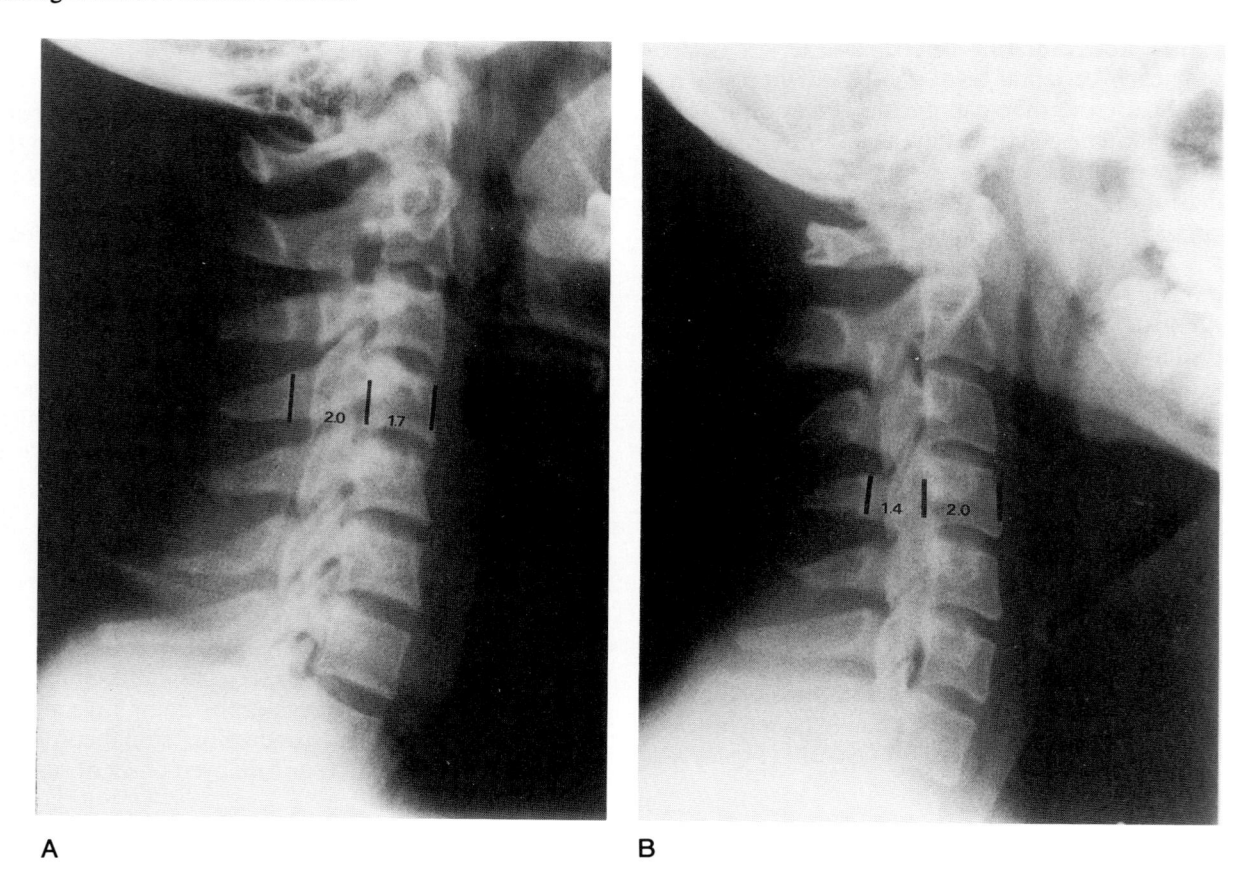

Fig. 49-3. Measurement of the sagittal diameter of the spinal canal and width of vertebral body. The ratio of spinal canal diameter to vertebral width is the Torg ratio and if < 0.8 is indicative of spinal stenosis. **(A)** Torg ratio 20/17 = 1.1. **(B)** Torg ratio 14/10 = 0.70. (From Rathbone et al.,[13] with permission.)

(Fig. 49-3). It is postulated that the spinal cord, suspended relatively freely within a column of fluid, is accelerated by kinetic energy delivered to the vertebral column sustaining a transient concussion against the canal wall. This would be potentiated in the presence of a hypermobile region of the spine or a narrowed spinal canal[13] accentuated by hyperflexion (Fig. 49-4). Magnetic resonance imaging provides excellent visualization of the spinal cord diameter and is the best method of determining the existence of spinal stenosis and cord impingement (Fig. 49-5 and Table 49-1).

Spinal Shock

Spinal shock refers to a complete cessation of function of the spinal cord distal to the level of injury. It is transient, lasting from minutes to weeks. Clinically, there is a total absence of sensation, motor power, and reflexes. It may resolve, rarely, with recovery of normal function or, more commonly, with incomplete or even complete loss of function. Generally, the more prolonged the duration, the poorer the outlook, however, prognostication should be avoided during this stage. The end of spinal shock is heralded by return of the bulbocavernosus and deep tendon reflexes, either with or without return of voluntary motor power and sensation (Fig. 49-6).

Spinal Cord Injury Without Radiologic Abnormality

Interpretation of spine radiographs is difficult in the pediatric age group, especially under 8 years of age. The incidence of spinal cord injury without radiographic abnormality is much higher in children than adults and must be carefully assessed. This topic is covered in Chapter 2.

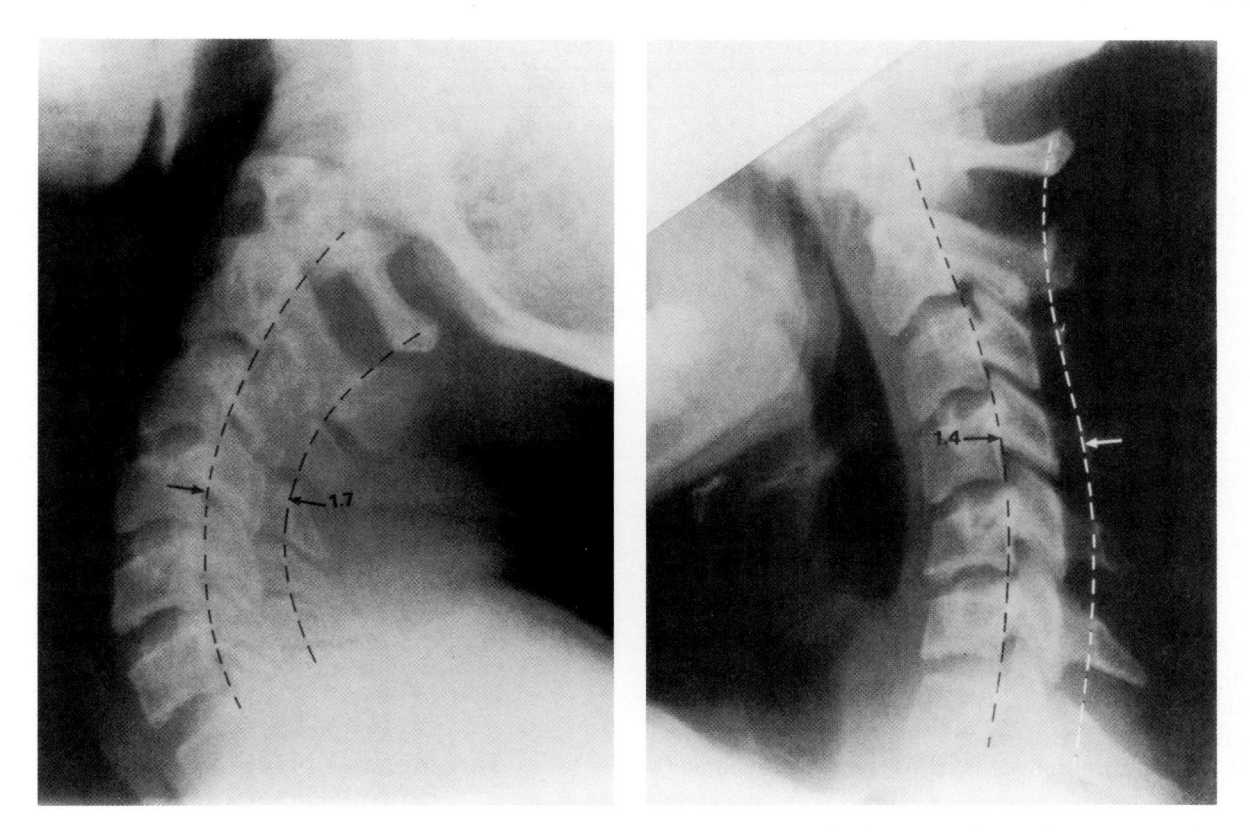

Fig. 49-4. Narrowing of spinal canal in flexion, which in the presence of spinal stenosis predisposes to cord impingement. (From Rathbone et al.,[13] with permission.)

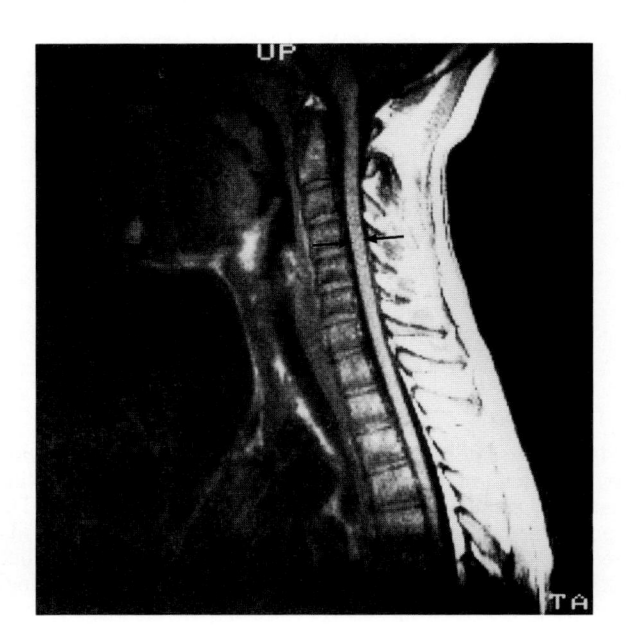

Fig. 49-5. Magnetic resonance imaging provides excellent visualization of spinal cord diameter and is the best method of determining the presence of cord injury or spinal stenosis in children.

TABLE 49-1. Sagittal Diameter of the Bony Cervical Spinal Canal in 120 Normal Children: Relation to Age

Age group	3–6 years			7–10 years			11–14 years		
	Boys 20 Mean mm	Girls 20 Mean mm	Total 40 Mean/SD mm	Boys 20 Mean mm	Girls 20 Mean mm	Total 40 Mean/SD mm	Boys 20 Mean mm	Girls 20 Mean mm	Total 40 Mean/SD mm
C1	20.2	19.6	19.9 ± 1.3	20.5	20.6	20.6 ± 1.3	21.2	21.4	21.3 ± 1.4
C2	18.2	17.6	17.9 ± 1.3	18.8	18.9	18.8 ± 1.0	19.3	19.5	19.4 ± 1.1
C3	16.3	15.8	16.0 ± 1.3	17.3	17.2	17.2 ± 1.0	17.8	17.7	17.8 ± 1.0
C4	16.0	15.6	15.8 ± 1.3	17.0	16.9	16.9 ± 0.9	17.3	17.2	17.3 ± 0.9
C5	15.9	15.5	15.7 ± 1.3	16.7	16.6	16.7 ± 0.9	17.1	16.9	17.0 ± 0.9
C6	15.8	15.3	15.6 ± 1.2	16.5	16.3	16.4 ± 0.9	16.8	16.6	16.7 ± 0.9
C7	15.6	15.0	15.3 ± 1.1	16.1	15.9	16.0 ± 0.9	16.3	16.2	16.2 ± 0.9

(From Markuske H: Pediatr Radiol 6:129, 1970.)

Delayed Onset of Neurologic Signs

A small number of cases are reported, more commonly in the pediatric literature, in which there is a delay in the onset of neurologic signs often associated with spinal cord injury without radiologic abnormality.[2] The child, having minimal signs or symptoms immediately postinjury, later evolves a pattern of spinal cord injury, usually over a period of 12 to 48 hours. It is tempting to explain this on a vascular basis, but there is little evidence to support this.

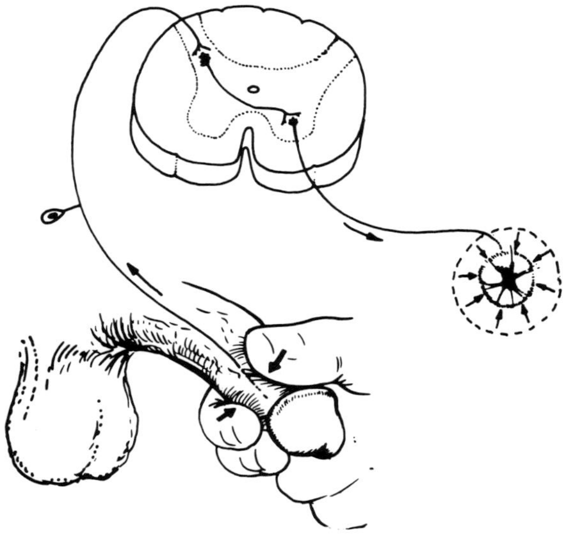

Incomplete Spinal Cord Injury: Brown-Séquard Lesion

Incomplete spinal cord injury presents as a hemisection of the cord, with ipsilateral loss of motor power and contralateral loss of pain and light touch. It is rare as a pure lesion clinically, but other incomplete cord syndromes may show some asymmetry. This incomplete cord injury has the best prognosis of approximately 90 percent chance of functional improvement.

Fig. 49-6. The bulbocavernosus reflex. Afferent stimulation, by compression of the glans penis, or a tug on the indwelling catheter, results in a contraction of the anal sphincter. This indicates an intact spinal reflex, occurring normally, but also returns following the stage of spinal shock. (From Hoppenfeld S: Orthopaedic Neurology: A Diagnostic Guide to Neurologic Levels. p. 100. JB Lippincott, Philadelphia, 1977, with permission.)

CENTRAL CORD SYNDROME

Typically, central cord syndrome occurs in the cervical area with more extensive loss of function in the upper extremities, usually of a lower motor neuron pattern. In the lower extremities, there is less extensive upper motor neuron loss. It is attributed to injury or spasm of the central sulcus vessels or direct bleeding or edema within the gray matter. There is about 50 percent chance of functional recovery with this pattern.

Anterior Spinal Cord Syndrome

The anterior spinal cord syndrome represents a more extensive involvement of the portion of the cord supplied by the anterior spinal artery. There is loss of motor power and pain and touch sensation below the level of the lesion. Deep touch (pressure) and position/vibration sense remain intact. Careful neurologic examination is required to differentiate this from a complete spinal cord injury.

Posterior Spinal Cord Syndrome

This is an extremely rare injury involving position, vibration, and pressure sensation below the level of the cord injury.

Complete Spinal Cord Injury

Complete spinal cord injury condition is evidenced by complete lack of all sensory modalities and voluntary muscle function with return of autonomous spinal cord function below the level of the injury—hyperreflexia, exaggerated superficial reflexes, and abnormal reflexes (Babinski). There is no hope of return of voluntary cord function.[14]

The underlying mechanism to explain the incomplete syndromes discussed above is usually explained on a vascular basis; however, Raynor and Koplik[15] have postulated that physical forces acting on the spinal cord may result in shearing stress within the cord, producing these typical clinical patterns.

SYSTEMIC EFFECT OF SPINAL CORD INJURY

Cardiac and Pulmonary

Mechanical trauma to the spinal cord, especially above the T5 level, may initially stimulate a massive sympathetic discharge with hypertension, marked increase in afterload, bradycardia, or dysrhythmia resulting in left ventricular strain or failure. There may be disruption of the pulmonary capillary endothelium with late cardiac or noncardiac pulmonary edema.

High circulating levels of β-endorphins have been implicated in left ventricular depression as well as diminished respiratory effort. Particularly during the stage of spinal shock, there is dilatation of the capacitance vessels and hypotension, which may also be accompanied by bradycardia with cord lesions above T6 due to loss of cardioaccelerator reflexes.[16] The child may experience shock to the extent that consciousness is lost.

IMAGING OF SPINAL CORD INJURIES

Plain Radiographs

Routine radiography is very helpful in localizing the level of the injury. Interpretation, particularly in the pediatric age group under 8 years, may be difficult and require special knowledge of the appearance or fusion of secondary ossification centers, variations in positioning of the spine, and the incidences and degree of pseudosubluxation (see Ch. 44).

Following reduction of dislocations and subluxations, plain films are necessary to document the adequacy of reduction and its maintenance. In the adult population, the restoration of position usually indicates decompression of the spinal cord and nerve roots. However, in children when the ring apophysis is not ossified, magnetic resonance imaging (MRI) is useful.

Myelography

Myelography is indicated if MRI is unavailable, in all cases of neurologic deterioration to determine whether this is on a vascular basis or is caused by residual or increasing mechanical compression. It is also useful in demonstrating the relief of compression following reduction of dislocations in children.

Myelography is essential in children demonstrating spinal cord injuries without radiologic abnormality (SCIWORA) to rule out compression by radiolucent soft tissues, such as disc or cartilaginous endplate. Also, myelography is helpful to demonstrate the level of the injury and the condition of the cord. Extradural leakage of the contrast has a very poor prognosis. Magnetic resonance imaging is rapidly replacing myelography in the assessment of spinal cord trauma in children.

Computed Tomography

Computed tomography is particularly useful in detecting small bony fragments and fracture lines when adequate slices are taken to give good detail on sagittal reconstruction.[17] When combined with metrizamide, information regarding the contour of the cord may also be seen.

Magnetic Resonance Imaging

The magnetic resonance imaging method of evaluation is available to most specialized centers for the management of spinal cord injuries. Experimentally, much information has been obtained regarding the pathogenesis of the cord injury using this technique. Subtle injuries to the osseous structures can be seen as a loss of high-signal intensity on T1-weighted images due to bleeding into the fat containing bone marrow and other soft tissue structures.[18] Imaging of the cord has shown areas of focal hemorrhage in both the gray as well as the white matter, cyst formation, and edema[19] (Fig. 49-5).

MANAGEMENT OF SPINAL CORD INJURIES

Awareness

Ambulance attendants, coaches, trainers, nurses, and physicians must be continually made aware of the potential of vertebral and spinal cord injuries in victims of high-velocity trauma, sports and recreation injuries, individuals suffering facial trauma, or unconscious following trauma. In each of these instances, the spine must be protected from movement until a thorough assessment has been completed.

General Management and Priority Setting

The first priority is to establish and maintain an adequate airway and ventilation. Great care must be taken in doing this to support the head and neck with a collar, sandbags, and tape, and manual traction as necessary. Patients with a high spinal cord injury (above C4) preexisting pulmonary disease, or facial or head injuries, may require early intubation and ventilation. Supplemental oxygen must also be given. The circulation must be supported. Spinal cord injury patients are generally hypotensive and bradycardic. Initially, maintaining the patient on a spine board in the reverse Trendelenburg position helps decrease venous pooling. Intravenous infusion of either crystalloid or colloid must be given to maintain perfusion of vital organs such as the brain and kidneys, and to maintain perfusion to the injured cord. Atropine is helpful in treating severe bradycardia. Small infusions of vasopressors, such as dopamine, may be necessary.[20,16] Patients who are hemodynamically unstable must be examined for concealed blood loss into the chest or abdomen.

Another possible cause of hypotension and bradycardia is hypothermia. These patients can neither vasoconstrict nor shiver and so must be kept covered and their temperature monitored.

Immobilization

Special care must be taken to completely immobilize the spine, generally in the anatomic position, unless significant traction or rotation are required. The head and neck should be supported in a cervical collar and sandbags, a small roll placed under the lordosis in both the cervical and lumbar area (Fig. 49-7). A short spinal board may be used for extrication, supplemented later by a long spinal board. In small children, the relatively large head size results in a forced flexion of the cervical spine with a standard spine board (Fig. 49-8). To avoid this dangerous position, a small mattress should be used to allow the head and neck to remain neutral or in slight extension. Care must also be exercised during intubation of the child to avoid excessive manipulation of the neck (Fig. 49-9). As soon as possible, the child should be removed from the spine board to relieve constant pressure on the sacral skin. Judicious log rolling for airway protection, skin care, and physical examination will not cause further injury.

Other General Measures

A nasogastric tube should be inserted in all spinal cord-injured children to protect against vomiting and aspiration. An indwelling bladder catheter is used initially until hemodynamic stability is achieved, thereafter intermittent catheterization should be instituted.

ASSESSMENT OF THE NEUROLOGIC INJURY

History

A thorough history is required, including the details of the accident (Fig. 49-10) preexisting neurologic abnormalities, loss of consciousness, movement of extremities following trauma and symptoms of numbness. It is important to note if the child was incontinent or voided voluntarily.

Physical Examination

Complete evaluation of motor power, including grading of all representative muscle groups must be per-

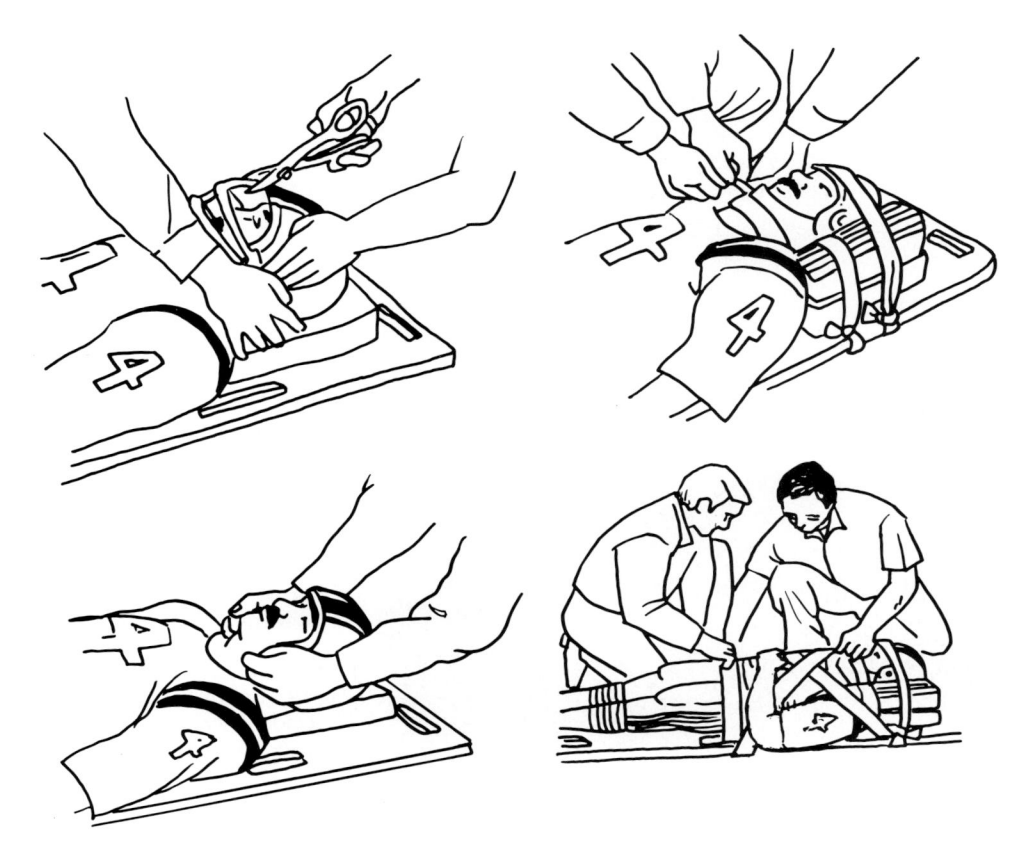

Fig. 49-7. Emergency immobilization of a suspected spinal injured athlete on the field to facilitate safe transport. (From Letts RM, MacDonald PB: Sport injuries to the pediatric spine. Spine-State of the Art Review 4:49, 1990, with permission.)

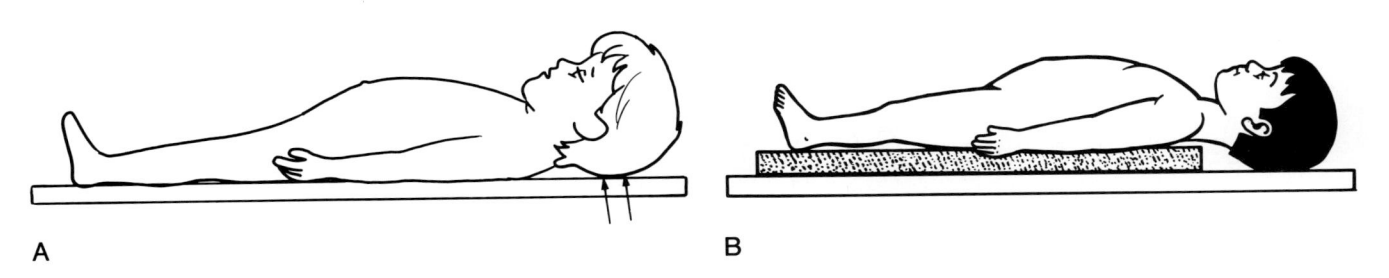

Fig. 49-8. **(A)** Infants and small children have large heads which result in cervical flexion when lying on a straight spine board. **(B)** To compensate for this large head size, a small mattress should be used for the torso and legs allowing the head and neck to be neutral or in slight extension thus avoiding the dangerous flexed position. (From Hezenberg J et al: J Bone Joint Surg [Am] 71:15, 1979, with permission.)

910 / Management of Pediatric Fractures

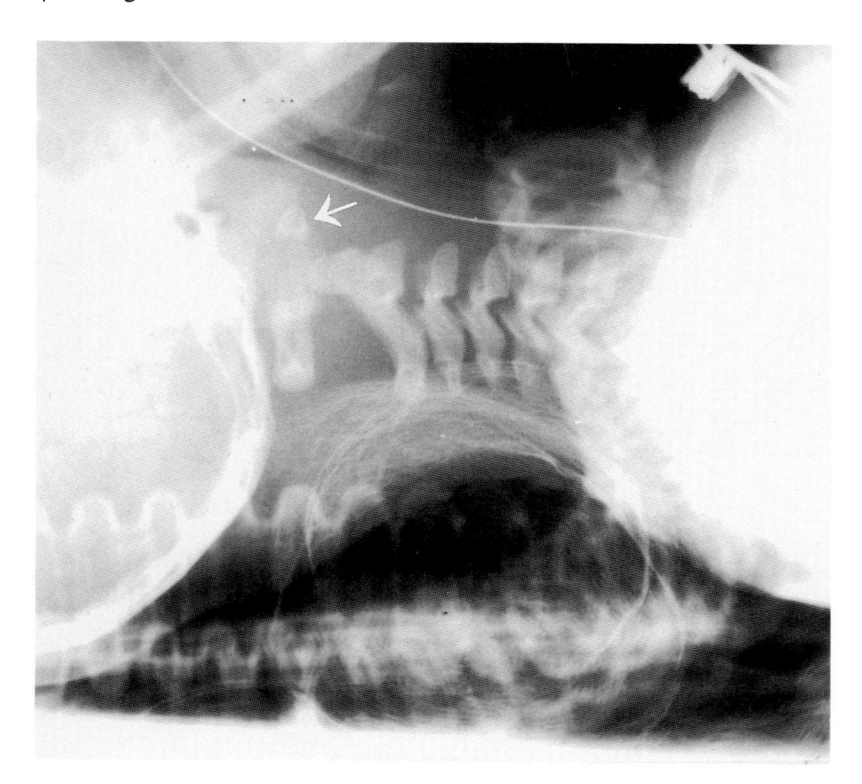

Fig. 49-9. Care must be taken during resuscitation and especially during intubation if cervical spine instability is suspected. *Arrow* points to a dislocation of C1 on C2 in a child injured in a motor vehicle accident, resuscitated at the accident scene but arrived completely quadriplegic to the emergency department.

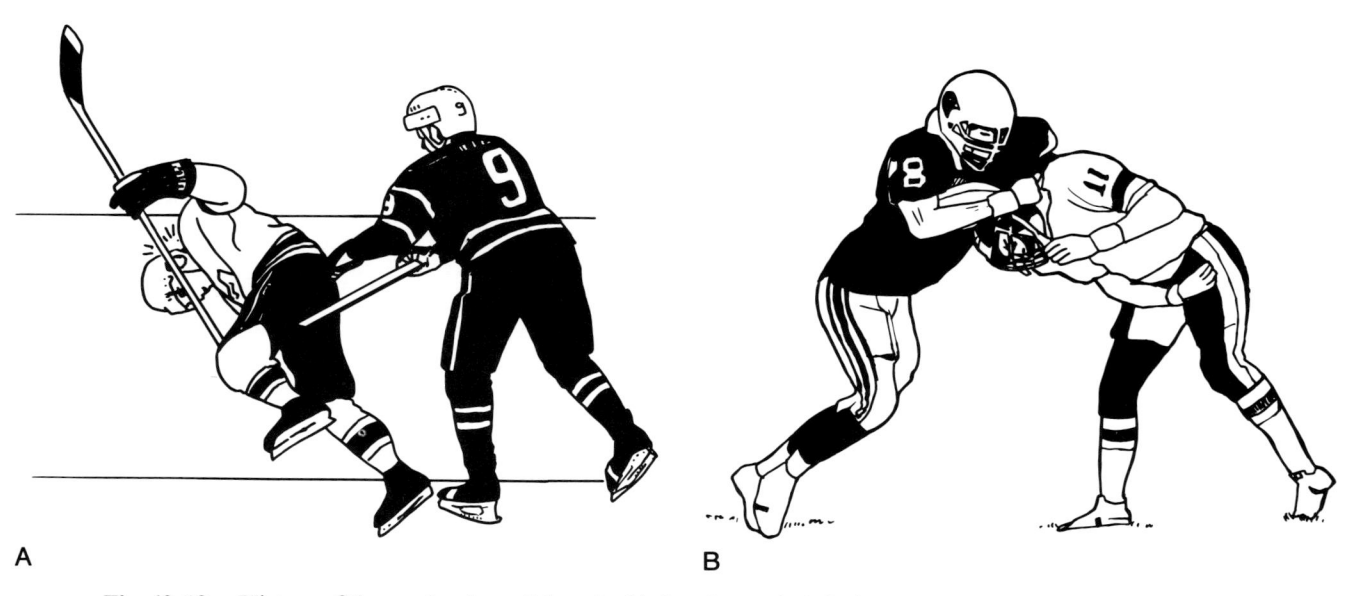

Fig. 49-10. History of the mechanism of the spinal injury is very helpful in localizing sites of spinal trauma. **(A)** A check from behind resulting in cervical hyperflexion. **(B)** Spearing resulting in a rotary flexion injury of the cervical spine. (From Letts RM, MacDonald PB: Sport injuries to the pediatric spine. Spine-State of the Art Review 4:49, 1990, with permission.)

formed and interpretated on a myotomal basis. This should include assessment of long toe flexors and voluntary anal sphincter contraction.

The sensory modalities of light touch, pain, pressure, position, and vibration must be tested as accurately as possible in accordance with the age of the child. The presence of sensation in the saddle area is an important indicator of an incomplete lesion.

A rectal examination is essential to assess resting tone of the anal sphincter, voluntary contraction, and performance of the bulbocavernosus reflex (Fig. 49-6). (The bulbocavernosus reflex is performed by tugging on the Foley catheter or squeezing the glans penis while palpating in the rectum.) The neurologic findings must be recorded on spinal injury protocol sheets allowing for serial documentation and comparison of results.

Specific Management

The first essential in management of the spinal cord injury is the provision of adequate flow of well-oxygenated blood. It has been clearly shown that the extent of spinal cord injury is directly proportional to the force applied and the duration of its application.[21] We cannot control the former, but must reduce the duration of physical compression on the cord as quickly as possible. In the cervical spine, dislocations can usually be reduced by halo traction. Thoracic and lumbar injuries reduction can also be achieved by closed postural means; however, this requires specialized nursing care in centers devoted to the management of spinal injuries.

Following reduction, relief of spinal cord compression must be demonstrated by myelography or an MRI in the pediatric patient.

Surgery

The indications for surgery in spinal cord injury are as follows:

1. Failed reduction or decompression by closed means
2. Increasing neurologic loss caused by residual compression
3. Prevention of late spinal instability or deformity

It is recognized that surgical decompression will not improve the outcome in children with neurologic signs indicative of a complete spinal cord injury. It is controversial whether surgical decompression improves recovery in the child with incomplete spinal cord injury. Surgery is indicated in these patients when there is radiologic evidence of continued cord compression by bone, soft tissue, or hematoma.[22] In the absence of neurologic injury, surgery may also be indicated to stabilize complex vertebral injuries where late instability and subsequent deformity may cause neurologic compression.

When surgical decompression is indicated, it must be performed by experienced spinal surgeons under optimal circumstances. The timing of surgery is controversial.[23] Certainly, with progressive neurologic deterioration, decompression is indicated. Otherwise, it is best accomplished either within 24 hours or after 7 to 10 days to avoid aggravation of the edema caused during the stage of ischemic injury. Decompression should be performed from the direction of the cord compression.[24] The approach must be studied carefully with a view to complete decompression as well as reconstruction to allow a stable construct. In most instances this will be an anterior decompression. Extensive posterior laminectomies should be avoided, especially in the cervical spine. If necessary it should be supplemented by spinal fusion to avoid spinal decompensation and future deformity.

Adjunctive Methods of Management

Many agents[25] (spinal cord cooling,[26] calcium channel blockers,[27] opioid receptor antagonists[28]) have been tried both experimentally and clinically, most of which were aimed at controlling the secondary injury. Until recently, the efficacy of these measures has been in question.

Steroids

Steroids are thought to act at several levels, by stabilizing cell membranes, correcting local electrolyte imbalance, minimizing edema, and decreasing the vasospastic effect of norepinephrine and other vasoactive amines.

Bracken and coworkers[29] have shown significant improvement in neurologic outcome in patients given methylprednisolone 30 mg/kg as a loading dose within 8 hours of injury, followed by infusion of 5.4 mg/kg/h for 23 hours. This study excluded patients under 13 years of age, and so information in the pediatric age group is lacking, but the same steroid protocol is recommended.

PROGNOSIS

In the pediatric group, there is some variation in the relative proportions of the different degrees of spinal cord injuries and outcome. This may be due to the variation in the maximum age between the different series, and therefore the proportion of patients under the age of 3.[30] Many series are reviews that had been conducted from rehabilitation institutions, which have therefore tended to look at the more seriously injured patients.

Children suffering spinal cord injury without radiologic abnormality (SCIWORA) are generally younger than those pediatric patients with vertebral injuries (average age 6 compared to 16, respectively). The incidence of complete lesions tends to be a little higher in those patients without vertebral injury.[31] When myelography is done in the group without vertebral injury, leakage of contrast is associated with a particularly poor prognosis. Magnetic resonance imaging will often demonstrate cord damage. In other age groups and in children with vertebral fracture, there is generally a similar prognosis for the cord injury as seen in adults.

COMPLICATIONS

Decubitus Ulceration

Avoidance of this complication begins the moment of injury. As soon as possible, the child should be moved from the spinal board to a regular hospital bed. Frequent turning every 2 hours and appropriate positioning must be carried out throughout the hospitalization by trained nursing staff. On a long-term basis, the most important factor in successful skin care is patient education in the technique of skin care. In children, it is extremely important to concentrate on good sitting balance, a well-fitted wheelchair and early treatment for hip contractures and spinal deformities. Use of standing frames and parapodiums assist in frequent position changes thus minimizing pressure concentration (Fig. 49-8).

Urinary Tract Infections

Spinal cord-injured children, with residual loss of voluntary bowel and bladder control, are perpetually at risk of urinary stasis, lithiasis, and infection. Although an indwelling bladder catheter is necessary during the acute phase of hemodynamic instability, this catheter should be removed as soon as possible and a regime of intermittent catheterization initiated. Later, Credés compression suprapubicly, bladder reflex emptying, and intermittent catheterization usually allow for regular bladder emptying at near capacity and small residual volumes of less than 100 cc. Close follow-up is required to prevent late urologic complications. These children are often best followed in the spina bifida clinic.

Heterotopic Bone Formation

Heterotopic bone formation occurs in approximately 10 to 20 percent of children, usually involving major joints, such as hips, knees, and elbows. It is usually associated with a spastic upper motor neuron lesion. The child presents with a swollen limb. Other possible diagnoses are venous thrombosis or fracture. Radiographs are usually normal initially but later demonstrate streaky ossification in the tissue planes about the involved joint. The bone scan is strongly positive and alkaline phosphatase often markedly elevated. Treatment consists of limiting the range of movement exercises but persisting at a lesser level. Residual serious limitation of range of movement may require surgical excision of the lesion when it becomes quiescent,[32] but there is risk of recurrence following excision.

Spinal Deformity

The risk and degree of developing spinal deformity following spinal cord injury is extremely high, depending on the age of the patient and the degree of spasticity[33] (Fig. 49-11). Scoliosis is the more common and severe deformity contributed to by asymmetrical muscle pull, plasticity of the pediatric spine and loading of the spine on sitting. Other causative factors may be deformity at the level of spinal injury, previous posterior surgical decompression (laminectomy), and hip contractures. The tendency to develop spinal deformity can be decreased by avoiding angular deformities at the level of the spinal injury and therapy to avoid joint contractures. Orthotic management with a well-fitted and lined polypropylene thoracolumbar spinal orthosis can be useful in delaying progression of the curve until the child is old enough for spinal fusion, although this is difficult due to spasticity and the risk of breakdown of insensitive skin. Although spinal fusion of these neurogenic curves is much more difficult and entails greater risk, spinal fusion is recommended for scoliotic curves greater than 40 degrees and kyphotic curves greater than 60 degrees (Fig. 49-12). Preoperatively, care must be taken to optimize pulmonary function, nutritional status, and skin care. The fu-

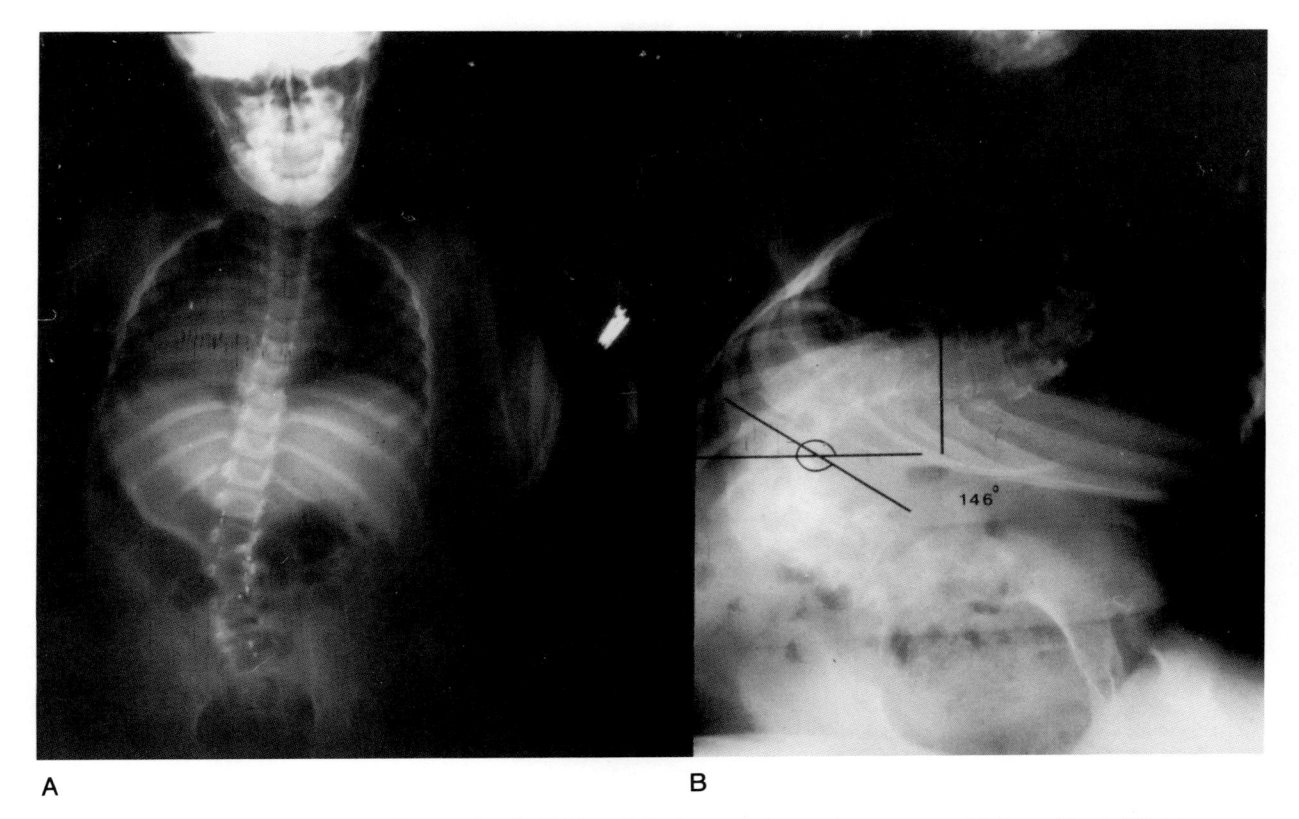

Fig. 49-11. (A) A 5-year-old girl sustained a T12 paraplegia at age 3 years in a motor vehicle accident. (B) At age 16, this untreated scoliosis has progressed to 146°. Scoliosis is an invariable development in children who sustain paraplegia under 10 years of age.

sion may have to be extended to include the sacrum and may require both anterior and posterior procedures. Segmental spinal instrumentation for posterior fusion (Luque) is the most satisfactory technique. Intraoperatively, meticulous attention to technique and the provision of autogenous bone graft are necessary.

Autonomic Dysreflexia

Patients with neurologic lesions above T6 may experience transient episodes of severe hypertension associated with vasodilatation in the head and upper extremities. Clinically the patient may complain of headache, nasal stuffiness, and profuse sweating above the neurologic lesion, nausea, vomiting, and bradycardia are also present.[34] This is usually caused by overstimulation of the sympathetic afferent spinal arc reflex by urologic manipulation, fecal disimpaction, or other stimuli, such as decubitus ulceration. Avoidance or removal of the noxious stimulus is the first line of treatment, but if hypertension is very severe, antihypertensive medication such as diazoxide may be lifesaving.

Deformity Secondary to Growth

In addition to the usual long-term sequelae in patients with residual neurologic deficit, the greatest problem facing the paraplegic or quadriplegic child is the effect of neurologic imbalance on the growing spine and hips. This results in a high incidence of spinal deformity and sitting imbalance with resultant decubitus ulceration and problems with toilet care (Fig. 49-12). Such children need close follow-up by a Seating Clinic team and are probably best managed in a Spina Bifida clinic setting[35] (Fig. 49-13). The management of the child paraplegic or quadriplegic is challenging and long term, but the rewards can be great (Fig. 49-14).

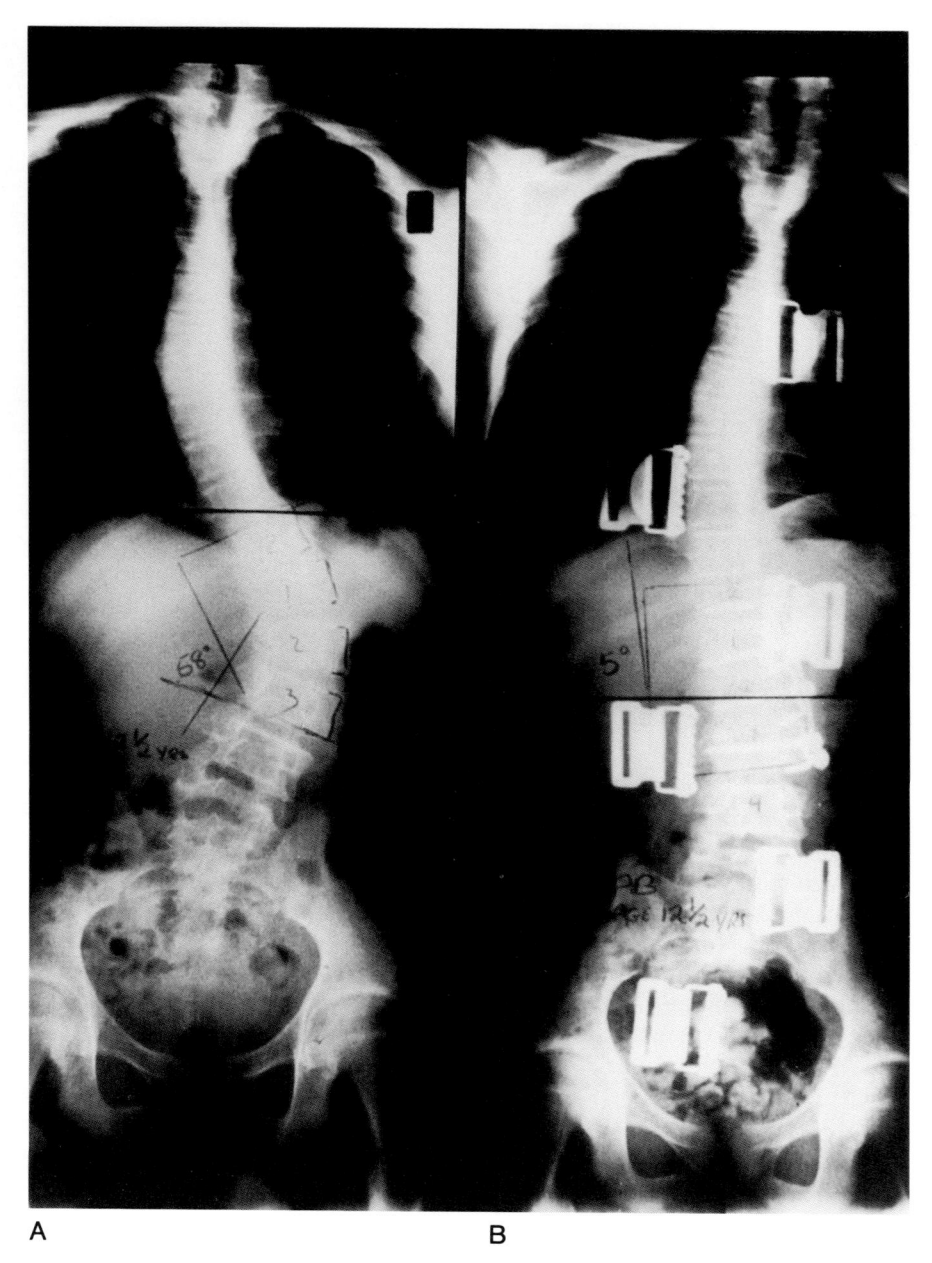

Fig. 49-12. (A) A 12.5-year-old boy who sustained a complete T12 paraplegia at age 6 years in a motor vehicle accident. (B) His increasing scoliosis was treated with an anterior fusion at age 12 which restored good sitting balance for him.

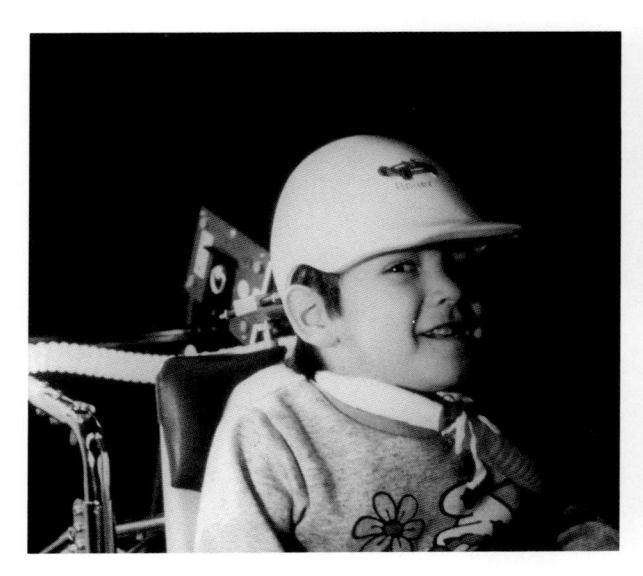

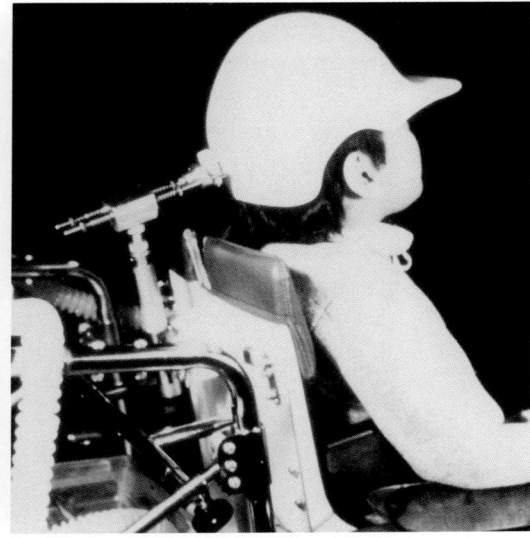

Fig. 49-13. Head support designed for this child with complete C1-C2 quadraplegia and no head control. This allowed him to sit upright in the wheelchair and facilitated the use of a tongue switch.

Spinal Cord Vascular Injury in Infants

Vascular injury is a rare cause of spinal cord injury secondary to vascular insufficiency of the cord, often due to thrombosis or embolism subsequent to umbilical artery catheterization. Infants predisposed to such ischemia are usually premature, infants of diabetic mothers, or polycythemic neonates. There is frequently associated vascular impairment of the extremities due to thrombosis of peripheral arteries. Prolonged hypotension of the infant is also felt to be a predisposing factor potentiating cord ischemia. Progressive neurologic impairment following an acute ischemia of the cord has been reported by Singer and colleagues[36] who attributed this phenomenon to increased thromboxanes potent vasoactive substances that may be involved in blood flow regulation, microvascular permeability, and inflammatory responses in the spinal cord.

Prognosis for cord recovery in these infants is marginal and most will have permanent paraparesis with resulting developmental orthopaedic malformations, including subluxation of the hip, scoliosis, and various foot abnormalities secondary to muscle imbalance. The acute management of the infant with such cord impairment requires the same careful monitoring as for any child with acute cord injury with care being taken to avoid pressure sores and institute regular intermittent catheterization.

SUMMARY

Acute spinal cord injury in children is unfortunately increasing in incidence. This is due to both increased exposure of children to high velocity trauma and improved methods of resuscitation for such injured children through cardiopulmonary resuscitation advances and improved access to pediatric intensive care units. The diagnosis of the extent of cord damage in children is somewhat more difficult both clinically and radiologically. With aggressive management in pediatric trauma centers, complications from this devastating injury can be minimized, or better yet prevented.

Spinal cord injuries, although rare in the pediatric population, are devastating injuries. The very young child, because of structural immaturity of the vertebral column, is predisposed to spinal cord injury. The diagnosis may be difficult due to radiologic peculiarities, the presence of spinal cord injury in the absence of lung injury and the delayed onset of neurologic signs.

There is probably little difference between the pediatric and adult patient with spinal cord injury with reference to proportion of degree of injury and recovery rates.

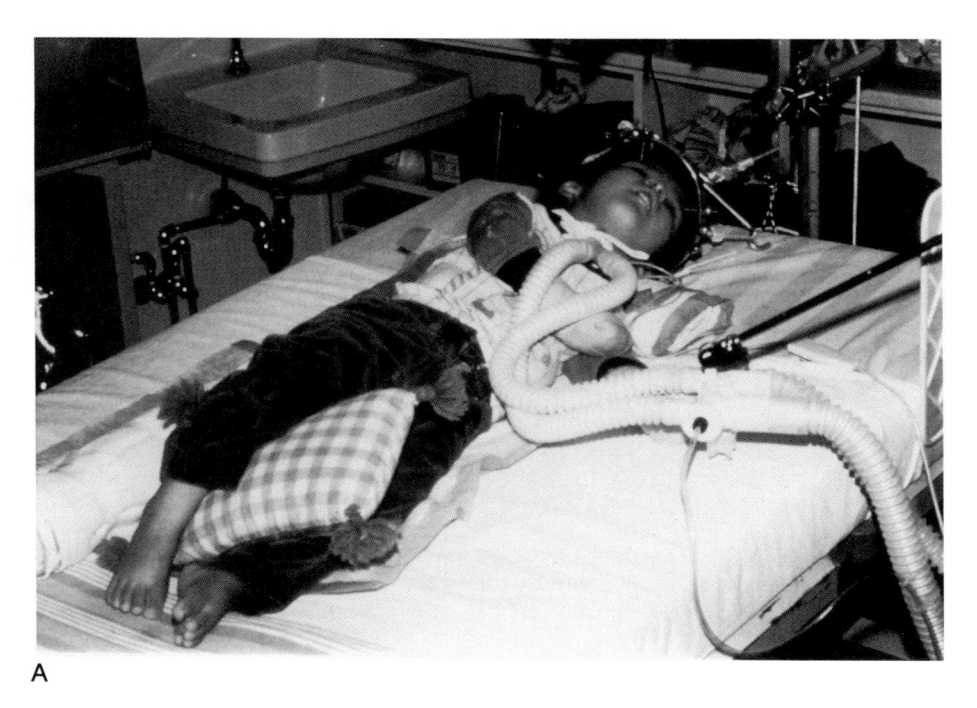

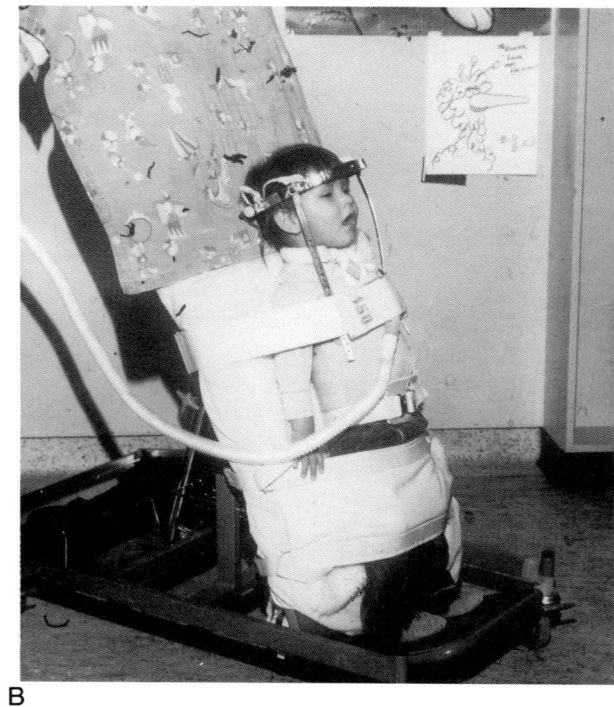

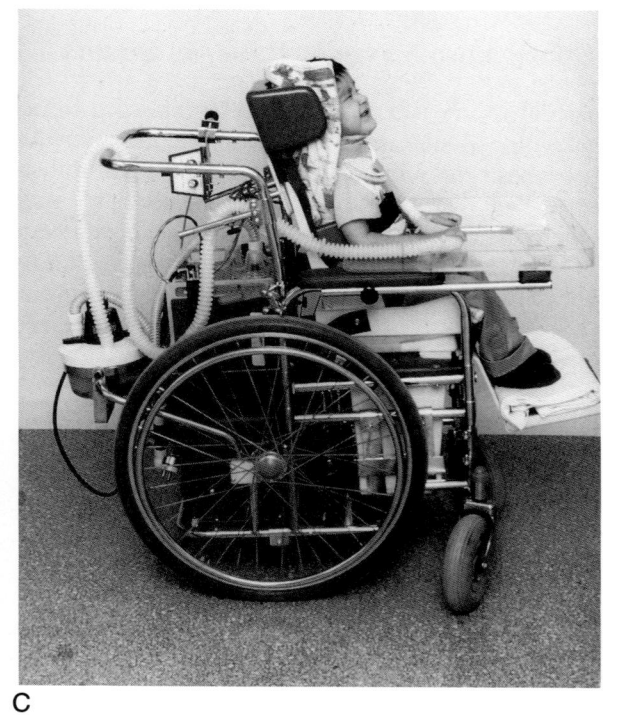

Fig. 49-14. (A) An 18-month-old boy with C1-C2 fracture dislocation and complete quadriplegia. Assisted ventilation and tracheostomy together with halo traction to reduce the cervical dislocation ultimately allowed this boy to be up in a (B) standing device and (C) wheelchair.

REFERENCES

1. Kewalramani LS, Kraus JF, Sterling HM: Acute spinal cord lesions in a paediatric population: epidemiological and clinical features. Paraplegia 18:206, 1980
2. Pang D, Wilberger JF: Spinal cord injury without radiographic abnormalities in children. J Neurosurg 57:114, 1982
3. Kewalramani LS, Turi JA: Spinal cord trauma in children. Spine 5:11, 1980
4. Crock HV, Yoshizawa H: The Blood Supply of the Vertebral Column and Spinal Cord in Man. Springer-Verlag, New York, 1977
5. Albin MD, Helsel P, Bunegin I: Axoplasmic transport patterns after experimental spinal crush injury. Anat Rec 190:603, 1978
6. Wagner F, Taslitz N, White RJ: Vascular phenomena in the normal and traumatized spinal cord. Anat Rec 163:281, 1969
7. Osterham JL, Mathews GJ: Altered non-epinephrine metabolism following experimental spinal cord injury. Part 1. Relationships to haemorrhagic necrosis and post-wounding neurological deficits. J Neurosurg 36:386, 1972
8. Osterham JL, Mathews GJ: Alteres non-epinephrine metabolism following experimental spinal cord injury. Part 2. Protections against traumatic spinal cord haemorrhagic necrosis by nonepinephrine synthesis blockade with alpha-methyltyronine. J Neurosurg 36:395, 1972
9. Faden AI: Opiate Antagonists and thyrotropin releasing hormone. JAMA 252:1452, 1984
10. McCord JM: Oxygen devoid free radicals in postischemic tissue injury. N Engl J Med 312:159, 1986
11. Del Bigio MR, Johnson GE: Clinical presentation of spinal cord concussion. Spine 14:37, 1989
12. Torg JS, Pavlov H, Genuario SE: Neuropraxin of the cervical spinal cord with transient quadriplegia. J Bone Joint Surg [Am] 68:1354, 1986
13. Rathbone D, Johnson G, Letts M: Spinal cord concussion in pediatric athletes. J Pediatr Orthop 12:616, 1992
14. Stauffer ES: Neurologic recovery following injuries to the cervical spinal cord and nerve roots. Spine 9:532, 1984
15. Raynor RB, Koplik B: Cervical cord trauma: the relationship between clinical syndromes and force of injury. Spine 10:193, 1985
16. Gilbert J: Critical care management of the patient with acute spinal cord injury. Crit Care Clin 3:549, 1987
17. Wittenberg RH, Boetel U, Beyer HK: Magnetic resonance imaging and computer tomography of acute spinal cord trauma. Clin Orthop 260:176, 1990
18. Yu S, Haughton VM, Rosenbaum AE: Magnetic resonance imaging and anatomy of the spine. Radiol Clin North Am 29:691, 1991
19. Flanders AE, Schaefer DM, Doan HT et al: Acute cervical spine trauma: correlations of MR imaging findings with degree of neurologic deficit. Radiology 177:25, 1990
20. Green BA, Eismont FJ, C'Heir JT: Spinal cord injury: a systems approach: prevention, emergency medical services, and emergency room management. Crit Care Clin 3:471, 1987
21. Rivlin AS, Tator CH: Effect of duration of acute spinal cord compression in a new acute cord injury model in the rat. Surg Neurol 10:38, 1978
22. Snowdy HA, Snowdy PH: Stabilization procedures in the patient with acute spinal cord injury. Crit Care Clin 3:569, 1987
23. Ducker TB, Bellegarrigue R, Salcmam M, Walleck C: Thinking of operative care in cervical spinal cord injury. Spine 9:525, 1984
24. Kostuik JP, Hurler RJ, Esses SI, Stauffer ES: The Adult Spine: Principles and Practice. Vol. 2. Raven Press, New York, 1991
25. De La Torre JC: Spinal cord injury review of basic and applied research. Spine 6:315, 1980
26. Albin MS, White RJ: Epidemiology, physiopathology and experimental therapeutics of acute spinal cord injury. Crit Care Clin 3:441, 1987
27. Guha A, Tabor CH, Smith CR, Piper I: Improvement in posttraumatic spinal cord blood flow with a combination of calcium channel blocker and a vasopressor. J Trauma 29:1440, 1989
28. Faden AI, Jacobs TP, Holaday JW: Opiate antagonist improves neurologic recovery after spinal cord injury. Science 211:493, 1981
29. Bracken MB, Shepard MJ, Collins WF et al: A randomized controlled trial of methyl-prednisolone or maloxan in the treatment of acute spinal cord injury. N Engl J Med 322:1405, 1990
30. Kewalraman LS, Tori JA: Spinal cord trauma in children, neurologic patterns, radiologic features and pathomechanics of injury. Spine 5:11, 1980
31. Ruge JR, Sinson GP, McLone DG et al: Paediatric spinal injury, the very young. J Neurosurg 68:25, 1988
32. Renshaw TS: The Paediatric Spine. Thieme, New York, 1985
33. Pouliquen JC, Beneux J, Pennecot GF: Progressive spinal deformity after spinal injury in children. Rev Chir Orthop 64:487, 1978
34. Jane MJ, Freehafer AA, Hazel C et al: Autonomic dysreflexia: a cause of morbidity and mortality in orthopaedic patients with spinal cord injury. Clin Orthop Rel Res 169:151, 1982
35. D'Astous JL, Kealey P, Mason B: Seating in Myelomeningocele in Principles of Seating the Disabled. p. 183. In Letts RM (ed): CRC Press, Boca Raton, FL, 1991
36. Singer R, Joseph K, Galai AN, Meyer S: Nontraumatic Acute neonatal paraplegia. J Pediatr Orthop 11:588, 1991

50

The SCIWORA Syndrome

Hubert Labelle
Claude Mercier

> Time heals what reason cannot.
> —SENECA

DEFINITION AND INCIDENCE

In the adult population, the syndrome of closed spinal cord injury without demonstrable skeletal injury has been clearly defined since the classic description by Taylor and Blackwood[1] in 1948. A similar syndrome in children was first delineated in 1977 by Cheshire[2] who proposed that a pediatric syndrome of traumatic myelopathy without visible skeletal injury should be recognized as a definite and separate clinical entity. Pang and Wilberger[3] in 1982 coined the name SCIWORA for *spinal cord injury without radiographic abnormalities* in children, a term now generally accepted for this distinct clinical syndrome characterized by clinical features and a prognosis different from children with spinal cord injuries and visible radiographic findings.

SCIWORA is defined as a syndrome of objective signs of traumatic myelopathy in children who show no radiographic evidence of skeletal injury or subluxation at the time of admission by plain radiographs of the spine, tomography, or myelography. Spinal cord injuries occurring during birth or after penetrating agents or electric shock are excluded from this definition.

The exact incidence of SCIWORA is difficult to establish with precision because most publications on the subject are small retrospective case series reported from specialized centers and do not properly reflect the incidence in the general population. All authors agree that spinal cord injury in children is not frequent, being reported in 0.6 to 13.2 percent[2,4-9] of traumatic injuries of the spine. SCIWORA accounts for 1.3 to 75 percent[2-17] of all spinal cord injuries in children with most series reporting around 20 to 30 percent. The only epidemiologic data available is the study of Kewalramani and colleagues,[4] which reported an annual incidence of spinal cord injury in children of 18.2 per million population and an annual incidence of SCIWORA of 1.6 per million population.

ANATOMY

The spine of a child is not simply a small adult spine. Its anatomy, physiology, radiographic appearance, and response to trauma differs greatly from the mature spine: this explains why SCIWORA is much more frequent between infancy and 16 years than in adults. Furthermore, neurologic injuries encountered in children younger than 8 years tend to be more frequent and much more serious than those seen in older children.[16]

The SCIWORA syndrome is a traumatic myelopathy produced by a self-reducing transient intervertebral subluxation of the spine. Several distinct anatomic characteristics of the pediatric spine increase its susceptibility to injury and allow momentary subluxation in response to deforming forces[3,5,7,12,16,18,19]:

1. The heavier infantile head is poorly supported by a proportionally weaker cervical musculature, rendering the upper cervical spine more vulnerable to injury.
2. In children, the ligaments, posterior joint capsules and cartilaginous structures are more elastic than in the adult spine, while the elastic recoil and plasticity of the spinal cord are limited by the pia mater. Leventhal has demonstrated that infantile spinal canals can be stretched 2 in. without structural damage, while the cervical spinal cord can be pulled down only 0.25 in. before rupturing.[3]
3. In children below the age of 8, there is normal hypermobility with anterior pseudosubluxation of C2 on C3.[19] This is explained by the relative horizontal configuration of the facet joints, the anterior wedged configuration of the growing vertebral bodies allowing anterior slipping, and hyperlaxity.
4. There is a lack of development of the uncinate processes, which normally limit lateral and rotational movements between adjacent vertebral bodies in the young child.
5. The infantile atlanto-occipital joint is inherently unstable due to hyperlaxity of ligaments and to flattening of the occipital condyles. This exposes the vertebral artery to compression: Gilles and colleagues have demonstrated bilateral occlusion of the vertebral arteries with the neck in extension at postmortem angiography.[18]
6. An increased vulnerability of the spinal cord in association with a decreased sagittal diameter of the cervical canal due to congenital cervical stenosis may be a contributing factor in some children. Torg and coworkers[20] have developed a ratio method comparing the sagittal diameter of the canal to the width of the vertebral body and have demonstrated that a ratio less than 0.8 is highly significant for stenosis. Hinck and colleagues[21] have shown that by age 13 years, the canal diameter should measure a minimum of 13.4 mm or should be classified as spinal stenosis.

These characteristic anatomic features explain why the majority of SCIWORA involve the cervical level, while thoracic lesions account for approximately 25 percent of cases, and lumbar lesions are infrequently reported. Younger children are more likely to have severe upper cervical lesions, while lower cervical lesions are evenly distributed through the ages of 6 months to 16 years. The young spine gradually matures to an adult status between 8 and 16 years, thus explaining the rarity of the SCIWORA syndrome in the adult population.

MECHANISM OF INJURY

While hyperextension injuries account for the vast majority of adult cases, 4 different mechanisms of injury[3] have been identified as responsible for the pediatric SCIWORA syndrome.

Hyperextension Injuries

Hyperextension of the cervical spine is a common mechanism involving mostly the lower cervical spine.[1] The spinal cord is compressed by the inward bulging of the interlaminar ligaments aggravated by a thickening of its cross section area during its simultaneous shortening. Elastic recoil of the hyperlax anterior ligamentous structures and reflex muscle spasm allow a spontaneous and relatively stable reduction and explain the normal radiologic appearance.

Flexion Injuries

The inherent instability of the upper juvenile spine,[22] coupled with a flexion injury, may produce sufficient temporary anterior subluxation to cause myelopathy without concomitant visible bony and ligamentous damage, after spontaneous reduction.

Distraction Injuries

Autopsy and surgical findings[23] as well as experimental studies support the concept that severe longitudinal distraction forces can stretch the spinal cord to rupture without severely disrupting bony and ligamentous structures in the cervical and thoracic spine.[3]

Ischemic Injuries

Spinal cord infarction[18] is a rare but well-documented event following trauma to the spine, most frequently in the lower thoracic area supplied almost exclusively by the unpaired great radicular artery of Adamkiewicz. Trauma may be minimal, and severe hypotension with suboptimal perfusion pressure to the traumatized cord may be an important factor.

The most frequent trauma responsible for SCIWORA are motor vehicle accidents in approximately 30 percent of cases, followed by falls from variable heights and sports-related injuries.[16] Some authors report that boys are more frequently affected than girls.[4]

CLASSIFICATION

Early SCIWORA

Early SCIWORA is the most frequent mode of presentation in over 50 percent of cases. Neurologic signs and symptoms of varying severity are manifest immediately after the traumatic event and do not recur.[3]

Delayed SCIWORA

A delayed onset of neurologic signs is reported in approximately one-third of subjects.[3] This "latent period" between injury and the appearance of neurologic deficits varies between 1 hour and as much as 4 days. Transient "warning symptoms" such as paresthesias, numbness, lightning sensation (L'hermitte's sign) and a generalized feeling of weakness are sometimes experienced immediately following trauma.[24] The latent period is followed by progressive sensorimotor paralysis, which presumably is the result of either (1) repeated insults to the spinal cord caused by repetitive movements on an "incipient" instability of the spine caused by the original traumatic event or (2) a slowly progressive ischemic injury of the cord.

Recurrent SCIWORA

In approximately 15 percent of reported cases, a second SCIWORA episode has followed an initial mild SCIWORA after a variable interval of 3 days to 10 weeks.[15] This recurrent syndrome is usually more severe and is associated with another traumatic episode, which may be trivial, such as a slight fall or throwing a ball. Since the initial neurologic deficit is mild, these children or adolescents are either improperly immobilized from the onset, do not comply to the prescribed immobilization, or return too soon to physiologic activities. A radiographically occult spinal instability to the spine from the initial trauma is the probable cause of this recurrent spinal cord injury. Repeated radiologic evaluations after the second episode are also within normal limits.

PHYSICAL EXAMINATION

A careful history to determine the cause and mechanism of injury and a detailed neurologic examination should be obtained for all patients with a suspected SCIWORA in order to establish the level, the pattern and the severity of the neurologic lesion. Three main patterns of injury are encountered[16]:

1. Complete spinal cord lesion (20 percent)
2. Incomplete spinal cord lesion
   A. Central cord syndrome (30 percent)
   B. Brown-Séquard syndrome (10 percent)
   C. Partial cord syndrome (35 percent)
3. Spinal cord concussion (5 percent)

The severity of each incomplete lesion is graded as *mild* if the child is able to ambulate and/or has mild to moderate hand weakness, or *severe* if ambulation is seriously impaired or profound weakness of hands or arms is present. There is no apparent correlation with the level of injury and the neurologic pattern of involvement.

Complete Physiologic Cord Transection

Complete anesthesia and absence of voluntary motor power distal to the level of injury will be evident on examination. Sacral sparing should be specifically sought for when spinal shock is over, as evidenced by the return of the bulbocavernous reflex, usually within 24 hours. As in adults, the prognosis for recovery is very poor.

Incomplete Spinal Cord Lesion

Central Cord Syndrome

Damage is mostly to the central gray matter and to the central portion of the corticospinal and spinothalamic tracts, producing a quadriparesis and affecting the upper extremities to a greater extent, with varying degrees of sacral sparing. Prognosis for recovery is good in mild lesions but fair to poor in severe lesions.

Brown-Séquard Syndrome

The Brown-Séquard syndrome is an infrequent pattern where the injury is mainly limited to either half of the spinal cord producing ipsilateral muscle paralysis and contralateral hypoesthesia to pain and temperature. Prognosis for recovery is good, especially in mild lesions.

Partial Cord Syndrome

The damage varies greatly both in severity and geographic distribution in this pattern, which regroups all incomplete lesions not included in the previous discus-

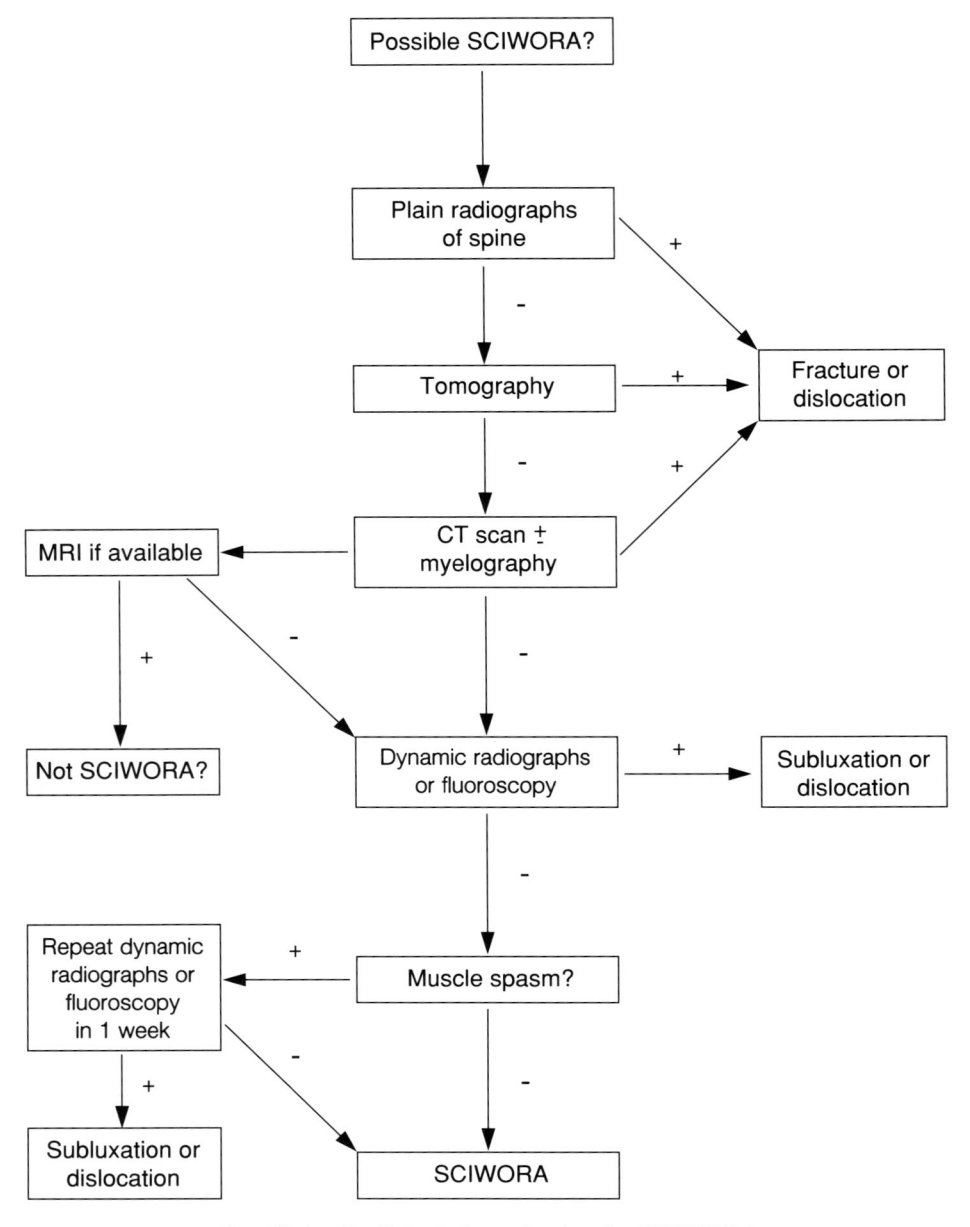

Fig. 50-1. Radiologic investigation for SCIWORA.

sion. Prognosis is good in mild lesions but poor in severe lesions.

Spinal Cord Concussion

A syndrome of neurapraxia of the cervical spinal cord with transient quadriplegia has been described by Torg and coworkers[20] in the young adult athlete. Recently, Rathbone and colleagues[25] have reported the occurrence of this syndrome during various sporting activities in 12 children between 8 and 16 years old. The episodes are transient, and complete recovery usually occurs in a few hours, although in some patients gradual resolution may extend over a period of 36 to 48 hours. Sensory and motor changes range from mild numbness or weakness to complete paralysis with eventually a complete recovery and return of full pain-free motion of the cervical spine. Congenital cervical stenosis is a contributing factor in a significant number of reported cases.[20,25]

Associated Injuries

Associated injuries such as head trauma, long-bone or pelvic fractures and thoracoabdominal injuries are frequently encountered, most commonly after motor vehicle accidents. They need standard evaluation and treatment as for any polytraumatized patient.

INVESTIGATION

Radiologic Investigation

By definition, radiologic investigation is negative for any bony or ligamentous abnormality: SCIWORA is a diagnosis that should only be made after a careful and standardized radiologic evaluation has excluded all other possible pathologic conditions. The suggested protocol for evaluation is outlined in Figure 50-1.

Standard anteroposterior and lateral radiographs of the entire spine and an open mouth view of the odontoid should be obtained for every polytrauma patient with a suspected SCIWORA, as soon as proper immobilization and emergency procedures have been established. For patients with isolated neurologic syndromes, radiologic evaluation can be limited to the symptomatic area (Fig. 50-2). If there is no evidence of fracture, dislocation, or subluxation with this initial investigation, anteroposterior and lateral linear tomograms of the involved area should be ordered next, to rule out an occult fracture or subluxation at any suspicious site or at the spinal level corresponding to the neurologic lesion. A search for congenital spinal stenosis should be done according to the criteria set by Torg and colleagues[20] and Hinck and colleagues.[21] If tomograms are normal, thin-sliced axial computed tomography (CT) is obtained. Whether a myelography should be done at the same time is still debated, some authors reporting that it is of little further value,[8] while others argue that traumatic disc herniations, hematomas, or cord rupture are better delineated by CT-myelography than plain CT with bony or soft tissue algorithms.[16,17,23] The diagnosis of SCIWORA is sustained even if slight abnormalities of the spinal cord, such as swelling or irregular contours, are identified, as long as no bony, discal, or ligamentous lesions are detected. If available, magnetic resonance imaging (MRI) should also be obtained in every suspected case, since it is the only test that allows direct visualization of intrinsic cord lesions: it is usually normal but may reveal focal high-intensity intrinsic lesion on sagittal T1-weighted images representing spinal cord contusion or hemorrhage.[26,27] Once again, the diagnosis of SCIWORA is sustained as long as no bony, discal, or ligamentous lesions are detected (Fig. 50-3).

If all static radiologic investigations are normal, the next step is to perform a dynamic assessment of the spine to rule out any occult instability. This can be achieved in two ways: dynamic plain radiographs or fluoroscopy with the patient's spine in maximum voluntary flexion and extension under the supervision of an experienced radiologist. In cases where no instability is detected, but spine motion is limited by secondary muscle spasm, the dynamic evaluation should be repeated later when muscle spasm has subsided.

The diagnosis of SCIWORA can finally be made only when all static and dynamic radiographs show no evidence of abnormality besides spinal cord contusion or hemorrhage. With the increasing quality of MRI and other techniques of medical imagery, it is probable that cord lesions will be detected with increasing frequency (Fig. 50-3). In this regard, SCIWORA might have to be more appropriately renamed SCIWOSRA or spinal cord injury without skeletal radiologic abnormality, to account for the detectable traumatic anomalies of the spinal cord.

Electrophysiologic Studies

Somatosensory evoked potentials (SSEP) have proven useful to document spinal cord dysfunction,[4] especially in children with associated craniocerebral trauma or young uncooperative children with questionable weakness on clinical examination. Abnormalities detected include prolongation of upper or lower extremity nerve latencies and decreased wave amplitudes. SSEPs are also useful to monitor neurologic recovery in the follow-up period and should be part of the routine investigation when available.

TREATMENT

Proper immobilization of the spine until the cord contusion and until the "incipient" instability of the spine have healed is the mainstay of treatment. In contrast to fractures and dislocations of the spine with neurologic injuries, which frequently require operative treatment, surgery has not proven useful in the management of SCIWORA.[28,29]

The suggested protocol of treatment is outlined in Figure 50-4.[16,24] The first priority goes to resuscitative maneuvers in polytraumatized patients. Reestablishment of an adequate airway, ventilation, and treatment of

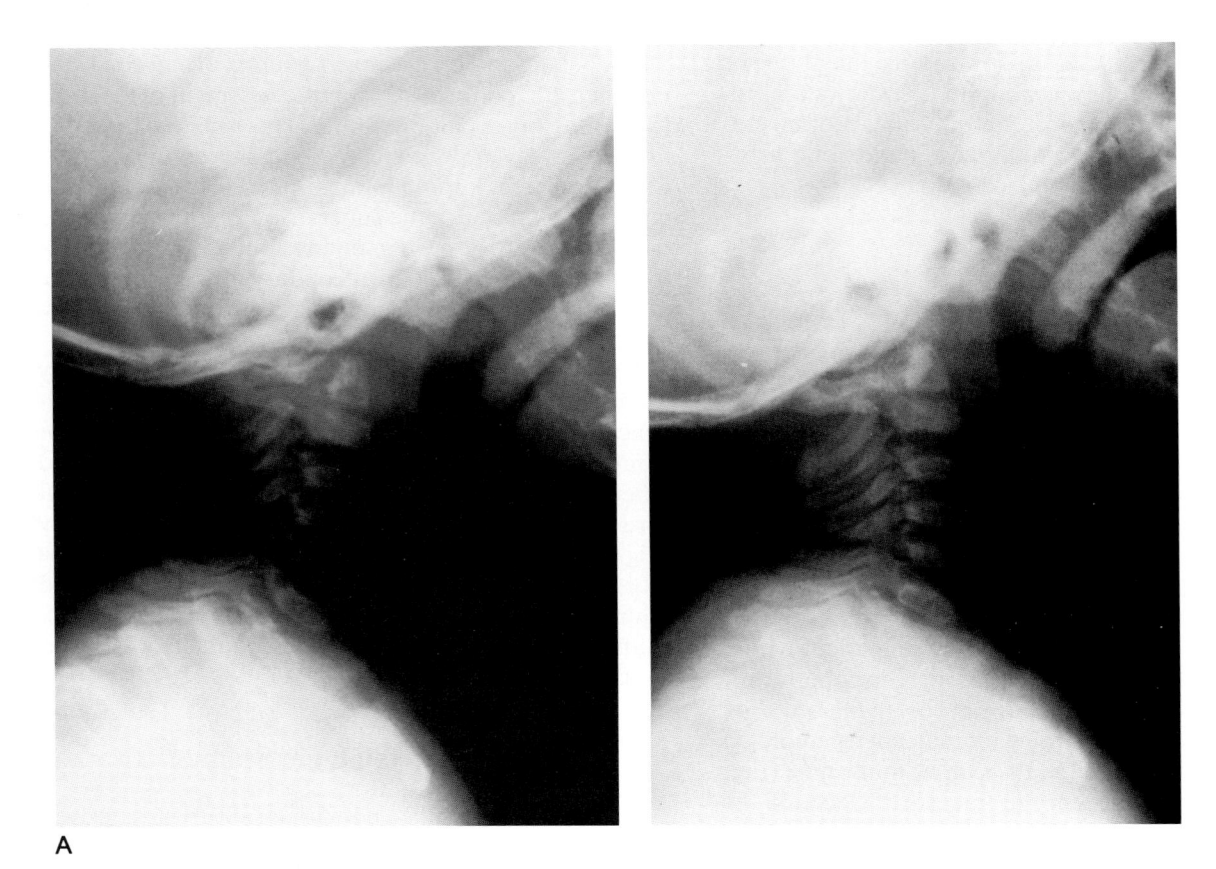

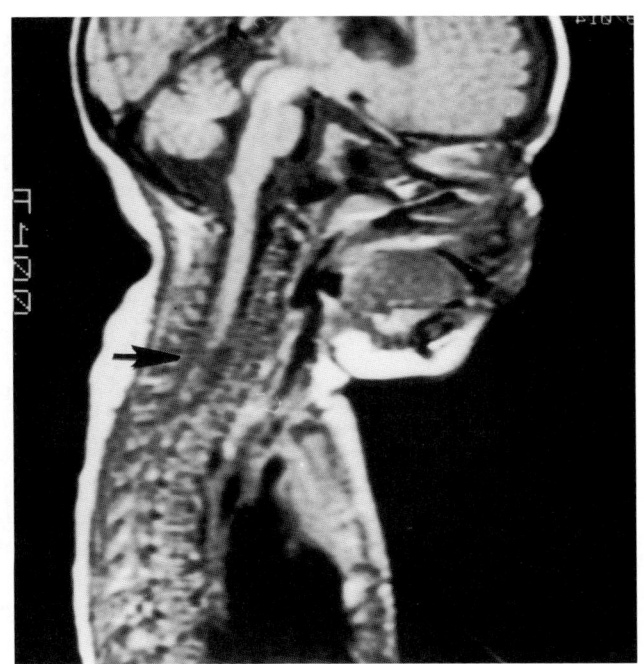

Fig. 50-2. (A) This 2-year-old boy was sitting in his car seat during a head on motor vehicle accident. He sustained immediate and permanent paraplegia, although his plain radiographs showed no fracture or dislocation. (B) An MRI of the spine revealed spinal cord hemorrhage and edema at the T2 level probably due to severe cord traction secondary to high-velocity flexion of the child's relatively large head at this age on the fixed torso. (Courtesy Eric Jones, M.D., West Virginia University School of Medicine.)

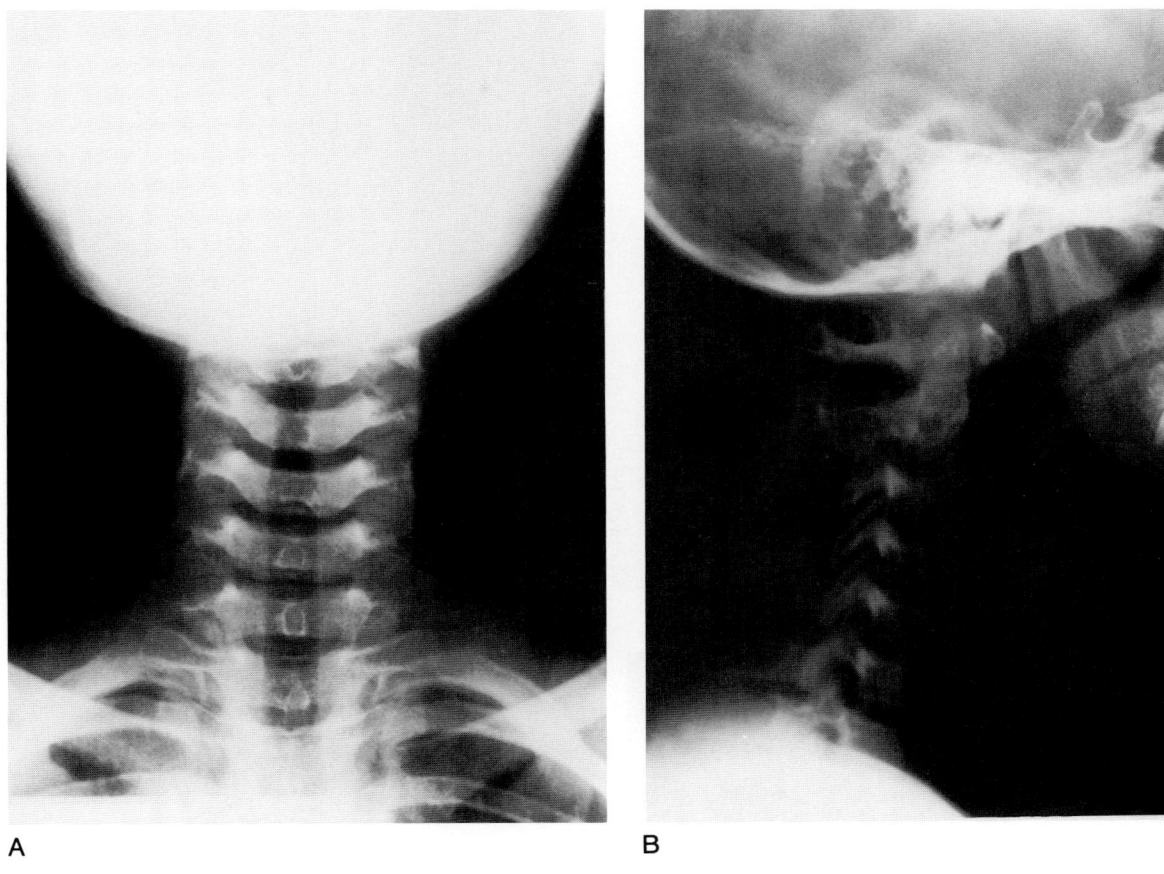

Fig. 50-3. (A) Anteroposterior, (B) lateral, (C) odontoid view of an 8-year-old girl who sustained a flexion injury of the neck after falling on her head in a playground. She developed an immediate Brown-Séquard syndrome. There is a slight physiologic subluxation of C2 on C3 and a loss of cervical lordosis seen on the lateral view (B) but the radiographic findings are essentially normal. *(Figure continues.)*

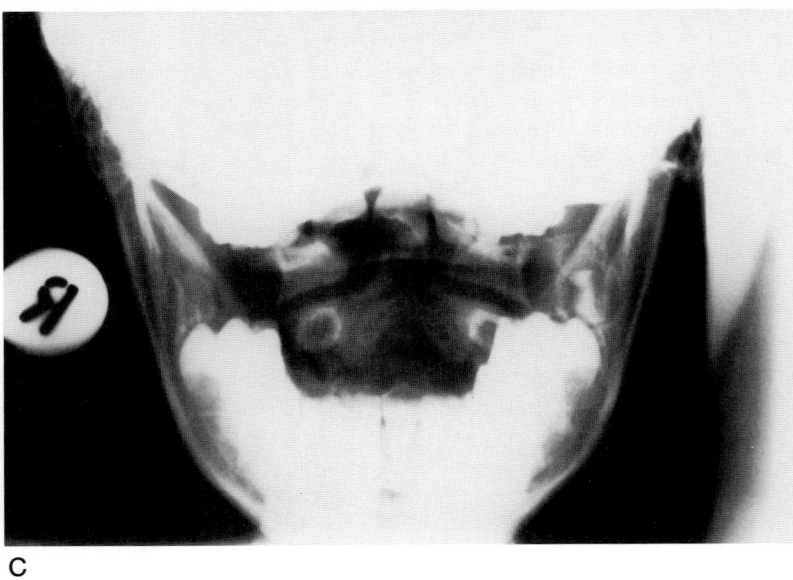

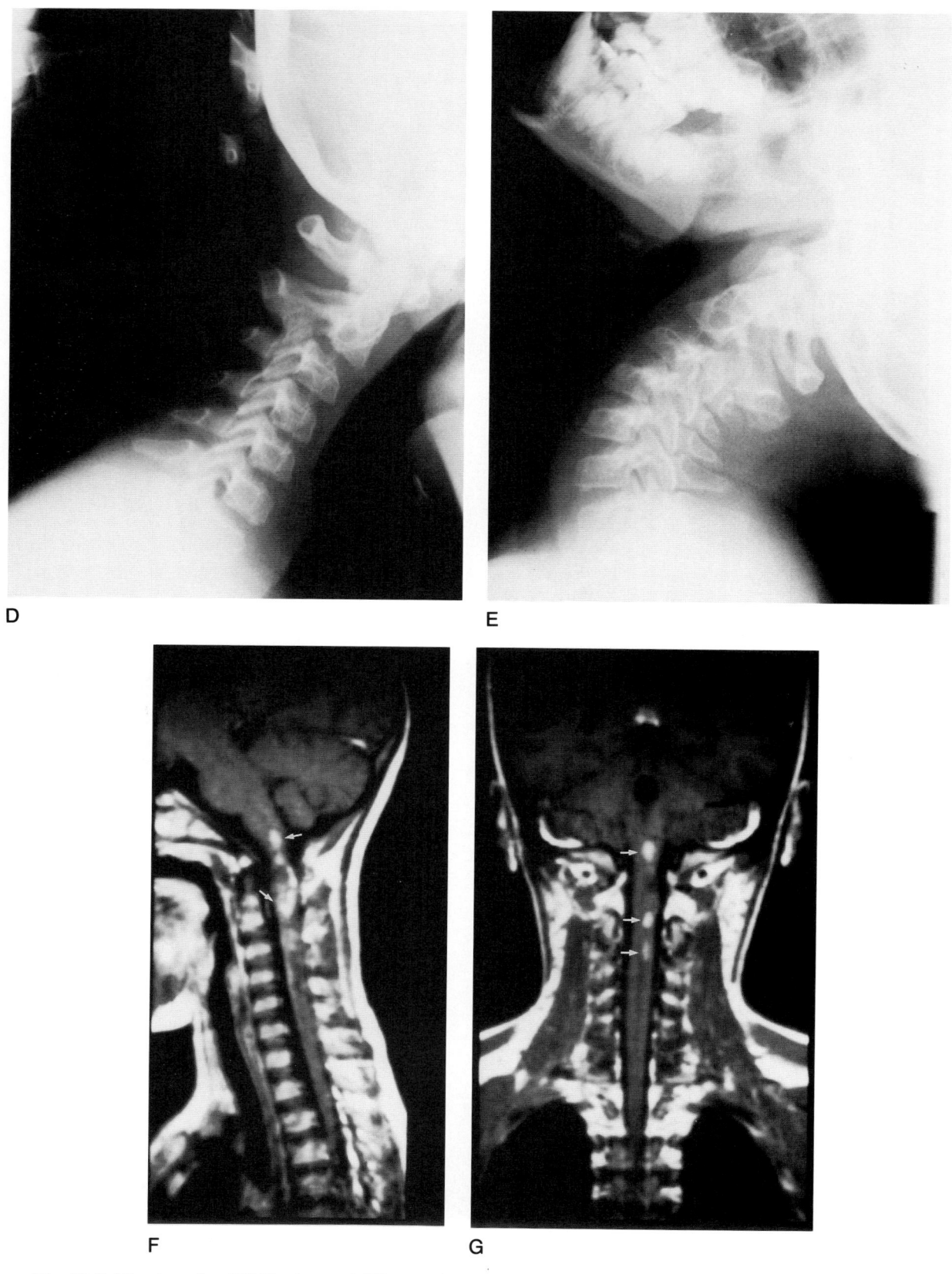

Fig. 50-3 *(Continued).* **(D)** Flexion and **(E)** extension lateral views of the cervical spine showed no evidence of fracture or dislocation, but flexion is limited by muscle spasm. **(F & G)** MRI scans revealed extensive areas of cord edema and hemorrhage in the upper cervical spine, possibly associated with an underlying vascular anomaly previously asymptomatic. The neurologic syndrome gradually disappeared a few months after the initial trauma.

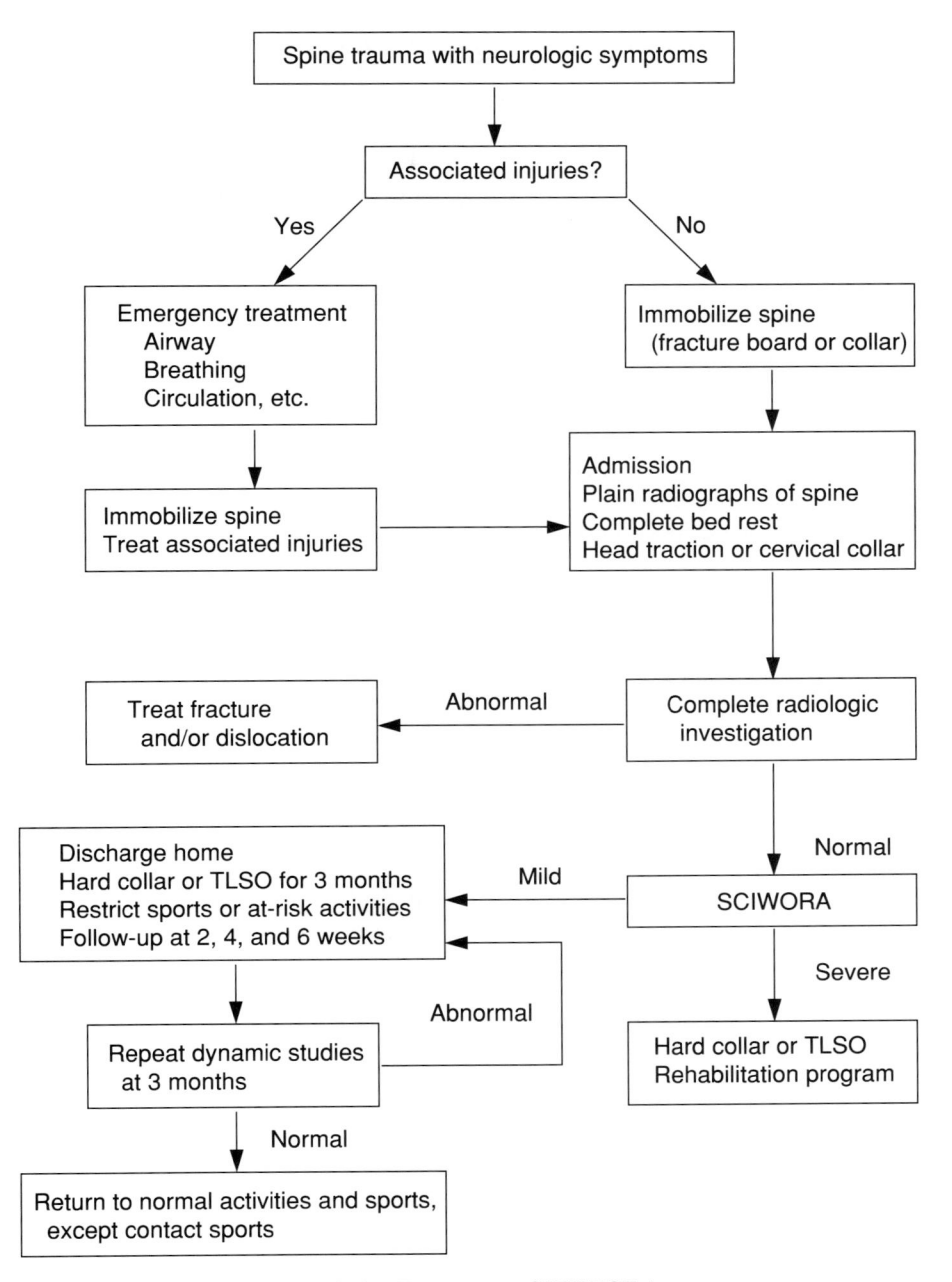

Fig. 50-4. Treatment of SCIWORA.

shock are done according to the standards of the American Trauma Society. The next priority is to immobilize the spine as soon as possible with a fracture board and a cervical collar for transportation, until appropriate anteroposterior and lateral radiographs of the spine can be performed. If the initial radiologic investigation is normal, patients should be admitted in the hospital and kept under close observation for a few days on complete bed rest with a rigid cervical collar or a head halter with light traction to immobilize the cervical spine. The radiologic investigation should then be completed as suggested in Figure 50-1. If a diagnosis of SCIWORA is confirmed, mild cases that are ambulatory or cases that have improved back to normal under observation, can be discharged home wearing a rigid cervical collar or a thoraco-lumbo-sacral orthosis (TLSO) on a full-time basis for 3 months. All sports and "at-risk" activities should be forbidden during this period, and follow-up evaluations with control radiography should be carried at 2, 4, and 6 weeks postdischarge from the hospital. Dynamic radiologic studies are repeated at 3 months posttrauma, and if normal, immobilization is discontinued and return to normal activities and sports is allowed. Some authors[25] feel that contact sports should be avoided for any child with a history of neurologic symptoms or signs following a cervical spine injury. If dynamic studies are abnormal, the diagnosis of SCIWORA should not be sustained, and further immobilization or surgical fusion should be considered.

In severe SCIWORA syndromes, immobilization with a rigid cervical collar or a TLSO is also recommended for 3 months and an appropriate rehabilitation program for paraplegics or quadriplegics should be instituted.

COMPLICATIONS AND PROGNOSIS

The most reliable predictor of neurological outcome is the initial neurologic status. The more severe the initial neural injury, the worse the prognosis. Most children with mild syndromes will recover partially or completely, while most children with severe syndromes will not recover. Children under 8 years old have a much poorer outcome because of the increased vulnerability of the immature spine.

Complications of the SCIWORA syndrome are mainly those of quadriplegia and include decubitus ulcers, respiratory failure, renal calculi, and so on. Treatment is the same as in other types of quadriplegia (see Ch. 49).

SUMMARY

The pediatric SCIWORA syndrome is a traumatic myelopathy in children who show no radiographic evidence of skeletal injury or subluxation by radiologic investigation. It accounts for 20 to 30 percent of traumatic injuries of the spine in children and it is caused by a self-reducing transient intervertebral subluxation of the juvenile spine, which is inherently more unstable due to increased laxity and certain anatomic characteristics.

A delayed onset of neurologic signs can be present in one-third of patients and the syndrome can recur in 15 percent of patients with a mild syndrome. The diagnosis can be established only after a careful radiologic evaluation has excluded any bony or ligamentous abnormalities. MRI may reveal evidence of spinal cord contusion or hemorrhage.

Treatment consists of adequate immobilization by a rigid cervical collar or TLSO and restriction of physical activities for 3 months. The prognosis for recovery of the neurologic injury is good in mild cases but poor in severe cases, and serious injuries are more frequent in children under age 8.

REFERENCES

1. Taylor AR, Blackwood W: Paraplegia in hyperextension cervical injuries with normal radiographic appearances. J Bone Joint Surg [Br] 30:245, 1948
2. Cheshire DJE: The paediatric syndrome of traumatic myelopathy without demonstrable vertebral injury. Paraplegia 15:74, 1977-78
3. Pang D, Wilberger JE Jr: Spinal cord injury without radiographic abnormalities in children. J Neurosurg 57:114, 1982
4. Kewalramani LS, Kraus JF, Sterling HM: Acute spinal-cord lesions in a pediatric population: epidemiological and clinical features. Paraplegia 18:206, 1980
5. Kewalramani LS, Tori JA: Spinal cord trauma in children: neurological patterns, radiologic features, and pathomechanics of injury. Spine 5:11, 1980
6. Osenbach RK, Menezes AH: Spinal cord injury without radiographic abnormality in children. Pediatr Neurosci 15:168, 1989
7. Ruge JR, Sinson GP, McLone DG, Cerullo LJ: Pediatric spinal injury: the very young. J Neurosurg 68:25, 1988
8. Scher AT: Trauma of the spinal cord in children. S Afr Med J 50:2023, 1976
9. Selecki BR, Roy R, Ness P: Neurotraumatic admissions to a teaching hospital: a retrospective study. Part 3. Spine and spinal cord injuries, with particular reference to the cervical region. Med J Aust p. 620, 1968
10. Burke DC: Spinal cord trauma in children. Proceedings of the Annual Scientific Meeting of the International Medical Society of Paraplegia, Stoke Mandeville Hospital, July 1970
11. Anderson JM, Schutt AH: Spinal injury in children: a review of 156 cases seen from 1950 through 1978. Mayo Clin Proc 55:499, 1980
12. Choi JU, Hoffman HJ, Hendrick EB et al: Traumatic infarction of the spinal cord in children. J Neurosurg 65:608, 1986
13. Glasauer FE, Cares HL: Traumatic paraplegia in infancy. JAMA 219:38, 1972
14. Glasauer FE, Cares HL: Biomechanical features of traumatic paraplegia in infancy. J Trauma 13:166, 1973
15. Pollack IF, Pang D, Sclabassi R: Recurrent spinal cord

injury without radiographic abnormalities in children. J Neurosurg 69:177, 1988
16. Pang D, Pollack IF: Spinal cord injury without radiographic abnormality in children: the SCIWORA syndrome. J Trauma 29:654, 1989
17. Walsh JW, Stevens DB, Young AB: Traumatic paraplegia in children without contiguous spinal fracture or dislocation. Neurosurgery 12:439, 1983
18. Ahmann PA, Smith SA, Schwartz JF, Clark DB: Spinal cord infarction due to minor trauma in children. Neurology 25:301, 1975
19. Pennecot GF, Gouraud D, Hardy JR, Pouliquen JC: Roentgenographical study of the stability of the cervical spine in children. J Pediatr Orthop 4:346, 1984
20. Torg JS, Pavlov H, Genuario SE et al: Neurapraxia of the cervical spinal cord with transient quadriplegia. J Bone Joint Surg [Am] 689:1354, 1986
21. Hinck BC, Hopkins CE, Savara ES: Sagittal diameter of the cervical spinal canal in children. Radiology 79:97, 1962
22. Stauffer ES, Mazur JM: Cervical spine injuries in children. Pediatr Ann 11:502, 1982
23. LeBlanc HJ, Nadell J: Spinal cord injuries in children. Surg Neurol 2:411, 1974
24. Bailes JE, Hadley MN, Quigley MR et al: Management of athletic injuries of the cervical spine and spinal cord. Neurosurgery 29:491, 1991
25. Rathbone D, Johnson G, Letts M: Spinal cord concussion in the pediatric athlete. J Pediatr Orthop 12:663, 1992
26. Hadley MN, Zabramski JM, Browner CM et al: Pediatric spinal trauma: review of 122 cases of spinal cord and vertebral column injuries. J Neurosurg 68:18, 1988
27. Matsumura A, Meguro K, Tsurushima H et al: Magnetic resonance imaging of spinal cord injury without radiologic abnormality. Surg Neurol 33:281, 1990
28. Andrews LG, Jung SK: Spinal cord injuries in children in British Columbia. Paraplegia 17:442, 1979
29. Hachen HJ: Spinal cord injury in children and adolescents: diagnostic pitfalls and therapeutic considerations in the acute stage. Paraplegia 15:55, 1978

51

Child Abuse Fractures

G. Brian Black

> In the little world in which children have their existence, who so ever brings them up, there is nothing so finely perceived and so finely felt, as injustice.
> —GREAT EXPECTATIONS

DESCRIPTION AND INCIDENCE

In this chapter the orthopaedic manifestations of child abuse will be discussed, emphasizing the radiologic features, differential diagnosis, and management as it affects the orthopaedic surgeon practicing today in North America. The thought of our weakest members of society being physically harmed by acts of commission and/or omission is distasteful to us all. Unfortunately, the incidence of child abuse has been found over the past two decades to be much higher than previously accepted. Normal child-rearing practices in the past by some elements of society are now defined as *abuse* and can no longer be condoned. All civilized countries must now deal with the problem by developing a comprehensive approach to the diagnosis and management of the abused child.

HISTORY OF CHILD ABUSE

Ours is not a proud history as a human race when abuse of our offspring is under discussion. A review of ancient literature contains many descriptions of children who were unwanted. Even in religious writings, violence toward children is recorded.[1] Nursery rhymes, such as "Humpty-Dumpty" and "Rock-a-bye-Baby" recited to us and by us to our children can be viewed as suggestive violence toward children. References to the "wicked stepmother" and "stepsisters" in such classic tales as *Cinderella* and *Snow White* are further reference to a violent theme toward children. Such classic novels as Dickens, *Oliver Twist*, Thomas Hardy's *Mayor of Casterbridge*, and Mark Twain's *Huckleberry Finn* show further evidence of unwanted children.[2] In the Orient, missionaries reported the practice of infanticide by destroying a surplus of infant girls.[3] Historical accounts from Britain, Russia, France, and the United States reveal children dying at the hands of their parents.[4,5] Although child abuse has existed probably since civilization began, brutalization of our children has received public attention only recently. According to English, in his book *Pediatrics and The Unwanted Child in History*, there were two periods in modern history in which society attempted to protect our children[5]:

> The first occurred just after the Civil War when unwanted children were gathered into large orphanages and foundling homes. The

philosophy guiding the children's institution was that the biological home was beyond saving and that only the foundling home provided a safe environment from further abuse and degradation. Examining physician records of children entering these institutions shows that many suffered fractures and bruises. The second period of attempted protection was the development of the concept of the foster home. Radiologists in the 1940s began to notice that biological homes, even if supported by a social welfare system, may not be safe homes.

Although society had long recognized that violence against children was occurring, it was not recognized as a criminal offense until the late 19th century[6]:

The first action brought on behalf of a battered child took place in New York City in 1870. Mary Ellen was being beaten daily by her parents. Attempts to correct this situation by appeals to the police and to the District Attorney's office were unsuccessful. Eventually an action was brought by the American Society for Prevention of Cruelty to Animals, which succeeded because Mary Ellen was certainly a member of the animal kingdom and was being cruelly used.

In 1946, Dr. John Caffey, a pediatric radiologist and pediatrician reported on six children who had chronic subdural hematomas in association with multiple fractures of the peripheral skeleton.[7] Furthermore, none of the six children had any history of trauma or evidence of skeletal disease to account for their fractures. In 1953, another radiologist, Dr. F. N. Silverman,[8] described the finding of metaphyseal fragmentation in the long bones implying willful abuse as the underlying etiologic event. It was Dr. C. Henry Kempe who introduced the term *"the battered child syndrome"* in 1962 and raised society's awareness of this social injustice.[9] Other terms have been used to identify this tragic entity such as *parent-infant trauma syndrome* (PITS), or *unexplained trauma of infancy* (UTI). Following Kempe's publication, laws were finally passed making it mandatory for health professionals to document cases of suspected abuse. In Manitoba, the first professional child abuse team was organized in Winnipeg in the 1960s. In 1974, The Child Abuse Protection Act was passed in the United States. The issue of child abuse had become a political, social, legal, and medical problem, and continues to be so.

DEFINITION

In Manitoba, and in most political jurisdictions, child abuse is defined as "the active and/or passive harming of a child by a person who is responsible for the child's care." It is important to remember that abuse may be generally categorized as emotional, physical, or sexual. In each of these broad categories the act may be active (commission) or passive (omission or neglect). For example, when discussing physical abuse there may be active abuse, that is, nonaccidental trauma (bruises, burns, fractures, etc.) or passive abuse, acts of neglect such as abandonment, malnutrition, or lack of supervision, which might lead to repeated accidents or a failure to provide adequate medical care. All individuals who have been entrusted to the care of the child are now responsible for reporting cases of abuse.

INCIDENCE

Exact figures on the frequency of child abuse cases are impossible to obtain. It is estimated that nearly 1,000 children die annually in the United States and that in 1988 approximately 1.6 million were abused or neglected.[10] In the province of Manitoba with a population of 100,000 children, in 1991, 2,237 children were referred to our SCAN (suspected child abuse or neglect) team with 1,886 proven to be abuse, an incidence of about 2 percent. Of these, 943 were involved in physical abuse: 20 children had sustained fractures of the peripheral skeleton, while 16 had skull fractures with or without intracranial hemorrhages; 5 children died as a direct result of the abuse.

The majority of abuse fractures occur in children under 3 years of age. It is possible that the older child might have developed a "means of escape." McClelland and Heiple[11] found that in children less than 1 year old, 56 percent of fractures were not accidental. Female children have been found to have had a higher incidence of abuse in Manitoba, by a ratio of 2:1. Abusers are frequently other caretakers and not always parents. Akbarnia and colleagues[12] have shown that if child abuse is missed in the emergency department, there is a 35 percent chance of reabuse and a 5 to 10 percent chance of death from child abuse. Abuse transcends all socioeconomic levels of our society, but tends to demonstrate a higher incidence in lower income groups in most studies. For every case reported, no doubt many others go undetected. Of those children sustaining a fracture caused by abuse, the initial contact physician in 20 to 30 percent of cases is the orthopaedic surgeon. It is clear that the orthopaedic surgeon must be cognizant of the possibility of child abuse when dealing with any fracture in a child, but especially in the infant.

DIAGNOSIS

A high degree of suspicion must be maintained by the orthopaedic surgeon when making a diagnosis of child abuse. The orthopaedist's role goes beyond the management of a child's fracture. Knowledge of the patterns of normal growth and development in children is essential. Unique anatomic features in the growing child and the mechanical forces applied to growing a bone must be appreciated when making a diagnosis of nonaccidental injury. Before a diagnosis is made, a detailed history and physical examination is paramount. The events and circumstances surrounding the injury should be recorded carefully. Injury investigators have more clearly defined the difference between injuries and accidents. Concepts of primary and secondary prevention have replaced the concept that accidents are random uncontrollable or unpredictable events.[13] The history obtained when dealing with child abuse is often vague and may not clearly explain all physical findings. It is important not to adopt a posture of confrontation, which only causes an alienation between surgeon and parents. The orthopaedic surgeon is a professional who is interested primarily in the well-being of the child and proper treatment of the orthopaedic injury. The orthopaedic surgeon must act as an advocate for the child. When assessing the child and families there are certain characteristics more typical of abusive parents (Table 51-1). These traits may add further evidence to an initial suspicion that the fracture was caused by abuse. No particular personality disorder is typical of an abusive parent. Remember that so-called "others," people in a position of trust, that is, babysitter, grandparents, or "boyfriends" may have harmed the child. Abused children, if old enough, should be asked if they understand why they are being examined. A straightforward approach is often helpful. Abused children may be aggressive or extremely passive in nature. All professionals need to combine their skills as a team if the interests of the child are to be served. This often necessitates involvement of social workers, psychologists, police, legal counsel, and other support groups. Such teams are referred to in different locales as child protection teams, SCAN teams, or trauma protection teams.

SKELETAL TRAUMA

Akbarnia and coworkers[14] found that one-third of all physically abused children required orthopaedic consultation. Fractures secondary to abuse are more commonly seen in children less than 3 years old. Conversely, according to Merten and colleagues,[15] less than 10 percent of children over 5 years old sustain fractures. Forces acting on the growing infant or child may be indirect (shaking, twisting) or direct (from blows). Any portion of the skeleton may be traumatized. Indirect forces are more common than direct blows. Merten and colleagues[15] have shown that extremity fractures are most common, followed by the skull with or without intracranial, retinal trauma, and, finally, rib fractures. The spine and pelvis are infrequently traumatized. However, traumatic injury to C1-C2 accompanied by retinal hemorrhage is now being more commonly appreciated as being secondary to violent shaking, the so-called "shaken baby syndrome." The most common cause of death is secondary to severe intracranial hemorrhage.[16] The initial evaluation of skeletal trauma fracture may not be readily apparent on radiograph. The acute signs of any bony injury must be searched for as tenderness, bruising, swelling, or redness. Careful observation of the child's face for signs of discomfort while gently palpating the extremities is helpful. Healed fractures are asymptomatic and may only be detected by proper radiologic examination.

EPIPHYSEAL FRACTURES

Injuries occurring at the epiphyseal-metaphyseal junction are highly suggestive of abuse. The periosteum surrounding the growing long bone is thick, well-vascu-

TABLE 51-1. Characteristics of Abusive Parents

- The abusing parent or parents generally have a background of deprivation and/or abuse in their own backgrounds. 'What kind of memories do you have of your childhood?'
- They tend to be self-oriented and from their perspective the child needs "fixing," rarely having insight as to their role in the situation.
- The abusing parent is often wary of authoritative professionals, especially those attached to the welfare system, who may have played a role in their own background.
- "Doctor shopping" is frequent, with the family moving from one physician or hospital to another with each abuse event.
- Their expectations for the child to behave are extraordinarily high, i.e., spanking the 6-month-old child so he won't cry.
- Spanking and other physically punitive disciplinary measures are used excessively and inappropriately.

(From McRae K: When to suspect child abuse. Medicine 2:185, 1989, with permission.)

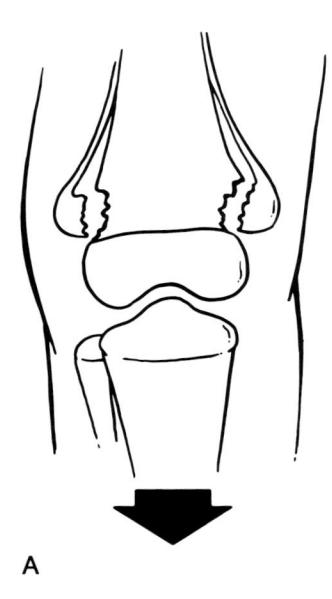

Fig. 51-1. (A) Dynamics of epiphyseal-metaphyseal fractures. Axial ligament and periosteal traction or torsion forces are generated by sudden traction of the extremity. Such injuries occur when the infant is held by the arms or legs and pulled or swung violently upward or forward. (Courtesy of Dr. J. Leonidas, Mount Sinai Medical Center, New York.) **(B)** Typical traction "corner" fracture pathognomonic of child abuse. *(Figure continues.)*

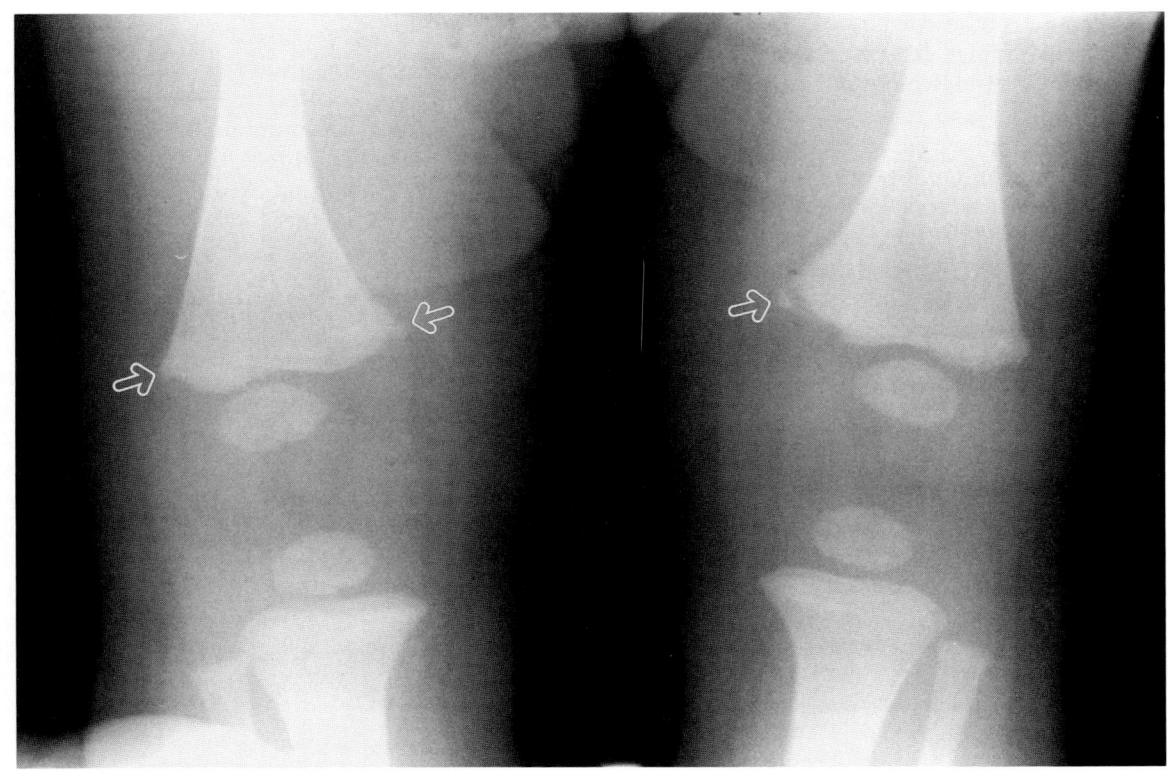

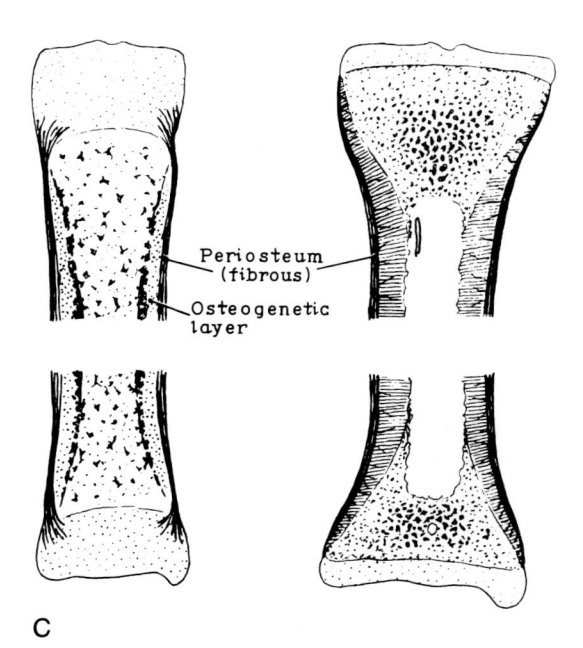

Fig. 51-1 *(Continued).* **(C)** Schematic drawings of the differences in periosteums and their attachments to the underlying cortex in young bones *(A)*, and adult bones *(B)*. In the growing younger bone, the fibrous external layer of the periosteum is relatively shallow and delicate with sparse and short Sharpey fibers; the osteogenic layer is thick *(stippled layer)*. In growing bones however, the periosteum is tightly anchored at both ends by heavy extensions into the epiphyseal cartilages. This loosely attached highly vascularized young periosteum is easily torn from its underlying cortex and free subperiosteal bleeding is common and copious which lifts the bone forming layers away from the cortex to form an external shell of new bone. In the adult bone, the periosteum is largely fibrous with reduced vascularization, but with many heavy and long Sharpey's fibers, which bind the periosteum tightly to the cortex the whole length of the shaft. As a result in the adult after injury, bleeding is rare under the periosteum and when it occurs, it does not lift the periosteum as in the case of young bone. (Fig. C from Caffey J: Pediatric X-Ray Diagnosis. Section 8: The Extremities. p. 1133, Year Book Publishers, Chicago, 1972, with permission.)

larized, and easily stripped from bone, as Sharpey's fibers are poorly developed in the diaphysis and metaphysis. The physeal plate is protected by a strong perichondrial ring. Forces applied to the ends of the long bones will result in a Salter-Harris type of growth plate injury.[17] Epiphyseal injuries are infrequently seen in child abuse but occur most commonly in the proximal and distal femur, tibia, and humerus.

METAPHYSEAL FRACTURES

Metaphyseal fractures in child abuse have received most attention in the orthopaedic literature and were thought to be almost pathognomatic of child abuse. Caffey[18] was the first to describe the metaphyseal fracture, which he felt represented an indirect avulsion injury to the metaphysis by the pull of the periosteum when a child was severely shaken (Fig. 51-1). It was Kleinman and Zito[19] who showed these to be transverse fractures through the metaphysis and only appear to be avulsion injuries because of radiographic projection (Fig. 51-2). Reed,[20] at Winnipeg Children's Hospital, has pointed out that these metaphyseal fractures can be seen in other orthopaedic conditions, including rickets, scurvy, multiple congenital contractures, and kinky-hair syndrome. Fractures occurring through the growth plate may lead to partial or complete growth arrest and permanent deformity. Kleinman and Zito[19] believed that metaphyseal fractures were most suggestive of abuse.

DIAPHYSEAL FRACTURES

King and colleagues[21] have emphasized that diaphyseal fractures of long bones are more common in child abuse cases and that they are often difficult to distinguish radiographically from accidental trauma. It was suggested by Akbarnia and Akbarnia[12] that diaphyseal fractures could be grouped into three broad categories:

1. Transverse, spiral, and oblique shaft fractures
2. Multiple fractures in various stages of healing
3. Bony deformity

Beals and Tufts[22] reported on a series of 80 femoral fractures in children less than 4 years old and found 30 percent were caused by child abuse. In 1986, we reviewed our musculoskeletal manifestations of child abuse and found that in a retrospective review of 105 fractures in 2,434 children, 50 percent of the long-bone fractures were diaphyseal in location.[23]

A spiral or oblique fracture of a long bone is produced by a twisting mechanism (Fig. 51-3). Whether accidental or nonaccidental a large amount of force is required to produce a femoral fracture. A direct blow causing a transverse fracture is also associated with major violence. Young children who are not ambulatory generally cannot produce violence enough to cause femoral fractures. Stories that the infant may have sustained a femo-

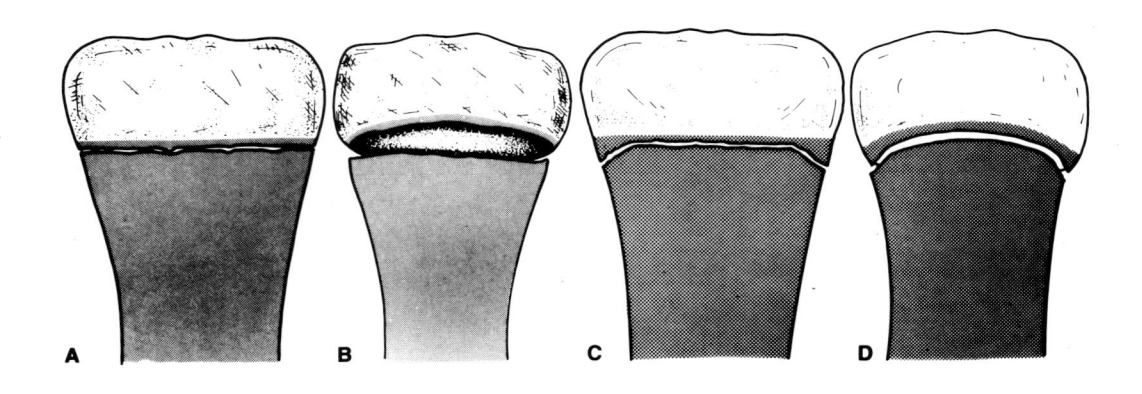

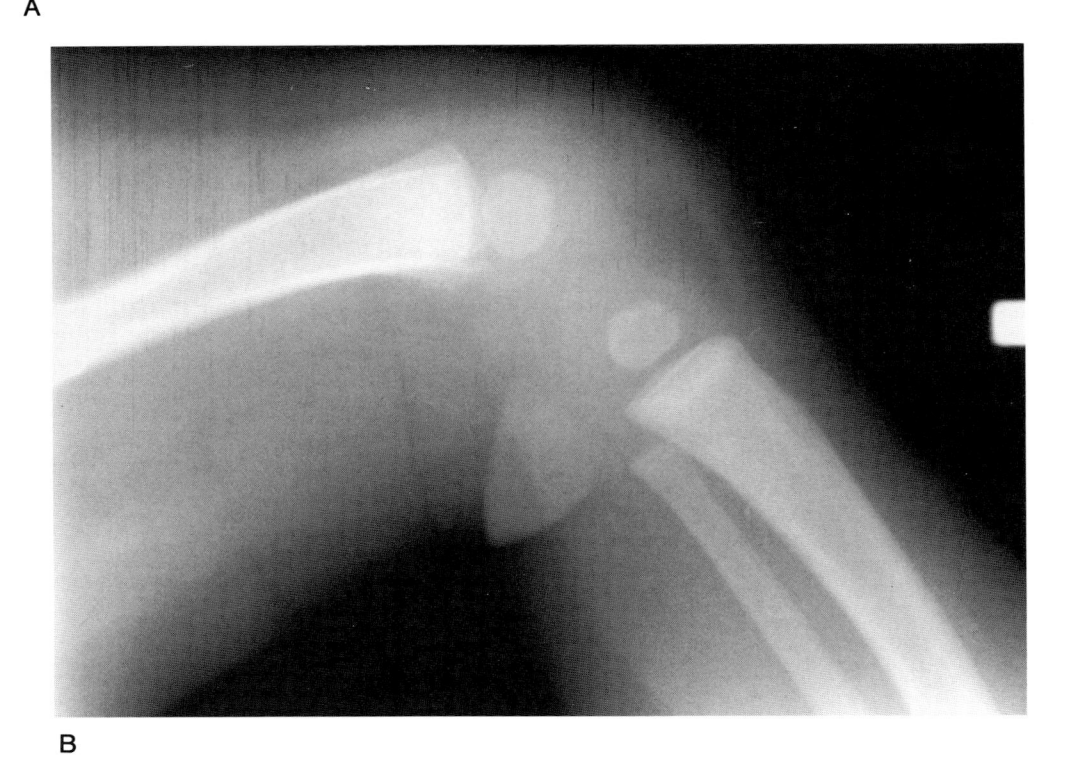

Fig. 51-2. **(A)** Model of metaphyseal lesion. *(A)* A planar fracture through the primary spongiosa produces metaphyseal lucency. *(B)* If the metaphysis is tipped or simply projected obliquely to the x-ray beam, the margin of the resultant fragment is projected with a bucket-handle appearance. *(C)* If the peripheral fragment is substantially thicker than the central fragment and the plane of injury is viewed tangentially, a corner fracture appearance results. *(D)* If the metaphysis is displaced or projected at an obliquity, as in Fig. B a thicker bucket-handle will be apparent. **(B)** Radiograph illustrating metaphyseal lesion. (Fig. A from Kleinman PK: Diagnostic Imaging of Child Abuse. Williams & Wilkins, Baltimore, 1987 with permission.)

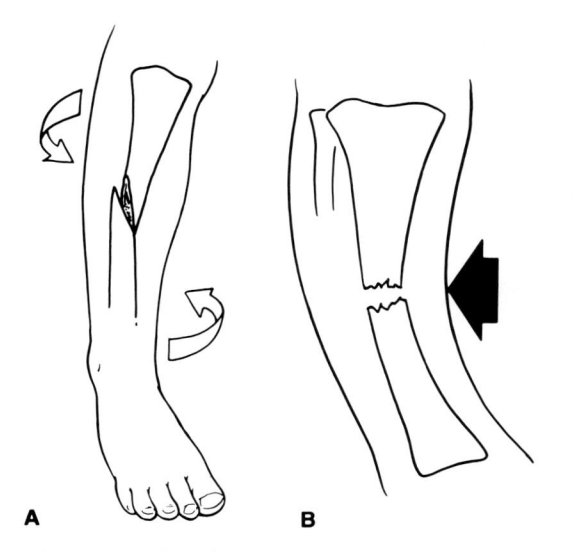

Fig. 51-3. Dynamics of diaphyseal fractures. **(A)** Spiral-oblique fracture results from torsion of the limb. **(B)** Transverse fracture results from more direct trauma such as sudden bending or a blow to the extremity. (From Pediatr Ann 12:12, 1983. Courtesy of Dr. J. Leonidas, Mount Sinai Medical Clinic, New York.)

ral fracture by getting his or her leg "caught in the crib rung" should be viewed with some suspicion.

RIB FRACTURES

Rib fractures are highly suggestive of abuse when seen in otherwise normal children less than 5 years old. The pediatric rib cage is extremely compliant and often will not fracture even during efforts of resuscitation. Indirect violence such as squeezing usually produces fractures of the posterolateral aspect of the ribs (Fig. 51-4). Direct pressure from shaking or choking a child has been shown to produce fractures anteriorly in the first or second ribs. These fractures may be difficult to diagnose early but become apparent on subsequent radiographic follow-up. Radionucleotide scanning has been useful in the early identification of rib fractures (Fig. 51-5).

SPINE FRACTURES

Spinal fractures, with or without associated spinal cord damage, are infrequently seen in child abuse cases. The exact incidence is difficult to estimate, as routine

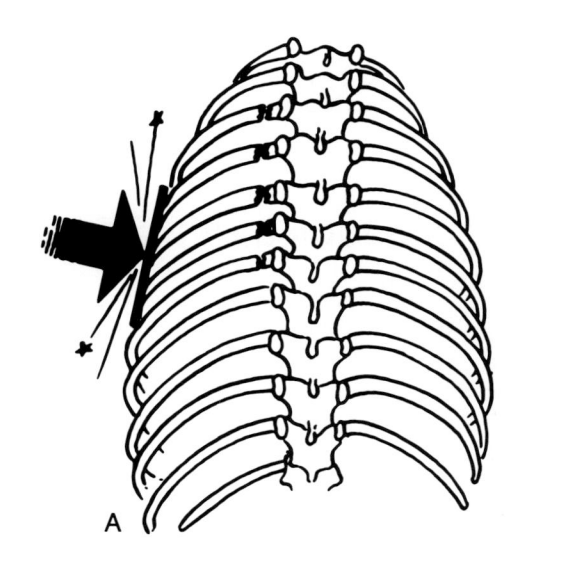

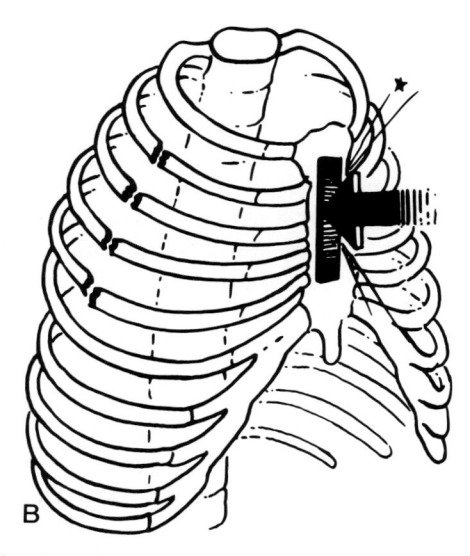

Fig. 51-4. Dynamics of rib fractures. Violent squeezing of the chest causes the ribs to spring and fracture at points of fixation or stress. **(A)** Side-to-side compression commonly results in posterior fractures, frequently adjacent to the costovertebral junction. **(B)** Direct blows may also cause rib fractures at this point of impact. (From Pediatr Ann 12:12, 1983. Courtesy of Dr. J. Leonidas, Mount Sinai Medical Center, New York.)

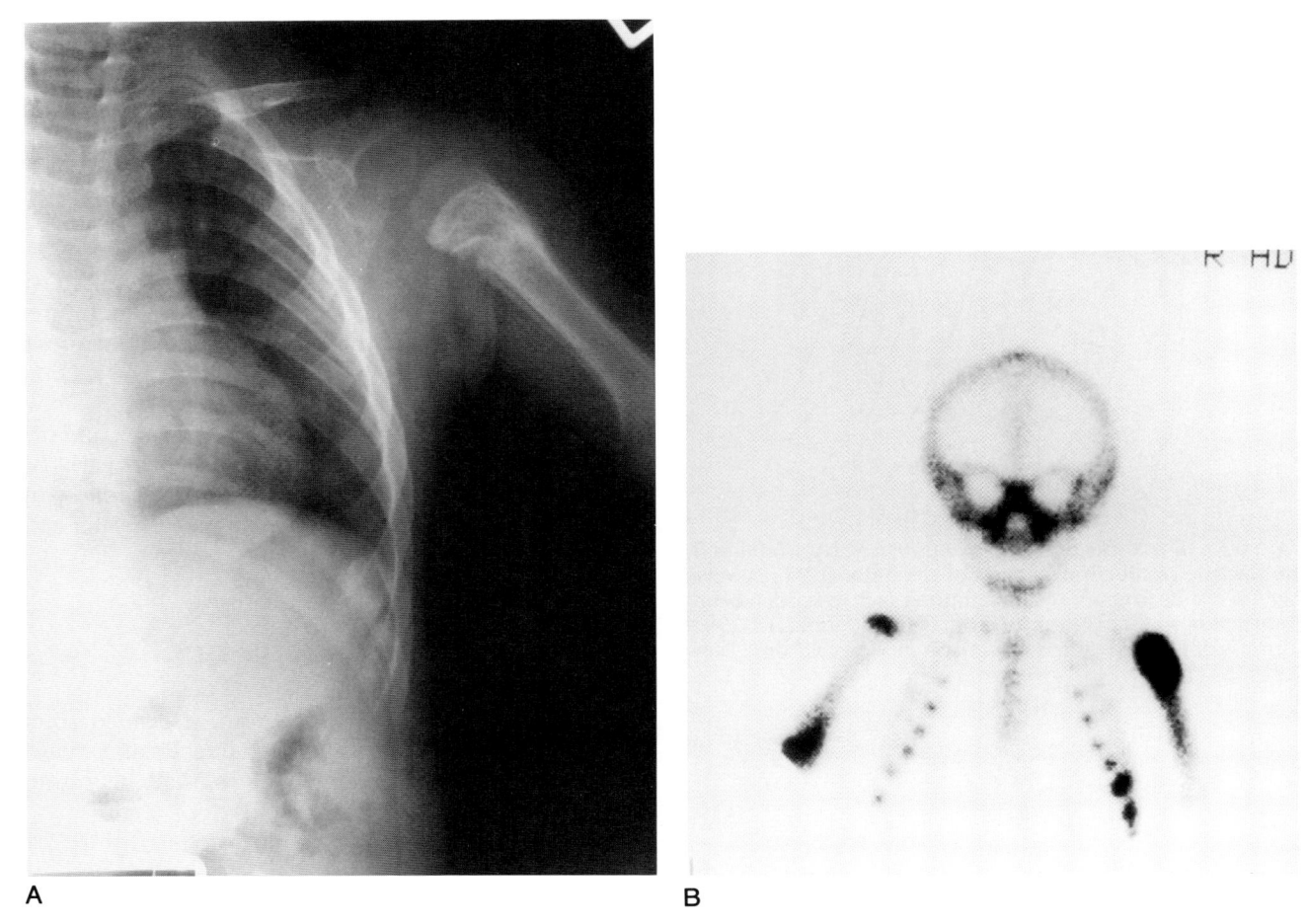

Fig. 51-5. (A) Chest film of an 11-month-old infant who presented with a fractured left humerus. No obvious rib fractures seen on plain film, although healing fracture of the left proximal left humerus is easily seen. (B) Technetium 99 bone scan of the same child illustrating increased uptake over left posterior lateral lower ribs as well as proximal left humerus and distal right humerus. All these areas were later shown to develop periosteal new bone confirming presence of fracture.

radiographs of the spine in a skeletal survey are not always routinely done. In abuse the vertebral bodies may show wedging anteriorly at multiple levels in the area of the thoracolumbar junction or lumbar spine. The mechanism is usually one of compression as the child is forcibly seated into a chair or onto a table top. Fractures of the spinous processes were reported by Kleinman and Zito[19] and felt to be secondary to extreme flexion-extension forces to the spine. It is important to remember that due to the extreme elasticity of the vertebral column in the young child, neurologic injury can occur without evidence of radiologic abnormality (SCIWORA).[24] As in the case of the spinal cord, the lack of hard evidence radiologically does not rule out that a child may have been the victim of physical abuse.

RADIOGRAPHIC ASSESSMENT

I have learned over the years that a radiologist with expertise in pediatric osseous assessment is invaluable when dealing with the subtle radiographic findings in possible skeletal abuse. The radiologist's input is critical to the overall assessment of the battered child syndrome. A skeletal survey is often diagnostic of the child abuse syndrome. The survey should include, as a minimum, two views of the skull, lateral view of the thoracolumbar spine, and anteroposterior views of both upper extremities, hands, pelvis, and both lower extremities, including the feet. The use of one 14-in. × 17-in. film, the so-called "baby gram" is to be discouraged, as detail is frequently lost while trying to position the baby. There are several

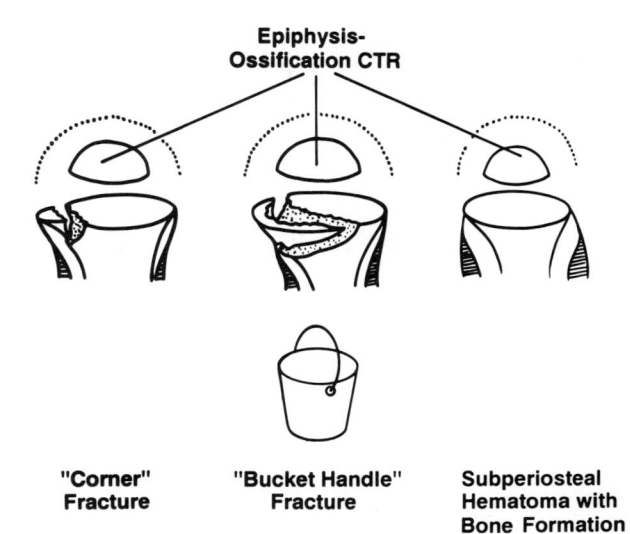

Fig. 51-6. (A) Pathologic features of typical radiographic appearances of child abuse. (B) A 4-month-old battered infant exhibiting a corner fracture and periosteal elevation. (Fig. A from Pediatr Ann 12:12, 1983. Courtesy of Dr. J. Leonidas, Mount Sinai Medical Center, New York.)

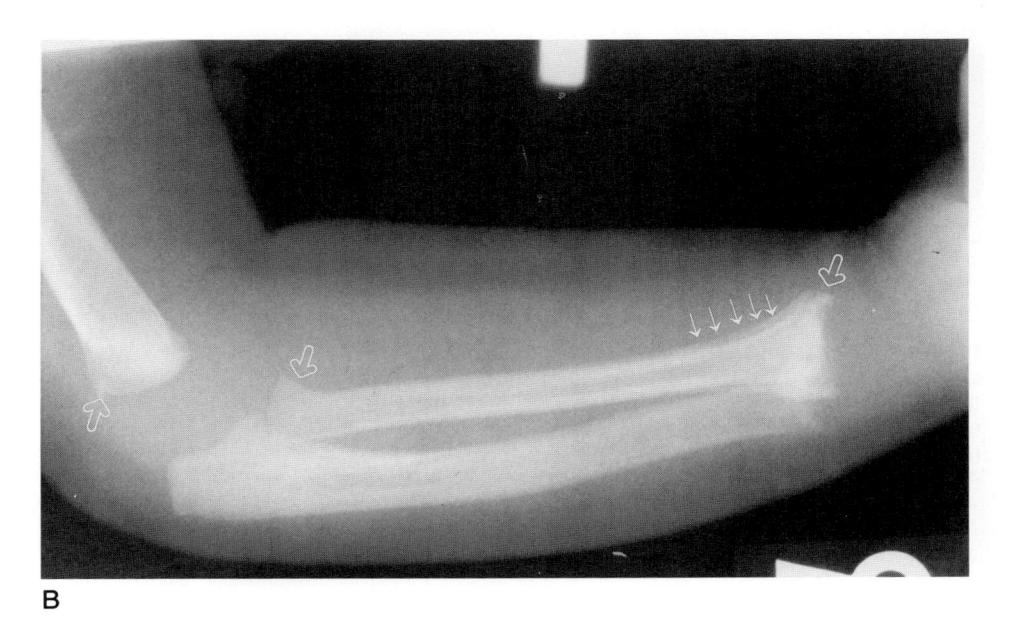

radiologic signs suggestive of abuse. These include healing fractures, multiple fractures, fractures in unusual locations, and metaphyseal fractures (Fig. 51-6). Other radiographic findings suggestive of abuse include posterior rib fractures, spinous process fractures, sternal fractures, complex skull fractures, and diaphyseal spiral and oblique fractures. Fractures of different stages of healing are almost pathognomatic of abuse. In a review of toddler's fractures at the Winnipeg Children's Hospital we found that fractures occurring in the tibia, which showed a fracture line distal and lateral, were almost always associated with child abuse[25] (Fig. 51-7). Any fractures which already show signs of healing suggests that the fracture is at least 10 days old (Figs. 51-8 to 51-10). The temporal relationship between stages of healing and radiographic features have been worked out by many investigators.[26] Technetium 99 bone scanning has been shown to be highly sensitive when used to assess skeletal injury, particularly in occult areas not easily accessible to clinical examination. The scan is frequently "hot" for many weeks during healing. Unfortunately, the scan has low specificity. We still favor the skeletal

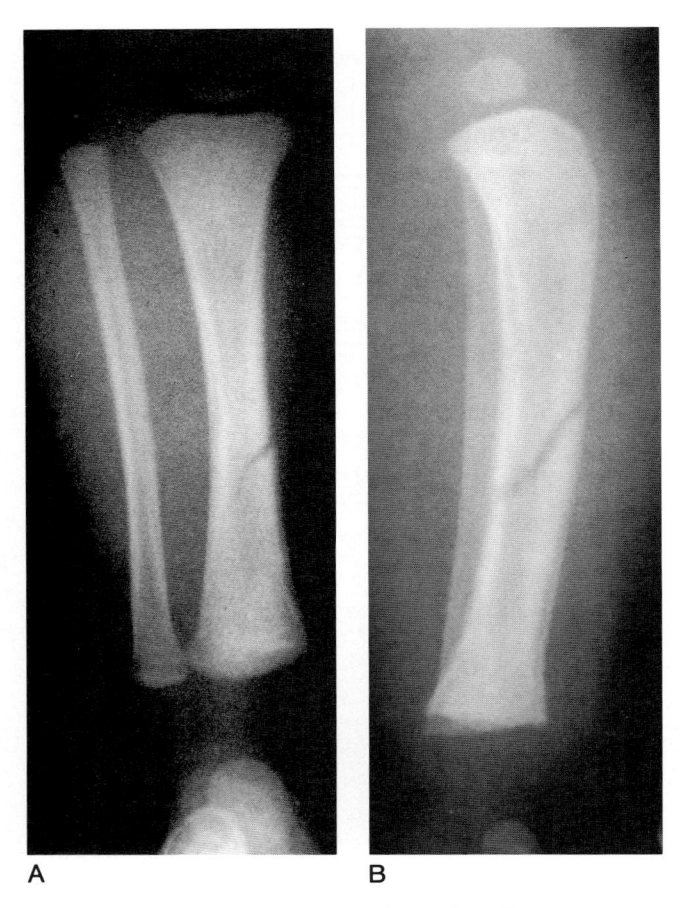

Fig. 51-7. (A) AP and (B) lateral views of the right lower leg of a 2-month-old boy, showing an undisplaced oblique fracture of the midshaft of the tibia, more proximal than the usual toddler's fracture. There is also slight irregularity of the distal tibial metaphysis and some mature periosteal reaction along the anterior aspect of the distal shaft in Fig. B.

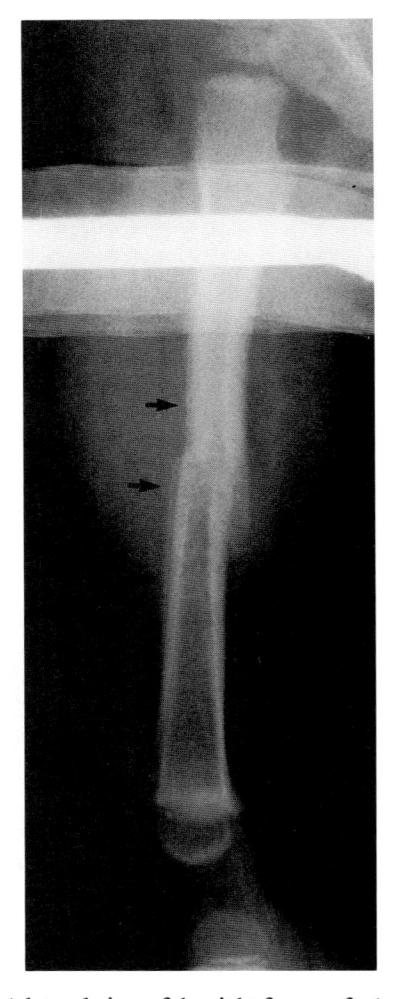

Fig. 51-8. A lateral view of the right femur of a 1-year-old girl shows an acute fracture of the midshaft. There is also periosteal reaction along the anterior aspect of the femur *(arrows)* indicating a previous injury.

survey, however, except in cases where a strong suspicion for abuse can be made and the initial survey is negative or nonconclusive. We have found the bone scan to be useful in identifying fractures of flat bones, such as the skull, ribs, and scapula, which may be missed on radiographic films (Fig. 51-11). Increased uptake of the radionucleotide in the areas of the physeal growth plate can obscure a subtle "corner" metaphyseal fracture. Magnetic resonance imaging (MRI) and computed tomography (CT) scans are modalities that are most useful in detecting subtle intracranial pathology. It is often said that the radiograph tells a story that the child either cannot tell or is too frightened to tell!

DIFFERENTIAL DIAGNOSIS

When assessing a child with radiologic features suggestive of abuse it is as important not to overdiagnose abuse as it is to detect abuse. A mistaken diagnosis can cause major pain and suffering to those falsely accused of abuse. We can all imagine the hurt of a parent when we find it necessary to apologize to parents for falsely suspecting them of abusing their child and then adding that a diagnosis of leukemia has been made. There are several conditions which should be included in the differential diagnosis (Table 51-2).

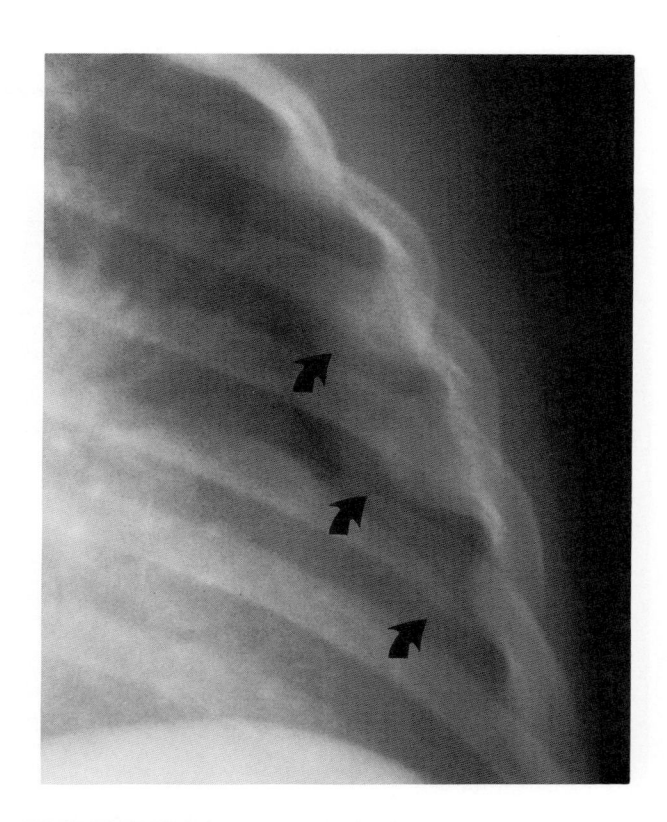

Fig. 51-9. A 7-month-old boy. There are healing fractures of the fourth, fifth, and sixth ribs of the left *(arrows)*.

A

B

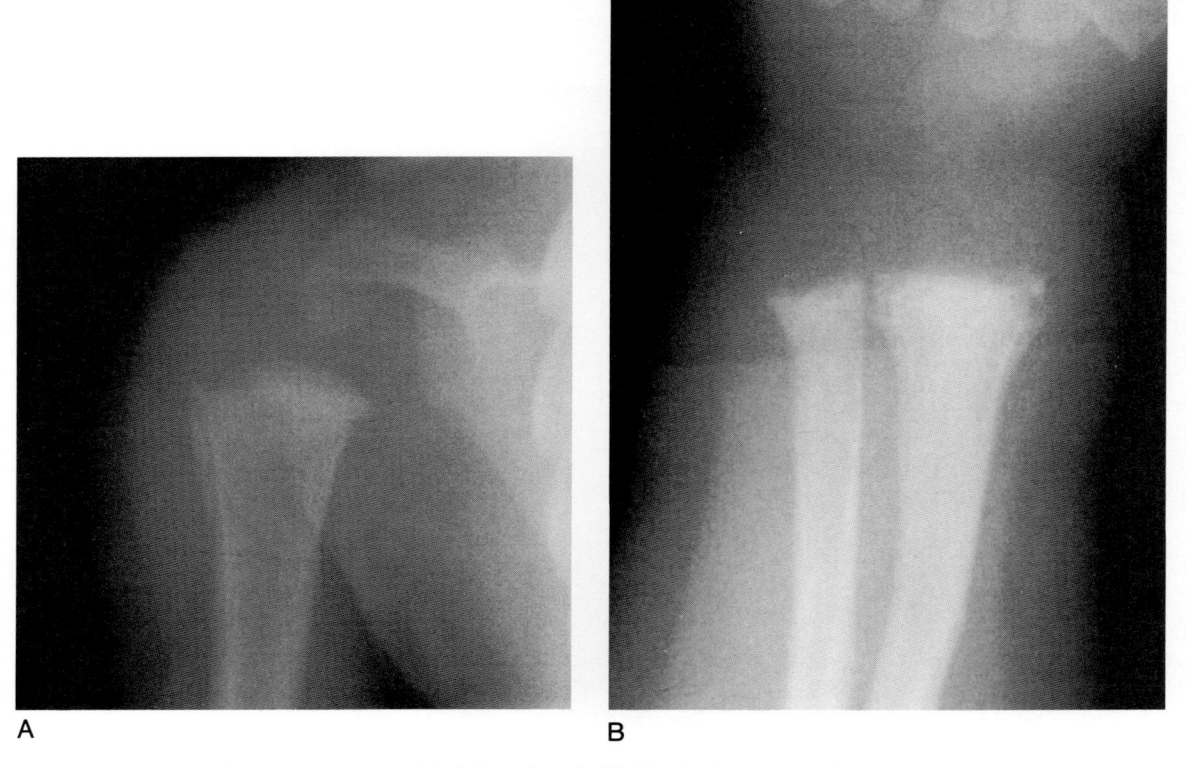

Fig. 51-10. **(A)** Right shoulder and **(B)** right wrist of a 3-month-old boy showing metaphyseal fractures typical of abuse in the proximal humerus and distal radius and ulna. There is periosteal reaction around the proximal humerus and distal radius, indicating that these fractures are a few weeks old.

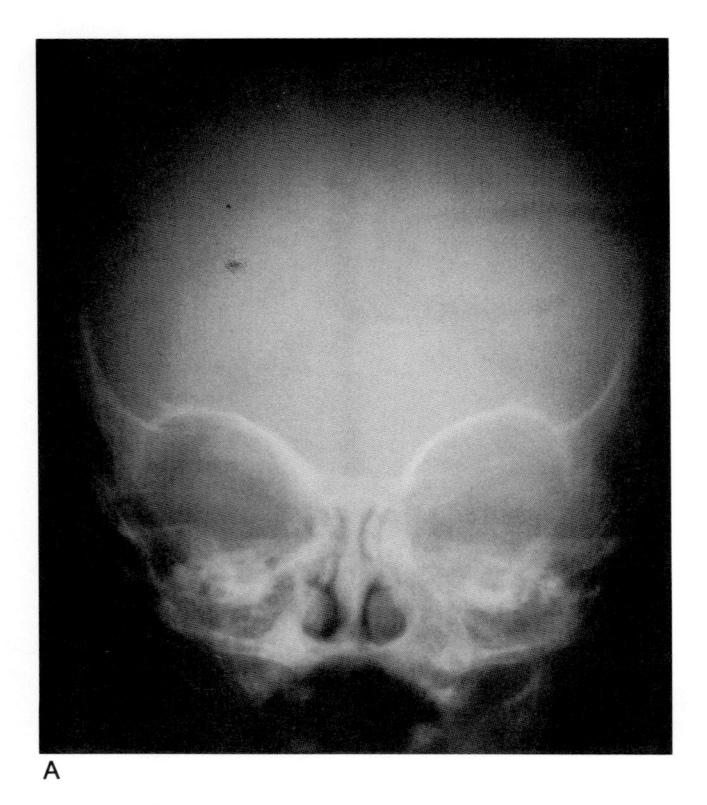

Fig. 51-11. (A) Frontal and (B) lateral views of the skull of a 3-month-old boy show a linear left parietal fracture extending from the coronal suture back to the region of the lambda.

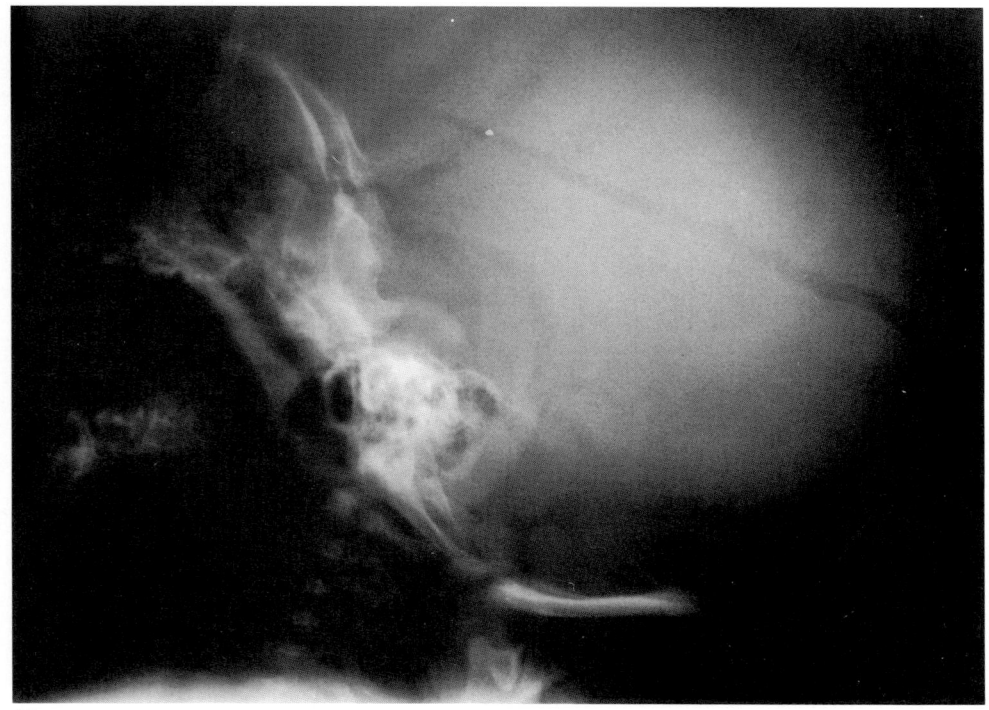

TABLE 51-2. Differential Diagnosis of Radiographic Signs Suggestive of Child Abuse

Rickets
Scurvy
Hypervitaminosis A
Osteomyelitis, including cytomegalovirus, syphilis
Infantile cortical hyperostosis (Caffey's disease)
Osteogenesis imperfecta
Bleeding disorders
Menkes syndrome (kinky-hair disease)
Congenital pseudoarthrosis of tibia, forearm, or clavicle
Neuromuscular disorders
Skeletal dysplasia
Neoplastic: leukemia, metastatic neuroblastoma or lymphoma

A thorough and careful history, radiologic investigation, and laboratory screening should help sort out your differential diagnosis.[27] A laboratory screen, including CBC, platelet count, PT, PTT, and bleeding time, should always be done.

MANAGEMENT AND PREVENTION

An orthopaedic surgeon's primary goal in the management of the abused child is the protection of that child. Beyond the careful management of the orthopaedic injury, Canadian and American law requires the recording and reporting of any suspected abuse. If the report is made in good faith the physician is protected by law. As the child's advocate, a report should be made in what you understand is in the best interest of the child and family. Children are frequently unable to speak for themselves. A significant number of children may be further abused if not protected and may even die from further injury. Admission to the hospital is recommended for any child suspected of having been abused. This allows proper orthopaedic treatment of the fractures, appropriate assessment by the SCAN team, and ensures a protected environment for the child. The etiology of the abuse is often very complex, requiring the assistance of other professionals, including social workers, legal counsel, and psychologists. The law under most Child and Family Services Acts clearly outlines the duty of all professionals to report an act of suspected child abuse, the consequences of not reporting, and stresses the protection of the informant. An orthopaedic surgeon is frequently asked to give legal testimony in abuse cases. Such information as type and location of fractures and the age of the fractures is frequently sought. Based on the radiographs, you will be asked to state mechanisms producing these injuries and whether or not underlying bone disease may be coexistent or whether the radiograph might represent a variation of normal. It is always wise to consult a pediatric radiologist who is experienced in the interpretation of radiographs as it relates to child abuse.

SUMMARY

If the orthopaedist is going to have a positive impact on reducing the incidence of nonaccidental trauma, we must support more comprehensive studies in defining injuries, their mechanism, and radiographic appearance that are most consistent with abuse. Support for more child protection workers to deal with the abused child and their families is a necessary step in reducing the incidence of child abuse in our society. Resources in the areas of prevention and treatment have not kept pace with the number of new cases presently being handled at children's hospitals. All orthopaedic surgeons must continue to play a critical role in the early diagnosis and treatment of the abused child and lending support to preventive and rehabilitative measures for child and family, which can only lead to the protection and care of our children.

ACKNOWLEDGMENTS

I would like to express my sincere gratitude to Miss Tammy Yacyshyn for her assistance in preparing the final manuscript. Also, to Dr. Martin Reed, Head of Pediatric Radiology, an expert in child abuse, who provided a description of the radiographic examples used in the text.

REFERENCES

1. Sari N, Buijukanal SNC: A study of the history of child abuse. Pediatr Surg Int 6:401, 1991
2. English PC, Grossman H: Radiology and the history of child abuse. Pediatr Ann 12:870, 1983
3. Bakan D: Slaughter of the innocents: A study of the Battered Child. Jossey-Boss, San Francisco, 1971

4. Langer WL: Infanticide: a historical survey. Hist Child Q 1:353, 1973
5. English PC: Pediatrics and the unwanted child in History: foundling homes, disease, and the origins of foster care in New York City 1860–1920
6. Rang M: Children's fractures. p. 51. JB Lippincott, Philadelphia, 1983
7. Caffey J: Multiple fractures in the long bones of infants suffering from chronic subdural hematoma. AJR 56:163, 1946
8. Silverman FN: The roentgen manifestations of unrecognized skeletal trauma in infants. AJR 69:413, 1953
9. Kemp CH et al: The battered child syndrome. JAMA 181:105, 1962
10. Christoffel KK: Violent death and injury in U.S. children and adolescents. Am J Dis Child 144:697, 1990
11. McClelland CO, Heiple KG: Fractures in the first years of life: a diagnostic dilemma? Am J Dis Child 136:26, 1982
12. Akbarnia BA, Akbarnia NO: The role of orthopedist in child abuse and neglect. Orthop Clin North Am 7:73, 1976
13. Hadden W, Baker S: Injury control in preventive and community medicine. p. 109. In Clark, McMahon (eds): Little, Brown, Boston, 1981
14. Akbarnia BA, Torg JS, Kirkpatach J et al: Manifestations of the battered child syndrome. J Bone Joint Surg [Am] 56:1159, 1974
15. Merten DF, Radkowski MA, Leonidas JC: The abused child: a radiological reappraisal. Radiology 146:377, 1983
16. Billmore ME, Myers PA: Serious head injury in infants: accidents or abuse? Pediatrics 75:340, 1985
17. Salter RB, Harris WR: Injuries involving the epiphyseal plate. J Bone Joint Surg 45:587, 1963
18. Caffey J: On the theory and practice of shaking infants. Am J Dis Child 124:161, 1972
19. Kleinman PK, Zito JL: Skeletal injury in the young battered infant: an expanded radiologic spectrum. Presented to the 26th annual meeting of the Society for Pediatric Radiology. Atlanta, April 1983
20. Reed MH: Pediatric skeletal radiology. Williams & Wilkins, Baltimore, 1992
21. King J, Dietendorf D, Apthorp J et al: Analysis of 429 fractures in 189 battered children. J Pediatr Orthop 8:585, 1988
22. Beals RK, Tufts E: Fractured femur in infancy: the role of child abuse and neglect. Pediatr Orthop 3:583, 1983
23. Black GB, McPherson J, Reed MH: Musculoskeletal manifestations of child abuse. Orthop Trans 10:616, 1986
24. Swishchuk LE: Spine and spinal cord trauma in the battered child syndrome. Radiology 92:733, 1969
25. Tenebein M, Reed MH, Black GB: The toddler's fracture revisted. Am J Emerg Med 8:208, 1990
26. O'Connor JF, Cohn J: Diagnostic imaging of child abuse. p. 112. In Kleinman PK (ed): Williams & Wilkins, Baltimore, 1987
27. Ragolsky RJ, Black GB, Reed MH: Orthopedic manifestations of leukemia in children. J Bone Joint Surg [Am] 68:494, 1986

52

Extremity Gunshot Fractures

Randall T. Loder

> The recognition of the existence of a problem is the first step to its solution.
> —Martin H. Fischer

INCIDENCE

The majority of pediatric gunshot wounds in the past occurred in rural areas, and were usually shotgun injuries.[1] With the rise in the underground drug culture and gang wars, gunshot injuries to children are becoming an urban violence problem of severe proportions.[2-5] The incidence of gunshot injury in children is rising, creating a new epidemic[4-11] in children of all ages.[3] More pediatric mortalities are being reported from gunshot wounds in Detroit than from polio when it was epidemic.[12]

It is difficult to obtain the true incidence of gunshot injuries in children; the mortality incidence is a more reliable figure. Firearm mortality in children increased from 18.1 (1979) to 22.1 (1988) per 100,000 children.[7] It is a staggering statistic when compared to mortality from natural causes. From 1984 to 1988 the firearm death rate for teenage black males doubled from 1.4 to 2.8 times the rate for natural diseases (e.g., cancer).[7] The morbidity for those children who survive is also high and it has been quoted that 25 percent of children shot result in permanent physical sequalae.[2] This is related to injuries involving both the musculoskeletal and other organ systems. Shotgun injuries can cause extensive multisystem damage and even more serious long-term sequelae.[13,14]

The number of children with gunshot injuries parallels the homicide rate. Victoroff and colleagues[5] showed a marked rise in extremity gunshot injuries treated at the Children's Hospital National Medical Center in Washington, D.C. This paralleled the rising annual murder rate in that city (Table 52-1). Thus the overall incidence of pediatric gunshot wounds can be estimated. Assuming the mortality of pediatric gunshot wounds to be approximately 5 percent (range: 2–13 percent)[2,6,15,16] and knowing the above incidence of firearm mortality as 22.1 (1988) per 100,000 children[7] it can be estimated that the overall annual incidence of gunshot injuries to children is 4.4 per 1,000 children.

The percentage of children with gunshot wounds sustaining extremity injuries ranges from 21 to 48 percent.[2,3,6,15-17] With the high incidence of gunshot wounds in children and from one-quarter to one-half involving the extremities, medical care personnel in trauma situations will be called upon to handle these injuries.

DESCRIPTION, MECHANISM OF INJURY, AND CLASSIFICATION

Gunshot injuries can be divided into powder and nonpowder weapons, with powder weapons divided into high- and low-velocity missiles, as well as shotgun and nonshotgun missiles. A high-velocity missile travels

TABLE 52-1. Annual Incidence of Extremity Gunshot Injuries Treated at the Children's Hospital National Medical Center, Washington, D.C.

Year	No. of Injuries	No. of Murders in Washington, D.C.
1985	1	148
1986	1	194
1987	8	225
1988	36	369
1989	30	434

(From Victoroff et al.,[5] with permission.)

more than 2,500 ft/s, and a low velocity less than 2,500 ft/s. A shotgun uses a large number of spheres, which form a spray pattern upon leaving the muzzle of the firearm. A nonshotgun is a single-missile firearm. Bullet diameter is defined as the bore diameter (in inches) and ranges from 0.17 to 0.45 for handguns. Thus a larger caliber gun has a larger diameter bullet.

Single-Missile Weapons

To understand the mechanism of injury in gunshot wounds, a simple knowledge of ballistics is necessary. Ballistics can assist the physician in determining injury severity, which is needed to institute appropriate treatment. Several thorough reviews of this subject have been published,[18-21] and are discussed in the following paragraphs.

Ballistics is the study of the natural physical laws governing projectile missiles and their predictable performances. The three main phases of ballistics are (1) *interior*, or actions within the weapon; (2) *exterior*, or from the end of the weapon to target impact (e.g., the child's extremity); and (3) *terminal*, or after entering the extremity. Wound ballistics specifically relates to the terminal phase, and is the study of the wounding capacity of missiles due to their interaction with the body.

The essential component of the interior phase is the kinetic energy (E_k) of the missile. The wounding capacity of the missile is related to the E_k of the missile. The total E_k of bullet entry into the tissues is divided into two components: (1) the velocity component, and (2) the rotational component. The velocity component is defined as

$$E_k = \frac{m(v_1 - v_2)^2}{2g},$$

where v_1 is the entrance velocity of the missile into the child, v_2 is the exit velocity of the missile from the child, and g is the gravitational constant. Thus doubling the velocity quadruples the E_k. A magnum shell adds extra gunpowder to the shell, increasing its velocity and imparting 20 to 60 percent more E_k than a standard shell. Since velocity is so key to the E_k, missiles have been classified as either high or low velocity. It is often hard to know the impact velocity, but the muzzle velocity is easy to determine. For practical purposes, the impact velocity equals the muzzle velocity at less than 50 yd distance for low-velocity missiles and 100 yd for high-velocity missiles. The rotational component is present only if the bullet is spinning. Rifling the gun barrel causes spinning. The energy of a rifle bullet is thus much greater than its equivalent handgun bullet, and a magnum rifle bullet may have up to 12 times the E_k of its equivalent handgun bullet.

The exterior phase is primarily dependent upon bullet shape, velocity, and its flow through the air. Aerodynamic factors alter the flight of the bullet, resulting in yaw (the angle between the long axis of the bullet and its path of flight) and tumbling (forward rotation of the bullet around its center of mass). Tumbling cannot usually occur in the air unless a bullet has lost so much velocity it will no longer penetrate the skin. Bullet motions increase air drag as more of the bullet's surface is presented to the airstream. This decreases bullet velocity and thus E_k. To inflict the greatest damage bullet velocity and mass need to be maximized. This can be done by modifying bullet composition. Most bullets are lead, which is high density and can carry more mass per volume than most metals. The drawback is that the melting point of pure lead causes melting at velocities of more than 2,000 ft/s. To bypass this, the bullet can be jacketed with another metal having a higher melting point. By this mechanism, high-speed bullets are possible.

Another important factor in the exterior phase is bullet shape, which is related to what is called the bullet ogive. The ogive is defined as the radius of bullet curve in the lateral projection. The ogive has an inverse relation to the ballistic coefficient, which quantifies the efficiency of a bullet in overcoming air resistance, similar to a coefficient of friction. A bullet with a low ballistic coefficient (or high ogive) will lose less velocity than one with a high ballistic coefficient (or low ogive). Pointed bullets have a higher ogive and a lower ballistic coefficient compared to blunt round-nosed bullets, and lose less velocity during air travel. This is exemplified by an M-16 bullet. This bullet has a high ogive and a high velocity (3,200 ft/s), which gives it the capability of killing a man at 300 yards. The ballistic coefficient is not a significant factor in close-range injuries less than 50 yd, and formerly was significant only to the hunter and soldier. However, the types of weapons seen in pediatric gunshot injuries are now involving M-16 and other high-velocity military weapons.[3]

The terminal phase is chiefly influenced by the factors that slow or retard the bullet in the target tissue. This decreases its E_k and transforms it into other types of energy. These other energies, such as heat, vibration, mechanical, and vacuum forces, cause tissue damage. Bullet retardation correlates with the drag coefficient, C_D, where $C_D = (K_D)(p)(v^2)(d^2)$, p is the specific gravity of the tissue, v the bullet velocity at impact, d the bullet diameter, and K_D the summation of other factors affecting the bullet.

As the tissue specific gravity (p) increases, bullet retardation increases, transferring more energy to the tissues and increasing damage. Bone, with it's high specific gravity, is able to slow a bullet more than muscle. Bone can thus be more severely damaged (Table 52-2). Bullet retardation is also dependent upon the impact velocity (v) and diameter (d). A high-velocity gunshot wound causes more tissue damage than a low-velocity gunshot wound, and a large shell (e.g., .357) causes more damage than a small shell. The factors that determine K_D are bullet composition, bullet shape and design, and aerodynamic parameters.

Bullet composition, shape, and design can be modified by jacketing and hollow pointing. Jacketed bullets maintain the bullet shape in both air and target tissue. This transfers less energy to the tissues than partially or nonjacketed bullets. Bullets with partial jackets (e.g., dumdum, mushroom, soft-nose) tend to increase their diameter in soft tissue. This increases tissue drag and imparts more energy to the tissues in a shorter distance. Partially jacketed bullets may also expand and stop when reaching tissues with high specific gravities (e.g., bone). This again transfers more energy and damage to the bone (e.g., fracture and comminution), whereas a jacketed bullet might pass through the bone. Nonjacketed bullets can expand up to three times their original diameter, transmitting more energy and creating a wider wound than even partially jacketed bullets. When comparing similar jacketed and nonjacketed bullets, the entrance wounds are similar, but the exit wounds are six times greater in diameter and the volumes of the wounds in one study[22] increased from 23.5 mm^3 to 917 mm^3 for jacketed and nonjacketed bullets of the same caliber and velocity. Another bullet design modification is the hollow-point, where its tip is hollowed out to form a concavity. This enhances bullet mushrooming while traveling through the target tissues, and increases destruction through a shorter distance than the unjacketed bullet. Thus these bullets are less prone to exit the body. Even more fatal modifications can be made, such as filling the hollows with gunpowder or phosphorus, which cause burns or explosions upon impact, or send showers of foreign objects into the wound.

While the aerodynamic parameters yaw and tumbling are not desirable in the exterior phase because they decrease bullet velocity, they are desirable in the terminal phase, for the same reason. These motions increase energy dissipation to tissues, which increases destruction. Perfect spheres have no yaw, and military bullets have minimal (3 percent) yaw. However, when the bullet hits the target tissue the yaw can vary, depending upon the angle of impact and tissue density. With a more acute angle of skin entry, more bullet surface area is presented to the tissues. This increases wounding energy and tissue destruction. Passing through variations in tissue density also changes the yaw, again causing increased bullet deceleration and destruction. Yaw also causes the exit wound to be greater than the entrance wound. Tumbling through the tissue also causes more tissue damage.

The actual tissue damage from the missile, the result of the C_D, is caused by three means: (1) laceration and crushing, (2) shock waves, and (3) cavitation. The direct force of the bullet causes laceration and crushing. This is the major means of damage with low-velocity gunshot wounds. If the bullet is traveling with 0 degrees of yaw (its pointed end forward and parallel to the longitudinal axis of flight), it will crush a tube of tissue no greater than its approximate diameter. If it yaws to 90 degrees, the entire long axis of the bullet strikes the tissue and may increase the amount of tissue crush up to three times. Bullet fragmentation, which commonly occurs when bone is struck, also increases tissue crushing.

Shock waves are generated by high-velocity missiles, due to compression of the tissue in front of the penetrating bullet. The region of compression moves away from

TABLE 52-2. Tissue Density and Wound Severity

Tissue	Specific Gravity	Wound Severity
Lung	0.4–0.5	Minimal
Fat	0.8	Moderate
Liver	1.01–1.02	Marked
Muscle	1.02–1.04	Marked
Skin	1.09	Marked
Bone	1.11	Extreme

(Adapted from DeMuth,[22] with permission.)

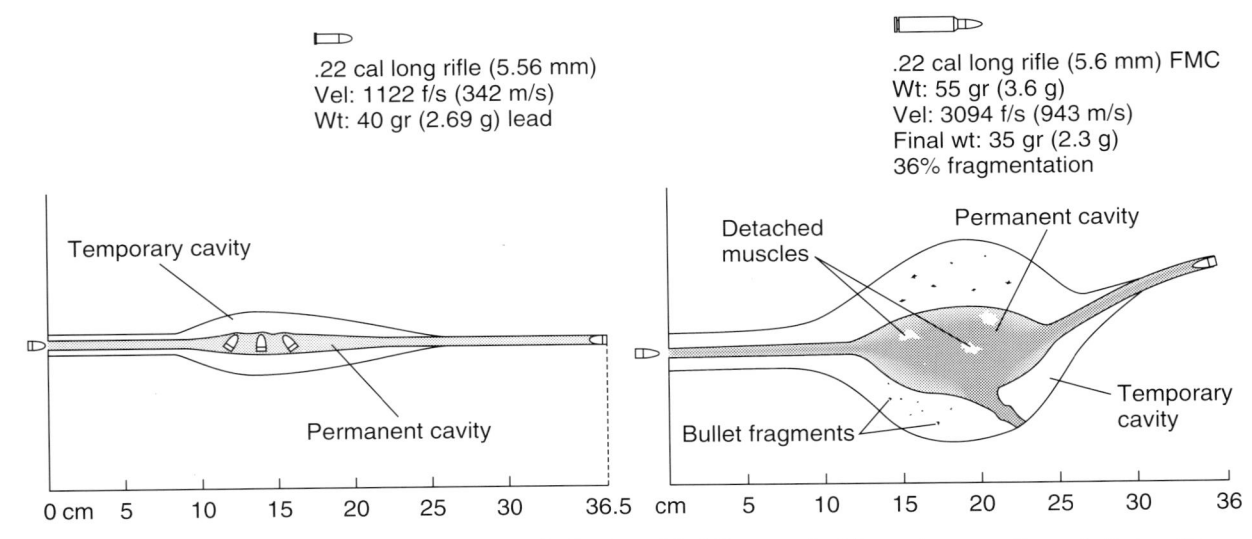

Fig. 52-1. Wound profiles of a same caliber missile, but with different velocities and masses. One missile is a .22 caliber long rifle bullet; the other is a .224 caliber missile from a military rifle (M-16A1) which is fully jacketed (FMC). Because of its much higher velocity, greater mass, and fragmentation in the tissue, the M-16 bullet can potentially create a much more severe wound. Note that both the temporary and permanent cavities are larger. (Adapted from Hollerman et al.,[19] with permission.)

the bullet at a velocity greater than the bullet itself. The shock waves are capable of creating high energy, up to more than 1,000 lb/in.^{2} of pressure. They are more destructive to gas-filled organs, and cause little damage to muscle or bone.

Cavitation, on the other hand, is much more destructive to all major body areas except for the abdomen. Cavitation occurs only when the bullet velocity is greater than 1,000 ft/s (Fig. 52-1). The bullet forces move the tissues forward and lateral to the bullet. The inertia of these forces exists for a few milliseconds after the bullet has passed through the tissue. This creates a temporary cavity of subatmospheric pressure, up to 30 to 40 times the bullet diameter. The cavity then collapses upon itself until it reaches atmospheric pressure, leaving a residual cavity that is much smaller than the temporary cavity before it collapsed. This aspect of tissue damage is similar to a diver entering the water. If the diver enters the water straight (0 degrees of yaw) the splash may be minimal. If the diver belly-flops (90 degrees of yaw), a large splash occurs. The splash of the diver is analogous to the temporary cavity in the tissue. There is a direct relationship between the maximum temporary cavity size, absorbed bullet energy, and irreversible tissue damage. The temporary cavity represents the area of devitalized tissue, which is important in rendering adequate care, since it has been rendered avascular by the cavitation. Cavitation also causes tissue damage by stretching smaller blood vessels as well as nerves and bones. Tissues near the density of water (e.g., bone) are more severely damaged when a large temporary cavity contacts them and more elastic tissue (e.g., skeletal muscle) is less affected.

Vascular injuries occur differently depending upon bullet velocity. Low-velocity missiles push the blood vessel ahead and stretch it before penetration. High-velocity missiles neatly shear the arterial wall, but the temporary cavity causes crushing trauma as well, extending up to 20 mm or greater, and involves all arterial layers.[23,24]

Bone fractures from bullets are different in metaphyses compared to diaphyses. "Drill hole" fractures are commonly seen in metaphyseal areas, and fragmentation and explosion seen in diaphyses.[25] This is because the more trabecular, spongy metaphyseal bone can absorb and dissipate much of the pressure in the temporary cavity. In the diaphyseal portions, the pressures in the temporary cavities are greater, with more fragmentation.

Overall, low-velocity weapons cause less damage. Common low-velocity weapons are all handguns, and the .22 caliber rifle. All other rifles are considered to be high-velocity weapons. The individual pellets from a shotgun are also considered to be high velocity when fired at a short range. Low-velocity bullets cause less damage because of their lower E_k. After skin penetration their energy is even less, and they tend to follow tissue planes from their entry point (rather than a straight line) to their final resting point. Because of these deviations, they may move around important structures without damaging them, and may also end up in locations completely unsuspected from the entry wound. When bone is encountered in their path and they cannot course around, they will most likely expend all of their energy in fracturing the bone, stopping in the periosseous space.

Shotguns

Shotgun wounds differ markedly from other missile wounds in their ballistics and mechanism of injury.[26] In certain cases they resemble war wounds from grenades with large body wall defects and massive extremity destruction, while at other times they produce only a few scattered small wounds of minimal significance.[27] Shotguns are smooth bore (not rifled) long-barreled guns, designed for killing fast-moving game birds and small animals. Today's shotgun shell is made of a plastic casing filled with a powder charge, followed by a wad upon which is placed the shot charge. The shot charge is a large number of small spheres that form a pattern upon leaving the muzzle. This overcomes the requirement for pinpoint accuracy needed in a single-bullet weapon. Shotguns are classified by their gauge. The number of spherical lead balls per pound able to fit the gun bore determines the gauge.

Upon firing, the shot charge and wad leave the muzzle. The shot pattern is determined by the shotgun choke, or a constriction at the muzzle end. The choke is much like a hose nozzle, funneling the shots in a specific pattern. The ideal pattern is an even distribution over the circle formed by the nozzle. In killing game, the effective range is from 20 to 40 yd. Under this range the dense pattern destroys so much of the animal that it is undesirable.

Unfortunately, under 20 yards is the range in which most shotgun wounds in children are inflicted, causing serious harm (Fig. 52-2). At this range the multiple shots act more like a single missile, and thus have a higher E_k than a single shot would. Although the muzzle velocities are usually low, injury can be substantial because of the combined mass of the shots. At a range of 10 yd, approximately 95 percent of the shots (using No. 6 shot) will be within a skin wound 9 in. in diameter when fired from a full-choke barrel. When the major portion of the charge is concentrated within a wound of entry less than 15 cm, there is sufficient velocity to produce a deep wound. Thus the wound of *entry* should be inspected for a shotgun wound, unlike the wound of *exit* for rifle wounds, to determine wound severity. In addition, the cotton wad and plastic casings used in the shotgun shell often penetrate deep into the wound. These are usually radiolucent and difficult to recognize, and their retention may lead to wound complications, primarily infection.

Nonpowder Weapons

The majority of this discussion on ballistics has focused on firearm-powder type weapons. Nonpowder weapons should not be forgotten as another cause of injury in children,[17,28,29] and may be involved in up to 66 percent of the cases of gunshot wounds in children.[17] Multiple-pump air rifles can inflict serious injuries and caused extremity wounds in 22 percent of nonpowder wounds in one series.[17] Air guns can produce a muzzle velocity from 400 to 900 ft/s,[29] but the velocity falls off rapidly once it leaves the muzzle. However, when fired at close range, they can maintain significant velocity, comparable to a .22 short rifle or a standard handgun, both having velocities of 800 ft/s.[18,29]

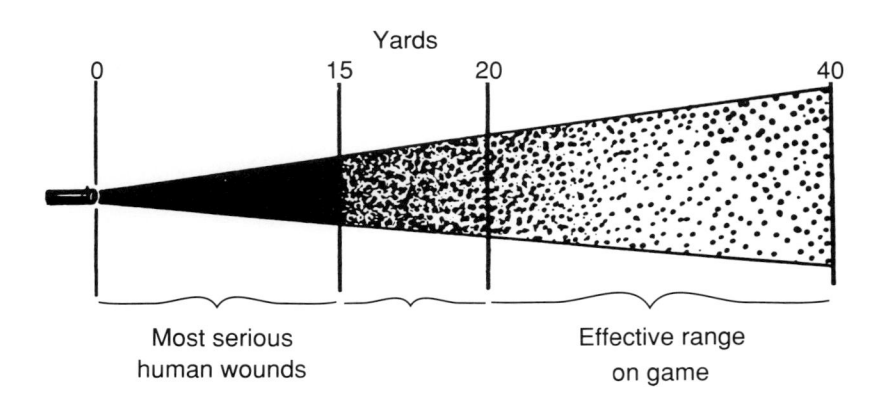

Fig. 52-2. A side view diagram of a shot pattern from a shotgun. (From DeMuth,[26] with permission.)

PHYSICAL EXAMINATION AND DIFFERENTIAL DIAGNOSIS

The initial physical examination and resuscitation treatment are carried out together. Do not forget the general ABCs of trauma. Valentine and coworkers[16] have developed a management schema for children with gunshot injuries (Fig. 52-3). Once this has been completed, attention can be directed to the extremity injury in particular.

The first extremity parameter to assess is vascular status (Fig. 52-3). If there is obvious vascular compromise clinically, immediate exploration and repair should be performed, bypassing arteriography. If, on the other hand, the injury is in proximity to vascular structures, but without clinical compromise, further study should be undertaken. Most authorities recommend arteriography.[6,12,16,30] A recent study suggests that ultrasonography may reduce the need for arteriography,[31] but further investigation is needed. This would be particularly welcome in children, since arteriography in children does have a higher morbidity.[32] It has been shown that clinical evaluation alone is accurate for identification of missile arterial injury in lateral thigh or upper arm wounds.[30]

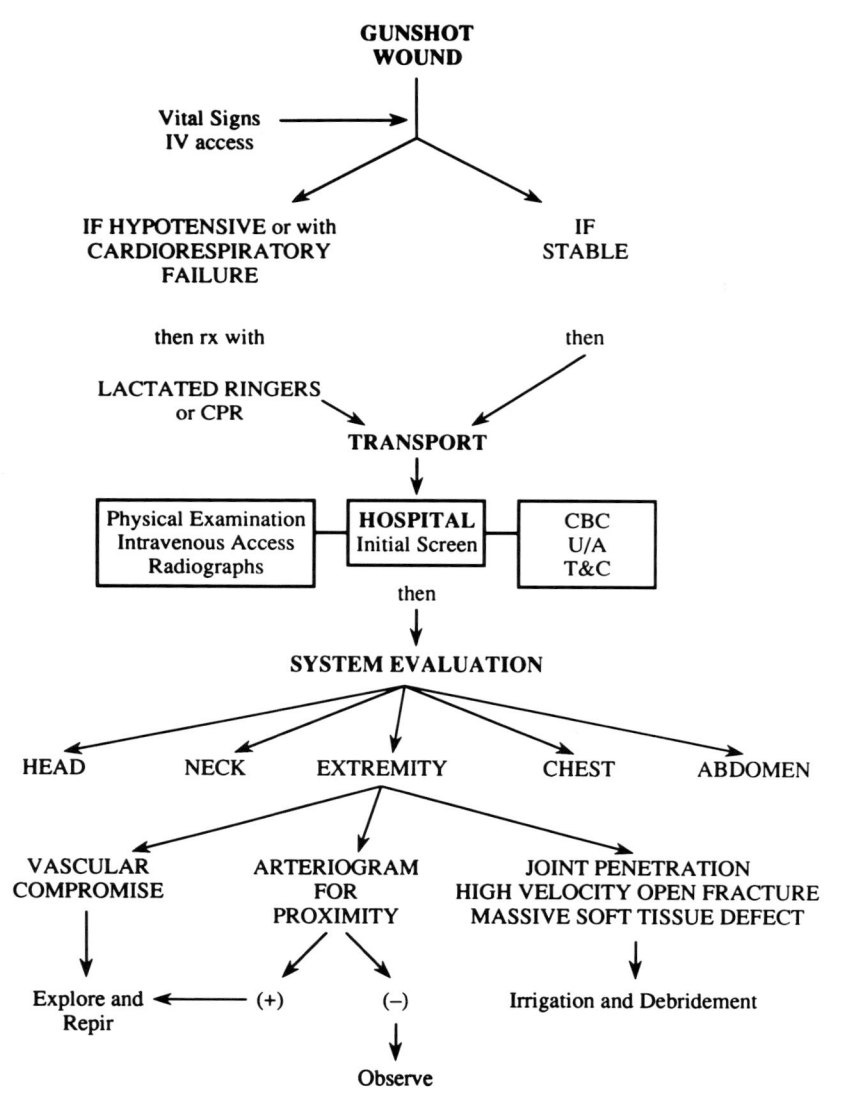

Fig. 52-3. Management schema for a child with a gunshot wound. (Adapted from Valentine et al.,[16] with permission.)

Areas at high risk for unsuspected arterial injuries are the calf (23 percent), forearm, and antecubital area (20 percent), popliteal fossa (9 percent), medial and posterior thigh (9 percent), and medial and posterior arm (8 percent).

The neurologic status of the extremity should also be determined, since the nerves run in close proximity to the vasculature. This examination will determine what deficits exist immediately after injury, and as a baseline with which to compare changes in the neurologic status. Although the development of a compartment syndrome is rare, low-velocity gunshot wounds to the proximal forearm, especially those with a concomitant fracture, are at high risk for development of a compartment syndrome.[33] Moed and Fakhouri,[33] in a series of 131 adult low-velocity gunshot wounds to the forearm documented a 36 percent incidence of compartment syndrome when a fracture in one of the proximal bones was present.

The entrance and exit wounds should next be assessed. The entrance wounds can be classified as simple (only one entrance site) or complex (more than one entry site with the same missile passing through more than one body part). In nonshotgun wounds the entrance wounds are usually relatively small. Depending upon the bullet velocity, design, and depth of tissue, the missile may or may not exit the child. Nonjacketed or partially jacketed bullets expand within the tissue and create large areas of tissue damage, even when of a low velocity. If the depth of tissue to penetrate is small, the bullet may have enough energy to exit the limb. These exit wounds are markedly larger than the entrance wounds. Fully jacketed high-velocity bullets will create both entrance and exit wounds, which are similar in size as long as there is little bullet tumbling. If the bullet tumbles through the tissue, however, as in an M-16 bullet, substantial tissue damage occurs (Fig. 52-1), and the exit wounds can be very large.

The wound locations are important in reconstructing the bullet path. It is important to know the child's position at the time of impact in order to reconstruct the missile tract. The wounds may be difficult to understand when examining the child in the emergency department in the anatomic position, but if the child is placed in the position at the time of injury, the entrance wound, bullet tract, and exit wounds will align properly (Fig. 52-4).

Shotgun wounds, on the other hand, often have large entrance wounds when shot at close range. At long ranges, shotguns produce minimal damage, due to dispersion of the smaller pellets resulting in a significant loss of projectile mass, as well as loss of velocity. The measure of shotgun wound severity is established by the entrance wound. When the major portion of the charge is concentrated within an entry wound of 15 cm or less, the velocity has been sufficient to produce a deep and severe wound.[26] This causes marked tissue shredding, which destroys bone, nerves, and vessels. Sherman and Parrish[34] have classified shotgun wounds into types I, II, and III. Type I is an injury that penetrates only the subcutaneous tissue and deep fascia; these are shot at long range. Type II, shot at close range, are injuries that penetrate structures beneath the fascia. Type III, shot at point blank, produce severe and extensive tissue damage.

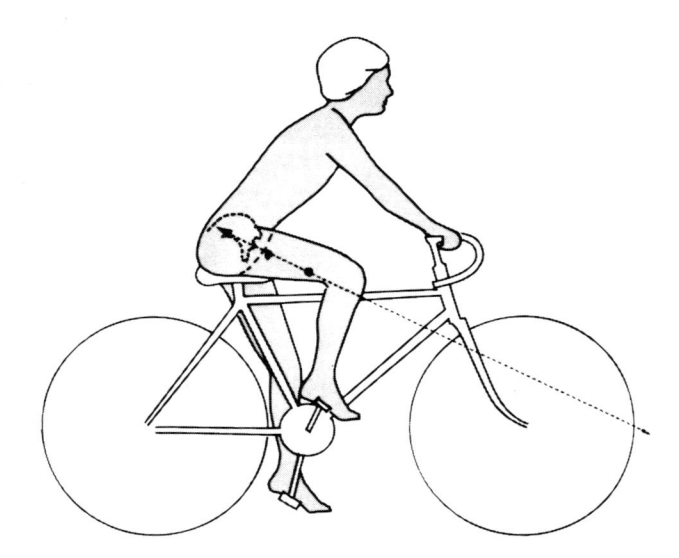

Fig. 52-4. The importance of recording the position of the child at the time of injury to determine the correct missile tract is illustrated by this bicyclist shot by a gun dropped by a friend riding in front of the child. (From Letts and Miller,[1] with permission.)

Radiographic examination of the involved areas should also be performed. This will determine the presence or absence of osseous injuries and can also be helpful in determining the bullet size.[21] If the bullet is still intact in the child, the missile was obviously low energy. Even if the bullet has partially fragmented, with an osseous fracture, and the bullet remains within the soft tissue, cavitation has probably not occurred. However, when there are metallic fragments at a large exit wound, with an explosion-type fragmentation fracture, cavitation has probably occurred. This is especially true if metallic fragments are widely distributed in the soft tissues. If no exit wound can be found on the child, then further radiographs of adjacent areas must be obtained until the bullet is found. Low-velocity bullets follow tissue planes with marked course deviations, and may end up in a body location completely unsuspected from the physical examination. Although it rarely occurs, missile embolism into the vascular system has been described.[35,36] The incidence was 0.3 percent in the Vietnam War. If the injury is periarticular, the radiographs will determine if the bullet is intra-articular, if there is proximity of the missile to the physis, or if the bullet violated the physis.

TREATMENT

To my knowledge, there are only three reviews specifically addressing extremity gunshot wounds in children.[1,5,12] The treatment guidelines below are both a compilation of these reviews as well as general suggestions from the adult literature, because many of the children are adolescents and their injuries and fracture treatment is often similar to adults.

The major tissues that must be treated with extremity gunshot wounds are (1) soft tissues, (2) osseous and articular structures, (3) neural structures, and (4) vascular structures. The first thing that must be determined is whether the injury is of a low or high velocity. As a usual rule, shotgun wounds in children occur from such close range that they should be considered high-velocity injuries.

Low-velocity injuries usually do not need formal operative debridement, unless a neural or vascular repair is required. The soft tissue wounds can be treated with either simple irrigation and sterile dressings in the emergency department, or with a simple debridement of superficial skin and subcutaneous tissue prior to irrigation and dressing. Although there has been no similar study of these two methods in children, in adults it has been shown that the simpler irrigation and dressing is all that is necessary.[37] If superficial debridement is felt to be needed, general anesthesia will usually be needed in younger children, whereas local anesthesia in the emergency department can be used in the more cooperative older child or adolescent.

The treatment of the gunshot fracture is mostly dependent upon the fracture character and location. Standard external immobilization means are usually adequate in younger children (e.g., splints, casts, or traction). In older adolescents the fractures should be treated as in adults (e.g., closed femoral nailings, open reduction and internal fixations of both bone forearm fractures, etc.), as well as in younger adolescents where appropriate. Closed, locked, intramedullary nails can be used in the adolescent femur fracture[38] if the femoral canal is large enough to accept the nail. Anatomic reduction should always be attempted in fractures which would normally require it, even in the absence of a gunshot wound (e.g., displaced intra-articular fractures). This usually requires open reduction and internal fixation. Rigid osseous stability may also be needed to protect neural or vascular repairs. This can be achieved with either external fixators or internal fixation, depending upon the fracture characteristics and wound contamination. Whatever the means of fixation, care should be taken to avoid the physis with the fixation devices. All intra-articular injuries should undergo a formal irrigation and debridement in the operating room to remove small fragments of bone and cartilage which can otherwise cause later joint destruction.[39,40] All intra-articular bullets and bullet fragments should be removed to prevent later joint destruction as well as systemic lead poisoning.[41,42] The synovial membrane should be closed.

Neural injuries in low-velocity gunshot wounds are quite rare, and when they do occur are usually neuropraxic-type contusions, which will spontaneously improve over time and require no formal operative exploration. Vascular injuries are also quite rare. However, when they do occur, immediate exploration and repair is indicated. If tissue ischemia has been prolonged for 4 to 6 hours or more prophylactic fasciotomy should be performed.

The role of antibiotics in low-velocity gunshot wounds, with or without fractures, is also controversial. Brunner and Fallon[37] used no antibiotics in 163 adult soft tissue wounds without fractures and had a 2.5 percent incidence of infection. All were superficial and responded to local therapy. Dickey and colleagues[43] demonstrated no significant prophylaxis with intravenous antibiotics in 96 adults with low-velocity gunshot fractures. In extremity gunshot wounds in children, my own series[12] had an infection rate of 2.4 percent, which included children with and without gunshot fractures as well as low- and high-velocity wounds. Intravenous antibiotics were given to 89 percent of the children. The infection rate in the series of Letts and Miller[1] was 11 percent, but they had a higher percentage of shotgun wounds in their series. All children in their series received prophylactic antibiotics. Victoroff and colleagues,[5] in a recent series from Children's National Medical Center in Washington, D.C., treated 62 percent of their children with prophylactic antibiotics, with all gunshot fractures given at least 48 hours of intravenous antibiotics. There were no known superficial or deep infections in any of their 75 children with extremity gunshot injuries. It thus seems plausible from these series that simple low-velocity soft tissue injuries in pediatric extremity gunshot wounds do not need intravenous prophylactic antibiotics. However, if there has been a gunshot fracture or intra-articular penetration intravenous antibiotics should be administered prophylactically for 24 to 48 hours. Tetanus toxoid should also be administered when appropriate.

High-velocity gunshot wounds and close-range shotgun wounds are associated with significant soft tissue and bone destruction (see Figs. 52-7, 52-8, and 52-9). The general principles of any serious open fracture apply to these high-velocity gunshot fractures. They may require multiple irrigation and debridements; immediate vascular repairs; internal fixation, external fixation and/or traction; skin grafts and other soft tissue coverage procedures; and occasionally delayed bone grafting for nonunion or segmental bone loss. In these children, a formal debridement and irrigation is needed in the operating room at least once, and often on several occasions to ensure that the wound remains clean, as areas of devitalized tissue from the cavitation effect demarcate.

At the time of debridement, neural lacerations, if encountered can be addressed. The causes of neural injury may be either contusion neuropraxia or traumatic laceration. Retained plastic shot containers in shotgun injuries can rarely cause compressive nerve palsies.[44] The timing of neural repairs is still open to debate. Luce and Griffin[45] in adult shotgun injuries of the upper extremity, noted that delay before intervention by nerve repair, grafting, or tendon transfers may well have compromised the ultimate functional results. However, those shotgun wounds that had neural injuries had more severe soft tissue and skeletal trauma with a higher incidence of vascular injuries. This may also have contributed to the poorer results. Hennessey and colleagues[46] recommended primary nerve repair in hand wounds if the amount of tissue damage and contamination allowed. They recommended withholding primary nerve repair in other areas, and stated that the nerve ends should be cleansed but not debrided, marked with clips and brought to lie in approximation with a single uniting suture, with definitive repair at a later time.

Deitch and Grimes[14] in a review of 112 extremity shotgun wounds have clearly shown that severity of injury increases as the Sherman and Parrish severity type increases. Soft tissue injuries occurred in 0, 0, and 100 percent of type I, II, and III injuries; bone and joint injuries occurred in 0, 50, and 48 percent of type I, II, and III injuries; neurologic injuries occurred in 1, 15, and 26 percent of type I, II, and III injuries; and vascular injuries in 0, 25, and 28 percent of type I, II, and III injuries. They recommend an aggressive approach to the soft tissues with immediate debridement, thoroughly searching for wadding. Arterial injuries should be rapidly treated, and venous injuries should be repaired when possible. Fasciotomy should also be readily performed in vascular injuries. Major long-bone fractures need stabilization, either internal or external. The major predictor of a fully functional extremity depends upon the presence or absence of major neural injury. They felt that any patient with a major neurologic injury not caused by ischemia or a compartment syndrome should undergo prompt operative exploration to determine if the nerve is intact. If only contused, the deficit can be followed over time with serial examinations. A delayed neurolysis may be necessary if improvement does not spontaneously occur. If transected, either a primary neural repair or marking of the nerve ends for a delayed repair should be done, based on the clinical condition of the patient and local wound conditions. Delayed wound closure should be performed as soon as the local wound contamination allows with skin grafts and flaps as needed.

The treatment required for these high-velocity and shotgun wounds is more aggressive and accounts for the increased time of hospitalization, number of operative procedures, and duration of intravenous antibiotics in these children. In the series of Stucky and Loder,[12] the average hospital stay, the number of operative procedures and time of intravenous antibiotics was 5.4 days, 0.5 procedures, and 4 days, respectively, for the nonshotgun injuries, and 21.8 days, 3.8 procedures, and 12 days, respectively, for the shotgun injuries.

Bullet removal, whether from a high- or low-velocity missile or shotgun or nonshotgun injury, is needed for all intra-articular injuries. In other areas removal is needed only if a debridement is being performed, the bullet is subcutaneous and causing skin problems, in tendon sheaths and causing tendon excursion difficulties, or causing neural compression.

Treatment of the social situation should not be forgotten. Over 70 percent of pediatric firearm fatalities occur in the home.[47] Many of these injuries when they occur accidentally, could have been easily avoided by proper parent education and gun storage means.[47,48] When they occur intentionally, appropriate social intervention should be instituted. A child who sustains a firearm injury is likely to know the perpetrator,[47] whether intentional or accidental. Input from social workers may improve the situation where the injury occurred. Most of the pediatric gunshot injuries could therefore be prevented by proper parent and child education and avoidance of certain social situations. Because of this, I strongly feel that all children with gunshot injuries should be admitted to the hospital so that appropriate education and social intervention be instituted.

Many of the children have relevant psychosocial or medical problems (43 percent in the series of Victoroff and colleagues[5]), which could also benefit from hospitalization and institution of appropriate therapy. These problems include drug use and distribution, incarceration and arrests, school difficulties, home runaways, teenage pregnancy, suicide attempts, and sexually transmitted diseases. In the Washington, D.C. series 25 percent of the children with gunshot injuries suffered from sexually transmitted diseases. If the sexually transmitted diseases in themselves could be treated, the hospital admission would have been worth its while from a public health viewpoint. Although no incidence figures are known for the population of pediatric extremity gunshot injuries, HIV infection should not be forgotten by the medical care team. This is due to (1) the high percentage of associated sexually transmitted diseases in these children, and (2) the risk of HIV with illicit drug use.

COMPLICATIONS

Neurologic

The incidence of neurologic complications ranges from 3 to 45 percent. In pediatric extremity series specifically, the incidence was 3 percent,[5] 9 percent,[12] and 38 percent.[1] All of the deficits resolved for Victoroff and colleagues,[5] whereas only 6 of the 11 sensory and 3 of the 12 motor deficits resolved for Letts and Miller.[1] In the series of Stucky and Loder[12] all three of the shotgun deficits were neuropraxias, whereas 2 of the 5 nonshotgun deficits were neuropraxias and 3 were lacerations. Since there are no series specifically addressing shotgun extremity injuries in children, it is difficult to get an incidence of neurologic injury as well as recovery. However, most authorities feel that shotgun injuries are associated with a higher incidence of neurologic deficit. In the only general series of pediatric shotgun injuries, Golladay and colleagues[48] noted a 10 percent incidence of permanent neurologic deficit. Schwartz and colleagues[44] recently described a sciatic nerve palsy caused by neural compression from a retained shot container in a 17-year-old boy with a shotgun thigh injury. The deficit slowly resolved after removal of the plastic shot container.

The incidence of neurologic complications in adults ranges from 3 to 58 percent. The highest incidence is that reported by Luce and Griffin[45] in a series of 77 adult upper extremity injuries. There were a total of 60 nerve injuries in 45 patients: 31 were explored and 14 (45 percent) were transected. Of the 29 that were observed, only 14 (48 percent) had a complete recovery. The next highest incidence (45 percent) was in a series of low velocity both bone forearm gunshot fractures, where 13 of 29 adults had 17 peripheral nerve injuries. The partial deficits had good recoveries, where as only 4 of 9 complete deficits had good recoveries, even after surgical exploration and repair at 6 to 8 weeks postinjury. It thus appears that forearm gunshot injuries, both shotgun and low-velocity nonshotgun types, carry a high risk of neurologic deficit with only moderate recovery. The incidence is lower for femoral gunshot fractures (9 percent).[38] Of the five neurologic deficits in that series, three involved the entire sciatic nerve with only one complete recovery, and two involved the peroneal nerve with only one complete recovery. None of those five injuries were surgically explored, either acutely or late. In the two general overall series of adult gunshot injuries where neurologic deficits were reported, the overall deficit was 3 percent in both.[49,50]

Vascular

The incidence of vascular complications ranges from 0 to 30 percent. The complications can be arterial, venous, or missile emboli. The incidence in the pediatric extremity gunshot series was 0 percent,[5] 1 percent,[12] and 16 percent.[1] The 16 percent incidence had a large number of shotgun injuries in the cases reviewed. The injury sites were the brachial (two children) or popliteal (three children) arteries. Golladay and colleagues[48] had a 30 percent incidence of vascular complications in shotgun wounds in children in a combined series of both truncal and extremity injuries. One of the vascular complications was arterial and two were pellet emboli.

In adult series of low-velocity gunshot wounds arterial injuries are rare, and range from 0 to 2 percent[33,49,51,52] with the exception of a recent series involving femoral fractures where it was 9 percent.[38] This is in sharp contrast to an earlier series[52] of femoral gunshot fractures where the incidence of vascular injury was less than 1 percent. The complication of compartment syndrome with low-velocity gunshot wounds should not be forgotten, especially if there are associated fractures of the proximal radius or ulna.[33,51] In the series of Dugas and D'Ambrosia,[53] which included both shotgun and nonshotgun injuries, the incidence rose to 12 percent; 17 were arterial and 3 were venous. In the series of Luce and Griffin,[45] which consisted solely of adult upper extremity shotgun injuries, the incidence of vascular injury was 23 percent. They also had two other arterial injuries in areas of the body not initially hit by the shot charge.

Gunshot arterial injuries are more commonly lower extremity (68 percent), have a low incidence of associated injuries (31 percent venous injuries, 8 percent neurologic, 6 percent osseous, and 13 percent in other organ systems), and are often repaired primarily (61 percent). The infection rate is low (13 percent) and functional recovery high (88 percent).

By contrast, shotgun arterial injuries are more evenly divided between the upper and lower extremity and result in multiple and lengthy lesions of extensive arterial trauma and thrombosis.[54] Since long stretches are involved by the blast, collateral circulation is low and palpable pulses present in only 10 percent of shotgun arterial injuries compared to 26 percent of gunshot vascular wounds to the extremities. Because of this, the repairs in shotgun injuries commonly require grafting, unlike primary repair in gunshot injuries. Bongard and Klein[13] have recently outlined a strategy for shotgun arterial injuries:

1. After hemodynamic resuscitation, stable patients undergo arteriography to define the anatomic origin of complex injuries.
2. Surgery commences with rapid proximal and distal control of disrupted segments.
3. Following vessel debridement, continuity is restored either by primary repair or by an autogenous graft, which is placed to allow coverage by viable soft tissues.
4. Completion arteriograms in the operating room evaluate the patency and provide evidence of distal arterial emboli if they exist.
5. Fractures are stabilized and disrupted nerves isolated for subsequent repair.
6. Fasciotomy is performed in the presence of distal swelling or prolonged ischemia.

In spite of this approach, the prognosis for shotgun arterial injuries of the extremities is poor. This is not due to the vascular repair, which is usually successful, but from neuromuscular and osseous injury with or without sepsis.[13,54] Raju[54] noted that only 12 of 39 patients with shotgun arterial injuries of the extremities had useful limbs.

A rare complication is that of bullet embolism.[35] For a bullet to embolize, the bullet must have very little kinetic energy remaining at the precise moment that it enters a blood vessel, and the diameter of that vessel must exceed that of the bullet. This allows the bloodstream to sweep the missile away, resulting in embolization. All of the reported cases involve low-velocity missiles. Shotgun injuries, due to their small missile size and large numbers of pellets are also predisposed to embolism.[55] The incidence of bullet embolism has increased fivefold in the last 14 years, reflecting both an increased awareness of the problem as well as increased societal violence.

Infection

Bullets are not sterilized by the heat of flight or discharge,[56] and thus gunshot injuries are contaminated, with a potential for infection. Nevertheless, the overall incidence of infection in adult low velocity gunshot wounds ranges from 0 to 4 percent.[37,38,43,45,50,51,53,57-59] Because of this low incidence, most authorities feel that simple soft tissue injuries in adult low-velocity gunshot wounds do not need antibiotics.[37] Some even feel that low-velocity gunshot fractures do not need antibiotics,[43,59] unless open reduction and fixation are performed.[38,49,58] Others feel that antibiotics should be used in all cases of gunshot fractures, including low-velocity injuries.[60] With regard to pediatric extremity gunshot injuries, it appears that antibiotics are usually used when a gunshot fracture is present, or any shotgun injury regardless of fracture.[1,5,12] As expected, the highest incidence of infection is with shotgun injuries.[1,54] The incidence of osteomyelitis is very low, with most series[5,12,37,38,40,43,50,57,58] reporting no cases, or occasionally a single case of osteomyelitis.[1,53,59]

It has recently been shown[61] that HIV seropositivity increases the risk of orthopaedic infections. This should not be forgotten, especially if a child's gunshot injury develops a sepsis beyond what is normally expected. This is therefore another reason to strongly consider the use of prophylactic antibiotics in gunshot fracture injuries.

Bone Loss and Nonunion

The incidence of segmental bone loss in pediatric extremity gunshot wounds was 4 percent in the series of Stucky and Loder,[12] and 28 percent in the series of Letts and Miller[1]; the 28 percent incidence is related to more shotgun wounds in that series. Bone grafts for either segmental loss or nonunion were required in 4 of 85 (5 percent) children in the series of Stucky and Loder. In spite of 28 percent having a bone loss of more than 10 percent in the series of Letts and Miller, all the fractures united.

The incidence of nonunion in adult gunshot fractures ranges from 0 to 16 percent.[38,45,50-53,57] As expected, the highest incidence was with shotgun injuries.[45] Parisien[50] had an overall nonunion rate of 3 percent, but it was 11 percent when looking at femoral and humeral fractures alone. This is contrasted by the 0 percent nonunion rate of Ryan and colleagues[52] where the femoral fractures were treated by closed immobilization means and the 4 percent delayed union and 0 percent nonunion rate of Wiss and coworkers[38] where the femoral fractures were treated by intramedullary nailing. Elstrom[51] clearly showed that displaced and/or comminuted both bone forearm fractures treated by open reduction, and internal fixation did much better than those treated with casts, with a 0 percent versus 20 percent delayed union rate. Open reduction and internal fixation of these fractures also improved joint motion.

Joint Contractures

When the exit wound involves a joint, contractures can develop. This occurred in 22 percent of the children in the series of Letts and Miller,[1] and most commonly involved the knee or areas where there was skin loss. Joint contractures in the adult series are rarely mentioned, except again as complications of delayed coverage. Luce and Griffin[45] in their series of adult upper extremity shotgun wounds noted that early wound coverage facilitated physiotherapy and splinting, with improved motion. We therefore recommend rapid coverage of wounds (as soon as the tissues are clean and permit such coverage) where loss of motion may be problematic, especially the upper extremity, knee, and periarticular locations. Contractures can also develop as complications of neurologic deficits. Here again early physiotherapy, splinting, and wound coverage (when needed) can minimize the development of permanent contractures.

Physeal Injuries

As with all fractures in growing children, trauma to the physis can cause late deformity. Only one series[1] has addressed this problem. The other two series of pediatric extremity gunshot wounds[5,12] had no long-term follow-up, due to the social milieu where the injuries occurred. Letts and Miller[1] noted 9 of 32 children (32 percent) who developed problems from physeal trauma (Fig. 52-5). In 6 children a complete arrest occurred secondary to physeal disruption from the bullet; 4 of these were around the knee. In 3 children the physis fused prematurely, even though the bullet did not pass through the physis but only in proximity to it. This indicates that the physis is vulnerable to indirect injury. We recommend close and frequent follow-up of all extremity gunshot wounds until skeletal maturity, especially those in periphyseal areas. Unfortunately, the social situations are such that many of these children never receive adequate follow-up. Bullet physeal complications should be handled as any other posttraumatic growth arrest.

Lead Intoxication

Lead poisoning from retained bullets can rarely occur. Although there has only been one report in children,[42] the incidence of this in children will probably rise due to the increasing incidence of pediatric gunshot wounds. Children also have a longer time to absorb the lead due to their younger age at injury.

Metallic lead is insoluble and most patients with retained lead missiles never develop systemic absorption. Most bullets lodge in soft tissue, become encapsulated in dense fibrous tissue, and are not likely to cause lead poisoning. In most cases of lead poisoning, the bullets lodge in joints.[7] Pseudocysts can also develop around bullets. It has been postulated that the cystic and synovial fluids dissolve the lead with diffusion into the general circulation.[41] The available surface area of retained lead particles also plays a role in developing lead poisoning. Buckshot injuries result in lead poisoning much more rapidly than a single retained bullet.[42,62]

The symptoms of lead poisoning are anemia, abdominal colic, nephropathy, encephalopathy, and neuropathy. Systemic lead is normally stored in bone, but it can be mobilized during periods of metabolic change affecting bone, the nervous system, or both. When this mobilization occurs, clinical symptoms can develop.[63]

If a child develops these symptoms, blood lead levels should be performed, keeping in mind technical laboratory difficulties with such levels.[63] When the level is elevated and the patient symptomatic, treatment should begin with chelation therapy using D-penicillamine. Once the patient has been stabilized to a blood lead level below 80 μg/dl, surgery can be safely performed to remove the lead. Surgical removal will prevent future episodes of lead poisoning. Surgery itself may mobilize lead bone stores creating severely symptomatic patients (and even death) if prior chelation therapy is not used.[63] Therefore chelation therapy prior to surgery is indicated for all patients with lead poisoning from retained bullets.

CASE EXAMPLES

Case 1

This 15-year-old boy was sprayed with bullets in a drive by shooting; the perpetrator and weapon type were unknown. Upon arrival to the emergency room he was hypotensive and moribund. Groin and buttock wounds were noted as were left forearm wounds. Mast trousers

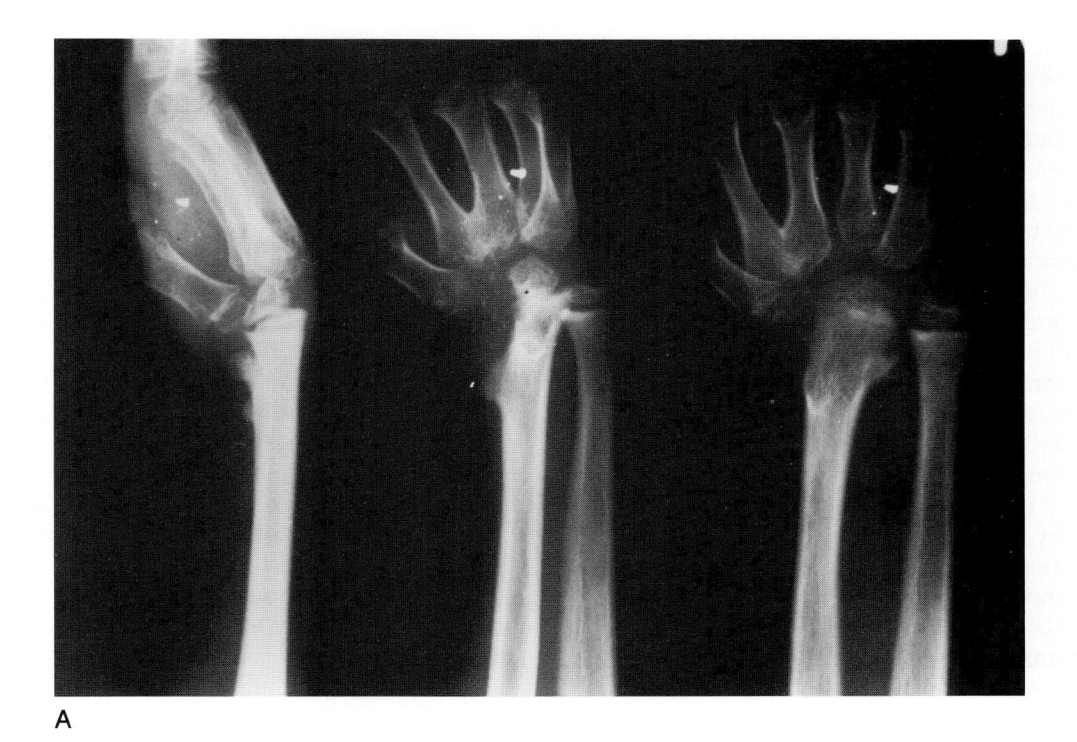

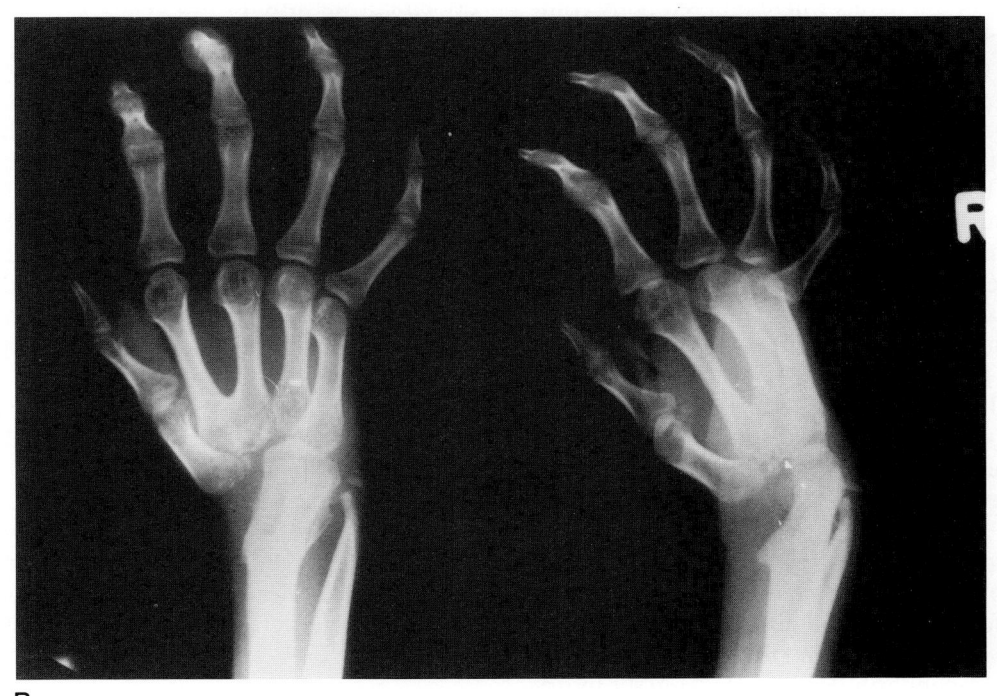

Fig. 52-5. (A) This 6-year-old boy was shot in the wrist with a shotgun, totally destroying his carpus. (B) The radiographs at 15 years of age, show a complete arrest of the distal radial physis but not the ulnar physis, which resulted in ulnar overgrowth and required a distal ulnar resection. (Courtesy of Dr. R. Mervyn Letts.)

had been placed at the scene and when attempting to deflate them he became markedly bradycardic and hemodynamically unstable. He was therefore taken immediately to surgery where an emergent thoracotomy with aortic cross-clamping was performed; this stabilized the blood pressure. Exploratory laparotomy was then performed with large amounts of free blood encountered in the peritoneal cavity. With continuing resuscitation the blood pressure again stabilized. Exploration revealed a left external iliac artery transection at the level of the inguinal ligament with multiple small bowel enterotomies from the bullet passages. Because of continuing massive hemorrhage the external iliac artery was ligated just proximal to the injury, and then the damaged small bowel resected. This was immediately followed by a four-compartment fasciotomy and a femoral artery–femoral artery bypass with Dacron graft (Fig. 52-6A). A sigmoidoscopy was also performed, which showed no distal colon injury. At this point the left hand was noted to be cool and arteriography showed a comminuted proximal radial shaft fracture (Fig. 52-6B&C) with radial artery transection (Fig. 52-6D); however, the hand was viable due to excellent collateral circulation. He then underwent an open reduction and internal fixation (Fig. 52-6E&F) of the radius where marked bony comminution as well as extensive destruction of the supinator muscle was noted. Irrigation and debridement of the entrance and exit wounds was also performed, which were noted to be on the left forearm dorsal laterally (exit) and volar proximally (entrance).

In total, four bullets were felt to have injured this child. One was a through-and-through passage of the left forearm, which resulted in the radius fracture. Another one was an entrance wound of the anterior abdomen, exiting the left buttock. It was this wound which caused the external iliac artery injury as well as an ilium fracture (Fig. 52-6G). The third was a through and through passage of the right buttock which caused no significant damage. The fourth was one which entered the left buttock and stopped just left of the anus (Fig. 52-6H), without causing any visceral or serious musculoskeletal damage.

The child survived his injuries. After he awakened a partial left peroneal palsy was noted, which was treated with an ankle-foot orthosis and observation, with gradual improvement. The left forearm wound remained clean and closed secondarily. Four weeks from the injury an autogenous iliac crest bone grafting of the radius was performed, which resulted in a rapid union (Fig. 52-6I&J) by 2 months from the time of injury with full flexion and extension but minimal pronation and supination due to the massive muscle and bone damage.

Case 2

This 14-year-old boy was shot at close range from a passing automobile while standing on a school sidewalk. Even though he stated that he did not know the assailant, the hospital received several threats to his life, requiring an admission under an alias name with visitor restriction.

Upon admission to the hospital, there was complete absence of sciatic nerve function, an entrance wound of 3 cm in the posterolateral left thigh, and intact dorsalis pedis and posterior tibial pulses. Because of the marked fracture comminution, bullet fragmentation and severe soft tissue injury it was felt that the injury was high energy in nature. Because the entrance wound was posterior, close to the popliteal fossa, and associated with a sciatic nerve palsy, an arteriogram was performed and the femoral artery noted to be intact (Fig. 52-7A). A formal irrigation and debridement with insertion of a proximal tibial traction pin was then done. The sciatic nerve was completely transected and the ends tagged in anticipation of a delayed repair. He was maintained in balanced skeletal traction, and two more repeat irrigations and debridements were performed. At the last debridement the wound was closed in a delayed primary fashion on the sixth postinjury day.

The wound remained clean, and 10 days after closure, an open reduction and internal fixation of the fracture, traction pin removal, and autogenous iliac crest bone grafting was performed. Note that the fixation devices did not violate the distal femoral physis (Fig. 52-7B&C). The neurosurgeons wished to wait until this wound had healed before repairing the sciatic nerve. This repair was done 1 week after the open reduction and internal fixation, followed by spica cast immobilization, which included the foot at the neutral position to prevent development of an equinus contracture.

The patient was lost to follow-up until 4 months postinjury when he presented for cast removal. The cast was removed, no skin ulcers were noted, and the fracture was healing. An ankle-foot orthosis was prescribed.

At 12 months postinjury the fracture was completely healed (Fig. 52-7B&C). There was no return of sciatic nerve function. However, he was able to ambulate without aids. There were no skin ulcers in spite of an insensate foot.

Case 3

This 10-year-old girl was sleeping at home in her bedroom. Her mother and brother became involved in a

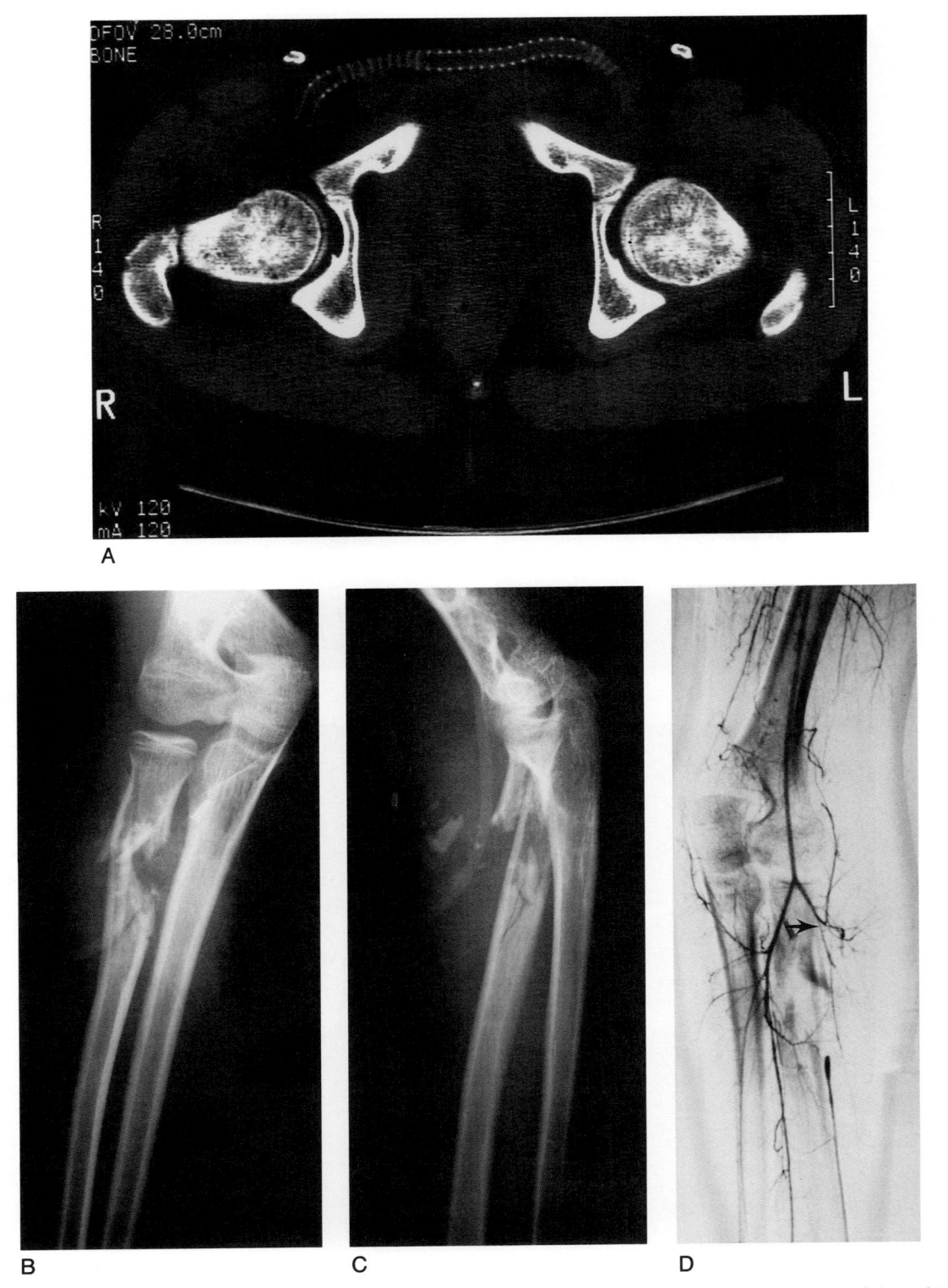

Fig. 52-6. **(A)** The pelvis CT scan postoperatively of the child in case 1 which shows the bypass graft (asterisk). **(B)** Anteroposterior and **(C)** lateral views showing the markedly comminuted proximal radial shaft fracture. **(D)** The angiogram showing the radial artery transection *(arrow). (Figure continues.)*

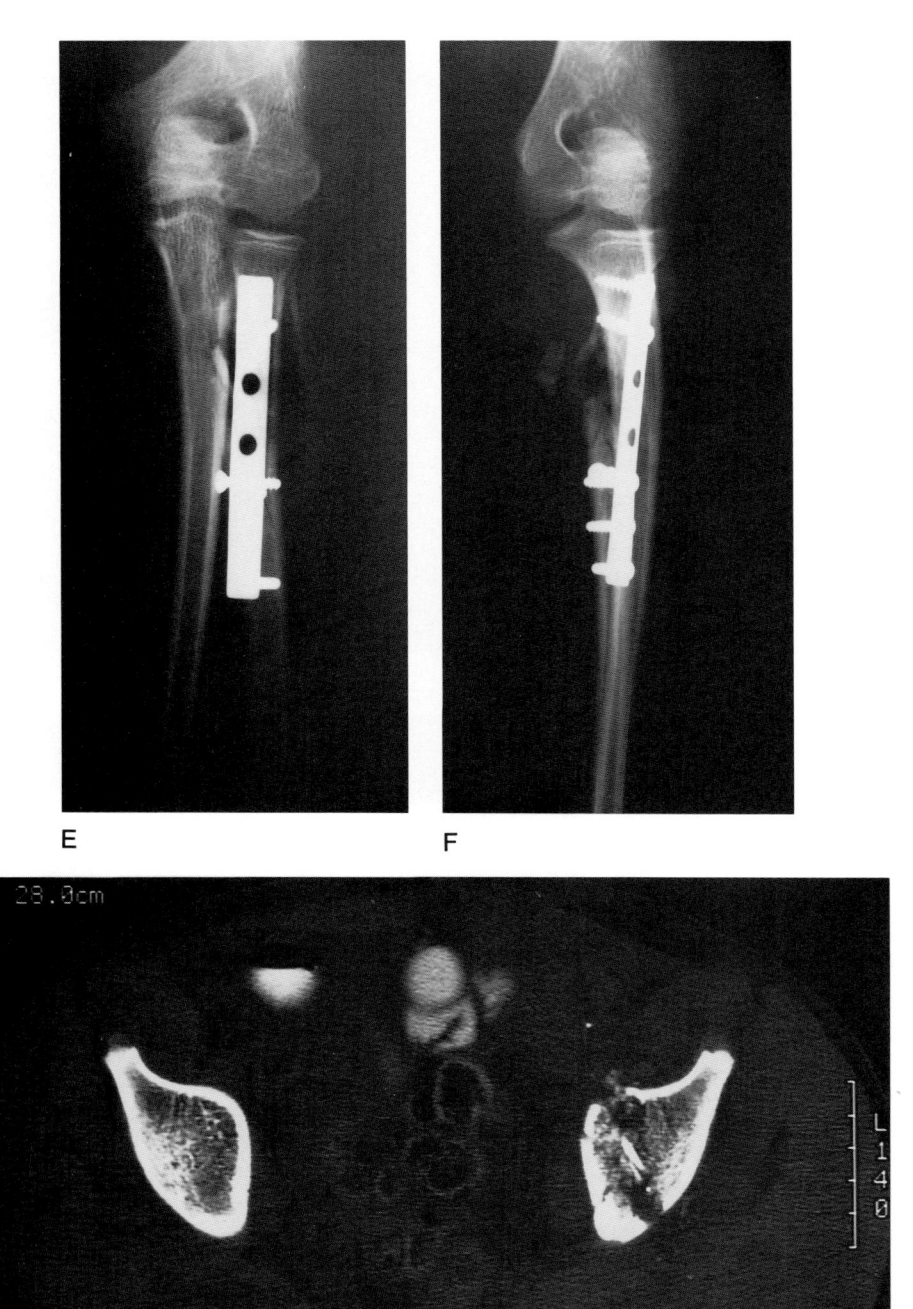

Fig. 52-6 *(Continued).* **(E)** Anteroposterior and **(F)** lateral views after open reduction and internal fixation. **(G)** A different level cut from the same CT scan as in Figure A showing the iliac fracture but without hip joint penetration. *(Figure continues.)*

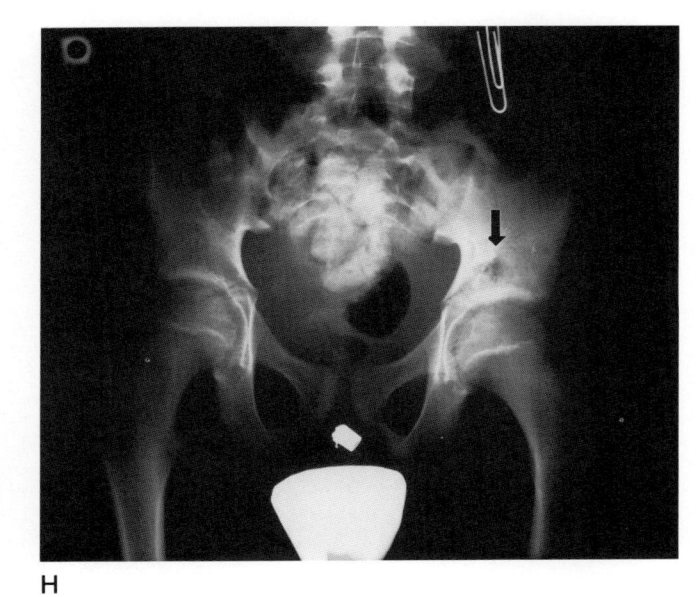

Fig. 52-6 *(Continued).* **(H)** An anteroposterior view of the pelvis 2 months after the injury showing the retained bullet as well as the healed iliac fracture *(arrow)*. **(I)** Anteroposterior and **(J)** lateral views 2 months after open reduction and internal fixation and 1 month after bone grafting, showing the fracture healed.

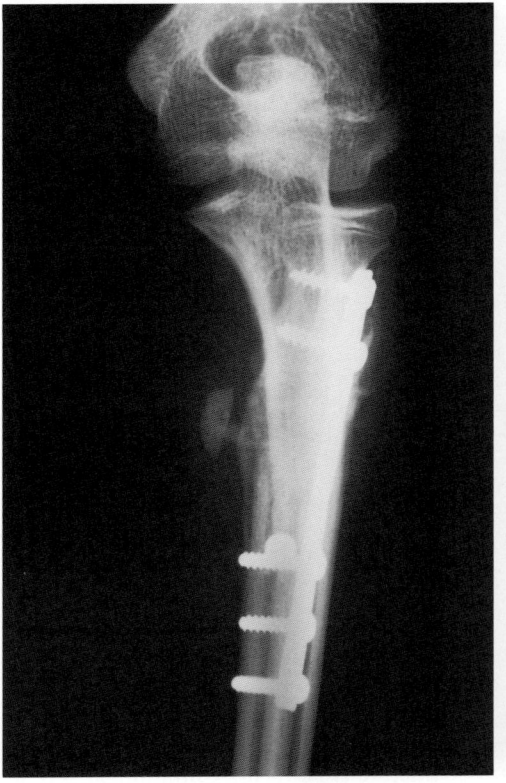

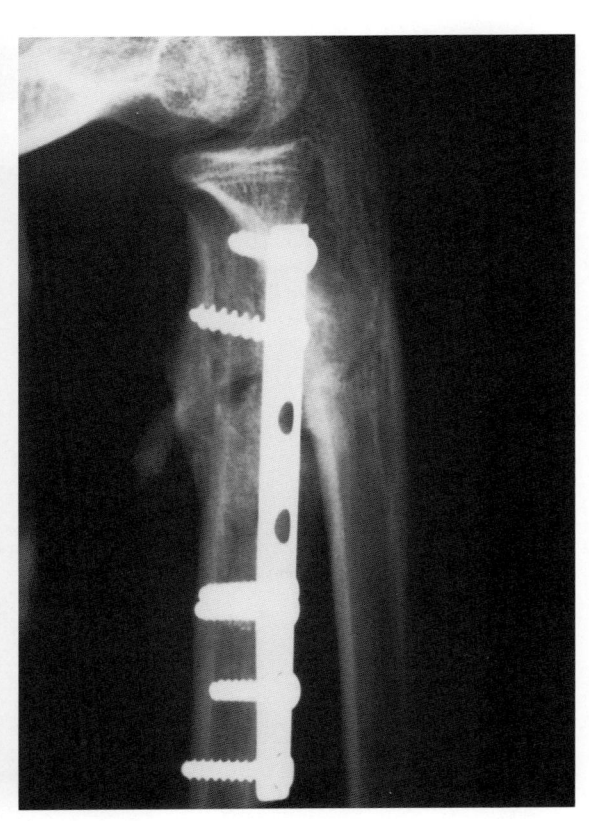

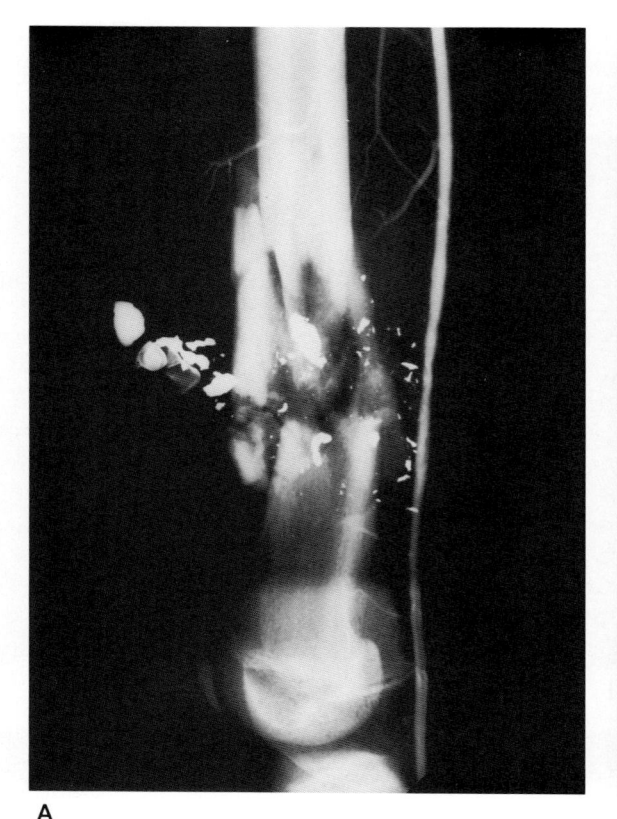

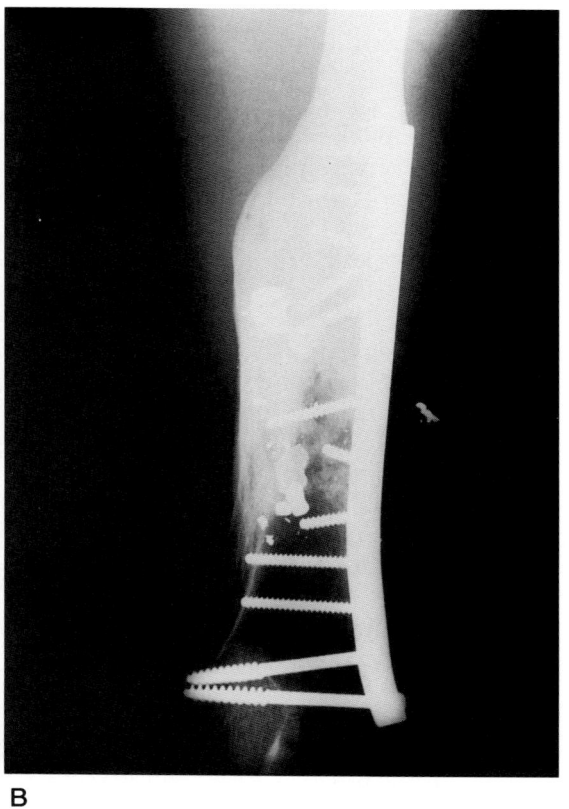

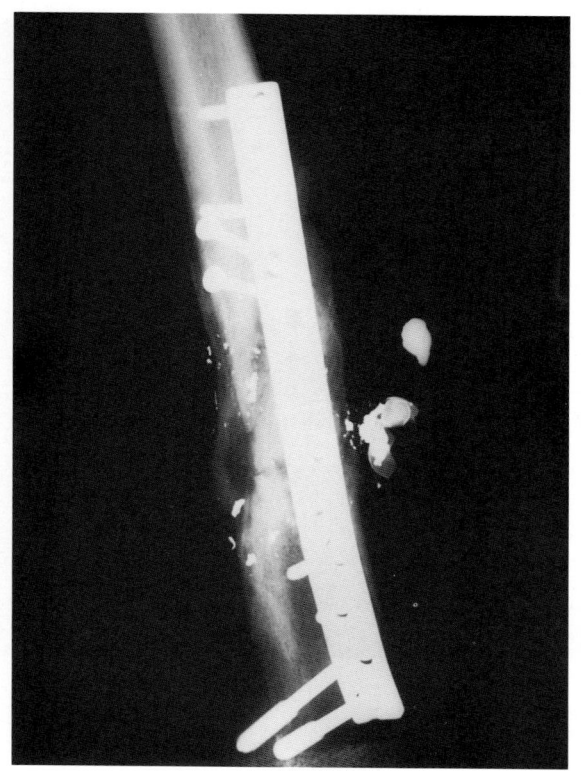

Fig. 52-7. (A) The arteriogram of a 14-year-old boy shot at close range with a high-velocity weapon. The distal femoral fracture is markedly comminuted with an intact arterial system. (B) Anteroposterior and (C) lateral radiographs showing complete healing of the fracture 12 months after injury. Note that the fixation devices did not violate the distal femoral physis. (From Stucky and Loder,[12] with permission.)

drug altercation at 3 A.M. in the living room, which was adjacent to the girl's bedroom. The brother assaulted the mother with a gun. The blast was deflected by the mother (which also required her hospitalization), penetrating the wall and hitting the child's left foot. This resulted in severe bone and soft tissue destruction (Figs. 52-8A–D).

On the morning of injury the wounds were formally irrigated and debrided in the operating room, along with multiple pin fixation. A repeat irrigation and debridement was performed on the third postinjury day and the wound was noted to remain clean with viable toes. Because of the large defect (Fig. 52-8E&F), it was felt that flap coverage was needed. An angiogram showed good digital vascularity and an adequate dorsalis pedis artery for soft tissue transfer (Fig. 52-8G&H). Therefore on the ninth postinjury day a lattissimus dorsi free flap was performed along with split-thickness skin graft coverage. The flap did well and the child was discharged in a short leg splint in the neutral position to prevent contracture development.

In 2.5 months after the injury the first metatrasal was reconstructed with an autogenous bicortical iliac crest graft (Fig. 52-8I&J). This was complicated by a *Serratia marcesens* infection in both the foot and iliac crest donor site, which resolved with incision and drainage, closure by secondary intention, and 6 weeks of intravenous gentamicin. After the 6-week course of antibiotics, the pins were removed and a short-leg cast was applied.

The cast was removed 3 months after the grafting reconstruction. All the wounds were healed and the graft was incorporating. At her last follow-up 12 months after injury, she ambulated with a plantigrade foot. Active ankle motion was from −20 to 45 degrees. There was no active extension or flexion of the great and second toes. All the wounds were closed with no drainage (Fig. 52-8K&L). Radiographs showed consolidation of the bone graft reconstruction (Fig. 52-8M).

Case 4

This 9-year-old boy was shot in the foot with a shotgun (Fig. 52-9A). He would give no details of the injury, although some of his acquaintances said that he had been "punished." He presented to the hospital 48 hours after the injury had occurred with a fever and wound contamination. He had tried to treat the wound himself by rubbing cooking oil over the injury. The injury was considered a Sherman and Salter-Harris type II to III injury. He was taken to the operating room immediately for an irrigation and debridement, as well as twice more. Eventually a clean wound was obtained (Fig. 52-9B), and covered with a split-thickness skin graft. After the graft had taken, he was discharged in short-leg cast but never returned again for follow-up.

SUMMARY

An aggressive approach to extremity gunshot wounds in children is needed. Institution of treatment requires differentiation between low-velocity or high-velocity and shotgun wounds. If it cannot be determined, then the injury should be considered high-velocity. Low-velocity wounds without fractures can be treated with simple dressings and emergency room irrigation. Prophylactic antibiotics should be used if there is an associated fracture. The fractures should be treated with standard means for each type. Internal or external fixation is not contraindicated, but rather encouraged, if that would normally be the standard treatment if it was not a gunshot fracture.

All high-velocity and shotgun wounds need a thorough irrigation and debridement in the operating room initially, and often sequentially until clean. Rapid soft tissue coverage should be obtained, using skin grafts and flaps if needed. Prophylactic antibiotics are necessary for all high-velocity and shotgun injuries.

Clinical vascular compromise should undergo immediate repair, including both major arterial and venous injuries. Arteriography should be performed whenever the bullet path has passed in proximity to major vessels and high-risk areas (calf, forearm and antecubital area, popliteal fossa, medial and posterior thigh, and medial and posterior arm). If the child has a neurologic deficit and the wound is being debrided in the operating room, the nerves should be explored. If a neural transection exists, either immediate or delayed repair should be done, depending upon the overall clinical status of the child and wound contamination. Reconstructive procedures (e.g., bone grafts) are performed whenever needed for segmental bone loss or nonunions. Long-term follow-up until skeletal maturity is recommended.

The epidemic proportions of pediatric gunshot wounds requires input not only from pediatric care teams, (orthopaedic surgeons, other surgical specialists, pediatricians) but also from public health officials, social workers, and child protection teams. I believe that all children with these injuries should be admitted to the hospital for appropriate social service and child protection team intervention. Associated psychosocial problems (e.g., truancy, school absences, law entanglements) and medical problems (drug use, sexually transmitted

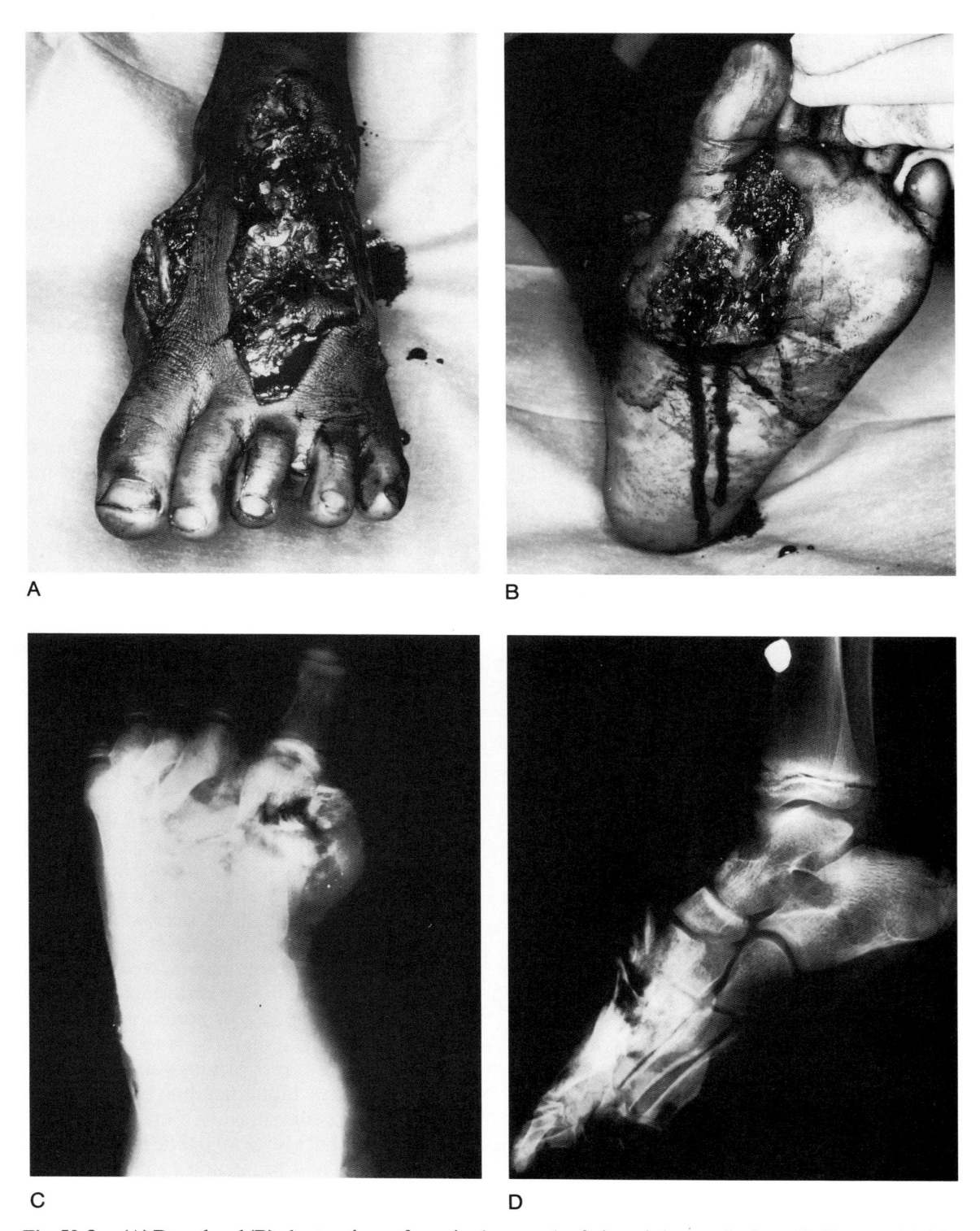

Fig. 52-8. (A) Dorsal and (B) plantar views of massive bone and soft tissue injury to the foot of a 10-year-old girl. (C) Anteroposterior and (D) lateral radiographs. *(Figure continues.)*

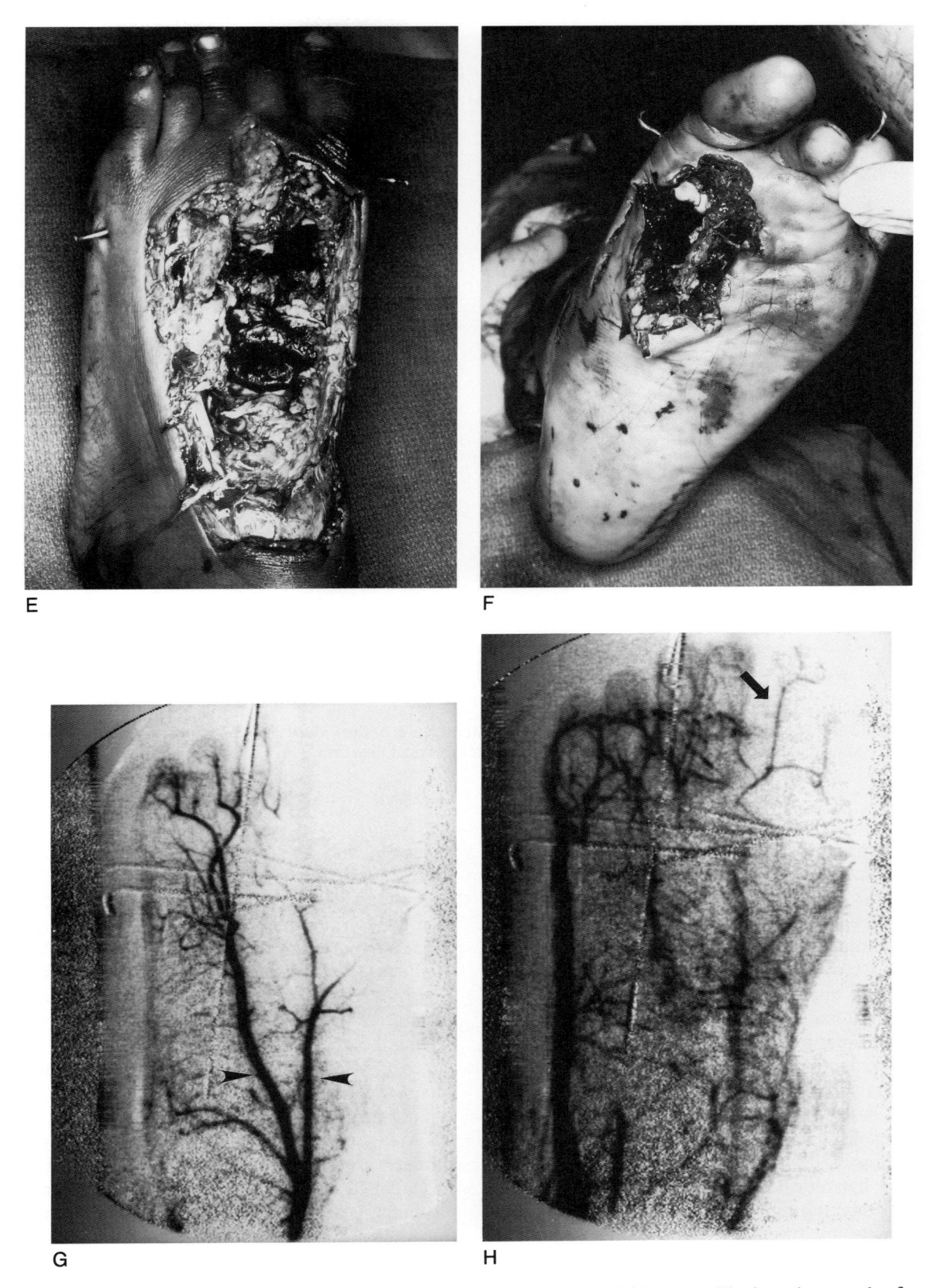

Fig. 52-8 *(Continued).* **(E)** Dorsal and **(F)** plantar views after radical debridements. The large bone and soft tissue defect is evident, and measured 5 × 4 × 3 cm. **(G&H)** Arteriograms **(G)** Note that the medial and lateral plantar arteries *(arrowheads)* are intact. **(H)** At a slightly later phase note that the toes are vascularized by the lateral plantar artery and collateral circulation. Although the vascularity to the great toe *(arrow)* was less than the other toes, it remained viable. *(Figure continues.)*

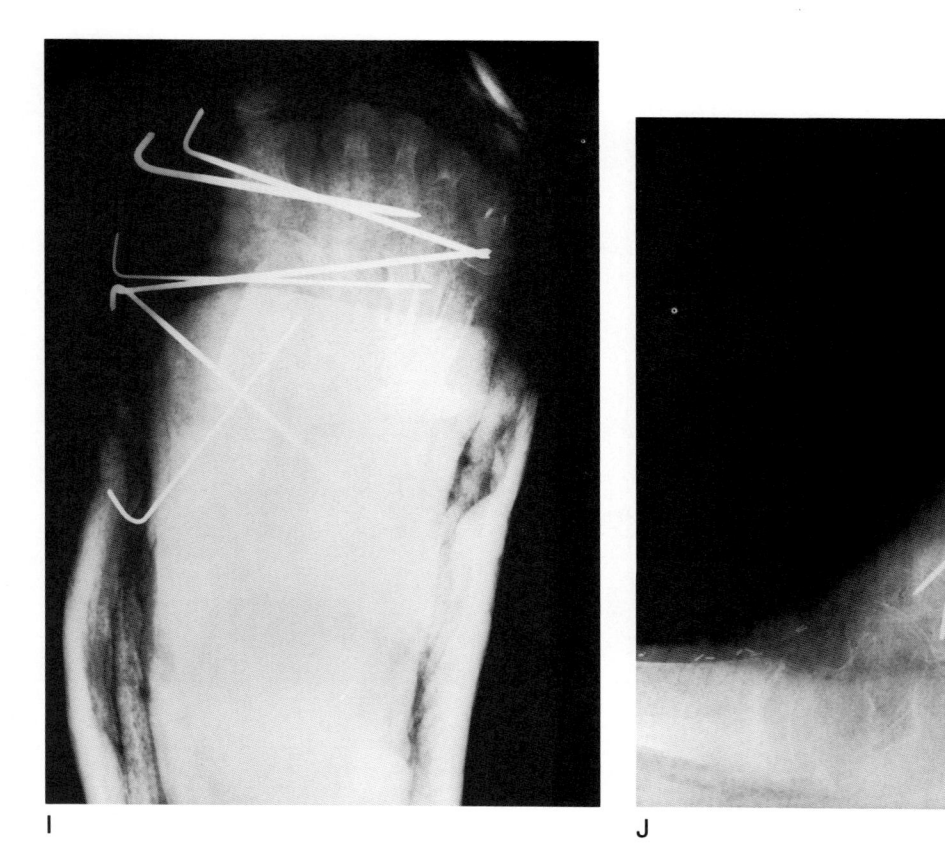

Fig. 52-8 *(Continued).* **(I)** Anteroposterior and **(J)** lateral views of the foot 2½ months after injury and immediately after reconstruction of the first metatarsal with a bicortical iliac crest graft. *(Figure continues.)*

diseases, teenage pregnancy) should be addressed. Child, parent, and public education for proper gun use should be given. Parents should be encouraged to remove the guns from their homes, since the majority of childhood gunshot wounds are the result of handguns in the home.[3] Education is strongly needed; in 51 percent of Canadian households in which there was a firearm, no member of the household had received instruction in the care and handling of firearms within the past 5 years.[64]

A new epidemic, that of intentional pediatric homicide, is also rising. The majority of these children are victims of street crime, often in the underground drug culture or gang retaliations. With these children not only are handguns used to commit the crimes but also modern warfare assault rifles, such as the M-16.[3] These rifles can cause devastating injuries and require war time (high-velocity) treatment.

The final question is that of prevention. In 1987 and 1988 alone, the last two years for which data are available, firearms accounted for 33,377 deaths between the ages of 0 and 34 years[7] in the United States. Nearly all were homicides and suicides. When isolating youths aged 15 to 29 years of age during 1987 and 1988 (which is similar to the age of the population involved in the 8½ year Vietnam War during which there were 62,897 casualties), 18,184 firearm deaths occurred. Extrapolating this death rate out to an 8½ year time span gives 77,282 deaths, or nearly 15,000 more than in the Vietnam War. Thus the United States is more dangerous for youths aged 15 to 29 years to die a firearm death than the Vietnam arena was during war time. Firearms are thus a major health hazard.

Areas of the country characterized by high rates of firearm ownership have the highest rates of homicide, aggravated assaults, and unintentional firearm deaths.[65] Handguns account for one-third of the 200 million firearms in use,[66] yet they are involved in 90 percent of criminal and firearm misuses. An estimated 200,000 handguns are stolen each year in the United States. Each year more than 90,000 U.S. citizens are assaulted,

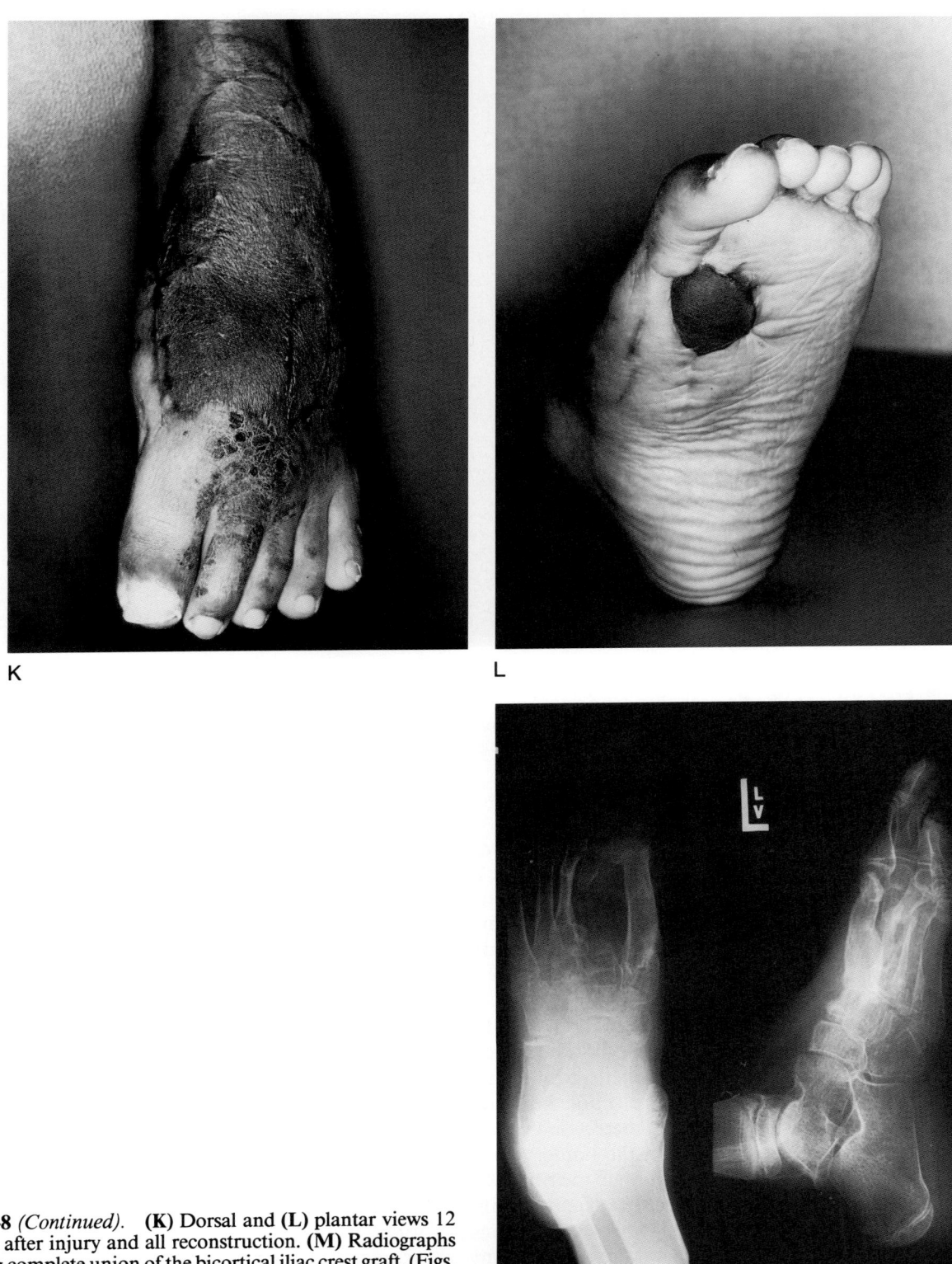

Fig. 52-8 *(Continued).* **(K)** Dorsal and **(L)** plantar views 12 months after injury and all reconstruction. **(M)** Radiographs showing complete union of the bicortical iliac crest graft. (Figs. A–F and I–M from Stucky and Loder,[12] with permission.)

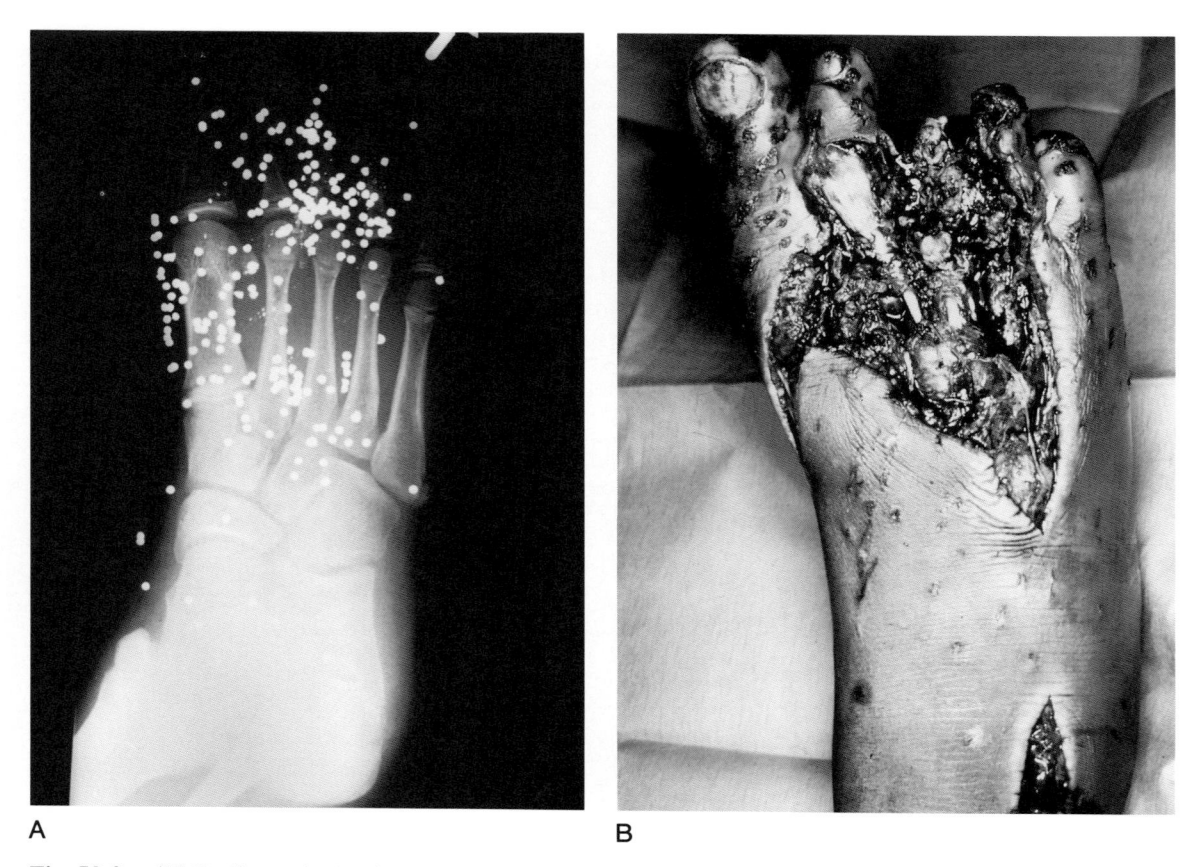

Fig. 52-9. (A) Radiograph showing many shot pellets without osseous injury. (B) The amount of debridement necessary to remove all the contaminated and nonviable tissue is shown. This was a Sherman and Parrish type II injury. After debridement coverage with a split-thickness skin graft was performed.

robbed, or raped by perpetrators armed with handguns. Nearly 10,000 are killed. Almost 20,000 people die in suicides committed with firearms each year, and the teenage and childhood suicide rate is markedly rising. This is also directly related to the accessibility of firearms in the home.[67] Clearly some type of firearm control is needed.

Critics of gun control argue that guns are needed for self-protection, but keeping a firearm in the home places the occupants in greater danger, rather than protecting them. For every one case of self-protection homicide involving a gun kept in the home, there are 43 more firearm deaths involving the gun in the home.[68] Even after deleting the suicides, a household member was killed 18 times as often as a stranger. The skeptics would argue that gun control won't work. However, Sloan and colleagues[69] have compared the firearm related homicide rate (Fig. 52-10) between Vancouver, British Columbia and Seattle, Washington. Both cities are quite similar in criminal activity and demographics, but Vancouver has a restrictive handgun law. The chance of being murdered in Seattle is 4.8 times higher than in Vancouver. Also, in a very recent study, Loftin and colleagues[70] clearly showed that restrictive licensing of handguns was associated with a prompt decline in homicides (25 percent) and suicides (23 percent) by firearms in the District of Columbia. They postulated that an average of 47 deaths each year in the District of Columbia were prevented. Clearly this is a start.

The health care professions, the government, and all of society, need to continue work on public education, gun control, and other preventive measures[71,72] to reduce this epidemic of destructive disease. Some states have now passed laws holding gun owners responsible for accidental shootings by children if the adult did not use reasonable care in storing the weapon.[73] Injury from firearms is now a public health problem whose toll is unacceptable. As has been so recently and succinctly

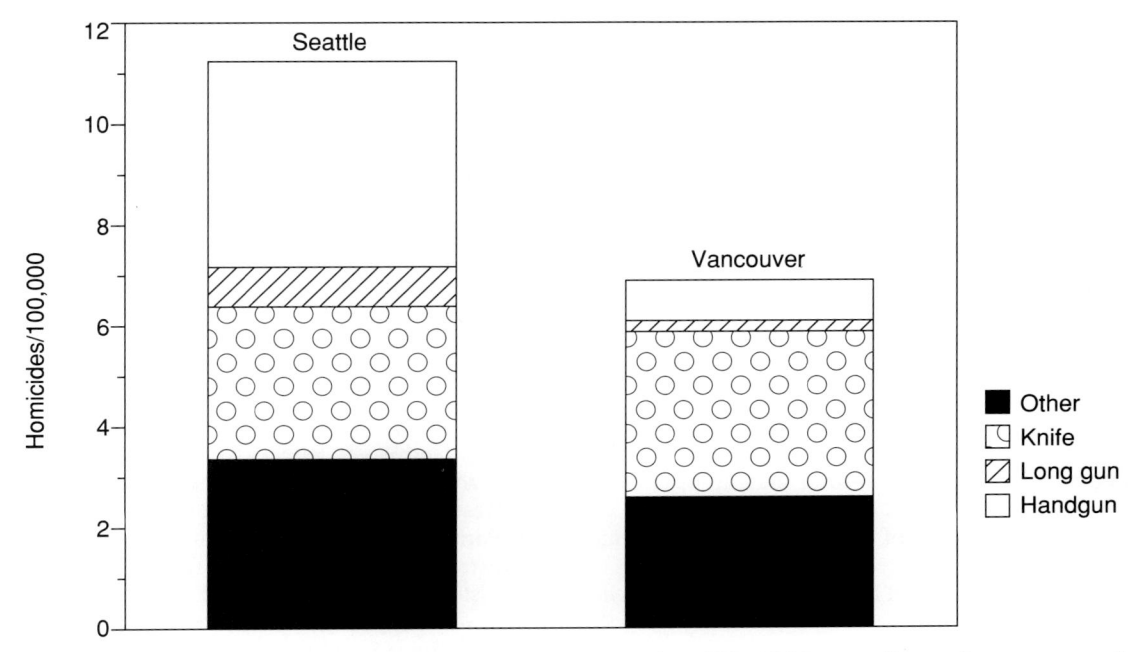

Fig. 52-10. Annual rates of homicide in Seattle and Vancouver for 1980–1986, according to the weapon used. "Other" includes blunt instruments, other dangerous weapons, and hands, fits, and feet. (From Sloan et al.,[69] with permission.)

stated,[66] the firearm "killing threshold" has exceeded the benefits.

REFERENCES

1. Letts RM, Miller D: Gunshot wounds of the extremities in children. J Trauma 16:807, 1976
2. Ordog GJ, Prakash A, Wasserberger J, Balasubramaniam S: Pediatric gunshot wounds. J Trauma 27:1272, 1987
3. Ordog GJ, Wasserberger J, Schatz I et al: Gunshot wounds in children under 10 years of age: a new epidemic. Am J Dis Child 142:618, 1988
4. Sanchez J, Lilac L, Holt RW: Gunshot wounds to legs in drug runners. N Engl J Med 320:1089, 1989
5. Victoroff BN, Robertson WW, Eichelburger M, Wright C: Extremity gunshot injuries treated in an urban children's hospital. Presented at the annual meeting of the Pediatric Orthopaedic Society of North America, Dallas Texas, May 12–15, 1991
6. Barlow B, Niemirska M, Gandhi RP: Ten year's experience with pediatric gunshot wounds. J Pediatr Surg 17:927, 1982
7. Fingerhut LA, Kleinman JC, Godfrey E, Rosenberg H: Firearm mortality among children, youth, and young adults 1-34 years of age: trends and current status: United States, 1979–88. Month Vital Stat Rep, suppl 39, 1991
8. Jason J: Child homicide spectrum. Am J Dis Child 137:578, 1983
9. Nelson KG: The innocent bystander: the child as unintended victim of domestic violence involving deadly weapons. Pediatrics 73:251, 1984
10. Rivara FP, Stapleton FB: Handguns and children: a dangerous mix. Dev Behav Pediatr 3:35, 1982
11. Schikler K, Jones MP: Gunshot wounds in children: a preventible disease. J Kent Med Assoc: 63, 1984
12. Stucky W, Loder RT: Extremity gunshot wounds in children. J Pediatr Orthop 11:64, 1991
13. Bongard FS, Klein SR: The problem of vascular shotgun injuries: diagnostic and management strategy. Ann Vasc Surg 3:299, 1989
14. Deitch EA, Grimes WR: Experience with 112 shotgun wounds of the extremities. J Trauma 24:600, 1984
15. Heins M, Kahn R, Bjordnal J: Gunshot wounds in children. Am J Public Health 64:326, 1974
16. Valentine J, Blocker S, Chang JHT: Gunshot injuries in children. J Trauma 24:952, 1984
17. Walsh IR, Eberhart A, Knapp JF, Sharma V: Pediatric gunshot wounds: powder and nonpowder weapons. Pediatr Emerg Care 4:279, 1988
18. Adams DB: Wound ballistics: a review. Milit Med 147:831, 1982
19. Hollerman JJ, Fackler ML, Coldwell DM, Ben-Menachem Y: Gunshot wounds: 1. Bullets, ballistics, and mechanisms of injury. Am J Radio 155:685, 1990

20. Mendelson JA: The relationship between mechanisms of wounding and principles of treatment of missile wounds. J Trauma 31:1181, 1991
21. Ordog GJ: Wound ballistics: theory and practice. Ann Emerg Med 13:1113, 1984
22. DeMuth WE Jr: Bullet velocity and design as determinants of wounding capability: an experimental study. J Trauma 6:222, 1966
23. Amato JJ, Billy LJ, Gruber RP et al: Vascular injuries: an experimental study of high and low velocity missile wounds. Arch Surg 101:167, 1970
24. Amato JJ, Rich NM, Billy LJ et al: High-velocity arterial injury: a study of the mechanism of injury. J Trauma 11:412, 1971
25. Huelke DF, Darling JH: Bone fractures produced by bullets. J Forensic Sci 9:461, 1964
26. De Muth WE Jr: The mechanism of shotgun wounds. J Trauma 11:219, 1971
27. Bell MJ: The management of shotgun wounds. J Trauma 11:522, 1971
28. Blocker S, Coln D, Chang JHT: Serious air rifle injuries in children. Pediatrics 69:751, 1982
29. Reddick EJ, Carter PL, Bickerstaff L: Air gun injuries in children. Ann Emerg Med 14:1108, 1985
30. Anderson RJ, Hobson RW II, Padberg FT Jr et al: Penetrating extremity trauma: identification of patients at high risk requiring arteriography. J Vasc Surg 11:544, 1990
31. Anderson RJ, Hobson RW II, Lee BC et al: Reduced dependency on arteriography for penetrating extremity trauma: influence of wound location and noninvasive vascular studies. J Trauma 30:1059, 1991
32. Shaker IJ, White JJ, Signer RD et al: Special problems of vascular injuries in children. J Trauma 16:863, 1976
33. Moed BR, Fakhouri AJ: Compartment syndrome after low-velocity gunshot wounds to the forearm. J Orthop Trauma 5:134, 1991
34. Sherman RT, Parrish RA: Management of shotgun injuries: a review of 152 cases. J Trauma 3:76, 1963
35. Patel KR, Cortes LE, Semel L et al: Bullet embolism. J Cardiovasc Surg 30:584, 1989
36. Rich NM: Missile injuries. Am J Surg 139:414, 1980
37. Brunner RG, Fallon WF Jr: A prospective, randomized clinical trial of wound debridement versus conservative wound care in soft-tissue injury from civilian gunshot wounds. Am Surgeon 56:104, 1990
38. Wiss DA, Brien WW, Becker V Jr: Interlocking nailing for the treatment of femoral fractures due to gunshot wounds. J Bone Joint Surg [Am] 73:598, 1991
39. Ashby ME: Low-velocity gunshot wounds involving the knee joint: surgical management. J Bone Joint Surg [Am] 56:1047, 1974
40. Livingstone RH, Wilson RI: Surgery of violence VI: gunshot wounds of the limbs. Br Med J 1:667, 1975
41. Leonard MH: The solution of lead by synovial fluid. Clin Orthop 64:255, 1969
42. Selbst SM, Henretig F, Fee MA et al: Lead poisoning in a child with a gunshot wound. Pediatrics 77:413, 1986
43. Dickey RL, Barnes BC, Kearns RJ, Tullos HS: Efficacy of antibiotics in low-velocity gunshot fractures. J Orthop Trauma 3:6, 1989
44. Schwartz JT Jr, Waters PM, Laurencin CT: Sciatic-nerve palsy associated with a retained plastic shot container in a shotgun injury. J Bone Joint Surg [Am] 73:607, 1991
45. Luce EA, Griffen WO: Shotgun injuries of the upper extremity. J Trauma 18:487, 1978
46. Hennessy MJ, Banks HH, Leach RB, Quigley TB: Extremity gunshot wound and gunshot fracture in civilian practice. Clin Orthop 114:296, 1976
47. Beaver BL, Moore VL, Peclet M et al: Characteristics of pediatric firearm fatalities. J Pediatr Surg 25:97, 1990
48. Golladay ES, Murphy KE, Wagner CW: Shotgun injuries in pediatric patients. S Med J 84:866, 1991
49. Howland WS Jr, Ritchey SJ: Gunshot fractures in civilian practice: an evaluation of the results of limited surgical treatment. J Bone Joint Surg [Am] 53:47, 1971
50. Parisien JS: The management of gunshot fractures of the extremities. Bull Hosp Joint Dis 28, 1981
51. Elstrom JA, Pankovich AM, Egwele R: Extra-articular low-velocity gunshot fractures of the radius and ulna. J Bone Joint Surg [Am] 60:335, 1978
52. Ryan JR, Hensel RT, Salciccioli GG, Pedersen HE: Fractures of the femur secondary to low-velocity gunshot wounds. J Trauma 21:160, 1981
53. Dugas R, D'Ambrosia R: Civilian gunshot wounds. Orthopedics 8:1121, 1985
54. Raju S: Shotgun arterial injuries of the extremities. Am J Surg 138:421, 1979
55. Bongard F, Johs SM, Leighton TA, Klein SR: Peripheral arterial shotgun missile emboli: diagnostic and therapeutic management-case reports. J Trauma 31:1426, 1991
56. Wolf AW, Benson Dr, Shoji H et al: Autosterilization in low-velocity bullets. J Trauma 18:63, 1978
57. Brettler D, Sedlin ED, Mendes DG: Conservative treatment of low-velocity gunshot wounds. Clin Orthop 140:26, 1979
58. Woloszyn JT, Uitvlugt GM, Castle ME: Management of civilian gunshot fractures of the extremities. Clin Orthop 226:247, 1988
59. Marcus NA, Blair WF, Shuck JM, Omer GE Jr: Low-velocity gunshot wounds to extremities. J Trauma 20:1061, 1980
60. Patzakis MJ, Harvey JP Jr, Ivler D: The role of antibiotics in the management of open fractures. J Bone Joint Surg [Am] 56:532, 1974
61. Hoekman P, Van de Perre P, Nelissen J et al: Increased frequency of infection after open reduction of fractures in patients who are seropositive for human immunodeficiency virus. J Bone Joint Surg [Am] 73:675, 1991
62. Stromberg BV: Symptomatic lead toxicity secondary to retained shotgun pellets: case report. J Trauma 30:356, 1990
63. Linden MA, Manton WI, Stewart M et al: Lead poisoning from retained bullets: pathogenesis, diagnosis, and management. Ann Surg 195:305, 1982

64. Chapdelaine A, Samson E, Kimberley MD, Viau L: Firearm-related injuries in Canada: issues for prevention. Can Med Assoc J 145:1217, 1991
65. Balser SP: Without guns, do people kill people? Am J Public Health 75:587, 1985
66. Kassirer JP: Firearms and the killing threshold. N Engl J Med 325:1647, 1991
67. Brent DA, Perper JA, Allman CJ et al: The presence and assessibility of firearms in the homes of adolescent suicides. JAMA 266:2989, 1991
68. Kellerman AL, Reay DT: Protection or peril?—an analysis of firearm-related deaths in the home. N Engl J Med 314:1557, 1986
69. Sloan JH, Kellermann AL, Reay DT et al: Handgun regulations, crime, assaults, and homicide: a tale of two cities. N Engl J Med 319:1256, 1988
70. Loftin C, McDowall D, Wiersema B, Cottey TJ: Effects of restrictive licensing of handguns on homicide and suicide in the District of Columbia. N Engl J Med 325:1615, 1991
71. Mercy JA, Houk VN: Firearm injuries: a call for science. N Engl J Med 319:1283, 1988
72. Christoffel KK: Toward reducing pediatric injuries from firearms: charting a legislative and regulatory course. Pediatrics 88:294, 1991
73. California man charged in death of grandson who shot himself. New York Times, 5Y, Saturday, January 4, 1992

53

Stress Fractures

Lyle J. Micheli
Allan F. Fehlandt, Jr.

> One of the surgeon's best remedies is tincture of time.
> —BÉLA SCHICK

CHALLENGE TO THE PEDIATRIC ORTHOPEDIST

Fatigue, or stress fractures, in children and adolescents have been relatively rare and only recently encountered in numbers that warrant review and classification. This increased occurrence of stress fractures in children and adolescents has paralleled their increased participation in organized sports. As with adult athletes engaged in repetitive training techniques, the young athletes have also now been presenting with stress fracture as part of the differential diagnosis of overuse injury and pain.

Devas,[1] in 1963, published the first review article on stress fractures in children. He discussed the clinical characteristics of approximately 40 cases that have been encountered in children. As with our more recent experience, the great majority of his children were engaged in repetitive sports training. He suggested that the different presentation of stress fractures in the pediatric patient can be traced to the different biomechanical characteristics of the child's bone. Since the child's bone is more plastic than the adult and is much more capable of rapid remodeling and healing, many of the stress fractures encountered in his series were characterized by proliferative callous. In many instances, the initial diagnosis was that of malignancy or infection. These early stress fractures in children contrasted with the adult pattern of stress fractures, where minimal callous occurred often well after the event, and after the pain has ceased.

In this initial review of 40 cases of stress fractures of the upper and lower extremity, Devas noted that the majority of these occurred in the proximal third of the tibia and fibula in the lower extremity, and in the first rib and humerus in the upper extremity. He emphasized that stress fracture must be included in the differential diagnosis of a child with painful limp, particularly if the child had been engaged in sports training.

Much of our information about the pathophysiology of stress fractures have come from observation of adults. Much of this information, in turn, has come from work in the military, where the early eponym for stress fracture was "march fracture" because they were seen so frequently in new recruits who had begun marching. In fact, the first known description of a stress fracture was by Breithaupt,[2] a Prussian military surgeon, who noted the occurrence of these painful injuries in the new recruits in his company.

DESCRIPTION

Stress fractures in children are receiving increased attention.[3] Stress fractures range from incomplete microfractures whose only symptom is pain to complete fractures of bone, and result from cyclic, repetitive physical stress below the threshold for single insult-induced bone failure or traumatic fracture[4] (Fig. 53-1).

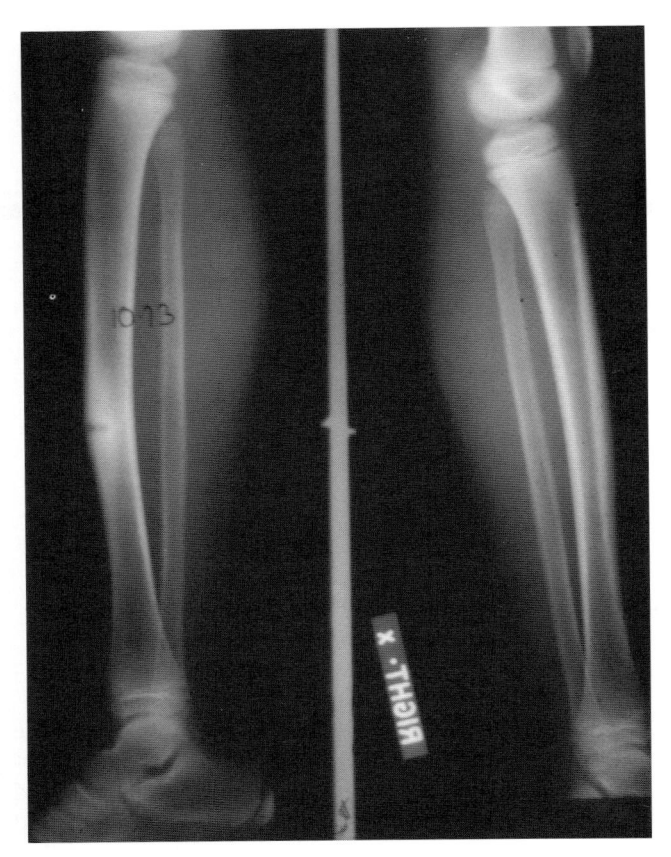

Fig. 53-1. Stress fracture of the anterior tibial diaphysis in an adolescent male.

Stress fractures in children and adolescents may be divided into two general categories: fatigue fractures, which occur when abnormal stress is applied to bone with normal elastic resistance, and insufficiency fractures, which occur when physiologic stress is applied to bones with abnormal elastic resistance.[5] Insufficiency fractures occur in bones weakened or altered by genetics, as in osteogenesis imperfecta; metabolic and endocrine disorders, as in renal osteodystrophy and hypoparathyroidism; acquired disorders, such as juvenile rheumatoid arthritis; nutritional disorders, as in rickets; and iatrogenically, as in steroid-induced osteomalacia.[5,6]

In healthy individuals with acquired conditions affecting bone metabolism, elasticity, or strength, a continuum between fatigue fractures and insufficiency fractures is evident. Examples are the amenorrheic ballet dancer[7] and distance runner,[8-11] or even individuals with decreased bone width.[12]

The term *fatigue fracture* has become synonymous with *stress fracture* in most medical literature, and will be used synonymously in this chapter unless otherwise stated. Spondylolysis, or stress fracture in the vertebral pars interarticularis, is discussed in detail in Chapter 67.

Stress fractures are a potentially debilitating subset of the family of overuse injuries.[13-15] Repetitive and specialized physical movement tasks are characteristic of organized sports and dance activities, and are the major etiologic factor in the occurrence of stress fractures in most children and adolescents. Repetitive movement patterns have no parallel in free play activities, as evidenced by the low incidence of overuse injuries in general, and especially stress fractures, in children and adolescents engaged in free play.[14,16]

INCIDENCE

The incidence of fatigue fractures in children and adolescents in the general population is not known. The apparent increase of these injuries parallels the increase of overuse injury in this population in general. This reflects an increase in participation in organized athletic training, competitive and recreational sports, and dance—activities that provide an environment for overuse injury, and stress fractures in particular, to occur with increased frequency.[3,14] Stress fractures in the pediatric population were previously a rare occurrence.[16-20] Stress fractures in competitive and recreational athletes are now common.[21,22] Stress fractures in the military have been documented for over 100 years.[2] Nonmilitary, nonathletic individuals are rarely afflicted with stress fractures; occurrence of stress fractures in this population may signal underlying, and possibly serious, medical problems.[23]

Improved awareness and understanding of fatigue fractures by the medical community have contributed to the increasing recognition of this overuse injury.[12,22] The understanding of pediatric stress fractures is evolving with advances in diagnostic aids, in particular [^{99m}Tc]methylene diphosphonic acid bone scans, which currently is the most sensitive test for diagnosing stress fractures.[6,22,24] Stress fracture studies in the past used plain radiographs as the primary diagnostic tool; interpretation of these in light of the current knowledge of the limitations of plain radiographs in assisting in the diagnosis of stress fractures suggests that the incidence of stress fractures in the past may have been underestimated.

The medical history of onset of extremity pain in association with repetitive training should alert the physician to include stress fracture in the differential diagnosis.[14,16]

Studies of the incidence of stress fractures arising from recreational and competitive sporting activities generally address an adult population or a mix of adult and adolescent patients. In a recent review of 131 athletes with stress fractures; 48.9 percent were between ages 10 and 19 years, with a higher incidence in girls.[25] While similar risk factors for the development of stress fractures affect both adults and children, the incidence of stress fractures in children and adolescents does not necessarily parallel that of adults, given similar risk factors and activities. The long bones of the child, with their greater bone elasticity and faster reparative ability, may be able to sustain high levels of repetitive stress without failure. However, stress injury to the epiphyseal plates or apophyses represent unique injuries to the child or adolescent.[14,26]

Prevention of stress fractures in the young may be facilitated by the identification of specific anatomic or physiologic risk factors, and the implementation of interventions based on these factors. There have been few studies attempting to identify risk factors in children or adolescents. Studies of risk factors for stress fracture in young military recruits, however, may be relatively more applicable to children and adolescents than to sedentary adults.[27] These military studies are similar to the sports medicine literature insofar as they attempt to identify the relationship between specific activities and stress fracture occurrence. Extrapolation of identifiable risk factors in young adult military populations to pediatric practice may decrease the morbidity from stress fractures in children and adolescents—if such preventive measures are instituted especially for the young athlete or dancer.

Examples of military data that relate to our clinical experience with pediatric stress fractures illustrate the importance of these studies. Protzman and Griffis[28] found that women had 10 times as many stress fractures as men during the same basic military training course, and Zahger and colleagues[29] also found stress fractures occurring with greater frequency in female soldiers undergoing military training. A higher incidence of stress fractures in athletically active girls was recently reported by Ha and coworkers.[25] Our clinic has seen increasing numbers of stress fractures in girls as they become more active in organized sports and dance activities. The expanded participation of girls in sports and dance camps, where activity levels often increase precipitously as in military training, gives us a seasonal increase in stress fracture cases in girls that is not matched by their male peers.

Interestingly, Giladi and colleagues[12] found in a young adult military population a correlation between tibial bone width and the total incidence of stress fractures, tibial stress fractures alone, and femoral stress fractures alone. This is the first report of a measurable physical parameter being identified as a risk factor for stress fractures. These authors also speculated that narrower bones in women, as demonstrated by Miller and Purkey,[30] contribute to their greater risk for incurring stress fractures. The basic mechanisms underlying these findings may be applicable to children and adolescents.

Military data also point to racial differences in the occurrence of stress fractures,[31] as illustrated in the report by Brudvig and colleagues[32] finding that white men had twice the incidence of stress fractures as black men during the same military training program. This matches our clinical impression that the pediatric black athlete, male and female, less commonly present with stress fractures than their white peers.

Earlier reports of stress fractures in athletic children include the nine patients in the report by Orava and colleagues[33] of 110 patients with stress fractures; the youngest child was 10 years old and all children were observed to exercise more than average. Stanitski and colleagues[34] discussed 7 athletically active children, aged 7 to 15 years, with stress fractures in their review. These and other reports correlate with our clinical impression that children and adolescents with stress fractures respond readily to conservative management and infrequently experience complications. A 10 percent incidence of delayed unions and nonunions of stress fractures was reported by Orava and Hulkko[35] in a series of 369 athletics-related stress fractures; half of these mostly adult patients were involved in endurance sports. We have not had this experience with growing patients, who incur fewer complications if given an appropriate environment for healing areas of stress injury.

ANATOMY

Children and adolescents differ from adults with respect to the strength, elasticity, remodeling potential of bones, richness of blood supply, and by the presence of growth plates and apophyses. These factors vary with the patient's age, determine the clinical course, site of lesion, and radiographic features of the stress fracture. The elasticity and plasticity of bone decreases with advancing age, increasing the predisposition for fractures. In the skeletally immature patient the mechanism of bone reaction to stress mirrors the same process in adults, but with greater intensity. When stress is applied to bone, resorption and subsequent remodeling occur to strengthen the bone; when the mechanisms of stress-induced strengthening are exceeded by the repetition of force, stress fractures can occur.

Devas[36] and others[31] classified fatigue fractures into compression and distraction types based on their radiographic appearance. Compression fractures are more common in younger patients.[6] Compression fractures are found at the ends of long bones (femoral neck, proximal tibia) or in short bones such as the calcaneous. These fractures occur with compression stress applied to the trabeculae of cancellous bone, often exhibiting sclerosis on plain radiographs. Microfracture of the trabeculae occurs with subsequent blastic repair. The secondary callus formation may never be demonstrated on plain radiographs. The midshaft of the tibia and femur are prototypical distraction fractures. These occur in cortical bone and appear in the shafts of long bones. Osteoclastic resorption is followed by endosteal and periosteal callous presenting as a lucency or break. These have a higher incidence of complete fracture with displacement and are more common in the older patient.[6] Radiographs may demonstrate a lucent line preceding any blastic repair.[36] Radiographs are frequently normal in the early phases of stress fractures because 30 to 50 percent loss of mineral is necessary before rarefaction, or resorptive processes are evident.

Lower Extremity and Pelvis

The lower extremity is most often affected in the child, adolescent, and in adults. The tibia and fibula are most commonly affected[37] (Figs. 53-1 and 53-2). Stress fractures to the midtibial diaphysis and femur, though uncommon, merit special consideration due to the potential for severe and protracted disability that can occur when they progress to complete fractures.[38-44] Stress fractures to the sacrum[45-47] and pubic rami[48,49] are rare. Progression to avulsion fracture of the iliac apophysis due to recurrent stress injury has been observed in our sports medicine clinic. Patellar stress fractures are also unusual[50,51] and distraction of the fragments may require surgical intervention.[52] Fibular stress fractures are common in the athletically active and occur most frequently in the distal two-thirds,[53] with proximal fibular stress fractures uncommon.[54]

Femur

Hip fractures account for fewer than 1 percent of all fractures in children.[41] Femoral neck stress fractures are rare under age 65,[55] and even less common in patients

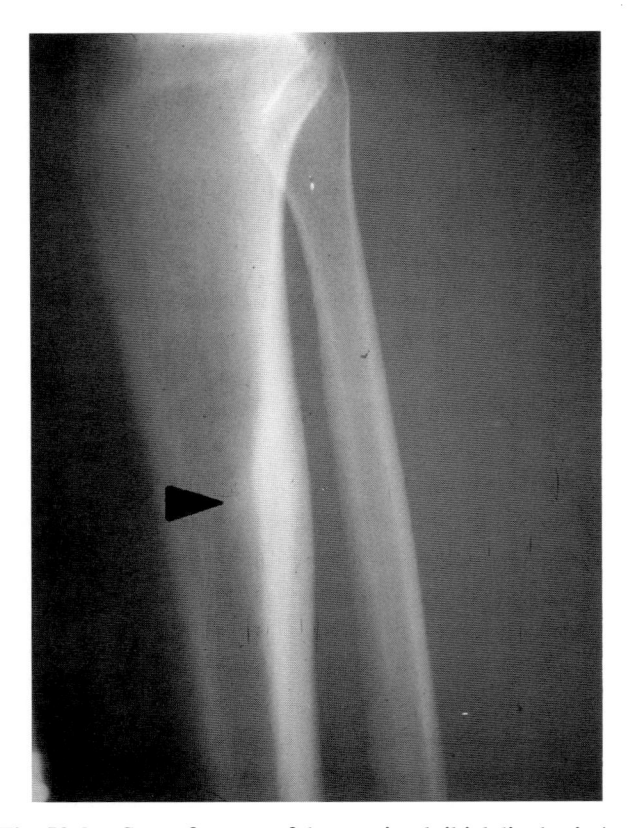

Fig. 53-2. Stress fracture of the proximal tibial diaphysis *(arrowhead)* in an adolescent athlete.

with open capital femoral epiphyses.[17,41-43] In a series of 936 stress fractures in soldiers, femoral stress fractures were found in 6 percent and high levels of motivation were identified as an additional risk factor to overuse.[56] Fullerton and Snowdy[31] identified a less than 5 percent incidence of femoral neck stress fractures in their series of 1,049 stress fractures in soldiers, and noted racial differences in occurrence. Femoral neck[57] stress fractures have been reported in runners. Wolfgang reported a femoral neck stress fracture in a 10-year-old girl who had the initial working diagnosis of traumatic synovitis. She had no specific injury but had been involved in vigorous jungle gym activities.[59] Femoral stress changes were observed with surprising frequency by Rosen and colleagues[60] in a review of pediatric stress fracture cases. Young ballet dancers constitute a subpopulation of adolescent females with a higher incidence of femoral neck stress changes apparent on plain radiographs and bone scans[61] (Fig. 53-3). We have observed femoral neck stress fractures in hyperactive children, as have others.[62] Avascular necrosis of the femoral head is a severe complication of femoral neck stress fractures and depends

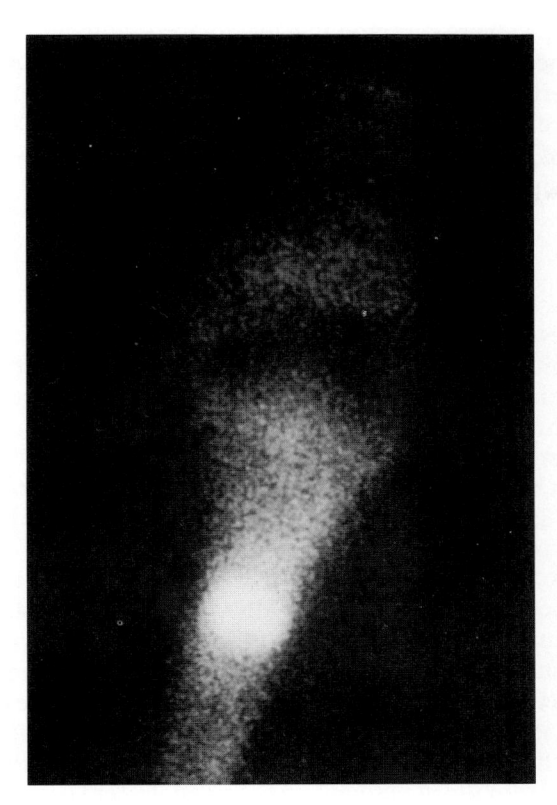

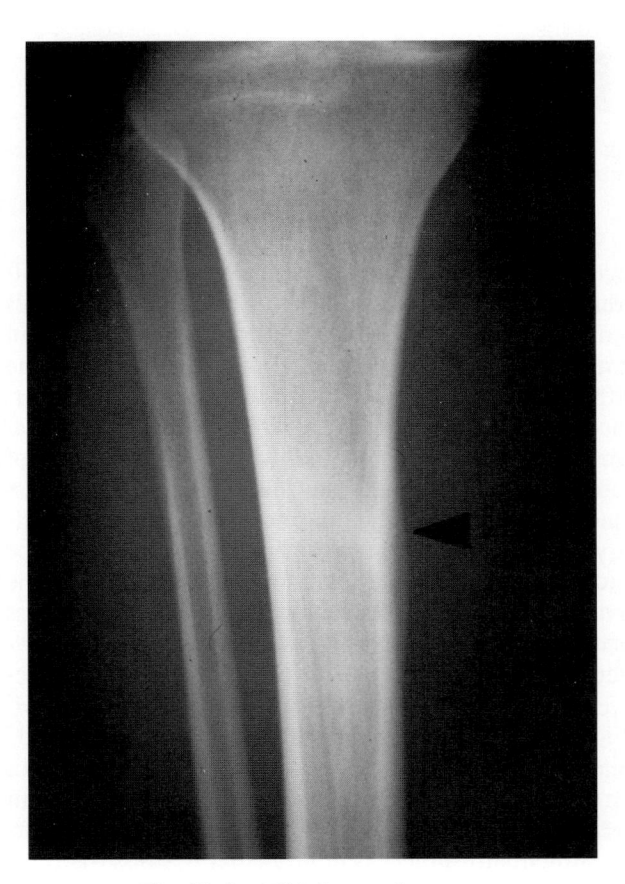

Fig. 53-3. Bone scan of tibial stress fracture.

more on the severity of the initial injury rather than the treatment.[41,63]

The femoral diaphysis and distal femur are uncommonly affected by stress fractures, as the report of a Salter-Harris type II stress fracture of the distal femoral epiphysis in a skeletally immature athlete as reported by Weber[64] illustrates. Displaced femoral-shaft[58] stress fractures and subtrochanteric[65] stress fractures have been reported in runners.

Tibia

Stress fractures of the proximal third of the tibia (Fig. 53-2) are far more common than anterior cortex fractures of the middle third (Fig. 53-1), with the latter comprising less than 5 percent of tibial stress fractures, and posing greater difficulty in treatment and proclivity for nonunion or complete fractures.[66-70] The case report by Brahms and colleagues[67] of a stress fracture in the anterior lateral cortex of the tibial midshaft in a football player that progressed to complete fracture despite being asymptomatic dramatically illustrates the potential morbidity from these fractures. Despite their relative infrequency, they must enter the differential diagnosis in the child or adolescent with anterior tibial pain (Fig. 53-4). Specific activities associated with this stress fracture include jumping sports, such as basketball[70] and ballet dancing.[68]

Foot and Ankle

Shelbourne and colleagues[71] reported stress fractures of the medial malleolus in runners, and suggested that this stress fracture be considered in the differential diagnosis of patients with an ankle effusion accompanied by chronic or subacute medial malleolar pain and a history of running activities causing the pain. Stress fractures of tibia or fibula accounted for 1.1 percent of the injuries in athletes attending one sports injury clinic.[72] Metatarsal stress fractures in children were rarely reported in the literature prior to bone scanning technology[73,74] (Fig. 53-5). Metatarsal mechanics underlie the high incidence of second and third metatarsal stress fractures in running and dancing activities, where these structures serve as rigid cantilevers, and forces are particularly high in the

Fig. 53-4. Tibial stress fracture.

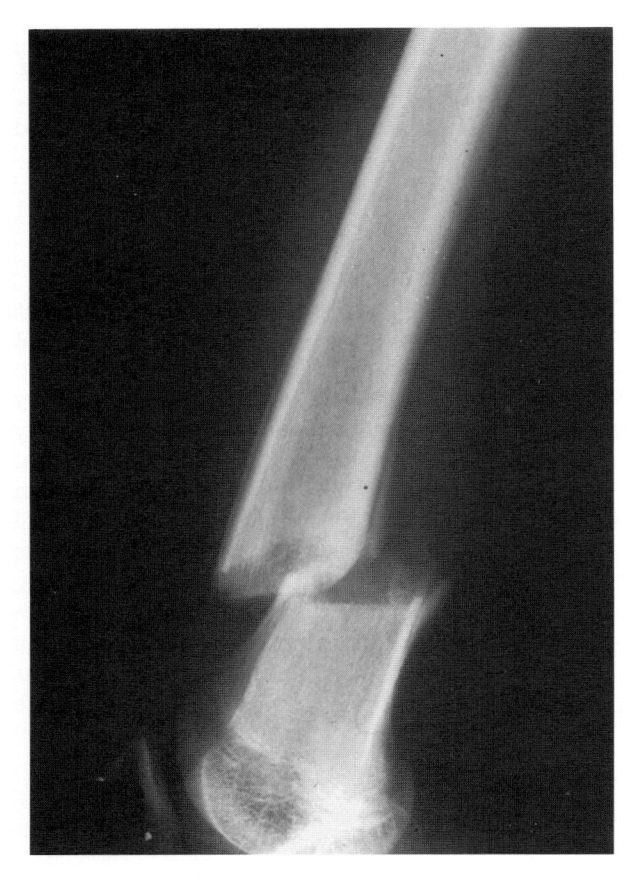

Fig. 53-5. Stress fracture with progression to complete fracture in an adolescent male distance runner.

second metatarsal[75]; factors as readily apparent in children and adolescents as in adults. Short first metatarsals cannot be implicated as a risk factor for stress fractures in runners.[76] The hallux sesamoid bone and the base of the fifth metatarsal are also sites of stress fractures in endurance athletes.[35] Stress fractures of the lateral metatarsal bones have been reported following reconstruction of hallux metatarsophalangeal joint.[77] Calcaneal stress fractures are relatively uncommon,[78] except in the military population where the mechanism of injury can be traced to overuse and marching techniques.[79,80] The proximal phalanx of the great toe was affected by a stress osteochondral fracture in a case report by Jones.[81] Navicular stress fractures usually are seen in physically active individuals,[21,35] particularly long-distance runners[82] (Fig. 53-5) but also have been reported in nonathletes.[83] Diagnosis of these fractures is commonly delayed, in part due to the common absence of findings on plain radiographs.[83] Failure of conservative treatment requiring subsequent surgery is not unusual.[35] Stress fractures in the foot are common in ballet dancers, both men and women. Particular attention must be paid to the young ballerina who is actively toe dancing, though male dancers suffer no less from stress injury to the feet.[84] Stress fractures at Lisfranc's joint are unique to toe dancing[85] (Fig. 53-6A&B).

Upper Extremity

Fewer stress fractures are observed in the upper extremity. Activities involving repetitive stress to the upper extremity include gymnastics and throwing sports. Gymnastics activities place substantial loads on the upper extremity as well as repetitive impacts to the wrist,[86] causing stress fractures of the carpal scaphoid[87] and Salter-Harris type I stress fractures of the distal radial and ulnar growth plates.[88]

Excessive throwing activities have produced well-described stress injuries to the elbow,[89,90] including stress fractures through the olecranon apophysis[91] with symptomatic nonunion,[92,93] and humeral stress fractures.[94] Repetitive forearm flexor activity in general can give rise to the relatively uncommon ulnar stress fracture,[95] which may require operative intervention.[35] A stress fracture in the ulnar diaphysis of an adolescent competitive tennis player, affecting the nondominant extremity in a player with a two-handed backhand stroke,[96] a stress fracture of the diaphysis of the ulna in a 22-year-old male body builder,[97] and ulnar stress fractures in a 19-year-old female softball pitcher and a 14-year-old volleyball player,[98] illustrate this unusual stress fracture.

The scapula is rarely affected, and we are unaware of any reports of children with scapular stress fractures. A stress fracture of the scapula in the superomedial portion in a jogger who ran with hand weights was reported by Veluvolu and coworkers.[99] Also infrequent are clavicular stress fractures. Dust et al reported a clavicular stress fracture complicated by nonunion after Dacron coracoclavicular reconstruction. The Dacron acted as a stress riser and then became interposed in the fracture.[100] Fractures in the hand are uncommon, as in the case of a metacarpal stress fracture in an adolescent tennis player,[101] and the stress fracture of the right ring finger in a young adult male bowler.[102]

Other Sites

Spondylolysis is a common stress fracture of the pars interarticularis[103-105] that is discussed elsewhere in this text (see Ch. 67). Stress fractures of the spinal pedicles are uncommon.[106] Sternal stress fractures are also un-

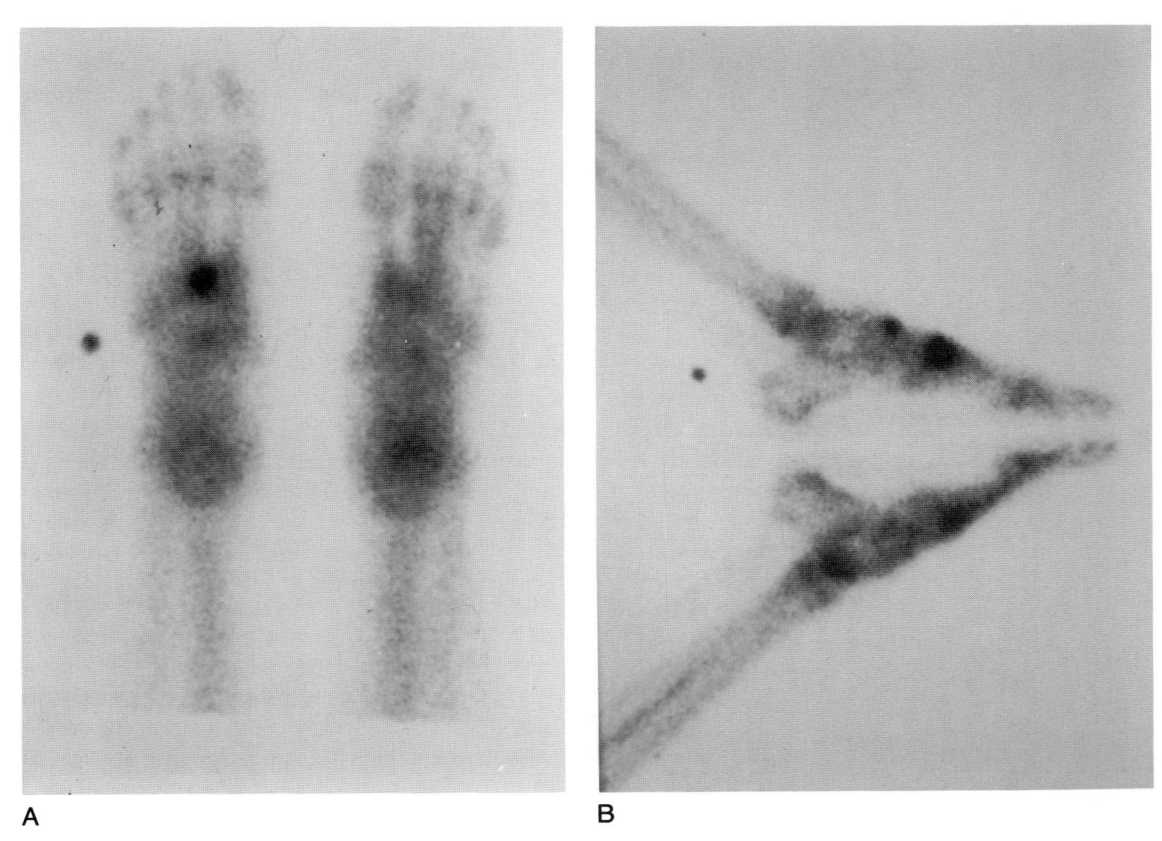

Fig. 53-6. (A) Anteroposterior bone scan of a stress fracture of the second metatarsal at Lisfranc's joint in an adolescent ballet dancer. (B) Lateral bone scan of a stress fracture of the second metatarsal at Lisfranc's joint in an adolescent ballet dancer.

usual.[107] Rib stress fractures are not uncommon,[108-111] and have been reported in male and female rowers,[113,114] tennis players,[115] golfers,[116] gymnasts,[113] basketball,[112] and baseball players,[117] and dancers.[118] Rib stress fractures also occur from coughing.[119] Lumbar back pain can arise from stress fractures of the lower ribs.[120]

MECHANISM OF INJURY AND RISK FACTORS

Animal studies are providing important insight to the pathomechanics of stress fractures. Rat studies reinforce the evidence that diffuse structural damage occurs to bone during repetitive loading.[121] A rabbit model has reinforced the concept that stress fractures are a sequential pathologic process that includes the periosteum, with the initial state of the stress fracture being accelerated absorption of bone followed by periosteal proliferation and compensatory new bone formation.[122] Repetitive stresses produced during running can cause acetabular stress fractures in racing greyhounds,[123] and racing thoroughbred horses are afflicted with stress fractures, of the forelimb.[124]

Ogden[37] emphasizes that pediatric stress fractures occur primarily from muscular activity and not impact, jarring injury. He outlines the general triad of causal factors underlying stress fractures in children: (1) a new or different activity, (2) strenuous activity, and (3) repetition of activity. A proposed mechanism is that physical exercise leads to muscle fatigue, causing altered movement patterns and distribution of stress, with resultant excessive concentration of forces being transmitted to underlying bone.[125] Others[34] argue that concentrated muscle forces, as opposed to fatigue per se, when acting across a specific bone with imposed repetitive tasks, enhance the loading that occurs from weightbearing on the particular part, with the rhythmic, subthreshold mechanical stresses summating beyond the stress bearing capacity of the bone. Lombardo and Benson[57] have also noted that the loading rate is more important that absolute load in the etiology of stress fractures. Skinner and Cook[126] calculated the number of cycles required to produce a femoral neck stress fracture in a runner; they recommended that runners beginning training limit their distance to no more than 100 miles over a 3-month period.

Specific mechanical stressors unique to the fibula have been examined in athletes; running on hard surfaces and powerful contraction of the extrinsic foot flexor muscles with subsequent stressful approximation of the fibula to the tibia accounted for most stress fractures in the lower part of the fibula.[53] Micheli[14] has outlined factors to check in the assessment of overuse stress fractures in the athletic pediatric patient; these include training errors, such as abrupt changes in intensity, duration or frequency of training; musculotendinous imbalance—of strength, flexibility or bulk; anatomic malalignment of the lower extremities, such as femoral anteversion, patella alta or lateral alignment, genu valgum, tibia vara, pes planus or cavo varus; footwear, including improper fit, inadequate impact absorbing material, excessive stiffness of sole, and/or insufficient support of the hindfoot; running surface—concrete pavement versus asphalt, running track, dirt or grass; associated disease states of the lower extremity; growth, and the growth spurt in particular. Paty[127] noted these factors, and that musculoskeletal injuries constitute over 60 percent of running injuries, stress fractures constituting a large portion of these.

Giladi and colleagues[128] identified narrow tibiae and higher degrees of external rotation at the hip as independent and cumulative risk factors for stress fractures in military recruits. Amenorrhea and associated hypoestrogenemia is associated with a higher incidence of stress fractures in runners[8,9,11] and ballet dancers,[7] with sustained history of oligomenorrhea a further predisposing factor.[10] Resumption of menses usually accompanies increased body weight or decreased training intensity in these athletes, with subsequent increase in bone mineral content and decreased incidence of stress fractures. Bone density has also been implicated as a factor in the development of femoral and calcaneal stress fractures in young adult males undergoing intense physical activity.[129]

Lysens and colleagues[130] identified a profile of factors which described the stress injury prone adolescent athlete; these included the physical traits of a combination of muscle weakness, ligamentous laxity, and muscle tightness. The effects of these factors were intensified by large body weight and length, high explosive strength, and malalignment of the lower limbs.[130] Recruits with running backgrounds suffered fewer fractures in a prospective study of marine recruits;[79] other studies have also reported a pretraining effect in helping prevent stress fractures in athletes.[80] Others have reported no protective effect of pretraining in military recruits.[131,132]

PHYSICAL EXAMINATION

Point tenderness and inflammation at the affected site in the absence of systemic symptoms are fundamental findings in the stress fracture patient.[34] In the younger child, particularly with lower extremity stress fractures, accompanying listlessness and a slight irregular fever may be exhibited, raising obvious concern for osteomyelitis or tumor.[37] Gentle provocative testing, a tuning fork,[25] or ultrasound induced pain[133] can augment the physical examination.

DIFFERENTIAL DIAGNOSIS

The differential diagnosis of the child with axial or appendicular skeletal pain must include malignant and benign neoplasm, monoarticular arthritis, infection, soft tissue injury, along with stress and traumatic fractures. These divergent problems underscore the importance of a careful and accurate history for narrowing the differential and arriving at the correct diagnosis. Children and adolescents engaged in repetitive activity with development of focal, mechanical pain, that is, pain aggravated with activity and relieved with rest, must engage a high index of suspicion for stress fracture.[14,34] The importance of recognizing stress fractures is evident considering that patients with stress fractures have undergone biopsy or even amputation.[134,135]

Examples of difficult to diagnose stress fractures include a case of bilateral symmetrical march fractures simulating juvenile rheumatoid arthritis in a young patient,[136] and a 10-year-old girl with a femoral neck stress fracture that on presentation initially was clinically similar to a traumatic synovitis.[59] Systemic disease may present as stress fractures, as in coelic disease with secondary malabsorption leading to osteomalacia and insufficiency-type stress fractures in young adults,[137] or recurrent metatarsal stress fractures in a patient with hypophosphatasia.[138] These reports suggest investigating for metabolic causes in patients with recurrent stress fractures.

DIAGNOSTIC IMAGING

Conventional Radiography

Radiography is performed at the time of the initial work up only to rule out nonstress injury such as complete fracture, fibrous dysplasia, osteomyelitis, or primary bone tumor. Conventional radiography can have a high rate of false negative results; 87 percent in one report of military recruits.[139] A stress fracture of trabecular bone will appear normal on radiographs for 10 to 21 days before resorption and proliferation associated with healing produce perceptible increase in density of the bone matrix.[140]

Osteoid osteomas, looser zones of osteomalacia, early osteogenic sarcomas, and chronic sclerosing osteomyelitis can have radiographic appearances similar to stress fractures.[141] Osteoid osteomas commonly have a lucent central nidus surrounded by thickened cortical bone on plain radiographs. These primary bone tumors most frequently occur in adolescent and young adult males. When they occur in the spine the posterior elements are usually involved.[142] Nocturnal pain is a common presentation of osteoid osteomas. Pain from osteoid osteomas is relieved by aspirin and is not necessarily activity-specific, whereas pain from stress fractures is activity related and often relieved completely by rest. Looser zones of osteomalacia are the radiographic manifestation of incompletely mineralized insufficiency fractures, which are generally seen in adults with concurrent findings of decreased mineralization, fractures, bowing of long bones, and characteristic spinal findings.[6] The axillary borders of the scapulae, femoral necks, and pubic rami constitute the most common areas of bilateral looser zones. Diffuse sclerosis without central lucency, and little change on serial radiographs characterize the radiographic findings of chronic sclerosing osteomyelitis. The radiographic appearance of osteogenic sarcomas includes aggressive periosteal reaction with spiculation, lamination and occasional Codman triangles, and a lytic component characterized by permeative, patchy destruction. These lesions are usually found in the metaphases of long bones.

Fatigue fractures along the soleal line of the posteromedial cortex of the proximal tibia in particular may be difficult to distinguish from malignant sarcomas, especially when historical risk factors for fatigue injury is equivocal; plain radiographs, bone scans, and computed tomography is useful in distinguishing between these two entities.[143] Stress induced changes can appear radiographically as osteochondromalike lesions.[144] Stress fractures, manifesting radiologically as symptomatic unilamellar periosteal appositions, highlight the importance of using multiple imaging techniques in distinguishing the periosteal reaction of tumors from stress fractures.[145]

Scintigraphy

Conventional radiography and bone scans form the cornerstone of diagnostic imaging for stress fractures in the pediatric and adolescent patient.[6] A focally abnormal scintigram, in the proper clinical setting, establishes the diagnosis of stress fracture, even in the presence of negative radiographs.[79] Rosen and colleagues,[60] in a review of 25 athletic patients aged 11 to 19, with an average age of 16, found 67 percent with scintigraphic abnormalities in the tibia and 25 percent involving the femur, and further concluded that extensive scintigraphic imaging of the pediatric patient with stress-related complaints essential to prevent potential permanent or prolonged disability from complete or displaced fracture.

Nuclear medicine skeletal imaging gains its sensitivity in evaluating skeletal and muscle abnormalities by detecting minor changes in metabolism and blood flow. Specificity and the ability to make an appropriate differential diagnosis is physician-dependent.[22] Nuclear medicine imaging techniques can be used to differentiate acute muscle injury, tibial stress syndrome, skeletal injury, periosteal reaction, stress fracture, traumatic fracture, joint abnormalities, connective tissue abnormalities, compartment syndrome and enthesopathy. Narrowing the differential may be assisted by performing procedure within a few days of the injury.

Using the classic methods of physical diagnosis in evaluating hip pain are the key to arriving at the diagnosis of stress fractures about the hip, but radiographic studies and particularly bone scans are necessary for confirmation.[146] Ammann and colleagues[24] in a series of 51 patients with hip pain and clinical suspicion of stress injury, demonstrated that stress abnormalities of the proximal femur, especially of the lesser trochanter, were depicted with greater clarity using a frog-leg view versus the standard anterior view.

A diagnostic delay averaging 3.5 months was observed in a large series of stress fractures complicated by nonunion and delayed union; isotope scans along with plain radiographs, tomography, and special radiographic views were used in the diagnosis of these fractures.[35] Bone scans are more sensitive than radiographs in detecting stress fracture of the medial malleolus.[71] Conventional radiology will frequently fail to reveal the cause of pain in dancers, and confirms the usefulness of scintigraphy in identifying stress fractures in this population.[147]

Scintigraphy requires the use of a radioactive label, and is time-consuming and expensive. Thermography combined with ultrasound-induced pain as a means of detecting the damaged periosteum in early stress fractures has been described.[148] Ultrasound-induced pain was found to be effective in detecting the damaged periosteum in early stress fractures.[133] Scintigraphy is clearly established as the most sensitive diagnostic tool for detecting bone stress injury, as well as the most widely accepted standard for detecting stress fractures in children and adolescents.

Magnetic Resonance Imaging

Magnetic resonance imaging (MRI) is proving useful in the detection of stress fractures.[149,150] It is more sensitive than radiography in the detection of stress fractures and shows characteristic changes earlier. MRI shows band like areas of very low signal intensity in the intramedullary space, continuous with cortex, at sites of stress fracture or new bone formation on radiographs. T1-weighted images show surrounding areas of decreased signal intensity in the marrow.[150]

MRI allowed distinction between an atypical healed stress fracture of the fibula that appeared via other imaging techniques to be chronic osteomyelitis.[151] MRI findings may prove useful in distinguishing between stress fractures and occult intraosseous fractures,[150] as illustrated in the case of a young gymnast with an occult tibial fracture.[152] MRI has also detected (the unusual) stress fracture missed by scintigraphy.[153]

MRI may be particularly useful in the pediatric population as it involves no ionizing radiation, is very sensitive in detecting stress fractures, and offers reliable differentiation from bone tumors. Unusual clinical courses may find its application essential when radiologic and bone scan diagnosis is equivocal and biopsy is considered.[154]

TREATMENT

Treatment varies with the age of the patient, location, and severity of the fracture. Early stress fractures are treated with relative rest for 2 to 4 weeks and with protective measures, including orthotics, splints, discontinuing the offending activity, or crutches and immobilization when necessary. Because physical stress constitutes the most important factor in modulating stress injury to bone, early cessation of stress forms the cornerstone of treatment and prevents prolongation of the recovery period by allowing bone repair to surpass resorption.[34] Loss of bony integrity mandates immobilization or fixation. Judicial modulation of stress, or "relative rest," in the patient who has not lost bony integrity can allow the motivated athlete to remain active while preventing further injury and promoting healing.[155] The highly motivated or overenthusiastic individual may be a candidate for casting or immobilization with an air cast boot to enforce activity restriction. We have also observed the difficulty in modifying activity-related stress in hyperactive children; these children in particular are candidates for more aggressive preventive intervention to prevent progression of stress fractures.

Correction of overuse injury risk factors is integrated into treatment protocols. Lower extremity malalignment illustrates the continuum between treatment and prevention in bone stress injury. Shock-absorbing insoles are effective in reducing the incidence of overuse injury.[14,156] In military recruits a higher prevalence of tibial and femoral stress fractures is observed in the presence of feet with high arches, and a higher incidence of metatarsal stress fractures in feet with low arches. Orthotics reduced the incidence of femoral stress fractures in recruits with high arches and the incidence of metatarsal fractures in those recruits with low arches, improving the shock absorbing capacity of the arch and reducing stress fractures.[156,157]

Adolescent females may require addressing nutritional factors, hormonal dysfunction, and amenorrhea to provide an optimum environment for stress fracture healing in a comprehensive treatment plan. These factors are emerging with greater frequency as the number of girls involved intense training in gymnastics, skating, and dance expands—and dysfunctional dieting in females starts at an early age.

Prolongation of the healing time for a stress fracture represents a relatively minor complication. Progression to complete fracture is a major complication. The diagnosis and treatment of most stress fractures is straightforward and simple. Several areas, however, merit special consideration because of their potential for prolonged morbidity and progression to complete fracture. Middiaphyseal tibial stress fractures and femoral neck stress fractures are most concerning. Medial malleolar and tarsal navicular stress fractures also represent possible management problems.

Proximal tibial stress fractures are common in children and adolescents and respond readily to conservative management.[14,135] Midshaft anterior tibial stress fractures are relatively uncommon, difficult to treat, prone to nonunion and have a high risk of progression to complete fracture with minimal trauma in the asymptomatic patient.[70] Patients with ununited stress fractures of the midtibia are not to return to athletics until there is definite and complete fracture union.[66] The increased chance of delayed union here can be traced to the subcutaneous location of the tibial cortex and its comparative hypovascularity. Rest and electrical stimulation for 3 to 6 months is recommended prior to surgical intervention.[70] Excision of a fibrous union at the stress fracture site and iliac bone graft is frequently necessary despite prolonged immobilization and augmentation with electromagnetic stimulation.[66]

Diagnostic delay in identifying femoral neck stress fractures can have severe consequences.[39] Exertional groin pain and pain at the extremes of hip movement in the patient who exercises vigorously mandates ruling out femoral neck stress fracture; scintigraphy should be utilized early,[31] despite the relative infrequency of this fracture in a young, healthy population.[158-162] Because of severe potential disability resulting from displaced femoral neck stress fractures, many authors have recommended early stabilization with internal fixating devices, particularly with tension side stress fractures.[39,160] Progression to frank femoral neck fractures with dislocation and subsequent avascular necrosis of the femoral head during the growth period has prompted recommendations for early open reduction and internal fixation because of the tendency for dislocation.[38,63] We have found open reduction and internal fixation rarely necessary at Children's Hospital in Boston, but we have occasionally applied spica casts in patients with projected compliance problems. Scintigraphy has allowed us to identify stress changes in the femoral neck earlier,[60] and subsequently intervene definitively, conservatively, and nonsurgically. Fullerton and Snowdy[31] developed a classification system of femoral neck stress fractures based on radiographic findings and treatment that may also be helpful in some patients with open capital femoral epiphyses.

Open reduction and internal fixation for medial malleolar stress fractures in young athletes is recommended to facilitate early range of motion.[71] Early immobilization, followed by progressive increases in activity are used for athletes with negative radiographs and positive bone scans, with full activity goals to be achieved in 6 to 8 weeks.

Nonunion of conservatively managed stress fractures of the tarsal navicular is not uncommon, and we have had to resort to operative management as have others.[35,163] Operative management is required when the patient remains symptomatic, and when there is separation or complete fracture noted on plain radiographs or computed tomography scan, extension of incomplete fracture, delayed healing, or presence of medullary cysts. Fitch and colleagues[65] recommended autologous bone graft after en bloc resection of the fracture surfaces.

In patients, such as professional dancers, with chronic, recurrent problems or difficult to heal fractures such as the tibial diaphysis, we are using galvanic bone stimulation with very encouraging results. More research is needed to establish guidelines for using bone stimulation in the healing of stress fractures.

CLASSIFICATION

Biomechanical,[162] radiographic,[161] scintigraphy-based,[22] and treatment-based[31] classification systems for femoral neck stress fractures have been proposed. Fullerton and Snowdy's classification involves division into compression-type, tension-type, and displaced femoral neck stress fractures, and practical application of the system via a proposed treatment algorithm.[31] These treatment protocols may not necessarily apply to the pediatric population, as consideration for open capital femoral epiphyses must be in the treatment protocol for the growing patient. It is most important to recognize that biomechanical forces on the tension side of the femoral neck are conducive to progression and displacement of a fracture in this area,[164] and that femoral neck fractures have a high degree of associated morbidity and protracted disability.

SUMMARY

Stress fractures are an important consideration in the differential diagnosis of extremity pain in the athletically active child or adolescent. The history and physical examination are most important in narrowing the differential diagnosis and ruling out tumor or infection, and are most effectively augmented by plain radiography and scintigraphy. Recognition of risk factors for stress-induced bone injury and understanding of activity-specific stressors allows integration of treatment protocols into preventive maintenance programs.

REFERENCES

1. Devas MB: Stress fractures in children. J Bone Joint Surg [Br] 45:528, 1963
2. Breithaupt ZVR: Pathologie monschuchew Fusser. Med Z 24:169, 1855
3. O'Neill DB, Micheli LJ: Overuse injuries in the young athlete. Clin Sports Med 7:591, 1988
4. Markey KL: Stress fractures. Clin Sports Med 6:405, 1987
5. Pentecost RL: Fatigue, insufficiency and pathologic fractures. JAMA 187:1001, 1964
6. Mandell GA, Harcke TH, Kumar JS: Stress fractures. p. 201. In Kricun ME (ed): Imaging strategies in pediatric orthopaedics. Aspen Publishers, Gaithersburg, MD, 1990
7. Warren MP, Brooks-Gunn J, Hamilton LH et al: Scoliosis and fractures in young ballet dancers: relation to delayed menarche and secondary amenorrhea. N Engl J Med 314:1348, 1986
8. Lindberg JS, Fears WB, Hunt MM et al: Exercise induced amenorrhea and bone density. Ann Intern Med 101:647, 1984
9. Marcus R, Cann C, Madvig P et al: Menstrual function and bone mass in elite women distance runners: endocrine and metabolic features. Ann Intern Med 102:158, 1985
10. Barrow GW, Saha S: Menstrual irregularity and stress fractures in collegiate female distance runners. Am J Sports Med 16:209, 1988
11. Olson BR: Exercised-induced amenorrhea. Am Family Physician 39:213, 1989
12. Giladi M, Milgrom C, Simkin A et al: Stress fractures and tibial bone width: a risk factor. J Bone Joint Surg [Br] 69:326, 1987
13. Stanish WD: Overuse injuries in athletes: a perspective. Med Sci Sports Exerc 16:1, 1984
14. Micheli LJ: Overuse injuries in children. p. 1103. In Lovell WW, Winter RB (eds): Pediatric Orthopedics. 2nd Ed. JB Lippincott, Philadelphia, 1986
15. Renstrom P, Johnson RJ: Overuse injuries in sports: a review. Sports Med 2:316, 1985
16. Micheli LJ: Sports injuries in the young athlete: questions and controversies. p. 1. In Micheli LJ (ed): Pediatric and Adolescent Sports Medicine. Little, Brown, Boston, 1984
17. Devas MB: Stress fractures in children. J Bone Joint Surg [Br] 45:528, 1963
18. Griffiths AL: Fatigue fracture of the fibula in childhood. Arch Dis Childhood 27:552, 1952
19. Berkebile RD: Stress fracture of the tibia in children. AJR 91:588, 1964
20. Zweymuller K, Frank W: Ermudungsbruche der Tibial im Kindesalter. Z Orthop 112:450, 1974
21. Torg JS, Pavlov H, Torg E: Overuse injuries in sport: the foot. Clin Sports Med 6:291, 1987
22. Matin P: Basic principles of nuclear medicine techniques for detection and evaluation of trauma and sports medicine injuries. Semin Nucl Med 18:90, 1988
23. Aspegren D, Cox JM, Benak DR: Detection of stress fractures in athletes and nonathletes. J Manipulative Physiol Ther 12:298, 1989
24. Ammann W, Matzinger J, Lloyd-Smith DR, Cohen PF, Clement DB: Femoral stress abnormalities: improved scintigraphic detection with frog-leg view. Radiology 169:844, 1988
25. Ha IK, Hahn SH, Chung M et al: A clinical study of stress fractures in sports activities. Othopedics 14:1089, 1991
26. Williams KE: The uniqueness of the young athlete: musculoskeletal injuries. Am J Sports Med 8:377, 1980
27. McBryde AM Jr: Stress fractures in athletes. J Sports Med 3:212, 1975
28. Protzman RR, Griffis CG: Stress fractures in men and women undergoing military training. J Bone Joint Surg [Am] 59:825, 1977
29. Zahger D, Abramovitz A, Zelikovsky L et al: Stress fractures in female soldiers: an epidemiological investigation of an outbreak. Milit Med 153:448, 1988
30. Miller GJ, Purkey WW Jr: The geometric properties of paired human tibiae. J Biomech 13:1, 1983
31. Fullerton LR Jr, Snowdy HA: Femoral neck stress fractures. Am J Sports Med 16:365, 1988
32. Brudvig TJ, Gudger TD, Obermeyer L: Stress fractures in 295 trainees: a one-year study of the incidence as related to age, sex, and race. Milit Med 148:666, 1983
33. Orava S, Puranen J, Ala-Ketola L: Stress fractures caused by physical exercise. Acta Orthop Scand 49:19, 1978
34. Stanitski CL, McMaster JH, Scranton PE: On the nature of stress fractures. Am J Sports Med 6:391, 1978
35. Orava S, Hulkko A: Delayed unions and nonunions of stress fractures in athletes. Am J Sports Med 16:378, 1988
36. Devas M: Stress Fractures. Churchill Livingstone, Edinburgh, 1975
37. Ogden JA: Skeletal Injury in the Child. Lea & Febiger, Philadelphia, 1982
38. King RE: Special problems of femoral neck fractures in adolescents and young adults. Hip 62, 1983
39. Johansson C, Ekenman I, To:rnkvist H et al: Stress fractures of the femoral neck in athletes: the consequence of a delay in diagnosis. Am J Sports Med 18:524, 1990
40. Blank S: Transverse tibial stress fractures: a special problem. Am J Sports Med 15:597, 1987
41. Canale ST: Fractures of the hip in children and adolescents. Orthop Clin North Am 21:341, 1990
42. Canale ST, Bourland W: Fracture of the neck and intertrochanteric region of the femur in children. J Bone Joint Surg [Am] 59:431, 1977
43. Coldwell D, Gross GW, Boal DK: Stress fracture of the femoral neck in a child. Pediatr Radiol 14:17, 1984
44. Friendenberg ZB: Fatigue fractures of the tibia. Clin Orthop 76:111, 1971

45. Hoang TA, Nguyen TH, Daffner RH et al: Case report 491: stress fracture of the right sacrum. Skelet Radiol 17:364, 1988
46. Volpin G, Milgrom C, Goldsher D et al: Stress fractures of the sacrum following strenuous activity. Clin Orthop 243:84, 1989
47. Carter SR: Stress fracture of the sacrum: brief report. J Bone Joint Surg [Br] 69:843, 1987
48. Pavlov H, Nelson TL, Warren RF et al: Stress fractures of the pubic ramus. J Bone Joint Surg [Am] 64:1982
49. Tehranzadeh J, Kurth LA, Elyaderani MK et al: Comboned pelvic stress fracture and avulsion of the adductor longus in a middle-distance runner: a case report. Am J Sports Med 10:108, 1982
50. Devas MB. Stress fractures of the patella. J Bone Joint Surg [Br] 42:71, 1960
51. Schranz PJ: Stress fracture of the patella. [Letter]. Br J Sports Med 1988 22:169, 1988
52. Jerosch JG, Castro WH, Jantea C: Stress fracture of the patella. Am J Sports Med 17:579, 1989
53. Devas MB, Sweetnam R: Stress fractures of the fibula: a review of fifty cases in athletes. J Bone Joint Surg 38:818, 1956
54. Blair WF, Hanley SR: Stress fracture of the proximal fibula. Am J Sports Med 8:212, 1980
55. Bindl G, Holz U: Fatigue fracture of the femoral neck in a recreational runner: a case report. Sportverletz Sportschaden 3:30, 1989
56. Meurman KO, Somer K, Lamminen A: Stress fractures of the femora of soldiers. ROFO 134:528, 1981
57. Lombardo SJ, Benson DW: Stress fractures of the femur in runners. Am J Sports Med 10:219, 1982
58. Luchini MA, Sarokhan AJ, Micheli LJ: Acute displaced femoral-shaft fractures in long-distance runners: two case reports. J Bone Joint Surg [Am] 65:1983
59. Wolfgang GL: Stress fracture of the femoral neck in a patient with open capital femoral epiphysis, a case report. J Bone Joint Surg [Am] 59:680, 1977
60. Rosen PR, Micheli LJ, Treves S: Early scintigraphic diagnosis of bone stress and fractures in athletic adolescents. Pediatrics 70:11, 1982
61. Schneider HJ, King AY, Bronson JL et al: Stress injuries and developmental change of lower extremities in ballet dancers. Radiology 113:627, 1974
62. Miller F, Wenger DR: Femoral neck stress fracture in a hyperactive child. J Bone Joint Surg [Am] 61:435, 1979
63. Kujat R, Suren EG, Rogge D, Twcherne H: Femoral neck fractures during the growth period: treatment principles, results, prognosis. Chirurg 55:43, 1984
64. Weber PC: Salter-Harris type II stress fracture in a young athlete: a case report. Orthopedics 11:309, 1982
65. Butler JE, Brown LS, McConnell BG: Subtrochanteric stress fractures in runners. Am J Sports Med 10:228, 1982
66. Green E, Rogers RA, Lipscomb BA: Nonunions of stress fractures of the tibia. Am J Sports Med 13:171, 1985
67. Brahms MA, Fumich RM, Ippolito VD: Atypical stress fracture of the tibia in a professional athlete. Am J Sports Med 8:131, 1980
68. Burrows HJ: Fatigue infraction of the middle of the tibia in ballet dancers. J Bone Joint Surg [Br] 38:83, 1956
69. Orava S, Hulkko A: Stress fracture of the mid-tibial shaft. Acta Orthop Scand 55:35, 1984
70. Rettig AC, Shelbourne DK, McCarroll JR et al: The natural history and treatment of delayed union stress fractures of the anterior cortex of the tibia. Am J Sports Med 16:250, 1988
71. Shelbourne KD, Fisher DA, Rettig AC et al: Stress fractures of the medial malleolus. Am J Sports Med 16:60, 1988
72. Orava S: Stress fractures. Br J Sports Med 14:40, 1980
73. Childress HM: March foot in a seven-year-old child. J Bone Joint Surg 28:1946
74. Zeitlin AA, Odessky IN: "Pied force" of Deutschlander's disease. Radiology 25:215, 935
75. Gross TS, Bunch RP: A mechanical model of metatarsal stress fracture during distance running. Am J Sports Med 17:669, 1989
76. Drez D, Young JC, Johnston RD et al: Metatarsal stress fractures. Am J Sports Med 8:123, 1980
77. Kitaoka HB, Cracchiolo A: Stress fracture of the lateral metatarsals following double-stem silicone implant arthroplasty of the hallux metatarsophalangeal joint. Clin Orthop 239:211, 1989
78. Ihmeidan IH, Tehranzadeh J, Oldham SA et al: Case report 443: florid cortical and periosteal reactions due to stress fractures of the right femur and left calcaneus in a "break dancer." Skelet Radiol 6:581, 1987
79. Greaney RB, Gerber FH, Laughlin RL et al: distribution and natural history of stress fractures in U.S. Marine recruits. Radiology 146:339, 1983
80. Leabhart JW: Stress fractures of the calcaneus. J Bone Joint Surg [Am] 41:1285, 1959
81. Jones P: Fatigue failure osteochondral fracture of the proximal phalanx of the great toe. Am J Sports Med 15:616, 1987
82. Ting A, King W, Yocum L, Antonelli D et al: Stress fractures of the tarsal navicular in long-distance runners. Clin Sports Med 7:89, 1988
83. Ehara S, el-Khoury GY: Bilateral stress fracture of the navicular in a non-athlete. Radiat Med 6:259, 1988
84. Hamilton WG: Foot and ankle injuries in dancers. Clin Sports Med 7:143, 1988
85. Micheli LJ, Sohn RS, Solomon R: Stress fractures of the second metatarsal involving Lisfranc's joint in ballet dancers: a new overuse injury of the foot. J Bone Joint Surg [Am] 67:1372, 1985
86. Markolf KL, Shapiro MS, Mandlebaum BR et al: Wrist loading patterns during pommell horse exercises. J Biomech 23:1001, 1990
87. Hanks GA, Kalenak A, Bowman LS et al: Stress fractures

87. of the carpal scaphoid: a report of four cases. J Bone Joint Surg [Am] 71:938, 1989
88. Carter SR, Aldridge MJ, Fitzgerald R et al: Stress changes of the wrist in adolescent gymnasts. Br J Radiol 61:109, 1988
89. Brogdon BJ, Crow NE: Little Leaguer's elbow. Am J Radiol 83:671, 1960
90. Pappas AM: Elbow problems associated with baseball during childhood and adolescence. Clin Orthop 164:30, 1982
91. Dehaven KE, Evarts CM: Throwing injuries of the elbow in athletes. Orthop Clin North Am 4:801, 1973
92. Pavlov H, Torg JS, Jacobs B et al: Non-union of olecranon epiphysis: two cases in adolescent baseball pitchers. Am J Radiol 136:819, 1981
93. Torg JS, Moyer RA: Non-union of a stress fracture through the olecranon epiphyseal plate observed in an adolescent baseball pitcher. J Bone Joint Surg [Am] 59:264, 1977
94. Tullos H, Fain R: Little league shoulder: rotational stress fracture of the proximal epiphysis. J Sports Med Phys Fitness 2:152, 1974
95. Evans DL: Fatigue fractures of the ulna. J Bone Joint Surg [Br] 37:618, 1955
96. Rettig AC: Stress fracture of the ulna in an adolescent tournament tennis player. Am J Sports Med 11:103, 1983
97. Hamilton KH: Stress fracture of the diaphysis of the ulna in a body builder. Am J Sports Med 12:405, 1984
98. Mutoh Y, Mori T, Suzuki Y et al: Stress fractures of the ulna in athletes. Am J Sports Med 10:365, 1982
99. Veluvolu P, Kohn HS, Guten GN et al: Unusual stress fracture of the scapula in a jogger. Clin Nucl Med 13:531, 1988
100. Dust WN, Lenczner EM: Stress fracture of the clavicle leading to nonunion secondary to coracoclavicular reconstruction with Dacron. Am J Sports Med 17:128, 1989
101. Murakami YT: Stress fracture of the metacarpal in a adolescent tennis player. Am J Sports Med 16:419, 1988
102. Fakharzadeh FF: Stress fracture of the finger in a bowler. J Hand Surg [Am] 14:241, 1989
103. Cyron BM, Hutton WC: The fatigue strength of the lumbar neural arch in spondylolysis. J Bone Joint Surg [Br] 60:234, 1978
104. Lamy, Clifford, Bazergui A et al: The strength of the neural arch and the etiology of spondylolysis. Orthop Clin North Am 6:215, 1975
105. Farfan HF, Osteria V, Lamy C: The mechanical etiology of spondylolysis and spondylolisthesis. Clin Orthop 117:40, 1976
106. Ireland L, Micheli LJ: Bilateral stress fracture of the lumbar pedicles in a ballet dancer: a case report. J Bone Joint Surg [Am] 69:140, 1987
107. Keating TM: Stress fracture of the sternum in a wrestler. Am J Sports Med 15:92, 1987
108. Powell RI: Fracture of the first rib: its occurrence and clinical diagnosis. Br Med J 1:282, 1950
109. Jenkins SA: Spontaneous fractures of both first ribs. J Bone Joint Surg [Br] 34:9, 1952
110. Curran JP, Kelly DA: Stress fractures of the first rib. Am J Orthop 8:16, 1966
111. Rademaker M, Redmond AD, Barker PV: Stress fracture of the first rib. Thorax 38:312, 1983
112. Sacchetti AD, Beswick DR, Norse SD: Rebound rib: stress induced first rib fracture. Am Emerg Med 12:177, 1983
113. Holden DL, Jackson DW: Stress fracture of the ribs in female rowers. Am J Sports Med 13:342, 1985
114. McKenzie DC: Stress fracture of the rib in an elite oarsman. Int J Sports Med 10:220, 1989
115. Devas MB: Stress fractures in athletes. Proc R Soc Med 62:933, 1969
116. Rassad S: Golfer's fractures of the ribs: report of three cases. AJR 120:901, 1974
117. Gurtler R, Pavlov H, Torg JS: Stress fracture of the ipsilateral first rib in a pitcher. Am J Sports Med 13:266, 1985
118. Brooke R: Jive fractures of the first rib. J Bone Joint Surg 41B:370, 1959
119. Derbes VJ, Harran T: Rib fracture from muscular effort with particular reference to cough. Surgery 35:294, 1954
120. Horner DB: Lumbar back pain arising from stress fractures of the lower ribs. J Bone Joint Surg [Br] 34:9, 1952
121. Forwood MR, Parker AW: Microdamage in response to repetitive torsional loading in the rat tibia. Calcif Tissue Int 45:47, 1989
122. Li G, Shang S, Chen G, Chen H et al: Radiographic and histologic analyses of stress fracture in rabbit tibias. Am J Sports Med 13:285, 1985
123. Wendelburg K, Dee J, Kaderly R, Dee L, Eaton-Wells R: Stress fractures of the acetabulum in 26 racing greyhounds. Vet Surg 17:128, 1988
124. Koblik PD, Hornof WJ, Seeherman HJ: Scintigraphic appearance of stress-induced trauma of the dorsal cortex of the third metacarpal bone in racing thoroughbred horses: 121 cases (1978–1986). J Am Vet Med Assoc 192:390, 1988
125. Baker J, Frankel VH: Fatigue fractures: biomechanical considerations. J Bone Joint Surg [Am] 54:1972
126. Skinner HB, Cook SD: Fatigue failure stress of the femoral neck: a case report. Am J Sports Med 10:245, 1982
127. Paty JG Jr: Diagnosis and treatment of musculoskeletal running injuries. Semin Arthritis Rheum 18:48, 1988
128. Giladi M, Milgrom C, Simkin A et al: Stress fractures: identifiable risk factors. Am J Sports Med 19:647, 1991
129. Pouilles JM, Bernard J, Tremolli:eres F et al: Femoral bone density in young male adults with stress fractures. Bone 10:105, 1989
130. Lysens RJ, Ostyn MS, Vanden Auweele Y et al: The accident-prone and overuse-prone profiles of the young athlete. Am J Sports Med 17:612, 1989

131. Swissa A, Milgrom C, Giladi M et al: The effect of pre-training sports activity on the incidence of stress fractures among military recruits: a prospective study. Clin Orthop Rel Res 245:256, 1989
132. Mustajoki P, Laapio H, Meurman K: Calcium metabolism, physical activity and stress fractures. Lancet 2:797, 1983
133. Moss A, Mowat AG: Ultrasonic assessment of stress fractures. Br Med J 286:1479, 1983
134. Engh CA: Stress fractures in children. J Trauma 10:532, 1970
135. Walter NE, Wolf MDP: Stress fractures in young athletes. Am J Sports Med 5:165, 1977
136. North AF Jr: Bilateral symmetrical march fractures simulating juvenile rheumatoid arthritis. Arthritis Rheum 9:77, 1966
137. Jerosch J, Jantea C, Geske B: Osteomalacia and fatigue fractures in celiac disease. Rheumatology 49:100, 1990
138. Harper MC: metabolic bone disease presenting as multiple recurrent metatarsal fractures: a case report. Foot Ankle 9:207, 1989
139. Volpin G, Petronius G, Hoerer D et al: Lower limb pain and disability following strenuous activity. Milit Med 154:294, 1989
140. Prather JL, Nusynowitz ML, Snowdy HA et al: Scintigraphic findings in stress fractures. J Bone Joint Surg 59:869, 1977
141. Daffner RH: Stress fractures: current concepts. Skelet Radiol 2:221, 1978
142. Cacayorin E, Hochlauser L, Petro GR: Lumbar and thoracic spine pain in the athlete: radiographic evaluation. Clin Sports Med 6:767, 1987
143. Davies AM, Evans N, Grimer RJ: Fatigue fractures of the proximal tibia simulating malignancy. Br J Radiol 61:903, 1988
144. Ballmer PE, Bessler WT: Case report 495: osteochondroma-like femoral lesions due to chronic professional stress in a Swiss cheese-maker. Skelet Radiol 17:382, 1988
145. Arrive L, Sellier N, Kalifa G et al: Diagnostic difficulties of isolated symptomatic unilamellar periosteal appositions: uncommon form of fatigue fracture in children. J Radiol 69:351, 1988
146. McBeath AA: Some common causes of hip pain: physical diagnosis is the key. Postgrad Med 77:189, 194, 198, 1985
147. Grahame R, Saunders AS, Maisey M: The use of scintigraphy in the diagnosis and management of traumatic lesions in ballet dancers. Rheum Rehab 18:235, 1979
148. Devereaux MD, Parr GR, Lachman SM et al: The diagnosis of stress fractures in athletes. JAMA 252:531, 1984
149. Mink JH, Deutsch AL: Occult cartilage and bone injuries of the knee: detection, classification, and assessment with MR imaging. Radiology 170:823, 1989
150. Lee JK, Yao L: Stress fractures: MR imaging. Radiology 169:217, 1988
151. Castillo M, Tehranzadeh J, Morillo G: Atypical healed stress fracture of the fibula masquerading as chronic osteomyelitis: a case report of magnetic resonance distinction. Am J Sports Med 16:185, 1988
152. Burks RT, Lock JR, Negendank WG: Occult tibial fracture in a gymnast: diagnosis by magnetic resonance imaging: a case report. Am J Sports Med 20:88, 1992
153. Keene JS, Lash EG: Negative bone scan in a femoral neck stress fracture: a case report. Am J Sports Med 20:234, 1992
154. Yousry T, Fink U, Breitner S et al: Magnetic resonance tomographic studies of stress fractures. Digitale Bilddiagn 9:69, 1989
155. Micheli LJ, Santopietro F, Gerbino P et al: Etiologic assessment of overuse stress fractures in athletes. Nova Scotia Med Bull 43:1980
156. Schwellnus MP, Jordaan G, Noakes TD: Prevention of common overuse injuries by the use of shock absorbing insoles: a prospective study. Am J Sports Med 18:636, 1990
157. Simkin A, Leichter I, Giladi M et al: Combined effect of foot arch structure and an orthotic device on stress fractures. Foot Ankle 10:25, 1989
158. Steinmuller L: Stress fracture of the femoral neck in a marathon runner: case report and review of the literature. Unfallchirurg 92:21, 1989
159. Kaltsas DS: Stress fractures of the femoral neck in young adults, a report of seven cases. J Bone Joint Surg [Br] 63:33, 1981
160. Volpin G, Hoerer D, Zaltzman S et al: Stress fractures of the femoral neck following strenuous activity. J Orthop Trauma 4:394, 1990
161. Blickenstaff LD, Morris JM: Fatigue fracture of the femoral neck. J Bone Joint Surg [Am] 48:1031, 1966
162. Devas MB: Stress fractures of the femoral neck. J Bone Joint Surg [Br] 47:728, 1965
163. Fitch KD, Blackwell JB, Gilmour WN: Operation for non-union of stress fracture of the tarsal navicular. J Bone Joint Surg [Br] 71:105, 1989
164. Black J: Failure of implants for internal hip fixation. Orthop Clin North Am 5:833, 1974

54

Avulsion Fractures

Jacques D'Astous

More is missed by not looking than by not knowing.

DEFINITION

The word avulsion comes from the latin *a*, which means "from," and *vellere,* which means "to pull." Avulsion injuries occur as a result of a traction force from muscle, tendon, or ligament on a bony insertion resulting in pulling away of a fragment of bone or apophysiolysis. These fractures are more common in children because of the presence of numerous apophyses not present in the mature skeleton. An apophysis can be defined as a bony prominence associated with an attachment of muscle or tendon connected to bone through a physeal plate. An apophysis does not contribute to longitudinal growth of the bone, hence an apophyseal growth arrest does not result in limb length inequality. Injury to the apophysis may, however, result in an alteration of the "contour" of the bone from either over or under growth.

Anatomy

Histologically, Sharpey's fibers at the bone tendon interface constitute an extremely strong muscle and tendon attachment to bone. Sharpey's fibers are intraosseous extensions of the collagen between the tendon or ligament and cortical bone. In adults, there is a tendency to avulse at the soft tissue/bone interface, while in children one usually sees cartilaginous or osseous failure.

For this reason, an injury that would lead to a cruciate ligament disruption or tearing in an adult would result in an avulsion of the tibial spine in a child.

Histologically, a traction physis is similar to pressure physis with the following differences: there is an increased number of longitudinal collagen fibers to help withstand traction forces and there is a decreased thickness of the proliferative layer with a slower rate of growth.[1] In certain instances, the thick periosteum can be completely avulsed off the bone such as one encounters in a sleeve fracture of the patella[2] (Fig. 54-1).

MECHANISM OF INJURY

Apophyseal injuries usually are the result of a substantial muscle/tendon/ligament pull such as occurs in landing from a jump, bracing from a fall, or tripping. This pull creates a traction force that is transmitted through the muscle/tendon interface to Sharpey's fibers, which insert into the cortical bone. Because the apophyseal growth plate is not as strong in resisting tensile forces as the bone/tendon interface, cleavage occurs through the apophyseal growth plate. The histologic layer of the cleavage plane in the human apophysis has not been documented but is probably similar to the growth plate fracture, that is, through the layer of hypertrophic cells.

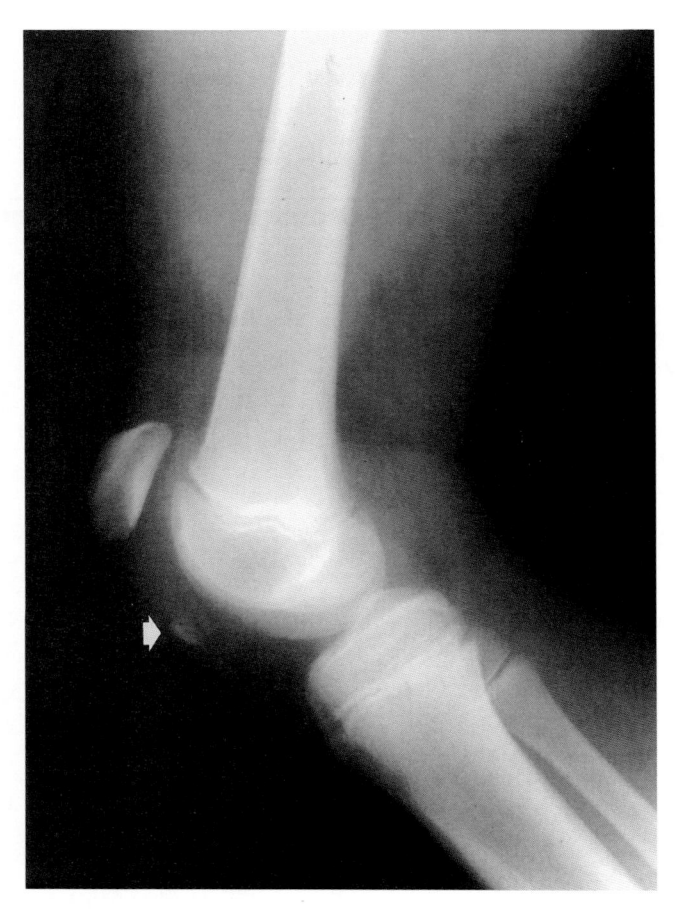

Fig. 54-1. Sleeve fracture of the patella in a 7-year-old boy who landed hard after jumping over a fence. This patient required an open reduction and internal fixation of his patellar fracture with a tension band and a repair of his extensor retinaculum.

CLASSIFICATION

Avulsion fractures may be classified biomechanically as shown in Table 54-1 or according to anatomic regions as illustrated in Table 54-2.

TREATMENT OF AVULSION FRACTURES

Nondisplaced avulsion fractures may be treated by simple immobilization and rest for a period of 2 to 3 weeks followed by progressive mobilization and resumption of activities.

The treatment of displaced fractures varies as to whether or not the displacement is minimal or if there is significant displacement. If the displacement is minimal, that is, less than 1 cm or if the fragment is not intra-articular, the treatment consists of simple immobilization or rest (Figs. 54-2 to 54-4). For those fractures that are significantly displaced or intra-articular, open reduction and internal fixation are indicated. Examples of fractures requiring open reduction and internal fixation are displaced fractures of the olecranon (Fig. 54-5), type III fractures of the tibial spine (Fig. 54-6), avulsion fractures of the tibial tuberosity (Fig. 54-7), and medial epicondyle fractures of the distal humerus with greater than 5 to 10 mm of displacement (Fig. 54-8).

COMPLICATIONS OF AVULSION FRACTURES

Avulsion fractures through an apophysis may lead to premature physeal plate closure. If this occurs in the late teens it is usually of no significance but, if it occurs early in life, there may be significant distortion of the anatomy such as a genu recurvatum following an avulsion fracture of the tibial tuberosity or a coxa valga following an avulsion fracture of the greater trochanter. Other complications are nonunion, which may lead to joint instability, for example, a nonunion of a fractured medial epicondyle of the distal humerus (Fig. 54-9) or a nonunion of an avulsed distal tip of fibula fracture (Fig. 54-10). Malunion, such as a malunited tibial spine fracture, may lead to a decreased range of motion of the knee and in

TABLE 54-1. Biomechanical Classification of Avulsion Fractures in Children

Type	Examples
Failure at the bone-tendon interface	Avulsion of the extensor digitorium longus insertion of the base of the distal phalanx in a mallet finger[3]
Intraosseous failure	Avulsion fracture of tibial spine[4-6]
Transapophyseal failure	Avulsion of ischial tuberosity, anterior inferior iliac spine[7]
Failure at the bone-periosteum interface	Sleeve fractures of the patella and olecranon[2]

TABLE 54-2. Classification of Avulsion Fractures in Children According to Anatomic Site

Site	Fracture
Spine	Endplate avulsions and fractures of the ring apophysis[8]
	Spinous process apophyseal avulsion (i.e., clay shoveller's, Chance fracture)
	Transverse process avulsion (most frequently seen in association with disruptions of the pelvic ring)
Upper extremity	
Scapula	Acromion, coracoid[9,10]
Humerus	Medial epicondyle, lateral epicondyle[11]
Ulna	Olecranon, ulnar styloid, coronoid process[12]
Radius	Radial styloid
Carpus	Trapezium, tuberosity of scaphoid, triquetrum[13,14]
Phalanges	Salter-Harris III fractures of the phalanges (i.e., skier's thumb with Salter-Harris type III fractures of the proximal phalanx and mallet finger with Salter-Harris type III fractures of the distal phalanx)[3]
Lower extremity	
Pelvis	Anterior superior iliac spine, anterior inferior iliac spine, ischium, iliac apophysis[7,15]
Femur	Lesser trochanter, greater trochanter, femoral head[16]
Patella	Sleeve fracture[2]
Tibia	Intercondylar eminence or tibial spine, tibial tuberosity, juvenile Tillaux and tip of the medial malleolus[5,6,17–22]
Fibula	Tip of the lateral malleolus
Tarsal bones	Flake avulsion fractures of the lateral body of the talus, os calcis, and cuboid[23]
Metatarsals	Base of the 5th metatarsal[24,25]
Phalanges	Type III fracture of the proximal phalanx of the great toe

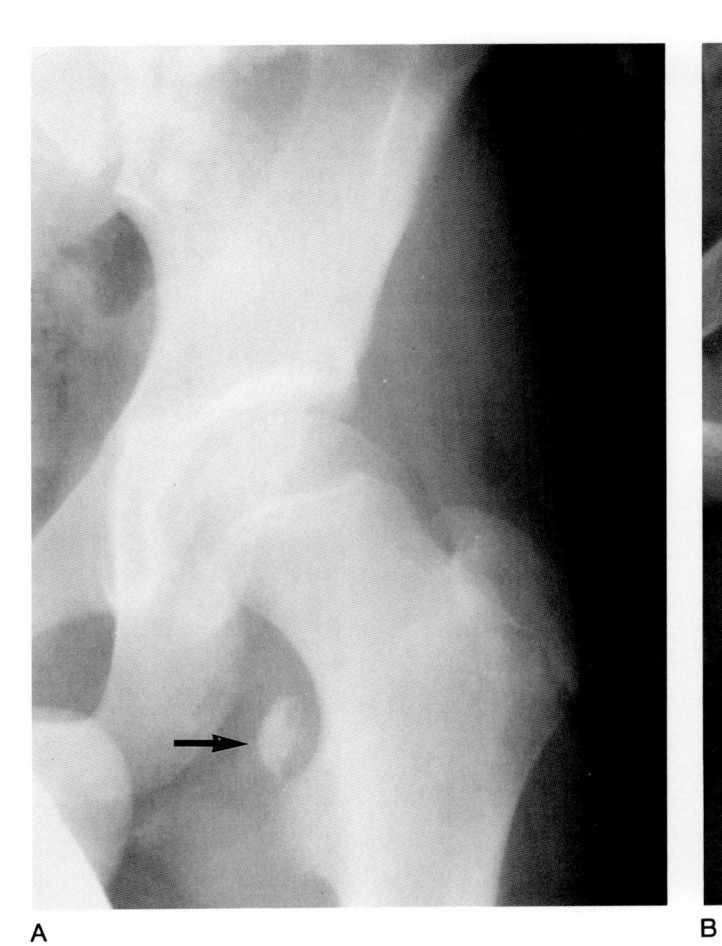

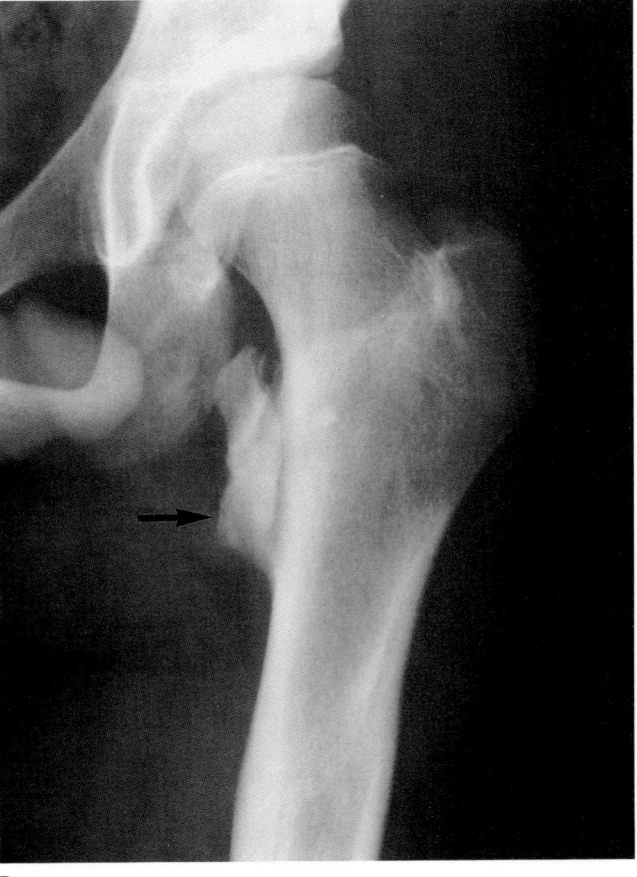

Fig. 54-2. (A) Avulsion fracture of the lesser trochanter by the iliopsoas in a 14-year-old boy, treated by bed rest, crutch walking, and reduced activity. (B) Same patient 4 months later, now asymptomatic. Note the periosteal new bone formation.

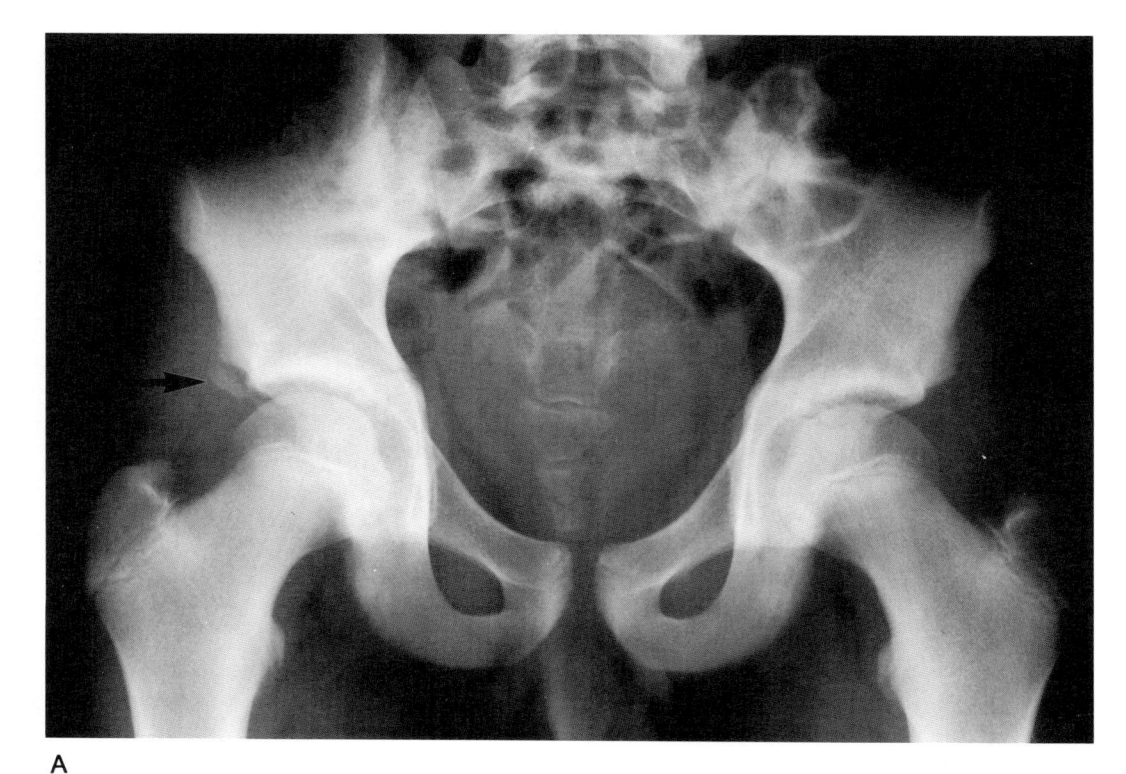

Fig. 54-3. (A) Rectus femoris avulsion fracture of anterior inferior iliac spine in a 12-year-old boy, treated symptomatically with reduced activity. (B) Same patient 1 month later. Note the periosteal new bone formation.

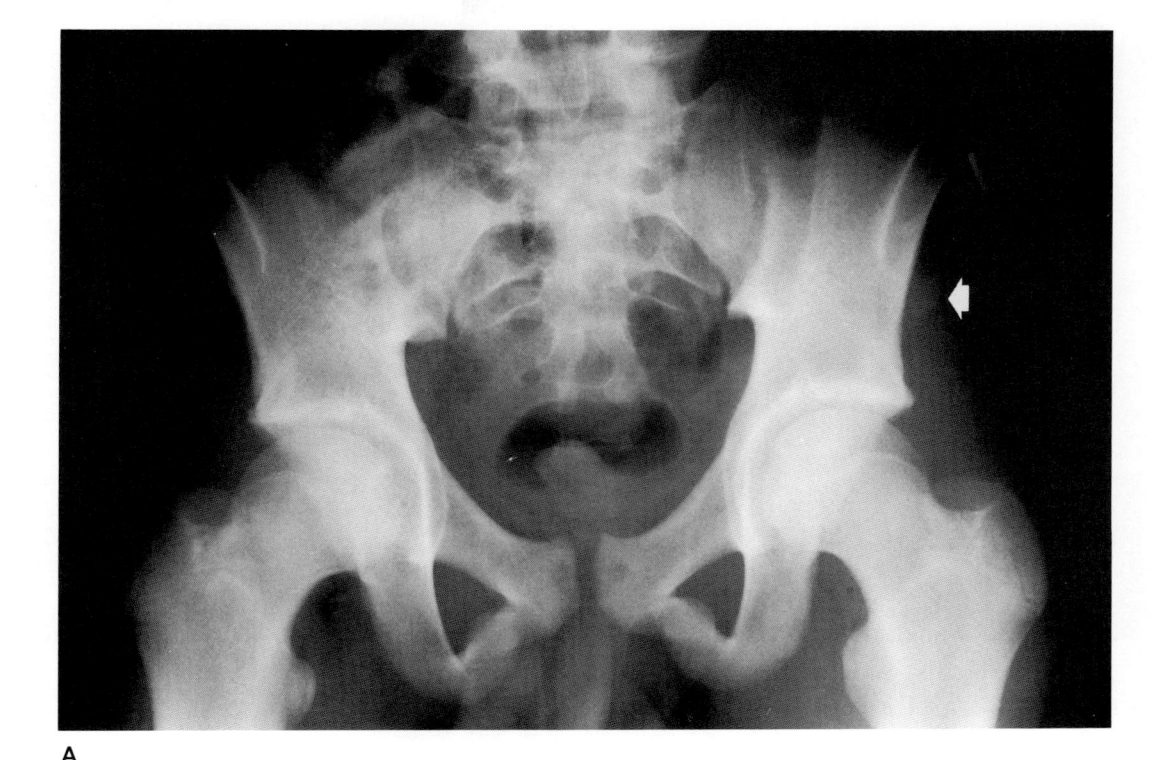

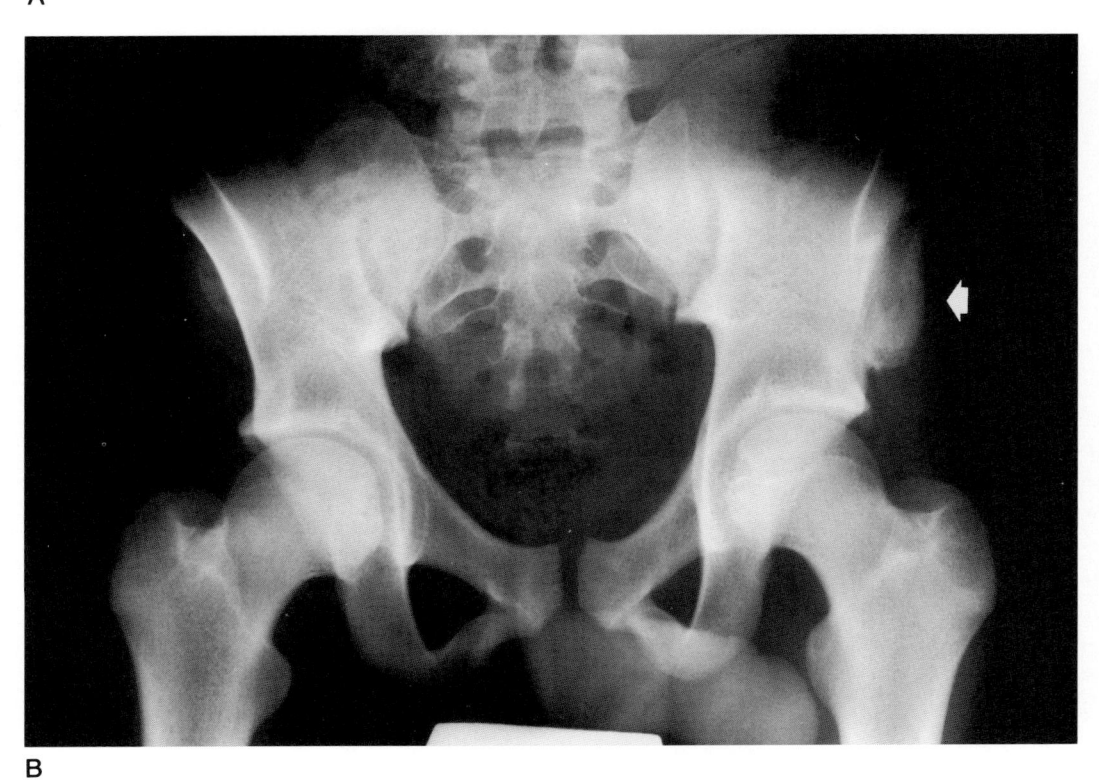

Fig. 54-4. (A) Avulsion fracture of anterior superior iliac spine in a 14-year-old track athlete by the sartorius attachment. (B) Same patient one year later. Note the abundant periosteal new bone on the left and a new fracture of the right anterior superior iliac spine!

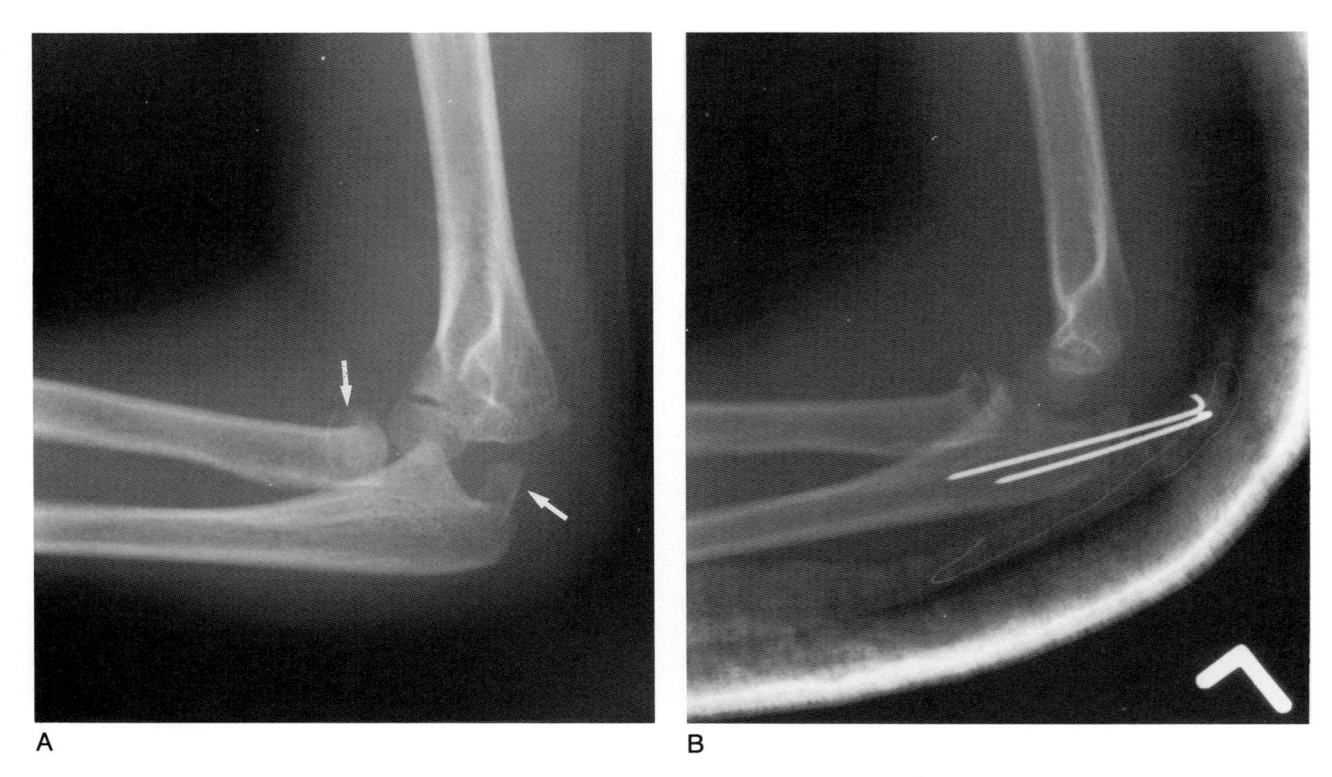

Fig. 54-5. **(A)** Avulsion of olecranon plus a fracture of the radial neck in a 7-year-old girl who fell off a slide. **(B)** Post closed reduction of the radial neck and open reduction with K-wire fixation of the avulsed olecranon fragment.

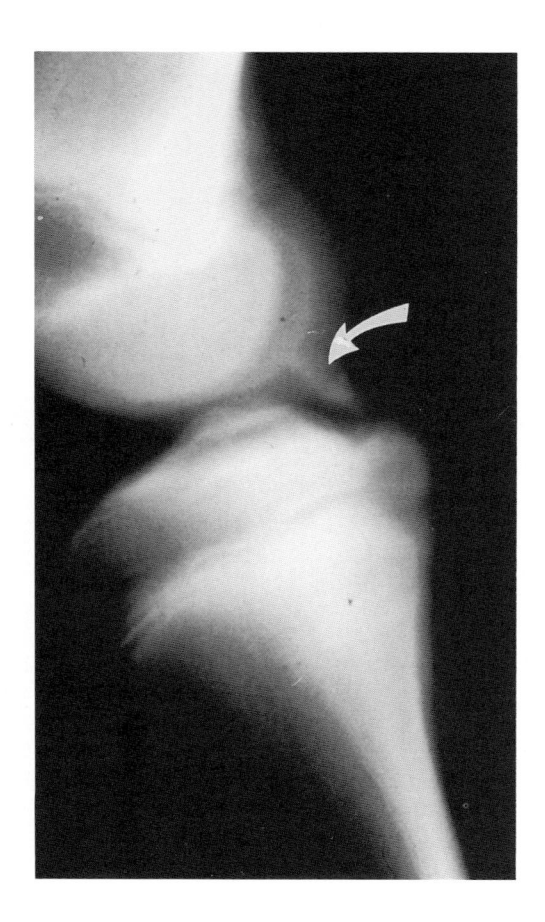

Fig. 54-6. Avulsion of the posterior tibial spine by the attachment of the posterior cruciate ligament.

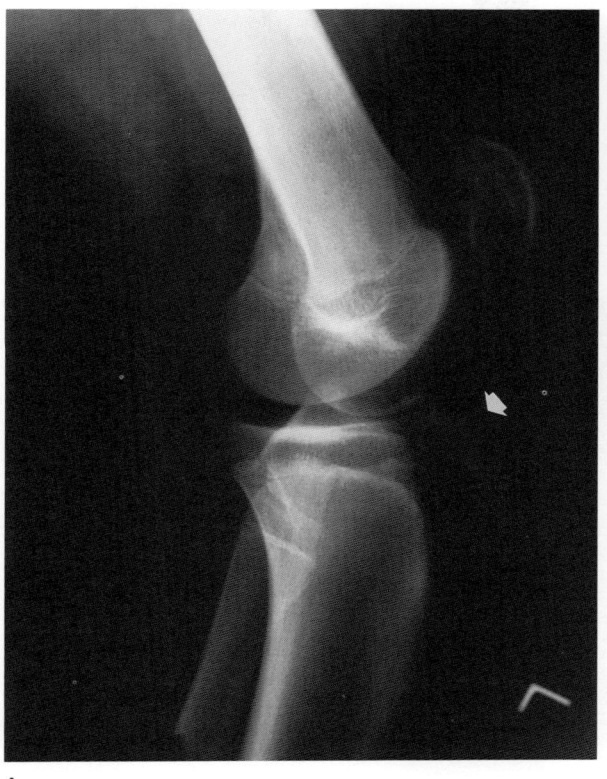

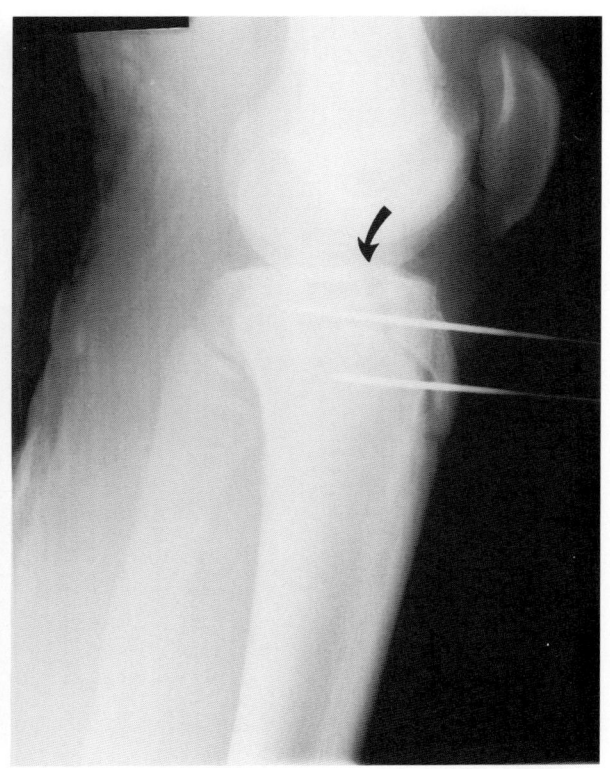

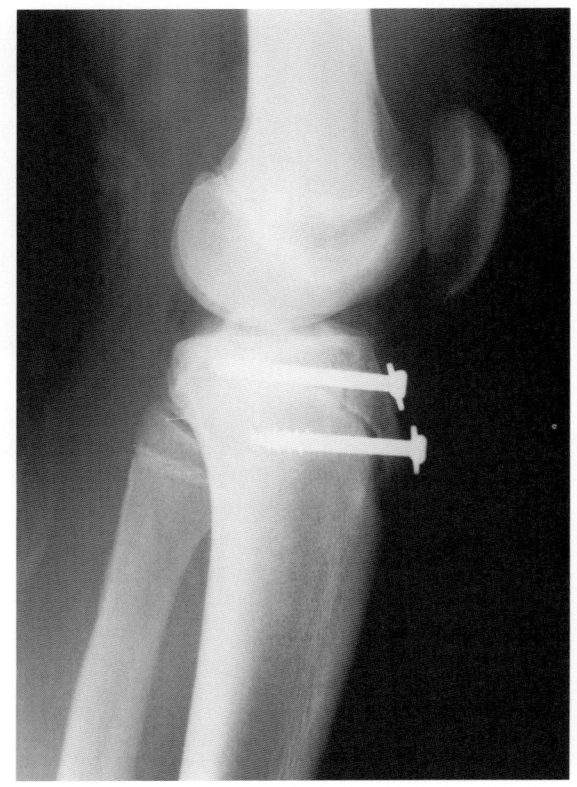

Fig. 54-7. (A) Avulsion of the tibial apophysis in a 15-year-old football player. (B) Reduction with K-wires was incomplete. (C) Reduction improved with two lag screws. Care must be taken in fusing the tibial apophysis in younger children or genu recurvatum will occur. In teenagers near skeletal maturity with minimal growth remaining, this can be done.

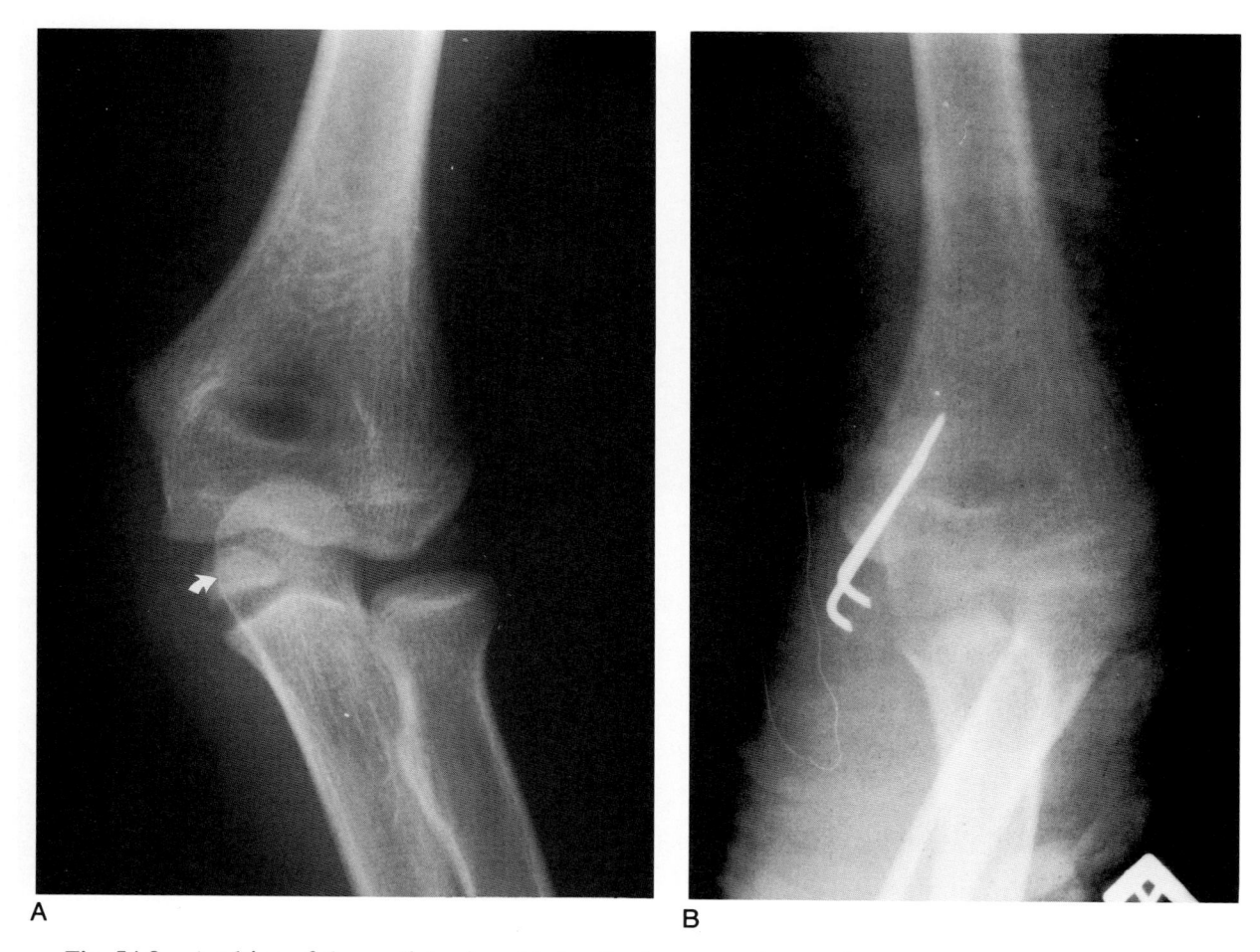

Fig. 54-8. Avulsion of the medial epicondyle by the flexor muscle mass is a common apophyseal avulsion fracture. **(A)** Occasionally the epicondyle becomes entrapped in the elbow during a concomittant dislocation of the elbow joint. The epicondylar fragment must be removed and fixed back in place usually with Kirschner wire fixation **(B)**.

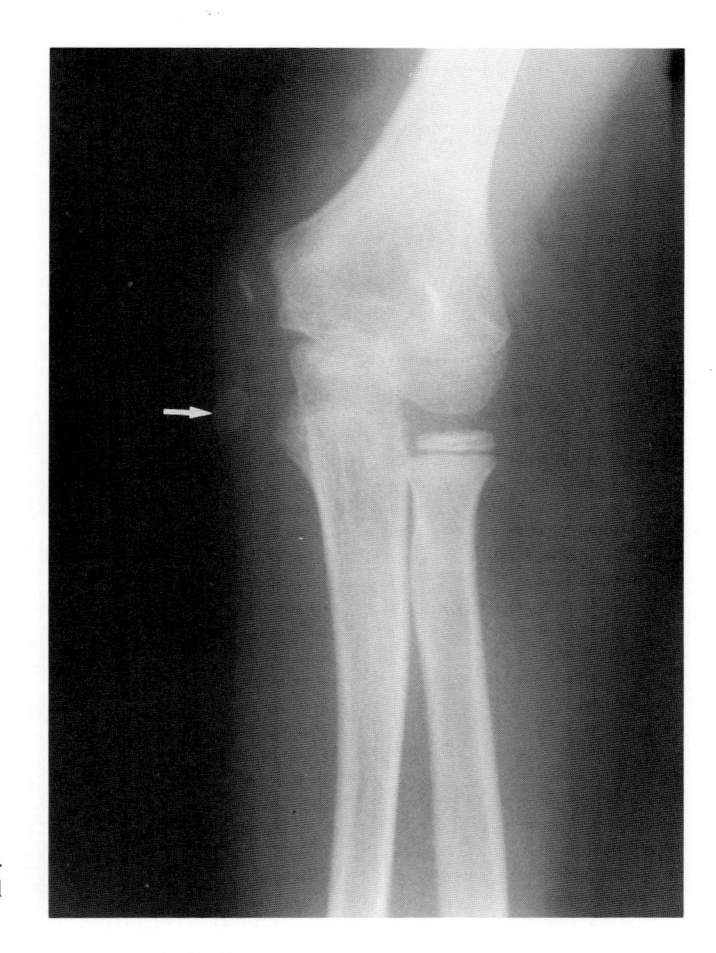

Fig. 54-9. Old untreated nonunion avulsion of medial epicondyle with reossification of residual remaining apophyseal cartilage.

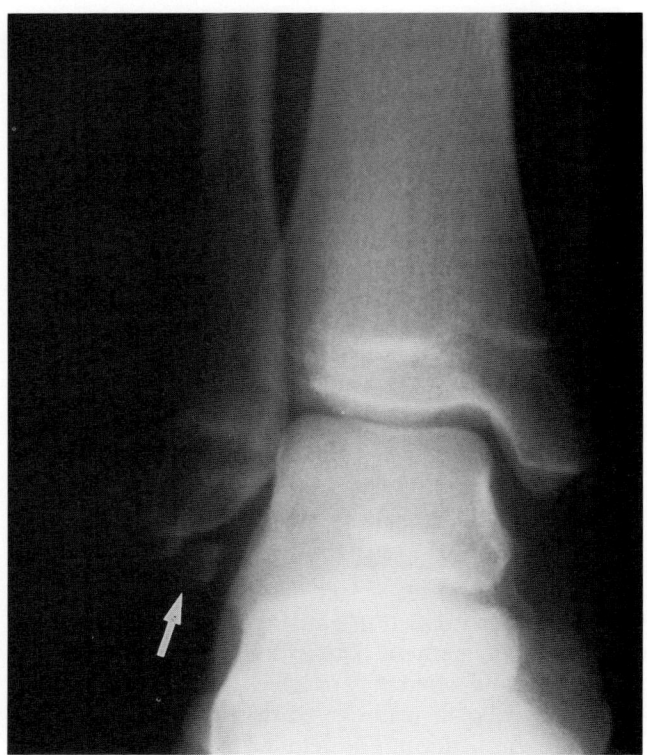

Fig. 54-10. Avulsion of tip of fibula by the anterior talofibular ligament and middle calcaneofibular ligament in a 15-year-old female basketball player. Although an old injury that has proceeded to nonunion, it caused recurrent pain and giving way due to intermittent impingement between the talus and fibula. Symptoms completely disappeared with removal of the fragment.

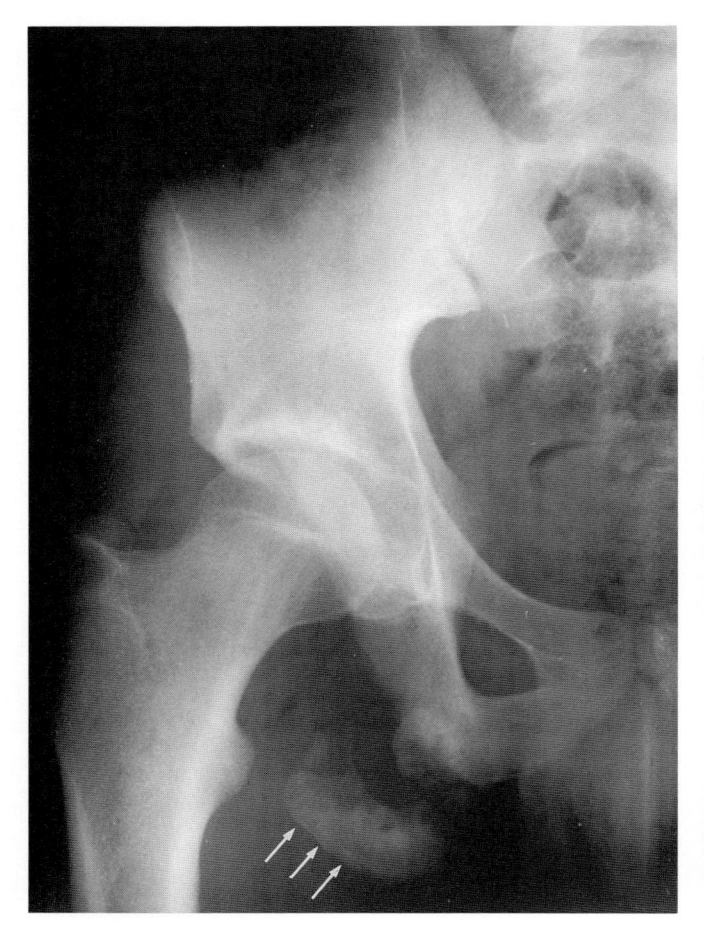

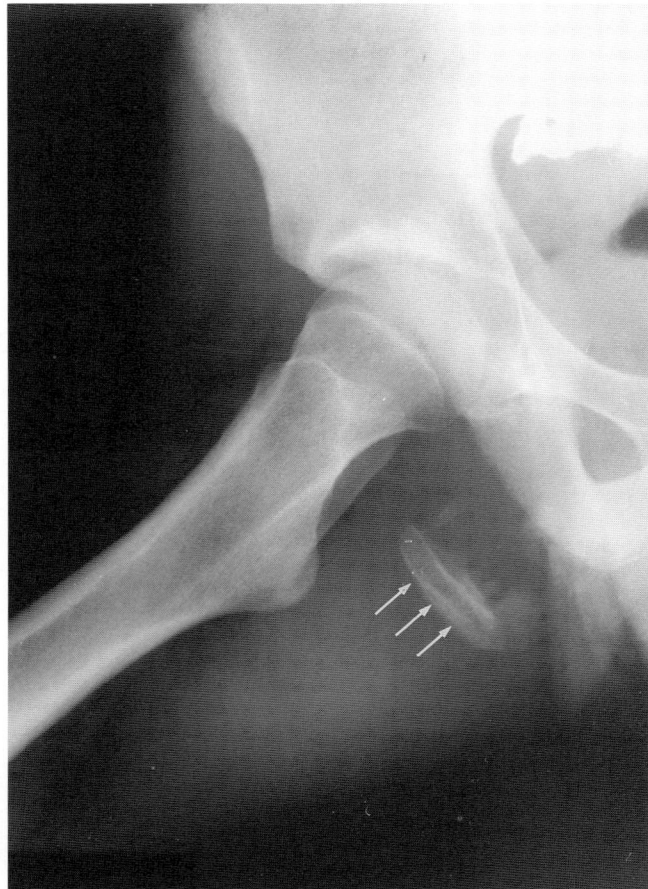

Fig. 54-11. Avulsion of ischial apophysis by the hamstrings in a 15-year-old sprinter.

particular, a block to full extension. Similarly, a malunited fracture of an avulsion fracture of the olecranon could lead to a decreased range of motion of the elbow and posttraumatic osteoarthritis. Finally, *excessive bone formation* may be seen as a consequence of apophyseal avulsion fracture, especially in the region of the ischial tuberosity (Fig. 54-11) and lesser trochanter (Fig. 54-2).

SUMMARY

Avulsion fractures result from excessive traction forces on a bony insertion transmitted through the muscle, tendon, or ligament. These fractures occur anywhere in the body and when they involve the apophysis, injury to the physeal plate leading to distortion of anatomy is a possible complication. The detailed treatment of specific avulsion injuries is covered in the chapters dealing with the specific anatomic regions.

REFERENCES

1. Bright RW: Physeal injuries. p. 170. In Rockwood CA, Wilkins KE, King RF (eds): Fractures in Children. 3rd Ed. JB Lippincott, Philadelphia, 1991
2. Grogan DP, Carey TP, Peffers D, Ogden JA: Avulsion fractures of the patella. J Pediatr Orthop 10:721, 1990
3. Seymour N. Juxta epiphyseal fracture of the terminal phalanx of the finger. J Bone Joint Surg [Br] 48:347, 1966
4. Ross AC, Chesterman PJ. Isolated avulsion of the tibial attachment of the posterior cruciate ligament in childhood. J Bone Joint Surg [Br] 68:747, 1986
5. Wiley JJ, Baxter MP: Tibial spine fractures in children. Clin Orthop Rel Res 255:54, 1990

6. Goodrich A, Ballard A: Posterior cruciate ligament avulsion associated with ipsilateral femur fracture in a 10-year-old child. J Trauma 28:1393, 1988
7. Wooton JR, Cross MJ, Holt KW: Avulsion of the ischial apophysis: the case for open reduction and internal fixation. J Bone Joint Surg [Br] 72:625, 1990
8. Dietemann JL, Runge M, Badoz A et al: Radiology of posterior lumbar apophyseal ring fractures: report of 13 cases. Neuroradiology 30:337, 1988
9. Montgomery SP, Loyd RD: Avulsion fracture of the coracoid epiphysis with acromioclavicular separation. J Bone Joint Surg [Am] 59:963, 1977
10. Eidman DK, Siff SJ, Tullos HS: Acromioclavicular lesions in children. Am J Sports Med 9:150, 1981
11. Fowles JV, Slimane N, Kassab MT: Elbow dislocation with avulsion of the medial humeral epicondyle. J Bone Joint Surg [Br] 72:102, 1990
12. Regan W, Morrey B: Fractures of the coronoid process of the ulna. J Bone Joint Surg [Am] 71:1348, 1989
13. Garcia-Elias M: Dorsal fractures of the triquetrum-avulsion or compression fractures? J Hand Surg [Am] 12:266, 1987
14. Cockshott WP: Distal avulsion fracture of the scaphoid. Br J Radiol 53:1037, 1980
15. Caudle RJ, Crawford AH: Avulsion fracture of the lateral acetabular margin: a case report. J Bone Joint Surg [Am] 70:1568, 1988
16. Barrett IR, Goldberg JA: Avulsion fracture of the ligamentum teres in a child: a case report. J Bone Joint Surg [Am] 71:438, 1989
17. Letts RM: The hidden adolescent ankle fracture. J Pediatr Orthop 2:161, -1982
18. Goldman AB, Pavlov H, Rubenstein D: The Segond fracture of the proximal tibia: a small avulsion that reflects major ligamentous damage. AJR 151:1163, 1988
19. Mirbey J, Besancenot J, Chambers RT et al: Avulsion fractures of the tibial tuberosity in the adolescent athlete: risk factors, mechanism of injury, and treatment. Am J Sports Med 16:336, 1988
20. Chow SP, Lam JJ, Leong JC: Fracture of the tibial tubercle in the adolescent. J Bone Joint Surg [Br] 72:231, 1990
21. Balmat P, Vichard P, Pem R: The treatment of avulsion fractures of the tibial tuberosity in adolescent athletes. Sports Med 9:311, 1990
22. Frankl U, Wasilewski SA, Healy WL: Avulsion fracture of the tibial tubercle with avulsion of the patellar ligament: report of two cases. J Bone Joint Surg [Am] 72:1411, 1990
23. Hawkins LG: Fractures of the lateral process of the talus. J Bone Joint Surg [Am] 47:1170, 1965
24. Canale ST, Williams KD: Iselin's disease. J Pediatr Orthop 12:90, 1992
25. Dameron TB: Fractures and anatomical variations of the proximal portion of the fifth metatarsal. J Bone Joint Surg [Am] 57:788, 1975

55

Osteochondral Fractures

Benoit Morin

The best diagnostic tool is a high index of suspicion.

An osteochondral fracture implies an intra-articular bony injury with associated chondral trauma. The diagnosis of chondral and osteochondral fractures in children, following an injury, must rely on a high index of suspicion, based on history and clinical evaluation, since initial radiographic investigation will frequently be negative.[1] Following the diagnosis of such an injury, the goal of treatment should be to restore joint congruity, to prevent mechanical joint dysfunction, and to delay cartilage destruction.

The optimal treatment should rely on a good understanding of bone and cartilage healing processes. Initially, the osteochondral defect will be filled by a clot from subchondral bleeding. The inflammatory phase is initiated via clot invasion by mesenchymal cells followed by fibroblasts with formation of granulation tissue. Progressively, this tissue will differentiate into hyaline cartilage[2] or fibrocartilage—usually the latter. The quality of the newly formed neochondrogenous tissue will be variable[3,4] in durability.

Many factors may influence the cartilage healing process. Noncontrollable factors include the velocity impact of initial trauma, the age of the patient,[2] the size of the defect[2,5] and its location,[4,5] the degree of initial displacement, and associated intra-articular or periarticular lesions. Other factors, mostly related to treatment, can be controlled and may influence the final outcome.

Although the "tolerable" loss of osteochondral surface has not been determined, it seems desirable, from experimentation results[2,5-7] to consider repositioning significant osteochondral fragments to minimize the extent of fibrocartilage formation, to reduce the radial contact stress at the junction with normal cartilage,[7] and possibly to prevent degenerative arthritis.

Mechanically, the restoration of joint congruity is also important. An osteochondral fragment of significant size will produce synovial irritation with subsequent synovitis, limited range of motion, and catching or locking. Joint incongruity will also produce stress on opposed articular surfaces progressing to chondramalacic changes of the adjacent cartilage, as shown experimentally by Convery and colleagues.[5] Osteochondral defects located in non-weight-bearing joints, or not adjacent to a major intra-articular structure such as a meniscus, are better tolerated and less prone to cartilage degeneration.

Finally, although mechanical stabilization is essential to promote solid bony union, early motion produces optimal cartilage regeneration and healing, while prolonged immobilization leads to joint contractures and intra-articular adhesions.[6] Thus, the ideal approach following an osteochondral fracture in children would be early motion of the injured joint by providing intrinsic stability of the fragment or its surgical stabilization.

INCIDENCE

The incidence of chondral and osteochondral injury is not known with precision and varies according to authors and locale. Furthermore, there is confusion as to the exact nature of osteochondritis dissecans with a significant number being considered to be related to microtrauma or undiagnosed previous injury.[1,8] Histologic studies of chronic loose bodies[9] have confirmed a traumatic origin in 40 percent of cases.

The incidence of osteochondral fractures related to injury in children is probably higher than would be suspected[10-12] and frequently underdiagnosed. Arthroscopic evaluation of the knee following posttraumatic acute hemarthrosis in athletic populations[13-15] has revealed an incidence of osteochondral fracturing between 6 and 14 percent. Haupt,[16] evaluating 12 children, found 4 instances of osteochondral fractures. Recently, Vellet and colleagues,[17] using magnetic resonance imaging in the evaluation of occult posttraumatic hemarthrosis of the knee, found an incidence of 72 percent of occult subcortical femoral or tibial fractures.

The talar dome is a common site for chondral or osteochondral fracture, although frequently overlooked.[18,19] Controversy also exists concerning the true nature of the lesion, especially those found on the medial aspect of the dome, many being considered as either an old undisplaced fracture, a stress fracture, or a true osteochondritis dissecans. The true incidence has not been firmly established in the literature, although many large series[18,20-25] have reported a history of trauma in 64 to 80 percent of cases. Anderson and colleagues,[26] using magnetic resonance imaging (MRI) examined 30 patients presenting a posttraumatic disability of the ankle with normal plain radiographs and discovered a 50 percent incidence of osteochondral lesions.

In children, the true relationship of osteochondral fracture with injury is even more controversial (Fig. 55-1). Gérard and associates,[23] reporting 15 children with osteochondral lesions of the talar dome, found a history of injury in only 5. Mazel and coworkers,[27] in a review of 23 fractures of the talus in children, reported 8 osteochondral lesions, with a precise history of trauma present in only 5 children.

An osteochondral fracture must, however, be suspected in any child presenting with a significant injury of the ankle. In his series of 40 acutely injured ankles surgically explored, Vahvanen and coworkers[28] reported a 32 percent incidence of osteochondral fragments avulsed either from the lateral malleolus or from the talus. Similarly, Schütze and Maas,[29] in a series of 130 children with lateral fibular ligament rupture, found at surgical exploration, an osteochondral fragment in 37 percent, one-third not visible on plain radiographs. Osteochondral fractures have been reported at many other sites, although much less frequently compared to the knee and ankle.

Hip dislocation has been clearly identified as a cause of osteochondral impaction or fracture, either from the acetabulum or the femoral head. More recently, the use of computed tomography (CT) has proven its usefulness[30,31] in assisting in the difficult diagnosis of an osteochondral fracture in the hip joint (see Ch. 28).

In children, traumatic hip dislocation is rare and osteochondral fractures are unusual.[32,33] Libri and colleagues,[34] in his series of 22 patients mentioned 9 cases with associated fractures of the acetabular rim. Harder and associates[35] reported 2 children with osteochondral fractures of the hip diagnosed with CT scan. Epstein,[36] reporting 44 hip dislocations in children, found 5 associated with a fracture of the acetabulum, while Stachel and coworkers[37] described 2 children with associated osteochondral fractures in his series of 8 traumatic hip dislocations.

In the upper limb, true osteochondral fractures are rare. In 1983, McElfresh and Dobyns[38] in a series of 103 intra-articular metacarpal head fractures, reported 8 osteochondral fractures. O'Brien[39] described osteochondral fractures related to phalangeal intra-articular fractures. Ogden[40] mentioned the possibility of an osteochondral fracture of the metacarpal epiphysis associated with metacarpophalangeal dislocation.

In the elbow, only 2 instances of true osteochondral fracture associated with dislocation of the elbow have been reported,[41,42] although McManama and colleagues,[43] reporting on osteochondritis dissecans of the capitellum in 14 patients, described 5 in whom a history of significant injury was present.

In the shoulder joint, only a few descriptions of osteochondral fractures have been published, all in adults following posterior dislocation.[44] In children, fractures involving the humeral head are classified as Salter-Harris type III or type IV injuries. The Bankart lesion of the glenoid rim in children following shoulder dislocation could be considered an osteochondral fracture.

ANATOMY

Osteochondral injuries involve a portion of the articular cartilage with a variable amount of subchondral bone. Less frequently, the avulsed fragment is limited to the cartilage itself, the fragment being sheared off the bone through the zone of uncalcified cartilage. The fragment may be variable in size and shape, from a few millimeters to as large as 5 cm in diameter, with a

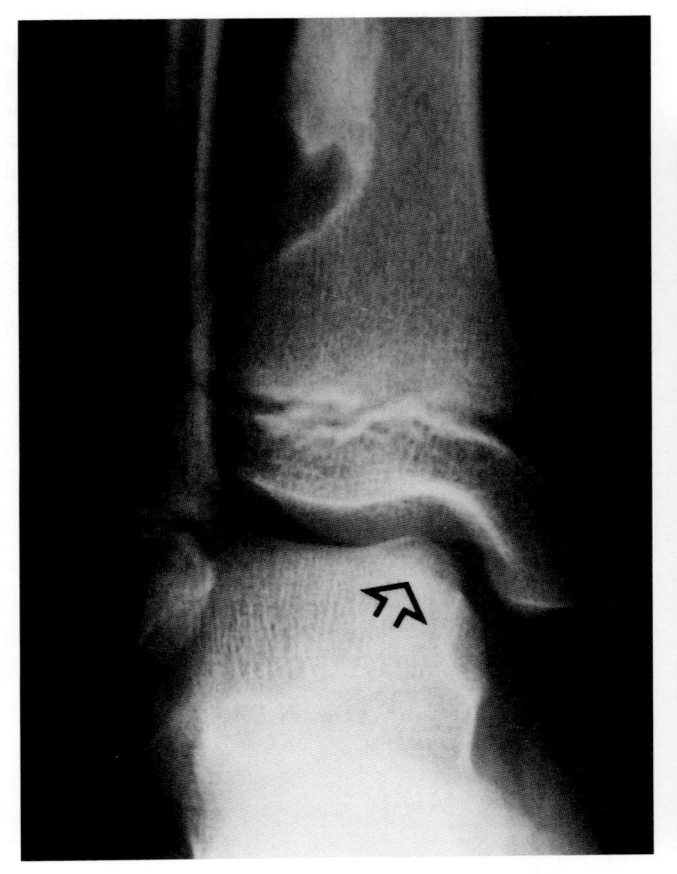

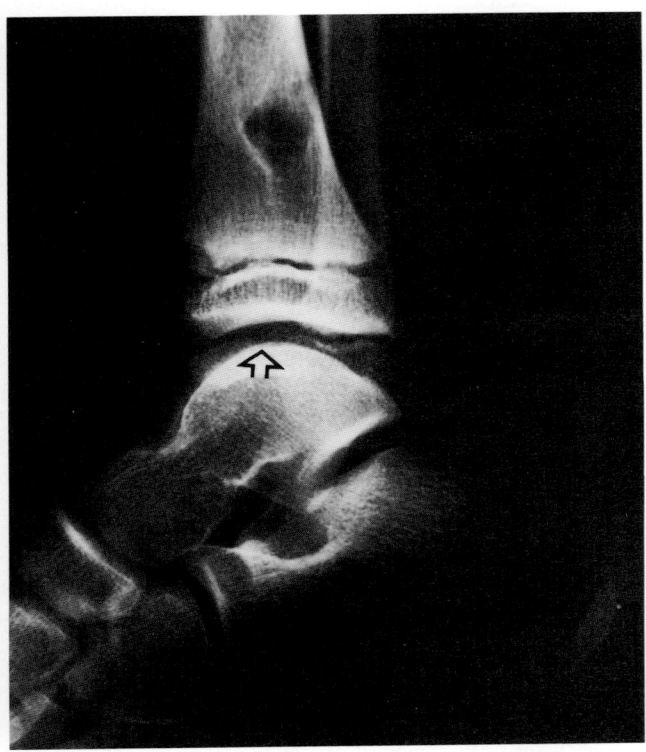

Fig. 55-1. This 11-year-old female gymnast sustained an inversion injury to her right ankle a few weeks before consultation. A diagnosis of ankle sprain was made and no specific treatment suggested, although radiographs showed an obvious osteochondral lesion of the medial talar dome. Note the fibrous cortical defect of the lateral tibial cortex which is in the process of resolving.

smooth, lacerated or multifragmented surface. Cartilaginous abrasion or even a "mirror image" fracture may be encountered on the opposite joint surface.

Following a knee injury, the osteochondral fragment is usually displaced, floating free in the joint. With delayed diagnosis, it may become embedded in the synovium[45] with progressive revascularization and resorption. The chondral fragment is often discovered only at surgery, as a loose body or still in its bed.[46,47]

At the ankle joint, the osteochondral lesion also varies in size and shape.[23,27,28] Significant trauma results in a radiologic thin fleck of subchondral bone, either from the lateral malleolus or lateral talar dome.[28] Histologically, the chronic loose bodies[45] may show proliferative changes of bone and cartilage, resorptive changes, or secondary degenerative calcification.

MECHANISM OF INJURY

Controversy exists concerning the mechanisms producing osteochondral injury. As proposed by Milgram and colleagues,[48] the basic mechanism is either an impaction or a rotatory or a shearing force acting tangentially to the joint surface, thus producing a chondral or osteochondral fracture of one or both joint surfaces in contact.

Osteochondral Fractures of the Knee

In 1966 Kennedy and colleagues[49] were the first to examine subchondral fractures in the biomechanical model. He described five possible ways of creating osteochondral fractures in the knee, resulting either from an exogenous or endogenous force (Fig. 55-2).

More recently, the "exogenous" mechanism (blow, fall) has been accepted by others[11,48] as responsible for some of the osteochondral fractures of the condyles or the patella. The "endogenous" mechanism from compressive and rotational forces has also been emphasized by Rosenberg[50] and Robert and colleagues,[11] although the most accepted cause is a patellar subluxation or dislocation.[48,50,53,58,60]

In our experience, the vast majority of osteochondral fractures of the knee occur in adolescents with a deficient extensor mechanism, the quadriceps generating extreme shearing forces while relocating the patella, resulting in an osteochondral fracture from either the patella, the lateral condyle, or both.

An unresolved question in the literature is the amount of flexion of the knee[49-51] at the time of the dislocation, most authors suggesting that dislocation occurs close to full extension. Conversely, according to Hughston and colleagues,[52] osteochondral fractures related to patellar dislocation occur at about 45 degrees of flexion. In our view, the location and extent of the osteochondral injury varies according to extensor mechanism tightness. In tighter patellofemoral joints, the relocation of the patella occurs closer to extension, more often with marginal or medial facet fracture of the patella. With a very dysplastic femoropatellar joint, the adolescent will report initial giving way and fall, followed by sudden and strong reflex contraction of the quadriceps. This leads to a forceful relocation of the patella, avulsing the lateral aspect of the lateral condyle close to or on weight-bearing surface, with associated scoring or frank osteochondral fracture of the patella (see Ch. 36).

Occasionally, with recurrent subluxations but without acute episodes of dislocation, the repetitive traction injury will produce a marginal osteochondral fragmentation of the medial facet of the patella (Fig. 55-3).

Osteochondral Fractures of the Ankle

In the ankle joint, the role of injury has been well established, mainly with osteochondral lesions involving the lateral aspect of the mortise. Berndt and Harty[20] were

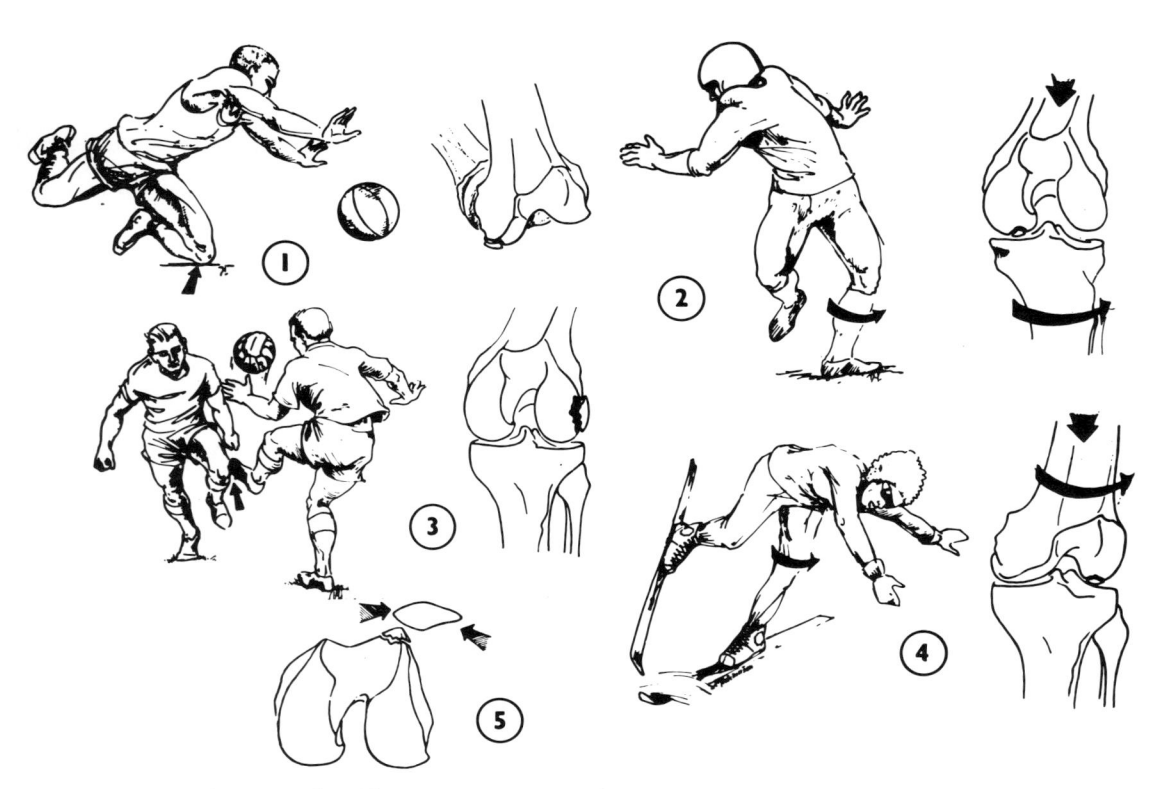

Fig. 55-2. The various ways in which the osteochondral fractures of the knee occur: *(1)* Direct shearing force on the medial condyle. *(2)* Rotatory compression force on the medial epicondyle. *(3)* Direct shearing force on the lateral condyle. *(4)* Rotatory compression force on the lateral condyle. *(5)* The action of the patella on the lateral condyle in dislocation or reduction. (From Kennedy et al.,[49] with permission.)

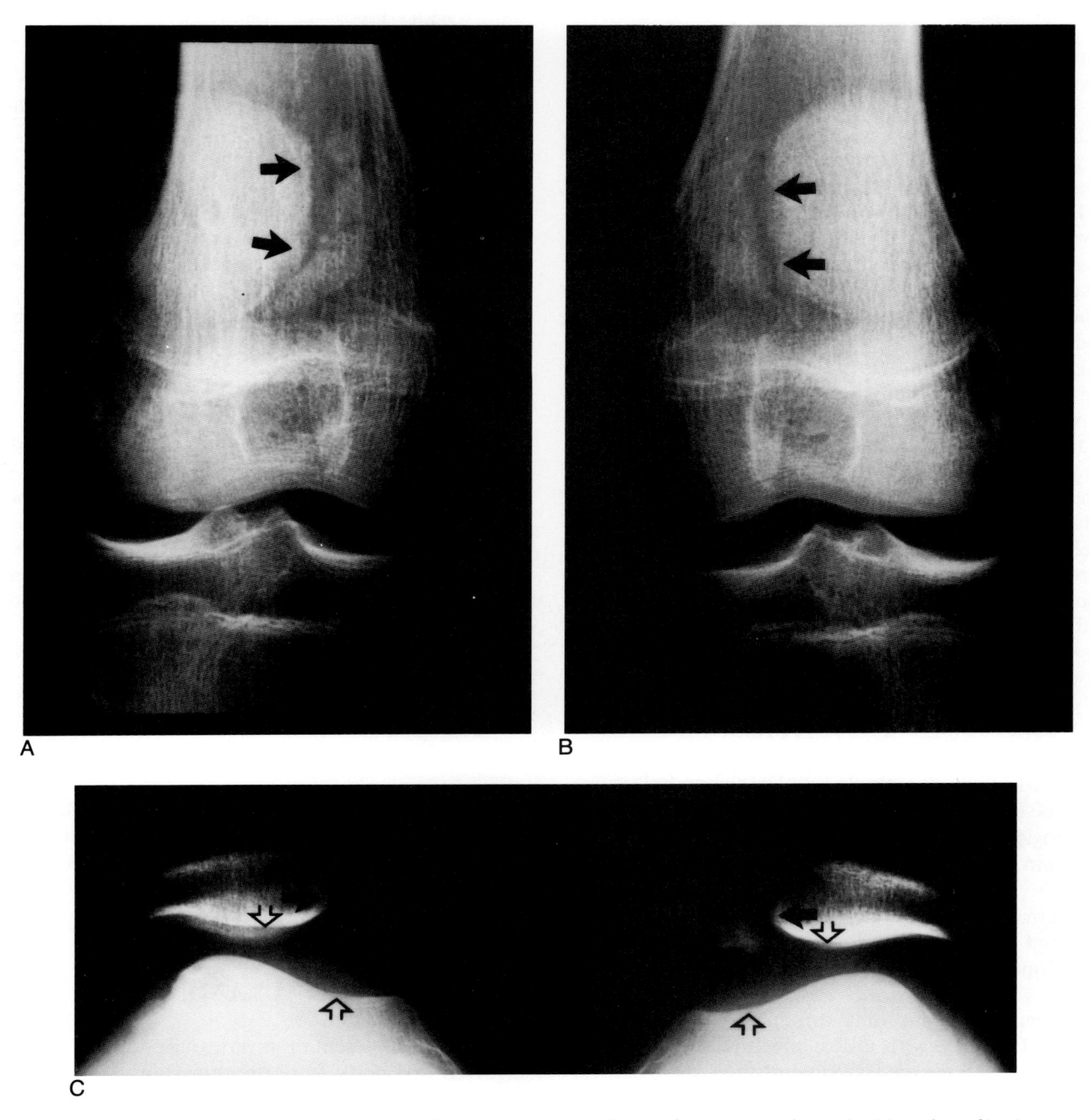

Fig. 55-3. **(A&B)** A 17-year-old patient with a long-standing history of a recurrent bilateral subluxation of both patellae. **(C)** Skyline views of the patellae show osteochondral fragmentation of medial facet and subluxed patellae.

the first to emphasize the traumatic nature of the lesion previously termed "osteochondritis dissecans" of the talus. From their clinical review and limited experiments on cadavers, these authors suggested that anterolateral dome lesions (44 percent) were secondary to inversion trauma on a dorsiflexed ankle. On the other hand, posteromedial lesions (56 percent) were attributed to forced inversion of the ankle with plantar flexion of the foot, calling this latter mechanism *torsional impaction* and responsible for so-called osteochondritis dissecans of the talus.

The series of Canale and Belding[22] confirmed inversion or inversion and dorsiflexion as the most frequent mechanisms causing osteochondral fractures, usually involving the lateral dome of the talus. In children, another reported mechanism was described by Vahvanen and colleagues,[28] where severe supination injury of the ankle resulted in an osteochondral fracture either from the lateral malleolus or from the lateral talar dome.

As described in the literature, osteochondral fractures of the lateral dome are the result of a shearing force, the dome hitting the articular surface of the lateral malleolus, while lesions of the medial aspect of the dome are related to a compression injury. This explains why lateral lesions are easier to recognize on plain films, while medial lesions are often diagnosed late, often requiring sophisticated imaging techniques such as tomography, arthrography, CT scan,[23] or MRI studies.[26]

CLASSIFICATION

In the knee joint, osteochondral and chondral lesions can be classified in several ways. Milgram[45] following histologic evaluation of loose bodies, proposed a classification in three groups:

1. From synovial osteochondromatosis
2. From surface joint disintegration
3. Secondary to osteochondral fracture

Macroscopically, the injury produces either an osteochondral fracture with visible subchondral bone, or a true chondral fragment if the fracture line passes entirely through uncalcified cartilage.

Based on the mechanism and the type of injury, in 1966, Kennedy and colleagues[49] were the first to propose a classification of osteochondral fracture of the femoral condyles (Table 55-1). More recently, with the advent of arthroscopy, unsuspected chondral fractures of the knee have been frequently identified and two arthroscopic

TABLE 55-1. Classification of Osteochondral Fractures of the Femoral Condyles

Site	Type	Mechanism
Medial condyle	Exogenous	Direct impact
	Endogenous	Rotation and compression forces
Lateral condyle	Exogenous	Direct impact
	Endogenous	1) Rotation and compression
		2) Patellar dislocation or reduction

(From Kennedy JC, et al.,[49] with permission.)

classifications of chondral fractures have been proposed. In 1988, Terry and coworkers[46] suggested two groups:

1. Incomplete chondral fracture with normal surface but shearing of the subchondral bone
2. Complete fracture, subdivided as a flap, stellate, or crater lesion

Bauer and Jackson,[47] following a review of 167 cases, found that chondral fractures were mainly caused by rotational forces, identifying six types of articular changes.

In 1959 Berndt and Harty,[20] after clinical and experimental observations of the ankle joint, proposed a classification of transchondral fractures of the dome of the talus as follows (Fig. 55-4):

Stage 1: Localized compression fracture
Stage 2: Incomplete avulsion
Stage 3: Complete avulsion
Stage 4: Inversion of the fragment

Recently, Anderson and colleagues[26] using MRI, frequently demonstrated a cystic formation in the type 1 lesion, adding a *Stage 2a* to Berndt and Harty's classification.

PHYSICAL EXAMINATION

The clinical presentation varies according to the joint involved and delay from the injury. With acute knee injury, it should be ascertained if there were contact, pivoting, twisting, or patellar hypermobility, or true dislocation, followed by collapse of the knee joint and the sensation of relocation of the patella. The rapidity of subsequent swelling indicative of bleeding should be recorded as well as any previous history of patellofemoral disorders.

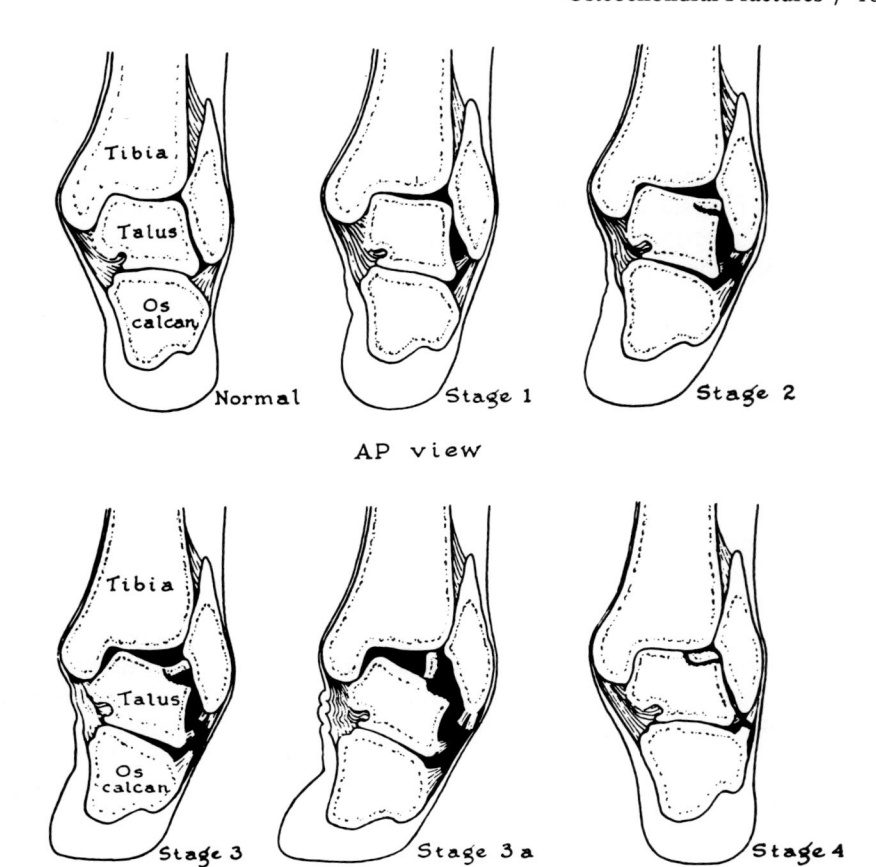

Fig. 55-4. Staging system of Berndt and Harty. *Stage 1:* The lateral border of the dome is compressed against the face of the fibula; *Stage 2:* Rupture of lateral ligament and partial avulsion of a chip. *Stage 3:* Complete avulsion but remain in place; *Stage 3a:* Fragment displaced; *Stage 4:* Displacement and inversion of the fragment. (From Berndt and Harty,[20] with permission.)

Objective evaluation should include examination of the noninjured knee to identify any suggestive signs of patellofemoral disorder such as patella alta, vastus medialis obliquus dysplasia, J sign, or frank patellar subluxation, lateral patellar laxity,[52] or the presence of an apprehension sign.

On inspection, the injured knee usually shows significant effusion and a flexed position. On palpation, tenderness is frequently found on the medial patellar facet, medial retinaculum, inferior border of the vastus medialis, and on the lateral condyle close to the weight-bearing surface. Occasionally, tenderness will be present over the medial capsular ligament and the femoral insertion of the medial collateral ligament if valgus stress occurred at the time of the injury. Patellar and ligamentous stability must be assessed.[52]

With subacute or chronic injury, the patient complains mainly of aching pain with exercise, intermittent swelling, locking, limited range of motion, and possibly a sensation of patellofemoral instability. Similarly, clinical evaluation of an ankle injury should include the history of mechanism of injury, presence of popping or cracking sensation at the time of injury, and subsequent rapid swelling.

Following an acute injury, inspection reveals swelling mainly over the lateral compartment of the ankle and effusion and tenderness on palpation of the lateral ligament and over the medial or lateral talar dome. Varus stress of the ankle and the anteroposterior drawer test should be performed to eliminate ligamentous instability.

Frequently, the initial diagnosis will have been a "simple" ankle sprain followed by persisting disability associated with swelling, catching, and giving way.[25] In such a chronic situation, clinical signs are subtle and may include tenderness over the talar dome, mild swelling of the ankle joint, and ligamentous laxity.

In other joints (hip, hand, elbow, shoulder), osteochondral fractures are usually secondary to dislocations. The examiner should bear this possibility in mind when faced with an acute dislocation or continued disability and pain after reduction of a dislocation.

DIFFERENTIAL DIAGNOSIS AND INVESTIGATION

The literature is unanimous on the difficulty in diagnosing the presence of an osteochondral fracture irrespective of the site and joint involved. The best diagnostic tool is probably a high index of suspicion of such a possibility when dealing with an acute injury[1] or with chronic posttraumatic disability of any joint.

In a child with a history of rapid swelling and clinical hemarthrosis after a knee injury,[11,12,54] one should suspect the possibility of an osteochondral fracture, frequently related to patellar dislocation. The differential diagnosis includes ligamentous injury, mainly the anterior cruciate ligament,[55,56] tibial spine avulsion, meniscal or capsular tears, and physeal fractures.

In children, the so-called "sprain" of the ankle joint should be viewed with suspicion, being frequently associated with an osteochondral fracture,[28,29] particularly following inversion injury. The differential diagnosis includes isolated ligamentous or physeal disruption, as well as triplane or Tillaux fractures in older teenagers.

Initial radiographic evaluation may be deceptive.[11,21,28,29,48,57] The osteochondral fracture is often very subtle and easily missed due to the poor quality of the initial radiograph[24] and the difficulty of evaluating the joint.[30,31] The lack of appreciation of the possibility of an associated osteochondral fracture by clinicians and radiologists also contribute to delay the diagnosis of this fracture.

In the presence of a significant hemarthrosis of the knee in children, plain films should include anteroposterior, lateral, obliques, tunnel and skyline views. One should search for a thin fleck only a "few osteocytes thick" free in the joint or irregularities in the normal contours of subchondral bone of the femoral condyles or patella in all views (Fig. 55-5). If an osteochondral injury is suspected, aspiration may be performed under sterile conditions to confirm the hemarthrosis, as well as to search for fat droplets in the aspirate. Arthrography has been of limited assistance as it is difficult to interpret.[57] The ultimate diagnostic step in investigation is arthroscopy, and its role in the diagnosis of osteochondral fracture has been reemphasized recently.[11,46,47]

In the ankle joint, if an osteochondral fracture is suspected, in addition to the standard AP and lateral views, a good mortise view will show the lateral talar dome as well as the articular surface of the lateral malleolus. Anteroposterior views in maximal plantar flexion and dorsiflexion may also reveal anteriorly or posteriorly located lesions. If clinical suspicion persists, a bone scan should be performed,[26] and, if positive, investigation completed either by arthrographic CT scan[24] or magnetic resonance imaging.[26]

Following reduction after hip dislocation, an osteochondral fracture may be suspected on plain films when nonconcentric reduction persists, compared to the opposite side, or, in a more chronic situation, when persisting pain is present. Every effort should be made to rule out such an osteochondral fragment. Arthrography will usually demonstrate a filling defect medial to the femoral head.[30,31] A tomogram, or better, a CT scan, will localize the position of the fragment as well as its origin from the femoral head or acetabulum (Fig. 55-6).

TREATMENT

The ideal treatment of osteochondral fractures in children remains somewhat controversial. There is no consensus in the literature as to the extent of osteochondral surface that can be safely removed, the delay between injury and surgery, the most appropriate type of surgery, and the best method of fixation. As stated by Henderson and Houghton[54] the restoration of joint contours is the aim of the treatment. The fragment should be preserved if possible and removed only if very small (Fig. 55-7), from a non-weight-bearing surface and purely cartilaginous. Even with a purely cartilaginous fragment, this should be preserved if significant in size and if the injury is recent. Optimal treatment is facilitated by "early" diagnosis,[1,10,11,12,49,54] no matter what the site. Arthroscopy has become an integral part of the treatment as well as diagnosis, since, depending on the arthroscopic findings, various therapeutic options can be considered.

Although infrequent, if the osteochondral fragment is still in its bed and undisplaced, it should be left intact, and the joint, kept in a cast or orthosis for 3 to 4 weeks. When the fragment is displaced and small (≤ 1 cm in diameter), or is multifragmented, or comes from a non-weight-bearing surface, or is already round, suggesting an old loose body, it is best treated by arthroscopic removal. The margin of the crater should be trimmed at a right angle to minimize the formation of a stress riser at the junction of normal and newly formed fibrocartilage.[5]

Knee

Controversy arises when large osteochondral fragments up to 5 cm in diameter are encountered. Milgram and colleagues[48] suggested excision because of the avascular nature of the fragment. Kennedy and colleagues[49]

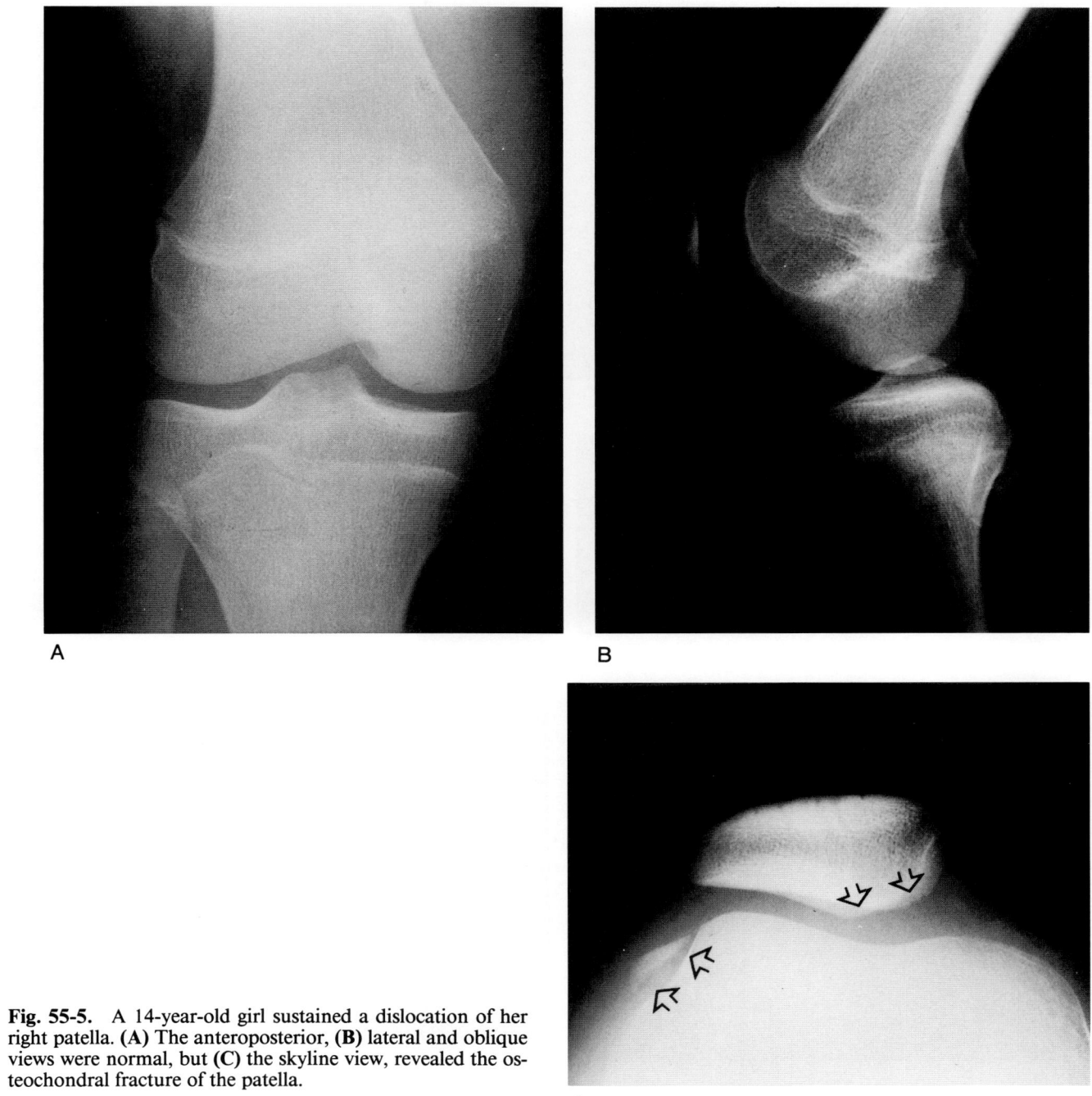

Fig. 55-5. A 14-year-old girl sustained a dislocation of her right patella. **(A)** The anteroposterior, **(B)** lateral and oblique views were normal, but **(C)** the skyline view, revealed the osteochondral fracture of the patella.

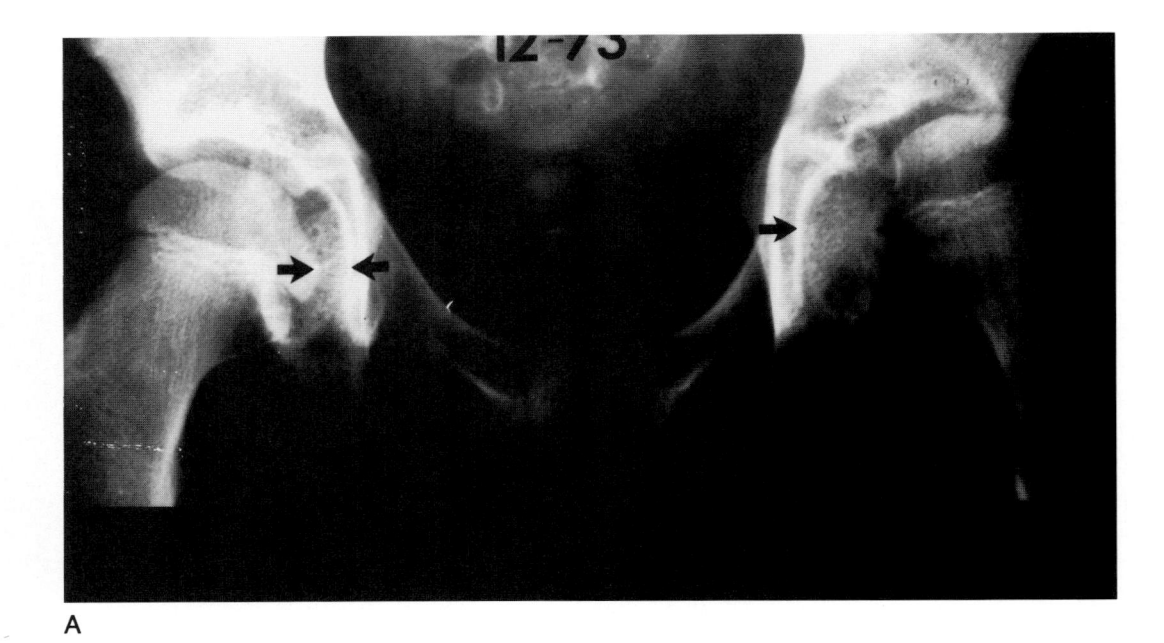

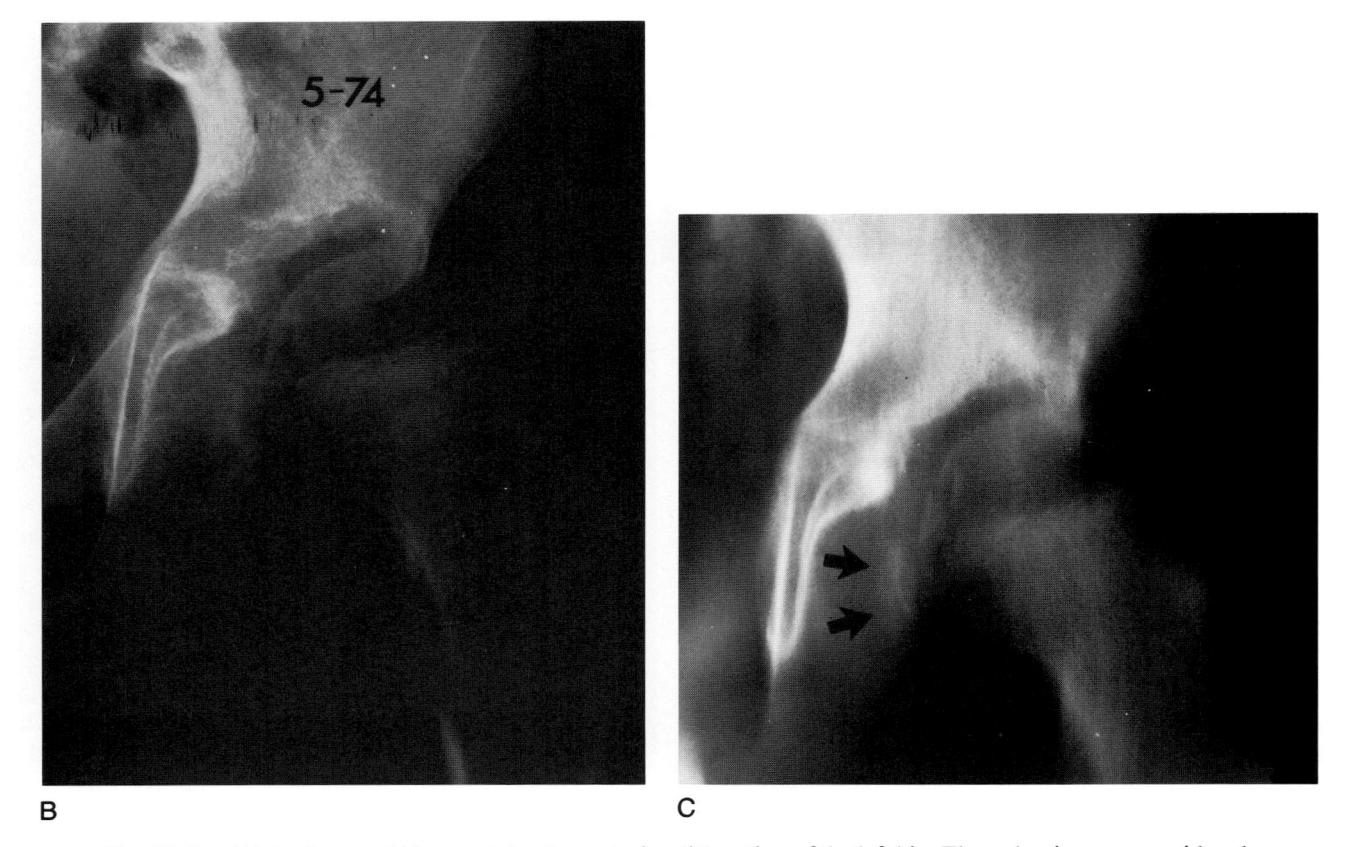

Fig. 55-6. (A) A 12-year-old boy sustained a posterior dislocation of the left hip. The reduction was considered adequate despite obvious residual subluxation. **(B&C)** Six months later, because of persisting pain, radiographs and tomograms were repeated, showing the suspicion of an osteochondral fragment. *(Figure continues.)*

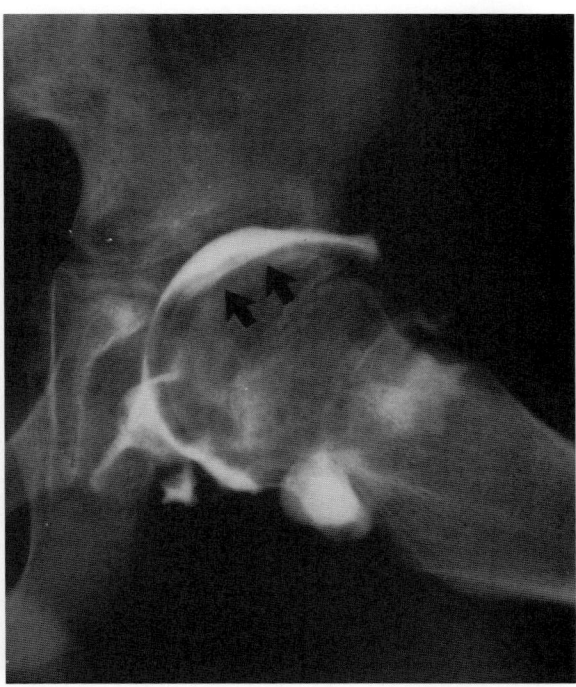

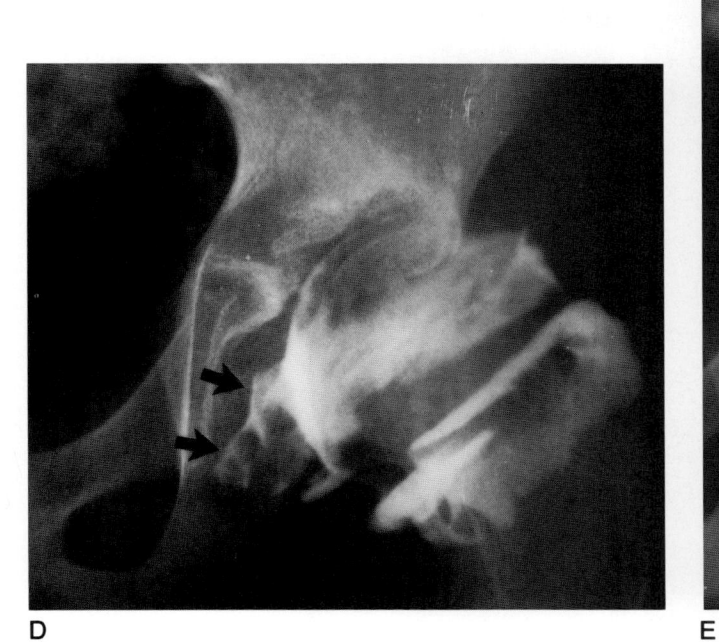

Fig. 55-6 *(Continued).* **(D&E)** An arthrogram was done showing clearly the osteochondral fracture originating from the femoral head. **(F)** At surgery, a large fragment was found and removed.

also suggested excision, but if the fragment is recent, large, and from a weight-bearing area, he favored fixation, as did Smillie[58] and Hammerle and Jacob.[59] Mathewson and Dandy[10] recommended open reduction and internal fixation if the injury was less than 2 weeks old, and removal if more than 2 weeks. Mayer and Seidlein[12] stressed the importance of early diagnosis and fixation of the fragment if sufficient in size and thickness, reporting better results compared to excision and late surgery. Milgram and colleagues[51] recommended the fixation of a fresh and large osteochondral fragment from the condyles with staples, reserving excision for fractures diagnosed "months late." Rorabeck and Bobechko[60] and Ahstrom[53] favored excision and extensor mechanism realignment, while Rosenberg[50] reported good short-term results with excision.

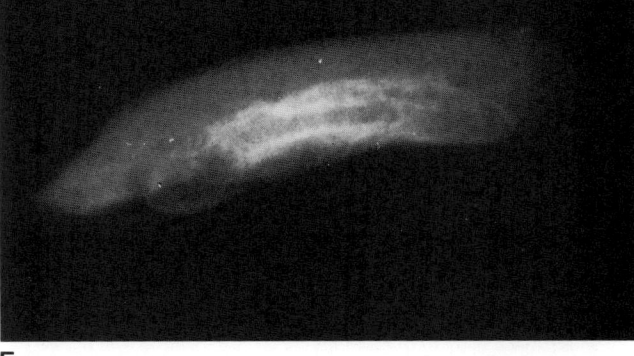

In children with large chondral or osteochondral fragments either from the condyles or the patella, we recommend open reduction and internal fixation as a first step if the lesion is less than 6 to 8 weeks old. With a fresh injury, reduction into the bed should not be difficult. With an older lesion, granulation tissue has to be curetted, the osteochondral bed drilled, and its margins carved. The chondral margins of the fragment must be carefully trimmed.

Many methods of osteochondral fragment fixation have been proposed: Smillie nails, K-wires, countersunk screws, bone pegs, and more recently, Herbert screws,

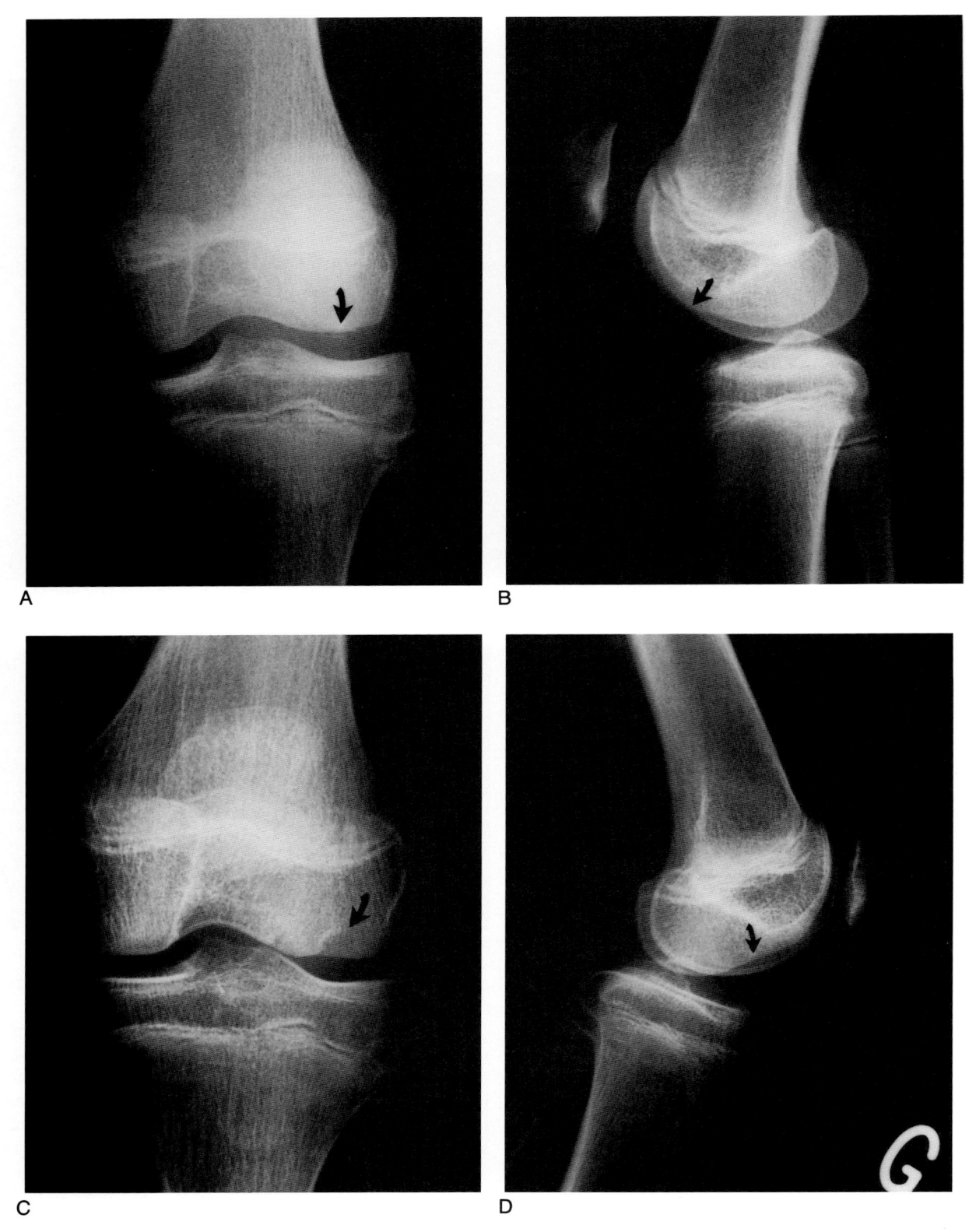

Fig. 55-7. **(A&B)** This 12-year-old girl sustained a dislocation of her left patella with spontaneous reduction. Initial radiographs show a small osteochondral fracture involving the weight-bearing aspect of the lateral femoral condyle. **(C&D)** Eight months postremoval of the osteochondral fragment with residual flattening of the lateral condyle.

biodegradable pins (Ortho Sorb) and fibrin glues. For many years, our favored method of fixation has been U-shaped stainless steel wires overlying the fragment in the sagittal plane, countersunk in cartilage by gradual tightening either on lateral aspect of the condyle (Fig. 55-8) or on the dorsum of the patella (Fig. 55-9). More recently, we have supplemented our fixation with fibrin sealant, which helps to stabilize the margin of the fragment (Fig. 55-10). This method of fixation has permitted early protected mobilization of the limb with satisfactory healing both clinically and radiographically, confirmed by arthroscopy in some cases.

As stated by Hughston and colleagues[52] a far more difficult question is the indication of simultaneous reconstruction of the extensor mechanism. Ahstrom,[53] however, does not hesitate to proceed to immediate reconstruction. In our experience, most of the children with osteochondral injury have an extensor mechanism imbalance. Decision of immediate or delayed treatment will depend on previous symptomatology, the age of the patient and the site of osteochondral avulsion. With a lateral condyle injury requiring a lateral approach, lateral release is done at the time of fixation, realignment of the extensor mechanism being performed subsequently if clinical instability persists. With an extensive patellar osteochondral fracture, the medial parapatellar approach is required. After reduction and fixation of the fragment, our approach is to perform lateral release and proximal realignment, as described by Hughston and colleagues.[52] In most cases, this has been sufficient to prevent patellar redislocation. With persisting disability from patellar instability, distal realignment should be performed.

Following surgery, continuous passive motion can be used as part of early and protected mobilization, although weightbearing should be restrained for 6 to 8 weeks to promote healing.

Talus

The treatment of an osteochondral fracture of the ankle joint is also controversial. Basically, irrespective of the location and stage, union of the fracture requires accurate reduction and immobilization.

Acute type I, II, and III talar dome fractures should be treated initially by 6 to 8 weeks of plaster immobilization, while type IV requires surgical exploration with either removal or fixation of the fragment.[21-23] With persisting symptoms in spite of adequate immobilization or following delayed diagnosis associated with chronic disability, the suggested treatment is excision of the fragment and curettage of the bed[18,21,22] either alone or associated with autogenous bone graft.[23,24,61]

Many recent publications on arthroscopic surgery for osteochondral lesions of the ankle have reported good results with fragment removal, curettage, and early mobilization.[62-65]

In children, the therapeutic approach is even more controversial, since history of trauma is uncertain in the majority of osteochondral lesions. Gérard and coworkers[23] reporting on 102 patients with osteochondral lesions, of whom 18 were children, found that most had a questionable history of trauma: 16 were treated conservatively and 4 lesions united, the remainder were stable both clinically and radiologically. Only 2 patients required surgery, both with a frank history of trauma. Mazel and associates[27] reviewed 23 fractures of the talus including 8 osteochondral fractures and proposed the following approach. With nondisplaced osteochondral fractures with a recent injury, the treatment should be conservative with plaster immobilization for 60 to 90 days, while with displaced fragment, the treatment should be surgical. With chronic injury, immobilization should be tried, but if disabling symptoms persist, surgical resection should be performed and the patient kept nonweightbearing for a 2- to 2½-month period.

Valvanen and colleagues[28] and Shütze and Maas[29] reviewing, respectively, large series of children with a talofibular ligament injury of the ankle, found at surgical exploration a high percentage of chondral and osteochondral fractures either from the lateral malleolus or the lateral talar dome. Treatment included excision or repositioning of the fragment and fixation with absorbable suture with good results. Recently, Angerman and Riegels-Nielson[66] reported on the use of fibrin sealant for fixation of six osteochondral fractures of the talus with uneventful healing and good functional results.

Our experience with osteochondral lesions of the ankle joint in children is limited, confirming the rarity of this pathology, even in a large pediatric practice. We agree with Mazel and coworkers[27] that acute undisplaced osteochondral fractures should be treated with prolonged immobilization, while displaced fragments from the lateral malleolus or lateral talar dome should be treated either by arthroscopy or arthrotomy. Small fragments should be excised, while larger ones should be fixed (Fig. 55-11). In chronic undisplaced lesions, we have used plaster immobilization with improvement in some (Fig. 55-12). On occasion, with persisting symptoms, arthroscopy was used for localized debridement and drilling of the osteochondral defect with subsequent good results. Rarely, the patient will present with a nonunion or malunion of a large osteochondral fragment

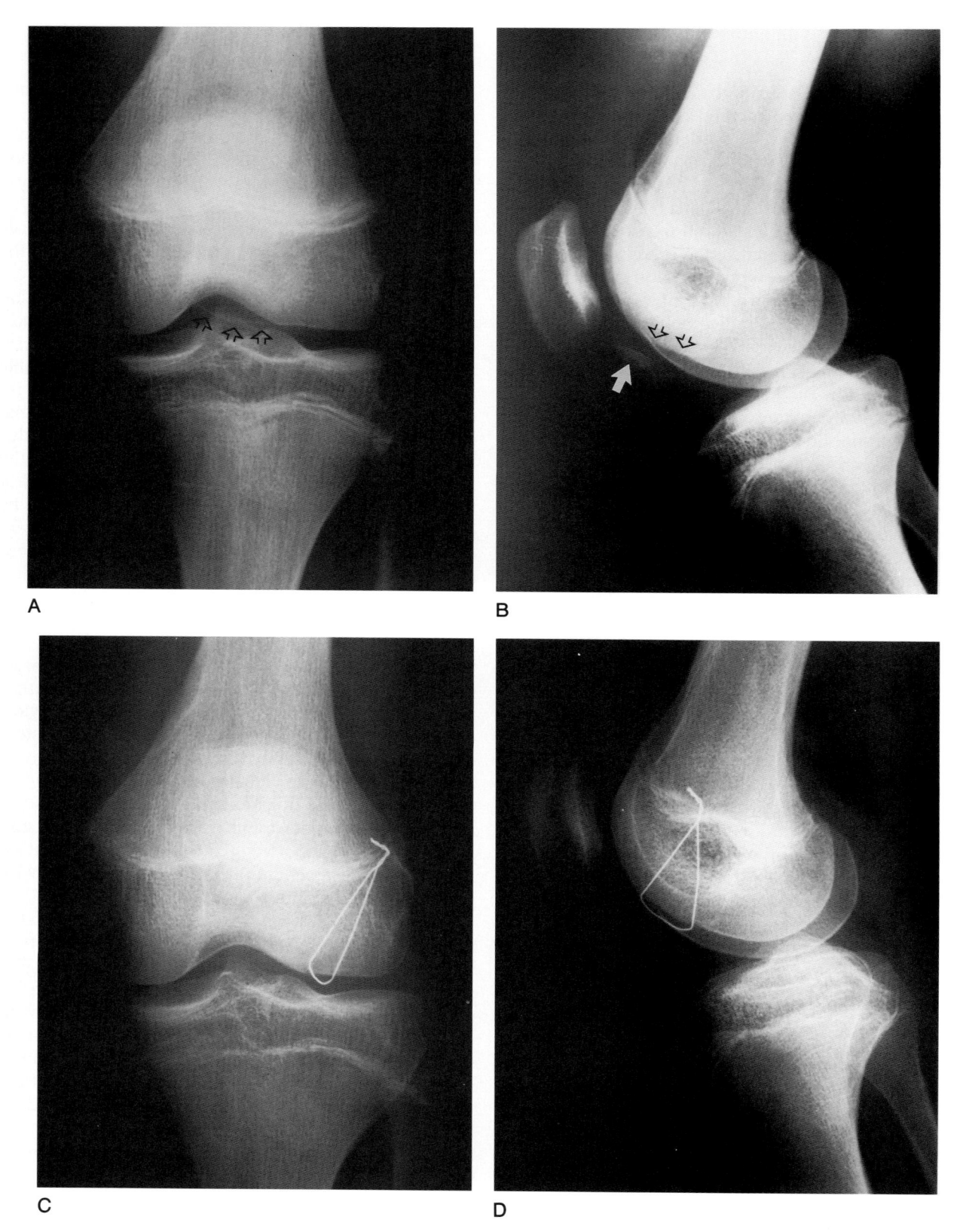

Fig. 55-8. **(A&B)** Following an acute dislocation of the left patella, this 15-year-old boy presented with this "few osteocytes thick" osteochondral fracture of the lateral condyle of the left knee. **(C&D)** An open reduction and internal fixation was achieved with a "U" shaped wire placed sagitally. Four months later, the patient is asymptomatic and the fracture appears healed on radiographs.

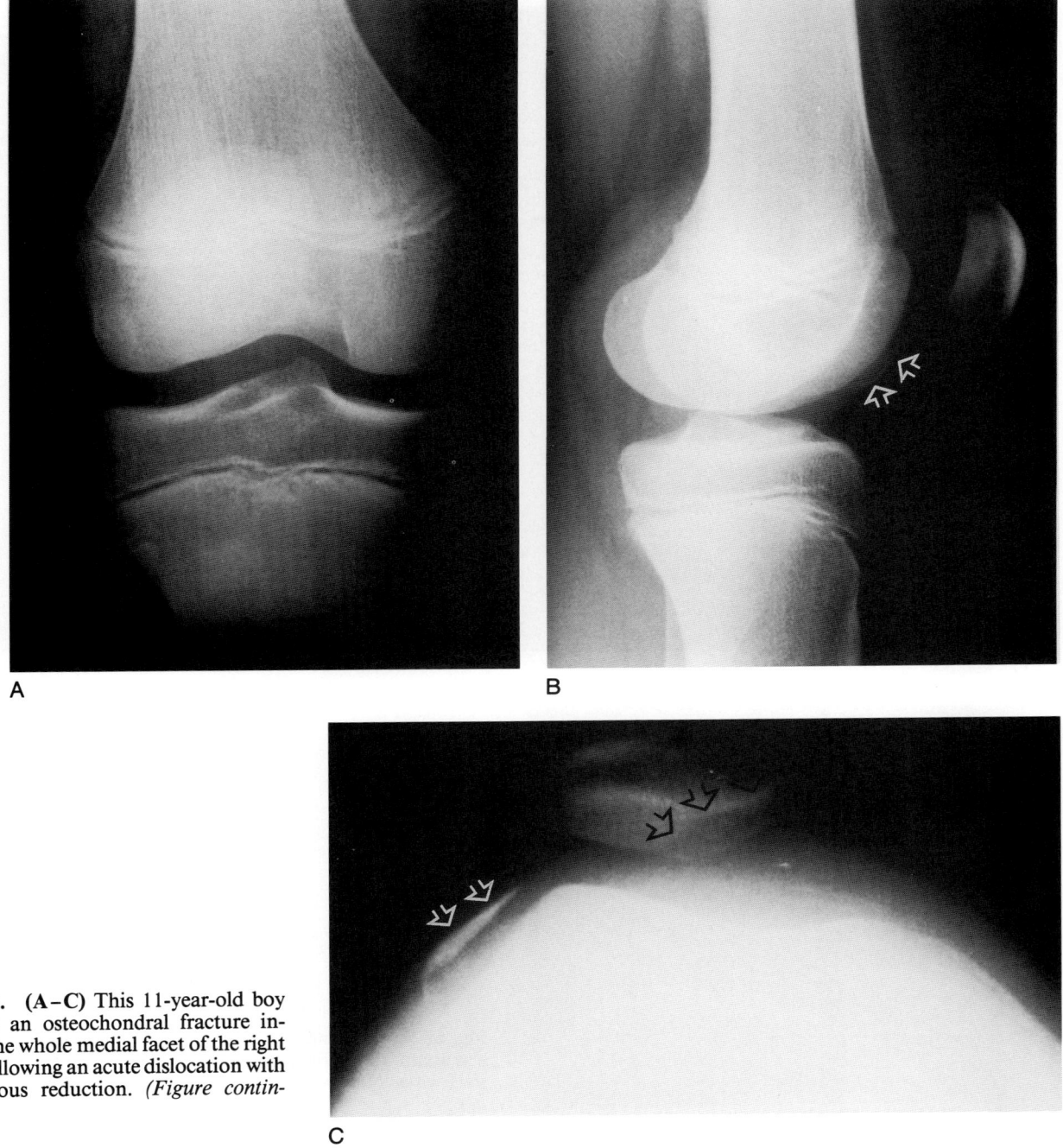

Fig. 55-9. (A–C) This 11-year-old boy sustained an osteochondral fracture involving the whole medial facet of the right patella following an acute dislocation with spontaneous reduction. *(Figure continues.)*

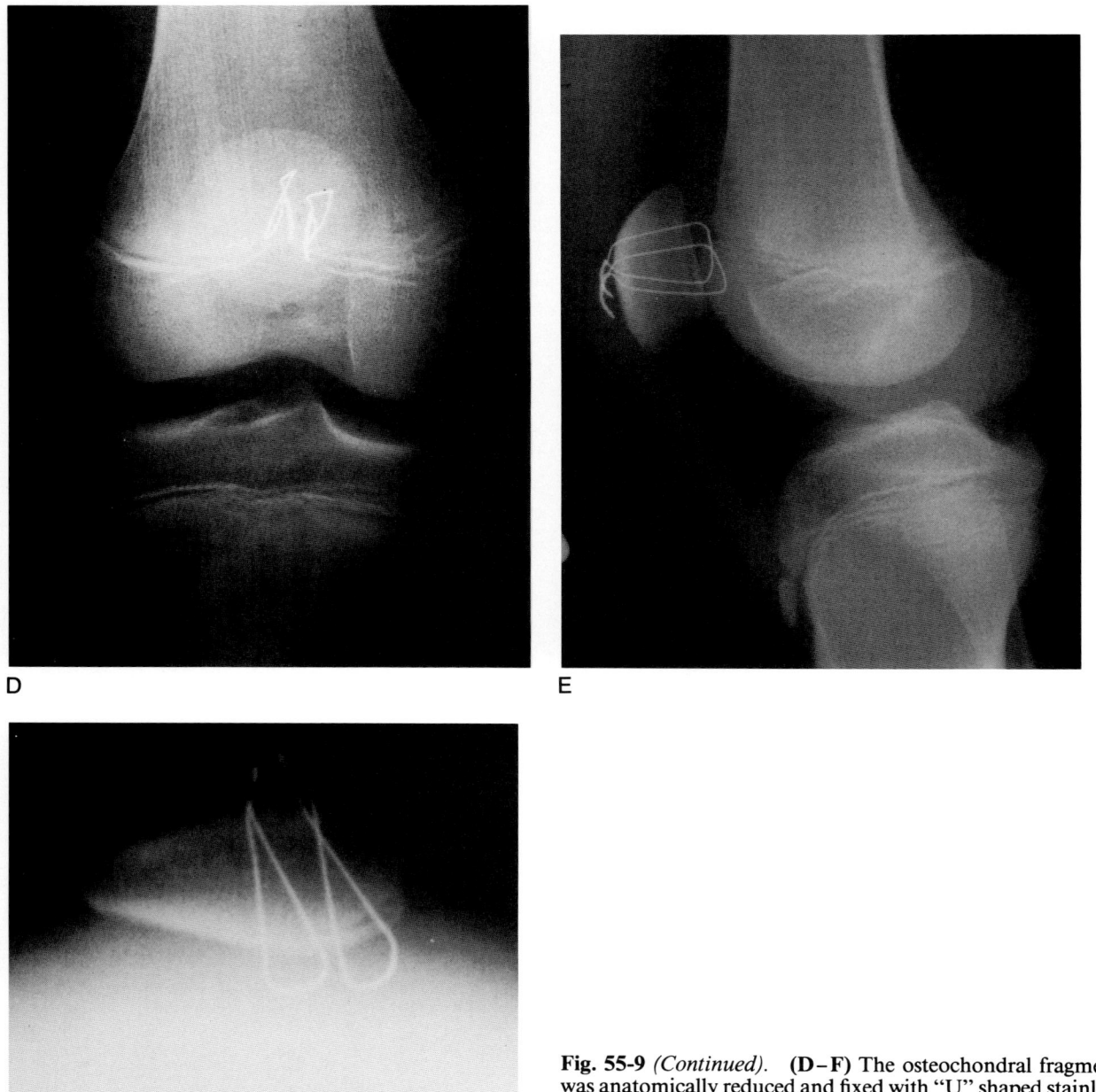

Fig. 55-9 *(Continued).* **(D–F)** The osteochondral fragment was anatomically reduced and fixed with "U" shaped stainless steel wires followed by V.M.O. advancement. *(Figure continues.)*

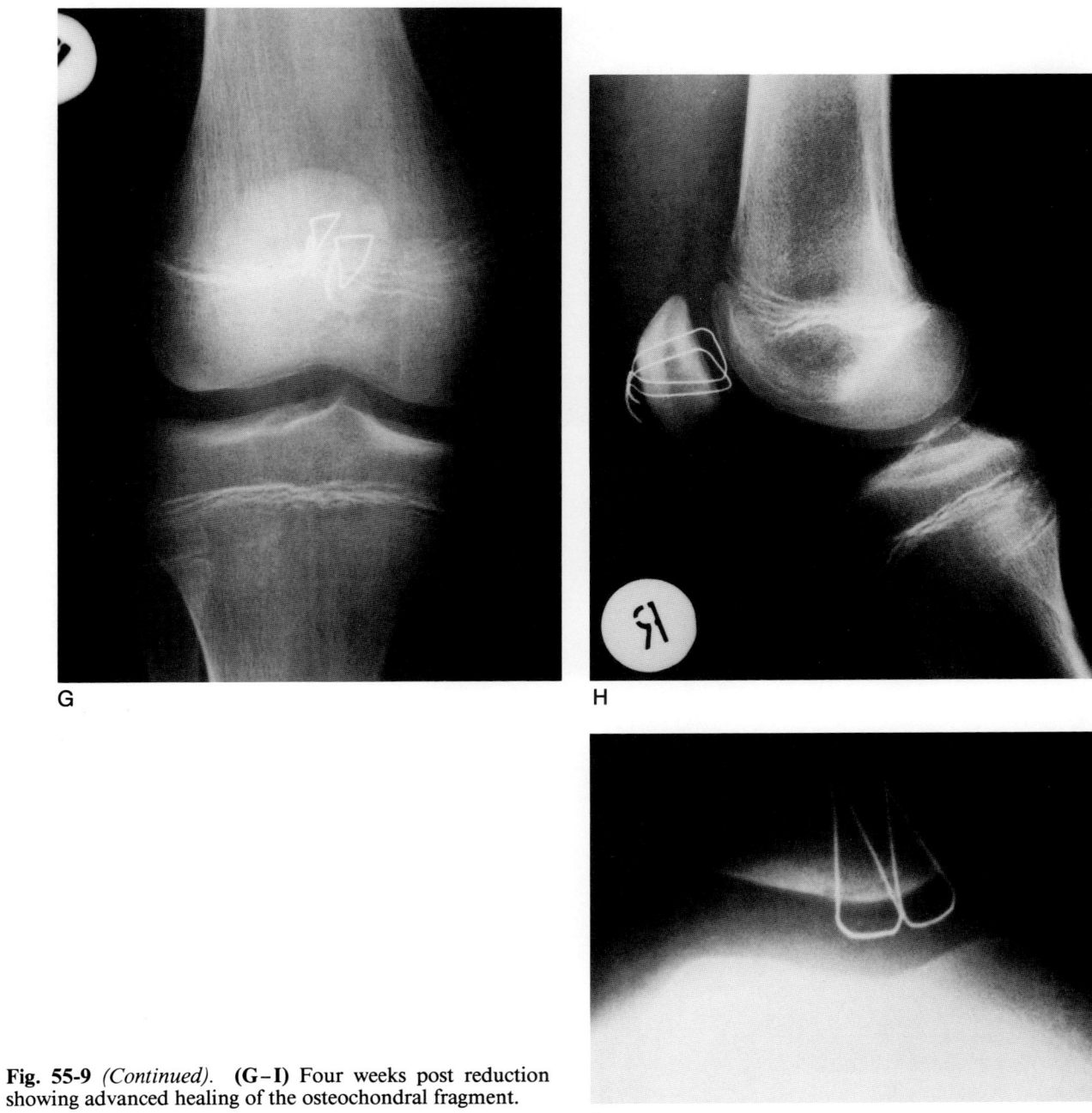

Fig. 55-9 *(Continued).* **(G–I)** Four weeks post reduction showing advanced healing of the osteochondral fragment.

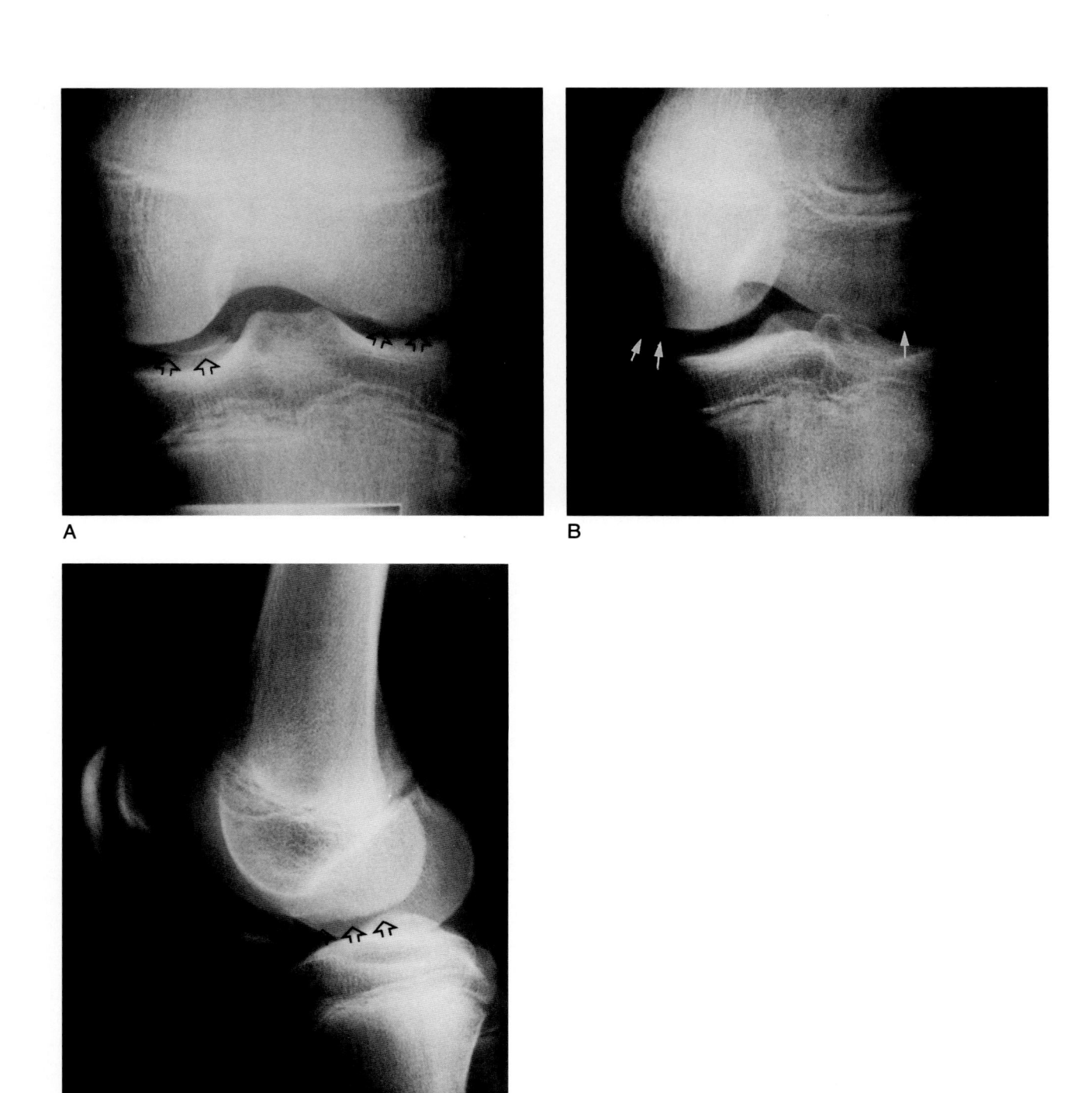

Fig. 55-10. (A–C) This 14-year-old boy sustained this extensive and comminuted osteochondral fracture of the lateral condyle of the left knee. *(Figure continues.)*

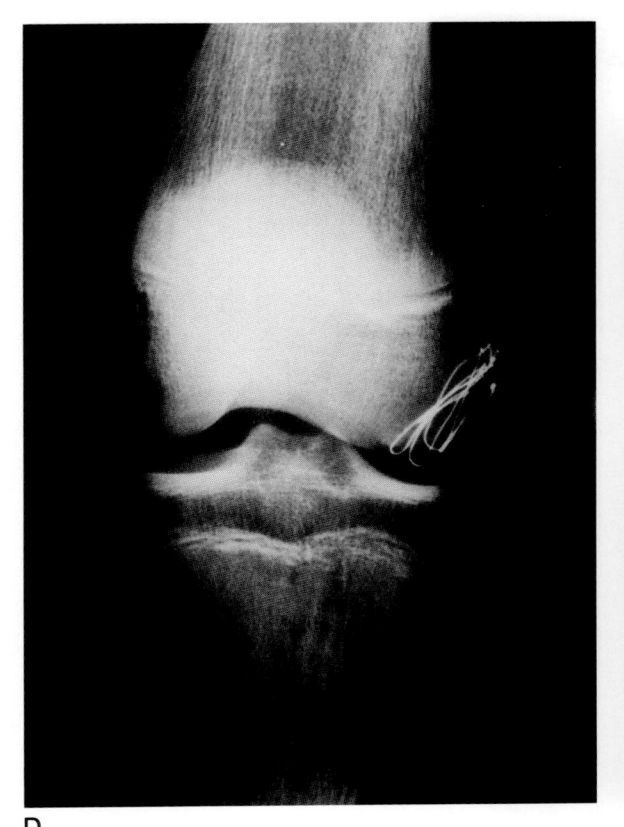

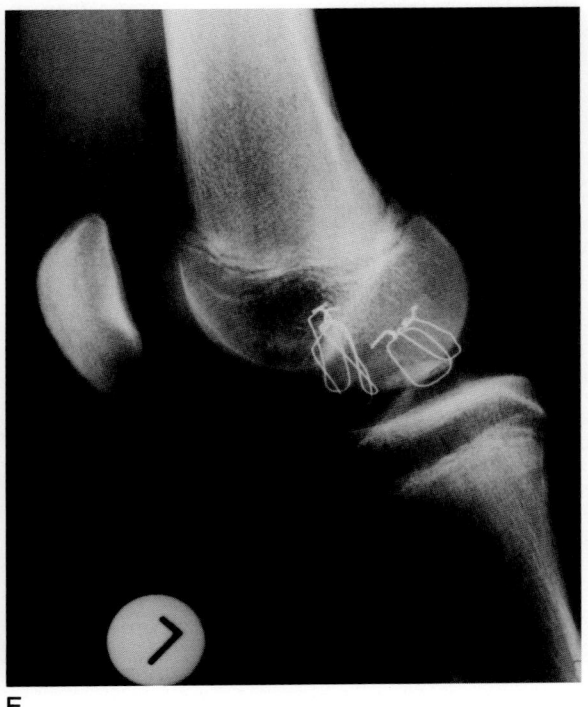

Fig. 55-10 *(Continued).* **(D&E)** At surgery, the fragment was multifragmented. The fixation was achieved by multiple "U" shaped stainless steel wires tightened over the lateral aspect of the condyle, supplemented with fibrin glue.

from the medial talar dome with significant secondary synovitis. In this situation, the fragment can be removed, although we prefer a more conservative attitude, which includes curettage of the bed to bleeding bone, autogenous bone grafting, meticulous trimming of the fragment, and fixation with countersunk screws.

Other Sites

For acute injury to other joints, the same basic principles of treatment apply. Following hip dislocation, early recognition of an osteochondral fragment is essential. The fragment should be excised or, if significant in size, reduced and fixed. In a more chronic situation, the only option is excision.

McElfresh and Dobyns[38] suggested that large osteochondral fractures of the metacarpals should be reconstructed with early mobilization. Zilch and Talke[67] reported their experience of reconstruction of the joint surface with fibrin sealant in 16 patients with osteochondral fragment at different locations in the upper limb. They suggested that this method may avoid early arthrodesis or oversized osteosynthetic material. Grant and Miller[42] reported a good result in a case report of an osteochondral fracture of the trochlea fixed with Smillie nails. From these reports, it appears that, as for the knee and ankle joints, and depending on the delay from injury, the site of the lesion and the size of the fragment, treatment consists either of open reduction and internal fixation of the fragment to restore joint congruity (Fig. 55-13), or excision of the fragment.

COMPLICATIONS

Short-term complications of undiagnosed and untreated children, depending on the joint involved, in-

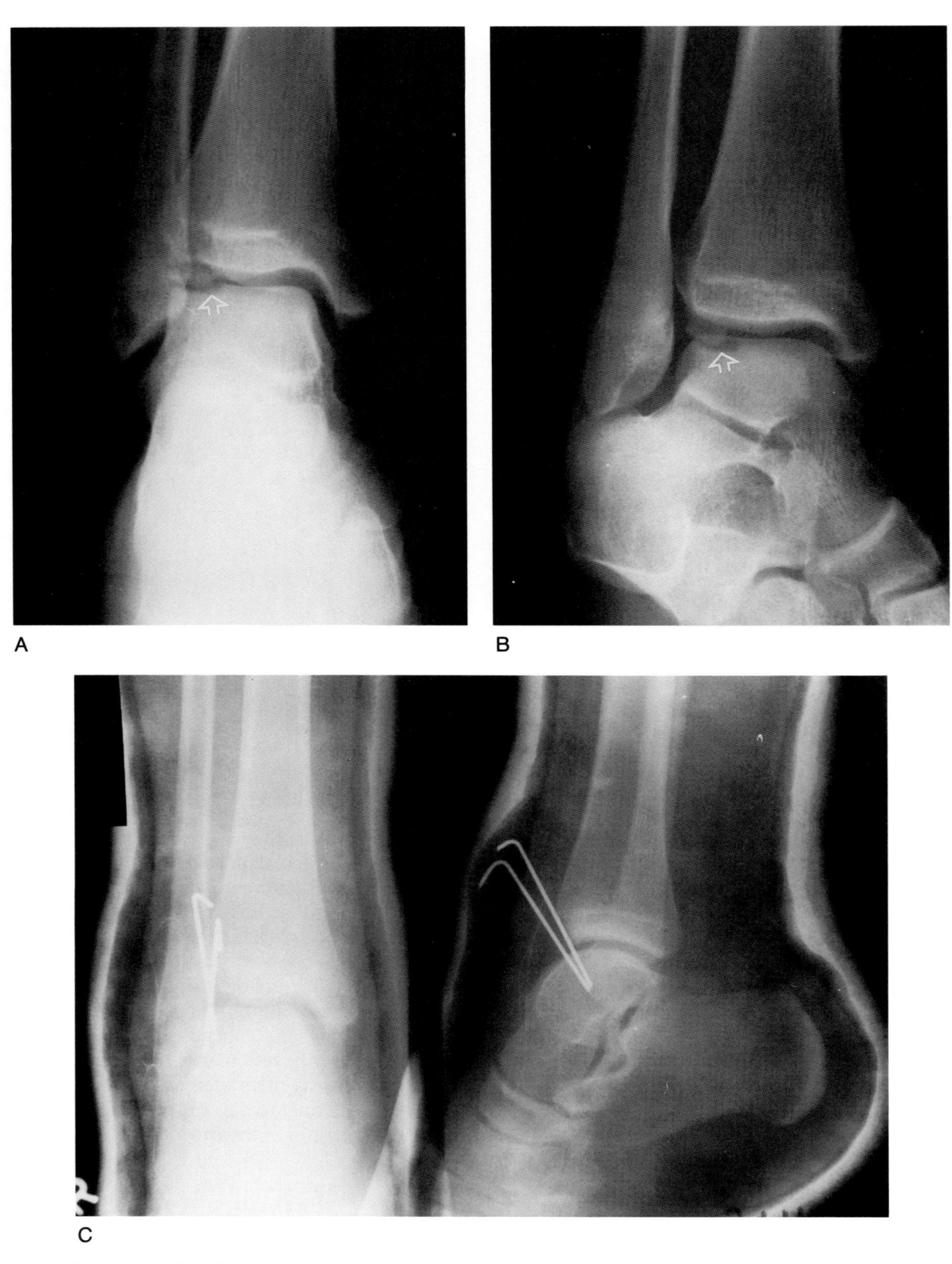

Fig. 55-11. **(A&B)** This 15-year-old boy sustained an osteochondral fracture of the lateral dome of the talus. At surgery, the fragment was found to be completely inverted with the cartilage opposed to the fracture bed. **(C)** The osteochondral fragment was anatomically reduced and held in place by two K-wires inserted percutaneously for easy removal 3 weeks later. *(Figure continues.)*

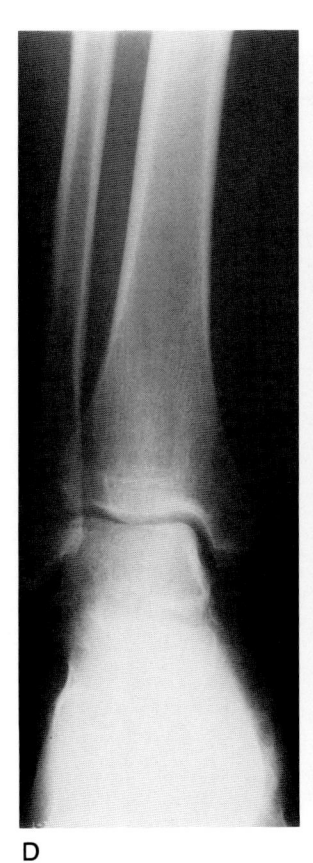

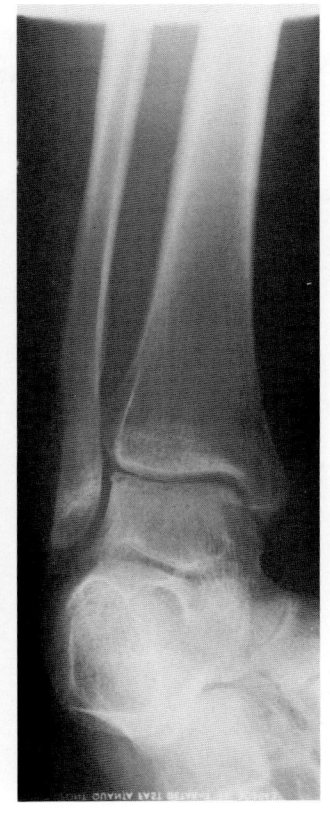

Fig. 55-11 *(Continued).* **(D)** Three months later, the fragment has healed with full pain free motion of the ankle.

clude intermittent or permanent pain, swelling, limited range of motion, or catching or locking, leading to permanent disability.[26] Short-term complications may also follow treatment. The effects of prolonged immobilization have been extensively studied.[2,6] They showed that this method of treatment leads to poor regenerated cartilage and to joint stiffness. Cartilage may also be damaged following ORIF, secondary to protruding osteosynthetic material or to material broken within the joint. In this respect, care should be taken to countersink screws or wires to avoid intra-articular protrusion of K-wires, screws, or nails. When using K-wires, placement should be such that later removal is facilitated without reentering the joint. Patients should be reviewed regularly for any displacement of osteosynthetic material (Fig. 55-14). Occasionally, this should be removed once the fracture has healed.[51] Deep infection and septic arthritis are also potential complications following surgery.

The unsolved problem related to long-term complications is potential degenerative osteoarthritis. As no long-term study exists for the knee joint, one should remember the similarity of the osteochondral fracture and the osteochondritis dissecans, in terms of the potential joint incongruity. The literature[68,69] suggests better long-term results following healing of osteochondritis dissecans of the femoral condyles treated before skeletal maturity, compared to excision of osteochondritis dissecans in a skeletally mature patient.

In the ankle joint, the prognosis seems to vary from one study to another. Bauer and colleagues[70] reported only 2 cases of osteoarthritis of 30 patients following osteochondritis dissecans, with an average follow-up of 21 years. Conversely, Canale and Belding,[22] reviewing 31 cases of osteochondral lesions of the ankle joint, mainly from the talar dome, found that approximately 50 percent had arthritic changes after an average follow-up of 11 years. From these data, it is difficult to propose any prophylactic approach to prevent degenerative arthritis, although it is our feeling that early diagnosis and reestablishment of cartilage integrity are the best ways to minimize short- and long-term complications.

SUMMARY

Although much has been written on osteochondral lesions, the diagnosis is often missed or delayed, leading to suboptimal treatment, chronic disability, and potential long-term sequelae. Following significant injury to any joint in children with rapid swelling, suggesting a hemarthrosis, an osteochondral fracture should be considered. Every effort should be made to rule out this possibility, including sophisticated radiographic methods or, better still, arthroscopic evaluation.

The therapeutic approach will vary with the joint involved, the location of the lesion and its size, and the time from injury. In our opinion, joint congruity should be restored when feasible, particularly when the defect is large or the lesion involves the weight-bearing surface.

The period of immobilization will vary with intrinsic stability of the fracture or its surgical stabilization. Weightbearing should be restrained until there is clinical and radiologic evidence of bony healing.

As significant disability may be associated with this injury, rehabilitation should be a part of the initial treatment to prevent muscle atrophy and subsequently to assist the patient in regaining a full range of motion, muscle strength, and endurance.

With early and adequate diagnosis and treatment, one may expect optimal clinical results, and hope to minimize long-term degenerative arthritis.

1022 / Management of Pediatric Fractures

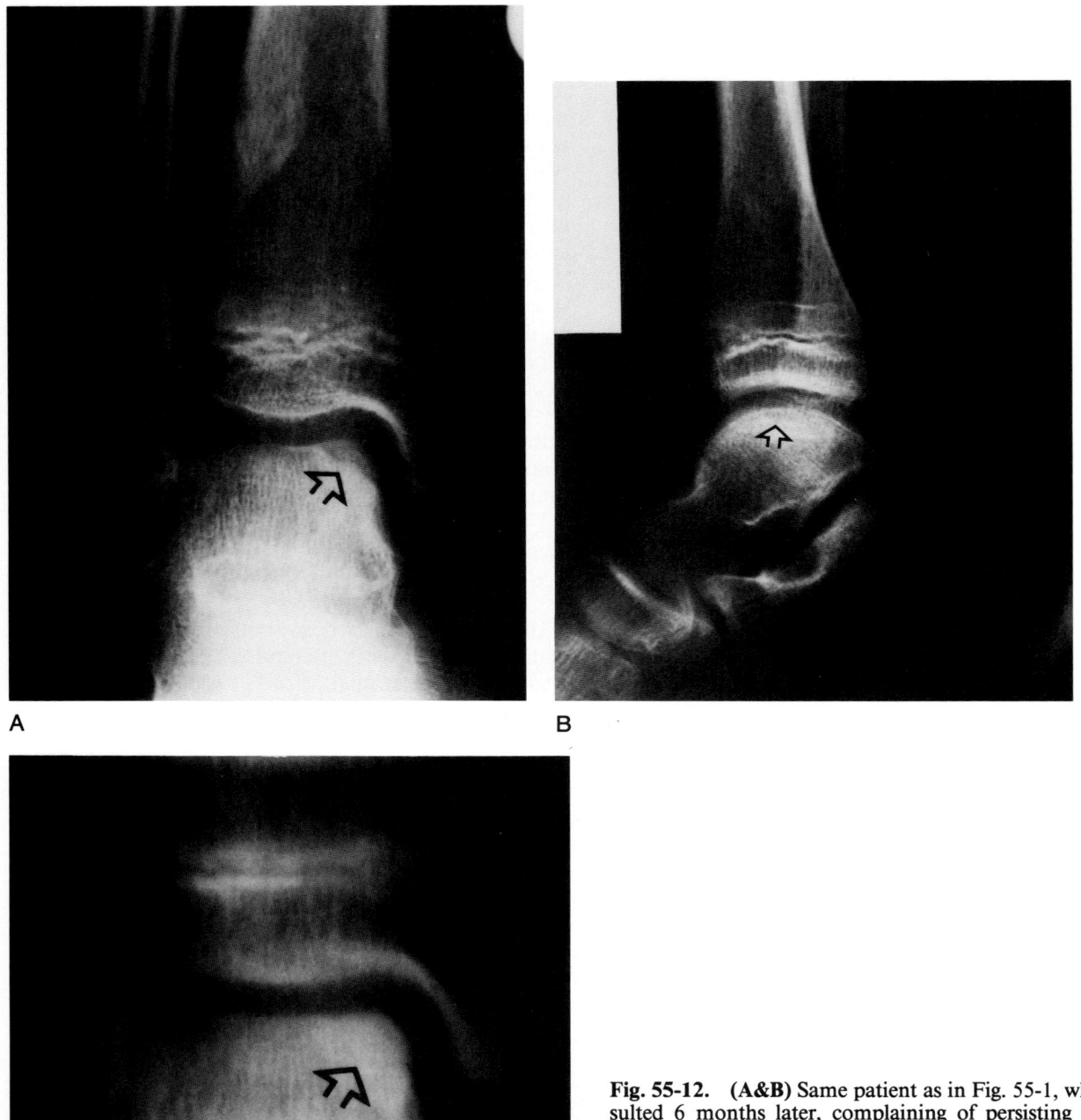

Fig. 55-12. (A&B) Same patient as in Fig. 55-1, who reconsulted 6 months later, complaining of persisting pain and swelling of the right ankle. Conservative treatment with prolonged immobilization with a walking cast followed by an AFO was employed. (C) Two years later, the patient is asymptomatic with radiographic evidence of healing of the osteochondral lesion.

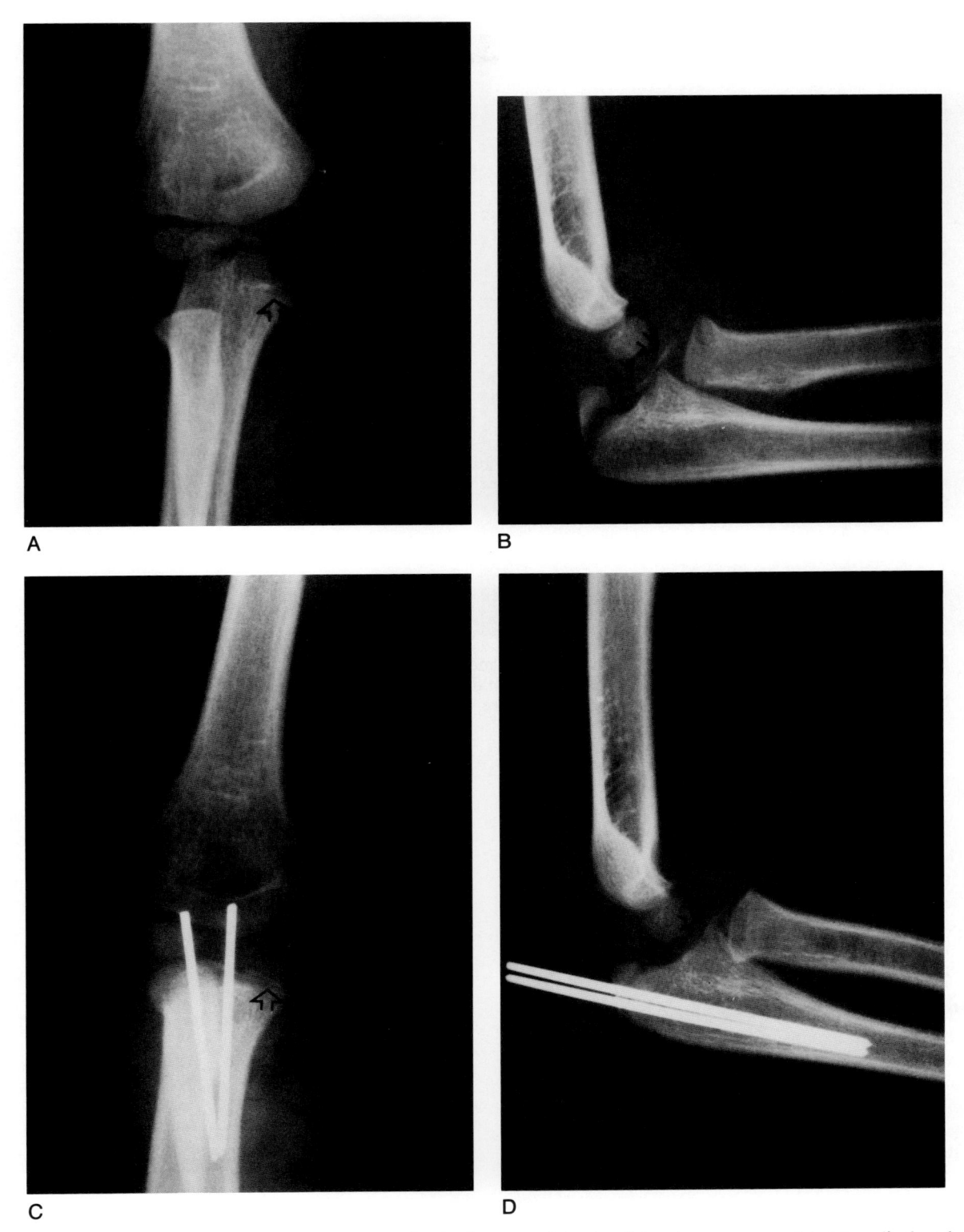

Fig. 55-13. **(A&B)** This 3-year-old girl sustained a fracture of the tip of the olecranon associated to a displaced osteochondral fracture of the lateral facet of the olecranon. **(C&D)** An open reduction of both fractures was performed without fixation of the osteochondral fragment, this latter being considered stable. One week later, radiographs show some displacement.

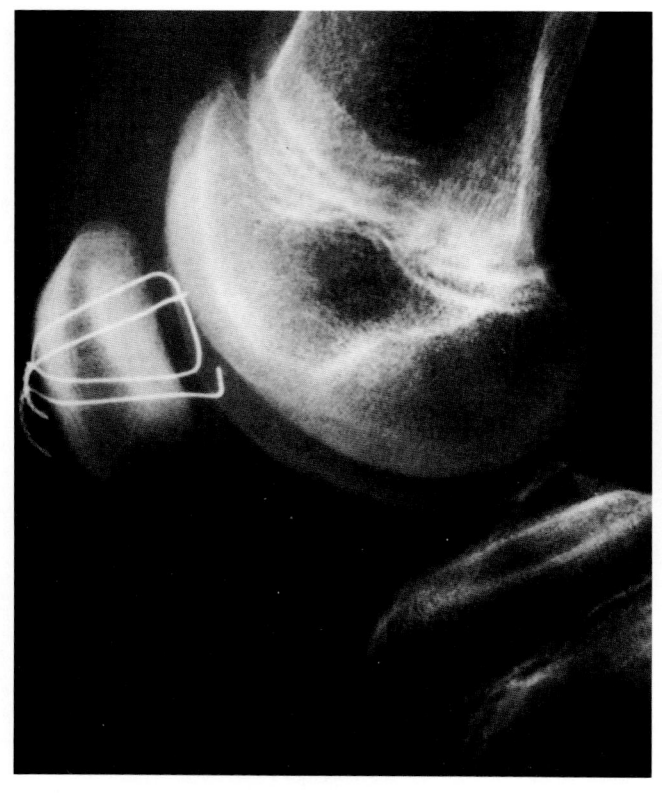

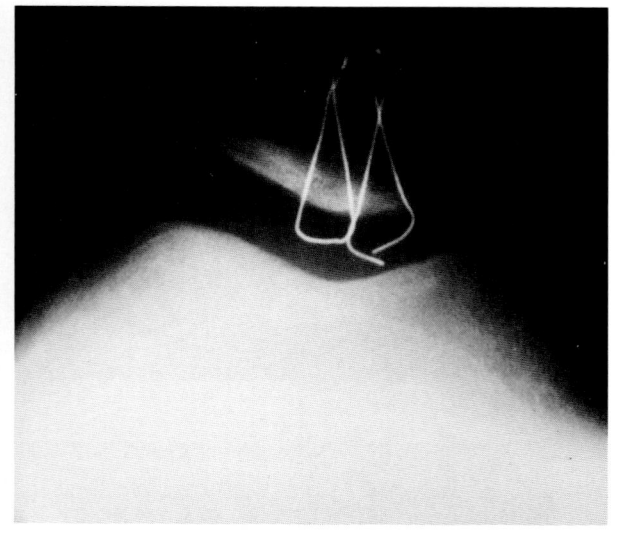

Fig. 55-14. Same patient as in Fig. 55-9 at follow-up, months after surgery. The radiographs showed a broken wire which required removal. Arthroscopy performed at the same time revealed a smooth surface of the patella, but abrasions of the femoral condyle by the broken wire.

REFERENCES

1. O'Donoghue DH: Chondral and osteochondral fractures. J Trauma 6:469, 1966
2. Salter RB, Simmonds DF, Malcolm BW et al: The biological effect of continuous passive motion on the healing of full-thickness defects in articular cartilage: an experimental investigation in the rabbit. J Bone Joint Surg [Am] 62:1232, 1980
3. Buckwalter JA, Mow VC: Cartilage repair as treatment of osteoarthritis. In Goldberg VM, Mankin HJ (eds): Osteoarthritis: Diagnosis and Management. 2nd Ed. WB Saunders, Philadelphia, 1990
4. Buckwalter JA, Rosenberg LC, Hunziker E: Articular cartilage: composition, structure, response to injury and methods of facilitating repair. p. 19. In Ewing JW (ed): The Science of Arthroscopy. Raven Press, New York, 1990
5. Convery FR, Akeson WH, Keown GH: The repair of large osteochondral defects: an experimental study in horses. Clin Orthop 82:253, 1972
6. O'Driscoll SW, Salter RB: The repair of major osteochondral defects in joint surfaces by neochondrogenesis with autogenous osteoperiosteal grafts stimulated by continuous passive motion: an experimental investigation in the rabbit. Clin Orthop 208:131, 1986
7. Mow VC, Ratcliffe A, Rosenwasser MP, Buckwalter JA: Experimental studies on repair of large osteochondral defects at a high weight bearing area of the knee joint: a tissue engineering study. J Biomech Eng 113:198, 1991
8. Pappas AM: Osteochondritis dissecans. Clin Orthop 158:59, 1981
9. Milgram JW: The classification of loose bodies in human joints. Clin Orthop 124:282, 1977
10. Matthewson MH, Dandy DJ: Osteochondral fractures of the lateral femoral condyle: a result of indirect violence to the knee. J Bone Joint Surg [Br] 60:199, 1978
11. Robert M, Govault E, Setton D et al: Les fractures ostéochondrales du genou chez l'enfant sportif. Ann Pediatr 34:287, 1987
12. Mayer G, Seidlein H: Chondral and osteochondral fractures of the knee joint: treatment and results. Arch Orthop Trauma Surg 107:154, 1988
13. Dehaven KE: Diagnosis of acute knee injuries with hemarthrosis. Am J Sports Med 8:9, 1980

14. Gillquist J, Hagberg G, Oreturp N: Arthroscopy in acute injuries of the knee joint. Acta Orthop Scand 48:190, 1977
15. Noyes FR, Bassette RW, Grood ES, Butler DL: Arthroscopy in acute traumatic hemarthrosis of the knee: incidence of anterior cruciate tears and other injuries. J Bone Joint Surg [Am] 62:687, 1980
16. Haupt PR, Reek A: Acute arthroscopy in children. Akt Traumatol 17:43, 1987
17. Vellet AD, Marks PH, Fowler PJ, Munro TG: Occult posttraumatic osteochondral lesions of the knee: prevalence, classification and short-term sequelae evaluated with MR imaging. Radiology 178:271, 1991
18. Yvars MF: Osteochondral fractures of the dome of the talus. Clin Orthop 114:185, 1976
19. Lantz BA, McAndrew M, Scioli M, Fitzrandolph RL: The effect of concomitant chondral injuries accompanying operatively reduced malleolar fractures. J Orthop Trauma 5:125, 1991
20. Berndt AL, Harty M: Transchondral fractures (osteochondritis dissecans) of the talus. J Bone Joint Surg [Am] 41:988, 1959
21. Pettine KA, Morrey BF: Osteochondral fractures of the talus: a long-term follow-up. J Bone Joint Surg [Br] 69:89, 1987
22. Canale ST, Belding RH: Osteochondral lesions of the talus. J Bone Joint Surg [Am] 62:97, 1980
23. Gerard Y, Bernier JM, Ameil M: Lésions ostéochondrales de la poulie astragalienne. Rev Chir Orthop 75:466, 1989
24. Koulvachouk JF, Schneider-Maunoury G, Rodineau J et al: Les lésions ostéochondrales du dôme astragalien avec nécrose partielle: leur traitement chirurgical par curetage et comblement. Rev Chir Orthop 76:480, 1990
25. Huylebroek JF, Martens M, Simon JP: Transchondral talar dome fracture. Arch Orthop Trauma Surg 104:238, 1985
26. Anderson IF, Crichton KJ, Grattan-Smith T et al: Osteochondral fractures of the dome of the talus. J Bone Joint Surg [Am] 71:1143, 1989
27. Mazel CH, Rigault P, Padovani JP et al: Les fractures de l'astragale de l'enfant: a propos de 23 cas. Rev Chir Orthop 72:183, 1986
28. Vahvanen V, Westerlund M, Nikku R: Lateral ligament injury of the ankle in children. Acta Orthop Scand 55:21, 1984
29. Schütze F, Maas V: Osteochondrale Mitbeteiligung bei fibulotalaren Bandrupturen. Z Kinderchir 44:91, 1989
30. Tehranzadeh J, Vanarthos W, Pais MJ: Osteochondral impaction of the femoral head associated with hip dislocation: CT study in 35 patients. AJR 155:1049, 1990
31. Ordway CB, Xeller CF: Transverse computerized axial tomography of patients with posterior dislocation of the hip. J Trauma 24:76, 1984
32. Barquet A: Traumatic hip dislocation in childhood. Acta Orthop Scand 50:549, 1979
33. Pennsylvania Orthopaedic Society: Traumatic dislocation of the hip joint in children: final report. J Bone Joint Surg [Am] 50:79, 1968
34. Libri R, Calderon JE, Capelli A, Soncini G: Traumatic dislocation of the hip in children and adolescents. Ital J Orthop Traumatol 12:61, 1986
35. Harder JA, Bobechko WP, Sullivan R, Danerman A: Computerized axial tomography to demonstrate occult fractures of the acetabulum in children. Can J Surg 24:409, 1981
36. Epstein HC: Traumatic anterior and simple posterior dislocations of the hip in adults and children. Instr Course Lect 22:115, 1973
37. Stachel P, Hofmann V, Kap-herr S, Schild H: Die traumatische huft Luxation im Kindesalter. Z Kinderchir 44:156, 1989
38. McElfresh EC, Dobyns JH: Intra-articular metacarpal head fractures. J Hand Surg 8:383, 1983
39. O'Brien ET: Fractures of the hand and wrist region. In Rockwood CA Jr, Wilkins KE, King RE (eds): Fractures in children. 3rd Ed. JB Lippincott, Philadelphia, 1991
40. Ogden JA: Wrist and hand. In: Skeletal Injury in the Child. 2nd Ed. WB Saunders, Philadelphia, 1990
41. Shankar NS, Craxford AD: Posterior dislocation of the elbow with osteochondral fracture. Br J Accident Surg 20:51, 1989
42. Grant IR, Miller JH: Osteochondral fracture of the trochlea associated with fracture dislocation of the elbow. Br J Accident Surg 6:257, 1975
43. McManama GB, Micheli LJ, Berry MV, Sohn RS: The surgical treatment of osteochondritis of the capitellum. Am J Sports Med 13:11, 1985
44. Blasier RB, Burkus JK: Management of posterior fracture-dislocations of the shoulder. Clin Orthop 232:197, 1988
45. Milgram JW: The development of loose bodies in human joints. Clin Orthop 124:292, 1977
46. Terry GC, Flandry F, Van Manen JW, Norwood L: Isolated chondral fractures of the knee. Clin Orthop 234:170, 1988
47. Bauer M, Jackson RW: Chondral lesions of the femoral condyles: a system of arthroscopic classification. J Arthrosc Rel Surg 4:97, 1988
48. Milgram JW, Rogers LF, Miller JW: Osteochondral fractures: mechanism of injury and fate of fragments. AJR 130:651, 1978
49. Kennedy JC, Grainger RW, McGraw RW: Osteochondral fractures of the femoral condyles. J Bone Joint Surg [Br] 48:436, 1966
50. Rosenberg NJ: Osteochondral fractures of the lateral femoral condyle. J Bone Joint Surg [Am] 46:1013, 1964
51. Milgram JE: Osteochondral fractures of the articular surfaces of the knee. In Helfet AJ (ed): Disorders of the Knee. JB Lippincott, Philadelphia, 1982
52. Hughston JC, Walsh WM, Puddu G: Patellar subluxation and dislocation. Monogr Clin Orthop p. 5. WB Saunders, Philadelphia, 1984
53. Ahstrom JP: Osteochondral fracture in the knee joint associated with hypermobility and dislocation of the patella. J Bone Joint Surg [Am] 47:1491, 1965

54. Henderson NJ, Houghton GR: Osteochondral fractures of the knee in children. In Problematic Musculo-skeletal Injuries in Children. Butterworth, London, 1983
55. Lipscomb AB, Anderson AF: Tears of the anterior cruciate ligament in adolescents. J Bone Joint Surg [Am] 68:19, 1986
56. McCarroll JR, Rettig AC, Shelbourne KD: Anterior cruciate ligament injuries in the young athlete with open physes. Am J Sports Med 16:44, 1988
57. Gilley JS, Gelman MI, Edson DM, Metcalf RW: Chondral fractures of the knee. Radiology 138:51, 1981
58. Smillie IS: Treatment of osteochondritis dissecans. J Bone Joint Surg [Br] 39:248, 1957
59. Hammerle CP, Jacob RP: Chondral and osteochondral fractures after luxation of the patella and their treatment. Arch Orthop Trauma Surg 97:207, 1980
60. Rorabeck CH, Bobechko WP: Acute dislocation of the patella with osteochondral fracture. J Bone Joint Surg [Br] 58:237, 1976
61. Ittner G, Jaskulka R, Fasol P: Treatment of flake fracture of the talus. Z Orthop Grenzgeb 127:183, 1989
62. Frank A, Cohen P, Beaufils P, Lamare J: Arthroscopic treatment of osteochondral lesions of the talar dome. Arthroscopy 5:57, 1989
63. Parisien SJ: Arthroscopic treatment of osteochondral lesions of the talus. Am J Sports Med 14:211, 1986
64. Baker CL, Andrews JR, Ryan JB: Arthroscopic treatment of transchondral talar dome fractures. Arthroscopy 2:82, 1986
65. Pritsch M, Horoshovski H, Farine I: Arthroscopic treatment of osteochondral lesions of the talus. J Bone Joint Surg [Am] 68:862, 1986
66. Angermann P, Riegels-Nielson P: Fibrin fixation of osteochondral talar fractures. Acta Orthop Scand 61:551, 1990
67. Zilch H, Talke M: Fibrinogen glue in osteochondral fractures with small fragments of the upper limb. Ann Chir Main 6:173, 1987
68. Hughston JC, Hergenroeder PT, Courtnay BG: Osteochondritis dissecans of the femoral condyles. J Bone Joint Surg [Am] 66:1340, 1984
69. Linden B: Osteochondritis dissecans of the femoral condyles. J Bone Joint Surg [Am] 59:769, 1977
70. Bauer M, Jonsson K, Linden B: Osteochondritis dissecans of the ankle. J Bone Joint Surg [Br] 69:93, 1987

56

Pathologic Fractures

Benoit Poitras
Charles H. Rivard

> Healing is a matter of time, but it is sometimes also a matter of opportunity.
> —HIPPOCRATES

Pathologic fractures occur with minimal trauma in bones weakened by some abnormal condition. The deficiency of the bone may be due to local changes or may be associated with a generalized skeletal disease.

True pathologic fractures occur in children from different causes than in adults. Paget's disease and Charcot's disease are seldom found in children. Metastatic malignancy is an unusual cause of fracture in childhood. On the other hand, osteogenesis imperfecta and congenital pseudarthrosis are infrequently a cause of fractures in adults.

CLASSIFICATION

Pathologic fractures may be classified as shown in Table 56-1.[1]

BIOMECHANICS OF BONE PREDISPOSING TO PATHOLOGIC FRACTURES

Bone fractures can be produced by a simple load that exceeds the ultimate strength of the bone or by repeated applications of a load of lower magnitude.[2] If the strength of the bone is modified by a local lesion or by a more generalized disease, then less force will be required to produce a pathologic fracture.

It has been demonstrated in several studies that a bone lesion in excess of 3.5 cm of destruction or greater than 50 percent of the cortex predisposes to pathologic fractures.[3] Since these are adult studies, smaller lesions may predispose children to pathologic fractures, depending upon in which bone they are located. Children's bones have the added advantage of possessing both elastic and plastic behavior. This tends to reduce the detrimental effects of the weakening effect of bone loss. The stress concentration factor of a material is based on the assumption that the material is somewhat homogeneous and has a linear elastic stress-strain curve. Children's bone is very elastic and usually requires a greater bone loss than adult bone to develop a pathologic fracture.

Biomechanical studies of drill holes in bone have suggested that the stress concentrating effect of any hole less than 30 percent of the bone diameter is approximately the same. Brooks and coworkers[4] have shown that the 2.8- or 3.6-mm drill hole in bone reduced the energy-absorbing capacity by 55 percent. Thus, it may be more important in children who are subjected to considerable torsion in their playtime activities to try to reduce these activities after a plate has been removed subsequent to fracture fixation or an osteotomy. Another factor that affects the forces exerted in bone is the presence of any sharp edges, notches, or cracks that may act as stress risers. Thus, lesions that erode bone in an eccentric

TABLE 56-1. Classification of Pathologic Fractures in Children

Local Causes	General Conditions

Benign tumors or tumorlike conditions
  Unicameral bone cyst
  Aneurysmal bone cyst
  Nonossifying fibroma
  Enchondroma
Malignant bone tumors
  Primary, e.g., osteogenic sarcoma (Fig. 56-1), Ewing's sarcoma
  Metastatic, e.g., neuroblastoma, Wilms' tumor
Infectious or inflammatory diseases
  Osteomyelitis (Fig. 56-2)
  Eosinophilic granuloma
Iatrogenic
  Removal of bone for bone graft
  Through screw holes
	Congenital affections
	  Osteogenesis imperfecta
	  Osteopetrosis
	  Pseudarthrosis in neurofibromatosis
	Developmental affections
	  Fibrous dysplasia
	Metabolic affections
	  Rickets and renal osteodystrophy
	  Scurvy
	  Hyperparathyroidism, primary and secondary
	  Cushing's syndrome from cortisone treatment
	  Drugs, e.g., methotrexate
	Disuse atrophy
	  Due to prolonged immobilization
	  Secondary to paralytic disease
	    Poliomyelitis
	    Cerebral palsy
	    Myelomeningocele
	    Muscular dystrophy

manner, such as a cyst or tumor, may predispose the bone to a concentration of forces at the pathology site due to the shape of the lesion itself and subsequently to the shape of the biopsy that is performed on the lesion. Clarke and coworkers[5] determined that the configuration that maximizes remaining bony strength following a biopsy is an oblong hole with rounded edges. Where possible, this type of biopsy lesion should be fashioned in children, although this is not always possible. Investigations of McBroom and coworkers[6] of the effects of metastatic bone lesions on the strength of bone suggested the possibility of a prediction of fracture based on the geometric properties of the bone lesions. The geometric effects are probably more significant with more rapidly expanding defects rather than slowly expanding defects such as are common in children, since with slower growing lesions, adaptive remodeling tends to restore the strength to the bone with appropriate remodeling in accordance with Wolf's law.

FRACTURE CHARACTERISTICS

Pathologic fractures have some common characteristics. These fractures generally are minimally displaced: they heal rapidly and nonunion is rare. The original pathologic lesions occasionally heal after the fracture without any further treatment, obliterated by the fracture callus.

The clinical history of pathologic fracturing is one of minimal trauma, causing the fracture. Usually, the child experiences a sudden onset of localized pain. Often, a twisting injury such as throwing a baseball will result in a rotatory torque of the upper extremity, which is often

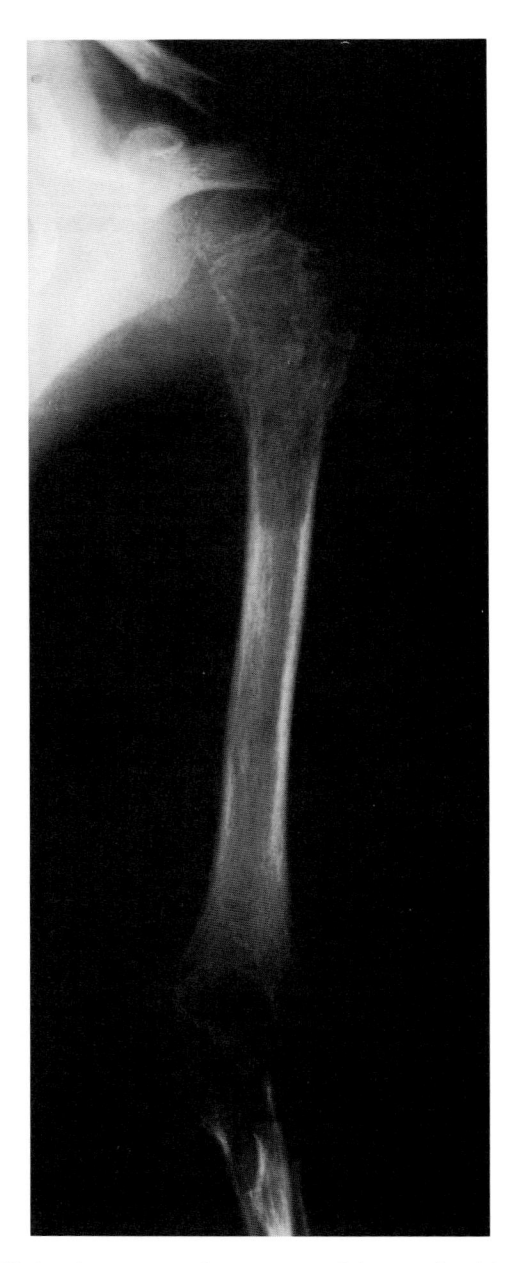

Fig. 56-1. An osteogenic sarcoma of the proximal humerus associated with a pathologic fracture.

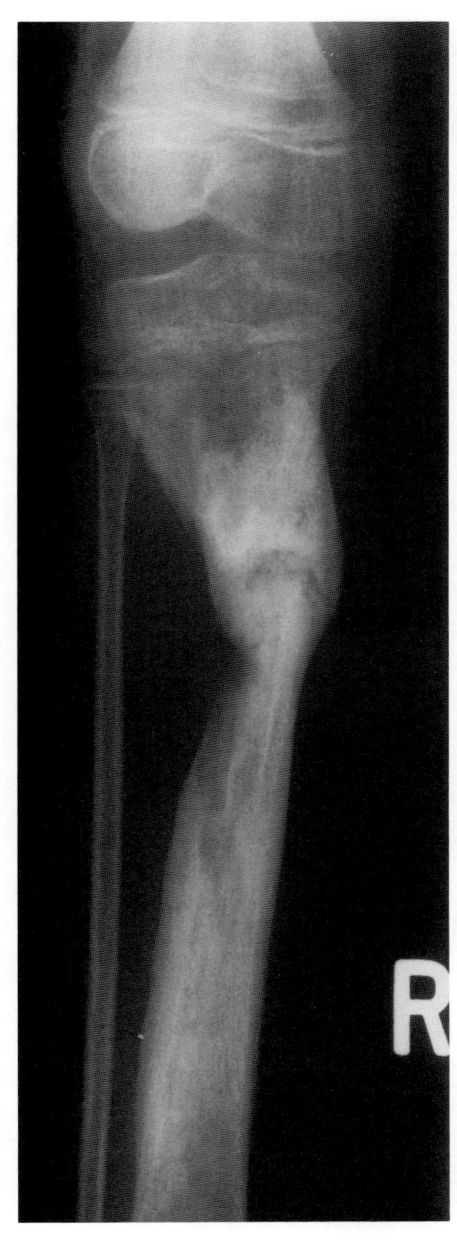

Fig. 56-2. Pathologic fracture through area of healing osteomyelitis.

sufficient to fracture through a defect in the humerus, or radius and ulna, resulting in a pathologic fracture.

TREATMENT

In general terms, treatment of pathologic fractures follows the same principles as other traumatic lesions: closed reduction when fractures are displaced, simple immobilization or cast, as needed, and for certain anatomic sites, such as the femoral neck, a more aggressive internal fixation may be required. When bony union is obtained, the original lesion, such as unicameral bone cyst and nonossifying fibroma, may need specific treatment.

Unfortunately, many children sustain pathologic fractures secondary to disuse osteoporosis either from prolonged immobilization in a cast or simply because they have other disabilities that make it difficult for them to weight bear. Wolf's law, which states that bone is laid down in direct proportion to the amount of stress that is exerted, is one of the best defences against fractures. Thus, as a general principle, it is best to have children ambulatory in casts and to avoid prolonged immobilization. In children who are relegated to wheelchair existence because of other disease processes or injuries, where possible, weightbearing in a standing frame or some other mobility device will greatly assist in preventing pathologic fracturing. In a recent study of the effects of weightbearing in osteogenesis imperfecta, Letts and coworkers[7] measured bone density in children with osteopenia secondary to osteogenesis imperfecta before and after supportive standing with a vacuum pants orthosis.[7] The bone mineral content as measured by the bone densitometer in the tibia showed significant increase in the bone density due to upright positioning.

In this chapter, common pathologic fractures associated with a number of predisposing factors that cause weakening of the bone structure are discussed. It is important to emphasize that in children, in contradistinction to adults, pathologic fracturing secondary to metastatic lesions are very uncommon.

Other conditions causing pathologic fractures such as myelomeningocele, osteogenesis imperfecta (Fig. 56-3), stress fractures, child abuse, severely handicapped children,[8] as well as pathologic fractures seen in the spine, are reviewed in more detail in other chapters.

UNICAMERAL BONE CYST

The unicameral bone cyst is a cavity within the bone containing serous fluid and lined by a thin membrane of connective tissue. The majority of these lesions are seen in the metaphysis of long bones and 90 percent are generally located in the proximal humerus or femur.[9] The lesion is radiolucent and centrally located, often immediately adjacent to the growth plate (Fig. 56-4) when the patient is 10 years of age or younger (as the patient

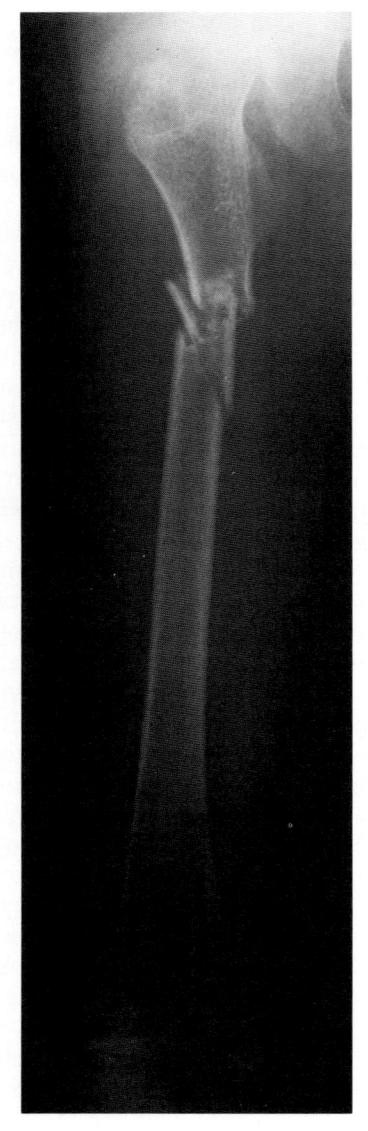

Fig. 56-3. A pathologic fracture of the proximal femur in a patient with osteogenesis imperfecta.

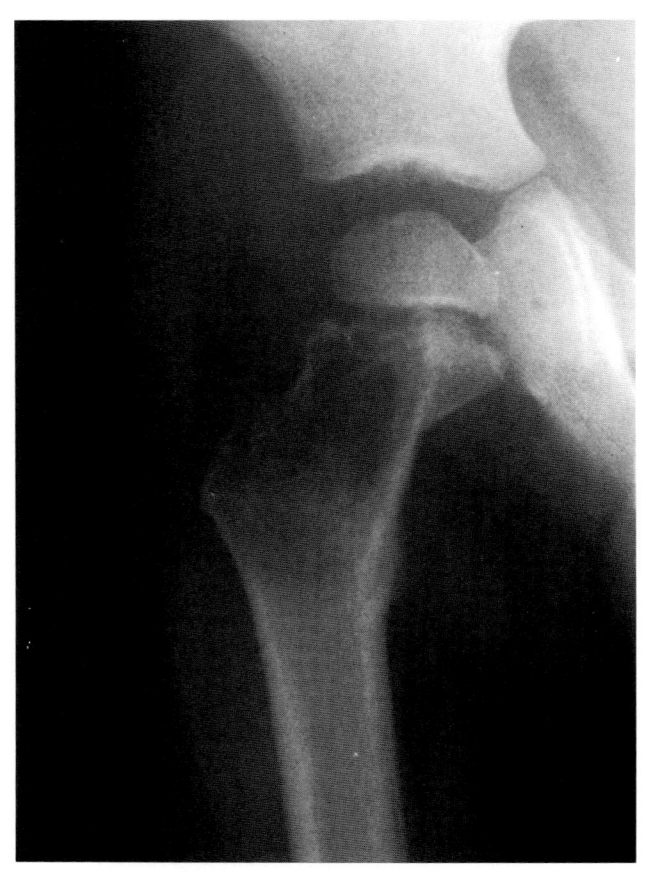

Fig. 56-4. Unicameral bone cyst of proximal femur in a 6-year-old girl. This lesion is immediately adjacent to the growth plate and is therefore considered very active. Pathologic microfractures and complete cortical fracturing is common in these cysts.

becomes older, the epiphysis grows away from the lesion).[10] Surrounding bone is not reactive, and there is no periosteal reaction. The unicameral bone cyst normally heals progressively during and after the second decade of life. Occasionally, it heals spontaneously after a pathologic fracture (Fig. 56-5).

The lesion is usually found when the patient sustains a pathologic fracture. In a series from Alfred Dupont Institute,[11] the diagnosis was made after pathologic fractures in 71 percent of 57 patients.

The cystic nature of this lesion can often be identified following a fracture when the "fallen fragment sign" is present (Fig. 56-6). A fragment of cortical bone "falls" into the cystic cavity, originating from the surface of the periosteum. Such migration of the fragment cannot be seen in a lesion that is filled with solid tissue.

Treatment of fractures in unicameral bone cysts includes simple immobilization in upper extremities and traction for fractures through femoral neck or shaft (Fig. 56-7). When bony union is obtained, new pathologic fractures must be prevented by eradicating the lesion. Only children who have a large cyst that is liable to develop a pathologic fracture require treatment.[12,13] Others should be observed until bony maturity, as many will regress and heal with growth and maturity.

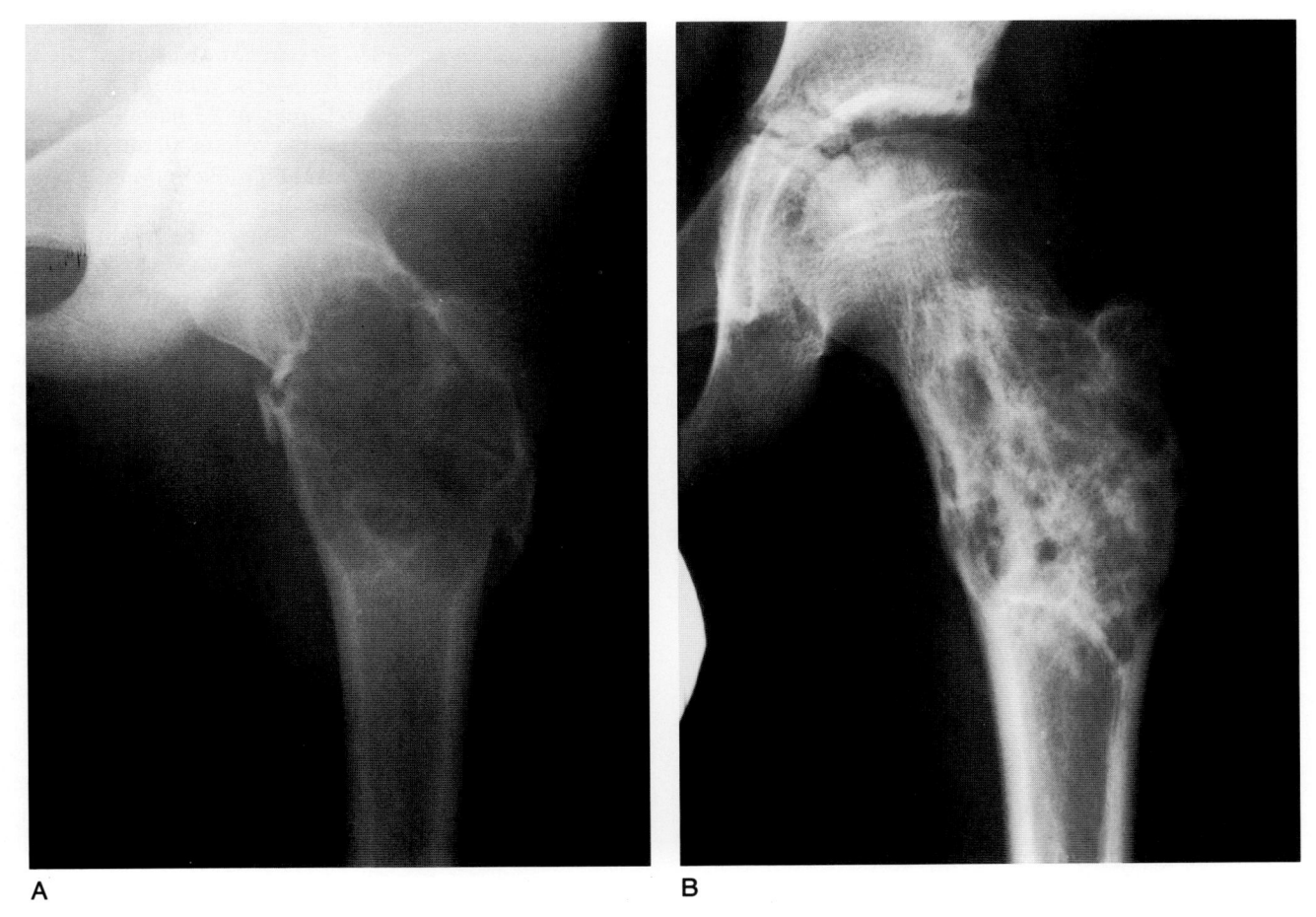

Fig. 56-5. **(A)** Pathologic fracture through an unicameral bone cyst of the femoral neck in an 11-year-old boy treated by skeletal traction for 4 weeks followed by spica cast for 3 weeks. **(B)** The same patient 2½ years later, with spontaneous healing without any other treatment.

ANEURYSMAL BONE CYST

Pathologic fractures through an aneurysmal bone cyst are less common than with the unicameral bone cyst. The lesion in aneurysmal bone cyst is eccentrically placed within the metaphysis of the involved long bone. Around 80 percent of such cysts occur during the second decade of life. More than 50 percent arise in the metaphysis of the humerus, femur, and tibia. Another 30 percent originates in the spine.

On plain radiographs, aneurysmal bone cyst is a radiolucent lesion located in the medullary canal of the metaphysis (Fig. 56-8). The lesion resorbs the cortex and elevates the periosteum to produce the aneurysmal appearance that could mimic that of a malignant tumor, but is always contained by the periosteum. Usually, a thin shell of reactive periosteum bone is seen.

If one could be sure of the benign nature of the lesions, the fractures could be treated by simple immobilization. When cortical integrity is restored, a biopsy, followed by an en bloc resection of the lesion and bone grafting, is recommended.

When the nature of the lesion cannot be determined by simple radiographs, CT scan studies may be helpful (Fig. 56-9). Hudson described a feature in which, when the patient lies still for 20 to 30 minutes, the cells in the fluid within the cyst cavity settle and a fluid level can be seen confirming the diagnosis of a cystic lesion.[14]

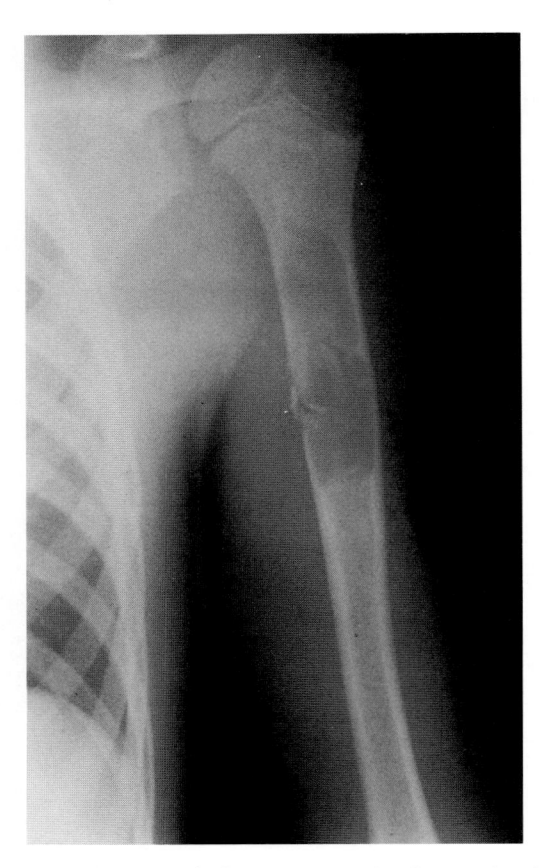

Fig. 56-6. A pathologic fracture through a humeral unicameral bone cyst. The fallen fragment sign is shown; that is, the cortical bone is angled inward toward the cyst cavity. This could not happen if the lesion was a solid tumor.

NONOSSIFYING FIBROMA

Nonossifying fibromas, nonosteogenic fibromas, and fibrous cortical defects are synonymous terms for the same basic histopathologic process in bone. There are two types of lesions seen on radiographs. The more common lesion is a small radiolucency within the cortex (<0.5 cm) with a sharply defined border. This is usually designated as a fibrous cortical defect. This type of lesion is rarely the site of a pathologic fracture (Fig. 56-10).

On the other hand, the typical appearance of the larger nonossifying fibroma is a metaphyseal lesion, eccentrically located within the medullary canal, the cortex bulging over the lesion, and surrounded by a well-defined thin rim of reactive bone. The radiologic appearance is usually typical enough that diagnosis can be made without bone biopsy.

Pathologic fractures occur in nonossifying fibromas when the lesion occupies 50 percent or more of the diameter of the bone in the transverse plane (Fig. 56-11). In a series from the Mayo Clinic, of 23 pathologic fractures reported in nonossifying fibromas, all but one were located in the lower extremity and most frequently in the distal part of the tibia.[15] The average age of the patients in this series was 12 years at the time of the fracture.

Treatment of pathologic fractures associated with this lesion consists mainly of cast immobilization with closed reduction, although displacement seldom occurs. Fracture healing occurs normally and is little impeded by the pathologic process. Drennan and colleagues[16] reported that the lesion can heal by itself after a fracture showing slow ossification from the periphery inward. In this study, some lesions were simply biopsied, others were biopsied, curetted, and grafted. The grafted lesions showed rapid healing of the defect.

Therefore, for fractures through nonossifying fibromas, it is recommended that patients be observed until complete healing of the fracture. If the lesion is still present after the fracture has healed and shows involvement of 50 percent or more of the diameter of the bone, curettage with bone grafting is indicated.

FIBROUS DYSPLASIA

Fibrous dysplasia is a developmental anomaly of bone in which the medullary canal is replaced by fibrous tissue. There are two forms of fibrous dysplasia: the monostotic and polyostotic form. Most patients (approximately 85 percent) have a single skeletal lesion and the remainder may have numerous lesions. The majority of patients with the polyostotic form have symptoms before the age of 10. Harris and colleagues[17] reported that 85 percent of patients with the polyostotic form have pathologic fracturing and 40 percent have 3 fractures or more. Extraskeletal manifestations similar to those of the Albright syndrome are seen in the most severe cases.

On plain radiographs, fibrous dysplasia presents a lucent area through the medullary canal with a variable ground-glass appearance (Fig. 56-12). There is cortical thinning, scalloping of the endosteal surface, and, occasionally, expansion of the bone. The periosteum is not disturbed unless there is a fracture.

Complete assessment of skeleton is essential for proper diagnosis and treatment and should be achieved by total body nuclear scan in preference to complete radiologic survey.

Pathologic fractures can occur in any affected bone,

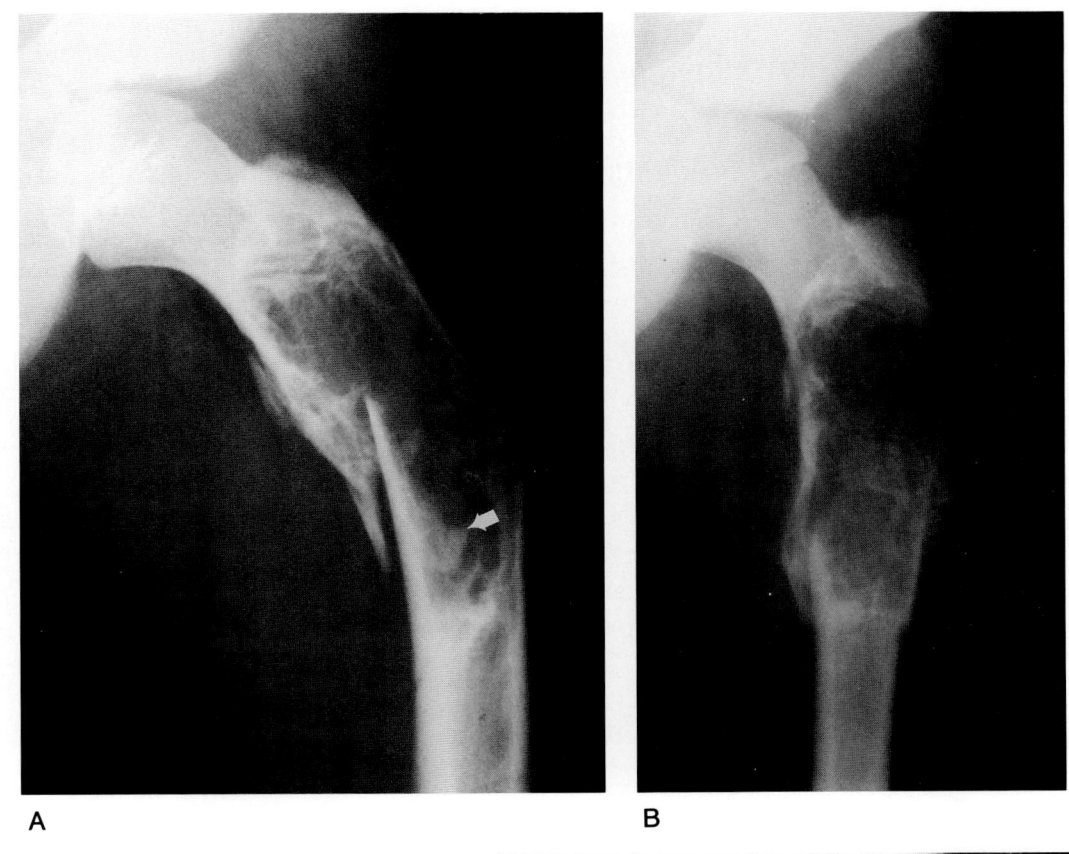

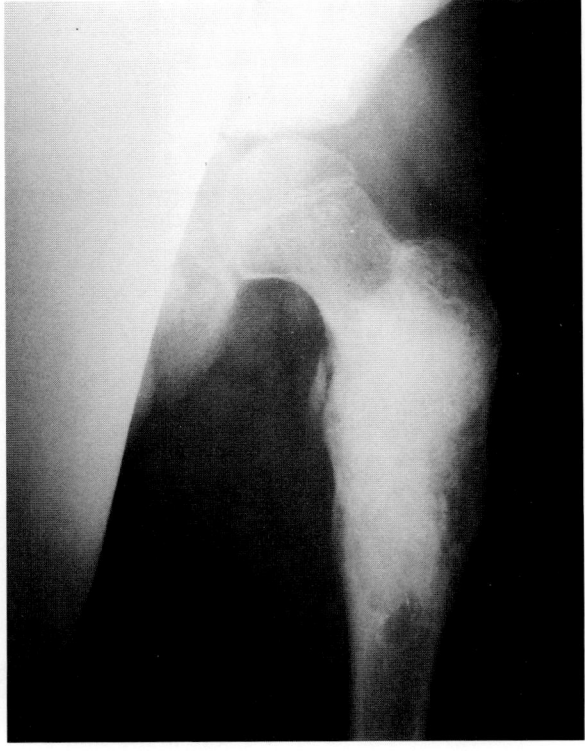

Fig. 56-7. (A) Pathologic fracture through an unicameral bone cyst of a 12-year-old boy. This patient sustained two fractures at ages 5 and 6. Corticosteroid injections were done 3 times at age 6. The lesion improved, and no further treatment was needed except follow-up radiographs every year until this new fracture. (B) Closed reduction was performed, followed by skin traction for a period of 4 weeks. (C) Curettage and grafting (bone bank) were performed, followed by 2 more weeks of traction and 4 weeks in a spica cast. This radiograph was taken 3 months after surgery.

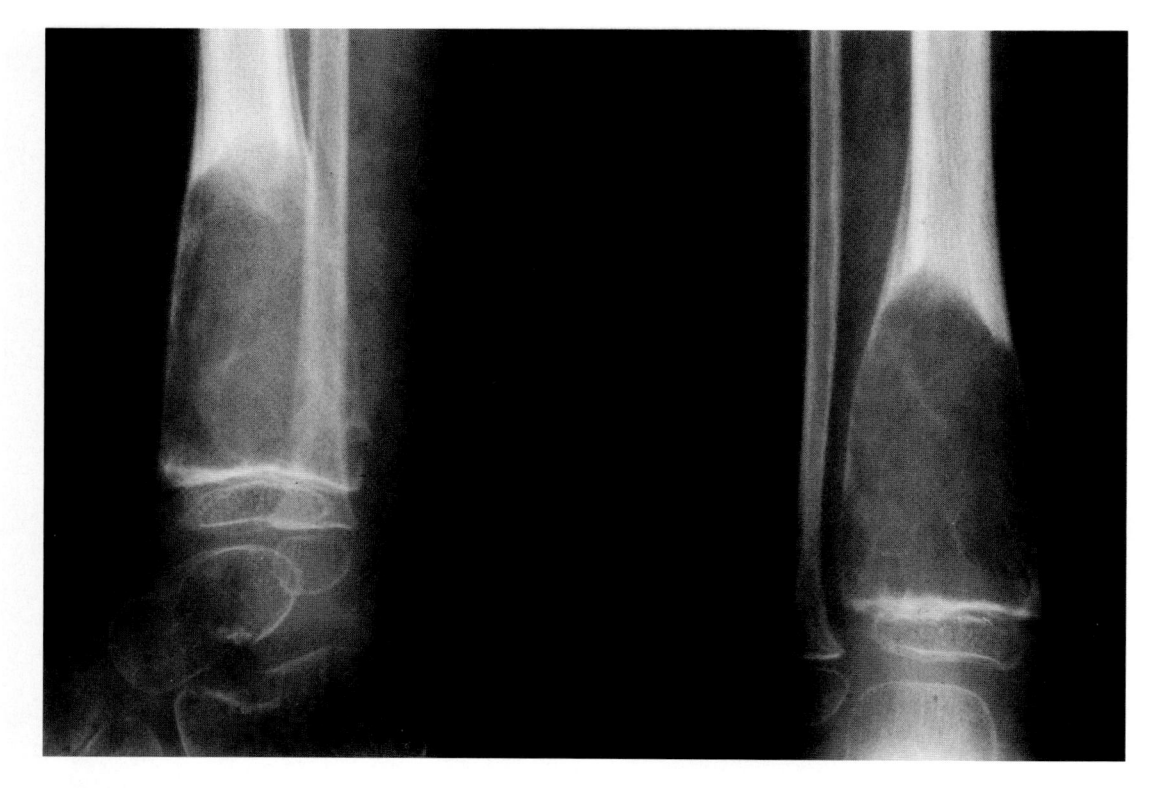

Fig. 56-8. Radiograph of a distal tibia with an aneurysmal bone cyst involving the entire metaphysis. This patient was treated by curettage and bone grafting with partial recurrence of the lesion.

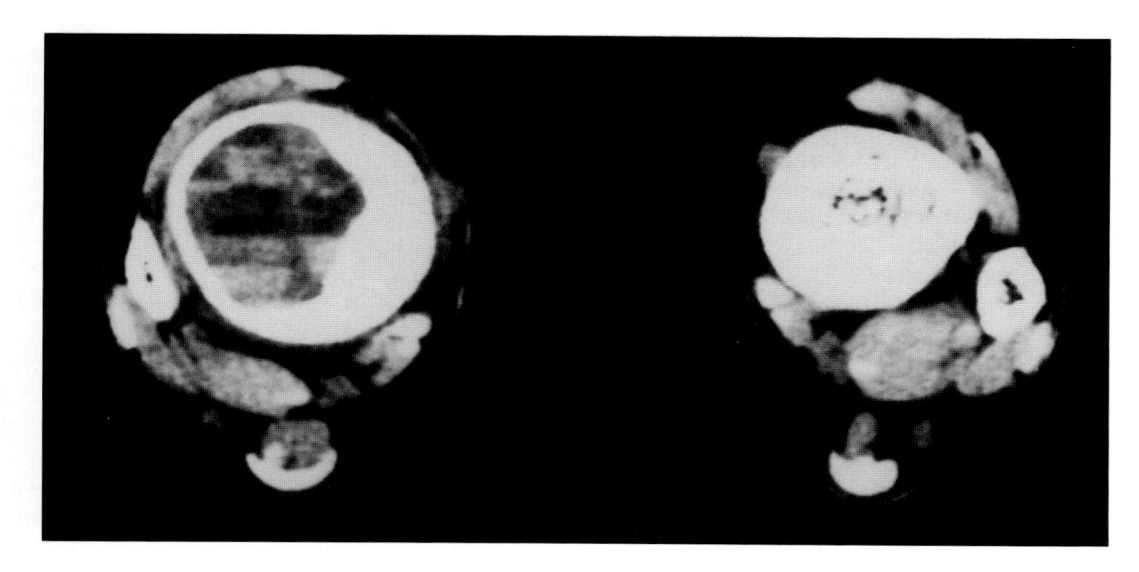

Fig. 56-9. CT scan of the same lesion shown in Fig. 56-8. Fluid level can be seen.

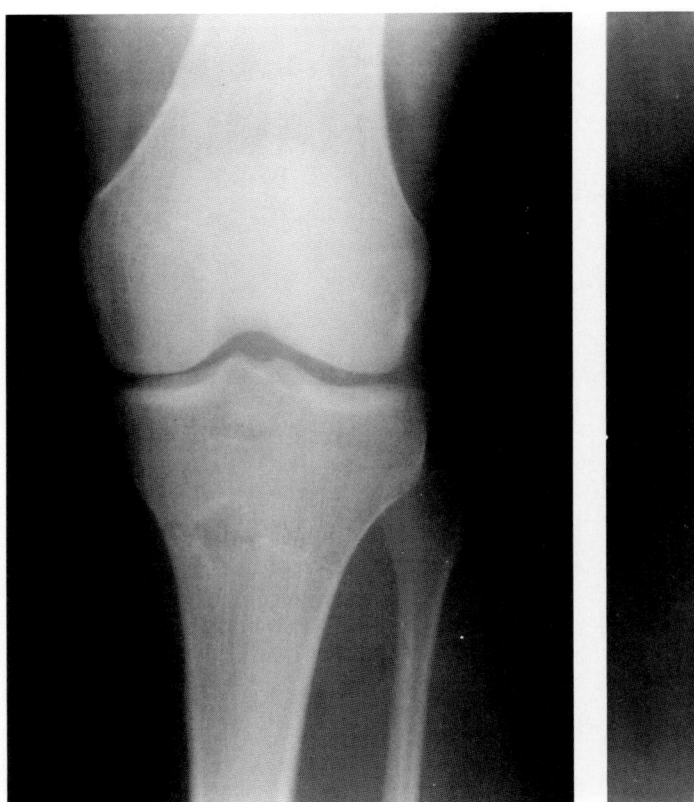

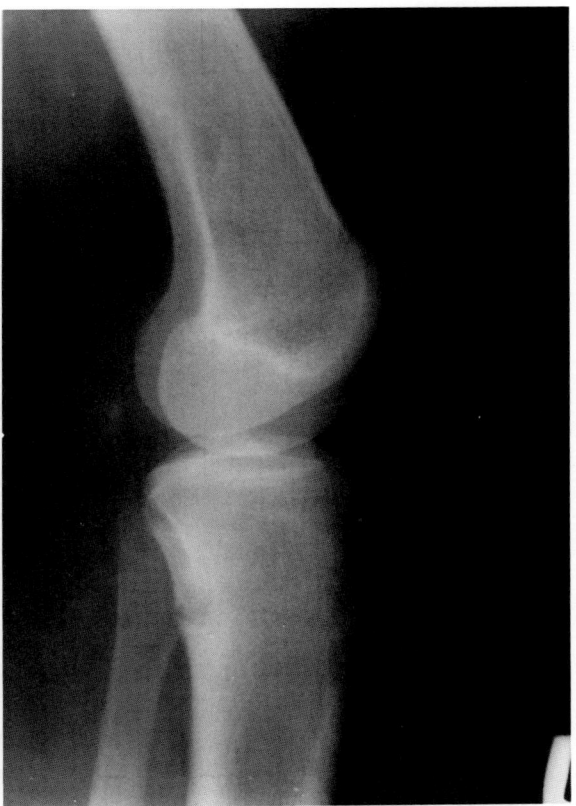

Fig. 56-10. Pathologic fracture through fibrous cortical defect.

but are more common in the polyostotic form of the disease. Dolher and Hughes[18] reported that polyostotic involvement may become evident in childhood and early infancy and represents a difficult therapeutic problem. Stephenson and associates[19] reviewed the results of treatment of 65 symptomatic lesions in 43 patients who had fibrous dysplasia. In the upper extremity (Fig. 56-13), fractures were less frequent than in the lower extremity, and a closed reduction with proper immobilization gave satisfactory results. In the lower extremity, for patients under 18 years of age, the results obtained by closed reduction or/and curettage and bone grafting were unsatisfactory, whereas, in children treated by internal fixation, the results were more satisfactory.

Pathologic fractures of the femoral neck secondary to fibrous dysplasia have the greatest potential of deformity (Fig. 56-14). Acute undisplaced fractures may be treated by skeletal traction followed by spica cast until bony union occurs. In younger children, if coxa vara is present, and in older children with an acute fracture, the femoral neck should be internally fixed with a valgus osteotomy and bone grafting if necessary. Enneking and Gearen[20] used fibular bone graft to bridge lesions of fibrous dysplasia in the femoral neck. Cortical bone is less likely to be resorbed than cancellous bone and is more likely to provide permanent structural support. Springfield[9] uses cortical allograft bone because of its availability and the theoretical assumption that allograft is less likely to resorb than autogenous bone.

DISUSE ATROPHY (POSTIMMOBILIZATION)

Loss of bone secondary to immobilization is a less common cause of pathologic fracture during childhood. Elsasser and colleagues[21] reported that immobilization between 3 and 6 weeks results in a reduction of bone mass at a mean value of 16 percent in the distal metaphysis of the radius. On the other hand, there was no significant change in the diaphysis of the same radius, and the loss was mainly in the trabecular bone.

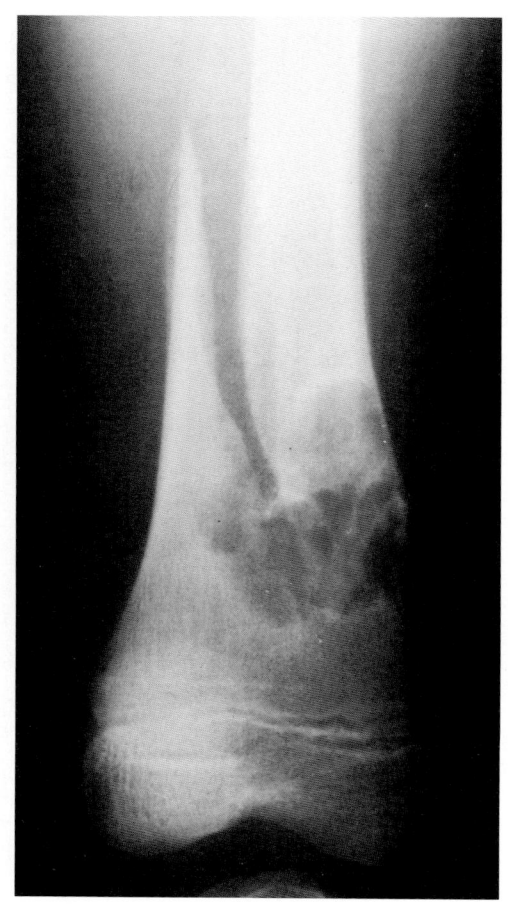

Fig. 56-11. Fracture through a nonossifying fibroma of the distal femoral metaphysis. This lesion occupies more than 50 percent of the diameter of the bone in the transverse plane.

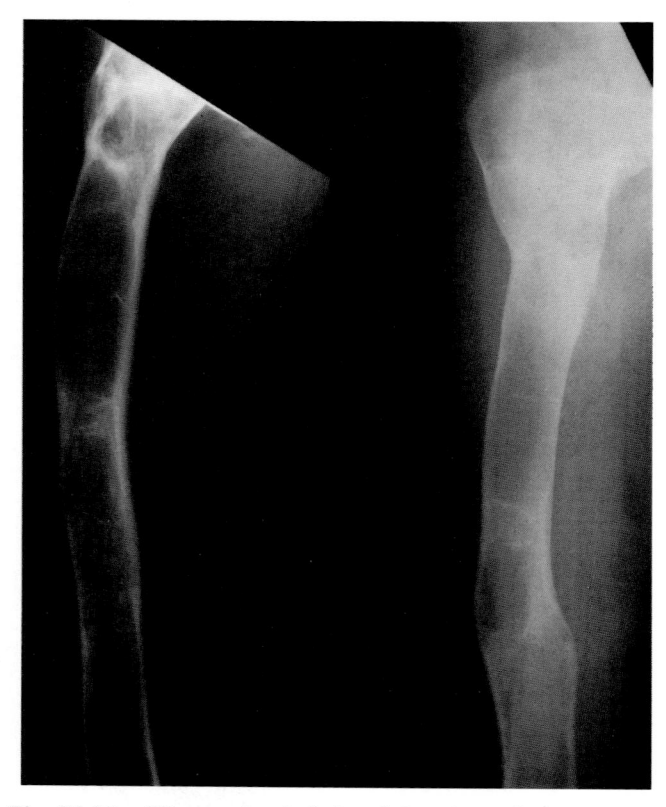

Fig. 56-12. Fibrous dysplasia involving the entire length of the femur with typical ground-glass appearance which weakens the bone predisposing to pathologic fracturing.

After prolonged cast immobilization, children often show some degree of osteoporosis, with a resultant weakening of the bone. Metaphyseal collapse can be seen during weightbearing, causing impaction fractures with pain about the knees and ankles may occur postimmobilization. Children with associated neuromuscular disease, such as cerebral palsy, muscular dystrophy, or myelomeningocele, are particularly prone to osteoporosis secondary to cast immobilization and subsequent pathologic fracturing. Therefore, cast immobilization should be reduced as much as possible for these patients.

Such fractures will heal rapidly and a minimum time of immobilization should be used in order to avoid the aggravation of osteoporosis. A gradual return to activity is therefore important in the rehabilitation of these children. These fractures should be managed with a weight-bearing cast or functional bracing to avoid a vicious circle of increased fragility, followed by recurrent fractures after removal of the cast or brace (see Ch. 60).

RENAL OSTEODYSTROPHY

Rickets may be due to poor nutrition, malabsorption, renal disease, the use of anticonvulsants as well as other more unusual disorders. Renal osteodystrophy refers to the osseous abnormality secondary to chronic renal failure. In general, it is a combination of rickets, secondary hyperparathyroidism, osteoporosis, and osteosclerosis.

The pathologic disturbance in rickets and renal osteodystrophy is a failure of mineralization of the osteoid. Radiographs demonstrate thinning of cortices, decrease in bone density, and widening and cupping of the metaphysis. The epiphyses are smaller, with a wide gap between the epiphysis and the metaphysis due to physeal thickening.

In renal osteodystrophy, there is a greater incidence of pathologic slipped epiphysis than true fractures. Mehls

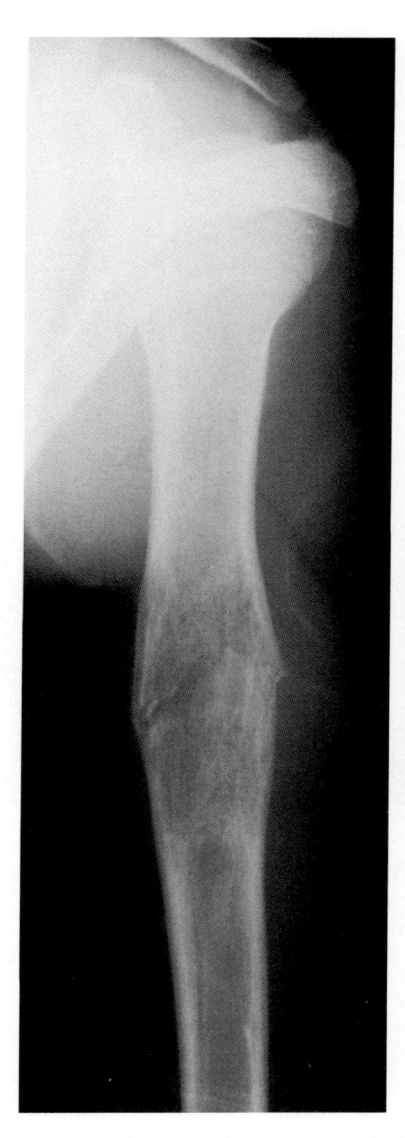

Fig. 56-13. Fracture through a fibrous dysplasia lesion in the humeral diaphysis.

and coworkers[22] reported this condition in 30 percent of their patients who were untreated and nondialyzed. The slippage usually occurs late in the terminal stages of osteodystrophy. The slips can be seen in distal radius, distal tibia, and proximal and distal femur. Slipped capital femoral epiphysis is also reported (Fig. 56-15). These are Salter-Harris type I fractures of the physis due to weakening of the epiphyseal plate secondary to the impaired ossification.

With appropriate treatment, including vitamin D, pathologic fractures and epiphyseal slippages in renal osteodystrophy usually heal well.[23] In children with slipped capital femoral epiphysis, internal fixation with 2 or 3 pins is recommended (see Ch. 27).

PATHOLOGIC FRACTURES OF THE SPINE

Pathologic fractures of the spine in children differ from that of adults in both etiology and treatment. In children the most common cause of pathologic fracture of the vertebrae is a primary benign tumor as opposed to malignancy and osteoporosis in adults. Pathologic fractures of the spine are also common in children being treated on high-dose steroids for malignancies at other sites in the body. Because the discs are very large in children and the vertebral bone is strong and well developed, considerable replacement of osseous tissue from a pathologic process has to occur before a pathologic fracture ensues. Usually this is in the form of a compression fracture, although some tumors, such as aneurysmal bone cyst, may involve the posterior elements as well and cause pathologic fatigue fractures in this area of the spine with resultant symptoms of pain and paraspinal muscle spasm.

Physical Signs and Symptoms

The main symptom of pathologic fracture of the spine in children is pain. The child may be able to mask this discomfort by splinting the spine very effectively through paraspinal muscle spasm. This creates the so-called "poker back," in which the child will not bend over to pick objects up off the floor, instead they squat down with the spine held rigidly straight.[24-26] Complaints of pain in the back and poor sitting tolerance because of discomfort in the spinal region always warrants aggressive investigation, since back pain is such an unusual complaint in a child, usually being secondary to underlying pathology. Plain radiographs may be deceptive in identifying a pathologic fracture unless it is quite gross. Often there is an initial period of microfracturing, which causes pain and discomfort, but which is seldom identifiable on plain films. This also occurs, for example, in the initial stages of eosinophilic granuloma before there is physical collapse of the vertebral body. Tomograms of the area of discomfort and CT scans are often diagnostic. If there is concern that the fracture is secondary to a neurologic tumor extending into the spine, an MRI will be helpful.[27-29] Most of the pathologic fractures seen in children occur between T2 and L2. Pathologic fractures may be responsible for the development of spinal curvature as children have very resilient

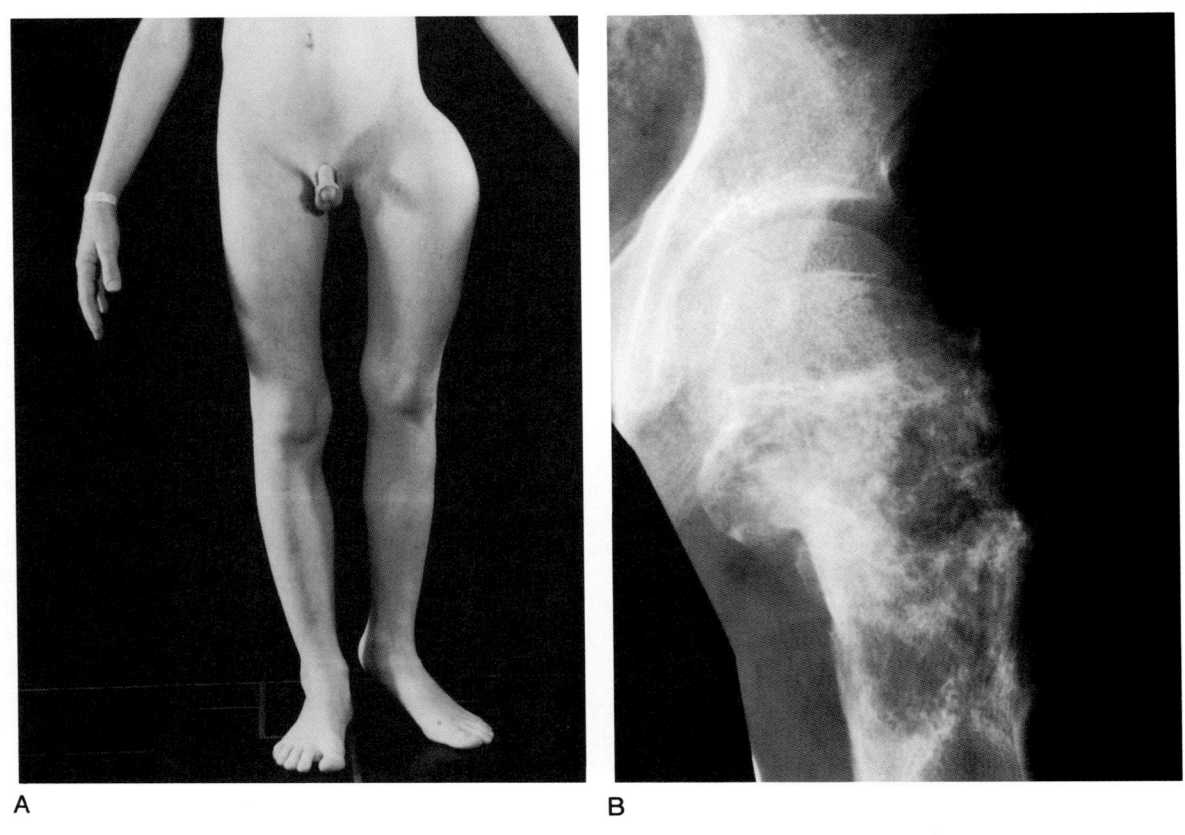

Fig. 56-14. (A) This 9-year-old patient presents the classical shepherd's crook deformity seen in fibrous dysplasia due to multiple recurrent fracturing of his left femoral neck. (B) The same patient 6 years later following valgus osteotomy of left hip and bone grafting. The shepherd's crook deformity has improved, and no further fractures have occurred following the surgery. The patient did not sustain any other pathologic fracture after surgery.

and mobile spinal columns and tend to pull away from areas of pain and discomfort, resulting in a scoliosis. Kyphosis is common in association with compression fractures of the spine and lordosis less common.

Causes of Pathologic Fractures of the Spine

Table 56-2 illustrates the common causes of pathologic fractures of the spine in the pediatric age group.

Benign Tumors

The most common benign tumors that result in pathologic fractures are aneurysmal bone cysts and eosinophilic granuloma.

ANEURYSMAL BONE CYSTS

Aneurysmal bone cysts are seen more frequently in girls and often involve more than one vertebra (Fig. 56-16). These tumors are usually quite visible on plain films and usually involve posterior elements but can result in vertebral body collapse as well. The child usually presents with pain and occasionally neurologic symptoms from cord impingement. Treatment by curettage and bone grafting is usually successful in eradicating this cyst, although recurrence is not uncommon. Unfortunately, the aneurysmal bone cyst often occur in rather inaccessible sites and may require innovative surgical approaches.[30-32] Treatment by radiation, although successfully reported,[33] should be avoided in children, due to the predisposition to develop future malignant degeneration and myelopathy.[34]

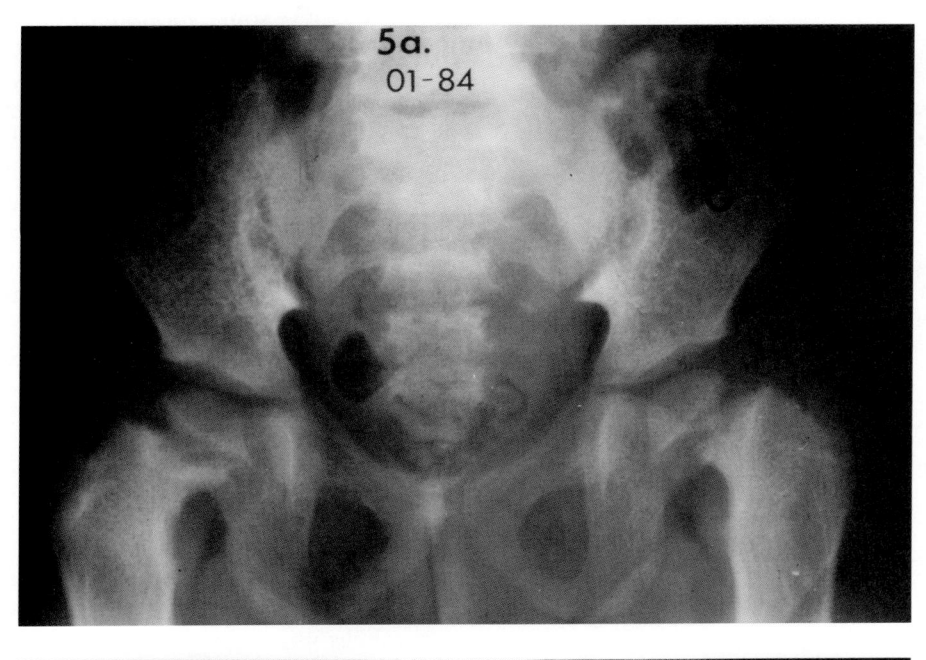

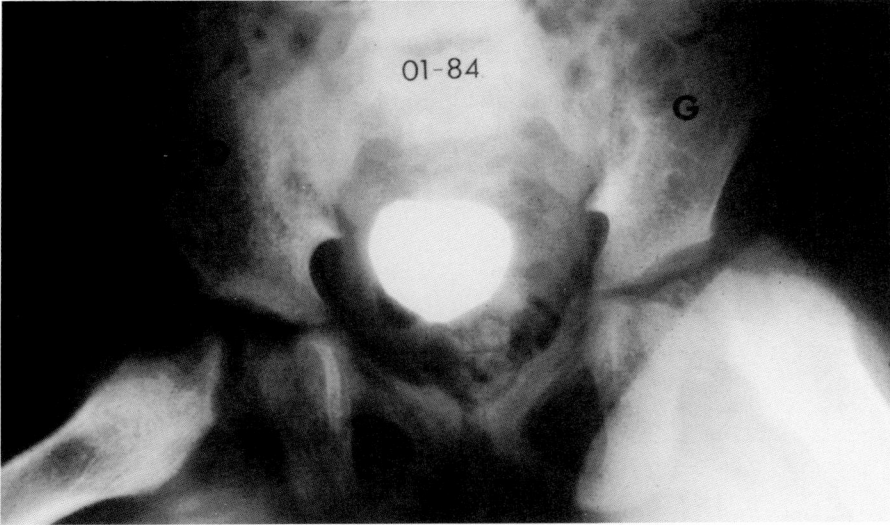

Fig. 56-15. The pelvis of a 5-year-old boy with renal osteodystrophy. Note the widening and cupping of both proximal metaphyses, widening of the epiphyseal growth plate and slippage of the left femoral head by almost 50 percent and the right by 25 percent.

TABLE 56-2. Pathological Causes of Vertebral Compression Fracture in Children

Benign tumors
    Aneurysmal bone cysts
    Eosinophilic granuloma
Metastatic tumors
    Neuroblastoma
    Ganglioneuroma
    Wilms' tumor
    Primary medulloblastoma
    Lymphoma and leukemia
Malignant tumors
    Ewing's sarcoma
    Osteosarcoma
Juvenile osteoporosis
    Osteogenesis imperfecta
    Juvenile rheumatoid arthritis
    Ankylosing spondylitis
    Gaucher's disease
    Osteoporosis
Metabolic diseases
    Rickets and scurvy
    Osteomalacia
    Cortisone osteoporosis
Infection:
    Tuberculosis
    Pyogenic infection

EOSINOPHILIC GRANULOMA

The eosinophilic granuloma not infrequently involves the vertebral body with complete collapse of the body resulting in so-called "vertebra plana." The eosinophilic granuloma is more common in boys and tends to involve only one vertebra, although involvement of two or more have been reported. The intervertebral disc is spared, and in younger children complete collapse of the vertebral body is more frequent. Needle biopsy of the lesion is usually diagnostic, and, with support with a spinal orthosis to relieve spinal motion, reconstitution of the vertebra usually occurs (Fig. 56-17). There may be a slight kyphosis persisting at the level of the vertebral collapse, especially if the vertebra does not completely reconstitute.[35] Aggressive management with chemotherapy may be indicated if there are extraspinal lesions indicating diffuse involvement. Radiation of the spinal lesion in children should be avoided due to the long-term increased incidence of malignant degeneration as well as dangers of asymmetrical growth of the spine.[36] In rare instances eosinophilic granuloma may cause spinal cord impingement necessitating open surgery and/or radiation.[37]

Metastatic Disease of the Spine

Metastatic disease of the spine contributing to pathologic fracturing is rare in the pediatric age group and not well documented. The most common primary tumors that metastasize to the axial skeleton in children are neuroblastoma, medulloblastoma, and Wilms' tumor. In children, approximately 25 percent of all spinal canal tumors are metastatic or from paravertebral extension.[38] The incidence of spinal involvement from neuroblastoma is about 20 percent, in medulloblastoma, 10 percent, and Wilms' tumor, about 6.5 percent[39,40] (Table 56-3).

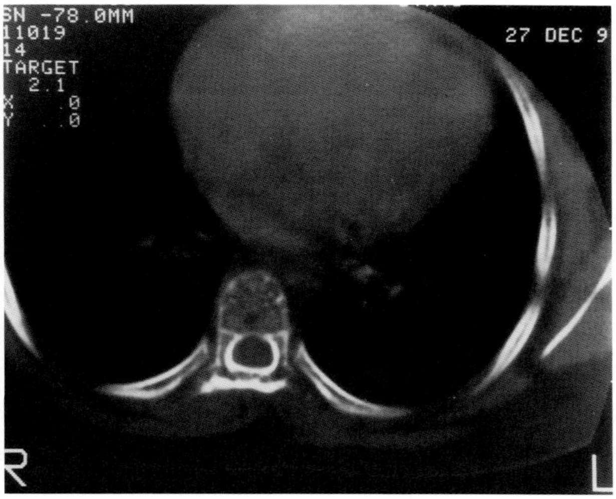

Fig. 56-16. Aneurysmal bone cyst recurrence in the body of T7 one year following bone grafting and posterior fusion in an 11-year-old girl.

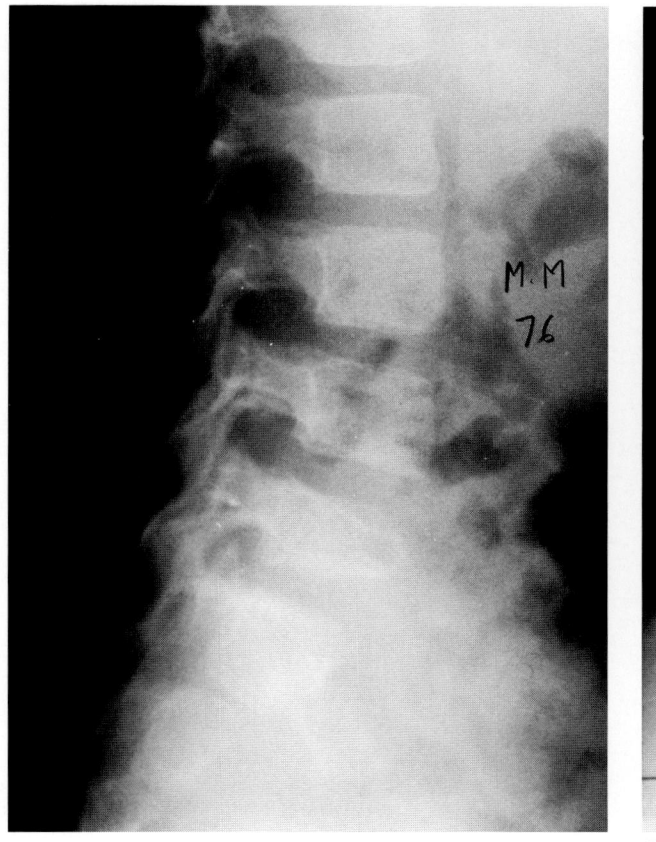

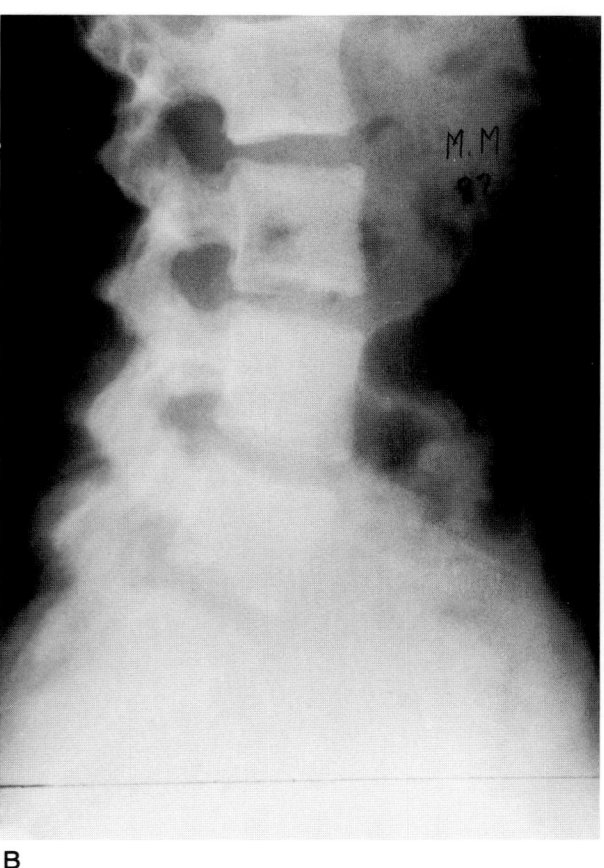

Fig. 56-17. (A) Eosinophilic granuloma. At L5 level with back pain without neurologic deficit. (B) Same patient 6 years later with complete restitution of the height of the vertebral body.

Basically there are three physiologic mechanisms that enable these tumors to involve the spine. The tumor mass may extend directly from its primary paravertebral region through lymphatic spread into the invertebral foramen or hematogenously deposited into the bone marrow via the Batson venous plexus.

TABLE 56-3. Common Tumors Metastatic to the Spine in Children

Neuroblastoma
Wilms' tumor
Medulloblastoma
Astrocytoma
Lymphoma
Sarcomas

The most consistent initial clinical presentation of a child with a metastic spinal lesion is localized back pain, which is often worse at night and tender to percussion. This may be associated with radicular pain, progressive weakness followed by sensory loss, and signs and symptoms of spinal cord involvement reflected as a change in gait pattern.

Plain radiographs are not often diagnostic in the initial stages of a metastatic spine lesion and may show only osteoporosis. In order for the plain film to unequivocally demonstrate vertebral body infiltration, 30 to 50 percent of bony destruction must take place. Technetium 99m bone scan may be helpful in localizing the lesion allowing vertebral biopsy either percutaneous or open (Fig. 56-18). The most useful method in identifying metastatic lesions of the spine is MRI (Fig. 56-19). In contrast to the CT scan, which is limited to a transaxial plain, the MRI is able to scan the entire spine sagittally and coron-

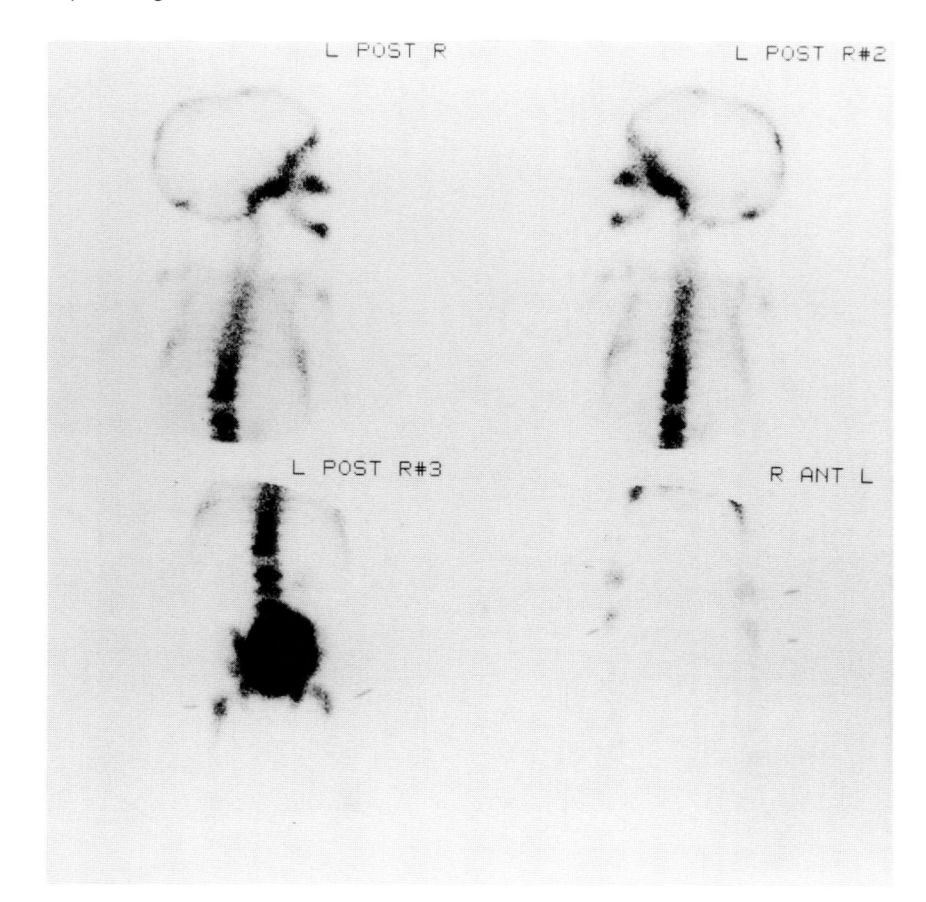

Fig. 56-18. Technetium 99m bone scan of 12-month-old child with multiple metastasis to the spine from a Wilms' tumor.

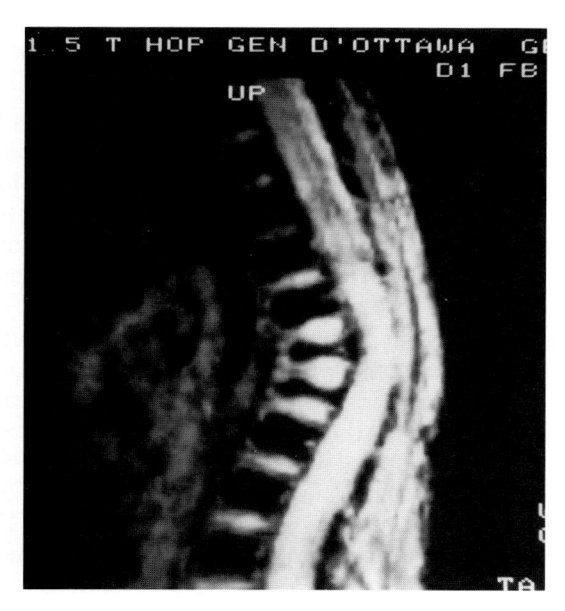

Fig. 56-19. Sagittal MRI of a 3½-year-old child with metastasis to spine from a neuroblastoma showing vertebral collapse of T11 and T12.

ally.[41] In children it allows superior resolution as compared to CT scan and without the use of ionizing radiation or contrast material. In children, the primary tumor diagnosis has usually been made, but occasionally a pathologic fracture of the vertebral body may be the first indication of an undiagnosed primary lesion.[42]

The treatment of the primary malignancy may in itself predispose to pathologic fracturing of the vertebra, especially when chemotherapy and steroids are utilized. In the presence of anterior vertebral collapse care must be taken to avoid a wide posterior laminectomy without concomitant spinal fusion since further collapse may result in spinal cord compromise. Harrington's classification of spinal metastases based on the amount of pathologic fracture is appropriate for children as well as adults[43] (Table 56-4).

With respect to therapeutic options, the basic triad of oncology options are chemotherapy, radiotherapy, and surgery. It has been suggested that, in the absence of extensive neurologic involvement or vertebral collapse with instability, chemotherapy should be used exclusively in the treatment of spinal metastases.[43,44] Some

TABLE 56-4. Harrington's Classification of Spinal Metastasis

Class I	No neurologic involvement
Class II	Involvement of bone without collapse or instability
Class III	Major neurologic involvement collapse or instability
Class IV	Vertebral collapse with mechanical pain but no neurologic involvement
Class V	Vertebral collapse with major neurologic involvement

investigations have clearly demonstrated the effectiveness of a multiagent regimen, which include a combination of cyclophosphamide, vincristine, cisplatin, VM-26, and Adriamycin[45] in the management of cord compression as a result of metastatic disease from childhood neuroblastoma.[46] Sanderson and colleagues[45] were able to report full restoration of neurologic function, including normal sphincter function and a 15 to 20 percent long-term survival rate when chemotherapy was used as the initial treatment. Similarly, Pritchard and associates[47] also showed that 22 percent of the children with bony metastasis from neuroblastoma survived a median of 61 months when only chemotherapy was administered. The concomitant use of high-dose corticosteroid, dexamethasone, may also be a major contributor in pain relief.[48]

Traditionally, radiotherapy with the standard dose of 3,000 to 4,000 rad has been advised if there was evidence of considerable neurologic impairment, but with no significant compromise to the integrity of the bony vertebral structures.[43] However, surgical excision may be indicated if irradiation has failed to provide adequate relief of neurologic impairment and prognosis of the child's tumor warrants such an approach.

An anterior approach is recommended as it allows resection of the anteriorly located tumor, decompression of the spinal cord, as well as the correction of kyphotic deformities. The collapsed vertebral bodies in cases of kyphosis repair may be replaced by bone grafts.[49]

The posterior laminectomy approach, on the other hand, is suitable for a multivertebral level decompression in the region of the lamina or pedicle. However, the removal of posterior bony elements, along with the stripping of supportive ligamentous structures, should be associated with spinal fusion and stabilization.

Postsurgical spinal deformity has been reported in 49 percent of children who underwent epidural tumor excision and laminectomy.[50] According to Lonstein, kyphosis is a result of bone loss as well as the loss of ligaments such as supraspinous ligament, interspinous ligament, ligamentum flavum, and joint capsule of facets, all of which contribute to the stability of the spinal column in the prevention of anterior collapse. Concomitant spinal fusion will avoid these serious complications.

Surgery, chemotherapy, and radiotherapy all may have a role in the management of the metastatic spine lesion in children, but the indications and contraindications, advantages, and disadvantages must be carefully considered in order to devise an effective treatment plan for both the spinal metastases and the child. To date, the factors that govern the development of an effective therapeutic strategy for complicated metastatic disease of the spine in children remain to be determined and must continue to be individualized.

Primary Malignant Tumors of the Spine

Although any of the mesenchymal elements contributing to spinal column development can result in a primary tumor in this area, the two most common primary malignant tumors seen in children's spines are Ewing's sarcoma and osteogenic sarcoma (Fig. 56-20). Either may present initially with a pathologic fracture, and diagnosis is usually confirmed by open or needle biopsy.[52] Generalized bone involvement by leukemia or lymphoma may also initially present with a pathologic fracture of the spine (Fig. 56-21).

Juvenile Osteoporosis

Many general pathologic conditions may result in osteoporosis of the spine to the extent that pathologic fracturing will ensue. Examples of this are osteogenesis imperfecta (Fig. 56-22) and Gaucher's disease. Pathologic fracturing of the vertebra in children emphasizes the need to ascertain the reason for the underlying fracture, bearing in mind that it may be symptomatic of a more generalized pathologic condition.[53,54]

Metabolic Diseases

Nutritional metabolic abnormalities are rare in modern affluent society but must be kept in mind in third world countries where malnutrition in children is rampant. In more affluent countries this malnutrition is being reflected in increasing numbers of adolescents

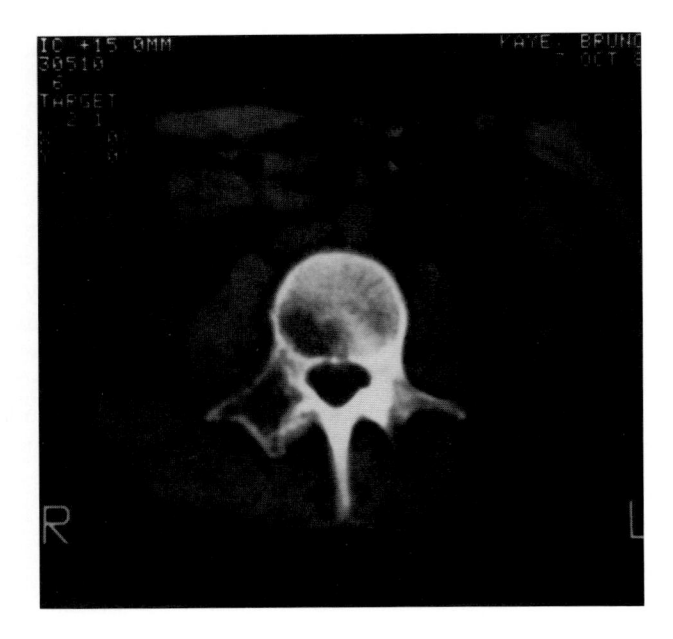

Fig. 56-20. Ewing's sarcoma involving T10 vertebra in a 15-year-old boy.

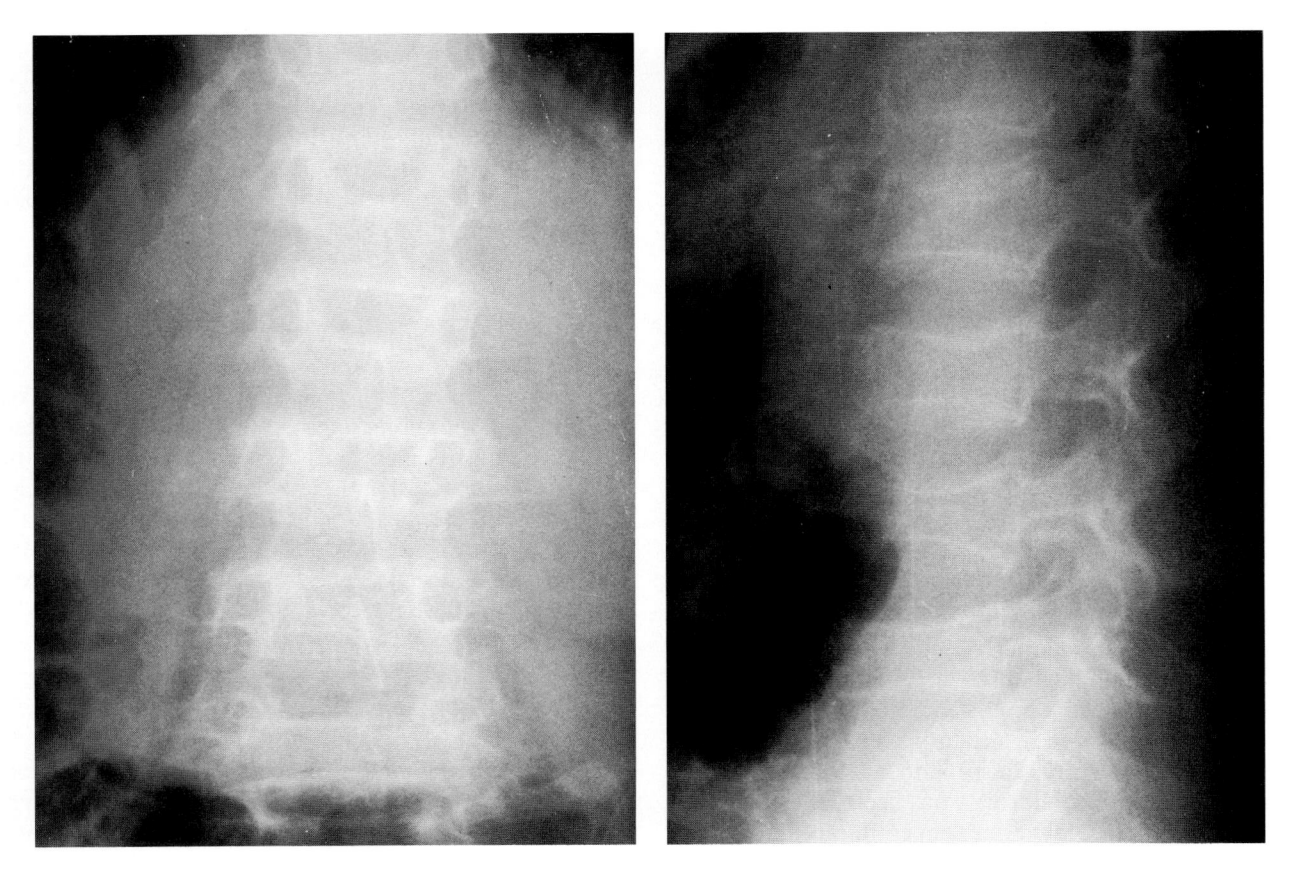

Fig. 56-21. Leukemic involvement of spine in child with acute lymphoblastic leukemia presenting with low back pain.

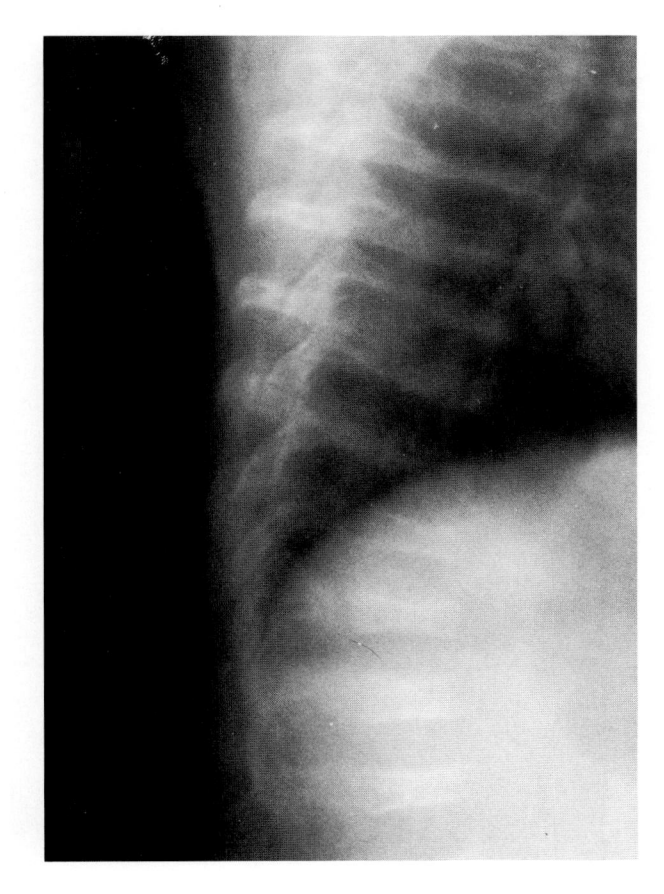

Fig. 56-22. Multiple pathologic compression fractures of the vertebral bodies in a 12-year-old girl with osteogenesis imperfecta.

with anorexia nervosa. This can result in severe osteoporosis and pathologic compression fractures of the spine.[53] Pathologic fracturing of the spine is probably most commonly associated with high-dose cortisone treatment of children for leukemia,[55] lymphoma, or severe juvenile rheumatoid arthritis.[56] Protection of the spine with an orthosis may assist in preventing pathologic fracturing until the cortisone therapy can be stopped.

Vertebral Infections

The most common infection resulting in pathologic fracturing of the spine in children is tuberculosis (Fig. 56-23). This is fortunately becoming less common throughout the world but is a type of infection that can cause a devastating pathologic fracturing of the vertebral bodies. In young children without spinal cord involvement treatment with antitubercular antibiotics—INH (isoniazid), rifampin, and pyrizinamide—the so-called "triple therapy," combined with a spinal cast or orthosis, is often effective in eradicating the infection. In older children and those with spinal cord involvement surgical extirpation of the infection usually from an anterior approach supplemented with antitubercular medication may be required.[57]

SUMMARY

Although pathologic fractures constitute an infrequent reason for bringing children to the emergency department, they must be considered especially where the fracture is secondary to minor trauma. One must keep in mind the biomechanics of bone predisposing to pathologic fractures, the common clinical characteristics, and the general principles of treatment of such fractures.

The common causes of pathologic fractures in children have been reviewed. It is important to recognize and to make the diagnosis of the basic lesion, as it will then be easier to manage the pathologic fracture and later on to definitively treat the lesion itself.

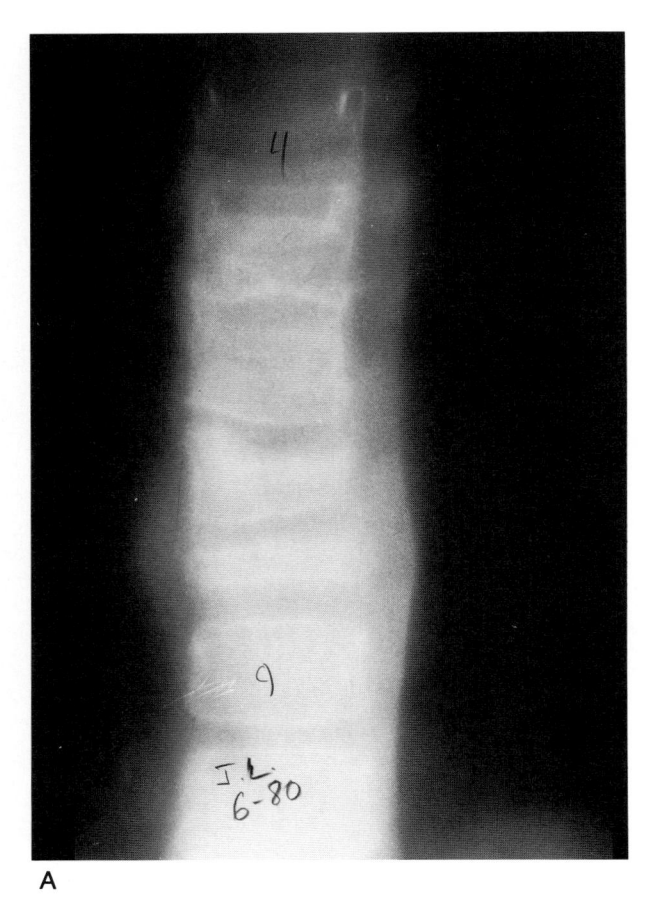

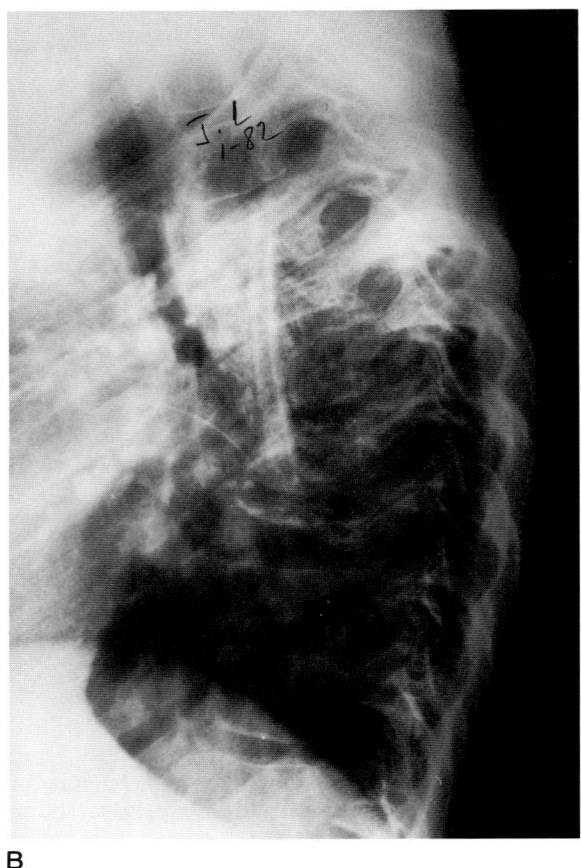

Fig. 56-23. (A) Tuberculosis infection of T5-T8 in a 12-year-old girl. (B) Treatment was by surgical drainage, strut grafting and antituberculosis medication shown 2 years later.

REFERENCES

1. Tachdjian MO: Pathologic fractures. p. 3366. In: Pediatric Orthopaedics. 2nd Ed. WB Saunders, Philadelphia, 1990
2. Nordin M, Frankel VH: Basic Biomechanics of the Musculoskeletal System. 2nd Ed. Lea & Febiger, Philadelphia, 1989
3. Leggon RE, Lindsay RW, Panjabi M: Strength reduction and effects of treatment of long bones with diaphyseal defects involving 50% of the cortex. J Orthop Res 6:540, 1988
4. Brooks DB, Burstein AH, Frankel VH: The biomechanics of torsional fractures; The stress concentration effect of a drill hole. J Bone Joint Surg [Am] 52:507, 1970
5. Clark CR, Morgan C, Sonstegard DA, Mathews LS: The effect of biopsy-hole shape and size on bone strength. J Bone Joint Surg 59:213, 1977
6. McBroom RJ, Cheal EJ, Hayes WC: Strength reductions from metastatic cortical defects in long bones. J Orthop Res 6:369, 1988
7. Letts M, Monson R, Weber K: The prevention of recurrent fractures of the lower extremities in severe osteogenesis imperfecta using vacuum pants. J Pediatr Orthop 8:454, 1988
8. Lee JJK, Lyne DL: Pathologic fractures in severely handicapped children and young adults. J Pediatr Orthop 10:497, 1990
9. Springfield DS: Bone and soft tissue tumors. p. 325. In Morrissy RT (ed): Lovell and Winter's Pediatric Orthopaedics. 3rd Ed. JB Lippincott, Philadelphia, 1990
10. Neer CS, Francis KC, Johnston AD, Kierman HA Jr: Current concepts on the treatment of solitary unicameral bone cyst. Clin Orthop 97:40, 1973
11. Kaelin AJ, MacEwen GD: Unicameral bone cysts: natural history and the risk of fracture. Int Orthop 13:275, 1989
12. Bleck EE, Kleinman RG: Special injuries of the musculo-

skeletal system. p. 173. In Rockwood C, Wilkins KE, King RE (eds): Fractures in Children. Vol. 3. JB Lippincott, Philadelphia, 1984
13. Scaglietti O, Marchetti PG, Bartolozzi P: Final results obtained in the treatment of bone cyst with methylprednisolone acetate (Depo-Medrol) and a discussion of results achieved in other bone lesions. Clin Orthop 165:33, 1982
14. Hudson TM: Fluid levels in aneurysmal bone cyst: a CT feature. AJR 141:1001, 1984
15. Arata MA, Peterson HA, Dahlin DC: Pathological fractures through non-ossifying fibromas. J Bone Joint Surg [Am] 63:980, 1981
16. Drennan DB, Maylahn DJ, Fahey JJ: Fractures through large non-ossifying fibromas. Clin Orthop 103:82, 1974
17. Harris WH, Dudley HR, Barry RJ: The natural history of fibrous dysplasia: an orthopaedic, pathological, and roentgenographic study. J Bone Joint Surg [Am] 44:207, 1962
18. Dohler JR, Hughes SPF: Fibrous dysplasia of bones and the Weil-Albright syndrome: a study of thirteen cases with special reference to the orthopaedic treatment. Int Orthop 10:53, 1986
19. Stephenson RB, London MD, Hankin FM, Kaufer H: Fibrous dysplasia: an analysis of options for treatment. J Bone Joint Surg [Am] 69:400, 1987
20. Enneking WF, Gearen PF: Fibrous dysplasia of the femoral neck: treatment by cortical bone-grafting. J Bone Joint Surg [Am] 68:1415, 1986
21. Elsasser U, Ruegsegger P, Anliker M et al: Loss and recovery of trabecular bone in the distal radius following fracture: immobilization of the upper limb in children. Klin Wochenschr 57:763, 1979
22. Mehls O, Ritz E, Krempien B et al: Slipped epiphyses in renal osteodystrophy. Arch Dis Child 50:545, 1975
23. Mankin HJ: Rickets, osteomalacia and renal osteodystrophy: Part II. J Bone Joint Surg [Am] 56:352, 1974
24. Bradford DS, Hensinger RN: Paediatric Spine. Thieme, New York, 1985
25. Samuda G, Cheng MY, Yeung CY: Back pain and vertebral compression: An uncommon presentation of childhood acute lymphoblastic leukemia. J Pediatr Orthop 7:175, 1987
26. Fraser RD et al: Orthopaedics aspects of spinal tumours in children. J Bone Joint Surg [Br] 59:143, 1977
27. Bale JF et al: Magnetic resonance imaging of the spine in children. Arch Neurol 43:1253, 1986
28. Kricun ME: Imaging Modalities in Spinal Disorders. WB Saunders, Philadelphia, 1988
29. Yuh WTC et al: Vertebral compression fractures: distinction between benign and malignant causes with MR imaging. Radiology 172:215, 1989
30. Sundaresan N et al: Tumors of the Spine, Diagnosis and Clinical Management. p. 553. WB Saunders, Philadelphia, 1990
31. McDonald P, Letts M, Sutherland G, Unruh H: Aneurysmal bone cyst of the upper thoracic spine: an operative approach through a manubrial sternotomy. Clin Orthop Rel Res 279:127, 1992
32. Caparna R, Albissini U, Picci P et al: Aneurysmal bone cysts of the spine. J Bone Joint Surg [Am] 67:527, 1985
33. Nobler MP, Higinbotham NL, Philipps RF: The cure of aneurysmal bone cyst. Radiology 90:1185, 1968
34. Hay MC, Paterson D, Taylor TKF: Aneurysmal bone cysts of the spine. J Bone Joint Surg [Br] 60:406, 1978
35. Copere EL et al: Vertebra plana calve's disease due to eosinophilic granuloma. J Bone Joint Surg [Am] 36:969, 1954
36. Neuhauser EBD et al: Radiation effects of roentgen therapy on the growing spine. Radiology 59:637, 1952
37. Green NE et al: Eosinophilic granuloma of the spine with associated neural deficit. J Bone Joint Surg [Am] 162:1198, 1980
38. Baten M, Vannucci RC: Intraspinal metastatic disease in childhood cancer. J Pediatr 90:207, 1977
39. Bever CT, Koeingsberger MR, Antunes JL et al: Epidural metastasis by Wilms' tumor. Am J Dis Child 135:644, 1982
40. Summer TE, Crowe JE, Parker MD et al: Solitary spinal metastasis from Wilms' tumour. Pediatr Radiol 9:175, 1980
41. Sarpel S, Sarpel G, Yu E et al: Early diagnosis of spinal-epidural metastasis by magnetic resonance imaging. Cancer 59:1112, 1987
42. Sim FM: Diagnosis and Management of Metastatic Bone Disease. Raven Press, New York, 1988
43. Harrington KD: Current concepts review: metastatic disease of the spine. J Bone Joint Surg 68:1110, 1986
44. Boland PJ, Lane JM, Sundarsean N: Metastatic disease of the spine. Clin Orthop Rel Res 669:95, 1982
45. Sanderson IR, Pritchard J, Marsh HT: Chemotherapy as the initial treatment of spinal cord compression due to disseminated neuroblastoma. J Neurosurg 70:688, 1989
46. Hayes FA, Thompson EI, Hvizdala E et al: Chemotherapy as an alternative to laminectomy and radiation in the management of epidural tumour. J Pediatr 104:221, 1984
47. Pritchard J, Kiely E, Rogers DW et al: Long-term survival after advanced neuroblastoma. N Engl J Med 317:1026, 1987
48. Allen JC: Management of metastatic epidural disease in children. J Pediatr 104:241, 1984
49. Perrin RG, McBroom RJ: Anterior versus posterior decompression for symptomatic spinal metastasis. Can J Neurol Sci 14:75, 1987
50. Lonstein JE: Post laminectomy kyphosis. Clin Orthop Rel Res 128:93, 1977
51. Wilkins RM et al: Ewing's sarcoma of bone. Cancer 58:2551, 1986
52. Flattey TJ et al: Spinal instability due to malignant disease. J Bone Joint Surg [Am] 66:47, 1984
53. Brotman AW, Stern TA: Osteoporosis and pathologic fractures in anorexia nervosa. Am J Psychiatry 142:495, 1985

54. Towbin R, Dunbar JS: Generalized osteoporosis with multiple fractures in an adolescent. Invest Radiol 16:171, 1981
55. Blatt J et al: Characteristics of acute lymphoblastic leukaemia in children with osteopenia and vertebral compression fractures. J Pediatr 105:280, 1984
56. Elsasser U et al: Bone rarefaction and crush fractures in juvenile chronic arthritis. Arch Dis Child 57:377, 1982
57. Louro JA: A spinal tuberculosis with neurological deficit: treatment with anterior vascularised rib grafts, posterior osteotomies and fusion. J Bone Joint Surg [Br] 72:686, 1990

57

Birth Fractures

Martin H. Reed
R. Mervyn Letts
Avrum N. Pollock

The future of a civilization may be judged by how it cares for its young.
—DANIEL PATRICK MOYNAHAN

There has been a trend toward a decrease in the incidence of birth injuries over recent years, presumably as a result of improving obstetrical practice.[1] Birth fractures, particularly fractures of the clavicle, comprise a significant proportion of birth injuries, although in general they are not the most serious.[2] Table 57-1 summarizes the experience with birth fractures at the Health Sciences Centre, Winnipeg during the last decade, and compares it to two other reported series.[2,3]

Most fractures occurring at birth, although disconcerting to parents, are usually more of a nuisance than a serious long-term problem for the infant. In most instances the fracture occurred because of some disproportion between the baby and the birth canal; occasionally because the baby had to be delivered rapidly due to fetal distress, or in some conditions such as arthrogryposis multiplex congenita or a congenital malformation rendering vaginal delivery impossible without a limb fracturing, or finally an abnormal presentation such as, an extended arm in a breech delivery, or a shoulder dystocia, resulting in more force having to be exerted simply to obtain a viable infant. Aside from treating the obvious fracture the orthopaedic surgeon should ensure that the parents realize the reason for the injury to their child and that the presence of the fracture may actually be the reason the family has a viable and otherwise normal infant. Since parents may wish to blame their obstetrician for unnecessary roughness, reassurance by the orthopaedic surgeon caring for the fracture will be of great benefit in ensuring the parents have a better appreciation and understanding of why such fractures occur.

Fractures occurring at birth may also be indicative of underlying pathology in the bone itself. The classical example of this is osteogenesis imperfecta, in which case the fractures may actually have occurred in utero. Children with myelomeningocele with paraplegia may have their lower extremities somewhat weakened by disuse osteoporosis, making them more prone to fracturing. Congenital abnormalities such as radiohumeral fusions or arthrogryposis may make limb flexion virtually impossible without a fracture occurring. In the majority of these instances, it is usually self-evident that there is an underlying pathologic process (Fig. 57-1).

FRACTURES OF THE CLAVICLE

Fractures of the clavicle are by far the most frequent type of birth fracture (Table 57-2), and, apart from soft tissue injuries such as cephalohematomas, are probably the most frequent of all birth injuries.[2] The reported incidences of clavicular fractures vary widely,[4] but the best studies, using either routine radiography or very

TABLE 57-1. Birth Fractures: Frequencies of Different Types

	Health Sciences Centre, Winnipeg (1980–1991)	Rubin[2]	Madsen[3]
Clavicle	37[a]	43	726
Limbs	11[a]	7	60
Spine	2		1

[a] One baby had a fracture of the clavicle and the ipsilateral humerus.

TABLE 57-2. Frequency of Birth Fractures in Descending Order

1. Fractures of clavicle (most common)
2. Fractures of humeral shaft
3. Fractures of femoral shaft
4. Epiphyseal fracture: humerus
5. Epiphyseal fracture: femur (least common)

careful clinical examination, have shown a frequency of between 1.7 and 2.9 percent of vaginal deliveries.[4] These fractures can occur in association with breech deliveries or in babies born by cesarean section,[3,5] but they are usually seen in babies who present in the vertex position and are born by vaginal delivery.[3-6] A high birth weight is considered to be a significant predisposing factor; in two studies the average birth weight of babies with clavicular fractures was significantly greater than the average birth weight of a control population (Table 57-3).[5,6] In our series 17 of 38 patients had a birth weight of 4.0 kg or more. Shoulder dystocia is also considered to be an important predisposing factor[2,5-7] (Table 57-3).

Fractures of the clavicle may also be sustained in breech babies, where there is some urgency to deliver the aftercoming head. In such instances, pressure may be exerted by the obstetrician's fingers over the clavicles with subsequent fracturing of the midshaft of the clavicle.

For complete fractures of the clavicle, the nursery staff should be made aware of the injury so that the baby can be handled judiciously. A short period of immobilization of the arm against the chest using stretchable mesh for holding on burn dressings is often sufficient. In several days, these fractures will form enough callus so that crepitus disappears and the baby can be handled with impunity.

Clavicular fractures occur more commonly on the right than on the left (Table 57-3)[3-6]; bilateral fractures are rare (Table 57-3).[3,5] It has been postulated that the right-sided predominance of these fractures is related to the fact that most vertex presentations are left occiput anterior, and that, in this position, there is either increased pressure on the right shoulder, particularly if there is dystocia,[5] or that the right shoulder, as the anterior shoulder, is delivered first[6] (Fig. 57-2).

A fracture of the clavicle is not usually recognized at the time of delivery,[6] and even after delivery it may not be obvious.[4] In a prospective study, which was undertaken to look specifically for these fractures, only 11 were found clinically during the initial hospitalization.[4] Another 7 were found at the time of the first office visit, when callus could be palpated at the fracture site.[4] In our series, clavicular fractures were not recognized clinically while the baby was in the nursery in 15 of the 38 patients; instead, they were noted incidentally on radiographs obtained for other reasons (Table 57-3). A number of fractures were undoubtedly never diagnosed.

TABLE 57-3. Birth Fractures of the Clavicle

	Health Sciences Centre, Winnipeg (1980–1991)	Oppenheim[5]	Gilbert[6]
Patients			
Total	38	57	60
Male:female	19:19		37:23
Average birth weight (g)	3,807	3,802[a]	3,768[b]
Shoulder dystocia	7	9	11
Breech delivery	4	2	
Cesarean section		3	1
Brachial plexus injury	1	3	
Fractures			
Right:left	22:15	38:18	41:19
Bilateral	1	1	

[a] Significantly higher than a control population ($p < .004$).
[b] Significantly higher than a control population ($p < .005$).

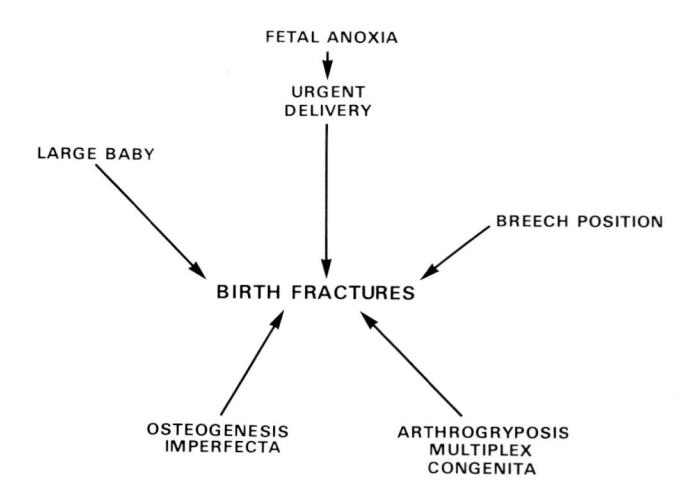

Fig. 57-1. Factors contributing to birth fractures in the newborn.

To examine the clavicles and neck in a newborn infant the thoracic spine should be gently hyperextended by a hand placed under the infant, allowing the head to fall back slightly, uncovering the neck and clavicles (Fig. 57-3). The clinical signs that suggest the presence of a fracture include edema and crepitus at the site, and, later, the presence of palpable callus.[3-5] At the time of the injury, lack of movement of the affected arm may also be noted. The differential diagnosis of this sign includes brachial plexus injury and humeral fracture.[5] Local signs should help to differentiate fractures at the two sites. In the case of a brachial plexus injury, there should be a true paralysis with no resistance to passive movement, whereas a fracture should produce a pseudoparalysis, and the baby will tend to resist passive movement. Rarely, a brachial plexus injury may complicate a fracture of the clavicle[5,7] (Table 57-3, Fig. 57-4).

Fractures of the clavicle are usually easily seen on radiographs. However, occasionally they may not be visible on standard views. Weinberg and colleagues[8] have described an apical oblique view of the clavicle, which they consider particularly effective for detecting an undisplaced fracture. These fractures usually occur in the middle third of the clavicle. They are usually complete fractures (Fig. 57-5), although greenstick fractures are sometimes seen (Fig. 57-6). If the fracture is complete, there is generally some displacement of the fragments, with the medial fragment elevated above the lateral fragment (Fig. 57-5). The main radiologic differential diagnosis is congenital pseudarthrosis of the clavicle. Like fractures, pseudarthroses occur more commonly on the right, and the medial segment always lies in front of and above the lateral segment.[9] In a pseudarthrosis, the adjacent ends of the clavicle are smoothly rounded, and may be slightly bulbous.[9] However, in the first few days of life it may be difficult to distinguish radiologically between a fracture and a pseudarthrosis. Ogden[10] has described a separation of the medial epiphysis of the clavicle, a very rare birth injury.

If the lesion is a fracture, callus should be evident clinically and radiologically by 2 weeks of age. Cumming[11] noted calcification in the callus around a clavicular fracture as early as 10 days after birth, but in another

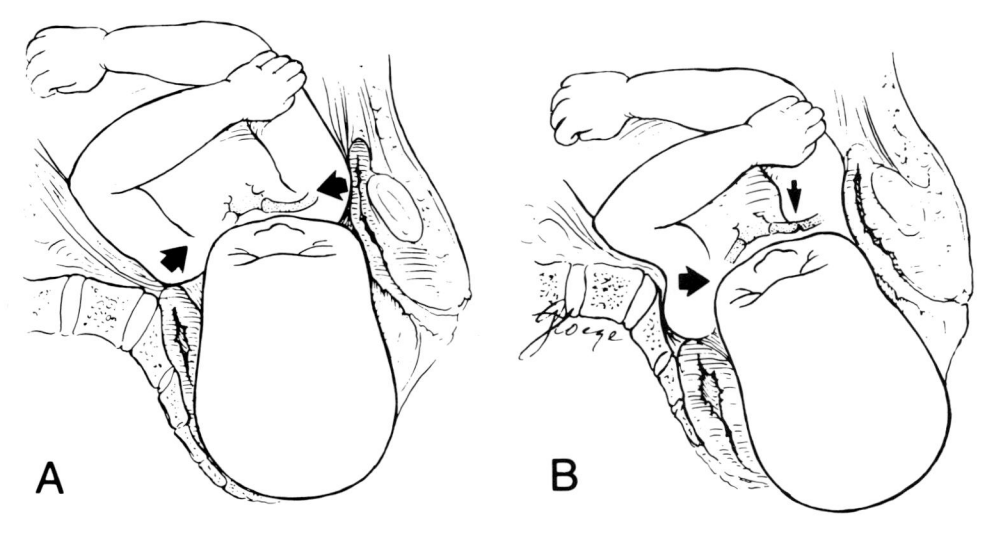

Fig. 57-2. (A&B) Shoulder compression and resultant clavicular fracturing in shoulder dystocia. (From Oppenheim et al.,[5] with permission.)

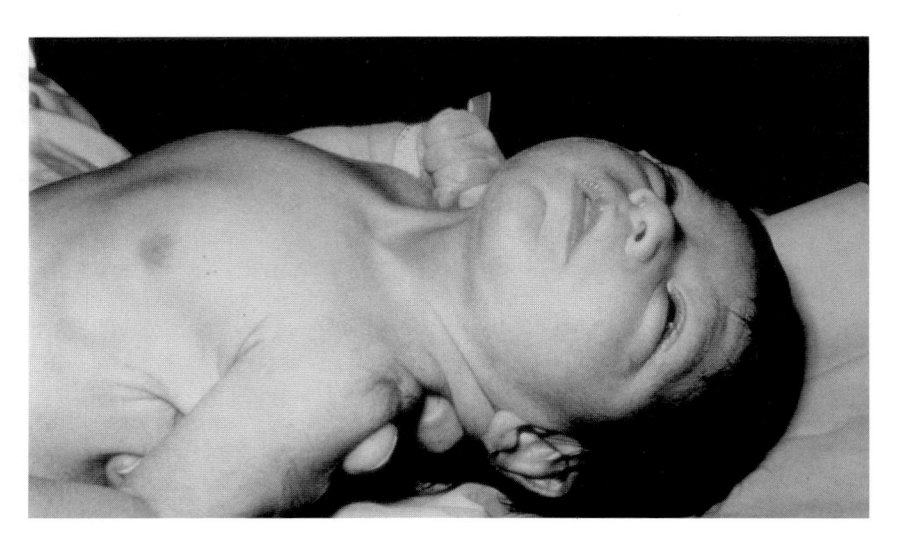

Fig. 57-3. Technique for examination of clavicles and neck in the newborn by arching the thoracic spine with a hand placed under the upper torso of the infant.

baby it was not visible even by 11 days of age. Callus develops rapidly, and the clavicle remodels, so that, by 6 months of age, there may be no sign of the previous fracture (Fig. 57-7). In general, fractures of the clavicle require little treatment, and they heal with no complications.[5]

LONG-BONE FRACTURES

Diaphyseal Fractures

Fractures of the long bones are far less frequent than fractures of the clavicle (Table 57-1). When they occur, they are usually diaphyseal, and, in most series, most frequently occur in the humerus[2,3] (Fig. 57-8; Table 57-4). The femur is the most common site of fracture in the lower extremity[3,11,12] (Table 57-4), but fractures of the tibia have been described.[3,11,13] A fracture of the distal radius has been reported in a baby who also had a fractured tibia.[13]

Fractures of the long bones usually involve the midshaft and are generally complete[11,12] (Fig. 57-7), although a plastic bowing type fracture of the femur resulting from birth trauma has been described.[14]

Humeral fractures are frequently associated with breech delivery (Table 57-4).[1,2,3,11] Fractures of the lower extremities are also often associated with breech presentation (Table 57-4), and may occur even when delivery is accomplished by cesarean section.[3,12,13] Neuromuscular diseases, such as myelomeningocele and spinal muscular atrophy, may predispose to birth fractures of the long bones[11,15]; babies with myelomeningoceles are also at increased risk of fracture in the neonatal period.[16]

Fractures of the midshaft of the humerus, often occurring during attempted deliveries of the extended arm in breech presentations, can be effectively managed by binding the arm to the torso using stretchable mesh. Occasionally, a small tongue depressor can be used to splint the humerus or a small strip of plaster. Healing is very rapid and usually within a week to 10 days the fracture is solid. Considerable angulation can be accepted as remodeling is rapid and complete (Fig. 57-8). Radial nerve palsy can occur in fractures at the junction of the distal and middle shafts, but is always a neuropraxia and will recover with time.

Fractures of the femur are a little more difficult to manage and usually demand splinting. This can usually be accomplished with plaster splints or two tongue depressors since most of these fractures are midshaft. If the fracture is more proximal, a small hip spica can be applied. Healing usually is sufficient by 2 weeks of age to discontinue all external splinting.

Physeal Fractures

Fractures involving the growth plates are less common than those involving the diaphyses (Table 57-4). The common sites are the proximal and distal humerus and the distal femur (Figs. 57-9 to 57-11), they have also been described in the proximal femur[19] and rarely in the distal tibia.[18] At all sites they are usually Salter-Harris type I fractures (Figs. 57-9 and 57-10), although type II fractures can also occur, particularly in the distal femur[18-20] (Fig. 57-11). Breech delivery is the most frequent predisposing factor for these fractures,[18-20] but, like diaphyseal fractures, they can also occur in babies with neuromuscular disorders (Fig. 57-11; Table 57-4).

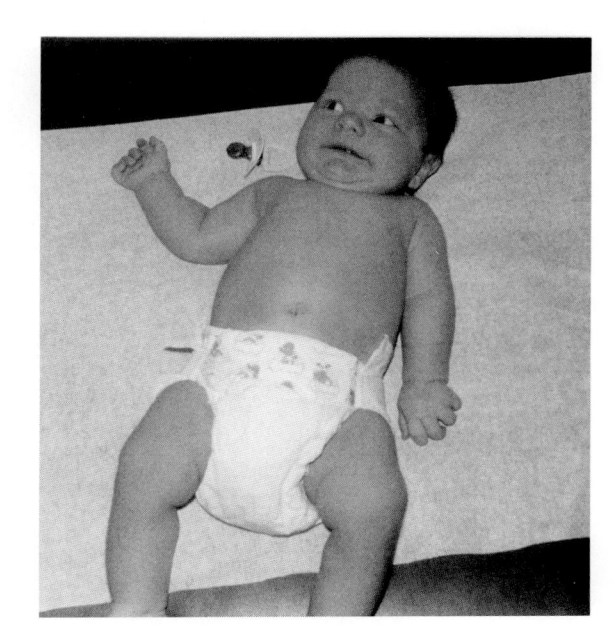

Fig. 57-4. A one-month-old infant with a fracture of the left clavicle and a left Erb's palsy sustained in a difficult breech delivery. The left arm remains extended and internally rotated.

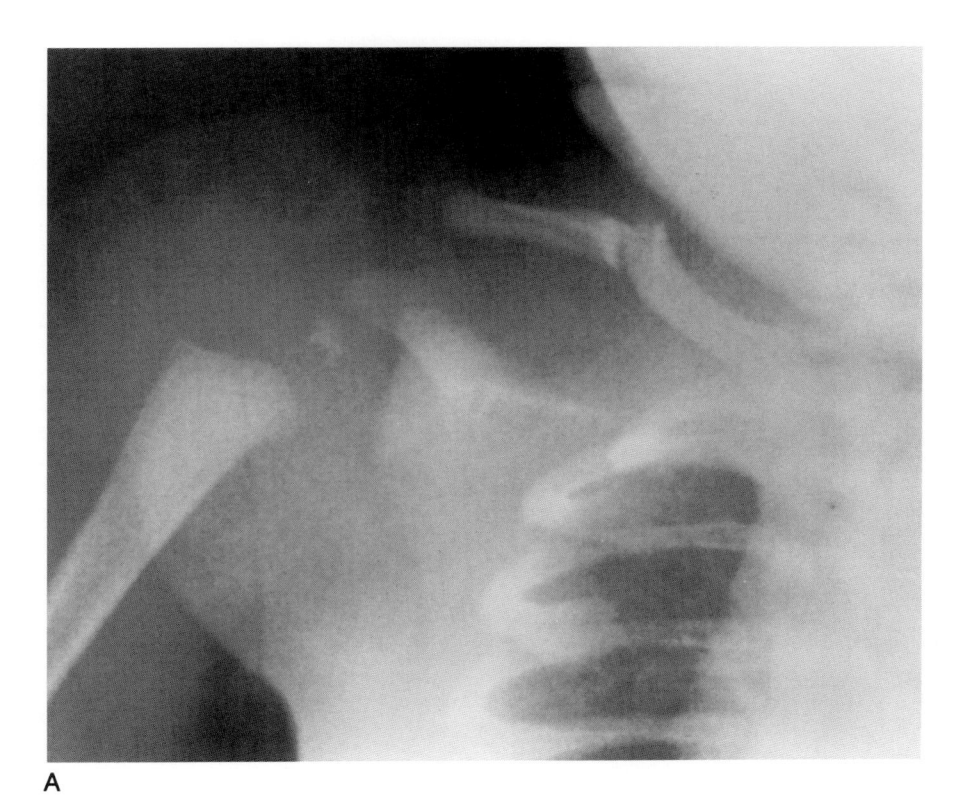

Fig. 57-5. Birth fracture of the right clavicle. **(A)** Day of birth. *(Figure continues.)*

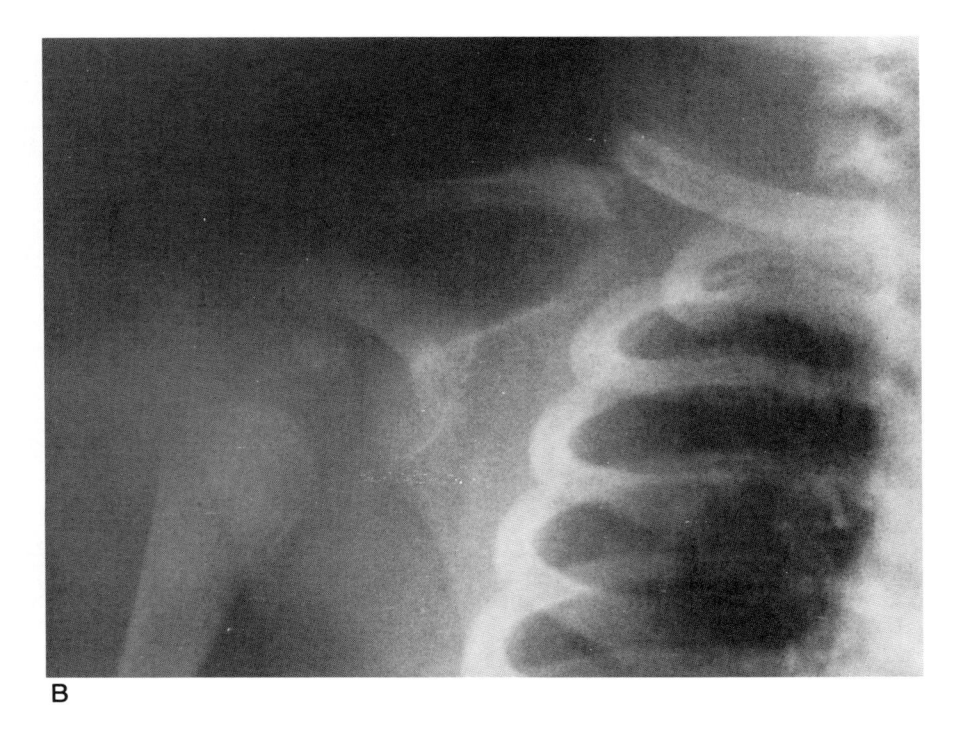

Fig. 57-5 *(Continued).* **(B)** At 10 days of age early callus is visible.

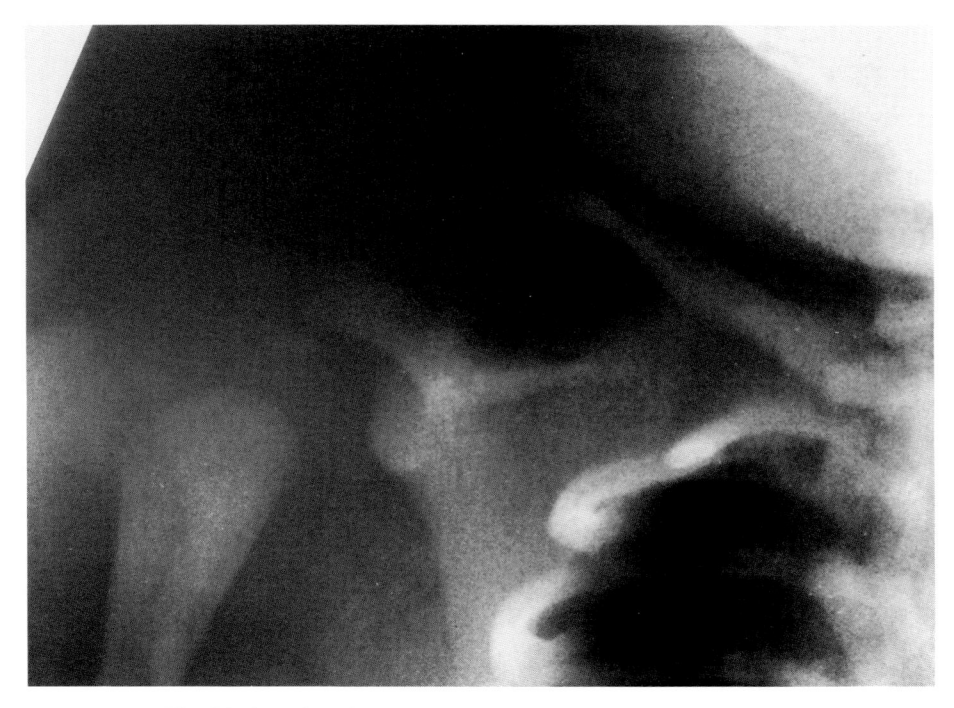

Fig. 57-6. Birth fracture of the right clavicle, greenstick type.

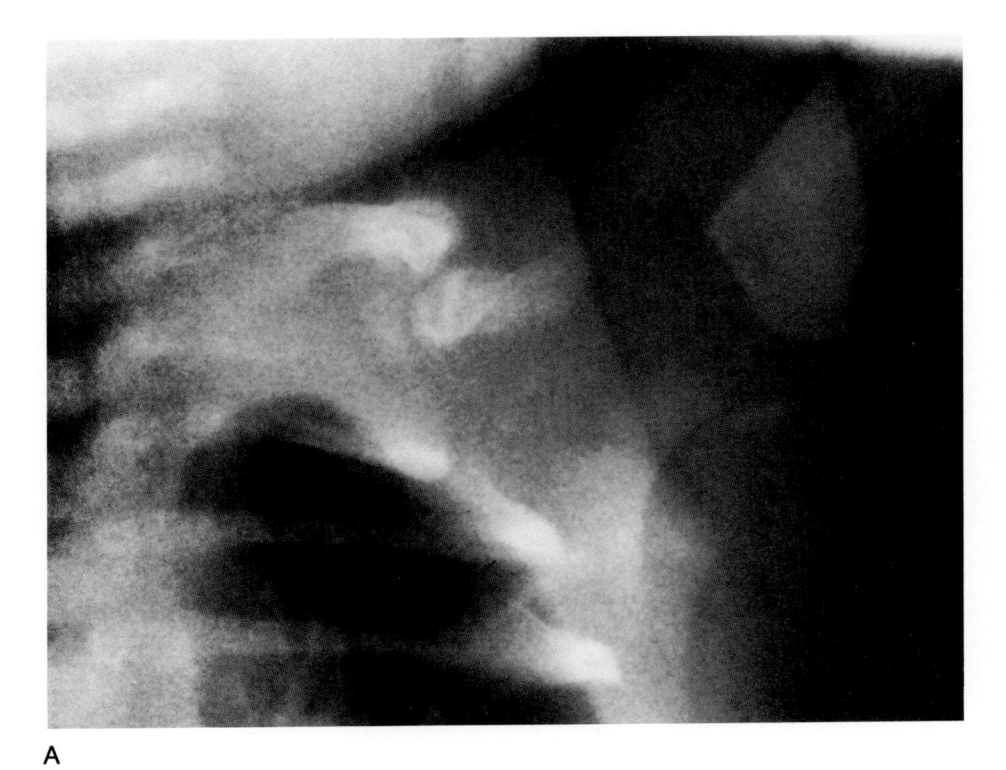

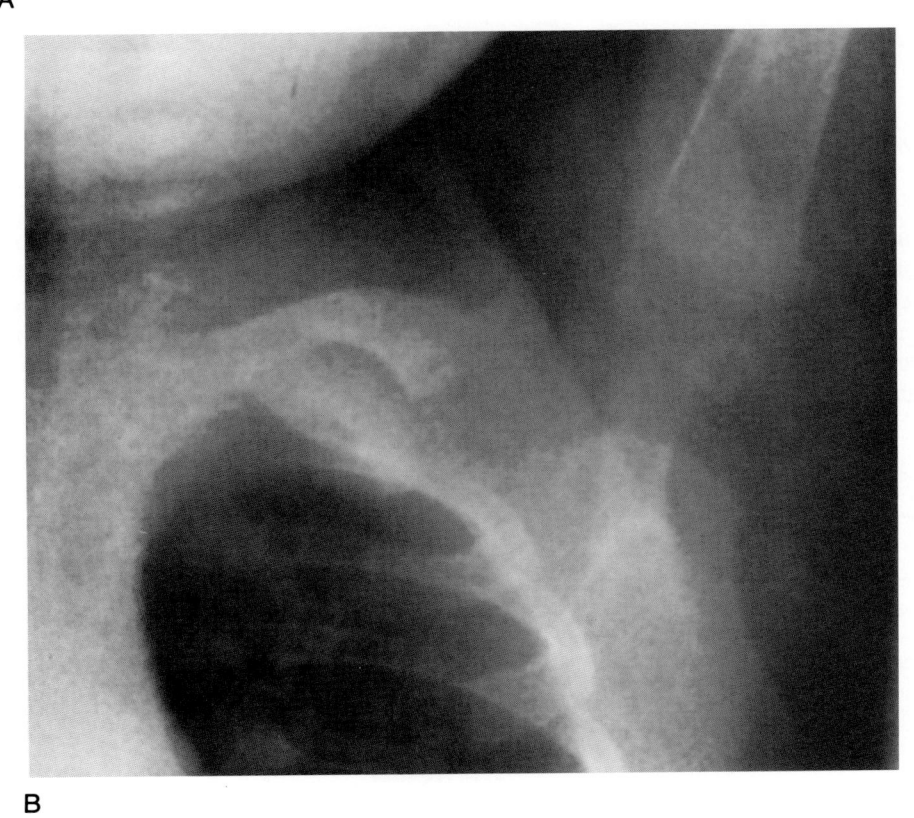

Fig. 57-7. Birth fracture of the left clavicle. **(A)** At 2 weeks of age there is early callus. **(B)** At 3 months of age the clavicle has largely remodeled.

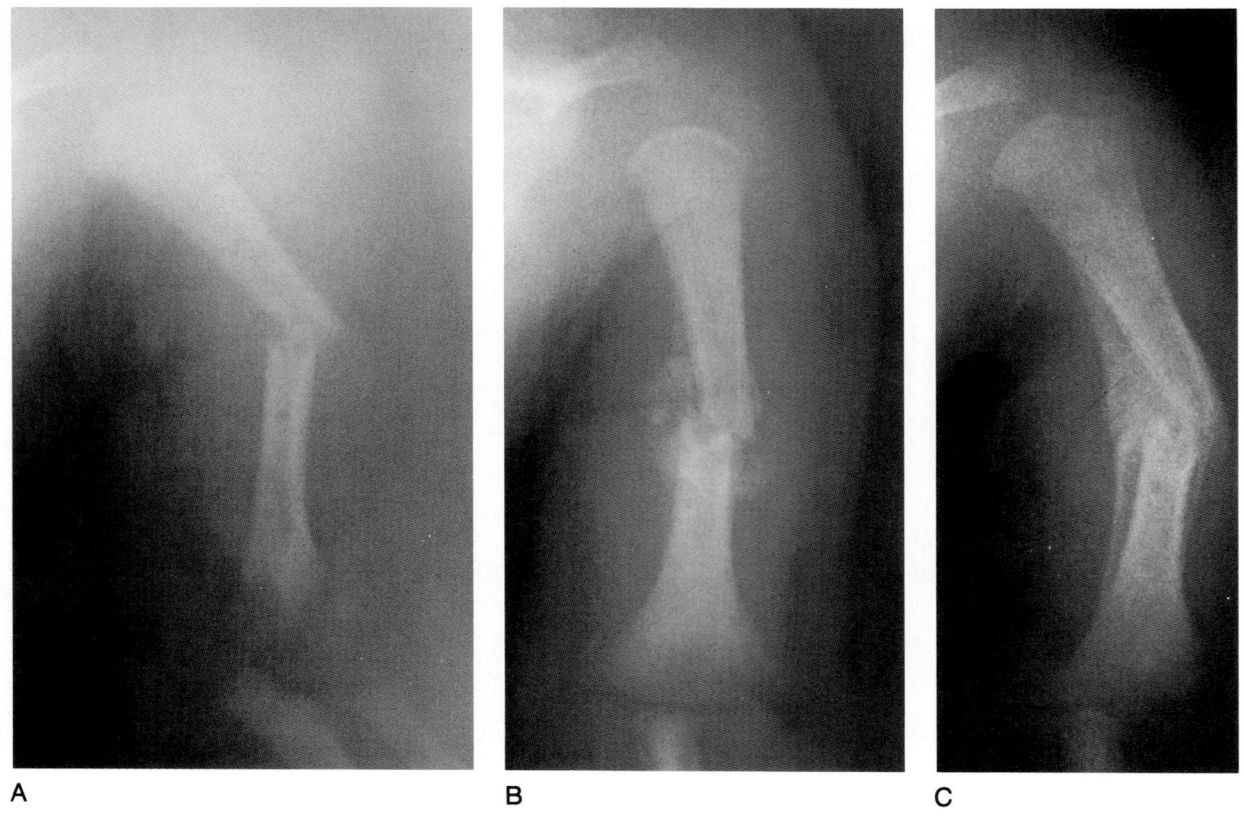

Fig. 57-8. Birth fracture of the middiaphysis of the left humerus. **(A)** First day **(B)** At 13 days of age there is well-developed callus. **(C)** At 5 weeks of age the fracture has healed and is starting to remodel.

The radiographic diagnosis of these injuries may be difficult. Proximal humeral epiphyses are frequently, and distal femoral epiphyses are usually, ossified in full-term babies, and, if the epiphysis is ossified, a displaced fracture at either site should be evident. However, if the fracture is minimally displaced or undisplaced, it may not be recognized on plain films. The epiphyses at other sites where these fractures occur, particularly the distal humerus and proximal femur, are not ossified at birth. If the epiphysis is not ossified, a fracture may be mistaken for a dislocation. However, traumatic dislocations related to delivery, have been described only rarely. At the proximal humerus and proximal femur, displacement of distal fragments is usually lateral and proximal. In the hip, this is the same direction as a congenital dislocation, but in the case of a fracture, the acetabulum should be normally developed. Septic arthritis should also be considered in the differential diagnosis of an epiphyseal fracture of the proximal femur, but systemic signs should help distinguish the two. The distal fragment is usually displaced medially in the case of an epiphyseal fracture of the distal humerus, opposite to the usual direction of displacement with a dislocation. As epiphyseal fractures heal, callus develops around the metaphysis (Figs. 57-9 and 57-11).

In the past, arthrography was usually used to confirm the diagnosis of these fractures acutely, if there was any

TABLE 57-4. Birth Fractures of the Extremities

	Total	Breech	Neuromuscular disorder
Humerus			
Diaphysis	5	3	
Epiphysis			
Proximal	1	1	
Distal	1		
Femur			
Diaphysis	1	1	
Epiphysis			
Proximal	1	1	
Distal	2		2

From the Health Sciences Centre, Winnipeg, 1980–1991.

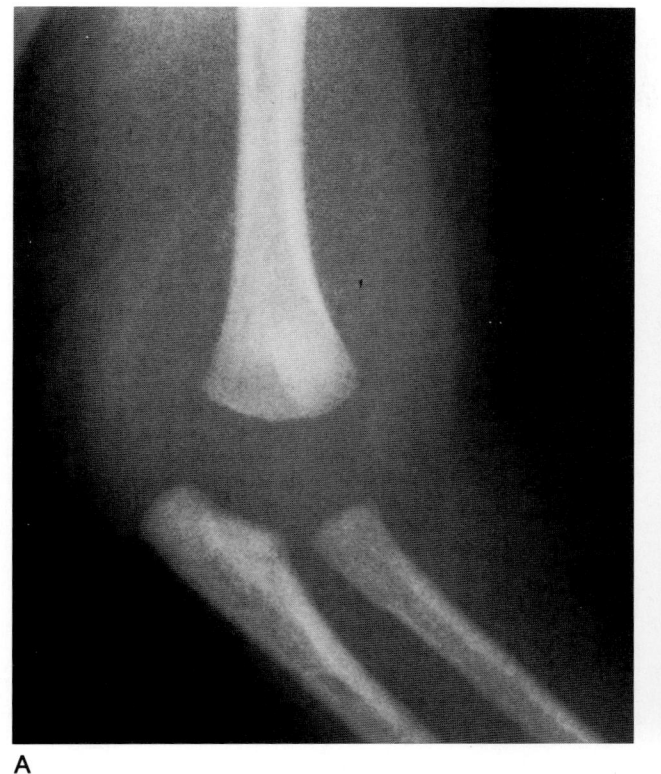

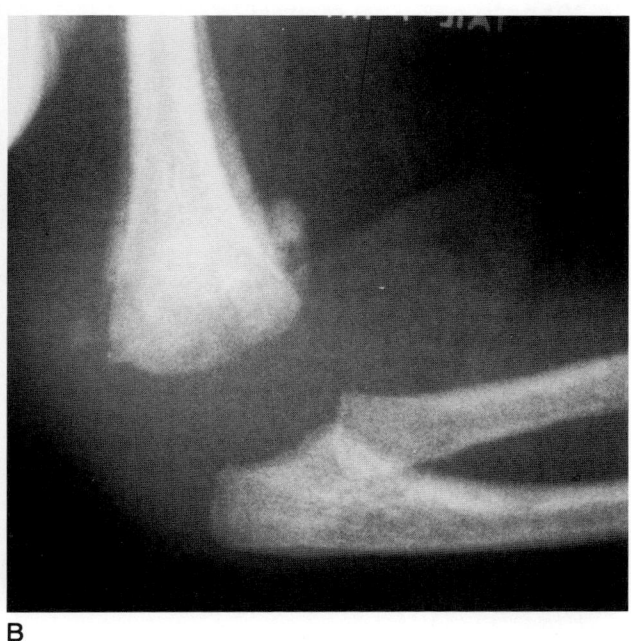

Fig. 57-9. Salter-Harris type I birth fracture of the distal humerus. **(A)** At 6 days of age there is minimal medial displacement. **(B)** At 2 weeks of age a metaphyseal callus is seen. (Courtesy of Dr. S. Miller, Department of Radiology, The Pas Health Complex, The Pas, Manitoba.)

doubt clinically.[19] However, sonography has recently been shown to be very effective in demonstrating them[20] (Fig. 57-10), and it is the best imaging modality to use after plain films, if further evaluation of these injuries is required.

The diagnosis of these fractures may not be made at the time of delivery, although in some instances, the obstetrician will have heard or felt a snap associated with the delivery of an extremity. Usually there has been associated obstetrical complications of the delivery, often associated with disproportion or abnormal presentation. Nursery staff are usually astute at picking up these injuries very quickly as the child does not use the extremity and there is the classic pseudoparalysis, especially noted during the startle or Moro reflex. Swelling around the joint occurs within hours and may be confused with a septic joint, since the area is warm and may even be somewhat inflamed looking. Since the epiphysis of the proximal humerus and distal femur is intra-articular in infancy, a hemarthrosis of the joint is always present. If there is considerable swelling, aspiration of the joint to relieve distention and concomitant pain is both therapeutic and diagnostic. Realignment of the epiphysis if displaced is recommended and will require a closed reduction under anesthesia. Immobilization of the joint with a miniature hip spica cast for the displaced proximal femoral epiphyseal injury may be necessary. Usually, the proximal humeral epiphyseal can be reduced and held in place with the arm immobilized with the chest wall.

Growth deformity of the humerus following a birth injury to the proximal epiphysis has been described,[21] but in general these fractures heal with no complications.[19]

DISLOCATIONS

Although dislocations can occur as congenital abnormalities, traumatic dislocations related to delivery are extremely rare. As mentioned in the previous section, epiphyseal fractures can mimic dislocations, and a limb deformity related to birth trauma, which resembles a

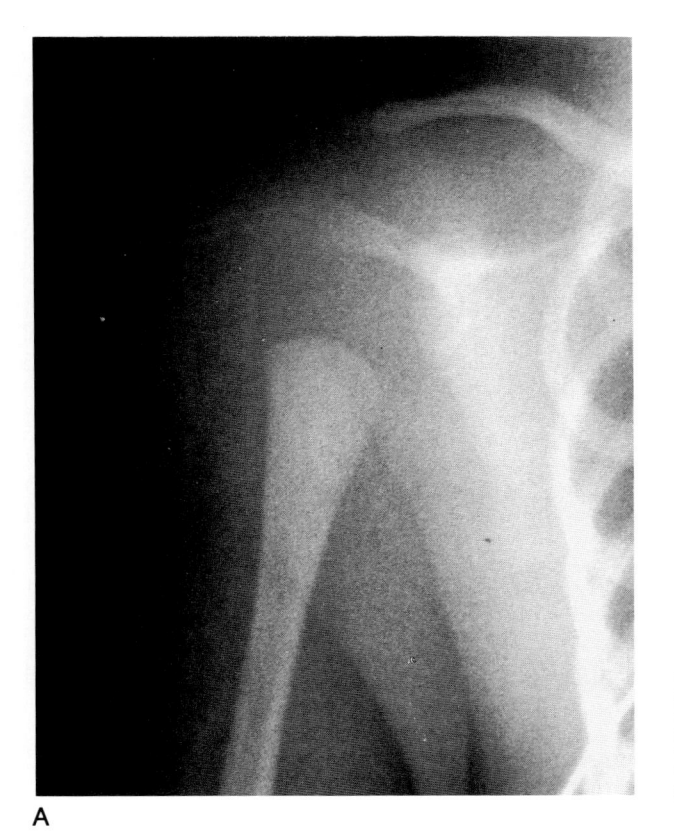

Fig. 57-10. Salter-Harris type I birth fracture of the proximal humerus. **(A)** Radiograph of the right shoulder is normal. **(B)** Ultrasound shows a slight malalignment of the proximal humeral epiphysis and the metaphysis, indicating a fracture. *(Figure continues.)*

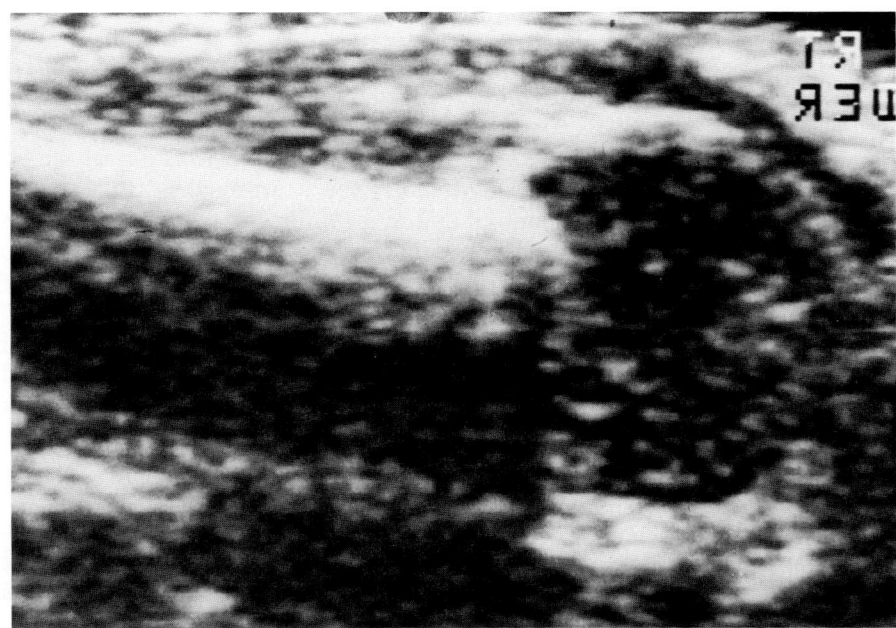

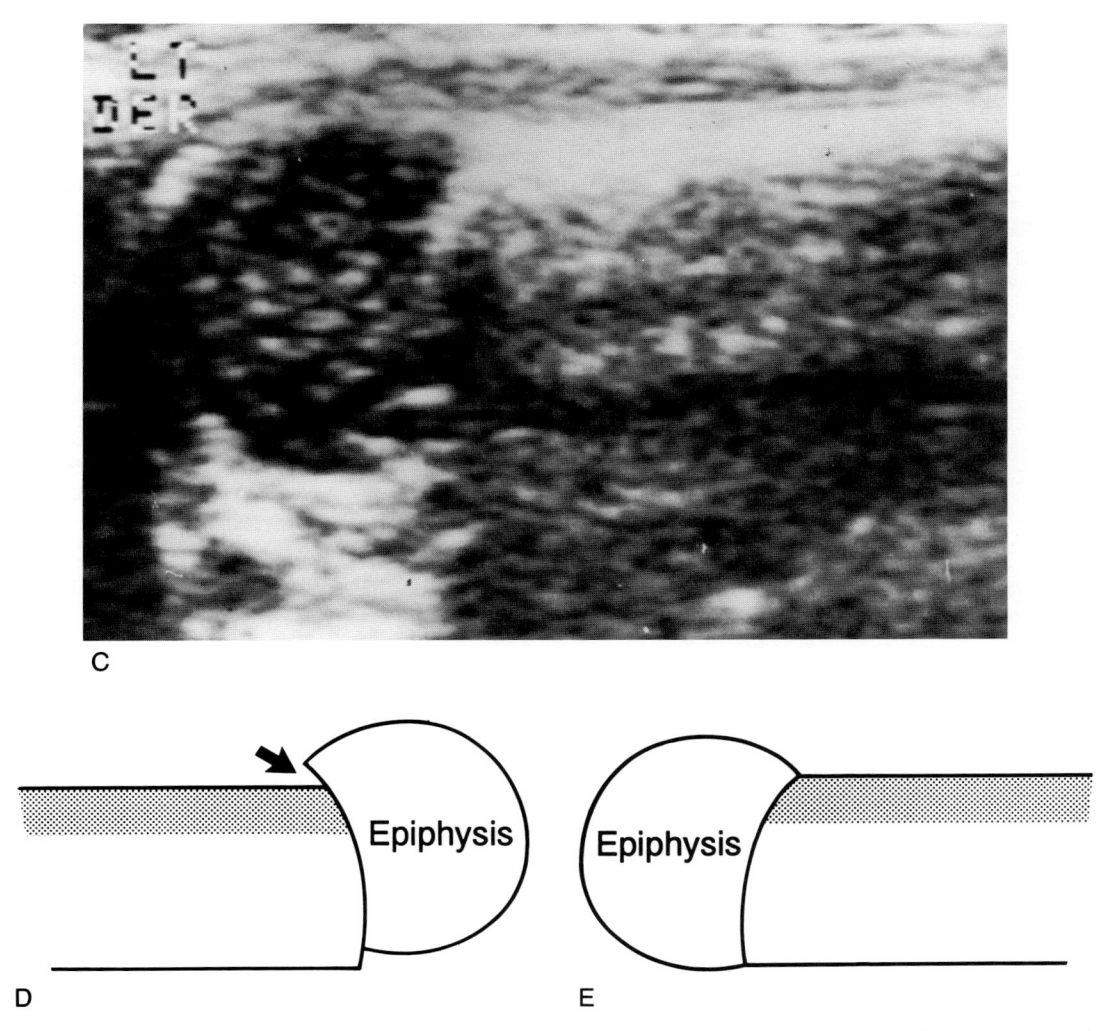

Fig. 57-10 *(Continued).* **(C)** Normal left shoulder for comparison. **(D&E)** Diagrams of ultrasound examinations showing **(D)** the right shoulder with the fracture *(arrow)* and **(E)** the normal left shoulder. (From Reed MH (ed): Pediatric Skeletal Radiology. p. 121. Williams & Wilkins, Baltimore, 1992, with permission.)

dislocation, will usually prove to be an epiphyseal fracture. An example of dislocation of the shoulder from birth trauma has been described.[22] Dislocation of the shoulder, particularly posteriorly, is a well-recognized complication of obstetrical brachial plexus paralysis,[23] and shoulder dislocation seen in association with this complication is probably always secondary and not the result of direct birth injury.[24]

Dislocation of the radial head as a result of birth trauma has been described rarely.[25]

SPINAL INJURIES

Spinal injuries as a result of birth trauma are, fortunately, rare (Table 57-1), but their consequences are devastating. They most commonly occur in association with breech presentation, particularly if the head is hyperextended.[1,26,27] In these situations, injury can occur at any level of the cord, but most frequently involves the lower cervical or upper thoracic region.[28] Spinal cord injury is a very rare complication of cephalic presenta-

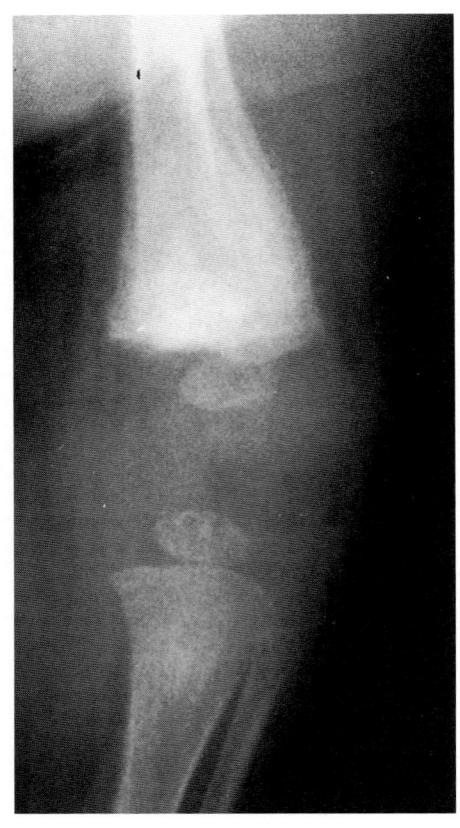

Fig. 57-11. Salter-Harris type II birth fracture of the distal femur in a baby with a myelomeningocele. At 1 month of age the fracture has healed.

tion, although it may occur if midforceps rotation is used; in this type of injury, the level of damage is usually high in the cervical cord. The pathologic features of spinal cord birth injuries include hemorrhage within and around the cord, edema and ischemia of the cord, and occasionally complete transection.[26,27]

In the majority of cases, ordinary radiographs demonstrate no abnormality, although dislocation or fracture of the cervical spine is occasionally seen.[26,28,29] Computed tomography (CT) myelography can be very useful in investigating these patients, and may show extradural hematoma or enlargement of the cord from edema or hemorrhage.[28] Ultrasonography may be useful in the early assessment of these patients, and may show more chronic abnormalities, such as cord atrophy, later.[28] The two patients in our series with spinal injuries (Table 57-1) both had cervical spine lesions related to forceps rotations. Neither had abnormalities on radiographs of the cervical spine; CT myelography was not performed on either one.

Thoracolumbar injury can also occur in the breech delivery from excessive pull on the legs or pelvis. This results in a stretching of the spinal cord with disruption at the T12 level. Radiographs are usually not helpful and the injury falls into the SCIWORA syndrome (spinal cord injury without evidence of any radiologic findings). Unfortunately, these injuries are usually permanent (see Chapter 50).

Some of these injuries are immediately fatal.[26] If the child survives, the diagnosis may be difficult because the clinical presentation is variable. Common signs include respiratory distress, and hypotonia or flaccid paralysis, but the clinical picture may be complicated by signs of concomitant intracranial injuries.[26-28] These injuries may be mistaken for other neuromuscular problems, such as amyotonia congenita, myasthenia gravis, or infantile spinal muscular atrophy.[1,26] No active forms of treatment have yet been shown to be effective.[1,27] These patients require supportive care, and their prognosis is usually poor.[1,26,27]

SUMMARY

Birth fractures are usually an indication of a difficult delivery secondary to malposition, disproportion, or congenital malformations.[30] Fortunately, most birth fractures heal rapidly and are not prone to serious complications. The role of the orthopaedic surgeon should be to assist in fracture immobilization, to reduce the child's discomfort until union has occurred, and to reassure the parents that the fracture usually does not cause any long-term disability for the child.

REFERENCES

1. Curran JS: Birth-associated injury. Clin Perinatol 8:111, 1981
2. Rubin A: Birth injuries: incidence, mechanisms, and end results. Obstet Gynecol 23:218, 1964
3. Madsen ET: Fractures of the extremities in the newborn. Acta Obstet Gynecol Scand 34:41, 1955
4. Joseph PR, Rosenfeld W: Clavicular fractures in neonates. Am J Dis Child 144:165, 1990
5. Oppenheim WL, Davis A, Growdon WA et al: Clavicle fractures in the newborn. Clin Orthop 250:176, 1990
6. Gilbert WM, Tchabo JG: Fractured clavicle in newborns. Int Surg 73:123, 1988
7. Gonik B, Hollyer VL, Allen R: Shoulder dystocia recognition: differences in neonatal risks for injury. Am J Perinatol 8:31, 1991

8. Weinberg B, Seife B, Alonso P: The apical oblique view of the clavicle: its usefulness in neonatal and childhood trauma. Skeletal Radiol 20:201, 1991
9. Manashil G, Laufer S: Congenital pseudarthrosis of the clavicle: report of three cases. AJR 132:678, 1979
10. Ogden JA: Chest and pectoral girdle. p. 313. In: Skeletal injury in the child. 2nd Ed. WB Saunders, Philadelphia, 1990
11. Cumming WA: Neonatal skeletal fractures: birth trauma or child abuse. Can Assoc Radiol J 30:30, 1979
12. Vasa R, Kim MR: Fracture of the femur at cesarean section: case report and review of literature. Am J Perinatol 7:46, 1990
13. Kaplan M, Dollberg M, Wajntraub G, Itzchaki M: Fractured long bones in a term infant delivered by cesarean section. Pediatr Radiol 17:256, 1987
14. Zionts LE, Leffers D, Oberto MR, Harvey JP: Plastic bowing of the femur in a neonate. J Pediatr Orthop 4:749, 1984
15. Burke SW, Jameson VP, Roberts JM et al: Birth fractures in spinal muscular atrophy. J Pediatr Orthop 6:34, 1986
16. Boytim MJ, Davidson RS, Charney E, Melchionni JB: Neonatal fractures in myelomeningocele patients. J Pediatr Orthop 11:28, 1991
17. Hagglund G, Hansson LI, Wibeg G: Correction of deformity after femoral birth fracture: 16-year follow-up. Acta Orthop Scand 59:333, 1988
18. Ekengren K, Bergdahl S, Ekstrom G: Birth injuries to the epiphyseal cartilage. Acta Radiol Diagn 19:197, 1978
19. Ogden JA, Lee KE, Rudicel A, Pelker RR. Proximal femoral epiphysiolysis in the neonate. J Pediatr Orthop 4:285, 1984
20. Broker FHL, Burbach T: Ultrasonic diagnosis of separation of the proximal humeral epiphysis in the newborn. J Bone Joint Surg [Am] 72:187, 1990
21. Lucas LS, Gill JH: Humerus varus following birth injury to the proximal humeral epiphysis. J Bone Joint Surg 29:367, 1947
22. Kuhn D, Rosman M: Traumatic, nonparalytic dislocation of the shoulder in a newborn infant. J Pediatr Orthop 4:121, 1984
23. Pollock AN, Reed MH: Shoulder deformities from obstetrical brachial plexus paralysis. Skeletal Radiol 18:295, 1989
24. Babbitt DP, Cassidy RH: Obstetrical paralysis and dislocation of the shoulder in infancy. J Bone Joint Surg [Am] 50:1447, 1968
25. Bayne O, Rang M: Medial dislocation of the radial head following breech delivery: a case report and review of the literature. J Pediatr Orthop 4:485, 1984
26. Dickman CA, Rekate HL, Sonntag VKH, Zabramski JM: Pediatric spinal trauma: vertebral column and spinal cord injuries in children. Pediatr Neurosci 15:237, 1989
27. Byers RK: Spinal-cord injuries during birth. Dev Med Child Neurol 17:103, 1975
28. Babyn PS, Chuang SH, Daneman A, Davidson GS: Sonographic evaluation of spinal cord birth trauma with pathologic correlation. AJNR 9:765, 1988
29. Stanley P, Duncan AW, Isaacson J, Isaacson AS: Radiology of fracture-dislocation of the cervical spine during delivery. AJR 145:621, 1985
30. Diamond LS, Alegado R: Perinatal fractures in arthrogryposis multiplex congenita. J Pediatr Orthop 1:189, 1981

58

Fractures in the Myelomeningocele Child

John V. Banta

The needs of children should not be made to wait.
—JOHN F. KENNEDY

The first report of undisplaced fractures of the tibial metaphysis by Gillies and Hartung[1] in 1938 called attention to the diagnostic pitfalls occasionally encountered in fractures in the paraplegic child. Fracture of osteopenic bone in an insensate limb may go unrecognized initially and present later with radiographic findings compatible with osteomyelitis or osteosarcoma, resulting in unnecessary biopsy[1-4] (Fig. 58-1). Following the introduction of successful valve shunts for the control of hydrocephalus[5] in 1957, there has been a marked increase in the survival of children with neural tube defects. Recent medical advances have also reduced the mortality of children sustaining spinal cord injury, and these children are also at risk for neuropathic fractures that have the same presenting features and potential complications.

The incidence of fractures in children with myelomeningocele is related to the level of paralysis, the age of the child, and indirectly to the rate of lower extremity reconstructive surgery. The overall incidence is reported to range from 8 to 30 percent.[4,6-10] Fractures have been commonly noted under 10 years of age[6,11] and usually occur distal to the level of neurologic involvement with femoral fractures common in thoracic levels of paraplegia and tibial fractures being more prevalent in children with lumbar levels.[11] Diaphyseal and metaphyseal fractures are common with higher levels of paralysis, whereas epiphyseal injuries are more frequently encountered in children who are ambulatory.[9,12,13] Recently, Boytim and colleagues[14] reported a 17 percent incidence of neonatal fractures in newborns with thoracic or upper lumbar levels of paralysis with associated contractures adjacent to the fracture sites (Figs. 58-2 and 58-3).

ANATOMY

Fractures characteristically present in the lower extremity below the level of sensory loss. Neuropathic fractures are best classified as diaphyseal, metaphyseal, or epiphyseal. Consideration of the anatomic location as well as the neurologic level allows the clinician to initiate the most appropriate treatment to both avoid complications and return the patient to his optimum mobility status. These fractures are characterized by rapid healing, often abundant callus formation, and painless swelling of the overlying soft tissues. The majority of such fractures can be best treated by nonoperative means.[6,15-18] Overriding, common in middiaphyseal fractures, can be accommodated for by a lift, but rotational alignment must be preserved for bracewear and optimum alignment for sitting in a wheelchair. Metaphyseal fractures are most common about the knee[6-9,19] and may result in joint contracture following healing, particularly in chil-

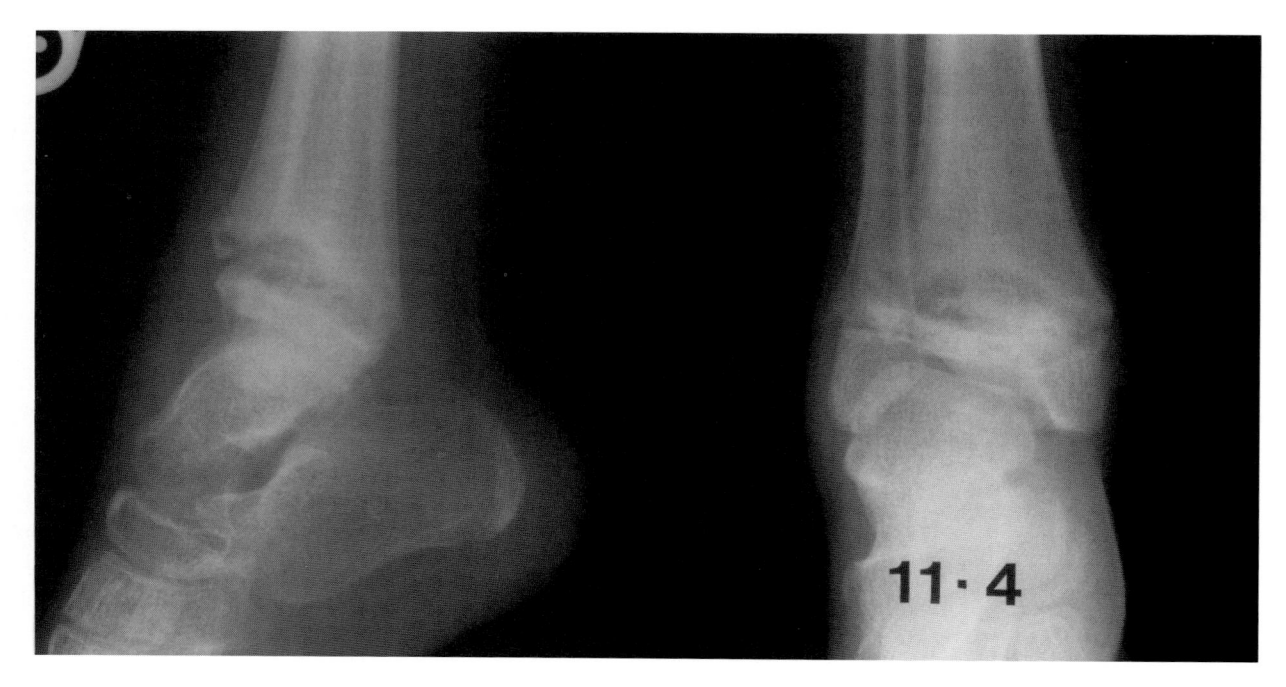

Fig. 58-1. An 11-year, 4-month-old girl with an L4 level developed epiphyseolysis of the distal tibial and fibular epiphyses demonstrating widening of the physis and metaphyseal sclerosis suggestive of infection.

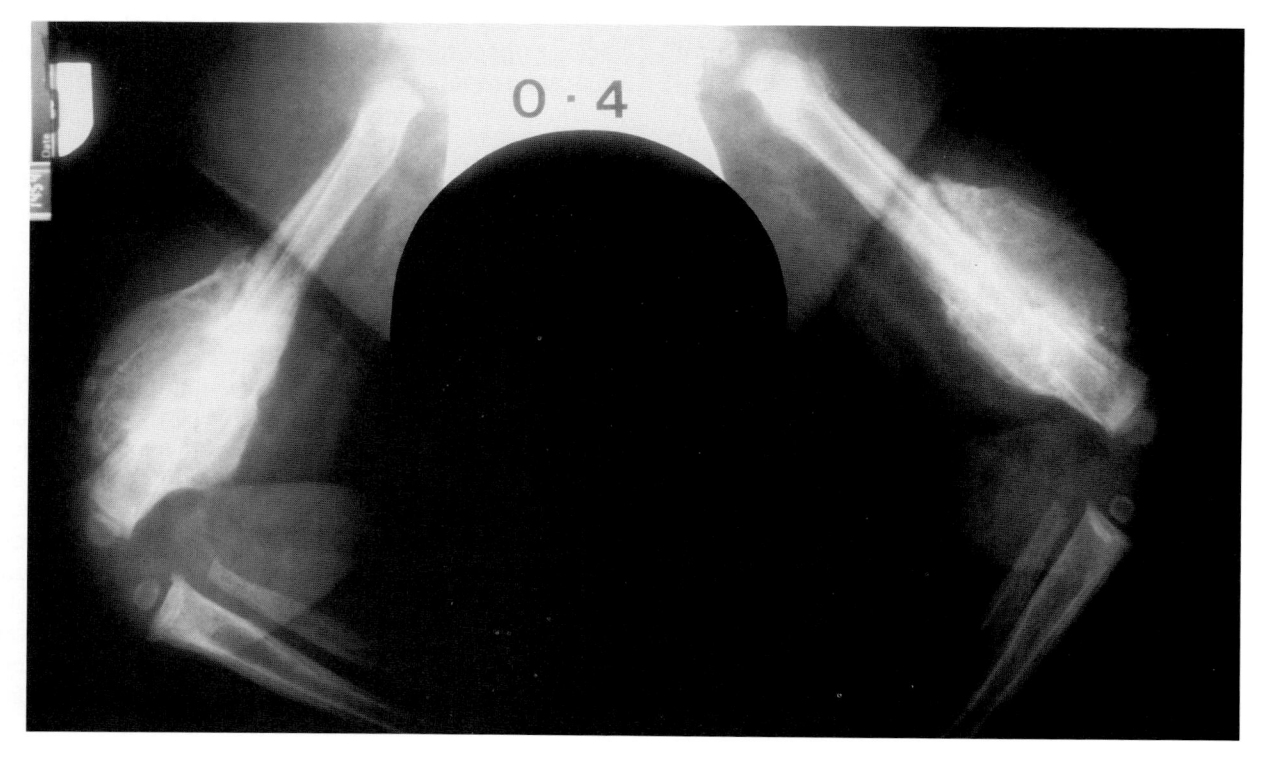

Fig. 58-2. A 4-month-old female with lower thoracic kyphosis sustained spontaneous bilateral femoral fractures following neonatal kyphectomy. Treatment was by application of bulky soft cast padding dressings.

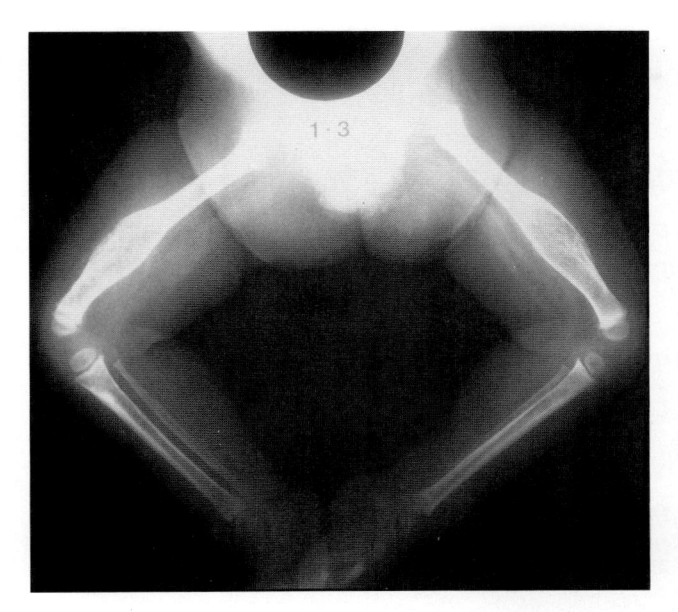

Fig. 58-3. The child in figure 2 at 1-year, 3 months of age with complete remodeling of the fractures. However, the knee contractures remain unchanged.

dren exhibiting reflex or spastic motor activity at the fracture site.

Epiphyseal injuries frequently demonstrate bizarre radiographic skeletal changes simulating infectious, metabolic, and neoplastic conditions and require special consideration.[3,13] Because of the delayed healing required for these injuries, prolonged immobilization of these fractures is required, and there is risk of Charcot arthropathy and premature growth arrest.[4] In contrast to the physeal injury of the distal femur and tibial epiphyses commonly encountered in children who are ambulatory, coxa vara, progressive femoral epiphyseolysis, and spontaneous femoral neck fracture can occur in children with thoracic or high lumbar levels of paraplegia (Fig. 58-4).

MECHANISM OF INJURY

Metaphyseal and diaphyseal fractures are commonly associated with cast immobilization[11] and are frequently recognized during the rehabilitation phase following reconstructive surgery.[6,7] Disuse osteopenia and joint stiffness with cast immobilization of paretic limbs too often lead to fracture with resultant prolonged rehabilitation. Following casting for one fracture, subsequent serial fractures of other long bones in association with abundant callus formation has been observed[11,20] (Fig. 58-5). The abundant proliferation of callus about multiple fracture sites is comparable to the radiologic changes seen in scurvy. This led McKibbin and coworkers[21] to suggest that a deficiency in ascorbic acid contributed to these fractured diaphyses in children with spina bifida. A subsequent study by Repasky and coworkers[22] demonstrated no differences in ascorbic acid uptake between spinal bifida children with and without fractures.

James[8] suggested that children with flail and insensate limbs sustain fractures due to inattention to their lower extremities during transfer activities. He suggested that epiphyseal displacement about the knee might be related to the insertion of the hamstring tendons and the origins of the gastrocnemius muscles about the knee joint. It is likely that shear forces are exerted at the distal femoral and proximal tibial physes in children with residual contractures when weightbearing in orthoses, especially in the presence of spasticity of reflex muscle activity in muscles crossing the knee joint (Fig. 58-6).

Epiphyseolysis was first described by Gyepes and colleagues[19] as irregularly widened metaphyses with widening of the epiphyseal plate accompanied by subperiosteal new bone formation. Impaired sensation was the most important factor contributing to these radiographic changes, which were not seen in a control group of children with paralysis due to poliomyelitis. Repetitive microtrauma without adequate immobilization delays the resorption of hematoma and disturbs normal ossification with a resultant increase in the zone of hypertrophied cartilage cells, which produces the widened physis commonly seen on radiographs.[4] Continued disruption of the normal healing process is accompanied by periosteal reaction and often abundant callus formation at the fracture site. Epiphyseal injury has been estimated to occur between 2 percent[4] and 9 percent[11] of children with spina bifida. However, due to the lack of acute symptoms, the exact prevalence of epiphyseal injury in this group of children is not known.

Proximal femoral epiphyseolysis and spontaneous separation of the upper femoral epiphysis is unusual, since it is most commonly observed in children with thoracic and high lumbar levels of paralysis. Weisl[23] speculated that this injury is caused by abnormal shear forces generated across the femoral neck during gait, whereas Shafer and Dias[18] speculated that it may be caused by repetitive stretching exercises to correct hip flexion and abduction contractures commonly seen in children with this level of paralysis (Fig. 58-7). Trueta's description[24] of the protective effect of the marrow cavities of the epiphysis upon the epiphyseal vessels in the developing femoral neck suggests that repetitive com-

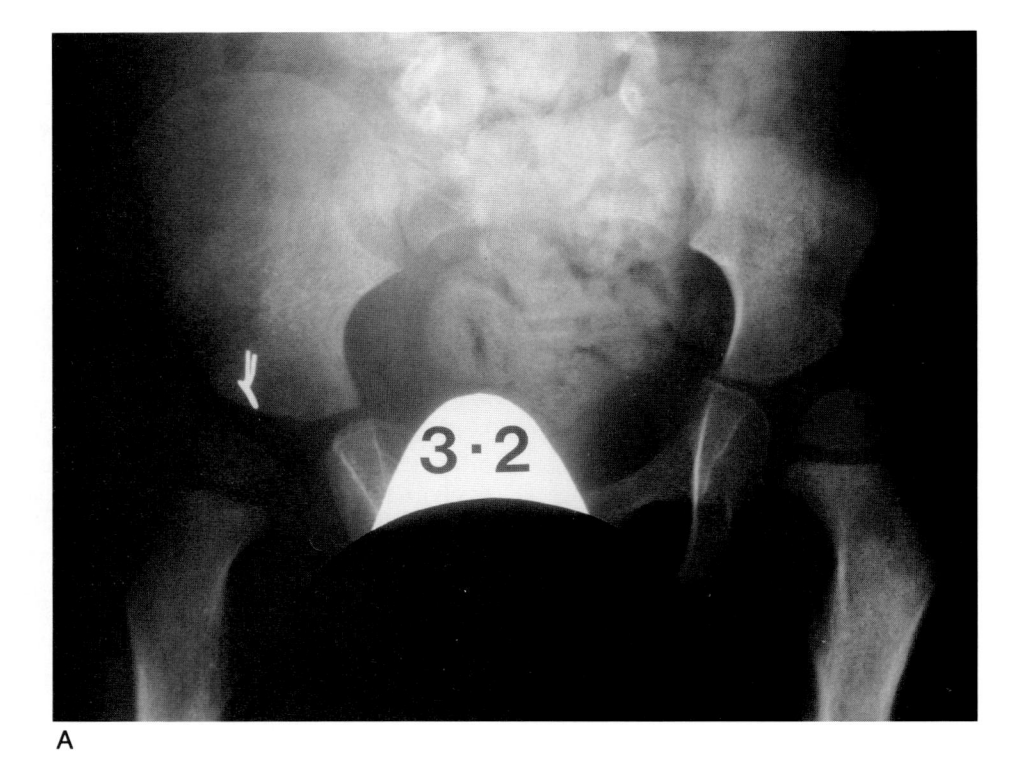

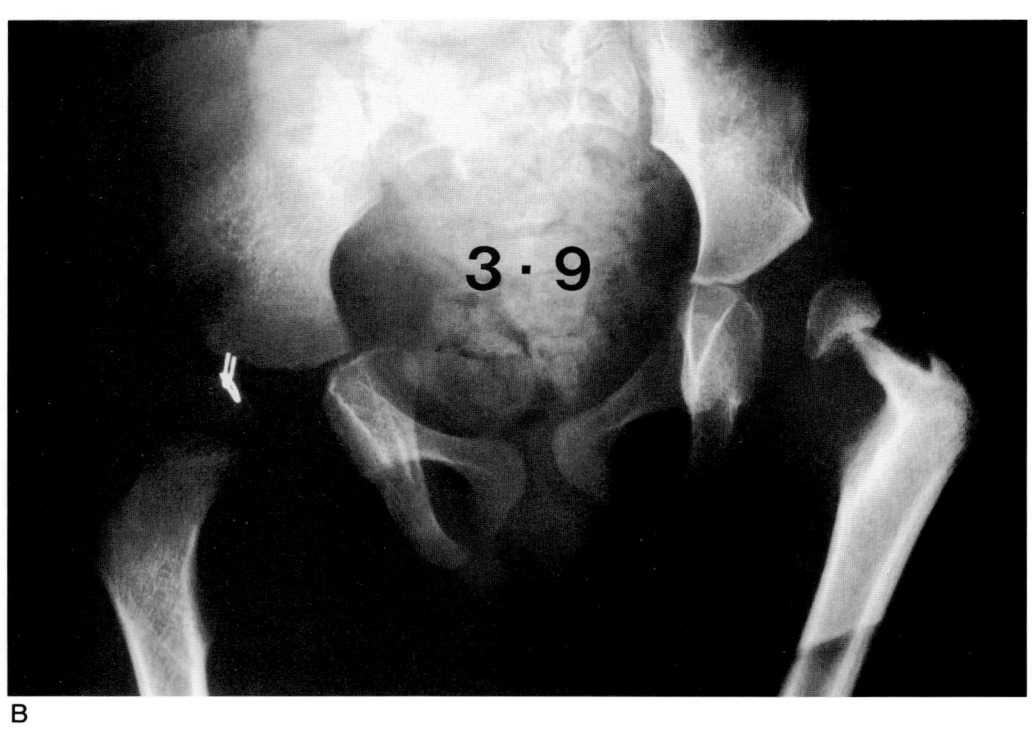

Fig. 58-4. (A) A 3-year, 2-month-old boy with a thoracic level 2 months following bilateral release of hip-flexion-abduction contractures with the vascular clips indicating the degree of proximal retraction of the transected psoas tendon of the right hip. (B) Seven months later, spontaneous lysis of the femoral neck of the left hip has occurred. *(Figure continues.)*

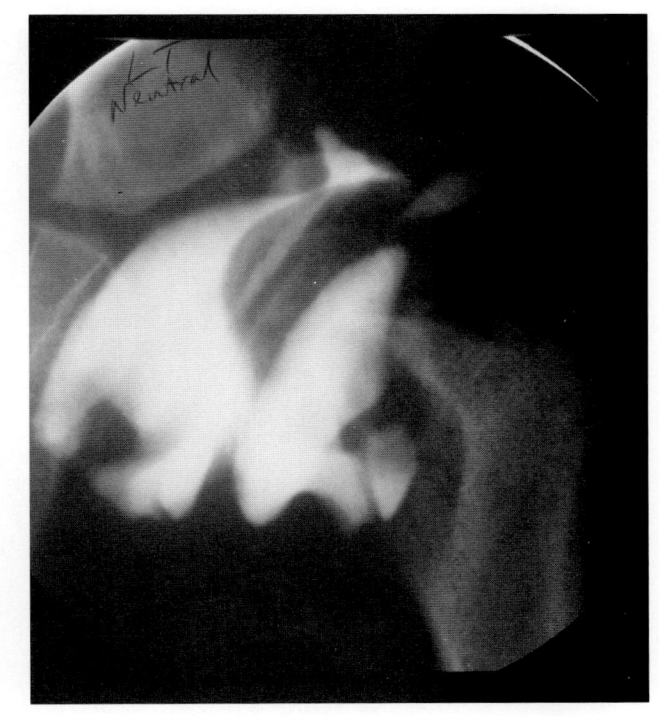

Fig. 58-4 *(Continued).* **(C)** Arthrogram reveals resorption of the cartilaginous neck with deossification at the periphery. **(D)** Four years later, progressive coxa vara has developed; however, the child remains ambulatory with a reciprocal gait orthosis with preservation of sagittal plane mobility of the left hip.

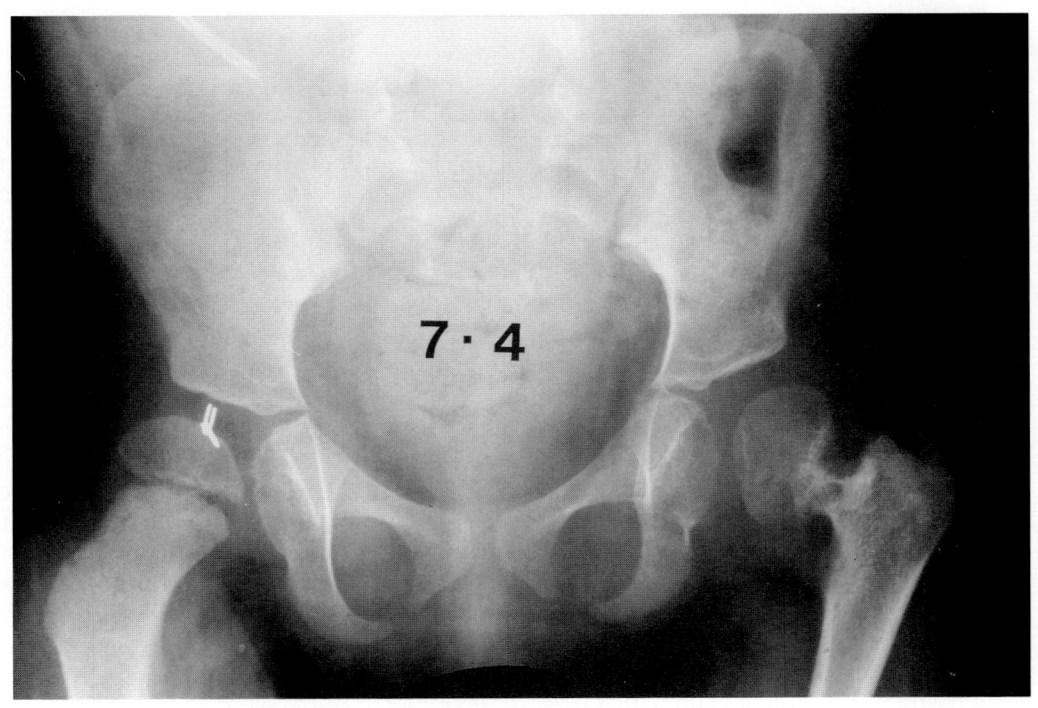

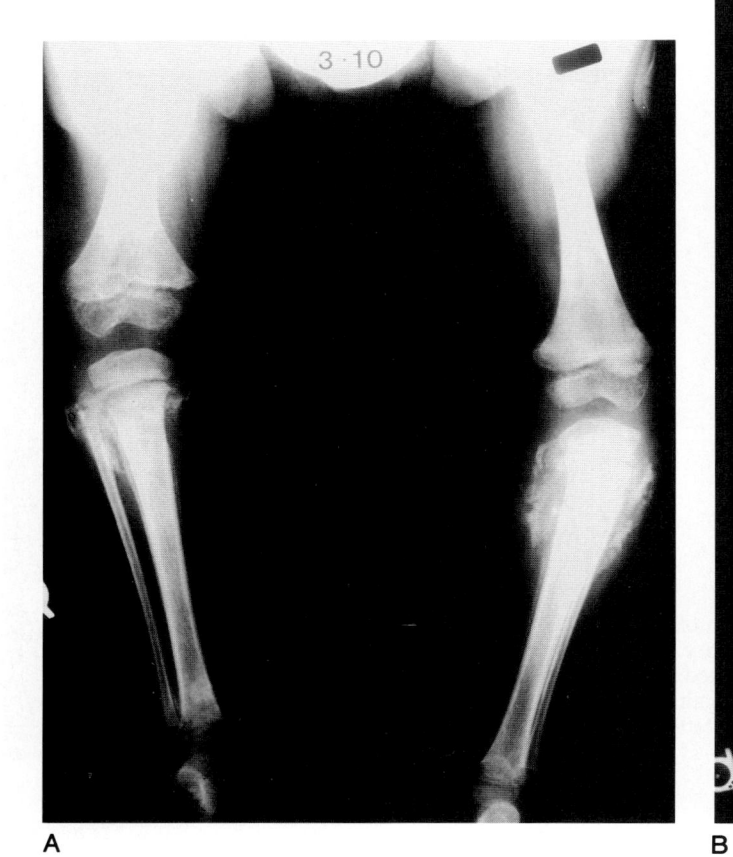

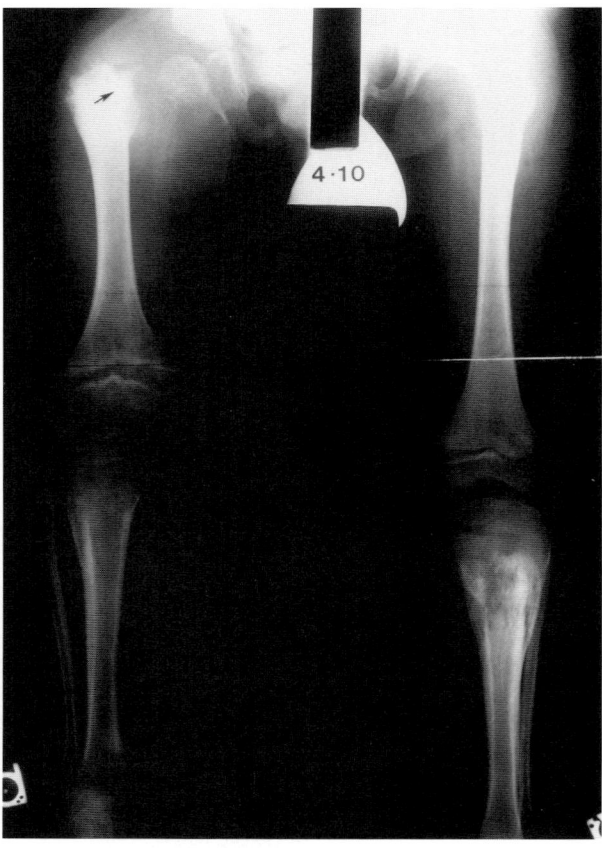

Fig. 58-5. (A) A 3-year, 10-month-old boy, L1 level, sustained fractures of both distal femoral and proximal tibial epiphyses following casting after soft tissue contracture releases of the hips and knees. (B) One year later, the fractures about the left knee and the right tibia have healed; however, the right distal femoral physis remains widened and he has sustained spontaneous epiphyseolysis of the right femoral neck. Limb length inequality was compensated for by a lift and he remained a household walker with a hip-knee-ankle-foot orthosis.

pressive and torque forces across the hip joint described above may lead to epiphyseolysis or femoral neck fracture with microfracture of the zone of provisional ossification from repetitive manipulation of the hip.

PHYSICAL EXAMINATION

The typical child presents several days following injury with unexplained painless swelling of the affected limb with redness of the overlying skin and local warmth. A common feature of a neuropathic fracture is the presence of a low-grade fever. In the absence of a urinary tract infection, a child with a fever of unknown etiology should be suspected to have sustained an occult fracture.[25] A low-grade leukocytosis and minimal elevation of the erythrocyte sedimentation rate is frequently observed.[13] If no abnormalities are evident on radiographic examination, stress views may reveal a classic Salter-Harris type I epiphyseal separation. Normally, healing is rapid, and early periosteal reaction and callus formation are evident within 7 to 10 days after injury.[25]

The differential diagnosis of neuropathic fracture in a child who presents only with fever must exclude occult infection of a central nervous system shunt, urosepsis, or pharyngitis or otitis. Swelling of a paretic lower extremity is common with cellulitis accompanying neurotrophic skin lesions. Deep vein thrombosis is uncommon in the child but must be considered in the older adolescent. Following recent skeletal injury with systemic signs of fever and mild leukocytosis, the radiograph should distinguish fracture from osteomyelitis.

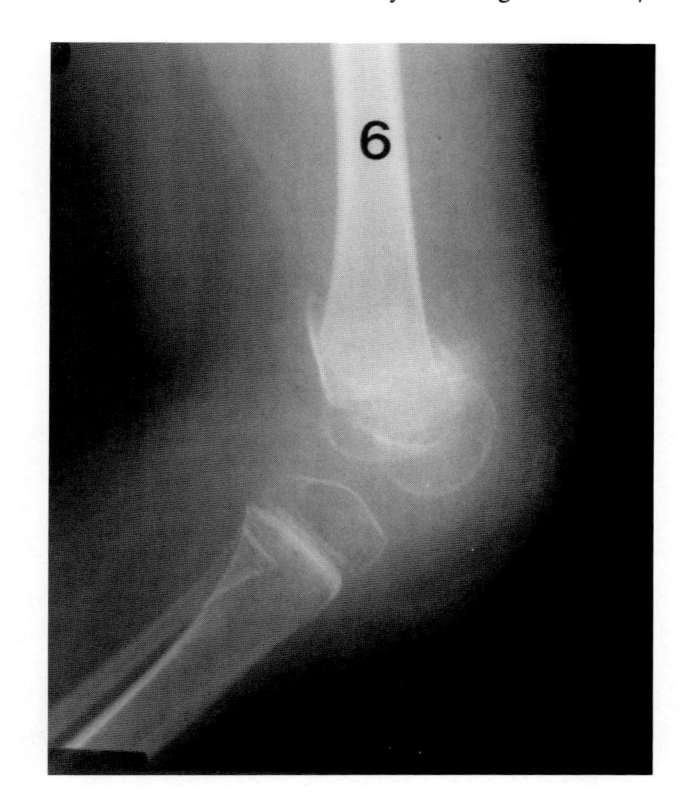

Fig. 58-6. A 6-year-old girl with a T12 level, with spastic hamstring function sustained this distal femoral metaphyseal fracture using a reciprocal gait orthosis. The fracture healed uneventfully but flexion contracture of the knee persisted.

A recent report by Anschuetz and associates[26] described "severe systemic dysfunction" in three children with thoracic paraplegia occurring after spica cast removal following spinal arthrodesis. Fever, tachycardia, tachypnea, and a drop in hematocrit level was noted, and radiographs revealed bilateral femoral fractures in all three cases. Prompt improvement in vital signs was noted in all cases following administration of intravenous fluids and application of posterior splints incorporating the lower trunk and extremities. Fat embolism syndrome was considered to be a possible contributing factor to this potentially life-threatening condition.

Long-standing epiphyseal injury, however, may present an alarming picture of bone resorption with a proliferative callus and periosteal reaction simulating scurvy, rickets, osteomyelitis, or malignancy.[4] Earlier reports noted the similarity of such fractures to other associated disorders including tabes dorsalis, congenital insensitivity to pain, and syringomyelia.[1] Charcot arthropathy is a recognized complication of myelomeningocele, but it is infrequent under 15 years of age (Fig. 58-8). Serial radiographs normally reveal progressive healing with remodeling of the bone at the fracture site and progressive resorption of the periosteal reaction. Epiphyseal lesions characteristically require a longer period of healing recognizable by the physis resuming its normal width. Delay in the normal healing process should alert the clinician to further diagnostic studies to rule out an occult septic process. Figure 58-9 illustrates a case in which there was delayed healing of a supracondylar fracture in a young girl who had sustained a supracondylar fracture of the femur 1 year following spinal fusion and motor rhizotomy for a thoracic level paraplegia with scoliosis. Osteomyelitis developed in the insensate extremity without systemic symptoms and was detected by abnormal bone scan.

TREATMENT INDICATIONS

In 1963, Eichenholtz[15] admonished, "encircling plaster casts are hazardous at best and skin traction is unacceptable" in the treatment of long-bone fractures in paraplegic patients. Freehafer and Mast[16] emphasized that, due to the rapid healing of fractures in cases of spinal cord injury, pillow splints in conjunction with well-padded casts provide the best treatment for fracture union with minimal complications in contrast to the many complications noted, following attempted open

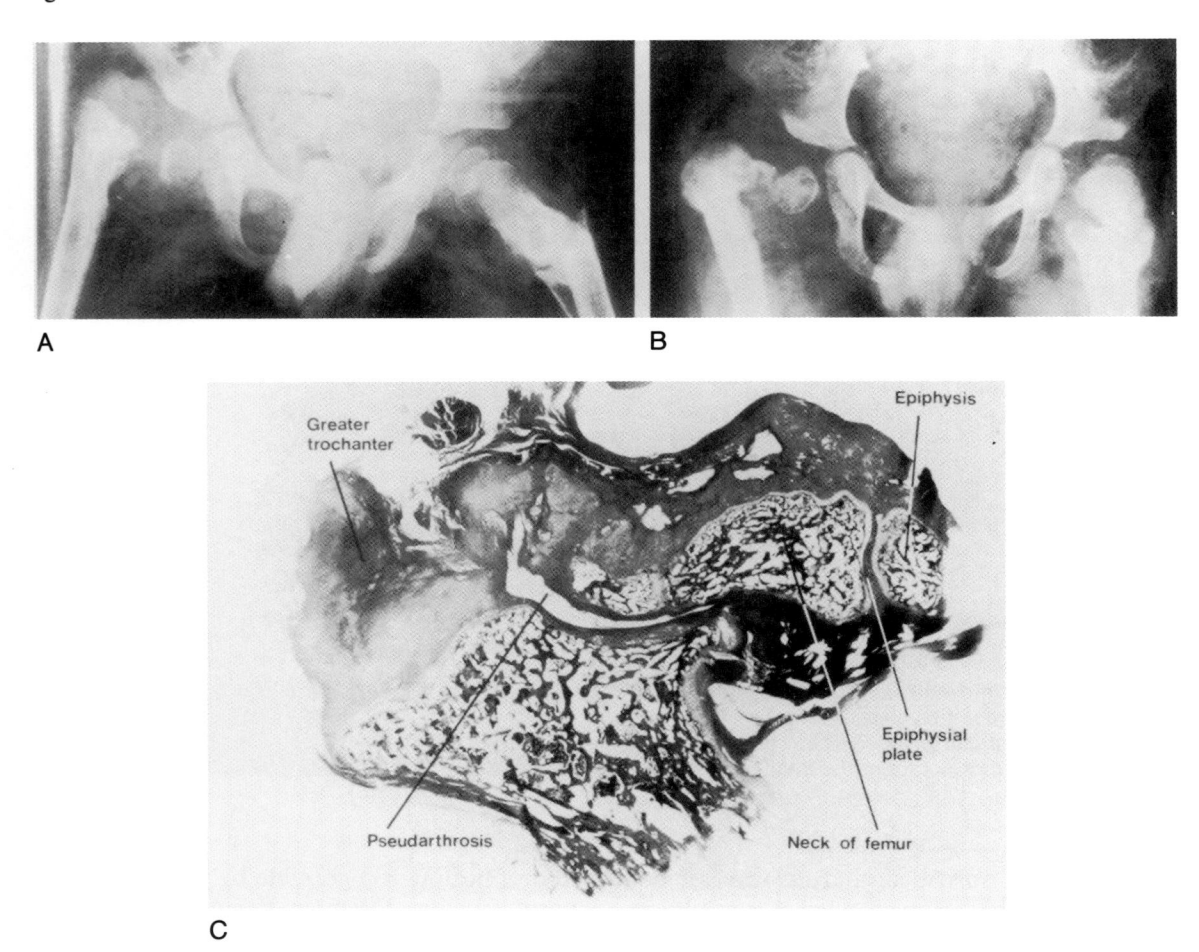

Fig. 58-7. (A) Initial radiograph showing a typical spontaneous epiphyseal lesion on the right side and a spontaneous fracture on the left side. (B) The spontaneous epiphyseal lesion on the right is healing with coxa vara and the fracture on the left is uniting in coxa valga. (C) Histologic section of the upper end of the right femur; the capital epiphysis lies at one edge of the section and the cartilaginous greater trochanter at the other. The epiphyseal plate and the pseudarthrosis at the base of the neck are clearly visible. (Histology by courtesy of Z. Rális.) (From Weisl,[23] with permission.)

reduction and internal fixation of long-bone fractures in patients with spinal cord injury. Subsequent reports[6,11,18] have confirmed the wisdom of conservative individualized treatment with temporary bulky soft dressings of sheet wadding followed by rapid transfer to orthoses, which provide the most practical method of treating most fractures in children with myelodysplasia (Fig. 58-10).

Rapid return to weightbearing to avoid the progressive deossification of disuse is a widely held precept in fracture management. Few controlled studies have been performed in the pediatric paraplegic population. A matched series of 72 children with high-level paraplegia in which half were treated by progressive ambulation with bracing and the other half were provided wheelchairs, revealed that the group who walked early had a average of 50 percent fewer fractures than the wheelchair group.[27] Rosenstein and coworkers[28] studied the effect of ambulation on bone density as measured by single photon absorptiometry. Bone density was most significantly related to the ambulatory status and the neurologic level. There was a suggestion that muscle activity was the more important factor, although weight-bearing stress did increase bone density in children lacking motor control through the lower extremities.

Physeal injury has not only a more guarded prognosis but requires prolonged immobilization in rigid well-padded casts for a minimum of 8 to 12 weeks.[13] In addi-

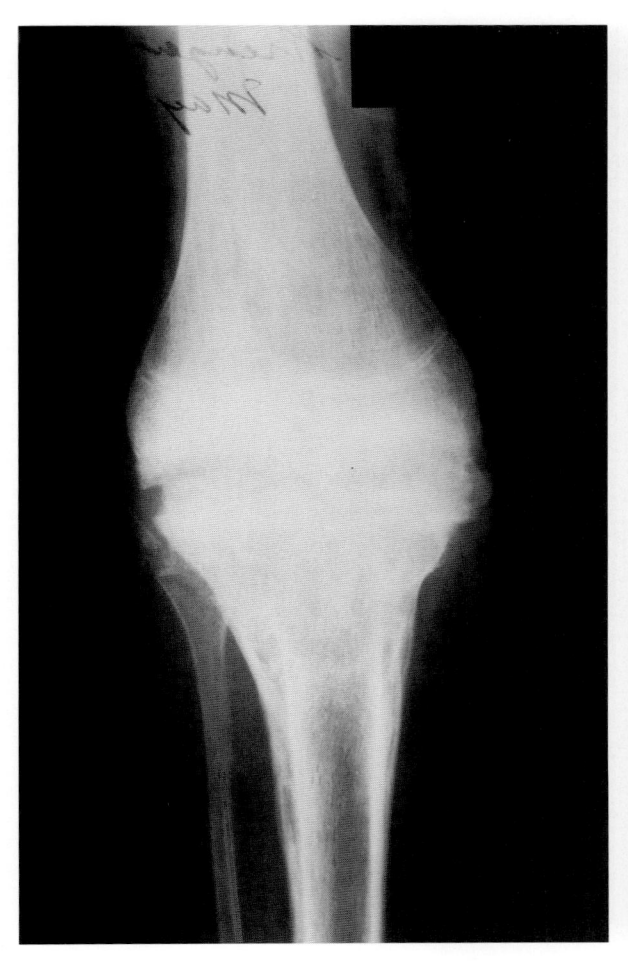

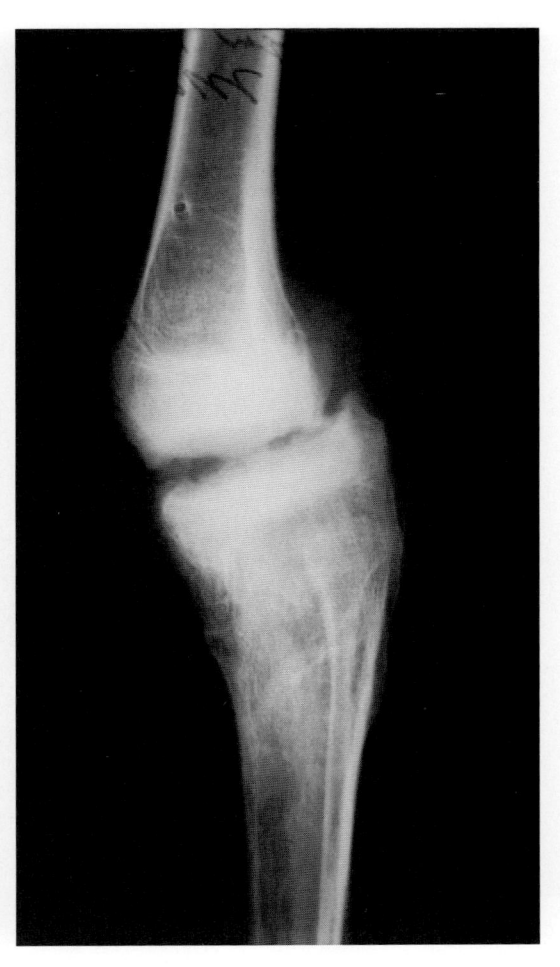

Fig. 58-8. A 14-year-old female with an L3 level paralysis who developed Charcot arthropathy of the right knee while ambulatory with a knee-ankle-foot orthosis (KAFO). (Courtesy of Dr. R. Mervyn Letts.)

tion to casting, others recommend the avoidance of weightbearing until there is both clinical and radiologic evidence of healing.[4,12]

My preferred method of treating neuropathic fractures is conservative, employing soft well-padded circumferential bulky webril dressings changed every 10 to 14 days to inspect skin integrity. Once callus is visible and the fracture is stable, the child is transferred to an appropriate orthosis to resume protected weightbearing or transfers at the preinjury level of activity. Diaphyseal fractures in thoracic level paraplegic children are allowed to override, since length discrepancy can easily be corrected by an appropriate lift. Rarely, a diaphyseal fracture in an older ambulatory patient is amenable to intermedullary fixation, but this technique should be reserved for patients with lower levels of paralysis with ambulatory potential.

Physeal injuries should be rigidly immobilized in well-padded casts and, if detected early, weightbearing is encouraged (Fig. 58-11). For those injuries detected late with widened and periosteal reaction, immobilization without weightbearing is preferred until healing is judged adequate by restoration of a normal physeal thickness.

The treatment of epiphyseolysis or femoral neck fracture in the child with a thoracic level paraplegia remains controversial. Reduction and pinning is recommended by Pfeil and colleagues,[10] but other authors recommend conservative treatment, since the lesion is most frequently encountered in children with thoracic level paralysis with only nonfunctional walking potential.[18,23,29] I agrees with these authors that this lesion does not impede the child's mobility. Any shortening can be corrected by a lift and any surgical intervention that

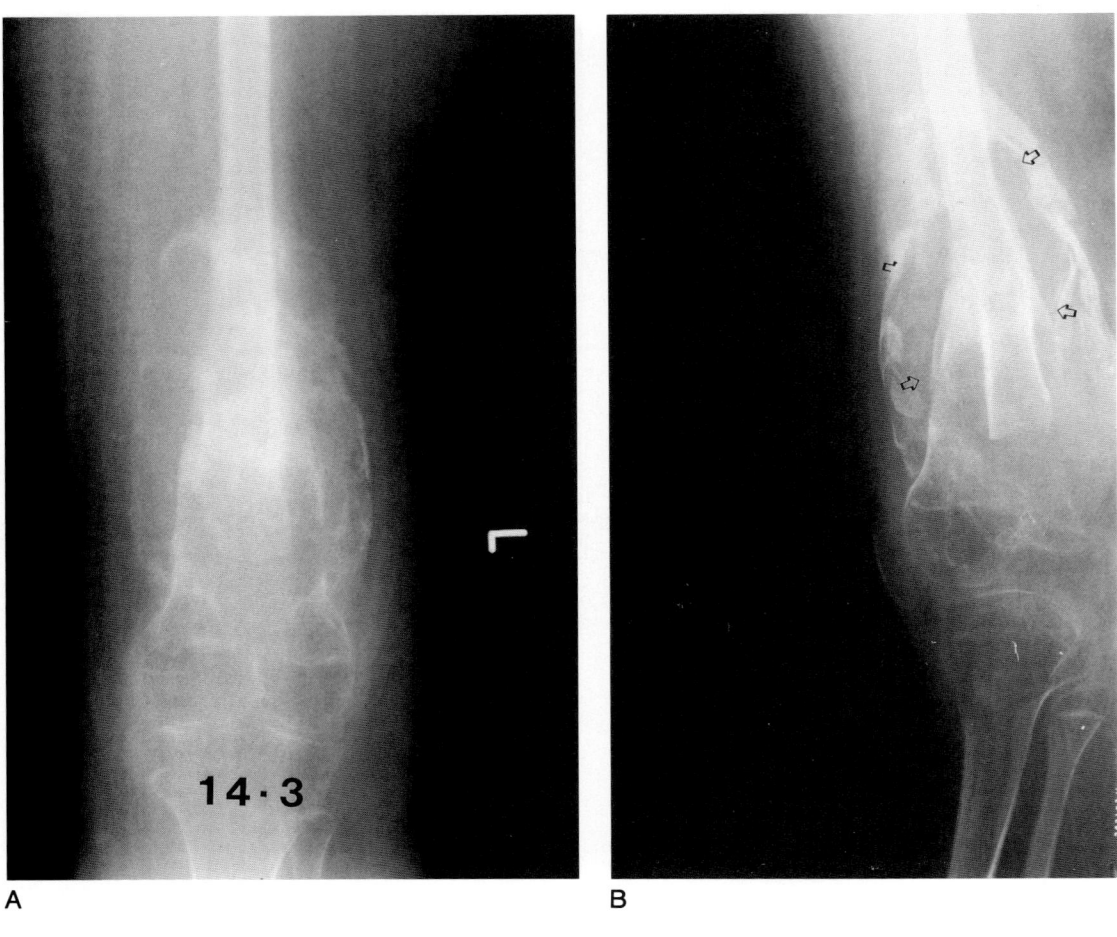

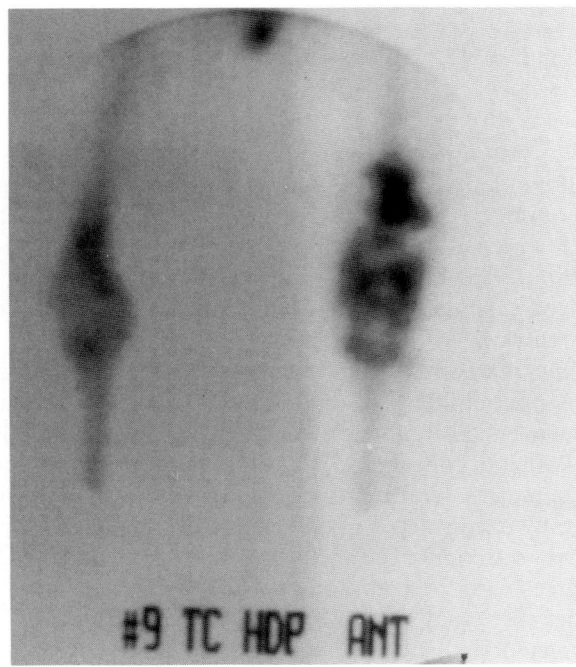

Fig. 58-9. (A) 14-year, 3-month-old girl with a T12 paraplegia 2 months following supracondylar fracture. She developed a pressure sore behind the heel in spite of a soft bulky dressing splint for this fracture. (B) At 1 month later. Note the persistent periosteal reactive bone in the absence of remodeling at the fracture site. The patient was entirely asymptomatic. (C) Bone scan shows intense uptake with a central "cold spot," representing the center of an abscess, which cultured β-hemolytic streptococci. *(Figure continues.)*

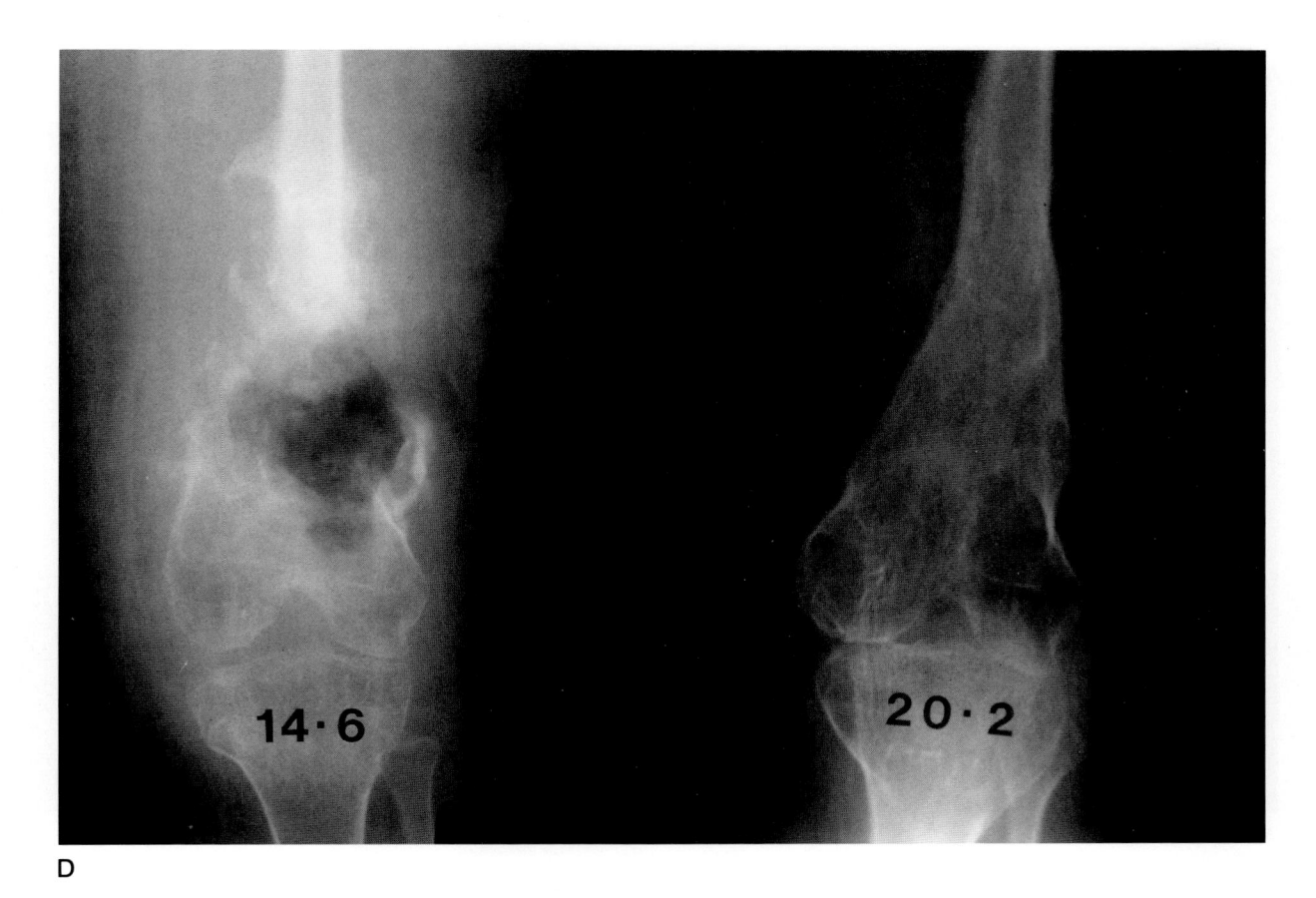

Fig. 58-9 *(Continued).* **(D)** Anteroposterior radiograph immediately following débridement *(left)* and remodeling 6 years following fracture *(right).*

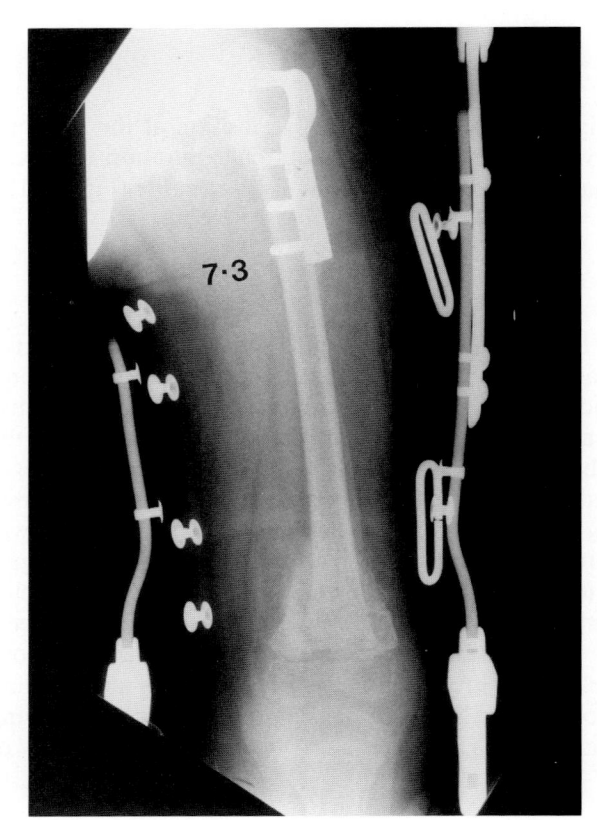

Fig. 58-10. A 7-year, 3-month-old boy with an L4 level 2 months following bilateral derotational intertrochanteric osteotomies sustained a supracondylar femoral fracture which was treated successfully with his hip-knee-ankle-foot orthosis without skin breakdown.

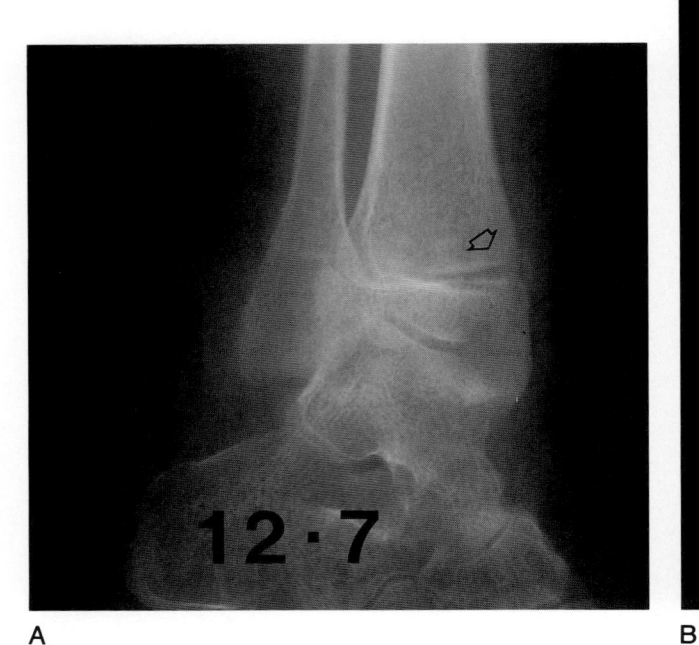

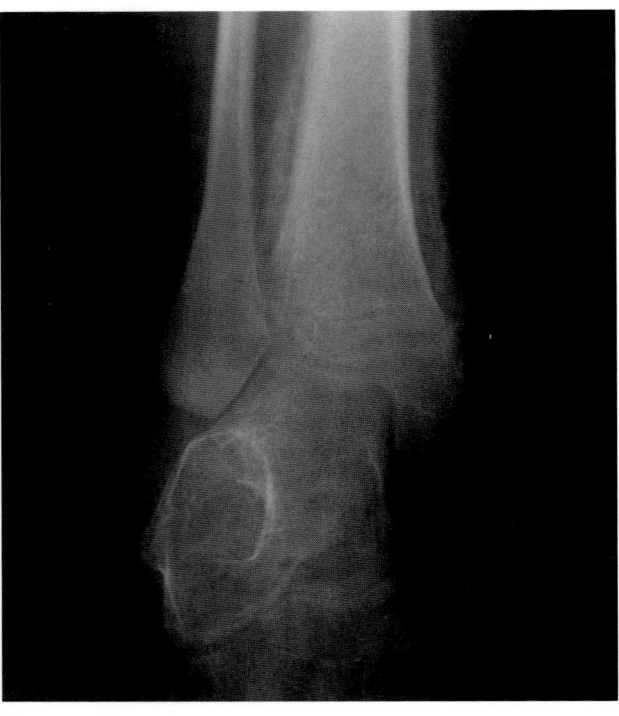

Fig. 58-11. (A) A 12-year, 7-month-old boy with an L5 level with early epiphyseolysis of the distal tibial epiphysis. His only symptom was painless swelling and slight warmth while fully ambulatory with ankle-foot orthoses. (B) One month later, the physis has restored to normal width, but abundant periosteal new bone is evident following nonweightbearing in a short-leg, well-padded, fiberglass cast.

might result in loss of passive motion at the hip joint would prove a serious functional limitation to wheelchair use and self-transfer skills in later life (Fig. 58-12).

COMPLICATIONS

The most common complications encountered in the management of these fractures are skin pressure sores and joint stiffness. Even with bulky soft splints, the child is at risk for pressure ulceration, particularly over the tuberosity of the os calcis. Frequent positional changes and prone lying for sleep combined with frequent dressing changes are recommended to avoid skin breakdown. Joint stiffness is common at the knee and may be aggravated in patients with reflexive motor activity. Spica casts are to be avoided whenever possible and, if necessary, should be removed early to allow the child controlled mobility in an appropriate orthosis until healing is complete. One study suggested that stiffness following fractures about the knee was present in the majority of patients but uniformly resolved within 3 years of injury.[30] However, the majority of the patients examined were ambulatory with a mean age of 5.6 years. In my experience, supracondylar femoral fractures accompanied by exuberant callus formation may result in permanent loss of motion, especially in children with thoracic level lesions.

The similarity of unrecognized epiphyseal injuries to Charcot arthropathy has been noted by many authors since Golding's description[2,9,17] in 1960. Neurotrophic degeneration, although uncommon, does occur at the hip, knee, ankle, and subtalar joints. Painless effusion of a joint should be thoroughly examined with appropriate radiographs. Rarely, a fresh injury with a large osteochondral fragment can be operatively repaired by replacing the fracture fragment in its bed in the epiphysis. Otherwise, intra-articular loose bodies should be removed and the joints protected by a limited motion orthosis to prevent coronal and transverse plane deforming forces (Fig. 58-13). Similarly, caution should be exercised in the arthrodesis of weight-bearing joints of

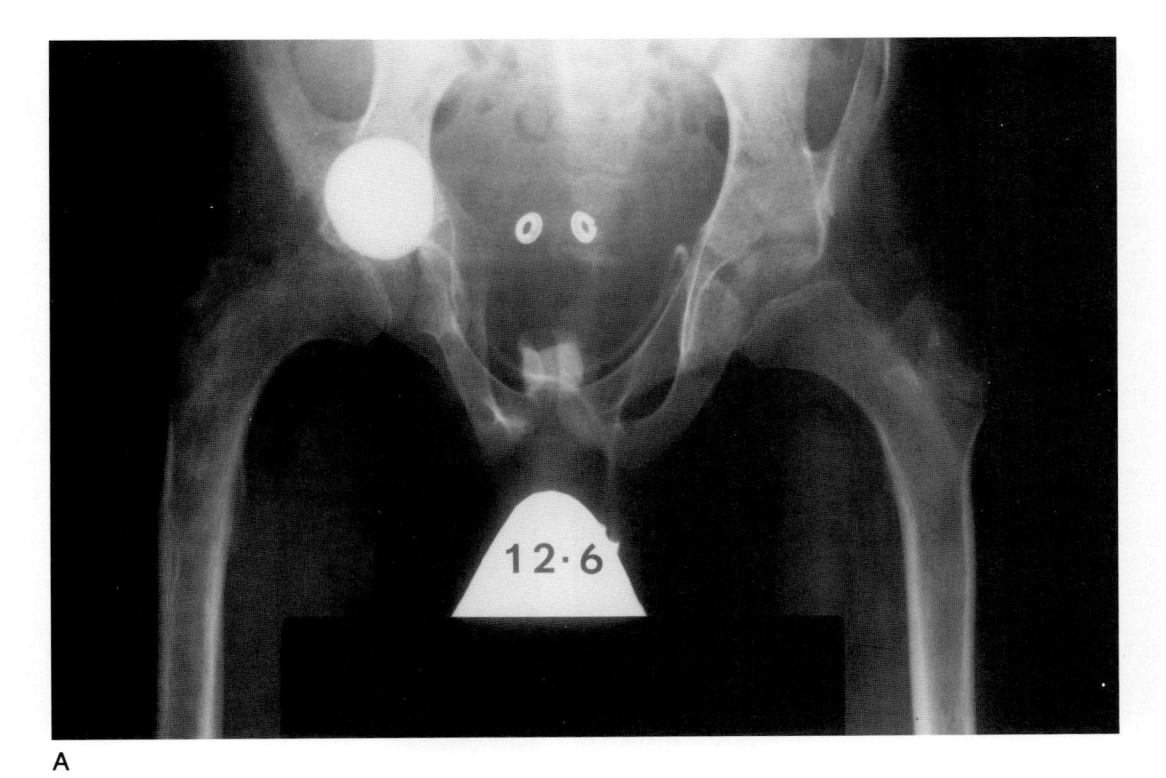

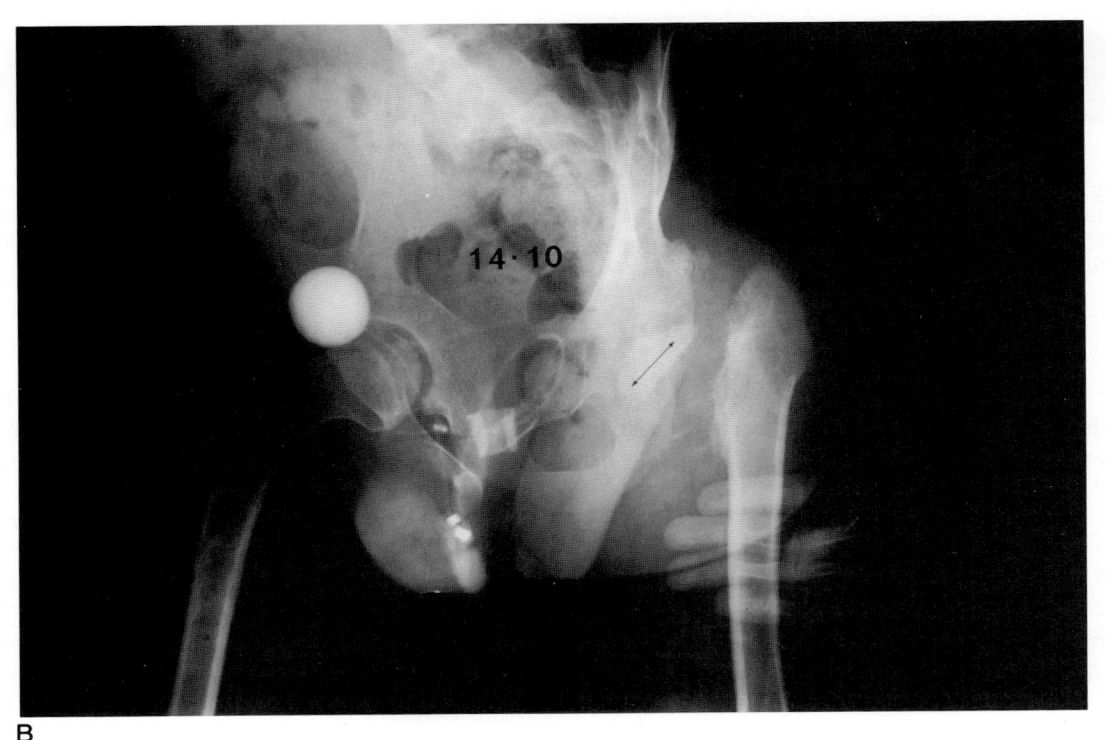

Fig. 58-12. (A) A 12-year, 6-month-old boy, L3, ambulatory 5 years following bilateral iliopsoas Sharrard transfers. (B) Two years later, he has sustained a spontaneous epiphyseal separation on the left, which is entirely asymptomatic.

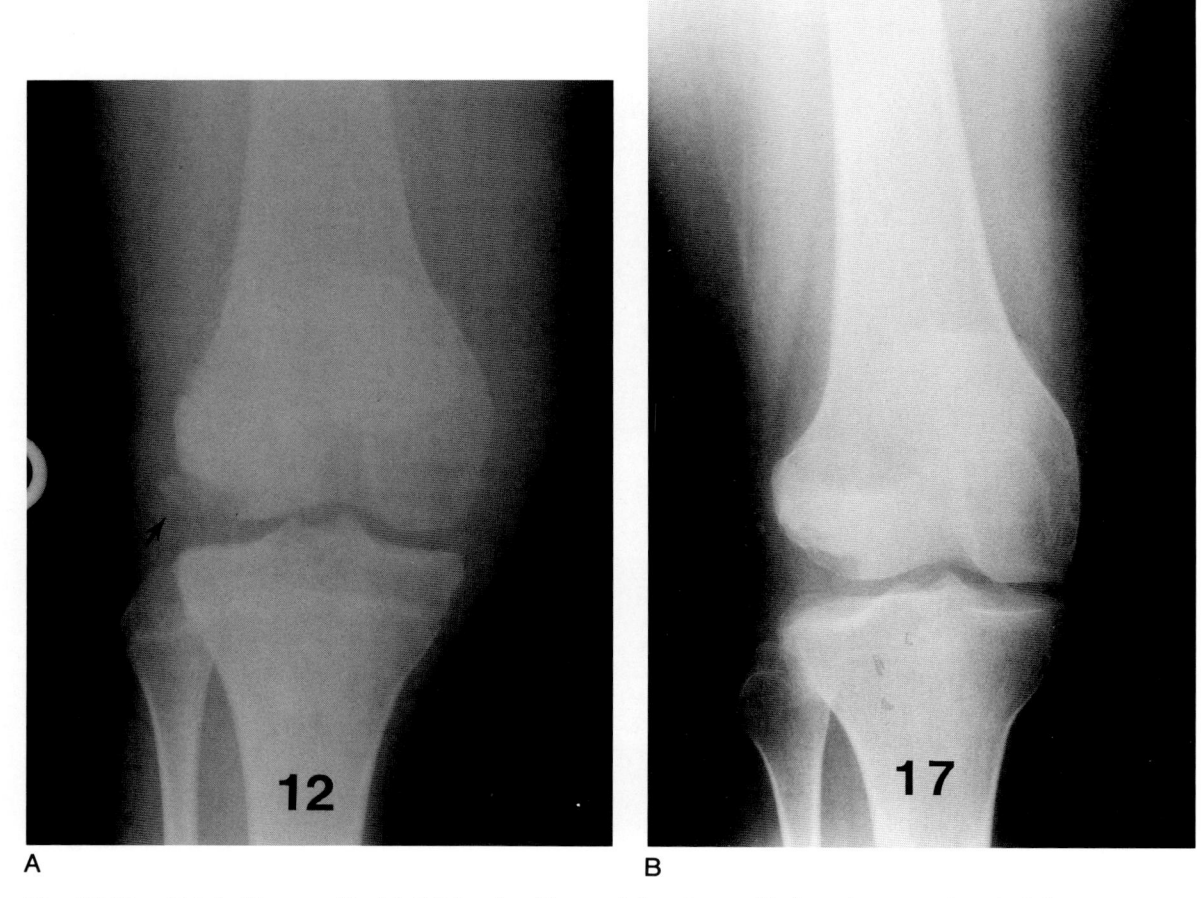

Fig. 58-13. (A) A 12-year-old girl, L5 level, with a painless knee effusion. An osteochondral fracture was removed athroscopically. She was placed in a knee-ankle-foot orthosis with full flexion-extension. (B) Five years later, she remains fully ambulatory with her brace, there has been no further loss of cartilage space, and her effusion has subsided.

the lower extremities since additional force will thereby be transmitted to the next mobile segment with increasing stress placed upon the articular joint surfaces (Fig. 58-14).

SUMMARY

Fractures are common in children with myelomeningocele and are directly related to the level of neurologic involvement. To reduce the previously reported high prevalence of fractures following reconstructive surgery, combined operations should be performed simultaneously by two teams, whenever possible, under one anesthetic, and postoperative immobilization should be kept to a minimum. Preoperative orthotic fabrication should be completed whenever possible to allow rapid removal of spica casts and transfer of the patient to a standing orthosis.

Fever of unknown etiology is a hallmark of unsuspected fracture in the absence of urinary tract infection. Ambulatory children are at risk for epiphyseal injury at the knee and ankle, which often goes undetected. A high index of suspicion and appropriate radiographic examination will allow early detection of neurotrophic fractures. The indications for surgical intervention are limited and most fractures respond well to conservative treatment with soft bulky dressings or well-padded casts with rapid return to orthotic wear to avoid pressure sore formation.

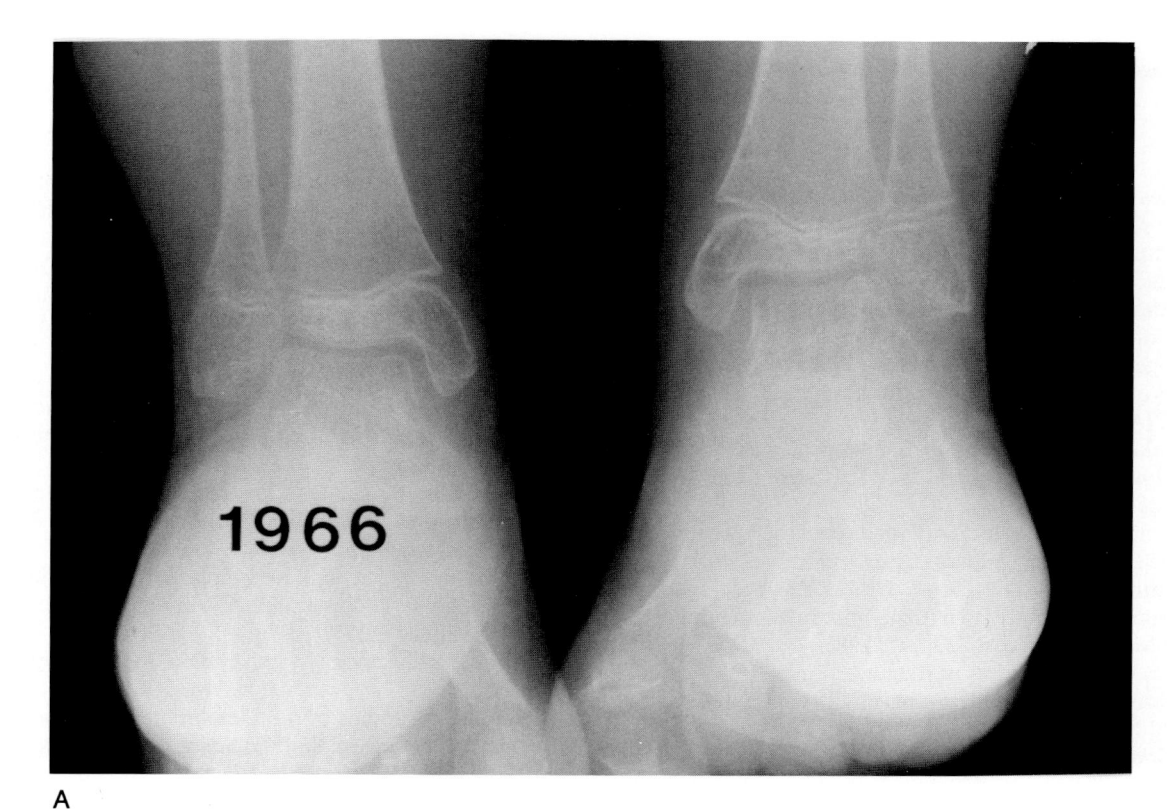

Fig. 58-14. **(A)** A 10-year-old girl 3 years following bilateral subtalar arthrodeses for hind-foot valgus deformity. **(B)** The patient in 1982 at age 26 has developed bilateral Charcot arthropathy with collapse of the dome of the talus, more advanced in the right ankle. She notes chronic, painless swelling, which is not relieved by an ankle-foot orthosis.

REFERENCES

1. Gillies CL, Hartung W: Fracture of the tibia in spina bifida vera: report of two cases. Radiology 31:621, 1938
2. Golding C: Museum Pages. III. Spina bifida and epiphysial displacement. J Bone Joint Surg [Br] 42:387, 1960
3. Soutter FE: Spina bifida and epiphysial displacement: report of two cases. J Bone Joint Surg [Br] 44:106, 1962
4. Wenger DR, Jeffcoat BT, Herring JA: The guarded prognosis of physeal injury in paraplegic children. J Bone Joint Surg [Am] 62:241, 1980
5. Guthkelch AN: Aspects of the surgical management of myelomeningocele: a review. Dev Med Child Neurol 28:525, 1986
6. Drennan JC, Freehafer AA: Fractures of the lower extremities in paraplegic children. Clin Orthop 77:211, 1971
7. Drummond DS, Moreau M, Cruess RL: Post-operative neuropathic fractures in patients with myelomeningocele. Dev Med Child Neurol 23:147, 1981
8. James CCM: Fractures of the lower limbs in spina bifida cystica: a survey of 44 fractures in 122 children. Dev Med Child Neurol, suppl 22:88, 1970
9. Korhonen BJ: Fractures in myelodysplasia. Clin Orthop 79:145, 1971
10. Pfeil J, Fromm B, Carstens C, Cotta H: Frakturen und Epiphysenverletzungen bei Kindern mit Myelomeningocele. Z Orthop 128:551, 1990
11. Lock TR, Aronson DD: Fractures in patients who have myelomeningocele. J Bone Joint Surg [Am] 71:1153, 1989
12. Evardsen P: Physeo-epiphyseal injuries of lower extremities in myelomeningocele. Acta Orthop Scand 43:550, 1972
13. Kumar SJ, Cowell HR, Townsend P: Physeal, metaphyseal, and diaphyseal injuries of the lower extremities in children with myelomeningocele. J Pediatr Orthop 4:25, 1984
14. Boytim MJ, Davidson RS, Charney E, Melchionni JB: Neonatal fractures in myelomeningocele patients. J Pediatr Orthop 11:28, 1991
15. Eichenholtz SN: Management of long-bone fractures in paraplegic patients. J Bone Joint Surg [Am] 45:299, 1963
16. Freehafer AA, Mast WA: Lower extremity fractures in patients with spinal-cord injury. J Bone Joint Surg [Am] 47:683, 1965
17. Menelaus M: The Orthopaedic Management of Spinal Bifida Cystica. 2nd Ed. p. 61. Churchill Livingstone, Edinburgh, 1980
18. Schafer MF, Dias LS: Myelomeningocele: Orthopaedic Treatment. p. 214. Williams & Wilkins, Baltimore, 1983
19. Gyepes MT, Newbern DH, Neuhauser EBD: Metaphyseal and physeal injuries in children with spina bifida and meningomyeloceles. AJR 95:168, 1965
20. Quilis AN: Fractures in children with myelomeningocele: report of 15 cases and a review of the literature. Acta Orthop Scand 45:883, 1974
21. McKibbin B, Toseland PA, Duckworth T: Abnormalities in vitamin C metabolism in spina bifida. Dev Med Child Neurol, suppl 15:55, 1968
22. Repasky D, Richard K, Lindseth R: Ascorbic acid and fractures in children with myelomeningocele. J Am Dietetic Assoc 69:511, 1976
23. Weisl H: Coxa vara in spina bifida. J Bone Joint Surg [Br] 65:128, 1983
24. Trueta J: Studies of the Development and Decay of the Human Frame. p. 86. WB Saunders, Philadelphia, 1968
25. Townsend PF, Cowell HR, Steg NL: Lower extremity fractures simulating infection in myelomeningocele. Clin Orthop 144:255, 1979
26. Anschuetz RH, Freehafer AA, Shaffer JW, Dixon MS, Jr: Severe fracture complications in myelodysplasia. J Pediatr Orthop 4:22, 1984
27. Mazur JM, Shurtleff D, Menelaus M, Colliver J: Orthopaedic management of high-level spina bifida: early walking compared with early use of a wheelchair. J Bone Joint Surg [Am] 71:56, 1989
28. Rosenstein BD, Greene WB, Herrington RT, Blum AS: Bone density in myelomeningocele: the effects of ambulatory status and other factors. Dev Med Child Neurol 29:486, 1987
29. Parsch K: Origin and treatment of fractures in spina bifida. Eur J Pediatr Surg 1:298, 1991
30. Drabu KJ: Stiffness after fractures around the knee in spina bifida. J Bone Joint Surg [Br] 67:266, 1985

59

Fractures in the Osteogenesis Imperfecta Child

Walter P. Bobechko

> No knowledge can be more satisfactory to a man than that of its own frame, its parts, their functions and actions.
> —THOMAS JEFFERSON

DESCRIPTION AND SPECTRUM

Osteogenesis imperfecta, otherwise known as brittle bone disease or fragilitas ossium, is a rare inherited connective tissue disorder with varying degrees of severity,[1] depending on the type of molecular defect (Table 59-1). It is an uncommon condition, of which most pediatric orthopaedic surgeons will usually have limited experience in management unless they work in a major center. The entire spectrum of the disease is based on the ever-recurring fractures[2-5] (Fig. 59-1).

In North America the Osteogenesis Imperfecta Society, has been formed and virtually all of osteogenesis imperfecta patients with their families inevitably belong to it. These families work with those specialists who have special interest and experience in osteogenesis imperfecta, thus assisting in the improvement of the long-term ongoing complexities of children with this major ossification abnormality.

The Spectrum of the Disease Process

In the severe forms of osteogenesis imperfecta, infants may sustain a fracture of one of their extremity bones on sudden movement of an extremity or when diapers are changed. Sudden muscle contractions may also precipitate fracturing. At the other extreme of the spectrum is the teenager who, with moderate trauma, may sustain five or six fractures during adolescence.[6] In those situations the bones may exhibit a vague osteoporosis but have a normal medullary cavity and a cortex that appears near-normal. In these very mild cases the diagnosis is made by exclusion, as there is no specific biochemical abnormality, nor is there a specific histologic picture in the pathology of mild osteogenesis imperfecta. The children with the most severe type of osteogenesis imperfecta at birth will have bones that often look thick radiographically (Fig. 59-2). The reason for the thickness of the bones at birth is callus deposition secondary to multiple intrauterine fractures. However, the bones remain very fragile. In some instances, such children will not survive more than a few months because of the multiple recurrent fractures and the associated anaemia. One must appreciate that virtually all the bones are involved in this process.

It is still not clearly understood whether it is a failure of deposition of bone or an increased osteoclastic activity with resorption of the trabeculae. It is recognized, however, that there is a difference in the periodicity of the collagen components, which results in an abnormal calcium deposition. In Figure 59-3 the thinness of the tra-

1080 / Management of Pediatric Fractures

TABLE 59-1. Classification of Osteogenesis Imperfecta

Type	Inheritance	Bone Fragility
I	Autosomal dominant	Fractures after birth
II	Autosomal recessive	Intrautero fractures, usually lethal
III	Autosomal recessive	Fractures at birth Progressive deformity
IV	Autosomal dominant	Fractures common but less frequent

(Modified from Sillence,[1] with permission.)

beculae in a typical case of osteogenesis imperfecta is shown, and the cortex, in this case of the tibia, is virtually nonexistent. The ability to form callus and to produce healing of a fracture or osteotomy remains excellent and usually very rapid healing occurs but always with poor quality bone.

At times in osteogenesis imperfecta a hyperabundance of callus may even form (Fig. 59-4). The degree of hyperplastic callus can be so great that at times it resembles a huge tumor[7,8] (Fig. 59-5).

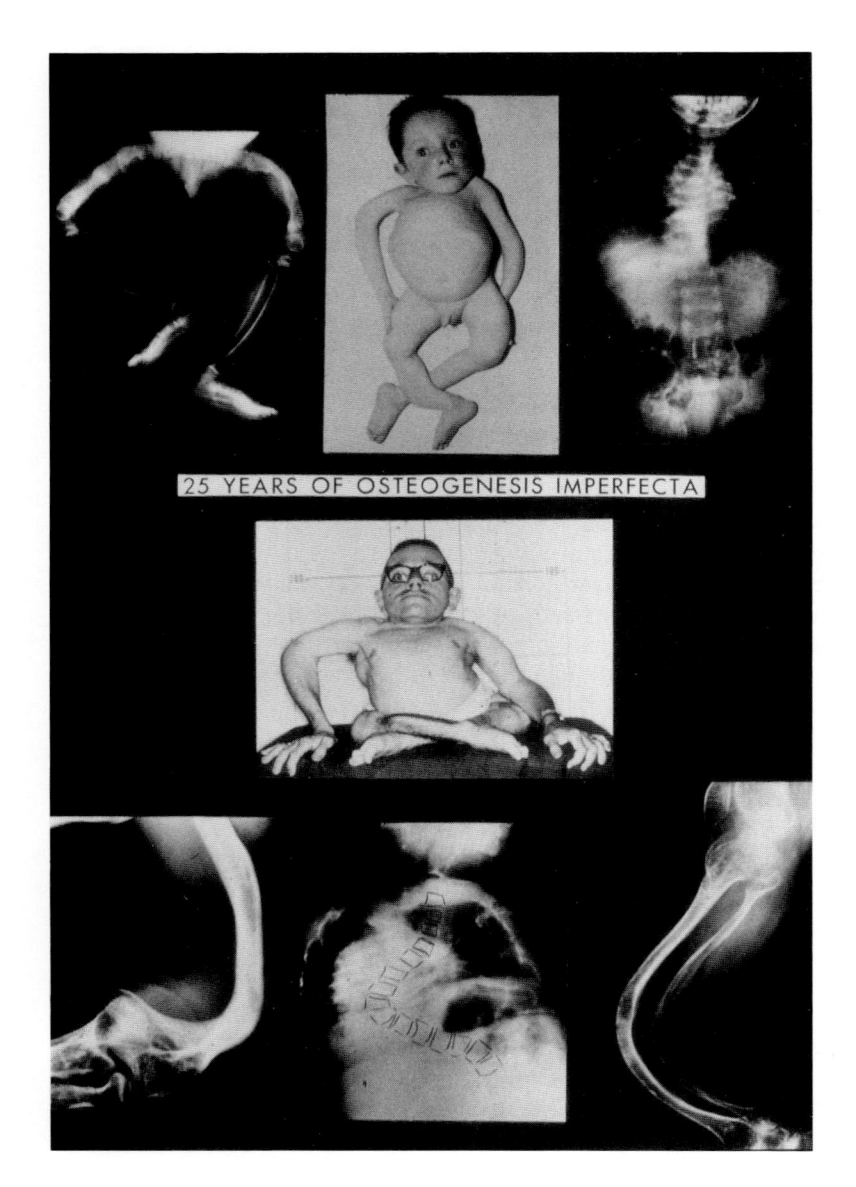

Fig. 59-1. The spectrum of untreated osteogenesis imperfecta from infancy to adulthood.

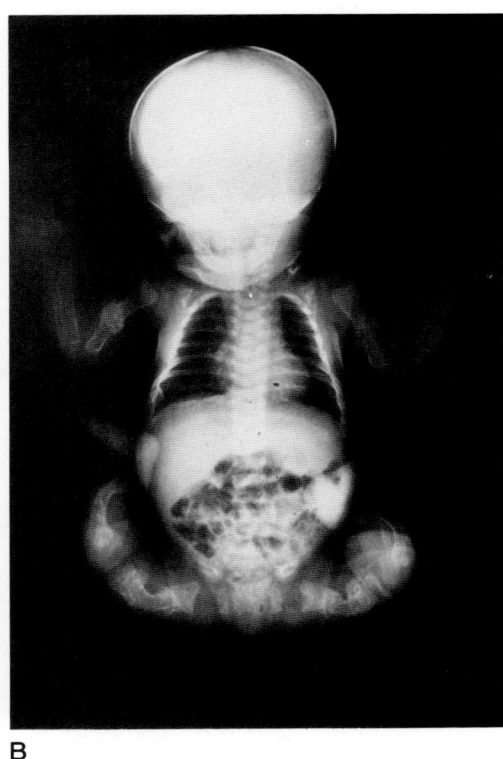

Fig. 59-2. (A) Newborn infant with severe "thick bone" type exhibiting multiple intrauterine fractures. (B) Osteogenesis imperfecta of a newborn infant. Many of the healed fractures occurred intrauterine, giving the bones a thickened appearance.

Histologically, this hyperplastic callus can resemble a malignant tumor (Fig. 59-6), resembling an osteogenic sarcoma. It may take many years before this hyperplastic callus eventually is resorbed, but, in most instances, the restoration of the extremity to normal does occur (Fig. 59-7).

Prior to the introduction of the Sofield technique of intramedullary nailing, osteogenesis imperfecta children developed grotesque deformities throughout their growing period.[9] The patient in Figure 59-8 at age 35 had a totally collapsed spine. Extremely severe fixed limb deformities is an example of the natural history of untreated fractures in osteogenesis imperfecta. It is the goal of modern treatment to prevent the occurrence of these deformities, since we are unable at present to alter the underlying biochemical aberration.

One of the still ill-understood phenomena is that with skeletal maturity the bones again become strong and solid and are no longer prone to fracture. It is thus the goal to maintain skeletal alignment in the osteogenesis imperfecta child until the onset of skeletal maturity.

Also not understood is the premature closure of epiphyseal plates in the children with osteogenesis imperfecta in the mild form. Thus the extremities, even if treated appropriately, will still always be considerably shortened resulting in short stature (Fig. 59-9). Adding to this loss of height is the development of serious spinal deformities in many osteogenesis imperfecta children. These deformities take the form of a collapsing scoliosis, kyphosis, and spondylolisthesis with intact neural arches (Fig. 59-10).

Osteogenesis Imperfecta or Child Abuse?

It is always a diagnostic dilemma when an infant presents in the first several months of life with several fractures. There have been numerous families that have been accused of child abuse, resulting in the osteogenesis imperfecta child being apprehended and placed under the protective custody of an agency. It is only after a

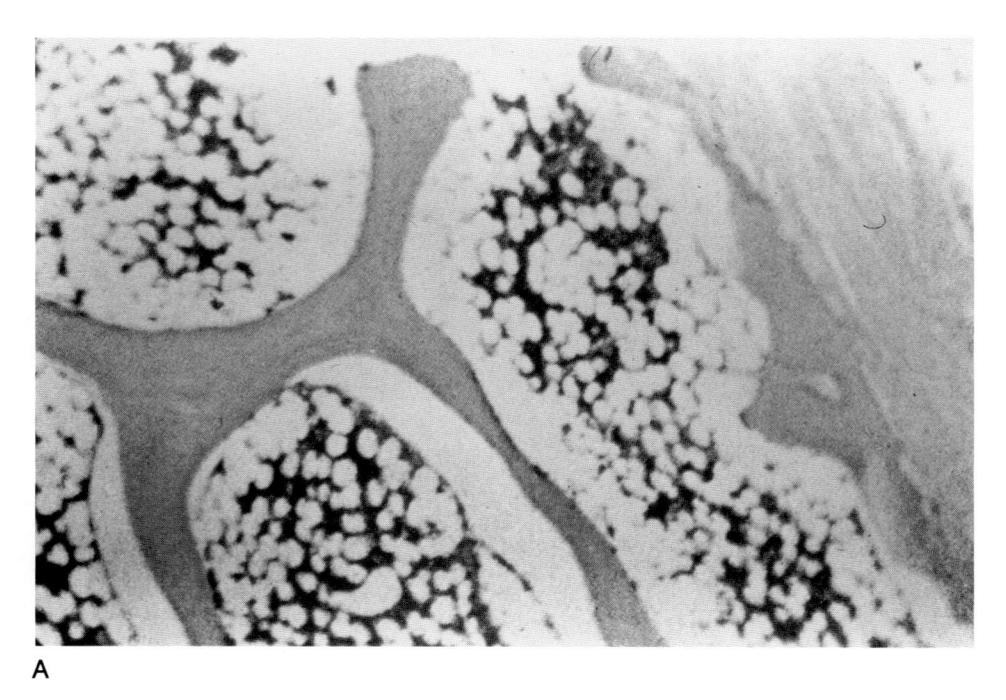

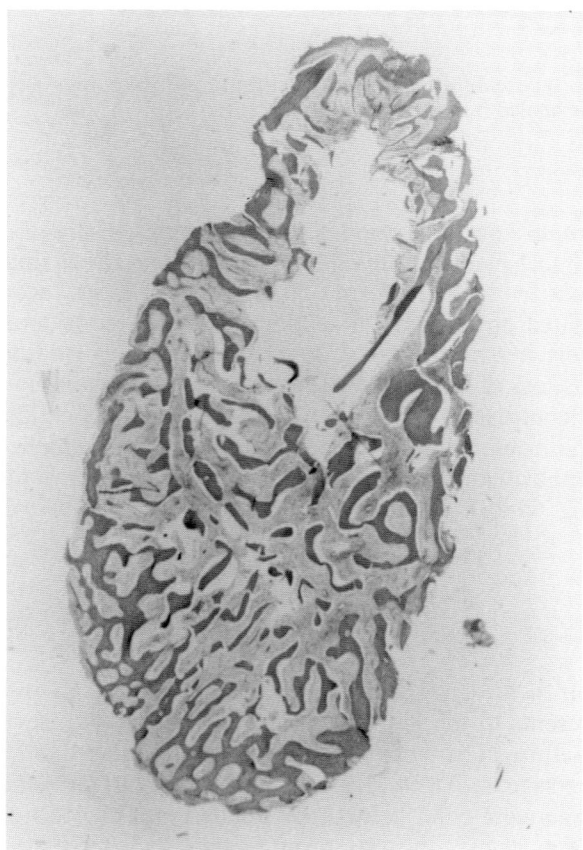

Fig. 59-3. (A) Scant thin trabeculae of osteogenesis imperfecta. (B) Cross section of tibia shows total lack of any cortex.

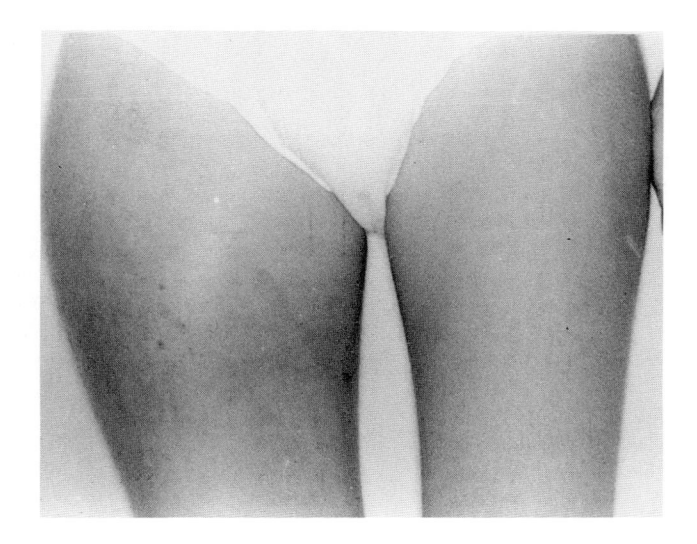

Fig. 59-4. Hyperplastic callus may resemble an osteogenic sarcoma but gradually matures.

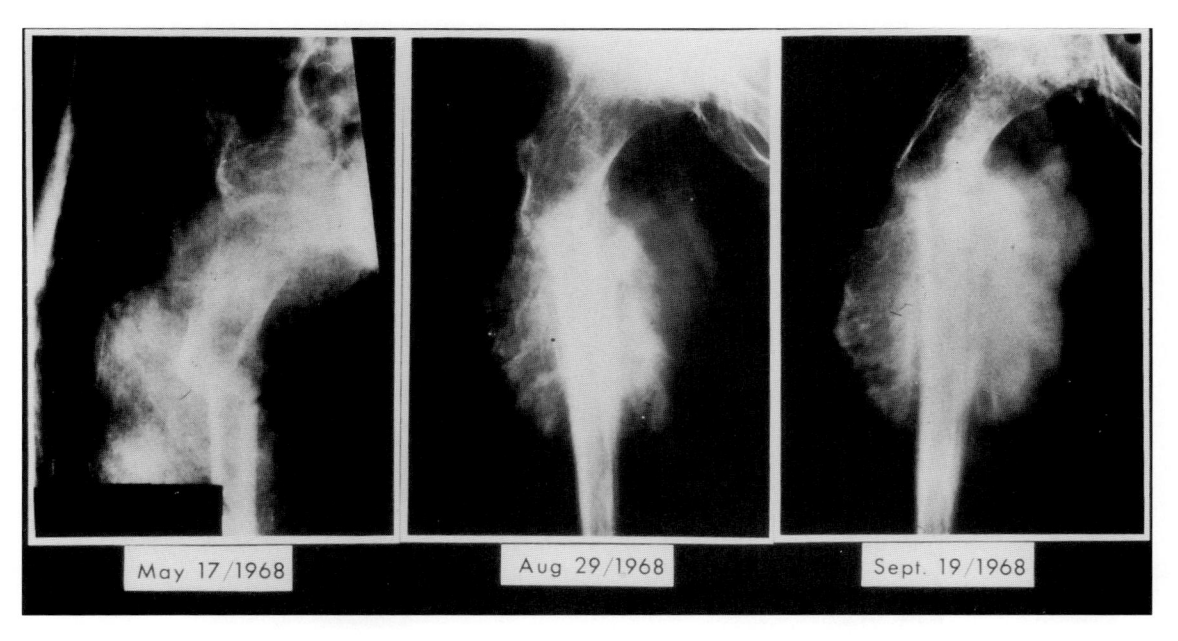

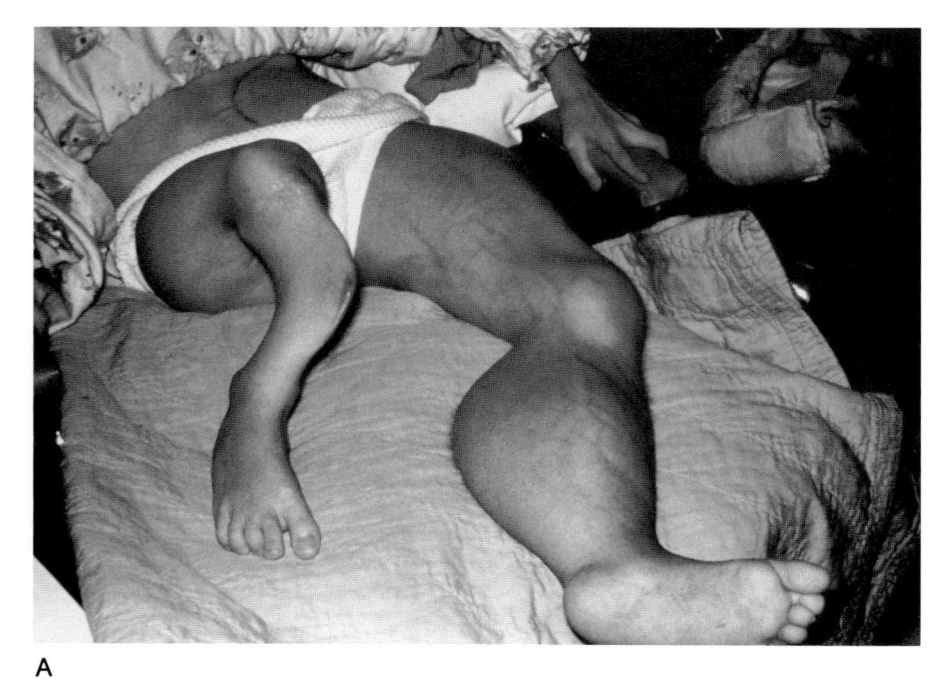

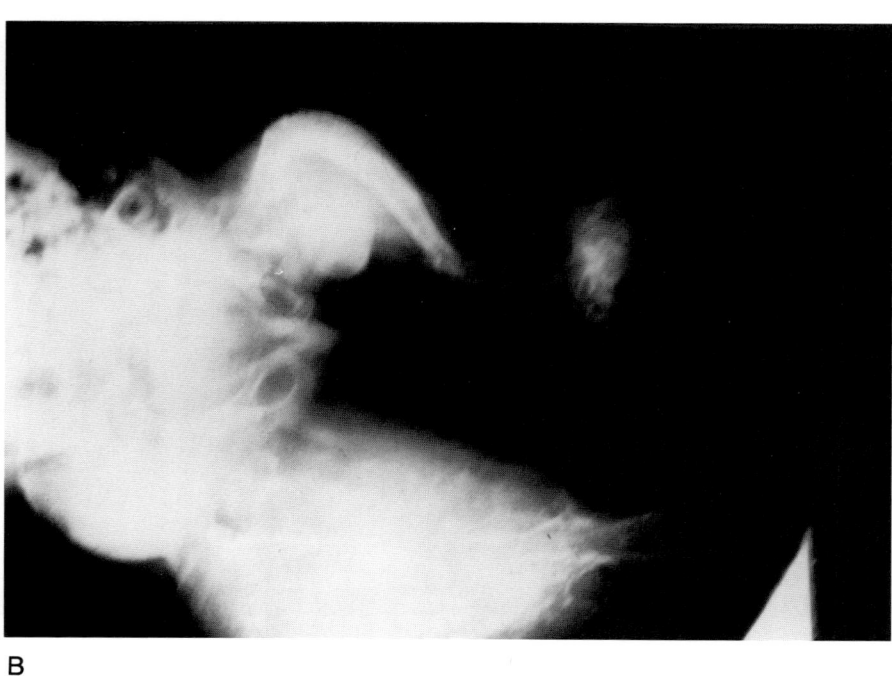

Fig. 59-5. (A) The clinical appearance of acute hyperplastic callus can resemble a highly malignant tumor. (B) The radiograph illustrates the extent of the hyperplastic callus. (Courtesy of Dr. R. Mervyn Letts.)

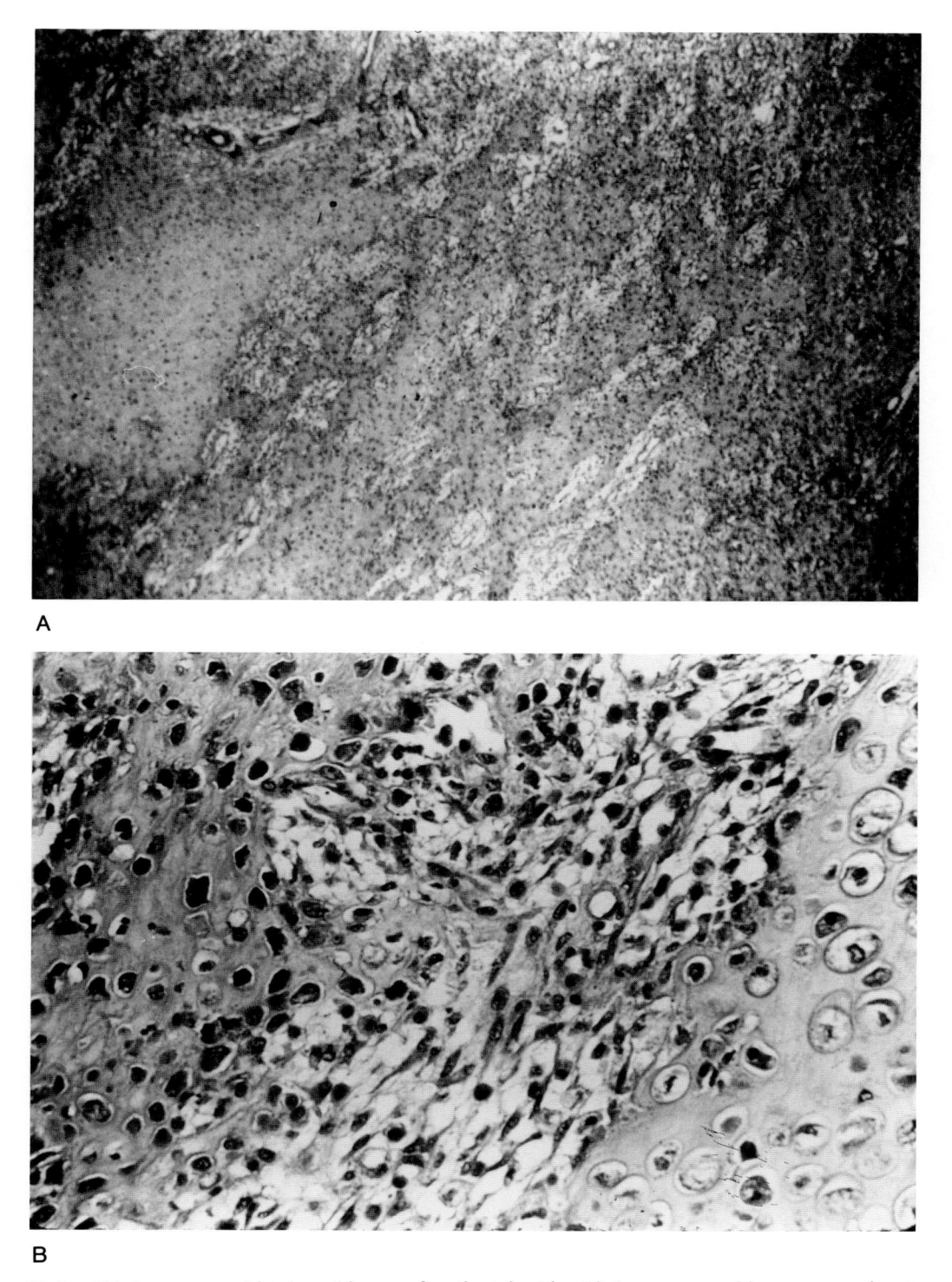

Fig. 59-6. (A) Low-power histology biopsy of patient in Fig. 59-4 may resemble an aggressive tumor. (B) High-power view of hyperplastic callus shows areas indistinguishable from a malignant tumor.

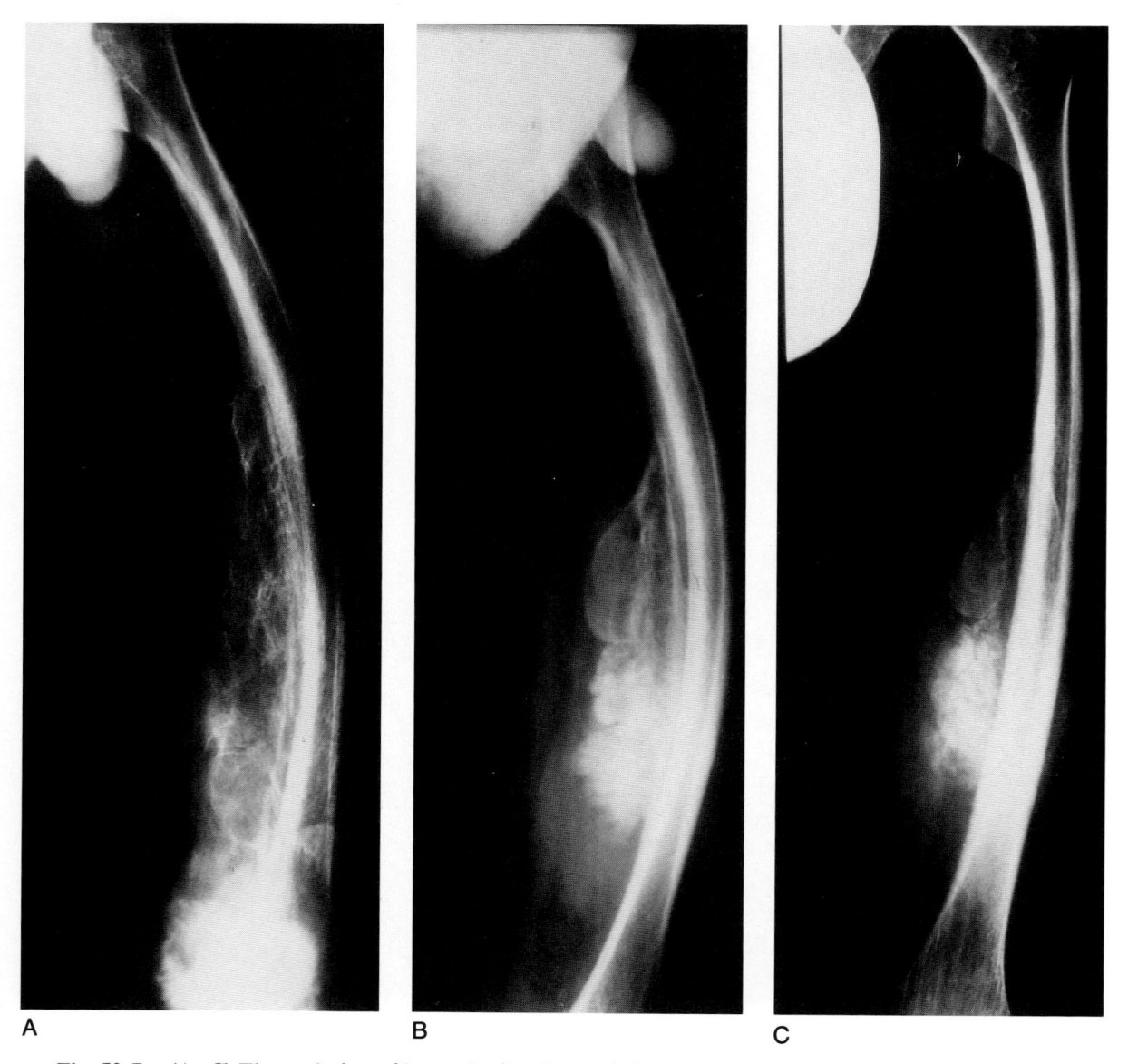

Fig. 59-7. (A–C) The evolution of hyperplastic callus and the eventual total resorption over several years.

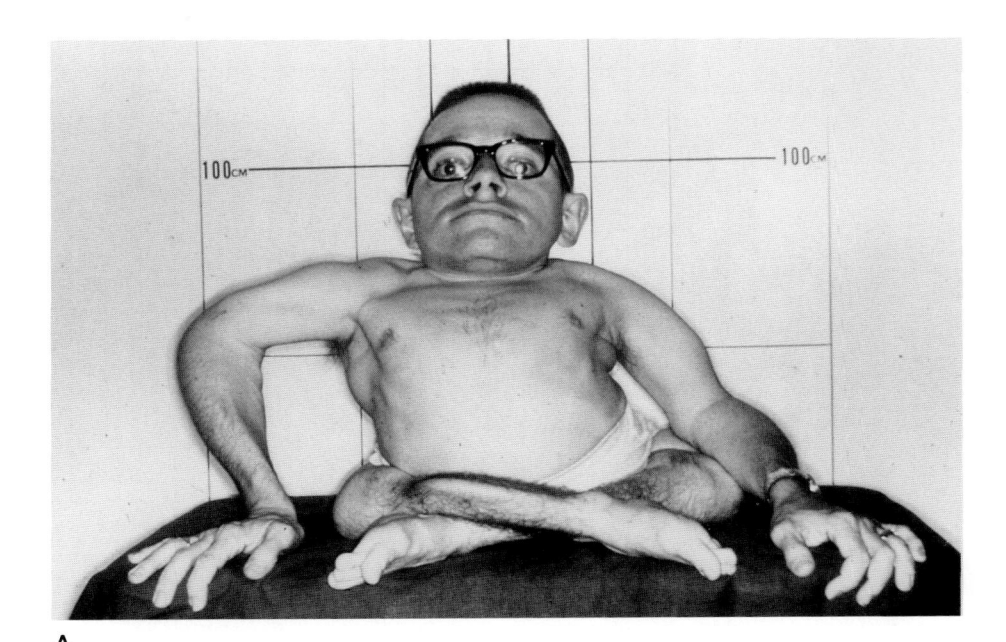

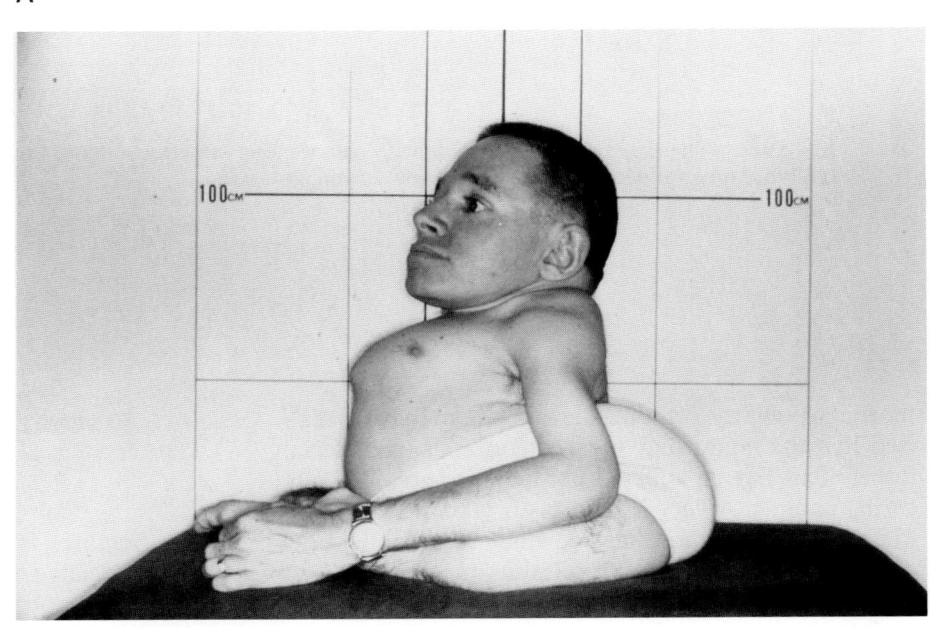

Fig. 59-8. (A&B) End result of untreated fractures of osteogenesis imperfecta at age 35. (Fig. A from King and Bobechko,[2] with permission.)

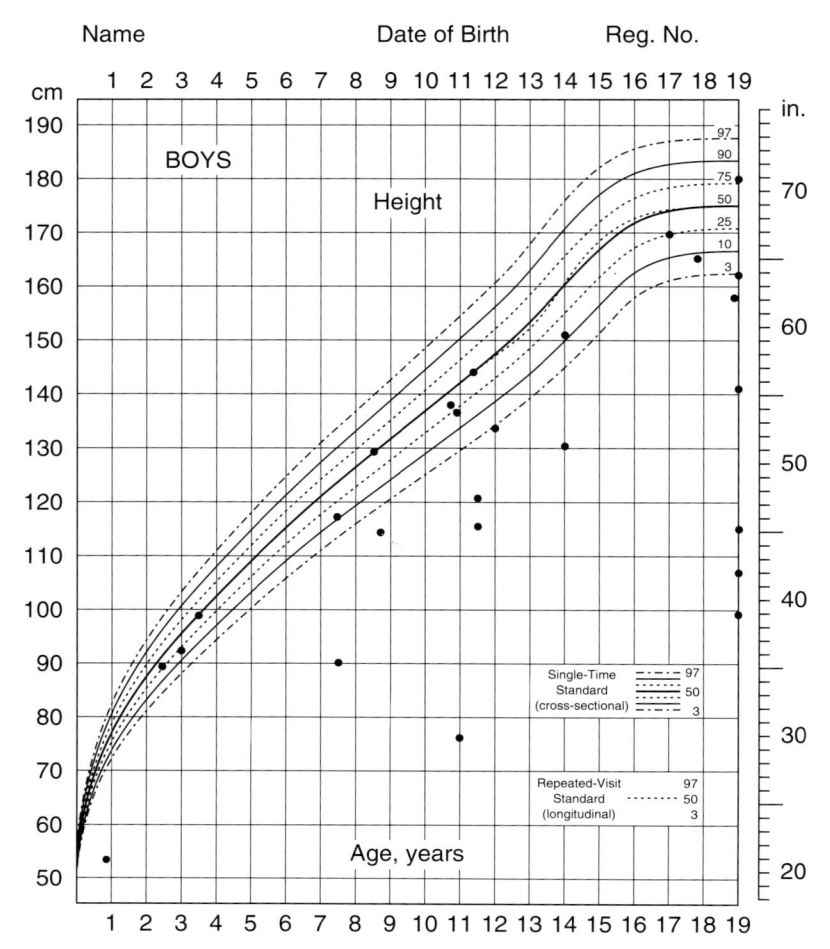

Fig. 59-9. The *dots* represent patients with osteogenesis imperfecta. Note how far below norm their heights remain. Some milder forms may be in low-normal group.

thorough pediatric orthopaedic assessment that it is realized that the infant may have osteogenesis imperfecta, rather than having suffered abusive fractures by truly caring parents. A very careful history and a babygram radiograph is usually indicated, which will usually show abnormal skeletal formation. It is thus imperative that in every case of infantile child abuse that osteogenesis imperfecta be considered in the differential diagnosis. In osteogenesis imperfecta traumatic epiphyseal slips do not occur, whereas they are frequently present in the typical trauma of child abuse with juxtaepiphyseal new bone formation.[10]

Fracture Patterns: The Bending of Bones

The fractures in osteogenesis imperfecta are of the variety associated with very minimal trauma. Not infrequently, over a period of several months the long bones gradually bend without an obvious fracture. These deformations are thought to represent microfractures that crack and heal without an actual fracture being obvious. The child may have minimal or no discomfort during this microfracture bending process. The deformities

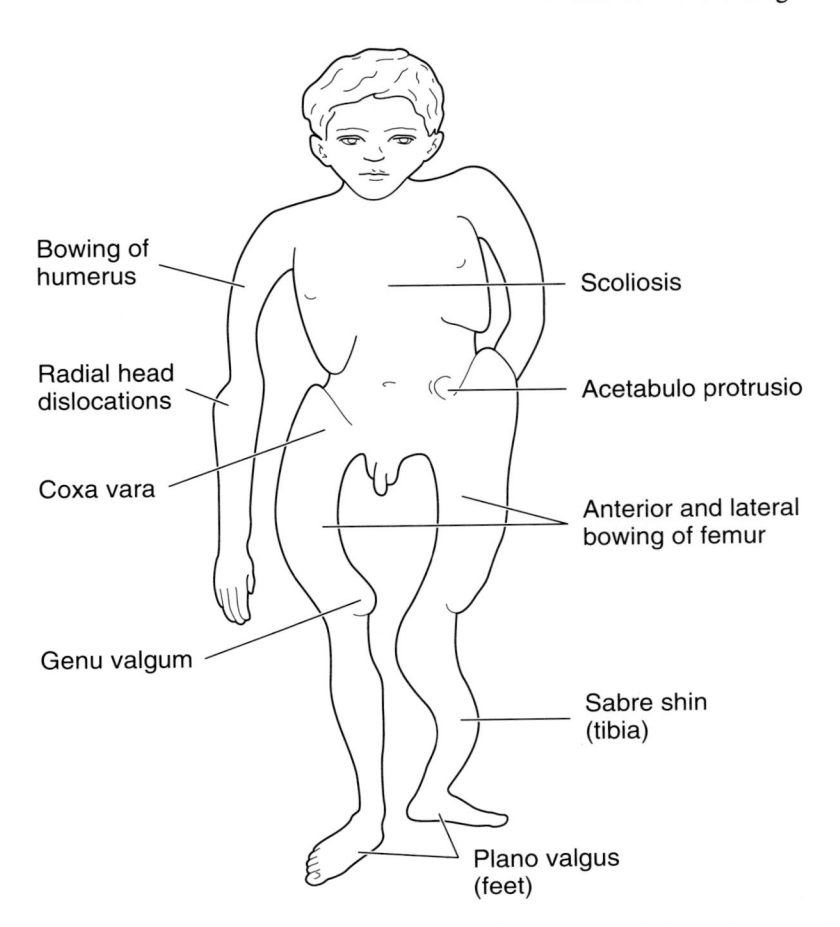

Fig. 59-10. The pattern of deformities in osteogenesis imperfecta. (Adapted from King and Bobechko,[2] with permission.)

over time become additive and the limb severely deformed without any acute single fracture.[6]

On physical examination, the children with osteogenesis imperfecta will be reluctant to let an unaccustomed examiner touch them, for they are apprehensive that other fractures will be sustained. The majority of the fractures that occur in osteogenesis imperfecta are frequently minimally undisplaced. It is amazing how such a series of undisplaced fractures can, over a period of years, lead to such grotesque deformities. The tibia and the femur have the greatest number of fractures (Fig. 59-11). Fortunately these are also the fractures that respond best to current methods of intramedullary fixation.

SURGICAL MANAGEMENT OF LONG-BONE FRACTURES

The Sofield concept and technique revolutionized the acute and long-term management of the fractures associated with osteogenesis imperfecta.[10]

The technique of multiple segmental osteotomy can be utilized (Fig. 59-12) to correct the more severe deformities. It is often necessary to remove some segments of bone, as when a length of curved bone is straightened and thus relatively lengthened, soft tissues will be stretched, and either the internal fixation pins will cut out or vascular problems may arise.

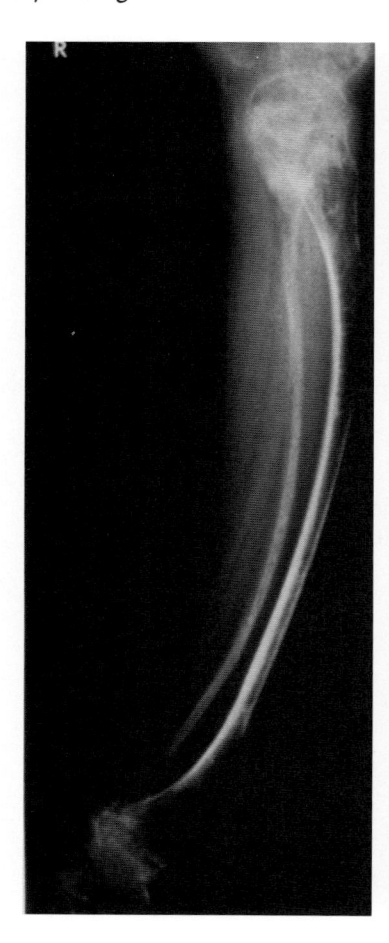

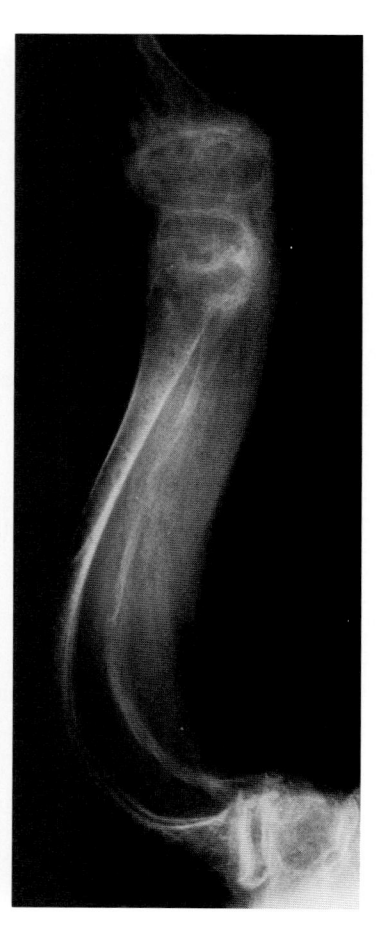

Fig. 59-11. Fractures occur most frequently in the femoral shaft and tibia. The marked bowing shown here predisposes to frequent fracturing.

In many instances, however, when a repeat Sofield osteotomy is done, such radical shortening and removal of segments of bone is unnecessary and only a small wedge needs to be removed. Since the bone is extremely soft, a simple rongeur can be utilized and a bone saw or mechanical power means are seldom required.

Lower Extremity Reconstruction

The Femur

In the lower extremity the femur can be readily fixed with intramedullary Rush pins. Utilizing an osteotomy and a retrograde hollow guide pin the Rush pin can be inserted in the pyriformis fossa adjacent to the greater trochanter under image intensification until it is just abutting, but not penetrating, the distal femoral epiphyseal plate (Fig. 59-13). After a variable period of time, usually between 12 and 24 months in a growing child, the pin will be outgrown as the distal femur grows away from it (Fig. 59-14). At that point, the femur will usually refracture and a new pin of longer length will have to be inserted. I feel that this is a preferable technique, rather than using the Bailey-Dubow sliding nail, even though Sofield Rush rodding requires multiple operative procedures.

The Bailey-Dubow sliding nail (Fig. 59-15) elongates and "grows" with the femur. The disadvantages are that, at the distal end, the T-bar of the nail has to fit into the intercondylar notch of the femur. The rod must transgress the epiphyseal plate exactly through the midcentral portion of the distal femoral epiphysis for the femur to grow without deformity. If the pin crosses the epiphyseal plate, not centrally but peripherally, premature epiphyseal plate closure may occur. As well the T-bolt often becomes loose in the knee joint no matter how securely it is tightened at the time of insertion.[11-14]

The average child with moderately severe osteogenesis

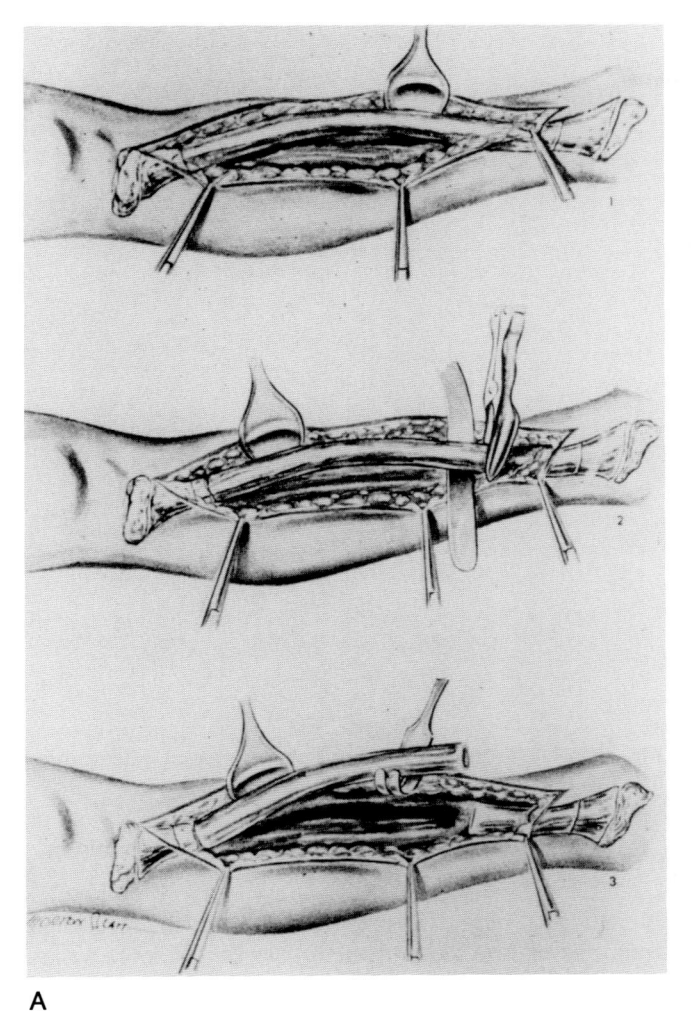

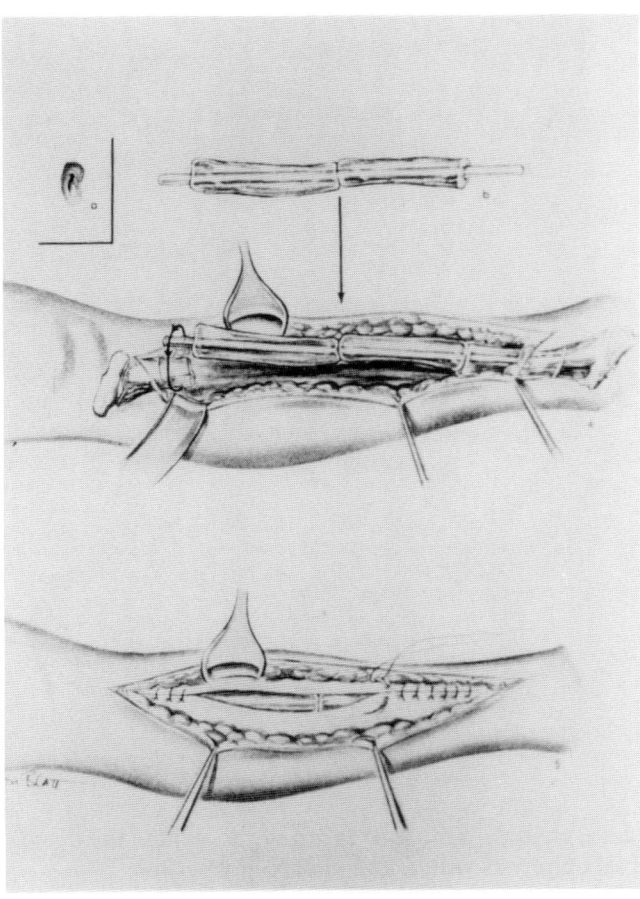

Fig. 59-12. (A) The total length of tibia need not be stripped of periosteum. The epiphyseal plate blood supply should be carefully preserved and not stripped of periosteum to minimize growth disturbance. (B) Technique of segmental osteotomies of tibia and use of circlage wire proximally to hold rod in position and yet not violating proximal tibia tubercle epiphysis.

imperfecta will require approximately three to six repeat Sofield femoral nailings during the course of their growth to maturity. At the end of growth the final Rush pin can be left permanently in situ (Fig. 59-16). The rod often results in a phenomenon known as *cortical decancellization,* as weight is transmitted through the rod rather than the cortex of the bone. In accordance with Wolff's law the cortex becomes very thin, contributing to refracture if the rod is removed and not replaced. At skeletal maturity the cortex usually reconstitutes (Fig. 59-17).

The Tibia

The tibia produces many more complex surgical technical problems of inserting a Rush pin. The proximal end the tibial epiphysis has a tonguelike projection for the tibial tubercle that must not be violated in the child, to avoid recurvatum of the proximal tibia. The Rush pin must be proximally inserted, often in a small channel along the medial side of the tibia, and then a circumferential wire used to hold it in position until it is placed distally through the segmental tibial osteotomy site.

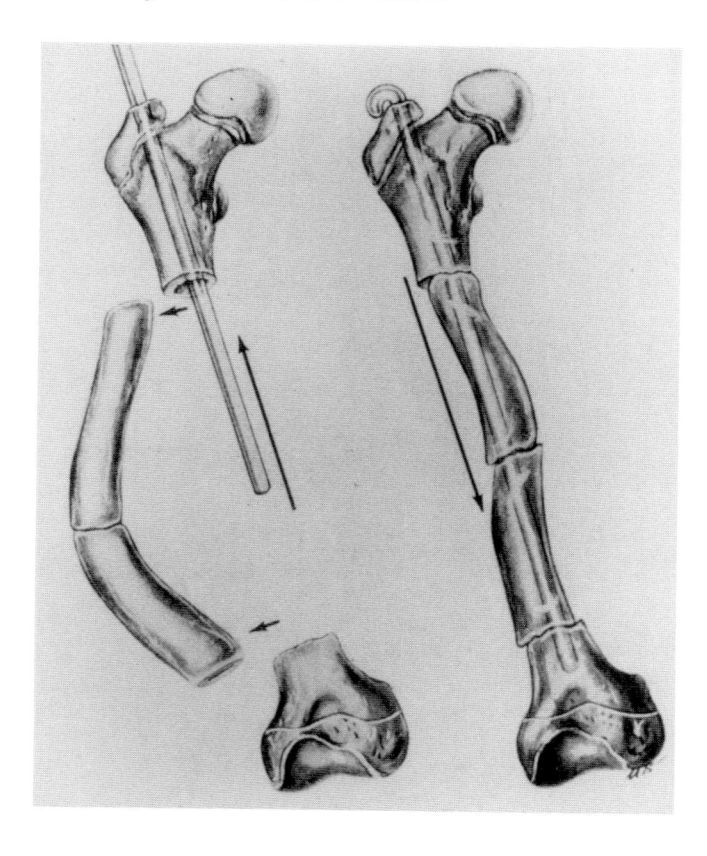

Fig. 59-13. Technique of multiple segmental osteotomies and intramedullary fixation.

Again, great care must be taken not to violate the distal tibial epiphysis with a long nail (Fig. 59-18).

Occasionally in a very tiny child in whom there is no other means to manage the recurring fractures of a tiny tibia, one may have to pass a fine K-wire retrograde through the os calcis and across the talus, violating the distal tibial epiphyseal plate. The fine K-wire should be passed up the tibial shaft just reaching, but not crossing, the proximal tibial epiphysis. This should be a technique of last resort because of the potential to cause growth disturbance of the distal tibial physis.

Postoperative Immobilization

Probably the most common error that is made in children with osteogenesis imperfecta is that, after an intramedullary nailing procedure or spontaneous fracture, the patient is immobilized like a typical fracture patient. This leads to very serious osteoporosis in the entire lower extremity, with the result that, after the immobilization is removed, there is an even greater tendency to fracture because of the iatrogenic disuse osteoporosis of immobilization. These fractures are commonly rotational fractures around the intramedullary pin. Fractures may also occur just proximal or distal to the pin termination due to the combination of cortical osteoporosis and the abnormal biomechanics that occurs at the function of the rigidly fixed bone and more mobile distal portion.

These children should preferably be immobilized in a very bulky cloth or soft tissue padded nonplaster hip spica or a similarly soft-padded long-leg immobilization type of splint. There should be no plaster immobilization, and the extremity should be immobilized for the least amount of time. After a few days, the soft cloth immobilization will gradually loosen and, in most instances, still provide sufficient protection while allowing early micromotion within the padded dressings.

Even the period of this bulky soft cloth immobilization should be very short. It usually should not be left on for more than 3 weeks to avoid the problems of postoperative immobilization osteoporosis and its very serious sequelae.

Once these soft tissue bulky dressings are removed, the child should not be totally mobilized, but kept partially

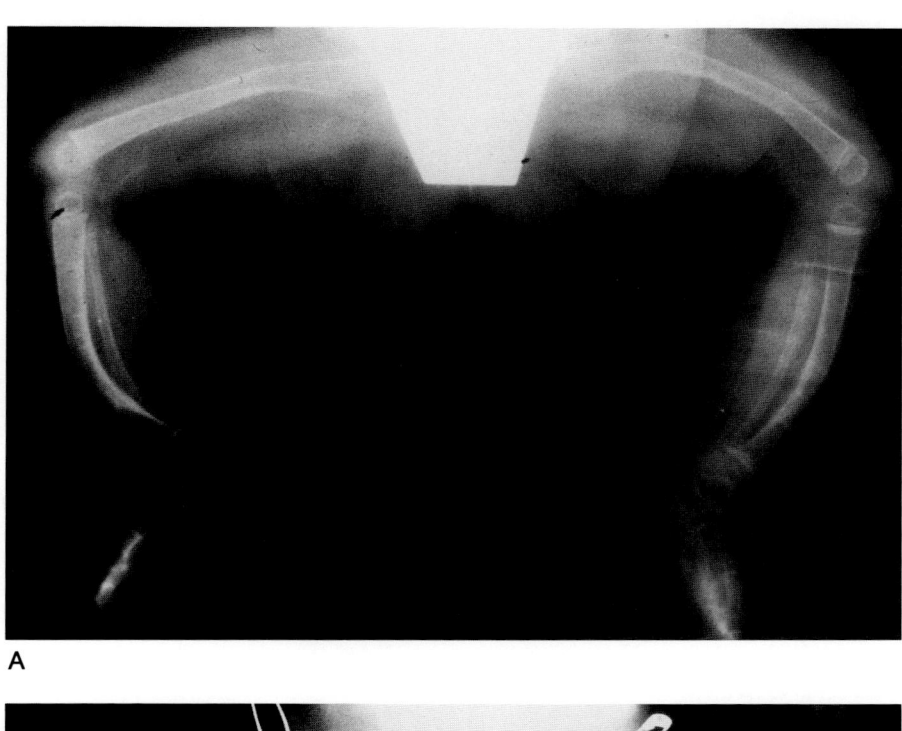

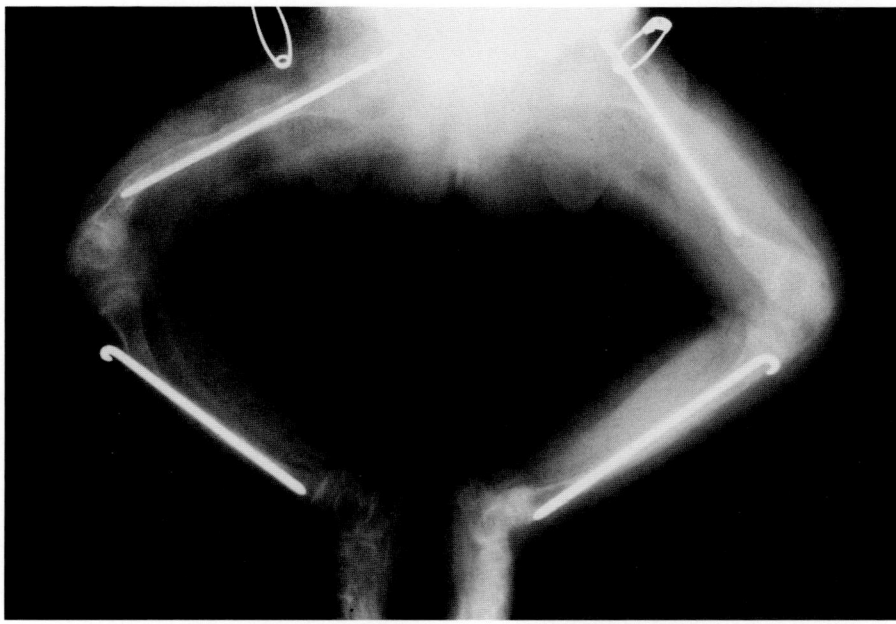

Fig. 59-14. (A) Preoperative status with frequent fractures. (B) Insertion of multiple intramedullary rods. *(Figure continues.)*

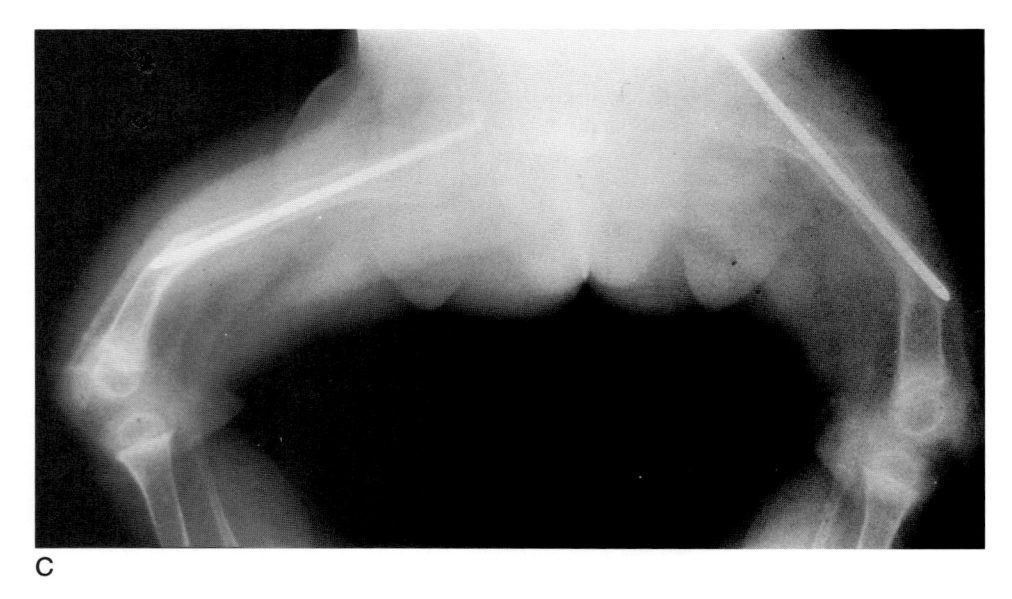

Fig. 59-14 *(Continued).* **(C)** Having outgrown the rods the femora tend to bend or break just beyond. The rods at this stage should be replaced.

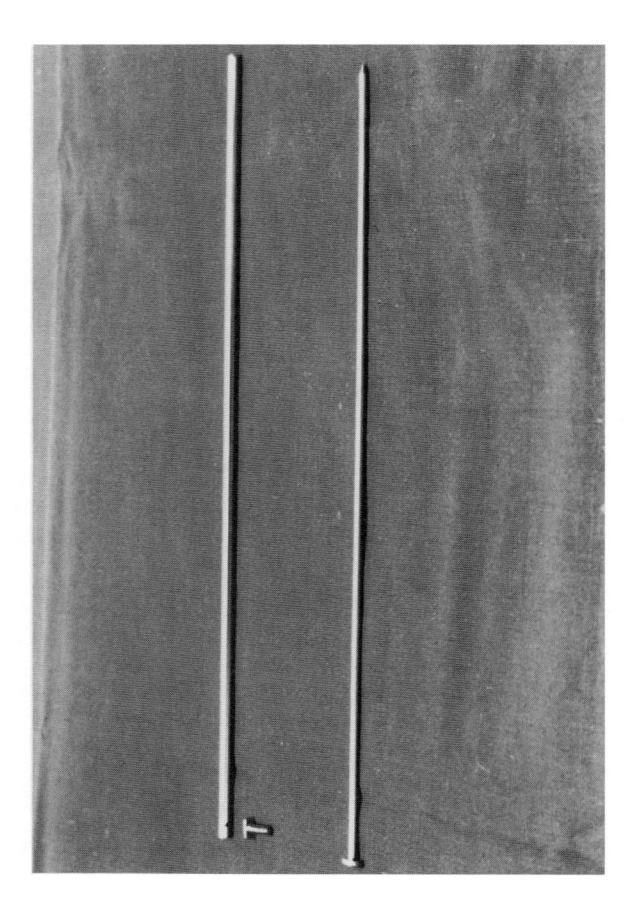

Fig. 59-15. The T-bar of the Bailey-Dubow sliding nail. The T component must fit in the intracondylar notch of the distal femur.

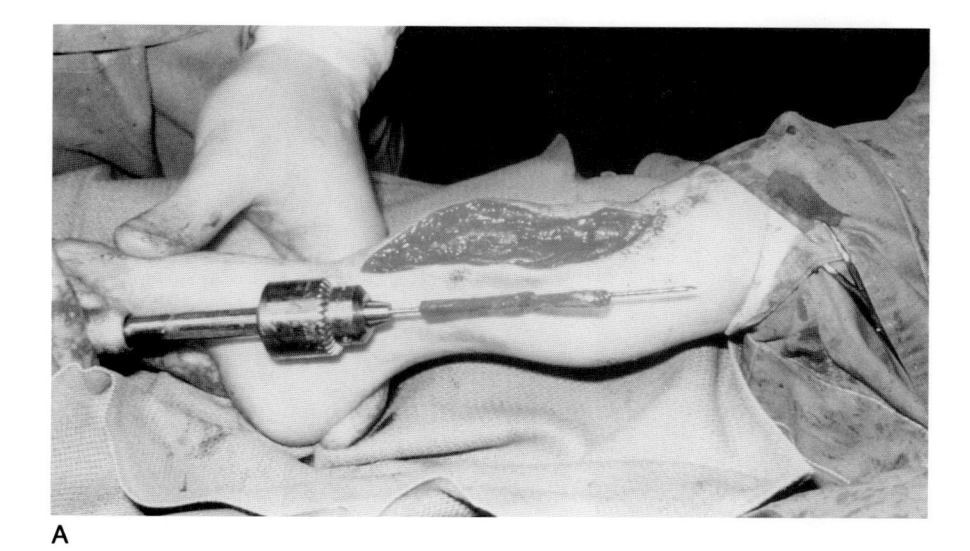

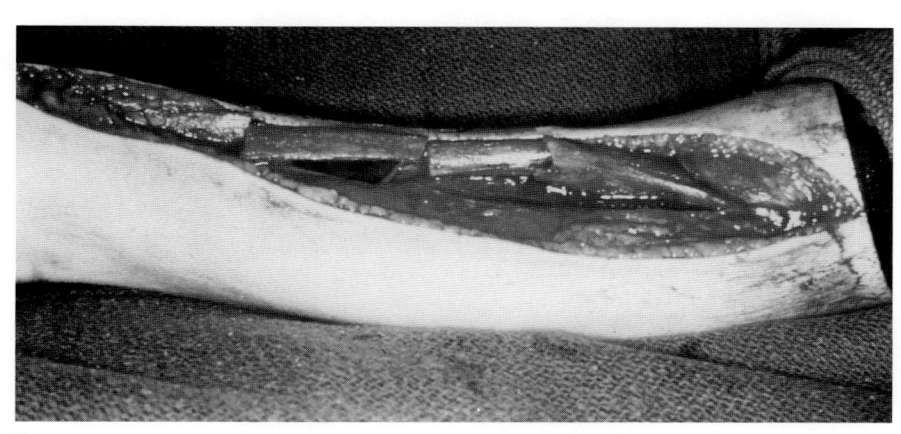

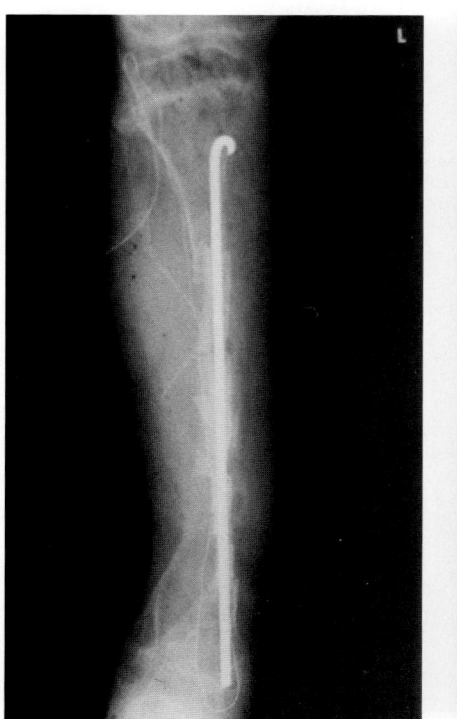

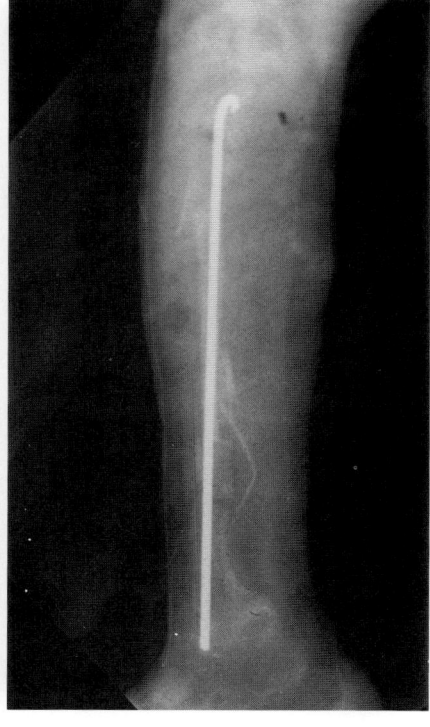

Fig. 59-16. **(A)** The Sofield technique in which the tibia is osteotomized and straightened on an intramedullary rod. **(B&C)** During segmental osteotomy the fragments can be left attached to their soft tissue blood supply.

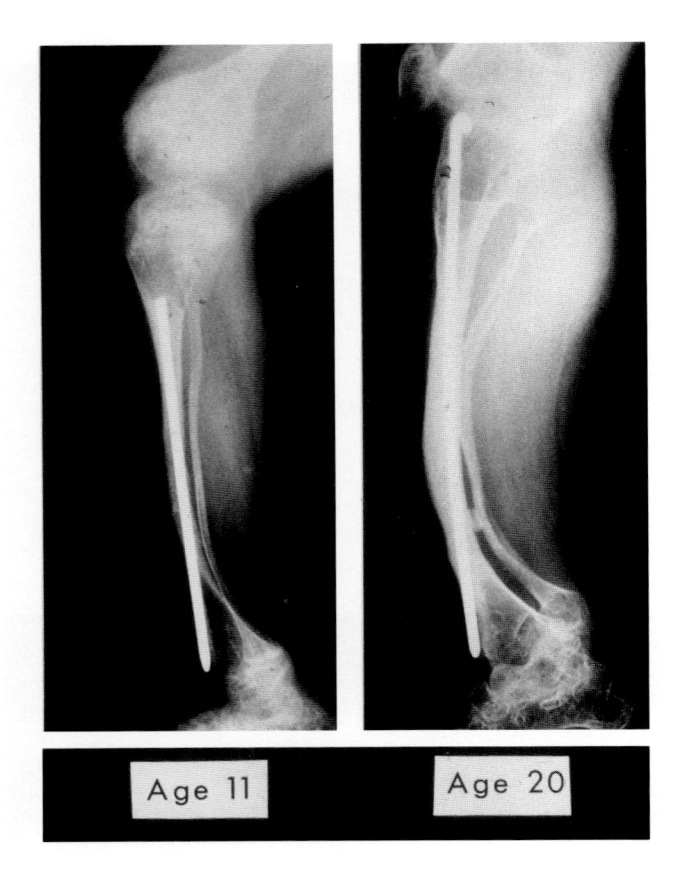

Fig. 59-17. Intramedullary rod in place. The cortex during growth becomes very thin or even disappears. Note reformation of a cortex around rod at skeletal maturity.

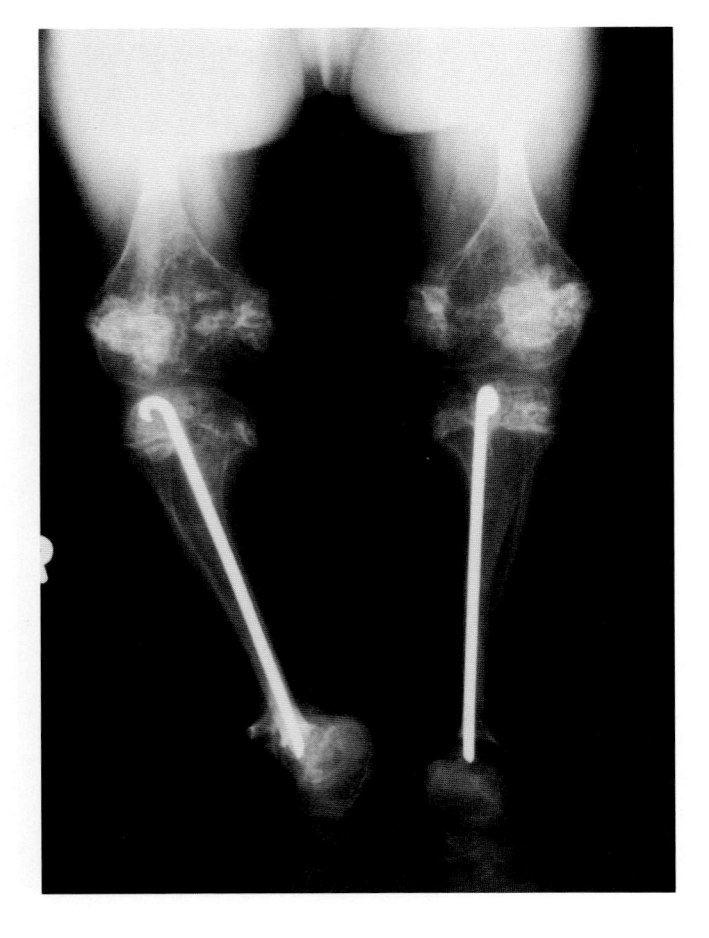

Fig. 59-18. The epiphyseal plates at both ends of tibia have been violated. This is a technique to avoid.

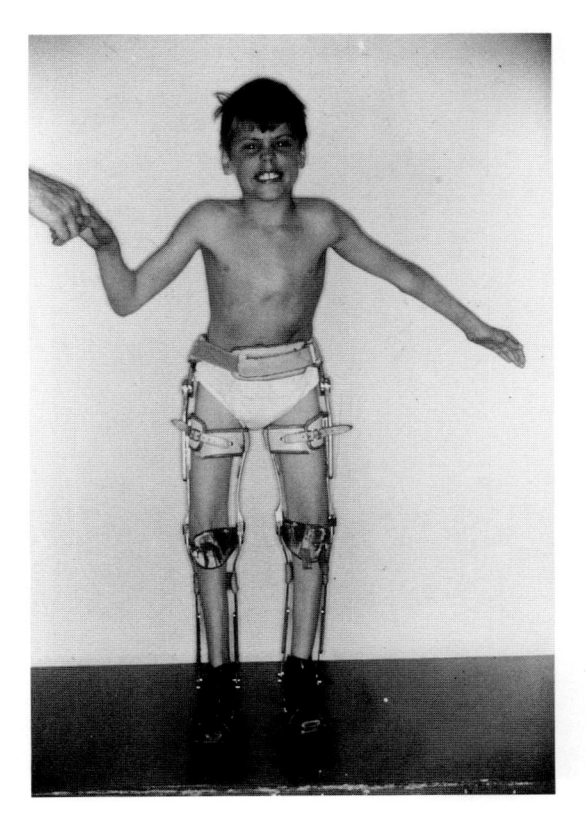

Fig. 59-19. Severe form of osteogenesis imperfecta. Long-leg bracing with pelvic band allows patient to ambulate at puberty.

osteoporosis and the vicious cycle of increasing fracture tendency.

It is fortunate that fractures of the femoral neck, for some unknown reason, are virtually unknown in osteogenesis imperfecta. Should such occur, internal fixation would be mandatory to prevent a severe coxa vara from occurring. Because of the extreme softness of the bone, skeletal traction is not recommended in lower extremity fractures due to migration of the traction pin. Epiphyseal plate injuries are very rare. In children with osteogenesis imperfecta the epiphyseal plate is stronger than the surrounding bone, in contradistinction to normal children where the physis is much weaker.

Joint injuries and dislocations in osteogenesis imperfecta are also uncommon, as the adjacent bone will usually break before the ligaments tear, the epiphyseal plate shears, or the joint dislocates.

The Upper Extremity

In the upper extremity, fractures of the distal half of the humerus are relatively common. In most instances, they can be treated by simple immobilization with the arm being held against the chest wall, either by bandaging or splinting for a period of approximately 10 days, at which time the fracture will have clinical stability. If the

recumbent. Several weeks later when there appears to be relatively solid union, hydrotherapy in a pool can usually be commenced. Most osteogenesis imperfecta patients will require some degree of splinting and bracing on a long-term basis (Fig. 59-19).

General Lower Extremity Problems

Many severe osteogenesis imperfecta patients will be totally unable, despite external bracing, to stand or walk until after they reach puberty, when spontaneous osteogenesis imperfecta-type fractures will cease.

Although osteogenesis imperfecta patients may have an intramedullary nail in satisfactory position in one of the long bones of the lower extremity, this still may not prevent all fractures. Rotational fractures around a rod usually requires no specific treatment, and the pain and discomfort of this type of undisplaced rotational fracture will usually spontaneously subside within a week, allowing return to their prefracture level of activity. Cast immobilization is still contraindicated, as it induces more

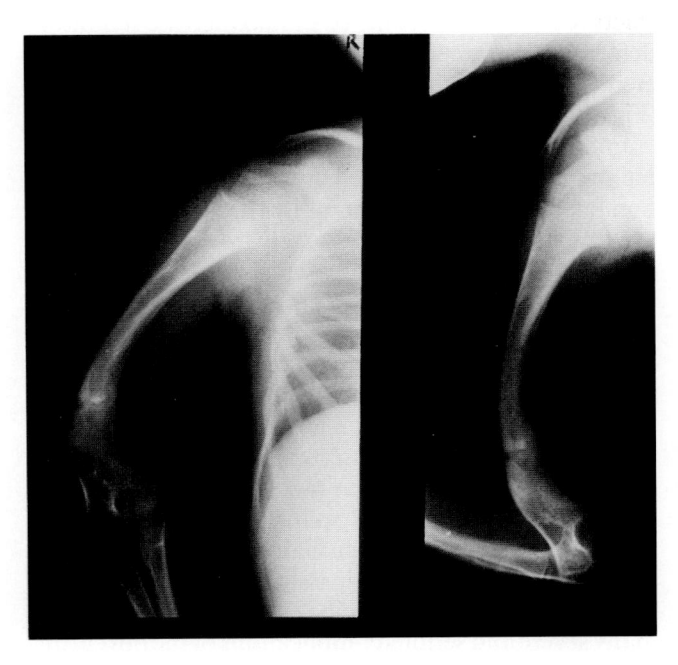

Fig. 59-20. Typical location of fracture and deformity of humerus in osteogenesis imperfecta.

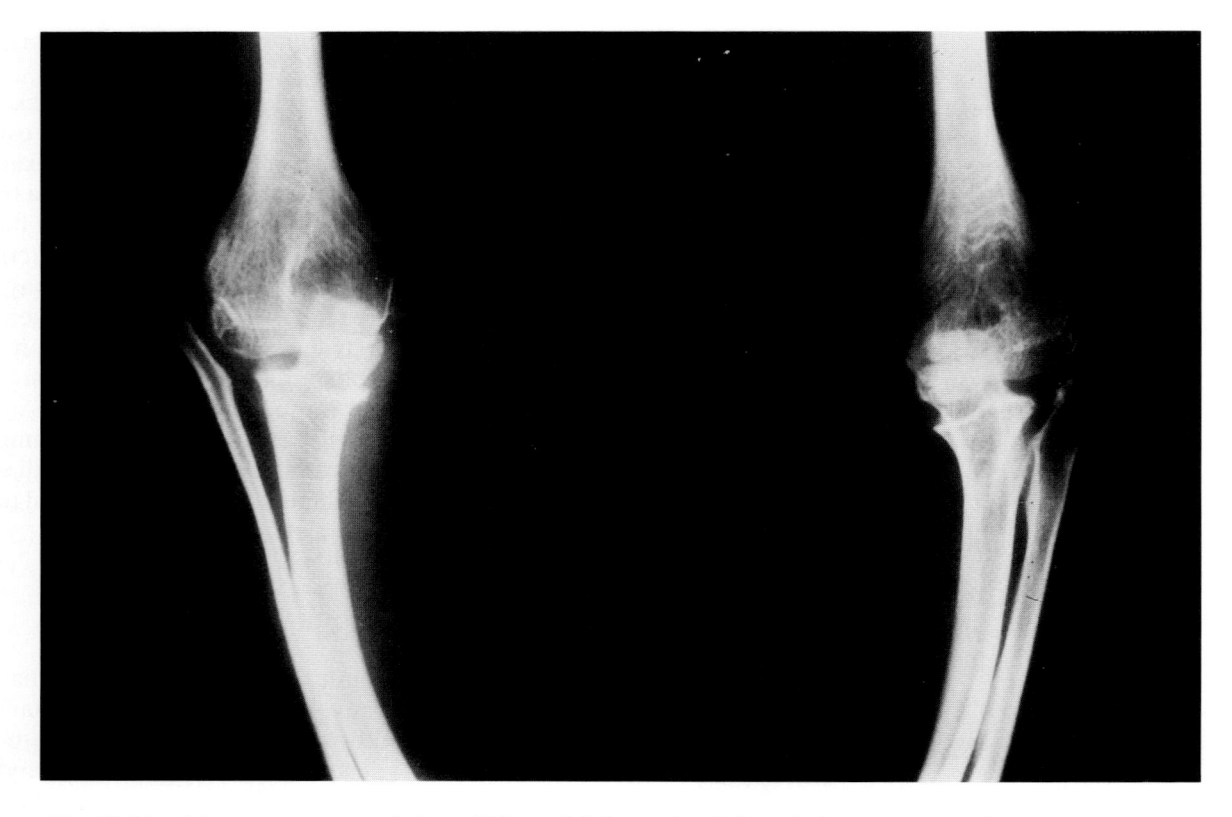

Fig. 59-21. Note common association of bilateral dislocated radial heads due to asymmetrical growth between the radius and ulna.

fracture is a recurrent one, or should there be significant deformity, intramedullary nailing again can be considered. This is also a not-uncommon site for a nonunion (Fig. 59-20).

In these instances, the pin can be passed often as blind nailing under radiographic control, through the olecranon fossa of the distal humerus up through the mid- and proximal shaft of the humerus, just reaching, but not crossing, the proximal epiphyseal plate. The hook of the Rush pin is then buried beneath the triceps tendon.

Deformities of the forearm bones in these children are often extremely difficult to manage because of their small size and frequent multiple three-plane deformities (Fig. 59-21). Occasionally, a fine Kirschner wire can be used to stabilize the ulna inserted via the olecranon. The radius can merely be broken by a closed osteoclasis and the fixed ulna is used as a splint to hold the radius in reasonable alignment. A transfixion pin should never be used to hold the radius by passing it through the distal humerus and crossing the elbow joint. This will lead to many severe and serious complications of the pin cutting through the joint and the distal humerus or possibly the head and neck of the radius. It is usually sufficient to stabilize the ulna with a pin from its proximal end at the olecranon going to, but not crossing, the distal ulna-epiphysis at the wrist level.

Spinal Deformities

Spinal deformities are the result of the multiple recurrent micro- and hairline subclinical fractures. They can, over time, lead to very serious spondylolisthesis with occasional multiple level cord compression. In this peculiar type of spondylolisthesis, the actual pars remains intact but is stretched out like toffee by recurrent microfractures and cyclic healing and refracture. These multiple microfractures of the spine also predispose to kyphosis and scoliosis.

Progressive spinal deformities should be fused early using homogeneous bank bone and an in situ fusion. Internal fixation is contraindicated due to the fragile bone. The fusion mass itself can also bend because of recurrent microfractures of the fusion mass.[15]

I have used a fine, thin, Luque rod, which is merely

contoured to the deformity and bone graft laid upon the internal fixation rod. The rod itself is totally unattached to any spine element. The purpose of this technique is to produce the effect of reinforced concrete where the bone graft will grow around the Luque rod adjacent to the lamina of the spine. This minimizes the biologic plasticity effect of the fusion mass and the slow progressive bending due to microfractures. The long-term results of this technique appear to be satisfactory.

Pseudarthrosis

Although pseudarthrosis after open osteotomy is rare, it can and does occur. Leaving soft tissues attached to some portion of the length of the long bone during surgical procedures, such as the Sofield technique, minimizes this complication.

A pseudarthrosis can, however, appear in osteogenesis imperfecta even without an open operative procedure. This is most common in the distal half of the humerus. Union can be achieved by excision of the pseudarthrosis with bone grafting and internal Rush pin fixation.[16]

The Limitations of Surgery for Multiple Fractures

There may come a point in the management of some of these extremely severe osteogenesis imperfecta patients where the fracture deformity, despite use of internal fixation cannot be prevented. The pins inevitably will cut out where the cortex is thin and fragile (Fig. 59-14C). In this situation, any type of internal fixation attempts become futile. One of the solutions is to perform a manual multilevel closed osteoclasis and align the limb visually to a relatively straight position. The limb is then immobilized in a soft bulky dressing for several weeks. This will at least allow the limb to look "humanoid" rather than end up as a grotesquely deformed extremity as seen in some untreated cases of osteogenesis imperfecta.

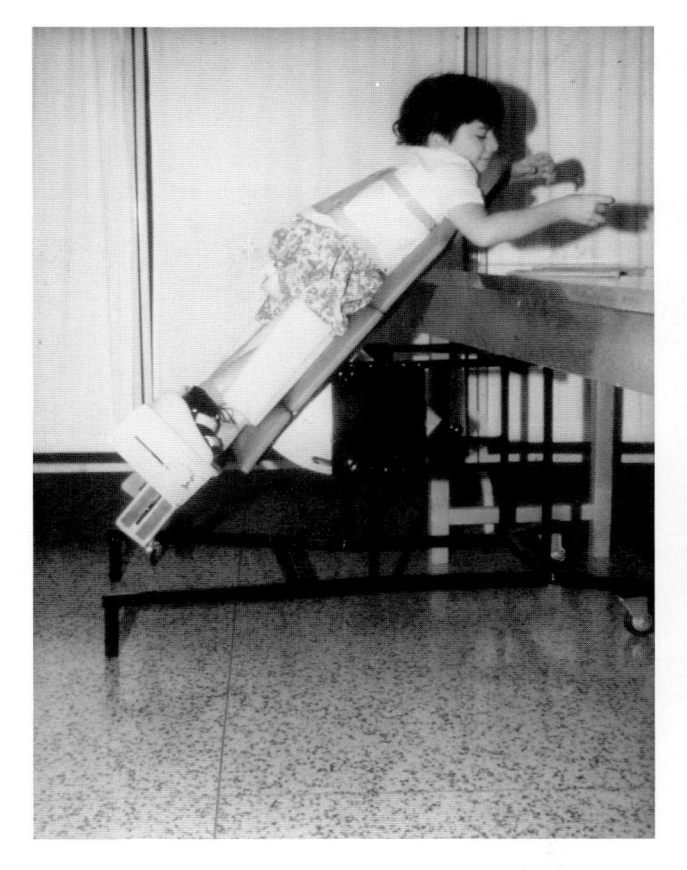

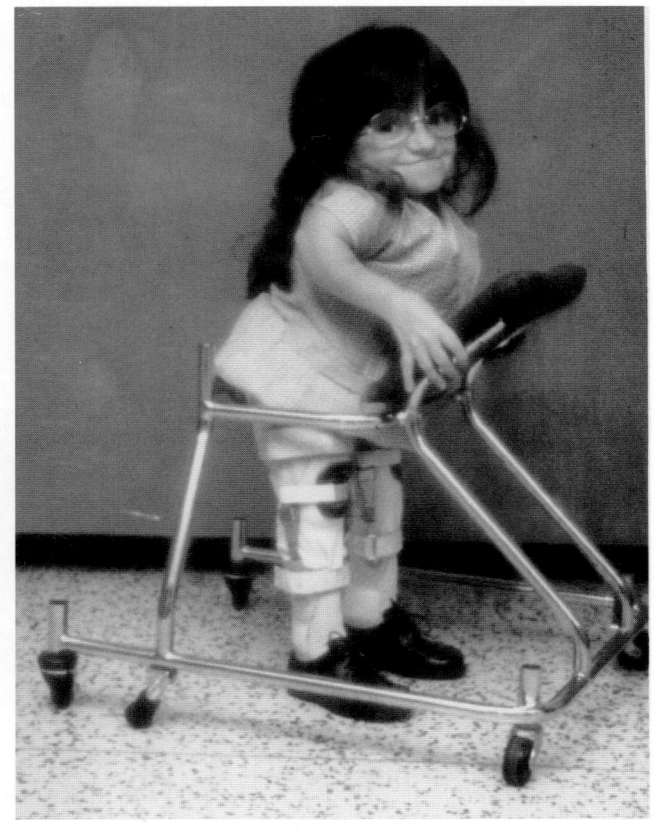

Fig. 59-22. Assistive standing and semiprone devices to allow partial weightbearing and stimulate bone formation in accordance with Wolff's law. (Courtesy of Dr. R. Mervyn Letts.)

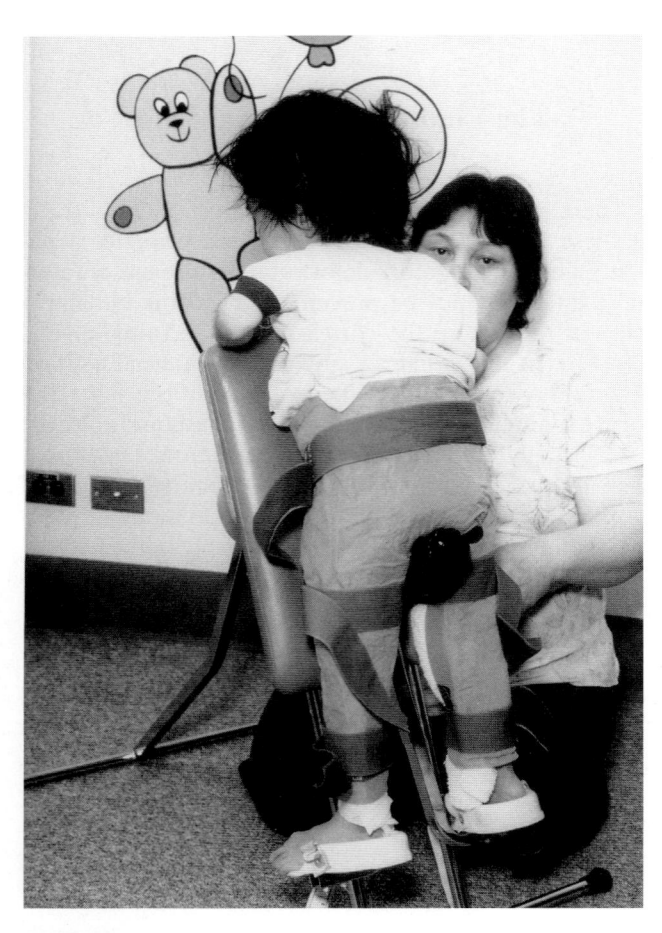

Fig. 59-23. Vacuum splints provide equalized pressure distribution and stability while simultaneously allowing protected yet limited motion. (Courtesy of Dr. R. Mervyn Letts.)

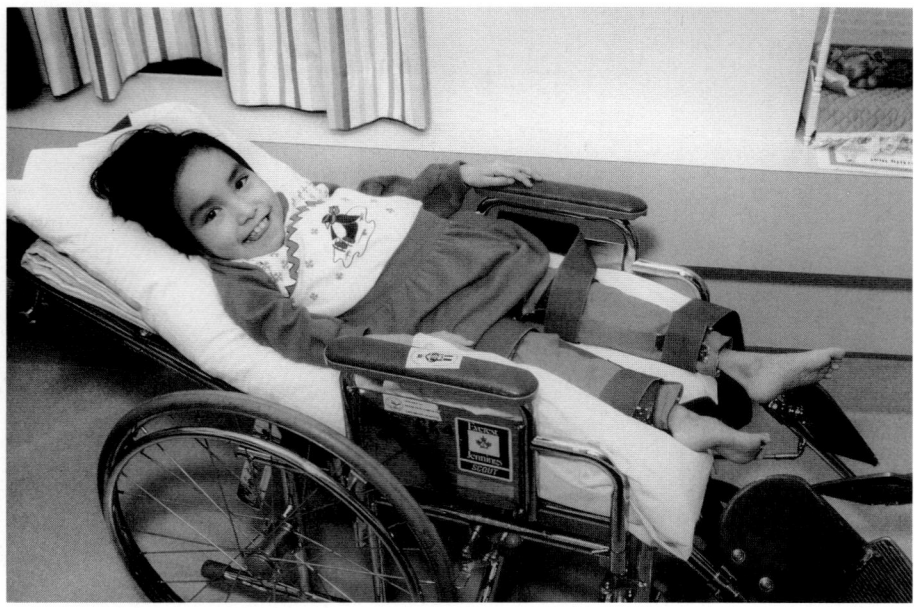

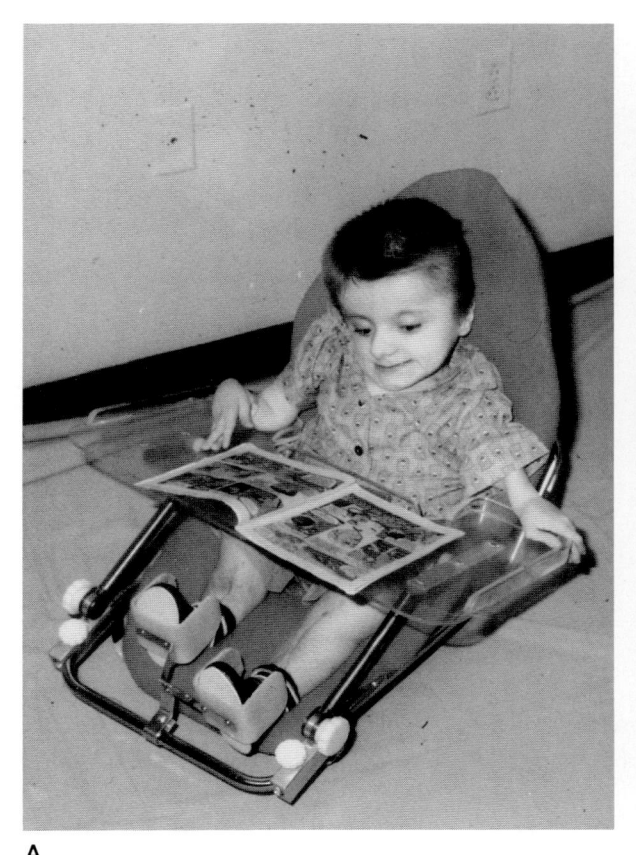

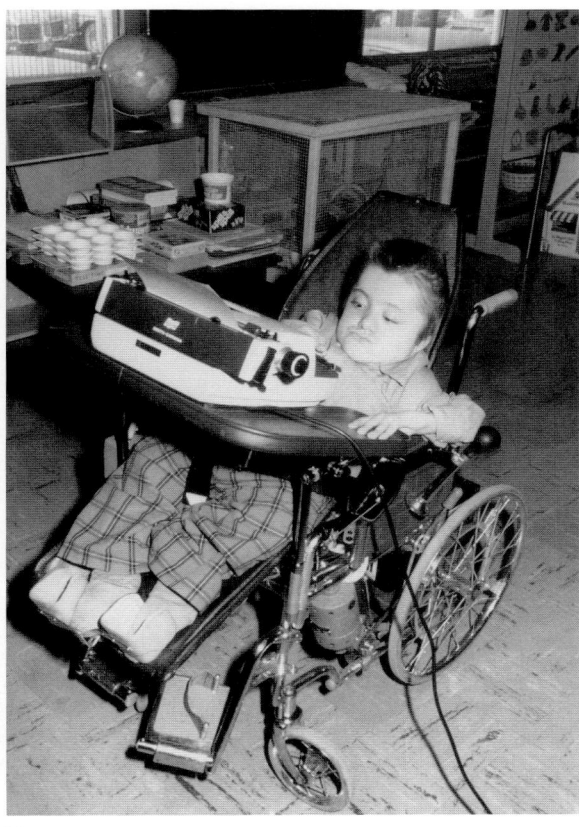

Fig. 59-24. (A) Custom-constructed inserts for strollers and (B) wheelchairs allow protective portability and yet will allow the child to be rapidly transferred to a mobility device. (Courtesy of Dr. R. Mervyn Letts.)

Special Devices

Although there are a multitude of special and custom-made devices and seating orthotic appliances, which are of value in osteogenesis imperfecta, these are beyond the scope of this chapter. Many custom-made devices can be fabricated for the individual patient to assist their activities of daily living and minimize fractures.[17]

Standing frames (Fig. 59-22) can be utilized to permit partial transfer of weight to the lower extremities and yet minimize fractures. This partial weightbearing appears to enhance the ossification process in accordance with Wolff's law.

Vacuum splints (Fig. 59-23) may serve as an alternate form of orthotic devices. These splints are light and can distribute pressure equally, enhancing bone deposition and yet permitting some protected motion.[18]

Eventually, in the older child, specially constructed and adapted protective seating inserts (Fig. 59-24A) and electric-powered wheelchairs (Fig. 59-24B) can be utilized prior to skeletal maturation of bone.

SUMMARY

The management of fractures secondary to osteogenesis imperfecta may be difficult, sometimes frustrating, but usually gratifying if the treatment team persists and limbs can be kept in a functional position until skeletal maturity.[19] The remarkable decrease in bone fragility that occurs at this time will even allow some osteogenesis imperfecta patients to ambulate at this age and all nonambulators will be good electric chair users (Fig. 59-25). The fracture management described in this chapter are techniques I have found to be most successful in dealing with osteogenesis imperfecta children in over 30 years of practice. However, the true future management of this

1102 / Management of Pediatric Fractures

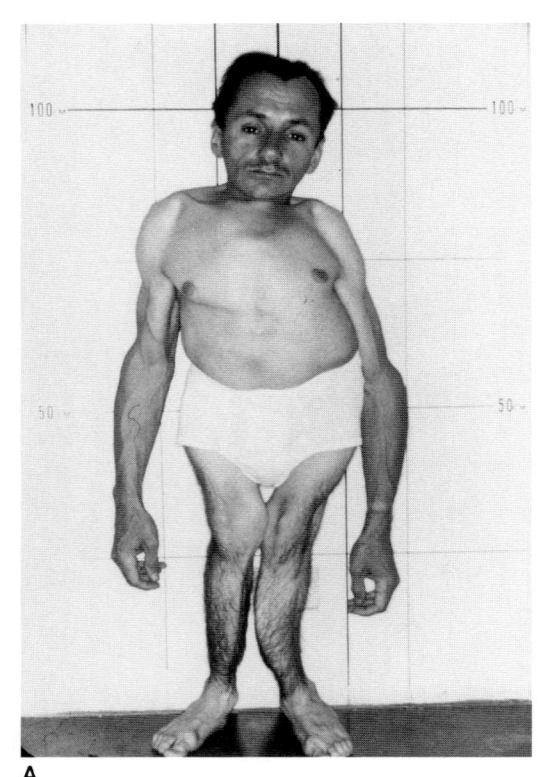

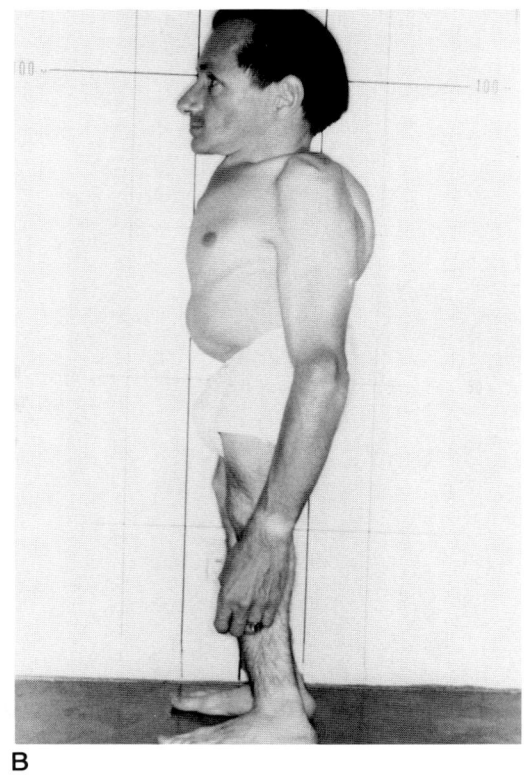

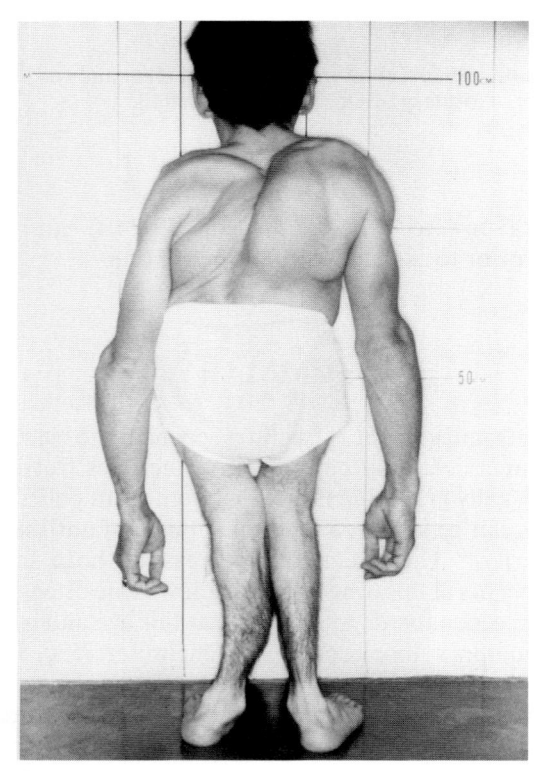

Fig. 59-25. (A–C) Adult patient who had segmental osteotomies as a child. Note asymmetrical growth of limbs and relative shortening of limbs. Note chest and spine deformity. The bones are no longer brittle and he is fully ambulatory. *(Figure continues.)*

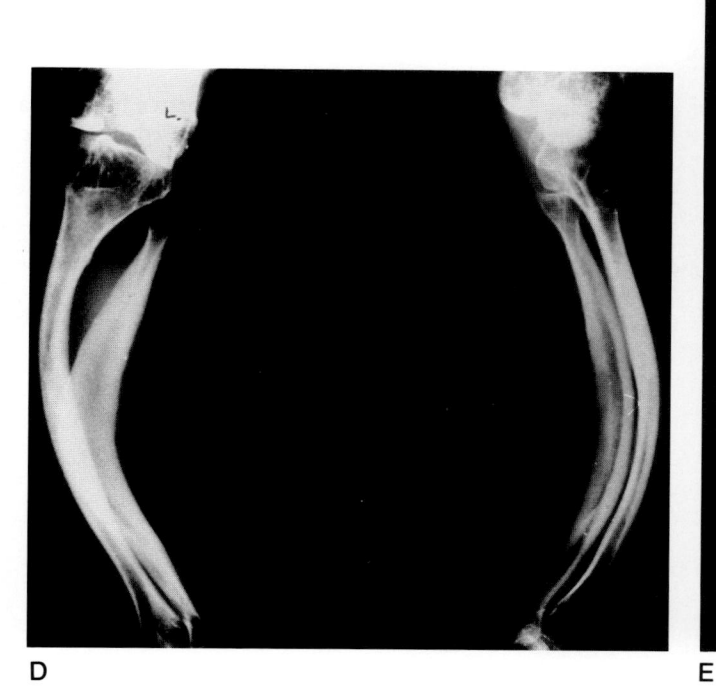

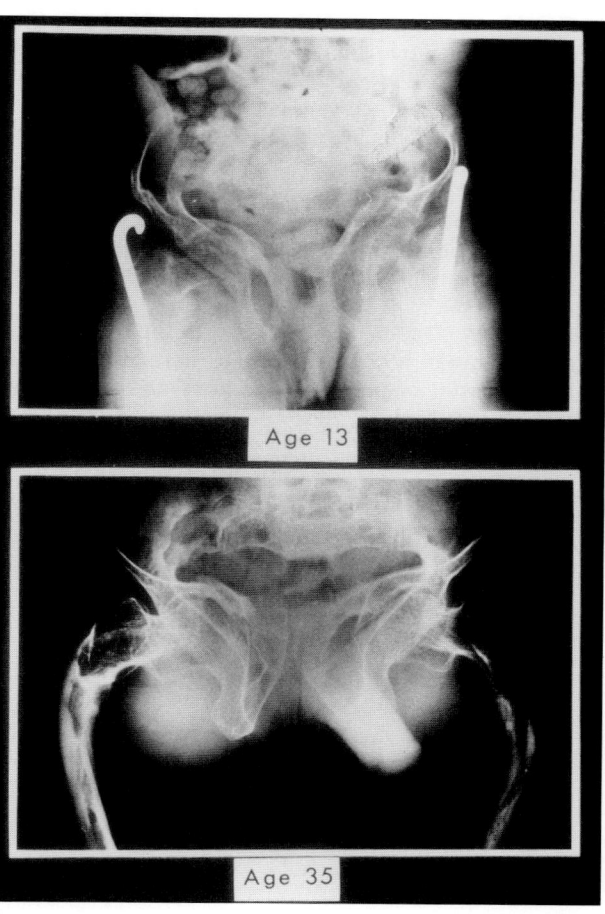

Fig. 59-25 *(Continued).* **(D&E)** The massive hypertrophy that occurs in adult life. Note the thickness of cortices.

fascinating disease process will not remain within the domain of the orthopaedic surgeon, but will be treated primarily by the biochemist or geneticist, who will, in the future, solve the riddle of the malfunction of the ossification process for these children.

REFERENCES

1. Sillence DO: Osteogenesis imperfecta: an expanding panorama of variants. Clin Orthop 159:11, 1981
2. King JD, Bobechko WP: Osteogenesis imperfecta: an orthopaedic description and surgical review. J Bone Joint Surg [Br] 53:71, 1971
3. Cole WG: The orthopaedic and medical treatment of osteogenesis imperfecta. Ann NY Acad Sci 543:157, 1988
4. Stoltz MR, Dietrich SL, Marshall GJ: Osteogenesis imperfecta: perspectives. Clin Orthop 242:1120, 1989
5. Gertner JM, Rott L: Osteogenesis imperfecta. Orthop Clin North Am 21:151, 1990
6. Frasca P, Alman B: Fracture failure mechanisms in patients with osteogenesis imperfecta. J Orthop Res 5:139, 1987
7. McCall RE, Bax JA: Hyperplastic callus formation in osteogenesis imperfecta following intramedullary rodding. J Pediatr Orthop 4:361, 1984
8. Burke TE, Crerand SJ, Dowling F: Hypertrophic callus formation leading to high-output cardiac failure in a patient with osteogenesis imperfecta. J Pediatr Orthop 8:605, 1988
9. Sofield HA, Miller EA: Fragmentation, realignment and intramedullary rod fixation of deformities of the long bones in children; a ten year appraisal. J Bone Joint Surg 41:1371, 1959
10. Dent J, Patternson C: Fractures in early childhood: osteogenesis imperfecta or child abuse? J Pediatr Orthop 11:184, 1991

11. Gamble JG, Strudwick WJ, Rinsky LA, Bleck EE: Complications of intramedullary rods in osteogenesis imperfecta: Bailey-Dubow rods versus non-elongating rods. J Pediatr Orthop 8:645, 1988
12. Lang-Stevenson AI, Sharrard WJW: Intramedullary rodding with Bailey-Dubow extensible rods in osteogenesis imperfecta: an interim report of results and complications. J Bone Joint Surg [Br] 66:227, 1984
13. Porat A: The results of operation in osteogenesis imperfecta: elongating and non-elongating rods. Pediatr Orthop 11:200, 1991
14. Bailey RW, Dubow HI: Evolution of the concept of an extensible nail accommodating to normal longitudinal bone growth: clinical considerations and applications. Clin Orthop 159:157, 1981
15. Hansom DA, Bloom BA: The spine in osteogenesis imperfecta. Orthop Clin North Am 19:2:449, 1988
16. Gamble JG, Rinsky LA, Strudwick J, Bleck EE: Nonunion of fractures in children who have osteogenesis imperfecta. J Bone Joint Surg [Am] 70:439, 1988
17. Letts RM: Seating in osteogenesis imperfecta in principles of seating the disabled. p. 203. CRC Press, Baton Rouge, FL, 1991
18. Letts RM, Monson R, Weber K: The prevention of recurrent fractures of the lower extremities in severe osteogenesis imperfecta using vacuum pants. J Pediatr Orthop 8:605, 1988
19. Shapiro F: Consequences of an osteogenesis imperfecta diagnosis for survival and ambulation. J Pediatr Orthop 5:456, 1985

60

Fractures in the Severely Handicapped Child

Dennis Lyne
Bernard A. Roehr

> O, then how quickly should this arm of mine now prisoner to the palsy, chastise thee.
> —William Shakespeare, Richard II

DESCRIPTION AND INCIDENCE

Children and young adults with multiple handicaps comprise a unique group of patients with respect to the diagnosis and management of pediatric fractures. They are susceptible to the development of pathologic fractures for a number of reasons, including poor bone quality, limb and joint deformity, and the lack of normal protective mechanisms.[1,2] The magnitude of the problem is such that the single most costly medical problem for the institutionalized seizure patient may be the treatment of pathologic fractures resulting from demineralized bone.[3]

Children and young adults with severe physical handicaps resulting in minimal ambulatory skills, mental deficiencies, and minimal self-care and feeding skills represent a large group of patients who are not well studied in the pediatric fracture literature. Reviews in large populations of severely physically and mentally handicapped institutionalized patients seem to indicate an incidence of fractures in the range of 1 percent.[2] In a review that we conducted during a 4-year period from 1985 to 1988 we found 19 patients with 32 fractures in a group of severely handicapped children numbering greater than 1,000 (Fig. 60-1).

ANATOMY

While all types of fractures peculiar to the pediatric population can be seen in the severely handicapped child, there seems to be a propensity of fractures in the lower extremities.[1] The majority of these occur in the femur and about the knee (Fig. 60-2). There seems to be a smaller group of patients with the more common physeal injuries seen in the normal child. In most patients with single fractures there is a significant traumatic episode such as a fall or forceful manipulation during therapy.

A special group for consideration is the patient who sustains multiple fractures either simultaneously or over a period of time. The history in these children is frequently more vague and the traumatic event less significant. History such as turning in bed, being transferred from bed to wheelchair, and waking up crying are fre-

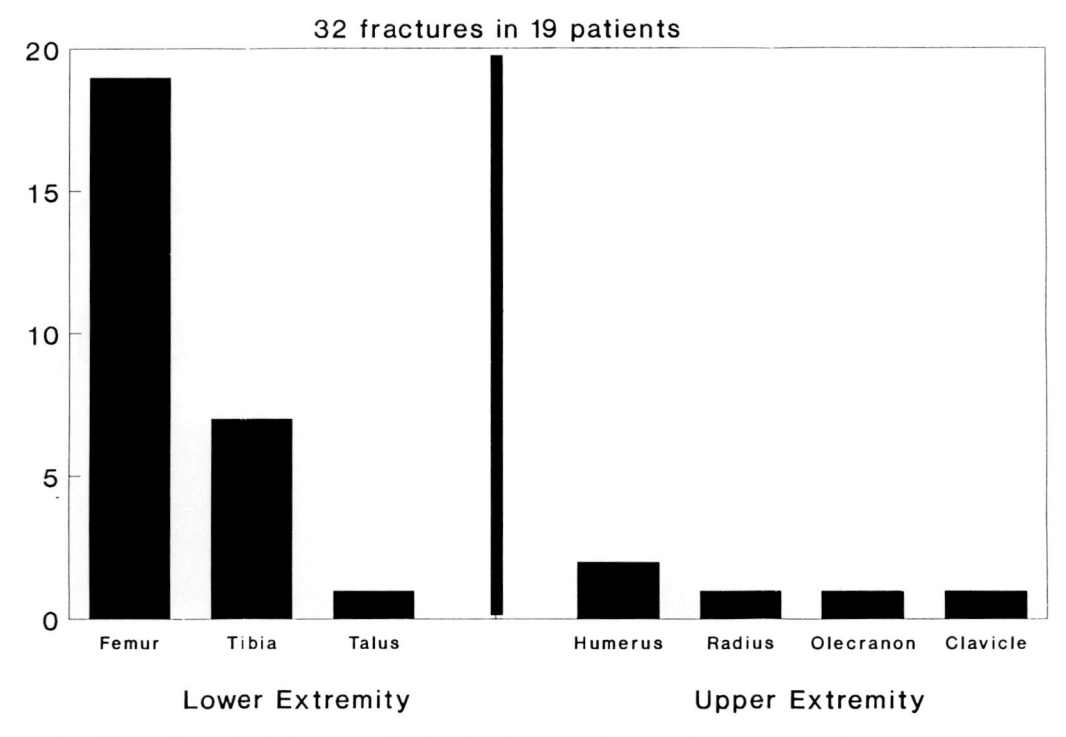

Fig. 60-1. Pathologic fracture distribution in a population of severely handicapped children.

MECHANISM OF INJURY

Usually the precise mechanism of injury is undetermined, as was the case in 70 of 134 fractures seen by McIvor and Samilson.[2] When a reliable history is obtained, the fractures frequently have occurred as a result of a fall or a direct blow such as striking the side rail of a bed. Many of the falls are associated with seizures. Fractures can also occur during bathing and radiographic examinations, or catching a limb in the siderails of a crib or door. Fractures may occur as a result of orthopaedic operations, through bone graft donor sites or as a result of stress risers created by orthopaedic implants or spica casts (Fig. 60-3). A distal femoral traction pin placed after femoral head resection can create sufficient cortical weakness to cause a supracondylar femur fracture.[1] Aggressive manipulation for contractures in therapy can cause fractures in both the upper and lower extremities.

quently noted and should lead the orthopaedic physician to consider investigating potential nutritional deficiencies.

As with the normal pediatric population, child abuse must always be considered when evaluating the multiple handicapped child with a fracture. Unfortunately, there is very little information on the subject, and, due to difficulty in documentation, these suspicions rarely lead to legal action.

CLASSIFICATION

Existing classification schemes for pediatric fractures apply in this group of patients but are not as helpful in planning treatment or predicting outcome as they are in the normal child. Perhaps more useful would be distinguishing between patients who sustain single fractures from a traumatic episode and patients who sustain multiple fractures for a pathologic reason.

We have found that fractures in severely handicapped children frequently occur because of poor bone quality. This has been attributed to a number of causes, including disuse due to minimal or nonambulatory status, nutritional deficiencies, and interference with normal bone

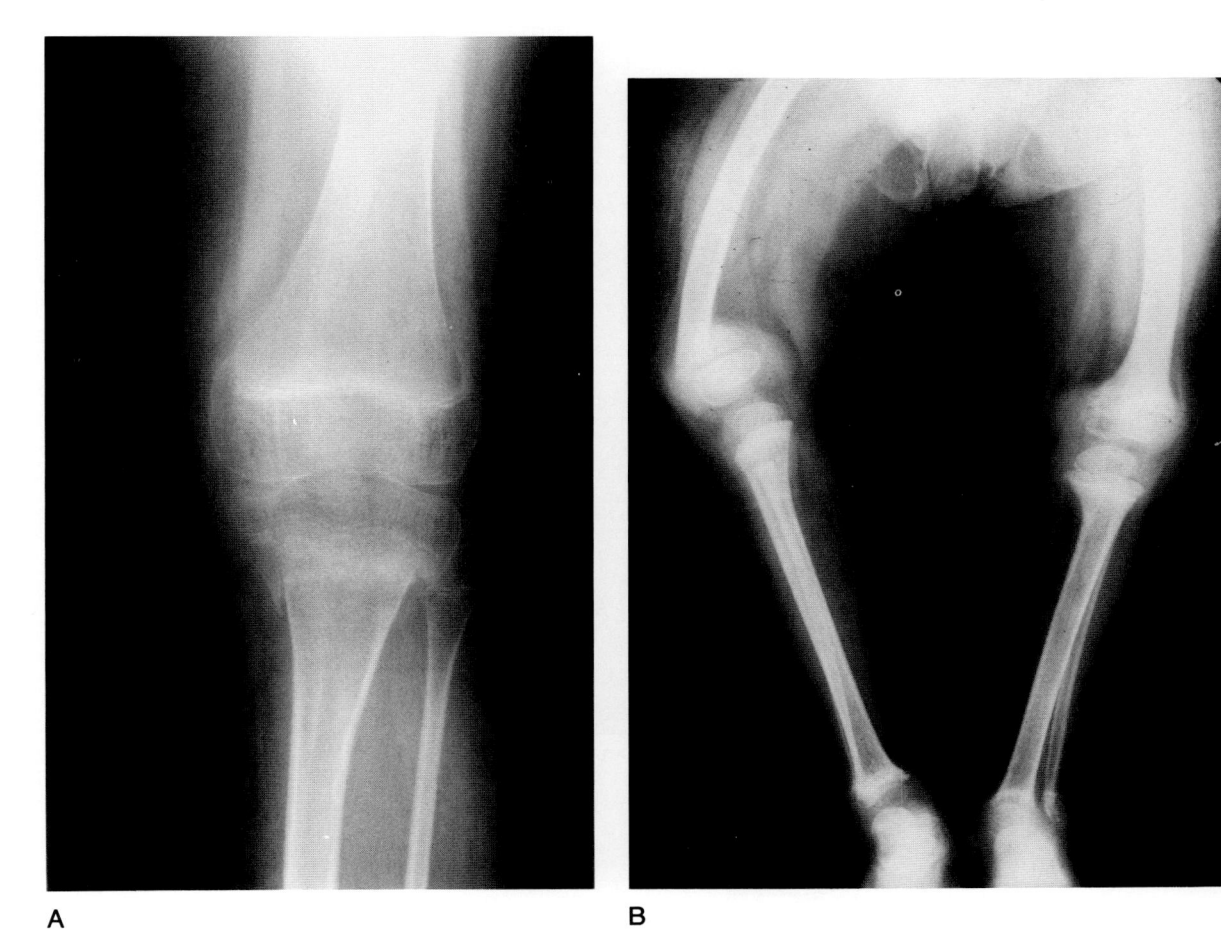

Fig. 60-2. **(A)** Typical radiographic appearance of a pathologic fracture of the left proximal tibial shaft in a 13-year-old boy with spastic quadriplegia. **(B)** A right distal fracture of the femur in a 7-year-old child on Dilantin for a seizure disorder.

mineral metabolism by drugs such as anticonvulsants and antacids.

The physiology of vitamin D was summarized by Mankin.[4] Vitamin D is derived from exogenous sources (ergosterol) and 7-dehydrocholesterol from cholesterol stored in the skin. These steroids undergo conversion by ultraviolet light to calciferol (D_2) and cholecalciferol (D_3); D_2 and D_3 first undergo hepatic conversion to 25-hydrocholecalciferol (25-OHD) and then renal conversion to 1,25-dihydrocholecalciferol (1,25-OH2D), the most biologically active form of vitamin D. The actions of vitamin D include increasing active calcium absorption from the gut, mobilization from bone, and reabsorption from the renal tubules.

Anticonvulsants alter vitamin D metabolism by induction of the hepatic microsomal mixed-function oxidase enzyme, which catabolizes 25-OHD and 1,25-OH2D to inactive metabolites. Some antacids may also block absorption of metabolites and thus induce rickets.

In addition to evaluating patients for the mechanism of injury, patients should be evaluated for dietary history. Frequently, dietary intake is found to be deficient. Patients should be evaluated with a biochemical profile; SMAC 21, and serum vitamin D levels, including 25-OHD and 1,25-OH2D. Calcium, phosphate, and alkaline phosphatase levels are not often useful in determining metabolic bone disease in this population but 25-OHD as a measure of body stores of vitamin D is very useful. 1,25-OH2D levels are unreliable because they can be normal, even though 25-OHD stores are significantly depleted. Interestingly, radiographic features of rickets such as widened physes are often not seen as the

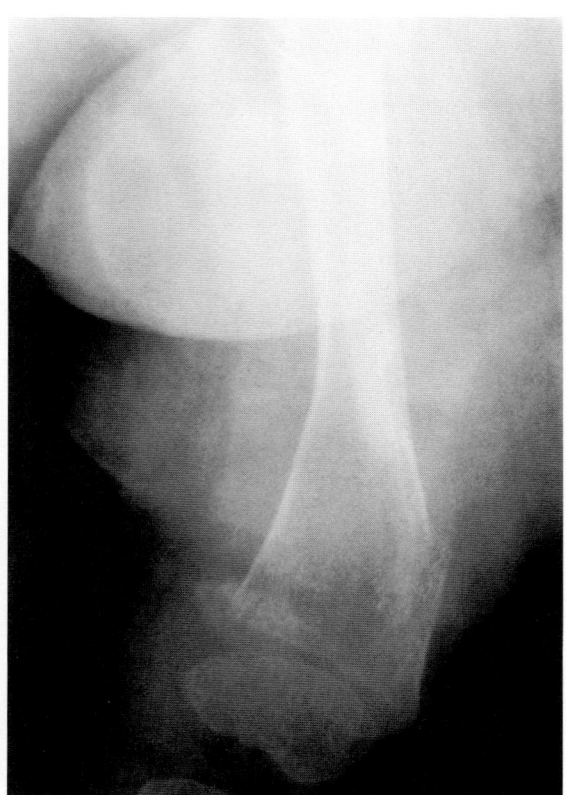

Fig. 60-3. (A) Subtrochanteric femur fracture in a 5-month-old spastic infant as a result of routine nursing care, after bilateral adductor tenotomies. The fracture was identified by the presence of redness, warmth, and swelling distal to an abduction orthosis in which the child was immobilized postoperatively. (B) The subtrochanteric fracture healed promptly with immobilization in a well-padded plaster splint and considerable remodeling has occurred at 3 months. This is typical of such fractures in severely handicapped osteoporotic children. (C) A skeletal survey revealed an ipsolateral supracondylar femoral fracture as well, most probably as a result of the stress riser created by the orthosis.

child is not growing due to the severely deficient nutritional state.

PHYSICAL EXAMINATION

The diagnosis of these fractures is frequently delayed because many of these children are unable to communicate effectively.[5] Physical findings play an important role in the diagnosis because the history is often either not available or quite vague. These physical findings include a range of symptoms from sudden change in personality to the typical swelling, redness, tenderness, and deformity of the fractured limb. Often pain can be reliably elicited upon gentle palpation of the long bones. Frequently these patients are referred with an incorrect diagnosis, because the redness, warmth, and swelling of a fracture hematoma can easily be confused with the clinical presentation of osteomyelitis and septic arthritis. If a fracture is not found on the initial radiographic examination, these entities need to be excluded in the usual manner and follow-up radiographs may be indicated. Bone tumors must also be kept in mind when evaluating these patients.

TREATMENT INDICATIONS

Closed Methods

Most fractures in the severely handicapped child can be treated by simple closed methods. It is important to try to maintain the overall alignment of the limb, but the treatment needs to be modified based on the individual patient's deformities and prefracture functional status. Shortening and angular deformities considered unacceptable in normal children can be accepted in the multiple-handicapped patient provided gross malunions that could affect patient seating and care are avoided.

Most fractures can be immobilized in well-padded plaster casts or splints. Treatment in plaster carries a significant risk of complications in this group of patients because of the high risk of skin ulcerations beneath the cast as well as stress risers created above and below the casts. For this reason well-padded splints, removed frequently for inspection of the underlying skin, are preferable.

The management of femoral shaft fractures can be problematic. Fractures of the femur can be treated by resting the involved lower extremity between pillows without traction or other immobilization.[5] Treatment of femoral shaft fractures with skeletal traction results in frequent complications with sacral decubiti and problems with the traction pin itself. Skin traction can be difficult because of skin fragility and low patient weight. Union occurs promptly and usually with abundant callous formation because even in nutritionally deficient patients necessary minerals are removed from the rest of the skeleton until body stores are virtually depleted.

Open Methods

Indications for open reduction and internal fixation in this population are quite rare and surgery is usually reserved for fractures about the hip.[2] Internal fixation can be considered in patients with severe acute or chronic spasticity who display unacceptable functional deformity despite closed treatment methods. Surgical intervention is fraught with complications because of the poor bone quality leading to loss of fixation and stress risers created about surgical implants.

Pitfalls to Avoid

Decubiti Ulcerations

The use of well-padded splints with frequent inspection of the underlying skin is important to avoid decubiti ulceration. It is important to be aggressive in turning the patients to avoid skin breakdown over the sacrum. Other areas of concern include the medial femoral condyle and the heel when dealing with femoral shaft fractures immobilized in plaster. In fractures with considerable deformity, it is not unusual for a closed fracture to develop an ulcer over the apex of the fracture angulation and become an open fracture. In these situations the open wound can be managed by debridement and dressing changes until fracture union, followed by definitive skin closure after the fracture has healed.[5] These wounds frequently appear 10 to 14 days after the fracture and are predicted by a visible and palpable prominence of a bony spike associated with a gradual discoloration and breakdown of the overlying skin.

Multiple Fractures

In the group of patients who sustain multiple fractures, it is important to treat the underlying cause, which is frequently vitamin D abnormalities. If these are discovered on the screening tests outlined, a therapeutic protocol consisting of nutritional supplementation and

TABLE 60-1. Treatment Protocol

1. Increased sunlight exposure (1–2 h/day)
2. Vitamin D
   A. Replacement: 25-OHD 20 µg/day
   B. Maintenance: vitamin D 1,000 U/day
3. Calcium 1,000–1,500 mg/day

maintenance therapy, calcium supplementation and increased sunlight exposure is instituted (Table 60-1). Response to treatment can be measured by monitoring serial 25-OHD levels and radiographic examinations. Results of this treatment are good, restoring calcium, phosphate and vitamin D levels to normal in most patients in 4 to 8 weeks. Most notable is the decreased incidence of multiple fractures, which did not recur in any of our patients at a mean follow-up of 1 year.[1]

COMPLICATIONS

In addition to the complications already outlined, these patients are susceptible to the same risks of the individual fractures as normal children, including neurologic and vascular injury. The two biggest complications to avoid are those of ulcerations and refracture, as outlined above.

Children and young adults with multiple handicaps are subject to a variety of medical problems that can complicate both the surgical and nonsurgical treatment of fractures. A multidisciplinary approach, including pediatric subspecialists, is useful to help identify and avoid difficulties such as ventriculoperitoneal shunt malfunction, pulmonary compromise, and aspiration. Special attention should be given to the management of gastroesophageal reflux, as this is a common condition in this population. In addition to the antecedent risks posed by general anesthesia, closed treatment, which prevents mobilization to a sitting position, can lead to aspiration pneumonitis.

SUMMARY

1. Sudden personality changes, such as crying, often indicates bony injury and should be investigated.
2. Careful examination of the extremities for swelling and tenderness should be performed, including gentle palpation of the long bones.
3. Short-term immobilization may be appropriate when a fracture is suspected clinically and initial radiographs are negative.
4. A thorough metabolic evaluation should be performed, especially in patients with a history of multiple fractures.
5. Appropriate decisions for treatment are based on the child's function and general medical condition.
6. Child abuse should be considered in certain circumstances, especially in light of repeated fractures without evidence of metabolic disease.

REFERENCES

1. Lee JJK, Lyne ED: Pathologic fractures in severely handicapped children and young adults. J Pediatr Orthop 10:497, 1990
2. McIvor WC, Samilson RL: Fractures in patients with cerebral palsy. J Bone Joint Surg [Am] 48:858, 1966
3. Tolman KG, Jubiz W, Sannella JJ, Madsen JA: Osteomalacia associated with anticonvulsant therapy in mentally retarded children. Pediatrics 56:45, 1975
4. Mankin JH: Rickets, osteomalacia, and renal osteodystrophy. Part I. J Bone Joint Surg [Am] 56:101, 1974
5. Miller PR, Galzer DA: Spontaneous fractures in the brain-crippled, bedridden patients. Clin Orthop Rel Res 120:134, 1976

61

Complications in Children's Fractures

R. Dale Blasier

You always regret the most the things you didn't do.

While most children's fractures have an excellent prognosis for healing and full return to function, some complications can be expected to occur. Complications can occur due to the nature of the fracture itself, the presence of associated injuries, delayed or improper treatment, infection, inadequate rehabilitation, psychologic factors, or even just plain bad luck.

Complications are best managed by avoidance. A constant vigil must be kept for potential complications and treatment must be instituted immediately to minimize ill effects.

If a complication is expected, or even possible, the child and family must be warned in advance. A few words of explanation beforehand will prevent a great deal of explanation afterward.

MALUNION

Basic Principles

Malunion may occur in any displaced fracture. Malunions tend to be a less frequent problem in children than in adults due to the child's capacity for remodeling. There are limitations, however, in how much correction of deformity can occur with growth. Good prognostic factors for remodeling include young age, small distance from the physis to the fracture, and a small amount of angulation (Table 61-1). Remodeling in children with 2 or more years of growth remaining, in fractures near the end of the bone and with the deformity in the plane of movement of the joint[1] is usually excellent. A poor prognosis for remodeling is noted in children older than 10 years, proximal fractures, especially in the forearm with rotational deformity, and a loss of the forearm radial bow.[2] Varus or valgus angulation will not usually correct completely, although radial forearm deviation has been noted to remodel almost as well as volar angulation if there are at least 2 years of growth remaining.[3] Rotational correction occurs to a minor degree, but this is usually less than 10 degrees.[4]

There are many problems that can occur as a result of malunion. Of concern to the family is the cosmetic appearance. There may be a peculiar bump in a highly visible area, such as in a malunion of a clavicle (Fig. 61-1). An abnormal limb positioning with cubitus varus or an unsightly asymmetry of the lower extremities in malunion of the femur or tibia is disconcerting.

Of major importance is any functional deficit that occurs as a result of malunion. For example, a unilateral external rotation gait may occur after rotational tibial malunion. Mechanical impingement can result from malunion of the proximal humerus, which limits glenohumeral abduction. Tibial valgus can cause the child to

TABLE 61-1. Good Prognosis for Remodeling

Young age (< 10 years)
Angulation close to physis
Physis is fast growing
Small amount of angulation
Angulation in plane of joint motion

become knockkneed, causing impingement during swingthrough. There is a significant potential for late degeneration of joints as a result of limb malalignment. Hemijoint overload of the knee can occur after varus or valgus deformity of the lower extremity. This may lead to pain or degenerative arthritis in some cases.

Several specific malunions tend to be poorly tolerated cosmetically or functionally. These include distal humeral varus deformity, femoral varus deformity, tibial valgus deformity, loss of radial forearm bow, and angulation of radius or ulna which limits rotation.[5,6]

Numerous factors can lead to malunion. These include unstable fracture patterns which tend to displace in spite of closed reduction. Inadequate patient follow-up or failure to return after initiation of fracture treatment predisposes to malunion. Malposition may be seen on radiographs but not corrected. Finally, a fracture may be malpositioned but the remodeling expected by the treating physician does not occur. A rare cause of malunion is the missed and untreated injury in the polytrauma patient.

Treatment Principles

Obviously the best treatment for malunion is prevention. However, in the established case, a definite treatment regimen must be planned. Treatment options include waiting if the fracture has a good prognosis for remodeling. If the fracture has a poor prognosis for remodeling it may be appropriate to go ahead and correct the malunion. The anteroposterior and lateral radiographic angulation of the fracture must be assessed. Comparison should be made with the normal contralateral limb radiograph. Rotational malunion is best determined by clinical examination. The appearance of the limb, the overall alignment of the limb, any obvious asymmetry, and the presence of a bump or protrusion should be assessed. The patient's functional deficit must be carefully determined. This includes loss of motion,

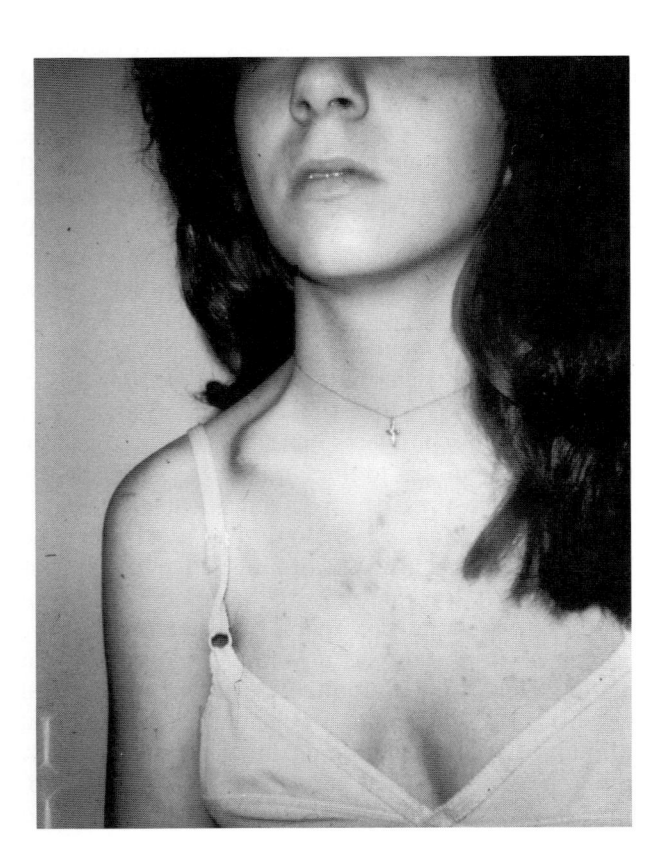

Fig. 61-1. Malunion. A 13-year-old girl had overriding of fracture of the clavicle. It went on to heal solidly, but left her with considerable deformity at the base of the neck. (Courtesy of Dr. R. Mervyn Letts.)

pain with use, and the potential for future adjacent joint degeneration. The concerns of the child and family must be considered. It is important to discuss with the family the exchange of a deformity for a scar. The family must also understand that there will be a cost in terms of hospitalization, recuperation, and possible repeat surgeries for removal of internal fixation devices (Table 61-2).

The treatment options must also be discussed with the child and the family. One option is to continue observation and allow more time for remodeling to occur. In many malunions, particularly in the forearm, the child may be completely asymptomatic.[7,8] If there are no perceived complaints and if the angulation is not severe, no treatment is indicated other than reassurance. Awaiting remodeling (Fig. 61-2) is practical if the fracture occurred near the end of a long bone, is in the plane of joint motion, and the child has considerable growth remaining. Adequate radiographs must be obtained to accurately document the magnitude of the angulation especially if an osteotomy is being planned (Fig. 61-2B). A drill osteoclasis with remanipulation and casting[9] has the advantage of not requiring an extensive surgical exposure, but does not necessitate an anesthetic and a period of casting. A formal osteotomy with internal fixation will require a second surgery for hardware removal (Fig. 61-3). There must be full consultation with the family and the older child regarding risks and benefits before this is undertaken. It is important to consider the deformity in three dimensions and assess rotation prior to the osteotomy. Gradual correction of the deformity by use of corticotomy and the techniques of Ilizarov may be appropriate if there is associated limb shortening.

In summary, the best means of dealing with malunion is prevention. Attention to detail and reasonable expectations for remodeling will be helpful in preventing deformity persisting into adulthood. When loss of bony alignment is observed on radiographs, specific and aggressive measures should be taken to obtain correction. It is sometimes difficult for the surgeon to explain to the family in the midst of treatment that an operation is necessary to correct a malunion, however it may be preferable and easier to accomplish at this time. It may be appropriate to warn the family early in the treatment that remanipulation or operation may be required in the treatment of unstable fractures. This will improve the understanding of the family should such treatment then be necessary. In established malunion, the use of well-described techniques for osteotomy or corticotomy will be helpful in obtaining the desired limb alignment.

Care should be exercised in malunions involving the growth plate to avoid physeal damage. It is preferable to allow healing to occur. If it is felt to be remodeling, and further growth will not correct the malunion, a metaphyseal osteotomy can be performed at a later date.

NONUNION

Fracture nonunion is very uncommon in children. If nonunion is encountered in the long bone of a child, it must be differentiated from congenital pseudarthrosis, especially in the tibia, fibula, and ulna.

Children's diaphyseal fractures are particularly resistant to nonunion due to the open physis[10] and very osteogenic periosteum.[11] Impediments to normal fracture healing are usually the cause of nonunion, such as soft tissue interposition,[11] infection after open procedure,[12] high-energy trauma, open fracture, soft tissue loss, inadequate fixation, fracture distraction, repeated manipulations, or marked fracture displacement[10] (Fig. 61-4; Table 61-3).

Articular fractures are more prone to nonunion than are shaft fractures in children. Probable causes include interposed periosteum,[11] circulatory insufficiency,[13] inhibition of callus and fibrin formation by joint fluid,[14] constant tensile forces,[15] displacement resulting in loss of bony continuity or rotation of the fragment to appose the articular surface to the metaphysis,[15] and excessive shearing force.[16] Nonunion of an intra-articular fracture is a serious malformation. It may be associated with pain, instability, or loss of motion.

The most common sites for intra-articular nonunion in children are the carpal scaphoid, the lateral humeral condyle, the radial neck, the femoral neck, and the medial malleolus.

TABLE 61-2. Factors in Decision-Making to Correct Malunion in a Child

Size of angular deformity
Cosmesis
Functional concerns
Family concerns
Pain
Potential joint degeneration
Scar formation
Repeat surgery for hardware removal
Surgical complications
Cost

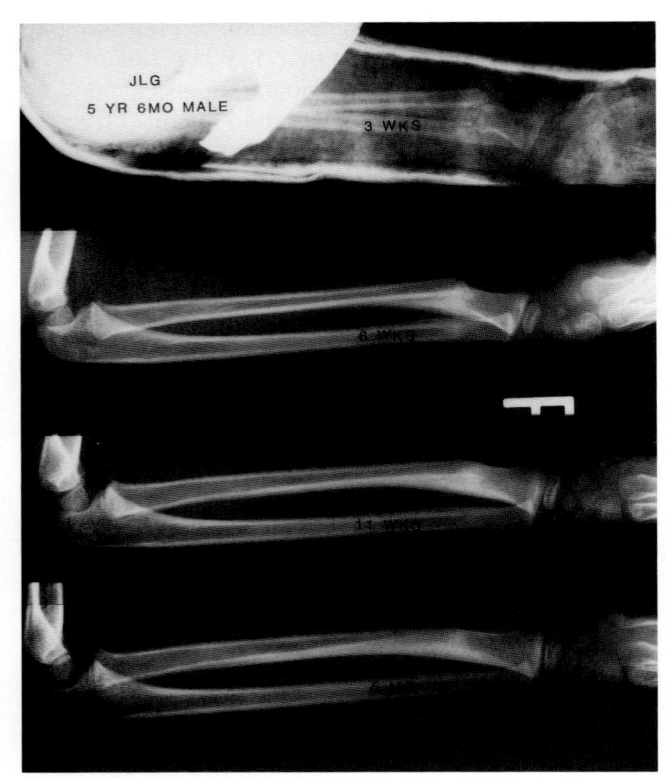

Fig. 61-2. **(A)** Remodeling. A 5-and-a-half-year-old boy sustained a displaced fracture of the distal radius and ulna. Due to inadequate follow-up, the fracture has consolidated in a malunited position at 3 weeks. At 6 weeks, new callus formation is seen on the concavity of the deformity. At 11 weeks, there is considerable remodeling. At 5 months, near normal alignment of the bone is seen. **(B)** Same ulnar fracture rotated several degrees prior to each film. Slight degrees of rotation "change" the apparent magnitude of the angulation. (Fig B from Pitt D, and Spears D. Radiologic reporting of skeletal trauma. Rad Clin N A 28:247 1990, with permission.)

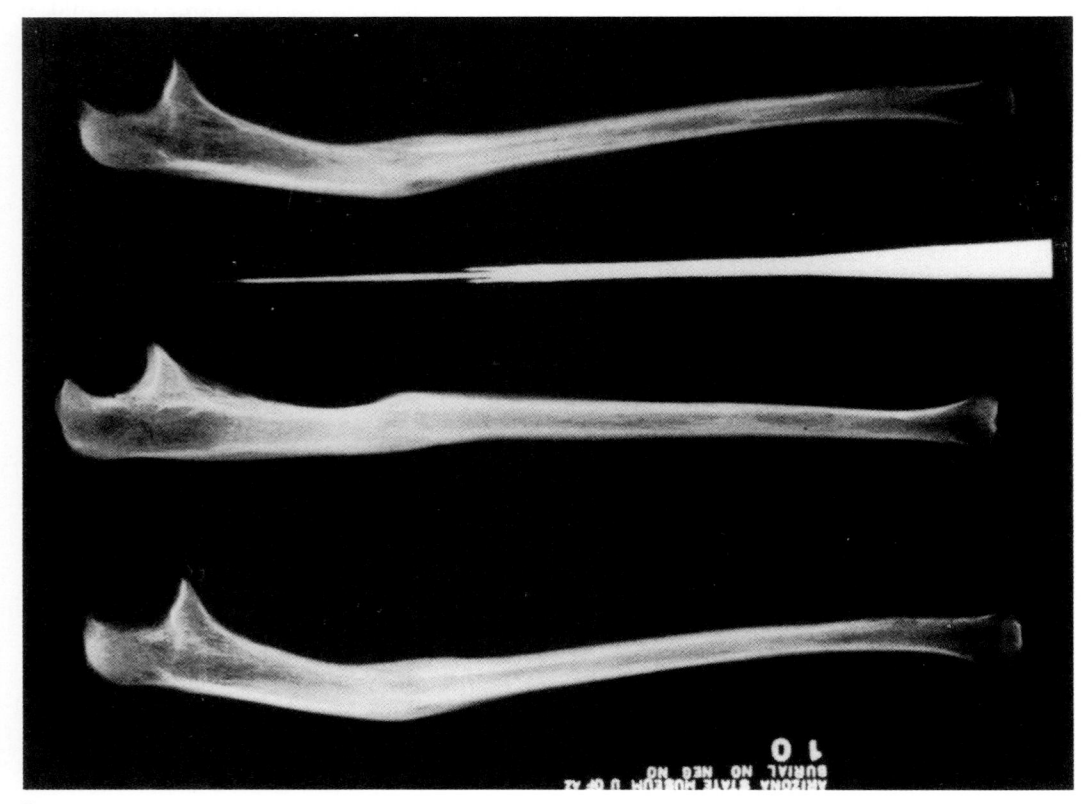

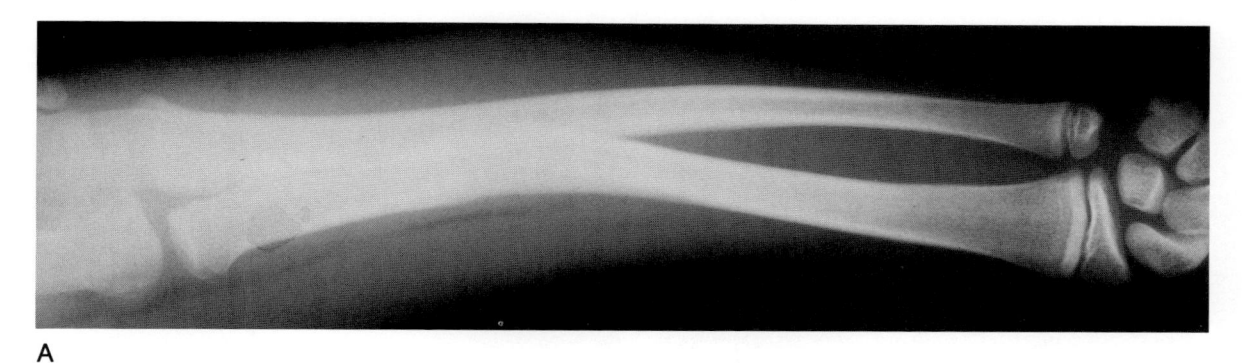

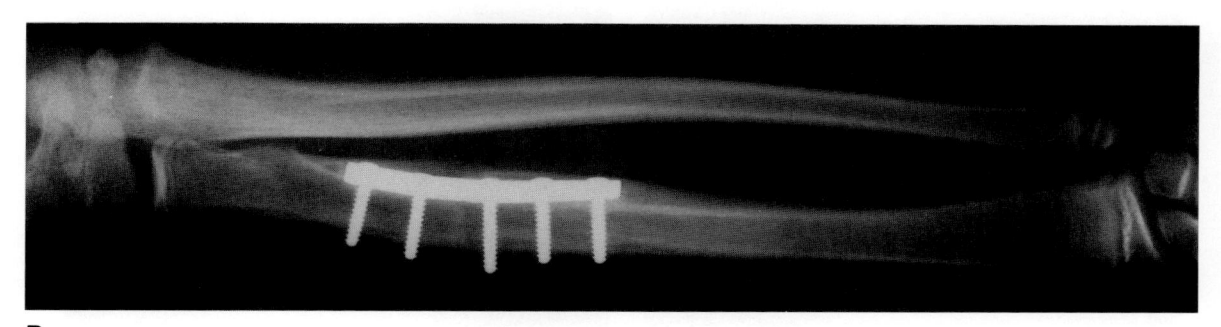

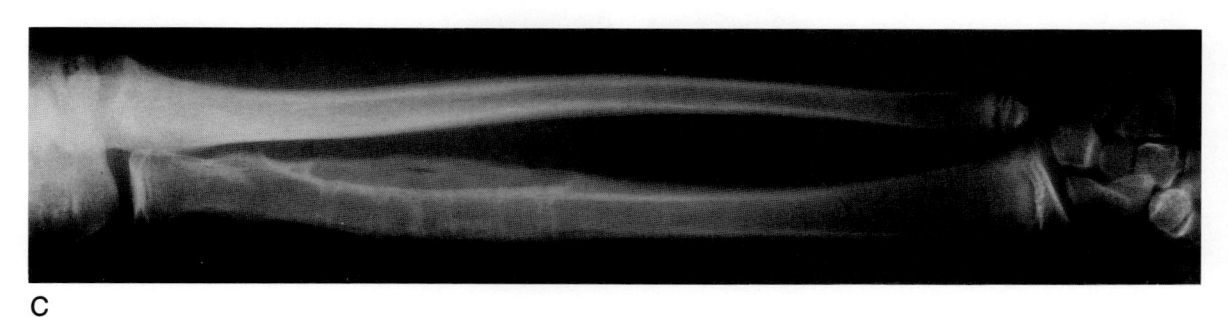

Fig. 61-3. Malunion requiring osteotomy. **(A)** This child had a malunion of proximal radius fracture which severely limited pronation. **(B)** Osteotomy with plate fixation improved function. **(C)** Result after plate removal.

The best method to treat nonunion of the child's fracture is prevention. Practical techniques include: (1) elimination of interposed tissue between bone ends by open reduction with coaptation of bone ends, (2) secure fixation of fracture fragments for an adequate duration of healing, (3) prevention of infection, and (4) ensuring soft tissue coverage.

Treatment of established nonunion includes eliminating pathologic causes such as congenital pseudarthrosis (Fig. 61-5). If it is clear that the benefits of union outweigh the morbidity, then surgery to include a combination of open reduction, resection of pseudarthrosis, internal fixation, and bone grafting is indicated.

Compression applied through external circular ring fixators has been effective in healing hypertrophic nonunion. Circular fixation may be combined with distraction histogenesis in cases of nonunion with bone loss, shortening or deformity[17,18] (Fig. 61-6).

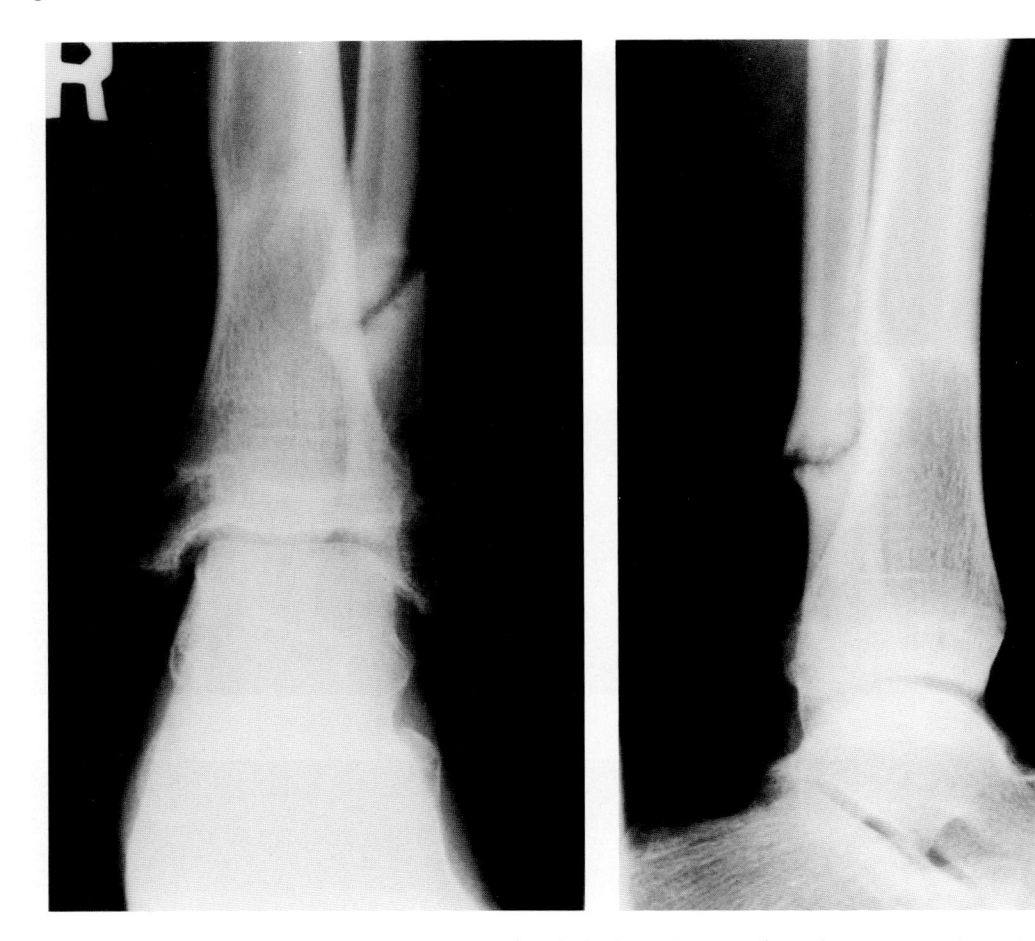

Fig. 61-4. Nonunion. A 16-year-old who previously had no abnormality prior to sustaining a fracture of the fibula. Fibular nonunion occurred in spite of adequate immobilization. (Courtesy of Dr. R. Mervyn Letts.)

TABLE 61-3. Causes of Delayed and Nonunion in Children

Soft tissue interposition
Infection
High-energy injury
Open fracture
Soft tissue loss
Inadequate immobilization
Fracture distraction
Repetitive manipulations
Marked fracture displacement
Intra-articular location
Circulatory insufficiency
Tensile forces
Shearing forces

PREMATURE PHYSEAL GROWTH ARREST

Growth arrest is known to occur after injury to the growth plate of long bones. Arrest may result in limb length discrepancy, disparate growth between parallel bones such as radius and ulna, and angulatory deformity if the physis is involved asymmetrically. Growth arrest may occur other than in long bones such as in fractures of the acetabulum with damage to the triradiate cartilage leading to acetabular growth disturbance.[19]

Growth arrest or slowdown may result from any one of several mechanisms after trauma. There may be direct damage to the epiphyseal plate due to dislocation or surgery.[20] Burns or electrical injuries may disturb growth. Excessive compression across a growth plate may cause growth retardation.[21] Prolonged immobiliza-

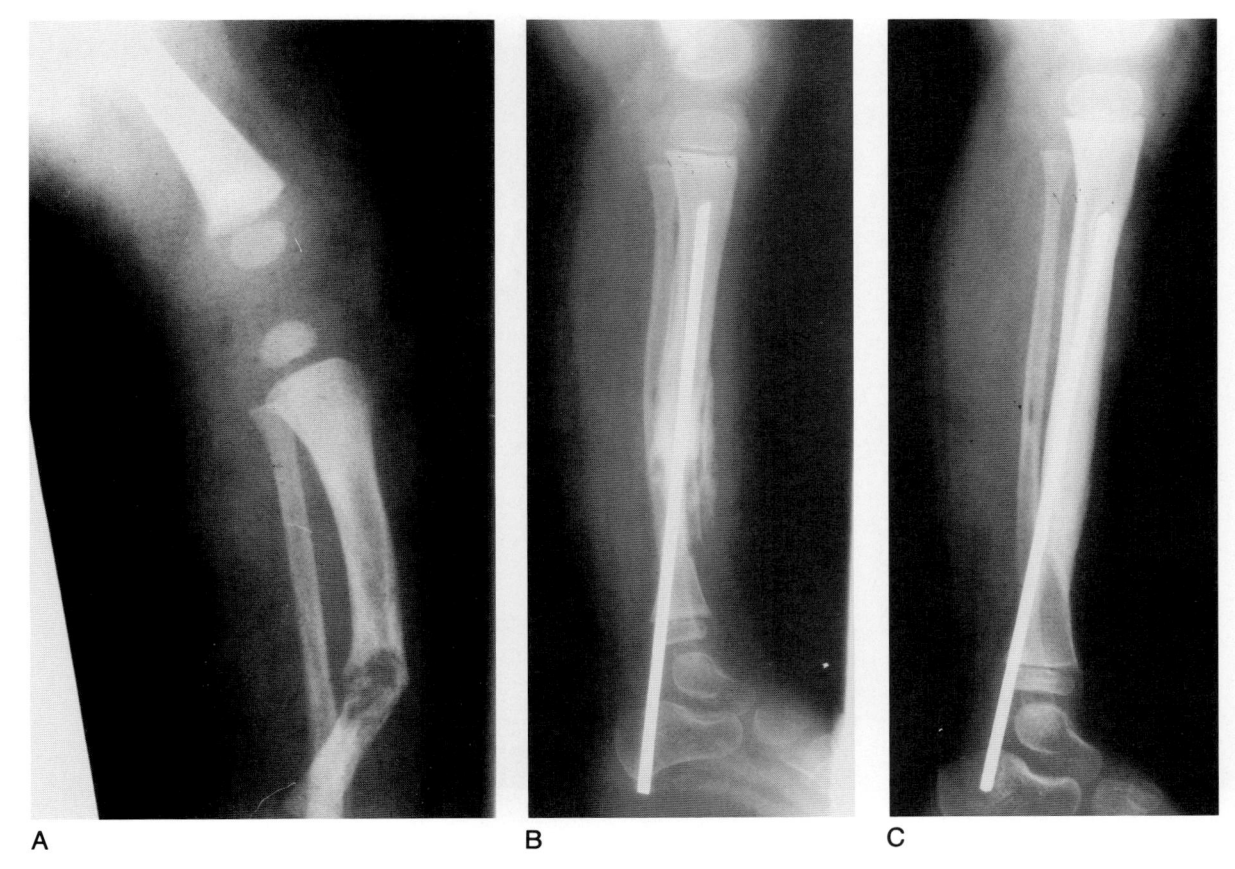

Fig. 61-5. Pseudarthrosis. Congenital pseudarthrosis must be considered in evaluating any child with nonunion. (A) A 1½-year-old child with pseudarthrosis of the tibia. (B) Closed reduction and intramedullary fixation using the Charnley technique. The rod was changed three times. (C) Pseudarthrosis consolidated with minimal leg length discrepancy at age 7 years. (Courtesy of Dr. R. Mervyn Letts.)

tion of the extremity may also slow growth.[20] Contiguous metaphyseal osteomyelitis may cause growth arrest.[20]

Mechanical damage to the growth plate is felt to result from one of two mechanisms: (1) the epiphyseal blood supply may be disrupted, and (2) there may be transverse and horizontal fissuring of the physis.[22] Mechanical damage to the growth plate can occur due to the injury itself or as a result of attempts to reduce the fracture.[22]

Common locations for growth derangement after fracture include the distal femur,[22] proximal tibia,[23] distal tibia, and distal radius,[24] although almost any physis may be involved. Physeal arrest may occur in long bones even in association with nonphyseal fractures.[23,25] The exact mechanism is unclear (Fig. 61-7).

Numerous mechanisms have been proposed for growth derangement after trauma. Compression injury to the physis may occur (Fig. 61-8). The perichondral ring may be injured,[23] allowing an osseous bridge to form at the periphery of the epiphysis.[26] The physis may be injured in such a way that the epiphyseal circulation with its osteoprogenitor cells comes into contact with the metaphyseal circulation resulting in formation of an osseous bridge.

In selected cases early intervention may be effective in preventing growth tethering or arrest. When there is compression damage to the physis, it is not likely that operative intervention can restore growth potential. The perichondral ring may be replaced if the avulsed tissue is not destroyed or lost.[27] The incidence of cross-healing between epiphysis and metaphysis can be decreased by anatomically reducing and fixing displaced Salter-Harris types III and IV injuries (Fig. 61-9).

After injury, the earliest sign of bony bridging may be a converging Harris line.[26] Complete growth arrest manifests as narrowing and then obliteration of the cartilagi-

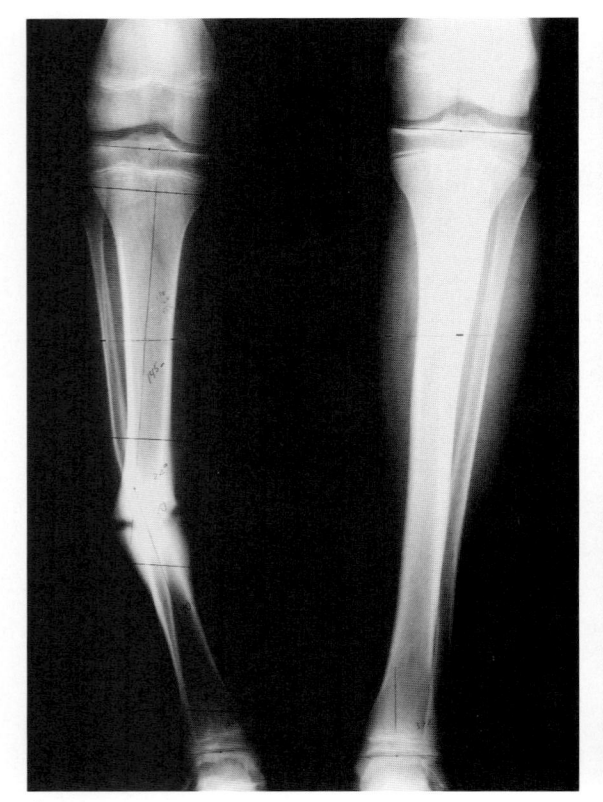

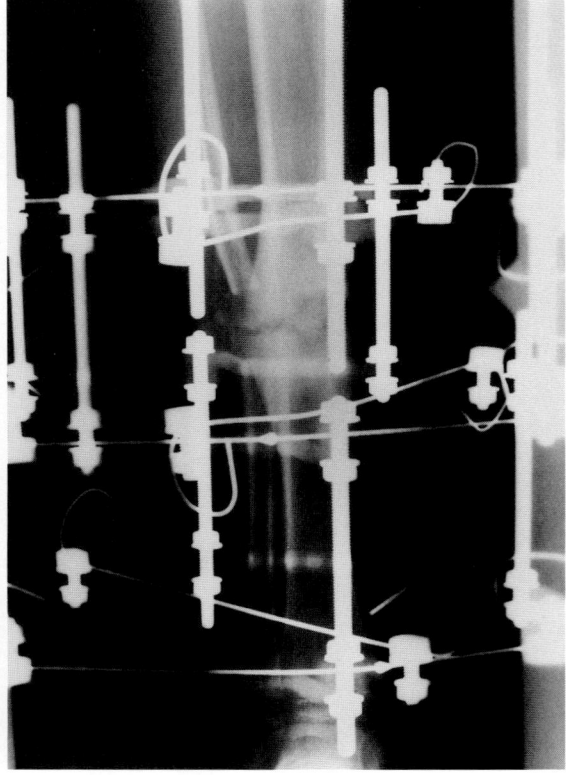

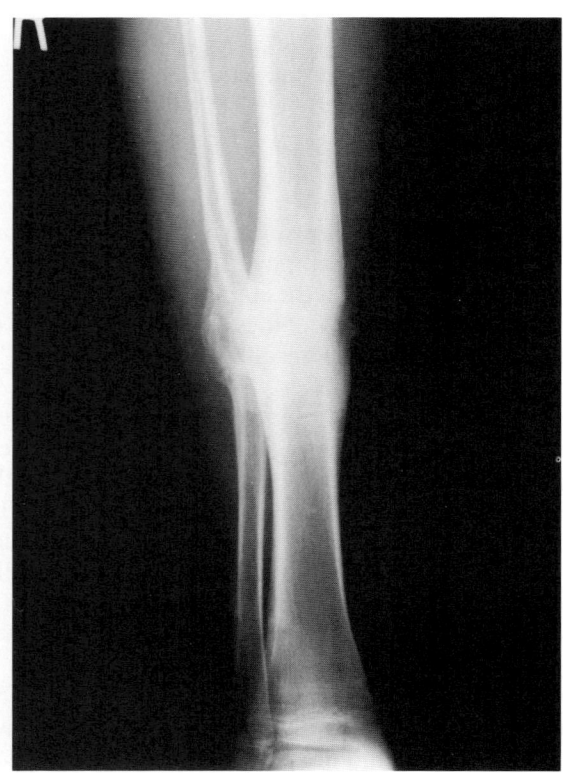

Fig. 61-6. Nonunion with angulation. **(A)** A 15-year-old boy with a painful, unstable nonunion of the midshaft of the right tibia. **(B)** He was treated with compression across the nonunion with an Ilizarov device. **(C)** He went on to solid healing with correction of the deformity. (Courtesy of Dr. Richard Pearce.)

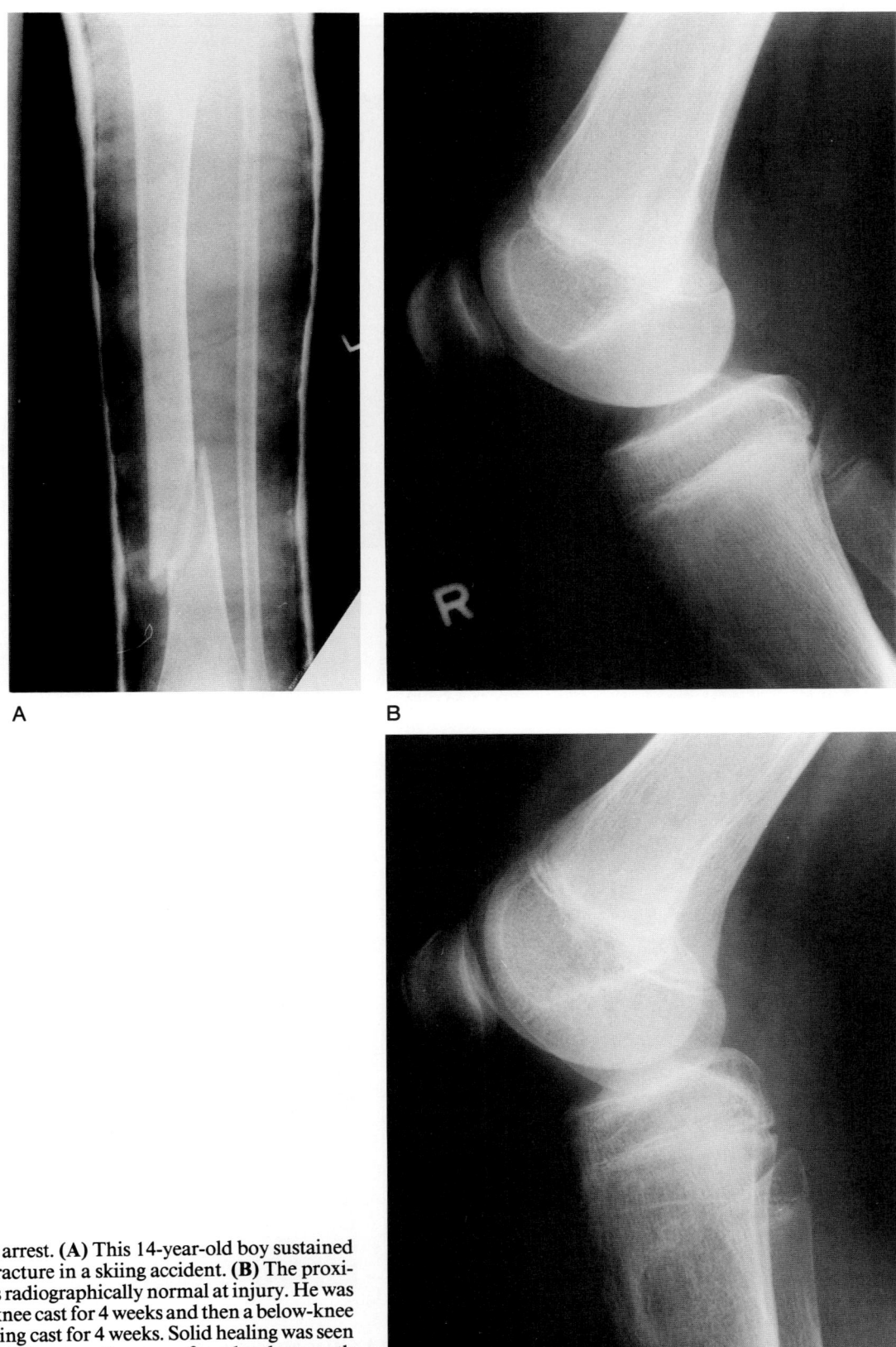

Fig. 61-7. Growth arrest. **(A)** This 14-year-old boy sustained a distal tibial shaft fracture in a skiing accident. **(B)** The proximal tibial physis was radiographically normal at injury. He was treated in an above knee cast for 4 weeks and then a below-knee patellar tendon bearing cast for 4 weeks. Solid healing was seen at 8 months. **(C)** At follow-up, there was found to be growth arrest of the proximal tibia. (Courtesy of Dr. R. Mervyn Letts.)

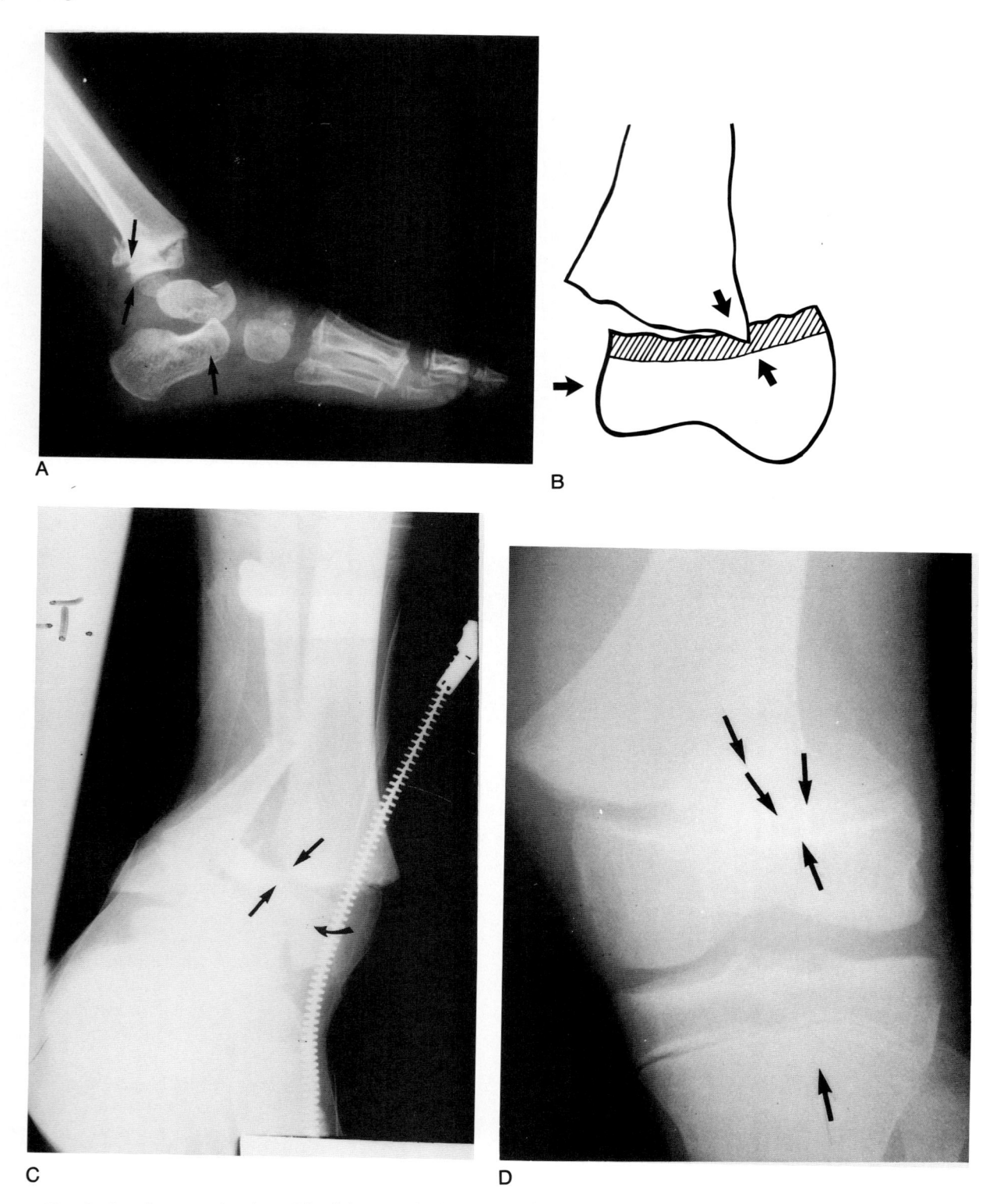

Fig. 61-8. Compression (type V) of the growth plate **(A&B)** in association with types I to IV physeal injuries at any site **(C&D)** can result in damage to the germinal cells of the growth plate **(E)** and resultant physeal arrest and limb shortening **(F)**. Arrows indicate areas of shear and compression damage to the physis caused by the sharp edge of metaphysis. *(Figure continues.)*

E　　　　　　　　　　　　　　F

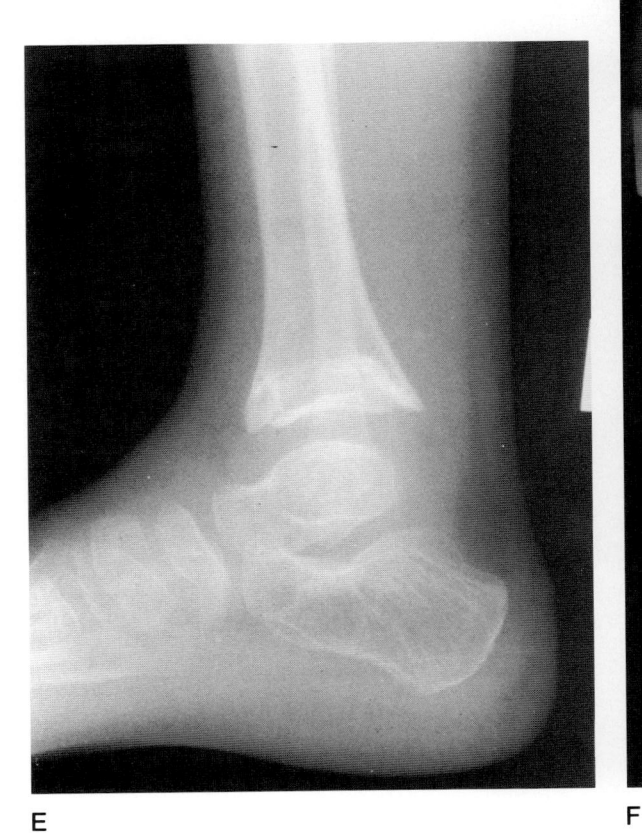

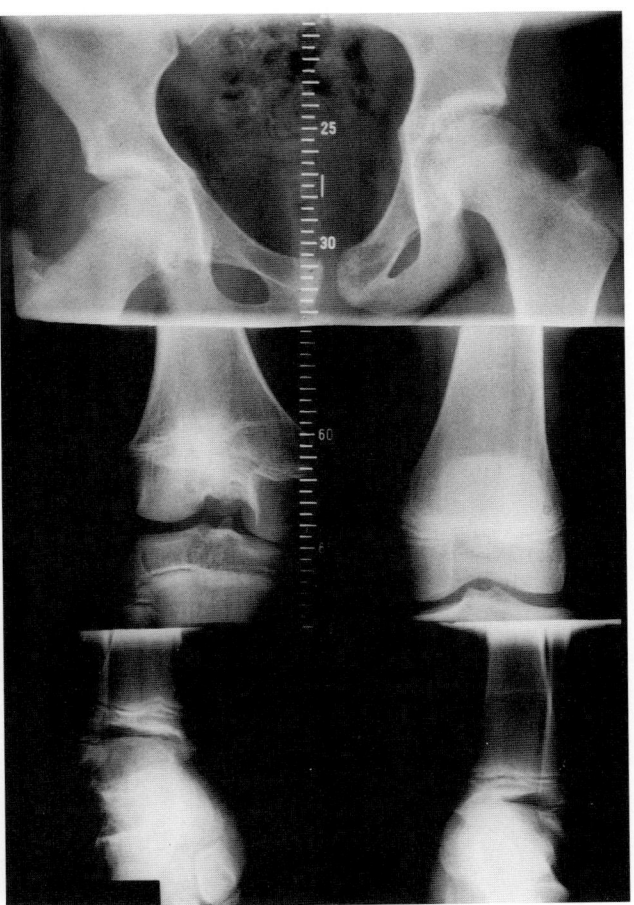

Fig. 61-8 *(Continued).*

nous physis as seen on radiographs. Established growth tethering may be amenable to resection with interposition of fat or an inert material[28,29] if the tether is small (see Ch. 62). Angular deformity may require osteotomy and arrest of growth on the opposite side of the physis to prevent recurrent deformity. For small limb length discrepancy (under 6 cm) contralateral epiphyseodesis may be considered. In the case of major limb length inequality (above 6 cm) or that associated with deformity, distraction osteogenesis techniques may be required (Fig. 61-10) (see Ch. 62).

POSTTRAUMATIC INFECTION

Infection occurs relatively rarely in children after musculoskeletal injury. Routes of inoculation include direct contamination through open traumatic wounds, surgical wounds, and by hematogenous inoculation to the site of injury.

An open fracture has a risk of contamination with subsequent development of wound infection or osteomyelitis. Irrigation and debridement is indicated as soon as possible to prevent the development of a wound environment that would allow supuration. After debridement, the wound should be left open to improve drainage. Cultures should be taken at the time of debridement to determine the type of microbial contamination.

Unlike adults, younger children are somewhat resistant to infection after open fracture. In our series of open forearm fractures,[30] 22 were followed for an average of 5 years. There were 18 grade I injuries, 2 grade II injuries, 1 grade IIIa injury, and 1 grade IIIb injury (Gustillo classification). Two deep wound infections occurred, which cleared with repeat incision drainage and intravenous antibiotics. There were no cases of osteomyelitis.

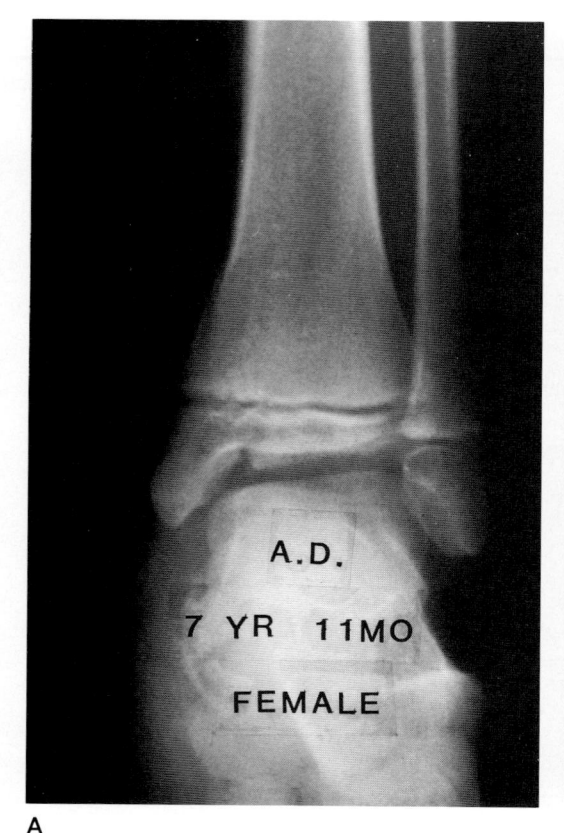

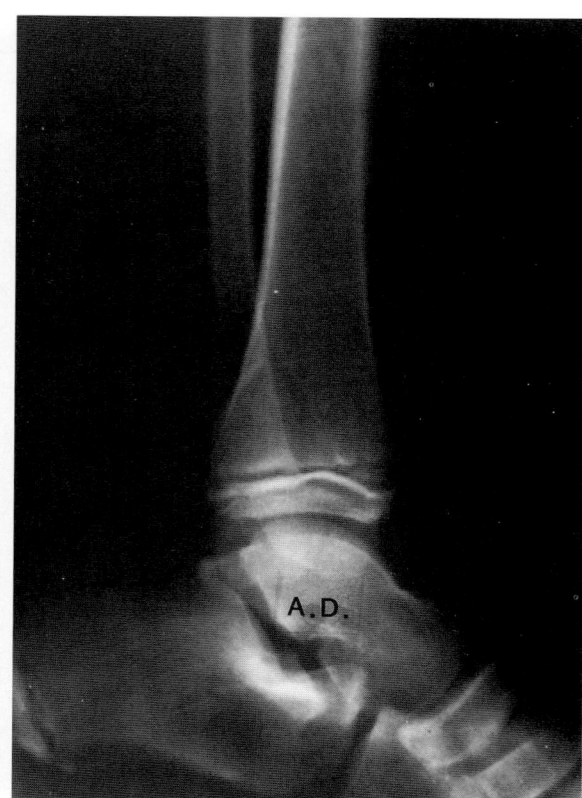

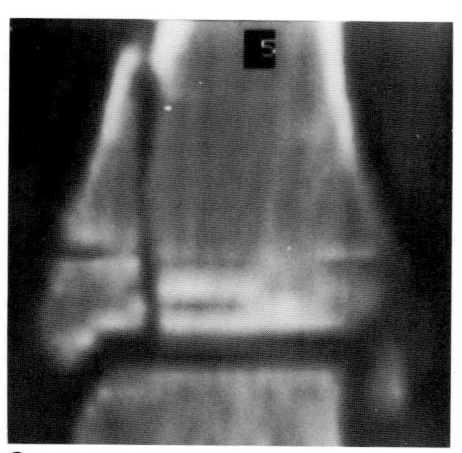

Fig. 61-9. Risk of arrest. A 7-year, 11-month-old girl had Salter-Harris type IV fracture of medial distal tibial physis. **(A&B)** Displacement appeared minimal. **(C)** Coronal CT reconstructions showed epiphyseal bone in contact with metaphysis. *(Figure continues.)*

D   E

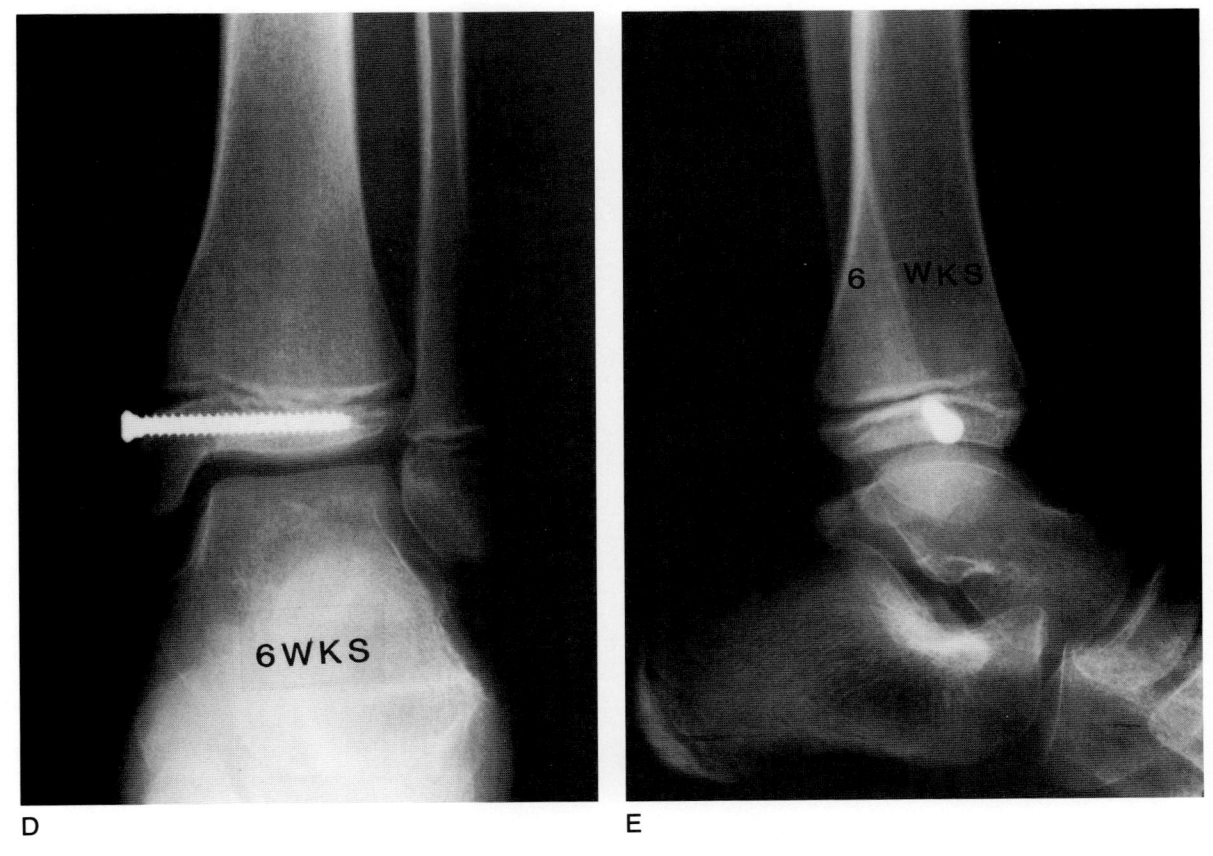

Fig. 61-9 *(Continued).* **(D&E)** Risk of growth arrest and joint incongruity lead to open reduction and internal fixation and undoubtedly avoided a physeal arrest. This case emphasizes the importance of a clear visualization of the fracture line.

In our series of open tibia fractures in children,[31] there were 31 open tibia fractures in children, consisting of 9 grade I, 6 grade II, and 16 grade III. In the 15 children under age 12, there was a 7 percent wound infection rate compared to 31 percent infection rate in the children age 12 or older. In children younger than age 12, there was no osteomyelitis compared to a 25 percent osteomyelitis rate in children older than age 12. These findings are supported by Song and colleagues[32] who found that deep infection did not occur in patients less than 12 years old, regardless of the grade of injury. This is in contradistinction to the work of Buckley and colleagues[33] and Yasko and Wilbur[34] who found that the morbidity of open fractures in children paralleled that in the adult population.

Although young children[30] have a special resistance to infection, the same initial debridement and wound toilet should be performed with skeletal stabilization by internal fixation, external fixation, or cast immobilization as necessary to prevent motion at the fracture site. Prophylactic broad-spectrum intravenous antibiotics should be started immediately. This should be changed if necessary to a specific antibiotic as soon as culture and sensitivity results are obtained. Repeat wound toilet should be performed where there is obvious residual contamination, positive culture, or a high-risk wound. Wound closure should not be performed until the wound is obviously sterile and healthy-appearing.

Hematogenous infection has been noted to occur after minor trauma. Children not infrequently present with infection adjacent to the epiphysis after a minor injury (Fig. 61-10). There may be no break in the skin or open wound, but the traumatic history is usually well documented. It is felt that bacteremia may seed the metaphyseal injury, causing a nidus of infection.[35,36] This phenomenon has been well demonstrated in a rabbit model.[37,38] While this has not been definitely proven as a predisposing etiologic factor in children, the similarities between the rabbit model and the observed clinical situ-

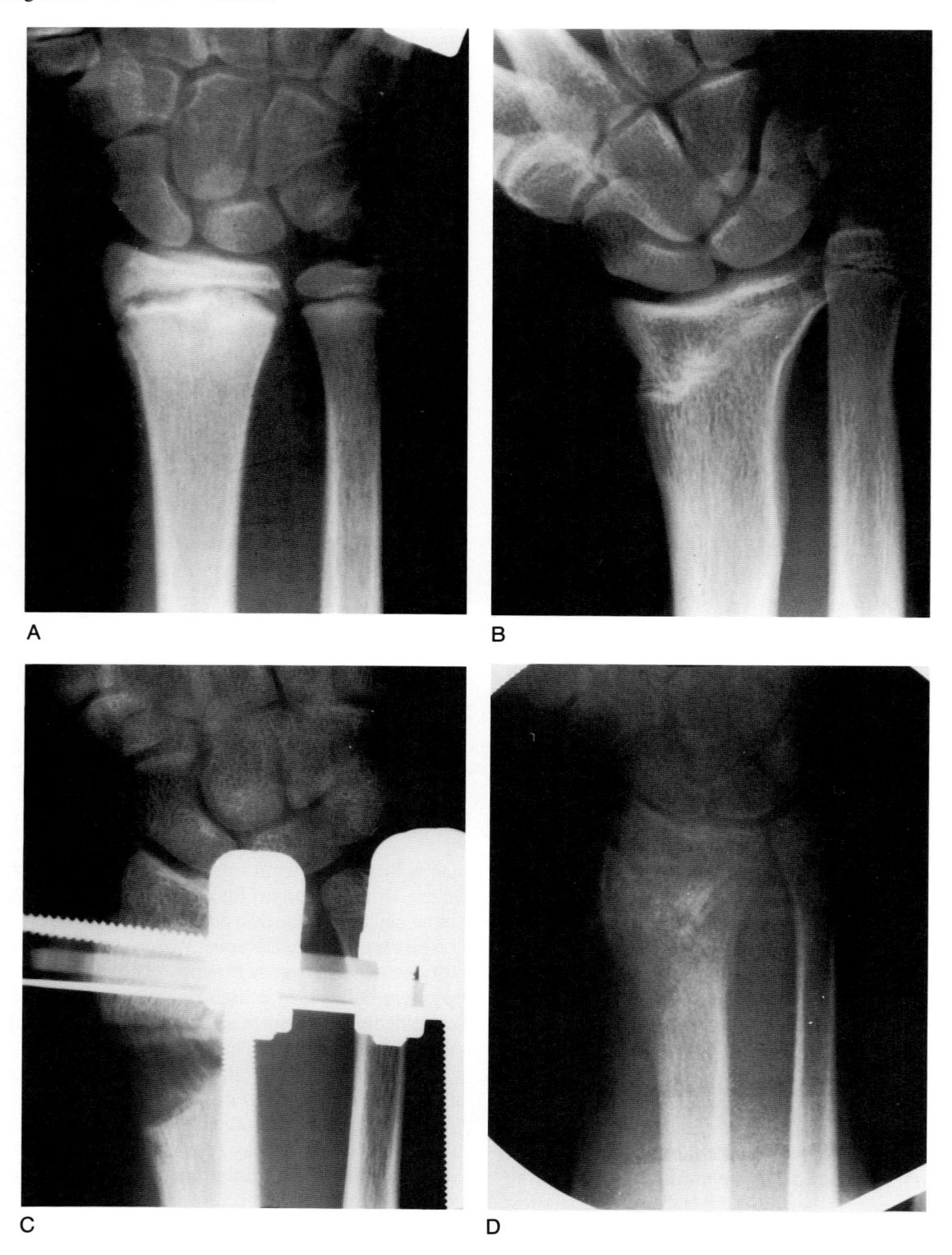

Fig. 61-10. Distal radial growth arrest. **(A)** This child had distal radial epiphyseal separation. **(B)** Growth arrest occurred with shortening and angulation. **(C)** Deformity correction and lengthening was performed with the Ilizarov device. **(D)** Result after consolidation. (Case courtesy of Dr. James Aronson.)

ation is striking. When a child complains of trauma and has residual pain and swelling, the presumed diagnosis of fracture or epiphyseal injury can be made. However, when a child presents with the same history followed by fever, redness, acute tenderness, and throbbing pain in spite of immobilization, consideration should be given to infection. An increased erythrocyte sedimentation rate or increased white count with left shift necessitates needle aspiration of the area for pus. If the diagnosis is made of posttraumatic hematogenous osteomyelitis, intravenous antibiotics to cover the common pathogens are indicated. Incision and drainage are necessary if lytic change can be seen on radiographs, if there is no improvement within a day or two of intravenous antibiotics, or if an obvious abscess is present. The family must be warned of the possibility of growth derangement when there is infection directly contiguous with the growth plate.

When infection occurs in the presence of an unstable skeletal segment, consideration should be given to external fixation of the segment to keep it immobilized while allowing access for wound toilet. If the infection occurs in the presence of an internal fixation device, the internal fixation device should remain in place as long as it provides rigid fixation and is not obviously the source of sepsis. Infection that occurs as a result of the surgical treatment of closed fractures should be treated in a similar manner.

GAS GANGRENE

Gas gangrene is a relatively unusual but devastating complication, which may occur following an open fracture in children. It is a process associated with a hypoxic wound environment that allows the infection to progress.[39] The bacteriologic agents usually associated with gas gangrene are large gram-positive anaerobic rods members of the genus *Clostridium*. Of six species, the most frequently cultured are *Clostridium perfringens, C. novyi,* and *C. septicum.* Gas gangrene can occur in a variety of clinical settings, the most frequent being posttraumatic after an open fracture. Anaerobic streptococci can also result in gas formation. This type of anaerobic infection is sometimes encountered in children after a fall from a bicycle or motor scooter resulting in large abrasions down to fascia. Gas gangrene may also occur postoperatively, particularly in the vascularly compromised patient. It may occur spontaneously or so-called "metastatic" to the extremities, although the primary problem lies in the gastrointestinal tract.[39,40] In children, it is most commonly encountered in contaminated open fractures of the limbs.

Historical Experience

In World War I, the incidence of clostridial myositis in the United States Army was 1 to 6 percent for extremity injuries. It was observed in World War II that clostridial myonecrosis occurred more commonly in the presence of arterial damage, when there was a large amount of muscle damage, when there was a delay in the treatment of the wound, or when inexperienced surgeons provided initial care. At the beginning of the Korean War, clostridial myonecrosis was relatively common, but the incidence dropped with the introduction and enforcement of a surgical policy that stressed debridement and delayed closure. These policies were started from the beginning of the Vietnam War where the incidence of clostridial myonecrosis in extremity injuries fell to 0.016 percent. It is felt that this was due to more prompt surgical treatment of wounds, thorough debridement, and an overall willingness to leave wounds open.[41]

Clostridial spores are ubiquitous. In order for gas gangrene to develop, there must be a unique wound environment. When tissue is damaged, its vascular supply is compromised and its oxygen tension lowered.[1] In this opportune environment of low oxygen tension, clostridia can multiply readily and rapidly.[39] Clostridia also release toxins, including alpha-toxin, a lecithinase that destroys the capillary cell membrane and cell wall. This leads directly to tissue destruction and increased capillary permeability producing the intense edema seen in myonecrosis. Alpha-toxin also has a myocardial depressant activity, which may cause shock and death. *Clostridium perfringens* also produces theta-toxin, which contributes to shock by releasing platelet-activating factor, which also has a mild myocardial depressing activity. Other toxins elaborated include K-toxin, a collagenase that contributes to the destruction of blood vessels. The elaboration of these toxins leads to the rapid and direct destruction of tissues and rapid spread of the infection proximally from the injured limb. Ultimately the activities of these toxins lead to hemolysis, anemia, hemoglobinuria, jaundice, oliguria, and to renal failure.[39]

Diagnosis

The diagnosis of gas gangrene is usually obvious when it is well established, but in early forms it may be more difficult to diagnose. The signs and symptoms of gas gangrene are many. Pain is most frequently seen and is usually out of proportion to the injury that has been sustained.[39] Fever is apparent and there is usually tachycardia out of proportion to fever.[39] Wound discharge is frequent and tends to be thin, dark brown, and foul smelling.[42,43] A Gram stain of the fluid will most often show gram-positive rods, which confirm the diagnosis. In the early stages, the skin about the wound is cool and edematous and later will develop a brownish discoloration and crepitation due to gas forming in the subcutaneous tissue and underlying muscle. Early on, the child may appear restless, anxious, or apprehensive.[40,41] As the patient becomes systemically ill, there is a paradoxical alertness despite profound hypotension and renal failure.[39] The muscle itself initially appears pale and superficially edematous. The deep muscle may appear beefy red but does not contract.[39] As the process becomes more established, the muscle may become frankly gangrenous, black, and friable.[39]

Any fluid elicited from the wound should be Gram-stained. The observation of large gram-positive rods confirms the diagnosis of clostridial necrosis. Clearly, cultures would take too much time to confirm the diagnosis and the Gram stain should provide enough evidence to initiate treatment.[39] Not all gas gangrene is caused by clostridial myonecrosis. The differential diagnosis includes necrotizing fasciitis, synergistic gangrene, which is caused by streptococcal and staphylococcal aerobes along with gram-negative rods, and streptococcal gangrene.[39]

The true incidence of clostridial myonecrosis has been estimated at about 0.1 cases per 100,000 per year in the United States.[39]

Treatment

The most effective method of dealing with gas gangrene is prevention. This can be achieved by minimizing the time between wounding and debridement, administration of proper antibiotics, debriding the wound thoroughly, and delaying closure of the wound.[41]

In the case of established clostridial myonecrosis, treatment may involve four modalities: surgical debridement, antibiotic therapy, hyperbaric oxygen therapy, and antitoxin administration. Immediate surgical debridement is the most important. All tissue that appears to be nonviable must be removed immediately as it represents an excellent culture medium for clostridia. Muscle of questionable viability can be retained if the opportunity for hyperbaric oxygen treatment is available, otherwise it must be removed. The wound should not be closed and must be packed opened. Fasciotomy of adjacent compartments should also be performed. The danger is of spread of the infection proximally toward the trunk. Amputation may be necessary to remove the source of sepsis.

Penicillin should be started immediately. The sodium salt is recommended rather than the potassium salt, which may aggravate hyperkalemia in the presence of hemolysis and renal failure.[39] The recommended dosage is 10 to 24 million units per day for 10 days.[39] Other effective antibiotics include tetracycline, chloramphenicol, and erythromycin. If the presence of a mixed infection is suspected or if a microbrial diagnosis has not been made, triple antibiotic coverage with penicillin G, aminoglycoside, and clindamycin are recommended.[39]

The use of hyperbaric oxygen therapy has been well described in the literature by Brummelkamp and colleagues[44] and more recently substantiated by Jackson and Waddell,[42] although its actual use in the clinical setting of clostridial myonecrosis has remained controversial. The relative inavailability of hyperbaric oxygen chambers has kept this treatment modality from becoming widespread.

The use of antitoxins may be considered when hyperbaric oxygen is not available.[39] The suggested dose of commercially available gas gangrene antitoxin is initially 75,000 units given intravenously and repeated every 6 hours.[39]

It must be remembered that the use of hyperbaric oxygen and antitoxins are only adjuncts in the treatment of the massive infection and muscle lysis. Surgical debridement and appropriate antibiotics are fundamental to eradicating the infection and the ensuing toxemia. The demise of the child will occur as a result of the toxic shock, and massive resuscitation efforts must be initiated. Efforts must be made at maintaining renal, hematologic, and systemic function in the septic patient.

Even with optimal treatment of clostridial myonecrosis, there is a 25 percent mortality[39] and even higher incidence of amputation.

The most important consideration in clostridial myonecrosis, of course, is prevention. Any wound or laceration that occurs in association with gross soil contamination, such as farmyard injuries, should be recognized as a high-risk injury and preventive measures toward gas gangrene should be undertaken.[39] In particular, the classic puncture wound of the forearm in children is particularly prone to this type of infection and should always be opened and the bone ends debrided. Water-contaminated wounds also should be treated with the same fervor.[41] In the case of established infection, recognition of the child with persistent pain, tachycardia, fever, and shock, especially in the presence of a draining wound, should alert the surgeon to consider the diagnosis of clostridial myonecrosis and immediately institute diagnostic and therapeutic measures. Emergent treatment should be undertaken to include immediate complete surgical debridement and appropriate antibiotic coverage with penicillin and to consider the use of adjunctive measures, such as hyperbaric oxygen and antitoxin, while immediately starting patient resuscitative efforts. Sound principles of wound management are paramount in preventing this deadly infection. Hampton[45] has stated "for clostridial myositis which develops in a primarily closed wound there is no excuse at all." Proper wound management is most important in both preventing and treating gas gangrene in association with open fractures in children.

ARTERIAL INJURY

Major arterial injury associated with closed fracture is unusual in the child.[46] Vascular injuries may occur more frequently with open fractures and near-amputations. Pulses must be checked routinely as part of the neurovascular examination after injury. Diminished intensity of the pulse is often attributed to vascular spasm but sustained limb ischemia is only rarely the result of vascular spasm.[47,48] When signs of vascular insufficiency accompany an extremity injury, vascular damage must be suspected and investigated promptly.[46] Early recognition and treatment may prevent late complications, such as compartment syndrome, limb undergrowth, and even limb loss. Altered blood flow may lead to central physeal growth arrest or the development of conical physes.[46]

Vascular injuries in children may be difficult to diagnose initially, thus delaying repair.[46] When a displaced fracture is associated with a decreased or absent pulse, immediate manipulative reduction of the fracture and reevaluation of the pulse and perfusion status should be performed (Table 61-4). If there is no improvement within an hour[47] or if there is specific evidence to suggest arterial injury, further investigation is warranted. Arteriography is helpful, but can lead to delay and occasionally arterial thrombosis in children.[49] Doppler pulse volume recording can provide a safe, noninvasive, dynamic evaluation of blood flow.[50] Digital subtraction angiography is an accurate method of evaluating arterial patency in which contrast is injected intravenously and subtraction imaging performed without the need for arterial puncture.[46,51] In the case of open injury, exploration of the vessels at wound toilet is indicated. Open arterial exploration has been suggested without angiography when circulation fails to improve after closed supracondylar humerus fracture,[52] since the site of the injury is known.

When a major arterial lesion is diagnosed, even if adequate collateral circulation is present to maintain a viable limb, vascular repair should be undertaken. This will prevent a late relative vascular insufficiency, which can occur as the limb musculoskeletal mass increases with growth and may exceed the capability of the remaining arterial supply to nourish the limb. This may result in limb length discrepancy or activity-induced ischemia.[46,53]

Operative fracture stabilization should be considered in order to protect the vascular repair and should precede the vascular repair in order to prevent disruption of the repair during manipulation. After vessel repair, consideration should be given to performing prophylactic fasciotomies distal to the site of repair, especially if the child's sensorium is impaired. If there has been considerable ischemic time, the risk of compartment syndrome after reperfusion is considerable.[54]

TABLE 61-4. Common Sites of Vascular Injuries in Children

Supracondylar humerus
Supracondylar femur
Ankle with dislocation
Proximal tibia

NERVE INJURY

Nerve injuries occur frequently in association with fractures in children. They are commonly seen after displaced supracondylar fractures in children. Most are the result of contusion or traction and will resolve spontaneously (Table 61-5).

TABLE 61-5. Common Nerve Injuries in Children

Anterior interosseus
Median nerve
Ulnar nerve
Radial nerve
Peroneal nerve
Sciatic nerve

Nerve injuries in children can be relatively silent. Children will commonly complain of numbness, but will rarely notice a motor loss, especially when it is painful to move.[55] The best way to diagnose a nerve injury is to have an index of suspicion and then to specifically test for each nerve function. This will lessen the likelihood of an awkward explanation of numbness or paralysis after fracture healing. Establishing that a nerve injury is present prior to the onset of treatment ensures that the nerve damage has not occurred secondary to the reduction.

Once a nerve injury has been diagnosed, a specific plan of action must be undertaken. A complete explanation of treatment and prognosis for recovery must be offered to the patient and family. If transection or laceration is suspected, repair should be undertaken as soon as practical. If neuropraxia is suspected, then a period of hopeful expectation is entered. The question exists of how long to wait after injury for functional return before exploring an injured nerve. For nerve injuries associated with supracondylar fractures of the humerus, it is suggested to wait at least 4 to 5 months before performing nerve exploration.[53,56]

Depending upon the findings at exploration, neurolysis, repair, or grafting may be required to regain nerve function. Nerve recovery after repair is dependent upon a number of factors, which have been clearly elaborated upon by Steinberg and Koman.[57]

1. Age. The prognosis for functional nerve recovery after injury or repair is better in children. In addition to achieving better results, children appear to recover more quickly. Age-related differences in recovery after nerve repair are due in part to enhanced cortical reorganization after nerve injury.

2. Level of injury. Distal injuries have a better prognosis for recovery than proximal.

3. Specific nerve injured. Radial nerve injuries are more likely to have functional motor return in the forearm than median or ulnar nerve lesions as the same level. Mixed motor-sensory nerves have a poorer recovery than primarily motor or primarily sensory. The incidence of nerve injury in the lower extremity is much lower than in the upper extremity. Return of motor function after peroneal repair is poorer than for the tibial.

4. Mechanism and nerve deficit. Recovery in clean or sharp nerve transection is superior to that after severe crushing or avulsion.

5. Rehabilitation and time to evaluation. Sensory and motor reeducation can improve functional recovery. Joint motion proximal and distal to the repair site must be maintained pending nerve recovery. When nerve regeneration occurs, 2 years may be required for recovery to plateau in young patients, compared to 5 years for adults.

6. Repair techniques. Primary neurorrhaphy offers the best prognosis for complete recovery. Nerve grafting diminishes manipulation and tension, but adds an additional suture line and the available nerve graft may not provide access for all of the proximal axons to the distal stump.

7. Associated injuries. More severe injuries with vascular damage, soft tissue damage, or contamination will adversely affect nerve regeneration.

8. Delay to repair. The functional results of neurorrhaphy become less satisfactory as the time between injury and repair increases. Clinically, 6 months represents a delay that significantly limits recovery.

In summary, clinical recognition is the first step in the management of nerve injury. Early repair is indicated for nerve transection. If transection is not suspected, a reasonable waiting period is warranted to allow for spontaneous nerve recovery prior to exploration. After nerve injury or repair, the prognostic factors noted above will be helpful in describing the functional prognosis for the family. Therapy to include sensory and motor reeducation and maintenance of joint motion should be undertaken pending return of nerve function. When motor nerve function cannot be effectively restored, tendon transfers are indicated.

POSTTRAUMATIC HETEROTOPIC OSSIFICATION

Heterotopic ossification is pathologic bone formation, which occurs in association with disease or trauma. It is frequently associated with central nervous system insult, such as traumatic brain injury or spinal cord injury; traumatic violent or surgical insult;[58] burns;[59] or tetanus.[60] The incidence increases with the severity of the injury.[61] It can also occur after contusion, muscle rupture, fracture, and dislocation around the hip joint.[62]

Heterotopic ossification tends to be para-articular but may be noted in the thigh,[63] hip, elbow, shoulder, finger joints, or clavicle[63,64] (Fig. 61-11). In children, such ossification is most common in the elbow and thigh.

The earliest signs of a focal area of heterotopic ossification are intense acute inflammation and pain on range of motion. Motion tends to decrease over the next few weeks and may progress to complete ankylosis.[63] In spi-

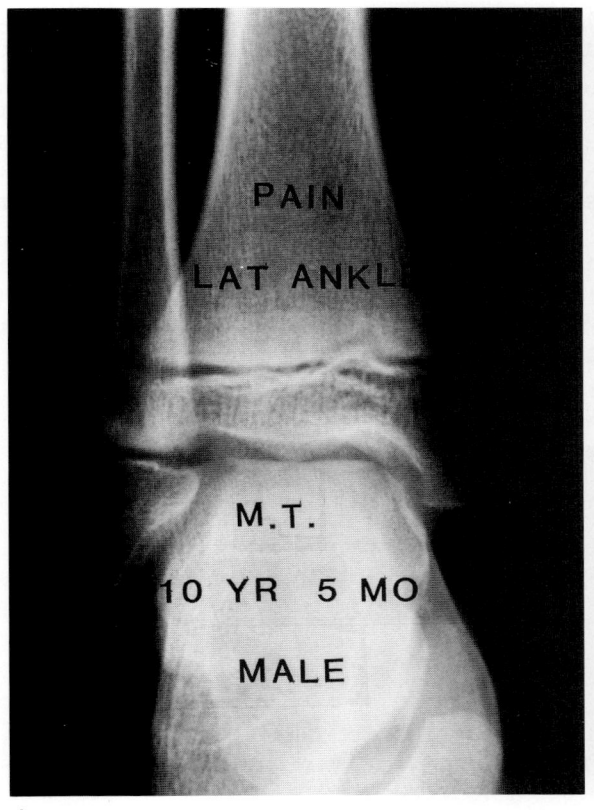

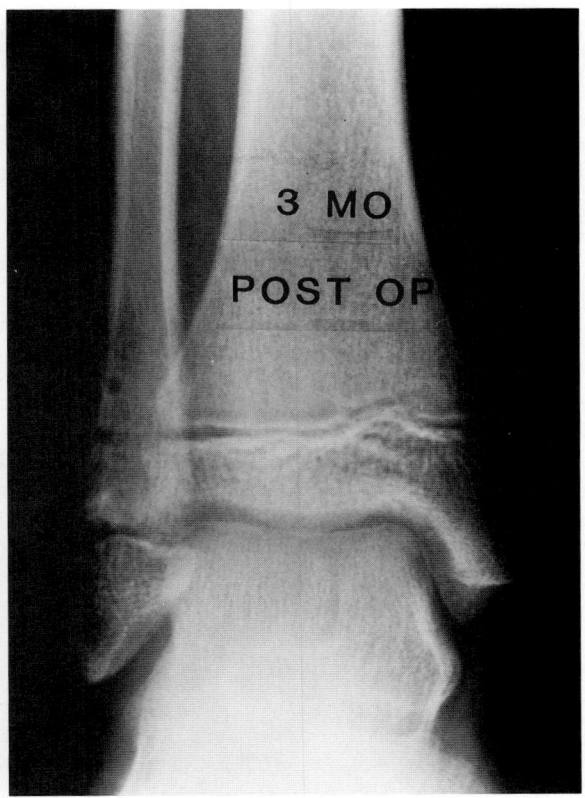

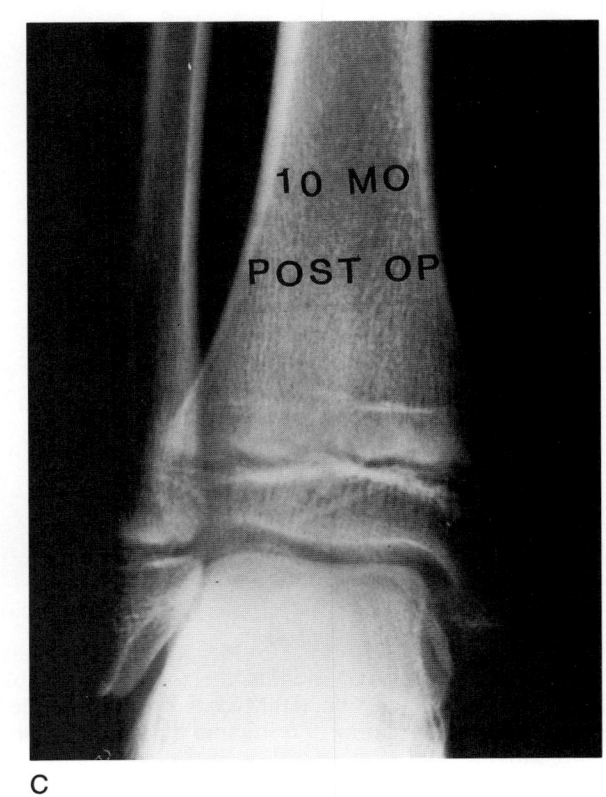

Fig. 61-11. Posttraumatic infection. **(A)** A 10-year-old boy had a recent history of a closed inversion injury to the ankle. He developed pain, swelling, and acute tenderness at the lateral malleolus. The sedimentation rate was elevated as was the patient's temperature. The patient underwent incision and drainage due to presumed sepsis. Pus was found at the site of the lateral malleolar physis, and a traumatic epiphysiolysis was confirmed. **(B)** The child was treated with intravenous antibiotics and immobilization. (Postoperative films show drill holes in the distal fibula.) **(C)** At long-term follow-up, physeal growth was normal.

nal cord-injured patients, decreased range of motion may be the only sign.[59] Limb swelling may occur that mimics thrombophlebitis.[59]

Heterotopic ossification may occur in normal children after significant trauma (Fig. 61-12). In neurologically compromised children, it can result from neurologic insult alone or as a result of local factors such as minor trauma or pressure sores.[59]

The onset of posttraumatic ossification in children ranges from 2 to 6 weeks after injury.

Serum alkaline phosphates is elevated in the majority of children who develop myositis ossificans and may be the earliest and most convenient test for its detection. Triple-phase bone scan is sensitive for detecting myositis ossificans within 2 to 4 weeks after injury.[65] Increased extraosseus uptake is highly suggestive. A decrease or steady state of the increased uptake on bone scan suggests that heterotopic ossification is mature.[65] Radiographs and CT scans are also useful in the diagnosis and in assessing maturity.

The morbidity is due to the acute pain and inflammation during the acute phase and in the limitation of joint motion in the late phase. The intense inflammation that marks the acute phase may be lessened by the use

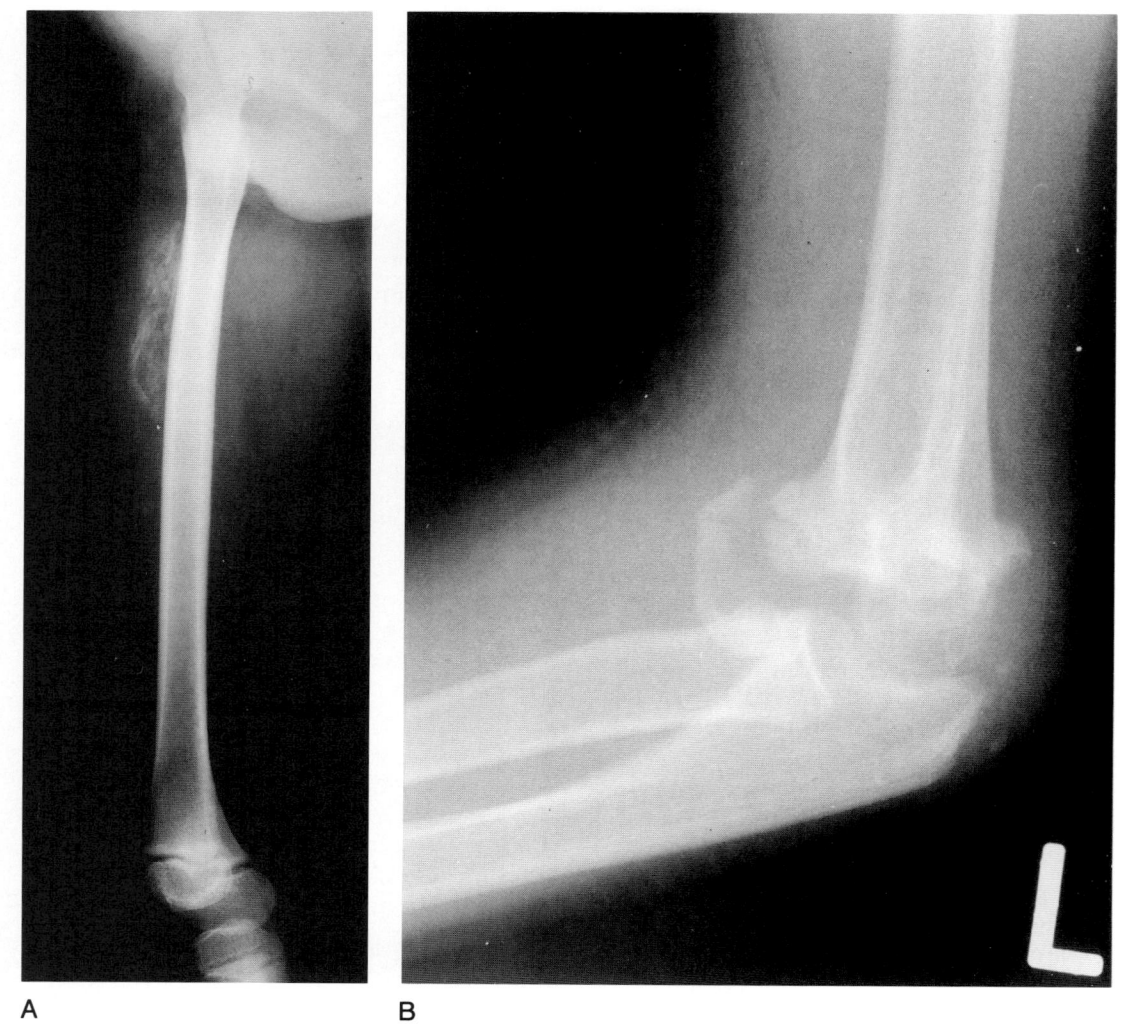

Fig. 61-12. Heterotopic ossification. **(A)** An 8-year-old boy sustained a blow to the anterior left thigh in a football game. At 3 months, there was considerable heterotopic ossification in the rectus muscle. It did not diminish his function. **(B)** Myositis ossificans of the brachialis muscle in a 14-year-old boy, 2 years after elbow dislocation resulting in restriction of elbow extension. This was resected resulting in improved range of elbow motion.

of nonsteroidal anti-inflammatory medications,[66] but these may have an inhibitory effect on fracture healing. Diphosphonates have been shown to be useful in inhibiting heterotopic bone formation[63] but is not desirable in the growing child or one with healing fracture. There also may be a rebound calcification effect after discontinuing diphosphonate therapy.[59] Radiation is known to be effective in preventing soft tissue ossification but is contraindicated in the growing child.[67]

During the period of formation, splintage of any involved joints in a functional position is indicated to avoid nonfunctional ankylosis.

In well-established heterotopic ossification, surgery may be indicated to maintain joint mobility or limb positioning (Fig. 61-12B). In minor cases that are asymptomatic, myositis ossificans is best left alone. Spontaneous resorption of the bone may occur in the extremities of young persons.[61] Timing for surgery is best in the quiescent state indicated by normal serum alkaline phosphatase, mature radiographic appearance, and baseline radionuclide bone imaging.[59] Metabolic quiescence does not assure that soft tissue ossification will not recur after resection.[58] After resection, prophylaxis with oral salicylates may be indicated to lessen the risk of recurrence.[63] Surgical timing varies according to etiology: the traumatic variety may be resected at 6 months, spinal cord injury type at 1 year, and traumatic brain injury myositis ossificans at 1.5 years.[65]

It must be emphasized that there are other serious causes of extraosseous ossification other than myositis ossificans, as illustrated in Figure 61-13.

JOINT STIFFNESS AFTER FRACTURE

Transient joint stiffness may occur after treatment of a fractured child's extremity, but long-term loss of joint motion is rare. Loss of joint motion is more frequent if surgery was a significant part of the treatment. Joint stiffness tends to improve with use of the extremity.

The child may or may not be aware of the restricted joint motion. Parents, however, may note that the child is not using the limb normally.

Joint stiffness may arise from many causes. After an injury to a limb the child may lose confidence in the extremity and be disinclined to use it until that confidence is regained. After immobilization, there may be a pain at the extremes of motion of a joint that discourages normal use (Fig. 61-14). The longer the immobilization, the more likely this is to occur. The knee and elbow are particularly prone to this phenomenon.

The majority of posttraumatic joint stiffness in children will respond to the child's normal play activities. Encouraging an early return to activity is the best means to achieve full motion and function of the extremity. A 6-week sentence of nightly dishwashing will help to loosen up a stiff wrist or elbow. Serial casting, dynamic hinged braces, or physiotherapy are rarely needed. When there is true soft tissue contracture causing joint stiffness, the use of therapeutic exercise or stretching may be of benefit. The need for surgical release of a joint to alleviate stiffness will almost never be necessary in a normal child.

Occasionally extra-articular bony ankylosis may occur, limiting joint motion such as the cross-union eliminating pronation supination in Figure 61-15. This was excised with a fat graft interposition with good return of function.

BEHAVIORAL CONSEQUENCES OF TRAUMA

Children involved with the physical trauma of a fracture are simultaneously plunged into emotional and social crisis as they and their families react to the emergency.[68] From accident to hospitalization to discharge, there are several predictable phases of the child's experience:[68]

1. Shock
2. Denial and panic
3. Protest and regression
4. Opportunism
5. Mourning
6. Readjustment

Children exposed to disaster have a modified sense of reality, increased vulnerability to future stresses, altered sense of the power of self, and early awareness of fragmentation and death.[69]

Posttraumatic stress disorder also occurs in children. The three basic diagnostic criteria are as follows:[70]

1. Persistent reexperiencing of the trauma
2. Avoidance of stimuli associated with the trauma or a numbing of responsiveness
3. Persistent symptoms of increased arousal

The severity of posttraumatic stress disorder in children may not parallel the nature of the disaster or the severity of injury.[70] The magnitude of effects of a frac-

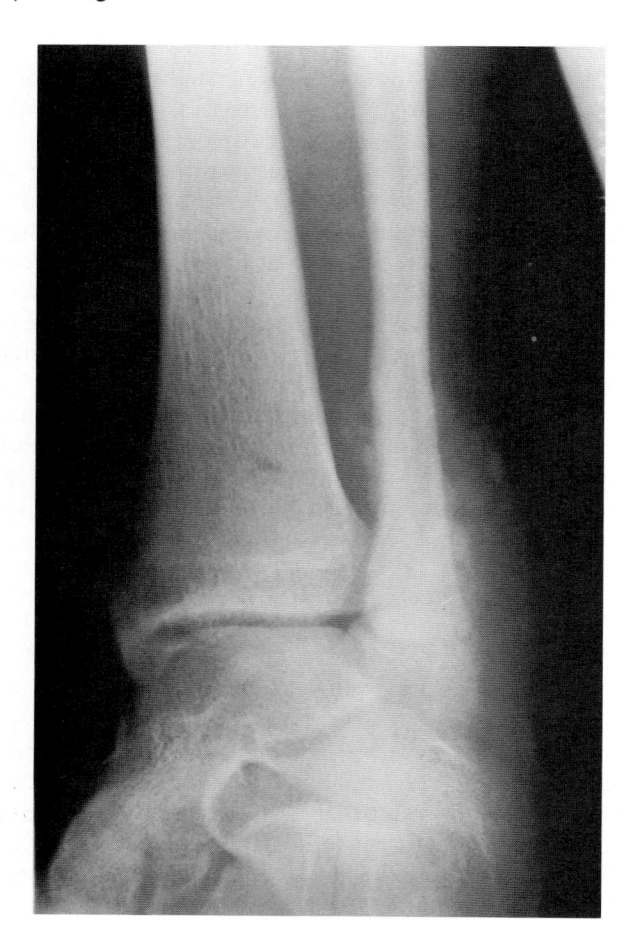

Fig. 61-13. Heterotopic ossification. This 14-year-old boy was hit in the left ankle by a hockey puck. Radiographs showed considerable ossification in the soft tissue. This was initially erroneously diagnosed as myositis ossificans. The child was ultimately diagnosed with osteogenic sarcoma at this location. Heterotopic ossification tends to occur proximally in extremities rather than distally where there is little muscle tissue. (Courtesy of Dr. R. Mervyn Letts.)

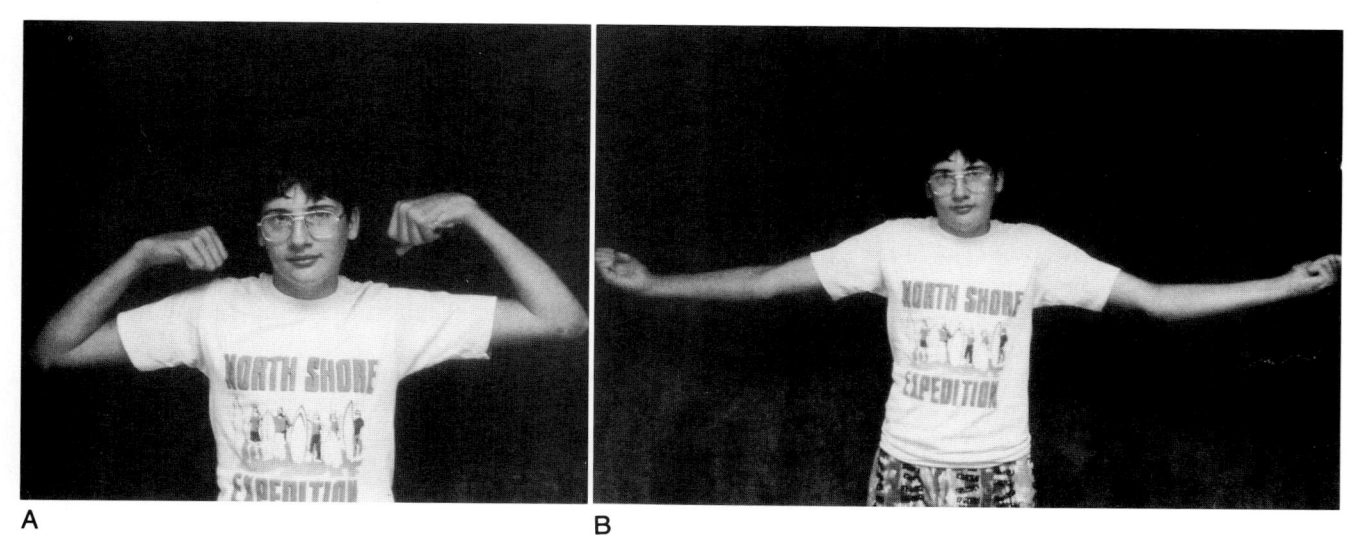

Fig. 61-14. Loss of motion. After healed extension supracondylar humerus fracture, **(A)** flexion is often limited, as is **(B)** full extension.

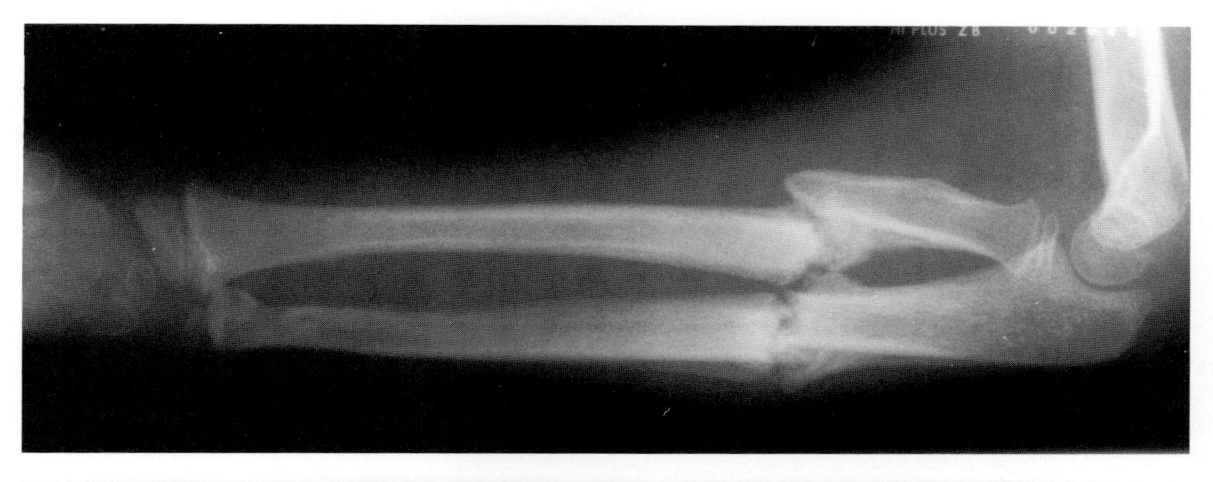

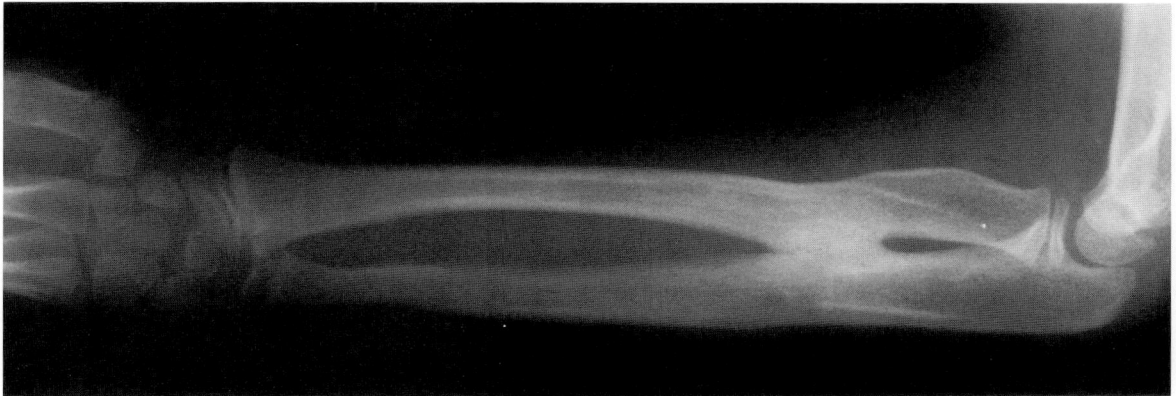

Fig. 61-15. Fracture proximal third radius and ulna in a 7-year-old boy that progressed to cross-union. Cross-union is very rare in fractures of the middle and distal thirds but more common in proximal third fractures of the radius and ulna.

ture on the child can be attributed to other major factors: (1) the child's developmental level at the time of injury, (2) the child's perceptions of the family's reactions to the injury, (3) the child's direct exposure to the injurious event,[69] (4) previous psychiatric history in child or family, and (5) the child's and family's experience in dealing with stress in the past.[70]

Trauma may adversely affect personality development in the child. Traumatized children are typically characterized by

1. Overcaution
2. Constriction of thought
3. Inhibition of action
4. Impairment of the ability to experience gratification

The change may be due to effect of the trauma not only on the child but also on the caretaking parent.[71] Though widely unrecognized, persistent behavioral disturbances may occur in up to 35 percent of traumatized children without head injury.[72] These dysfunctions include phobias, major scholastic difficulties, rage attacks, and episodic depression.

Detrimental effects may occur in other members of the family as well. For example, 66 percent of uninjured siblings may develop emotional disturbances, school problems, and aggressive personality changes. Parents reported worsening of the marital relationship in 32 percent of cases and new social and financial problems in 60 percent.[72]

Young children establish a certain mental representation of their bodies, referred to as "the body image." After severe injury, the child's image of his damaged body will be altered. The surgeon must help the child to heal not only the body but the mind's image as well.

Doll play and puppetry can be utilized by child life

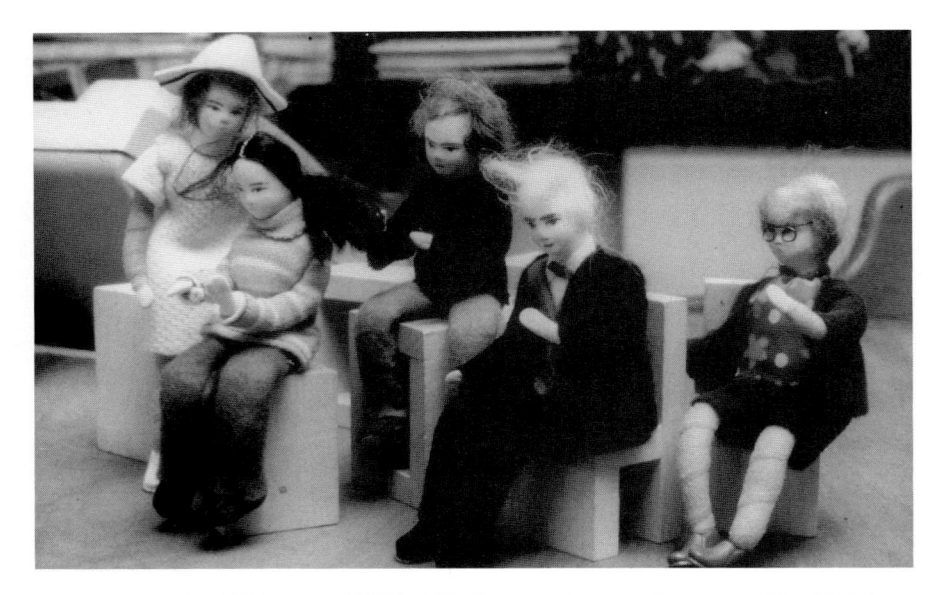

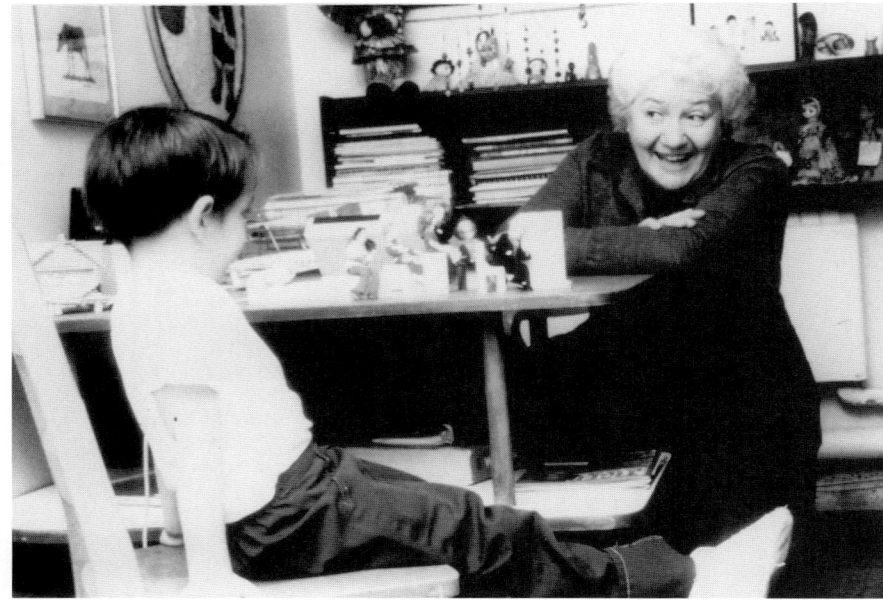

Fig. 61-16. Doll play. Figures depicting the child's own family assist the therapist in play-acting to remove guilt and anger in traumatized children. (Courtesy of Dr. R. Mervyn Letts.)

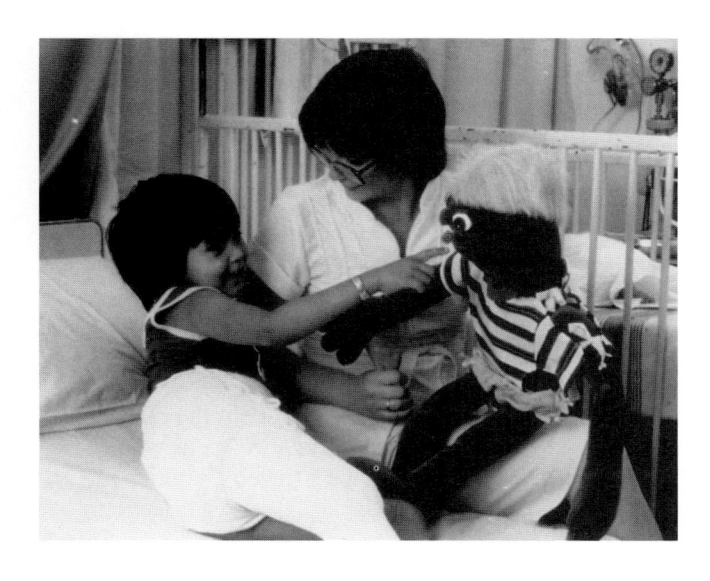

Fig. 61-17. Puppetry. Puppets can be utilized to allay anxiety, explain surgical procedures, and casts. (Courtesy of Dr. R. Mervyn Letts.)

Complications in Children's Fractures / 1135

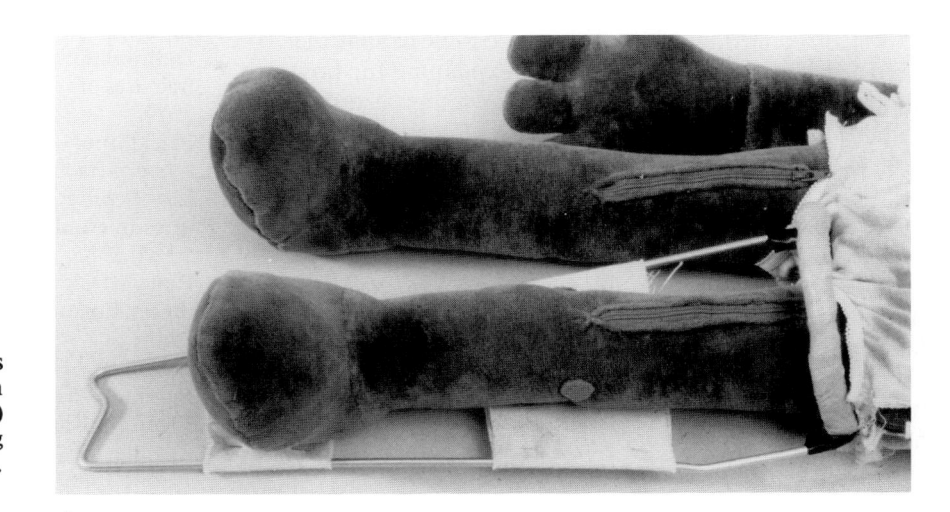

Fig. 61-18. Puppet with Thomas splint. **(A)** Puppet is used to explain traction to young children. **(B&C)** Fractures can be revealed by opening zippers and treatment explained. (Courtesy of Dr. R. Mervyn Letts.)

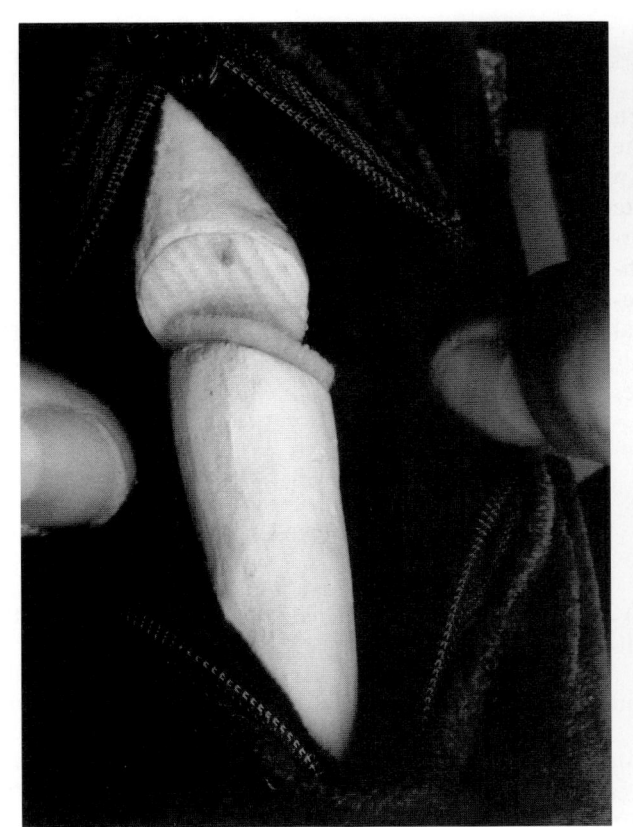

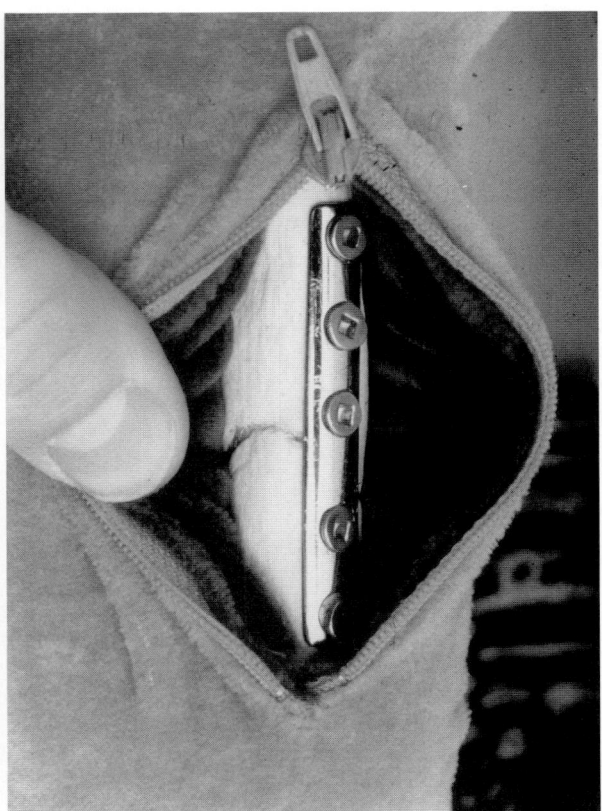

therapists or other trained support staff[73] (Fig. 61-16). Discussions in which children act out with dolls or puppets and ventilate their anxieties about their bodies often relieve them of unrealistic fears or expectations (Fig. 61-17). By using dolls or puppets it is possible to allay the child's anxiety of hospitalization by explaining the hospital routine (Fig. 61-18), the reasons for procedures, and the course of impending surgery. This technique has been shown to be useful in the preoperative psychological preparation of young children facing amputation or major musculoskeletal procedures.[73]

Behavioral changes should come to be expected in the traumatized child. The hidden morbidity of pediatric trauma lies in these psychosocial disabilities. Changes in family interactions and cognitive and behavioral symptoms should be expected in the patient and family members.[74] An awareness of potential problems and an availability of multidisciplinary assistance should help to lessen the effects of the trauma.

SUMMARY

Complications of fractures in children are often unique and quite distinct from those encountered in the adult population. Restriction of joint motion is seldom a major complication, whereas injury to the growth plate can be a devastating permanent and increasing deformity. Fractures in children fortunately remodel significantly, and nonunion is rare. The recovery of nerve injury in young children is excellent. The psychological component of injury is often a neglected area of treatment by orthopaedic surgeons and one that deserves more attention.

REFERENCES

1. Bright R: Remodeling following injury. p. 61. In Rockwood CA, Wilkins KE, King RE (eds): Fractures in Children. Vol. 3. JB Lippincott, Philadelphia, 1984
2. Creasman C, Zaleske DJ, Ehrlich MG: Analyzing forearm fractures in children. Clin Orthop 188:40, 1984
3. Davis DR, Green DP: Forearm fractures in children. Clin Orthop 120:172, 1976
4. Hägglund G, Hansson LI, Norman O: Correction by growth of rotational deformity after femoral fracture in children. Acta Orthop Scand 54:858, 1983
5. Fuller DJ, McCullough CJ: Malunited fractures of the forearm in children. J Bone Joint Surg [Br] 64:364, 1982
6. Tarr RR, Garfinkel AI, Sarmiento A: The effects of angular and rotational deformities of both bones of the forearm: an in vitro study. J Bone Joint Surg [Am] 66:65, 1984
7. Price CT, Scott DS, Kurzner ME, Flynn JC: Malunited forearm fractures in children. J Pediatr Orthop 10:705, 1990
8. Daruwalla JS: A study of radioulnar movements following fractures of the forearm in children. Clin Orthop 139:114, 1979
9. Blackburn N, Ziv I, Rang M: Correction of the malunited forearm fracture. Clin Orthop 189:54, 1984
10. Lewallen RP, Peterson HA: Nonunion of long bone fractures in children: a review of 30 cases. J Pediatr Orthop 5:135, 1985
11. Rang M: Children are not just small adults. p. 1. In: Children's Fractures. 2nd Ed. JB Lippincott, Philadelphia, 1983
12. Blount W: Fractures in Children. Williams & Wilkins, Baltimore, 1955
13. Flynn JC, Richards JF: Non-union of minimally displaced fractures of the lateral condyle of humerus in children. J Bone Joint Surg [Am] 53:1096, 1971
14. Hardacre JA, Nahigian SH, Froimson AI, Brown JE: Fractures of the lateral condyle of the humerus in children. J Bone Joint Surg [Am] 53:1083, 1971
15. Wilkins KE: Fractures and dislocations of the elbow region. p. 363. In Rockwood CA, Wilkins KE, King RE (eds): Fractures in Children. Vol. 3. JB Lippincott, Philadelphia, 1984
16. Canale ST, King RE: Pelvic and hip fractures. In Rockwood CA, Wilkins KE, and King RE (eds): Fractures in Children. JB Lippincott, Philadelphia, 1984
17. Paley D, Catagni MA, Argnani F et al: Ilizarov treatment of tibial nonunions with bone loss. Clin Orthop 241:146, 1989
18. Maiocchi AB, Aronson J: Operative Principles of Ilizarov. Williams & Wilkins, Baltimore, 1991
19. Heeg M, Klasen HJ, Visser JD: Acetabular fractures in children and adolescents. J Bone Joint Surg [Br] 71:418, 1989
20. Morscher E: Etiology and pathophysiology of leg length discrepancies. In Hungerford DS (ed): Leg Length Discrepancy: The Injured Knee. Springer-Verlag, New York, 1977
21. Bright RW: Physeal injuries. In Rockwood CA, Wilkins KE, and King RE (eds): Fractures in Children. JB Lippincott, Philadelphia, 1984
22. Riseborough EJ, Barrett IR, Shapiro F: Growth disturbances following distal femoral physeal fracture-separations. J Bone Joint Surg [Am] 65:885, 1983
23. Hresko MT, Kasser JR: Physeal arrest about the knee associated with non-physeal fractures in the lower extremity. J Bone Joint Surg [Am] 71:698, 1989
24. Lee BS, Esterhai JL, Das M: Fracture of the distal radial epiphysis. Clin Orthop 185:90, 1984
25. Hunter LY, Hensinger RN: Premature monomelic growth arrest following fracture of the femoral shaft. J Bone Joint Surg [Am] 60:850, 1978

26. Rang M: Injuries of the epiphysis, the growth plate, and the perichondrial ring. In: Children's Fractures. 2nd Ed. JB Lippincott, Philadelphia, 1983
27. Brunner CH: Fractures in and around the knee joint. In Weber BG, Brunner C, Freuler F (eds): Treatment of Fractures in Children and Adolescents: Springer-Verlag, New York, 1979
28. Langenskiöld A: An operation for partial closure of an epiphysial plate in children, and its experimental basis. J Bone Joint Surg [Br] 57:325, 1975
29. Bright RW: Operative correction of partial epiphyseal plate closure by osseous-bridge resection and silicone-rubber implant. J Bone Joint Surg [Am] 56:655, 1974
30. Klasson SC, Blasier RD: Open pediatric forearm fractures. 56th Annual Meeting, Western Orthopedic Association, Monterey, California, October 10-14, 1992
31. Blasier RD, Barnes CL, Puskarich C: Open tibia fractures in children. Annual Meeting, American Acadamy of Pediatrics-Orthopedic Section, New Orleans, Louisiana, October 26-27, 1991
32. Song KM, Sangeorzan BJ, Benirschke SK et al: Open fractures of the tibial shaft in skeletally immature patients. 58th Annual AAOS Meeting, Anaheim, California, March 7-11, 1991
33. Buckley SL, Griffin PP, Smith G et al: Open tibia fractures in children. 58th Annual AAOS Meeting, Anaheim, California, March 7-11, 1991
34. Yasko A, Wilbur J: Open tibia fractures in children. Orthop Trans 13:761, 1989
35. Morrissy RT, Haynes DW: Acute hematogenous osteomyelitis: a model with trauma as an etiology. J Pediatr Orthop 9:447, 1989
36. Morrissy RT, Shore SL: Acute hematogenous osteomyelitis. p. 271. In Gustilo RB, Gruninger RP, Tsukayama DT (eds): Orthopaedic Infection: Diagnosis and Treatment. WB Saunders, Philadelphia, 1989
37. Morrissy RT, Haynes DW, Nelson CL: Acute hematogenous osteomyelitis: the role of trauma in a reproducible model. 26th Annual ORS Meeting, Georgia, February 1980
38. Whalen JL, Fitzgerald RH, Morrissy RT: A histological study of acute hematogenous osteomyelitis following physeal injuries in rabbits. J Bone Joint Surg [Am] 70:1383, 1988
39. Present DA, Meislin R, Shaffer B: Gas gangrene. Orthop Rev 19:33, 1990
40. Chetta SG, Weber MJ, Nelson CL: Non-traumatic clostridial myonecrosis: a report of two cases. J Bone Joint Surg [Am] 64:456, 1982
41. Brown PW, Kinman PB: Gas gangrene in a metropolitan community. J Bone Joint Surg [Am] 56:1445, 1974
42. Jackson RW, Waddell JP: Hyperbaric oxygen in the management of clostridial myonecrosis (gas gangrene). Clin Orthop 96:271, 1973
43. Fee NF, Dobranski A, Bisla RS: Gas gangrene complicating open forearm fractures. J Bone Joint Surg [Am] 59:135, 1977
44. Brummelkamp WH, Boeream I, Hogendijk J: Treatment of clostridial infections with hyperbaric oxygen drenching: a report on 26 cases. Lancet 1:235, 1963
45. Hampton OP: Wounds of the Extremities in Military Surgery. CV Mosby, St. Louis, 1951
46. Friedman RJ, Jupiter JB: Vascular injuries and closed extremity fractures in children. Clin Orthop 188:112, 1984
47. Bliss B, Bradley JWP, Fairgrieve J et al: Vascular injuries. [Editorial]. J Bone Joint Surg [Br] 71:738, 1989
48. Burnett HF, Parnell CL, Williams GD, Campbell GS: Peripheral arterial injuries: a reassessment. Ann Surg 183:701, 1976
49. Shaker IJ, White JJ, Signer RD et al: Special problems of vascular injuries in children. J Trauma 16:863, 1976
50. Broudy AS, Jupiter JB, May JW: Management of supracondylar fracture with brachial artery thrombosis in a child. J Trauma 19:450, 1979
51. Wagner ML, Singleton EB, Egan ME: Digital subtraction angiography in children. AJR 140:127, 1983
52. Clement DA, Phil D: Assessment of a treatment plan for managing acute vascular complications associated with supracondylar fractures of the humerus in children. J Pediatr Orthop 10:97, 1990
53. Ogden JA: Skeletal Injury in the Child. Lea & Febiger, Philadelphia, 1982
54. Mubarak SS, Carroll NC: Volkmann's contracture in children: aetiology and prevention. J Bone Joint Surg [Br] 61:285, 1979
55. Jones ET, Louis DS: Median nerve injuries associated with supracondylar fractures of the humerus in children. Clin Orthop 150:181, 1980
56. Culp RW, Osterman AL, Davidson RS et al: Neural injuries associated with supracondylar fractures of the humerus in children. J Bone Joint Surg [Am] 72:1211, 1990
57. Steinberg DR, Koman LA: Factors affecting the results of peripheral nerve repair. p. 349. In Gelberman RH (ed): Operative Nerve Repair and Reconstruction. Vol. 1. LB Lippincott, Philadelphia, 1991
58. Garland DE, Orwin JF: Resection of heterotopic ossification in patients with spinal cord injuries. Clin Orthop 242:169, 1989
59. Garland DE, Shimoyama ST, Lugo C et al: Spinal cord insults and heterotopic ossification in the pediatric population. Clin Orthop 245:303, 1989
60. Chantraine A, Véry JM, Baud CA: A biophysical study of posttraumatic ectopic ossification: a case report. Clin Orthop 255:289, 1990
61. Puzas JE, Miller MD, Rosier RN: Pathologic bone formation. Clin Orthop 245:269, 1989
62. Keret D, Harcke TH, Mendez AA et al: Heterotopic ossification in central nervous system-injured patients following closed nailing of femoral fractures. Clin Orthop 256:254, 1990
63. Mital MA, Garber JE, Stinson JT: Ectopic bone formation in children and adolescents with head injuries: its management. J Pediatr Orthop 7:83, 1987
64. Mital MA, Garber JE, Stinson JT: Management of ectopic

bone formation in the head-injured child and adolescent, abstracted. Orthop Trans 7:518, 1983
65. Garland DE: A clinical perspective on common forms of acquired heterotopic ossification. Clin Orthop 263:13, 1991
66. Mital MA, Garber J: Ectopic bone formation and its management in the head-injured child and adolescent, abstracted. Orthop Trans 7:187, 1983
67. Coventry MB, Scanlon PW: The use of radiation to discourage ectopic bone: a nine-year study in surgery about the hip. J Bone Joint Surg [Am] 63:201, 1981
68. Ravenscroft K: Psychiatric consultation to the child with acute physical trauma. Am J Orthopsychiatry 52:298, 1982
69. Newman JC: Children of disaster: clinical observations at buffalo creek. Am J Psychiatry 133:306, 1976
70. Martini DR, Ryan C, Nakayama D, Ramenofsky M: Case study: psychiatric sequelae after traumatic injury: the Pittsburgh regatta accident. J Am Acad Child Adolesc Psychiatry 29:70, 1990
71. Gislason IL, Call JD: Case report: dog bite in infancy: trauma and personality development. J Am Acad Child Psychiatry 21:203, 1982
72. Basson MD, Guinn JE, McElligott J et al: Behavioral disturbances in children after trauma. J Trauma 31:1363, 1991
73. Letts M, Stevens L, Coleman J, Kettner R: Puppetry and doll play as an adjunct to pediatric orthopaedics. J Pediatr Orthop 3:605, 1983
74. Harris BH, Schwaitzberg SD, Seman TM, Herrmann C: The hidden morbidity of pediatric trauma. J Pediatr Surg 24:103, 1989

62

Posttraumatic Physeal Arrest

John G. Birch

> Most human beings have an almost infinite capacity for taking things for granted.
> —ALDOUS HUXLEY

DESCRIPTION AND INCIDENCE

Physeal fractures are a common form of skeletal injury in children.[1-4] A relatively uncommon complication of physeal injuries is the formation of a physeal bar (also called bony bridges or physeal arrests).[4-6] Whenever a bridge of bone develops across a portion of physis, tethering of the metaphyseal and epiphyseal bone together can occur. These partial physeal bars can result in angular deformity, joint distortion, limb length inequality, or a combination of these, depending on the location of the arrest, the rate and extent of growth remaining in the physis involved, and the health of the residual affected physis. Although these partial bars are not common, their presence usually demands preventive or corrective treatment to minimize the long-term sequelae of the disturbance of normal growth that they can create.

ANATOMY

Partial physeal bars have fairly typical plain radiographic characteristics (Fig. 62-1). The bar itself will usually be quite sclerotic. It will bridge the normal physis, connecting the epiphyseal and metaphyseal bone. Usually, an asymmetric growth arrest line will be seen tapering to the bar itself, which replaces the original physis, indicating that no growth is occurring in the region of the bar. There will be a variable distortion of the joint surface, angular deformity, and loss of length. The severity of these deformities depends on the location of the bar, how long it has been present, and how extensive growth of the remaining physis has been.

Partial physeal bars can be classified anatomically[7] based on the relationship of the bar to the residual "healthy" physis (Fig. 62-2). "Central" arrests are those that are completely surrounded by a perimeter of normal physis, so that they are like islands within the remaining physis. Characteristically, a central arrest will distort the joint surface by causing tenting of the physis (and epiphysis), and loss of normal longitudinal growth. If a central type of arrest is eccentrically located, it can cause angular deformity as well.

"Peripheral" bars are eccentrically located at a margin of the affected physis. They primarily cause progressive angular deformity, usually with loss of length as well. Typically, they cause less joint surface disturbance than central arrests.

"Linear" bars are "through-and-through" lesions, which share characteristics of central and peripheral arrests. They typically occur as a result of Salter-Harris type III or IV physeal fractures.[3]

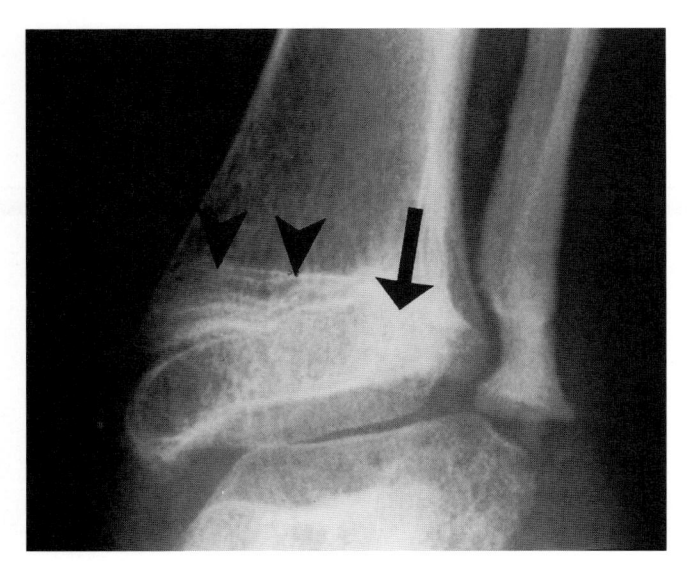

Fig. 62-1. Peripheral arrest of posterolateral distal tibia after lawnmower injury. Note growth arrest line *(arrowheads)* tapering to the bar itself *(arrow)* seen as a sclerotic area of bone replacing the physis.

MECHANISM OF INJURY

Partial physeal bars most commonly result from partial destruction of the physis after physeal fracture, with a portion of the physis replaced by bone connecting the epiphyseal and metaphyseal bone. Physeal fractures that cross the physis (such as Salter-Harris types IV and V fractures) are more likely to result in partial physeal bars than are type I or II fractures. However, other anatomic considerations are equally important.[4,8] For example, distal femoral fractures of any physeal fracture pattern are much more likely to be complicated by physeal bar than other locations. On the other hand, while distal radial physeal injuries are common, partial physeal bars there are relatively uncommon. True partial physeal bars after trauma are also unusual in the proximal humerus or elbow. Most clinical series show bars to be most common in the distal femur, proximal tibia, and distal tibia.[8-11]

While physeal fractures are the usual mechanism of injury resulting in partial physeal bars, any injury to the physis may cause them. Other causes include infection[12] (especially neonatal multifocal osteomyelitis or as a sequela of meningococcemia), infantile Blount's disease, asymmetric radiation to the physis, enchondromatosis, direct surgical trauma, and, occasionally, without known antecedent cause.[8]

PHYSICAL EXAMINATION

Physical examination will demonstrate the sequelae of the disturbance of growth. Limb length inequality and angular deformity will be obvious, when present. Although the joint surface may be distorted radiographically, there is usually no pain, crepitus, or loss of range of motion of the affected joint. If the potential for the development of a partial physeal bar has been recognized, it may be detected early radiographically, even though there may be no abnormal physical findings.

DIFFERENTIAL DIAGNOSIS

Angular deformity and shortening may result after malunion of diaphyseal or metaphyseal fractures. These will be essentially static deformities, and are easily differentiated on plain radiographs of the affected extremity.

Proximal tibial metaphyseal fractures may result in progressive valgus angular deformity. However, there will be no shortening clinically, and once again, the nature of the growth disturbance is easily differentiated on plain radiographs. There may be an asymmetric growth arrest line, but this arrest line will be moving away from the physis in all locations, indicating no location where there is cessation of growth.

Lesions such as osteochondromata, enchondromata, or unicameral bone cysts can influence physeal growth adversely, usually by disrupting a portion of normal physis. In such cases, the lesions themselves are usually easily identified on plain radiographs, and there is no radiographic evidence of true partial physeal bars (sclerotic bar spanning the physis, growth arrest line tapering to the physis itself, tenting of the physis with joint distortion). These lesions are not amenable to partial physeal bar resection, but they may require other physeal surgical modalities. If excision is required, and growth of the residual physis is desired, handling of the excision may need to follow the guidelines outlined below for partial physeal bar resection. We have had no success restoring normal growth by resection surgery in these conditions, however.[8]

Occasionally, physeal fracture will result in an asymmetric disturbance of growth, without frank complete arrest of growth at any point. In these cases, angular deformity may develop, but no true sclerotic bony bar will be identifiable. Furthermore, the growth arrest line will be asymmetric, but will not taper to the physis itself. Rather, the entire line will have grown away from the physis after injury. In such rare cases, spontaneous correction may occur.

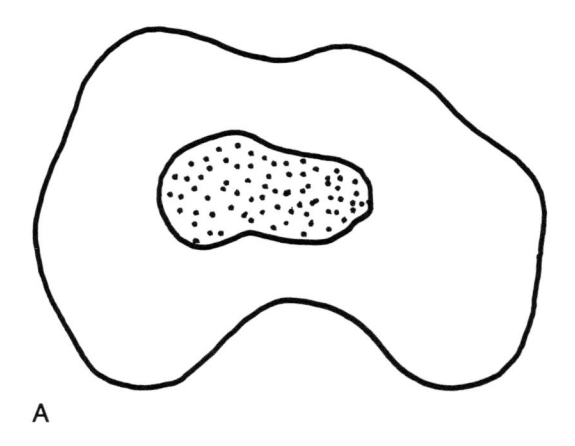

Fig. 62-2. Morphologic classification of partial physeal arrests. **(A)** Central physeal arrest. The area of arrest *(stippled)* is completely surrounded by healthy physis (here shown as an outline of the distal femoral physis). The area of arrest does not contact the perimeter of the physis at any point. **(B)** Peripheral physeal arrest. The area of arrest is eccentrically located at the periphery of the physis, so that it is bounded by normal physis on one side, and periosteum (transformed from perichondrium normally present) on the perimeter of the bone. **(C)** Linear physeal arrest. The area of arrest is bounded on either side by normal physis, but its ends are in contact with the perimeter of the bone. Typically, this pattern is seen after Salter-Harris type III or IV physeal fractures, especially of the distal tibia.

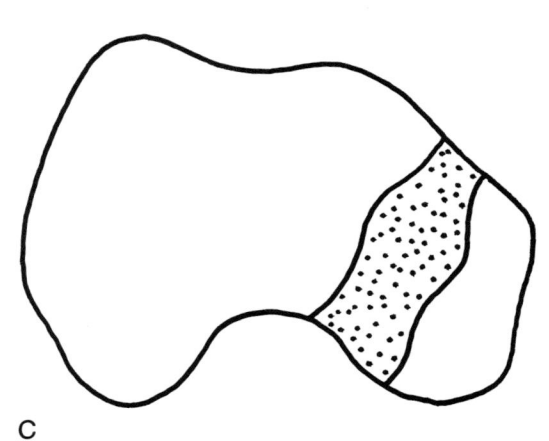

TREATMENT INDICATIONS

The presence of a partial physeal bar will almost always demand treatment. Very occasionally, no appreciable deformity will result from a bar, and thus no treatment is necessary. This can occur when the bar develops so close to maturity that the remainder of normal physeal growth is too minimal to create deformity or appreciable limb length inequality. The treating surgeon should determine the skeletal age of the patient and calculate the growth remaining for the physis involved to evaluate this possibility. This is frequently the case after triplane fracture of the ankle, for example.[5] Alternatively, so much of the physis may be damaged that what little normal physis remains is unable to create angular deformity or joint distortion (epiphysiodesis effect). When this occurs, one only needs to prevent progressive limb length discrepancy in an appropriate manner.

In virtually all other cases, the presence of a partial physeal bar will demand treatment. The amount of difficulty that the bar will create depends on the location of the arrest, the rate of growth of the remaining physis, and the amount of absolute growth to be expected of the involved physis prior to maturity.

The treatment alternatives include the following:

1. Prevention of bar formation
2. Partial physeal bar resection
3. Physeal distraction
4. Repeated osteotomies for angular deformity performed throughout growth
5. Completion of the epiphysiodesis of the involved physis, angular deformity correction if necessary, and treatment of the limb length inequality resulting from the epiphysiodesis

Prevention of Bar Formation

Some experimental work has suggested that indomethacin given for a period of time after injury to a physis may prevent formation of a partial physeal bar.[13]

There has been no clinical investigation that supports this experimental evidence, and its use remains empirical.

Some authors have suggested that open reduction of physeal fractures should be undertaken with a view toward preventing future physeal bar formation.[14] Specifically, in addition to accurate and secure reduction of the fracture, if damaged physis is encountered at the time of open reduction, the area should be protected by immediate fat graft interposition in the hopes of preventing subsequent bar formation, which might otherwise occur. The absence of bar formation in small series of fractures in short follow-up has been encouraging that this preventative treatment is warranted.

Partial Physeal Arrest Resection

Conceptually, resection of a partial physeal bar (or epiphysiolysis, as the operation is sometimes called) to allow resumption of normal growth is the ideal procedure to manage patients with this condition.[8,9,11,14-22] However, the operation can be very demanding technically, and our results[8] have been uneven and uncertain. Specifically, we have seen restoration of useful growth across a physis treated by partial physeal bar resection in only 33 percent of our cases. We have been unable to reliably predict successful resection. In almost all cases where we were successful in restoring growth, that growth ceased prior to skeletal maturity, allowing some portion of limb length inequality, angular deformity, or both to recur. Finally, we had significant complications in some patients. Thus, the decision to undertake this procedure must be made very carefully. Consideration of the factors discussed below will help the treating surgeon decide if this procedure is indicated.

1. *Etiology of the arrest.* Arrests due to infection or irradiation are less likely to respond to resection, presumably because the remainder of the physis is "unhealthy."
2. *Anatomic type of the arrest.* Central and linear arrests tend to respond more favorably than peripheral types.
3. *Physis affected.* Proximal humeral and femoral lesions cannot be exposed under tourniquet intraoperative hemostasis, which will make visualization of the physis much more difficult. Distal femoral bars tend to have a poorer prognosis for resumption of growth after resection than those of the distal tibia.
4. *Extent of the arrest.* Lesions affecting more than 25 percent of the surface area of a particular physis are thought not as likely to respond to resection.
5. *Amount of growth remaining in the physis affected.* The treating surgeon must determine that an appropriate amount of growth remains in the affected physis to warrant an (unpredictable) attempt to restore that growth. In general, at least 2 years of growth remaining is a minimum requirement.

Once the surgeon has determined to attempt physeal bar resection based on the considerations given above, the surgical procedure must be carefully planned. This planning includes (1) making a precise localization of the bar; (2) determining the optimum surgical exposure of the bar; (3) deciding whether to perform simultaneous osteotomy for exposure, preexisting deformity correction, or both; and (4) deciding which interpositional material will be used to retard reformation of the bar.

Precise Determination of the Location and Size of the Bar

This is an essential preoperative evaluation. Surgical descriptions of this procedure are deceptively simple, whereas the surgery itself is often very tedious. Resecting the bar without inadvertently damaging healthy physis is almost always quite difficult. A very firm concept of the size and location of the bar within the circumference of the affected physis helps the surgeon a great deal to remove the bar successfully. There are four basic methods to help localize the bar more accurately than plain anteroposterior (AP) and lateral radiographic views allow.

MULTIPLE VIEW PLAIN RADIOGRAPHS

This is the least useful method of definitive evaluation, but in certain peripheral lesions, such as those associated with infantile Blount's disease where the bar is quite typically located in the posteromedial peripheral portion of the proximal tibial physis, they will suffice.

POLYTOMOGRAPHY

Tomograms are the classical method used to determine the location and extent of the bar. With serial AP and lateral view tomograms, the location and extent of the lesion can be estimated by the mapping method of Carlson and Wenger.[23] Good imaging of the bar can be enhanced by having the radiologist take the tomographic cuts perpendicular to the physis itself, taking into consideration the shape of the physis including any deformity the arrest has created; taking narrow (3 mm) cuts; and using hypocycloidal polytomograms, which provide a sharper image than linear tomograms.

CT Scan of the Affected Physis, With or Without Sagittal Reconstruction

Properly oriented computed tomography (CT) scan cuts (perpendicular to the physis) can provide a clear image of a physeal bar,[24-26] and with sagittal reconstruction, be analyzed similar to polytomograms with respect to mapping the extent of physis involvement (Fig. 62-3). However, it can be difficult to orient the patient properly in the gantry to obtain cuts perpendicular to the lesion.

Magnetic Resonance Imaging

Magnetic resonance imaging (MRI) has tantalizing potential for preoperative evaluation of partial physeal bars.[27-29] Patient positioning in the gantry is not a problem, as it can be for CT scanning. The quality of physeal signals may help differentiate between "sick" physes, which are unable to respond to partial physeal bar resection and those in which the remaining physis has a more normal signal and thus, at least theoretically, be more likely to respond favorably to surgery. The method of image acquisition is important to maximize the value of this modality. Typical T1- and T2-weighted images, which image the bone perimeter and physis fairly well, tend not to differentiate normal cortex, normal physis, and bar very well. On the other hand, gradient echo 3DFT imaging or short T1 inversion recovery (STIR) techniques much more clearly differentiate between bar and abnormal tissue in and around normal physis (Fig. 62-4). To date, most surgeons will feel comfortable only with more distinct radiographic imaging preoperatively.

Selection of the Optimum Surgical Exposure of the Arrest

In general, central lesions are approached "blindly" from the metaphyseal side via either a metaphyseal window or a metaphyseal osteotomy. Before deciding whether or not to use an osteotomy approach, consider whether corrective osteotomy is required (see below), in which case, transosteotomy exposure may be advantageous. Which bone is affected is also an important consideration. Proximal tibial lesions usually are not amenable to transosteotomy approach, since osteotomies below the tibial tubercle will leave the surgeon at the end of a funnel a long distance from the bar. Also, distal tibial and distal radial lesions would require osteotomy of both bones in the segment involved, which might produce more morbidity to the patient than is desirable.

Peripheral lesions are usually approached directly, resecting the bar and the overlying periosteum. One exception to this is posterior peripheral lesions of the distal femur. Posterior fossa approaches for these lesions are difficult and have been associated with peroneal nerve palsy.[9,30] An alternative is to perform metaphyseal osteotomy and rotate the femur until the posterior periosteum can be elevated distally to the level of the peripheral bar.

For any metaphyseal osteotomy approach, the soft tissues may have to be decompressed to allow adequate rotation of the distal fragment to allow the surgeon to see into the medullary canal. Usually, the best method to accomplish this is to resect a small segment of metaphysis, that is, perform a small shortening osteotomy, to adequately relax the soft tissues. When an osteotomy approach in the distal femur is selected, it is usually easier to rotate the distal fragment into the surgeon's line of vision from a medial approach.

Decision Regarding the Need for Simultaneous Osteotomy

If an osteotomy for exposure purposes has not already been decided upon, the surgeon must consider whether the extent of existing deformity warrants simultaneous osteotomy. While anecdotal cases of spontaneous correction of angular deformity are known to occur after successful physeal bar resection, such corrections are by no means universal. Furthermore, successful bar resection is unpredictable, and resumption of growth is not

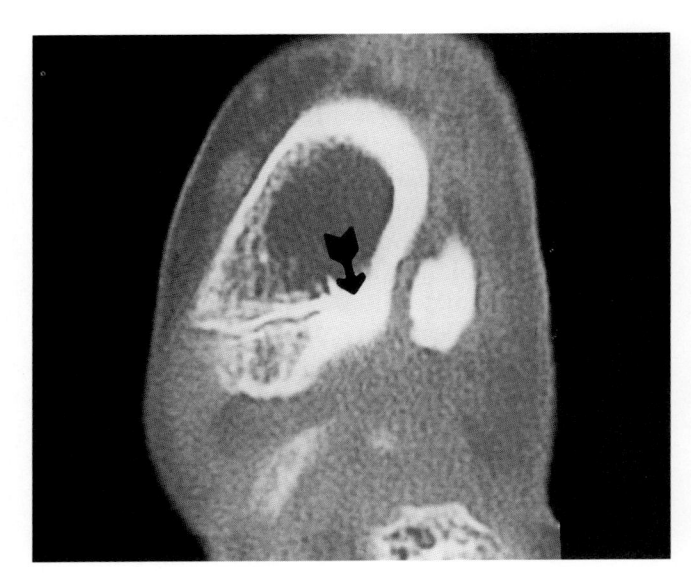

Fig. 62-3. Frontal plane axial CT scan of the distal tibia of the same patient as in Figure 62-1. When the patient can be positioned to obtain CT cuts perpendicular to the physis, the physeal bar can be readily demonstrated *(arrow)*.

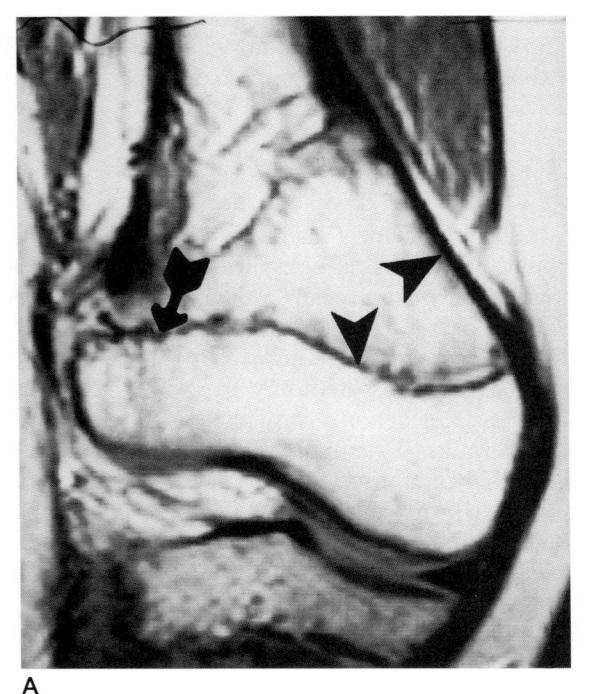

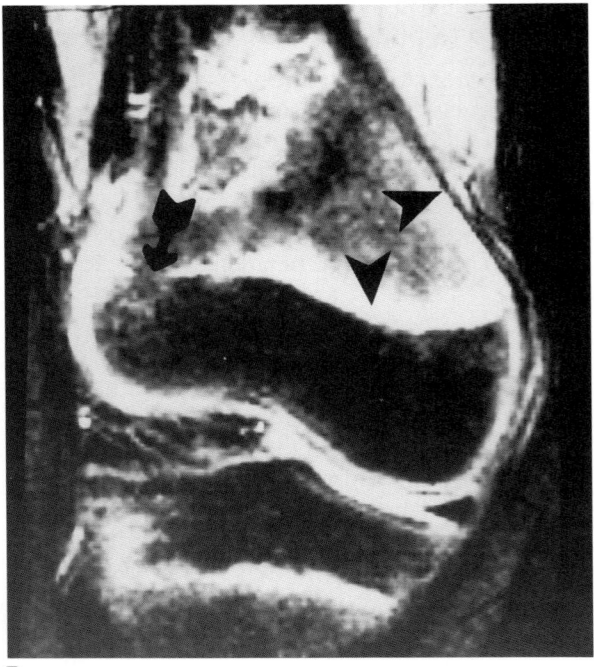

Fig. 62-4. Use of magnetic resonance imaging to localize partial physeal bars. (A) T1-weighted MRI of a patient with partial physeal arrest of the lateral portion of the distal femur after a Salter-Harris type II fracture. While there is obvious disruption of the normal physis *(arrow)* and angular deformity, it is difficult to distinguish the area of bony arrest from the normal physis and the femoral cortex *(arrowheads)*. (B) MRI of the same region of the distal femur, using STIR sequencing technique (see text). Using this method of imaging, the area of physeal arrest *(arrow)* is easily differentiated from the remaining physis and the femoral cortex *(arrowheads)*.

ensured by good surgical technique or excellent indications (such as a discrete posttraumatic central arrest in a young patient). For these reasons, I prefer to perform corrective angular osteotomy in any patient in whom the preoperative deformity is not acceptable on a permanent basis. When, based on these criteria, osteotomy is deemed necessary, I prefer to perform it after bar resection, unless of course, the osteotomy is to be used as the method of physeal bar exposure. Delaying the osteotomy until the bar resection has been completed will minimize intraoperative blood loss from the osteotomy site, and the surgeon does not have to contend with instability of the limb created by the osteotomy while trying to perform the physeal bar resection.

Selection of Interpositional Material

After the bony bar has been removed, a cavity will exist across the physis where the bar was. This cavity must be filled with some material to retard the redevelopment of a bony tether between the metaphysis and epiphysis within that cavity.[15,20,31] Experimental surgery has confirmed the need for this interpositional material to enable subsequent resumption of normal growth. Experimental and clinical experience has documented the effectiveness of four interpositional materials: autogenous fat,[9-11,15,20] methyl methacrylate (Cranioplast),[17] silicone rubber,[18] and hyaline cartilage[19] (experimentally only). The inert materials are felt to conform better to the cavity and are less likely to be displaced by immediate postoperative bleeding. Silicone rubber has always been considered investigational for this purpose, and is not currently commercially available.

Fat has the advantages of being readily available, either locally or from the buttock, and autogenous. There is experimental and clinical evidence that, in at least some cases, the fat graft remains viable and hypertrophies with growth[32,33] (Fig. 62-5). On the other hand, the fat graft can be more easily displaced from its location within the cavity at the level of the physis, and pre-

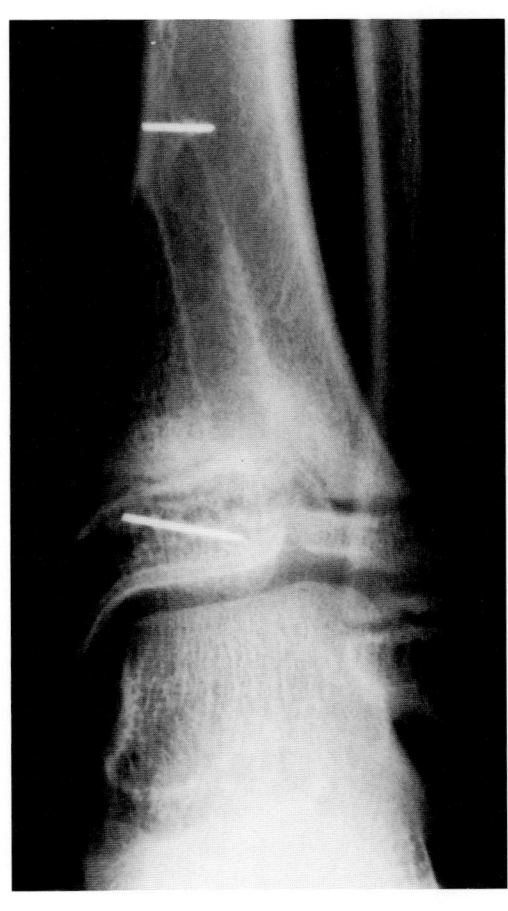

Fig. 62-5. AP view of an ankle, 5 years after successful resection of a central arrest of the distal tibia, with fat interposition. The original surgically created cavity is still evident, indicating viability of the fat graft.

cautions to prevent this should be taken at the time of surgery.

Surgical Technique

Several basic tools will be required to make the actual procedure of bar resection as simple and effective as possible. The fundamental technical difficulty is adequate visualization of the bar itself and the portions of the physis to be exposed by the resection. Several tools and preparations will help greatly in this regard.

Bleeding significantly reduces the surgeon's ability to see physis and differentiate it from bone. Whenever possible, the surgery should be performed under tourniquet hemostasis. The surgeon should expect a great deal more difficulty if tourniquet hemostasis is not possible, for example, in the proximal humerus.

A brilliant light source should be available. A headlight, light source from an operating microscope, or a fiberoptic lighted sucker tip can be used. Magnification should also be available, either by using an operating microscope or loupes.

During the surgery, the bone cavity should be frequently flushed with irrigation, sucked dry, and the physis "polished" with a gauze. Coupled with a brilliant light source and magnification, this procedure will significantly enhance the surgeon's ability to see the physis, and differentiate it from the bone in the cavity being created.

A high-speed bur will facilitate the gentle removal of the sclerotic bone which usually makes up the bulk of a bar, while minimizing the injury to the residual physis, which will be exposed during the removal of the bar itself.

The basic technique of the resection is to identify, enter, and gradually remove the bone which has replaced the physis, without unduly exposing or injuring the remaining healthy physis. Periodic radiographic or, preferably, fluoroscopic confirmation that the surgeon is working at the level of and making progress toward exposing the residual physis is absolutely essential to accomplish this.

Finally, in all central types of arrest, it is impossible to see the entire circumference of the cavity directly, and some aid must be used to look into the cavity. A small dental or ENT (ears, nose, and throat) mirror can be used for this purpose. Alternatively, an angled arthroscope can be inserted into the cavity for this purpose.

Technique of Central Physeal Bar Resection

Central arrests will be approached from the metaphyseal marrow cavity either via a metaphyseal cortical window or osteotomy. The surgical approach must be selected with care, with the purpose of maximizing the surgeon's ability to see into the cavity that will be created.[30] If a window approach is decided upon, then its location should be as close as possible to the bar itself, to maximize visualization of the bar through it, which is almost always difficult. If a metaphyseal osteotomy is used for exposure, then it too should be as close to the physis as possible, again to minimize the difficulty of visualization of the bar itself.

With either technique, the initial procedure is to create a metaphyseal marrow cavity directed at the bar itself

1146 / Management of Pediatric Fractures

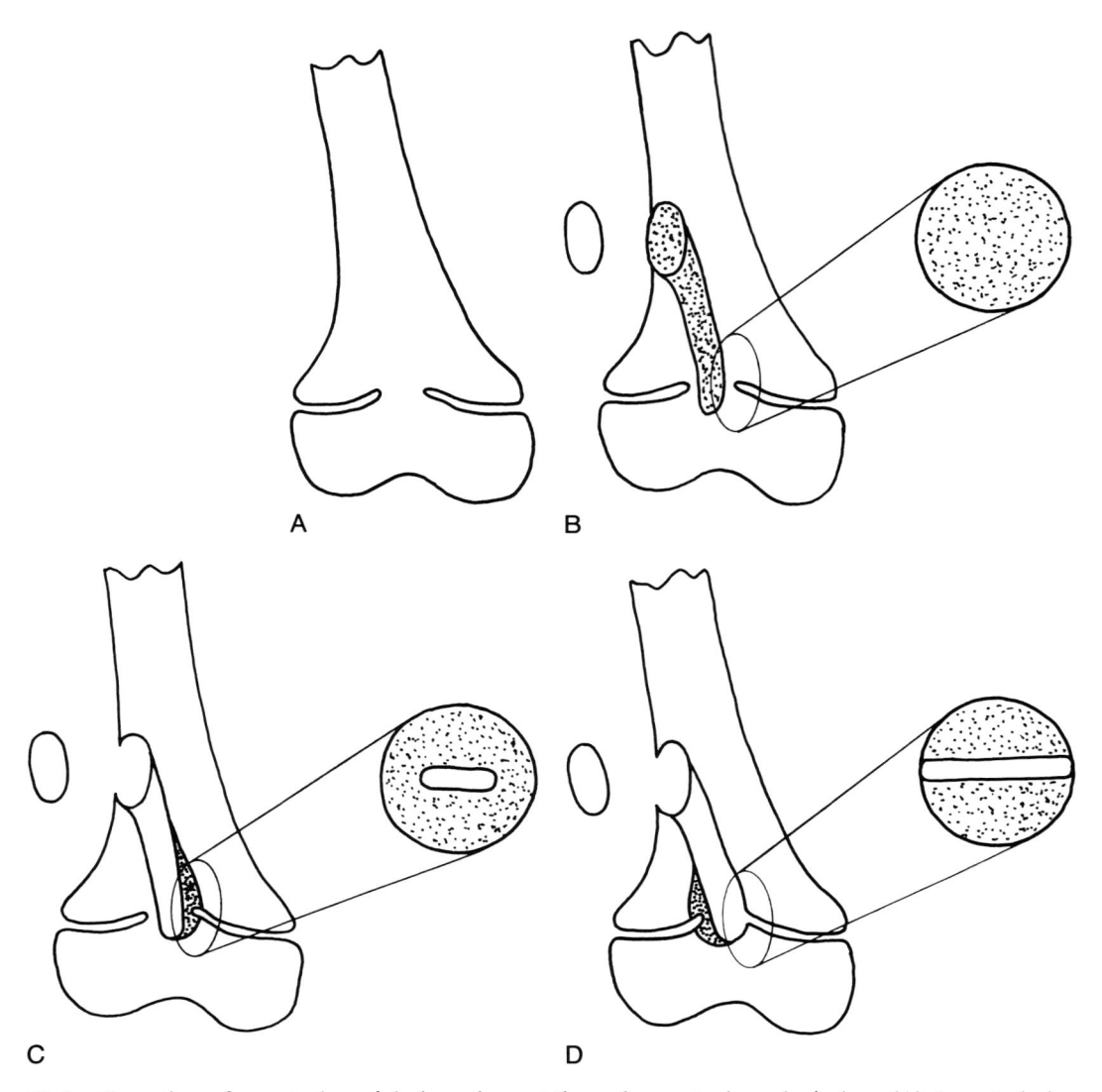

Fig. 62-6. Resection of a central partial physeal arrest through a metaphyseal window. **(A)** A central physeal arrest of the distal femur. **(B)** The initial steps of the operation are to remove an oval window of metaphyseal cortex near the arrest, and to create a cavity extending from the window beyond the physis through the arrest under fluoroscopic control. At this point, no physis should be evident *(inset)*. **(C)** Under fluoroscopic control, the cavity is gradually enlarged at the level of the physis until the physis becomes visible within the cavity *(inset)*. **(D)** The cavity is then gradually expanded following the portion of physis that was exposed initially, until the physis can be identified circumferentially within the cavity *(inset)*. *(Figure continues.)*

(Fig. 62-6). This must be done under fluoroscopic control. The bar itself is usually sclerotic, with a consistency distinctly firmer than the normal cancellous bone; this can aid the surgeon's orientation. This cavity should be extended within the substance of the bar beyond the level of the residual physis into the epiphysis. Ideally, at this point, no physis is yet visible (see inset, Fig. 62-6B). Next, using a high-speed bur, the cavity is expanded at the level of the physis. Fluoroscopic confirmation that this expansion is occurring at the level of the physis, rather than above or below it is essential at this point. Eventually, the cavity will be enlarged until it contacts the physis at some point (Fig. 62-6C). The cavity should then be gradually enlarged circumferentially from the point where the physis is visible, until the physis can be seen to completely ring the cavity (Fig. 62-6D). During this portion of the procedure, the bur should be worked in a to-and-fro fashion, perpendicular to and at the level of the

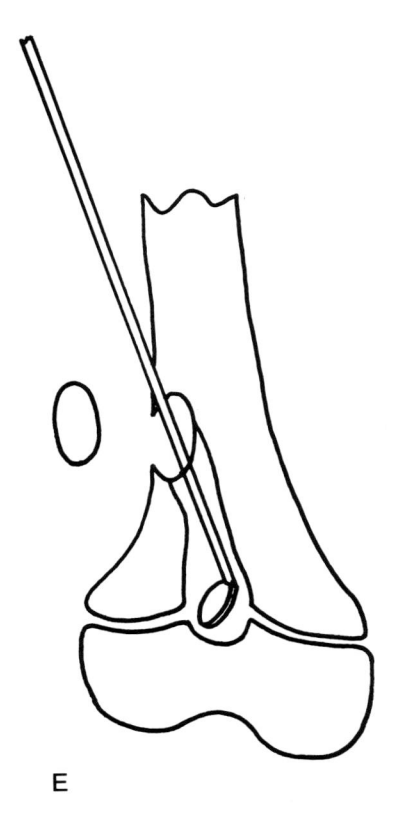

Fig. 62-6 *(Continued)***(E)** A small dental mirror or arthroscope can be inserted into the cavity to allow circumferential viewing of the physis.

physis, to minimize the amount of injury to the physis itself. Either a small mirror or arthroscope will be necessary to confirm that the physis is visible around the entire perimeter of the cavity, indicating complete resection of the bar (Fig. 62-6E).

Once the resection is complete, the interpositional material of choice should be inserted into the cavity. If an inert material such as Cranioplast is to be used, it is necessary to anchor it to the epiphyseal side of the cavity by means of a K-wire or small Steinmann pin inserted through the epiphyseal bone into the cavity prior to inserting the cement. This will help keep the material in proximity to the physis should normal growth occur. Also, the material should cover the exposed physis while simultaneously having as little contact with the metaphyseal bone as possible (Fig. 62-7A). This prevents the interpositional material itself from acting as a tether between the metaphyseal and epiphyseal bone and from migrating with the metaphysis away from the physis should normal growth resume. A small K-wire can be inserted into the metaphyseal cortex to serve as a marker. If normal growth occurs postoperatively, that fact as well as the extent of growth over time can be readily appreciated by measuring the distance between the metaphyseal marker and the epiphyseal anchoring pin.

If fat is used as the interpositional material, it is not necessary to anchor it to the epiphysis. However, the fat may be washed away from the physis by postoperative bleeding into the cavity. To prevent this, I prefer to pack the entire cavity with fat, and to seal it into the cavity by either replacing the metaphyseal window or covering the window with soft tissue (Fig. 62-7B). Remember to insert a wire marker into the epiphysis in place of the anchoring pin used for inert materials, so that growth across the affected physis can be documented (Fig. 62-8).

If osteotomy is necessary and has not been used as the route of bar exposure, it can be performed at this time.

Technique of Peripheral Physeal Bar Resection

Peripheral bars will usually be exposed directly by the surgical approach which will expose the bone at the level of the physis directly over the bar itself. Even if osteotomy will be necessary to correct angular deformity, it is usually preferable to delay this until after bar resection is complete. The exception to this may be peripheral posterior distal femoral bars, as discussed above.

The normal perichondrium and perichondral ring are replaced by periosteum over peripheral bars. This periosteum is usually easily stripped from the underlying bar, and along with fluoroscopy, serves as a landmark to identify the location of the bar. This periosteal tissue should be excised to help prevent reformation of the bar peripherally. Next, the bar is gradually removed with a high-speed bur, creating a cavity in the metaphyseal-epiphyseal bone at the level of the residual physis (Fig. 62-9).

There are two ways for the surgeon to confirm the proper level for the resection. One method is to begin the resection in the middle of the bar, and create a cavity directed toward the residual physis under fluoroscopic control. Initially, no physis at all will be visible (see inset, Fig. 62-9A). Resection will continue, directed toward the physis until a small portion of the residual physis will be seen in the depths of the cavity (Fig. 62-9B). From the point where the physis has been exposed, the remaining bar should be gradually removed toward the periphery of the bone, until healthy perichondrial ring has been identified at the extreme margins of the resection. During this exposure, the same to-and-fro technique of using the bur perpendicular to the physis should be used.

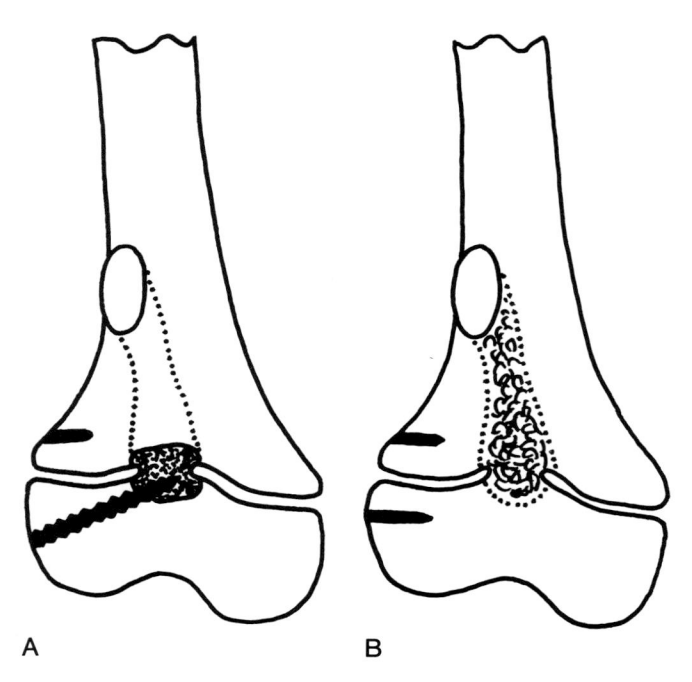

Fig. 62-7. Interpositional material location to prevent reformation of the arrest. **(A)** If an inert material such as Cranioplast is used as the spacer material, it should be pressed into the epiphyseal cavity, cover the physis, and encroach on the metaphyseal side of the cavity as little as possible. The material should be anchored to the epiphysis by means of a Steinmann pin placed in the epiphyseal bone extending into the epiphyseal cavity. A second wire is inserted into the metaphysis to serve as a marker. **(B)** If autogenous fat is used, it is not necessary to anchor it to the epiphysis. The entire cavity should be filled with fat, and the window sealed with the original bone or soft tissue to prevent displacement of the fat. K-wires are inserted into the epiphysis and metaphysis to serve as markers only.

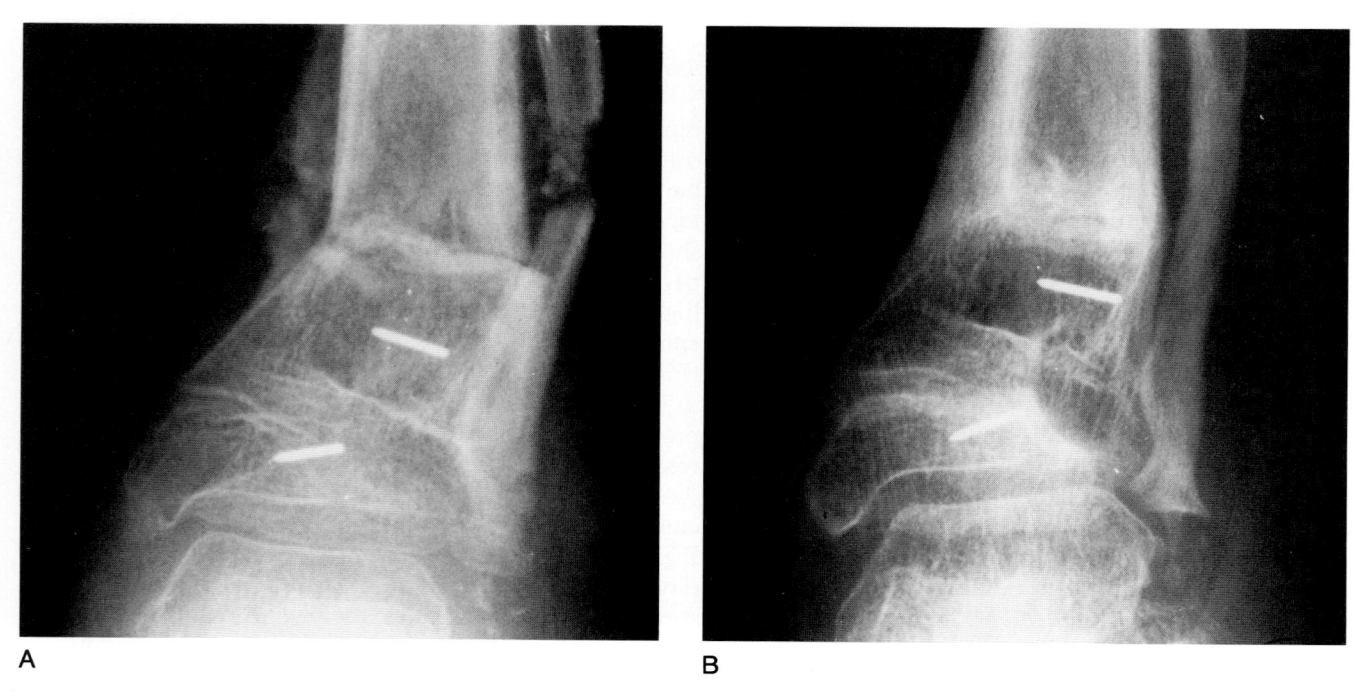

Fig. 62-8. Use of metaphyseal and epiphyseal markers to detect early resumption of normal growth after physeal bar resection. **(A)** Same patient as Figure 62-1, 4 weeks after physeal bar resection with fat interposition and distal tibial osteotomy. Note that the sclerotic bar seen in Figure 62-1 has been removed. Fine K-wire markers have been inserted into the metaphyseal and epiphyseal bone at the time of surgery. **(B)** At 4 months later, the markers have separated 3 mm. without change in their angular relationship. This serves as an early indication of resumption of longitudinal growth after physeal bar resection.

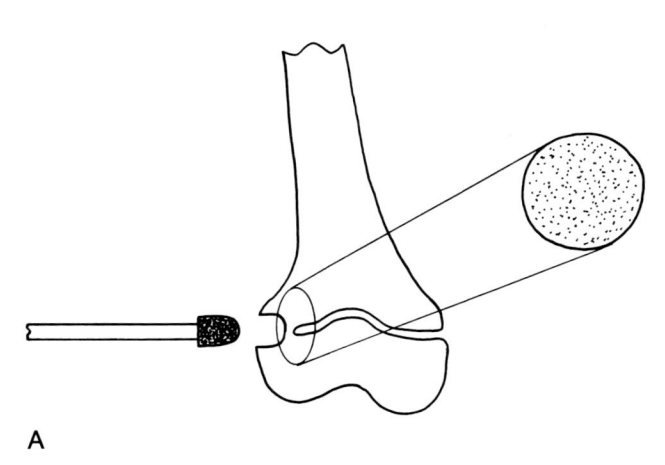

Fig. 62-9. Surgical resection of a peripheral physeal arrest. **(A)** The periosteum overlying the physeal bar is exposed. A high-speed bur is used to gradually remove the bone that has replaced the physis. Resection is directed toward the normal physis, under fluoroscopic control. At this stage, only bone will be evident in the surgically created cavity *(inset)*. **(B)** Eventually, the cavity will extend to contact the normal physis at some point. The physis will appear as a small cartilage band in the depths of the cavity *(inset)*. **(C)** Using the exposed rim of physis and under fluoroscopic control, the cavity is gradually enlarged by the bur until the physis can be traced to the perimeter of the bone.

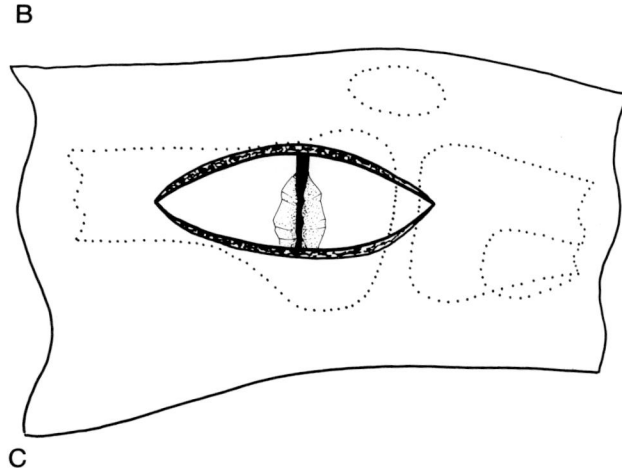

An alternative method is to identify the periosteum over the bar and strip it circumferentially until healthy physis and perichondral ring is identified at one extreme edge of the bar (Fig. 62-10). Resection begins at this known endpoint into the depths of the bar and the opposite extreme, again using fluoroscopy to confirm that resection is directed at the level of the physis.

With either technique, once the bar has been completely resected, the residual physis should be visible as a rim of cartilage within the cavity, which extends from the extremes of the healthy perimeter of normal physis and perichondral ring (Fig. 62-9C). At this point, osteotomy can be performed as desired. Anchor pin, interpositional material, and marker wire should be inserted as for central bars (see above). If fat is used as the interpositional material, then the overlying soft tissue should be closed over the fat graft to help hold the graft in place. The surgeon may wish to release the tourniquet prior to graft placement to achieve hemostasis with bone wax or gelfoam.

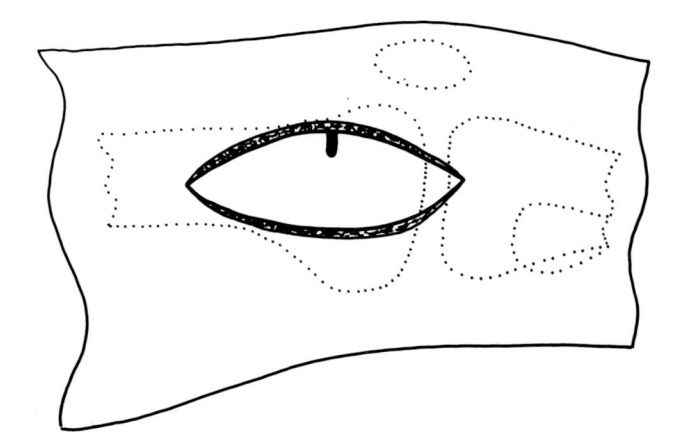

Fig. 62-10. An alternative method of preparing for surgical resection of a peripheral physeal arrest (see text). The periosteum which has replaced the normal perichondrium is exposed, and elevated peripherally until the normal perichondrial ring is identified. Resection of the bony bar is then performed as diagrammed in Figure 62-9, commencing from this normal landmark.

Technique of Linear Physeal Bar Resection

The surgical technique of linear bar resection is a combination of central and peripheral bar resection techniques. The bar should be exposed at one end as for peripheral lesions, and gradually "cored out," working across the bone within the bar to the opposite end of the arrest. Visualization of the exposed physis should be prepared for similar to central arrests. Interpositional material and markers should be used as for peripheral and central arrests.

Physeal Distraction

This technique consists of mounting an external fixator (Ilizarov, Orthofix, or other) across the physeal arrest in an epiphyseal-metaphyseal or epiphyseal-diaphyseal configuration and commencing gradual distraction.[34,35] After a period of distraction varying from a few days to several weeks, the physis will usually separate (often as an acutely painful episode) thereby "breaking" the bar. Angular deformity and lengthening can then continue as desired by manipulating the external fixator (Fig. 62-11).

The advantages of this technique include the fact that it is a more certain way to correct deformity and limb length equality, and that the correction is performed at the level of the deformity (the epiphyseal-metaphyseal junction). One potential disadvantage is that the external fixation of the epiphyseal portion of the bone, particularly of the distal femur, may be intra-articular with some attendant risk for septic arthritis. Furthermore, subsequent growth of a physis so treated is unlikely. Thus, in general, this technique should be reserved for a patient approaching skeletal maturity, and in whom this anatomic level of correction is desirable.

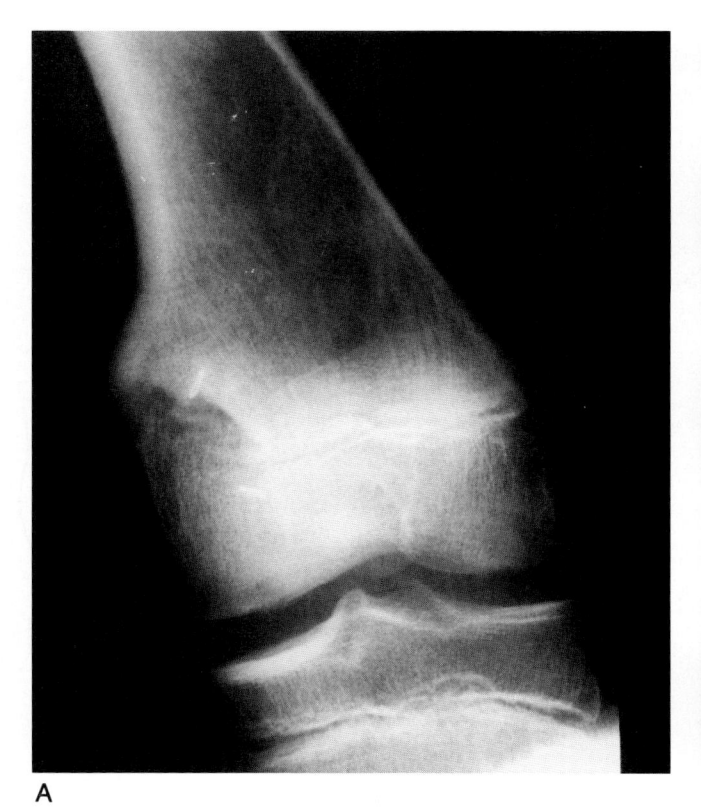

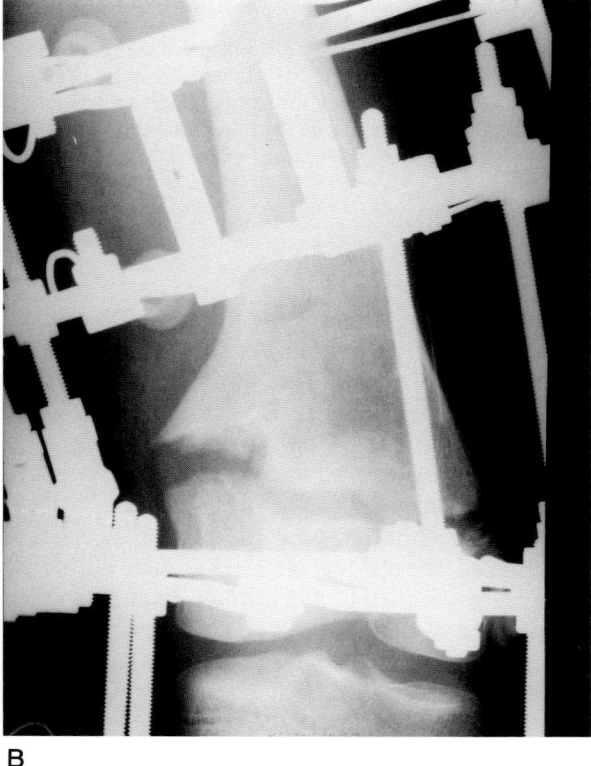

Fig. 62-11. Management of a partial physeal bar by external fixation and physeal distraction. **(A)** Distal femoral physeal bar after physeal fracture with angular deformity and shortening in a 14-year-old boy. **(B)** Radiographic appearance after Ilizarov external fixation with distraction across the physis until the bar was disrupted with further lengthening and angular deformity correction. (Courtesy Dr. C. E. Johnston, Texas Scottish Rite Hospital, Dallas, Texas.)

Repeated Osteotomies During Growth

The simplest method to correct angular deformity produced by partial bars (usually of the peripheral type) is to perform repeated osteotomies of the affected bone as required during growth. This method obviously will not correct limb length inequality, which may also be present, nor affect possible joint distortion, which may result from the arrest. In young patients with a great deal of growth remaining in whom previous physeal bar resection has been unsuccessful or is technically impossible, there may be no reasonable treatment alternative.

Completion of the Epiphysiodesis and Management of Resulting Limb Length Discrepancy

Sometimes, the presence of a partial physeal bar is well recognized, but its resection is deemed unwarranted or impossible. Typically, this is the case when insufficient growth remains to warrant unpredictable efforts to salvage that growth (by partial physeal bar resection), attempted physeal bar resection has failed to restore normal growth, or physeal bar resection is not otherwise advisable (too large a bar, too inaccessible, or the residual physis is unhealthy, such as occurs after radiation or

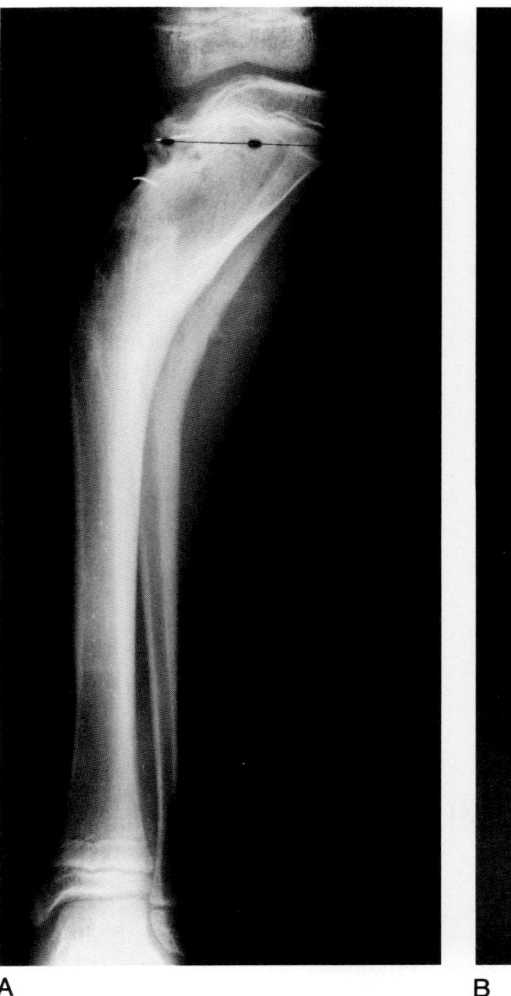

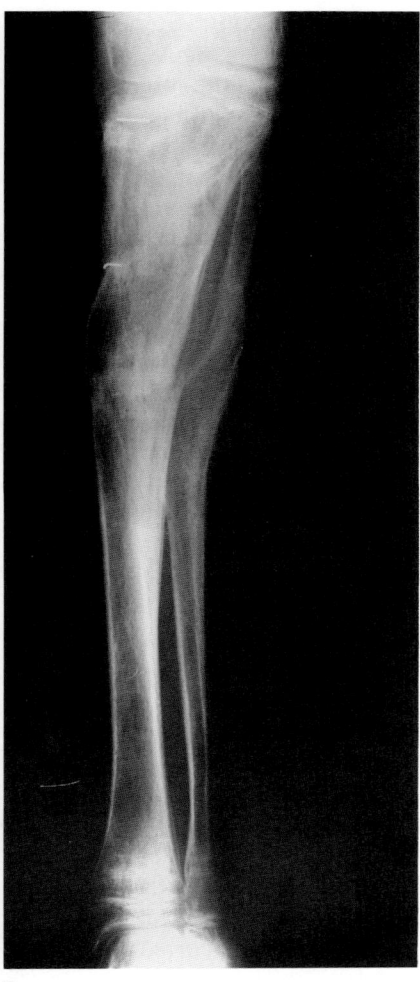

Fig. 62-12. Management of partial physeal bar by completion of epiphysiodesis, external fixation and metaphyseal deformity correction and lengthening. **(A)** 11-year-old boy with infantile Blount's disease, after three previous tibial osteotomies, and two previous attempts at partial physeal bar resection. Recurrent physeal bar and varus deformity, persistent postsurgical valgus deformity, and 4 cm of shortening. **(B)** After completion of proximal tibial epiphysiodesis, angular deformity correction and lengthening of the metaphysis. Tibia was overlengthened 1 cm to compensate for loss of length due to epiphysiodesis.

infection). The technique is to simply complete the epiphysiodesis of the affected physis, so that no further (distorted) growth will occur. The surgeon must then consider correction of existing angular deformity and limb length inequality and subsequent limb length discrepancy that will develop during the remainder of growth.

One method to control progressive limb length discrepancy caused by completing the epiphysiodesis of a damaged physis is to perform epiphysiodesis of the same physis in the opposite extremity. Remember that this procedure will result in no correction of a preexisting discrepancy, since both physes will be closed. If a discrepancy is to be reduced (generally, those greater than 2 cm), then other physes in the contralateral limb will also have to undergo epiphysiodesis. Acute angular corrective osteotomy by the method of the surgeon's choice may be combined with completion of the epiphysiodesis whenever preexisting angular deformity is deemed unacceptable. Again, opposite extremity epiphysiodesis will need to be considered to manage existing and projected discrepancy due the completion of the epiphysiodesis.

Completion of the epiphysiodesis may be combined with limb lengthening with an external fixation device, such as the Ilizarov apparatus, either simultaneously or in a staged fashion. In general, lengthening should be considered when the projected discrepancy will be 4 cm or greater. When the discrepancy at maturity will be less than 20 percent of the total bone length (or not more than 6–7 cm), delaying the lengthening until the completion of growth may be appropriate. When the discrepancy will be greater than 20 percent of the total length of the involved bone at maturity, either staged lengthenings or a combination of lengthening and contralateral epiphysiodesis should be considered.

When osteotomy for angular deformity is considered, an a attractive alternative is to perform simultaneous lengthening for existing or projected discrepancy, even when that discrepancy will be less than 4 cm. This spares the opposite limb from epiphysiodesis, but will extend the treatment program commensurate with the amount of lengthening required. In theory, the treating surgeon may simultaneously perform angular correction, correct existing limb length inequality, and overlengthen to offset the loss of length due to the completion of the epiphysiodesis (Fig. 62-12). However, such "overlengthenings" can be difficult because of the resistance of the soft tissues, and in general, should not be attempted beyond 1 or 2 cm.

SUMMARY

Since partial physeal bars can produce severe deformity and be very vexing to treat, it is fortunate that they are a relatively rare consequence of physeal injury. Surgeons should be vigilant to their presence, as early recognition will allow treatment to begin before severe deformity has resulted. Ideally, an established bar may be resected, allowing resumption of normal growth. In practice, however, this is only a modestly and unpredictably successful procedure, and the surgeon is often left with more traditional methods to try to control deformity produced by the partial arrest. Recent advances in external fixation, deformity correction, and limb lengthening such as by the Ilizarov method will prove a useful advance in the management of these deformities.

REFERENCES

1. Peterson CA, Peterson HA: Analysis of the incidence of injuries to the epiphyseal growth plate. J Trauma 12:275, 1972
2. Ogden JA: Injury to the growth mechanism of the immature skeleton. Skeletal Radiol 6:237, 1981
3. Salter RB, Harris WR: Injuries involving the epiphyseal plate. Instr Course Lect 45A:587, 1963
4. Mizuta T, Benson WM, Foster BK et al: Statistical analysis of the incidence of physeal injuries. J Pediatr Orthop 7:518, 1987
5. Cass JR, Peterson HA: Salter-Harris type IV injuries of the distal tibial epiphyseal growth plate, with emphasis on those involving the medial malleolus. J Bone Joint Surg [Am] 65:1059, 1983
6. Landin LA, Danielsson LG, Jonsson K, Pettersson H: Late results in 65 physeal ankle fractures. Acta Orthop Scand 57:530, 1986
7. Bright RW: Physeal injuries. p. 87. In Rockwood CA, Wilkins KE, King RE (eds): Fractures in Children. Vol. 3. JB Lippincott, Philadelphia, 1984
8. Birch JG: Surgical technique of physeal bar resection. Instr Course Lect 41:445, 1992
9. Langenskiold A: Surgical treatment of partial closure of the growth plate. J Pediatr Orthop 1:3, 1981
10. Williamson RV, Staheli LT: Partial physeal growth arrest: treatment by bridge resection and fat interposition. J Pediatr Orthop 10:769, 1990
11. Broughton NS, Dickens DRV, Cole WG, Menelaus MB: Epiphyeolysis for partial growth plate arrest results after four years or at maturity. J Bone Joint Surg [Br] 71:13, 1989
12. Langenskiold A: Growth disturbances after osteomyelitis of femoral condyles in infants. Acta Orthop Scand 55:1, 1984

13. Sudmann E, Husby OS, Bang G: Inhibition of partial closure of epiphyseal plate in rabbits by indomethacin. Acta Orthop Scand 53:507, 1982
14. Foster BK: The experimental basis for growth plate surgery. p. 109. In Menelaus MD (ed): The Management of Limb Inequality. Churchill Livingstone, Edinburgh, 1991
15. Langenskiold A: The possibilities of eliminating premature partial closure of an epiphyseal plate cause by trauma or disease. Acta Orthop Scand 38:267, 1967
16. Ogden J: The evaluation and treatment of partial physeal arrest. J Bone Joint Surg [Am] 69:1297, 1987
17. Peterson AH: Partial growth plate arrest and its treatment. J Pediatr Orthop 4:246, 1984
18. Bright RW: Operative correction of partial epiphyseal plate closure by osseous-bridge resection and silicone-rubber implant: an experimental study in dogs. J Bone Joint Surg [Am] 56:655, 1974
19. Lennox DW: Cartilage as an interposition material to prevent transphyseal bone bridge formation: an experimental model. J Pediatr Orthop 3:207, 1983
20. Osterman K: Operative elimination of partial epiphyseal closure: an experimental study. Acta Orthop Scand, suppl 147:7, 1972
21. Broughton NS, Cole WG: The management of growth plate arrest. p. 121. In Menelaus MD (ed): The Management of Limb Inequality. Churchill Livingstone, Edinburgh, 1991
22. Burke SW: Principles of physeal bridge resection. Barr JS (ed): Instr Course Lect 38:337, 1989
23. Carlson WO, Wenger DR: A mapping method to prepare for surgical excision of partial physeal arrest. J Pediatr Orthop 4:232, 1984
24. Young JWR, Bright RW, Whitley NO: Computed tomography in the evaluation of partial growth plate arrest in children. Skeletal Radiol 15:530, 1986
25. Murry K, Nixon GW: Epiphyseal growth plate: evaluation with modified cornal CT. Radiology 166:263, 1988
26. De Campo JF, Boldt DW: Computed tomography of partial growth plate arrest: initial experience. Skeletal Radiol 15:526, 1986
27. Havranek P, Lizler J: Magnetic resonance imaging in the evaluation of partial growth arrest after physeal injuries in children. J Bone Joint Surg [Am] 73:1234, 1991
28. Jaramillo D, Hoffer FA, Shapiro F, Rand F: MR imaging of fractures of the growth plate. AJR 155:1261, 1990
29. Gabel GT, Peterson HA, Berquist TH: Premature partial physeal arrest: diagnosis by magnetic resonance imaging in two cases. Clin Orthop 272:242, 1991
30. Birch JG, Herring JA, Wenger DR: Surgical anatomy of selected physis. J Pediatr Orthop 4:224, 1984
31. Friedenberg ZB: Reaction of the epiphyseal to partial surgical resection. J Bone Joint Surg [Am] 39:332, 1957
32. Langenskiold A: The fate of fat transplants in operations for partial closure of the growth plate: clinical examples and an experimental study. J Bone Joint Surg [Br] 68:234, 1986
33. Mayer V, Marchisello PJ: Traumatic partial arrest of tibial physis. Clin Orthop 183:99, 1984
34. de Pablos J: Bone lengthening methods in the treatment of angular deformities of the long bones. p. 331. In de Pablos and Canadell J (eds): Bone Lengthening Current Trends and Controversies. The University of Navarro, Pamplona, Spain, 1990
35. Foster BK: Interpositional and distractional physiolysis: clinical results. p. 243. In Uhthoff HD, Wiley JJ (eds): Behavior of the Growth Plate. Raven Press, New York, 1988

63

Reflex Sympathetic Dystrophy

Maureen P. Baxter

> Example is not the main thing in life it is the only thing.
> —Albert Schweitzer

DESCRIPTION AND INCIDENCE

Reflex sympathetic dystrophy (RSD) is the commonly accepted term describing a complex clinical entity typically affecting one extremity. Other terms, such as Sudeck's atrophy, algoneurodystrophy, causalgia, reflex neurovascular dystrophy, reflect the broad spectrum of clinical symptoms and the poorly understood pathophysiology. The characteristics of the syndrome include moderate to severe limb pain with swelling, dysesthesia to light touch, and autonomic nerve dysfunction with vasomotor instability and dystrophic skin changes.

RSD is generally considered less common in children than in adults. There is no actual incidence reported in the literature, since the disorder is frequently unrecognized. In a review of all patients seen in the Orthopedic Clinic at the Children's Hospital of Eastern Ontario during a 1-year period, only 10 new cases were diagnosed.

In 1990, Dietz and colleagues[1] reviewed 80 cases of RSD in children published in the English literature and added 5 cases of their own. Their review showed a male:female ratio of 1:6. The mean age of reported cases was 11 years (range: 3 to 17 years). Although this disorder is most frequently encountered in the teenage population, it can occasionally affect young children. Dysesthesia to light touch was the most common physical finding (87 percent). Signs of vasomotor instability were present in 83 percent of cases, including color changes (60 percent), decreased temperature (58 percent), altered sweating (14 percent), and decreased pulses (16 percent). Local swelling was noted in 70 percent of their cases. The regional distribution was foot and ankle (52 percent), arm (21 percent), knee (14 percent), hand (8 percent), and shoulder (5 percent).

ANATOMY

There has been no universally accepted theory to explain the pathogenesis of this syndrome. The specific site of the neural system that propagates the disease is still disputed.[2,3] The two most widely accepted proposals include those of Livingston[4] and of Melzak and Wall.[5] Livingston proposed an abnormal state of heightened activity in the internuncial neuron pool in the spinal cord, which propagates the continuous stimulation of sympathetic nerve fibers. Melzak and Wall's gate-control theory suggests that certain cells in the substantia gelatinosa of the spinal cord act to direct incoming afferent impulses. The large myelinated fibers act to inhibit the control system. The small fibers, such as the afferent sympathetic fibers, tend to stimulate the substantia gelatinosa to open the gate, thereby increasing the transmission of pain impulses to the brain.

MECHANISM OF INJURY

The mechanism of injury may vary from trivial to severe trauma. Neither a fracture nor a crush injury need occur. In fact, only half of the children reported by Dietz and colleagues[1] recalled a precipitating episode of trauma. Lower extremity involvement was more common in children, and the knee was a frequent site of pathology. RSD affecting the knee of adolescent females was frequently misdiagnosed as chondromalacia patellae.

CLASSIFICATION

The clinical manifestations of the disease in children can be divided into three stages, according to Lankford:[6]

Stage I: Represents the condition during the first 3 months and is marked by deep burning and persistent pain, dysesthesia of skin, swelling, and vasomotor instability, predominantly vasodilatory.

Stage II: The continuation of the symptoms from 3 to 9 months, is marked by gradual relief of pain and the appearance of vasoconstrictive symptoms such as progressive stiffness and deformity as the swelling subsides; trophic changes appear in the skin.

Stage III: Represents the presence of symptoms in excess of 9 months and features intractable progressive atrophy of skin, muscle, and bone.

PHYSICAL EXAMINATION

The typical child with RSD will show intense preoccupation with the affected limb. (Fig. 63-1). The findings on clinical examination will vary depending on the stage of the disease. There is no one pathognomonic sign; however, Dietz and colleagues[1] found the *tache cerebrale,* a sign of autonomic dysfunction originally de-

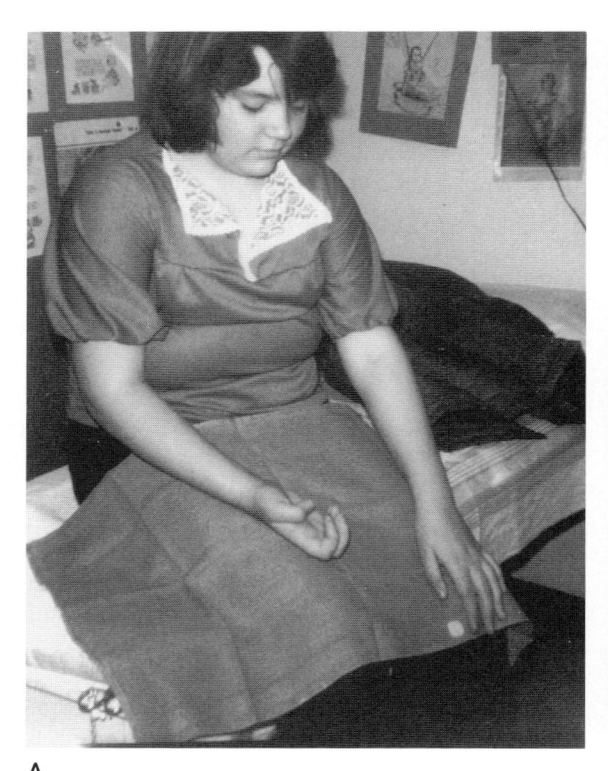

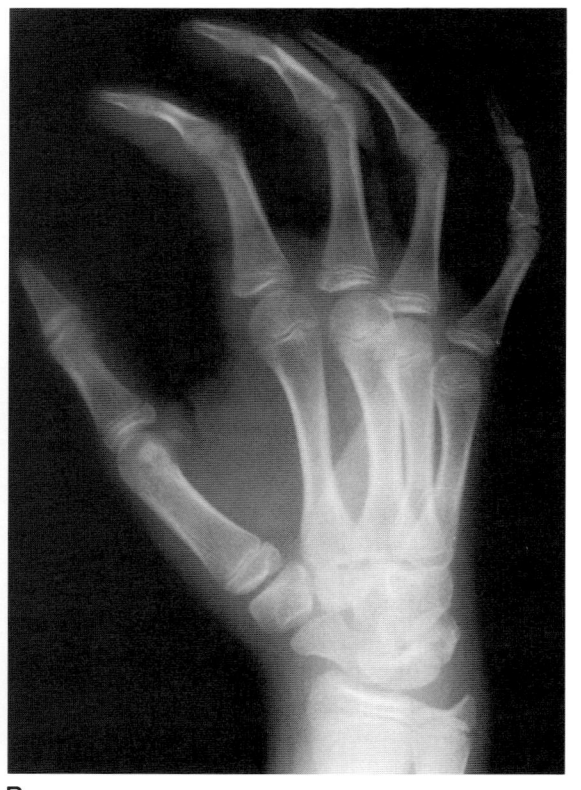

Fig. 63-1. (A) This 13-year-old girl shows the classic "oculopalmar syndrome" typical of upper extremity RSD. She had a minor crush injury to hand sustained when a friend closed a locker door on her hand. (B) The radiograph shows only a nonspecific, diffuse osteopenia.

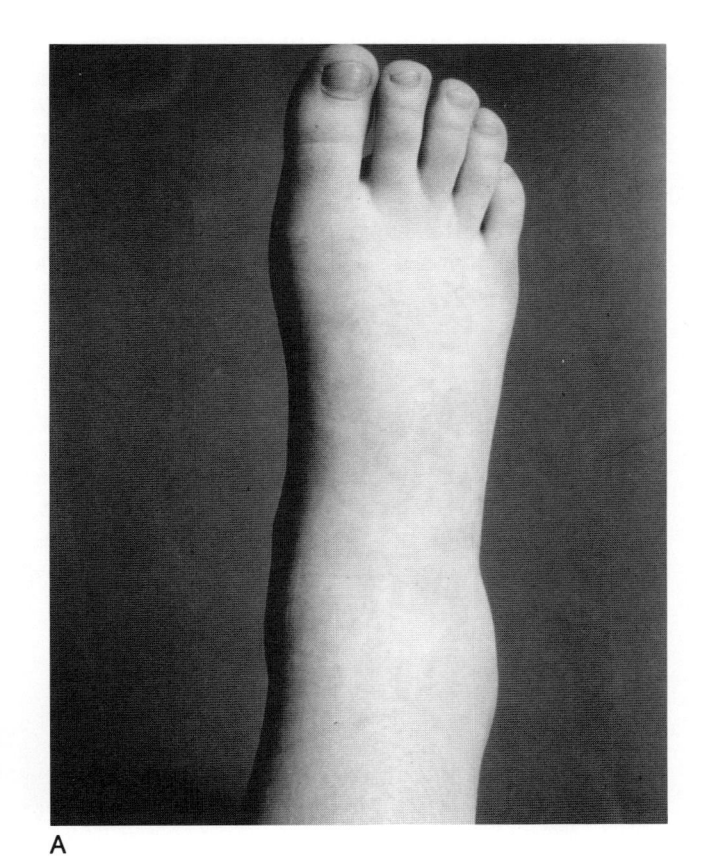

Fig. 63-2. **(A)** This 16-year-old boy suffered a minor ankle sprain with no initial swelling or ecchymosis. Three months later, his ankle is edematous, cold, and mottled. He has been unable to weight bear for 6 weeks. **(B)** The radiograph shows only a nonspecific, diffuse osteopenia.

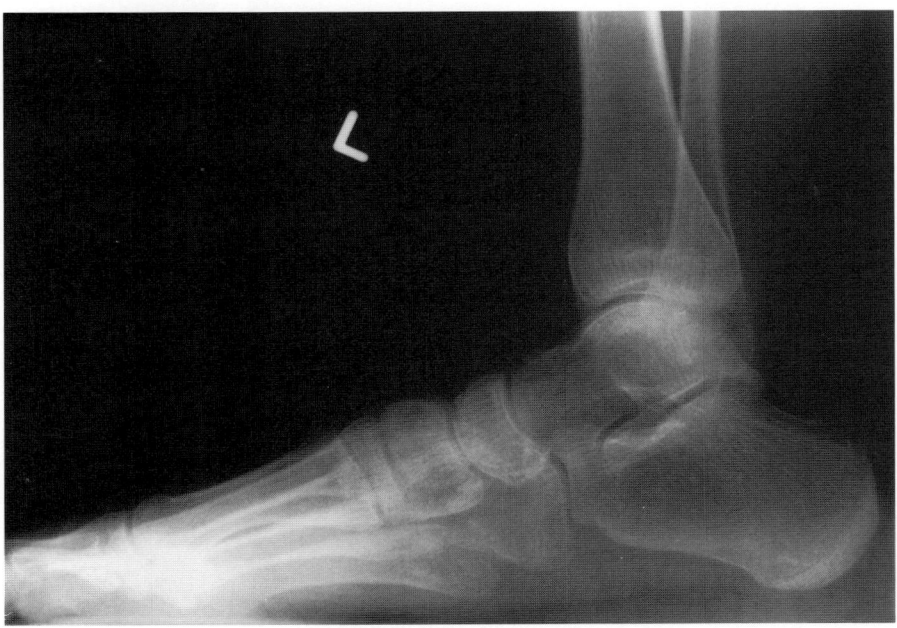

scribed in children with acute central nervous system disease,[7] to be helpful in the diagnosis of RSD. The tache cerebrale is elicited by stroking the skin in the affected area with a blunt object such as the head of a safety pin, using the contralateral limb as a control. Autonomic dysfunction is demonstrated by the appearance of an erythematous line 15 to 30 seconds after the stimulus.[8] These authors found the tache cerebrale was present in all 5 of their reported cases. In 2 patients, the sign was present before other signs of autonomic dysfunction appeared.

DIFFERENTIAL DIAGNOSIS

The average delay in diagnosis is usually about 6 months.[1] A somatic origin for the pain must be ruled out. Radiographic studies are not frequently helpful. Nonspecific diffuse osteopenia occurs in only a small percentage of affected children[1] (Fig. 63-2). The spotty or patchy osteopenia typical of adults with RSD is rare in children (Fig. 63-3). Perhaps the higher turnover rate of a child's metabolically active bone may rapidly repair the atrophic bony changes of RSD and therefore prevent the pattern of patchy osteopenia. Several authors report a lack of sensitivity and specificity for bone scanning in this disorder in children.[9,10] Patterns of increased uptake, decreased uptake or normal were fairly evenly distributed.[1] These findings may reflect the duration of the disease or represent a manifestation of the vasomotor instability of the affected extremity. Routine laboratory studies, including complete blood count, sedimentation rate, biochemistry profile, and rheumatologic and immunologic tests, are all negative.

A recent report by Bryan and colleagues[11] describes a technique for early diagnosis of RSD. The authors measured pressure-pain thresholds with an instrument called a dolorimeter developed by Atkins and Kanis.[12] Their study examined adult patients with persistent pain after

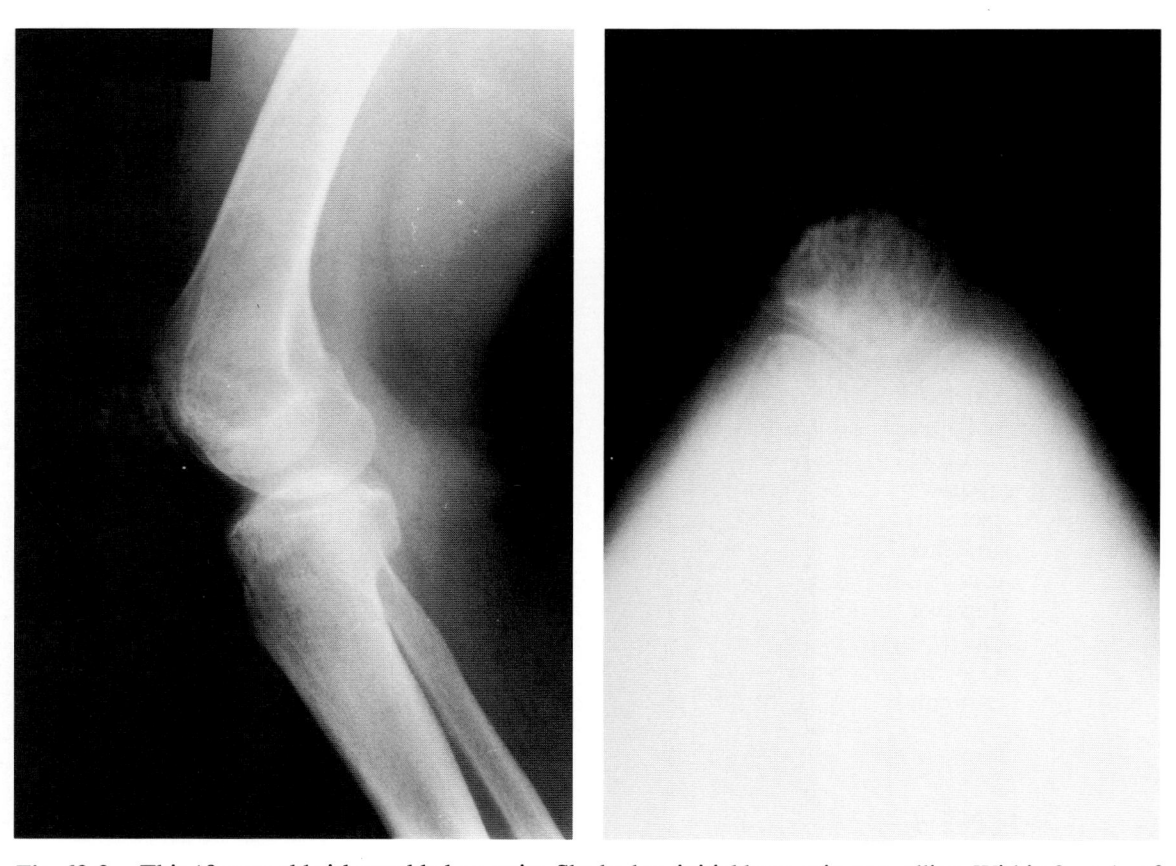

Fig. 63-3. This 18-year-old girl stumbled on stairs. She had no initial knee pain or swelling. Within 2 weeks of injury, her knee became progressively stiff and sore. Her disability progressed to the point where she was unable to weight bear at all. Her radiographs 5 months after the injury showed the spotty pattern of osteopenia seen more frequently in adults with RSD.

an injury and objective findings of RSD. The examining instrument consisted of a clamp with rubber-tipped jaws attached to a pistol grip handle. The jaws were placed over the dorsal and volar surfaces of an interphalangeal joint of the thumb in the upper extremity and the great toe in the lower extremity. Pressure was increased in a controlled fashion. The patient was asked to press a button switch when the perceived sensation changed from pressure to pain. The mean pressure-pain threshold was lower on the affected side with a gradual return to normality on repeated testing during the course of the disorder. This noninvasive, clinically reproducible test deserves further evaluation, especially in the pediatric population, as a potential aid to earlier diagnosis.

Disturbances in psychological function in children with RDS may represent an important component of the disorder.[10,13-16] Situations involving family dysfunction, including loss of a parent, alcohol and substance abuse, or psychiatric illness in the family, physical or sexual abuse of the patient, and divorce and remarriage must be considered as precipitating factors.

In 1989, Seale[17] published a helpful algorithm to assist in the definitive diagnosis of RSD (Fig. 63-4). A technique of modified differential spinal blockade was described to determine whether the pain is sympathetic, somatic, or central in origin. Saline is used as a placebo, and 5 percent procaine, as a pharmacologic spinal blockade. If the patient's pain is relieved by saline, the pain is possibly of psychogenic origin because no pharmacologic blockade has been administered. However, 5 percent procaine effectively blocks all somatic and sympathetic fibers. If its introduction does not provide pain relief, the pain may be considered to be central (malingering, psychogenic, or encephalized due to extended duration of pain). If patients obtain relief with procaine, then they are monitored for return of pinprick sensation and motor function, skin temperature, and changes in blood pressure. If the pain returns simultaneously with the return of pinprick sensation, then it may be assumed to be somatic in origin, since the larger somatic neural fibers recover from the anesthesia faster than the smaller sympathetic fibers. However, if the pain relief persists after the return of motor function and pinprick sensation, but while the sympathetic functions remain blocked, the pain is sympathetic in origin.

TREATMENT INDICATIONS

It is generally agreed that early recognition and prompt treatment provide the greatest chance of a favorable outcome. Since the average delay in diagnosis of this condition is 6 months, patients and parents are often hostile and frustrated. They have frequently seen many physicians and undergone extensive testing before feeling that their complaints have been taken seriously. Therefore, extra time and patience are required to fully explain the nature of the condition and the treatment plan as well as to provide emotional support and encouragement.

Physical therapy is the mainstay of treatment. Dietz and coworkers[1] reported 78 percent success with noninvasive, nonpharmacologic therapy. Edema is controlled by frequent limb elevation and the use of compression bandages. Distal-to-proximal massage provides desensitization as well as reducing edema. Mobilization of joints and soft tissues and massage to desensitize the areas of dysesthesia are part of the initial treatment regimen. Weightbearing despite discomfort is an integral part of the rehabilitation program. Unfortunately, immobilization is a commonly used treatment for extremity pain of unclear etiology. Most patients have already undergone prolonged periods of inactivity through the use of casts, splints, wheelchairs, crutches, and even bed rest. Therefore, a detailed explanation of the disorder to the patient and the parents is crucial to obtain compliance with the program. Perhaps all physicians involved in the treatment of children and adolescents with extremity pain of unknown etiology would be well advised to opt for earlier referral to physical therapy rather than immobilizing the unknown.

Massage therapy should be performed by the patient using lanolin skin cream three times a day. This technique has already been described for use in RSD by Frazer.[18] According to the gate control theory of Melzak and Wall,[5] massage therapy would stimulate the large type A afferent fibers, thereby increasing inhibitory control by the cells in the substantia gelatinosa to block the abnormal pain reflex emmanating from the small type C afferent fibers.

Transcutaneous nerve stimulation (TNS) has been described as a useful adjunct in treating RSD.[19-21] It is believed to activate both the small and large fibers, thereby inhibiting synaptic activity in the substantia gelatinosa and dorsal gray matter and reducing the transmission of pain sensation to higher centers. However, two authors have presented conflicting evidence with respect to the effect of TNS on sympathetic tone. Owens and colleagues[22] claimed a decrease in sympathetic tone, which would be beneficial to the disease process. However, Abram[23] described an increase in sympathetic tone, which would be deleterious rather than beneficial. TNS therapy is considered safe and noninvasive with only minor complications of skin irritation, dysesthesias, and dependence on the unit. As long as the patient is

1160 / Management of Pediatric Fractures

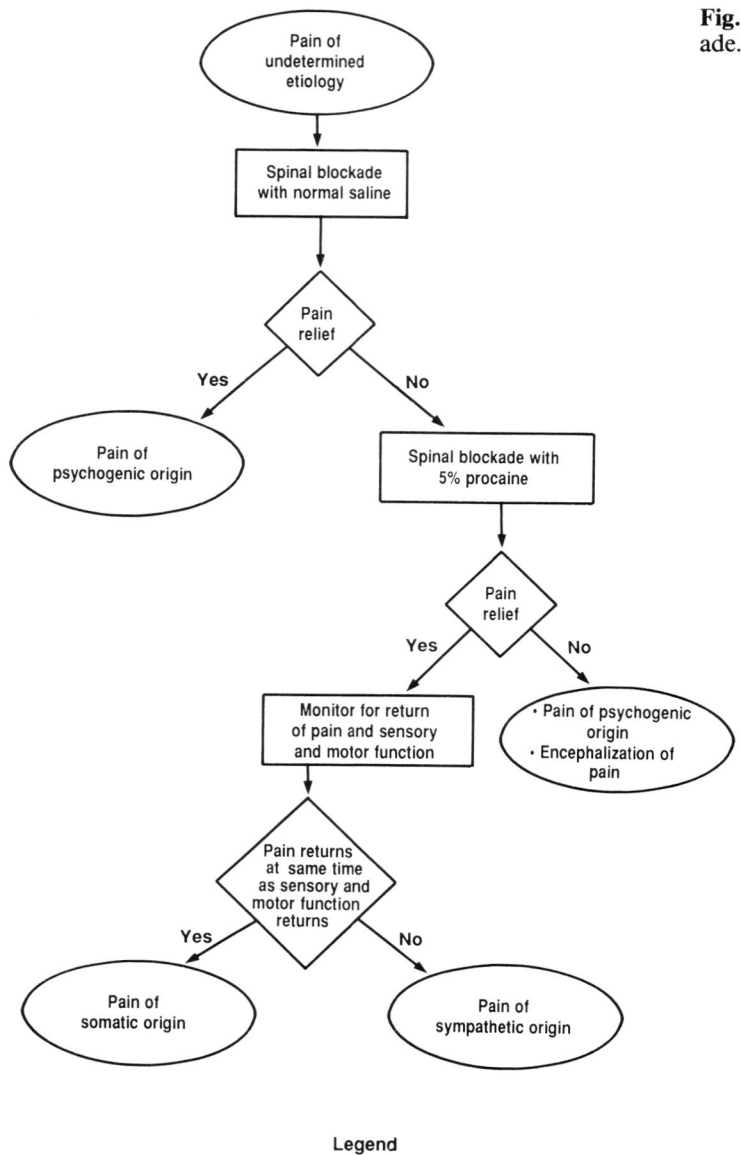

Fig. 63-4. A technique of modified differential spinal blockade. (From Seale,[17] with permission.)

```
Pain of undetermined etiology
        ↓
Spinal blockade with normal saline
        ↓
    Pain relief
   /          \
 Yes           No
  ↓             ↓
Pain of      Spinal blockade with
psychogenic   5% procaine
origin            ↓
              Pain relief
             /          \
           Yes           No
            ↓             ↓
  Monitor for return    • Pain of psychogenic
  of pain and sensory     origin
  and motor function    • Encephalization of
            ↓             pain
  Pain returns at same
  time as sensory and
  motor function returns
       /         \
     Yes          No
      ↓            ↓
   Pain of      Pain of
   somatic      sympathetic
   origin       origin
```

Legend
Oval = starting or finishing condition
Rectangle = action to be taken
Diamond = question, test result, or condition answered by "yes" or "no"

showing a positive response to this modality, its use can be continued.

Pharmacologic therapy appears to contribute no discernible effect on the clinical course of RSD. Aspirin and indomethacin were of no benefit in one study of 23 children.[15] The use of corticosteroids in children is controversial in terms of both efficacy and side effects.[10,15,24]

Since stress has been suggested as a contributing factor to the development of RSD in childhood, some investigation of the family situation is warranted in patients who are refractory to simple management of RSD before embarking on more invasive courses of therapy. If an adequate trial of physical therapy fails to resolve these symptoms, more aggressive treatment may be required. The safest and most simple intervention involves the use of a intravenous regional Bier block. While the affected limb is under regional anesthesia, the patient can be shown that full range of motion of the joints is possible and pain-free. Although not therapeutic, this technique frequently overcomes some of the emotional blocks to successful therapy.

True therapeutic sympathetic blockade can be achieved in three ways: intravenous regional chemical block, pharmacologic spinal block, and surgical sympathectomy. Intravenous regional block can be performed using either guanethidine or reserpine as sympathetic blocking agents. Guanethidine displaces norepinephrine from intraneuronal storage granules to produce a prolonged sympathetic blockade. Reserpine reduces the reuptake of catecholamines. Hannington-Kiff[25] described considerable success with the former and Benzon and associates[26] reported results with the latter. Neither study included pediatric patients. Neither drug is currently approved for intravenous infusion in Canada or the United States.

Pharmacologic spinal blockade is obtained by infiltrating the region of the lumbar sympathetic chain with a long-acting anesthestic agent such as bupivacaine hydrochloride. There has been no study of this technique in children. It has a major disadvantage in that the blocks need to be repeated daily or every other day until pain is controlled.

Surgical sympathectomy is considered in adults if the blocks become less effective over time. Its use in children is discouraged since RSD in this group seems self-limited and up to 25 percent of adult patients treated with this

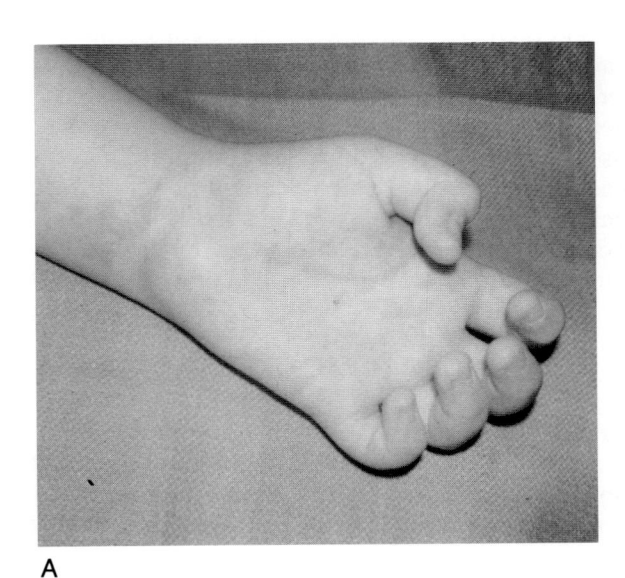

Fig. 63-5. (A) Hand of child with RSD following a minor crush injury of her forearm 3 months prior to this photograph. (B&C) Following a Bier block with Solucortef injection with 0.5 percent xylocaine.

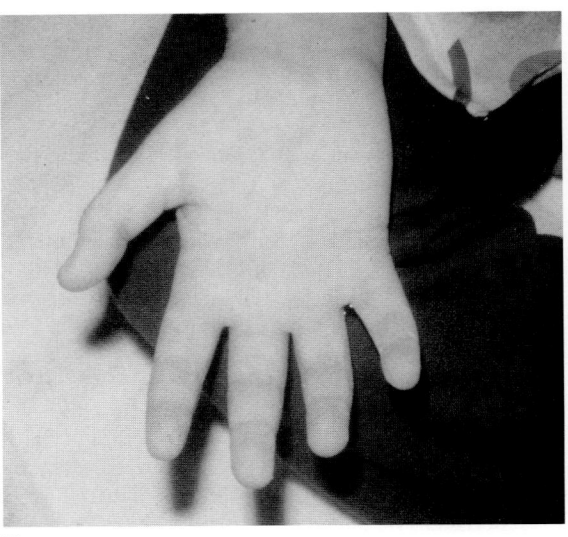

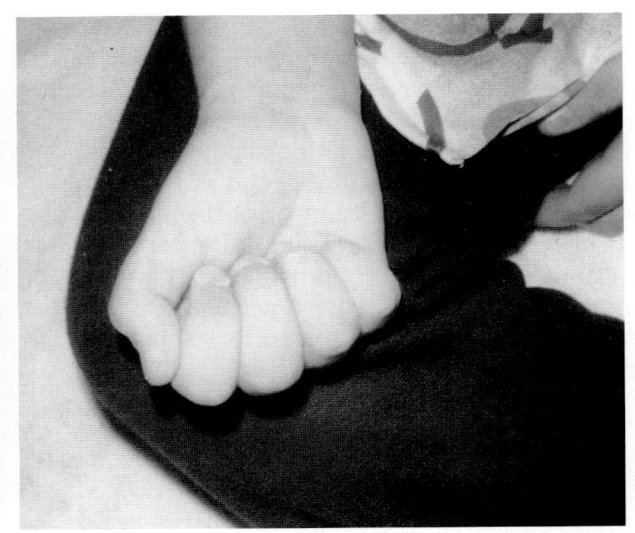

technique remain with persisting problems. Its effect on skeletal growth, if any, is not known.

Another surgical technique recently described for treatment of RSD is that of bilateral ablation of the cingulate gyrus. This procedure has been used in neurosurgery to treat a variety of neuropsychiatric disorders and intractable pain associated with cancer, phantom limb, and thalamic disease. Santo and coworkers[27] reported a case of one adult patient who underwent the procedure with an early encouraging result, but the benefits were short-lived.

My preferred method of treatment is aggressive physical therapy, usually on an outpatient basis. Hospital admission is required in severe or refractory cases to ensure compliance, or where the patient's physical location does not permit regular attendance in therapy. Physician support is crucial to the success of the conservative program. Frequent follow-up is required to monitor the patient's progress. Early referral for psychological assessment, counseling, and therapy is beneficial in refractory cases. An invasive procedure I have found useful is a Bier block with local anesthetic to demonstrate to the child that painless joint mobility was possible (Fig. 63-5). This is only rarely indicated. I have not found medication or immobilization very helpful with children with RSD.

COMPLICATIONS

Permanent disturbances in growth have been reported as a result of RSD.[28] Chronic underuse of the affected limb or the underlying disease mechanism may lead to growth impairment. Previous reports have indicated that either increased or decreased uptake on bone scans can be seen depending on the phase of RSD.[9,15] Transient growth arrest may follow a period of decreased blood flow to open physes. Similarly, a period of increased blood flow to open physes may result in premature growth arrest via early physeal closure.

In comparison to the adult population, chronic trophic changes with joint stiffness, and skin and muscle atrophy are only rarely seen (2 percent).[1] A delay in diagnosis and prolonged immobilization are contributing factors. The recurrence rate in the same location or in another location is reported as 5 percent.[1] Recurrences have been reported up to 5 years after resolution of the initial complaints.

SUMMARY

RSD in children is generally considered to carry a more favorable prognosis than in adults, with most children's complaints resolving without any permanent sequelae.[1,13,15,29] However, the morbidity, both physical and psychological, associated with the disorder is significant. Early recognition generally results in a more rapid resolution of symptoms. Chronic trophic changes and contractures characteristic of adults are not commonly seen in children. Noninvasive, nonpharmacologic therapy is the mainstay of treatment. The typical patient is an adolescent female with no history of trauma. This disorder should be considered in any child who presents with a chronic painful extremity.

REFERENCES

1. Dietz FR, Mathews KD, Montgomery WJ: Reflex sympathetic dystrophy in children. Clin Orthop Rel Res 258:225, 1990
2. Bonica JJ: Causalgia and other reflex sympathetic dystrophies. p. 141. In Bonica JJ, Lindbloom U, Iggo A (eds): Advances in Pain Research and Therapy. Vol. 3. Raven Press, New York, 1979
3. Schutzer SF, Gossling HR: The treatment of reflex sympathetic dystrophy syndrome. J Bone Joint Surg [Am] 66:625, 1984
4. Livingston WK: Pain Mechanisms: A Physiologic Interpretation of Causalgia and Its Related States. p. 83. Macmillan, New York, 1943
5. Melzac R, Wall PD: Pain mechanisms: a new theory. Science 150:971, 1965
6. Lankford LL: Reflex sympathetic dystrophy. p. 145. In Evarts CM (ed): Surgery of the Musculoskeletal System. Vol. 1. Churchill Livingstone, New York, 1983
7. Martin GI: The significance of tache cerebrale in neonatal meningitis. J Pediatr 87:321, 1975
8. Gellis SS, Feingold M, Steinhoff MC: Picture of the month. Tache cerebrale. Am J Dis Child 3:709, 1977
9. Laxer RM, Allen RC, Malleson PN et al: Technetium 99m-methylene-diphosphonate bone scans in children with reflex neurovascular dystrophy. J Pediatr 106:437, 1985
10. Ruggeri SB, Athreya BH, Doughty R et al: Reflex sympathetic dystrophy in children. Clin Orthop 163:225, 1982
11. Bryan AS, Klenerman L, Bowsher D: The diagnosis of reflex sympathetic dystrophy using an algometer. J Bone Joint Surg [Br] 73:644, 1991
12. Atkins RM, Kanis JA: The use of dolorimetry in the assessment of posttraumatic algodystrophy. Br J Rheumatol 28:404, 1989
13. Ashwal S, Tomasi L, Neumann M, Schneider S: Reflex sympathetic dystrophy syndrome in children. Pediatr Neurol 4:38, 1988
14. Sherry DD, Weisman R: Psychologic aspects of childhood reflex neurovascular dystrophy. Pediatrics 81:572, 1988
15. Bernstein H, Singsen BH, Kent JT et al: Reflex neurovascular dystrophy in childhood. J Pediatr 93:211, 1978

16. Aftimos S: Reflex neurovascular dystrophy in children. N Z Med J 99:761, 1986
17. Seale KS: Reflex sympathetic dystrophy of the lower extremity. Clin Orthop Rel Res 243:80, 1989
18. Frazer FW: Persistent post-sympathetic pain treated by connective tissue massage. Physiotherapy 64:211, 1978
19. Steig RL: New methods for achieving pain control with transcutaneous nerve stimulation. Neurology 26:356, 1976
20. Richlin DM, Carron H, Rowlingson JC et al: Reflex sympathetic dystrophy: successful treatment by transcutaneous nerve stimulation. J Pediatr 93:84, 1978
21. Loeser JD, Black RG, Christman A: Pain relief by transcutaneous stimulation. J Neurosurg 42:308, 1975
22. Owens S, Atkinson ER, Lees DE: Thermographic evidence of reduced sympathetic tone with transcutaneous nerve stimulation. Anesthesiology 50:62, 1979
23. Abram SE: Increased sympathetic tone associated with transcutaneous electrical stimulation. Anesthesiology 45:575, 1976
24. Forster RS, Fu FH: Reflex sympathetic dystrophy in children: a case report and review of the literature. Orthopedics 8:475, 1985
25. Hannington-Kiff JG: Relief of Sudeck's atrophy by regional intravenous guanethidine. Lancet 1:1132, 1977
26. Benzon HT, Chomka CM, Brunner EA: Treatment of reflex sympathetic dystrophy with regional intravenous reserpine. Anesth Analg 59:500, 1980
27. Santo JL, Arias LM, Barolat G et al: Bilateral cingulumotomy in the treatment of reflex sympathetic dystrophy. Pain 41:55, 1990
28. Rush PJ, Wilmot D, Saunders N et al: Severe reflex neurovascular dystrophy in childhood. Arthritis Rheum 28:952, 1985
29. Fermaglich DR: Reflex sympathetic dystrophy in children. Pediatrics 60:881, 1977

64

Compartment Syndrome

Kenneth L.B. Brown

> Nature is always hinting at us. It hints over and over again. Finally we realize and take the hint.
>
> — ROBERT FROST

Compartment syndrome occurs when the effects of increased pressure from within or without a confined space leads to a diminution of perfusion and function of the tissues within that space. This condition may be a cause of increased morbidity following trauma, burns, surgery, and revascularization in children. If the increased intracompartmental pressure is not decompressed by early fasciotomy, permanent damage to the muscles and nerves in the compartment will result. The changes in these damaged tissues result in severe contractures of the extremity. An unrecognized compartment syndrome has the potential to be permanently physically disabling for the child and devastating for the caregivers.

PATHOGENESIS OF COMPARTMENT SYNDROME

Irrespective of the underlying cause, the pathogenetic mechanism is the development of increased tissue pressure in an enclosed fascial space, which compromises the circulation to nerves and muscles within it (Table 64-1). There are three theories to explain the decreased tissue perfusion.[1] Eaton and Green[2] believed that compartment syndromes are caused by arterial spasm, which results from injury or increased intracompartmental pressure. This is an uncommon cause since many children with compartment syndrome have a normal distal pulse, and there is no evidence of arterial spasm seen on their arteriograms. Another theory is the alteration in arteriole critical closing pressure. Arterioles have a small radius and relatively thick smooth muscle walls, resulting in a high mural tension. This necessitates a high transmural pressure difference to maintain flow. If this critical pressure difference does not exist because of increased tissue pressure or decreased arterial pressure, the arterioles close.[3] Veins will collapse when the tissue pressure is greater than the venous pressure because of their thin flaccid walls. If the blood continues to flow from the capillaries the venous pressure will again rise until it is greater than tissue pressure and the venous flow is reestablished. This increased venous pressure causes a decreased arteriovenous gradient and therefore a decreased tissue blood flow. The normal capillary pressure is 20 to 30 mmHg.[4]

When increased tissue pressure reduces the local arteriovenous gradient by any of the above mechanisms, blood flow decreases to the extent that the metabolic demands of the tissue are no longer met. This causes a loss of function and compartment syndrome ensues. The critical tissue pressure necessary to cause compartment syndromes is not defined.[4-8] The amount of pressure that the tissues can tolerate before functional abnormalities are produced is decreased by factors affecting local blood flow such as the position of the limb,[9] underlying medical conditions,[10,11] the state of the circulation and the time of exposure to the increased pressure. The influence of limb position on intracompartmental pressure was demonstrated in an experimen-

TABLE 64-1. Pathogenesis of Compartment Syndrome

Arterial Spasm	Critical Closing Pressure Change	Decreased Venous Pressure
Pathogenesis		
↓ Venous Inflow	High transmural pressure to maintain flow in muscle arterioles	ICP Venous pressure causes of collapsed veins
↑ Endothelial permeability causes progressive intramuscular edema	↑ ICP or ↑ Arterial pressure	↑ Capillary flow causes ↑ Venous pressure
↑ Compartment pressure	↓ Transmural pressure and arterioles close	↑ Venous pressure causes ↑ Arteriovenous gradient

tal study in humans.[7] Standing on both feet raised the anterior tibial compartment pressure to 20 mmHg. Standing on one foot increased the pressure to 40 mmHg, heel standing raised it to 65 mmHg, and isometric contracture increased the pressure to 95 mmHg. Certain underlying medical problems, such as sickle cell trait may lower the threshold for the occurrence of compartment syndrome.[12]

An experimental study in dogs demonstrated that nerves are very susceptible to permanent damage by increased intracompartmental pressure.[13] Pressure greater than 50 mmHg caused nerve conduction failure. Complete conduction block correlated with the axonal degeneration seen on histologic examination. At higher pressures less time was required to abolish conduction, and histologic findings showed a worsening of axonal degeneration. The damage was proportional to the pressure. Large fast-conducting fibers are more susceptible to increased intracompartment pressures than smaller slower conducting fibers. This selectivity may be due to difficulties in maintaining nutrient diffusion in the larger fibers and the increased sensitivity to mechanical compression due to their larger size.

The time factor has been examined by Rorabeck and associates.[14,15] It is not only the absolute pressure but the duration of increased pressure that is important. For example, 60 mmHg for 2 hours is less damaging than 40 mmHg for 14 hours. Nerve shows functional abnormalities such as paresthesia and hyperesthesia within 30 minutes. Irreversible functional loss occurs after 12 to 24 hours of total ischemia. In muscles there is change within 2 to 4 hours, which becomes irreversible after 4 to 12 hours. When ischemia lasts longer than 4 hours, there may be a significant myoglobinuria, which reaches a maximum about 3 hours after the circulation is restored and persists up to 12 hours.[16,17]

Capillary endothelium is damaged by prolonged ischemia. This damage results in an increased capillary permeability. When the circulation is restored, there is an extravasation of fluid, which causes increased extracellular volume and then intercompartment pressure. The capillary endothelium is sufficiently affected after 3 hours of ischemia to cause postischemia swelling of 30 to 60 percent.[17] This mechanism is particularly important following revascularization of limbs following arterial repair[18] or after prolonged tourniquet application. Elevated pressures for greater than 12 hours are most likely to produce permanent functional deficits.

CAUSES OF COMPARTMENT SYNDROME

The underlying features of all compartment syndromes are the same regardless of etiology (Table 64-2). Increased tissue intracompartmental pressure is the central pathogenetic factor, and it can be caused by a decreased compartmental size (extrinsic factors) or an increased volume of compartment contents (intrinsic factors). Extrinsic factors cause a decreased volume and distensibility of a compartment. Encircling casts and padding have been shown to decrease intracompartmental volume by approximately 40 percent.[19] It is not only the rigidity of the cast itself that is important, but the padding beneath the cast can also cause constriction. Even air splints have been shown to cause compartment syndromes.[19,20,21] All of these external devices lead to decreased compliance of the fascial envelope of the compartment or limb. The application of traction on the limb also increases tension on the fascial envelope. Skin traction may be particularly dangerous because traction and the constrictive dressings are additive. This situation is worsened when the limb is elevated such as with "gallows" or Bryant's traction. These factors may account for the occasional compartment syndrome encountered during the treatment of femoral fractures in children.[22]

TABLE 64-2. Etiology of Compartment Syndrome in Children

1. Trauma—fractures
2. Tight dressings and casts
3. Traction—gallows or Bryant's
4. Tibial osteotomy
5. Burns
6. Hauser procedure
7. Coagulation defect

Another important cause of extrinsic pressure producing a compartment syndrome is in a comatose or anesthetized patient whose limb is positioned beneath the body. Care must be taken in positioning patients for surgery to avoid prolonged pressure on the underlying limb.[23]

These extrinsic effects are compounded by factors that increase the compartment contents, such as edema caused by fluid loss from injured capillaries, the addition of exogenous fluids such as infiltrating intravenous fluid from intravenous or intraosseous infusions, or bleeding from fractures or other injuries.[24,25] There is minimal compliance to the enclosing fascial envelope, that is, as the compartmental contents are increased due to swelling, pressure within the compartment increases exponentially because the elasticity of the fascial envelope diminishes with increasing distension.

DIAGNOSIS OF COMPARTMENT SYNDROME

The critical clinical symptoms and signs of compartment syndrome are as follows:

1. Pain out of proportion to the injury
2. Tenderness to palpation
3. Painful passive stretch
4. Hypesthesia of the nerve and muscles transversing the compartment

These are the four key signs. The "5 P's," that is, pain, pallor, pulselessness, paresthesia, and paralysis, should be deemphasized because they can be dangerously misleading. Unless there has been a transection of a major vessel (Holden type I),[26] distal pulses are usually still present even in limbs with markedly elevated compartmental pressures. This has been well documented in several studies.[2,4,27,28] The time taken to obtain an arteriogram may further delay the diagnosis and treatment of a compartment syndrome,[26] and the cannulation of the artery may further interfere with the blood supply, especially in children with small arteries.[29] In those with an absent peripheral pulse in whom arterial damage is suspected, an intraoperative arteriogram can be obtained by the percutaneous injection of radiopaque dye through a small butterfly needle proximal to the suspected site of injury. Capillary fill is also usually normal in children with established compartment syndromes because of collateral flow and good distal runoff. Paralysis is a late sign, and permanent damage has already occurred.

The child at risk must be examined at frequent intervals and the findings and time of examination carefully documented in the chart. Sensory examination, motor power, passive stretch, and palpation should each be documented clearly. The nurse's notes should be consulted and any discrepancies discussed. On physical examination of movement, beware of the "springy" toes or fingers. For example, when the toes are voluntarily wiggled there may be lack of dorsiflexion power, but after plantar flexion the toes spring back, giving the appearance of a functioning anterior compartment. Similarly when the fingers are extended, they may rebound, making it appear that there is active flexion. In children with a nerve injury, the paralysis may make the clinical diagnosis of compartment syndrome versus nerve paralysis difficult.[30,31] The clinical signs may also be masked in children with tourniquet paralysis.[32] Direct nerve stimulation with an anesthetist's nerve stimulator can be used to differentiate them. The myoneural junction is the part of the motor unit most sensitive to ischemia. When muscles are paralyzed by compartment syndrome they do not have the normal response to direct stimulation of the motor nerve; however, if there is nerve damage proximal to the compartment, stimulation of the nerve will cause muscle contraction. Entrapment of muscles in a fracture site can also mimic a compartment syndrome, since the child is unable to flex and extend the fingers, and passive stretch causes pain.[33]

The usual sequence of events is as follows: pain during passive stretch, then paresthesias, then paresis, and finally anesthesia.[4] Pain on passive stretch is not always a reliable sign because the child may exhibit pain due to the injury itself, and in the case of nerve paralysis proximal to the compartment, this sign may be completely absent. Likewise, paresis may be difficult to evaluate because of guarding due to pain.[17] This is particularly true in young children who are fearful and not always cooperative. For these reasons, a sensory deficit, which is the earliest neurologic sign,[34] may be a more reliable sign.

Beware of the frightened child who reacts by crying as

you enter the room even before beginning your examination. The opposite extreme is the frightened, stoical child who does not cry or complain of pain but lies motionless and suffers in silence. When muscle paralysis supervenes, the pain decreases, and the child's behavior returns to normal. It is only later when contractures of the toes or fingers are noted that the diagnosis is made. Both of these scenarios are dangerous because these children are likely to be ignored and not examined completely. In these circumstances or in a comatose or spinal injury patient, a careful gentle clinical examination may not be possible and more objective methods such as compartment pressure measurements are necessary.

COMPARTMENT PRESSURE MEASUREMENTS

It is best to give the child some sedation before measuring the compartment pressures. A combination of pethidine (1 mg/kg to a maximum dose of 30 mg), hydroxyzine (1 mg/kg to a maximum dose of 30 mg), and droperidol (0.1 mg/kg to a maximum dose of 3 mg) has been a very effective "cocktail" for minor procedures such as this. It is best to avoid injection of local anesthetic into the deep compartment lest it affect the compartmental pressure. All methods of recording are acceptable. The Whitesides method[8] or its variation with an arterial pressure transducer[5] uses materials readily at hand and, while not as accurate as the wick catheter, it gives reliable indications of compartmental pressure.[7,35,36] The Whitesides method is not as satisfactory for long-term monitoring, since saline must be injected to keep the needle from blocking. Some authors feel that this may contribute to increased pressure,[7] but others have calculated the effects and found them not to be significant.[6] Even proponents of the wick catheter technique admit that continued pressure monitoring is not always practical, since only one compartment is monitored and often more than one compartment in a limb is involved. The wick catheter has been very valuable as a research tool to study the effects of compartment syndromes on different tissues and to monitor the effects of treatment on the intracompartmental pressures. No matter which method of measurement is chosen, one should become experienced in the measurement of compartmental pressures. There are several sources of error, such as blockage of the catheter, leaking connections, bubbles, improperly calibrated transducer, improper placement of the needle, and improper monitoring of the compartment at risk—for example, a needle in the superficial posterior compartment rather than the deep posterior compartment of the leg. Newer technology has provided more simplified kits for the measurement of compartment pressures.

There is no single pressure value that is applicable for all individuals. Whitesides and colleagues[8] stated that fasciotomy should be related to the difference between the compartment pressures and the diastolic blood pressure. However, this does not necessarily correlate with muscle blood flow.[37] Compartment pressure measurements have shown that pressures in excess of 45 mmHg are usually associated with compartment syndromes, and pressures greater than 60 mmHg consistently cause compartment syndromes.[35] The duration of the intracompartmental pressure increase is as important as the magnitude, and a continuous monitoring gives a trend. Triffitt and colleagues[38] measured pressures in the anterior and posterior compartments continuously for up to 72 hours in 20 patients with closed tibial shaft fractures. Although 7 patients (35 percent) had pressures above 40 mmHg and 14 (70 percent) above 30 mmHg, in the absence of symptoms the monitored pressures did not relate to outcome. They concluded that continuous monitoring in this type of patient was of doubtful benefit. The issue is not the decreased perfusion but what is the pressure that causes irreversible damage. The threshold appears to be about 30 mmHg for about 8 hours,[27] or 40 mmHg for 6 hours.[39] Remember that these values do not apply to patients with a low perfusion state in the limb. Mubarak and colleagues[7] made control measurements in patients who had undergone tibial osteotomy. They showed that pain and paresthesias first appeared when the pressure measured 30 mmHg.[7] Individuals vary in their tolerance for increased tissue pressure, so there cannot be an absolute value that is applicable to all patients.[40] It appears that the pressure tolerance of children is not significantly different from that of adults.[5] As a guide, pressures less than 30 mmHg require repeated examination and continued monitoring. Depending on circumstances, 30 to 45 mmHg is a gray zone, and pressures greater than 45 mmHg require urgent fasciotomy to avoid permanent damage to tissue (Fig. 64-1).

There appears to be a subacute form of compartment syndrome in which apparent full recovery of function occurs even when fasciotomy is performed late. These cases have only been described in children and are poorly documented.[2,41-43] I have treated a child with an undisplaced radial neck fracture who had a decompressive fasciotomy 9 days after her fracture. After her fracture was splinted, the family made several trips to the emergency department because of her pain, and on one of her visits she was admitted for observation and later

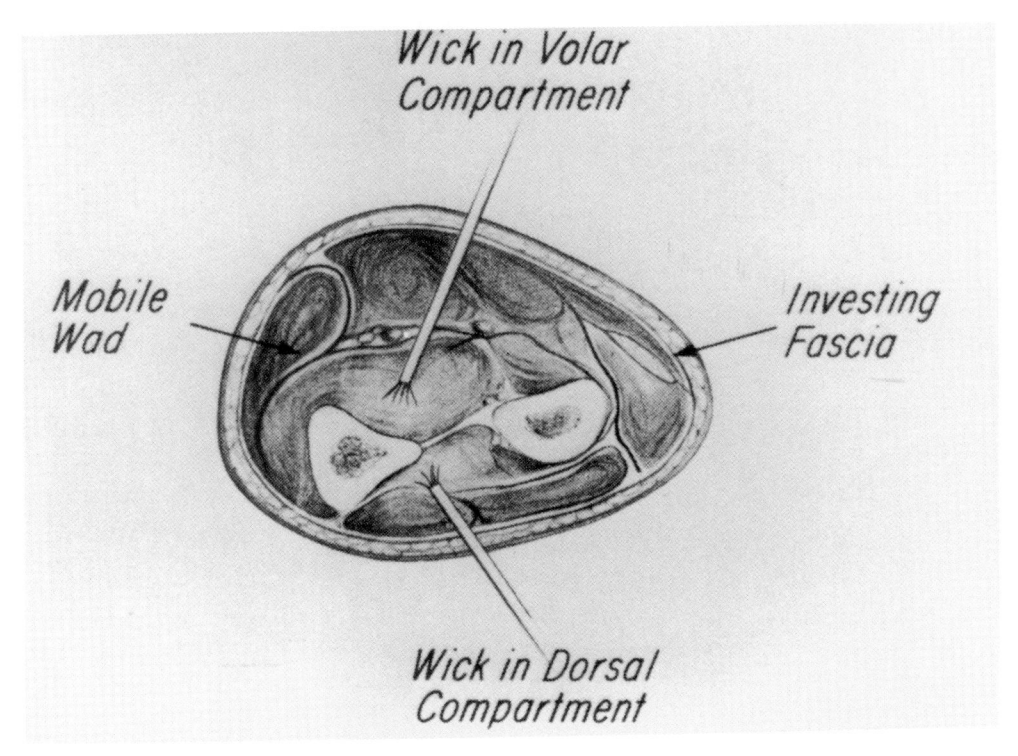

Fig. 64-1. Cross section of the proximal forearm demonstrating catheter placement. (From Gelberman et al.,[65] with permission.)

discharged after her symptoms improved. On a subsequent visit to the emergency unit, her volar forearm compartment pressure was 40 mmHg, as measured by the Whitesides method.[8] Following volar fasciotomy, her symptoms were relieved in the immediate postoperative period, and she made a full and uneventful recovery.

COMPARTMENT SYNDROMES IN SPECIFIC SITES

Volar Compartment Syndrome of the Forearm

The volar compartment of the forearm is bordered by the radius, ulna, and interosseous membrane and is enveloped by the antebrachial fascia.[44] The principle muscles contained are flexor pollicis longus, flexor digitorum profundus, flexor carpi ulnaris, flexor digitorum superficialis, palmaris longus, and flexor carpi radialis. The median and ulnar nerve traverse the compartment. The symptoms and signs of a volar compartment syndrome are hypesthesia on the volar aspect of the fingers, tenseness of the volar fascia, pain on passive extension of the fingers and wrist, and weakness of flexion of the fingers and wrist. Fasciotomy can be accomplished via an ulnar border incision or a lazy S incision starting above the elbow crease and ending just distal to the transverse carpal ligament, which allows decompression of the median nerve in the carpal tunnel. This more extensive incision allows improved access to the neurovascular structures, but both approaches are equally effective for decompression of the compartment.[12] Volar decompression also decreases the pressure in the dorsal compartment, but in severe cases this compartment should be decompressed by a separate dorsal fasciotomy (Fig. 64-2).

Compartment Syndromes in the Hand and Foot

Paresthesia is not a reliable sign when dealing with a compartment syndrome of a hand or foot because no sensory nerve traverses the compartment.[43,45-48] Paresthesias in the hand only occur when there is involvement

Dorsal   *Volar – Ulnar*   *Volar*

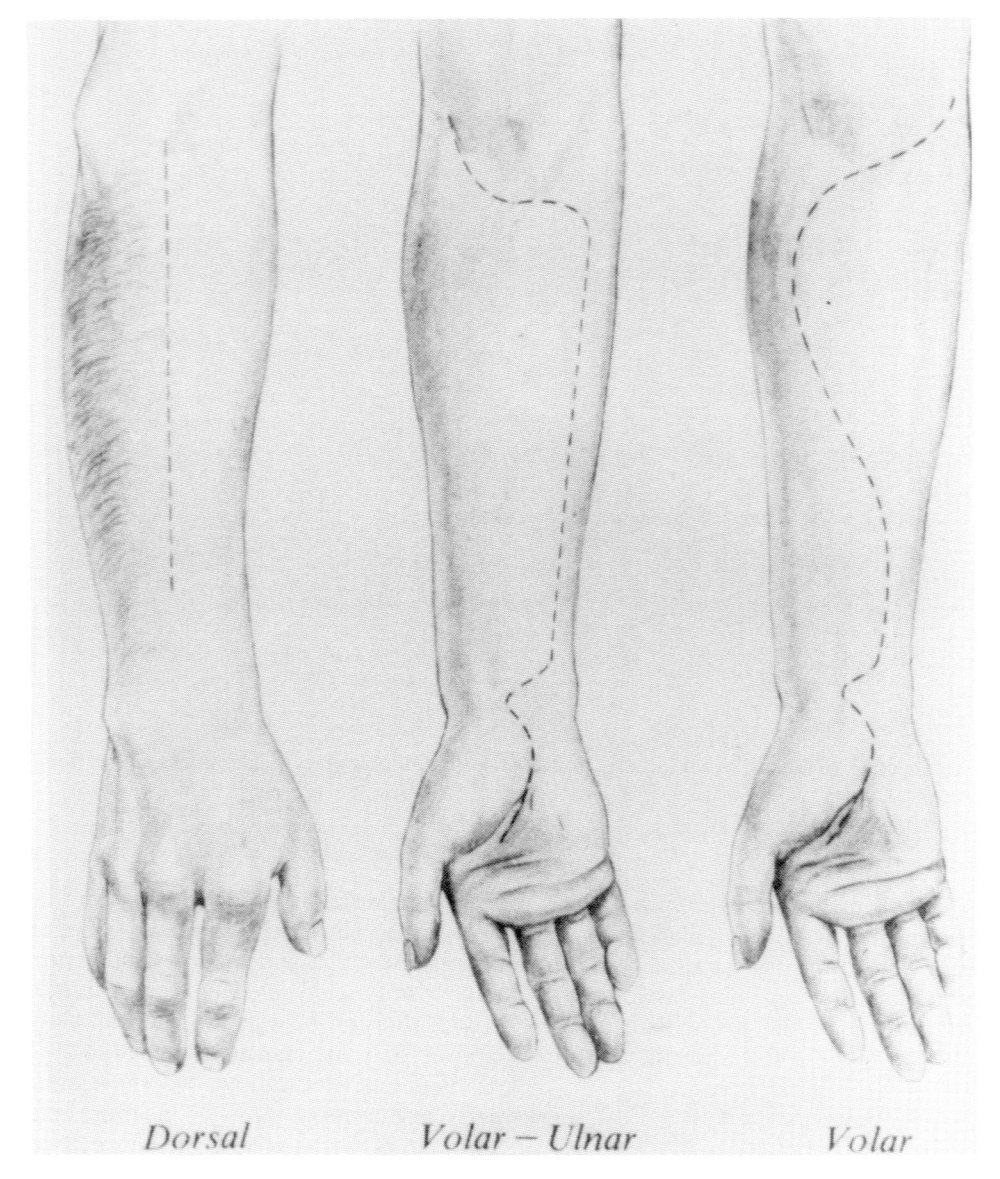

Fig. 64-2. Dorsal, volar-ulnar, and curvilinear volar incisions recommended for fasciotomy of the volar or dorsal compartments to relieve compartment pressure. (From Gelberman et al.,[65] with permission.)

of Guyon's canal (ulnar nerve) or the carpal tunnel (median nerve symptoms). This is an important finding because these areas will have to be decompressed as well during fasciotomy of the intrinsics. It is imperative to examine all of the interosseous compartments separately, since there may be selective involvement. An important physical finding is pain on passive stretching of the involved interosseous muscle. This is done by gently deviating each finger radially and ulnarly to alternately test the intrinsics on both sides of the digit. These compartments can be effectively decompressed by dorsal incisions to incise the investing fascia.

Anterior Compartment Syndrome of the Leg

The anterior compartment of the leg is bounded by the tibia, fibula, interosseous membrane, and anterior crural fascia. It is separated from the lateral compartment by

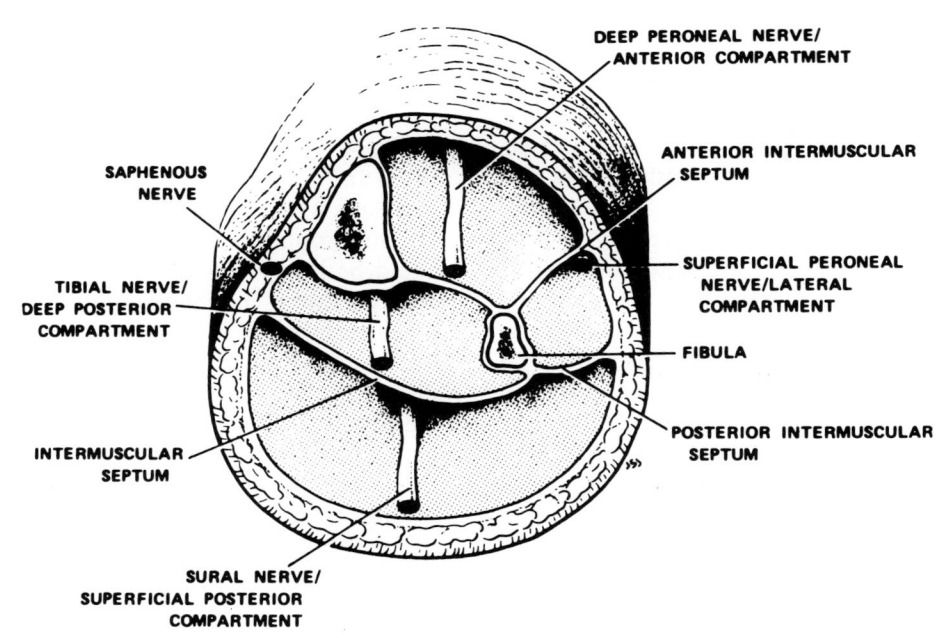

Fig. 64-3. Cross section at the junction of the middle and distal thirds of the leg illustrating the four compartments and their respective nerves. (From Mubarak and Owen,[27] with permission.)

the anterior crural intermuscular septum. The main muscles include the tibialis anterior, extensor hallucis longus, and extensor digitorum longus with the deep peroneal nerve coursing throughout (Fig. 64-3). The symptoms and signs of anterior compartment syndrome are: hypesthesia in the first dorsal web space; tenderness along the anterior compartment fascia; pain on passive toe and foot plantar flexion; and weakness of toe extension and foot dorsiflexion. This compartment is adequately decompressed by an incision in the lateral-proximal part of the leg[27] (Fig. 64-4).

Posterior Compartment Syndrome

The deep posterior compartment of the leg is bounded by the tibia, fibula, interosseous membrane, and transverse crural intermuscular septum. The muscles included are the flexor digitorum longus, tibialis posterior, and the flexor hallucis longus. The posterior tibial nerve courses through the compartment. Clinically, the deep posterior compartment syndrome is identified by hypesthesia on the plantar aspect of the foot, tenseness of the deep posterior compartment fascia, which lies between the Achilles tendon and the tibia in the distal part of the leg,[49] pain on passive toe extension and foot eversion, and weakness of toe flexion and foot inversion. The superficial posterior compartment is bounded by the deep crural fascia and the transverse crural intermuscular septum. This compartment is rarely if ever involved in isolation. This compartment can be decompressed by a 15-cm incision in the distal part of the leg, 2 cm posterior to the posteriomedial edge of the tibia.[27]

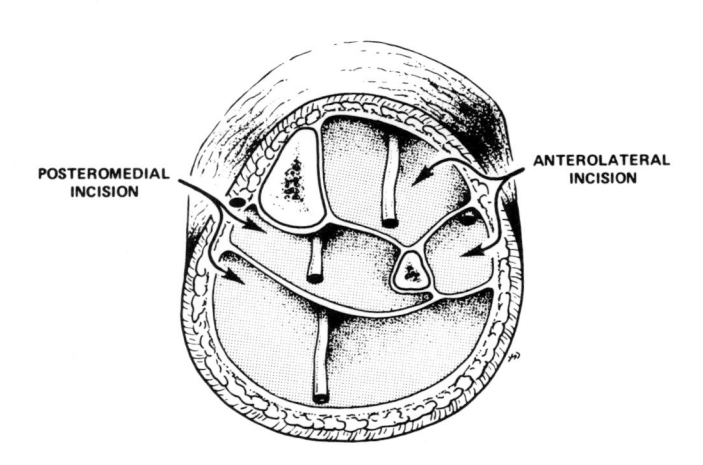

Fig. 64-4. Composite illustrating four compartment decompression using the double incision method. (From Mubarak and Owen,[27] with permission.)

Compartment Syndrome of the Thigh

This compartment syndrome is a rarely described entity most commonly seen in patients suffering multiple trauma. In about half of the cases there is an associated femur fracture,[50] often open. In most other cases the compartment syndrome is secondary to a severe contusion. In many of the children compartment syndrome may develop in another anatomic site in addition to the thigh. Risk factors include severe hypotension requiring large volumes of intravenous fluids, use of antishock trousers, vascular injuries, and coagulopathies.[51,52]

There are two groups of patients encountered. One group is made up of conscious patients with severe thigh pain and a tense compartment. The other group is in unconscious children whose only physical finding is a tense compartment. There are three compartments of the thigh: anterior or quadriceps, posterior or hamstring, and medial or adductor compartments. Any or all of the compartments may be involved at one time. In all cases the child complains of severe pain, which is increased when the compartment contents are stretched passively. For example, in an anterior thigh compartment syndrome, there is a tense quadriceps muscle. Pain is increased when the knee is bent with the hip extended. There is hypesthesia in the femoral nerve distribution, that is, the lateral, intermediate, and medial cutaneous nerves of the thigh and in the saphenous nerve distribution below the knee. In the posterior thigh compartment syndrome, the hamstring muscles are tense, and pain is increased when the knee is extended with the hip flexed. There may be decreased sensation around the foot. The adductor compartment is tested with passive leg abduction. There may be decreased sensation on the proximal-medial aspect of the thigh in the obturator nerve distribution. The anterior and posterior compartments can be decompressed by a single lateral incision. If the pressure in the medial compartment is still elevated, then a separate medial incision can be used to decompress it.

PREVENTION OF COMPARTMENT SYNDROME

A surgeon must maintain a high index of suspicion whenever treating children with injured extremities. The level of monitoring is high for certain injuries, such as supracondylar fractures, but it is important to realize that compartment syndromes have been described following many otherwise innocuous injuries, even undisplaced fractures[53-57] and soft tissue injuries.[33,58-60,62] These conditions may be more dangerous, since the elevated pressures may not be recognized early enough to institute appropriate treatment.

In conditions such as supracondylar fractures where a lot of swelling is to be expected, tight encircling dressing and casts should be avoided. If a child must be transported and supervision will be difficult or treatment impossible, it is better to transport the child with the injured extremity supported by a splint, or, if casted, the plaster should be bivalved with the padding cut as well. It is better to lose a reduction than to lose the extremity! Remember, if evacuating children by air, that if the aircraft is nonpressurized, a pressure gradient will develop between the limb and the environment. This may aggravate a compartment syndrome, especially if the limb is encircled by a rigid support that prevents the expansion of the limb.

When treating displaced fractures with hematoma blocks, one should be aware of the possibility of contributing to intracompartmental pressure by the injection of the local anesthetic.[63] There is some concern by surgeons that regional anesthetic blocks by anesthetists may mask an underlying or impending compartment syndrome.[64] Although the block may interfere with the early detection of subtle sensory changes,[9] a careful physical examination will reveal pain that is unrelieved by the anesthetic agent and a tense swollen compartment.

Parents and supervising nursing staff should be educated on the important physical signs of impending compartment syndromes. It is a wise policy to give an instruction sheet to parents explaining what signs to look for and to demonstrate some of the examination points such as the passive muscle stretch prior to discharge home. As a routine policy, parents should be required to return the child to the hospital for a "cast check" within 12 hours of any reduction.

If an impending compartment syndrome is suspected, constricting bandages should be removed and the limb placed at the level of the heart. In an experimental study in dogs Garfin and coworkers[19] showed that splitting the cast on one side decreases compartmental pressure by 30 percent. Spreading the cast decreases pressure by 65 percent and cutting the padding decreases it a further 10 percent. If there has not been any improvement within the hour, compartment pressures should be measured and, if necessary, fasciotomy should be scheduled.

TREATMENT OF COMPARTMENT SYNDROME

The goals of treatment are early diagnosis, prompt decompression, and uncomplicated recovery. Sympathetic nerve blocks have not been very effective in preventing compartment syndromes, probably because ischemic tissue is already a potent stimulator for vasodilatation. The indication for surgical decompression is the presence of definite clinical signs, or even equivocal ambiguous signs, when there is an increase of the intracompartmental pressure greater than 45 mmHg.[6] As a general rule when performing a fasciotomy, a tourniquet is not recommended, since it prolongs ischemia and makes it difficult to assess bleeding muscle for viability. It is acceptable to use a tourniquet during the initial exposure to decrease bleeding and identify the neurovascular structures and then to deflate it. Nonviable muscle does not bleed when cut or contract when pinched, but these findings are not very reliable for determining viability, especially in children. Therefore it is better not to resect muscle, which appears to be nonviable at the time of fasciotomy, since in some cases it may recover.[5,42,65] It is safer to have a second look under general anesthesia 2 to 3 days following fasciotomy. At this time obviously nonviable tissue can be debrided, and some of the wound may be closed or skin grafted. If the compartment syndrome is treated early and the tissues do not bulge much following fasciotomy, it may seem reasonable to close the skin.[66] However, it is safer to leave the skin open because postischemic swelling may cause a recurrence of the compartment syndrome due to the constriction of the tight skin.[67] Consideration should be given to the internal fixation of fractures in children with compartment syndrome, since the stabilizing effects of the soft tissues is often lost following decompression. Since a cast is not necessary, it allows access to the limb for monitoring and decreases the chance of recurrent compartment syndrome because of an encircling cast.[34]

Factors affecting the results are (1) the incision length, (2) whether an incision is left open or closed, (3) the timing of surgery, either early or late, (4) the amplitude of the underlying tissue pressure, and (5) predisposing patient factors such as hypertension, shock or vascular disease. Percutaneous decompression should only be considered to help prevent compartment syndrome after surgery. In cases of established compartment syndrome, the skin must be opened widely to adequately decompress the compartment. The length of skin incision necessary to decompress a compartment has been looked at by Cohen and coworkers.[68] Tissues do not flow like a liquid therefore a small opening in a compartment will not be adequate to allow decompression. Compartment syndromes still occur in the presence of fascial defects such as open fractures.[56,69,70] Mubarak and colleagues[4] also noted that epimysiotomy had little additional effect after fasciotomy in the arm and leg. The exception is the deltoid and gluteal area where the fascia was is blended with the epimysium. Subperiosteal subtotal fibulectomy alone is inadequate for decompression of the leg.[27] This procedure only decreases the intracompartmental pressures by 10 to 15 mmHg, and the pressures only fall to normal when the whole periosteal bed is opened in each compartment.[27] Fibulectomy has an added disadvantage in children. It may result in further destabilization of the fracture or in a progressive valgus deformity of the ankle. Elevation of a limb to increase the venous drainage is not a good idea when the intracompartmental pressure is increased. Elevation of the limb causes decreased blood pressure and decreased transmural pressure gradients, which then favors vascular closure.[71] Vascular perfusion must exceed the tissue pressure therefore elevation cannot augment venous drainage once the intracompartmental pressure is elevated.[17] This may have been a mechanism for the development of compartment syndromes in children who were in traction.[22,55]

When a compartment has been decompressed, the muscles often bulge through the fascial defect and leave the skin incision gaping. This defect may require split thickness skin grafts when the limb has recovered. A technique has been described to decrease the necessity of skin grafting and its esthetic consequences. After fasciotomy, skin staples are applied to both edges of the wound like the eyelets of a shoe. Elastic vessel loops are threaded through the staples and each day on the ward the "laces" are tightened, thus gradually opposing the skin edges.[72,73]

SUMMARY

The development of a compartment syndrome is a common complication of injury and surgery on a limb. A surgeon must develop a high index of suspicion for this complication because the list of conditions that cause it is growing. When a child appears to be developing a compartment syndrome, constrictive dressings must be removed and the compartment palpated. Sensory, motor, and passive movements must be carefully examined and documented in the chart. Compartmental pressure measurements can be useful to clarify ambiguous cases or to monitor the changes over the period of observation. If there is not significant improvement in the child's symptoms after 1 to 2 hours, decompressive fasciotomies should be performed.

REFERENCES

1. Willis RB, Rorabeck CH: Treatment of compartment syndrome in children. Orthop Clin North Am 21:401, 1990
2. Eaton RG, Green WT: Epimysiotomy and fasciotomy in

the treatment of Volkmann's ischemic contracture. Orthop Clin North Am 3:175, 1972
3. Ashton H: The effect of increased tissue pressure on blood flow. Clin Orthop 113:15, 1975
4. Mubarak SJ, Owen CA, Hargens AR et al: Acute compartment syndromes: diagnosis and treatment with the aid of the wick catheter. J Bone Joint Surg [Am] 60:1091, 1978
5. Matsen FA III, Veith RG: Compartmental syndromes in children. J Pediatr Orthop 1:33, 1981
6. Matsen FA III, Winquist RA, Krugmire RB: Diagnosis and management of compartmental syndromes. J Bone Joint Surg 62:286, 1980
7. Mubarak SJ, Hargens AR, Owen CA et al: The wick catheter technique for measurement of intramuscular pressure: a new research and clinical tool. J Bone Joint Surg [Am] 58:1016, 1976
8. Whitesides TE, Jr, Haney TC, Morimoto K, Harada H: Tissue pressure measurements as a determinant for the need of fasciotomy. Clin Orthop 113:43, 1975
9. Montgomery CJ, Ready LB: Epidural opioid analgesia does not obscure diagnosis of compartment syndrome resulting from prolonged lithotomy position. Anaesthesiology 75:541, 1991
10. Knezevich S, Torch M: Streptococcal toxic shocklike syndrome leading to bilateral lower extremity compartment syndrome and renal failure: a case report. Clin Orthop 254:247, 1990
11. Nixon RG, Brindley GW: Hemophilia presenting as compartment syndrome in the arm following venipuncture: a case report and review of the literature. Clin Orthop 244:176, 1989
12. Hieb LD, Alexander AH: Bilateral anterior and lateral compartment syndromes in a patient with sickle cell trait. Clin Orthop 228:190, 1988
13. Hargens AR, Romine JS, Sipe JC et al: Peripheral nerve-conduction block by high muscle-compartment pressure. J Bone and Joint Surg [Am] 61:192, 1979
14. Rorabeck CH, Clarke KM: The pathophysiology of anterior tibial compartment syndrome: an experimental investigation. J Trauma 18:299, 1978
15. Rorabeck CH, McNab I: The pathophysiology of the anterior tibial compartment syndrome. Clin Orthop 113:52, 1975
16. Goodman MJ: Isolated lateral-compartment syndrome. J Bone Joint Surg [Am] 62:834, 1979
17. Matsen FA III: Compartment syndrome: an unified concept. Clin Orthop 113:8, 1975
18. Wolf YG, Reyna T, Schropp KP, Harmel RP: Arterial trauma of the upper extremity in children. J Trauma 30:903, 1990
19. Garfin SR, Mubarak SJ, Evans KL et al: Quantification of intracompartmental pressure and volume under plaster casts. J Bone Joint Surg [Am] 63:449, 1981
20. Aprahamian C, Gessert G, Bandyk DF et al: MAST-associated compartment syndrome (MACS): a review. J Trauma 29:549, 1989
21. Bingold AC: On splitting plasters: a useful analogy. J Bone Joint Surg [Br] 61:294, 1979
22. Mubarak SJ, Carroll NC: Volkmann's contracture in children: aetiology and prevention. J Bone Joint Surg [Br] 61:285, 1979
23. McLaren AC, Ferguson JH, Miniaci A: Crush syndrome associated with use of the fracture table. J Bone Joint Surg [Am] 69:1447, 1987
24. Wall JJ: Compartment syndrome as a complication of the Hauser procedure. J Bone Joint Surg [Am] 61:185, 1979
25. Wiggins HE: The anterior compartmental syndrome: a complication of the Hauser procedure. Clin Orthop 113:90, 1975
26. Holden CEA: The pathology and prevention of Volkmann's ischaemic contracture. J Bone Joint Surg [Br] 61:296, 1979
27. Mubarak SJ, Owen CA: Double-incision fasciotomy of the leg for decompression in compartment syndromes. J Bone Joint Surg [Am] 59:184, 1977
28. Schreiber SN, Liebowitz MR, Bernstein LH: Limb compression and renal impairment (crush syndrome) following narcotic and sedative overdose spectrum of disease. J Bone Joint Surg [Am] 54:1683, 1972
29. Williams PH, Bhatnagar HK, Wisheart JD: Compartment syndrome in a five-year-old child following femoral cannulation for cardiopulmonary bypass. Eur J Cardiothorac Surg 3:474, 1989
30. Davies JAK: Peroneal compartment syndrome secondary to rupture of the peroneus longus: a case report. J Bone Joint Surg [Am] 61:783, 1979
31. Gibson MJ, Barnes MR, Allen MJ, Chan RNW: Weakness of foot dorsiflexion and changes in compartment pressures after tibial osteotomy. J Bone Joint Surg [Br] 68:471, 1986
32. Luk KDK, Pun WK: Unrecognized compartment syndrome in a patient with tourniquet palsy. J Bone Joint Surg [Br] 69:97, 1987
33. Hussain S, Barja RH: Interposition of extensor digitorum tendon in distal radius fracture mimicking a compartment syndrome. J Hand Surg 14A:255, 1989
34. Rorabeck CH: The treatment of compartment syndromes of the leg. J Bone Joint Surg [Br] 66:93, 1984
35. Matsen FA III: Compartmental Syndromes. Grune & Stratton, New York, 1980
36. McDermott AGP, Marble AE, Yabsley RH: Monitoring acute compartment pressures with the S.T.I.C. catheter. Clin Orthop 190:192, 1984
37. Clayton JM, Hayes AC, Barnes RW: Tissue pressure and perfusion in the compartment syndrome. J Surg Res 22:333, 1977
38. Triffitt PD, König D, Harper WM et al: Compartment pressures after closed tibial shaft fracture: their relation to functional outcome. J Bone Joint Surg [Br] 74:195, 1992
39. Allen MJ, Stirling AJ, Crawshaw CV, Barnes MR: Intracompartmental pressure monitoring of leg injuries: an aid to management. J Bone Joint Surg [Br] 67:53, 1985

40. Matsen FA III, Mayo KA, Krugmire RB et al: A model compartmental syndrome in man with particular reference to the quantification of nerve function. J Bone Joint Surg [Am] 59:648, 1977
41. Dolich BH, Aiache AE: Drug-induced coma: a cause of crush syndrome and ischemic contracture. J Trauma 13:223, 1973
42. Geary N: Late surgical decompression for compartment syndrome of the forearm. J Bone Joint Surg [Br] 66:745, 1984
43. Spinner M, Aiache A, Silver L, Barsky AJ: Impending ischemic contracture of the hand: early diagnosis and management. Plast Reconstr Surg 50:341, 1972
44. McDougall CG, Johnston GHF: A new technique of catheter placement for measurement of forearm compartment pressures. J Trauma 31:1404, 1991
45. Bednar DA: Post-traumatic compartment syndrome of the foot. Can J Surg 34:179, 1991
46. Bonutti PM, Bell GR: Compartment syndrome of the foot: a case report. J Bone Joint Surg [Am] 68:1449, 1986
47. Mittlmeier T, Machler G, Lob G et al: Compartment syndrome of the foot after intraarticular calcaneal fracture. Clin Orthop 269:241, 1991
48. Vigasio A, Battison B, De Filippo G et al: Compartmental syndrome due to viper bite. Arch Orthop Trauma Surg 110:175, 1991
49. Matsen FA III, Clawson DK: The deep posterior compartmental syndrome of the leg. J Bone Joint Surg [Am] 57:34, 1975
50. Schwartz JT, Brumback RJ, Lakatos R et al: Acute compartment syndrome of the thigh: a spectrum of injury. J Bone Joint Surg [Am] 71:392, 1989
51. Ebraheim NA, Hoeflinger MJ, Savolaine ER, Jackson WT: Anterior compartment syndrome of the thigh as a complication of blunt trauma in a patient on prolonged anticoagulation therapy. Clin Orthop 263:180, 1991
52. Tarlow SD, Ackterman CA, Hayhurst J, Ovadia DN: Acute compartment syndrome in the thigh complicating fracture of the femur: a report of three cases. J Bone Joint Surg [Am] 68:1439, 1986
53. Hernandez J, Peterson HA: Fracture of the distal radial physis complicated by compartment syndrome and premature physeal closure. J Pediatr Orthop 6:627, 1986
54. Matthews JG: Fractures of the olecranon in children. Injury 12:207, 1981
55. Naito M, Ogata K: Acute volar compartment syndrome during skeletal traction in distal radius fracture: a case report. Clin Orthop 236:234, 1989
56. Royle SG: Compartment syndrome following forearm fracture in children. Injury 21:73, 1990
57. Santoro V, Mara J: Compartmental syndrome complicating Salter-Harris type II distal radius fracture. Clin Orthop 233:226, 1988
58. Aerts P, De Boeck H, Casteleyn PP, Opdecam P: Deep volar compartment syndrome of the forearm following minor crush injury. J Pediatr Orthop 9:69, 1989
59. Brumback RJ: Compartment syndrome complicating avulsion of the origin of the triceps muscle. J Bone Joint Surg [Am] 69:1445, 1987
60. Brumback RJ: Traumatic rupture of the superior gluteal artery, without fracture of the pelvis, causing compartment syndrome of the buttock. J Bone Joint Surg [Am] 72:134, 1990
61. Kym MR, Worsing RA: Compartment syndrome in the foot after an inversion injury to the ankle. J Bone Joint Surg [Am] 72:138, 1990
62. Owen CA, Woody PR, Mubarak SJ, Hargens AR: Gluteal compartment syndromes: a report of three cases and management utilizing the wick catheter. Clin Orthop 132:57, 1978
63. Younge D: Haematoma block for fractures of the wrist: a cause of compartment syndrome. J Hand Surg 14B:194, 1989
64. Strecker WB, Wood MB, Bieber EJ: Compartment syndrome masked by epidural anesthesia for postoperative pain: report of a case. J Bone Joint Surg [Am] 68:1447, 1986
65. Gelberman RH, Zakaib GS, Mubarak SJ et al: Decompression of forearm compartment syndromes. Clin Orthop 134:225, 1978
66. Sheridan GW, Matsen FA III: Fasciotomy in the treatment of the acute compartment syndrome. J Bone Joint Surg [Am] 58:112, 1976
67. Gaspard DJ, Kohl RD, Jr.: Compartmental syndromes in which the skin is the limiting boundary. Clin Orthop 113:65, 1975
68. Cohen MS, Garfin SR, Hargens AR, Mubarak SJ: Acute compartment syndrome: effect of dermotomy on fascial decompression in the leg. J Bone Joint Surg [Br] 73:287, 1991
69. Brostrom L-A, Stark A, Svartengren G: Acute compartment syndrome in forearm fractures. Acta Orthop Scand 61:50, 1990
70. DeLee JC, Stiehl JB: Open tibia fracture with compartment syndrome. Clin Orthop 160:175, 1981
71. Matsen FA III, Krugmire RB, King RV: Increased tissue pressure and its effects on muscle oxygenation in level and elevated human limbs. Clin Orthop 144:311, 1979
72. Cohn BT, Shall J, Berkowitz M: Forearm fasciotomy for acute compartment syndrome: a new technique for delayed primary closure. Orthopaedics 9:1243, 1986
73. Fassier F, Elbaz A, Gagnon S, Stanciu C: Technical note: delayed primary closure of fasciotomy wounds without skin grafting, abstracted. Proceedings of the Pediatric Orthopedic Society of North America, 1992

65

Fat Embolism Syndrome

Alan Gurd

> The essence of wisdom is the ability to make the right decision on the basis of inadequate evidence.
> —ALAN GREGG

DEFINITION AND INCIDENCE

The fat embolism syndrome is a well-recognized complication of major trauma in adults but rarely encountered in its typical form in children. Fat embolism, in its strict sense, merely describes the presence of circulating macroglobules of fat (10 μm or larger in diameter). Pathologic fat emboli found at autopsy (usually in the lung) may have no relationship to the patient's symptoms or to the cause of death. Evidence of pulmonary fat embolism at postmortem is reported from 70 to 100 percent in all patients dying after trauma.[1-3]

HISTORICAL REVIEW

Fat embolism was first described in autopsy material[4,5] in 1862. However, it was 1873 before the first classical clinical features were described in a patient who had sustained a fractured femur and subsequently died.[6] Since these early days, fat embolism (usually at postmortem) has most frequently been reported in association with fractures but also following trauma without fracture.[3,7] It has also been described (again at postmortem) in association with numerous nontraumatic conditions, such as operative trauma,[8] after liposuction,[9] and lipectomy,[10] low-pressure decompression,[11] diabetes,[12] acute hemorrhagic pancreatitis,[13] fatal *Clostridium welchii* toxemia,[14] chronic alcoholism and the nephrotic syndrome,[15] certain poisoning deaths, including carbon tetrachloride, mercury chloride, chloroform, arsphenamine, and strychnine,[16] and following lymphography.[17] In 1969, Drummond and colleagues[18] discussed nine cases of fat embolism in children and noted a relationship to collagen disease. In 1962 Simon Sevitt[3] wrote the first book on this subject in English, which marked the centenary of the original German papers. In his book, Sevitt noted the paucity of cases of fat embolism in children, which he believed to be the result of various factors:

1. The fat in children contained less oleic acid than in adults.
2. The fat in children is more viscous and therefore less liable to become embolic.
3. The marrow in children's long bones is dominantly red marrow, and there is therefore less fatty marrow for embolization.

Sevitt did study some children who were trauma victims and found pulmonary fat. He finally concluded that children could develop fat embolism and that the infrequency of clinical fat embolism syndrome in this age group probably relates more to the low incidence of their sustaining severe and multiple fractures. It now appears that it is the development of the "respiratory distress syndrome" that is rare in the child, since the presence of fat emboli can be found in children who have sustained multiple trauma if searched for diligently.

PATHOGENESIS

Fat normally exists in the blood as glycerides (usually triglycerides), cholesterol, esters, phospholipids, and acids and travels either in solution attached to β-lipoproteins or as a minute suspension of particles (chylomicrons) that measure less than 1 μm in diameter.

There are two classical theories as to where the circulating fat (globules of larger than 10 μm) in the fat embolism syndrome originates. The early belief was that the circulating globules are merely released from a fatty depot, usually the bone marrow of a fractured long bone. Peltier[19] remains a major proponent of this "mechanical theory of intravasation of preexisting fat."

Lehman and Moore[20] first postulated that some of the fat already circulating as minute chylomicrons coalesces to form larger pathologic fat globules. It is suggested that this phenomenon occurs in response to the presence of toxic substances released at or soon after major trauma. This has become known as the "metabolic theory of pathologic fat embolism."

CLINICAL FEATURES

The "classical" features of the fat embolism syndrome are nonspecific and inconsistent. Because of the variability in clinical presentation and the lack of an absolutely reliable diagnostic test, guidelines were drawn up that proved to be useful.[21] Surgeon "awareness" of this complication of major trauma remains the most important aspect in diagnosis. Certain clinical and laboratory features were looked for in association with finding evidence of fat macroglobulinemia:

1. Evidence of major injury
2. A latent period defined as that time following injury to the onset of one of the presenting "major" features (usually 24 to 48 hours)

In a series of 100 cases, the diagnosis was accepted on finding a minimum of one major feature plus four minor or laboratory features along with demonstrating a fat macroglobulinemia.[22] The majority, 93 cases, had major trauma with at least one major bone fracture; 7 had major trauma but with no fractures or a very minor one (calcaneum, patella). In every case a latent period was noted prior to the onset of symptoms (4 hours to 15 days; average: 46 hours) (Table 65-1).

Respiratory involvement was the predominant feature in 75 patients with dyspnea, tachypnea, and moist-

TABLE 65-1. Diagnostic Features of Fat Embolism Syndrome in Children

Major features
  Respiratory insufficiency
  Cerebral involvement
  Petechial rash

Minor features
  Significant pyrexia
  Tachycardia
  Retinal changes
  Jaundice
  Renal changes

Laboratory features
  Anemia
  Thrombocytopenia
  High ESR
  Decreased Pao_2

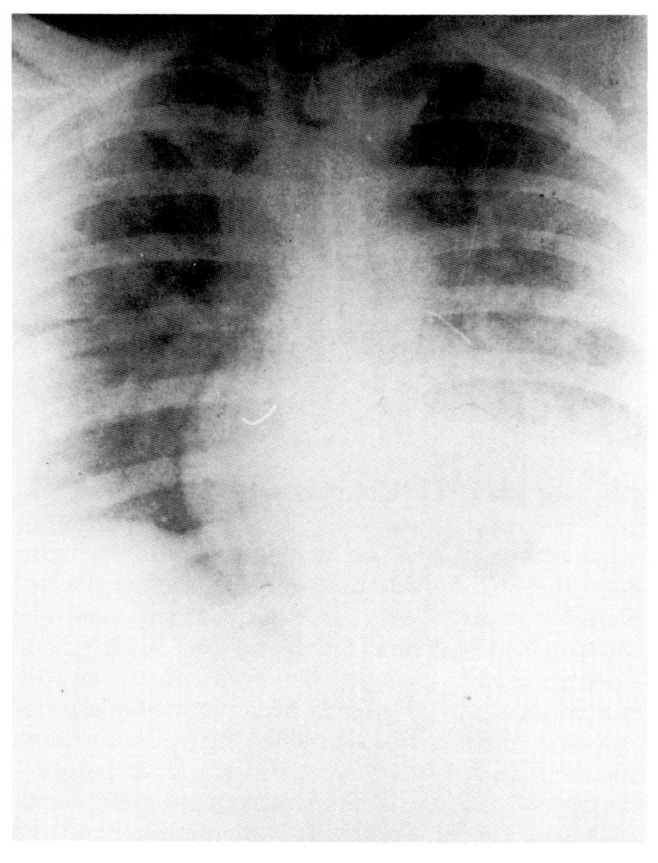

Fig. 65-1. The typical "snowstorm lung" seen in patients suffering from severe fat embolism and resulting in a low Po_2 and respiratory distress.

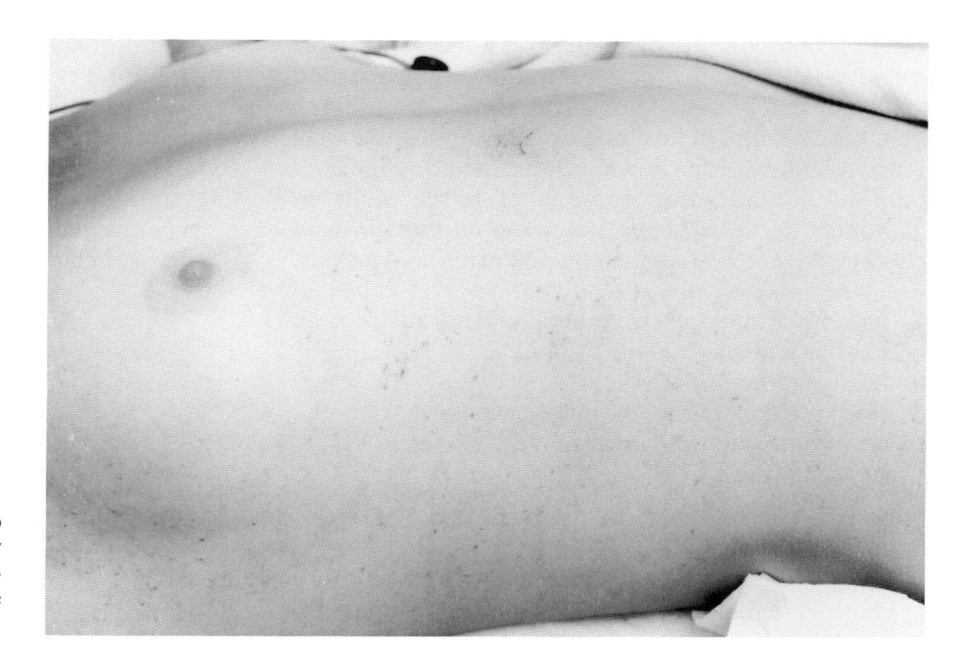

Fig. 65-2. An 11-year-old girl who developed multiple petechia, mostly on her neck and chest 36 hours following a femur fracture. There were no pulmonary signs or symptoms.

rales noted over the whole-lung fields. The classical radiograph finding is of bilateral, generalized lung involvement with patchy consolidation (Fig. 65-1). Cyanosis was uncommon, even in the presence of marked arterial hypoxia, because of the associated anemia. Serial blood gas analysis is indicated. Lindeque and colleagues[22] will make the diagnosis of posttraumatic pulmonary fat embolism if the Pao_2 falls below 60 mmHg.

Cerebral manifestations, typically confusion, are usually secondary to respiratory insufficiency; however, there are cases described where confusion and even coma has developed in the absence of either a head injury or respiratory distress.

The petechial rash (Fig. 65-2), often described as pathognomonic for the fat embolism syndrome, was found in only 57 patients. Typically this rash needs to be looked for carefully, in a good light, once or twice daily with a magnifying glass. The rash is usually found over the anterior axillary fold and the root of the neck. It is useful to check the buccal muscosa and the retina where it may also be seen (Fig. 65-3).

A significant pyrexia of greater than 39.4°C and tachycardia greater than 120 per minute was noted in almost 100 percent of patients. Retinal changes, such as exudates and petechial hemorrhages (7 patients), jaundice (5 patients), and renal changes, such as oliguria and hematuria (22 patients), were less commonly observed.

Laboratory evidence of a concomitant disseminated

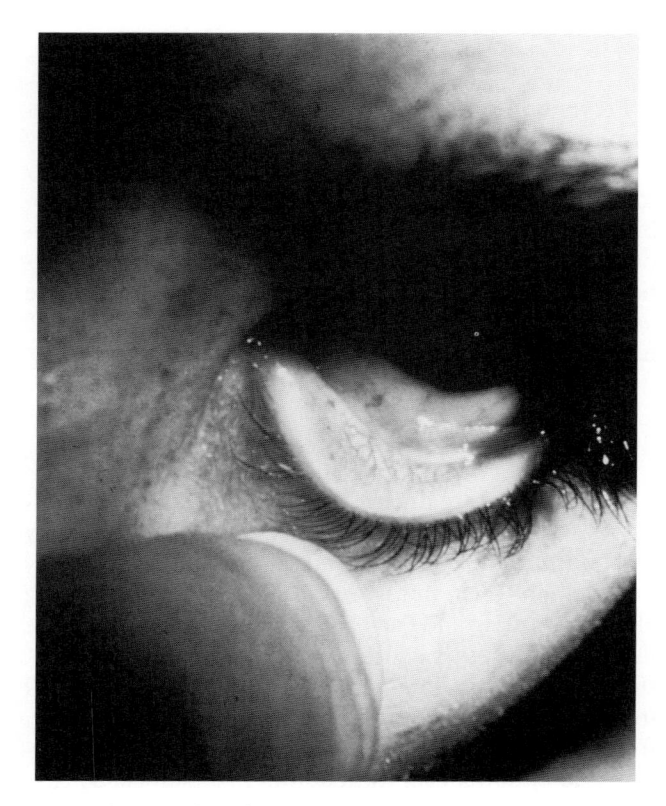

Fig. 65-3. Conjunctival petechiae in a 14-year-old boy 48 hours after sustaining an ipsilateral fracture of the tibia and femur.

intravascular coagulation (DIC) was almost invariable (rapidly developing anemia, thrombocytopenia, and very high ESR).

In the 100 cases of fat embolism syndrome there were only 5 children. The clinical features noted in the children did not differ from those found in the adults. In Toronto[23] 21 cases of posttraumatic fat embolism in children were reviewed, with the following conclusions:

1. Fat embolism occurs in children under similar conditions as adults.
2. Most cases are mild.
3. Hemorrhagic shock or gram-negative bacteremia may be contributing factors.

TREATMENT

Management of the traumatized child should involve methods that may prevent the fat embolism syndrome developing or, if necessary, treatment of the established condition.

Prophylaxis

Prevention of fat embolism basically means the prevention of posttraumatic shock. This will include early and adequate volume substitution, correction of any metabolic acidosis, analgesics, and early fracture immobilization. There are reports of less fat embolism in patients subjected to immediate internal fixation than patients whose fractures are treated conservatively.[24] The use of prophylactic protease inhibitors[7,25] and steroids[26] have been described, but their value is not yet proven.

Established Case

The essential treatment is for the respiratory insufficiency. The surgeon must ensure an adequate airway and administer oxygen (nasal or face mask). Respiratory involvement is monitored and levels of $Paco_2$ rising above 50 mmHg and Pao_2 below 60 mmHg indicates the need for ventilatory assistance. The arterial oxygen tension should be maintained at 70 mmHg or higher. All modalities for respiratory assistance must be available, from simple suction and oxygen to mechanical ventilation and endotracheal intubation. The established case should be managed in some form of intensive care unit.

The rapidly developing anemia and increasing blood viscosity should be corrected with fresh blood and physiologic substitutes such as low molecular weight dextran, which improves microcirculatory flow.[27,28]

There is no known specific medication; however, there are reports of the beneficial effects of massive intravenous steroid therapy[29] and intravenous heparin.[30] Digoxin may be used to manage arrhythmias or early heart failure, and antibiotics are usually given to prevent a bacterial pneumonia developing in a damaged lung.

SUMMARY

The fat embolism syndrome is a well-recognized complication of major trauma, especially when there is major bone involvement. Features vary from the very mild to fulminant respiratory involvement, which can be fatal. Although the literature largely deals with the adult, there is no doubt that fat embolism occurs in children, probably more frequently than is appreciated. In children, the circumstances resulting in its occurrence, the clinical features, and the principles of treatment are similar to those described for the adult. Surgeon awareness is important for early diagnosis and early treatment. Management is basically that of total respiratory care and posttraumatic shock.

REFERENCES

1. Warren S: Fat embolism. Am J Pathol 22:69, 1941
2. Grant RT, Reeve EB: Observations on the general effects of injury in man. MR Council Special Report, series 277. Her Majesty's Stationary Office, London, 1951
3. Sevitt S: Fat Embolism. Butterworth, London, 1962
4. Wagner E: Capillarembolie mit flussigem Fett, eine Ursache der Pyaramie. Arch Heilkd 3:241, 1862
5. Zenker FA: Beitrage zur normalen und pathologischen Anatomie der Lunge. J Braunsdorf 31, Dresden, 1862
6. Bergmann E von: Zur Dehr von der Fetemboli. Inaug Diss Dorpat Katow, EJ, 1873
7. Gurd AR, Wilson RI: The fat embolism syndrome. J Bone Joint Surg [Br] 56:408, 1974
8. Peltier LF: Fat embolism following intra medullary nailing. Surgery 32:719, 1952
9. Laub DR Jr, Laub DR: Fat embolism syndrome after liposuction: a case report and review of the literature. Ann Plast Surg 25:48, 1990
10. Boezaart AP, Clinton CW, Braun S et al: Fulminant adult respiratory distress syndrome after lipectomy: a case report. S Afr Med J 78:693, 1990
11. Haymaker W, Davison E: Fatalities resulting from exposure to simulated high altitudes in decompression chambers. J Neuropathol Exp Neurol 9:29, 1950

12. Kent SP: Fat embolism in diabetic patients without physical trauma. Am J Pathol 31:399, 1955
13. Lynch MJG: Nephrosis and fat embolism in acute haemorrhagic pancreatis. AMA Arch Intern Med 94:709, 1954
14. Cook WT, Frazer AC, Peeney ALP et al: Clostridial infections in war wounds. Lancet 1:487, 1945
15. Lynch MJG, Raphael SS, Dixon TP: Fat embolism in chronic alcoholics. AMA Arch Pathol 67:68, 1959
16. Grosskloss HH: Fat Embolism. Yale J Biol Med 8:59, 175, 297, 1935–36
17. Nelson B, Rush EA, Takasugi M, Wittenberg J: Lipid embolism to the brain after lymphogram. N Engl J Med 273:1132, 1965
18. Drummond DS, Salter RB, Boone UJ: Fat embolism in children: its frequency and relationships to collagen disease. Can Med Assoc J 101:200, 1969
19. Peltier LF: The mechanism of parenchymatous embolism. Surg Gynaecol Obstet 100:612, 1955
20. Lehman EP, Moore RM: Fat embolism including experimental production without trauma. AMA Arch Surg 14:621, 1927
21. Gurd AR: Fat embolism: an aid to diagnosis. J Bone Joint Surg [Br] 52:732, 1970
22. Lindeque BGP, Schoeman HS, Dommisse GF et al: Fat embolism and the fat embolism syndrome: a double-blind therapeutic trial. J Bone Joint Surg [Br] 69:128, 1987
23. Weiss GM, Rang M, Salter RB: Post traumatic fat embolism in children: review of the literature and of experience in the Hospital for Sick Children, Toronto. J Trauma 13:529, 1973
24. Saikku LA: Fat embolism in connection with treatment of fractures. Acta Chiur Scand 108:275, 1954
25. Armis CJ, Hilden H: Inhibition of thromboplastic activity by Trasglov. Scand J Haematol 4:13, 1967
26. Ashbaugh DG, Petty TL: The use of corticosteroids in the treatment of respiratory failure associated with massive fat embolism. Surg Gynaecol Obstet 123:493, 1966
27. Evarts CM: Low molecular weight dextran. Med Clin North Am 51:1285, 1967
28. Bergentz SE: Fat embolism. Prog Surg 6:85, 1968
29. Evarts CM: Complications. p. 184. In Rockwood CA, Green DP (eds): Fractures. Vol. 1. JB Lippincott, Philadelphia, 1975
30. Sage RH, Tudor RW: Treatment of fat embolism with heparin. Br Med J 1:1160, 1958

66

Operative Fixation of Children's Fractures

Kenneth J. Guidera
John A. Ogden

> The most important person in the operating theatre is the patient.
> —RUSSELL HOWARD

There are a number of biologic factors that affect why the utilization of internal and external fixation has not been emphasized or utilized as frequently, prior to skeletal maturity, as it has been in adults.[1] Principally, fractures in children usually result from relatively simple injurious causes, rather than the complex mechanical forces that frequently cause adult skeletal injury. This results in less comminution of a fracture involving the diaphysis or metaphysis. In comparison, many problematic adult fractures, such as hip fractures and multiple, comminuted injuries, are much less common in children. Accordingly, the methods of treatment are generally simpler when dealing with the disrupted immature skeleton. The appropriate emphasis is on *closed* reduction for a much larger percentage of fracture patterns when compared to similar, although not necessarily comparable, anatomic injuries in the mature skeleton. About 20 percent of skeletal injuries prior to skeletal maturity involve the physis, a structure obviously not found in the normal adult. Most growth plate fractures, which principally involve types 1 and 2 patterns, are usually treated effectively by nonoperative methods.

The basic principle of most fracture reductions in children is the "reversal" of the mechanism of injury, which is usually carried out as painlessly as possible. It is axiomatic that if a fracture is produced by an external force, it should be reduced by making the distal fragment "retrace its steps" back to a normal anatomic configuration. Reduction by this method, however, relies on the presence of partial soft tissue (periosteal) linkages. These are more likely to be present (intact) in the child with his or her characteristically thicker periosteum. Another axiom of fracture treatment is to align the fracture fragment that may be most easily controlled. The proximal fragment usually adopts a position dictated by the pull of muscles attached to it. Accordingly, the distal fragment may be more easily controlled, and should be aligned longitudinally and axially with the displacing proximal fragment. The smaller arms and legs of children make manipulation and subsequent control easier in the child than the adult.

Closed methods are usually successful in children because of (1) rapid fracture healing, (2) minimal problems with postimmobilization stiffness, and (3) progressive fracture remodeling. Subsequent growth, particularly, may allow acceptance of less than complete anatomic alignment. However, such physiologic changes generally need at least 2 years of remaining growth, a fracture near the end of the bone, and angulation in the plane of mo-

---

This work was supported in part by the Skeletal Educational Association and the Foundation for Musculoskeletal Research and Education.

tion of the contiguous joint. Remodeling does not "correct" intra-articular fractures, displaced physeal/epiphyseal fractures, angulated or rotated diaphyseal fractures, and certain displaced fractures, each of which often requires more aggressive (i.e., operative) approaches for effective reduction.

Except in those chondro-osseous fractures involving joints, physes, and epiphyses, absolute anatomic reduction of the metaphyseal and diaphyseal bone fragments is not always necessary and sometimes should be avoided. Angulation in the middle third of long bones is not ideal and should be corrected as close to normal as possible. In girls under 10 and boys under 12 years of age, however, angulation of fragments near the joints is more acceptable.

Remodeling usually occurs *only* if the deformity is in the plane of motion of the contiguous joint. Proximity to a joint is also essential. A middiaphyseal angulation of 15 to 20 degrees may not remodel at all, whereas a 45- to 50-degree metaphyseal angulation adjacent to the physis may remodel completely. The patient's age is extremely important. There must be enough growth remaining to allow such remodeling. Concomitant with the age concept is the fact that physeal regions contributing most to elongation are likely to progressively correct (e.g., the proximal humerus, distal radius, distal femur, and proximal tibia in older children; proximal femur and distal humerus in the younger child). These physeal growth rate factors change with time. For example, considerable longitudinal growth occurs in the proximal femur in the first 8 to 10 years. In contrast, the distal femur becomes the more dominant growth region after 10 years.

After injury, the bones of children may grow at an accelerated rate for months to years.[2] Accordingly, overgrowth is a concomitant of many childhood fractures, especially those involving the femur or tibia, although any longitudinal bone may be involved. Further, even a seemingly noninjured bone in the ipsilateral leg may undergo some overgrowth, probably because of the temporarily increased blood flow to the leg following a major injury.

Closed reduction is adequate to maintain relatively normal alignment of most fractures in children because the plastic remodeling of their bones generally renders good final anatomic and functional results. In contrast, certain fractures, especially those near the elbow, may require prompt open reduction.

Unnecessary surgery has been undertaken, sometimes resulting in permanent disability, because a treating physician has failed to appreciate the recuperative and remodeling powers of the child. *Such circumstances do not enhance the acceptance of the role of skeletal fixation, by whatever means, in children.*

Another factor is that children are not initially as "stiff" following immobilization, nor do they remain so, when compared to an adult immobilized for a similar period of time. The rapidity of healing in children obviously decreases the time of immobilization, and may also allow progressive mobilization of joints while the fracture itself is still specifically immobilized (e.g., the progression from long-leg cast to short-leg cast). Children are much more eager to resume activities ("natural" physical or occupational therapy) and usually have a very positive desire to resume their normal preinjury life-style. Adults, in comparison, usually come out of a cast stiffer, require programmed therapy and often have other factors such as workers' compensation that may significantly affect the rate of rehabilitation and recovery.

The physeal morphology changes with maturation. Initially this structure (in three dimensions) is a relatively flat planar structure. However, as the skeleton matures and the child grows in length and weight, the physis changes to an undulated structure adapted to "resist" angular stress/strain. The size of the epiphyseal ossification center also affects the absorption of "fracture energy" in the immature skeleton. Both of these morphologic changes affect fracture patterns. Type 1 physeal injuries are more common in infants and young children with none to minimal ossification within the epiphysis. In contrast, as the ossification center enlarges and matures (i.e., responds to mechanical stimuli), the type 2 pattern becomes more prevalent, and types 3 and 4, with physeal disruption become more likely to occur.

The porosity of the metaphysis changes with time. This is rapidly formed bone (modeling) that is eventually replaced by mechanically responsive bone formation (remodeling). The changing corticalization of the diaphysis also affects fracture failure patterns and responsiveness. The initial cortex is a combination of endochondral bone formation and subperiosteal membranous bone formation. This combination is in a constant state of biologic flux, remodeling in response to applied biologic/biomechanical demands of the individual child. This constant remodeling affects healing and recovery from deformity. It also affects the choice of fixation device and the need for removal.

Rapid healing rates are characteristic of young children. This reflects the osteogenic capacity of the developing periosteum. However, as the child gets older, especially into adolescence, this periosteal reactive capacity for making a circumferential stabilizing callus becomes progressively less.

Since different treatment techniques may achieve similar outcomes, making the appropriate decision becomes an extremely important step. An adequate approach should include (1) a definition of the specific fracture problem, particularly the complexity of the fracture and the extent of cartilaginous (i.e., radiologically invisible) involvement, (2) exploration of the various appropriate options for treatment, (3) the choice of the best treatment alternative for the given circumstances, and (4) basing the choice on the alternative carrying the least risk to the patient.

CONCEPTS OF SKELETAL FIXATION

Some physicians emphatically condemn internal fixation of almost all fractures in children, suggesting that consequences such as nonunion, delayed union, altered growth, infection, and ugly scars may arise. Blount,[3] in particular, was a staunch advocate of closed reduction. His philosophy has been "championed" by many as a reason not to undertake operative fixation in fractures in children.

It is certainly correct that the thoughtless use of internal or external fixation should be strongly discouraged in treating fractures in children, but it is also incorrect to deny its appropriate, skilled application. A useful guide is that operative treatment for a child's fracture is indicated when conservative treatment does not or probably will not achieve an acceptable result (Table 66-1).

While most fractures in children may be managed with closed techniques, rigid adherence to this implied "rule of nonsurgical treatment" of children's fractures may be counterproductive, in either the severely injured child or the one with an isolated fracture that is (or should be) appropriately treated with some type of skeletal fixation. When adhering to reasonable indications and good technique, percutaneous, internal, and external fixation are extremely helpful in preventing both early and late complications of fracture treatment and effectively treating the fracture.

There has been an increasing emphasis on the use of open reduction in children and adolescents, especially in the European literature.[1,2,4-41] Certainly, the trend in the treatment of skeletal injuries in adults is toward operative intervention, resulting, in part, from advances in the techniques of fixation, the specific implants available, and increases in the understanding and control of perioperative wound infection.

The drawbacks of closed treatment may be a relatively long period of immobilization, prolonged hospitalization, muscular atrophy, and joint stiffness, all of which may be lessened, if not eliminated, by active, aggressive open treatment. However, restoration of function in muscles and joints is not as problematic in children, and, even if perfect alignment cannot be achieved and maintained by external immobilization, remodeling and longitudinal growth often correct certain degrees of angular malalignment.

Closed or open reduction with internal fixation are commonly indicated as an appropriate method of treating fracture-separations of the capitellum, trochlea, and the medial epicondylar regions. In certain situations it may be more appropriate to accept a less than ideal closed reduction and undertake elective operative correction later when local or general conditions of the patient are normal (i.e., he or she has recovered from other injuries). It should also be remembered that surgeons have little reservation about using internal fixation to stabilize an osteotomy (i.e., a controlled surgical "fracture"), but yet often appear reluctant to use comparable fixation for a spontaneous fracture in the same anatomic region.

Thompson and colleagues[31] reviewed 4,411 pediatric fractures. Only 3.6 percent (170) of these patients underwent skeletal fixation. Group 1 included 90 skeletally immature children, while Group 2 involved 66 skeletally mature adolescents. Upper extremity fractures (especially those involving the distal humerus) were the major indication for open reduction and internal fixation (ORIF) in Group 1, whereas intra-articular fractures predominated in Group 2. Minor complications were found in 18 percent of Group 1 and 12 percent Group 2. They believed, however, that these complications were fewer than the number that would have occurred had operative intervention *not* been undertaken. Most external fixation devices were used in the lower extremity fractures.

At any age, complicating factors, such as burns, spasticity (developmental or due to head injury), or multiple

TABLE 66-1. Indications for Reduction and Fixation Prior to Skeletal Maturation

Displaced epiphyseal or physeal fracture; realignment of the physis
Displaced intra-articular fracture; realignment of joint surface
Unstable fracture (e.g., hip, spine, lateral condyle of distal humerus); fractures with a "bad reputation" for displacement (adolescent both bones forearm, medial malleolus)
Multiply injured patient, especially one with neurologic or head injury
Open injury, especially with extensive muscle or soft tissue loss
Delayed union after closed treatment; prevention of nonunion
Nonunion after closed treatment
"Floating" joints; challenging combinations of injury in the same limb
Economics of hospitalization
Pathologic fractures
Segmented bone loss
Avulsion (traction) injuries
Neglected fractures
Segmental bone loss
Interposition of soft tissues

osseous injuries, may significantly affect treatment decision-making. For instance, fractures of the femoral shaft may be treated more satisfactorily by fixation in cases involving severe hypertonicity resulting from head trauma. The potential calamities of nonunion and infection should be reasonably avoidable through good surgical technique along with appropriate prophylactic antibiotic treatment. Growth abnormalities should not occur if the vulnerability of the physes, both peripherally and centrally, is respected.

Advances in radiographic imagery have also greatly facilitated the specific anatomic diagnosis and, accordingly, treatment of pediatric fractures. Fluoroscopy may be used preoperatively to assess potential instability (e.g., lateral condylar fracture of the distal humerus). Intraoperative imaging may allow closed reduction with percutaneous fixation to minimize hardware (e.g., the relatively undisplaced lateral condylar fracture). Such technology also allows reasonably accurate external fixator pin placement and closed reduction with appropriate fixator adjustment. The role of magnetic resonance imaging (MRI) has yet to be defined. However, recent papers show the possibility of better defining fracture anatomy (therefore, better treatment basis) and the more diffuse extent of injury (e.g., the metaphyseal or epiphyseal bone bruise). Unfortunately, metallic implants preclude postoperative MRI evaluations (e.g., to evaluate the possibility of ischemic necrosis following a femoral head or neck fracture).

More detailed studies of the failure patterns of the child's skeleton suggest that "simplicity" of propagation does not always prevail. Microcomminution not readily evident on routine radiography may increase the need for stabilization. Physeal fractures, in particular, must be carefully analyzed. With increasing fracture anatomic definition, the indications for operative intervention will become more clearly defined.

Changes in technology may be both beneficial as well as detrimental to children's bones. For example, titanium pins in slipped capital femoral epiphysis (SCFE) may be extremely difficult to remove and may even break during such an attempt. However, they have the advantage of potentially allowing some degree of magnetic resonance imaging.

The development of external fixation devices in the adult with polytrauma has been expanded to comparable situations in the child. These devices, whether uniaxial or ring (polyaxial) fixators, are increasingly sophisticated in design and applicable to the immature skeleton. However, the nuances of the child's bone, especially physeal anatomy and metaphyseal porosity, must be respected during application.

Changing economic factors have also become important. These have arisen in many sectors, especially from the insurance industry, the availability of health insurance, and the drive of health maintenance organizations (HMO). The use of fixation allows the child to leave the hospital much sooner. Six to eight weeks of traction for a femoral fracture leads to considerable per diem costs. Young parents have variable degrees of medical insurance (or none at all). Insurance companies and health maintenance organizations exert pressure to decrease hospitalization. In many families both parents work, or there may be a single parent (separated, divorced) who is working.

Changing concepts of rehabilitation have been applied to handicapped (e.g., neuromuscular disorders) and normal children who have sustained fractures. Fixation obviously allows more rapid, albeit appropriately paced and protected, resumption of motion than the fracture allowed to heal without hardware.

Another reason to undertake fixation of fractures in children is to avoid "fracture illness" in which a long period of casting leads to porosis and atrophy, phenomena that are more likely in children with neuromuscular diseases who would probably benefit from more aggressive fracture management so that they may be mobilized to decrease the rapidity of onset of porosis.

Finally, better medical care in pediatric intensive care units has led to increased survival of multiply injured patients. Comatose children wake up with greater regularity than head-injured adults. However, while comatose, they may have severe decerebrate rigidity that makes fracture control difficult. External fixators may be placed under local anesthesia if the neurosurgical situation precludes general anesthetic techniques. This avoids a patient with "iatrogenic" deformity and the need for reconstructive surgery when they recover from the head injury.

It is equally important to remember that closed treatment is not without hazard. Cast sores may develop when there is insufficient padding, when swelling creates pressure, or when there is an indentation in the cast. Compartment syndromes may develop with closed injuries. A compressive cast may increase the extent of damage. Loss of position may occur when soft tissue swelling progressively dissipates, allowing the development of looseness within the cast. Traction tape allergy may develop, especially in myelodysplastic children with latex allergies.[42]

INDICATIONS FOR FIXATION

Several concepts regarding the utilization of skeletal fixation prior to skeletal maturity may be considered. It is better to undertake gentle, controlled open reduction of a physeal fracture rather than resorting to multiple, forceful closed reductions. Fixation should be temporary; whenever possible, the fixation should be easy to remove (pins, K-wires, screw). Temporary internal stabilization should be supplemented with a cast. Rigid (i.e., compressive) fixation rarely is necessary, since the initial (primary) union is going to progressively disappear with subsequent growth and remodeling. Further, such rigidity may decrease the prolific subperiosteal callus formation that is typical (and important) to fracture stability in a child. Anatomic reduction and maintenance of physeal (especially types 3 and 4) and articular injuries is usually necessary and appropriate. External fixators should be removed as soon as possible after some initial fracture stability is evident radiographically or to manipulation. A cast or orthosis may be used to protect the child while further healing and remodeling occur. The primary use of external fixation is for children with open injuries, especially those with extensive soft tissue injuries. This allows "aggressive" management of soft tissue injuries. In polytrauma patients, with or without head injury, stabilizing the multiple fractures enables earlier mobilization, often facilitating recovery of nonorthopaedic injuries. However, less than 5 percent of children admitted with polytrauma probably require operative fracture therapy, or some type of skeletal fixation, especially the application of external fixation. External fixation is also recommended for children with an open fracture associated with skin loss or burns, in children with head injury with resultant increased motor tone, and in polytrauma patients to facilitate care, transport for diagnostic modalities, and therapeutic procedures. ORIF should be used for challenging combinations of fractures, such as both bones of the forearm combined with a distal humeral fracture or fractures of both sides of the knee to create a floating knee. This methodology of fixation should also be considered in potentially unstable fracture cases, such as a Chance injury of the spine. ORIF is also indicated when there is loss of bone substance, such as in the tibia, to allow subsequent bone transport later without loss of length due to soft tissue contractures. Contraindications to internal fixation may include contaminated wounds, or whenever such fixation is unnecessary or inappropriate. A list of general indications for the use of fixation devices in children and adolescents is included in Table 66-1.

Internal fixation of nonarticular fractures in children does not have to be absolutely anatomically perfect. However, articular fractures require as much dilligence in reduction as in the adult. Because of the variability allowed in the necessary extent of anatomic reductions, small flexible rods and flexible plates may be used as temporary expedients, but should be coupled with some external splinting to allow controlled healing and rapid rehabilitation.

External devices in children are primarily used for open fractures, skin loss, or burns, and those that cannot be treated effectively by internal fixation which should be the preferred method of treatment. These devices are also useful for children with polytrauma and multiple fractures, those requiring fasciotomy, and those with extensive contaminated wounds that require debridement and maintenance of an open wound until it may be safely closed secondarily or skin grafted. External fixators allow maintenance of limb length during initial treatment, particularly when there is extensive bone loss. Meticulous pin care is necessary to avoid necrosis either from heat of insertion or infection (ring sequestrum).

Many types of fractures of the physis and epiphysis are best treated by open reduction and internal fixation. However, open reduction may be dangerous if performed several days or weeks after an epiphyseal injury, because the danger of damage to the physis may increase. If displacement is still severe and open reduction is necessary, the surgeon may lessen, if not altogether avoid, these risks by handling the region around the physis with extreme care.

When internal fixation is used in the immature skeleton, it is *not* always necessary to observe the same principles of "rigid" fixation generally applied to fractures in adults. The more porous, elastic bone of the child requires fixation for *alignment purposes,* rather than to enhance the process of healing itself. Rotational deformities *must* be corrected, whether the child is treated by operative or nonoperative methods.

When applying an external fixator one must attempt to avoid the physis during pin placement. In general, pins should be at least 1 to 2 cm from the physis. Sometimes pins may be placed in the epiphyseal ossification center (transversely). Pins also should not be so close to the physis that a pin tract infection could extend to the physis. Cortical bone porosity in the metaphysis may affect "purchase" of pins. Meticulous pin care is requisite. Half-pins may also be used with a cast or orthosis.

The physis may not be particularly "forgiving" to transphyseal hardware. Any fixation device crossing the physis invariably should be smooth and of a small diameter. Larger diameter devices increase risk of bridge formation through the residual defect left after hardware removal. Threaded devices are contraindicated, presumably because of compression restraint whether or not the threads continually traverse the physis or are placed beyond in the metaphyseal bone, as in a malleolar screw. However, even smooth pins, particularly if left an extended time may be associated with physeal bridging.

Perhaps one of the most important goals in the treatment application of open reduction and external fixation (OREF) is to *minimize the amount of hardware.* The next goal is to rely on cast augmentation as well as soft tissues that are intact. For instance, the periosteum is often incompletely disrupted and can be used as an effective internal splint that allows less hardware than might be necessary in an adult.

METHODS OF FIXATION

Pins

External fixation pins incorporated into a cast represent a simple technique that also requires adequate reduction of the bone fragments as part of the application of the cast. It is relatively lacking in flexibility and adjustability.

K-wire fixation usually must be supplemented with a cast or splint. A smooth wire is less likely to disrupt growth if the physis has to be crossed. Pins may be placed percutaneously and, if put in the proper position, usually do not interfere with neurovascular function. The drawbacks are that they are not rigid, especially the smaller diameter wires. They sometimes lack stability. They do not compress and they may preclude early motion. The goal should be to use the smallest diameter that allows anatomic reduction to be obtained and maintained, and then to use cast supplementation for stability until there is sufficient "stickiness" in the fracture. Good examples for this include supracondylar fracture of the distal humerus. However, these types of fixation in a hip fracture are usually contraindicated.

One may decide whether these should be kept subcutaneous or not. If left penetrating the skin there can be some reactivity around the skin penetration sites that can lead to hypertrophic granulation tissue as well as infection.

When the growth plate must be traversed it is important to use smooth pins and try to get these as close as possible to the anatomic center of the physis. Damage to peripheral tissue such as the zone of Ranvier is more likely to lead to angular growth deformity.[43] Threaded pins are more likely to be associated with growth plate damage if they must cross the physis. With type 2 or 4 growth mechanism injuries efforts should be made to transversely fix the metaphyseal fragment to the rest of the metaphysis, and, in the case of type 4, epiphyseal ossification center to epiphyseal ossification center and thus avoid any angularly directed pin fixation across the physis.

Screw Fixation

Screw fixation allows secure fixation, even of small fragments. It is of particular benefit in periarticular and physeal fractures leading to stable interfragmentary fixation. There is a potential for growth arrest if the threads cross the physis. Screw fixation may be done with the fluoroscope utilizing cannulated screws after initial pin fixation of the fracture. The smooth pin may thus function as the guidewire for the subsequent screw. It may be subject to breakage from shear stress and, accordingly, when used in the lower extremities should be coupled with adequate protection with either a cast or brace and graduated weight bearing.

Blades and Plates

Plate fixation produces relatively to completely rigid internal fixation, depending upon the type of device used. Again, it often should be supplemented with a cast in a child. Such augmentation allows the use of smaller plates. Rigid compression is not usually necessary because of the remodeling potential of the developing skeleton. These plates do give stable, definitive skeletal fixation. The drawbacks are that one must strip the periosteum and periosteal blood supply. This may lead to a decrease in bone mass beneath the plate either from increased cortical porosity or increased endosteal resorption. Periosteal stripping may also encourage new bone formation that envelops the plate, making removal difficult.

The AO technique relies heavily on dynamic compression to enhance primary bone healing with osteon remodeling. This is not as important in children as you want to encourage the formation of the reactive callus in the subperiosteal region and allow remodeling. In many children in whom a plate is used that particular cortex may no longer be "existent" in 2 or 3 years as the child grows the bone latitudinally (in width or diameter) as well as length.

Medullary Techniques

Intramedullary rods allow axial alignment to be maintained without undue stress to the surrounding bone. This is a stable axial alignment. It does allow progressive load sharing and weightbearing, since most shaft fractures that are treated with these types of devices tend to be simple fractures rather than comminuted fractures. They are generally not disruptive of the periosteal blood supply. Extensive reaming, however, may affect endosteal circulation and is less necessary in the child. The problems relate to using care with the insertion when you are near the growth plate. They may still allow angular rotatory deformation. This again may be addressed by temporary application of a cast or brace.

Intramedullary techniques should not violate the growth plate.[44] The increasing utilization of medullary rods in femoral shaft fractures in children has led to a lower and lower age for suggested application. However, the growth plate of the greater trochanter as well as any residual epiphysis and physis along the superior and posterior femoral neck may be damaged by insertion of such a rod and can lead to trochanteric growth arrest with a valgus deformity. Flexible intramedullary devices such as Matev or Enders nails or rods are more appropriate to use as these can be inserted through metaphyseal windows and kept away from the growth plate.

External Fixators

The unilateral frames are relatively simple to apply and lead to stable fixation. Half-pins may be placed with minimal soft tissue damage or neurovascular entrapment. There is an adjustable aspect to these. Nonunion rates may be higher but some of the newer methods utilizing dynamic compression on a progressive basis may avoid this, particularly since nonunion is so rare in children. The circular external fixation frame, such as the Ilizarov, again are extremely stable. They do allow bone transport when there is bone loss. They do allow angular adjustment. However, they are relatively complicated to apply and may be restrictive to soft tissue reconstructions.

Biodegradable Materials

Smooth pins, screws, and plates are being constructed of various biodegradable materials.[45] The benefit is presumably not having to subsequently remove the hardware. However, the smooth pins do not allow compression of a fragment to the rest of the skeleton. More importantly there are a number of reported osteolytic reactions to these implants, often many months after the fracture has been fixed and has healed. The appearance is comparable to osteomyelitic changes.

COMPLICATIONS OF FIXATIONS

Reliance on the implanted hardware is often a problem. Children have an occupation known as play. They will try to get back to it as soon as possible. The child, through his or her parents, must be discouraged from resuming activity when the fracture pain dissipates. The initial concern of parents as to what the posttreatment limitations are quickly changes to "should my child be doing . . . ?". As such, if one follows the dictum of minimizing the amount of hardware, one must supplement this with external restraint or constraint devices such as cast, braces, and splints.

The overall problems with internal fixation include the incarceration of the hardware, soft tissue stripping that may lead to dysvascular fragments, fixation devices that are too rigid, which lead to bone atrophy and growth arrest, or growth stimulation from the surgical approach as well as possibly from the presence of the device.

Inappropriate utilization of fixation devices may lead to delayed union or nonunion. Large, rigid fixation devices are generally unnecessary, as is extensive reaming of the medullary cavity to fit a larger rod. Large, rigid plates in children may actually deter healing and contribute to delayed union, if not nonunion. Children's fractures rely extensively on subperiosteal new bone formation, which is deterred by both the rigidity of fixation and the stripping of the periosteum to apply such a device. Small, thin plates are less likely to cause such a problem.

During and following reduction with either external or internal fixation it is imperative that radiographs be obtained to document the position of the fragments. This may involve a portable radiograph or a "hard copy" from the image intensifier. It is difficult to justify a film 1 to 2 weeks later that shows malposition if none was obtained intraoperatively to show acceptability of the reduction.

Unnecessary performance of open reduction is never indicated. Common fractures, such as the distal radial metaphysis, are appropriately treated by closed means. The routine application of ORIF (is contraindicated), except in the rare case that cannot be manipulated into position because of herniation through muscle or periosteum.

When an external fixation device is removed, the child still needs to be protected. Our preference is a full contact orthosis coupled with progressive mobilization. Refracture may also be a complication of plate removal.

Growth damage may occur from inappropriate application of hardware. A malleolar screw or any other threaded device that crosses the physis substantially increases the risk of causing or worsening growth plate damage.

Infection is a serious complication of any operative procedure. The use of prophylactic antibiotics is appropriate, even in a closed fracture treated with external fixation or percutaneous pinning. The child's skeleton is at greater risk for hematogenous infection than that of the adult.

Delayed union and nonunion are rare complications of children's fractures. Rigid fixation and excessive periosteal stripping may increase the risk. If either develops after ORIF, removal of the device and more conservative methods (i.e., casting, orthotic bracing) are indicated.

Pin migration may occur, often to a distant site. This is more likely with a smooth pin.

Vascular damage may occur when fixation pins are near a major blood vessel. Similarly, protruding screws or plates may also damage vessels.[46]

REMOVAL OF FIXATION DEVICES

Obviously any external fixation device pin, or percutaneous (protruding) pin should be removed. The use of percutaneous pinning to stabilize fractures such as a supercondylar distal humerus or a lateral condylar distal humerus allow rapid removal of the extraneous or subcutaneous fixation device. However, it is also important, with the use of internal fixation, to consider removing the implanted device as soon as healing and remodeling of the fracture permits. Fixation devices effectively function as stress risers and may affect the normal remodeling of the enlarging skeleton.[47–49] There are instances of refracture. If there are deformities that require subsequent reconstruction the overgrowth of bone may make removal of the devices difficult and may actually add to the morbidity of the subsequent operative procedure. The stress shielding that the devices indubitably cause may inhibit normal bone remodeling. They do not generally interfere with appositional growth in a young child. In fact, this process may continue to the point of complete envelopment (incorporation) of the plate. The device may also be a focus of late infection.

The fabrication of fixation devices, especially pins and screws, from biodegradable materials may preclude the need for removal of metallic devices. However, these operative fixation methods are not without actual or potential problems. The most significant is a dramatic osteolysis around the implant. This is probably an inflammatory reaction (foreign body reaction) to the implant. However, when it occurs the obvious concern is the presence of an infected implant and osteomyelitis. This reaction may occur soon after surgery, but may also occur over a year later.

IMMOBILIZATION

Because children devise ingenious methods for destroying immobilization devices, casts or splints that supplement fixation methods must be applied securely. As a general rule, one or more joints on either side of the fracture should be immobilized initially. Follow-up radiographs should be obtained at about 5 to 10 days after reduction. During this time, the reactive swelling and pain are subsiding and the child's activity level is increasing, so the cast may become loose and put increased stress on the implant. In comparison to closed reduction the use of fixation minimizes loss of reduction when the cast loosens. However, small fixation devices are subject to bending, and small intramedullary rods do not rigidly control rotation.

Functional fracture bracing has been shown to be effective in children 16 years of age or younger.[50] The method probably should be restricted to fractures in the distal third of the femur or the entire tibia. Midshaft femoral fractures should *not* be treated by this method. For children, the only significant advantage of fracture bracing is the greater freedom afforded to both the child and the parents, although this advantage is difficult to evaluate quantitatively. This methodology also has merit in conjunction with limited internal fixation. In fact, combination of cast or cast-brace with limited or temporary internal or percutaneous fixation may be highly effective in the child to minimize hospitalization and maximize the rapidity of rehabilitation.

SEDATION AND ANESTHESIA

Before satisfactory operative treatment can be provided, the fears and apprehensions of the child (and often the parents) must be dispelled, and pain should be alleviated. If reduction is necessary, proper levels of sedation or anesthesia or both are essential.

Children present unique anesthetic considerations related not only to their small size but also to physiologic differences. An inverse relationship exists between age and anesthetic requirements. The changes in anesthetic requirements with age parallel changes in cerebral oxygen consumption, cerebral blood flow, and neuronal density.

In any fracture requiring muscle relaxation for reduction, a general anesthetic is more useful. This is particularly true for supracondylar humeral and dorsally displaced distal radial fractures. If general anesthesia is used, the child may be admitted to the hospital for observation, not only of the recovery from anesthesia but also of the peripheral neurovascular response to the injury, since displacement and manipulative reduction, which may be difficult, certainly constitute further trauma to the already injured tissues.

ASSOCIATED SOFT TISSUE AND VASCULAR INJURIES

The determination of possible vascular injury to the extremity is a critical step in the initial evaluation of the patient. Injury with profuse bleeding and fractures or dislocations that have a high risk of vascular injury should be assessed appropriately, regardless of the presence of peripheral pulses. An arteriogram is especially important in children with suspected popliteal artery damage following displaced epiphyseal fractures or dislocation above the knee. By the time clinical signs of vascular impairment become obvious, the extremity may not be salvageable. Similar consideration should be given to brachial arterial injury.

Severe soft tissue injuries associated with open fractures are the result of high-energy trauma. The external fixator is especially helpful in providing stabilization of the fracture, while concomitantly allowing access to the soft tissue injury. In the case of vascular injury needing surgical repair, bone fixation is needed to decrease risk of postoperative damage to the vascular repair, particularly in children with associated head trauma. The external fixator is ideal for this situation. Children tolerate these devices well, as they also do in leg-lengthening procedures. The external fixator also permits early mobilization of the multiply injured patient with unstable fractures, therefore reducing possible metabolic and pulmonary morbidity.

COMPARTMENT SYNDROME

Arm or leg compartment syndromes and their complications may occur following open reduction and internal fixation and may be a major cause of long-term disability. Elbow and knee injuries are particularly associated with this complication.

A period of ischemia followed by resurgent blood flow may cause increased intramuscular swelling. Similarly, an impaired venous overflow may increase interstitial edema. Bleeding (extraosseous) may also cause compartment syndrome. The classic signs of compartment syndrome include pain not relieved by sedation, tenseness of affected compartments, hypesthesia, weakness, and significant pain on passive stretch of the involved muscles. The presence of a peripheral pulse (palpable or Doppler) does *not* rule out the diagnosis of compartment syndrome. In the young child or any child with central nervous system injury, the diagnosis of compartment syndrome may be quite difficult; therefore, compartmental monitoring is recommended. When compartment syndrome is suspected, appropriate decompression of the involved compartment should be performed to prevent long-term complications. Such decompression may often be done electively (prophylactically) at the time of open reduction.

HEAD INJURY

The physician must be aware of some of the basic principles of treating head injuries in children, although fracture of the skull is generally less significant than the comparable injury in an adult. The prime consideration is not the fracture, but damage to the brain and intracranial fluid accumulation. In the young child with an elastic skull, much of the blow is absorbed by the osseous plates. Despite considerable depression of the bone, there may be little actual brain injury. Even the skull of an older child with closing sutures absorbs a good deal of the blow, transmitting less force to the brain itself. However, injuries to the tips of the frontal or temporal lobes may cause prolonged unconsciousness, extending for weeks or even months, *but usually with complete recovery ultimately.*

Head trauma adds to the difficulties of skeletal traction and casts. Patients with altered states of consciousness following central nervous system injury may have spastic muscle posturing that often requires rigid stabilization of fractures. Femoral fractures in children with head injury may be extremely difficult to control in traction.

The child's ability to survive severe head injury makes maintaining adequate alignment of any fracture critical, regardless of the severity of the initial injury. When alignment cannot be readily and easily maintained by traction, stabilization with internal or external fixation is indicated.[51,52] The external fixator may be applied with relative ease, even under local anesthesia, and is helpful in preserving the alignment of long bone fractures in children. External fixation allows mobilization of the patient out of traction while maintaining osseous alignment, even in cases involving spastic patients. Internal fixation is less indicated in these patients, and often contraindicated because of the physiologic alterations of brain function, cerebral edema, and so on that could adversely effect anesthetic risks. The risks of infection at the fracture site complicate open fracture management. External fixation also allows the treatment of such soft tissue injury.

Intramedullary nailing of femoral fractures in children has been successful in preventing alignment complications in the brain-injured child. The significant danger of injury to the vascular supply of the femoral head or to the trochanteric epiphysis, with growth arrest in either instance, markedly increases the risks of this procedure. Closed intramedullary nailing of femoral fractures in children aged 10 to 15 years has excellent results. When the procedure is properly performed, operative trauma and complications are minimal, and early mobilization is possible.

REFERENCES

1. Ogden JA: Skeletal Injury in the Child. 2nd Ed. WB Saunders, Philadelphia, 1990
2. Kirby RM, Winquist RA, Hansen ST Jr: Femoral shaft fractures in adolescents: a comparison between traction plus cast treatment and closed intramedullary nailing. J Pediatr Orthop 1:193, 1981
3. Blount W: Fractures in Children. Williams & Wilkins, Baltimore, 1955
4. Alonso JE, Horowitz M: Use of the AO/ASIF external fixator in children. J Pediatr Orthop 7:594, 1987
5. Aronson J, Tursky EA: External fixation of femur fractures in children. J Pediatr Orthop 12:157, 1992
6. Baijal E: Instances in which intramedullary nailing of a child's fracture is justifiable. Injury 7:181, 1976
7. DeBrunner AM: Frakturen im Kindesalter: Konservative oder operative Therapie? Zentralbl Chir 99:641, 1974
8. Ecke H: Traumatische Veranderungen an der Wachstumsfuge, ihre Behandlung und Prognose. Z Kinderchir, suppl 11:699, 1972
9. Editorial: Internal fixation for fractures in childhood. Br Med J 1:1301, 1976
10. Ehalt W: Verletzungen bei Kindern und Jugendlichen. Enke, Stuttgart, 1961
11. Gregory RJH, Cubison TCS, Pinder IM, Smith SR: External fixation of lower limb fractures in children. J Trauma 33:691–3, 1992
12. Haas SL: Restriction of bone growth by pins through the epiphyseal cartilaginous plate. J Bone Joint Surg [Am] 32:338, 1950
13. Hackenbroch MH: Die Indikation zur Osteosynthese bei der frischen Kindlichen Verletzung. Z Kinderchir, suppl 11:671, 1972
14. Hecker WC, Daum R: Grundsatzliche Indikationsfehler bei Kindlichen Frakturen. Lagenbecks Arch Chir 327:864, 1970
15. Jonasche E, Bertuel E: Verletzungen bei Kindern bis zum 14 Lebensjahr. Hefte Unfallheilkd 150:1, 1981
16. Jungbluth Kh, Daum R, Metzger E: Schenkelhalsfrakturen im Kindesalter. Z Kinderchir 6:392, 1968
17. Kehr H, Hierholzer G: Technik der Osteosynthese bei Kindlichen Frakturen. Monatsschr Unfallheilk 78:199, 1975
18. Kirschenbaum D, Albert MC, Robertson WW et al: Complex femur fractures in children: treatment with external fixation. J Pediatr Orthop 10:588, 1990
19. Kumer EH, Weyland F: Indikation zur operativen Behandlung Kindlicher Frakturen. Aktuel Traumatol 1:63, 1971
20. Lehmann L, Ferber WN: Die Anwendung des Fixateur externe in der Behandlung Kindlicher Schaft Frakturen. Monatsschr Unfallheilkd 78:401, 1975
21. Leonard MH, Dubravcik P: Management of fractured fingers in the child. Clin Orthop 73:160, 1970
22. Ligier JN, Metaizeau JP, Prevot J: Elastic stable intramedullary nailing of femoral shaft fractures in children. J Bone Joint Surg [Br] 70:74, 1988
23. Metaizeau J-P: Osteosyntheses chez l'enfant. Sauramps Medical, Paris, 1988
24. Probst J: Nachbehandlung und Beobachtung Kindlicher Frakturen. Langenbecks Arch Chir 342:319, 1976
25. Quinten J, Evrad H, Govat P, Cornil C, Burny F: External fixation in childhood traumatology. Orthopedics 7:463, 1984
26. Rab GT: Operative treatment of children's fractures. In Chapman MW (ed): Operative Orthopaedics. 2nd Ed. JB Lippincott, Philadelphia, 1993
27. Reff RB: The use of external fixation devices in the management of severe lower extremity trauma and pelvic injuries in children. Clin Orthop 188:21, 1984
28. Schranz PJ, Gultekin C, Colton CL: External fixation of fractures in children. Injury 23:80, 1992
29. Schweizer P: Indikationen zur operativen Knochenbruch Behandlung in Kindesalter. Med Welt 27:187, 1976
30. Spiegel PG, Mast JW: Internal and external fixation of fractures in children. Orthop Clin North Am 11:405, 1980
31. Thompson GH, Wilber JH, Marcus RE: Internal fixation of fractures in children and adolescents: a comparative analysis. Clin Orthop 188:10, 1984
32. Tolo VT: External skeletal fixation in children's fractures. J Pediatr Orthop 3:435, 1983
33. Tolo VT: External fixation in multiple injured children. Orthop Clin North Am 21:393, 1990
34. Vinz H: Operative Behandlung von Knochenbruchen bei Kindern. Zentralbl Chir 97:1377, 1972
35. Vinz H, Grobler B: Osteosynthese in Kindesalter: biomechanische Aspekte und alter physiologische Osteosyntheseverfahren. Zentralbl Chir 100:455, 1975
36. Weber BG: Das Besondere bei der Behandlung der Frakturen im Kindesalter. Monatsschr Unfallheilkd 78:193, 1975
37. Weber BG, Brunner C, Freuler F: Die Frakturenbehand-

lung bei Kinder und Jugendlichen. Springer-Verlag, Berlin, 1978
38. Weller S: Spezielle Gesichtspunkte bei der Behandlung Kindlicher Frakturen. Z Kinderchir, suppl 11:655, 1972
39. Wilkins KE: Changing patterns in the management of fractures in children. Clin Orthop 264:136, 1991
40. Witt AN, Walcher K: Korrekturoperationen nach Kindlichen Verletzungen. Z Kinderchir, suppl 11:841, 1972
41. Ziv I, Blackburn N, Rang M: Femoral intramedullary nailing in the growing child. J Trauma 24:432, 1984
42. Meeropol E, Frost J, Pugh L, Roberts J, Ogden JA: Latex allergy in children with myelodysplasia: a survery of Shriners Hospitals. J Pediatr Orthop 13:1–4, 1993
43. Siffert RS: The effect of staples and longitudinal wires on epiphyseal growth. J Bone Joint Surg [Am] 38:1077–88, 1956
44. Bjerkreim I, Langard O: Effect upon longitudinal growth of femur by intramedullary nailing in rats. Acta Orthop Scand 54:363, 1983
45. Partio EK: Absorbable screws in the fixation of cancellous bone fractures and arthrodeses: a clinical study of 318 patients. Thesis, University of Helsinki, 1992
46. Paul MA, Patka P, van Heuzen EP, Koomen AR, Rauwerds J: Vascular injury from external fixation: case reports. J Trauma 33:917, 1992
47. Beaupre GS, Carter DR: Warping of cross sections in the torsion of long bones with internal fracture fixation plates. J Orthop Res 5:296, 1987
48. Berjesen T, Benum P: The stress-protecting effect of metal plates on the intact rabbit tibia. Acta Orthop Scand 54:810, 1983
49. Moyen BJ, Lahey PJ, Weinberg EH, Harris WH: Effects on intact femora of dogs of the application and removal of metal plates. J Bone Joint Surg [Am] 60:940, 1978
50. McCullough NC III, Visant JE Jr, Sarmiento A: Functional fracture-bracing of long-bone fractures of the lower extremity in children. J Bone Joint Surg [Am] 60:314, 1978
51. Porat S, Milgrom C, Myska M, Whisler JH, Zoltan JD, Mallin BA: Femoral fracture treatment in head injured children: use of external fixation. J Trauma 26:81, 1986
52. Ziv I, Rang M: Treatment of femoral fracture in the child with head injury. J Bone Joint Surg [Br] 65:276, 1983

67

Traumatic Spondylolysis and Spondylolisthesis

Thomas S. Renshaw

> When you have eliminated the impossible whatever remains, however improbable, must be the truth.
> —A. Conan Doyle

Spondylolysis is the term used to describe a defect in the pars interarticularis region of the posterior elements of a lumbar vertebra (Fig. 67-1). The *pars interarticularis* is the area that joins the pedicle, transverse process, and superior facet process of its vertebra to its lamina, spinous process, and inferior facet process. Spondylolysis occurs only in humans and has not been described as a congenital finding, although it has been documented radiographically in a 4-month-old infant who had a clinical deformity at birth and L4 on L5 spondyloptosis.[1] It has not been reported in individuals who have never walked.[2]

Spondylolisthesis is the forward or anterior translation or slipping of the spondylolytic vertebra relative to the vertebra immediately caudal to it (Fig. 67-2). When L5-S1 slipping occurs, the spinous process, laminae, and inferior articular processes of L5 remain with the posterior sacral elements while the superior articular processes, transverse processes, pedicles, and vertebral body translate forward.

ETIOLOGY

The spondylolytic defect is the result of a pars interarticularis fracture possibly caused by an acute traumatic event but far more commonly by chronic stress repeatedly applied to this structurally inadequate part of the vertebra during upright activities.[3-6] As one would expect, this condition is seen more often in vigorous athletes such as weight lifters,[7] football linemen,[8] and gymnasts.[9] Spina bifida occulta is seen in from 22 to 65 percent of patients with pars defects and may contribute to stress concentration at that region.[10-12] Genetic factors can also be important, since spondylolisthesis has been found in up to 45 percent of some Eskimo tribes and in from 15 to 50 percent of relatives of patients with this condition.[13-15] Mechanical factors that concentrate stress at the pars interarticularis and predispose it to failure are the rotation of a lumbar spine in a lordotic or hyperlordotic posture and the compression of the lumbar spine in a flexed or straight posture.[5,16,17] Acute fractures of the pars interarticularis often result from seemingly minor trauma and very likely represent the final mechanical insult to an already weakened structure (Fig. 67-3).

PREVALENCE

Spondylolysis occurs most commonly at the fifth lumbar vertebra (approximately 97 percent of cases[18]), next most often at the fourth, and much less commonly at L3, L2, and L1, respectively. Its prevalence at L5 is

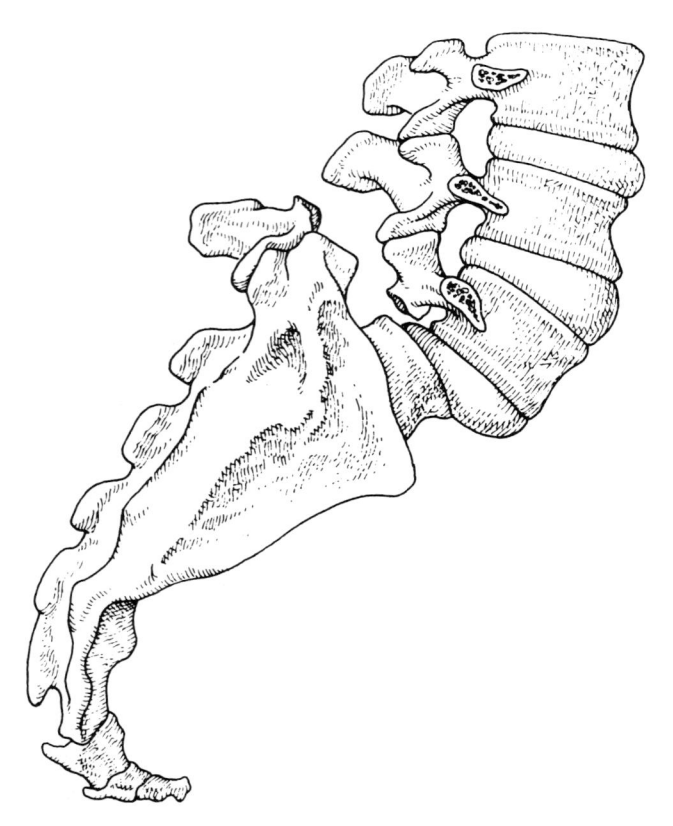

Fig. 67-1. Lateral drawing of the lumbar spine showing spondylolysis, a defect in the pars interarticularis, and mild spondylolisthesis.

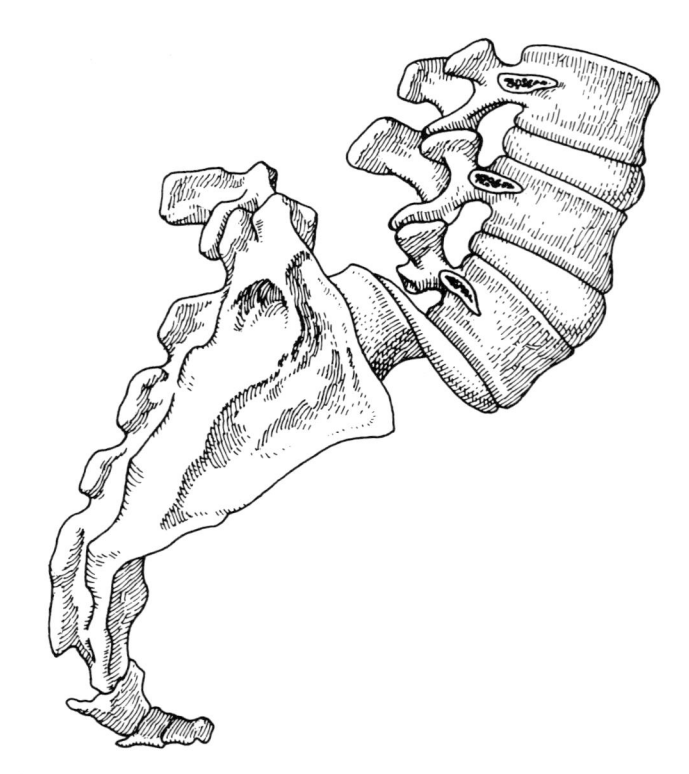

Fig. 67-2. Spondylolisthesis with forward displacement of L5 in relation to S1. Spondylolysis is also present.

zero at birth and has been reported to be approximately 4 percent in 6-year-olds and 5 to 6 percent in adults.[11] The prevalence in adults is lowest in black females (1.1 percent), high in white males (6.4 percent),[19] and, as noted, can reach 45 percent in certain Eskimo tribes because of genetic factors.[14] After the second decade, the prevalence probably remains constant in all populations.[13,20,21] Spondylolysis has been reported to occur in as high as 40 to 50 percent of patients with Scheuermann's kyphosis.[17] The reasons for this are unknown, but may relate to transient osteopenia during the pubertal growth spurt. The prevalence of isthmic spondylolisthesis is 2 to 3 percent in the general population, meaning that about one-half of patients with spondylolysis can be expected to develop a slip.[11]

TABLE 67-1. Classification of Causes of Spondylolisthesis

Type I (Dysplastic)
  Congenital dysplasia or absence of the lumbosacral facet joints without pars interarticularis defect.
Type II (Isthmic)
  A lesion of the pars interarticularis: either a stress fracture, an acute fracture, or the elongation of an intact pars interarticularis.
Type III (Degenerative)
  Long-standing degenerative changes with remodeling of the facet joints.
Type IV (Traumatic)
  Fractures of the vertebrae in areas other than the pars interarticularis.
Type V (Pathologic)
  Localized bone destruction or generalized bone disease.

CLASSIFICATION OF SPONDYLOLISTHESIS

Spondylolisthesis has been classified by Wiltse et al.[22] into five categories (Table 67-1). Type 1, the dysplastic type, is a congenital deficiency of the superior sacral and/or inferior L5 facets that allows anterior translation of L5 on S1. Type 2, the isthmic type discussed in this chapter, is caused by a fracture of the pars interarticularis from either acute or chronic stress, or from an elongation of the pars, most likely the result of repeated pars micro-

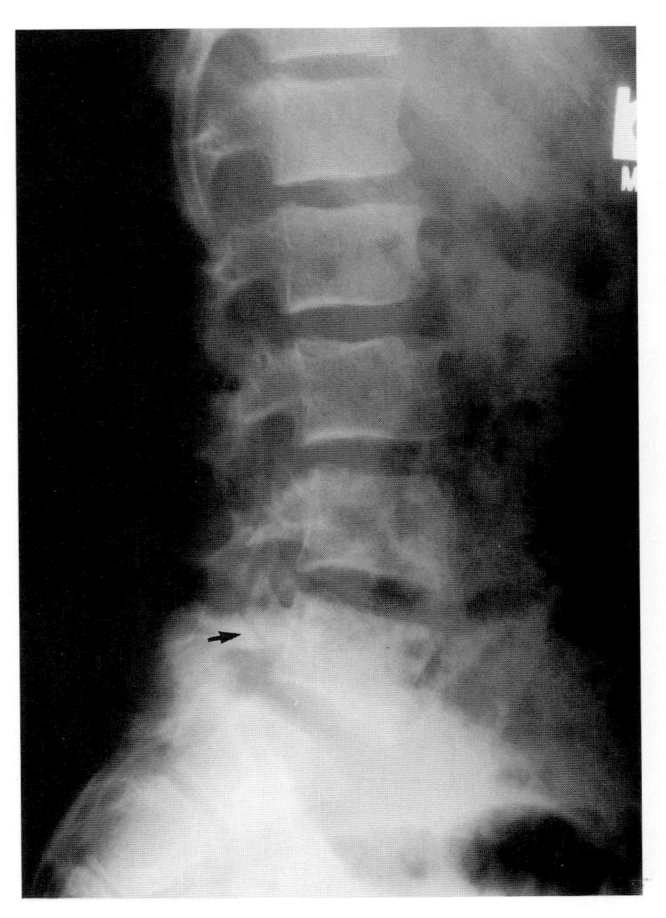

Fig. 67-3. Lateral view of the lumbar spine in a 12-year-old boy with acute low back pain following a fall on the ice. The arrow points to an oblique fracture of the L5 pars interarticularis.

fractures with healing and remodeling. The isthmic type accounts for 97 percent of spondylolisthesis in children or adolescents.[18] Type 3, the degenerative type, is the result of degenerative arthritis of facet joints and/or degenerative disc disease. Type 4, traumatic spondylolisthesis, is the result of acute fractures in other parts of the vertebra, such as facets, laminae, pedicles, or vertebral bodies. Type 5, the pathologic type, may be caused by neoplastic processes or generalized metabolic bone disease.

PATHOLOGY

Spondylolysis is really a nonunion or pseudarthrosis of a pars interarticularis fracture. The pars defect is filled with fibrocartilaginous callus,[23] which sometimes becomes attenuated or disappears when spondylolisthesis occurs.

When spondylolisthesis reaches 50 percent or more, substantial adaptive changes are seen, including erosion or rounding of the anterosuperior corner of S1 and erosion or compression of the posterior body of L5, imparting a trapezoidal shape to that vertebra (Fig. 67-4).[12] A true kyphotic relationship between L5 and S1 occurs, so that the greater the slip, the more likely it is for further slipping to occur. As L5 translates forward, the L5-S1 intervertebral disc becomes deformed, and stretching, fragmentation, and often splitting occur in multiple areas of the annulus fibrosis and nucleus pulposus. Later, the degenerated olisthetic disc seems to provide spontaneous segmental stabilization.[18] Despite these changes, the abnormal disc rarely causes nerve root compression.[24] Nerve compression can occur by stretching of the cauda equina over the posterosuperior corner of the sacrum, by S1 root compression at the lateral recess, or by L5 root compression by the fibrocartilaginous mass surrounding the pars defect.[25] Other unrelated causes of back pain, such as tumors or infections of the spine, may occur but are no more common than in the general population.

CLINICAL CHARACTERISTICS

Most people with spondylolysis or spondylolisthesis are asymptomatic. Although most cases of spondylolysis are thought to begin between ages 6 and 10 years, very few children become symptomatic before their second decade. Only 23 percent of a large series reported symptoms before age 20; and less than half of these sought medical attention.[20,26]

Historically, approximately 80 percent of patients present with pain, almost always localized to the lumbosacral region and mild to moderate in intensity.[27] Often the discomfort radiates into the buttocks and/or thighs and is exacerbated by physical activities and decreased by rest. Much less common is back pain associated with more severe unilateral or bilateral radicular pain extending to the leg or foot. The nerve root pain may be caused by foramenal stenosis at the site of the pars defect or hypertrophy of the ligamentum flavum. Although the severity of pain does not always relate to the severity of the deformity, patients with more intense pain tend to have greater degrees of slipping. The history should include known episodes of trauma, specific athletic activities, and any known occurrence of spondylolysis or spondylolisthesis in family members.

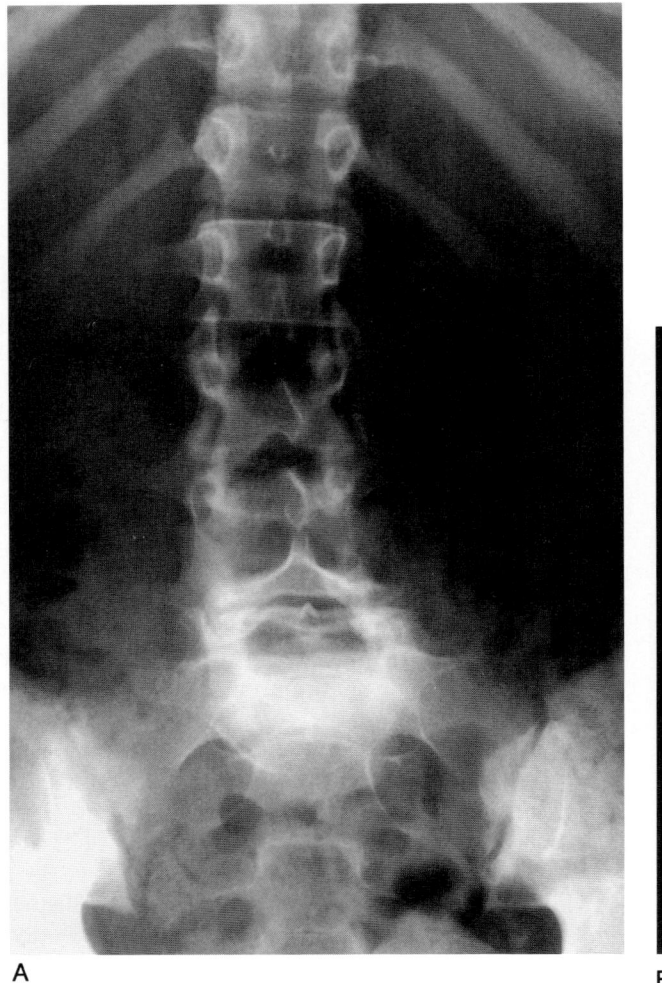

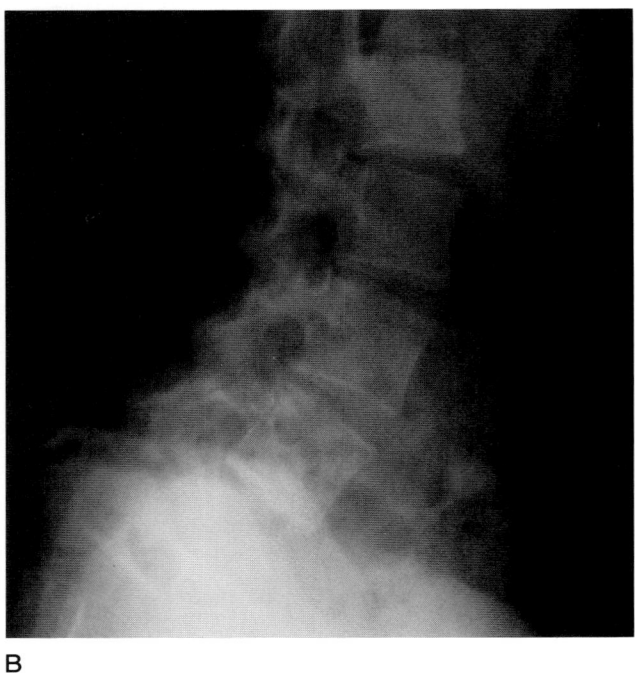

Fig. 67-4. Anteroposterior and lateral radiographs of severe spondylolisthesis. **(A)** The anteroposterior view shows foreshortening of the lumbar spine with superimposition of L4, L5, and the upper sacrum. **(B)** Lateral view of the same patient showing severe displacement of L5 on S1.

Physical examination should include assessment of gait, hamstring tightness, neurologic status, spinal contours, paraspinal muscles, and evaluation for possible scoliosis. While most patients will have a normal gait, those with more severe involvement often show a shortened stride length, posterior pelvic rotation in the sagittal plane, and decreased knee motion, resulting in a somewhat stiff-legged waddle. Hamstring tightness, also known as the Phalen-Dickson sign, occurs in approximately 80 percent of patients (Fig. 67-5).[10] Its cause is unknown. It may be a compensatory mechanism to attempt to stabilize the lumbosacral region and is probably not caused by nerve root irritation.[28] Whereas physical signs may correlate with severity of slip, patients with minimal slips usually do not have positive physical findings and, indeed, patients with severe slips may have very few detectable physical signs. In patients with spondylolisthesis of greater than 50 percent, abnormal neurologic findings may be detected in up to 35 percent.[10] Positive neurologic findings can include lower extremity weakness, hypesthesias or paresthesias, and a decrease or asymmetry in the magnitude of deep tendon reflexes. Such findings are more likely to be seen in patients with greater degrees of slippage. Neurologic evaluation should include assessment of the cauda equina, including peroneal sensation and a history of any bowel or bladder disturbances.

Patients with greater than 50 percent slips often show a posterior pelvic tilt with a more vertical sacrum when standing. A palpable step-off at L5-S1 may be detectable.

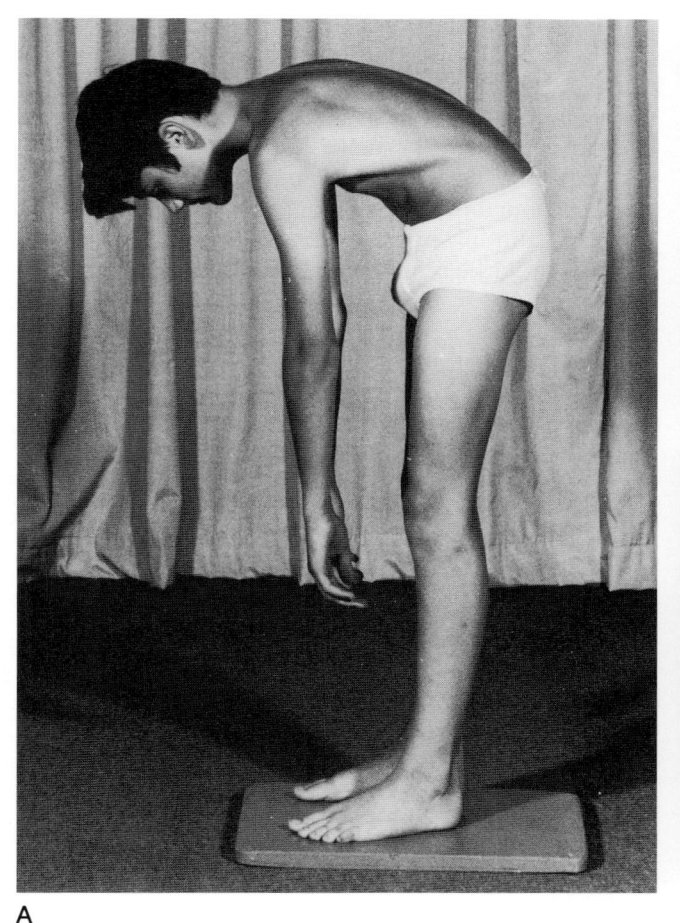

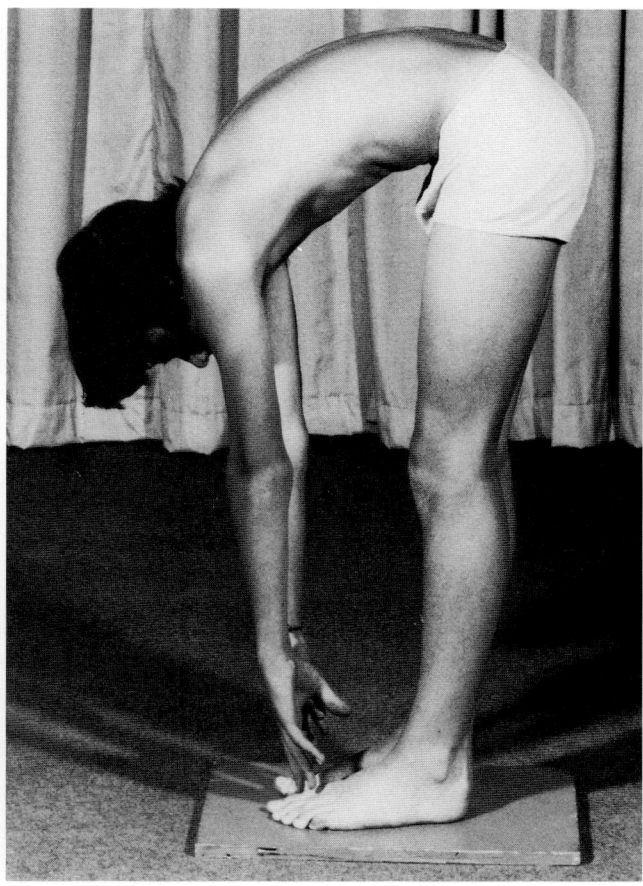

Fig. 67-5. A boy with spondylolisthesis and tight hamstrings. **(A)** Preoperatively, an attempt to touch his toes shows severe restriction of forward lumbar flexion caused by hamstring tightness. **(B)** Postoperatively, the hamstring tightness has spontaneously resolved.

With range of motion of the lumbar spine there may be dysrhythmia, guarding, and/or spasm of the paraspinal muscles.

In severe slips, the center of gravity is displaced forward, resulting in a long lordotic hyperextension of the lumbar and thoracic spine, extending to near the shoulders. This causes an apparent foreshortening of the trunk. In patients with spondyloptosis (complete dislocation of L5 which descends anterior to the body of S1), true trunk shortening occurs.

Approximately 40 percent of patients with spondylolisthesis will show some signs of at least mild scoliosis (Fig. 67-6).[29] These are often functional lumbar curves that disappear with recumbency.[27,30] Such curves can become structural and progressive. In addition, scoliosis may result from malrotation of L5 as it translates forward on S1. Scoliosis should be followed in all patients with spondylolisthesis and should be treated independently, if treatment is necessary.

RADIOGRAPHIC EVALUATION

Plain radiographs obtained in the coronal and lateral projections with the patient standing are the baseline studies required for evaluation of a child with back pain. When spondylolisthesis is present, the pars defect is usually easily visible on the lateral view so that oblique radiographs are unnecessary (Fig. 67-7). Oblique views, however, should be obtained if a pars defect is not clearly seen on the lateral view, as these lesions are best seen in the oblique projection, particularly unilateral pars defects. Approximately 20 percent of patients with spon-

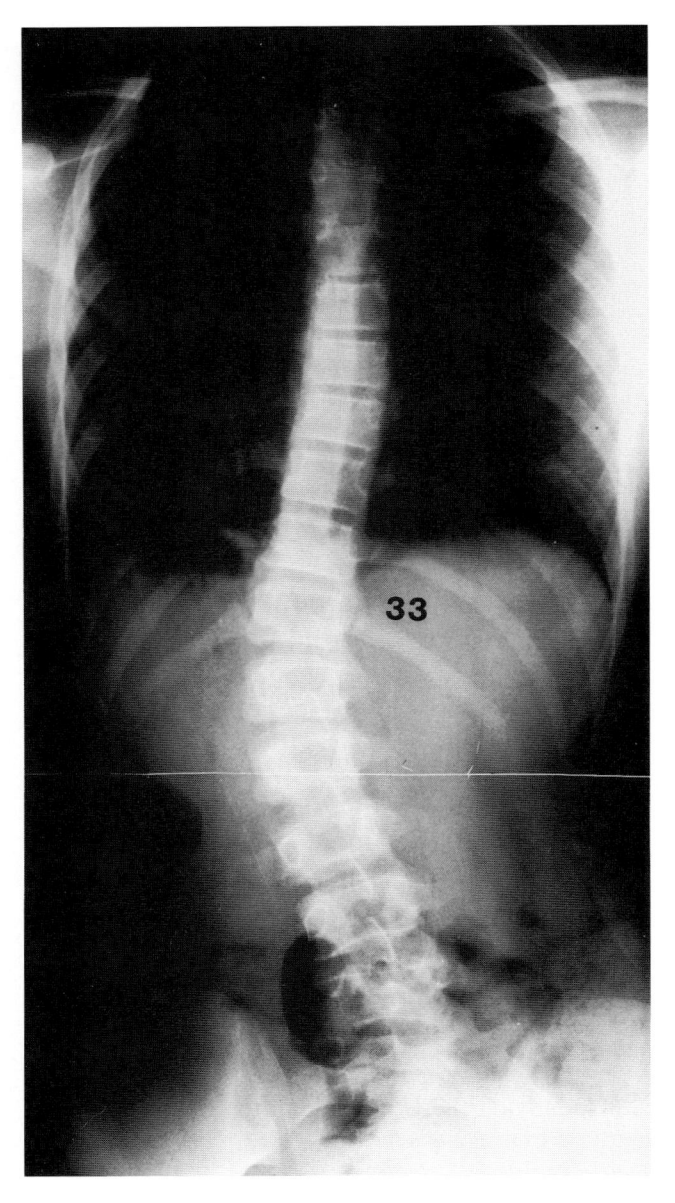

Fig. 67-6. Radiograph showing 33-degree left thoracolumbar scoliosis in a patient with an asymptomatic L5-S1 spondylolisthesis of 20 percent.

If pars defects are not seen on standard plain radiographs, including obliques, then oblique tomography, a computed tomography (CT) scan of the pars area, or a technetium bone scan should be considered. Plain radiographs or CT will usually show a small pars fracture, whereas a bone scan will show increased activity around an acute fracture or an impending fracture, which is probably multiple microfractures with attempts at healing. It should be remembered that bone scans may be negative in established (greater than 6 to 12 weeks) pars defects.

Lateral radiographs are the most useful views for following lesions of the pars to detect slipping or progression of established slips. Such films should always be taken in the standing position to prevent recumbency from allowing varying degrees of spontaneous reduction.[34] Lateral plain films in supine hyperextension and traction can be valuable in determining whether postoperative closed reduction of a slip can be successful.

Myelography has very little value in spondylolisthesis. With slips of less than 50 percent, a narrowing of the dural sac is noted at the level of the step-off. Once a slip exceeds 50 percent, the sac is usually completely blocked.[35] The primary indication for a myelogram in a patient with spondylolisthesis is to rule out other unusual causes of back pain, such as tumors or herniated discs occurring in the area cephalad to the slip. Such unusual lesions should be suspected when pain is disproportionate to the magnitude of the slip or when there are unusual neurologic findings such as unilateral radicular pain, weakness, atrophy, depressed reflexes, or cauda equina deficiency. Disc herniations occur in 0 to 6 percent.[36] Magnetic resonance imaging (MRI) is now probably more valuable than myelography in detecting associated pathologic lesions, especially disc herniation, and in assessing the spinal cord and lower lumbar nerve roots.

CT is effective for visualizing the L5 and S1 nerve roots when radicular symptoms are present, in determining the degree of spinal stenosis, particularly on the sagittally reconstructed views, and in demonstrating subtle pars fractures.[37]

dylolysis have unilateral defects.[21,31,32] The suspicion of a unilateral defect is further heightened by noting hypertrophy and/or sclerosis of the opposite pars area or pedicle as a response to increased stress opposite the defect.[33] Other findings occasionally associated with unilateral spondylolysis are lateral wedging of the vertebral body in the coronal plane and asymmetry of the posterior vertebral arch.

QUANTIFYING SPONDYLOLISTHESIS

Amount of Slipping

The amount of forward displacement is traditionally determined by assessing the amount of anterior translation of the posterior surface of L5 in relation to the top of

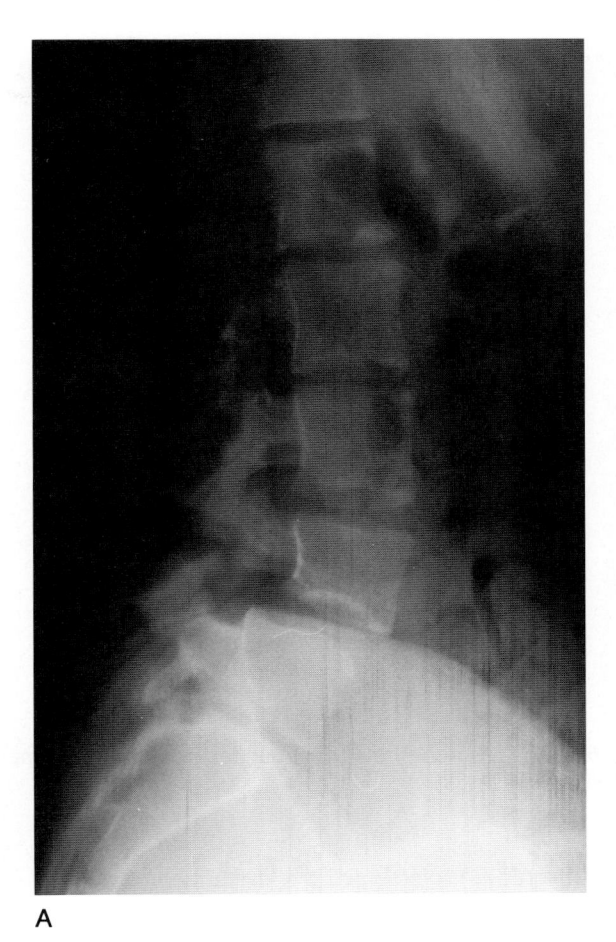

Fig. 67-7. The radiographic appearance of spondylolysis. **(A)** Lateral view showing spondylolysis at L4 with spondylolisthesis of L4 on L5. **(B)** Oblique view of the same patient. Arrows indicate the defect in the pars interarticularis. **(C)** The patient was treated with a posterior bilateral transverse process fusion from L4 to S1. The solid fusion mass has obliterated the pars defect.

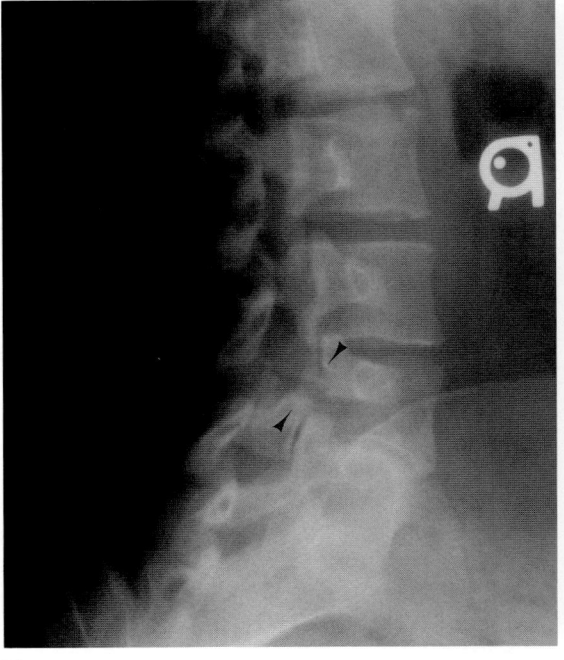

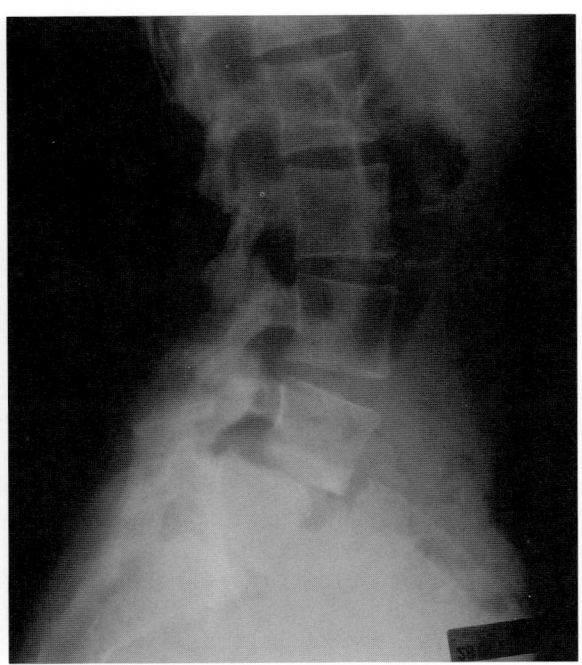

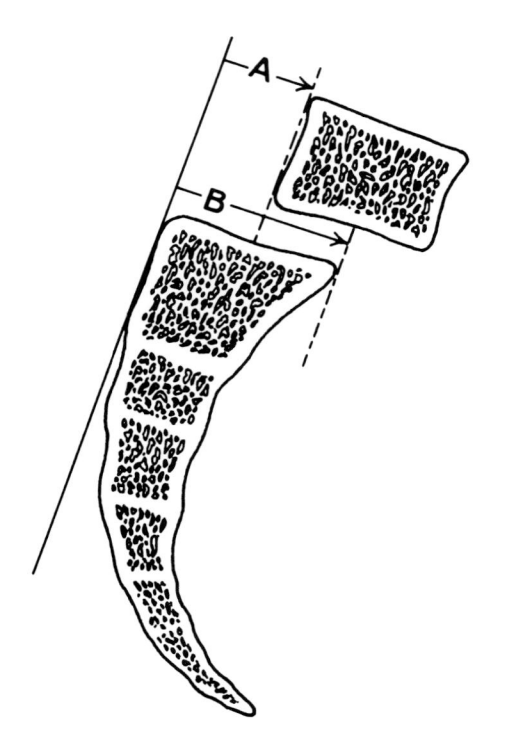

Fig. 67-8. The appropriate technique for measuring percent slippage (A/B × 100).

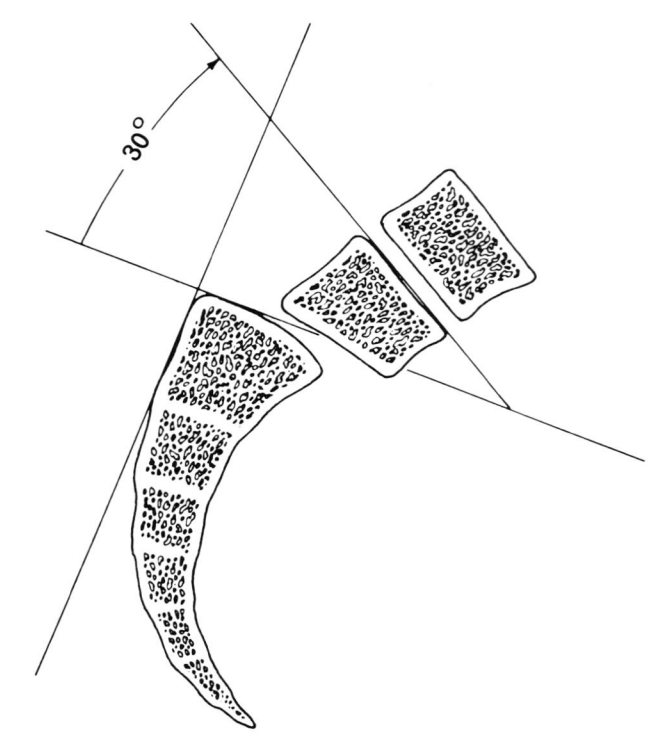

Fig. 67-9. Technique for measurement of the slip angle. In this case, the cephalad end plate of L5 was most appropriate.

S1. Meyerding[38] developed a classification system by dividing the top of S1 into four quadrants. In this classification, a grade 1 slip is less than 25 percent; grade 2, 25 to 50 percent; grade 3, 50 to 75 percent; grade 4, 75 to 100 percent; and grade 5, complete spondyloptosis. More recently, Taillard[39] described the amount of slipping as the percentage of the superior surface of S1 that remains uncovered, measured from its posterior edge to the tangent to the posterior surface of L5 as related to the entire superior surface of S1. When there is erosion of the anterosuperior corner of S1, the widest diameter of S1 on the lateral view is used (Fig. 67-8).

Angular Deformity

The angular deformity, known as the slip angle, is a measure of lumbosacral kyphosis. This is determined by measuring, on a standing lateral radiograph, the angle formed by the perpendicular to a line drawn along the posterior cortex of the body of S1 and a second line parallel to an end plate of L5 or L4 (Fig. 67-9). While there is not universal agreement regarding which end plate should be used, the cephalad end plate of L5 or L4 is probably more accurate, particularly if there is erosion of the caudal end plate of L5.[40] In the normal spine, there is no forward translation of L5 on S1 and the slip angle is zero degrees or less.

Sacral Inclination

The sacral inclination is determined by measuring the angle formed by the posterior surface of the first sacral vertebra and a vertical line perpendicular to the floor (Fig. 67-10). This should always be done on a standing radiograph. Normal sacral inclination is usually greater than 30 degrees.

NATURAL HISTORY

Although the prevalence of spondylolysis in the general population is approximately 5 to 6 percent, with spondylolisthesis occurring in 2 to 3 percent, most people with these lesions are either completely unaware of their situation or never become symptomatic enough to visit a physician.[11] Some risk factors for the development

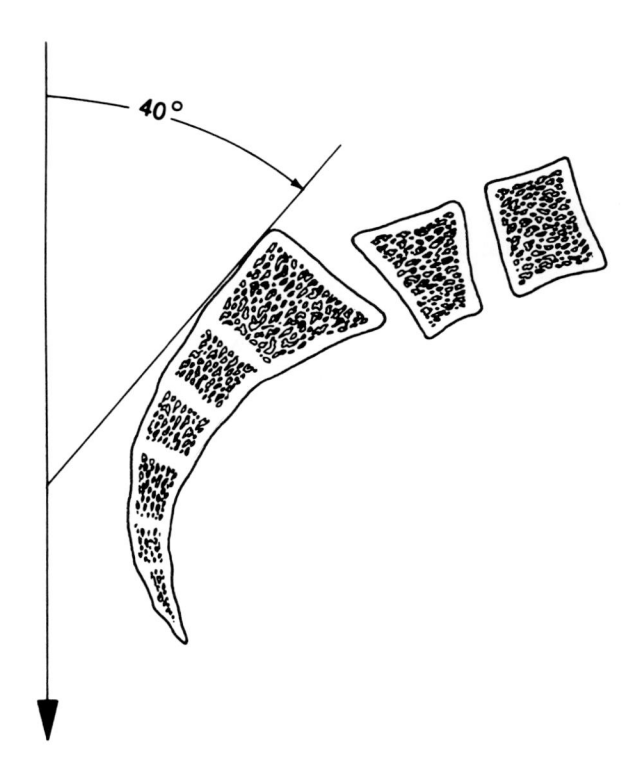

Fig. 67-10. Technique for measuring sacral inclination.

of pain or further slipping of spondylolisthesis are as follows (Table 67-2):

1. The greater the slippage, particularly with slips of 50 percent or more, the greater the risk for further progression.[12,18,41]
2. The greater the slip angle, especially when it exceeds 30 degrees, the greater the risk of pain and/or further slip[10]
3. Patients under 15 years of age and those undergoing the preadolescent growth spurt are at higher risk[12,21]

TABLE 67-2. Risk Factors for a Poor Prognosis in Spondylolisthesis

1. Greater degree of slipping (50% or more)
2. A larger slip angle (>30 degrees)
3. Younger age (<15 years of age)
4. Females have a worse prognosis than males
5. Dysplastic spondylolisthesis is more likely to cause continuing pain than isthmic spondylolisthesis
6. Greater anterior sagittal plane imbalance necessitating more compensatory hyperlordosis cephalad to the spondylolisthesis
7. Long established pain or neurologic deficit

4. Females, particularly children, have a worse prognosis than males. Girls are more likely than boys to have earlier onset of spondylolisthesis, more severe symptoms, and a more severe slip[10,18,42]
5. Patients with spondylolisthesis with dysplastic lumbosacral facets are more likely to have continued pain[12,27,42]
6. Patients with greater anterior sagittal plane imbalance necessitating more compensatory hyperlordosis above the slip are more likely to be symptomatic.[12,21,43]
7. Patients with established pain or neurologic deficit are less likely to respond to nonsurgical treatment.[44]

TREATMENT

Treatment of spondylolysis and spondylolisthesis must be individualized and may range from no follow-up to complex reconstructive surgery.

No Follow-up

A skeletally mature individual with asymptomatic pars defects, with or without a slip of less than 50 percent, is best advised to seek medical attention only if symptoms arise or a deformity is noted. In this situation, the risk of a slip developing or progressing is extremely small.

Serial Observation

Skeletally immature patients with asymptomatic pars defects and/or slips of less than 50 percent are well advised to have annual evaluation, including a standing lateral radiograph of the lumbosacral region. It may be appropriate to see the patient every 6 to 9 months from age 10 through 15 years, when the risk for further slipping is greatest and the growth spurt is occurring.[41,45] Restriction of activities in this group is probably unnecessary.

Nonoperative Treatment

Patients with symptomatic spondylolysis and spondylolisthesis of less than 50 percent are appropriate for a nonoperative program including restriction of activities, even to the point of temporary bed rest if necessary while symptomatic, and/or the use of a body cast or an orthosis. If the symptoms have been present for less than 3 months, if a technetium bone scan shows increased uptake at the site of the defect, and if there is no or little slip, then the defect has a reasonable chance of healing with cast or orthotic immobilization.[9] Incorporation of one thigh in the immobilization device is probably not necessary. Lesions that meet these criteria but are of longer duration are unlikely to heal with immobilization. A nonoperative program of restricted activities and flexion (not extension) exercises,[46] and, if these fail, a trial of casting or orthotic management are indicated. If nonoperative treatment has not been successful within 6 months, further persistence is probably futile. Approximately 60 percent of appropriately selected symptomatic patients will respond to nonoperative treatment with resolution of their symptoms.[26,46]

Surgical Treatment

The indications for surgery include patients with mild slips but intractable pain and failure of nonoperative treatment; any slip of greater than 50 percent, because the risk of further slipping is high; documented progression of slipping; a high slip angle (greater than 45 degrees) with substantial postural deformity or gait abnormality; and patients with any amount of slip and objective neurologic deficit.

Repair of the Lytic Defect

Repair of the defect is intuitively attractive and has been successful for patients with symptomatic pars defects, but no slipping, at the levels of L4 or above. At L5, the low morbidity of a one-level fusion of the transverse processes of L5 to the sacral ala and the high success rate of such a procedure make this the treatment of choice, rather than attempting to repair the defect.

A commonly used repair technique for pars lesions at L4 or above includes bilateral tension-band wiring across the pars defect from the transverse process to the spinous process and bridging the defect with autogenous iliac bone graft. Bradford[47] reported on 22 patients treated with the Scott wiring technique, and in his series, all patients less than 18 years of age had satisfactory healing of their defects. Screw fixation across the pars, described by Buck,[48,49] is technically more difficult. A newer technique involves compression arthrodesis with Cotrel-Dubousset rods and bilateral pedicle screws and offset laminar hooks.[41]

One-Level L5-S1 Fusion

One-level L5-S1 fusion is indicated for patients with symptomatic L5 pars defects that have not responded to nonoperative treatment or in patients with the symptomatic L5-S1 slip of less than 50 percent. The technique is a posterior lateral fusion of the transverse processes of L5 to the sacrum. Most surgeons use a single vertical midline incision through the skin and subcutaneous fat but make separate lateral incisions through the paraspinal muscle fascia with muscle splitting down to the transverse processes and sacral alae.[22] The transverse processes are decorticated, and a window and small tunnel are created in the top of the sacral alae. A cortical or cancellous graft can then be inserted into the sacrum through the window and positioned either anterior or posterior to the L5 transverse process. Abundant strips of iliac bone are then added to augment the fusion mass, which should extend to the tips of the transverse processes; bone should be laid over the facet joints after removing their capsules. Removal of the facet joints themselves is probably not necessary. Postoperatively, most surgeons would immobilize a child or adolescent in an ambulatory lumbosacral cast or orthosis for 3 to 6 months, after which radiographic evidence of solid union and a clinical report of absence of pain should be noted. Mild gait abnormalities, hamstring tightness, and radicular symptoms without objective neurologic deficit can be expected to resolve with a solid lumbosacral arthrodesis.[43,50-52]

Two-Level L4-S1 Fusion

Two-level L4-S1 fusion is indicated for any slip of greater than 50 percent, painful or not, because pain, further slipping, or neurologic problems are likely.[21,27] In slips of this magnitude, it is technically not possible to expose adequately only the L5 transverse processes, because of their more severe anterior translation. The transverse processes of L4 must also be exposed to get to the L5 transverse processes. L4 to S1 fusions are also indicated with slip angles of greater than 30 degrees and in cases in which compensatory retrolisthesis at L4-L5 is noted. The technique is similar to that described for the L5-S1 fusion, except that bone grafting extends to the transverse processes and facet joints of L4. Postoperatively, most patients are treated for 3 to 6 months with an ambulatory orthosis or a cast, which often includes one hip and thigh. Most surgery for spondylolisthesis should be one- or two-level in situ fusions, and good results may be expected in more than 80 percent of cases (Fig. 67-11).[43,52-54]

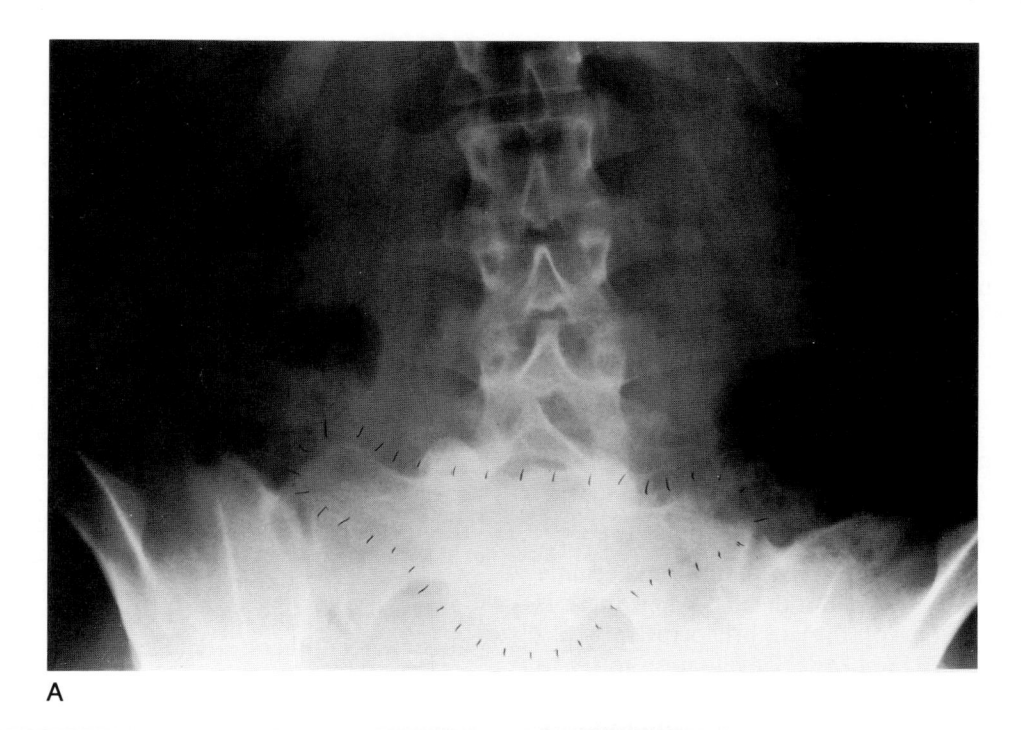

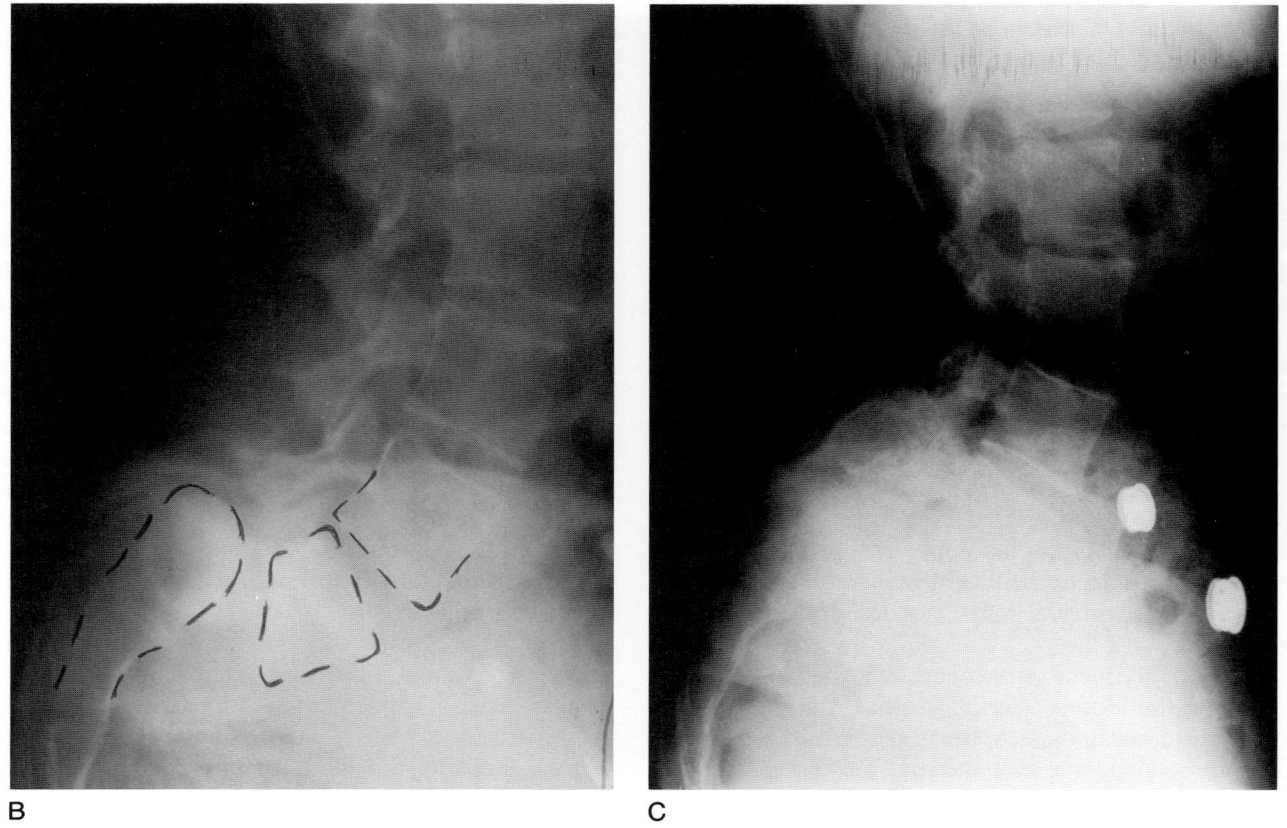

Fig. 67-11. Severe spondylolisthesis. **(A)** Anteroposterior view of a 100-percent slip in a patient with isthmic spondylolisthesis. The so-called inverted Napoleon's hat outline of the 5th lumbar vertebra rotated into the transverse plane is seen. **(B)** Lateral view of the same patient showing the complete spondylolisthesis. **(C)** Postoperative lateral view showing solid arthrodesis from L4 to the pelvis.

Anterior Fusion In Situ

In the past, anterior fusion in situ has been used, particularly in Europe, with mixed results.[55] This approach is technically more difficult than posterolateral transverse process in situ arthrodesis and carries with it the risk of damage to major vascular structures or the presacral sympathetic nerve plexus. It also has a higher pseudarthrosis rate. The majority of surgeons now prefer combining anterior fusion with posterior stabilization and fusion.

Decompression and Fusion

Decompression is appropriate for patients with objective neurologic deficit, including weakness, atrophy, reflex changes, documented hypesthesia, and cauda equina symptoms.[56] It is also indicated when there is severe radicular pain. Appropriate preoperative workup would include MRI and/or CT evaluation to try to identify precisely the neuropathologic lesion. Decompression is not indicated simply for symptoms of sciatica or tight hamstrings, as these resolve following solid in situ fusions. When decompression is indicated a midline approach is best, with removal of the posterior lamina and the bone and fibrocartilage from the pars defect, the attachment of the pars to the pedicle, and exploration of the nerve root. Occasionally, removal of more of the pedicle, the transverse process, and the intervertebral disc will be necessary. The nerve root should be totally decompressed. Then an autogenous fat graft is placed about the nerve root, and a posterolateral transverse process spinal fusion from L4 to the sacrum is always performed. Following decompression the spine is less stable and immobilization (either by means of internal fixation, such as plates or rods and pedicle screws, or in a body cast, including one thigh), is necessary. As long as further slipping does not occur, ambulation may be started as soon as tolerated. Should further slipping be apparent, then the patient should remain recumbent with a bilateral pantaloon hip spica cast with the hips extended until the fusion is solid.

Attempts to decompress neurologic signs by simply removing the loose posterior laminae, the Gill procedure,[57] are contraindicated, because this is inadequate to decompress the nerve root and may only serve to make the spondylolisthesis more unstable.[51,58] Adequate decompression must always be accompanied by spinal fusion.[55,59]

Reduction of the Slip and Fusion

The principles involved in reduction include correcting the lumbosacral kyphosis and decreasing the anterior translation of L5 on S1 to balance the spine in the sagittal plane. This can be accomplished by closed or open methods.

CLOSED REDUCTION

Closed reduction has gained popularity because of its safety. The method most commonly used was described by Scaglietti et al.[60] The patient is placed supine on a fracture table, distraction is applied to the pelvis with the hips hyperextended, and a body cast, including both thighs, is applied. After this casting technique, Scaglietti et al.[60] performed an in situ fusion in the cast. Currently, most surgeons prefer to do the in situ fusion and then, a few days later, apply the corrective cast and maintain the patient in recumbency for at least 3 months, followed by ambulation in a unilateral pantaloon spica for another 1 to 3 months. This technique is particularly valuable for lesions that demonstrate reasonable correctability on maximum flexion and extension preoperative radiographs (Fig. 67-12).

OPERATIVE REDUCTION

Lesions that are more severe and/or less flexible, including complete spondyloptosis, may be considered for operative reduction and stabilization. These are usually slips of greater than 75 percent with slip angles of greater than 45 degrees. A particular indication for operative reduction is for the patient who has substantial forward translation of the upper body's center of gravity such that a long, severe, compensatory lordosis is present above the lesion. If decompression of nerve roots is necessary, reduction may also be considered because further slipping could result in recurrent nerve root compression. Some physicians now believe reduction is indicated in all slips of greater than 50 percent to attempt to decrease the pseudarthrosis rate.[54]

Most of the current reduction techniques employ pedicle screw fixation of the lumbosacral spine to posterior plates or rods to gain and maintain reduction. The theoretical advantages of reduction are the restored sagittal plane balance of the spine, an improved cosmetic appearance for the patient, a decreased likelihood of further slipping, and a decrease in the pseudarthrosis rate. At present, multiple studies with long-term experience

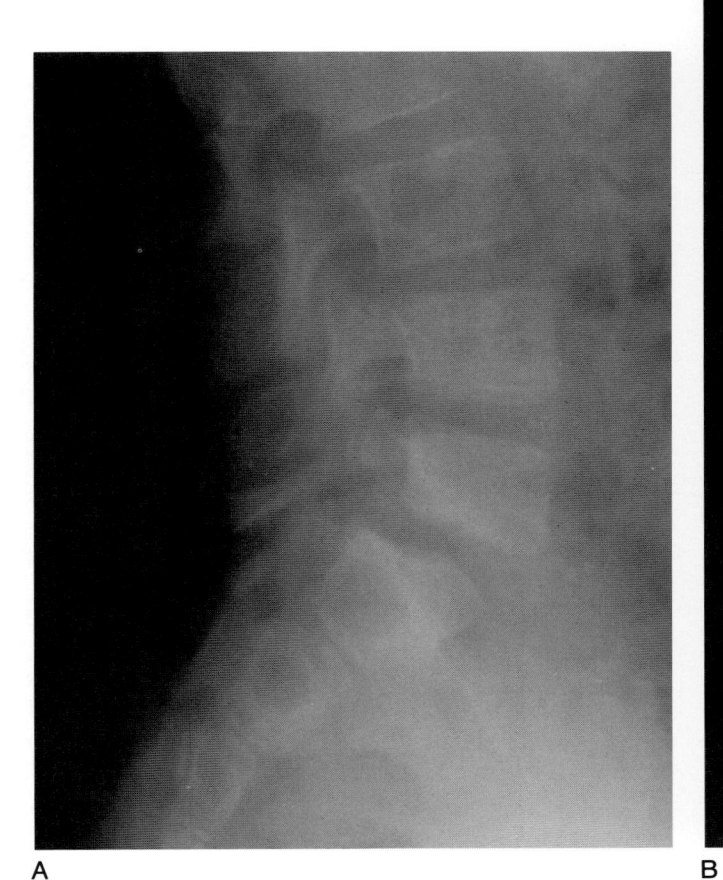

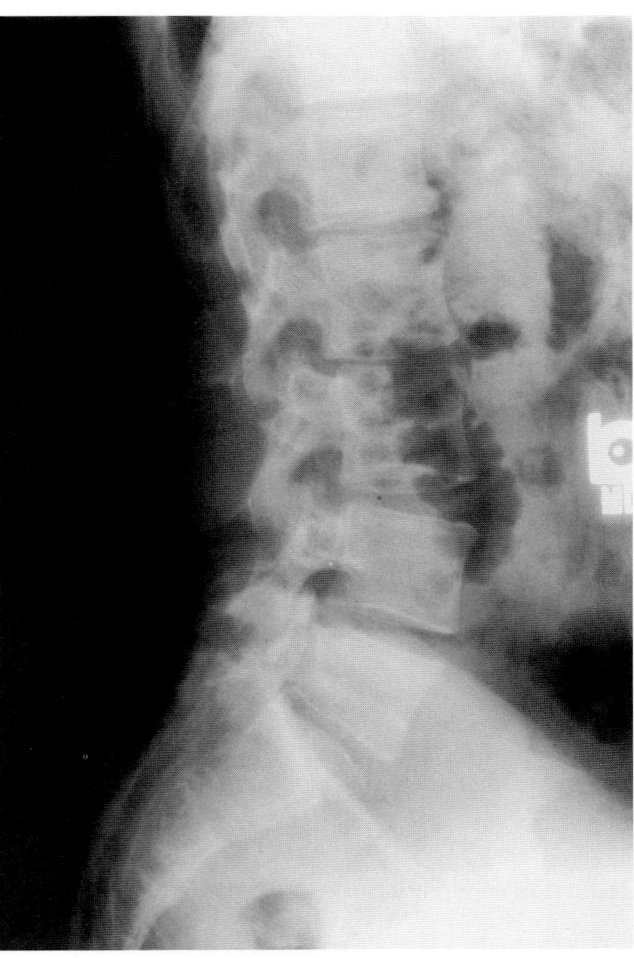

Fig. 67-12. Surgical treatment of spondylolisthesis of L5 on S1. **(A)** Lateral view of a 14-year-old boy with refractory low back pain and a grade I, L5 on S1 spondylolisthesis. **(B)** Lateral view following posterior bilateral transverse process in situ fusion from L5 to S1 with postoperative reduction cast treatment using the Scaglietti method.

with operative reduction and internal fixation are lacking. The indications, risks, and benefits of this technically demanding treatment program have yet to be firmly defined. The disadvantages of operative reduction of spondylolisthesis are the morbidity of the extensive surgical procedure required and the risk of neurologic damage, particularly L5 nerve root injury or cauda equina injury, which may be temporary or permanent. With anterior surgery, injury to the presacral nerve plexus may lead to retrograde ejaculation in males and the potential exists for life-threatening major vascular complications.[61,62]

REDUCTION WITHOUT INTERNAL FIXATION

In children with severe slips and little flexibility, correction can be obtained by performing posterior decompression of the L5 nerve roots and an L4 to S1 transverse process fusion and by placing the patient in straight halo-femoral traction. Traction is carried out for 1 or 2 weeks to increase the correctability of the kyphotic lesion, and then an anterior fusion with strong tricortical iliac or fibular bone strut grafting is performed, followed by treatment by a single pantaloon hip extension spica cast in recumbency for 4 months. This is followed by ambulation in a single leg spica cast for an additional 2 to 6 months. This technique can be safely monitored during the correction process of traction and does not require the use of large metallic implants in small children.[63]

REDUCTION WITH INTERNAL FIXATION

In adolescents and adults, a commonly used technique for the reduction of severe lumbosacral spondylolisthesis consists of posterior decompression of the L5 nerve roots and a single-stage posterior fusion from L4 to the sacrum using pedicle screws to gain purchase on the vertebral bodies and rods or plates to maintain the reduction. After insertion of the screws and other fixation, slow constant leverage is maintained, often for several hours, to gain the soft-tissue creep and relaxation necessary to correct the kyphosis and gain the posterior translation of L5.[54] Following completion of the reduction, plates or rods are applied and an abundant posterior lateral fusion mass is created with autogenous iliac graft. It is wise to then augment the fixation with a postoperative pantaloon cast and allow the patient to be ambulatory. Cast immobilization is maintained until the fusion is radiographically solid, usually in 3 to 6 months. Some surgeons augment this technique with an anterior fusion.[41,64]

Reduction of Severe Slips and Spondyloptosis

When the slip is nearly complete or spondyloptosis has occurred and the kyphotic deformity is rigid with a slip angle of greater than 45 degrees, particularly in patients who are skeletally mature or nearly so, a combined anterior and posterior approach may be necessary to accomplish reduction. There are many different techniques for accomplishing combined anterior and posterior reduction and fusion. These include

1. Preliminary halo-femoral traction for reduction, and if this is achieved, an anterior L5-S1 diskectomy and fusion using tricortical iliac crest bone blocks, followed by posterior bilateral transverse process fusion
2. Preliminary posterior distraction and posterior translation with internal fixation and transverse process fusion, followed by second-stage anterior diskectomy and fusion
3. Posterior bilateral transverse process fusion done concomitantly with a posterior approach to an anterior interbody fusion at L5-S1
4. Preliminary anterior vertebrectomy of L5 (in complete spondyloptosis) with excision of the L4-L5 and L5-S1 disks. This is followed, usually 1 to 2 weeks later, by a second-stage posterior fusion, reducing the body of L4 over the sacrum and performing posterolateral arthrodesis with internal fixation. The patient is usually kept in recumbency until the fusion is solid.[65,66]

All of these techniques carry the risk of cauda equina or nerve root damage, pseudarthrosis, loss of correction, severe blood loss, and disruption of the presacral nerve plexus. Technically, it is extremely difficult to perform an anterior strut graft fusion unless the slip has been reduced to 25 percent or less.

At present one cannot recommend one means of reducing severe spondylolisthesis over another. Longer follow-up with series containing more patients treated by single techniques is necessary before the benefits and risks of each method can be clearly defined. It may be, however, that for spondyloptosis, anterior resection of L5 and posterior reduction of L4 on the sacrum has a lesser risk of cauda equina injury than attempts at distraction to pull the body of L5 up out of the pelvis. It is important to re-emphasize that the goal in spondylolisthesis surgery is to obtain and maintain sagittal plane balance, reducing the lumbosacral kyphosis or slip angle, and balancing the spine. Complete reduction of a slip is not necessary. Again, currently the vast majority of spondylolisthesis surgery should be one- or two-level in situ posterior lateral arthrodeses.

Pitfalls and Complications

Problems with the surgical treatment of spondylolisthesis include the development of a pseudarthrosis, progression of slipping despite a solid fusion, and the risk of neurologic injury. The risk of pseudarthrosis is low in slips of less than 50 percent treated by uncomplicated posterior lateral transverse process fusions with autogenous bone grafting. The pseudarthrosis rate increases as the magnitude of the slip increases beyond 50 percent. The likelihood of successful fusion probably can be enhanced in severe slips by reduction of the slip and either the use of internal fixation or the accomplishment of an anterior interbody fusion in addition to the posterolateral fusion. When pseudarthroses occur in severe slips treated by posterolateral fusion only, strong consideration should be given to an anterior interbody fusion in addition to repairing the posterior pseudarthrosis.[67]

Since the forces producing the slip and the lumbosacral kyphosis do continue to act on the spine despite solid arthrodesis, progression of deformity via remodelling and plastic deformation of the fusion mass can and

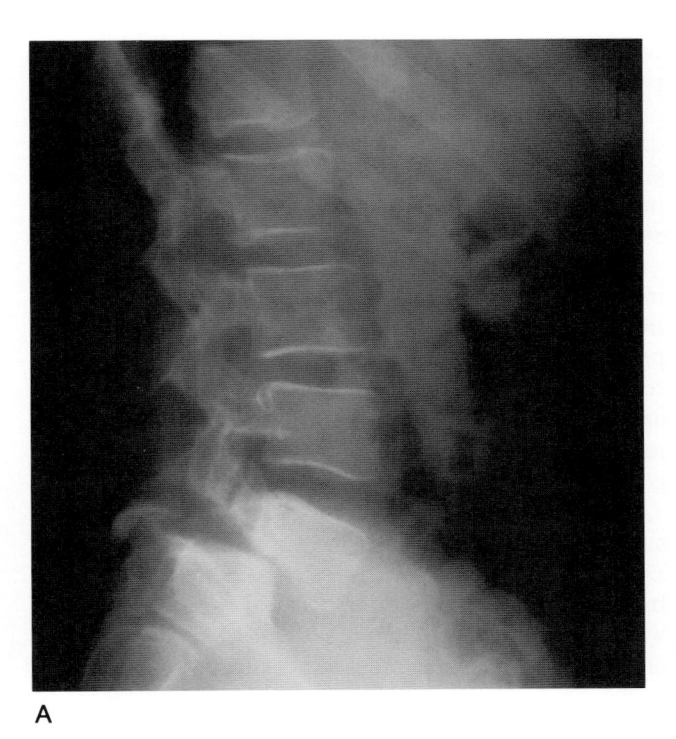

Fig. 67-13. Further slipping despite a solid fusion. **(A)** Preoperative radiograph of an L5-S1 spondylolisthesis of approximately 50 percent. Note the slight retrolisthesis of L4 on L5. **(B)** Postoperative anteroposterior view showing a solid fusion from L4 to S1. **(C)** Postoperative lateral view demonstrating further progression of the slip to 80 percent, despite the solid fusion. The progression occurred during the first postoperative year. Since then, no further slipping has occurred.

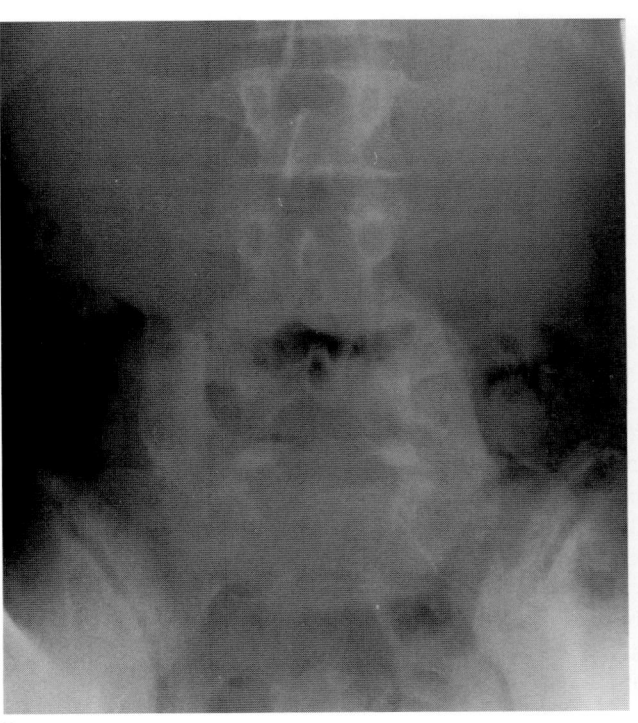

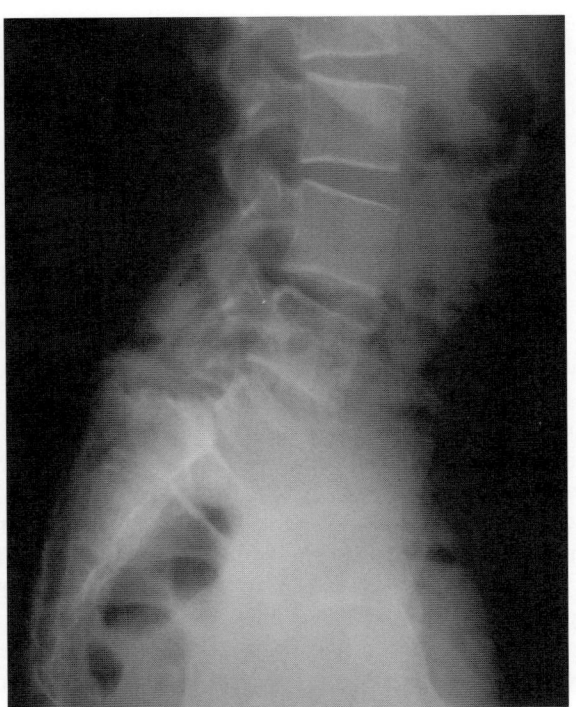

sometimes does occur (Fig. 67-13). Edwards[54] cites an average risk of further slip progression of 33 percent and of increased lumbosacral kyphosis of 15 to 20 percent in patients with apparent solid fusions. In Seitsalo's report,[18] the risk of further slipping was about 23 percent, but on average it did not exceed another 10 percent displacement. The risks are greater with deformities of greater magnitude, and it may be that reduction with internal fixation will eventually become standard treatment for such slips.

Neurologic injury related to spondylolisthesis surgery may be caused by either unavoidable or injudiciously traumatic (1) traction on a nerve root during decompression, (2) neuropraxia or edema of nerve roots during reduction of a severe slip,[62,68] (3) cauda equina syndrome associated with in situ fusion of severe slips,[69] and (4) injury to the presacral nerve plexus during anterior surgery.[61]

Postoperative cauda equina syndrome following in situ fusion can often be ruled out in the recovery room. Detection of this neurologic lesion is best accomplished by testing perineal or saddle sensation, as many patients will have a catheter in their bladder. The suspected cause is neuropraxia and edema resulting from the stretching of the cauda equina over the posterosuperior corner of the sacrum. When this is detected, the patient should be returned to the operating room and, via a posterior approach with retraction of the dura, a sacroplasty should be performed to remove the posterosuperior bony corner of S1 to allow anterior decompression of the cauda equina.

SUMMARY AND CONCLUSIONS

Spondylolysis, an acquired defect of the pars interarticularis in a lower lumbar vertebra, is caused by repeated mechanical stress on that structurally inadequate area of the posterior bony arch. Hereditary factors and certain specific physical activities play a role in increasing the risk of developing this lesion. Spondylolysis occurs in approximately 5 to 6 percent of the population, and 80 percent of these people remain asymptomatic.

Spondylolysis is one of many lesions that can lead to spondylolisthesis, often with subsequent spinal deformity and pain. Spondylolisthesis occurs most frequently between the ages of 6 and 15 years and the risk for continued progression is greatest during that period. The diagnosis is confirmed radiographically, most often after a history of low back and sometimes buttock and thigh pain and the physical findings of tight hamstrings, paraspinal muscle guarding, and occasionally an alteration in gait. A palpable lumbosacral step-off and a compensatory, long, thoracolumbar lordosis are seen with more severe grades of slipping.

The treatment for acutely fractured spondylolysis consists of immobilization, in an attempt to heal the lesion. When a symptomatic pars defect is of long standing, but slipping has not occurred, conservative treatment by restriction of activities, flexion exercises, or occasionally an orthosis or cast is often successful. Surgery may be necessary for individuals with intractable pain, progressive slipping, positive signs of neurologic deficit, a large slip angle, substantial postural deformity or gait disturbance, or for a skeletally immature individual with spondylolisthesis greater than 50 percent. The majority of surgically treated patients do best with a posterior lateral transverse process fusion. Reducing severe spondylolisthesis is sometimes indicated but may increase the risk of neurologic damage and other problems. The goal of surgery is to produce a solid arthrodesis at the lumbosacral junction with a balanced spine in the sagittal plane and the absence of neurologic injury. When this is accomplished, signs and symptoms are alleviated in the great majority of patients.

REFERENCES

1. Borkow SE, Kleiger B: Spondylolisthesis in newborn. A case report. Clin Orthop 81:73, 1971
2. Rosenberg NJ, Bargar WL, Friedman B: The incidence of spondylolysis and spondylolisthesis in nonambulatory patients. Spine 6:35, 1981
3. Newman PH: A clinical syndrome associated with severe lumbosacral subluxation. J Bone Joint Surg [Br] 47:472, 1965
4. Cyron BM, Hutton WC, Troup JDG: Spondylolytic fractures. J Bone Joint Surg [Br] 58:462, 1976
5. Farfan HF, Osteria V, Lamy C: The mechanical etiology of spondylolysis and spondylolisthesis. Clin Orthop 117:40, 1976
6. Lafferty JF, Winter WG, Gambaro SA: Fatigue characteristics of posterior elements of vertebrae. J Bone Joint Surg [Am] 59:154, 1977
7. Bradford DS: Treatment of severe spondylolisthesis: A combined approach for reduction and stabilization. Spine 4:423, 1979
8. Ferguson RJ: Low-back pain in college football lineman. J Bone Joint Surg [Am] 56:1300, 1974
9. Jackson DW, Wiltse LL, Cirincione RJ: Spondylolysis in the female gymnast. Clin Orthop 117:68, 1976
10. Boxall D, Bradford DS, Winter RB, Moe AJH: Management of severe spondylolisthesis in children and adolescents. J Bone Joint Surg [Am] 61:479, 1979

11. Fredrickson BE, Baker D, McHolick WJ et al: The natural history of spondylolysis and spondylolisthesis. J Bone Joint Surg [Am] 66:699, 1984
12. Blackburne JS, Velikas E: Spondylolisthesis in children and adolescents. J Bone Joint Surg [Br] 59:490, 1977
13. Baker DR, McHollick W: Spondyloschisis and spondylolisthesis in children. J Bone Joint Surg [Am] 38:933, 1956
14. Tower SS, Pratt WB: Spondylolysis and associated spondylolisthesis in Eskimo and Athabascan populations. Clin Orthop 250:171, 1990
15. Wynne-Davies R, Scott JHS: Inheritance and spondylolisthesis. A radiographic family survey. J Bone Joint Surg [Br] 61:301, 1979
16. Krause H: Effect of lordosis on the stress in the lumbar spine. Clin Orthop 117:56, 1976
17. Neithard FB: Scheuermann's disease and spondylolysis. Orthop Trans 7:103, 1983
18. Seitsalo S: Spondylolisthesis in children and adolescents. A long-term clinical and radiographic study. Acta Orthop Scand 62 (suppl 246):80, 1991
19. Rowe GG, Roche MB: The etiology of separate neural arch. J Bone Joint Surg [Am] 35:102, 1953
20. Lafond G: Surgical treatment of spondylolisthesis. Clin Orthop 22:175, 1962
21. Laurent LE, Osterman K: Spondylolisthesis in children and adolescents: a study of 173 cases. Acta Orthop Belg 35:717, 1969
22. Wiltse LL, Newman PH, MacNab I: Classification of spondylolysis and sponydylolisthesis. Clin Orthop 117:23, 1976
23. McAfee PC, Yuan HA: Computer tomography in spondylolisthesis. Clin Orthop 166:62, 1982
24. Birch JG, Herring JA, Maravilla K: Splitting of the intervertebral disc in spondylolisthesis: a magnetic resonance imaging finding in two cases. J Pediatr Orthop 6:609, 1986
25. Shook JE: Spondylolysis and spondylolisthesis. Spinal disorders in the child and adolescent. In Hsu JD (ed): Spinal Disorders in the Child and Adolescent. Hanely & Belfus, Philadelphia, 1990
26. Pizzutillo PD, Hummer III CD: Nonoperative treatment for painful adolescent spondylolysis or spondylolisthesis. J Pediatr Orthop 9:538, 1989
27. Hensinger RN, Lang JR, MacEwen GD: Surgical management of spondylolisthesis in children and adolescents. Spine 1:207, 1976
28. Phalen GS, Dickson JA: Spondylolisthesis and tight hamstrings. J Bone Joint Surg [Am] 43:505, 1961
29. Fisk JR, Moe JH, Winter RB: Scoliosis, spondylolisthesis and spondylolysis: their relationship as reviewed in 539 patients. Spine 3:324, 1978
30. Risser JC, Norquist DM: Sciatic scoliosis in growing children. Clin Orthop 21:137, 1961
31. Porter RW, Park W: Unilateral spondylolysis. J Bone Joint Surg [Br] 64:344, 1982
32. Murray RD, Colwill MR: Stress fractures of the pars interarticularis. Proc R Soc Med 61:555, 1968
33. Sherman FC, Wilkinson RH, Hall JE: Reactive sclerosis of a pedicle and spondylolysis in the lumbar spine. J Bone Joint Surg [Am] 59:49, 1977
34. Lowe RW, Hayes TD, Kaye J et al: Standing roentgenograms in spondylolisthesis. Clin Orthop 117:75, 1976
35. Newman PH: Stenosis of the lumbar spine in spondylolisthesis. Clin Orthop 115:116, 1976
36. Bradford DS: Spondylolysis and spondylolisthesis. In Bradford DS et al (eds): Moe's Textbook of Scoliosis and Other Spinal Deformities. WB Saunders Philadelphia, 1987
37. Rothman SLG: Computed tomography of the spine in older children and teenagers. Clin Sports Med 2:247, 1986
38. Meyerding HW: Spondylolisthesis. Surg Gynecol Obstet 54:371, 1932
39. Taillard W: Le spondylolisthesis chez l'enfant et l'adolescent. Acta Orthop Scand 24:115, 1955
40. Wiltse LL, Winter RB: Terminology and measurement of spondylolisthesis. J Bone Joint Surg [Am] 65:768, 1983
41. Taddonio RF: Isthmic spondylolisthesis. p. 565. In Bridwell KH, DeWald RL (eds): The Textbook of Spinal Surgery. Vol. 1. JB Lippincott, Philadelphia, 1991
42. Dandy DJ, Shannon MJ: Lumbo-sacral subluxation. J Bone Joint Surg [Br] 53:578, 1971
43. Harris IE, Weinstein SL: Long-term follow-up of patients with grade III and IV spondylolisthesis. Treatment with and without posterior fusion. J Bone Joint Surg [Am] 69:960, 1987
44. Pizzutillo PD, Mirenda W, MacEwen GD: Posterolateral fusion for spondylolisthesis in adolescence. J Pediatr Orthop 6:311, 1986
45. Wiltse LL, Jackson DW: Treatment of spondylolisthesis and spondylolysis in children. Clin Orthop 117:92, 1976
46. Sinaki M, Lutness MP, Hstrup DM, Chu CP, Gramse RR: Lumbar spondylolisthesis: retrospective comparison and three-year follow-up of two conservative treatment programs. Arch Phys Med Rehabil 70:594, 1989
47. Bradford DS: Spondylolysis and spondylolisthesis in children and adolescents. In Bradford DS, Hensinger RN (eds): Pediatric Spine. Thieme and Stratton, New York, 1985
48. Buck JE: Direct repair of the defect in spondylolisthesis. J Bone Joint Surg [Br] 52:432, 1970
49. Buck JE: Further thoughts on direct repair of the defect in spondylolisthesis. J Bone Joint Surg [Br] 61:123, 1979
50. Barash HL, Galante JO, Lambert CN, Ray RD: Spondylolisthesis and tight hamstrings. J Bone Joint Surg [Am] 52:1319, 1970
51. Bosworth DM, Fielding JW, Demarest L, Bonaquist M: Spondylolisthesis: a critical review of a consecutive series of cases treated by arthrodesis. J Bone Joint Surg [Am] 37:767, 1955
52. Johnson JR, Kirwan EO: The long-term results of fusion in situ for severe spondylolisthesis. J Bone Joint Surg [Br] 65:43, 1983
53. Velikas EP, Blackburne JS: Surgical treatment of spondylolisthesis in children and adolescents. J Bone Joint Surg [Br] 63:67, 1981

54. Edwards CC: Reduction of spondylolisthesis. p. 605. In Bridwell KH, DeWald RL (eds): The Textbook of Spinal Surgery. Vol. 1. JB Lippincott, Philadelphia, 1991
55. Harms J, Boehm H, Ziekle K: Surgical treatment of spondylolisthesis. p. 585. In Bridwell KH, DeWald RL (eds): The Textbook of Spinal Surgery. Vol. 1. JB Lippincott, Philadelphia, 1991
56. Johnson LP, Nascu RJ, Dunham WK: Surgical management of isthmic spondylolisthesis. Spine 13:93, 1988
57. Gill GG, Manning JG, White HL: Surgical treatment of spondylolisthesis without spine fusion. J Bone Joint Surg [Am] 37:493, 1955
58. Marmor L, Bechtol CO: Spondylolisthesis. J Bone Joint Surg [Am] 43:1068, 1961
59. Osterman K, Lindholm TS, Laurent LE: Late results of removal of the loose posterior element (Gill's operation) in the treatment of lytic lumbar spondylolisthesis. Clin Orthop 117:121, 1976
60. Scaglietti O, Frontino C, Bartolozzi P: Technique of anatomical reduction of lumbar spondylolisthesis and its surgical stabilization. Clin Orthop 117:164, 1976
61. Flynn JC, Hoque MA: Anterior fusion of the lumbar spine. J Bone Joint Surg [Am] 61:1143, 1979
62. DeWald RI, Faut MM, Taddonio RF et al: Severe lumbosacral spondylolisthesis in adolescents and children. J Bone Joint Surg [Am] 63:619, 1981
63. Bradford DS, Boachie-Adjei O: Treatment of severe spondylolisthesis by anterior and posterior reduction and stabilization. A long-term follow-up study. J Bone Joint Surg [Am] 72:1060, 1990
64. Boos N, Marchesi D, Aebi M: Treatment of spondylolysis and spondylolisthesis with Cotrel-Dubousset instrumentation: a preliminary report. J Spinal Dis 4:472, 1991
65. Gaines RW, Nichols WK: Treatment of lumbar spondyloptosis by spondylectomy and reduction. p. 593. In Bridwell KH, DeWald RL (eds): The Textbook of Spinal Surgery. Vol. 1. JB Lippincott, Philadelphia, 1991
66. Huizenga BA: Reduction of spondyloptosis with two-stage vertebrectomy. Orthop Trans 7:21, 1983
67. Verbiest H: The treatment of lumbar spondyloptosis or impending lumbar spondyloptosis accompanied by neurologic deficit and/or neurogenic intermittent claudication. Spine 4:68, 1979
68. Bradford DS: Management of spondylolysis and spondylolisthesis. p. 151. In American Academy of Orthopaedic Surgeons: Instructional Course Lectures XXXII. CV Mosby, St Louis, 1983
69. Schoenecker PL, Cole HO, Herring JA, Capelli AM, Bradford DS: Cauda equina syndrome (CES) following in situ arthrodesis for severe spondylolisthesis at the lumbosacral junction. J Bone Joint Surg [Am] 72:369, 1990

APPENDIX

Computer Indexing of Fractures

Jacques D'Astous

> Happiness lies in the absorption in some vocation which satisfys the soul.
> —Sir William Osler

Accurate diagnostic coding of fractures is an essential part of accurate record keeping. We have all experienced the frustrations of going to medical records to obtain a list of patients with a specific injury, for example, a supracondylar fracture of the humerus, only to discover, that the ICD9 code "812" includes all fractures of the humerus from the tip of the greater tuberosity down to the medial epicondyle. As well as facilitating data retrieval for clinical research projects, an accurate coding system would be useful for determining the incidence of a certain type of fracture in our patient population.

In 1985, at the time we implemented computerized billing, there was a need to develop a "user-friendly" system of coding orthopaedic diagnoses that would not require the constant looking up of numerical codes and could be easily inserted on the patients chart at the time of the clinic visit. The idea was to code the fracture one time only for billing purposes as well as for data retrieval at a later date. In order to be a useful research tool, the coding system had to be more anatomically specific than the ICD9 system that existed at the time. The present ICD9.CM Expanded, published in 1988 now provides us with the anatomic specificity but requires looking up a numerical code in the code book.[1] It was also important for this indexing system to be compatible with the ICD9 codes to permit comparison to other databases and to be compatible with the government or insurance company billing systems.

Although this indexing system developed at the Children's Hospital of Eastern Ontario, was for all pediatric orthopaedic diagnoses, only the section that deals with fractures is outlined here.

The CHEO Fracture Coding System in itself is quite simple and is based on the clinical description of the fracture (see the code listings at the end of this chapter). The code for a particular fracture can be broken down into three sections. The first section describes the injury (i.e., fracture or dislocation), the second section describes the bone involved (i.e., humerus, radius) and the third section describes the anatomic region of the bone involved (i.e., medial condyle, distal radius). The computer was used to sort all of the codes alphabetically in order to ensure that there were no duplicate codes. A suffix may be added to indicate that the fracture is compound (CPD), and a second suffix describes the treatment (NR = no reduction, OR = open reduction, ORIF = open reduction internal fixation, PP = percutaneous pinning). For example, a closed supracondylar fracture of the humerus, treated by closed reduction and percutaneous pinning is coded as follows: FHSC.CR.PP (**F**racture **H**umerus **S**upra**C**ondylar **C**losed **R**eduction **P**ercutaneous **P**inning). Because this is the language we use every day in fracture management, there is no need to look up a code in the ICD9.CM Expanded and code this same injury as 812.41, which only describes this as a supracondylar fracture of the humerus and tells us nothing about the treatment. This simplified coding system is also very easy to modify and may be expanded by adding codes for areas of special interest such as the mechanism of injury. For example, it would be possible to retrieve tibial shaft fractures resulting from All-Terrain Vehicles as FTS.ATV, and all tibial shaft fractures resulting from ski injuries as FTS.SKI. Similarly, the code **TEACH** might be added as a suffix to highlight all interesting fractures that could be used for teaching purposes.

The CHEO system has proven to be very useful for data retrieval for use in teaching or research. For example, if the number of fractures treated in a particular year was required, the computer would be asked to print all codes beginning with the letter **F**. To pull out all of the humeral fractures, all codes beginning with **FH** would be requested, and if all supracondylar fractures of the humerus were required, all codes matching **FHSC** would be printed.

Table A-1 illustrates how this simple coding system can be fully compatible with the ICD9.CM Expanded.

HARDWARE AND SOFTWARE REQUIREMENTS

The CHEO Fracture Coding System may be used in most commercial billing packages providing that there is at least one field available for diagnosis and that this field can accept text (alpha) entries. Also, the length of the diagnosis field should be a minimum of 8 characters long or longer if the treatment codes are to be included in the diagnosis field (e.g., FHSC.CR.PP, 10 characters to describe closed reduction and percutaneous pinning of a supracondylar fracture of the humerus).

The CHEO coding system has also been used in database programs such as DBase (Borland), Paradox 3.5 (Borland), and Executive Card Manager (Hewlett-Packard). Typically, a patient record, using separate fields for diagnosis, treatment, and mechanism of injury would allow the database to sort and retrieve records according to the diagnosis, treatment, or mechanism of injury (Figs. A-1 to A-3).

The minimum hardware requirements to run most commercial billing programs and the above-mentioned database programs would be an 80286 AT-compatible computer with 640K of RAM. However, an 80386 IBM-compatible computer with 4 megabytes of RAM would allow faster search and retrieval functions as well as the possibility of multitasking.

SUMMARY

A simple coding system, fully compatible with the ICD9.CM Expanded was developed at the Children's

TABLE A-1. CHEO Fracture Coding System Analysis

ICD9.CM Expanded	CHEO Alpha Code	Description
812.4 Fracture Distal End of humerus/Elbow Closed		
812.40 Lower end, unspecified part	FHD	Fracture Humerus Distal
812.41 Supracondylar fracture of humerus	FHSC	Fx Humerus SupraCondylar
812.42 Lateral condyle (Capitellum)	FHLC	Fx Humerus Lateral Condyle
812.43 Medial condylar (Trochlea)	FHMC	Fx Humerus Medial Condyle
812.44 Condyle(s) unspecified	FHC	Fx Humerus Condyle(s)
812.49 Other Trochlea		
812.491 T-Condylar	FHTC	Fx Humerus T-Condylar
812.492 Multiple fractures		
812.499 Other fracture lower end, closed		
	FHCAP	Fx Humerus Capitellum

Fig. A-1. Typical database screen for a patient who suffered a S-H type II fracture of the distal femur (FFD2) resulting from a ski injury (SKI) and treated by a closed reduction and percutaneous pinning (CR.PP).

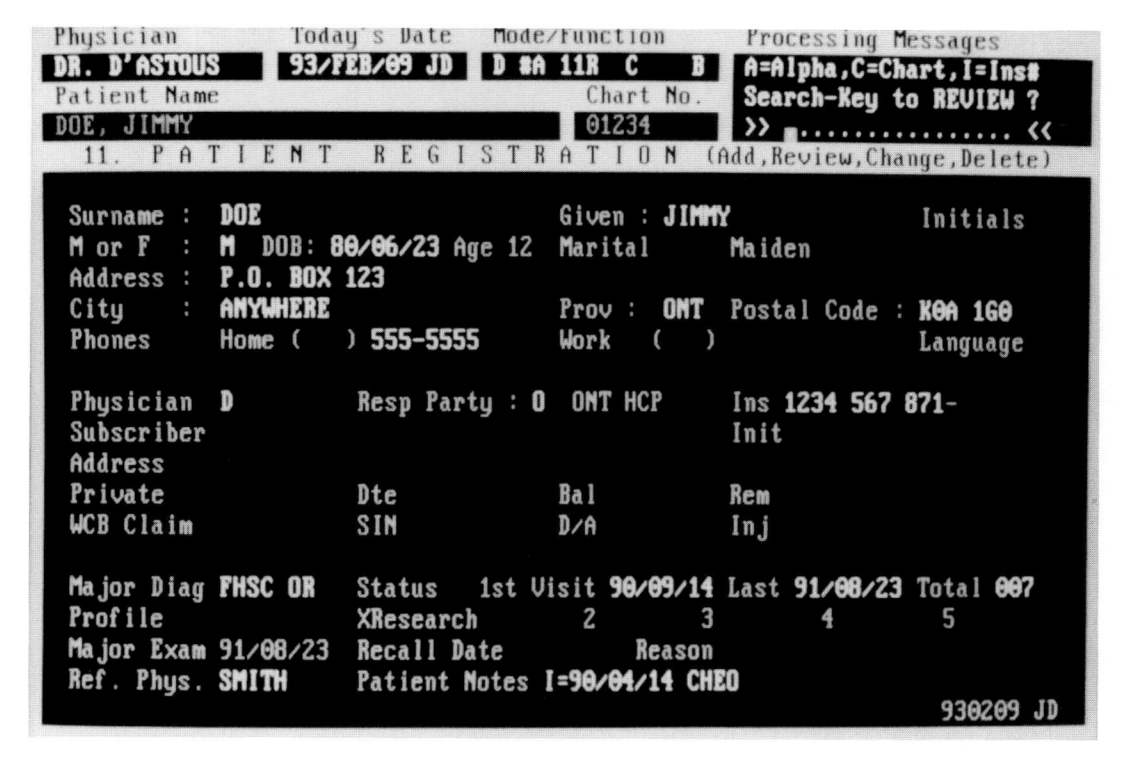

Fig. A-2. Typical patient registration screen from a commercial billing program (MD 5000) who suffered a supracondylar fracture of the humerus (FHSC) treated by an open reduction (OR).

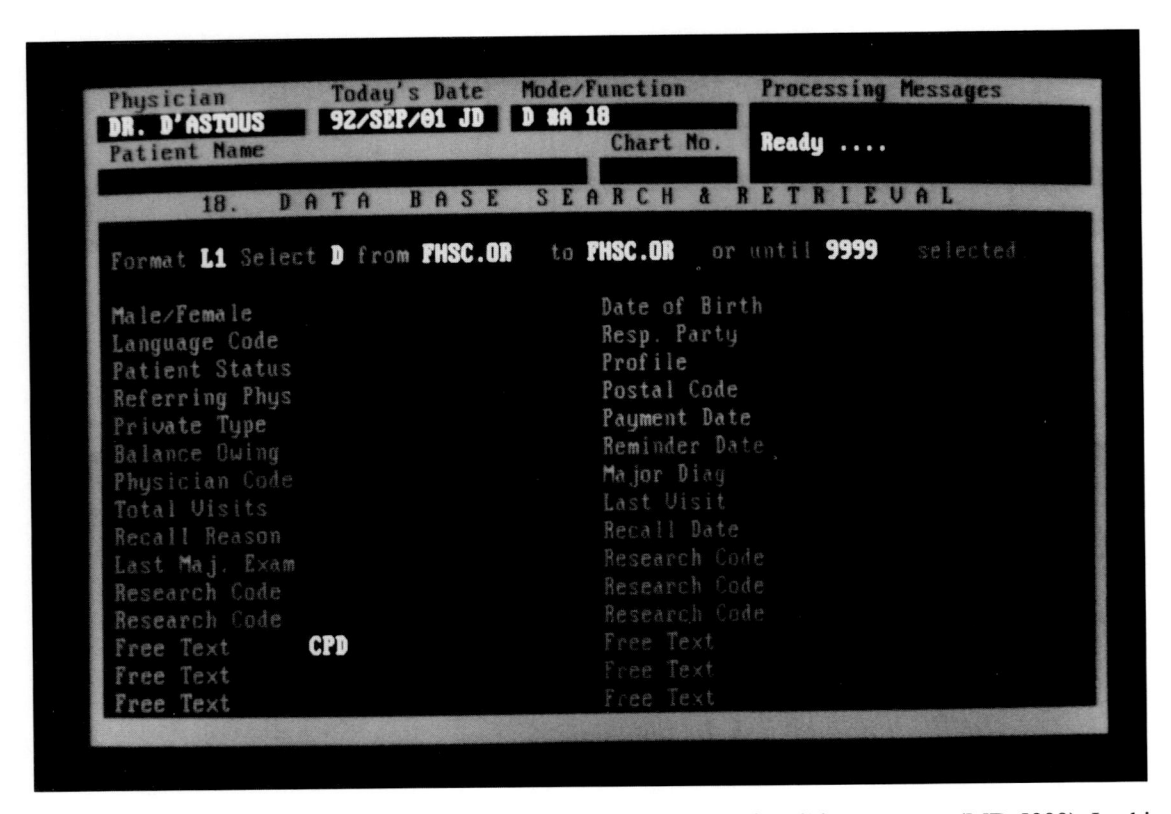

Fig. A-3. Database and search and retrieval screen from a commercial billing program (MD 5000). In this example, the search is for patients with a diagnosis (D) of a compound (CPD) supracondylar fracture of the humerus (FHSC) treated by open reduction (OR).

Hospital of Eastern Ontario to allow coding by the orthopaedic surgeon in the clinic or office without having to look up the codes in a reference manual. The CHEO Fracture Coding System permits more accurate coding as the billing/coding clerk does not have to figure out which ICD9.CM code applies to "fractured wrist." Nevertheless, it does require some effort on the part of the orthopaedic surgeon. The other major advantage is that the data are inputed only once and can be used for both billing and data-retrieval purposes.

The implementation of this system in our group of six pediatric orthopaedic surgeons has been relatively straightforward and the secretarial staff have been very supportive.

REFERENCE

1. Orthopaedic ICD9.CM Expanded; American Academy of Orthopaedic Surgeons, 1986, American Academy of Orthopaedic Surgeons, 222 South Prospect Avenue, Park Ridge, IL 60068

Cheo Fracture Coding System

Fractures (F)

Spine: (805) (without cord damage)
FSPC	Fx cervical spine (C1–C7)
FSPT	Fx thoracic\dorsal spine (D1–D12 or T1–T12)
FSPL	Fx lumbar spine (L1–L5)
FSPS	Fx sacrum (S1–S4)
FSPCO	Fx coccyx

Spine: (806) (with cord damage) P = paralysis
FSPPC	Fx cervical spine (C1–C7)
FSPPT	Fx thoracic\dorsal spine (D1–D12 or T1–T12)
FSPPL	Fx lumbar spine (L1–L5)

Pelvis: (808)
FP	Fx Pelvis unspecified
FPIL	Fx Ilium, Iliac crest
FPIS	Fx Ischium
FPP	Fx Pubis, Pubic rami
FPAC	Fx Acetabulum
FPAV	Avulsion fx.— Ischial tuberosity, Anterior superior iliac spine, Anterior inferior iliac spine
FPD	Fracture dislocation of pelvis, disruption of pelvis, diastasis of pubic symphysis

Femur: (821)
FF	Fx femur unspecified
FFD	Fx femur distal unspecified
FFN1	Type 1 fx proximal femur
FFN	Fx femoral neck
FFI	Intertrochanteric fx femur
FFST	Subtrochanteric fx femur
FFS	Fx femoral shaft
FFSC	Supracondylar fx femur
FFD1	Type 1 fx distal femur (FFD2\3\4\5—for Types 2,3,4,5)
FFMC	Fx medial condyle femur
FFLC	Fx lateral condyle of femur
FFTC	T-condylar fx femur, Y-condylar fx femur
FFO	Osteochondral fx distal femur
FFLT	Fx femur lesser trochanter
FFGT	Fx femur greater trochanter

Patella: (829)
- FPA — Fx patella
- FPAO — Osteochondral fx patella
- FPAOD — Fx dislocation patella
- FPAS — Sleeve Fx patella

Tibia: (823)
- FT — Fx tibia unspecified
- FTSP — Fx tibial spine, intercondylar eminence
- FTM — Fx proximal tibia metaphysis
- FTP — Fx tibia proximal unspecified
- FTP1 — Type 1 — fx proximal tibia (FTP2\3\4\5)
- FTS — Fx tibial shaft
- FTD — Fx distal tibia unspecified, or distal tibial metaphysis
- FTDE — Fx distal tibia epiphysis
- FTD1 — Type 1 fx distal tibia (FTD2\3\4\5)
- FTT — Triplane fx distal tibia or ankle
- FTMM — Fx medial malleolus

Fibula: (823)
- FFIB — Fx fibula unspecified
- FFIBP — Fx fibula proximal
- FFIBLM — Fx lateral malleolus
- FFIBD — Fx fibula distal
- FFIBD1 — Type 1 — fx distal fibula
- FFIBD2 — Type 2 — fx distal fibula
- FFIBAV — Fx fibula avulsion
- FTFIBD — Fx tib-fib distal unspecified

Ankle: (824)
Includes FTD1, FTT, FTMM, FFLM
- FA — Fx ankle unspecified
- FAB — Fx ankle bimalleolar
- FAT — Fx ankle trimalleolar

Foot: (829)
- FN — Scaphoid, navicular, tarsal
- FTA — Fx talus
- FCUB — Fx cuboid
- FCA — Fx os calcis, calcaneus
- FCUN — Fx cuneiform
- FMT — Fx metatarsal (1 to 5)
- FSES — Fx sesamoid

Foot: (816)
- FTOE — Fx toe unspecified
- FTOEP — Fx phalanx of foot or toe
- FTOEPA — Fx toe phalanx great toe
- FTOEPB — Fx toe phalanx 2nd
- FTOEPC — Fx toe phalanx 3rd

Closed Reduction	CR
Open Reduction	OR
Open Reduction Internal Fixation	ORIF
Percutaneous Pinning	PP

Dislocations (D)

Spine:
DSPC	Dislocated C-spine
DSPT	Dislocated thoracic-dorsal spine
DSPL	Dislocated lumbar spine

Pelvis:
DP	Fx dislocation pelvis, Malgaigne fx
DSI	Dislocated scro-iliac joint

Hip:
DH	Dislocated hip (traumatic)

Knee:
DK	Dislocated knee
DPA	Patellar dislocation
DPAR	Recurrent dislocation of patella

Ankle:
DA	Dislocated ankle
DAF	Dislocated ankle with fracture

Feet:
DFOOT	Dislocated tarsal, joint
DT	Dislocated toe, IP joint, MTP joint

Shoulder: (831)
DS	Dislocated shoulder, glenohumeral dislocation
DSR	Recurrent dislocation shoulder
DAC	Acromio-clavicular (A.C.) dislocation
DSC	Sternoclavicular (S.C.) dislocation

Elbow: (832)
DE	Dislocated elbow
DEF	Fracture dislocation elbow
DEM	Monteggia fx dislocation
DEHR	Dislocated radial head

Finger: (834)
DFIN	Dislocated finger, IP or MCP joint

Subluxations (Su)

Spine:
- SUSPC   Subluxation C-spine, atlanto-axial rotatory subluxation
- SUSPT   Subluxation T-spine
- SUSPL   Subluxation L-spine

Pelvis:
- SUSI   Sacroiliac subluxation

Hip:
- SUH   Hip subluxation (traumatic) (not congenital or paralytic)

Knee:
- SUPA   Patellar subluxation, patello-femoral subluxation
- SUPAR   Recurrent subluxation, patello-femoral subluxation

Ankle:
- SUA   (Recurrent) subluxation ankle
- SUAP   Subluxation of peroneal tendons

Shoulder:
- SUS   Shoulder or glenohumeral subluxation
- SUSR   Recurrent subluxation of shoulder or glenohumeral joint

Elbow:
- SUE   Elbow Subluxation
  Recurrent elbow subluxation
  Recurrent pulled elbow
  Pulled elbow
  Radial Head Subluxation

Finger:
- SUFIN   Subluxation finger unspecified

Wrist:
- SUW   Subluxation wrist unspecified

Sprains and Strains (S)

Spine: (847)
- SSPC   Sprain cervical spine
- SSPT   Sprain thoracic, dorsal
- SSPL   Sprain lumbar

Hip:
- SH   Sprain hip
- SSI   Sprain S.I. joint

Muscle:
SMQ	Sprain muscle quadriceps
SMH	Sprain muscle hamstring
SMD	Sprain muscle deltoid
SMGM	Gluteus maximus strain

Knee: (844)
SKMC	Sprain, strain, tear medial collateral ligament
SKLC	Sprain, strain, tear lateral collateral ligament
SKAC	Sprain, strain, tear anterior cruciate
SKPC	Sprain, strain, tear posterior cruciate

Knee: (718)
SKMM	Tear medial meniscus
SKLM	Tear lateral meniscus

Ankle: (845)
SA	Sprained ankle, strain, tear
	—ant.post., talofibular
	—calcaneofibular
	—tibiofibular lig.
	—diastosis

Foot:
SAACH	Sprain, tear Achilles tendon
SFOOT	Sprain foot
STARSUS	Sprain tarsus, ligzfrang

Toes: (845)
STOE	Sprain toe (collateral ligament)

Shoulder: (840)
SS	Sprain shoulder
SSAC	Sprain AC joint
SSSC	Sprain SC joint

Elbow: (840)
SE	Sprain elbow

Wrist: (842)
SW	Sprain wrist, distal radioulnar joint

Index

Page numbers followed by f indicate figures; those followed by t indicate tables.

A

Abbreviated Injury Scale (AIS), 32–33
Abdominal injuries
  anesthesia considerations in, 84
  in multiply injured child, 28
    evaluation of, 32
  resulting from seat belt usage. *See* Seat belt fractures.
Accessory centers of ossification
  bipartite patella and, 78
  in differential diagnosis of fractures, 44, 46f–47f, 67
Accessory ossicles, in differential diagnosis of fractures, 45, 50f, 67
Acetabular fractures, 468–469, 471f–474f
  classification, 471, 474t
  treatment, 471, 474–475, 475t
  triradiate cartilage injury, 475, 475f, 476f, 477f
Acute slipped capital femoral epiphysis
  anatomy, 513, 514f, 515f
  classification, 514, 515f
  complications, 518, 519f, 520
  description and incidence, 513
  differential diagnosis, 516, 518
  injury mechanism, 513, 514
  physical examination, 514, 516, 516f, 517f
  treatment, 520f, 520–521
    indications for, 518, 518f
Airway management, in multiply injured child, 28–29
AIS (Abbreviated Injury Scale), 32–33
All-terrain vehicles (ATVs), accident-related injuries, 6–7
  management of. *See* Multiply injured child.
Anesthesia
  adverse reactions to, 84
  assessing child for, 83
  conscious sedation, 85
  fasting prior to, 84
  general, 85
  local, 88, 91, 91t
  and malignant hyperthermia, 85
  in multiply injured child, 83–84
  postoperative care and, 91
  preexisting medical conditions and, 84
  psychological preparation for, 84–85
  regional. *See* Regional anesthesia.
Aneurysmal bone cysts, 1031, 1034f, 1038, 1040f
Angular deformity(ies)
  following intra-articular proximal tibial epiphysis fracture (Salter-Harris types III & IV), 602
  management by Ilizarov technique. *See* Ilizarov technique.
  in spondylolisthesis, 1202, 1202f
  in tibial fractures, 651–652
Angulation, progressive
  following distal femoral epiphyseal fracture, 585, 590, 590f
  following intra-articular fracture of knee (Salter-Harris types III & IV), 596
Ankle
  anatomy, 755
  fracture dislocations. *See* Ankle fractures.
  regional anesthesia for, 89–90, 90f
Ankle fractures
  anatomy, 713–714, 714f, 715f–717f
  classification, 714, 718, 718f–719f, 720, 720f–721f
  complications, 733f, 734
  description and incidence, 712
  differential diagnosis, 722
  injury mechanism, 714, 717f
  nontraumatic pathology mimicking, 80
  normal anatomy and variants mimicking, 79f, 79–80
  osteochondral, 1004, 1006
    injury mechanism, 1004, 1006
  physical examination, 720, 722
  radiologic diagnosis of, 79f, 79–80
  stress type, 977–978, 979f
  technical factors, 79
  transchondral, 1006
  treatment
    direct axial compression, 731, 731f
    dorsiflexion injuries, 722, 722f
    eversion injuries, 723, 724f–725f
    inversion injuries, 723, 725f, 726, 726f–728f
    plantar-flexion injuries, 722–723, 723f
    rotational injuries, 726
    special considerations, 731, 732f, 734
    Tillaux fracture, 726, 728, 728f–729f
    triplane fractures, 728, 730f, 731
Anxiolytics, for conscious sedation, 86
AOD. *See* Atlanto-occipital dislocations (AOD).
Apophysis, tibial, avulsion of, 625, 626f, 627f
Apophysitis, tibial. *See* Osgood-Schlatter disease.
Apprehension tests, 161

1225

Arterial injury(ies)
  as complicating factor, 1127, 1127t
  distal femoral epiphyseal injuries associated with, 585, 589f
Arthritis, septic, of hip, 61f, 76–77
Arthrography
  of the elbow, 275
  in fracture diagnosis, 40, 43f
Asoma, mimicking spinal trauma, 72–73, 73f
Atlantoaxial displacements
  rotatory, 822, 823f
    classification, 822, 822t, 824f
    clinical findings, 822
    complications, 825–826
    injury mechanism, 822, 824f
    radiologic evaluation, 824, 825f
    treatment, 824–825, 825f
    traumatic ligamentous disruption, 826
Atlantoaxial instability, mimicking spinal trauma, 68, 69f, 72
Atlanto-occipital dislocations (AOD)
  anatomy, 797–798, 798t, 799f
  classification and radiology, 800, 800f–801f, 800t
  complications, 803, 805
  description and incidence, 797, 798f
  differential diagnosis, 801
  injury mechanism, 798, 800, 800f
  physical examination, 801
  treatment
    closed methods, 801–802
    halo fixation, 802, 802f
    open methods, 802, 803f
    pitfalls, 802–803, 804f–805f
Atlas vertebra
  congenital defects of, 55f
  development and normal ossification of, 809
  fracture dislocations. See Atlanto-occipital dislocations (AOD); Jefferson fracture.
Atrophy, immobilization causing, 1035–1036
ATVs. See All terrain vehicles (ATVs).
Autonomic dysreflexia, as spinal cord injury complication, 913, 915, 915f, 916f
Avascular necrosis
  as epiphyseal plate injury complication, 23–24
  as femoral head fracture complication, 500, 502, 502f–504f, 505–506
  as hip dislocation complication, 534
  of lateral condylar humerus, 256, 256f
  in talar fractures, 757, 758f
  of trochlea, 194, 194f
Avulsion fractures
  anatomy, 989, 990f
  classification
    anatomic, 990, 991t
    biomechanical, 990, 990t
  complications, 990, 997f–998f, 998
  definition, 989
  of fifth metatarsal base, 772
  of inferior pole of the patella, 679, 680f
    medial margin, 682–683, 683f
  injury mechanism, 989
  of the olecranon, 271, 274f
    treatment, 280
  of tibial apophysis, 625, 626f, 627f
    treatment, 990, 991f–996f
Avulsive cortical irregularity, of femoral metaphysis, 78
Axis vertebra
  development and normal ossification of, 809
  fractures of
    C2 ring
      complications, 822
      hangman's, 819, 820f–821f
      injury mechanism, 819
      physical examination, 819
      radiologic evaluation, 819
      treatment, 822
    odontoid process (dens), 817
      classification, 817, 817t
      complications, 819
      injury mechanism, 817, 817t
      physical examination, 817–818
      radiologic evaluation, 818, 818f
      treatment, 818–819

B

Bailey-Dubow sliding nail technique, 1090, 1094f
Battered child syndrome, 932
Bed, falls from, injuries resulting from, 5
Bennett's fracture, 415
Bicycle accidents, injuries seen in, 6
  management of. See Multiply injured child.
Bier block, 88t, 88–89
  for treatment of reflex sympathetic dystrophy, 1160–1161, 1161f
Bipartite patella, 78
  traumatic separation of, 681–682, 681f, 682f
Birth fractures
  clavicular, 114–116, 1049–1052, 1050t, 1051f–1055f
  description and incidence, 1049, 1050t
  diaphyseal. See Diaphyseal fractures.
  and dislocations, 1057, 1059
  of the extremities, 1056t
  frequency and types, 1050t
  long-bone
    diaphyseal, 1052, 1056f, 1056t
    physeal, 1052, 1056–1057, 1057f–1060f
  and spinal injuries, 1059–1060
Bleeding disorders, misdiagnosed as child abuse, 940, 943, 943t
Blockades. See Bier block; Regional anesthesia, techniques; Spinal blockade.
Blood loss, systemic responses to, 30t
Blood replacement, in multiply injured child, 31
Blood supply, to epiphyses, 12
  growth disturbance prognosis and, 20
Bloodwork, in evaluation of multiply injured child, 31
Bone cysts, and pathologic fractures
  aneurysmal, 1031, 1034f, 1038, 1040f
  unicameral, 1029–1030, 1030f–1033f
Bone formation. See Ossification.
Bone grafting
  radial growth arrest and, 364, 364f
  scaphoid fractures, 395f, 396
Bone scans, in fracture diagnosis, 40, 43f
Brachial plexus block, 89
Brachial plexus palsy, obstetrical, 164–165
Bradford frame traction, 542–543
Breathing management, in multiply injured child, 29
Brown-Séquard lesion, 906
  in SCIWORA syndrome, 921
Bryant's traction, 542, 542f
Buckle (Torus) fracture, of distal radius and ulna, 348
  treatment indications, 351
Bulbocavernosus reflex, 904, 906f
Bunk bed, falls from, injuries resulting from, 5
Bupivacaine, pharmacology of, 91, 91t
Burst fractures of thoracolumbar spine
  classification (Denis), 857, 858f
  treatment of, 864, 868
  unique characteristics of, 870, 871f, 872, 872f–873f

C

Caffey's disease. See Hyperostosis.
Calcaneus
  anatomy, 757, 759
  degloving injury to, 649–650, 650f
  fractures of
    case example, 762f–763f, 764
    classification, 760t
    injury mechanism, 760
    signs and symptoms, 760f–761f, 760–761
    treatment, 764
Calve's disease, 73, 74f
Capitate fractures, 401f, 401–402, 402f
Capitellum of humerus, fractures of. See Humeral fractures, capitellum.
Cardiac disease, anesthesia considerations in, 84
Cardiac system, effects of spinal cord injuries on, 907
Carpal bone fractures
  bipartite condition, 386, 388, 388f
  capitate fractures, 401f, 401–402, 402f
  CHEO coding system for, 1220
  description and incidence, 385
  dislocations associated with, 402, 403f

embryology, 385–386, 386f–387f, 386t
injury mechanism, 388–389
misinterpretation of accessory bones as, 388, 389f
radiologic diagnosis, 67, 68f
of the scaphoid. *See* Scaphoid fractures.
of the triquetrum. *See* Triquetral fractures.
Carpus
  fractures of. *See* Carpal bone fractures; *specific bones.*
  ligamentous injuries of, 396–398
Cartwheel injuries. *See* Distal femoral epiphyseal injuries.
Cast(s). *See also* Immobilization.
  for distal radial and ulnar fractures, 360
  as external cause of compartment syndrome, 1166
  for femoral shaft fractures, 547
  Minerva, 828, 828t
  for proximal tibial physis fractures, 617
  for supracondylar nonphyseal femoral fractures, 565
Cauda equina syndrome, postoperative, 1210
Centers of ossification
  in differential diagnosis of fractures
    accessory. *See* Accessory centers of ossification.
    irregular, 44–45, 49f
    multipartite, 44, 48f–49f
  knee, 78
Central cord syndrome, 906–907
  in SCIWORA syndrome, 921–922
Cerclage wiring, transverse patellar fractures and, 673
Cerebrocostomandibular syndrome, 75
Cervical spine fractures and dislocations
  of abnormal spine, 826, 827f, 827t
  atlantoaxial. *See* Atlantoaxial displacements.
  atlanto-occipital. *See* Atlanto-occipital dislocations (AOD).
  of atlas vertebra. *See* Jefferson fracture.
  of axis vertebra. *See* Axis vertebra, fractures of.
  C1-C2 vertebrae
    anatomy, 807–809, 809f
      atlantoaxial motion, 810f, 810–811, 811f
      development and normal ossification, 809
      normal variations, 811
      occipitoatlantoaxial complex stability, 809–810
    congenital malformations, 812, 812f
    description and incidence, 807, 808f, 808t
    fusion of, 829
    injury mechanism, 811–812, 812t
    neck immobilization, 828f, 828t, 828–829
    patient transportation, 827–828
    physical examination, 812–813

    radiologic evaluation, 813f, 813–814, 814t
  C2-C3 displacement, 826
  C3-C7 vertebrae
    anatomy, 832, 834f–837f, 837, 838f–840f
    clinical assessment, 838, 841, 843
    description and incidence, 833
    diagnostic pitfalls, 844–845, 845t
    injury mechanism, 837–838, 841f–843f
    radiographic interpretation, 843–844, 844f, 845f, 846f, 847f–848f
    treatment, 845–846, 849f
  congenital malformation, 850
  Klippel-Feil syndrome, 850
  obstetrical injuries, 846, 850
  orthoses, types of, 828t, 828–829
    halo fixation, 828t, 828–829
    Minerva cast, 828, 828t
  transport of patients with, 827–828
Cervical spondylolisthesis, 55f
Chemical block (intravenous regional), for treatment of reflex sympathetic dystrophy, 1161
CHEO fracture coding system, 1213–1214, 1214t, 1215f–1216f, 1217–1223
  compatibility with ICD9.CM Expanded coding system, 1214t
  for dislocations, 1221–1223
  for fractures, 1217–1221
  hardware and software requirements, 1214
  for sprains and strains, 1223
  for subluxations, 1222
CHEOPS pain scale, 91, 91t
Child abuse
  common conditions misdiagnosed as, 940, 943, 943f
  definition, 932
  differential diagnosis, 940, 943, 943t
  fractures resulting from
    description and incidence, 931
    diagnosis, 933, 933t
    diaphyseal, 935, 937, 937f
    epiphyseal, 933, 935
    femoral shaft, 540
    incidence, 932–933
    management and prevention, 943
    metaphyseal, 934f–935f, 935, 936f
    radiographic assessment, 938–940, 939f–943f
    of rib(s), 937, 937f–938f
    skeletal trauma, 933
    of spine, 937–938
  history, 931–932
  legislation
    Child Abuse Protection Act, 932
    Child and Family Services Acts, 943
  osteogenesis imperfecta misdiagnosed as, 1081, 1088
  parental characteristics, 933t
Child Abuse Protection Act, 932

Child and Family Services Acts, child abuse and, 943
Chondral fractures and lesions, of the knee, 1006
Cingulate gyrus, bilateral ablation of, 1162
Circulation management, in multiply injured child, 29–30
Clavicle
  CHEO fracture coding system for, 1219
  cleidocranial dysplasia of, 61
  congenital pseudarthrosis of, 61, 65f
    misdiagnosed as child abuse, 940, 943, 943t
  dislocations of. *See* Clavicular dislocations.
  fractures of. *See* Clavicular fractures.
Clavicular dislocations
  classification, 130–131
  medial end
    anatomic considerations, 123–124, 124f
    classification
      direction, 125
      displacement, 125
      types, 125
    complications, 127
    description and incidence, 123
    diagnosis, 125
    injury mechanism, 124f, 124–125
    management, 126
      closed reduction. *See* Closed reduction.
      open reduction technique, 127
    physical examination, 125
  outer end
    anatomic considerations, 127f–129f, 129–130
    complications, 133–134
    description and incidence, 127, 129
    diagnosis, 132, 132f
    injury mechanism, 130, 130f, 131f
    physical examination, 131–132
    treatment, 132–133, 133f
Clavicular fractures, 113
  at birth, 114–116, 1049–1052, 1050t, 1051f–1055f
  complications, 119
    brachial plexus injury, 119–120
    nonunion, 119
    other, 120
    pneumothorax, 120
    vascular injury, 120
  conditions mimicking
    cleidocranial dysostosis and neurofibromatosis, 120
    congenital pseudarthrosis, 120
    coracoid process growth plate mistaken for, 61, 64f
  development and anatomic considerations, 113, 114f
  in head trauma patients, 119
  injury mechanism, 114
  lateral end, 117, 119, 119f
  medial end, 117

Clavicular fractures *(Continued)*
  midclavicular segmental (Z fracture), 117, 118f
  midclavicular shaft, 115f–117f, 116–117
  spurious, 60, 64f
  as subchondral resorption site, 64
  surgical treatment, 119
Cleidocranial dysplasia, clavicular manifestations, 61
Closed reduction. *See also* Repeat reduction; Skeletal fixation.
  for ankle injuries
    dorsiflexion, 722
    eversion and inversion, 723
    osteochondral fractures, 1013
  for atlanto-occipital dislocations, 801–802
  CHEO fracture coding system and, 1221
  for clavicular dislocation
    anterior, 126
    posterior, 126–127
  for complete mid-shaft radial and ulnar fractures, 329, 332, 332f–334f
  for epiphyseal plate injuries, 20
  for femoral injuries
    distal epiphyseal, 580f–583f, 580–581
    supracondylar fractures, 565–566, 566f
  for fibular fractures, 637–638
  for first metatarsal fractures, 773
  for knee injuries
    floating knee, 668, 668f
    transverse patellar fractures, 673
  for metatarsal shaft and neck fractures, 769, 770f–771f, 771
  for pathologic fractures, 1029
  in proximal tibiofibular joint management, 628
  for seat belt injuries to spine and abdomen, 882, 884f
  in severely handicapped children, 1109
  in spondylolisthesis, 1206, 1207f
  for tibial fractures, 637–638
    isolated proximal, 621
    proximal physis, 615, 617f, 617–618
    triplane, 742, 747f–748f
  for toe fractures, 782, 784f
  for transcondylar fractures of distal humerus, 205–206, 207f
Clostridial myonecrosis. *See* Gas gangrene.
Clostridial myositis. *See* Gas gangrene.
Clostridium sp., 1125
Coccydynia, traumatic. *See* Traumatic coccydynia.
Coccygodynia. *See* Traumatic coccydynia.
Compartment syndrome, as injury complication
  description, 1165
  diagnosis, 1167–1168
  etiology, 1166–1167, 1167t
  in floating knee, 669
  of the foot, 1169–1170
    anatomy, 790–791
    classification, 791

    description and incidence, 789–790, 790f
    differential diagnosis, 791
    injury mechanism, 791
    physical examination, 791, 792f
    treatment indications, 793, 793f
      fasciotomy, 793–794, 794f
      pitfalls, 794
  of the forearm volar compartment, 1169, 1170f
  of the hand and foot, 1169–1170
  of the leg
    anterior, 1170–1171, 1171f
    posterior, 1171
  pathogenesis, 1165–1166, 1166t
  pressure measurements, 1168–1169, 1169f
  prevention, 1172
  and skeletal fixation, 1191
  of the thigh, 1172
  in tibial fractures, 650–651
  treatment, 1172–1173
Compound fractures, CHEO coding system for, 1220
Compression
  spinal cord, 903–904, 904f, 905f, 906t
  of vertebral bodies, 73–74, 74f, 75f
Computed tomography (CT), in fracture diagnosis and assessment, 39–40, 42f
  craniocervical junction, 40, 42f
  partial physeal arrest resection, 1143, 1143f
  patellar dislocation, 687–688
  pelvis, 75
  ribs, 74
  in SCIWORA syndrome, 922f, 923, 924f–926f
  spinal cord injuries, 907
  spine, 68, 69f
  spondylolytic defect, 1200
Computer indexing of fractures, 1213
  CHEO coding system, 1213–1214, 1214t, 1215f–1216f, 1217–1223
  compatibility of coding systems, 1214t
  hardware and software requirements, 1214
  ICD9.CM Expanded coding system, 1213–1214
Concussion, spinal cord. *See* Spinal cord injuries, concussion.
Congenital coxa vara, 77, 78f
Congenital osseous defects, 53, 55f
  pseudarthrosis, 53, 56f
  skeletal deformities, 53–54
Congenital pseudarthrosis, 53, 56f
  of clavicle, 61, 65f
  of forearm bones, 66
  misdiagnosed as child abuse, 940, 943, 943t
  of subtrochanteric region, 77, 77f
  of tibia, 79, 656, 656t, 657f
Congenital syphilis, metaphyseal lucent bands in, 54, 58f
Congenital wedge vertebra, mimicking spinal trauma, 73, 74f

Congruence angle, patellar, measurement of, 687, 688f
Conscious sedation, 85
Coronoid fractures. *See also* Olecranon fractures.
  anatomic considerations
    developmental, 260–262, 261f
    structural, 259–260, 260f
  differential diagnosis, 274–275
  injury mechanisms, 262, 266, 272f–273f
  treatment, 275
    direct-blow, 280
    extensor avulsion injuries, 280
    intra-articular, 279–280
    metaphyseal injuries
      extension, 277–279, 278f
      flexion, 277
      shear, 279, 279f
    methods, 275–277, 276f, 277f
    open, 280
    physeal injuries, 277
    stress, 280
Cortical irregularity, of femoral metaphysis, 78
Cotrel-Dubousset rods, 1204
Coxa vara, congenital, 77, 78f
Craniocervical junction, CT imaging of, 40, 42f
Crush injuries
  of the foot, complication of. *See under* Compartment syndrome.
  of the hand. *See under* Phalanges (hand), fractures and dislocations of.
Cryer classification, 460–461, 462t
CT. *See* Computed tomography (CT).
Cutdown, common sites for, 30
Cysts, of the bone. *See* Bone cysts.
Cytomegalovirus, misdiagnosed as child abuse, 940, 943, 943t

D

Dacron coracoclavicular reconstruction, stress fractures following, 978
"Dancer's fracture," 40f
Decompression
  gastric, in multiply injured child, 29
  in spondylolisthesis, 1206
Decubitus ulceration
  in severely handicapped child, 1109
  as spinal cord injury complication, 912
Deformity(ies)
  following intra-articular proximal tibial epiphysis fracture (Salter-Harris types III & IV), 602
  skeletal, 53–54
  spinal, following spinal cord injury, 912–913, 913f, 914
Degloving injuries
  heel, 649–650, 650f
  with tibial fractures, 643, 644f

degloving lesion, 643, 646, 646f, 647f
  management, 648f, 648–649, 649f, 649t
Delayed SCIWORA, 921
Delayed union
  causes, 1116t
  CHEO fracture coding system and, 1220
Delivery, injuries to neonate during. *See* Birth fractures.
Depuytren's fracture. *See* Galeazzi and Galeazzi-equivalent fractures.
Diaphyseal fractures
  at birth
    of femur, 1052, 1056t
    of humerus, 1052, 1056f, 1056t
    of long bones, 1052, 1056f, 1056t
  in myelomeningocele child. *See* Myelomeningocele child, fractures in.
Digital nerve block, 89, 89f
Dirt bikes, accident-related injuries, 6–7
Discitis, mimicking spinal trauma, 68, 70f
Dislocation(s). *See also specific sites and types.*
  CHEO fracture coding system for, 1221–1223
  nontraumatic causes, 58, 61f
Distal femoral epiphyseal injuries
  anatomy, 569–570, 570f, 571f
  classification
    by direction of displacement, 576, 576f
    Ogden, 575, 576f
    Salter-Harris, 571, 572f, 574f, 574–575, 575f. *See also* Intra-articular fractures, of knee.
  complications, 585, 586, 586f, 587f
  description and incidence, 569
  differential diagnosis, 577
  examination
    physical, 576–577
    radiologic, 577, 578f–579f
  injury mechanism, 570
    direct, 570, 571f
    hyperextension force, 571
    hyperflexion forces, 571
    valgus, 570–571
    varus force, 571
  treatment
    associated arterial injury, 585, 589f
    displaced fractures
      closed reduction, 580f–583f, 580–581
      open reduction, 581, 583–584, 584f–588f
    general principles, 577, 580, 580f
    open fractures, 584
    undisplaced fractures, 580
Distraction injuries, SCIWORA syndrome and, 920
Dorsal hemivertebra, 73, 73f
Downhill skiing, injuries associated with, 7, 7f
Down syndrome, atlantoaxial instability in, 72
Dyschondrosteosis, 67

Dysplasia
  fibrous, and pathologic fractures, 1032, 1035, 1036f–1038f
  skeletal, misdiagnosed as child abuse, 940, 943, 943t
Dysreflexia, autonomic, as spinal cord injury complication, 913, 915, 915f, 916f

E

Early SCIWORA, 921
ECG. *See* Electrocardiography (ECG).
Elbow
  arthrography of, 275
  dislocations of. *See* Elbow dislocations.
  floating, 358f, 359
  fractures of. *See* Elbow fractures.
  unique features, 262
Elbow dislocations
  anatomy, 225, 227, 230f, 231f
  CHEO fracture coding system and, 1221
  complications, 234
    heterotopic calcification, 235
    neurovascular injury, 234f, 234–235
    pulled elbow, 235, 237f, 238
    recurrent dislocations, 235, 236f
    unreduced dislocations, 235
  incidence, 225
  injury mechanism
    most common types, 227, 231f
    other types, 227–228
  Monteggia fracture-dislocation, 310, 311–312, 313f
  neurovascular considerations, 228
  treatment, 228, 230, 232f–233f
    preferred method, 230
Elbow fractures
  CHEO coding system for, 1219
  of coronoid and olecranon. *See* Coronoid fractures; Olecranon fractures.
  joint stiffness after, 1131, 1132f–1133f
  Monteggia fracture-dislocation, 310, 311–312, 313f
  radiologic diagnosis of
    nontraumatic pathology mimicking, 66, 66f
    normal anatomy and variants mimicking, 65f, 66
    technical pitfalls, 64, 66
Elbow sprain, CHEO fracture coding system and, 1223
Elbow subluxations, CHEO fracture coding system and, 1222
Electrical stimulation, as treatment of nonunion in tibial fractures, 653
Electrocardiography (ECG)
  evaluating multiply injured child, 31
  monitoring patient undergoing regional anesthesia, 87
Electrophysiologic studies, in SCIWORA syndrome, 923

Eosinophilic granuloma, and pathologic spinal fractures. *See under* Spinal fractures.
Epidemiology, of fractures, practical applications, 1
Epidural block, 90
Epiphyseal plate
  histology, 11–12, 12f
  injuries to. *See* Epiphyseal plate injuries.
  nutritional mechanisms, 12
  relative growth at ends of long bones, 13
  relative strength of, 12
Epiphyseal plate injuries
  age of patient determining growth disturbance prognosis, 20
  blood supply and, 20
  classifications
    Salter-Harris, 13f–19f, 15–19
    other schemes, 19
  closed versus open, 20
  complications
    avascular necrosis, 23–24
    failure to diagnose early, 21
    malunion, 21–22, 22f
    neurologic, 22–23
    nonunion, 22, 23f
    osteomyelitis, 22, 24f
    premature growth cessation, 24–25, 25f
    vascular, 23
  diagnosis, clinical and radiographic, 13
  growth disturbance following, 14
    premature cessation, management of, 24–25, 25f
    prognostic factors, 19–20
  incidence, 3–5, 4f, 4t
    by age and sex, 13
    by site, 13–14
  in myelomeningocele child. *See* Myelomeningocele child, fractures in.
  severity of, 20
  treatment principles, 20–21
    follow-up observation, 21
    immobilization, 21
    prognosis estimation and discussion, 21
    reduction. *See* Reduction, of epiphyseal plate injury.
Epiphyseal plates, in differential diagnosis of fractures, 44, 45f, 46f
  irregular margins, 45, 51, 51f
Epiphyses
  avascular necrosis of, 23–24
  blood supply to, 20
Epiphysiodesis, completion in linear physeal bar resection, 1151f, 1151–1152
Epiphysis, femoral involvement. *See* Acute slipped capital femoral epiphysis.
Equestrian injuries, 8
Extension injuries, of the olecranon, 262f–268f, 262–263
Extensor avulsion fractures, of the olecranon, 271, 274f
  treatment, 280

External fixation. *See also* Ilizarov technique; Skeletal fixation.
  and excessive shortening in cast, 555
  femoral shaft fractures, 550, 551f
  fibular fractures, 639–640, 640f–642f, 642–643
  ipsilateral femoral/tibial fractures, 552–553, 553f
  multiple trauma and, 551–552
  open fractures, 550–551
  pathologic fractures, 554f, 555
  tibial fractures, 639–640, 640f–642f, 642–643
  vascular injury and, 552, 552f
External fixators, 1189
Extremity(ies). *See* Lower extremity; Upper extremity.

F

Fall(s), injuries caused by, 5, 5t
  management of. *See* Multiply injured child.
Fasciotomy, of foot compartments, 793–794, 794f
Fasting, preoperative, 84
Fat embolism syndrome
  description and incidence, 1177
  diagnostic features, 1178f, 1178t, 1178–1180, 1179f
  history, 1177
  pathogenesis, 1178
  treatment, 1180
    for established case, 1180
    prophylactic, 1180
Femoral condyles, 1006, 1006t
Femoral fractures
  birth-induced, 1052, 1056–1057, 1057f–1060f
  CHEO coding system for, 1217
  distal epiphyseal. *See* Distal femoral epiphyseal injuries.
  ipsilateral. *See* Floating knee.
  of the midshaft, 90
  in myelomeningocele child. *See* Myelomeningocele child, fractures in.
  radiologic diagnosis of, 78
    nontraumatic pathology mimicking, 79
    normal anatomy and variants mimicking, 78–79, 79f
  in severely handicapped child. *See* Severely handicapped child, fractures in.
  of the shaft. *See* Femoral shaft fractures.
Femoral nerve block, 90
Femoral shaft fractures
  anatomy, 539–540
  child abuse, 540
  classification, 540
  complications
    growth arrest, 556
    leg length discrepancy, 555–556
    malunion, 555, 556f, 557f
  description and incidence, 539
  injury mechanism, 540
  neonatal, 540
  pathologic, 540
  physical examination, 541
  stress, 540–541
  stress type, 976–977, 977f
  supracondylar
    nonphyseal. *See* Supracondylar femoral fractures, nonphyseal.
    physeal. *See* Distal femoral epiphyseal injuries.
  treatment, 541–542
    bracing, 1190
    Bradford frame traction, 542–543
    Bryant's traction, 542, 542f
    cast bracing, 547, 1190
    hip spica, early application of, 543f, 543–544
    operative management, 547, 548f–549f, 550–553, 551f–554f, 555. *See also* External fixation, of femoral shaft fractures.
    Russell's traction, 546, 546f
    skeletal traction, 546f, 546–547
    skin traction, 544, 544f–545f, 546
Femur
  acute epiphyseal separation. *See* Acute slipped capital femoral epiphysis.
  deformity correction by Ilizarov technique, 699f, 700
  and intra-articular fractures of knee. *See* Intra-articular fractures, of knee.
  overgrowth of, as floating knee complication, 669
Fibroma, nonossifying, and pathologic fractures, 1032, 1035f, 1036f
Fibular fractures
  anatomy, 631–632, 636f
  CHEO coding system for, 1218
  classification, 633, 638t
  and degloved lower limb. *See* Degloving injuries.
  description and incidence, 631, 632f, 633f–635f
  injury mechanisms, 632, 637f, 638f
  in mangled extremity, 650, 651t
  physical examination, 633–634
  radiographic evaluation, 634, 636
  of shaft, 654
  treatment
    closed methods, 637–638
    external fixation, 639–640, 640f–642f, 642–643
    of open fractures, 639, 639t
    operative indications, 638–639
Fingers. *See* Phalanges (hand), fractures and dislocations of.
Fixation. *See* External fixation; Ilizarov technique; Internal fixation; Skeletal fixation.
Flexion injuries
  of the olecranon, 263, 266, 268f
  SCIWORA syndrome and, 920
Floating elbow, 358f, 359
Floating knee
  anatomy, 661–662, 663f
  classical presentation, 662f
  classification, 663f
  complications, 668–669
  description and incidence, 661, 662f
  injury mechanism, 662, 664f, 665f
  physical examination, 663, 665f
  treatment, 663, 666f–667f, 668
Fluid resuscitation, in multiply injured child, 30–31
Follow-up observation, in epiphyseal plate injuries, 21
Foot
  crush injury to. *See under* Compartment syndrome.
  eversion and inversion movements, 755
  fractures of
    metatarsal involvement. *See* Metatarsus, fractures and dislocations of.
    phalangeal involvement. *See* Phalanges (foot), fractures and dislocations of.
    radiologic diagnosis of
      nontraumatic pathology mimicking, 80
      normal anatomy and variants mimicking, 79f, 79–80
      technical factors, 79
    stress type, 977–978, 978f, 979f
    tarsal involvement. *See* Tarsal bones, fractures and dislocations of.
Forearm. *See also* Radius; Ulna.
  CHEO fracture coding system for, 1220
  compartment syndrome in, 1169, 1170f
  congenital pseudarthrosis of, 940, 943, 943t
  radiologic diagnosis of trauma to
    nontraumatic pathology mimicking, 66, 66f
    normal anatomy and variants mimicking, 65f, 66
    technical pitfalls, 64, 66
Fracture fragments, 67
Fracture(s)
  birth-induced. *See* Birth fractures; *specific sites.*
  care principles, 35
  CHEO coding system for, 1217–1221
  commonest, 3, 3f
  computer indexing of. *See* Computer indexing of fractures.
  epidemiology, practical applications, 1
  falls causing, 5, 5t
  incidence
    by age, 2, 2t
    by site of injury, 2t, 2–3
  resulting from child abuse. *See* Child abuse, fractures resulting from.

road and off-road accidents causing, 5–7. *See also* Seat belt fractures.
  soft tissue injury and. *See* Soft tissue injury(ies).
  sports and recreation activities causing, 7f, 7–8, 8t
Fusion, vertebral
  cervical spine fractures and dislocations, 829
  in spondylolisthesis, 1204, 1205f, 1206–1208, 1207f

G

Galeazzi and Galeazzi-equivalent fractures
  clinical appearance, 317
  complications, 319f, 320
  description and incidence, 313f, 313–314
  diagnosis, 317–318
  distal radio-ulnar joint anatomy, 314, 314f, 316
  injury mechanism, 314f–316f, 316, 317t
  treatment, 317f, 318, 320
Gangrene, from puncture wounds, 359
Gas gangrene, 1125
  diagnosis, 1125–1126
  history, 1125
  treatment, 1126–1127
Gastric decompression, in multiply injured child, 29
GCS (Glasgow Coma Scale), 31–32, 32t
General anesthesia, 85
Genu recurvatum, following intra-articular proximal tibial epiphysis fracture (Salter-Harris types III & IV), 602
Glasgow Coma Scale (GCS), 31–32, 32t
Glenohumeral joint, 159
Glenohumeral translation, 160–161, 161f, 162f
Glenoid fossa. *See* Coronoid fractures; Olecranon fractures.
Graham and Kiernan classification, 267
Graves classification, 267
Greenstick fractures
  involving radius and ulna
    distal, 348, 348f, 351–352
    midshaft, 334, 336, 338f–341f
    proximal ulna, 268, 268f
  of tibia and fibula, treatment of, 772, 772f
Growth arrest
  as epiphyseal plate injury complication, 24–25, 25f
  physeal. *See* Physeal growth arrest.
  radial, osteotomy to correct deformity secondary to, 364, 364f
Growth disturbance
  and cessation of growth. *See* Growth arrest.
  following epiphyseal plate injuries. *See* Epiphyseal plate injuries, growth disturbance following.

in odontoid process, 819
Growth plates. *See* Epiphyseal plates.
Gunshot fractures of the extremities
  case examples, 956, 958, 959f–961f, 962–963, 964f–966f, 968f
  complications
    bone loss and nonunion, 955–956
    infection, 955
    joint contractures, 956
    lead intoxication, 956
    neurologic, 954
    physeal injuries, 956, 957f
    vascular, 954–955
  description, injury mechanism, and classification, 945–946
    nonpowder weapons, 949
    shotguns, 949, 949f
    single-missile weapons, 946–949, 947t, 948f
  incidence, 945, 946t
  physical examination and differential diagnosis, 950f, 950–952, 951f
  treatment, 952–954
Gustilo classification, 614

H

Halo fixation, 802, 802f
Hamstring tightness, 1198, 1199f
Hand
  carpal and metacarpal injuries. *See* Carpal bone fractures; Metacarpal fractures.
  compartment syndrome in, 1169–1170
  finger and nail bed injuries. *See* Phalanges (hand), fractures and dislocations of.
  radiologic diagnosis of trauma to, 67, 68f
Hand-foot syndrome, subperiosteal new bone in, 57, 60f
Handicapped child. *See* Severely handicapped child.
Hand-Schüller-Christian disease, flattened vertebral bodies in, 73
Hangman's fracture, 819, 820f–821f, 822, 855f–856f. *See also* Cervical spine fractures and dislocations.
  pseudosubluxation simulating, 68, 71f
Harrington's classification, of spinal metastasis, 1042, 1043t
Head injury(ies)
  anesthesia considerations in, 84
  distal radial and ulnar fracture treatment and, 359
  Glasgow Coma Scale in evaluation of, 31–32, 32t
  in multiply injured child. *See* Multiply injured child.
  skeletal fixation in patient with, 1191–1192
Heel. *See* Calcaneus.
Height, falls from a. *See* Fall(s).

Hematoma block, 88
Hemoglobinopathies, anesthesia considerations in, 84–85
Hepatic disease, anesthesia considerations in, 85
Heterotopic bone formation
  posttraumatic, 1128, 1129f, 1130f, 1130–1131, 1132f
  as spinal cord injury complication, 912
Hip
  immature, biomechanical concepts of, 486f–488f, 486–487
  subluxations affecting, 1204
    nontraumatic, 58, 61f
    traumatic, 76–77. *See also* Traumatic dislocation of hip.
  traumatic dislocations of. *See* Traumatic dislocation of hip.
Hip fractures
  and biomechanical concepts of immature hip, 486f–488f, 486–487
  classification, 488t, 488–489, 489f–492f
  complications
    coxa vara, 506
    femoral head
      avascular necrosis of, 500, 502, 502f–504f, 505–506
      traumatic osteochondral fracture of, 506, 507f, 508, 508f
    nonunion, 506
    premature closure of physis, 506
    triradiate cartilage injuries, 508, 508f–511f, 511
  description and incidence, 483
  differential diagnosis, 489, 493f
    pathologic fracture, 489
    stress fractures, 489, 493
  mechanism of, 487
  physical examination, 489
  radiologic diagnosis of
    nontraumatic pathology mimicking, 76–77, 77f, 77t, 78f
    normal anatomy and variants mimicking, 75–76, 76f
    technical factors, 75
  treatment, 493
    closed reduction and pinning, 498
    extracapsular, type IV, 496, 501f–502f
    intracapsular
      type I, 493, 494, 495f
      types II and III, 494, 495f–496f, 496, 497f–500f
    open arthrotomy, 498, 500
    stress fractures, 498
  vascular supply and drainage considerations in, 483, 484f, 485f
    extracapsular arterial ring, 483–485, 485f
    intra-articular subsynovial arterial ring, 485, 485f
    intraosseous arterial supply, 485, 486f
    ligamentum teres artery, 485–486
    venous, 486

History, of patient, in trauma management, 28
Horseback riding, injuries associated with, 8
Humeral fractures
  capitellum
    anatomic considerations, 283, 284f–288f, 287–288
    classification, 288, 291f
    description and incidence, 283
    differential diagnosis, 288–289
    injury mechanism, 288, 289f, 290f
    physical examination, 288
    treatment, 289–290, 292f, 293
  CHEO coding system for, 1219
  complications, 154–156
  distal, at birth, 1052, 1056–1057, 1057f–1060f
  lateral condylar
    anatomic considerations, 241
    classifications
      by degree of displacement, 245–246, 246f
      by site, 244f, 245, 245f
    complications
      associated fractures, 257, 257f
      avascular necrosis of capitellum, 256, 256f
      delayed union, 254
      infection, 257
      late degenerative arthritis, 257
      malunion, 254, 255f
      nonunion, 253, 253f–254f
      physeal arrest, 254–255
      prominence of lateral condyle, 255, 256f
      tardy ulnar nerve palsy, 255–256
      varus deformity, 255
    description and incidence, 241, 242f
    differential diagnosis, 248
    injury mechanism, 241–243, 243f, 244f, 245
    management pitfalls
      diagnostic, 252, 252f
      operative decision-making, 252–253
    physical examination and radiographic appearance, 246, 248
    treatment indications, 248
      nonoperative management, 247f, 248f, 248–249, 249f
      operative management, 249–251, 250f, 251f
  medial condylar
    classification, 220, 223f
    complications
      avascular necrosis, 225, 227f, 228f
      loss of motion, 222
      nonunion, 223
      overgrowth, 225, 229f
    incidence, 218
    injury mechanism, 218, 220, 222f
    radiology, 220–221, 224f–225f
    treatment, 221–222, 226f
  medial epicondylar
    anatomy, 212
    classification (Rang), 213, 215f, 217t
    injury mechanism, 212–213, 213f–216f
    radiology, 213–214, 217f
    treatment, 214–215, 218f
      preferred method of, 215–218, 219f–221f
  metaphyseal
    anatomic considerations, 146
    classification, 146, 149t
    complications, 148
    description and incidence, 144, 146, 148f
    injury mechanism, 146, 148f, 149f
    physical examination, 146–147, 149f
    treatment, 147, 150f–151f
  proximal
    anatomic considerations, 137, 138f
    at birth, 1052, 1056–1057, 1057f–1060f
    classification, 138, 138t
    complications
      humeral shortening, 144, 147f
      limitation of motion, 144
      neurologic injury, 144
      varus angulation, 144, 146f–147f
      vascular injury, 144
    description and incidence, 137
    differential diagnosis, 138
    injury mechanisms, 137–138, 138t
    physical examination, 138
    radiologic examination, 138, 139f–140f
    treatment indications, 141f–142f, 142, 143f–144f, 144, 145f–146f
  in severely handicapped child. See Severely handicapped child, fractures in.
  shaft
    anatomic considerations, 152, 152f
    classification, 152, 156t
    complications
      malunion, 154, 157f
      radial nerve injury, 154, 156f
      vascular injury, 154
    description and incidence, 148, 152
    injury mechanism, 152, 153f, 154f, 155f–156f
    physical examination, 152–153
    radiologic examination, 153
    treatment, 153–154
  supracondylar. See Supracondylar humeral fractures.
  transcondylar distal
    anatomic considerations, 199–200
    classification, 200f, 201, 201f, 202f
    complications, 207–208, 208f
    description and incidence, 199
    diagnostic features, 202–203, 204f–205f, 205, 206f
    differential diagnosis, 202, 203f
    injury mechanism, 200–201
    management, 205
      closed reduction, 205–206, 207f
      open reduction, 206–207
      pitfalls of, 207
      traction, 206
    physical examination, 201–202
Humerus
  deformity correction by Ilizarov technique, 700, 700f–702f
  fractures of. See Humeral fractures.
Hyperextension injuries
  distal femoral epiphyseal fracture and, 571
  SCIWORA syndrome and, 920
Hyperflexion injury, distal femoral epiphyseal fracture and, 571
Hyperostosis
  clavicular/scapular sites for, 64
  misdiagnosed as child abuse, 940, 943, 943t
  rib site for, 75
  subperiosteal new bone in, 57–58, 60f
Hyperthermia, malignant, 85
Hypervitaminosis A, misdiagnosed as child abuse, 940, 943, 943t
Hypothermia, prevention in multiply injured child, 31

I

ICD9.CM Expanded coding system, compatibility with CHEO fracture coding system, 1214t
Ilizarov technique, 695–696
  advantages of, 696
  disadvantages of, 696
  hinge placement in, 703, 706f–710f, 711
  in posttraumatic angular deformity management, 696, 698
    femur, 699f, 700
    hinge placement types, 703, 706f–710f, 711
    humerus, 700, 700f–702f
    radius and ulna, 700, 703, 703f–705f
    tibia, 697f–698f, 698
Immobilization
  atrophy through disuse and, 1035–1036
  in epiphyseal plate injuries, 21
  following lower extremity reconstruction, 1092, 1097, 1097f
  of neck (C1-C2 vertebral fractures), 828f, 828t, 828–829
  of patient with spinal cord injuries, 908, 909f–910f
  skeletal fixation and, 1190
  in spondylolysis, 1208, 1210
Infantile cortical hyperostosis. See Hyperostosis.
Infection(s)
  posttraumatic, 1121, 1123, 1125
  vertebral, pathologic spinal fractures and, 1045, 1046f
Injury(ies). See Fracture(s).
Injury Severity Score (ISS), 32–33
Internal fixation. See also Skeletal fixation.

open reduction, CHEO fracture coding system and, 1221
for scaphoid fractures, 395f, 396
in spondylolisthesis, 1208
for transverse patellar fractures, 673–674, 674f
Interosseous wire loop technique, 674, 674f
Intra-articular fractures
  of knee
    central patellar, 691, 691f
    distal femoral epiphysis (Salter-Harris III & IV)
      anatomy, 593–594
      classification, 594
      complications, 595–596
      differential diagnosis, 594
      incidence, 593
      injury mechanism, 594, 595f
      physical examination, 594
      treatment indications, 594–595, 595f–597f
      unique characteristics, 596, 598
    intercondylar eminence of the tibia
      anatomy, 602–603, 603f
      classification, 603, 604f
      complications, 606
      description and incidence, 602
      injury mechanism, 603
      physical examination, 603
      posterior tibial spine avulsions, 603–604
      treatment, 604–606, 606f, 607f
      untreated, 606
    osteochondral, 606–607, 682–683
    proximal tibial epiphysis (Salter-Harris III & IV)
      anatomy, 598
      classification, 598, 599f–601f
      complications, 602
      differential diagnosis, 599
      incidence, 598
      injury mechanism, 598
      physical examination, 598–599
      treatment indications, 599, 601
  of the olecranon, 271
Intramedullary nailing
  of femoral fractures in brain-injured child, 1192
  Sofield concept and technique, 1081, 1089–1090, 1091f
  tibial fractures, 643
Intramedullary rods, 1188–1189
Intravenous regional anesthesia, 88t, 88–89. *See also* Bier block.
  for treatment of reflex sympathetic dystrophy, 1161
Intubation, tracheal, in multiply injured child, 29
Ipsilateral fractures, of tibia and femur. *See* Floating knee.
Irreducible fractures, treatment of distal radius and ulna, in, 358

Irregular centers of ossification, in differential diagnosis of fractures, 44–45, 49f
Iselin's disease, 772
ISS (Injury Severity Score), 32–33

J

Jefferson fracture, 814
  complications, 817
  CT imaging of, 39, 42f
  injury mechanism, 814
  physical examination, 814
  radiologic diagnosis and evaluation of, 68, 814, 815f–816f
  treatment, 816f, 817
Joint dislocations, nontraumatic causes, 58, 61f
Joint stiffness
  after fracture, 1131, 1132f–1133f
  following elbow injury, 281
  following intra-articular distal femoral epiphysis fracture (Salter-Harris types III & IV), 598
Jones fracture, 772
Juvenile kyphosis, mimicking spinal compression fractures, 73, 75f

K

Kinky-hair disease. *See* Menkes syndrome.
Kirner's deformity, 67, 68f
Kirschner-wire fixation, transverse patellar fractures, 673–674, 674f
Klippel-Feil syndrome, 850
Knee dislocations. *See also* Patellar dislocations.
  complications, 628
  congenital, 79
  management, 626, 628
  pathogenesis, 626, 627f
Knee fractures. *See also* Patellar fractures.
  chondral, 1006
  ipsilateral, of femur and tibia. *See* Floating knee.
  joint stiffness following, 1131, 1132f–1133f
  in myelomeningocele child. *See* Myelomeningocele child, fractures in.
  osteochondral, 606–607, 682–683
    injury mechanism, 1003–1004, 1004f, 1005f
    Milgram classification, 1006
    treatment, 1008, 1011, 1013, 1014f–1019f
  radiologic diagnosis of
    nontraumatic pathology mimicking, 79
    normal anatomy and variants mimicking, 78–79

technical factors, 78
  in severely handicapped child. *See* Severely handicapped child, fractures in.
Kyphosis
  juvenile, mimicking spinal compression fractures, 73, 75f
  lumbosacral, in spondylolisthesis, 1202

L

Lankford classification, 1156
Lateral retinacular release, in patellar reconstruction, 690
Lead poisoning, resulting from retained bullets, 956
Leg, compartment syndrome in
  anterior, 1170–1171, 1171f
  posterior, 1171
Leg length discrepancy. *See* Limb length; Shortening.
Leukemia, neoplastic, 940, 943, 943t
Lidocaine
  for local/hematoma block, 91, 91t
  pharmacology of, 91, 91t
Ligamentous injury, as floating knee complication, 669
Limb length. *See also* Shortening.
  managing discrepancy following linear physeal bar resection, 1151f, 1151–1152
  restoring through distraction osteogenesis. *See* Ilizarov technique.
Limbus fractures of thoracolumbar spine
  causes of, 857, 865f–867f
  differential diagnosis, 864
  treatment, surgical, 869
  unique characteristics of, 872
Linear physeal bar resection
  distraction, 1150, 1150f
  managing outcome conditions of, 1151f, 1151–1152
  repeated osteotomies, 1151
Local anesthesia/anesthetics
  local/hematoma block, 88
  pharmacology, 91, 91t
Long bone fractures. *See also* Myelomeningocele child, fractures in; *specific bones.*
  birth-induced, 1052, 1056f, 1056t
  treatment by Ilizarov technique. *See* Ilizarov technique.
Lower extremity. *See also individual limbs.*
  gunshot fractures of. *See* Gunshot fractures of the extremities.
  mangled, 650, 651t
  stress fractures of
    femoral, 976–977, 977f
    foot and ankle, 977–978, 978f, 979f
    pelvis and, 976
    tibial, 977, 977f

Lucent bands, metaphyseal. *See* Metaphyseal lucent bands.
Lumboscaral kyphosis, following spondylolisthesis surgery, 1208, 1209f, 1210
Lymphoma, neoplastic, 940, 943, 943t

M

Madelung deformity, 67
Magnetic resonance imaging (MRI)
 in fracture diagnosis, 40–41
 of knee, 68, 70f
 for partial physeal arrest resection, 1143, 1144f
 in SCIWORA syndrome, 923, 924f, 926f
 of spinal cord injuries, 905f, 907–908
 of spine, 68, 70f
 of spondylolytic defect, 1200
 of stress fracture, 982
Malignant hyperthermia, 85
Malignant tumors, and pathologic spinal fractures, 1043, 1044f
Mallet finger, 433
Malrotation, in tibial fractures, 652
Malunion
 basic principles, 1111–1112, 1112f, 1112t
 CHEO fracture coding system and, 1220
 as complication following injury
  C2 (hangman's) fractures, 822
  distal femoral epiphyseal fracture, 590
  to epiphyseal plate, 21–22, 22f
  floating knee, 668
 treatment principles, 1112–1113, 1113t, 1114f–1115f
Mangled extremity, 650, 651t
Mangled Extremity Severity Score (MESS), 650, 651t
Massage therapy, for treatment of reflex sympathetic dystrophy, 1159
Menkes syndrome
 metaphyseal spurs in, 57, 59f
 misdiagnosed as child abuse, 940, 943, 943t
MESS (Mangled extremity severity score), 650, 651t
Metabolic diseases, and pathologic spinal fractures, 1043, 1045
Metacarpal fractures
 anatomic considerations, 407–408, 408f, 409f
 CHEO coding system for, 1220
 classification, 409, 409f
 complications, 417–418
 description and incidence, 407
 differential diagnosis, 411
 injury mechanism, 408–409
 physical examination, 410, 410f
 treatment indications, 411, 413
  Bennett's fracture, 415
  carpometacarpal fractures-dislocations, 415
  intra-articular fractures, 414f, 414–415
  metacarpophalangeal joints, dislocations of
   complex, 417
   thumb joint, 415, 416f, 417
  neck fractures, 413f, 414
  shaft fractures, 411f–412f, 413
Metaphyseal fractures
 of distal radius and ulna, treatment indications, 351–352, 352f, 353f
 of humerus. *See* Humeral fractures, metaphyseal.
 in myelomeningocele child. *See* Myelomeningocele child, fractures in.
 of the olecranon, 269–271
Metaphyseal irregularity, in differential diagnosis of fractures, 51, 52f
Metaphyseal lucent bands
 causes of, 53t
 pathologic, 54, 57, 57f, 58f
 physiologic, in radiographic differential diagnosis of fractures, 51, 53f
Metastasis, spinal, Harrington's classification of, 1043t
Metastatic disease, and pathologic spinal fractures, 1040–1043, 1041t, 1042f, 1043t
Metatarsus, fractures and dislocations of
 anatomy
  bones, 767, 768f
  joints, 767–768, 768f
  muscles, 768
  surface, 768
 complications
  neurologic, 782
  premature physeal closure, 782
  vascular, 782
 description and incidence, 767
 differential diagnosis, 769
 fifth metatarsal, 771–772, 772f–774f
 first metatarsal, 773, 775f
 injury mechanism, 769
 open fractures, 775
 physical examination, 769
 sesamoid fractures, 779–781, 781f
 stress fractures, 775, 778, 780f
 treatment indications, 769, 769f
  for shaft and neck
   closed methods, 769, 770f–771f, 771
   open methods, 771
Midazolam, for conscious sedation, 86
Milgram classification, 1006
Minerva cast, 828, 828t
Minibikes, accident-related injuries, 6–7
"Missed-Monteggia lesion," 303–304, 310f
Monteggia-equivalent lesions, 298, 300f–301f
Monteggia fracture-dislocation, 295
 classification, 296, 297f–298f, 298, 299f
 clinical course, 299, 302f, 303f, 304f
 complications, 307
  associated nerve injuries, 310, 312f
  cross-union, 311, 312f
  elbow, 310, 311–312, 313f
  myositis ossificans, 310–311
  persistent subluxation of radial head, 308, 310
  redislocation of radial head, 307–308
 equivalent lesion types, 298, 300f–301f
 fascial reconstruction of annular ligament, 304, 311f
 in forearm, 305
 of triceps, 304–305, 311f
 injury mechanism, 295–296, 296f, 297f
 long-standing untreated, 305, 307
 "missed," 303–304, 310f
 treatment, 299, 302–303, 305f–310f
Morphine, for conscious sedation, 86
Motor vehicle accident(s), 5–7
 injury management following. *See* Multiply injured child.
MRI. *See* Magnetic resonance imaging (MRI).
Multipartite centers of ossification, in differential diagnosis of fractures, 44, 48f–49f
Multiply handicapped child. *See* Severely handicapped child.
Multiply injured child
 abdominal trauma evaluation in, 32
 anatomic considerations, 28
 anesthesia considerations, 83–84
 approach to, 27
 chest trauma evaluation in, 32
 determining injury severity in, 32–34
 head injuries in, 27
  closed, Glasgow Coma Scale in evaluation of, 31–32, 32t
 injury patterns in, 27–28
 management of
  injury severity determination, 32–34
  orthopedic care principles, 34–35
  primary survey and resuscitation, 28–31
  secondary survey and definitive care, 31–32
 physiologic response of, 28
 spine trauma evaluation in, 32
Muscle sprains and strains, CHEO fracture coding system and, 1223
Myelography
 of spinal cord injuries, 907
 spondylolytic defect and, 1200
Myelomeningocele child, fractures in
 anatomy, 1063, 1065, 1066f–1067f
 complications, 1074, 1076, 1076f, 1077f
 description and incidence, 1063, 1064f–1065f
 injury mechanism, 1065, 1068, 1068f–1070f
 physical examination, 1068–1069, 1071f–1073f
 treatment indications, 1069–1071, 1073f, 1074, 1074f, 1075f

Myositis ossificans
  following elbow injury, 281
  in Monteggia fractures-dislocations, 310–311
  in radial head and neck fractures, 380

N

Nail bed injuries. *See under* Phalanges (hand), fractures and dislocations of.
Nailing, intramedullary. *See* Intramedullary nailing.
Narcotics, for conscious sedation, 86
Neck injuries. *See* Cervical spine fractures and dislocations.
Necrosis, avascular. *See* Avascular necrosis.
Neonate, injuries suffered during birth. *See* Birth fractures.
Neoplastic leukemia, 940, 943, 943t
Neoplastic lymphoma, 940, 943, 943t
Neoplastic metastatic neuroblastoma, 940, 943, 943t
Nerve injury(ies), 1127t, 1127–1128
  common, 1127t
  peroneal, following proximal tibiofibular joint dislocation, 629
Neural arch defects, mimicking spinal trauma, 73, 73f. *See also* Spondylolysis.
Neural grooves, in differential diagnosis of fractures, 51, 52f
Neuroblastoma, neoplastic metastatic, 940, 943, 943t
Neurologic damage
  as injury complication
    to epiphyseal plate, 22–23
    to intra-articular proximal tibial epiphysis, 602
    to olecranon, 280
  spinal cord injury
    assessment, 908, 910f, 911
    delayed onset of signs, 906
  in spondylolisthesis
    decompression attempts and, 1206
    postoperative, 1210
Neurologic disease, anesthesia considerations in, 85
Neuromuscular disorders, misdiagnosed as child abuse, 940, 943, 943t
Nonsteroidal anti-inflammatory drugs (NSAIDs), traction tendinitis and, 679
Nonunion, as injury complication, 1113, 1115, 1116f–1118f, 1116t
  CHEO fracture coding system and, 1220
  C2 ring (hangman's) fractures, 822
  epiphyseal plate injury, 22, 23f
  odontoid process (dens) fractures, 819
  olecranon fractures, 281
  scaphoid carpal bone, 393–394, 394f, 396
  tibial fractures, 652–653, 654f

electrical stimulation of, 653
Nutrition. *See* Blood supply.

O

Observation
  follow-up, in epiphyseal plate injuries, 21
  of patient undergoing regional anesthesia, 87
Obstetrical brachial plexus palsy, 164–165
Obstruction, airway, in multiply injured child, 29
Odontoid process
  fracture complications, 819
  in radiologic diagnosis of spinal fractures, 68, 71f, 71–72, 72f
Off-road vehicle accidents
  injuries associated with, 6–7
  injury management following. *See* Multiply injured child.
Ogden classification, 575, 576f
Olecranon fractures. *See also* Coronoid fractures.
  anatomic considerations
    developmental, 260–262, 261f
    structural, 259–260, 260f
  arthrographic examination, 275
  classifications, 266–268, 269t
    direct blow, 271
    extensor avulsion, 271, 274f
    intra-articular, 271
    metaphyseal, 270–271
    open, 271
    physeal, 269–270, 274f
    stress, 271
  complications
    joint stiffness, 281
    myositis ossificans, 281
    nonunion, 281
    varus deformity, 281
    vascular and neurologic, 280
  description and incidence, 259
  differential diagnosis, 274–275
  injury mechanisms
    direct trauma, 266, 268f–271f
    extension, 262f–268f, 262–263
    flexion, 263, 266, 268f
  physical examination, 272, 274
  treatment, 275
    direct-blow, 280
    extensor avulsion injuries, 280
    intra-articular, 279–280
    metaphyseal injuries
      extension, 277–279, 278f
      flexion, 277
      shear, 279, 279f
    methods, 275–277, 276f–277f
    open, 280
    physeal injuries, 277
    stress, 280
Open fractures

of the olecranon, 271
treatment for
  distal radius and ulna, 350, 358
  fibula, 639, 639t
  tibia, 639, 639t
Open reduction. *See also* Repeat reduction; Skeletal fixation.
  of the ankle
    eversion and inversion injuries, 723, 726, 726f–728f
    triplane fractures, 731
  for atlanto-occipital dislocations, 802, 803f
  CHEO fracture coding system and, 1221
  for distal femoral epiphyseal injuries, 581, 583–584, 584f–588f
  for epiphyseal plate injuries, closed versus, determining growth disturbance prognosis, 20
  for fibular fractures
    indications, 638–639
    proximal tibiofibular joint management and, 629
  for fractures in myelomeningocele children, 1069
  for fractures occurring in severely handicapped children, 1109
  for lesser tarsal bone fractures, 765
  for metatarsal shaft and neck fractures, 771
  for osteochondral fractures of the ankle, 1013, 1019, 1020f–1021f
  for osteochondral fractures of the knee, 1011, 1013, 1014f–1019f
  for prevention of physeal bar formation, 1142
  for radial and ulnar fractures
    complete mid-shaft, 332, 334, 335f–336f, 337f
    distal, 356, 356f–357f, 358
  for seat belt injuries to the spine and abdomen, 882, 885f
  in spondylolisthesis, 1206–1207
    with internal fixation, 1208
    without internal fixation, 1207–1208
  for supracondylar femoral fractures, 566, 567f, 568
  for talar fractures, 756f, 757
  for thoracolumbar spine fractures and dislocations, 855f–856f, 868
  for tibial fractures
    indications, 638–639
    isolated proximal, with intact fibula, 621
    proximal physis, 618, 618f
    proximal tibiofibular joint management and, 629
  for tibial triplane fractures, 742, 745f–746f
  in tibiofibular joint management, 629
  for Tillaux fracture, 726
  for toe fractures, 782, 785f, 787
  for transcondylar distal humeral fractures, 206–207
  for transverse patellar fractures, 673–674, 674f

Osgood-Schlatter disease, 625, 626f
  trauma to knee and, 79
Os odontoideum, 819
Ossicles, accessory, in differential diagnosis of fractures, 45, 50f
Ossification
  centers of. *See* Accessory centers of ossification; Centers of ossification.
  heterotopic. *See* Heterotopic bone formation.
  of proximal femur, 486, 486f
  subperiosteal. *See* Subperiosteal new bone.
  vertebral, normal development and, 809
Osteochondral fractures
  classification, 1006, 1006t, 1007f
  complications, 1019, 1021, 1024f
  description, 1001
  differential diagnosis, 1008, 1009f–1011f
  incidence, 1001–1002, 1003f
  injury mechanisms, 1003–1004, 1004f, 1005f, 1006
  physical examination, 1006–1007
  treatment, 1008, 1011, 1012f, 1013, 1014f–1023f, 1019
Osteochondritis dissecans, trauma to knee and, 79
Osteogenesis imperfecta
  description and spectrum of, 1079, 1080f, 1080t
  fracture patterns and bending of bones in, 1088–1089, 1090f
  long bone surgical management in, 1089–1090, 1091f
  lower extremity reconstruction in
    Bailey-Dubow sliding nail technique, 1090, 1094f
    femur, 1090–1091, 1092f–1096f
    general problems, 1097
    postoperative immobilization, 1092, 1097, 1097f
    Sofield concept. *See* Sofield concept and technique.
    tibia, 1091–1092, 1096f
  misdiagnosed as child abuse, 940, 943, 943t, 1081, 1088
  skeletal maturity in, 1101, 1102f–1103f
  special devices for, 1099f–1101f, 1101
  spectrum of disease process in, 1079–1081, 1081f–1089f
  spinal deformities in, 1098–1099
  surgical limitations for multiple fractures in, 1099
  upper extremity fractures in, 1097f, 1097–1098, 1098f
Osteomyelitis
  as epiphyseal plate injury complication, 22, 24f
  misdiagnosed as child abuse, 940, 943, 943t
Osteoporosis, juvenile, and pathologic spinal fractures, 1043, 1045f
Osteotomy
  in linear physeal bar resection, 1151

  in partial physeal arrest resection, 1143–1144
Overgrowth, as injury complication
  femoral and tibial, 669
  humeral, 154–156
    medial condylar, 225, 229f

P

Pain
  postoperative, 91
  scales measuring, 91, 91t
Palsy, obstetrical brachial plexus, 164–165
Papavasiliou classification, 267
Paraplegia, management of, 914f, 915, 916f
Parent-infant trauma syndrome (PITS), 932
Parents, child abuse and. *See* Child abuse.
Pars interarticularis, spondylolytic defect in. *See* Spondylolisthesis; Spondylolysis.
Partial cord syndrome, in SCIWORA syndrome, 921
Partial physeal arrest resection
  bar location and size for, 1142–1143, 1143f, 1144f
  interpositional material for, 1144–1145, 1145f
  optimum surgical exposure for, 1143
  simultaneous osteotomy need for, 1143–1144
Passenger, accident-related injuries seen in, 6
  management of. *See* Multiply injured child.
Patella
  bipartite, 78
    traumatic separation of, 681–682, 681f, 682f
  dislocations of. *See* Patellar dislocations.
  fractures of. *See* Patellar fractures.
Patella alta, measurement of, 687, 687f
Patellar dislocations
  acute
    redislocation following, 689–690, 690t
    treatment, 688–689
  central intra-articular, 691, 691f
  CHEO coding system for, 1221
  congenital versus habitual, 684
  diagnosis, 685–686
  lateral, 684–685
  predisposing factors, 685
  radiographic assessment, 686–688, 687f, 688f
  results, 690t
  and traumatic separation of bipartite patella, 681–682, 681f, 682f
  treatment, 686, 686f
    in acute injury, 688–689
    nonoperative therapy, 690–691
    operative repair, 690, 690t
Patellar fractures
  anatomy, 671–672
  CHEO coding system for, 1218

  comminuted, 674, 675f–676f
  description and incidence, 671
  inferior pole, 676–680, 677f, 678f
  injury mechanisms, 672, 672t
  lateral marginal, 683, 684f
  medial margin, 682f, 682–683, 683f
  osteochondral, 606–607, 682–683
  superior pole, 680–681
  transverse, 672, 673f
    diagnosis, 672–673
    treatment, 673–674, 674f
  and traumatic separation of bipartite patella, 681–682, 681f, 682f
Patella tilt, measurement of, 687, 688f
Pathologic fracture(s)
  aneurysmal bone cysts, 1031, 1034f
  characteristics, 1028–1029
  CHEO coding system for, 1220
  classification, 1027, 1028t
  description, 1027
  of distal radius and ulna, 350
  disuse atrophy (postimmobilization), 1035–1036
  fibrous dysplasia, 1032, 1035, 1036f–1038f
  nonossifying fibroma, 1032, 1035f, 1036f
  predisposing bone biomechanics, 1027–1028
  of proximal tibia, 624, 624f.625f
  renal osteodystrophy, 1036–1037, 1039f
  of spine, 1037
    benign tumors, 1038
    aneurysmal bone cysts, 1038, 1040f
    eosinophilic granuloma, 1040, 1041f
    causes, 1038, 1040t
    characteristics, 1037–1038
    juvenile osteoporosis, 1043, 1045f
    malignant tumors, 1043, 1044f
    metabolic diseases, 1043, 1045
    metastatic disease, 1040–1043, 1041t, 1042f, 1043t
    vertebral infections, 1045, 1046f
  treatment, 1029, 1030f
  unicameral bone cysts, 1029–1030, 1030f–1033f
Patient history, in trauma management, 28
Pedestrian accidents, injuries sustained in, 6
  management of. *See* Multiply injured child.
Pediatric Trauma Score (PTS), 33t, 33–34
Pelvic dislocations, CHEO fracture coding system and, 1221
Pelvic fractures. *See also* Sacrum and coccyx, fractures of.
  acetabular. *See* Acetabular fractures.
  anatomic considerations, 453, 454f, 455–456
  CHEO coding system for, 1217
  classification, 458
    Cryer, 460–461, 462t
    Tile, 458, 458t
    Torode and Zieg, 458f–461f, 458t, 458–460

complications
    abdominal injuries, 480
    musculoskeletal, 480f, 480–481
    neurologic, 478
    urologic, 478, 478f–479f, 480
description and incidence, 453
external fixation, 467–468, 469f–471f
injury mechanism, 461–462
investigation and radiologic assessment, 463–464,465f–466f
maltreatment, 476, 478
misdiagnosis, 475–476
physical examination and diagnosis, 462–463, 463f, 464f
radiologic diagnosis of trauma to
    nontraumatic pathology mimicking, 76–77, 77f, 77t, 78f
    normal anatomy and variants mimicking, 75–76, 76f
    technical factors, 75
stress type, 976
treatment indications (Torode and Zieg classification)
    type I (avulsion), 464, 466
    type II (iliac wing), 466–467
    type III (simple ring), 466–467
    type IV (ring disruption), 467, 468f
Pelvic subluxation, CHEO coding system for, 1222
Pelvis
    fractures of. See Pelvic fractures.
    unique features of, 456f, 456t, 456–458, 457f
Percutaneous pinning, CHEO fracture coding system and, 1221
Peroneal nerve injury, following proximal tibiofibular joint dislocation, 629
Phalanges (foot), fractures and dislocations of
    incidence and description, 782, 783f
    treatment, 782, 784f–787f, 787
Phalanges (hand), fractures and dislocations of
    adolescent mallet finger, 433
    anatomic considerations, 421, 422f–423f, 423
    classification, 425, 427, 428f, 429f
    complications, 437f, 438f–439f, 439
    description and incidence, 421
    differential diagnosis, 428, 430f, 431f
    distal, 429–430, 431f–432f
        volar avulsion of, 430, 432f
    distal physeal (Seymour fracture), 431, 433
    injury mechanism, 423, 423f–425f, 425, 426f–427f
    middle, 433f, 433–434, 434f
    nail bed and crush injuries
        anatomic considerations, 441–442, 443f–444f
        classification, 445–446, 446f, 446t, 447f
        complications, 450
        description and incidence, 441, 442f, 443f

    injury mechanism, 442, 444f–445f, 445
    physical examination, 446, 448
    treatment
        crushed hand, 448
        fingertip injuries, 448, 448f–449f, 449–450
        wringer injury, 450
    physical examination, 427–428, 430f
    proximal, 438
        intra-articular, 436, 438
        of phalanx neck, 436
        physeal injuries
            type II, 434–435, 435f
            types III and IV, 435–436, 436f
        of the shaft, 436
    regional anesthesia for, 89, 89f
    thumb joint, 415, 416f, 417
    treatment indications, 428–429
Phalen-Dickson sign, 1198, 1199f
Physeal bars
    anatomy of, 1139, 1140f, 1141f
    description and incidence, 1139
    differential diagnosis, 1140
    injury mechanism, 1140
    physical examination, 1140
    treatment indications, 1141
        prevention, 1141–1142
        resection
            central, 1145–1147, 1146f–1148f
            linear, 1150f, 1150–1152, 1151f
            for partial physeal arrest, 1142–1145, 1143f–1145f
            peripheral, 1147, 1149, 1149f
            surgical technique, 1145
Physeal fractures
    birth-induced, 1052, 1056–1057, 1057f–1060f
    of distal radius and ulna, 348–350, 349f–350f
        treatment indications, 352–353, 353f–355f, 356
        treatment pitfalls, 359
    gunshot related, 956, 957f
    of the olecranon, 269, 274f
Physeal growth arrest
    as floating knee complication, 669
    posttraumatic. See Physeal bars.
    premature, 1116–1117, 1119f–1124f, 1121
Physical therapy, for treatment of reflex sympathetic dystrophy, 1159
PITS (Parent-Infant Trauma Syndrome), 932
"Plastic fracture," 53
Platyspondyly, 73–74, 74f, 75f
Polytomography, for partial physeal arrest resection, 1142
Postoperative cauda equina syndrome, 1210
Posttraumatic events
    heterotopic ossification, 1128, 1129f, 1130f, 1130–1131, 1132f
    infection, 1121, 1123, 1125
    physeal growth arrest. See Physeal bars.

    stress disorder, 1131, 1133, 1134f–1135f, 1136
Preexisting medical conditions, anesthesia considerations, 84
Preiser's disease of the scaphoid, 391
Premature physeal growth arrest, 1116–1117, 1119f–1124f, 1121
Preventative measures, epidemiological studies contributing to, 1
Progressive angulation. See Angulation, progressive.
Pseudarthrosis
    congenital. See Congenital pseudarthrosis.
    following spondylolisthesis surgery, 1208
Pseudosubluxation, simulating hangman's fracture, 68, 71f
Psychological preparation, for anesthesia, 84–85
PTS (Pediatric Trauma Score), 33t, 33–34
Pulmonary system, effects of spinal cord injuries on, 907
Pulse oximetry, monitoring patient undergoing regional anesthesia, 87
Puncture wounds, treatment of distal radius and ulna in, 359

Q

Quadriplegia, management of, 915, 915f, 916f

R

Radial and ulnar fractures. See also Coronoid fractures; Olecranon fractures.
CHEO coding system for, 1219–1220
distal
    anatomic considerations, 345–346, 346f
    classification, 348, 348t
        buckle (Torus) fracture, 348
        complete fractures, 348, 349f
        Greenstick fracture, 348, 348f
        open fractures, 350
        pathologic fractures, 350
        physeal fractures, 348, 349f–350f, 350
    complications
        cross-union, 365
        growth arrest of radius, 361f–364f, 364
        growth arrest of ulna, 364–365
        malunion, 360, 364
        neurologic injury, 360
        nonunion, 365
        refracture, 365
        vascular injury, 360, 360f
    description and incidence, 345
    differential diagnosis, 351
    injury mechanism, 346, 347f, 348
    pathology of, misinterpreted, 365, 365f, 366f

Radial and ulnar fractures *(Continued)*
  physical examination, 350, 351f
  treatment indications
    closed methods, 351–356, 352f–355f
    open methods, 356, 356f–358f, 358–360
  head of radius. *See* Radial head fractures.
  midshaft
    anatomy, 323, 324, 324f
    classification, 324
    complete shaft, 327f–329f, 329, 329t, 330f–334f, 332, 334, 335f–336f, 337
      closed reduction, 329, 332, 332f–334f
      indications, 327f–329f, 329, 329t, 330f–331f
      open reductions, 332, 334, 335f–337f
    complications
      malunion, 336, 338, 341f
      nerve injury, 341
      other, 341, 342f
      refracture, 338, 340
      synostosis, 340–341
    description and incidence, 323
    differential diagnosis, 326, 326f
    Greenstick type. *See* Greenstick fractures, involving radius and ulna.
    injury mechanism, 324, 325f
    physical examination, 324, 326
  neck of radius. *See* Radial neck fractures.
Radial head fractures, 369
  anatomic considerations, 369–370, 370f
  classification, 371, 373, 374f
  complications, 380
    forearm compartment syndrome, 383
    loss of motion, 380
    misdiagnosis, 383
    myositis ossificans, 380
    neurovascular, 380, 383
    osteonecrosis of, 380, 382f
    premature physeal closure, 380
    proximal radioulnar synostosis, 380, 381f
    upper limb alignment, alteration of, 380
  differential diagnosis, 373
  fixation techniques, 378–379
  injury mechanism, 370–371, 371f–373f
  physical examination, 373
  postoperative management principles, 379
  protuberance of radial head, 383
  radiographic examination, 373–374, 375f
  treatment indications, 374–376, 376f, 377f, 378
  treatment pitfalls, 379–380
Radial neck fractures, 369
  anatomic considerations, 369–370, 370f
  classification, 371–373, 374f
  complications, 380
    forearm compartment syndrome, 383
    loss of motion, 380
    misdiagnosis, 383
    myositis ossificans, 380
    neurovascular, 380, 383
    nonunion of, 380
    premature physeal closure, 380
    proximal radioulnar synostosis, 380, 381f
    upper limb alignment, alteration of, 380
  differential diagnosis, 373
  fixation techniques, 378–379
  injury mechanism, 370–371, 371f–373f
  physical examination, 373
  postoperative management, principles of, 379
  radiographic examination, 373–374, 375f
  treatment indications, 374–378, 376f, 377f, 378
  treatment pitfalls, 379–380
Radiographic examination
  alternative imaging modalities to, 39–41
  comparative views, 37–38, 38f, 39f
  distal femoral epiphyseal injuries, 577
  elbow and forearm, 64–67
  femur, knee, and lower leg, 78–79
  foot and ankle, 79–81
  hand and wrist, 67
  injury patterns suggesting additional investigation by, 39
  of multiply injured child, 31
  nontraumatic pathology mimicking traumatic injury, 53–58
  normal variants mimicking traumatic injury, 41, 44–53
  partial physeal arrest resection and, 1142
  pelvis and hip joints, 75–78
  in SCIWORA syndrome, 922f, 923, 924f–926f
  seat belt fractures, 882, 883f–884f
  shoulder and shoulder girdle, 60–61, 64, 161, 163f
  of spinal cord injuries, 907
  spine, 67–74
  stress fractures, 981
  symptom patterns aiding progression of, 38–39, 40f
  thoracic cage, 74–75
  tibial fractures and dislocations, 78–79, 634, 636
  traumatic injury mimicking disease processes, 58, 62f
Radius
  deformity correction by Ilizarov technique, 700, 703, 703f–705f
  dislocation of. *See* Monteggia fracture-dislocation.
  fractures of
    Galeazzi type. *See* Galeazzi and Galeazzi-equivalent fractures.
    radial head. *See* Radial head fractures.
    radial neck. *See* Radial neck fractures.
    and ulna. *See* Radial and ulnar fractures.
Recreational activities, injuries associated with, 7f, 7–8, 8t
Recurrent dislocation, of proximal tibiofibular joint, 629f, 629–630
Recurrent SCIWORA, 921
Reduction
  closed. *See* Closed reduction.
  of epiphyseal plate injury
    determining growth disturbance prognosis, 20
    principles of
      gentleness, 20
      method, 20–21
      time, 20
  and fixation, indications for, 1185t
  open. *See* Open reduction.
  repeat, 359, 359f
Reflex sympathetic dystrophy (RSD)
  anatomic considerations, 1155
  classification (Lankford), 1156
  description and incidence, 1155
  differential diagnosis, 1157f, 1158f, 1158–1159, 1160f
  injury mechanisms, 1156
  physical examination, 1156, 1156f, 1158
  treatment indications, 1159–1162, 1161f
    Bier block, 1160–1161, 1161f
    bilateral ablation of the cingulate gyrus, 1162
    intravenous regional chemical block, 1161
    massage therapy, 1159
    pharmacologic spinal blockade, 1160f, 1161
    pharmacologic therapy, 1160
    physical therapy, 1159
    surgical sympathectomy, 1161–1162
    transcutaneous nerve stimulation, 1159–1160
Regional anesthesia
  monitoring, 87
  patient selection, 87
  risks, 87t, 87–88
  techniques
    ankle block, 89–90, 90f
    brachial plexus block, 89
    digital nerve block, 89, 89f
    epidural block, 90
    femoral nerve block, 90
    intravenous block. *See* Bier block.
    local/hematoma block, 88
    spinal block. *See* Spinal blockade.
    sympathetic nerve block, 90–91
Remodeling
  in malunion, 1111–1113
  operative fixation and, 1183–1184
Renal disease, anesthesia considerations in, 85
Renal osteodystrophy, and pathologic fractures, 1036–1037, 1039f
Repeat reductions, of physeal injury in radial and ulnar distal fractures, 359, 359f
Respiratory disease, anesthesia considerations in, 84

Revised Trauma Score (RTS), 34, 34t
Rib fractures, 104
  anatomic considerations, 104–105
  child abuse causing, 107
    osteogenesis imperfecta versus, 105–106, 106f, 107f
  classification, 105, 105t
  classification and complications, 107–108
  diagnosis, 105–106, 106f, 107f
  major versus minor trauma causing, 107–108
  pathologic, 107
  stress type, 979
  treatment, 106–107
Rickets, 940, 943, 943t
Road accidents, injuries sustained in, 5–6
  management of. See Multiply injured child.
RSD. See Reflex sympathetic dystrophy (RSD).
RTS (Revised Trauma Score), 34, 34t
Russell's traction, 546, 546f

S

Sacrum and coccyx, fractures of
  anatomy, 889–890, 890f, 891f, 892
  classification, 891f, 892
  complications, 893
  description and incidence, 888
  differential diagnosis, 892–893, 893f
  injury mechanism, 892
  physical examination, 892
  traumatic coccydynia. See Traumatic coccydynia.
  treatment, 893, 894f, 895f–896f
Scaphoid fractures, 389–390, 390f, 391f
  bipartite, 391
  of carpal bone, 389, 390f, 391f
    site, 390, 391f
  distal avulsion fractures, 392, 392f
  Preiser's disease of, 391
  site of, 390, 391f
  treatment, 392–393, 393f
    bone grafting and internal fixation, 395f, 396
    clinical appearance, 396, 397f
    nonunion, 393–394, 394f, 396
Scapular fractures, 96
  anatomic considerations, 96
  CHEO coding system for, 1219
  classification, 97, 99f, 99t
  complications, 103–104
  description, 96
  diagnosis
    physical examination, 99, 100t
    radiographic techniques, 100, 100f, 101f
  embryology, 96, 97f, 99t
  incidence, 96
    by site, 99, 100t
  injury mechanism, 97
  treatment
    of acromion fractures, 103
    of body fractures, 100
    of coracoid fractures, 103
    displaced scapular fractures, 101t
    of glenoid fractures, 102–103
    of neck fractures, 101–102, 102f
    of scapular spine fractures, 103
    scapulothoracic dissociation, 103
Scheuermann's disease, mimicking spinal compression fractures, 73, 75f
Scintigraphy, stress fracture diagnosis, 981–982
SCIWORA syndrome, 904
  anatomic features, 919–920
  classification, 921
  complications and prognosis, 928
  definition and incidence, 919
  delayed, 921
  early, 921
  electrophysiologic studies, 923
  injury mechanism in, 920
  physical examination, 921–923
  prognosis for, 912
  radiologic investigation, 922f, 923, 924f–926f
  recurrent, 921
  treatment, 923, 927f, 927–928
Scoliosis, in spondylolisthesis patients, 1199, 1200f
Scott wiring technique, 1204
Scurvy
  metaphyseal lucent bands in, 54, 57f
  misdiagnosed as child abuse, 940, 943, 943t
Seat belt fractures
  anatomy, 877–878, 878f, 879f, 879t
  classification, 879, 881f
  complications
    neurologic, 884
    osseous, 884, 885f
  description and incidence, 877, 878f
  imaging, 882, 883f–884f
  injury mechanism, 878–879, 880f
  physical examination, 879, 882, 882f
  pitfalls, 882
  prevention, 884
  treatment
    closed methods, 882, 884f
    open methods, 882, 885f
Sedation, conscious, 85
Segmental fractures, treatment of distal radius and ulna, in, 358f, 358–359
Septic arthritis, of hip, 61f, 76–77
Severely handicapped child, fractures in
  anatomic considerations, 1105–1106, 1107f
  classification, 1106–1107, 1109
  description and incidence, 1105, 1106f
  injury mechanisms, 1106, 1108f
  physical examination, 1109
  treatment indications
    closed methods, 1109
    open methods, 1109
  pitfalls
    decubitus ulcerations and, 1109
    multiple fractures, 1109–1110, 1110t
  vitamin D deficit, 1107, 1109–1110
Severity of injury, classification schemes, 32–34
  Pediatric Trauma Score, 33t
  Revised Trauma Score, 34t
Seymour fracture, 431, 433
Shortening. See also Growth arrest.
  following distal femoral epiphyseal fracture, 590, 591f
  following floating knee injury, 661
  following intra-articular fracture of knee (Salter-Harris types III & IV)
    distal femoral epiphysis, 596
    proximal tibial epiphysis, 602
  and restoration of limb length. See Ilizarov technique.
Shotgun injuries. See Gunshot fractures of the extremities.
Shoulder
  dislocation of. See Shoulder dislocation(s).
  in obstetrical brachial plexus palsy, 164
    nonoperative treatment, 165
    operative treatment, 165
    prognosis, 164
  and shoulder girdle, radiologic diagnosis of trauma to
    nontraumatic pathology mimicking, 61, 65f
    normal anatomy and variants mimicking, 61, 64f
    technical pitfalls, 60, 64f
Shoulder dislocation(s)
  anatomic considerations
    glenohumeral joint, 159
    proximal humerus, 159
  classification, 160, 160t
  complications, 164
  description and incidence, 159
  injury mechanism, 160
  physical examination
    apprehension tests, 161
    atraumatic dislocations, 160
    differential diagnosis, 161–162
    glenohumeral translation, 160–161, 161f, 162f
    radiographic examination, 161, 163f
    traumatic dislocations, 160
  treatment indications
    closed methods, 162
    open methods, 163f, 163–164, 164f
Sickle cell disease, subperiosteal new bone of hand-foot syndrome in, 57, 60f
Sinding-Larsen-Johansson disease, 679
Sitting imbalance, spinal cord injuries and, 913, 915
Skateboarding, injuries associated with, 8, 8t

Skeletal fixation
  associated soft tissue and vascular injuries, 1191
  compartment syndrome and, 1191
  complications, 1189–1190
  concepts of, 1185tt, 1185–1186
  description, 1183–1185
  head injury and, 1191–1192
  immobilization, 1190
  indications for, 1185t, 1186–1188
  methods
    biodegradable materials, 1189
    blades and plates, 1188
    external fixators, 1189
    medullary techniques, 1188–1189
    pins, 1188
    screw, 1188
  remodeling and, 1183–1184
  removal of devices, 1190
  sedation and anesthesia, 1190–1191
Sleeve fractures, of inferior pole of the patella, 676, 677f, 678f, 679
Snowmobiles, accident-related injuries, 6–7
Soccer, injuries associated with, 7
Sofield concept and technique, 1089–1090, 1091f
  Sofield Rush rodding vs. Bailey-Dubow sliding nail, 1090–1091, 1092f–1096f
Soft tissue injury(ies)
  abdominal, resulting from seat belt usage. See Seat belt fractures.
  skeletal fixation and, 1191
  and tibial fractures, 643, 644f
Somatosensory evoked potentials (SSEPs), documenting spinal cord dysfunction, 923
Spina bifida occulta, mimicking spinal trauma, 73
Spinal blockade, 90
  for treatment of reflex sympathetic dystrophy, 1160f, 1161
Spinal cord injuries, 903f
  anatomy, 901, 902f, 903
  assessing neurologic damage in
    history, 908, 910f
    physical examination, 908, 911
  central cord syndrome, 906–907
  clinical presentation, 903
  complete, 907
    SCIWORA syndrome and, 921
  complications
    autonomic dysreflexia, 913, 915, 915f, 916f
    decubitus ulceration, 912
    heterotopic bone formation, 912
    spinal deformity, 912f, 912–913, 914f
    urinary tract infections, 912
    vascular injury and, 915
  compression, 903–904, 904f–906t
    juvenile kyphosis and, 73, 75f
  concussion, 903–904, 904f–906t
  in SCIWORA syndrome, 922
  definition and incidence, 901
  delayed onset of neurologic signs in, 906
  imaging of, 907–908
  incomplete, 906
    SCIWORA syndrome and, 921–922
  management
    adjunct methods, 911
    general measures, 908, 909f–910f
    specific measures, 911
    steroids, 911
    surgery, 911
  primary, 903
  prognosis, 911–912
  secondary, 903
  spinal shock, 904, 906f
  systemic effect of, 907
  vascular injury causing, 915
  without radiologic abnormality. See SCIWORA syndrome.
Spinal cord syndrome
  anterior, 906–907
  posterior, 907
Spinal dislocations, CHEO coding system for, 1221
Spinal fractures
  anesthesia considerations in, 84–85
  CHEO coding system for, 1217
  pathologic, 1037
    causes of, 1038, 1040t
    characteristics, 1037–1038
    Harrington's classification of metastasis, 1043t
    metastatic disease, 1040–1043, 1041t, 1042f, 1043t
    resulting from benign tumors, 1038
      aneurysmal bone cysts, 1038, 1040f
      eosinophilic granuloma, 1040, 1041f
  radiologic diagnosis of trauma to
    nontraumatic pathology mimicking, 71–74, 73f–75f
    normal anatomy and variants mimicking, 68, 71, 71f, 72f
    technical factors in, 67–68, 69f–70f
  resulting from seat belt usage. See Seat belt fractures.
Spinal shock, 904, 906f
Spine
  birth injuries to, 1059–1060
  cord injuries. See Spinal cord injuries.
  deformity of, as spinal cord injury complication, 912f, 912–913, 914f
  fractures of. See Spinal fractures.
    cervical. See Cervical spine fractures and dislocations.
    thoracolumbar. See Thoracolumbar spine fractures and dislocations.
  metastasis of, Harrington's classification, 1042, 1043t
  myelomeningocele of. See Myelomeningocele child, fractures in.
Spondylolisthesis
  asymptomatic, treatment indications, 1203
  cervical, 55f
  classification, 1196t, 1196–1197
  clinical characteristics, 1197–1199, 1199f
  defined, 1195, 1196f
  etiology, 1195, 1197f
  measurements techniques in, slippage amount, 1200, 1202, 1202f
  measurement techniques in
    sacral inclination, 1202, 1203f
    slip angle, 1200, 1202f
  natural history, 1202–1203, 1203t
  pathology, 1197, 1198f
  poor prognosis in, risk factors for, 1203t
  prevalence, 1195–1196
  radiographic evaluation, 1199–1200, 1201f
  restricted activities, as treatment indication, 1203–1204
  serial observation of, as treatment indication, 1203
  surgical treatment, 1204
    anterior fusion in situ, 1206
    decompression and fusion, 1206
    lytic defect repair, 1204
    one-level L5-S1 fusion, 1204
    pitfalls and complications, 1208, 1209f, 1210
    reduction methods
      closed and open, 1206–1208, 1207f
      for severe slips and spondyloptosis, 1208
    two-level L5-S1 fusion, 1204, 1205f
Spondylolysis
  asymptomatic, treatment indications, 1203
  clinical characteristics, 1197–1199, 1199f
  defined, 1195, 1196f
  etiology, 1195, 1197f
  fractures mistaken for, 58, 62f–63f
  mimicking spinal trauma, 73
  natural history, 1202–1203
  pathology, 1197, 1198f
  prevalence, 1195–1196
  radiographic evaluation, 1199–1200, 1201f
  restricted activities, as treatment indication, 1203–1204
  Scott wiring technique for, 1204
  serial observation of, as treatment indication, 1203
  surgical correction of. See Spondylolisthesis, surgical treatment.
Spondyloptosis, surgical reduction of, 1208
Sports, injuries associated with, 7f, 7–8, 8t
Sprains and strains, CHEO fracture coding system and, 1223
Spurs, metaphyseal, mimicking fractures, 57, 59f
Stairs, falls down. See Fall(s).
Sternum, fractures of
  anatomic considerations, 93, 94f
  classification, 95, 95f
  description and incidence, 93
  embryology, 93–95

injury mechanism, 95
physical examination, 95
treatment, 95–96
Steroids, in management of spinal cord injury, 911
Stiffness. See Joint stiffness.
Stress fracture(s), 972
 anatomy, 975–976
  femur, 976–977, 977f
  foot and ankle, 977–978, 978f, 979f
  lower extremity, 976, 976f
  other sites, 978–979
  pelvis, 976
  tibia, 977, 977f
  upper extremity, 978
 CHEO coding system for, 1220
 classification, 983
 description, 973, 974f
 diagnostic imaging
  conventional radiography, 981
  magnetic resonance imaging, 982
  scintigraphy, 981–982
 differential diagnosis, 980
 of fibular shaft, 654
 in hip
  differential diagnosis, 489, 493
  treatment, 498
 incidence, 974–975
 injury mechanism and risk factors, 979–980
 in military personnel, 974–975
 in olecranon, 271
 physical examination, 980
 in proximal tibia, 623f, 624
 in sacrum, 892
 sports training and, 973, 974, 975
 treatment, 982–983
Subchondral resorption site, clavicle as, 64
Subluxations
 CHEO fracture coding system for, 1222
 nontraumatic causes, 58, 61f
 traumatic causes. See specific sites.
Subperiosteal new bone
 pathologic, mimicking fractures, 57–58, 60f
 physiologic, in radiographic differential diagnosis of fractures, 51, 54f
Sulcus angle, patellar, measurement of, 687, 688f
Supracondylar femoral fractures
 nonphyseal
  anatomy, 563, 564f
  classification, 565, 565f
  complications
   knee stiffness, 568
   malunion, 568
   neurovascular, 568
  description and incidence, 563
  injury mechanism, 563, 564f, 565
  physical examination, 565
  treatment
   closed reduction, 565–566, 566f

open reduction, 566, 567f, 568
   simple plaster immobilization, 565
 physeal. See Distal femoral epiphyseal injuries.
Supracondylar humeral fractures
 anatomic considerations, 167, 168t
 classification, 171, 172f, 173f–175f, 173–175
  treatment decisions, 174–175
 complications, 191
  early
   infection, 193
   neurologic deficits, 191
   vascular injury, 191, 193
  late
   avascular necrosis of trochlea, 194, 194f
   cubitus varus, 194, 195f, 196
   elbow stiffness, 194
   hyperextension of the elbow, 196f, 197–197
   neurologic deficits, 193
   vascular, 193
 description and incidence, 167
 diagnostic features, 167–171
  carrying angle, 168–169
  periosteal hinge, 167–168
  radiologic measurements, 169, 170f–171f, 171
  varus or valgus tilt, 168, 169f
 injury mechanism, 171, 172f
 physical examination, 175
 differential diagnosis, 175, 176f
 treatment, 175, 177
  closed reduction technique, 181–182
  management plans, types 1 and 2, 177, 177f–179f, 179, 180f–181f, 181
  open reduction, 183–184
  percutaneous pinning, 184, 185f–187f, 189–190
  pitfalls in, 190–191, 192f–193f
  supracondylar cast-splint, 177
  traction, 188f–189f, 190, 190f
  of type 3 fractures, 182–183, 183f, 184f
Sympathectomy, surgical, for treatment of reflex sympathetic dystrophy, 1161–1162
Sympathetic nerve block, 90–91
Symphysis pubis, widening of, 76, 77t
Synchondroses, in differential diagnosis of fractures, 41, 44, 44f
Syphilis
 congenital, metaphyseal lucent bands in, 54, 58f
 misdiagnosed as child abuse, 940, 943, 943t

T

Talus
 anatomy, 755
 fractures of

classification, 757, 757t, 758f–759f
  osteochondral, treatment for, 1013, 1019, 1020f–1022f
  signs and symptoms, 755, 756f, 757
  treatment, 764
Tarsal bones, fractures and dislocations of
 anatomy, 751, 755
 description and incidence, 750, 752f–754f
 lesser forms, 765f, 765–766
Tarsometatarsal dislocations, fractures associated with, 773, 775, 776f–778f
^{99m}Tc-methylene diphosphonate (Tc-MDP) bone scans, 40, 43f
Temperature, patient's, during regional anesthesia, 87
Tendinitis, traction, at inferior pole of the patella, 679–680
Thigh, compartment syndrome in, 1172
Thoracic trauma. See also Rib fractures.
 anesthesia considerations in, 84
 radiologic diagnosis of fractures in
  nontraumatic pathology mimicking, 75
  normal anatomy and variants mimicking, 74–75
  technical factors, 74
Thoracolumbar spine fractures and dislocations. See also Vertebra(e).
 anatomy, 854
 characteristics, 853, 855f–857f
 classification, 857, 858f–867f
 complications
  delayed, 872
  neurologic, 870
  vascular, 870
 description and incidence, 853
 differential diagnosis, 858, 864
 injury mechanism, 854
 physical examination, 857–858
 treatment
  of burst type, 864, 868
  of limbus type, 869
  pitfalls, 869–870
  surgical, 868
   preoperative planning, 868–869
 unique characteristics, 870, 872
  burst type, 870, 871f, 872, 872f–873f
  limbus type, 872
 vertebral maturation, 853, 855f–857f
Thumb joint, dislocation of, 415, 416f, 417
Tibia
 congenital pseudarthrosis of, 656, 656t, 657f
  misdiagnosed as child abuse, 940, 943, 943t
 deformity correction by Ilizarov technique, 697f–698f, 698
 dislocations and fractures of. See Tibial fractures and dislocations.
 overgrowth of, as floating knee complication, 669
Tibial apophysis, avulsion of, 625, 626f, 627f

Tibial apophysitis. *See* Osgood-Schlatter disease.
Tibial fractures and dislocations
  anatomy, 631–632, 636f
  CHEO coding system for, 1218
  classification, 633, 638t
  complications
    angular deformities, 651–652
    compartment syndrome, 650–651
    delayed union and nonunion, 652–653, 654f
    electrical stimulation in nonunions, 653
    malrotation, 652
    vascular injuries, 651
  degloving injuries associated with. *See* Degloving injuries.
  description and incidence, 631, 632f–635f
  and extensive soft tissue injury, 643, 644f
  injury mechanisms, 632, 637f, 638f
  intra-articular, of knee. *See* Intra-articular fractures, of knee.
  ipsilateral. *See* Floating knee.
  in mangled extremity, 650, 651t
  in myelomeningocele child. *See* Myelomeningocele child, fractures in.
  physical examination, 633–634
  proximal
    isolated, with intact fibula, 620f, 621
      complications, 621–624, 622f
      management, 621
    pathologic, 624, 624f.625f
    stress, 623f, 624
  proximal physis, 615, 616f–617f
    complications, 619, 619f
    management, 615
      closed reduction, 615, 617f, 617–618
      open reduction, 618, 618f
    physical examination, 615
    radiologic assessment, 615
  proximal shaft
    anatomy
      muscles, 612–613
      physis, 613, 613f
      tibia and fibula, 611
      vessels and nerves, 611–612, 612f, 613f
    classification, 613–614
    incidence, 611
    injury mechanism, 613–614
    management
      closed fractures, 614
        general principles, 614–615
        open fractures (Gustilo classification), 614
  radiographic diagnosis and evaluation of, 634, 636
    nontraumatic pathology mimicking, 79
    normal anatomy and variants mimicking, 78–79
    technical factors, 78
  in severely handicapped child. *See* Severely handicapped child, fractures in.
  shaft
    associated with paralysis, 654–655
    pathologic, 655, 656f
    stress, diagnosis and treatment of, 653–654
    in toddlers, 653
  stress type, 977, 977f
  Tillaux type, 739, 744f
  treatment
    closed methods, 637–638
    external fixation, 639–640, 640f–642f, 642–643
    intramedullary nailing, 643
    of open fractures, 639, 639t
    operative indications, 638–639
    in presence of degloving, 648f, 648–649, 649f, 649t
  triplane
    anatomy, 735–736, 737f
    classification, 737
    complications, 747
    description and incidence, 735, 736f
    differential diagnosis, 739, 744f
      Tillaux fracture, 739, 744f
    examination, 739
    four-part, 739
    injury mechanism, 736, 737, 737f
    medial, 739, 743f
    three-part lateral, 739, 741f–742f
    treatment of
      closed reduction, 742
      open reduction, 742, 745f–746f
      treatment pitfalls, 742, 746f–748f
    two-part lateral
      extra-articular, 739, 740f
      intra-articular, 738f, 739, 739f
Tibiofibular joint, proximal, dislocation of, 628
  complications, 629f, 629–630
  management, 628–629
  recurrent, 629f, 629–630
Tile classification, 458, 458t
Tillaux fracture
  in ankle, 726, 728, 728f–729f
  in tibia, 739, 744f
TNS. *See* Transcutaneous nerve stimulation (TNS).
Toes. *See* Phalanges (foot), fractures and dislocations of.
Tomography, in fracture diagnosis
  computed. *See* Computed tomography (CT).
  conventional, 39, 41f
Torode and Zieg classification, 458f–461f, 458t, 458–460
Torus fracture. *See* Buckle (Torus) fracture.
Tracheal intubation, in multiply injured child, 28–29
Traction
  as external cause of compartment syndrome, 1166
  in management of floating knee injury, 668, 668f
  in treatment of femoral shaft fractures, 542
    Bradford frame, 542–543
    Bryant's traction, 542, 642f
    Russell's traction, 546, 546f
    skeletal, 546f, 546–547
    skin, 544, 544f–545f
Traction tendinitis, at inferior pole of the patella, 679–680
Transcutaneous nerve stimulation (TNS), for treatment of reflex sympathetic dystrophy, 1159–1160
Trauma
  acute. *See* Multiply injured child.
  behavioral consequences of, 1131, 1133, 1134f–1135f, 1136
  injury resulting from, mimicking disease processes, 58, 62f
  patient history in management of, 28
  unexplained, in infancy, 932
Traumatic coccydynia
  complications, 897f–898f, 898
  differential diagnosis, 897
  etiology and classification, 893–894, 896f
  physical examination, 896–897
  treatment, 897f, 897–898
Traumatic dislocation of hip, 76–77
  anatomy, 523
  associated fractures, 533t, 533–534
  classification, 524, 524t, 525t
    anterior, 529, 530, 530f, 531f
    fracture-dislocation
      central type, 533
      Stewart & Milford scheme, 532f, 533
    obturator, 530, 531f
    posterior, 525f, 525–526, 526f, 526t, 527f–529f, 529, 530f
    postoperative management, 529
  complications, 534
    avascular necrosis, 534
    chronic or neglected, 536
    coxa magna, 536, 536f
    early osteoarthritis, 536
    heterotopic ossification, 536
    neurologic injury, 534, 536
    nonconcentric reduction, 534, 535f
    prognostic factors, 536–537
    recurrent, 534
  differential diagnosis, 525
  epidemiology, 523
  in myelomeningocele child. *See* Myelomeningocele child, fractures in.
  soft tissue injuries associated with, 533, 533t
  vascular supply, 524, 524f
Triplane fractures
  of ankle, 728, 730f, 731
  of tibia. *See* Tibial fractures and dislocations, triplane.
Triquetral fractures, 398, 398f
  clinical diagnosis, 399–400, 400f
  injury mechanism, 398–399, 399f
  treatment, 400–401

Tuberculosis, and pathologic spinal fractures, 1040t, 1045, 1046f
Tumors, and pathologic spinal fractures
  benign, 1038, 1040, 1040t
  infections, 1040t, 1045, 1046f
  juvenile osteoporosis, 1040t, 1043, 1045f
  malignant, 1040t, 1043, 1044f
  metabolic diseases, 1040t, 1043, 1045
  metastatic, 1040t, 1040–1043, 1041t, 1042f, 1043t

U

Ulceration, decubitus. *See* Decubitus ulceration.
Ulna
  deformity correction by Ilizarov technique, 700, 703, 703f–705f
  dislocation of. *See* Galeazzi and Galeazzi-equivalent fractures.
  fractures of
    CHEO coding system for, 1219
    distal. *See* Radial and ulnar fractures, distal.
    midshaft. *See* Radial and ulnar fractures, midshaft.
    Monteggia type. *See* Monteggia fracture-dislocation.
    radius and. *See* Radial and ulnar fractures.
Ultrasound, in fracture diagnosis, 40, 41
Unexplained trauma of infancy (UTI), 932
Union, delayed
  in C2 ring (hangman's) fractures, 822
  in tibial fractures, 652–653, 654f
Upper extremity. *See also* individual bones.
  gunshot fractures of. *See* Gunshot fractures of the extremities.
  stress fractures of, 978
Urinary tract infections, as spinal cord injury complication, 912
UTI. *See* Unexplained trauma of infancy (UTI).

V

Valgus deformity, as proximal tibial fracture complication, 622f, 622–624
Valgus injury, distal femoral epiphyseal fracture and, 570–571
Varus injury
  deformity following, 281
  distal femoral epiphyseal fracture and, 571
Vascular grooves, in differential diagnosis of fractures, 51
Vascular injury(ies)
  arterial, distal femoral epiphyseal injuries associated with, 585, 589f
  causing spinal cord injuries, 915
  common sites, 1127t
  as complication in tibial fractures, 651
  as complication of olecranon fracture, 280
  epiphyseal plate injury and, 23
  intra-articular proximal tibial epiphysis fracture (Salter-Harris types III & IV) and, 602
  skeletal fixation and, 1191
Vastus medialis advancement, in patellar reconstruction, 690
Vehicular accidents, injuries sustained in, 5–7
  management of. *See* Multiply injured child.
Venous access, for circulation management, 30
Vertebra(e)
  absence or hypoplasia of mimicking spinal trauma, 72–73, 73f, 74f
  apical center of, development and normal ossification, 809
  atlas. *See* Atlas vertebra.
  axis. *See* Axis vertebra.
  congenital wedge, 73, 74f
  flattened, 73–74, 74f, 75f
  fractures of
    cervical spine. *See* Cervical spine fractures and dislocations.
    radiologic diagnosis, 71
    thoracolumbar spine, Thoracolumbar spine fractures and dislocations
  infections of, pathologic spinal fractures and, 1045, 1046f
  ossification of, normal development and, 809
  spondylytic defect. *See* Spondylolisthesis; Spondylolysis.
Vertebra plana, 73, 74f
Vital signs, normal pediatric values, 30t
Vitamin D, 1107, 1109–1110

W

Weapons
  and gunshot injuries. *See* Gunshot fractures of the extremities.
  and homicide rates for Seattle and Vancouver (1980-1986), 969t
Wedge vertebra, congenital, mimicking spinal trauma, 73, 74f
Wilkins classification, 267, 268, 269t
Wrist, fractures of. *See* Carpal bone fractures.

Z

Z fracture, clavicular, 117, 118f